T0294987

Principles of Neonatology

Principles of Neonatology

Edited by

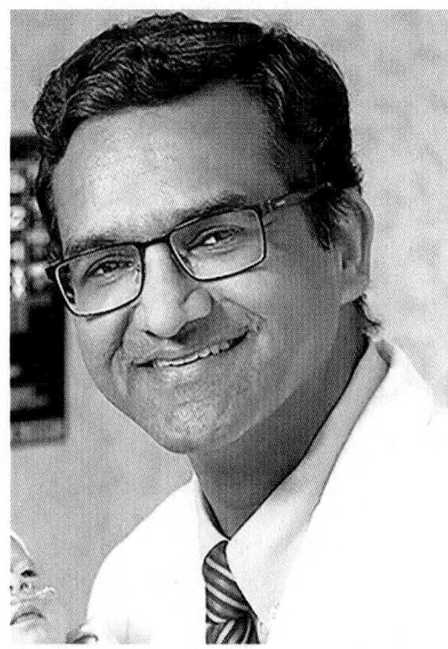

Akhil Maheshwari, MD, FAAP, FRCP (Edin)

Professor (Clinical) of Pediatrics and of Molecular & Cellular Physiology
Chief, Division of Neonatal Medicine
Vice-Chair of Translational Research in Pediatrics
Director, Fellowship Program of Neonatal-Perinatal Medicine
Louisiana State University Health Sciences Center—Shreveport
Shreveport, Louisiana

Founding Chair, the Global Newborn Society
Founding Editor-in-Chief, the journal Newborn
CEO of the non-profit organization, GNS, LLC (publishing for public health)
Managing Partner of the non-profit organization, CogniVantage, LLC (medical tools needed for public health)
Member, Forum for Children's Health, Louisiana

Section Editors: Nitasha Bagga, Cynthia Bearer, John Benjamin, Shazia Bhombal, Renee Boss, Waldemar Carlo, Robert Christensen, Wendy Chung, David Cooke, Jonathan Davis, Sharon Groh-Wargo, David Hackam, Naveen Jain, Eric Jelin[†], Sheela Magge, Frances Northington, Prabhu Parimi, Karen Puopolo, Michael Repka, Paul Sponseller, David Tunkel

[†]Deceased

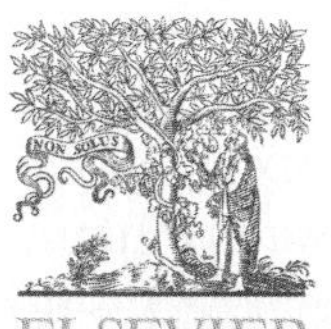

ELSEVIER

Elsevier
1600 John F. Kennedy Blvd.
Ste 1800
Philadelphia, PA 19103-2899

PRINCIPLES OF NEONATOLOGY, FIRST EDITION ISBN: 978-0-323-69415-5

The cover illustration: Our cover shows a young infant in whom the damaged body fabric is being knitted back to recovery. Some threads look loose, possibly reflecting both the still-incomplete process of development and also the unraveling that may have occurred during the illness. The infant is holding one of these threads and is contributing to the repair. The right hand is close to the mouth for self-soothing. The density of the threads is more in the limbs than in the head, a well-documented upward sequence of neurological development.

The background shows a gradual transition in the shades of blue. Appropriate, timely care can pull an infant up from the dark depths of an ocean of illness towards a lighter surface illuminated by the lights of recovery.

International Standard Book Number: 978-0-323-69415-5

Content Strategist: Sarah Barth
Senior Content Development Specialist: Priyadarshini Pandey
Publishing Services Manager: Catherine Jackson
Senior Project Manager: Daniel Fitzgerald
Designer: Patrick C. Ferguson

Printed in India

Last digit is the print number: 9 8 7 6 5 4 3 2 1

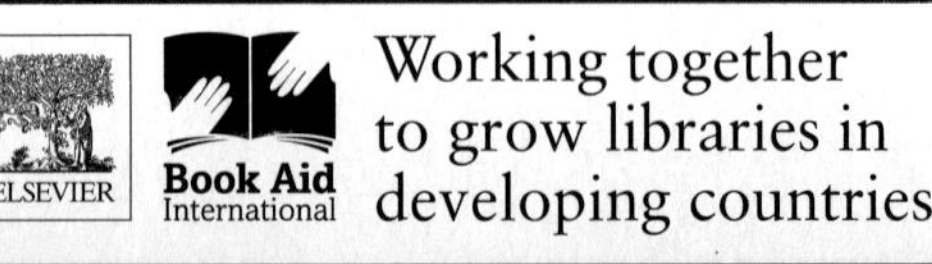

I dedicate this book to my parents, Dr. Parmatma Sharan and Gayatri Mahesh, who brought me into this world and taught me how to live; all my elder siblings – Sharad, Purnima, Deepshikha, and Kuldeep, Sanjeev, and Sadhana, who have inspired, motivated, and tolerated their brat younger brother; and my new parents who have adopted me here in the United States, Bob and Wendy Christensen. I could not have asked for more.

—Akhil Maheshwari, MD, FAAP, FRCP (Edin)

List of Contributors

Pankaj B. Agrawal, MD
Chief of Neonatology, University of Miami, Jackson Health System
Professor of Pediatrics and Genetics, University of Miami
Miami, Florida
Chair, Project Newborn
Visiting Professor Boston Children's Hospital and Harvard Medical School
Boston, Massachusetts

Yasmin Akhtar, DO, MPH
Clinical Associate of Pediatrics
Division of Pediatric Endocrinology
Johns Hopkins University School of Medicine
Baltimore, Maryland

Jubara Alallah, MD, ABP, SBP
Neonatologist, Assistant Professor of Pediatrics
King Abdulaziz Medical City-WR, Ministry of National Guard
King Abdullah International Medical Research Centre
King Saud bin Abdulaziz University for Health Sciences (KSAU-HS)
Jeddah, Kingdom of Saudi Arabia

Ziad Alhassen, MD
Assistant Clinical Professor of Pediatrics
Department of Pediatrics
University of California Irvine
Orange, California

Gabriel Altit, MDCM, MSc, FRCPC, FAAP
Assistant Professor
Department of Pediatrics
McGill University
Neonatologist
Division of Neonatology
Montreal Children's Hospital
Montreal, Quebec, Canada

Abbas AlZubaidi, PhD
Sigma Lambda Technologies
Biomedical Prototyping
Carleton, Gatineau, Quebec, Canada

Lahin M. Amlani, BS
Medical Student
Johns Hopkins University School of Medicine
Baltimore, Maryland

Martin Antelo, MD
Cardiac Surgeon
Centro Cardiovascular, Hospital de Clínicas
University of the Republic
Montevideo, Uruguay

Gayatri Athalye-Jape, MD, FRACP, CCPU, PhD
Consultant Neonatologist
Neonatal Paediatrics
King Edward Memorial Hospital
Clinical Lead, Neonatal Follow Up Program
King Edward Memorial Hospital
Clinical Senior Lecturer
School of Medicine
University of Western Australia
Honorary Research Fellow Neonatal Paediatrics
Telethon Kids Institute
Perth, Western Australia, Australia

Jargalsaikhan Badarch, MD
Associate Professor
Department of Obstetrics and Gynecology
Mongolian National University of Medical Sciences
Ulaanbataar, Mongolia

Gerri Baer, MD
US Food and Drug Administration
Center for Drug Evaluation and Research, Office of New Drugs
Silver Spring, Maryland

Nitasha Bagga, MBBS, DNB, Fellowship in Neonatology
Consultant Neonatologist
Rainbow Children's Hospital
Hyderabad, India

Timothy M. Bahr, MS, MD
Assistant Professor of Pediatrics
Intermountain Healthcare
University of Utah
Salt Lake City, Utah

Yaniv Bar-Cohen, MD
Director, Electrophysiology
Department of Pediatrics & Cardiology
Children's Hospital Los Angeles
University of Southern California
Los Angeles, California

Stephanie M. Barr, MS, RDN, LD
Neonatal Dietitian
Department of Pediatrics
MetroHealth Medical Center
Adjunct Lecturer
Department of Nutrition
Cass Western Reserve University School of Medicine
Cleveland, Ohio

Andrew J. Bauer, MD
Director
The Thyroid Center
Division of Endocrinology & Diabetes
The Children's Hospital of Philadelphia
Professor of Pediatrics
The Perelman School of Medicine
The University of Pennsylvania
Philadelphia, Pennsylvania

Cynthia F. Bearer, MD, PhD, FAAP
Professor of Pediatrics
Department of Pediatrics
Rainbow Babies and Children's Hospital
Cleveland, Ohio

Ross M. Beckman, MD
Pediatric Surgery Fellow
Baylor College of Medicine
Texas Children's Hospital
Houston, Texas

Marc Beltempo, MD, FRCPC, MSc
Department of Pediatrics
Montreal Children's Hospital – McGill University
Health Centre
Montreal, Quebec, Canada

Melania M. Bembea, MD, MPH, PhD
Associate Professor
Anesthesiology and Critical Care Medicine
Johns Hopkins University School of Medicine
Baltimore, Maryland

Sheila Berlin, MD
Associate Professor and Vice Chair
Department of Radiology
University Hospitals of Cleveland
Director of Pediatric CT
Department of Radiology
Rainbow Babies and Children's Hospital
Cleveland, Ohio

Shandeigh N. Berry, PhD, RN
Assistant Professor of Nursing
Saint Martin's University
Olympia, Washington

Vineet Bhandari, MD, DM
Professor of Pediatrics, Obstetrics & Gynecology, and Biomedical Sciences
Cooper Medical School of Rowan University
The Children's Regional Hospital at Cooper
Camden, New Jersey

Shaifali Bhatia, MD, MRCPCH
Metro Multispeciality Hospital
Sector 11, NOIDA
Uttar Pradesh, India

Shazia Bhombal, MD
Clinical Associate Professor of Pediatrics
Division of Neonatal and Developmental Medicine
Stanford University School of Medicine
Palo Alto, California

Elaine O. Bigelow, MD
Resident Physician
Department of Otolaryngology—Head and Neck Surgery
Johns Hopkins University School of Medicine
Baltimore, Maryland

Carley Blevins, BS
Laboratory Assistant
Department of Thoracic Surgery
Johns Hopkins University School of Medicine
Baltimore, Maryland

Suresh Boppana, MD
Professor of Pediatrics & Microbiology
University of Alabama at Birmingham
Birmingham, Alabama

Renee Boss, MD, MHS
Associate Professor of Pediatrics
Division of Pediatrics
Johns Hopkins University School of Medicine
Core Faculty
Berman Institute of Bioethics
Baltimore, Maryland

Sandra Brooks, MD, MPH, FAAP
Associate Medical Director—Neonatal Intensive Care Unit
Department of Pediatrics
Division of Neonatology
Johns Hopkins All Children's Hospital
St. Petersburg, Florida

Giuseppe Buonocore, MD
President, EURope Against Infant Brain Injury
Secretary of the Union of European Neonatal and Perinatal Societies
Siena, Italy

Jennifer Burnsed, MD, MS
Department of Pediatrics
University of Virginia
Charlottesville, Virginia

Andrew C. Calabria, MD
Clinical Director
Division of Endocrinology & Diabetes
The Children's Hospital of Philadelphia
Associate Professor of Clinical Pediatrics
Department of Pediatrics
Perelman University School of Medicine at the University of Pennsylvania
Philadelphia, Pennsylvania

Melisa Carrasco, MD, PhD
Section of Pediatric Neurology
Department of Neurology
University of Wisconsin School of Medicine and Public Health
Madison, Wisconsin

Brian S. Carter, MD
Professor of Pediatrics, Medical Humanities & Bioethics Pediatrics—Neonatology
University of Missouri—Kansas City School of Medicine
Bioethicist Bioethics Center
Children's Mercy Hospital
Kansas City, Missouri

Praveen Chandrasekharan, MD, MS
Associate Professor of Pediatrics
Neonatologist, Oishei Children's Hospital of Buffalo
University of Buffalo
Buffalo, New York

Raul Chavez-Valdez, MD
Department of Pediatrics—Division of Neonatology
Laboratory of Neonatology
Neuroscience Intensive Care Nursery
Johns Hopkins University School of Medicine
Baltimore, Maryland

Lauryn Choleva, MD, MSc
Instructor of Pediatrics
Division of Pediatric Endocrinology
Icahn School of Medicine at Mount Sinai
New York, New York

Robert D. Christensen, MD
Professor of Pediatrics
Department of Pediatrics
University of Utah
Salt Lake City, Utah

Wendy K. Chung, MD, PhD
Kennedy Family Professor of Pediatrics and Medicine
Pediatrics, Division of Molecular Genetics
Columbia University Irving Medical Center, New York
New York, New York

Sarah A. Coggins, MD
Attending Neonatologist
Division of Neonatology
The Children's Hospital of Philadelphia
Philadelphia, Pennsylvania

David W. Cooke, MD
Associate Professor of Pediatrics
Division of Pediatrics
Johns Hopkins University School of Medicine
Baltimore, Maryland

Laura Cummings, PharmD, BCPS, BCPPS
Clinical Pharmacist
MetroHealth Medical Center
Cleveland, Ohio

Erin R. Currie, PhD, RN, CPLC
Assistant Professor
School of Nursing
University of Alabama at Birmingham
Birmingham, Alabama

Joanne O. Davidson, PhD
Associated Professor
Department of Physiology
The University of Auckland
Auckland, New Zealand

Jonathan M. Davis, MD
Vice-Chair of Pediatrics and Chief of Newborn Medicine
Tufts Medical Center
Boston, Massachusetts

Colby L. Day-Richardson, MD
Assistant Professor of Pediatrics
Division of Neonatology
University of Rochester Medical Center
School of Medicine and Dentistry
Rochester, New York

Diva D. De Leon, MD, MSCE
Professor of Pediatrics
Division of Pediatrics
The Children's Hospital of Philadelphia/
Perelman School of Medicine at the
University of Pennsylvania
Chief
Division of Endocrinology and Diabetes
Department of Pediatrics
Director
Congenital Hyperinsulinism Center
The Children's Hospital of Philadelphia
Philadelphia, Pennsylvania

Kavita Dedhia, MD
Assistant Professor
Otolaryngology Head and Neck Surgery
Division of Pediatric Otolaryngology
University of Pennsylvania/Children's
Hospital of Philadelphia
Philadelphia, Pennsylvania

Alvaro Dendi, MD
Neonatologist
Department of Neonatology, Centro
Hospitalario Pereira Rossell School of
Medicine
University of the Republic, Montevideo
Montevideo, Uruguay

Anita Deshpande, MD
Assistant Professor of Pediatric
Otolaryngology
Emory University School of Medicine,
Children's Healthcare of Atlanta
Atlanta, Georgia

Janis M. Dionne, MD
Clinical Associate Professor
Division of Nephrology, Department of
Pediatrics
University of British Columbia
Vancouver, British Columbia, Canada

Keyur Donda, MBBS
Assistant Professor of Pediatrics
University of South Florida
Tampa, Florida

Lee Donohue, MD, FAAP
Associate Clinical Professor
Department of Pediatrics
UC Davis Children's Hospital
Sacramento, California

Jefferson J. Doyle, MBBChir, PhD, MHS
Assistant Professor of Ophthalmology and
Genetics
Wilmer Eye Institute
The Johns Hopkins Hospital
Baltimore, Maryland

Susan J. Dulkerian, MD
Associate Professor of Pediatrics
Neonatology/Pediatrics
University of Maryland School of Medicine
Baltimore, Maryland

Vikramaditya Dumpa, MD
Associate Professor of Pediatrics
University of Arkansas for Medical Sciences
Arkansas Children's Hospital
Little Rock, Arkansas

Andrea F. Duncan, MD, MSClinRes
Associate Professor of Pediatrics, Division
of Neonatology
Associate Chief, Diversity, Equity and
Inclusion, Division of Neonatology
Associate Chair, Diversity and Equity,
Department of Pediatrics
Diversity Search Advisor, Department of
Pediatrics
University of Pennsylvania Perelman
School of Medicine
Medical Director, Neonatal Follow-up
Program
Children's Hospital of Philadelphia
Philadelphia, Pennsylvania

Alexandra M. Dunham, MD
Resident of Orthopaedic Surgery
Johns Hopkins University School of
Medicine
Baltimore, Maryland

DiAnn Ecret, PhD, MSN, RN, MA cert
Assistant Professor
School of Nursing
Ave Maria University
Ave Maria, Florida

Kelstan Ellis, DO, MSCR, MBe
Clinical Assistant Professor at the University
of Missouri—Kansas City School of
Medicine
Department of Pediatrics, Division of
Palliative Care at Children's Mercy
Hospital
Kansas City, Missouri

Dina El-Metwally, MD, PhD
Chief
Division of Neonatology
Professor of Pediatrics
Department of Pediatrics
University of Maryland School of Medicine
Baltimore, Maryland

Eric W. Etchill, MD, MPH
Resident of Cardiothoracic Surgery
Johns Hopkins University School of Medicine
Baltimore, Maryland

Yahya Ethawi, MD, CABPed, Neonatal Perinatal Fellowship
Consultant and Head of NICU
Department of Pediatrics
Saudi German Hospital Ajman
Ajman, United Arab Emirates

Allen D. Everett, MD
Professor of Pediatrics
Department of Pediatrics & Cardiology
Johns Hopkins University
Baltimore, Maryland

Jorge Fabres, MD, MSPH
Associate Professor of Neonatology
Department of Neonatology
Pontificia Universidad Católica de Chile
Santiago, Chile

Ryan J. Felling, MD, PhD
Associate Professor of Neurology
Johns Hopkins University School of Medicine
Baltimore, Maryland

Tanis R. Fenton, MHSc, PhD, RD, FDC
Professor
Cumming School of Medicine
University of Calgary
Calgary, Alberta, Canada

Dustin D. Flannery, DO, MSCE
Assistant Professor of Pediatrics
Department of Pediatrics
University of Pennsylvania Perelman
School of Medicine
Attending Physician
Neonatology
Children's Hospital of Philadelphia
Philadelphia, Pennsylvania

Joseph T. Flynn, MD, MS
Chief
Division of Nephrology
Seattle Children's Hospital
Professor of Pediatrics
Department of Pediatrics
University of Washington School of Medicine
Seattle, Washington

Michaelene Fredenburg, LHD
President and CEO
Institute of Reproductive Grief Care
San Diego, California

John Fuqua, MD
Professor of Clinical Pediatrics
Division of Pediatric Endocrinology
Indiana University School of Medicine
Indianapolis, Indiana

Alejandro V. Garcia, MD
Assistant Professor of Surgery
Department of Surgery
Johns Hopkins University School of Medicine
Baltimore, Maryland

Steven Garzon, MD
Assistant Professor of Clinical Pathology
University of Illinois
Chicago, Illinois

Estelle B. Gauda, MD
Professor of Pediatrics, University of Toronto
Head, Division of Neonatology
Women's Auxiliary Chair in Neonatology at SickKids
Senior Associate Scientist, SickKids Research Institute
Director, Toronto Centre for Neonatal Health
The Hospital for Sick Children
Toronto, Ontario, Canada

Marisa Gilstrop Thompson, MD
Maternal Fetal Medicine and Clinical Genetics
Delaware Center for Maternal Fetal Medicine
Newark, Delaware

Barton Goldenberg, BSc (Econ), MSc (Econ)
President & Founder
ISM/CRM Consultants, Inc.
Bethesda, Maryland

Andres J. Gonzalez Salazar, MD
General Surgery Resident
Department of Surgery
The Johns Hopkins Hospital
Baltimore, Maryland

Julie E. Goodwin, MD
Associate Professor of Pediatrics (Nephrology)
Department of Pediatrics, Section of Nephrology
Yale University School of Medicine
New Haven, Connecticut

Steven L. Goudy, MD
Professor of Pediatric Otolaryngology
Division Chief of Pediatric Otolaryngology
Emory University School of Medicine
Children's Healthcare of Atlanta
Atlanta, Georgia

Ernest Graham, MD
Associate Professor of Gynecology & Obstetrics
Johns Hopkins University School of Medicine
Baltimore, Maryland

Kathryn Grauerholz, MSN, ANP-C, ACHPN
Director of Healthcare Programs
Healthcare Education
Institute of Reproductive Grief Care
San Diego, California

Mari L. Groves, MD
Assistant Professor of Neurosurgery
Department of Neurosurgery
Johns Hopkins University School of Medicine
Baltimore, Maryland

Mireille Guillot, MD, MSc
Department of Pediatrics, Faculty of Medicine, CHU de Québec-Université Laval
Quebec, Canada

Alistair J. Gunn, MBChB, PhD
Professor of Physiology and Paediatrics
Department of Physiology
University of Auckland
Auckland, New Zealand

Arjun Gupta, BS
Clinical Research Fellow
Department of Orthopaedics
Johns Hopkins University School of Medicine
Baltimore, Maryland

David J. Hackam, MD, PhD
Chief of Pediatric Surgery
Professor of Surgery
Johns Hopkins University School of Medicine
Pediatric Surgeon in Chief and Co-Director
Johns Hopkins Children's Center
Baltimore, Maryland

Joaquin Hidalgo, MD
Neurosurgeon
North Mississippi Health System
Tupelo, Mississippi

Erin Honcharuk, MD
Assistant Professor of Orthopaedic Surgery
Orthopaedic Surgery
Johns Hopkins University School of Medicine
Baltimore, Maryland

Zeyar Htun, MD
Fellow
Pediatrics/Neonatology
Rainbow Babies & Children's Hospital
Cleveland, Ohio

Mark L. Hudak, MD
Professor and Chair of Pediatrics
Chief, Division of Neonatology
University of Florida College of Medicine—Jacksonville
Jacksonville, Florida

Colleen A. Hughes Driscoll, MD
Assistant Professor of Pediatrics
Department of Pediatrics
University of Maryland School of Medicine
Baltimore, Maryland

Thierry A.G.M. Huisman, MD, PD, EDiNR, EDiPNR
Radiologist-in-Chief and Edward B. Singleton Chair of Radiology
Department of Radiology
Texas Children's Hospital and Baylor College of Medicine
Houston, Texas

Mireille Jabroun, MD
Assistant Professor of Ophthalmology
Department of Ophthalmology and Vision Science, University of Arizona College of Medicine
Tucson, Arizona

Eric M. Jackson, MD
Associate Professor of Neurosurgery
Pediatrics, and Plastic and Reconstructive Surgery
Johns Hopkins University School of Medicine
Baltimore, Maryland

Naveen Jain, MBBS, MD, DNB, DCH, DM
Senior Consultant
KIMSHEALTH Thiruvananthapuram
Kerala, India

Rajesh Jain, MBBS, MD, PG Diploma Diabetes
Chair
Diabetology
DiabetesAsia
Jain Hospital and Research Centre Pvt Ltd
Kanpur, Uttar Pradesh, India

Angie Jelin, MD
Associate Professor of Gynecology & Obstetrics
Department of Gynecology & Obstetrics
The Johns Hopkins Hospital
Baltimore, Maryland

Eric Jelin, MD†
Associate Professor of Pediatric Surgery
Surgery, Gynecology & Obstetrics
Johns Hopkins University School of Medicine
Baltimore, Maryland

Sandra E. Juul, MD, PhD, FAAP
Professor of Pediatrics and Neuroscience
Co-Director, Intellectual and Developmental Disabilities Research Center
University of Washington
Seattle, Washington

David A. Kaufman, MD
Professor of Pediatrics
Department of Pediatrics
University of Virginia School of Medicine
Charlottesville, Virginia

†Deceased

Haluk Kavus, MD
Medical Geneticist
Postdoctoral Research Scientist
Pediatrics
Division of Molecular Genetics Columbia University
New York, New York

Alison Kent, BMBS, FRACP, MD
Head of Unit, Neonatology, Women and Babies Division
Women's and Children's Hospital
Adelaide, South Australia, Australia
Honorary Professor, Australian National University College of Health and Medicine
Canberra, Australia
Adjunct Professor of Pediatrics, Department of Pediatrics
University of Rochester School of Medicine and Dentistry
Golisano Children's Hospital at URMC
Rochester, New York

Sundos Khuder, MD, CABP
Arab Board of Pediatrics, Neonatal Intensive Care Fellowship
Neonatologist/Head of Pediatric Department
NICU
Imam Zain El Abidine Hospital
Karbala, Iraq
Pediatrician/Head of NICU Department
NICU
Al Zahrawi Hospital
Damascus, Syrian Arab Republic

Mark L. Kovler, MD
Surgical Resident
Department of Surgery
Johns Hopkins University School of Medicine
Baltimore, Maryland

Courtney L. Kraus, MD
Assistant Professor of Ophthalmology
Johns Hopkins Medical Center
Baltimore, Maryland

Ganga Krishnamurthy, MBBS
Department of Pediatrics
Columbia University Medical Center
New York, New York

Stephanie K. Kukora, MD
Assistant Professor
Division of Neonatal-Perinatal Medicine
Department of Pediatrics
University of Michigan
CS Mott Children's Hospital
Ann Arbor, Michigan

Ashok Kumar, MD
Professor and Head
Department of Pediatrics
Banaras Hindu University
Varanasi, India

Shaun M. Kunisaki, MD, MSc
Associate Professor of Surgery
Pediatric Surgery
Johns Hopkins Children's Center
Baltimore, Maryland

Margaret Kuper-Sassé, MD, FAAP
Assistant Professor of Pediatrics
Department of Pediatrics-Neonatology
Rainbow Babies and Children's Hospital
Cleveland, Ohio

David M. Kwiatkowski, MD, MS
Associate Professor
Department of Pediatric Cardiology
Stanford University School of Medicine
Palo Alto, California

Satyan Lakshminrusimha, MBBS, MD, FAAP
Professor of Pediatrics
Department of Pediatrics
UC Davis Children's Hospital
Sacramento, California

Naomi T. Laventhal, MD, MA
Associate Professor
Department of Pediatrics
Division of Neonatal-Perinatal Medicine
Center for Bioethics and Social Sciences in Medicine
University of Michigan
Ann Arbor, Michigan

Shelley M. Lawrence, MD, MS
Associate Professor of Pediatrics
Department of Pediatrics
Division of Neonatal-Perinatal Medicine
University of Utah
Salt Lake City, Utah

Angela E. Lee-Winn, PhD
Assistant Professor of Epidemiology
Department of Epidemiology
Colorado School of Public Health
Aurora, Colorado

Steven Leuthner, MD, MA
Professor of Pediatrics and Bioethics
Division of Neonatology and Palliative Care
Medical College of Wisconsin
Medical Director
Palliative Care
Children's Wisconsin
Wauwatosa, Wisconsin

Laura Lewallen, MD
Assistant Professor of Pediatrics
Orthopedic Surgery
University of Chicago
Chicago, Illinois

Tamorah R. Lewis, MD, PhD
Associate Professor of Pediatrics
Department of Pediatrics
University of Missouri—Kansas City School of Medicine
Kansas City, Missouri

Hillary B. Liken, MD
Pediatric Cardiology Fellow
University of Michigan
Ann Arbor, Michigan

Arūnas Liubšys, MD, PhD
Associate Professor
Director of Neonatology Center
Vilnius University Hospital Santaros Klinikos
Vilnius, Lithuania

Kei Lui, MB BS UNSW, MD UNSW, FRACP
Senior Clinical Academic Neonatologist and Professor
School of Clinical Medicine
Discipline of Paediatrics and Child Health
University of New South Wales
Chair, Global Newborn Society
Chair, Australian and New Zealand Neonatal Network
Member, Board of Directors of the iNEO International Neonatal Network
Sydney, Australia

Akhil Maheshwari, MD, FAAP, FRCP (Edin)
Professor (Clinical) of Pediatrics, and of Molecular & Cellular Physiology
Louisiana State University Health Sciences Center—Shreveport
Shreveport, Louisiana

Nathalie L. Maitre, MD, PhD
Professor
Director of Early Development and Cerebral Palsy Research
Division of Neonatology
Department of Pediatrics
Emory University School of Medicine
Children's Healthcare of Atlanta
Atlanta, Georgia

Kartikeya Makker, MBBS
Division of Neonatal-Perinatal Medicine
Assistant Professor of Pediatrics
Johns Hopkins University School of Medicine
Baltimore, Maryland

Cherry Mammen, MD, FRCPC, MHSc
Pediatric Nephrologist
Department of Pediatrics
BC Children's Hospital
Vancouver, British Columbia, Canada

Richard J. Martin, MBBS
Professor
Pediatrics, Reproductive Biology, and Physiology & Biophysics
Case Western Reserve University School of Medicine
Drusinsky-Fanaroff Chair in Neonatology
Pediatrics/Neonatology Rainbow Babies & Children's Hospital
Cleveland, Ohio

María Mattos Castellano, MD
Neonatologist
Centro Hospitalario Pereira Rossell
Montevideo, Uruguay

Jessie R. Maxwell, MD
Associate Professor of Pediatrics & Neurosciences
Department of Pediatrics
University of New Mexico
Albuquerque, New Mexico

Renske McFarlane, BMBS, BA (Hons)
Department of Neonatology
University Hospitals Sussex
Brighton, United Kingdom

Gabrielle McLemore, PhD
Associate Professor of Biology
Department of Biology, SCMNS
Morgan State University
Baltimore, Maryland

Kera M. McNelis, MD, MS
Assistant Professor of Pediatrics
Department of Pediatrics
Cincinnati Children's Hospital Medical Center, University of Cincinnati College of Medicine
Cincinnati, Ohio

Christopher McPherson, PharmD
Clinical Pharmacy Specialist
St. Louis Children's Hospital
Associate Professor of Pediatrics
Department of Pediatrics
Washington University School of Medicine
St. Louis, Missouri

Ulrike Mietzsch, MD
Clinical Associate Professor of Pediatrics
Department of Pediatrics
Division of Neonatology
University of Washington, Seattle Children's Hospital
Seattle, Washington

Rachel R. Milante, MD
Strabismus & Pediatric Ophthalmology
Wilmer Eye Institute
Baltimore, Maryland
Strabismus & Pediatric Ophthalmology
Legazpi Eye Center
Albay, Legazpi City, Philippines

Jena L. Miller, MD
Assistant Professor of Gynecology & Obstetrics
Division of Gynecology & Obstetrics
Assistant Professor of Surgery
Division of Surgery
The Johns Hopkins Center for Fetal Therapy
Baltimore, Maryland

Vinayak Mishra, MBBS
General Practice Registrar
Blackpool Teach Hospitals NHS Foundation Trust
Lancashire, United Kingdom

Sagori Mukhopadhyay, MD, MMSc
Assistant Professor of Pediatrics
Department of Pediatric Medicine
University of Pennsylvania
Philadelphia, Pennsylvania

Sara Munoz-Blanco, MD
Assistant Professor of Pediatrics
Division of Neonatology
Assistant Professor of Internal Medicine
Section of Palliative Care
University of Texas Southwestern
Dallas, Texas

Mimi L. Mynak, MD
Department of Pediatrics
Jigme Dorji Wangchuck National Referral Hospital
Thimphu, Bhutan

Isam W. Nasr, MD
Assistant Professor of Surgery
Johns Hopkins University School of Medicine
Baltimore, Maryland

Niranjana Natarajan, MD
Associate Professor of Neurology
Department of Neurology
Division of Child Neurology
University of Washington
Seattle, Washington

Hema Navaneethan, MD
Assistant Professor of Pediatrics
Department of Pediatrics
University of Nebraska Medical Center
Omaha, Nebraska

Shannon N. Nees, MD
Assistant Professor of Pediatrics
Nemours Cardiac Center
Nemours Children's Health
Wilmington, Delaware

Jessie Newville, BS
Neurosciences
University of New Mexico School of Medicine
Albuquerque, New Mexico

Mai Nguyen, MD
Assistant Professor
John Peter Smith Hospital
Burnett School of Medicine, Texas Christian University
Fort Worth, Texas

Shahab Noori, MD, MS CBTI
Professor of Pediatrics
Fetal and Neonatal Institute
Division of Neonatology
Children's Hospital Los Angeles
Department of Pediatrics
Keck School of Medicine, University of Southern California
Los Angeles, California

Namrita J. Odackal, DO
Assistant Professor of Pediatrics, Ohio State University
Division of Neonatology, Nationwide Children's Hospital
Columbus, Ohio

Robin K. Ohls, MD
August L "Larry" Jung Presidential Endowed Chair
Chief, Division of Neonatology
Department of Pediatrics
University of Utah
Salt Lake City, Utah

Betsy E. Ostrander, MD
Assistant Professor of Pediatrics
Division of Pediatric Neurology
University of Utah
Salt Lake City, Utah
Director, Fetal and Neonatal Neurology Program
Primary Children's Hospital
Salt Lake City, Utah

Mohan Pammi, MD, PhD, MRCPCH
Professor of Pediatrics
Department of Pediatrics
Baylor College of Medicine
Houston, Texas

Prabhu S. Parimi, MD, MBA
Professor of Pediatrics
Case Western Reserve University
Division Chief of Neonatology
Department of Pediatrics
Metro Health Medical Center
Cleveland, Ohio

Albert Park, MD
Professor
Otolaryngology Head and Neck Surgery
Division of Pediatric Otolaryngology
University of Utah
Salt Lake City, Utah

Monika S. Patil, MD
Assistant Professor of Pediatrics
Department of Pediatrics
Baylor College of Medicine
Houston, Texas

Elaine M. Pereira, MD
Assistant Professor of Pediatrics
Department of Pediatrics
Columbia University Irving Medical Center/New York Presbyterian
New York, New York

Muralidhar H. Premkumar, MBBS, DCH, DNB, MRCPCH, MS
Associate Professor of Pediatrics & Neonatology
Baylor College of Medicine
Houston, Texas

Webra Price-Douglas, PhD, NNP-BC, IBCLC
The Johns Hopkins Hospital
University of Maryland Medical Community Medical Groups
Baltimore, Maryland

Karen M. Puopolo, MD, PhD
Professor of Pediatrics
University of Pennsylvania Perelman School of Medicine
Section Chief
Newborn Medicine
Pennsylvania Hospital
Attending Physician
Neonatology
Children's Hospital of Philadelphia
Philadelphia, Pennsylvania

Heike Rabe, MD, PhD
Professor of Perinatal Medicine
Academic Department of Paediatrics
Brighton & Sussex Medical School
University of Sussex
Honorary Consultant Neonatologist
Neonatology
Brighton and Sussex University Hospitals
Brighton, United Kingdom

Mohammad M. Rahman, MBBS, DCH, FCPS (Neonatology)
Fellow of the Institute of Child and Mother Health and of the Institute of Education and Research
Dhaka University
Dhaka, Bangladesh

Kristina Reber, MD
Professor of Pediatrics
Department of Pediatrics
Baylor College of Medicine
Division Chief of Neonatology
Texas Children's Hospital
Houston, Texas

Venkat Reddy Kallem, DrNB Neonatology
Consultant Neonatologist
Paramitha Children's Hospital
Hyderabad, Telangana, India

Michael X. Repka, MD, MBA
David L. Guyton MD and Feduniak Family Professor of Ophthalmology
Professor of Pediatrics
Johns Hopkins University School of Medicine
Baltimore, Maryland

Daniel S. Rhee, MD, MPH
Assistant Professor of Surgery
Johns Hopkins University School of Medicine
Baltimore, Maryland

Megan L. Ringle, MD, MPH
Assistant Professor of Neonatology
Division of Neonatology
Department of Pediatrics
Wake Forest School of Medicine
Winston Salem, North Carolina
Clinical Medicine Fellow
Division of Neonatal and Developmental Medicine
Department of Pediatrics
Stanford University
Clinical Neonatal-Perinatal Medicine Fellow
Neonatal and Perinatal Medicine
Stanford University, School of Medicine
Palo Alto, California

Allison Rohrer, MS, RD, LD
Neonatal Dietitian
Department of Pediatrics
Medical University of South Carolina
Charleston, South Carolina

Christopher J. Romero, MD
Associate Professor of Pediatrics
Division of Pediatric Endocrinology and Diabetes
Icahn School of Medicine at Mount Sinai
New York, New York

Marisa A. Ryan, MD, MPH
Pediatric Otolaryngologist—Head & Neck Surgeon
Peak Pediatric
Ear Nose & Throat
Lehi, Utah

Maame E.S. Sampah, MD, PhD
Research Fellow
Department of Surgery
The Johns Hopkins Hospital
Baltimore, Maryland

Amarilis Sanchez-Valle, MD
Professor of Pediatrics
University of South Florida
Tampa, Florida

Guilherme M. Sant'Anna, MD, PhD, FRCPC
Full Professor of Pediatrics
Pediatrics—Neonatology
Associate Member
Department of Medicine—Division of Experimental Medicine
McGill University
Montreal, Quebec, Canada

Ola D. Saugstad, MD, PhD
Department of Pediatric Research
University of Oslo and Oslo University Hospital
Oslo, Norway
Anne and Robert H. Lurie Children's Hospital of Chicago, Feinberg School of Medicine, Northwestern University
Chicago, Illinois

John P. Schacht, DO
Division of Clinical Genetics, Columbia University
New York, New York

Robert L. Schelonka, MD
Professor and Chief
Division of Neonatology
Department of Pediatrics
Oregon Health and Science University
Portland, Oregon

Erin E. Schofield, MD
Assistant Professor
Department of Pediatrics/Division of Neonatology
University of Maryland School of Medicine
Baltimore, Maryland

David T. Selewski, MD, MSCR
Associate Professor of Pediatrics
Department of Pediatrics
Medical University of South Carolina
Charleston, South Carolina

Prakesh S. Shah, MD, MRCP, FRCPC, MSc
Professor of Pediatrics
Division of Pediatrics
Mount Sinai Hospital and University of Toronto
Toronto, Ontario, Canada

Jessica G. Shih, MD
Department of Plastic & Reconstructive Surgery
Johns Hopkins University School of Medicine
Baltimore, Maryland

Erica M.S. Sibinga, MD, MHS
Associate Professor of Pediatrics
Division of Pediatrics
Johns Hopkins University School of Medicine
Baltimore, Maryland

Winnie Sigal, MD
Assistant Professor of Pediatrics
Department of Pediatrics
Division of Endocrinology and Diabetes
The Children's Hospital of Philadelphia/ Perelman School of Medicine at the University of Pennsylvania
Philadelphia, Pennsylvania

Brian Sims, MD, PhD
Professor of Pediatrics
Division of Neonatology
UAB Women and Infant Center
University of Alabama at Birmingham
Birmingham, Alabama

Rachana Singh, MD, MS
Associate Chief, Newborn Medicine
Department of Pediatrics
Tufts Children's Hospital
Professor of Pediatrics
Tufts University School of Medicine
Boston, Massachusetts

Srijan Singh, MD, DM
Assistant Professor
Department of Pediatrics
Grant Government Medical College and Sir JJ Group of Hospitals
Mumbai, Maharashtra, India

Donna Snyder, MD, MBE
US Food and Drug Administration
Office of the Commissioner Office of Pediatric Therapeutics
Silver Spring, Maryland

Helena Sobrero, MD
Adjunct Professor
Neonatologist
Department of Neonatology
Centro Hospitalario Pereira Rossell
School of Medicine, University of the Republic
Montevideo, Uruguay

Paul D. Sponseller, MD, MBA
Professor, Orthopaedic Surgery
Chief, Division of Pediatric Orthopaedics
Department of Orthopaedics
Johns Hopkins University School of Medicine
Baltimore, Maryland

Carl E. Stafstrom, MD, PhD
Director
Division of Pediatric Neurology
Department of Neurology
Johns Hopkins University School of Medicine
Baltimore, Maryland

Heidi J. Steflik, MD, MSCR
Assistant Professor of Pediatrics
Department of Pediatrics
Medical University of South Carolina
Charleston, South Carolina

Lisa R. Sun, MD
Assistant Professor of Neurology
Division of Neurology
Johns Hopkins University School of Medicine
Baltimore, Maryland

Sripriya Sundararajan, MBBS, MD
Associate Professor of Pediatrics
Department of Pediatrics
Division of Neonatology
University of Maryland School of Medicine
Baltimore, Maryland

Sarah N. Taylor, MD, MSCR
Professor of Pediatrics
Section of Neonatal Perinatal Medicine
Yale University School of Medicine
New Haven, Connecticut

Norma Terrin, PhD
Tufts Clinical and Translational Science Institute and the Institute for Clinical Research and Health Policy Studies
Tufts Medical Center
Boston, Massachusetts

Prolima G. Thacker, MBBS, MS, DNB
Observer
Pediatric Ophthalmology and Strabismus
Wilmer Eye Institute
Baltimore, Maryland

Bernard Thébaud, MD, PhD
Department of Pediatrics, Children's Hospital of Eastern Ontario and CHEO Research
Institute, Regenerative Medicine Program Ottawa Hospital Research Institute
Department of Cellular and Molecular Medicine, University of Ottawa
Ottawa, Ontario, Canada

Rune Toms, MD, MSc
Associate Professor of Pediatrics
Department of Pediatrics
University of Alabama at Birmingham
Birmingham, Alabama

Benjamin A. Torres, MD
Associate Professor of Pediatrics
Department of Pediatrics
University of South Florida
Tampa, Florida

David E. Tunkel, MD
Professor of Otolaryngology-Head and Neck Surgery
Johns Hopkins University School of Medicine
Director of Pediatric Otolaryngology
The Johns Hopkins Hospital
Baltimore, Maryland

Christine H. Umandap, MD
Medical Geneticist
DMG Children's Rehabilitative Services
Phoenix, Arizona

Diana Vargas Chaves, MD
Assistant Professor of Pediatrics
Division of Neonatology
Columbia University Medical Center
New York, New York

Maximo Vento, MD, PhD
Professor of Neonatology
Division of Neonatology
University & Polytechnic Hospital La Fe
Professor
Neonatal Research Group
Health Research Institute La Fe
Valencia, Spain

Jonathan Walsh, MD
Associate Professor of Otolaryngology-Head and Neck Surgery
Department of Otolaryngology
The Johns Hopkins Hospital
Baltimore, Maryland

Jolan Walter, MD, PhD
Robert A. Good Endowed Chair, Division of Pediatric Allergy & Immunology
Associate Professor, College of Molecular Medicine
Associate Professor, College of Medicine Pediatrics
Tampa, Florida

Meaghann S. Weaver, MD, MPH, FAAP
Chief Division of Pediatric Palliative Care Pediatrics
Children's Hospital and Medical Center—Omaha
Omaha, Nebraska

Kristin Weimer, MD, PhD, MHS
Assistant Professor of Pediatrics
Department of Pediatrics
Duke University
Durham, North Carolina

Jennine Weller, MD, PhD
General Surgery Resident
Department of Surgery
The Johns Hopkins Hospital
Baltimore, Maryland

Lindy W. Winter, MD
Medical and Quality Officer for Pediatric Services
Medical Director
Regional Neonatal Intensive Care Unit
Medical Director
Continuing Care Nursery
Director of Neonatology Quality Improvement
Department of Pediatrics
University of Alabama, Birmingham
Birmingham, Alabama

Tai-Wei Wu, MD
Assistant Professor of Pediatrics
Fetal and Neonatal Institute
Division of Neonatology
Children's Hospital Los Angeles
Department of Pediatrics
Keck School of Medicine, University of Southern California
Los Angeles, California

Mabel Yau, MD
Assistant Professor of Pediatrics
Adrenal Steroid Disorders Program
Mount Sinai School of Medicine
New York, New York

Preface

Newborn infants are a high-risk population with mortality rates similar to those in 58–60-year-olds. They can have many acute problems, which require timely management to ensure survival, and chronic issues that may have lifelong consequences. If appropriately treated, the practice is rewarding. If not, the consequences can be physically and emotionally devastating for both parents and care-providers.

There is many a medical textbook focused on problems seen in newborn infants. But we still need one that (a) can cover the needs of both the East and the West, and so we requested help from more than 220 experts from all over the world; (b) is comprehensive, but the chapters are sized according to the likely needs of a practicing care-provider; and (c) contains enough useful information but is still convenient to carry and is not so large that it becomes just a decorative piece in the office. We planned sections focused on the care of premature and critically-ill neonates; resuscitation and respiratory illness; feeding; nutrition; endocrine disorders; infections; cardiac defects and disorders; blood disorders; skin conditions; neurological disorders; immunology; sections on renal, eye, auditory, and orthopedic conditions; inborn errors and other genetic conditions; surgical issues; palliative care; follow-up; organization; and leadership. We have tried to size these sections based on the probability/frequency of need in clinical practice. Thinking further, we moved the section on skin conditions towards the end because of the higher likelihood of need during active patient care to facilitate quick access during clinical rounds.

Acknowledgments

I want to express gratitude to our section editors, Drs. Nitasha Bagga, Cynthia Bearer, Waldemar Carlo, Sharon Groh-Wargo, David Cooke, Sheela Magge, Karen Puopolo, Shazia Bhombal, Robert Christensen, Frances Northington, John Benjamin, Michael Repka, David Tunkel, Paul Sponseller, Wendy Chung, David Hackam, Renee Boss, Naveen Jain, Jonathan Davis, and Prabhu Parimi. Many authors participated in this book because of their commitment to the Global Newborn Society (https://www.globalnewbornsociety.org/), a rapidly-growing public service organization that is now active in 122 countries. There are other leaders from the Rotary Club. I have learnt so much here—to each one, thank you!

We want to take a moment of silence. We lost one of our dearest section editors, Dr. Eric Jelin, while this book was still in development. He will be missed but never forgotten.

I wish to thank Sarah Barth, Priyadarshini Pandey, Daniel Fitzgerald and the entire Elsevier publishing team for making this book possible. I would also like to thank Drs. Sue Aucott and Tina Cheng at the Johns Hopkins University for supporting me in all times, good and bad.

Contents

SECTION 1

Care of the Premature and Critically-Ill Neonate

OUTLINE

Section 1

CHAPTER

1 Design of Neonatal Intensive Care Units

Margaret Kuper-Sassé, Cynthia F. Bearer, Dina El-Metwally

KEY POINTS

1. Historically, neonatal intensive care units (NICUs) have been designed as open-bay units with multiple patient beds in a room. However, the trend has shifted toward designing units with single-patient or single-family rooms.
2. Single-family rooms have facilitated a reduction in auditory and noxious stimuli and improvement in positive stimuli to support appropriate development.
3. Parents and families have reported increased engagement in the care of their infants.
4. In NICUs with single-family rooms compared with open-bay NICUs, maternal feeding and infant growth seem to have improved.
5. Care in single-patient rooms was expected to reduce infection rates, but the evidence for such improvement is uncertain.
6. Single-family rooms have improved parent involvement but may have created new challenges for caregivers. The introduction of alarms may help by alerting staff members about changes in the clinical status of the patients and facilitating timely intervention.

Introduction

Historically, neonatal intensive care units (NICUs) have been designed as open-bay units with multiple patient beds in a room, a design that was introduced in the 1940s.[1] The trend has shifted toward the inclusion of parents with neonatal care. Thus units consisting of single-patient or single-family rooms (SFRs; many of which include a reserved space for parents inside the patient room) required new construction. This configuration for neonatal care units was introduced as the ideal design in the 1990s.[2] The new design reflected the general trend in healthcare toward patient and family satisfaction by emphasizing privacy and a feeling of individualized care, but by design, it neglects the elements that aid staff in caring for the patients, such as visibility, ease of access to patients, and efficiency of caring for multiple patients.[1] The movement represented a change in focus away from the needs of staff and toward families' needs, which in many cases are contradictory.[3]

Patient Safety

Alarms are designed to alert staff members to patient status changes and allow for intervention as necessary. Caregiver alarm fatigue, caused by sensory overload and resultant decreased or delayed responsiveness to alarms, can have adverse effects on patient safety.[4] Exposure of nurses and patients to alarm sounds was found to be 44% higher in the open-bay style NICU (Fig. 1.1) than in the SFR-style NICU (Figs. 1.2–1.4), potentially with effects on both patients and staff. Excessive alarm exposure may also cause nurses to increase upper alarm limits to decrease the frequency of alarms, resulting in patient oxygen saturations being outside of the recommended ranges. Infants experience greater than 80% of their noxious noise exposure from alarms, which can be harmful in many ways, including affecting patient cardiopulmonary stability and sleep-wake cycles.[5,6]

Decrease Stressful Stimuli and Increase Positive Stimuli

In the NICU environment, the needs of multiple parties must be balanced. Newborn and infant patients require minimal noxious stimuli (Figs. 1.5 and 1.6) and the presence of positive stimuli to support appropriate development. Parents want to be able to assist with the care of their infants and to have privacy while living in the unit with their infants (see Fig. 1.4). The staff needs to have the ability to care for patients in a low-stress and amicable working environment (see Fig. 1.6).[7] By the 1990s, preterm infants were increasingly found to be uniquely vulnerable to the effects of negative sensory stimuli, stress, and sleep-cycle disturbances.[8]

One negative sensory stimulus is noise, compared with sound. The goal for the sound environment in the NICU, especially when considering preterm infants whose auditory organs and neurologic pathways are still developing and maturing, should always be a minimization of noxious noise while maintaining exposure to positive sounds as would happen within the womb[8a] (see Fig. 1.5). The negative effects of noise, especially high-frequency noise,[8b] on preterm infants include short-term effects on the stability of cardiovascular and respiratory systems,[8c,8d] disruption of sleep patterns,[8e] and potential long-term harm to the auditory and nervous systems.[8b,8f]

There has long been a recommendation to reduce sound exposure in the NICU so that it does not exceed a level greater than 45 dB for preterm infants and term infants who are ill.[8a] As was intended from the design, sound exposure is decreased in SFRs compared with open-bay NICUs.[8g,8h] An unintended consequence of the reduced sound environment appears to be delayed language development at 2 years of age in former preterm infants from SFRs compared with their open-bay counterparts.[8a]

There is a positive correlation between preterm infants' exposure to parental speech and their quantity and quality of vocalizations at postmenstrual ages of 32 and 36 weeks,[8h] indicating

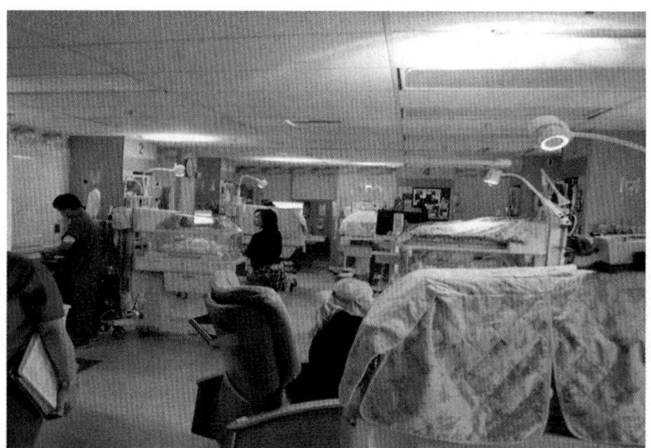

Fig. 1.1 An Open-Bay Newborn Intensive Care Unit With Eight Beds. Parents are provided comfortable chairs to spend time close to their infants. (2011, University of Maryland Hospital.)

that positive sound is beneficial to their development. Evidence shows enhanced development of the auditory cortex after exposure to recordings of maternal voice and heartbeat in infants born extremely prematurely, compared with routine NICU sound exposure.[8i]

The modification of noise in the NICU environment has been shown to decrease transitory noise after the implementation of clinical mobility communication systems (CMCS) such as smartphones and the elimination of overhead pages. In one study, the percentage of sounds that exceeded the thresholds recommended by the Environmental Protection Agency and International Noise Council decreased from 31.2% to 0.2% after the implementation of CMCS.[8j]

The benefit of music as a positive stimulus has also been explored. In one study, playing Brahms' lullaby sung by a female vocalist to late preterm infants was noted to reduce sleep interruptions and increase brain maturation patterns measured by amplitude-integrated electroencephalogram.[8k] This study suggests that singing to preterm babies may have implications for their brain development. The SFR NICU plan reduces infants' exposure to harmful noise. Future areas of study will need to examine how to provide positive auditory stimuli, more closely mimicking the environment in the womb, to the developing infant.

Infection

Outcome studies comparing infection rates between open-bay and SFR NICUs are conflicting and controversial. No difference in hospital-acquired infections (HAI) was found in one study.[8l] In contrast, catheter-associated bloodstream infections were decreased from 10.1 per 1000 device-days to 3.3 per 1000 device-days over 9 months after the transition from an open-bay to an SFR-style layout in one US NICU.[1] A systematic review and meta-analysis through August 2018 that included 13 separate patient populations (N = 4793) of preterm infants showed a reduction in rates of sepsis with no change in long-term neurodevelopmental outcome in the SFR design versus open bays.[9] A retrospective review of medical records of infants admitted to open-bay versus single-family units, including 1823 infants and 55,166 patient-days, showed similar rates of methicillin-resistant *Staphylococcus aureus* (MRSA) colonization, late-onset sepsis, and mortality. Further analysis showed hand hygiene compliance was associated with decreased MRSA colonization, with hazard ratios of 0.83 and 0.72 per 1% higher compliance. The increased daily census was associated with increased MRSA colonization only in SFRs and not open-bay setups, with a hazard ratio of 1.31 (P = .039).[10]

Family-Centered Care and Improved Parent-Infant Interactions

SFRs are an improvement in many aspects of family-centered care in the NICU (see Fig. 1.4). One of the most important attributes of

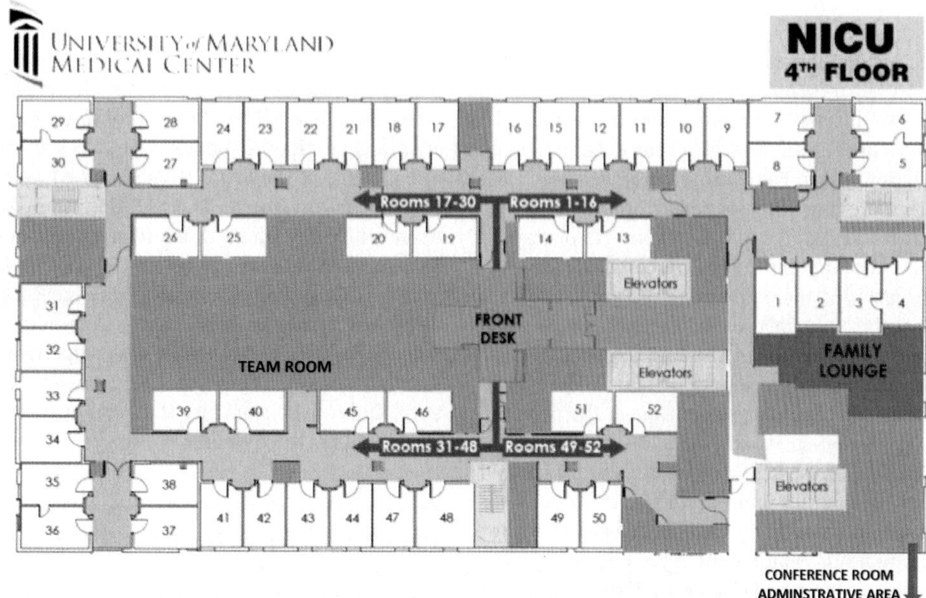

Fig. 1.2 Architectural Plan of the Single-Family-Room Newborn Intensive Care Unit at the University of Maryland Hospital. The single-family rooms allow the families to have some privacy. There is a family lounge where the parents can try to relax and at least transiently lower their anxiety levels from having a premature or critically ill infant with increased risk of mortality.

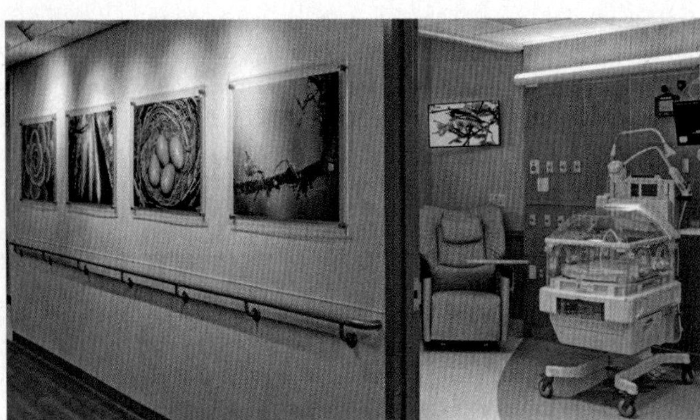

Fig. 1.3 Newborn Intensive Care Unit at the University of Maryland Hospital. Single-family rooms have community-based artwork, an attempt to create a pleasant environment.

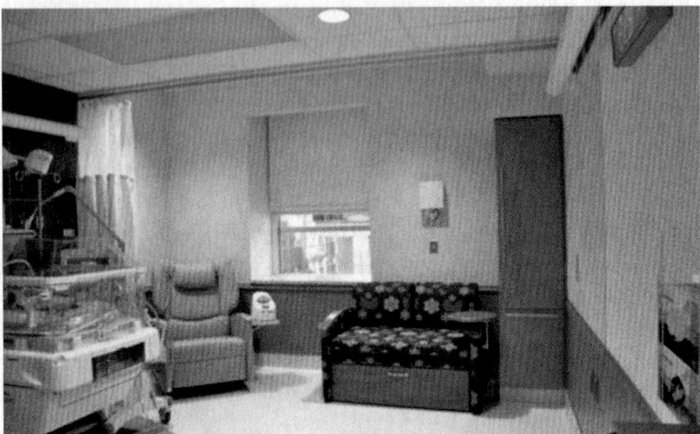

Fig. 1.4 A Single-Family Room in the Newborn Intensive Care Unit at the University of Maryland Hospital. The parents are provided with a recliner, breast pump, sleeping couch, and locker.

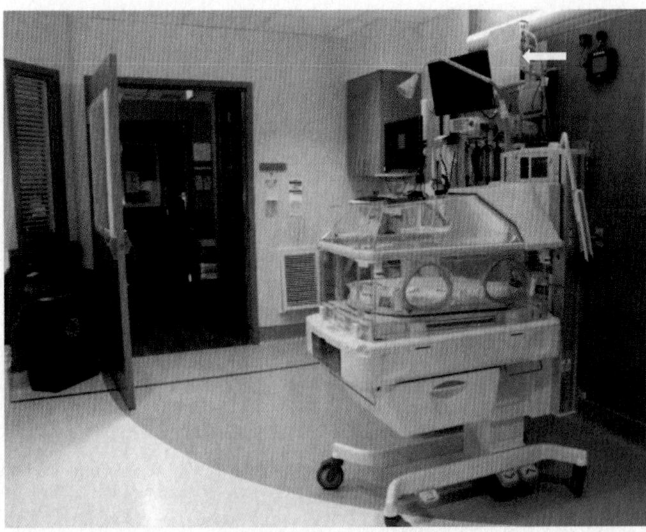

Fig. 1.5 Newborn Intensive Care Unit at the University of Maryland Hospital. A noise meter *(arrow)* has been placed on the top of the isolette.

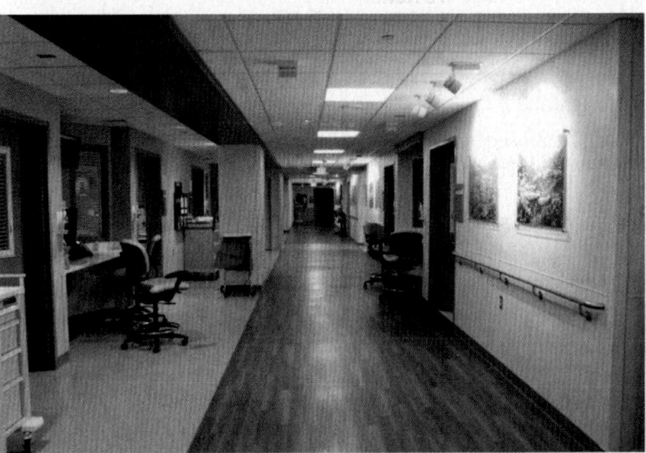

Fig. 1.6 Newborn Intensive Care Unit at the University of Maryland Hospital. The unit features spacious hallways, comfortable lighting, and rubber floors to minimize undue visual or auditory stimulation.

SFRs is parents' ability to participate in decision-making and help with bedside caregiving.[11] SFRs provide a feeling of increased privacy for families, as was shown in one NICU in the United States that conducted a survey during a 6-month period after moving from an open-bay style to an SFR style. Parents felt more involved in care and less like visitors and felt they had privacy to experience their emotions of happiness and distress with their infant.[12] SFRs with space for families to stay have been shown in multiple studies to improve family satisfaction.[13–15,15a] Families are more involved in care, including spending more time in the patient's room,[16,16a] maternal breastfeeding rates are higher,[9,14] and the total length of stay is shortened,[17] likely all because families feel more comfortable with a private, dedicated space within the patient room.[3] Parents' ability to be present and involved from admission to discharge likely also increases their confidence in caring for their infant long before discharge, contributing to the decreased length of stay.[18] However, contrary to the expectation that spending more time at the bedside would reduce anxiety, maternal stress related to NICU admission was slightly increased in the SFR setting.[19] To counter this difficulty, many centers have included family lounges within the NICUs to provide some space where parents can try to relax and at least transiently lower their anxiety levels from having a premature or critically ill infant who may be at increased risk of mortality (Fig. 1.7).

Patient- and family-engaged care is defined as "care planned, delivered, managed, and continuously improved in active partnership with patients and their families (or care partners as defined by the patient) to ensure integration of their health and healthcare goals, preferences, and values"[20] and is considered the culture of care. There is a direct relationship between NICU design and the culture of care.[21] The benefits of the SFR NICUs are owed to increased maternal and paternal involvement. The SFR setting provides the privacy and opportunity for maternal involvement; for example, increased rates of breastfeeding and human milk provision at 4 weeks was higher in SFR NICUs. Every 10 mL/kg/day increment of breast milk at 4 weeks was associated with increased cognitive, language, and motor Bayley scores (0.29, 0.34, and 0.24, respectively).[24] The SFR provides a private space that promotes parental involvement, extensive presence, and skin-to-skin care that cannot be accomplished in a traditional and crowded open-bay unit.[21]

Staffing Patterns, Nursing Workload, and Communication

The trend toward SFR structure in NICUs, despite solving some problems regarding parent involvement, creates a shift in challenges to caregivers, with inconsistent impressions among different groups. In

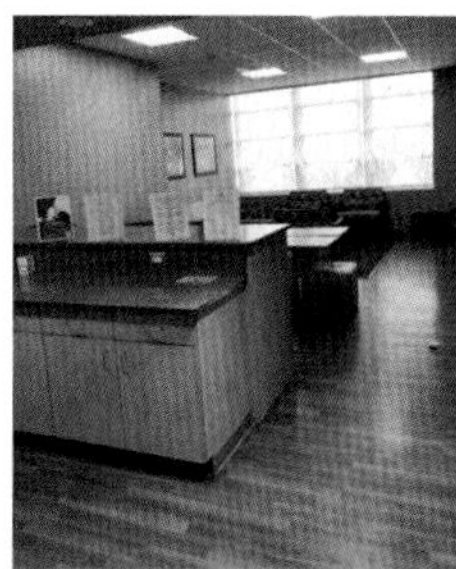
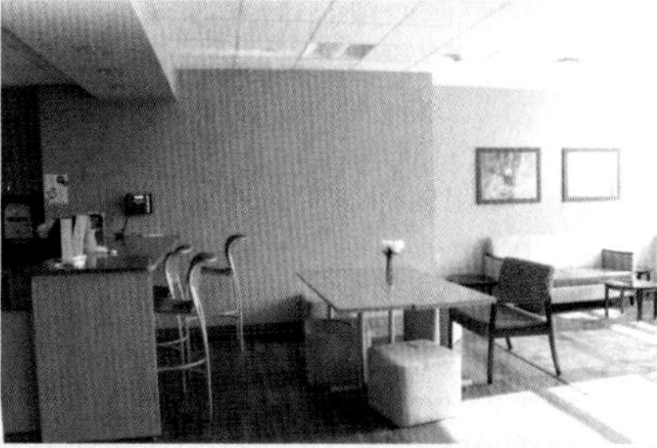
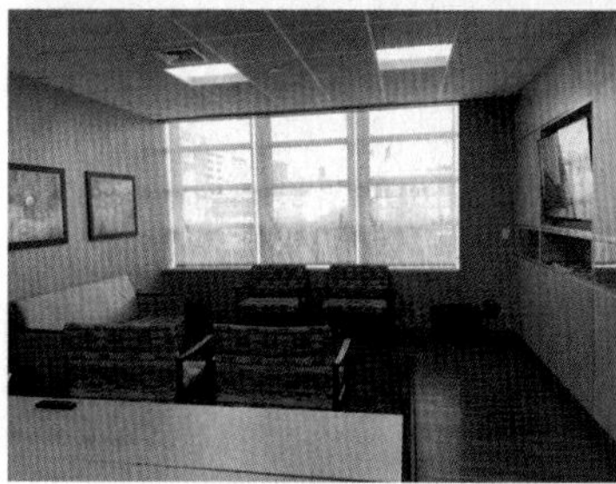
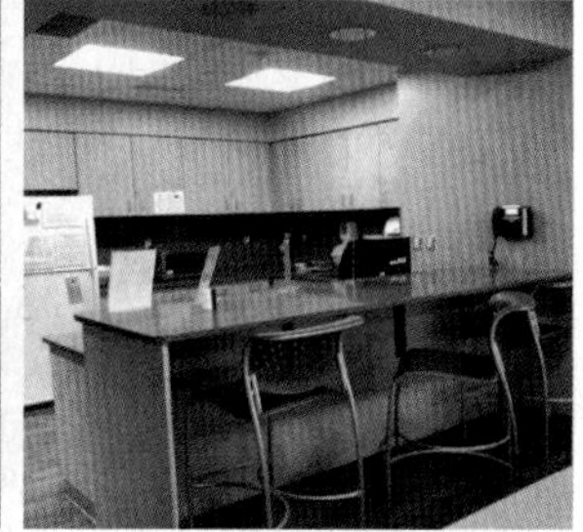

Fig. 1.7 Family Lounge in a Newborn Intensive Care Unit at the University of Maryland Hospital.

a study of a group of 127 nurses conducted before and after the transition from open-bay to SFR NICUs, 70% of the nurses felt that they had an increased workload in the single-family layout owing to increased physical difficulty with more walking required and an inability to see all patients at once or from other patients' bedsides.[1] Nurses in single-family units found it troubling that there was not a centralized location from which all their patients could be seen, thus making it difficult to know the status of all their patients at all times.[1,22] The reduced visibility of patients to their nurses and reliance on mechanical monitoring raises concerns about patient safety in an SFR-style unit.[7] A study of 21 staff members conducted 1 year after transitioning from an open-bay to a single-family design found that the staff felt they had less interaction with one another and thus had fewer opportunities for assistance and learning from colleagues.[22] In contrast, a survey of interdisciplinary staff conducted as quality improvement 1 year after the transition to an SFR structure found that staff had a perception of improved patient care, an improved environment for patients, families, and caregivers, and lower workplace stress.[23] There may be other factors that influence caregivers' impressions of workload and patient safety between sites, potentially including strategies (e.g., video monitors, communications systems, etc.) to adapt to these challenges.

Growth and Weight Gain

Growth is improved in SFR NICUs compared with open-bay NICUs in preterm infants <30 weeks' gestation and <1250 g at birth.[24] Infants in SFR NICUs had higher rates of human milk provision at 1 and 4 weeks and higher human milk volume at 4 weeks. Vohr et al. reported that increments of 10 mL/kg/day in human milk at 4 weeks were associated with increases of 0.29, 0.34, and 0.24 in Bayley cognitive and language scores.[24] Lester and colleagues compared patients in the same unit from before and after the transition to SFRs and found greater and faster weight gain among 123 preterm infants in SFRs compared with 93 patients in an open-bay unit (23.9 ± 3.8 g/day versus 22.2 ± 4.7 g/day, respectively; $P < .003$). However, other growth parameters such as head circumference were not significantly different between groups.[25] The results may have had multiple confounders because rates of sepsis were higher in the SFR NICU group. In contrast, necrotizing enterocolitis rates were lower compared with the open-bay group (sepsis, 25.8 versus 17.9; necrotizing enterocolitis, 4.3 versus 10.6, respectively). Another published study compared two populations of infants with a gestational age of 28 to 32 weeks at birth in SFR versus open-bay NICUs that both used the same feeding protocols and found no significant differences in weight, length, or head circumference at 34 weeks' postmenstrual age and 4 months' chronologic age. Consistent with other studies, the SFR parents spent significantly more time with their babies and provided more skin-to-skin care than did the parents of babies in the open-bay unit, but developmental milestones achieved were not significantly different between the two.[21]

Neurodevelopment Outcome

Neurodevelopment of preterm infants may be affected by placement in an SFR NICU. Vohr et al. reported in 2017 that Bayley III language composite scores were significantly higher and cognitive scores were marginally higher in preterm infants with a birth weight ≤1250 g at 18–24 months' chronologic age in SFR NICUs, after adjusting for covariates.[24] Interestingly, infants grouped by the amount of skin-to-skin care, breastfeeding, and maternal care and not by room type had greater cognitive, language, and communication scores, implying that maternal involvement had a more significant impact on outcomes than the site of care did. Lester et al. found that the number of days of maternal involvement was greater in the SFR than the open-bay NICU ($P < .002$), suggesting that the effect of the SFR was actually related to increasing maternal involvement. In this study, for every 1-day increase in the number of days per week of maternal involvement, the cognitive composite score increased by 1.6 points ($P = .002$), the language composite score increased by 2.9 points ($P < .000$), and both the receptive and expressive communication scores increased by 0.5 points ($P < .000$).[26]

In contrast, Pineda et al. reported lower Bayley language scores, a trend for lower motor scores, and lower amplitude integrated electroencephalography cerebral maturation in 2-year outcomes of 86 infants born at <30 weeks' gestational age and nursed in an SFR room compared with an open-bay NICU.[19] The low developmental scores were attributed to the lower sensory exposure and stimulation in the SFR NICU. Of note, in the study by Pineda et al., the parents had less visitation during the length of stay (25.5 ± 25.4 hours/week for SFR infants versus 16.9 ± 13.5 hours/week for open-bay infants), leading to consequently decreased holding, cuddling, skin-to-skin care, and breastfeeding and further supporting the argument that outcomes may be owed to maternal or paternal involvement.[27] Although the observations from the studies by Pineda et al. and Vohr et al. appear to present conflicting outcomes, they support the literature that upholds the importance of maternal presence and involvement in infants' care.

A systematic review and metanalysis of 13 study populations comparing outcomes at 18 to 24 months of age in preterm infants cared for in an SFR NICU versus an open-bay NICU, found no difference in cognitive Bayley III scores among the two NICU designs.[9]

Hybrid Model

Some NICU designers advocate for a hybrid model of SFRs and group-care spaces that is used selectively based on each infant's clinical status and the developmental and social needs of infants and families.[28] Some NICUs in Sweden and Turkey transition infants (also known as "feeders and growers") from the traditional open-bay room to the SFR as they become more mature and require less intensive care.[28] Also, there are differences in the use of SFRs depending on the stay and visitation policies of each setting. Some SFR NICUs require parents to "live in" and stay 24 hours a day from admission until discharge.[17] However, most SFR NICUs in the United States do not mandate a similar requirement; instead, they have an open-door policy where rooming-in is encouraged but at the convenience of parents.

Impact of the COVID-19 Pandemic

The pandemic of SARS-COV-2 in 2020 altered the standard family visitation policies in all healthcare facilities. During the peak of the pandemic, policies for visitation of parents in the NICU varied from no visitation to the standard preoutbreak 24/7 visitation policies.[29,30,30a] Most NICUs across the nation had some visitation restrictions that allowed one parent or caregiver, who was the same every day, at the bedside during the daytime.[31] A few policies were stringent and only allowed the same family-designated parent or caregiver throughout the duration of the infant's hospitalization. The NICUs with SFR designs were privileged to provide a private and closed environment, thus making infection control measures such as physical barriers, distancing, and separate air supplies attainable.[32] More NICUs with SFRs were able to maintain a 24-hour parental presence with babies and caregivers compared with open-bay units (64% versus 45%).[33] The majority of NICUs across the United States used technology such as teleconferencing to keep parents involved in their baby's care during limited visitations.[29] The plateauing of the pandemic enabled most NICUs to relax the visitation rules, allowing two caregivers at the bedside during the day, and some allowed one parent or caregiver to stay overnight.[34]

Summary

The transition of NICU design from open bay to SFRs has advantages that overall outweigh the disadvantages. Open-bay NICUs have improved parent satisfaction and involvement, increased breastfeeding rates, allowed for more visitation during a pandemic, decreased noxious noise stimuli, and improved short- and long-term medical outcomes for infants. SFR NICUs have caused obstacles for staff in hindering visibility and the ability to take care of multiple infants at once, decreased interaction among nursing staff, increased sensory deprivation of infants, and showed evidence of increased maternal stress and rates of MRSA colonization during times of high census. The shift in care model is considered an improvement, although more work remains to be done to correct the issues that have been brought to light, with a hybrid model as a possible solution for the future that will encompass the best of both models.

Advantages and Disadvantages of a Single-Family Room Design Neonatal Intensive Care Unit

Advantages	**Disadvantages**
Reduction in mortality and morbidity[14]	Isolation and sensory deprivation of infants[19]
Reduction in adverse medical outcomes[25,35]	Increased feelings of isolation of mother and family[27,36]
Improved hand hygiene	Delayed language development[19]
Reduction in infection[1,9,14,17,25]	Difficult interaction with the families[36]
Decreased length of hospital stay[17,18,26,37]	Increase in nurses' workload[36]
Lower rates of rehospitalization[17,26,35]	Decreased visibility in the NICU[1,7,22,36]
Fewer episodes of apnea of prematurity[14]	Difficulty of staff communication and less interaction among staff[1,22]
Decreased bronchopulmonary dysplasia (BPD)[17]	More maternal stress[27]
Fewer medical procedures[25]	Increased MRSA colonization with increased daily census[38]
Optimal provision of human milk and breastfeeding at discharge[9,14,24]	
Shorter interval to full enteral feeds and rate of growth[25]	
Better neurobehavioral stability at discharge[25,39]	
Decreased noise level[1,8g,8h,8j]	
Increased family-centered care and enhanced maternal rooming-in and involvement[11,16,21,26,27,40]	
Lower parental stress, anxiety, and depression[26]	
Greater parent satisfaction[15,37]	
Increased walking per shift by nurses and nurse practitioners[15]	
Decreased alarm fatigue, thus enhancing patient safety[6,7]	
Increased perception of quality and safety[23,41]	
Decreased rate of sepsis[9]	
Decreased catheter-associated bloodstream infections[1]	
Improved Bayley cognitive, language, and motor scores[24]	
Higher breastfeeding rates[9,14]	
Increased family satisfaction[13–15,15a]	
Able to accommodate parent visitation during a pandemic[33]	

MRSA, Methicillin-resistant *Staphylococcus aureus*; *NICU*, neonatal intensive care unit.

CHAPTER 2

NICU Environment for Parents and Staff

Angela E. Lee-Winn, Dina El-Metwally, Erica M.S. Sibinga

KEY POINTS

1. The admission of a premature or critically ill infant to a neonatal intensive care unit (NICU) is a stressful event for parents.
2. Parents in the NICU experience stress-induced emotional problems related to infant hospitalization, loss of control, and loss of contact with their infant.
3. The NICU staff can help develop strategies and interventions to help parents feel more comfortable and involved.
4. There is a need for mindful, cost-effective interventions to reduce parental distress.

The neonatal intensive care unit (NICU) is an emotionally charged environment both for parents and for healthcare providers. Having a newborn who needs to be in the NICU may come as an unexpected and traumatic event for parents. Furthermore, their infant's medical issues requiring the NICU may lead to higher levels of distress, symptoms of depression, anxiety, and trauma, along with increased sleep disturbance and fatigue, compared with parents with full-term, healthy newborns.[1] Nurses in the NICU provide critical round-the-clock care and services for vulnerable newborns and their families. Because their constant presence in the NICU is a requirement of the job, NICU nurses not only frequently witness parents' suffering and loss but also have their own and their fellow nurses' emotional turmoil ("contagious grief").[2,3] There is a great need to address the mental health and well-being of both parents and nursing staff in the NICU. In this section, we review literature on the impact of the NICU environment on parents and nursing staff and recommendations for meeting the unique needs of NICU parents and nursing staff.

NICU Parents

Many parents are unprepared to face the challenges of the NICU experience because most parents imagine having a healthy baby, who will be in the well-baby nursery for a day or two and be discharged home. Stemming from fears of their infant's medical problems and the possibility of losing their baby, parents with infants in the NICU experience greater feelings of sadness and anxiety. Because of the medical needs of infants in the NICU, parents also experience interrupted contact and reduced time being physically close to their newborn in the NICU, which also contributes to delayed parent–infant bonding.

A systematic review of qualitative studies on parental experiences in the NICU showed stress-induced emotional problems, stress of infant hospitalization, and loss of control or contact with babies as the top concerns of NICU parents.[4] These parents report experiencing extreme stress owing to feelings of restlessness, worry, fear, shame, guilt, and nervousness from their infant's admission to the NICU. As a likely contributor to these feelings, the physical NICU environment includes issues with complex staff communication and hospital equipment and technology that may overwhelm NICU parents.[5,6] Experiencing good communication with staff and longer interaction times with their infants in a welcoming and quiet atmosphere can compensate for some of these stressors and may, at least for short, intermittent periods, improve the NICU experience (Fig. 2.1).[7]

Very few studies have explored fathers' or both parents' experiences in the NICU, possibly because fathers typically spend fewer hours in the NICU. Fathers with infants in the NICU often experience similar or lower levels of stress than mothers do, but they show the tendency to cope with their stressful NICU experiences by withdrawing and becoming disconnected.[8,9] Younger fathers and fathers of infants with extremely low birth weight or infants who are very preterm reported increased stress in the NICU.[9] Fathers with newborns in the NICU face difficulties carrying out double duties as caretaker and breadwinner, including job loss owing to changes in family dynamics and interruption in their routine life.[10]

Opportunities in the NICU for Reducing Distress

Parents

The staff and environment in the NICU can have a positive impact on parents. Negative feelings and stress that mothers experience in the NICU are the main factors of delayed transition to parenthood.[4] The NICU staff could play a crucial role in developing and carrying out strategies and interventions that aim to help parents feel more comfortable and involved. The NICU staff can help parents by providing emotional support and, perhaps most importantly, actively engaging parents to participate in their infant's care in any way appropriate for their medical condition.

Because the experience of separation from their infant evokes stress among NICU parents,[5] the NICU management could develop parent-oriented approaches to infant care, including involving parents in caring for their newborn infants in the NICU in any way possible. Involving parents directly in their infant's care, even in small ways, has the

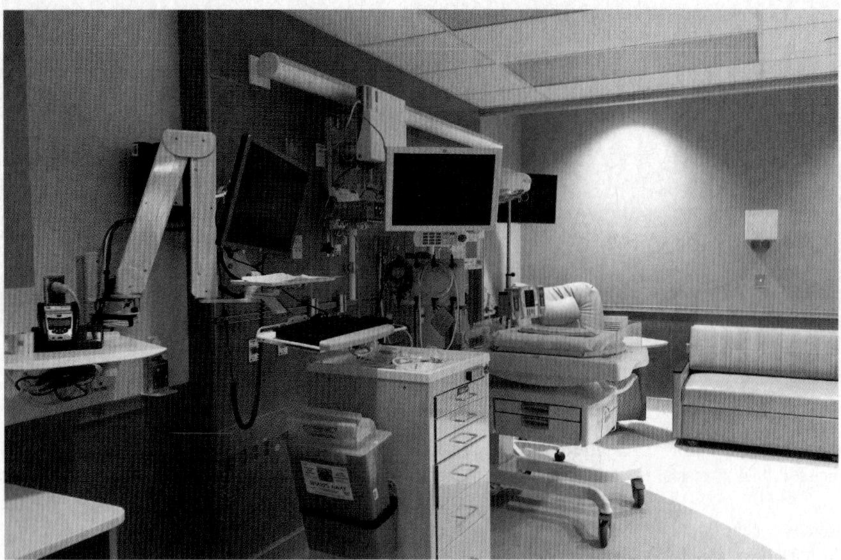

Fig. 2.1 A Single-Family Room Provides Parents With Privacy and Opportunities to Interact With Their Infant. (2011, NICU at the University of Maryland Medical Center.)

potential to increase parent-infant bonding and empower parents to gain confidence in their capability to take care of their infant, especially as their infant approaches discharge from the hospital. The availability of novel electronic devices to improve communication between parents and care providers can also be helpful (Figs. 2.2 and 2.3). Such a strategy will likely have the added benefit of strengthening the relationship between NICU parents and healthcare team members and lead to achieving optimal health of the whole family.

Acknowledging fathers' emotional states and stressors in the NICU is a step to help them feel included and valued. The NICU staff's early assessment of fathers' perceptions of potential environmental stressors in the NICU and their coping strategies can be valuable in engaging fathers in their infant's care. Being alert and quick to link fathers with available resources, particularly for younger fathers and fathers with low birth weight or preterm infants, is also crucial.

A growing number of NICU-based interventions for parents have been found to reduce long-term distress, particularly depressive symptoms.[11,12] Mindfulness-based interventions are gaining popularity owing to their cost-effective implementation[12] and growing evidence for their effectiveness for stress reduction,[11] which is a critical concern for NICU parents (Figs. 2.4 and 2.5). A pilot study of a mindfulness intervention delivered via video and audio recordings for mothers whose babies are in the NICU showed promising preliminary results in reducing maternal psychological distress and stress symptoms and improving sleep.[13] The individual and flexible nature of an audio-video program that can be used flexibly by parents offers significant potential for future implementation and dissemination in the NICU setting.

NICU Nursing Staff

The major focus for NICU settings has been more about emotional strain on families and less on NICU nursing staff. Working in a NICU can be both taxing and gratifying. Nurses in a NICU provide unwavering support, stay at the bedside along with families, and witness both agony and happiness. Many families bond with their NICU nurses and build trusting relationships. Nurses who establish stronger relationships with infants and families show higher levels of self-compassion, which in turn is associated with lower compassion fatigue, secondary traumatic stress, and burnout.[14]

However, a number of barriers contribute to challenges faced by NICU nurses. A survey among 72 NICU nurses from three Magnet facilities in North Carolina reported inadequate staffing as the most common stressor, which also has been identified as a national issue.[15] The importance of adequate staffing is also made clear in an ethnographic study of NICU nurses revealing that well-resourced and well-staffed institutions can buffer NICU nurses' emotional labor and hardship.[3]

The cultural norm for NICU nurses is often to suppress and numb their emotions when providing services to newborns and their families. Impossible demands for nurses to be "superhumans" who have no body or heart and receive too few rest breaks and too little support have emerged as a concern among NICU nurses.[2] Nurses' day-to-day emotional burden from their everyday work in NICUs has often been underrecognized.[3] A report showed 49% of survey respondents who were members of the National Association of Neonatal Nurses indicated moderate to severe secondary traumatic stress (i.e., stress results from helping or wanting to help a traumatized or suffering person).[2] Such work stress can have a negative impact on NICU nurses' professional and personal well-being, which in turn can negatively impact patient outcomes.[16]

Nurses in the NICU also rely on and can effectively support each other (the "sisterhood of nurses").[3] Studies have shown that NICU nurses who experienced errors or adverse events (e.g., mistakes, close calls, and incidents involving patient injury or harm resulting from medical care)[17] but also reported high levels of perceived coworker support showed lower levels of anxiety, depression, burnout, and secondary traumatic stress than did nurses who reported low levels of perceived coworker support.[18] Therefore, the peer support of NICU nurses can buffer the negative effects of NICU stress. Additionally, lack of respect and appreciation from their direct supervisors and physicians was also a concern and stressor among NICU nurses.[16]

Recommendations to Medical Institutions and Organizations

Few NICUs have programs for supporting and providing resources for NICU nurses.[19] The lack of institutional attention to NICU nurses' emotions and emotional labor can eventually lead to burnout and

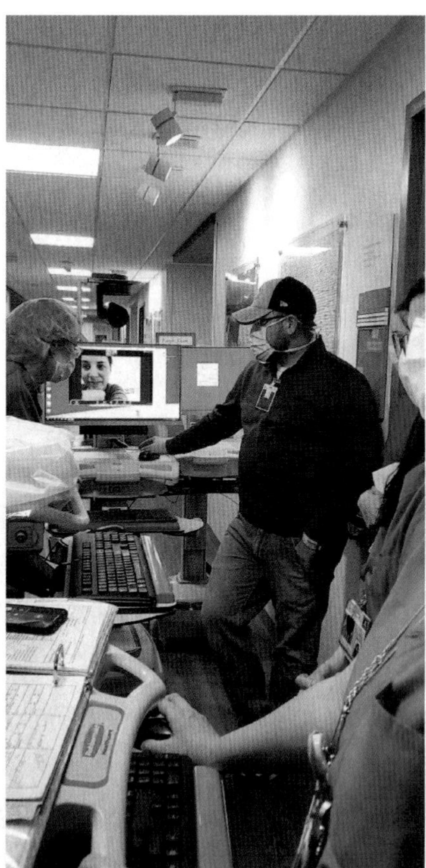
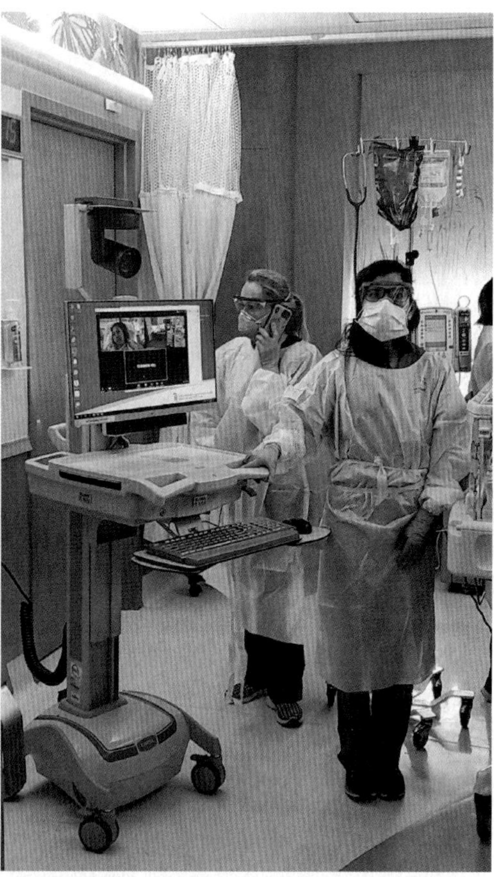

Fig. 2.2 NICU Zoom Telecart. This device allows virtual communication with parents who are not present on site during rounds in the neonatal intensive care unit. The device combines electronic medical records with the video platform Zoom. (2011, University of Maryland Medical Center.)

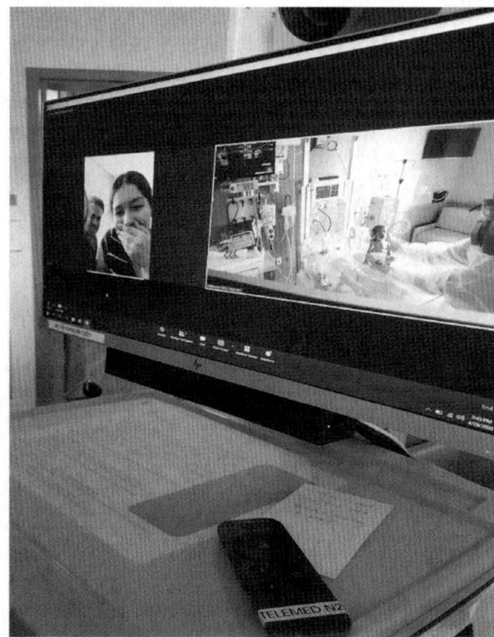
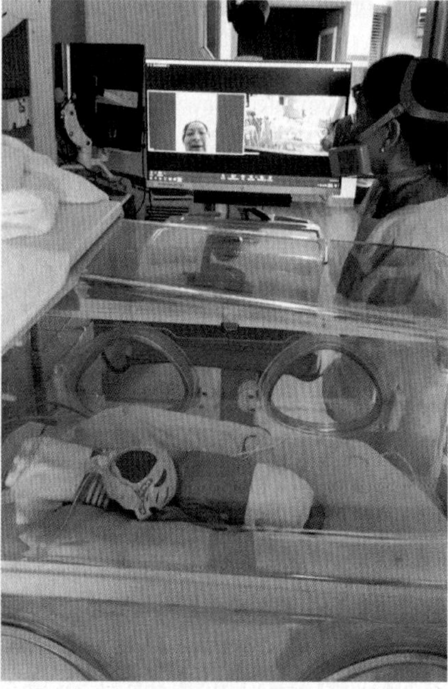

Fig. 2.3 A Mother With COVID-19 Pneumonia Sees Her 10-Day-Old Premature Infant (26 Weeks' Gestational Age) After She Herself Recovered Sufficiently to Be Extubated. (2021, University of Maryland Medical Center.)

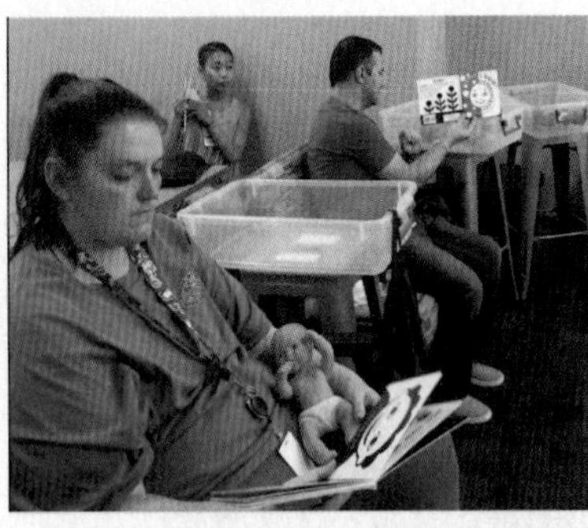
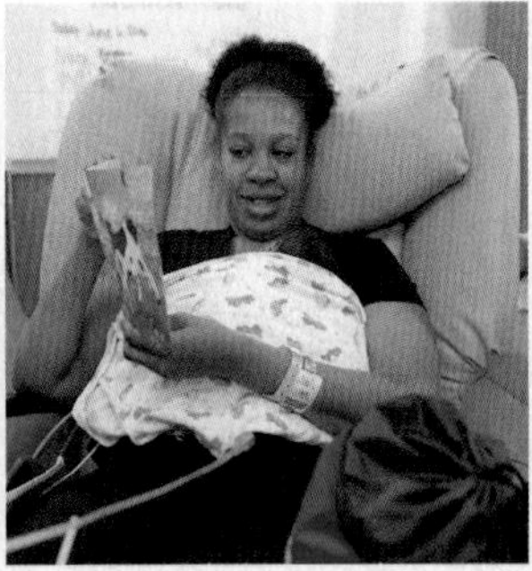
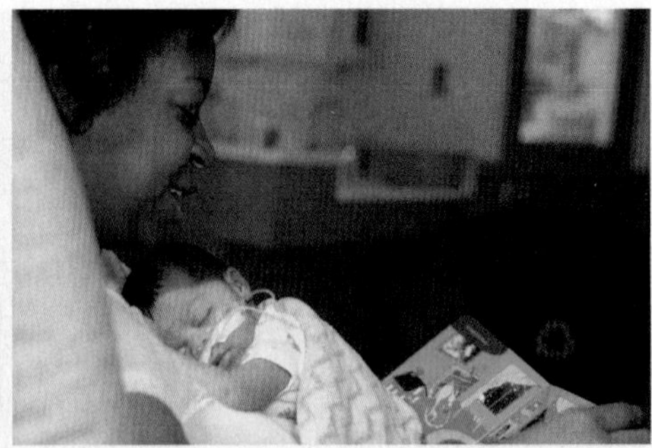

Fig. 2.4 Parents Engaged in the Mini-Gosling Early Language and Literacy Program in a Neonatal Intensive Care Unit. Such programs can support parents through mindfulness and stress reduction. This particular program was named to remind everyone about the intellectual potential of these young infants; the goose is one of the most intelligent birds, known for its memory. (2021, University of Maryland Medical Center.)

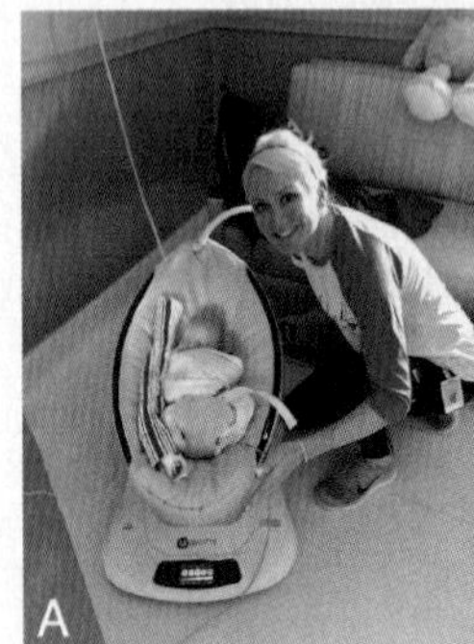

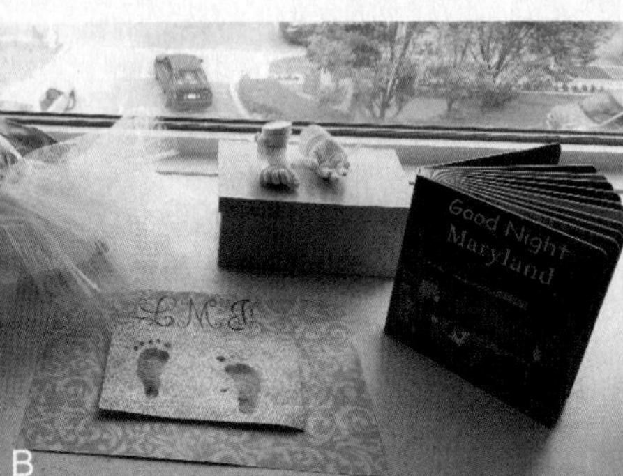

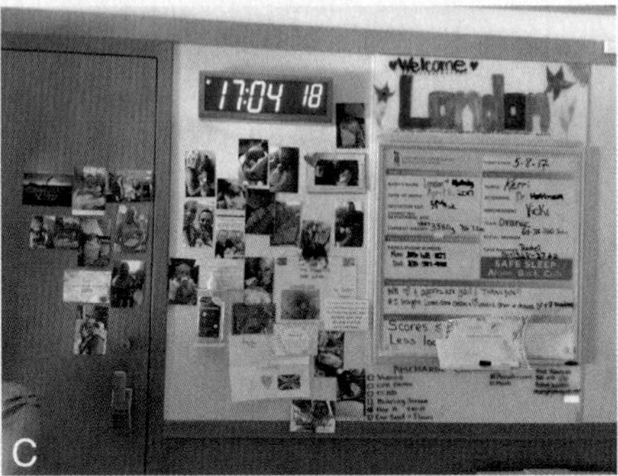

Fig. 2.5 A Friendly Environment in the NICU May Possibly Lower Some of the Stress That Parents of These Critically Ill Infants Continuously Endure. (A) A mother watching her baby, who only recently began to recover from critical illness, in a swing. (B) the windowsill in a patient room, featuring a customized casting of an infant's hand and foot, designed by the NICU Child-life Services. (C) A picture-board in an infant's room allows parents to save pictures, visitors' autographs, and other memorabilia. (2017, University of Maryland Medical Center.)

high turnover rates, costing institutions financially and impairing the quality of care provided. Continued efforts to improve quality of life among NICU nurses is vital to promote a healthy and safe work environment, which in turn will allow NICU nurses to provide the best possible care to infants and their families in NICUs.

Safe, flexible, and collaborative staffing should be considered and implemented to reduce NICU nurses' stress.[16] Future efforts to create and implement cost-effective strategies that allow for sufficient staffing, with breaks and training time for NICU nurses for better-quality patient care, are necessary. The availability of support programs, such as with cuddlers who can allow nurses to have brief breaks from the emotionally taxing environment, can also help (Fig. 2.6).

Building positive professional relationships with infants and their families in the NICU and collegial relationships with physicians are key actions administrators and managers could take to support NICU nurses.[14] Group cohesion, teamwork, and

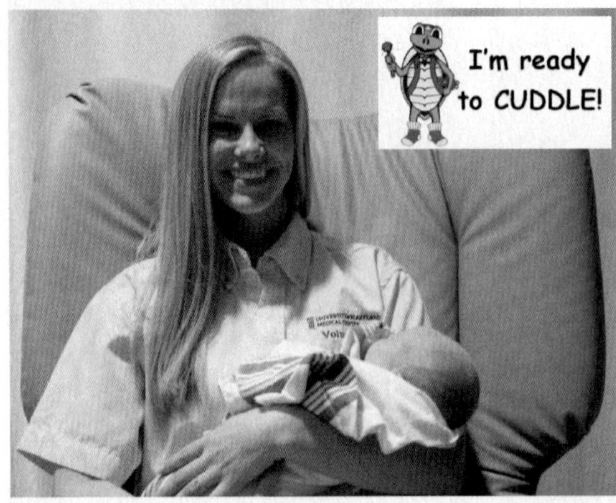

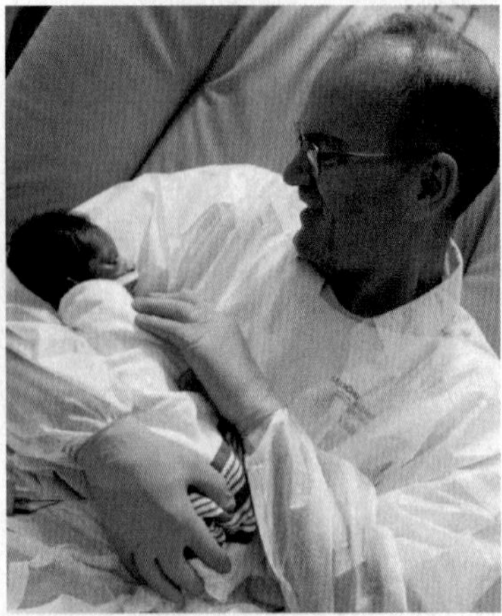

Fig. 2.6 A "Ready to Cuddle" Magnet Program in the Neonatal Intensive Care Unit. Volunteers (seen here in yellow shirts) who have been screened and trained spend time with the babies to provide some of the affectionate human interaction that healthy term infants would normally receive at their homes. Parents have the choice to accept it or to opt out. (2015, University of Maryland Medical Center.)

communication among healthcare providers have been suggested as keys to providing the highest possible quality of care in the NICU.[19–21] Creating and maintaining a collegial atmosphere that can promote respect and collaboration among all healthcare team members in NICUs can also be a first step toward creating a workspace that buffers NICU nurses' stress. Team-building and relationship-building activities for NICU staff on a regular basis could be beneficial.

Recognizing NICU nurses' everyday emotional labor and providing an outlet for their emotional distress and resources to cope with such burdens should be a priority for leadership to consider. Meeting the NICU staff's unique needs and promoting nurses' quality of life can be a sustainable approach to achieving decreased burnout and increased job satisfaction and well-being among nurses, ultimately improving the care of newborns and their families in the NICU and worker and patient safety.[3,22,23]

Setting up a supportive environment for all NICU nurses from the beginning of their employment and making efforts to increase perceived support (i.e., availability of support and a recipient's satisfaction with received support) rather than just received support (i.e., the quantity of support one receives) is beneficial.[24] Management should strive to meet the need for providing support for NICU care providers, especially after an event,[25] not only to reduce their emotional distress but also to improve overall patient safety.

Being aware of one's emotions and having skills to address negative emotions could help avoid traumatization and burnout among NICU nurses. Brief mindfulness interventions, for example, may be effective in improving provider well-being.[26] At an organizational level, providing tools and training sessions to reduce stress and manage emotional labor could benefit NICU nurses. Careful development and rigorous testing of mindfulness programs on their effectiveness and sustainability are necessary.

Section 1

CHAPTER

3 Safe Use of Health Information Technology

Yahya Ethawi, Abbas AlZubaidi, Akhil Maheshwari

KEY POINTS

1. Information technology (IT) can improve healthcare in its (1) efficiency in terms of economical achievement of goals, (2) effectiveness by improving the capacity to do so, and (3) efficacy with the capacity to achieve success under ideal, controlled circumstances.
2. IT can improve the safety of healthcare delivery with continuous quality improvement, sociotechnical approaches in hardware and software, and improved use of personnel.
3. Electronic health record (EHR) systems need monitoring in eight dimensions for the possibility of harm: human-computer interface, workflow and communication, clinical content, organizational policies, processes, hardware and software problems, external and vendor-related problems, and system management.
4. A Health IT Safety measurement framework has been developed to follow (1) continuous quality improvement and sociotechnical approaches, (2) use of health IT, and (3) healthcare safety concerns.
5. EHR alerts provide careful oversight of personnel allocation, errors, adequacy of resources, care quality, and education in various systems.
6. EHR systems can provide continuous access to and integrity of confidential patient data.

Introduction

Information technology (IT) is an important tool that can be used to improve productivity in various systems, including healthcare. In addition to improving workflow, IT can help assess interventions for both efficiency (the capacity to achieve a goal in the most economical way) and effectiveness (the capacity to do so given all variables). The eventual goal is to enhance and refine procedures to reach the best possible efficacy (capacity to achieve success under ideal, controlled circumstances).

Health IT aims to provide customized solutions, support clinical decisions, and record alerts (Fig. 3.1). The most important challenges have been in the design and acceptance of interventions and the tracking and evolution of outcomes (the DATE paradigm). The Institute for Healthcare Improvement suggests that reliability of healthcare is a three-part cycle of failure prevention, failure identification, and process redesign and defines *reliability* as "failure-free operation over time."[1] Information systems can provide continuous monitoring with real-time or nearly real-time reporting as a means of achieving reliability.[2] As such, it makes sense to think about the role of health IT in reliability as it relates to healthcare quality and patient safety.

As in any other organization, there has been a need for fiscal and human-resource planning and for managing expectations relative to cost, scope, and outcomes. We also need to identify reportable events before these turn into actual impediments in patient care and establish preventive methods. These ideas, described in the *Sentinel Event Alert 42*,[3] elaborate on the safe implementation of health information. In many events that have hitherto been perceived as unavoidable, sociotechnical interaction can improve safety. In any system, the goal is to develop and promote a culture of process improvement. We structure all our programs to develop goals that are specific, measurable, achievable, relevant, and time-framed (SMART). We have structured our thinking about health IT in the following sections.

The Need to ACT: A Focus on *A*ccess, *C*ommunication, and *T*racking

Access to Information

Health IT has improved access to medical records and has improved patient safety. Each patient has an interconnected, complex set of documents in his or her electronic health record (EHR), which is frequently created using multiple externally developed software applications.[4] These records originate from diverse stakeholders with specific requirements for documentation, including physicians, nurses, and other auxiliary personnel. They may dictate or use a specialty-specific template and clinical management, and then either they or others may add information codes that inform about real-time clinical decision support, quality reporting, and billing.[5,6] Families may also want a comprehensible explanation of the medical problems of their infant.[5] The revenue cycle departments of hospitals typically require a specifically designed note to include the necessary data elements to support the bill.[5] Auxiliary services such as the pharmacy use health IT to execute antimicrobial stewardship and to monitor pharmaceutical use, and the hospital administration may also want an unambiguous track of the patient's hospital stay.[7] The quality-control surveillance personnel may want to track records for any typing errors, inconsistencies, or redundancies. Scientists may also want information about specific events to determine outcomes based on clinical interventions.[6] Payer-sponsored quality-based incentive programs may seek evidence on key performance metrics.[1,8]

The evaluation of EHRs shows a need to address both technical and nontechnical contextual factors such as care providers and the workflow to improve the quality of care.[9] There are at least eight dimensions where EHRs can possibly cause sentinel events and actual harm (Fig. 3.2).[10] Ensuring EHR safety requires shared responsibility between several entities, including EHR developers and individuals within the local healthcare organization; this can fail[10,11] and cause important errors.[5] The 21st Century Cures Act promises to address

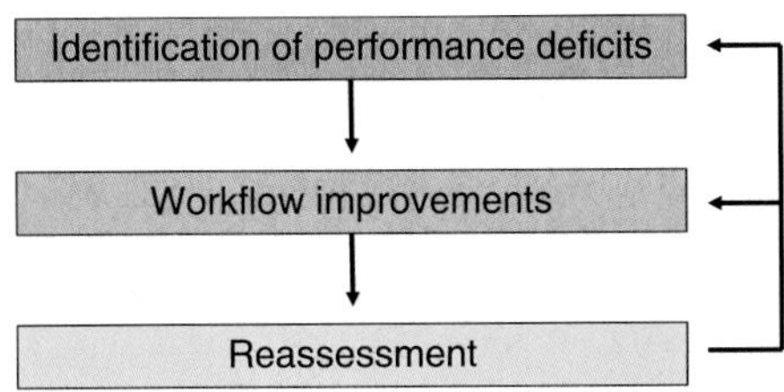

Fig. 3.1 The Standard Paradigm of Continuous Identification of Performance Deficits, Workflow Improvement, and Reassessment. Similar to other performance-focused systems, healthcare information technology follows this paradigm. Understanding this cycle helps create awareness and system reliability, aiming to improve healthcare quality and patient safety.

many of these concerns through the promulgation of new rules and regulations governing EHR interoperability, usability, and security.[12] EHRs introduce new kinds of risks into an already complex healthcare environment where both technical and social factors must be considered. An analysis of sentinel event reports received by The Joint Commission between January 1, 2010, and June 30, 2013, identified 120 sentinel events that were health IT–related. Factors contributing to the 120 events were placed into categories corresponding to eight sociotechnical dimensions necessary to consider for safe and effective health IT, as described by Sittig and Singh.[13] Listed by order of frequency, factors potentially leading to health IT sentinel events involved the following eight dimensions (see Fig. 3.2).

To address patient safety needs and regulations, a Health IT Safety measurement framework has been developed that follows both continuous quality improvement and sociotechnical approaches in three areas: (1) technological issues in hardware or software, (2) inappropriate use of health IT, such as deliberate suppression of alerts in EHRs, and (3) potential healthcare safety concerns such as medication errors and care delays before the occurrence of actual harm. The framework seeks to solve identified problems by integrating safety programs with organizational learning, comprehensive 360-degree assessment of safety in high-risk areas such as those with vendor involvement, and other factors that rely heavily on automated measurements. In 2011 an Institute of Medicine (IOM) report on health IT and patient safety emphasized the shared responsibility between key stakeholders including vendors, care providers, healthcare organizations, health IT departments, and public and private agencies.[14] These stakeholders have complementary roles in improving EHR safety.

The EHR safety measures should be synchronized with safety guidelines and quality-management scopes developed by international organizations such as the International Electrotechnical Commission, because the EHR and its subsequent derivations (application, platform, software, and management tools) are considered medical software and should abide by regulatory and directive items.

Communication

In 2011 the IOM report *Health IT and Patient Safety: Building Safer Systems for Better Care* highlighted that building health IT for safer use is a shared responsibility between "vendors [EHR and clinical content developers], care providers, provider organizations and their health IT departments, and public and private agencies."[14] Another IOM report, *Improving Diagnosis in Health Care*, again emphasizes "collaboration is needed among the health IT vendors, Office of the National Coordinator for health IT, and users" to ensure that health IT supports patients and healthcare professionals.[15,16]

In the past few years, Health IT has been deployed on a large scale, and thus the consequences of health IT–related safety concerns can rapidly affect not only a single department or institution but possibly an entire healthcare system.[17] As IT-enabled patient care is rapidly becoming the norm, it is essential to (1) refine the science of measuring health IT–related patient safety, (2) make health IT–related patient safety an organizational priority by securing commitment from organizational leadership and refocusing the

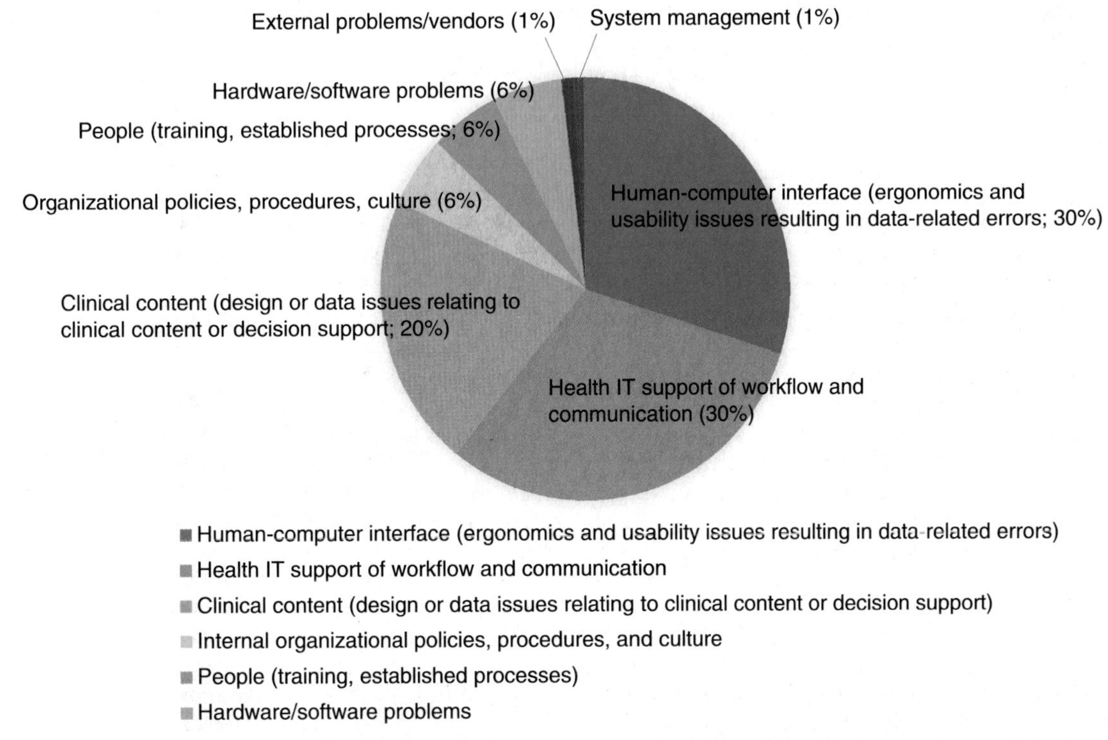

Fig. 3.2 Eight Dimensions in Which Electronic Health Record Deficiencies Can Cause Sentinel Events and Actual Harm.

organization's clinical governance structure to facilitate measurement and monitoring, and (3) develop an environment that is conducive to detecting, fixing, and learning from system vulnerabilities.[11,16,18]

Tracking

The intersection of health IT and patient safety involves three overlapping domains:

1. Use of health IT hardware and software
2. Use of technology by clinicians, staff, and patients and identification and mitigation of unsafe changes in workflows that emerge due to technology use
3. Identification and monitoring of patient safety events, risks, and hazards

Each domain is supported by principles adapted from the SAFER (safety assurance factors for electronic health record resilience) guides (Table 3.1).[19,20] Measurement in all three domains typically involves both retrospective and prospective measurements. Good measures should meet certain criteria: being impactful, such as demonstrating the importance of measurement and reporting; scientific acceptance, such as reliability and validity; feasibility, from a clinical, technical, and financial standpoint; usability, or easy extraction from existing EHRs; and transparency, with reviewability by all stakeholders.

The tracking of patient safety events requires continuous communication between multiple stakeholders including healthcare providers, patient safety professionals, and EHR vendors to collaboratively develop tools and strategies to optimize the safety of health IT.[21] Improved measurement is needed to create feedback for organizational learning, which in turn should lead to development of more refined measurement tools, clear definitions, and rigorous assessments of the types of safety concerns the organization should focus on. Monitoring for risks and hazards requires a heterogeneous group of experts, including technicians such as EHR developers, user interface designers, database administrators, and hardware and networking infrastructure personnel; experts on healthcare delivery systems such as clinical medicine and quality improvement; and leaders who continuously observe organizational change, risk management, and patient safety. Such a framework shares responsibility for improvement.

In any healthcare system, IT use should aim high to prevent *any* adverse quality and safety event from happening. Early success of automated reminders and alerts has raised expectations.[13] The development of alerts in EHRs is increasingly becoming a standard mechanism to prevent potential missed quality and patient-safety events. The aim of healthcare IT should be to provide careful oversight of the overall PEACE (Personnel allocation, Errors, Adequacy of resources, Care quality, and Education) in the system:

- Personnel allocation: The health IT service framework assumes that organizations will modify their existing patient-safety structures and processes to include the skill mix needed for the provision of comprehensive care.[22,23] There may be some variability in the needs of different organizations.[24] An EHR system allows for a development acuity score based on the physiologic data on a predefined time frame for the nursing leaders to allocate appropriate staff to provide safe care. A similar paradigm can be used

Table 3.1 Development, Use, and Safety of Electronic Health Records

Safety Area	Issues for EHR Developers	Issues for Healthcare Organization
EHR Interoperability	Develop and establish formats for transmitting clinical data	Families may choose not to share information about infant or themselves
	Develop standard technologies needed for specific patient populations	Share information with outside organizations
	Develop standard formats for exchanging data with external systems	Ensure computer systems and software are compatible
EHR Usability	Easy-to-use design and functions	Maintain hardware and software
	Use unambiguous text and actionable items	Consistent screen configuration
	Maintain usability principles for building user-customizable screens	Ensure adequate training of operators, appropriate resourcing, customization, and proper use of EHRs
	Respond to user feedback promptly	
EHR Security	Systems for adverse event reporting and clinical database management	Ensure clinical data are accurately recorded, stored, and communicated
	Develop robust procedures to improve EHR usability in clinical settings	Identify areas for usability improvement of EHR end-user interactions
	Enable complete, incremental, integrated, encrypted backups	Single sign-on to facilitate data access
	Create read-only downtime access	Software protection for EHR operations
	Log user actions and provide reporting tools to monitor and investigate suspicious behavior	Conduct periodic security risk assessments of confidentiality, integrity, and availability of protected EHRs
	Ensure backward-compatible data access for new versions	Develop, follow, and routinely update IT disaster recovery plans consistent with HIPAA Security Rule
	Provide role-based access to users	
	Enable multifactor authentication	
	Enable data-level access rights	
	If EHRs are cloud-based, developers provide disaster recovery plan to the organization	

The idea is to build safety assurance factors for electronic health record resilience (SAFER) guides.

EHR, Electronic health record; *HIPAA*, Health Insurance Portability and Accountability Act.

Modified from Gettinger A, Csatari A. Transitioning from a legacy EHR to a commercial, vendor-supplied, EHR: one academic health system's experience. *Appl Clin Inform.* 2012;3(4):367–376.

to assign an appropriate mix of patients to an advanced nurse practitioner to provide safe care. Such an approach will enhance safe care and improve staff satisfaction. However, healthcare organizations might need informaticians or clinicians trained in clinical informatics to collaborate with a multidisciplinary clinical oversight committee to help identify risks, prioritize interventions, and review IT-related solutions and patient outcomes. They might also create multidisciplinary EHR safety teams with human factors and informatics expertise to investigate safety events with potential "health IT involvement."[25] These teams could work within the protections of patient safety organizations during investigations and solution development and be integrated with an organization's existing risk management infrastructure.

- Monitoring for errors: Successful organizations need to be prepared for continuous, rigorous assessment of measurement readiness in all three domains of organizational readiness and how these are integrated within their existing patient safety infrastructure.[26] This requires the health IT systems to be closely involved in safety events. Risk managers and other quality personnel need to be continuously aware of the risk indicators for safety issues.[27] They may consider using proactive risk assessments using SAFER guides and integrate these activities within their existing patient safety programs.
- Adequacy of resources: Comprehensive data on resources needed for patient care and for IT-related services are critical.[28] Voluntary reporting alone may not be adequate because this may detect only a fraction of problems and be fraught with biases and not-latent errors and near misses.[28] Moreover, very few organizations are reporting safety issues related to health IT or EHRs. Thus alternative approaches to automated data collection need to be used to capture and respond appropriately to the full scope of health IT–related safety risks. Organizations need to consider additional methods of measurement beyond reporting, such as the use of automated triggers to detect wrong patient orders, helpdesk logs, triggers for ordering recovery medications, real-time observations, and feedback from users. There is also a need for framework components such as data on the turnaround time for resolving vendor-reported EHR safety concerns (for shared responsibility). Better measurement will also promote the development of a comprehensive taxonomy of health IT system concerns.[28]
- Quality of care: The system needs to identify top priorities for measure development. The National Quality Forum is currently developing a comprehensive approach to assess health IT measurement and conduct measure gap analyses. Such a framework could help identify priorities for measure developments. The health IT frameworks can help conceptualize patient safety related to health IT, both in terms of risks emanating from health IT and its uses and how health IT might be harnessed to enhance patient safety. A key risk in any new measurement initiative, which this framework could help overcome, is leaving out one or more essential concepts that are fundamental to improvement initiatives, which could lead the initiative to fail. The framework proposes to integrate both retrospective and prospective measurement of health IT systems within an organization's existing clinical risk management and safety programs and aims to facilitate organizational learning, comprehensive 360-degree assessments, refinement of measurement tools and strategies, and shared responsibility to identify problems and implement solutions.[29] This approach would enable achievement of the safety benefits of health IT in real-world clinical settings.
- Education: The shared responsibility framework requires regulators to work together to establish safety standards, report problems, investigate accidents, and disseminate their findings. There is a need for a sociotechnical approach that includes addressing the technical aspects of patient care, the maintenance requirements, and the social components of the policies and procedures that govern issues all the way from healthcare training and health to assigning the roles and responsibilities of maintenance crews.[29] This type of multistakeholder, dynamic collaboration has been tremendously successful not only in building trust between stakeholders but also in reducing the number of accidents.

Shared Responsibility in EHR Safety

A well-designed EHR built with appropriate feedback loops can strengthen multidisciplinary collaboration with improved efficiency, fewer errors, lower costs, and improved outcomes.[29,30] Many IT deficiencies can alter outcomes (Table 3.2). Such EHR systems can simultaneously cater to multiple needs in patient care, staffing, drug dispensation, and administration.[30] Improved sectional communication can also help clinical care providers in configuring, implementing, and maintaining records.[24] An ideal system would also allow the local EHRs to extract data from external laboratories, prescription clearinghouses, and medical records.[19,31,32] The three basic safety areas to monitor are interoperability, usability, and security (see Table 3.1).[33]

Usability of EHRs

EHR usability is an important determinant of safety of care. It can be affected by factors related to both the software and the hardware. Software developers should measure real-world EHR usability for product innovation and improvement.[4,11,32] Poorly built user interfaces can obscure important patient information and integration of data from procedures and can cause errors in the entering of orders.[6,34] In routine care, the development of task lists, text boxes, alerts, notifications, and graphic elements can facilitate monitoring and diagnosis and can improve patient safety.[24,30] EHR hardware is also

Table 3.2 Health IT Failure Can Alter Outcomes

Health IT Failure	Problem	Adverse Outcome
Lack of health IT communication systems	Difficulty in communication between the family and care providers	Wrong alerts
Lack of adequate patient identifying systems	Treatment prescribed to wrong infant	Unnecessary drug administration with toxic effects
Lack of drug dosing options	Dosing errors	Drug toxicity
Erroneous interaction with external systems	Errors during transfer to another hospital	Repeated drug administration
Software safety features not implemented	Misidentification	Procedures delayed

IT, Information technology.

important: larger and better high-resolution and flat-screen displays and high-performance servers can improve user efficiency and data-management flexibility. Appropriate hardware and netware can improve the visualization of alerts in order entry as well as drug-drug, drug-allergy, and drug-condition interaction alerts and alarm functionalities.[6,34]

EHR developers can improve health systems by customizing the default configurations to match local needs. Local experts can guide the development of appropriate EHR configuration settings, customization decisions, and monitoring of local user activities. They can teach clinician-users about the use of EHRs, which can form a feedback loop for appropriate, need-based customization.[29] However, there is a need for a balance; excessive changes in EHRs can also create safety hazards that may not have been imagined by the original developers of the EHR or in the ancillary systems with which these programs are interfaced.[11,24] There may be a need to form multisystem teams for knowledge gathering and dissemination of information on usability-related safety issues, possibly from all three arms—formative, summative, and postimplementation usability.

EHR Security

EHR systems can facilitate continuous access to and integrity of confidential patient data.[17,31] EHR security breaches have been seen all over the world.[17] In most cases, EHR data may be at risk when the users fail to observe security protocols or when third-party vendors can access a health system's computer network but appropriate security controls are not in place. Health systems must maintain appropriate controls for access, wherein users have to be certified to gain entry, short-term users have limited, role-based access, there are protection systems in place to prohibit inappropriate access, and there are encrypted, off-site, backup procedures to prevent loss of data.[31] Similarly, there is a need to ensure the privacy and security of protected health information with appropriate administrative, physical, and technical safeguards.[17]

Despite its numerous advantages, healthcare IT is not without risks. In the ECRI Institute's 2013 list of hazards, 4 of the top 10 hazards were directly related to health IT. According to Miller and Tucker, "Technology-related adverse events can be associated with all components of a comprehensive technology system and may involve errors of either commission or omission. These unintended adverse events typically stem from human-machine interfaces or organization/system design."[35] There is a need for systemwide adoption of shared responsibility principles.[5] Appropriate policy initiatives and legislation can help and are needed.[36] The recently passed "21st Century Cures Act of 2016 aims to improve EHR interoperability, usability, and security,[37] but the specific rules that emanate from it will need to adopt shared responsibility principles (see Table 3.1).[37]

Coiera (2009) described a "middle-out" approach to encourage EHR developers and health systems to work together to improve EHR safety.[38] In these suggestions, payers can support health systems and EHR usability by modifying reimbursement guidelines for evaluation and management services to reduce dependence on unnecessarily detailed structured documentation.[39] Payers could also promote information-sharing activities between organizations to minimize safety issues.[38] Similarly, cybersecurity clearinghouses and cyberinsurance carriers can help health systems improve their data-loss prevention programs.[40]

There is a need for shared responsibility in EHR software license agreements with nondisclosure provisions and intellectual-property protections, performance warranties, and indemnity and limitation of liability provisions.[5,10,13,41–43] Health systems could strengthen intellectual-property provisions to ensure sharing of information such as EHR-related adverse events.[9,18] Health systems and EHR developers can play complementary roles by following the tort law, which provides that each party is responsible for its own acts and omissions, rather than including indemnification and limitation of liability provisions, which typically favor the developer.

The Institute for Healthcare Improvement suggests that reliability with regard to healthcare is a three-part cycle of failure prevention, failure identification, and process redesign, and it defines reliability as "failure-free operation over time."[44,45] Information systems can provide continuous monitoring with real-time or nearly real-time reporting as a means of achieving reliability.[44,45] As such, it makes sense to think about the role of health IT in reliability as it relates to healthcare quality and patient safety.

Actions Suggested by The Joint Commission

The Joint Commission emphasizes three crucial areas: safety culture, process improvement, and leadership.[46] The safety culture emphasizes the maintenance of an organization-wide culture of safety, high reliability, and effective change management. There is a need to recognize the importance of early identification, reporting, analysis, and reduction of health IT–related hazardous conditions, close calls, or errors.

Each adverse event should be analyzed to determine whether health IT contributed to the event in any way. If so, consider the eight dimensions (see Fig. 3.1) to understand how health IT contributed to the event and what can be done to prevent a similar event from recurring. Health IT as a contributing factor may not be evident initially, and hence, all eight dimensions should be investigated.

The system needs a proactive, methodical approach to health IT process improvement that includes assessing patient safety risks. The SAFER guide can be used to develop checklists or use a failure mode and effects analysis or a similar method to identify potential system failures before they occur. Once a new IT system is implemented, there is a need for extensive testing including downtime drills with frontline staff end-users. The EHR needs to be carefully integrated. Families should be provided access to electronic records. Key EHR safety metrics may be monitored via dashboards.

The use of multidisciplinary representation and support can help in providing leadership and oversight to health IT planning, implementation, and evaluation.[47] The workflow processes should be carefully analyzed. The information management chapters of the accreditation manuals cover electronic information. Users should consider the use of any technology in relation to the standards and be aware of potential risks to the safety of patients, as in any clinical situation, particularly with regard to the ability to send and receive critical information.

Information on the website https://www.jointcommission.org (*Sentinel Event Alert*, Issue 54, p. 5) is useful, as are other important resources including the webpage Safe Health IT Saves Lives (https://www.jointcommission.org/resources/patient-safety-topics/sentinel-event/safe-health-it-saves-lives/), which includes an infographic and a free online course, "Investigating and Preventing Health Information Technology-Related Patient Safety Events,"[48] to learn how to identify, report, and address health IT–related safety concerns in an organization (continuing education credit is available for physicians, nurses, healthcare administrators, and healthcare quality professionals [ACCME, ANCC, ACHE, CPHQ]). Another important resource is the Safer guides.[2]

Conclusions

Health IT has become an integral part of the practice of medicine.[49] As with any new technology, health IT brings many benefits and applications as well as potential concerns and risks. Most of the current literature reflects outcomes at single sites or institutions, and national estimates are extrapolations from these single-site studies. As the implementation and use of health IT systems increase, it will be increasingly important to keep patient safety and quality as a major focus. Indeed, with the advancement of new data analytics and management technologies such as machine learning, deep learning, higher order statistical analysis, and quantum computing, health IT becomes more diverse and involves multidisciplinary integration with many clinical settings and application fields. This will boost the research and development of this technology to cover most healthcare specialties.

Section 1

CHAPTER

4 Pharmacologic Management of Neonatal Pain and Agitation

Christopher McPherson

KEY POINTS

1. Preterm neonates are exposed to frequent painful and agitating stimuli during intensive care. Pain and agitation have a negative impact on long-term outcome.
2. Laboratory tests and invasive procedures should be used judiciously in neonates.
3. A systematic scoring system should be used prior to, during, and after acute painful procedures.
4. Neonatal intensive care units should develop an algorithm for the treatment of pain, including standardized nonpharmacologic and pharmacologic interventions.
5. Nonpharmacologic interventions such as facilitated tucking should be consistently used prior to mild to moderately painful procedures.
6. Sucrose may be used to mitigate behavioral responses to minor painful procedures; clinicians can safely use the lowest effective doses ≤10 times every 24 hours.
7. Rapidly acting opioids with short durations of action (fentanyl or remifentanil) should be administered before moderately painful procedures, including nonemergency intubations. Benzodiazepines provide anxiolysis but may cause hypotension in preterm neonates.
8. Continuous multimodal analgesia and sedation (such as morphine/fentanyl and dexmedetomidine) should be used to promote ventilator synchrony and minimize oxygen consumption in ventilated term neonates. These agents may be avoided for short durations of mechanical ventilation.
9. Currently, no pharmacologic therapy has shown benefit in preterm neonates requiring prolonged, invasive mechanical ventilation. Low-dose morphine may be used selectively on the basis of clinical judgment. In the setting of insufficient sedation from low-dose morphine infusion, dexmedetomidine infusion may be considered, titrated carefully to effect while monitoring closely for adverse reactions.

Introduction

Optimal and compassionate neonatal care demands the prevention and treatment of acute pain and chronic agitation. The traditional definition of pain relies on self-report, presenting challenges in nonverbal populations including neonates.[1] Late into the 20th century, preterm neonates underwent major surgical procedures without perioperative or postoperative analgesia.[2] However, extensive research has elucidated the developmental physiology of nociception, documenting completion of ascending pathways connecting peripheral sensory neurons to the thalamus between 20 and 24 weeks of gestation, which is at or below lower limits of viability.[3] Additionally, clinical research clearly documents the unique susceptibility of preterm neonates to adverse metabolic, behavioral, and clinical effects from acute painful procedures in the absence of appropriate analgesia.[4] In fact, pain has emerged as an important modifiable risk factor for altered brain maturation and neurodevelopmental disability after preterm birth.[5,6]

Despite these data, sedation and analgesia are still not used consistently in painful procedures in neonatal care.[7,8] More than 40 acute-pain assessment tools exist, combining vital signs and behavioral responses in an attempt to quantify the subjective experience of the neonate.[9] Research continues regarding more objective measures of pain and modalities to assess chronic pain and agitation in neonates. Nonpharmacologic comfort measures represent the standard of care for procedural pain. The provision of analgesia prior to moderate and major procedures ranging from endotracheal intubation to invasive surgery is now increasingly accepted, but further work is needed.[10] Specifically, the selection of the optimal cocktail of analgesic, sedative, and/or anesthetic agents for specific clinical situations represents an ongoing challenge for clinicians.[7] Finally, the optimal approach to neonates requiring invasive mechanical ventilation requires careful consideration of clinical status and available evidence.[8]

Pathophysiology

Nociception, derived from the Latin *nocere*, or to harm or hurt, defines the transmission of noxious stimuli from peripheral sensory neurons to the brain, triggering physiologic and behavioral responses. Contrary to historical misconceptions, ascending pathways mediating nociception connect peripheral sensory neurons to the thalamus before neonatal viability whereas descending inhibitory pathways do not mature until far later in gestation.[3] Peripheral sensory neurons first develop in the perioral area of the human fetus during the seventh week of gestation. The face, palms, and soles of the feet are populated by the 11th week of gestation, followed by the trunk, arms, and legs in the 15th week, with all cutaneous and mucous surfaces populated by the 20th week of development. Importantly, complete myelination of these neurons is not necessary, with conduction of nociceptive signals occurring via unmyelinated C fibers and thinly myelinated A delta fibers (Fig. 4.1). In fact, incomplete myelination slows conduction velocity, but neonates have shorter interneuron length. On balance, preterm neonates have lower flexor reflex thresholds compared with older patients.[11]

Peripheral sensory neurons synapse with the dorsal root ganglion of the spinal cord via dorsal horn interneurons on formation.[12] However, laminar arrangement and synaptic interconnection (along with a significant degree of myelination) does not begin until 30 weeks of gestation, partially explaining the inability of neonates to attenuate noxious stimuli. Within the spinal cord, glutamate and tachykinin stimulate N-methyl-D-aspartate (NMDA) and tachykinin

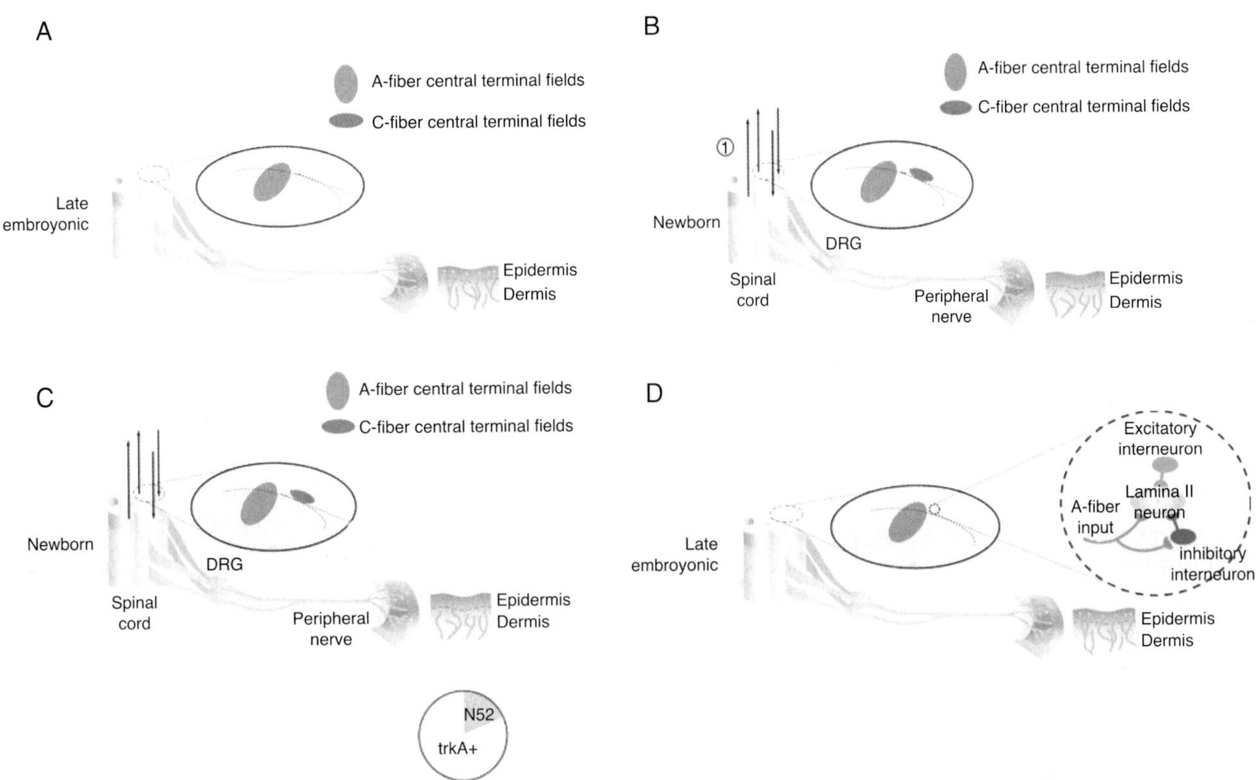

Fig. 4.1 Development of Pain Fibers. (A) A-fibers enter the dorsal horn gray matter during the last few embryonic days and are the first primary afferents to do so. These fibers are diffusely distributed and the superficial projections gradually retract in the first 3 weeks after birth. C-fibers can be seen in the dorsal horn during late embryonic stages but enter the gray matter only 2 to 3 days before birth. Unlike A-fibers that are distributed in a more diffuse fashion, the C-fibers enter the lamina II of the spinal cord in topographically appropriate regions. The connectivity may be weak at birth, but it strengthens within 2 weeks. (B) Primary afferent innervations occur in the skin earlier than central projections. By late embryonic stages, primary afferents of all classes have reached the skin and innervate through the dermis into the epidermis. These projections die back during the immediate perinatal period to leave the full adult situation of dermal innervations present soon after birth. (C) In early postnatal life, descending fibers are structurally similar but are still not functionally active. The neuronal activity is seen at the end of the third week At birth, nearly 80% of the dorsal root ganglion (*DRG*) neurons express the nerve growth factor receptor trkA. During the first postnatal week, half of these neurons lose trkA expression and begin expressing receptors for glial cell line-derived neurotrophic factor. (D) The excitatory and inhibitory activities in the superficial dorsal horn become balanced after birth, through changes in both local interneuron circuitry and descending fibers. A-fiber input weakens as the influence of C-fiber input increases. (From Beggs S, Fitzgerald M. Development of peripheral and spinal nociceptive systems. In Anand KJ, Stevens BJ, McGrath PJ, eds. Pain in Neonates and Infants. 3rd ed. Philadelphia, PA: Elsevier; 2007:15.)

receptors, amplifying sensory inputs. The NMDA receptor fields in the dorsal horn are larger than adult fields through the newborn period. Additionally, γ-aminobutyric acid (GABA), a primary inhibitor of the action of glutamate in adults, induces neuronal depolarization in neonates due to overexpression of the sodium-potassium-chloride cotransporter NKCC1 and resultant elevation in baseline intracellular chloride concentrations.

The thalamus relays sensory input from the spinal cord to the cerebral cortex. Lateral spinothalamic connections appear in the fetus at the time of initial peripheral sensory neuron formation. Thalamocortical connections occur by 24 weeks of gestation, completing the link between peripheral sensory neurons and the cerebral cortex, which develops neurons itself beginning at 8 weeks of gestation with arborization by 20 weeks.[13] Unfortunately, descending inhibitory pathways originating in the brainstem do not connect to the dorsal horn until late in the third trimester of human gestation. This immaturity appears to have both anatomic and chemical origins due to delayed interneuron maturation in the substantia gelatinosa and delayed expression of noradrenaline, dopamine, serotonin, and other neurotransmitters.[14] More specifically, descending projections appear late in fetal life but do not begin to express neurotransmitters vital to the inhibitory functionality of the pathway until at least 42 weeks postmenstrual age, with full functionality delayed until 48 weeks.[15]

These unique aspects of nociception in immature neonates contribute to the significant consequences of untreated pain. Preterm neonates experience prolonged hyperalgesia and allodynia after tissue damage, leading to chronic periods of nociception and stress.[16] Early tissue damage results in persistent dendritic sprouting in peripheral sensory nerve terminals and within the dorsal root ganglion, resulting in hyperinnervation of injured areas and their spinal projections that persist in adulthood.[17] The rapidly maturing fetal and neonatal central nervous system is also susceptible to long-term epigenetic alteration from noxious stimuli.[18] Repeated painful procedures enhance perceptual sensitivity and lower flexor reflex thresholds into childhood.[19,20] Finally, repetitive pain in infancy appears to impact brain morphology in clinically important ways, a subject discussed in more detail in the Long-Term Outcomes section of this chapter.

Clinical Features

Neonates demonstrate a complex behavioral, physiologic, and hormonal response to painful stimuli, further reinforcing the necessity of optimal approaches to prevention and treatment (Table 4.1). Behavioral responses have historically been divided into four general categories: simple motor responses, facial expressions, crying, and complex behavioral responses.[3] Simple motor responses include flexion and adduction of extremities in response to a focal painful stimulus.[11,21] Neonates produce similar facial responses to acute pain compared with older patients, including brow bulge, eye squeeze, nasolabial furrow, and open mouth.[22] Crying is the primary method of neonatal communication; however, crying owed to pain, hunger, or fear can be distinguished by both the subjective evaluation of trained observers and by spectrographic analysis.[23] Common complex behavioral responses to acute pain in the neonate include alterations of the sleep-wake cycles, decreased attentiveness, and increased irritability compared with neonates who undergo a similar painful procedure after local anesthesia.[24]

Physiologically, neonates respond to painful stimuli with decreased oxygen saturations, tachycardia with increased variability in heart rate and blood pressure, and consequent fluctuations in intracranial pressure, increasing the risk for intraventricular hemorrhage (IVH) in preterm neonates.[25–27] Hormonally, neonates demonstrate increases in plasma cortisol, catecholamines (both epinephrine and norepinephrine), β-endorphins, insulin, glucagon, aldosterone, and growth hormone in response to acute noxious stimuli.[28] Chronic stress also suppresses the immune system in the already susceptible neonatal host.[29] Importantly, both physiologic and hormonal responses to acute pain can be attenuated with appropriate analgesia or anesthesia.[4,30]

Table 4.1 Clinical Features of Neonatal Pain

Physiologic	Hormonal	Behavioral
↓Oxygen saturation	↑Cortisol	Simple motor
↕Heart rate	↑Epinephrine	Flexion and adduction
↕Blood pressure	↑Norepinephrine	Facial expressions
↕Intracranial pressure	↑β-Endorphins	Brow bulge
	↑Insulin	Eye squeeze
	↑Glucagon	Nasolabial furrow
	↑Aldosterone	Open mouth
	↑Growth hormone	Crying
		Complex
		Altered sleep–wake cycle
		↓Attentiveness
		↑Irritability

Evaluation

Clinical pain scoring systems are used to assess procedural pain, acute distress associated with handling, or postoperative pain. Neonatal pain assessment tools generally include physiologic (e.g., heart rate, blood pressure, respiration rate, oxygen saturation, and skin color), behavioral (e.g., crying, facial expression, and bodily reactions), and contextual (e.g., gestational age and behavioral state) components. The five most commonly used neonatal assessment tools include the Neonatal Facial Coding System–Revised,[31] Premature Infant Pain Profile–Revised,[32,33] Neonatal Pain, Agitation and Sedation Scale (N-PASS),[34,35] Neonatal Infant Pain Scale,[36] and Bernese Pain Scale for Neonates (Table 4.2).[37] The interrater reliability of these five scales is very high (intraclass coefficients >0.96) for venipuncture in late preterm and term infants, and all the tools discriminate between a painful and stressful stimulus.[38] Behavioral items (specifically body tenseness, restlessness, and extremity tone) more consistently indicate pain compared with physiologic measures. It is important for individual neonatal units to choose one tool and rigorously train caregivers to consistently

Table 4.2 Assessment Scales of Neonatal Pain and Agitation

	Gestational Age, Weeks	Tool	Score
ACUTE PAIN			
Neonatal Facial Coding System–Revised	25–40	Physiologic: none Behavioral: brow bulge, eye squeeze, nasolabial furrow, horizontal mouth stretch, taut tongue Contextual: none	0–5
Premature Infant Pain Profile–Revised	25–40	Physiologic: heart rate, oxygen saturation Behavioral: brow bulge, eye squeeze, nasolabial furrow Contextual: gestational age, behavioral state (active or quiet, awake or asleep)	0–18
Neonatal Infant Pain Scale	26–47	Physiologic: breathing pattern Behavioral: facial expression, cry, arm tone, leg tone Contextual: behavioral state	0–7
Bernese Pain Scale for Neonates	27–41	Physiologic: respiratory pattern, heart rate, oxygen saturation, skin color Behavioral: duration of cry, time to calm, brow bulge with eye squeeze, posture Contextual: behavioral state	0–27
ACUTE PAIN OR PROLONGED PAIN OR AGITATION			
Neonatal Pain, Agitation and Sedation Scale	23–40	Physiologic: vital sign changes (choice of heart rate, respiratory rate, blood pressure, oxygen saturation) Behavioral: crying or irritability, facial expression, extremities tone Contextual: gestational age, behavioral state	7–13 for preterm; 10–10 for term
PROLONGED PAIN OR AGITATION			
COMFORTneo	25–43	Physiologic: none Behavioral: calmness or agitation, respiratory response to mechanical ventilation or crying, body movement, facial tension, body and muscle tone Contextual: alertness	6–30

assess before, during, and after painful procedures. Of these tools, only the N-PASS has been evaluated to assess chronic pain and agitation during mechanical ventilation.[34] The COMFORTneo tool was also developed and validated for this purpose.[39] These tools may be used for regularly scheduled assessments such as those during routine care of neonates receiving mechanical ventilation.

Objective markers of neonatal pain have been targeted by investigators for decades. Electroencephalography, near-infrared spectroscopy (detecting increases in oxygenated hemoglobin in the contralateral somatosensory cortex), skin conductance (reflecting autonomic function), and salivary cortisol have all been documented to discriminate noxious painful stimuli from touch.[40–45] In term neonates, near-infrared spectroscopy, heart rate, and oxygen saturation appear to capture an acute response to pain, whereas skin conductance and salivary cortisol represent a more prolonged stressful response.[46] These objective measures moderately correlate with behavioral assessment (r = 0.20–0.42). Further research is required to determine the optimal measure or combination of measures of acute and chronic pain and stress in infancy.

Management

Nonpharmacologic Therapy for Pain and Agitation

Optimal treatment of pain and agitation in neonates requires a multimodal approach, including both nonpharmacologic and pharmacologic strategies. Nonpharmacologic therapies are underused in clinical practice.[47] Nonpharmacologic strategies with documented efficacy before acute mildly to moderately painful procedures such as needle sticks include nonnutritive sucking, breast milk, skin-to-skin contact, kangaroo care, and facilitated tucking.[48] Facilitated tucking improves both pain reactivity (immediately after the painful stimulus) and immediate regulation (at least 30 seconds after the painful stimulus) in preterm neonates, whereas nonnutritive sucking positively impacts both domains in term neonates, emphasizing the importance of tailoring nonpharmacologic therapy bundles based on neonatal maturity.[49] Although the optimal bundle of nonpharmacologic interventions remains undefined, individual neonatal units should select the most feasible interventions with supporting evidence and consistently use those interventions prior to all mildly to moderately painful procedures.[10]

Sucrose

Clinical trials in neonates consistently document reduction of crying, facial grimacing, and motor activity after oral administration of sucrose prior to mildly to moderately painful procedures including heel lance, venipuncture, and intramuscular injection.[50] The effective dose varies substantially in trials (range, 0.05–3 mL of 12%–50% sucrose), although a recent randomized trial suggested 0.1 mL of 24% solution reduces the behavioral response to heel lance as effectively as higher doses.[51] The balance of evidence supports the use of sucrose in neonates; however, outstanding questions remain regarding the efficacy, mechanism, and long-term impact.

Oral sucrose does not consistently impact objective measures of neonatal pain, including oxygen consumption or energy expenditure, salivary/plasma cortisol concentrations, and neural activity of nociception-evoked circuits in the spinal cord or brain.[50,52,53] Most strikingly, sucrose does not prevent the development of remote hyperalgesia in neonates.[54] Sucrose alters the behavioral response to painful stimuli by an unclear mechanism, which may include stimulation of some combination of endogenous opioid, dopaminergic, cholinergic, or serotonergic pathways.[55–58]

The limited understanding of the objective efficacy and mechanism of oral sucrose should promote great caution regarding long-term neurodevelopmental outcomes of preterm neonates exposed to sucrose repeatedly in the early stages of brain development. Data regarding chronic *in utero* alterations in opioid, dopamine, acetylcholine, or serotonin signaling suggest the potential for negative neurologic impact on motor function and attention.[59] Sucrose (0.1 mL of 24% solution) prior to all invasive procedures in a population of preterm neonates in the first week of life had no impact on measures of motor development or attention/orientation at term-equivalent follow-up.[60] However, increased sucrose exposure (greater than 10 doses per day) was associated with poorer scores, an association not observed in the placebo group, suggesting this finding was not attributable to increased exposure to painful procedures.[9,60] Additionally, a retrospective study found no protective effect from glucose prior to painful procedures on brain growth, functional connectivity, and neurodevelopmental impairments at 18 months of age.[61] These findings have been replicated in animal models, with the addition of long-term alterations in white and gray matter volumes.[62,63] In this setting, sucrose must be used judiciously in neonatal care, only prior to mildly to moderately painful procedures and at the minimum effective dose, and prescribed, documented, and reported as a medication.[10]

Premedication for Endotracheal Intubation

Endotracheal intubation is a common invasive procedure in neonatal intensive care required for ventilation and/or oxygenation of immature or acutely ill neonates. Endotracheal intubation facilitates stabilization of the neonate but causes acute distress and disturbs physiologic homeostasis. Direct laryngoscopy produces injury to the tongue, gums, and arytenoids in as many as half of procedures.[64] Disturbances in physiologic homeostasis are common, including hypoxemia (mean decrease of 27 torr), bradycardia from vagal stimulation (mean decrease of 52 beats per minute), and systemic, pulmonary, and intracranial hypertension.[65–69]

The neonate must be effectively oxygenated with bag-mask ventilation before, during, and after premedication. Administration of medications may prolong the time period before intubation; however, premedication reduces procedure time and number of attempts while minimizing airway trauma and disturbances of physiologic homeostasis.[64,70,71] Various analgesics, sedatives, vagolytics, and muscle relaxants have been evaluated for this purpose; careful review of efficacy, safety, and pharmacokinetic data and consideration of the practical aspects of delivery allow selection of the most appropriate agents (Table 4.3).

Analgesia

Opioids provide analgesia through agonism of G protein–coupled μ-opioid receptors, inhibiting presynaptic and postsynaptic peripheral neuron membrane potentials, neuronal firing in the dorsal horn of the spinal cord, and ascending pathways in the brainstem. The ideal opioid for premedication has a rapid onset and short duration of action with minimal impact on respiratory mechanics. Remifentanil distributes within 1 minute of intravenous administration and undergoes

Table 4.3 Pharmacokinetic and Clinical Data Regarding Premedications for Endotracheal Intubation

Drug	Pharmacokinetic Data[a]	Clinical Data
ANALGESICS		
Remifentanil	Onset within 1 minute, half-life 5.4 minutes (Intranasal dosing: onset ~3 minutes)	Produces good or excellent intubating conditions; extubation possible in ~20 minutes Produces stiff chest with rapid administration
Fentanyl	Onset within 1 minute, half-life 9.5 hours (Intranasal dosing: onset 5–10 minutes)	Produces superior intubating conditions to remifentanil when given with muscle relaxant Produces stiff chest with rapid administration May prolong time required to successful extubation
Morphine	Onset in 5–15 minutes, half-life 10 hours	No impact on physiologic adverse effects when given ≤5 minutes before intubation
SEDATIVES		
Midazolam	Onset in 1–2 minutes, half-life 6.3 hours (Intranasal dosing: onset ~5 minutes)	Improves pain scores and reduces physiologic changes when added to fentanyl Produces clinically significant hypotension in high proportion of preterm neonates
Propofol	Onset within 1 minute, half-life 13 minutes	Improves oxygen saturations and minimizes procedure time compared with opioid Produces clinically significant hypotension in high proportion of preterm neonates
Ketamine	Onset in 1–2 minutes, duration of 15–30 minutes	Improves pain scores and reduces vagal bradycardia compared with no premedication Direct negative inotropic effects
VAGOLYTICS		
Atropine	Onset within 1 minute, duration of ~2 hours (Intramuscular dosing: onset 15–30 minutes)	Eliminates vagal bradycardia during intubation
Glycopyrrolate	Onset within 1 minute, duration of ~2 hours	Neonatal clinical data lacking
MUSCLE RELAXANTS		
Succinylcholine	Onset within 1 minute, duration of 6–8 minutes (Intramuscular dosing: onset 4 minutes, duration 16 minutes)	With atropine, reduces physiologic disturbances and facilitates more rapid successful intubation
Pancuronium	Onset in 2–5 minutes, duration of 2–3 hours	With atropine, reduces physiologic disturbances
Vecuronium	Onset in 2–3 minutes, duration of 50–70 minutes	With opioid, produces good intubating conditions
Rocuronium	Onset in 1–3 minutes, duration of 40–60 minutes (Intramuscular dosing: onset 7 minutes, duration ~2 hours)	With opioid and atropine, improves success rate on first attempt
Cisatracurium	Onset in 2–3 minutes, duration of 35–45 minutes	Neonatal clinical data lacking

[a]Pharmacokinetic data are presented as mean values in studies of preterm neonates after intravenous administration when available and were extrapolated from older patient populations when neonatal data were unavailable.

elimination by blood and tissue esterases with an elimination half-life of 5.4 minutes in neonates.[72] Remifentanil produces good or excellent intubating conditions in neonates and improves the rate of first-attempt success compared with placebo or a longer-acting opioid (morphine).[73,74] Like remifentanil, fentanyl distributes almost immediately on intravenous administration but has a relatively long elimination half-life in both preterm neonates (mean 9.5 hours) and term neonates (mean 5.2 hours).[75,76] Although fentanyl effectively produces favorable intubation condition, use of this agent in conjunction with the INSURE (Intubation, SURfactant therapy, Extubation) approach may prolong the need for mechanical ventilation.[77,78] Rapid infusion of concentrated fentanyl or remifentanil should be avoided due to the potential for chest wall rigidity.[79] Neonatal units must have easy access to dilute remifentanil (20 mcg/mL stable for 24 hours) or fentanyl (5 mcg/mL stable for 90 days) prepared sterilely in a pharmacy and avoid bedside manipulation of the commercially available 50 mcg/mL intravenous solutions. Administration of either agent must occur via a syringe pump over a minimum of 3 minutes.[80,81] In some circumstances, neonates without intravenous access require intubation. Fortunately, intranasal administration of intravenous remifentanil or fentanyl produces a similar clinical effect to intravenous administration.[82–85] Mucosal atomization devices (MADs) have been documented to improve acceptance of intranasal medications in young pediatric patients while increasing effect and decreasing the time to onset of analgesia.[86,87] Critically, MADs require 0.1 mL overfill to account for drug lost in the device during delivery. Failure to account for this excess volume in prescribing and administration may lead to subtherapeutic doses.

Sedation

Midazolam, a benzodiazepine, produces sedation by binding to $GABA_A$ receptors, promoting hyperpolarization of the neuron via chloride influx. Midazolam produces hypnotic activity in 1 to 2 minutes with a median plasma elimination half-life of 6.3 hours in preterm neonates.[88,89] Midazolam further improves intubating conditions, lowers pain scale scores, and reduces physiologic disturbances when used in conjunction with analgesia.[90] However, benzodiazepines should not be used alone for endotracheal intubation and should not be included in the premedication sequence for preterm neonates with a corrected gestational age <34 weeks due to an unacceptable risk of desaturation and/or hypotension.[91–93] For appropriately selected patients without intravenous access, intranasal midazolam allows for provision of sedation.[94,95] As with intranasal fentanyl, administration via a MAD may improve efficacy and tolerability.

Identification of a single anesthetic agent to safely provide analgesia and sedation in neonates prior to intubation remains an outstanding goal. Propofol agonizes $GABA_A$ receptors and antagonizes NMDA receptors, resulting in analgesia, sedation, and amnesia.[96]

Propofol distributes almost immediately into the central nervous system with a median elimination half-life of 13 minutes, despite prolonged distribution and terminal elimination from adipose tissue.[97] In a small randomized trial, propofol reduced desaturation and facilitated successful intubation in neonates with a short recovery time compared with a cocktail including morphine.[98] Unfortunately, neonates have a highly variable response to propofol with regard to both efficacy and adverse effects, with clinically significant hypotension common.[99,100] Ketamine, an NMDA antagonist with sedative and analgesic effects, has a rapid onset of action (1–2 minutes) and relatively short duration (15–30 minutes). Pilot observational data in preterm neonates demonstrated lower pain scores and less vagal bradycardia with ketamine compared with no premedication.[101] Of concern, ketamine has direct negative inotropic effects, which are generally overcome by augmentation of cardiovascular function through stimulation of endogenous catecholamine release. The relevance of this adverse effect to neonates remains unknown but has been previously associated with cardiac arrest in patients with exhausted catecholamine stores. Considering all data, midazolam remains the sedative of choice for premedication of neonates ≥34 weeks' postmenstrual age.

Vagolytics

Atropine reduces or eliminates vagal bradycardia by antagonizing acetylcholine, secreted by the efferent postsynaptic membrane of the vagus nerve in the sinoatrial node. Atropine rapidly distributes after intravenous injection with a relatively prolonged duration of action (approximately 2 hours). As part of an appropriate premedication cocktail, atropine eliminates procedural bradycardia in neonates.[102] In patients without intravenous access, atropine may be given intramuscularly, although the delayed onset of action (mean 15–30 minutes) limits the utility of this route.[103] Clinicians should pay specific attention to the dosing of atropine, using an appropriate weight-based dose of 0.02 mg/kg. In the early 1970s, an observational study including term infants found an association between extremely low doses of atropine (0.0036 mg/kg or less) and mild heart rate slowing (approximately 9 beats per minute).[104] In their discussion, the authors shared their clinical practice of giving "a minimum dose of 0.1 mg of atropine to our patients." Despite a lack of validation, this approach was widely adopted by tertiary references and international guidelines.[105] This recommendation is specifically dangerous for small neonates because toxic reactions including lethargy, periodic breathing, and seizures have been documented after administration of two flat doses of 0.1 mg in a 2.2 kg patient, equaling 4.5 times the recommended weight-based dose.[106] Multiple prospective observational studies in preterm neonates, the largest including 253 neonates, have refuted the concept of paradoxical bradycardia from low doses of atropine.[107–109] Changing local culture may be more difficult but must be prioritized given the implications of appropriate dosing of atropine for the safety of the smallest neonates.

Muscle Relaxation

Muscle relaxation with depolarizing or nondepolarizing neuromuscular blockers improves intubating conditions and blunts the rise in intracranial pressure associated with endotracheal intubation.[66,110] Succinylcholine, a depolarizing neuromuscular blocker, depolarizes the muscle membrane by binding to acetylcholine receptors. It has a rapid onset (20–40 seconds) and short duration of action (6–8 minutes).[111] However, it needs to be used cautiously in neonates with hyperkalemia, as it may increase serum potassium levels.[112] There is a need for cautious use after surgical trauma, when most infants have some inflammation with increased expression of membrane acetylcholine receptors in the muscles. There may also be a need for caution in neonates receiving concomitant medications that may increase plasma potassium levels, including β-adrenergic blockers and angiotensin-converting enzyme inhibitors.[113] Succinylcholine is a well-described trigger of malignant hyperthermia, although this autosomal dominant susceptibility occurs in only 0.5 per 10,000 of the general population.[114] Finally, succinylcholine has been associated with significant bradycardia and even asystole in a setting of concomitant vagal stimulation, suggesting the potential utility of concurrent atropine administration.[115–117] Succinylcholine can be given intramuscularly in patients without intravenous access. However, this route alters the pharmacokinetic properties of succinylcholine, extending the onset and duration of action to a mean of 4 minutes and 16 minutes, respectively.[118] Dose-response studies demonstrate more reliable muscle relaxation using double the standard intravenous dose for intramuscular administration.[119]

Pancuronium, vecuronium, rocuronium, and cisatracurium are nondepolarizing neuromuscular blockers, competitively inhibiting acetylcholine at the motor endplate. Pancuronium has the most robust clinical data in neonates, reducing bradycardia and mitigating increased intracranial pressure from endotracheal intubation.[66,120] However, pancuronium does not possess ideal pharmacokinetic properties for procedural muscle relaxation, with a slow onset (2–5 minutes) and long duration of action (2–3 hours).[121,122] Alternative nondepolarizing neuromuscular blockers are used widely but have very limited data in neonates.[123,124] Vecuronium is hepatically metabolized, with an intermediate onset (2–3 minutes) and duration of action (50–70 minutes).[125] Rocuronium is also metabolized in the liver, but it may act more quickly (1–3 minutes) and for shorter periods (40–60 minutes).[126,127] The strength of rocuronium over vecuronium is its stability as an intravenous solution (vecuronium needs reconstitution before administration). Cisatracurium is another emerging agent that may be useful in patients with renal and/or hepatic dysfunction.[128] Of all these nondepolarizing neuromuscular blockers, rocuronium could be administered intramuscularly if needed, although the effects are less predictable.[129]

Conclusions Regarding Premedication for Endotracheal Intubation

In the absence of an absolute contraindication, neonates should receive analgesia with consideration of sedation, a vagolytic, and a muscle relaxant before endotracheal intubation (Table 4.4).[116] Remifentanil appears to be the most appropriate opioid for analgesia, although fentanyl may be used due to the prolonged stability of a dilute preparation. Neonatal units must ensure the availability of an appropriate formulation and use of infusion pumps to avoid chest wall rigidity. Intranasal fentanyl may be used in patients without intravenous access. Midazolam can be a useful adjunct, although concerns remain about hypotension in infants with hemodynamic instability. Atropine effectively minimizes vagal bradycardia; weight-based dosing of this agent can be useful. Succinylcholine may also improve intubating conditions and success rates but must be avoided in patients with hyperkalemia and/or a family history of malignant hyperthermia. In the absence of this information, providers may prefer rocuronium.

Analgesia and Sedation for Other Major Procedures

High-quality evidence supports the provision of analgesia for male circumcision.[130] Subcutaneous ring block with 1% lidocaine is the

Table 4.4 Protocol for Premedication Before Endotracheal Intubation

Medication Class	Medication	Route	Dose	Concentration	Volume	Onset
Analgesia	Fentanyl[a]	Intravenous	2 mcg/kg Give on pump over 3 minutes to avoid chest wall rigidity[b]	5 mcg/mL	0.4 mL/kg	1 minute
		Intranasal	2 mcg/kg	5 mcg/mL	0.4 mL/kg	5–10 minutes
Sedation	Midazolam for neonates ≥34 weeks' corrected gestational age	Intravenous	0.1 mg/kg Give on pump over 2 minutes	1 mg/mL	0.1 mL/kg	1–2 minutes
		Intranasal	0.2 mg/kg	1 mg/mL	0.2 mL/kg	5 minutes
Vagolytic	Atropine	Intravenous	0.02 mg/kg Rapid intravenous push	0.05 mg/mL[c]	0.4 mL/kg	1 minute
		Intramuscular	0.02 mg/kg	0.4 mg/mL	0.05 mL/kg	15–30 minutes
Muscle relaxants[d]	Rocuronium	Intravenous	1 mg/kg Intravenous push	10 mg/mL	0.1 mL/kg	1–3 minutes
	Succinylcholine	Intramuscular	4 mg/kg	20 mg/mL	0.2 mL/kg	4 minutes

[a]Fentanyl was chosen over remifentanil due to extended stability of dilute formulation.

[b]Chest wall rigidity may be treated with rocuronium 1 mg/kg intravenous push.

[c]To prepare 0.05 mg/mL dilution, combine 1 mL (0.4 mg) atropine + 7 mL sterile water for injection = 8 mL.

[d]Only to be ordered by attending physician or fellow; patient must be supportable with bag mask ventilation before paralytic administration.

Table 4.5 Advantages and Disadvantages of Available Agents for Continuous Sedation of Preterm Neonates During Mechanical Ventilation

Agent	Advantages	Disadvantages
Morphine	Increased ventilator synchrony Decreased adrenaline concentrations No impact on incidence of severe intraventricular hemorrhage, periventricular leukomalacia, or death	Hypotension Prolongation of mechanical ventilation Prolongation of time to full enteral feedings Tachyphylaxis
Fentanyl	Decreased adrenaline and cortisol concentrations Less impact on gastrointestinal motility compared with morphine	Prolongation of mechanical ventilation Delayed meconium passage Rapid tachyphylaxis
Midazolam	Decreased pain scores during endotracheal suction	Increased severe intraventricular hemorrhage, periventricular leukomalacia, or death Hypotension Myoclonus Frequent delirium Tachyphylaxis
Dexmedetomidine	Decreased adjunctive sedation compared with fentanyl Decreased incidence of delirium compared with benzodiazepine Minimal respiratory depression Minimal impact on gastrointestinal motility	Potential hypotension and bradycardia

preferred strategy and may be augmented with positioning and oral sucrose. Less evidence exists to guide analgesia for major bedside procedures such as chest drain insertion and removal; infiltration of the insertion site with local anesthetic such as lidocaine 1% could be combined with a short-acting opioid such as fentanyl 1 to 4 mcg/kg.[131] Intraoperative anesthesia is beyond the scope of this chapter, but ongoing research has been clearly supportive.[132] Studies support the use of opioids in infusions or scheduled boluses, such as morphine 10 mcg/kg/hour or 30 mcg/kg/dose every 3 hours, for postoperative pain.[133] Scheduled acetaminophen administration may be useful[134]; intravenous acetaminophen is preferable to rectal therapy, which shows erratic absorption and unclear efficacy.[135,136] Intravenous acetaminophen is relatively expensive, but its use should be supported for appropriate indications.[137] To control cost and ensure continued availability, intravenous acetaminophen may be restricted to evidence-based indications such as postoperative pain and treatment of patent ductus arteriosus (not heel lance, postbirth pain, or eye examination).[138,139]

Continuous Analgesia and Sedation During Mechanical Ventilation

Neonates produce high levels of stress hormones during mechanical ventilation.[140–142] The asynchrony in self-breathing and mechanical ventilation may increase the need for higher peak airway pressures and tidal volumes and contribute to lung damage.[143] Nonpharmacologic therapy, including appropriate containment and an optimal sensory environment, may help. Continuous, multimodal analgesia and sedation may be needed to achieve ventilator synchrony and minimization of oxygen consumption in ventilated term neonates.[144] Conversely, continuous analgesic or sedative medications can possibly be avoided for short durations of assisted ventilation such as in respiratory distress syndrome.[144] The use of continuous sedation or analgesia in ventilated preterm neonates who exhibit agitation is controversial (Tables 4.5 and 4.6).[8,145]

Table 4.6 Data Regarding Early Sedative or Analgesic Exposure and Long-Term Outcome

Agent	Preclinical	Clinical
Opioids	Neuroapoptosis Reduced neuronal density and dendritic length Reduced brain growth Persistently decreased motor activity Persistently impaired learning ability	Reduced cerebellar growth[a] Increased tone at 36 weeks' postmenstrual age[a] Impaired cognitive and motor outcome at 18 months of age[a] Lower scores on the visual analysis domain of intelligence quotient at 5 years of age[b] Superior executive function by parent report at 8–9 years of age[b]
Benzodiazepines	Neuroapoptosis Suppressed neurogenesis Delayed motor development	—
Dexmedetomidine	Neuroprotection and decreased lesion size in models of periventricular leukomalacia Neuroprotection and improved developmental outcome in models of hypoxia-ischemia and isoflurane exposure	—

[a]Retrospective and prospective studies of relatively high-level opioid exposure.
[b]Prospective study of relatively low-level opioid exposure.

Benzodiazepines

Continuous infusion of midazolam to sedate ventilated preterm neonates may increase the incidence of severe IVH, periventricular leukomalacia, or death.[93] Some of these effects may be driven by bolus doses of midazolam and consequent transient episodes of hypotension with reduced mean cerebral blood flow velocity.[92] Preclinical studies show neuroapoptosis and long-term functional deficits after early exposure to benzodiazepines, raising further concerns about these medications in the absence of long-term outcome data.[146]

Opioids

Opioid therapy in preterm neonates requiring mechanical ventilation has limited documented benefit and clear adverse effects. Continuous morphine infusion does not impact the composite incidence of IVH, periventricular leukomalacia, or death (in the absence of preexisting hypotension).[93,147] Acute adverse effects include a longer duration of ventilation, lower tolerance of enteral feedings, and subtle tone abnormalities at a postmenstrual age of 36 weeks.[148–150] Preclinical data indicate possible adverse neurodevelopmental effects.[146] However, follow-up data in preterm human neonates treated with low-dose morphine infusion (100 mcg/kg bolus followed by 10 mcg/kg/hour for ≤7 days; median duration of exposure 77 hours) seems more reassuring.[151–153] Until more data confirm safety, it may be prudent to limit cumulative doses to minimize the possibility of adverse effects.[154–156]

Data regarding a pharmacokinetically different opioid emphasize the importance of considering the degree of exposure when evaluating the potential long-term implications of therapy. When infused continuously in immature preterm neonates, fentanyl accumulates significantly.[157] Fentanyl infusion has short-term adverse effects similar to morphine but may have more frequent adverse neurodevelopmental effects at a corrected age of 24 months (1 mcg/kg bolus followed by 1 mcg/kg/hour for ≤7 days; the median duration of treatment was 151.5 hours).[158,159] A retrospective cohort study supported this concern, associating increased cumulative fentanyl exposure with impaired cerebellar growth.[160] A pharmacokinetic study in preterm infants suggested that a cautious dosing of continuous infusion fentanyl may be safer (0.5 mcg/kg/hour for the first 4 days of life; 0.75 mcg/kg/hour from 5–9 days of life).[161] However, the efficacy of low-dose continuous morphine or fentanyl infusions in mechanically ventilated preterm neonates has not been clearly documented. In this setting, doses are frequently escalated, producing the acute adverse effects inherent to opioid exposure along with long-term risk.

Alpha-2 Receptor Agonists

Alpha-2 receptor agonists can augment sedation in chronically ventilated preterm neonates while minimizing both short- and long-term adverse effects. Dexmedetomidine is a selective alpha-2-adrenergic receptor agonist that provides analgesia, anxiolysis, and sedation through reduced sympathetic outflow from the locus coeruleus and increased release of substance P from the dorsal horn of the spinal cord. Clinical data suggest there is a potential for short-term benefits compared with opioids, including superior efficacy, less respiratory depression, and no impact on gastrointestinal motility.[162,163] Unlike benzodiazepines and opioids, preclinical data examining alpha-2 agonists suggest neuroprotection of the immature brain.[164] Cautious use of dexmedetomidine is indicated pending robust safety and efficacy data. However, use may be warranted considering the adverse effects of benzodiazepines and opioids.

Conclusions Regarding Continuous Analgesia and Sedation During Mechanical Ventilation

Multimodal continuous-infusion analgesia and sedation should clearly be provided to late preterm or term neonates with hypoxia and respiratory failure requiring aggressive mechanical ventilation. However, continuous analgesic or sedative medications can possibly be avoided when the clinicians expect a short duration of mechanical ventilation; no pharmacologic therapy has demonstrated benefit in prolonged, invasive mechanical ventilation. Low-dose morphine (≤10 mcg/kg/hour and/or 50 mcg/kg/dose as needed at least 5 minutes before agitating stimuli) may be used at the discretion of the medical care team in normotensive preterm neonates. In the setting of insufficient sedation, dexmedetomidine infusion may be cautiously considered.

Long-Term Outcomes

Preterm neonates exposed to more procedural pain demonstrate long-term effects on brain development with smaller volumes of the white matter, corticospinal tract, and subcortical gray matter.

Thalamic volumes are also decreased, particularly in the somatosensory thalamus, at term equivalent age.[5,165,166] Greater neonatal stress predicts decreased frontal and parietal brain width and altered maturation and functional connectivity in the temporal lobes at term equivalent age.[167] Exposure to greater procedural pain predicts lower cognitive and motor composite scores at 8 months, 18 months, and 3 years of age.[5,168] Neonates exposed to more skin-breaking procedures demonstrate greater internalizing behaviors, such as anxiety and depression, at 8 years.[169] Neonatal pain also predicts thinner cortex in multiple brain regions, particularly the frontal and parietal lobes, and smaller regional volumes in the limbic system and basal ganglia at school age.[170,171] The association between pain and dysmaturation of superior white matter also persists and is associated with intelligence quotient.[172] Furthermore, cumulative neonatal pain-related stress also relates to brain function, reflected in changes to background cortical rhythmicity at school age, negatively predictive of visual-perceptual abilities.[173] Unfortunately, as previously described, pharmacologic interventions to treat pain have no or a negative impact on long-term outcome. Research in this field must continue, prioritizing compassionate care in the newborn period while focusing on optimal long-term neurodevelopment.

Section 1

CHAPTER 5

Neonatal Transport

Webra Price-Douglas, Susan J. Dulkerian

KEY POINTS

1. Transport is not a benign event for the neonate, the family, and the transport team.
2. Transport is a significant transition in care and has risk and safety concerns beyond the physical movement of the neonate.
3. Decompensation is not uncommon due to the movement, vibration, noise, and change in environment during transport and must be anticipated and addressed as needed.
4. Neonatal transport is complex and labor and equipment intensive.
5. Management may vary based on environment.

Introduction

Advances in neonatology and technology have led to increased survival rates of neonates, especially low birth weight infants. The neonatal period is defined as the first 4 weeks of life and is the period of greatest mortality in childhood. The mortality rate in infancy is 5.96 per 1000 infants, with a mortality rate during the neonatal period of 4.04 per 1000 neonates. Infants may be born outside a regional center and require transport to a neonatal intensive care unit due to low birth weight, congenital anomalies, or multisystem problems.[1] Neonatal transport is a frequent, daily occurrence in which the process, workforce, resources, and quality of care may vary widely[2] (Box 5.1).

Evaluation

Clinical Evaluation

When a referral is made for a neonatal transport, it is important and useful to make an initial brief assessment or brief clinical assessment and evaluation of the infant, his or her most likely diagnosis, and the urgency for the transport team to arrive at the referring facility. A transport referral or intake sheet is a tool commonly used by transport teams to obtain certain clinical data in order to better assess the acuity and potential urgency for transport. The personnel, equipment, and resources available at the referring facility may vary widely depending on the level of perinatal care designation and the services provided there. Assessment of this variability allows for triage and appropriate use of the transport team.

■ Box 5.1 Conditions Requiring Neonatal Transport

The primary reasons for neonatal transport often mirror the common causes of death in the neonatal period, followed by the need for subspecialty consultation, evaluation, and management.

1. Prematurity and low birth weight
2. Congenital and chromosomal anomalies
3. Maternal complications (preeclampsia, maternal abruption, placenta previa, cord prolapse, or accidents)
4. Sepsis
5. Respiratory distress secondary to respiratory distress syndrome, transient tachypnea of the newborn (TTN), and metabolic derangements
6. Necrotizing enterocolitis with or without bowel perforation
7. Intrauterine hypoxia and birth asphyxia

Initial Management Assessment

During the initial call, the accepting neonatologist or physician should make an initial management assessment and suggest any additional treatments to initiate while the team in en route. It is important to professionally suggest alternative therapies if an assessment is made for which initial management or therapies are not optimal.

Laboratory

If not already done, request that vital signs are assessed, including temperature, blood pressure of all four extremities, and respiratory rate. The initial laboratory evaluation will vary depending on the diagnosis but always should include a blood glucose level. If the glucose level is assessed by an automated bedside analyzer and is less than 50 to 110 mg/dL, recommend that a serum glucose sample be sent. Recommend immediate intravenous treatment if the blood glucose level is less than 50 to 110 mg/dL, depending on the clinical scenarios.[3] A recommendation to obtain other laboratory analyses will depend on the suspected or confirmed diagnosis(es).

For respiratory symptoms, appropriate initial laboratory testing includes glucose, ABG/CBG, and serum electrolytes. For suspected infection, laboratory testing should include NEC, glucose, complete blood cell count (CBC), CRP if available, and a blood culture. An inquiry about history of maternal herpes simplex virus infection (HSV) should be made.

Imaging

Access to timely radiology testing can be a challenge at some facilities, but when available, a chest x-ray and/or an abdominal x-ray is recommended, depending on the presentation of the neonate. If the infant has been intubated, recommend a chest x-ray (with an orogastric tube in place before obtaining the film). Imaging for other less common diagnoses may be beyond the scope of this chapter but include a suspected subgaleal hematoma and thus an urgent need for further studies. Confirm endotracheal tube placement by at least two methods including chest x-ray, direct laryngoscopy, capnography, and auscultation.[4]

Management

Temperature Regulation

One of the principles of a successful transition to extrauterine life is maintained thermoregulation.[3,5] Cold stress can mimic and indeed worsen other possible comorbidities such as hypoglycemia and respiratory distress syndrome and has been implicated in an increased risk factor for intraventricular hemorrhage and other long-term outcomes in the very low birth weight infant.[6] The infant should be managed with appropriate support to ensure normothermia. The infant should be transported in a temperature-controlled isolette with additional thermal support when indicated, including but not limited to the use of a disposable, gel-filled warmer mattress, polyethylene bags, and blankets whenever cold stress is a concern during transport.[3,5]

Respiratory Considerations

Pulse oximetry is an essential and useful tool in monitoring a transitioning or sick infant.[5] An infant with respiratory symptoms (e.g., tachypnea, apnea, periodic breathing, grunting, flaring, or retractions) should have a chest x-ray and blood gas analysis to assess for hypoxia, hypercarbia, and acidosis. Recommendations should be made to the referring provider pending results of testing in order to support the infant until the transport team arrives to assist in care, stabilization, and transfer.

Infectious Disease

Sepsis should always be considered in an infant who is not transitioning well. A good history should be obtained and initial screening should be done. A blood culture and CBC with manual differential with or without CRP should be obtained, and antibiotics should be started. Ampicillin and an aminoglycoside should be initiated, with additional gram-negative and anaerobic coverage in the incidence of suspected intestinal pathology (NEC, bowel perforation, or obstruction).[3,7]

CVS

Cardiovascular pulse oximetry should be initiated and preductal and postductal saturation recorded if the infant is in respiratory distress with or without cyanosis to screen for congenital ductal-dependent cyanotic heart disease.[8] A blood gas measurement can be helpful in diagnosis, and an exhocardiogram (ECHO) is indicated but may not be available at the referring facility. The transport team should anticipate and have available all life-saving medications: for example, prostaglandin E1 and other vasoactive agents. The transport team must be prepared for any untoward side effects from any medications administered. Frequently seen during transport are complications such as apnea necessitating intubation, vasodilation resulting in hypotension, or vasoconstriction resulting in hypertension.

Hematology

Assessment for anemia in incidences of maternal hemorrhage at the time of delivery can be quickly assessed with hematocrit or a CBC. Emergent PRBCs may be indicated in incidences of severe maternal abruption or neonatal anemia.[3] The transport team needs a mechanism for obtaining for the release of O-negative, leukocyte-washed, and irradiated PRBCs.

Metabolism

There are multiple diagnoses that lead to metabolic derangements. An initial assessment of acid–base status is key to ruling out an inborn error of metabolism that results in severe acidosis. Blood gas and serum electrolyte values should be obtained. Recommend that a state metabolic screen is obtained prior to transfer of the infant.

Neurology

Seizures can be an initial presenting symptom for infants with several diagnoses: infection, intracranial hemorrhage, or systemic or metabolic derangements such as hypoglycemia, hypocalcemia, hyponatremia, or hypoxia or opioid withdrawal. Initial treatment should be phenobarbital, with adjunctive treatment with lorazepam or midazolam. Secondary treatment depends on the underlying diagnosis. Hypoglycemia should always be ruled out and promptly treated if present.

Hypoxic-Ischemic Encephalopathy

With a history of a suspected perinatal hypoxic event, hypoxic-ischemic encephalopathy (HIE) should be considered. Cord blood analysis should be performed and an infant blood gas measurement obtained within the first hour of life (ideally) to be used in assessing an indication for neonatal cooling.

Recommend contacting the referral center for specific recommendations regarding eligibility for cooling and stabilization and ongoing management while awaiting the transport's arrival. Instructions may be given regarding passive cooling, including turning off the radiant warmer bed heat source.[9–12] A servo-controlled device should be used during the transport. There are ongoing clinical trials that may alter inclusion and exclusion criteria.

Cranial Hemorrhages

There are presently no universally accepted treatments for cranial hemorrhages, and the main strain of therapy in the transport arena is supportive care. Nonaccidental trauma is unusual in the immediate neonatal period but must be considered if the situation warrants.

Social/Emotional Considerations

The neonate is the newest member of the family, and the need for separation and transfer to another facility is often traumatic. The transport team should greet the family and give an update on the infant's status and plan of care. The team should share information about the neonatal intensive care unit to which the infant will be transferred, including contact numbers. If feasible, the mother and family should be able to see the infant before he or she is transferred out of the facility. Whenever possible, the mother should be transferred to that facility so that she may be with her infant.

Communication

Transitions in care increase the possibility for miscommunication and errors to occur. The Joint Commission National Patient Safety Goals mandate implementing the use of handoffs within each institution.[13] Safety programs such as Team Strategies and Tools to Enhance Performance and Patient Safety between staff and teams suggest standardized tools and strategies to avoid errors.[14] In transport situations, there are more opportunities for errors and miscommunications because there is a transition of not only healthcare providers but also institutions.

Communication for transport consists of three major components: (1) the healthcare team, (2) the transport team, and (3) the family. Communication between the healthcare team and the transport team is ideally completed on a recorded telephone line for quality and safety purposes. Communication with the family may be in person at the bedside, on a recorded telephone line, or via other digital communications.

All communication must be clear, concise, comprehensive, and timely and documented appropriately. Communication that reflects these attributes is vital to the safety and well-being of the patient and the transport team.

Documentation

The purpose of documentation is to ensure ongoing optimal patient care and communication regarding the continuity of care during transport. Documentation must be complete, legible, dated, timed, and signed. Documentation must be completed to provide the most complete, clear assessment of the patient and the care that is provided. In the medical–legal arena, when subsequent providers, reviewers, and juries are unable to get a clear view of the patient and the care that was provided, there is often a negative impression or assessment of the care overall. Documentation must be factual and void of judgment, criticism, or editorial comments. If there is a concern about the adequacy or quality of care, there should be an internal process for review and feedback. Standardized documentation is also highly encouraged and may be mandated by the institution.[15]

Consent

Written consent for transport must be obtained from the parents or legal guardian or designee. In a situation in which the mother is unable to consent and the referral and accepting physician deem the transport life-saving, a medical emergency consent can be obtained and signed by both providers (referring and accepting). This situation is known as the *emergency exception rule* or the *doctrine of implied consent.* Often the names of the physicians are documented on the consent form and signed by a witness on a recorded call. As soon as the mother, parent, or legal guardian is available, the signature is added to the written consent form signed by the physicians. Each facility that participates in transport must have a policy, procedure, or guideline to outline this situation or practice.

Consultation/Medical Director's Role

The transport team, the medical control physician, and/or the consultant may not be privileged to practice medicine, nursing, or respiratory therapy in the referral facility. The transport team functions as a consultation service under the direction of the physician present. Recommendations should be made when appropriate. The transferring physician must remain involved in the care of the infant, has legal responsibility for care of the infant, and is responsible for signing the transfer certificate at the time of transfer.

If there is a disagreement regarding care that cannot be resolved at the time, the transport team may be instructed to depart as soon as possible and change care or management when the infant is loaded into the transport vehicle. Most often the patient becomes a patient of the accepting hospital at the time of transfer and/or when the patient departs the premises of the referral hospital. All decisions or disagreements should be documented by all caregivers.[15]

Safety

The safety of the team, patient, and others must be paramount in all transport decisions.[16] The transport team is exposed to additional risks including but not limited to weather, time of day, geography, traffic, natural and unnatural disasters, and physical conditions. For this reason, the transport team must have policies, procedures, and guidelines to address all of the above risks. Education and competencies must be included to address the specific conditions that may include but are not limited to altitude, extreme weather, natural and unnatural disasters, water egress, and cold weather survival. Transport is physically demanding, and some teams have specific fitness requirements. Chronic health issues that include but are not limited to diabetes, allergies, and hypertension must be considered. Self-limiting conditions such as pregnancy and injuries must also be addressed in transport policies, procedures, and guidelines and may differ from institutional requirements. There are often guidelines provided by professional associations or regulatory agencies.

Types of Transport and Other Considerations

Transport may become necessary to a higher level of care including but not limited to subspecialty care, diagnostic testing, and evaluation. Transport to a lower level of care is also considered to facilitate recovery and reunification with family to build ongoing support. There are several types of transport, each with advantages and disadvantages. The primary concern is the safe, efficient transport of the neonate with the most appropriate personnel and equipment (Fig. 5.1).

One-way transport uses services of personnel, equipment, and vehicles dispatched by the referral hospital to the receiving center. The primary advantages are time saved and knowledge of the patient by the referral center, which reduces a transition in care. A disadvantage is the cost of maintaining necessary experienced staff and equipment. Studies have shown that there is increased morbidity and mortality when neonates are transported by an untrained versus a trained neonatal team.

Two-way transport uses the services of personnel, equipment, and vehicles dispatched by the receiving center. This is the most common for neonatal and pediatric transport. This type of transport is cost-effective and most often provides more experienced transport staff, trained specifically in neonatal transport, with the most sophisticated equipment and techniques. Disadvantages include the potential delay in transfer and the expense of maintaining a skilled neonatal transport program.

In three-way transport, a transport service without affiliation to the referral or receiving center is used. This is most frequently used with a less common mode of transport, such as fixed wing, boat, or ferry. An evaluation process must be completed to determine the cost–benefit ratio. Additional attention to the skill set and expertise of staff, age-appropriate supplies and equipment, cost, and an established transport agreement is suggested.[15,17]

Back/return/convalescent transport is used when neonates are transferred back to the local or birth hospital when they no longer require the resources of the regional neonatal intensive care center. The receiving facility should consider back-transport after completion of the treatment or procedure. The neonate may be transported by a team from the receiving hospital, the referring hospital, or a third facility or company. The level of care during transport must remain the same as the highest level of care provided. The family should be involved in the decision of transferring the infant, including a visit to the hospital prior

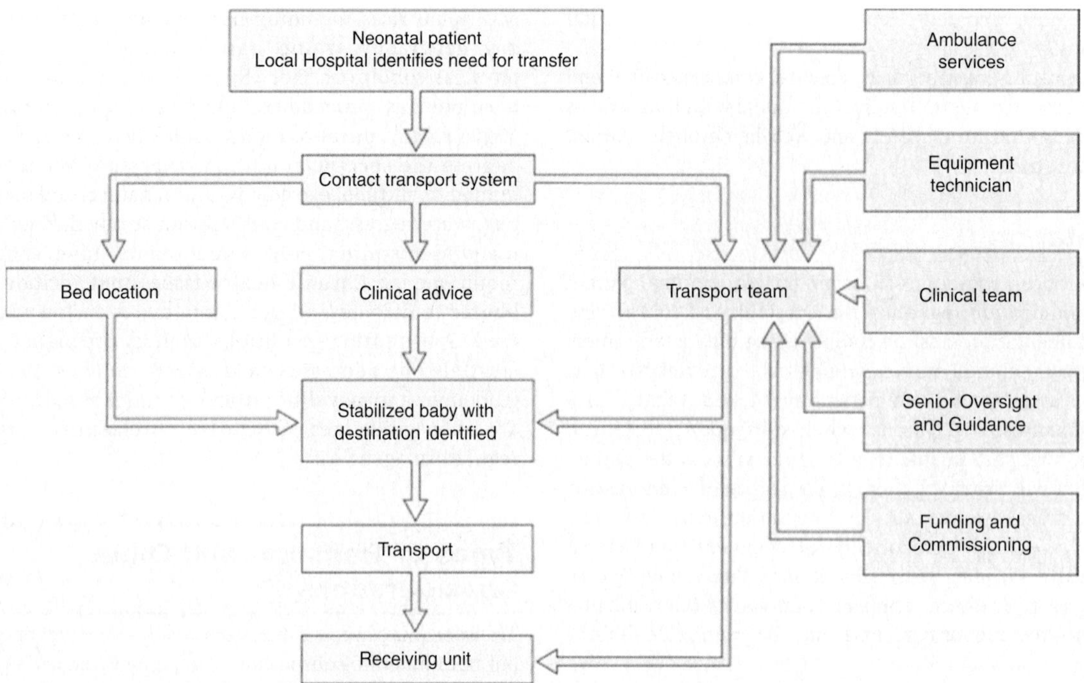

Fig. 5.1 Resuscitation and Transport of a Sick Neonate. (Reproduced with permission from O'Donnell et al. *Rennie and Roberton's Textbook of Neonatology*. 2012:223–243.)

to the transfer. Parental anxiety and loss of continuity of care may be evident when leaving the neonatal intensive care unit. This strategy provides the most efficient use of resources, improves relationships, and increases opportunities for involvement of parents and primary care providers in care. This may not be possible due to managed care or insurance contractual agreements. There is the potential need for transport back to a higher-care facility if the patient's condition deteriorates at the community hospital.[18]

Mode of Transport

Two primary modes of transport are used—ground ambulances and rotor or fixed-wing aircrafts (Figs. 5.2 and 5.3). In some locales, boats and ferries may be used. The selection of mode depends on the patient's condition, the level of medical care available, the transport staff required, distance, traffic, and weather. An ideal transport vehicle should be safe, quiet, comfortable, and appropriately equipped. The transport vehicle must provide the same resources available in the neonatal intensive care unit (blended gases, climate control, electricity with redundant backup, etc.). Careful consideration of the risk and benefits of different modes of transportation must be considered prior to each transport. Speed is never a priority over safety.[15,17]

Decompensation

Decompensation often occurs during transitions in care and may be the most common management challenge. Unnecessary decompensations can often be avoided with preplanning and education. The following situations may result in decompensation that could delay

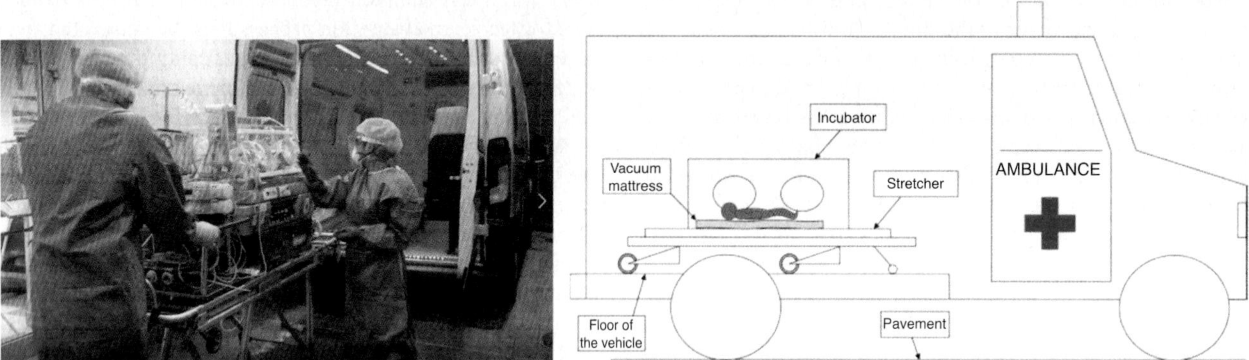

Fig. 5.2 The Vehicle–Road Interface Is an Important Consideration in the Transport of Premature and Critically Ill Infants. (Reproduced with permission from Bellini and Gente. *Air Med J*. 2020;39:154–155; and Bouchut et al. *Air Med J*. 2011;30:134–139.)

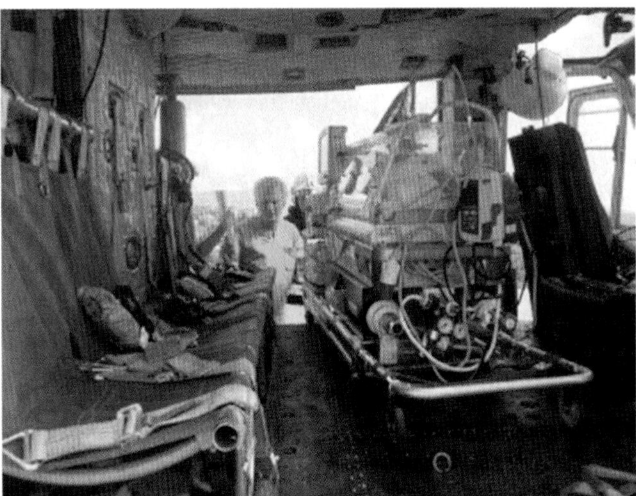

Fig. 5.3 Air Transport of a Sick Neonate. (Reproduced with permission from Bellini et al. *Air Med J.* 2020;39:24–26.)

or derail a transport. These situations must be discussed regularly to remain in a state of preparedness.

- Unplanned extubation
- Equipment transition
- Change in environment
- Climate or weather
- Temperature
- Noise
- Vibration
- Potential accidents
- Traffic

Unique Challenges

Transport offers unique challenges not found in other healthcare settings. The first is consent, which the mother may not be capable of providing. The father of the baby might not be allowed to provide consent, depending on marital status and the laws of the jurisdiction. The best practice is to ask the referral hospital that has a relationship with the mother and family to obtain the transport consent. When this is not possible, other options must be available.

The ethical principles apply in transport. The expectation and hope that transport will provide additional solutions and resources is not always met. In a situation when transport may not be in best interest of the patient and family, the transport team is on the front line of addressing those unmet expectations. This can be stressful for everyone involved. Transparent communication is always the best approach to create situational awareness for all healthcare team members. When the prognosis has changed, the ability to offer the family realistic choices is imperative. Those choices may include palliative or comfort care, providing chosen death rituals, or even transport when death is inevitable. The parents are the ultimate decision-makers for their infant. The transport team may provide support for the referral center staff, who may not have the opportunity to care for families who experience the death of their infant.[19]

When care appears to be futile, transport can be challenging for the transport team because of the potential for the complication of death during transport. Certain questions must be addressed prior to departure, such as who will pronounce the infant's death and who will have jurisdiction of the body if the transport team is en route at the time of death. Depending on the distance, teams often must continue resuscitation efforts during the entire transport until arrival to the accepting center.

Education and Training

Education and training should include the following:

1. Clinical competence
2. Procedural skill mastery
3. Transport procedure and equipment
4. Administrative details
5. Documentation
6. Transport environment versus hospital
7. Motion sickness
8. Public relations/customer service
9. Outreach education
10. Other
    A. Stress management
        1. Potential of vehicular accidents
        2. Being (or the sense of being) the only one to perform lifesaving skills or make lifesaving decisions
        3. Having to practice in unfamiliar surroundings or with limited resources
        4. Erratic work schedules and late calls
        5. Physical stress—moving, vibrating, noisy environment (Fig. 5.4)
            a. Moving—motion sickness, limited assessment
            b. Vibration—dehydration, fatigue
            c. Noise—fatigue
        6. Care of the transport team
            a. Critical incident management (CISM)
            b. Resiliency
            c. Informal support
    B. Air medical physiology
        1. The sum of partial pressures of individual gases in the atmosphere defines the barometric pressure; an inverse relationship exists between altitude and barometric pressure
        2. Dalton's law—the sum of the partial pressures of individual gases in a mixture is equal to the total pressure of that mixture
        3. Boyle's law—at constant temperature, the volume of a gas varies inversely with the pressure

As altitude increases, the resultant decrease in barometric pressure will result in alveolar hypoxemia and increase pulmonary vascular resistance unless one adjusts the FiO_2 to compensate for the change. In addition to hypoxia, there are dysbarisms or a disturbance from a difference between pressures in other areas of the body. Any closed space or body cavity may be affected; for example: pneumothorax, bowel obstruction, air splints. *A balloon will double its volume from sea level to 18,000 ft.*

Cabin pressurization in fixed wing can help reduce effects, but care must be taken to avoid rapid depressurization or decompression. High altitude will potentiate effects of drugs or alcohol, sleep deprivation, fatigue, and hypoglycemia. It is illegal for any person to act as a crew member within 8 hours of consumption of any alcoholic beverage or using any drug that affects the person's faculties in any way contrary to safety. Night vision is impaired at altitudes greater than 5000 ft.

Quality

Neonatal transport is essential and lifesaving. Each program, regardless of size, must have a total management quality process for continually

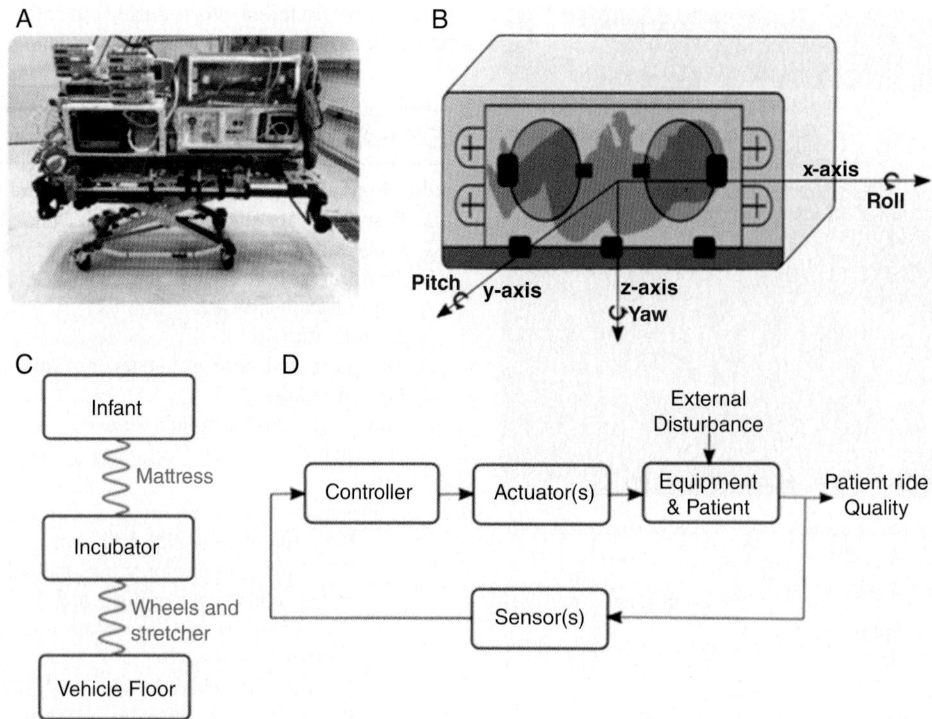

Fig. 5.4 Infant Incubator Design and Vibration Isolation Systems. (A) A typical neonatal transport system. (B) A standard vehicle coordinate system applied to the transport equipment incubator. (C) Passive vibration isolators act by altering the natural frequency of the system to produce a vibration attenuation. (D) Active vibration isolation systems comprise a sensor attached to the stationary object that detects vibration and a controller that analyzes the frequency and amplitude of the vibration and outputs a feedback signal to an actuator that converts the incoming energy into movement, thus creating an opposing force that cancels out the vibration. (Reproduced with permission from Goswami et al. *Early Hum Dev*. 2020;146:105051.)

evaluating and improving the services provided.[4–16,18] Some measure of patient and process outcome must be completed and include all members, especially medical care providers, and the other healthcare providers involved in the transport process. A written plan with parameters and measures that are transparent and communicated and integrated into a larger intuitional hospital safety and quality program is imperative. The American Academy of Pediatrics, the National Association of Neonatal Nurses, and other professional organizations offer minimal standards for transport teams. There is now the ability to track, report, and compare transport data with similar programs internationally. The Ground Air Medical Quality Transport (GAMUT) Quality Improvement Collaborative uses the GAMUT database as a free resource for transport teams to track, report, and analyze their performance on transport-specific quality metrics by comparing it to that of other programs (2019). Additional information can be found at https://www.gamutqi.org/.

CHAPTER 6

Radiation Safety in Premature and Critically-Ill Neonates

Sheila Berlin

KEY POINTS

1. Digital radiography is a frequently used imaging technique in neonatal intensive care units (NICUs), with many infants having multiple radiographs during their stays.
2. High-energy photons in ionizing radiation can damage DNA, particularly with repeated natural background exposures and diagnostic medical imaging.
3. Radiation dose is a measure of the amount of exposure of the tissues of the body to radiation; it is determined by the energy, duration, and area of beam exposure.
4. In NICUs, the highest reported total radiation doses are fortunately less than the annual natural background effective dose. However, caregivers need to remain cognizant of the risks. The significance of scatter or secondary radiation in the vicinity of a radiographic exposure also needs to be considered. Several guidelines have been established to minimize these risks.
5. A key concept that guides imaging use in the NICU is the As Low as Reasonably Achievable (ALARA) principle. The ALARA principle is the offspring of the linear no-threshold hypothesis, which implies that there is no safe dose of ionizing radiation.

Introduction

The benefit of medical imaging in saving lives and improving treatment for the premature and critically-ill neonate is well established. Digital radiography is the most frequently used imaging technique in the neonatal intensive care unit (NICU), with many infants having multiple radiographs during their stays. These images, largely of the chest and abdomen, provide critical information about life-support device placement, acute life-threatening conditions such as tension pneumothorax and bowel perforation, and disease response to medical and surgical interventions. To generate these important diagnostic images, digital radiography—along with fluoroscopy and computed tomography (CT)—use low doses of ionizing radiation.

Substantial scientific data show that high-energy photons from ionizing radiation can damage DNA when delivered at high doses; however, these effects occur at many multiples of the doses received in diagnostic medical imaging and natural background exposure.[1] All humans are exposed to low doses of ionizing radiation from ubiquitous sources such as cosmic and terrestrial radiation; the degree of exposure depends on variables such as altitude and home ventilation. Although children are more radiosensitive than adults (i.e., the cancer risk per unit dose of radiation is higher) and have longer lifetimes over which to express a radiation-induced genetic mutation, adaptive DNA repair mechanisms appear to function well in children exposed to low doses of radiation.[2] We know that delivering doses at increments rather than all at once allows tissues to recover, and the risk from multiple serial exams is not cumulative.[3] Most important, the radiation doses to which even the most frequently imaged critically-ill neonates are exposed remain a fraction of the annual natural background radiation. Because ionizing radiation is one of the potential iatrogenic harms to which neonates and their parents and caregivers may be exposed, it is important to understand how dose is measured and optimized in neonatal radiographic, fluoroscopic, and CT imaging.

Quantifying Radiation Exposure

Radiation dose is a measure of the amount of exposure of the tissues of the body to radiation. The dose of radiation to which a patient is exposed is determined by three factors: the energy of the x-ray beam, the duration of beam exposure, and the area over which the beam is applied. There are several methods used to quantify radiation dose; the most useful are calculations of absorbed dose, equivalent dose, and effective dose. Absorbed dose, expressed in milligrays (mGy), is the amount of energy deposited by radiation into an absorbing medium; the mass can be anything—people, water, air, or a rock. Equivalent dose, measured in millisieverts (mSv), is calculated for individual organs. Effective dose, also measured in mSv, is calculated for the whole body; it is the summation of equivalent doses to all organs, each adjusted according to the organ sensitivity to radiation. Effective dose is the preferred metric for reporting radiation dose and is widely used in the scientific community to compare different techniques for dose optimization. It is important to recognize that the International Commission on Radiological Protection introduced the use of effective dose for the targeted purpose of setting limits for radiation protection—not to predict cancer risk among exposed persons. The formula for calculating effective dose incorporates weighting factors for radiation quality and organ sensitivity across all ages and both sexes; as a result, this formula does not apply to any specific individual or radiosensitive subpopulations such as children.[4]

The average annual effective dose of natural background ionizing radiation in the United States is 3 mSv, with a range from 1 to 20 mSv. At these background doses, there is no direct evidence of harm.[5] A person might accumulate an effective dose from natural background of about 50 mSv in the first 17 years of life and about 250 mSv during an average 80-year lifetime.[6] For healthcare workers with occupational exposure, the International Commission on Radiological Protection recommends a dose limit of 20 mSv/year.[7] In the United States, the National Council on Radiation Protection and Measurements sets a dose limit of 50 mSv/year for these individuals.[8]

Estimation of exposure to medical radiation in the NICU has been reported using modern digital radiographic techniques. These studies report effective dose ranges from 0.012 to 0.016 mSv per radiograph.[9–12] Total effective doses for some highly imaged infants has been reported to be as high as 1.5 mSv for patients with chronic lung disease or necrotizing enterocolitis.[13] Even the highest reported total radiation doses are less than the annual natural background effective dose. In order to help caregivers better understand dose metrics, use of a relative risk descriptor comparing medical radiation dose to natural background dose is helpful. Because of the complexity of scientific dose metrics, the background equivalent radiation time was designed to educate the general public about radiation dose without complex concepts or terminology. Using the background equivalent radiation time relative risk descriptor, a single portable radiograph of the chest would be the equivalent of approximately 1 day of natural background radiation[14] (Table 6.1).

Another concern that arises in the NICU is the significance of scatter or secondary radiation in the vicinity of a radiographic exposure.[15,16] Scatter radiation occurs when the beam intercepts an object—most frequently the patient's body—that causes the x-rays to be scattered. The radiation dose from scatter is a very small fraction of the dose received from the primary x-ray beam. An important principle of dose reduction is the inverse square law; this property of physics states that if one doubles the distance from the primary radiation source, dose is reduced by a factor of four. To minimize the amount of scatter radiation dose to caregivers, parents, and neighboring patients in the NICU, these individuals should be positioned at least 1 meter from the irradiated field; at this distance, the primary scatter radiation is estimated to represent approximately 0.1% to 0.2% of the incident radiation.[17] If healthcare personnel are required to be within 1 meter of the radiation field, they should wear a lead apron.

Another key concept that guides imaging use in the NICU is the As Low as Reasonably Achievable (ALARA) principle. The ALARA principle is the offspring of the linear no-threshold hypothesis, which implies that there is no safe dose of ionizing radiation.[18] The ALARA principle is based on the assumption that low doses of radiation might be harmful and therefore should be minimized for medical imaging procedures.

Image Acquisition to Optimize Dose and Adhere to the ALARA Principle

Recommendations for adhering to the ALARA principle and minimizing the use of ionizing radiation in medical imaging require healthcare providers to answer the following questions. First, is the imaging medically necessary? Radiographs should only be obtained if the information they provide is likely to impact the care of the patient—not simply as a daily default routine. Second, are there alternatives such as sonography or magnetic resonance imaging that could serve as appropriate diagnostic alternatives? Bedside point-of-care ultrasound is emerging as a quick and inexpensive imaging modality in the NICU. Diagnostic applications for point-of-care ultrasound in the NICU include the evaluation and monitoring of common pulmonary diseases, hemodynamic instability, patent ductus arteriosus, persistent pulmonary hypertension of the newborn, necrotizing enterocolitis, and intraventricular hemorrhage.[19] Third, does the imaging facility "child-size" their imaging protocols to minimize radiation dose? Although doses for radiographic examinations in the NICU are low, technical factors of imaging protocols may not be optimized for low birth weight neonates.[20] Digital radiography can compensate for exposure technique errors with powerful postprocessing and display tools. For example, an erroneously overexposed (and higher dose) chest radiograph may appear of diagnostic quality; this automatic adjustment function of digital radiography prevents any visual feedback for dose errors. In fact, overexposure will increase the signal-to-noise ratio and likely decrease the complaints from radiologists regarding image quality. These factors have resulted in a phenomenon known as "dose creep." To prevent dose creep, technical factors such as kilovoltage peak (kVp) and milliamperes (mAs) should be optimized for the size of the neonate, and standardized protocols should be established for modern digital radiography equipment. Dose reduction can be achieved by using weight or body circumference parameters and adopting high kVp and low mAs techniques.[20]

Unintentional radiation exposure can be minimized by adhering to standard collimation techniques, optimal patient positioning, and artifact removal. The American Society of Radiologic Technologists, American College of Radiology, and Society for Pediatric Radiology support preexposure collimation of the x-ray field; this limits the beam to the area of interest and defines the field of view.[21] Proper collimation reduces patient dose, minimizes scatter radiation, and improves image quality (Fig. 6.1). Many radiographs are exposed with nonrelevant body parts in the field of view; this unintentionally exposed anatomy includes the head, abdomen, and upper extremities for chest radiographs and the lower extremities and chest for abdominal radiographs.[22] Masking (applying a black border) or cropping should not be used as substitutes for appropriate preprocedure collimation; all captured image data are part of the patient's permanent medical record and should be presented to the radiologist to determine whether any unintentionally exposed anatomy is of diagnostic value. Proper positioning for anteroposterior views, cross-table lateral views, and decubitus views—with particular attention to avoiding patient rotation—can prevent the need for repeat radiographs (Fig. 6.2). Collaboration between the radiology technologist and care providers in the NICU to clear the relevant anatomy from overlying leads and other temporarily removable artifacts will also result in decreased repeat exposures.

Once a mainstay of patient radiation protection, gonadal shielding has been reexamined by the scientific community. In light of the most current scientific literature, the American Association of Physicists in Medicine (AAPM), American College of Radiology, Health Physics Society, Radiological Society of North America, and Image Gently and Image Wisely recommend discontinuation of the use of patient gonadal shielding as a routine practice.[23] Use of these shields during x-ray–based diagnostic imaging may obscure anatomic information, compromise the diagnostic efficacy of the examination, and result in a second exposure. Furthermore, shields that are detected

Table 6.1 Background Dose Equivalent Radiation Time

Radiation Source	Radiation Dose Estimate	Estimates of Equivalent Amount of Background Radiation
Natural background radiation	3 mSv	1 year
Airline passenger for cross country travel	0.04 mSv	4 days
Newborn chest x-ray	0.01–0.02 mSv	1 day
Upper gastrointestinal series	0.5 mSv	2 months
VCUG	0.3 mSv	5 weeks
Computed tomography of the head	0.5–2 mSv	2–8 months

VCUG, voiding cystourethrogram.

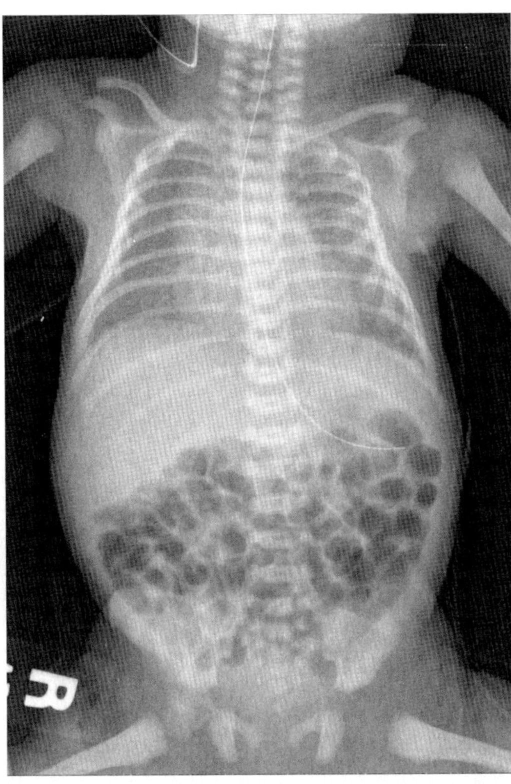

Fig. 6.1 Optimal Collimation for Anteroposterior Portable Chest and Abdominal Radiograph.

by automatic exposure controls of an imaging system can result in an *increase* in the patient's radiation dose. According to the AAPM, "Because of these tangible risks and minimal to nonexistent benefit associate with fetal and gonadal shielding, the AAPM recommends that the use of such shielding should be discontinued."[3] Because patient shielding has been used for more than 70 years, this shift in practice may result in questions from healthcare providers and parents. The AAPM has prepared a list of frequently asked questions

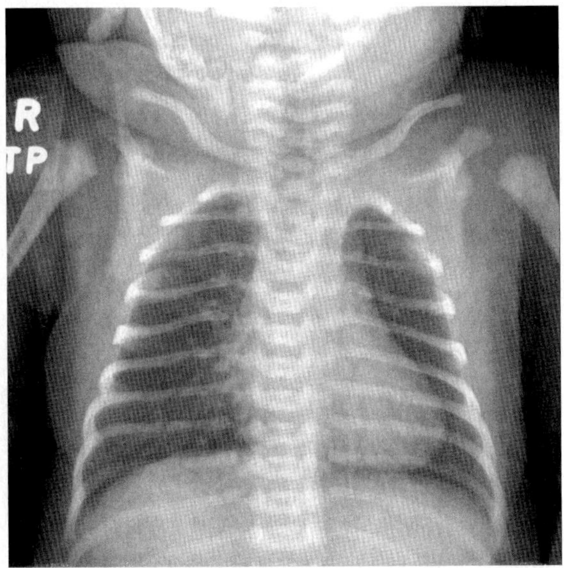

Fig. 6.2 Optimal Positioning for an Anteroposterior Portable Chest Radiograph.

to help healthcare providers address common concerns about the discontinuation of lead shielding[3] (Appendix 6.1).

This departure from the use of patient shielding also applies to fluoroscopy and CT imaging—two modalities that may provide helpful diagnostic information in the premature or critically-ill neonate. The most commonly performed fluoroscopy exams in the newborn are the upper gastrointestinal series, contrast enema, and voiding cystourethrogram. These exams are performed using pulsed fluoroscopy techniques to minimize radiation dose; reducing the number of frames from 30 per second (continuous fluoroscopy) to 4 per second results in a dose reduction of 75%.[24] Another technique to minimize radiation exposure during fluoroscopic exams is the use of the last image hold capture tool rather than additional digital radiographic exposures. This tool displays the last fluoroscopic image on the monitor when the fluoroscopy pedal or hand switch is released to terminate the fluoroscopic run. Each of these "saved" captures is less than 10% of the dose of a conventional digital radiographic exposure.[25] These images are not only obtained at no additional dose to the patient but also can be recorded and stored in the patient's digital imaging records. Since the first patient scan in 1971, CT use has increased rapidly because of this modality's excellent diagnostic accuracy, availability, short acquisition time, and cost-effectiveness. With this expansion in application, CT scientists have created technology to child-size protocols, automatically adjust exposure based on patient size, and reduce dose using features such as iterative reconstruction.[26] Using current dose optimization techniques, effective doses for fluoroscopy and CT imaging remain near or below that of a year of natural background radiation (see Table 6.1). Furthermore, there remains no definitive scientific proof that the small doses of radiation from CT increase cancer risk. It is clear that all hypothetical predicted cancer risks from CT are extremely low.[5] Therefore anticipated benefits to the patient of a medically necessary fluoroscopic examination or CT scan are "highly likely to outweigh any small potential risks."[27]

Healthcare providers play a critical role in the education of parents and other caregivers of neonates in the NICU. Sensationalistic reports in the public media may lead some parents to fear or refuse safe and appropriate medical imaging. To address such radiophobia, the most recent position of the medical imaging community should be shared, which "recognizes that the risk for the majority of imaging exams is either too small to be determined or may even be zero."[3] Parents and providers should be reassured that although the hypothetical risk is extremely small, medical imaging professionals aim to use the dose that is as low as reasonably achievable, and many tools can be used to minimize radiation exposure to their child.

Appendix 6.1

Why Is My Child Not Shielded Now?

Shields have been used in the past, but we know more about radiation now and have imaging equipment that uses much less radiation than in the past. We have also seen that shields can cover up parts of your child's body that are important for the doctor to see.

Why Is My Child Not Shielded If I Am Required to Wear a Lead Apron While I Am in the Room With Them?

Your child's doctor wants an image so that he or she can better see what is going on inside your child's body. This exposes your child to a little bit of radiation. Your doctor has thought about the benefits and risks to your child. He or she has decided that the benefit from having the information from the image is much higher than the risk from the radiation, which is very small or zero. Because you aren't being imaged, there is no need for you to get any radiation, so we give you an apron to wear to make sure that you don't get any dose.

My Child Previously Had an Imaging Exam Where Shielding Was Used. Why the Change in Practice?

Patient shields have been used for more than 70 years. A lot has changed since then. We have better machines that use much less radiation. We also know more about how radiation affects the human body. Some parts of the body—like the testicles and ovaries—are much less sensitive to radiation than we used to think; thus there is no benefit from placing shields on your child.

Can I Ask for a Shield for My Child?

We do not recommend using lead shielding during imaging exams. Some exams can never be done using a shield because it would cover parts of the body we need to see. But, if you insist that we use a shield, we will honor your request if it is possible to do so without compromising the exam your child is having.

SECTION 2

Neonatal Resuscitation and Respiratory Care

OUTLINE

Section 2

CHAPTER 7

Placental Transfusion in the Newborn

Sripriya Sundararajan, Renske McFarlane, Heike Rabe

KEY POINTS

1. Delayed cord clamping (DCC) is a very powerful yet simple, no-cost intervention practice that can transform the lives of children and mothers around the world.
2. DCC is a practice of waiting to cut the umbilical cord until sufficient time (3–5 minutes) has elapsed to permit blood flow from the placenta to the newborn while the baby is transitioning to extrauterine life.
3. DCC facilitates placental transfusion and maintains systemic cardiac output until the newborn lungs establish lung circulation with the initiation of spontaneous breathing.
4. Placental transfusion can also be accomplished by umbilical cord milking or cord milking through an intact umbilical cord.
5. Placental transfusion volume to the newborn depends on the time to clamp the cord after birth, the position of the newborn relative to the location of the placenta, placental contractions, and the onset of spontaneous breathing in the newborn.
6. DCC is an easily implemented intervention that requires joint cooperation among healthcare providers involved in childbirth and a participatory culture change in public health.
7. Major benefits of DCC include improved cardiopulmonary transition, improved survival rates with reduced hospital mortality for preterm infants, reduction in iron-deficiency anemia in term infants during the first year of life through improved iron stores, and positive impact on neurodevelopment at 4 years of age.

Introduction

The transition from fetal to newborn life is characterized by both initiation of spontaneous breathing and changes to circulation. Delayed cord clamping (DCC) is a practice of waiting to cut the umbilical cord until sufficient time (3–5 minutes) has elapsed to permit blood flow from the placenta to the newborn while the baby is transitioning to extrauterine life. DCC facilitates placental transfusion,[1] or the transfer of warm oxygenated blood from the placenta to the newborn at a slow rate, facilitated by uterine contraction.[2,3] DCC permits placental transfusion, and a passive transfer of stem cells, antibodies, and iron-rich blood from the placenta to the newborn occurs. DCC has enormous proven benefits for both premature and term infants. In the preterm infant, DCC assists with improved cardiopulmonary transition with stable blood pressures, reduction in intraventricular hemorrhages (IVH), reduced infection rates, reduced use of blood products in the neonatal intensive care unit, and improved survival rates.[4] In the term infant, DCC is associated with reduction of both iron-deficiency anemia and improved neurodevelopmental outcomes at 4 years of age.[5]

DCC is an age-old practice that has shifted to immediate clamping during the decades since the 1950s without conducting randomized controlled trials on this change.[6,7] Currently, the umbilical cord is clamped early, from immediately to within 15 seconds of birth,[7] while there is still a significant circulation occurring through the umbilical vessels. The newborn is then quickly transferred to the pediatric provider in an effort to avoid delayed resuscitation. Immediate clamping of the cord is both a nonphysiologic and avoidable intervention that abruptly interrupts the natural process of placental transfusion. Immediate cord clamping prevents acquisition of adequate blood volume and thus may cause more harm than benefit to the baby. Reports from a systematic review and meta-analysis of delayed versus early umbilical cord clamping for preterm infants report a 28% to 30% increase in hospital deaths for preterm infants who had their cords clamped immediately after birth.[4,8]

It has been reported that 80 to 100 mL of blood transfers from the placenta in the first 3 minutes after birth.[1,9,10] Clamping the umbilical cord while significant circulation is still occurring through the umbilical vessels drops the cardiac output by approximately 40%.[11] This deprives the newborn of the benefit of added circulating blood volume (up to 100 mL) from continuing placental transfusion. Sick and preterm infants are especially likely to benefit from the additional blood volume achieved by DCC, besides term infants.[2,12,13] Despite endorsements for DCC by numerous governing bodies and stakeholders (Table 7.1) including the International Federation of Gynaecology and Obstetrics (2003), European Confederation of Midwives (2003), Society of Obstetricians and Gynaecologists of Canada (2009, 2016), International Liaison Committee on Resuscitation (2010, 2015), International Consensus on Cardiopulmonary Resuscitation (2011), World Health Organization (2014), National Institute for Health and Care Excellence (NICE) of the United Kingdom (2015), Royal College of Obstetricians and Gynaecologists (2016), *Textbook of Neonatal Resuscitation*, 7th edition (2016), Helping Babies Breathe, 2nd edition (2016), American Academy of Pediatrics (2017), American College of Obstetricians and Gynecologists (2017), and European Association of Perinatal Medicine, the practice of DCC has been slow to be adopted.[14]

Pathophysiology of Placental Transfusion

In the fetus, the lungs are filled with fluid. No gas exchange occurs, and this results in approximately 15% of the right ventricular cardiac output entering the fetal lungs. The oxygenated umbilical

Table 7.1 Recommendations for Delayed Cord Clamping by Major Stakeholders

Organization	Preterm (<37 Weeks)	Term (>37 Weeks)
WHO (2014)	Delayed umbilical cord clamping (not earlier than 1 minute after birth) is recommended for improved maternal and infant health and nutrition outcomes	
RCOG (2015)	Umbilical cord should not be clamped earlier than 1 minute if there are no concerns over cord integrity or the baby's well-being	In healthy term babies, practice deferred cord clamping (delay clamping for at least 2 minutes)
ILCOR (2015)	For uncompromised babies, a delay in cord clamping of at least 1 minute from the complete delivery of the infant is recommended for term and preterm babies; as yet, there is insufficient evidence to recommend an appropriate time for clamping the cord in babies who require resuscitation at birth	
ACOG (2017)	Delay umbilical cord clamping in vigorous term and preterm infants for at least 30–60 seconds after birth	
AAP (2017)	Endorse recommendations of ACOG 2017	
NICE (2019)	If a preterm baby needs to be moved away from the mother for resuscitation or there is significant maternal bleeding, consider milking the cord and clamp the cord as soon as possible; wait at least 30 seconds, but no longer than 3 minutes, before clamping the cord of preterm babies if the mother and baby are stable; position the baby at or below the level of the placenta before clamping the cord (2019)	Do not clamp the cord earlier than 1 minute from the birth of the baby unless there is concern about the integrity of the cord or the baby has a heart rate less than 60 bpm that is not getting faster; clamp the cord before 5 minutes to perform controlled cord traction as part of active management; if the woman requests that the cord is clamped and cut later than 5 minutes, support her in her choice (2015)
SOGC	Delayed cord clamping by at least 60 seconds is recommended irrespective of mode of delivery	The risk of jaundice is weighed against the physiologic benefits of delayed cord clamping

AAP, American Academy of Pediatrics; *ACOG*, American College of Obstetricians and Gynecologists; *ILCOR*, International Liaison Committee on Resuscitation; *NICE*, National Institute for Health and Care Excellence; *RCOG*, Royal College of Obstetricians and Gynaecologists; *SOGC*, Society of Obstetricians and Gynaecologists of Canada; *WHO*, World Health Organization.

venous blood from the placenta that enters the right atrium is shunted across the foramen ovale to enter the left atrium. This serves as a preload for the left ventricle to supply oxygenated blood to the head and neck vessels. The umbilical venous blood that enters the right ventricle and pulmonary artery is then shunted across the ductus arteriosus to supply the rest of the body tissues. However, soon after birth, when the baby initiates breathing, the lungs are filled with air that assists with the drop in pulmonary vascular resistance and increases blood flowing into the pulmonary circulation. Thereafter, blood returns to the left ventricle to maintain systemic cardiac output. The newly accelerated pulmonary blood flow now replaces the umbilical venous blood as the source of the preload. This results in improved left ventricular output and systemic blood flow.

Clamping the umbilical cord resulted in a drop of right ventricular output and thereafter the systemic cardiac output in preterm lamb studies.[15–17] If immediate clamping of the umbilical cord is performed before breathing is established, this blocks the acquisition of added blood volume from the placenta. This results in hypovolemia in a newborn, especially when compromised by asphyxia. Experimental studies in preterm lambs have shown positive effects for both systemic and cerebral hemodynamic parameters, including oxygen saturation when respiratory support is initiated prior to clamping the umbilical cord.[18–20] The drop in right ventricular output is mitigated when the cord is clamped after breathing is established. The umbilical venous blood now serves as a source of left ventricular preload until the pulmonary venous return is established with breathing and systemic blood flow is thereafter maintained.

Thus establishing lung inflation and pulmonary circulation through effective breathing prior to the clamping of the umbilical cord could lead to smoother cardiovascular transition and reduce the risk of IVH.[21] Therefore placental transfusion is an effective method of enhancing arterial oxygen content from the additional blood volume, maintaining cardiac output and increasing oxygen delivery during the transition period while the baby is attempting to establish breathing and pulmonary circulation. In addition, placental transfusion has been associated with lower incidences of sepsis and necrotizing enterocolitis in preterm infants. Placental blood remains an untapped physiologic reservoir of hematopoietic and pluripotent stem cell lines.

Factors That Determine Placental Transfusion

Several important factors determine the volume of residual placental blood that is transferred to the neonate (Fig. 7.1). They are as follows.

Time of Cord Clamping

The volume of blood that is being transferred from the placenta to the infant is proportional to the timing of the cord clamping. DCC ranging from 30 seconds to the cessation of cord pulsations will transfer blood volumes ranging from 16 to 45 mL/kg[9] as opposed to immediate cord clamping in both vaginal and cesarean births.

Uterine Contractions

The mode of delivery (vaginal versus cesarean birth) influences the volume of placental transfusion. The uterine pressure gradient between the intrauterine umbilical vein and neonatal right atrium facilitates placental transfusion. In vaginal births, the uterine contractions during the third stage of labor can facilitate up to 50% of placental transfusion volume.[22]

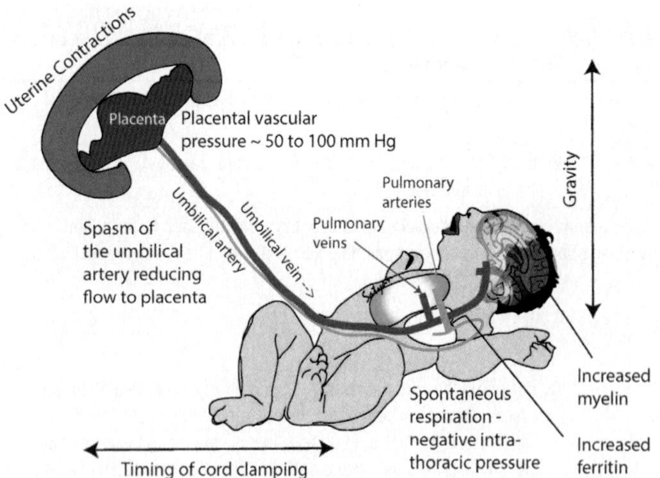

Fig. 7.1 Factors That Influence Placental Transfusion With Delayed Cord Clamping. The volume of placental transfusion is influenced by the timing of the cord clamping, strength of the uterine contractions, source of umbilical blood flow, time to establishment of spontaneous respiration, and effect of gravity. (Courtesy AC Katheria et al.)

Source of Umbilical Blood Flow

The umbilical arteries constrict (usually within approximately 30–45 seconds), preventing a net backflow from the infant to the placenta.[21] The umbilical vein remains patent during the third stage of labor and facilitates placental transfusion.

Time to Establishment of Spontaneous Breathing

Spontaneous breathing and crying result in lung aeration that establishes pulmonary circulation. Until spontaneous breathing is established, the umbilical venous blood serves as a source of left ventricular preload. Allowing babies to breathe with an intact umbilical cord that is still attached to the mother permits continued placental transfusion to the right atrium and subsequent left ventricular filling until the left ventricle blood is replaced with pulmonary blood flow. This allows a smooth cardiovascular transition from placental to neonatal circulation while mitigating wide swings of systemic and cerebral blood flow, especially in premature infants.[23,24]

The Effect of Gravity

The position of the infant influences the amount of placental transfusion volume through the effect of gravity.[25] Placental transfusion occurs during DCC when infants are held below the level of the vaginal introitus in vaginal births or below the level of the uterine incision in cesarean deliveries. Term infants assigned to DCC for 5 minutes and placed on the mother's abdomen received a larger placental transfusion volume compared with those with a 2-minute delay, as reported by Mercer et al.[26] Mothers could safely be allowed to hold their baby on their abdomen or chest while blood continued to flow from the placenta to the newborn.[26,27] This practice enhances maternal–infant bonding.

Methods of Cord Management After Birth

Immediate Cord Clamping

Immediate cord clamping (ICC) refers to the clamping of the umbilical cord immediately, or usually within 15 seconds, after birth. ICC results in one-third of the total blood volume remaining in the placenta. ICC is still very common in hospital settings throughout the world.[28] ICC deprives the infant of iron stores[29–33] and contributes to iron deficiency in infancy.[28] In fact, early umbilical cord clamping (less than 1 minute after birth) is not recommended by the World Health Organization unless the neonate is asphyxiated and needs to be moved immediately for resuscitation.[3,34]

Delayed Umbilical Cord Clamping

DCC is the practice of delaying the cutting of the umbilical cord until sufficient time has elapsed to permit placental transfusion to the infant. There is great variation in the timing of DCC, ranging from 30 seconds to 5 minutes to until the cord pulsations stop. The World Health Organization, International Liaison Committee on Resuscitation, and other organizations recommend waiting for at least 30 to 60 seconds after birth for the most vigorous term and preterm newborns.[14,34–36] This practice facilitates a physiologic passive transfer of warm, oxygenated, iron-rich blood from the placenta at a slow rate to the newborn. DCC prevent iron-deficiency anemia during the first 6 months of life.[37] It also reduces anemia at 8 and 12 months of age in high-risk populations.[38]

Intact Umbilical Cord Milking

DCC should not be confused with umbilical cord milking (UCM). Milking refers to the manual expression of blood from the umbilical cord. Intact UCM is the active practice of gently squeezing or milking blood down a short segment of intact umbilical cord (20–30 cm) that is attached to the placenta toward the baby 3 to 4 times at a rate of 10 cm/sec before clamping the cord. UCM is another method of transfusing placental blood to the newborn that is not physiologic but contributes to added neonatal blood volume.[39] UCM offers the added benefit of not delaying resuscitation in an unstable and compromised neonate who needs to be timely resuscitated.[21] UCM can be performed in any setting in 15 to 20 seconds, equivalent to the time it takes for ICC.[40] Thus UCM may serve as an alternative to DCC by providing equivalent benefits to preterm infants but without delaying resuscitation. In a post hoc analysis of a prematurely terminated randomized clinical trial of UCM versus DCC for 45 to 60 seconds among preterm infants born at <32 weeks of gestation, there was a statistically significant higher rate of severe IVH in the UCM subgroup in infants born at <28 weeks of gestation that led to early study termination for this age group.[41] Retrospective analysis of extremely preterm infants (<29 weeks of gestation) from the National Institute of Child Health and Human Development Neonatal Research Network suggests that DCC is the preferred practice for placental transfusion, because UCM exposure was associated with an increase in the adverse outcome of severe IVH (grade 3 or 4).[42] Three other randomized clinical trials comparing DCC for 30 to 60 seconds with UCM performed four times did not show a significant difference for rates of IVH in preterm infants born at <33 weeks of gestation.[42a,42b,42c] Effects on reducing mortality in preterm infants are similar to those reported for DCC. Intact UCM is considered an alternative method for providing placental transfusion if DCC is not feasible in term infants.

Cut Umbilical Cord Milking

Cut UCM is the practice of actively squeezing the residual blood down a long segment of an umbilical cord that is cut soon after birth

Table 7.2 Summary of Immediate and Long-Term Benefits of Delayed Cord Clamping for Infants (Term, Preterm, or Low Birth Weight) and Mothers From Individual Studies

Immediate Benefits			**Long-Term Benefits**	
Preterm/Low Birth Weight Infants	Full-Term Infants	Mothers	Preterm/Low Birth Weight Infants	Full-Term Infants
Decreases risk of • Intraventricular hemorrhage, all grades • Necrotizing enterocolitis • Late-onset sepsis	Provides adequate blood volume and birth iron stores	No effect on maternal bleeding or length of the third stage of labor	Increases Hb at 10 weeks of age	Improves hematological status (hematocrit/Hb) at 2–4 months of age
Decreases need for • Blood transfusions for anemia or hypotension • Surfactant • Mechanical ventilation	Increases hematocrit/Hb	Indication from "cord drainage" trials that less blood-filled placenta shortens the third stage of labor and decreases the incidence of retained placenta	Improves neurodevelopmental outcomes in male infants	Improves iron status until up to 6 months of age
Increases • Hematocrit/Hb • Blood pressure • Cerebral oxygenation • Red blood cell flow				

Hb, Hemoglobin.

and detached from the mother but still attached to the baby. The neonatal provider subsequently milks the blood into the baby after untwisting the long segment of the cord.[43]

Placental Transfusion

What Are the Benefits of Placental Transfusion?

There are immediate and long-term benefits of placental transfusion for both preterm and low birth weight infants and term infants (summarized in Table 7.2).[3,4,36,38,44] Immediate benefits of placental transfusion for preterm or low birth weight infants that have been reported include the following:

- Decreased risk of IVH of all grades
- Decreased risk of necrotizing enterocolitis and late-onset sepsis
- Decreased need for blood transfusions for anemia or low blood pressure
- Improved iron stores with reduction in infant anemia as demonstrated by higher hematocrit and hemoglobin
- Higher mean blood pressure during the transition soon after birth and improved cerebral oxygenation and red blood cell volume

Immediate benefits of placental transfusion for full-term infants include the following:

- Increased hematocrit and hemoglobin
- Reduction of infant anemia from added blood volume and iron stores

Long-term benefits of placental transfusion for preterm or low birth weight infants include the following:

- Increased hemoglobin at 10 weeks of age
- Potential beneficial long-term neurodevelopmental outcomes in male infants

Long-term benefits of placental transfusion for full-term infants include the following:

- Improved hematologic indices at 2 to 4 months of age
- Improved iron status at up to 8 months of age
- Improved neurodevelopment at 4 years of age

What Are the Perceived Risks Associated With Placental Transfusion?

Perceived risks of placental transfusion include the following:

- Jeopardizing timely resuscitation in an unstable compromised neonate
- Risk of hypothermia
- Hypertransfusion and associated polycythemia
- Prolonged hyperbilirubinemia
- Maternal postpartum hemorrhage

All of these risks have been recently refuted by randomized controlled trials.

When Is Placental Transfusion Indicated?

DCC facilitates placental transfusion. DCC (performed approximately 1–3 minutes after birth) is recommended for all births while initiating simultaneous essential neonatal care (see Table 7.1). Early umbilical cord clamping (at less than 30 seconds) is not recommended unless the neonate is asphyxiated and needs to be moved immediately for resuscitation.

What Are the Contraindications to Placental Transfusion?

Unstable Infant. For any newborn requiring immediate resuscitation and/or infants prenatally diagnosed with hydrops fetalis, placental transfusion is contraindicated unless resuscitation with the intact cord can be facilitated.

Unstable mother. Placental transfusion is contraindicated if there is maternal bleeding or another condition necessitating immediate intervention (abruption, cord prolapse).

How to Set Up a Quality Improvement Project on Implementation of Placental Transfusion Protocol

Any curriculum design or educational planning is a longitudinal process aimed at developing a relevant and meaningful educational experience to achieve a desired outcome. Methods of traditional curriculum development extended to medical education incorporate adult learning concepts that center on motivation, experience, engagement, and application. The following are steps for implementing DCC in a hospital setting.

Recruit and Motivate the Potential Stakeholders

- Create a participant list including obstetricians, neonatologists, pediatricians, nurse practitioners, midwives, and nursing staff.
- Discuss a step-by-step approach for implementing DCC in a hospital setting (Fig. 7.2).
- Have a written protocol with agreement from the major stakeholders.
- Clarify operational definitions such as time of birth, assignment of Apgar scores, and immediate clamping of the cord, and define DCC.
- Take a leadership role in advocacy.
- Educate through repeated teaching and motivate stakeholders.

Address Concerns Raised Regarding DCC

- Develop an educational initiative and an online audit tool with video material to address these concerns.
- Assess and address logistical and operational issues.
- Discuss timely assessment of 1-minute Apgar scores when the infant is still attached to the umbilical cord on the mother's abdomen or perineum.
- Discuss decreasing hypothermia in the delivery room through meticulous attention to thermoregulation guidelines while simultaneously performing DCC.
- Discuss the timely provision of a preheated radiant warmer and prewarmed hats, blankets, and towels, drying and stimulating the infant during DCC, and having a warm ambient temperature (70°F–72°F) in the operating room to decrease hypothermia in infants.

Evaluate Readiness for DCC

- Perform simulation exercises to promote confidence among the healthcare team.
- Establish high-quality communication between delivery and stabilization teams.
- Disseminate information about DCC through grand rounds and integrate in weekly multidisciplinary meetings.
- Document the practice of DCC (including the duration of cord-clamping time) in delivery and resuscitation notes in electronic health records and monitor outcome data through quality improvement projects.
- Periodically monitor adherence to the protocol through quality improvement initiatives within the institution.
- Revise the protocol as needed.

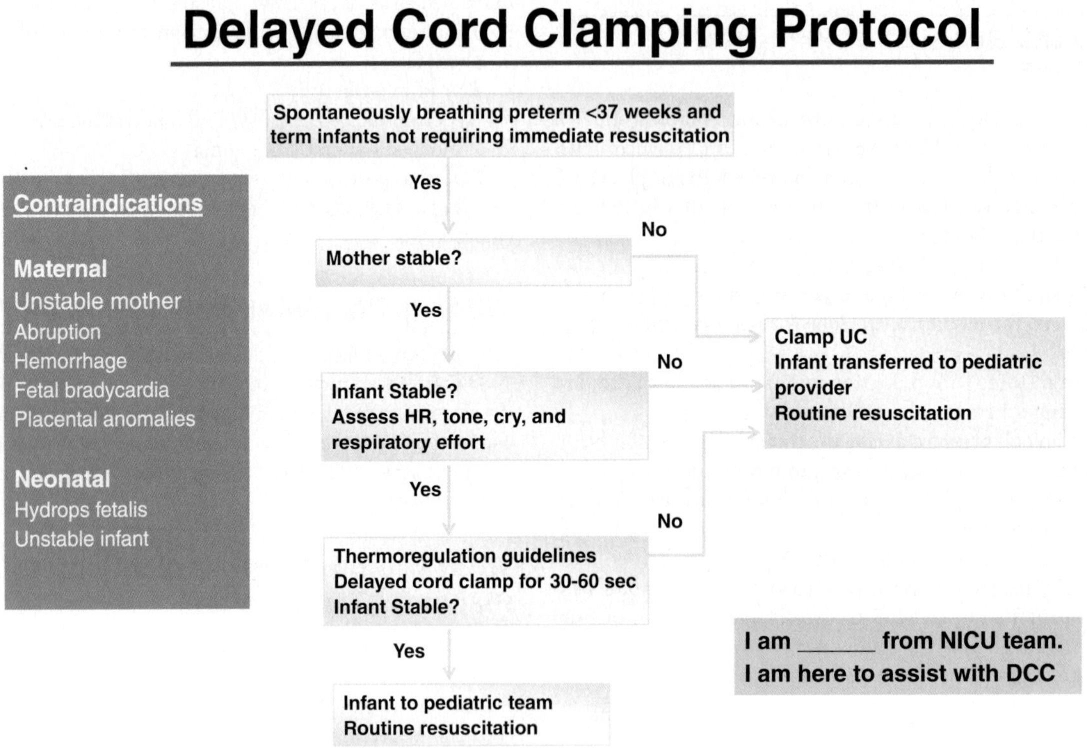

Delayed Cord Clamping Protocol

Spontaneously breathing preterm <37 weeks and term infants not requiring immediate resuscitation

Yes

Mother stable?

No

Yes

Infant Stable?
Assess HR, tone, cry, and respiratory effort

No

Yes

Thermoregulation guidelines
Delayed cord clamp for 30-60 sec
Infant Stable?

No

Yes

Infant to pediatric team
Routine resuscitation

Clamp UC
Infant transferred to pediatric provider
Routine resuscitation

Contraindications

Maternal
Unstable mother
Abruption
Hemorrhage
Fetal bradycardia
Placental anomalies

Neonatal
Hydrops fetalis
Unstable infant

I am ______ from NICU team.
I am here to assist with DCC

Fig. 7.2 Guidelines for Delayed Cord Clamping (DCC) in Spontaneously Breathing Preterm Infants (<37 Weeks) and Term Infants Who Do Not Require Immediate Resuscitation. *NICU*, Neonatal intensive care unit; *UC*, umbilical cord. (Courtesy University of Maryland School of Medicine.)

Long-Term Outcomes

Reduction of Infant Anemia

DCC is a safe and effective method to reduce infant anemia until up to 6 months of age.[37] Several studies worldwide have demonstrated higher ferritin levels and increased total body iron stores up to 6 months after DCC compared with immediate cord clamping.[31,32,45–49]

In cesarean births, a less invasive method of DCC of shorter duration compared with the active cord milking could offer the same potential benefit of improved iron stores from placental transfusion. DCC for 30 seconds after elective cesarean birth resulted in higher iron stores at up to 4 months of age compared with vaginal births with early cord clamping.[44] The hematologic parameters at 4 months of age that were achieved from a DCC of 30 seconds in cesarean births were comparable to those from a DCC of >180 seconds in vaginally born infants.

Reduction in Infant Death Before Discharge

A Cochrane review of the effect of the timing of umbilical cord clamping and other strategies to influence placental transfusion at preterm birth on maternal and infant outcomes was performed with data available from 40 studies involving 4884 babies and their mothers.[4] Preterm infants, predominantly from high-income countries and including multiple births between 24 and 36 6/7 weeks of gestation at birth, received DCC ranging from 30 to 180 seconds, with most studies delaying for 30 to 60 seconds. Early clamping ranged from immediately to less than 30 seconds after birth, and UCM mostly occurred before cord clamping, but some were clamped after cord milking. A major finding from this Cochrane review was that compared with early cord clamping, DCC may reduce the risk of infant death up to the time of hospital discharge (average risk ratio, 0.73; 95% CI, 0.54–0.98; 20 studies, 2680 babies), with little or no effect on severe IVH (grades 3 and 4) or on chronic lung disease.[4] Whereas the current evidence supports not clamping the cord before 30 seconds for preterm births, future studies comparing varying lengths of delay are warranted.

Effect on Neurodevelopmental Impairment

DCC appears to protect very low birth weight male infants against motor disability at a corrected age of 7 months.[50] Rabe et al. found in their prospective follow-up study of developmental outcomes at 2 and 3.5 years that in babies born very preterm who received cord milking at birth, cord milking did not have any long-term adverse effect on neurodevelopment compared with DCC for 30 seconds.[51] This suggests that cord milking could be offered as a safe practice and as an alternative to DCC in preterm births while offering the same benefits from placental transfusion in this vulnerable premature population when immediate care of the preterm baby is needed. Andersson et al. showed that DCC (≥180 seconds after delivery) compared with early cord clamping (≤10 seconds after delivery) was associated with improved fine motor function at 4 years, especially in boys, indicating that the amount of time before clamping the cord has an impact on neurodevelopment.[5,52]

Conclusions

Placental transfusion through DCC has become the standard in newborn care, with multiple benefits to both the preterm and term population. These benefits predominantly include improved cardiopulmonary transition, reduced incidences of IVH and necrotizing enterocolitis, decreased need for blood transfusion, decreased mortality in preterm infants,[53] and a reduction in infant anemia and improved developmental outcomes in term infants.[5,52] Placental transfusion must be considered in the management of every newborn not requiring immediate resuscitation.

CHAPTER 8 Neonatal Resuscitation

Lee Donohue, Ziad Alhassen,
Satyan Lakshminrusimha

KEY POINTS

1. Knowledge of the normal physiologic transition from fetal to neonatal life and potential disruptions of this process is vital to a comprehensive understanding of neonatal resuscitation.
2. Preparation of personnel and equipment prior to resuscitation is essential.
3. The first steps in resuscitation include stimulating the infant, maintaining a normal body temperature through management of heat gain and loss, and assessment of breathing and heart rate.
4. Infants who do not establish adequate respirations following the initial resuscitative steps are in secondary apnea. These infants will require respiratory support with positive pressure ventilation.
5. The adequacy of positive pressure ventilation should be assessed by change in heart rate and chest rise. Ventilation corrective steps should be performed if needed.
6. Chest compressions are started when the heart rate is below 60 beats per minute despite effective ventilation for 30 seconds and are performed using a 3:1 compression to ventilation ratio. Newborn infants who receive chest compressions have a high incidence of mortality and short-term neurologic morbidity.
7. Epinephrine should be given to infants who have a heart rate less than 60 beats per minute despite adequate ventilation and chest compressions for 30 seconds. Epinephrine is more effective when given via the intravenous route versus the endotracheal route.
8. Volume resuscitation is potentially lifesaving in the setting of hypovolemic shock, acute blood loss, or sepsis.
9. The choice to withhold aggressive resuscitation in the delivery room involves complex ethical considerations and should result from a collaborative decision involving both healthcare providers and parents.

Introduction

Most babies successfully transition from fetal to neonatal life without any support. Approximately 15% will require some type of resuscitation, although only 5% will require resuscitation beyond drying and stimulation.[1] These percentages may seem small, but with an estimated 3.8 million births in the United States in 2017[2] and 136 million worldwide,[3] there are 190,000 babies in the United States and 6.8 million worldwide each year who require resuscitative measures beyond the initial basic steps.

Birth attendants with neonatal resuscitation training can decrease neonatal mortality.[4,5] Two of the most common neonatal resuscitation training programs are the Neonatal Resuscitation Program (NRP) and Helping Babies Breathe, both from the American Academy of Pediatrics. However, although these programs are a good start, being truly prepared for resuscitation necessitates regular practice of skills. Neonatal death rates are higher at hospitals with a lower number of annual births.[6] A study of rural hospitals revealed that many providers had not performed neonatal resuscitation in the past year.[7] There was also a correlation between frequency of skill performance and comfort level.[7]

Additionally, it is helpful to be aware of the physiology of neonatal transition, resuscitation, and postresuscitation care. This knowledge is particularly important during complex resuscitation when the newborn is not improving after standard resuscitative actions.

The Transition From Fetal to Neonatal Life

The essential step during transition from fetal to neonatal life is ventilation to establish the lungs as the site of gas exchange. In utero, the fetus receives oxygen and nutrients from the placenta through the umbilical vein. The oxygenated blood traverses the ductus venosus, right atrium, patent foramen ovale, left atrium, left ventricle, and aorta to the carotid and coronary arteries supplying the brain and heart. Some of the less oxygenated blood returning to the heart from the superior and inferior vena cava goes to the pulmonary circulation, but most crosses the ductus arteriosus and goes to the lower body and back to the placenta (Fig. 8.1A).

At the time of birth, the infant initiates breathing and aerates its lungs because the lungs must now be the site of gas exchange, rather than the placenta. The transition from fluid-filled to air-filled airways is mediated both by active sodium absorption by the respiratory epithelium and the increase in airway pressure that occurs with the onset of breathing. Air replaces fluid, the lung becomes inflated, and the functional residual capacity (FRC), with air and an air–fluid interphase, is created. This, along with the increase in oxygenation that accompanies adequate ventilation, causes a significant decline in pulmonary vascular resistance. If umbilical cord clamping is delayed past ventilation of the lungs, two sources of oxygenated blood (the umbilical vein and pulmonary veins) contribute to left ventricular preload (see Fig. 8.1B). Subsequently the umbilical cord is clamped and blood stops flowing to the low-resistance placenta, causing an increase in systemic vascular resistance. The pressure in the left atrium then exceeds that of the right owing to both the increased systemic vascular resistance and the increase blood return to the left atrium, which leads to the functional closure of the foramen ovale (see Fig. 8.1C). The elevated left-sided pressure also causes the flow from right to left across the ductus arteriosus to switch to left to right. The increase in oxygenation causes closure of this shunt during the first days of life in term infants.

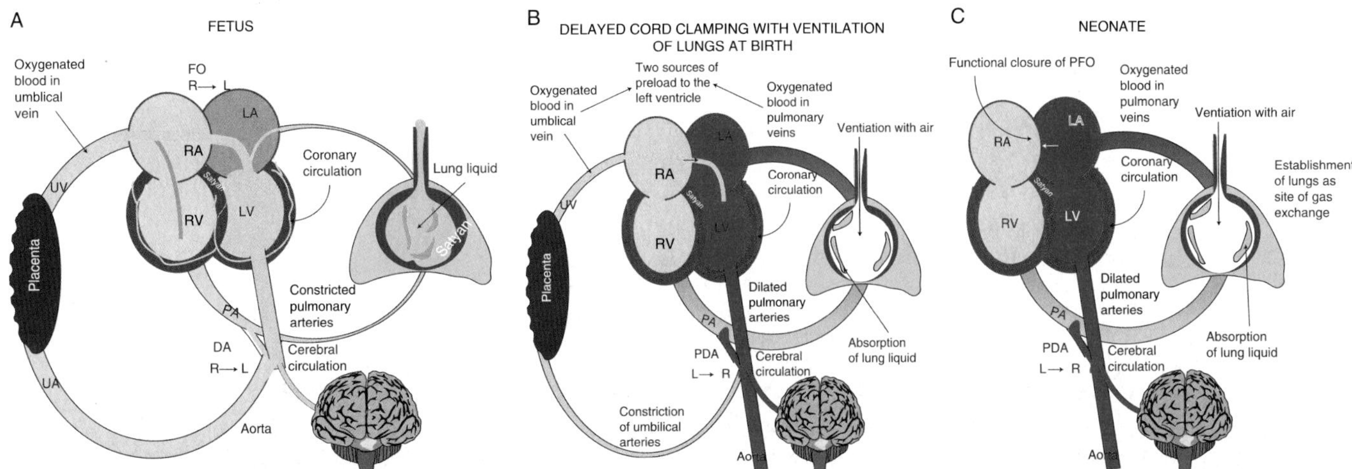

Fig. 8.1 Transition From Fetal to Neonatal Physiology. (A) Fetal circulation with liquid-filled lungs. The placenta serves as the organ of gas exchange, with deoxygenated blood coming from the umbilical arteries (UAs) and oxygenated blood leaving the placenta to the fetus through the umbilical vein (UV). Oxygenated blood enters the right atrium (RA) and crosses through the foramen ovale (FO) right to left (R→L) to perfuse the cerebral and coronary circulations. Deoxygenated blood from the systemic veins enters the RA and the right ventricle (RV) to the pulmonary artery (PA). As the pulmonary vasculature is constricted with high resistance, blood enters the aorta through the ductus arteriosus (DA) and reaches the placenta. (B) Transitional circulation during delayed (physiologic) cord clamping. Oxygenated blood from the umbilical vein and from the newly ventilated lungs (through the pulmonary veins) enters the left atrium and contributes to the left ventricular (LV) preload. (C) Neonatal circulation after removal of the placenta is characterized by reduced pulmonary vascular resistance (due to ventilation of the lungs) and increased systemic vascular resistance (due to removal of the placenta), resulting in a left to right (L→R) shunt at the patent ductus arteriosus (PDA) and eventual closure of PDA and patent foramen ovale (PFO). Ventilation of the lungs is the key step in this transition. The lungs are established as the site of gas exchange. (Copyright Satyan Lakshminrusimha.)

Pathophysiology of Perinatal Asphyxia

This process of neonatal transition can be disrupted by alteration of placental blood flow to the fetus or due to neonatal factors impairing the establishment of pulmonary gas exchange, such as impaired ventilation, airway anomalies, birth asphyxia, or parenchymal lung disease (respiratory distress syndrome [RDS] or meconium aspiration syndrome). The term *asphyxia* describes this lack of sufficient gas exchange resulting in hypoxemia, hypercapnia, and acidosis. The fetus first attempts to redistribute blood flow to vital organs including the brain and heart. However, prolonged asphyxia leads to severe injury to these organs, causing hypoxic-ischemic encephalopathy (HIE).

Asphyxia causes distinctive patterns of breathing and hemodynamic changes. Geoffrey Dawes first described these patterns in 1968 based on his animal model of asphyxia.[8] A similar phenomenon has been described in infants.[9] After a period of acidosis, there is an initial attempt to recover with respiratory efforts to improve gas exchange followed by a period of primary apnea. During primary apnea, bradycardia is observed with preservation of blood pressure by several compensatory mechanisms. Stimulation during this time could result in recovery of normal respirations. As asphyxia progresses without stimulation and recovery, gasping respirations develop, followed by a period of secondary apnea. During secondary apnea, blood pressure drops, resulting in myocardial dysfunction.[10] During this period, positive pressure ventilation (PPV) is required for resuscitation, and stimulation alone is not adequate (Fig. 8.2).

In addition, asphyxia can modify the circulatory changes that occur at the time of birth. Hypoxia and acidosis inhibit the normal decrease in pulmonary vascular constriction and closure of the ductus arteriosus, so right-to-left blood flow continues. There may also be persistence of the right-to-left flow through the foramen ovale due to pulmonary hypertension that causes increased right atrial pressure.[11]

Prompt resuscitation may be able to reverse these alterations, especially if the period of asphyxia was recent and brief. The subsequent portions of this chapter will discuss how to prepare and carry out newborn resuscitation.

Preparation

The most important part of a successful resuscitation is what happens prior to delivery. Five questions (Table 8.1) with the pneumonic GRASP should be communicated between obstetric and pediatric providers. The team should be informed about gestational age, possible risk factors (such as diabetes, hypertension, and history of prior pregnancy or delivery problems), color of the amniotic fluid, number of fetuses, and plans for placental transfusion. The neonatal providers must have the appropriate resuscitation skills, and all resuscitation equipment should be functional and located nearby. Although risk factors are present in many babies requiring extensive resuscitation, the need for resuscitation can also be a surprise. It is thus important to be prepared at every delivery.

Personnel

It is essential that the teams responsible for neonatal resuscitation are able to expertly perform their respective tasks and communicate effectively. In a review of 47 cases of perinatal death or permanent disability reported to the Joint Commission under the Sentinel Event Policy, communication, staff competency, and training were identified as the top root causes.[12] The traditional method of neonatal resuscitation certification is the NRP from the American Academy of Pediatrics, which requires providers to complete training every

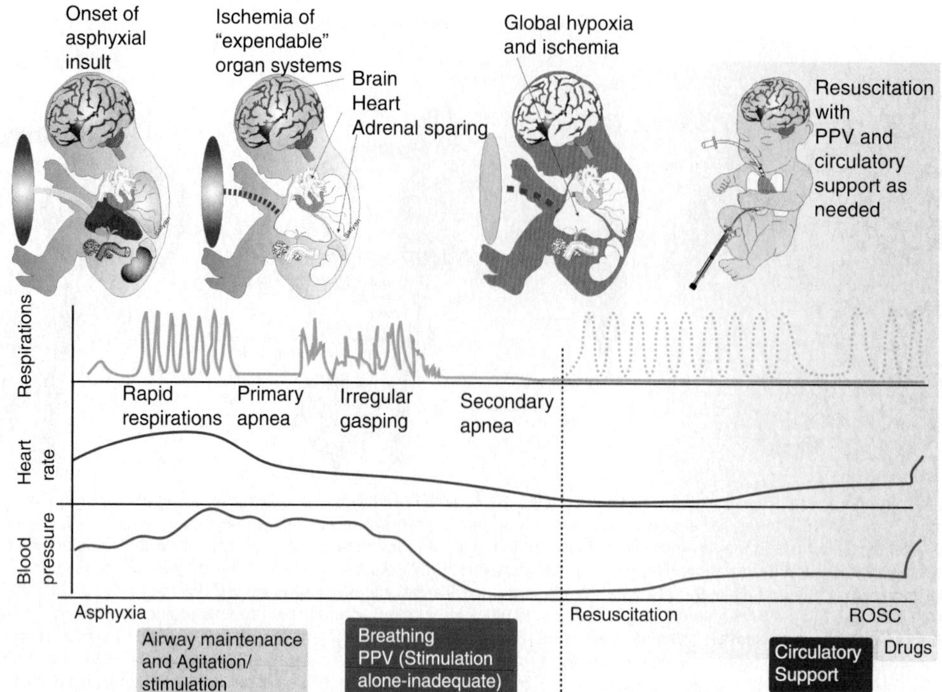

Fig. 8.2 Pathophysiology of Asphyxia and Resuscitation. Respiratory *(green line)*, heart rate *(purple line)*, and systemic blood pressure *(red line)*. Soon after an asphyxial insult, rapid respirations are observed as a compensatory phenomenon. Subsequently, primary apnea associated with bradycardia is noted. At this phase, blood flow to nonexpendable organs such as the brain, heart, and adrenals is maintained, and blood pressure remains within normal limits. Maintaining the airway and agitation (stimulation) is required at this stage. However, if stimulation is not provided or if asphyxial insult is severe and ongoing, irregular gasping followed by secondary apnea and hypotension occur. Breathing with positive pressure ventilation (PPV) is required in the presence of secondary apnea because global ischemia can deprive blood flow to the brain and heart. The hyphenated *blue line* overlapping respirations depicts PPV. Circulatory support in the form of chest compressions is necessary in the presence of persistent bradycardia despite effective PPV. Drugs—epinephrine (or volume)—are indicated when PPV and chest compressions are ineffective. Effective resuscitation results in return of spontaneous circulation (ROSC). (Copyright Satyan Lakshminrusimha.)

Table 8.1 Questions to Ask Before Delivery (GRASP)
Gestational age—What is the expected gestational age?
Risk factors—Are there any additional risk factors?
Amniotic fluid—Is the amniotic fluid clear?
Single/multiple—How many babies are expected?
Placental transfusion—Are there any plans for delayed cord clamping or cord milking?

2 years. However, this program does not ensure competence. The most recent International Liaison Committee on Resuscitation consensus statement that addresses timing for advanced resuscitation retraining presents evidence that there is a decay in skills and knowledge within months after initial training.[13] This statement also states that more frequent training is needed, although the optimal frequency and method of training remain undetermined.[13] Personnel should also be capable of working together as a team. The use of interdisciplinary simulation including mock code drills on a continual basis helps to maintain skills and develop coordination among staff.[14]

One individual whose sole responsibility is the infant and who is capable of initiating resuscitation should attend every delivery. They or another person in the immediate vicinity should be capable of the complete process of neonatal resuscitation. If there are risk factors, at least two people should be at the delivery and prepared to resuscitate the infant. A team briefing should occur prior to the delivery during which the leader is identified, roles of each member are assigned, equipment is checked, and anticipated resuscitation needs are discussed.[15]

Equipment

Resuscitation equipment should be checked on a regular basis and just prior to each delivery for both availability and function. A standardized equipment checklist can be helpful, and an example of this is provided in the NRP textbook.[15]

Initial Assessment and Management

An initial assessment of the infant should be made upon delivery. The infant can stay with the mother for the resuscitation if he or she appears to be of term gestation, has good tone, and is breathing or crying (Fig. 8.3).

Drying and Stimulation

After the infant is born, the infant should be dried (or if premature, the infant's body should be placed in a plastic bag or wrap) to prevent evaporative heat loss. Drying also provides stimulation and is often sufficient for an infant that is in primary apnea to begin breathing. Additional stimulation by flicking the soles of the feet and rubbing the back can also be provided. Warmth should be provided by placing vigorous babies skin to skin with their mother or moving them to a radiant warmer.

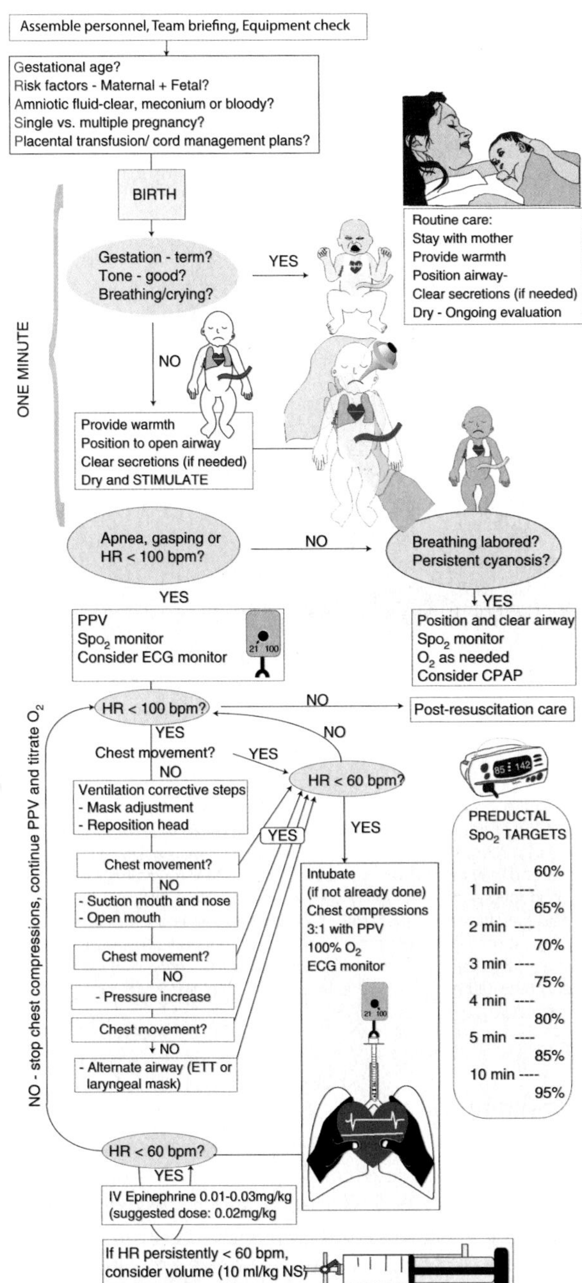

Fig. 8.3 Pictorial Flow Diagram of Neonatal Resuscitation. Resuscitation begins prior to delivery with team assembly, equipment check, and briefing. Initial questions follow the GRASP mnemonic (see Table 8.1). After delivery, an initial assessment of gestational age, muscle tone, and breathing occurs. If the infant is term with good tone and normal respirations, the infant should stay with the mother and routine resuscitation should be provided. If these three criteria are not met, routine resuscitation is provided in addition to further assessment. Additional respiratory support can be provided to infants who are having breathing difficulty or cyanosis via oxygen or pressure, but an infant who remains apneic or bradycardic requires support with positive pressure ventilation. Monitoring of oxygen saturation and heart rate with pulse oximetry (Spo_2) and electrocardiogram (ECG) should also be considered at this point. The target preductal (right upper extremity) Spo_2 values at each time point should be the range between the numbers above and below the time point in the inset. Positive pressure ventilation (PPV) should continue for an infant who remains bradycardic or apneic. The effectiveness of ventilation should be assessed, and ventilation corrective steps (mnemonic—MR SOPA, Fig. 8.6) should be performed if needed. Finally, if the heart rate (HR) decreases to less than 60 beats per minute (bpm) and does not improve with adequate ventilation, then intubation, chest compressions, and 100% oxygen should be provided. At this time, further therapy with medications and assessment for additional confounding issues such as a pneumothorax or hypovolemia (correcting with normal saline [NS]) should be considered. *CPAP,* Continuous positive airway pressure; *ETT,* endotracheal tube; *IV,* intravenous. (Modified from Perlman et al.[1] Copyright Satyan Lakshminrusimha.)

Thermal Management (Fig. 8.4)

Term infants should be placed skin to skin after delivery, if they meet the criteria above or in a radiant warmer to avoid excessive heat loss. They should be dried and the wet blankets should be removed to prevent evaporative heat loss.[15] The temperature of nonasphyxiated infants should be measured and be kept between 36.5°C and 37.5°C because both hypothermia and hyperthermia are associated with increased morbidity and mortality.[1]

Additional measures should be taken if a preterm infant is expected. There was a 28% increase in mortality and 11% increase in late-onset sepsis for each 1°C decrease in temperature at neonatal intensive care unit admission in a 2007 analysis.[16] Prior to the birth of a preterm infant, the temperature in the delivery and resuscitation room should be adjusted so it is 74°F to 77°F (24°C–25°C).[15] There is also evidence that the use of plastic covers or bags and a combination of measures including the addition of plastic caps and thermal mattresses from resuscitation through admission prevents hypothermia in preterm infants[17] and is the recommendation of the NRP.[15]

Respiratory Effort and Heart Rate

The infant's head and neck should be positioned such that the neck is slightly extended in the "sniffing" position.[15] If the infant is with the mother, a trained observer should be able to see the infant's nose and mouth, and the head should be turned to one side (see Fig. 8.3).[18] The NRP continues to recommend suctioning the mouth before the nose (*M* comes before *N*) to ensure that oral secretions are not aspirated if the newborn gasps when the nose is suctioned if the infant appears to be having difficulty breathing due to secretions or is apneic, although there is a lack of supportive evidence.[19]

If the infant remains apneic at 30 seconds of life, PPV should be initiated and heart rate should be monitored by either auscultation or placement of electrocardiogram (ECG) leads[15]; palpation of the umbilical cord may not be reliable,[20] although assessment by auscultation may also be inaccurate.[21,22] At the time PPV is initiated, the recommendation by the NRP is to place a pulse oximeter and consider placing ECG leads for monitoring of the infant's heart rate and oxygen saturation.[15] However, ECG detects the heart rate faster than pulse oximetry,[23,24] and pulse oximetry may underestimate the heart rate.[25,26] A pulse oximeter can also be used to measure oxygen saturation of an infant who is breathing with a normal heart rate but remains cyanotic, because it has been shown that it is difficult for providers to make an assessment of color.[27] Advantages and disadvantages of various modes of heart rate assessment in the delivery room are shown in Fig. 8.5.[28]

Ventilation

When the initial steps of resuscitation fail to produce spontaneous respiration, the infant is likely in secondary apnea and will need respiratory support (see Fig. 8.2). The provision of ventilation in the delivery room is crucial to a successful resuscitation of a depressed infant. It is through ventilation and establishment of FRC that both the respiratory and cardiovascular changes occur in the transition from fetal to neonatal life.

Positive Pressure Ventilation (PPV)

PPV should be initiated by 60 seconds of life if the baby is apneic, gasping, or has ineffective respirations or if the heart rate is less than 100 beats per minute.[15] Initially, PPV is given by a face mask

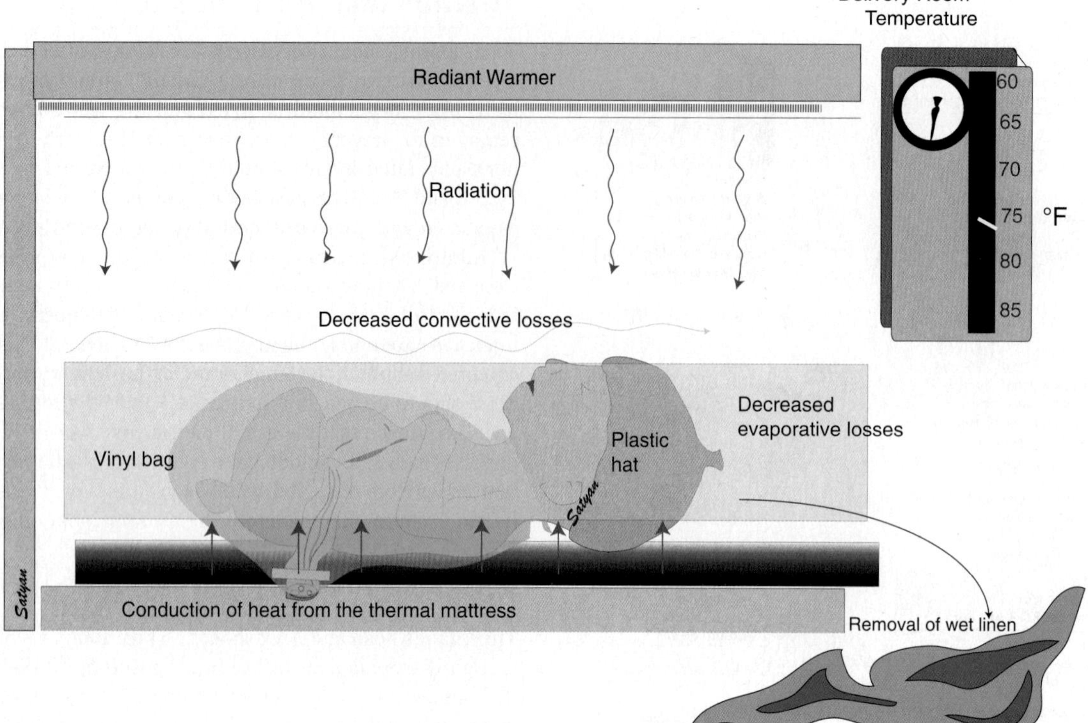

Fig. 8.4 Mechanisms of Heat Loss During Resuscitation. The newborn infant has the potential to gain or lose heat by four mechanisms: radiation, conduction, convection, and evaporation. Heat is lost to surrounding surfaces that are not in direct contact with the infant via radiation and is proportional to the temperature difference between the infant's body and the environmental sources. A radiant warmer provides a source of radiant heat to counteract heat losses. Increasing the temperature of the delivery room can also decrease the amount of heat loss by radiation. Conduction is the second way infants can gain or lose heat. Conduction heat energy is transferred between surfaces that are in direct contact with each other. An infant can lose heat via conduction if placed on a cooler surface and can gain heat if in contact with a warmer surface such as a heated mattress. Heat can also be transferred via convection by air passing over the infant. The delivery room is cooler than the infant, so the infant loses heat by this mechanism. This source of heat loss can be minimized by increasing the room temperature and ensuring the sides of the radiant warmer are up and surrounding the infant. Finally, the infant can lose heat by evaporation. This can be reduced by drying in a term infant or the use of a polyurethane hat placed on the head and polyurethane bag or wrap covering the infant's body in preterm infants. (Modified from Mathew et al.[127] Copyright Satyan Lakshminrusimha.)

and a pressure-generating device (discussed in more detail below). There should also be an oxygen blender to titrate the fraction of inspired oxygen, which should be set at 0.21 for term infants and 0.21 to 0.3 for preterm infants. The recommendation is to set the equipment used to provide PPV at a peak inspiratory pressure (PIP) of 20 to 25 cm H_2O and a positive end-expiratory pressure (PEEP) of 5 cm H_2O, if the device allows PEEP, and to give breaths at a rate of 40 to 60 per minute, which approximates the normal respiratory rate of a normal term newborn.[15]

The use of PEEP during PPV in resuscitation is common in most centers in the United States.[29] Animal studies suggest that PEEP is beneficial, including in the establishment of FRC.[30] Without PEEP, there is the potential of losing FRC and alveolar collapse with each breath. However, studies in infants have not shown a change in the number of infants requiring intubation when PEEP is added.[31] Nevertheless, it is generally thought that PEEP should be used if available, and the NRP recommends a resuscitation device that is capable of administering PEEP for the resuscitation of preterm infants.[15]

Pressures Delivery Devices

There are several different types of devices used to generate positive pressure in the delivery room. The choice of device is largely made based on availability of equipment. Providers should familiarize themselves with the equipment in each of their workplaces.

Self-Inflating Bag

Self-inflating bags are intermittently compressed to provide ventilation. They inflate spontaneously after compression. This type of device cannot provide a consistent amount of oxygen, does not provide PEEP unless equipped with a special valve, and cannot be used to provide continuous positive airway pressure (CPAP). It is difficult to accurately provide consistent PIP[32,33] and PEEP even with the addition of the valve.[33] The advantage of the self-inflating bag is that is can be used without a source of compressed air. This makes it useful in resource-limited areas.

Flow-Inflating Bag

A source of compressed air is required for flow-inflating bags. These bags also are compressed to provide ventilation, and a lower degree of compression is maintained between ventilations to provide PEEP. The bag then inflates through the flow from the gas source. The pressures delivered are highly dependent on the operator. Many experienced providers like this type of bag because they believe it is possible to feel the compliance of the lungs and adjust the pressures accordingly. However, anesthesiologists ranging from inexperienced residents to experienced pediatric trained attending physicians were unable to identify intermittent occlusion of the endotracheal tube (ETT) when providing ventilation using a flow-inflating bag and test lungs corresponding to that of a term neonate.[34] Flow-inflating bags can be used to provide CPAP.

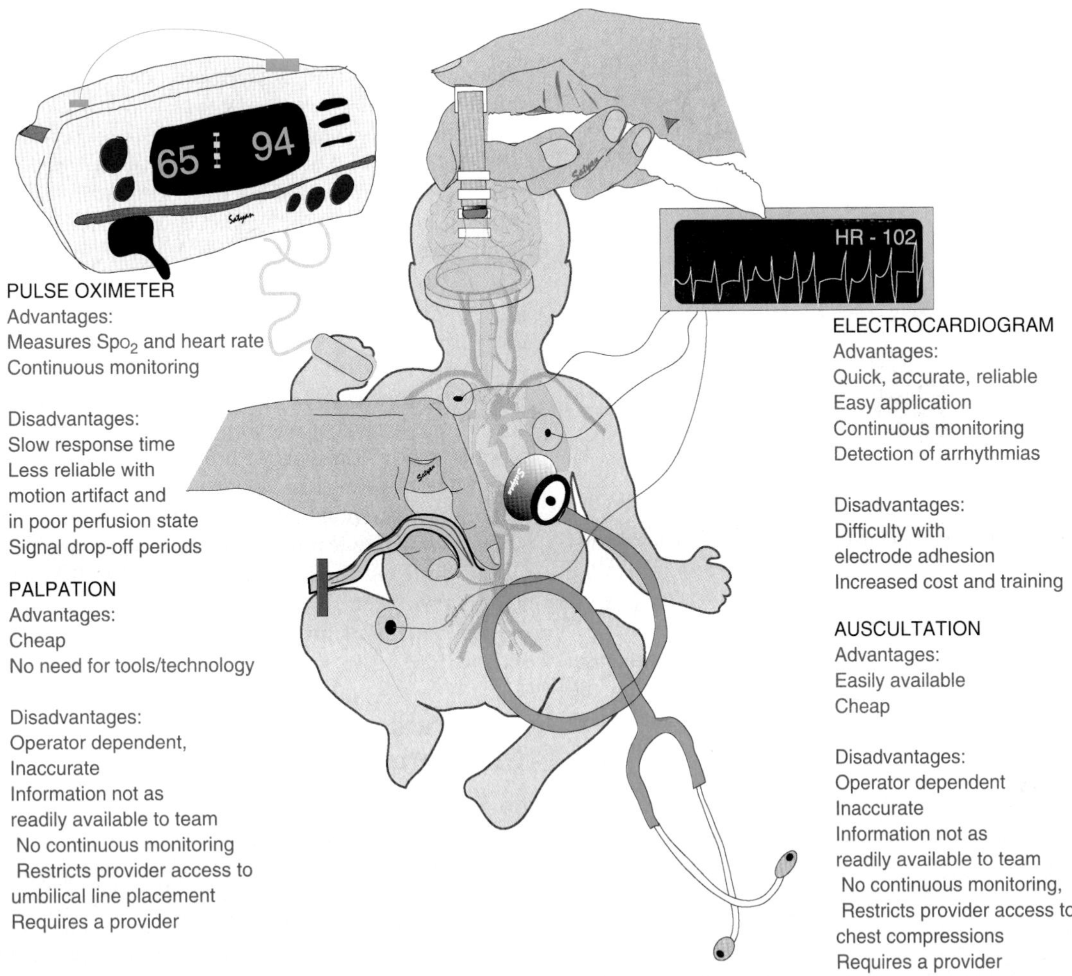
65 94
HR - 102
PULSE OXIMETER
Advantages:
Measures Spo_2 and heart rate
Continuous monitoring
Disadvantages:
Slow response time
Less reliable with motion artifact and in poor perfusion state
Signal drop-off periods
PALPATION
Advantages:
Cheap
No need for tools/technology
Disadvantages:
Operator dependent,
Inaccurate
Information not as readily available to team
No continuous monitoring
Restricts provider access to umbilical line placement
Requires a provider
ELECTROCARDIOGRAM
Advantages:
Quick, accurate, reliable
Easy application
Continuous monitoring
Detection of arrhythmias
Disadvantages:
Difficulty with electrode adhesion
Increased cost and training
AUSCULTATION
Advantages:
Easily available
Cheap
Disadvantages:
Operator dependent
Inaccurate
Information not as readily available to team
No continuous monitoring,
Restricts provider access to chest compressions
Requires a provider

Fig. 8.5 Methods of Heart Rate Assessment in the Delivery Room. There are four methods of heart rate assessment in the delivery room, each with advantages and disadvantages. The method to be used should be chosen based on availability of equipment and training of providers. Electrocardiography is the most accurate method and is most widely recommended for use in the delivery room, but this resource is not always available. Pulse oximetry is more reliable than other methods, but it can take some time to display an accurate heart rate and requires adequate perfusion. Pulse oximeter monitors also may not be available in every delivery room. Umbilical cord palpation and auscultation with a stethoscope are both not as accurate as pulse oximetry or electrocardiography and do not provide continuous monitoring but only require equipment that is readily available in most delivery rooms. (Modified from Vali et al.[28] Copyright Satyan Lakshminrusimha.)

T-Piece Resuscitation Device

T-piece resuscitation devices also require a gas source. The PIP and PEEP are set using dials, and a hole on the top or side of the device is covered intermittently to provide ventilations. PEEP is delivered when the hole is uncovered. CPAP can be given simply by leaving the hole uncovered. These devices have been shown in many studies to be the most consistent in the delivery of both PIP and PEEP.[32,33] Studies of the use of these resuscitation devices in newborn infants requiring PPV have shown a decrease in the need for intubation,[35,36] a shorter duration of PPV, and less supplemental oxygen during resuscitation.[35]

Assessment of Efficacy

The best measurement of adequate ventilation is improvement in the heart rate. The NRP recommends assessing the heart rate after 15 seconds of PPV and continuing to use heart rate and chest rise to make repeated assessments.[15] There are several studies indicating that clinician assessment of chest rise as a surrogate for appropriate tidal volume may not be accurate[37] and may result in hypocarbia.[38] Respiratory function monitors can be used to measure and display tidal volume delivery and can aid in the detection of a leak around the mask[39–41] or an airway obstruction,[40] but they are not widely available. A colorimetric CO_2 detector can also be used to aid in detection of adequate ventilation,[42] and the NRP recommends its use for this purpose.[15]

Corrective Steps (Figs. 8.3 and 8.6)

Providing adequate ventilation with a mask and resuscitation device requires skill. If the infant is not improving with PPV, it is important to assess all components. The mask must be appropriately sized, and a good seal between the mask and the infant's face must be maintained. One study showed that the typical leak around the mask placed on a manikin was approximately 55% but could be improved with instruction.[43] The two-person ventilation technique, in which one person positions the mask on the face and performs maneuvers to help open the airway if necessary while the other person delivers the breaths, decreases mask leak.[44] The infant must be positioned with the neck slight extended so the airway is open. It is very easy, especially in preterm infants, to overextend or flex the neck and cause airway obstruction. Performing the jaw-thrust maneuver can

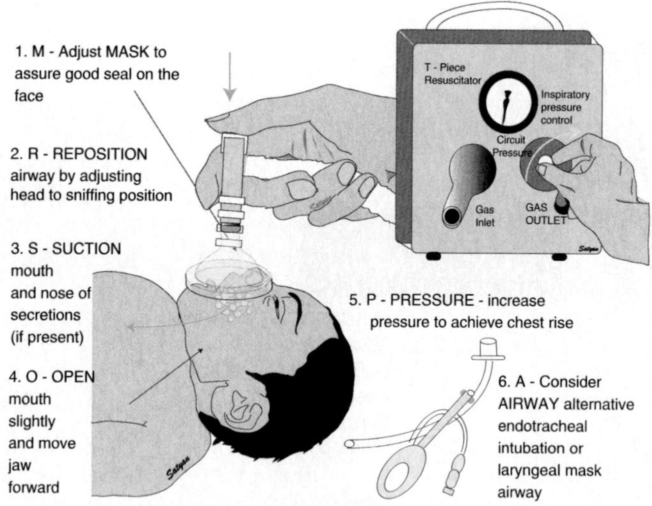
1. M - Adjust MASK to assure good seal on the face
2. R - REPOSITION airway by adjusting head to sniffing position
3. S - SUCTION mouth and nose of secretions (if present)
4. O - OPEN mouth slightly and move jaw forward
5. P - PRESSURE - increase pressure to achieve chest rise
6. A - Consider AIRWAY alternative endotracheal intubation or laryngeal mask airway
T - Piece Resuscitator
Inspiratory pressure control
Circuit Pressure
Gas Inlet
GAS OUTLET

Fig. 8.6 Corrective Steps to Improve Efficacy of Ventilation. These steps use the mnemonic MR SOPA. Please see text for details. (Copyright Satyan Lakshminrusimha.)

also aid in maintaining an open airway. The mouth, then the nose, can be suctioned to ensure secretions are not contributing the obstruction. It is also important to make sure that the mouth stays in the open position so that air can easily flow into the oropharynx. Once there is a good mask seal and the airway is open, if PPV is still not effective, the pressure administered can be augmented by increasing the squeeze of the self-inflating or flow-inflating bag or adjusting the dial on the t-piece device.

Alternative Airways

If appropriate PPV is being delivered after the corrective steps mentioned above and the infant fails to improve or continues to have ineffective respirations, an alternative airway should be placed to provide more efficient and consistent pressure delivery. A secure airway also should be immediately placed before initiation of chest compressions (CCs) if the heart rate is less than 60 beats per minute and is not improving.[15] The 2 common types of alternative airways are ETTs and laryngeal mask airways (LMAs).

Endotracheal Tubes (ETTs)

The intubation procedure requires skill to perform proficiently. Neonatal ETTs are usually uncuffed and straight and range in size from 2.0 to 4.0 mm in internal diameter. The laryngoscope blade used is a straight or Miller blade in sizes 000 to 0 for preterm infants and 0 or 1 for term infants. There are potential complications including bradycardia due to vagal stimulation and trauma to the oral and pharyngeal structures and the trachea. Mask ventilation must be paused for the attempt, and the infant's heart rate and saturations can decline during attempts.[45] This can be minimized by limiting the duration of the attempt to 30 seconds,[46] and this is now recommended.[15] Videolaryngoscopy can be useful in assisting with ventilation, particularly for experienced providers.[47–50]

Correct placement of the ETT can be verified by an increase in heart rate, equal breath sounds by auscultation, mist in the ETT, and detection of CO_2 by an end-tidal CO_2 detector. Several studies have shown that the use of a CO_2 detector reduces the time to verification of ETT location.[51,52] There is no difference in outcomes with quantitative (such as mainstream or side-steam end tidal CO_2) devices or qualitative (colorimetric) devices.[53] Although the tidal volume threshold for detection of CO_2 is sufficiently low to detect CO_2 during PPV using appropriate tidal volume in extremely low birth weight infants,[54] the detector may not show color change if insufficient tidal volume is being provided or cardiac output is low[55] (Fig. 8.7). Tracheal or bronchial obstruction[56] and severe cardiorespiratory compromise (often with extreme prematurity) can result in false negative results with CO_2 detectors in spite of tracheal intubation.[51,57]

Laryngeal Mask Airway

ETT placement is not possible in some cases due to provider inexperience or airway anomalies such as Pierre Robin sequence. An alternative is the LMA, a soft mask with an inflatable rim that covers the laryngeal opening connected to an airway tube. The LMA is inserted through the oropharynx and onto the airway. The inflatable rim can then be expanded with a small amount of air through an external balloon. One LMA is available in size 0.5 for infants weighing less than 4 kg, but most available LMAs are size 1 and designed for infants weighing 2 to 5 kg, although these LMAs have been studied in infants weighing >1.5 kg.[58,59] The current recommendation for use is in late preterm and term infants.[1,58,59]

Continuous Positive Airway Pressure (CPAP)

The distending airway pressure provided by CPAP may be useful in the establishment of FRC during resuscitation in infants who are breathing spontaneously, because the pressure may prevent collapse during expiration. Its use is recommended in infants who have increased work of breathing or low oxygen saturations and particularly in preterm infants who may be surfactant deficient.[15]

Sustained Inflation

Sustained inflation (SI), which is when PIP is provided for a period longer than what is customary in normal intermittent PPV, has been theorized to potentially be a method for initial lung recruitment and establishment of FRC while minimizing lung injury in the delivery room for apneic infants. There is both animal[60,61] and some human infant[62–65] data to support the use of SI in resuscitation. One meta-analysis showed improvement in the need for mechanical ventilation,[66] whereas another showed no difference in short or long-term outcomes. A recent randomized controlled trial of SI in the resuscitation of preterm infants (SAIL study) was stopped early due to increased mortality in the first 48 hours of life in the intervention group and is outlined in Fig. 8.8.[67] Consensus statements recommend against the use of SI outside of clinical trials until further evidence arises.[1]

Support of Circulation

Chest Compressions

It is estimated that 0.1% of term infants and up to 5% of preterm infants will receive CCs in the delivery room. Newborn infants who receive CCs have 41% mortality and a high incidence of short-term neurologic morbidity.[1,68–70]

There are currently two widely accepted theories that explain the mechanism of blood flow during CCs: the cardiac pump theory

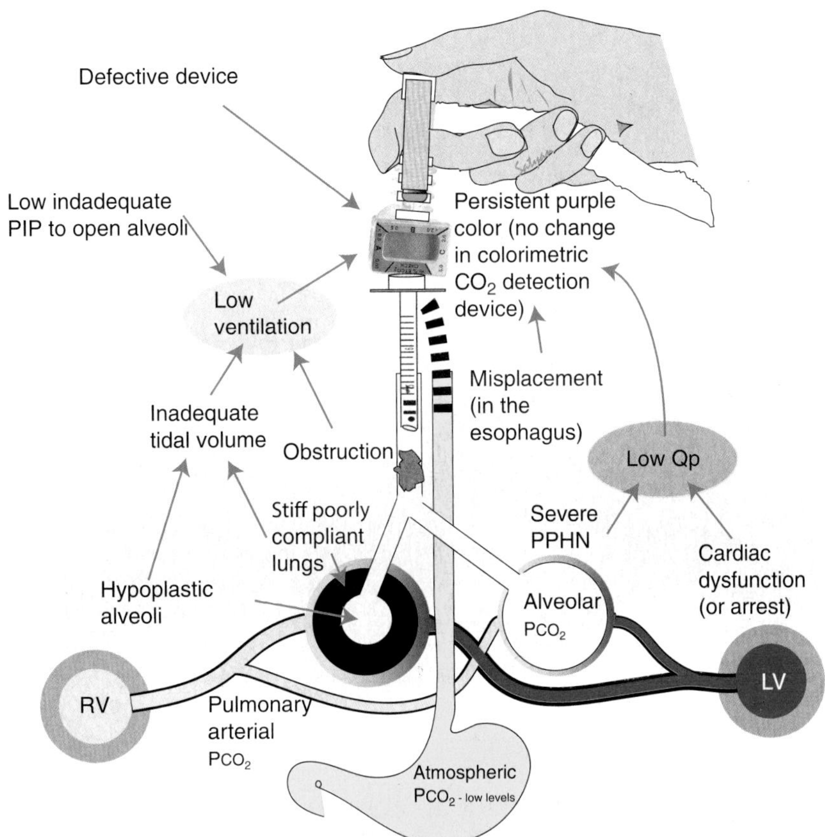

Fig. 8.7 Causes for Persistent Purple Coloration of a Colorimetric CO_2 Detector in Neonates. The most common reason is esophageal intubation. The other causes can be classified into inadequate ventilation and poor perfusion. Extreme prematurity can be associated with both hypoventilation and low pulmonary flow. *LV*, Left ventricle; *PIP*, peak inspiratory pressure; *PPHN*, persistent pulmonary hypertension of the newborn; *Qp*, quantum potential; *RV*, right ventricle. (Copyright Satyan Lakshminrusimha.)

and the thoracic pump theory. The cardiac pump theory, described by Kouwenhoven et al.[71] in the 1960s, suggests that blood flow during CCs is produced by the compression of both ventricles. During a compression, intraventricular pressure rises, the atrioventricular valves close, and the aortic and pulmonary valves open, allowing for anterograde blood flow. During release, the intraventricular pressures rapidly fall, which causes the atrioventricular valves to open and allow blood flow into the ventricular cavities.[72] Alternatively, the thoracic pump theory was first described in the 1980s by Rudikoff et al.[73] and was supported by other studies during that era.[74,75] During a CC, the increase in intrathoracic pressure allows blood to flow from the thoracic vessels through the heart and into the systemic circulation, and the heart acts as a conduit and not a pump for flow. Retrograde flow is prevented by venous valvular closure and collapse of the thoracic veins. Anterograde flow requires the mitral valve to remain open during the whole cardiac cycle. During release, the thoracic circulation fills, to be moved into the heart again during a second compression. There are also a number of newer theories that have been developed: the lung pump theory,[76] the left atrial pump theory,[77] and the respiratory pump theory.[78] In reality, the intricate dynamics of blood flow during cardiopulmonary resuscitation (CPR) is not fully explained by a single theory and is most likely supported by a combination these theories. Newly born infants in the delivery room have high pulmonary vascular resistance and a large ductus arteriosus, preventing the buildup of high diastolic blood pressure during CCs to increase coronary perfusion.[79] The exact mechanism of blood flow during CCs in newly born infants is not known.

The current NRP guidelines specify to start CCs if the heart rate remains under 60 beats per minute despite effective ventilation for 30 seconds. High-quality CCs require at least two trained personnel and a combination of an optimal compression-to-ventilation (C:V) ratio, rate, depth, technique, and chest recoil between CCs.[80] Adequate CCs lead to increased cardiac output and improved outcomes. CCs are best achieved using the two-thumbs technique, where both thumbs are placed on the lower third of the sternum along the nipple line of the infant with the remaining fingers placed around the back and chest.[1,81] The chest should be compressed to a depth of approximately one-third of the anterior–posterior diameter of the chest.[1,81] Incomplete chest wall recoil from overcompressing the chest may lead to decreased cardiac output, rib fractures, cardiac contusions, and other thoracic and liver injuries.[80]

It is recommended to perform CCs using a C:V ratio of 3:1, which consists of 90 CCs and 30 inflations per minute with a pause after every third CC to deliver a breath. Inflations and CCs should be synchronized to avoid inadequate ventilation during CCs. This approach may not optimize cardiac output during CPR, because every interruption in CCs results in a drop in coronary perfusion pressure that needs to be regenerated with the next compression cycle. During CPR, in pediatric and adult patients, the CC rate in patients with an advanced airway is 100 CCs per minute, which is higher than the 60- to 100-beats per minute baseline heart rate at rest. Using the 3:1 C:V ratio results in 90 beats per minute, which is significantly lower than the physiologic newborn heart rate of 120 to 160 beats per minute. However, bradycardia or asystole in the neonate is usually caused by asphyxia and hypoxia

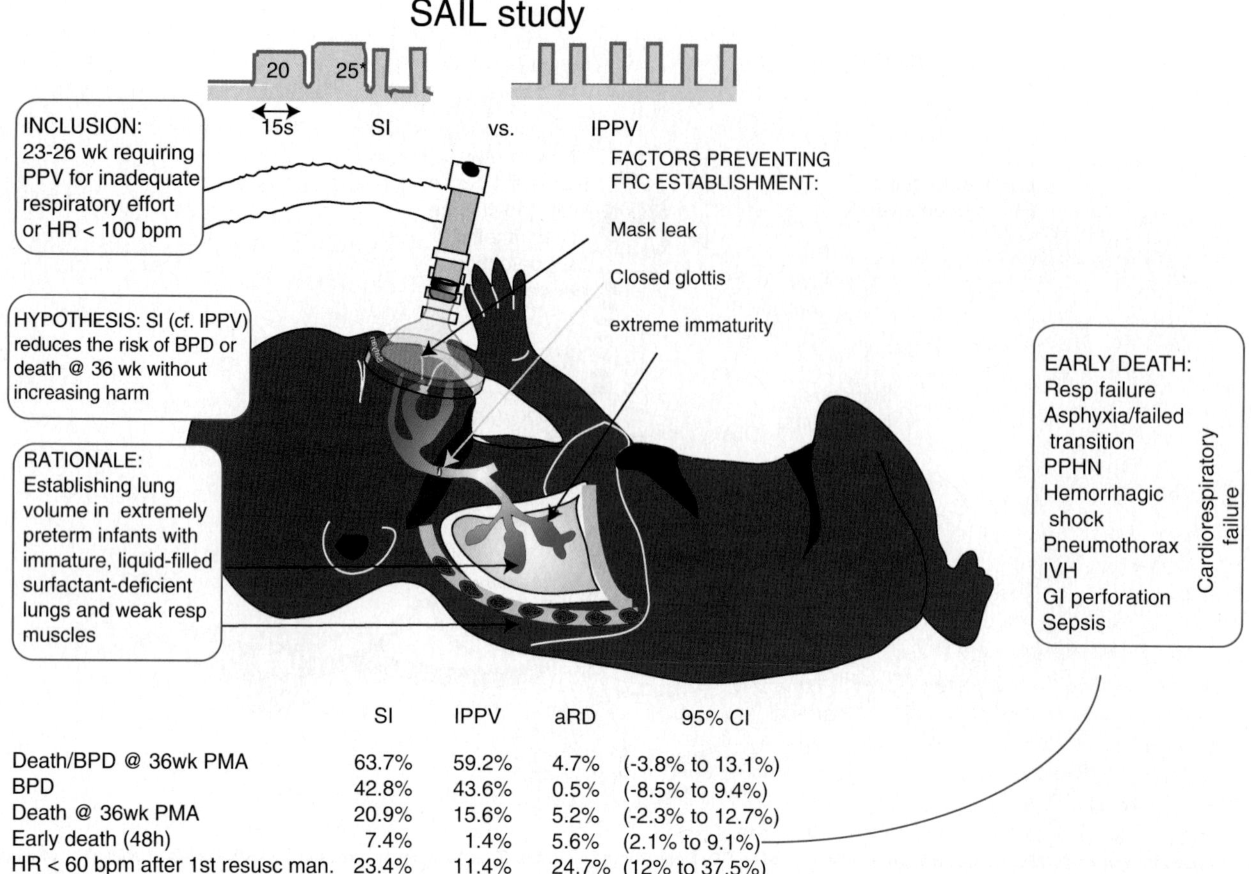

Fig. 8.8 A Graphic Abstract Outlining the SAIL Study by Kirpalani et al.[67] Evaluating Sustained Inflation (SI) Versus Positive Pressure Ventilation (PPV) During Initial Resuscitation. Inclusion criteria, hypothesis, rationale, and results are shown. Early death (during the first 48 hours after birth) was observed to be higher in preterm neonates randomized to SI. Causes of early death are listed in the inset. *BPD,* Bronchopulmonary dysplasia; *GI,* gastrointestinal; *HR,* heart rate; *IPPV,* intermittent positive pressure ventilation; *IVH,* intraventricular hemorrhage; *PPHN,* persistent pulmonary hypertension of the newborn; *PMA,* post menstrual age. (Copyright Satyan Lakshminrusimha.)

rather than a primary cardiac etiology. Therefore, providing ventilation during neonatal CCs is more likely to be beneficial than in pediatric and adult patients.[80,82,83] In addition, continuous compressions result in higher diastolic pressure and coronary perfusion in children and adults, but a similar phenomenon may not occur in newly born infants because of ductal steal.[79] The current recommendation of a 3:1 C:V ratio is based on expert consensus without strong evidence.[1,81]

Schmölzer et al.[84] used an alternative approach of performing CCs with continuous SI. Their technique allowed for maintaining a constant high airway pressure while CCs were delivered continuously at a rate of 120 per minute. Passive ventilation occurred during the compression with the increase in thoracic pressure. Results showed the group receiving CCs with SI had improved hemodynamic variables, minute ventilation, decreased mortality, decreased epinephrine administration, and time to return of spontaneous circulation (ROSC) compared with the group receiving 3:1 C:V CPR. A randomized trial was performed that compared CCs with SI at CC rates of 90 per minute versus 120 per minute. Both groups had similar times of ROSC, survival rates, and hemodynamic and respiratory parameters. However, carotid blood flow, mean arterial pressure, and cardiac output were higher in the group receiving 90 CCs per minute with SI versus the group receiving 120 CCs per minute with SI.[85] However, with a recent association found between increased early mortality with SI in extremely preterm infants,[67] positive results from further studies would be necessary before SI during resuscitation can be recommended.

The initial oxygen concentration is set to 21% for term infants and 21% to 30% for preterm infants.[86] However, during CCs, current NRP guidelines recommend increasing the oxygen concentration to 100%.[1,81] High oxygen concentrations may be necessary to promote oxygen delivery to the brain and heart during CCs[87] but may lead to the formation of free radicals, which play a major role in reperfusion/reoxygenation injury after asphyxia. Therefore, when the patient has been successfully resuscitated, the oxygen concentration must be weaned as rapidly as tolerated to minimize oxidative stress.[83]

Finally, during a prolonged resuscitation with the delivery of CCs, it is important to allow for constant rotation of CC providers. Enriquez et al. showed CC quality decreased and fatigue was frequent before 10 minutes had elapsed on a neonatal simulator.[88] Provider fatigue was associated with both a lack of aerobic activity and a body mass index ≥ 25. This finding supports the need for guidelines requiring frequent rotation of CC providers during prolonged neonatal resuscitations. Optimal positioning of providers during CC and umbilical venous catheter placement is shown in Fig. 8.9.

Epinephrine

For asphyxiated neonates who develop asystole or severe bradycardia, the administration of epinephrine is sometimes an essential step to

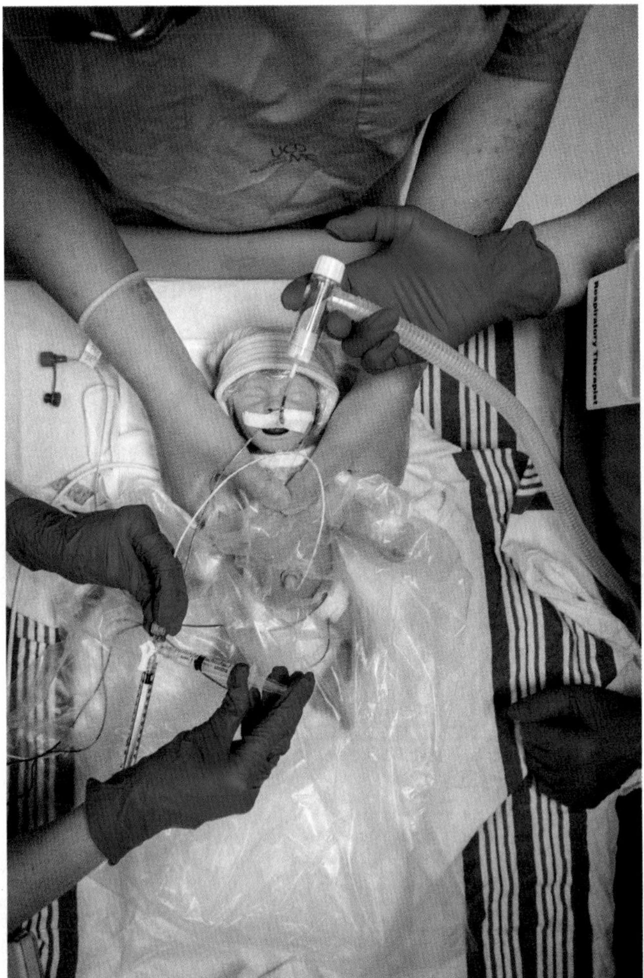

Fig. 8.9 Optimal Positioning of Neonatal Resuscitators During Resuscitation Involving Positive Pressure Ventilation (PPV), Chest Compressions, and Umbilical Venous Catheter Placement. Chest compressions are delivered from the head-end of the baby so that an additional resuscitator can place an umbilical venous catheter and administer epinephrine.

attain ROSC. Epinephrine is the only medication for neonatal resuscitation currently recommended by the International Liaison Committee on Resuscitation to be given if the heart rate is less than 60 beats per minute despite effective ventilation and CCs for 30 seconds.[1,81] Epinephrine can be delivered via an intravenous (IV), intraosseous (IO), or endotracheal (ET) route. The current recommended dose range is 0.01 to 0.03 mg/kg (0.1–0.3 mL/kg—suggested initial dose 0.02 mg/kg or 0.2 mL/kg) of 1:10,000 epinephrine solution via an IV or IO route followed by a 3-mL normal saline flush, or 0.05 to 0.1 mg/kg (0.5–1 mL/kg—suggested initial dose 0.1 mg/kg or 1 mL/kg) via an ET route while attempting vascular access.[89] However, a recent paper suggests that simplifying the recommendation to a single dose of 0.02 mg/kg IV or 0.1 mg/kg ET as the suggested initial dose may decrease administration errors.[90] These authors also suggest increasing the normal saline flush volume to 3 mL to ensure that the medication reaches the right atrium.[90] These changes were included in the *Textbook of Neonatal Resuscitation*, 8th edition.[91] A summary of changes outlined in that textbook are shown in Fig. 8.10.

Multiple animal and human studies have demonstrated that the IV route is more effective than the ET route.[92–97] This is thought to be due to increased bioavailability and the potential to bypass hepatic metabolism if the drug enters the inferior vena cava through the ductus venosus and bypasses the lung with direct access to the systemic circulation through the foramen ovale.[98] Halling et al. performed a retrospective study looking at the efficacy of IV versus ET epinephrine administration in neonates.[97] They demonstrated that IV and ET epinephrine administrations frequently needed to be repeated before ROSC was achieved. Of the 30 infants in the study who received initial ET epinephrine, 6 (20%) responded to a single ET dose alone. Among the 24 infants who did not respond to initial ET epinephrine and subsequently received IV epinephrine, 17 (71%) achieved ROSC after the addition of one or more IV doses.[97] Furthermore, the overall total dose of epinephrine received before ROSC was lower in infants receiving only IV epinephrine compared with those who received a combination of IV and ET doses before ROSC.[97] It is important to achieve early intravenous access to improve efficacy of epinephrine during neonatal resuscitation.[98]

Volume Resuscitation

In the infant who is not responding to the above measures of circulatory support, a trial of intravascular volume repletion may be warranted. It can be quite challenging to determine which infants will benefit from volume resuscitation. Increasing intravascular volume is potentially lifesaving in the setting of hypovolemic shock or sepsis; however, it can be detrimental in the setting of poor cardiac function or an asphyxiated infant who is usually euvolemic.[99]

Infants with a history of acute fetal blood loss from placental abruption, umbilical cord prolapse, fetal-maternal hemorrhage, or recent history of fetal blood sampling may be candidates for volume resuscitation.[100] It is imperative to assess infants undergoing resuscitation for signs of hypovolemia such as a weak pulse, pallor, and prolonged capillary refill time. For volume expansion, an isotonic crystalloid solution such as normal saline or blood may be used. The current recommended dose is 10 mL/kg, which may be repeated if necessary.[101] Careful consideration is important in the premature infant, because rapid infusion of volume has been associated with intraventricular hemorrhage.[89]

If significant blood loss has occurred, an infusion of packed red blood cells may be warranted to provide sufficient oxygen-carrying capacity. This can be achieved emergently by transfusing non-cross-matched O-negative blood, blood from the placenta, or blood drawn from the mother. It is important to discuss this with the blood bank and have O-negative blood prepared ahead of time when acute blood loss is suspected. In a newborn piglet model of asphyxia and moderate hemorrhage, Mendler et al. compared packed red blood cell transfusion with isotonic crystalloid solution during resuscitation.[102] There was no difference in time to ROSC and no difference in epinephrine use between the two groups. Although there was no difference in the groups in the resuscitation phase, the benefits of replacing lost blood may have a larger role in postresuscitation care.

Telemedicine

Telemedicine, the delivery of care over a distance using telecommunication technologies, offers the opportunity to immediately bring a more experienced team from a tertiary center to newborns at rural or community nurseries to provide support or even to lead resuscitation. Telemedicine assistance provided during neonatal resuscitation and stabilization was shown to improve providers' perception of teamwork as well as patient safety and quality of

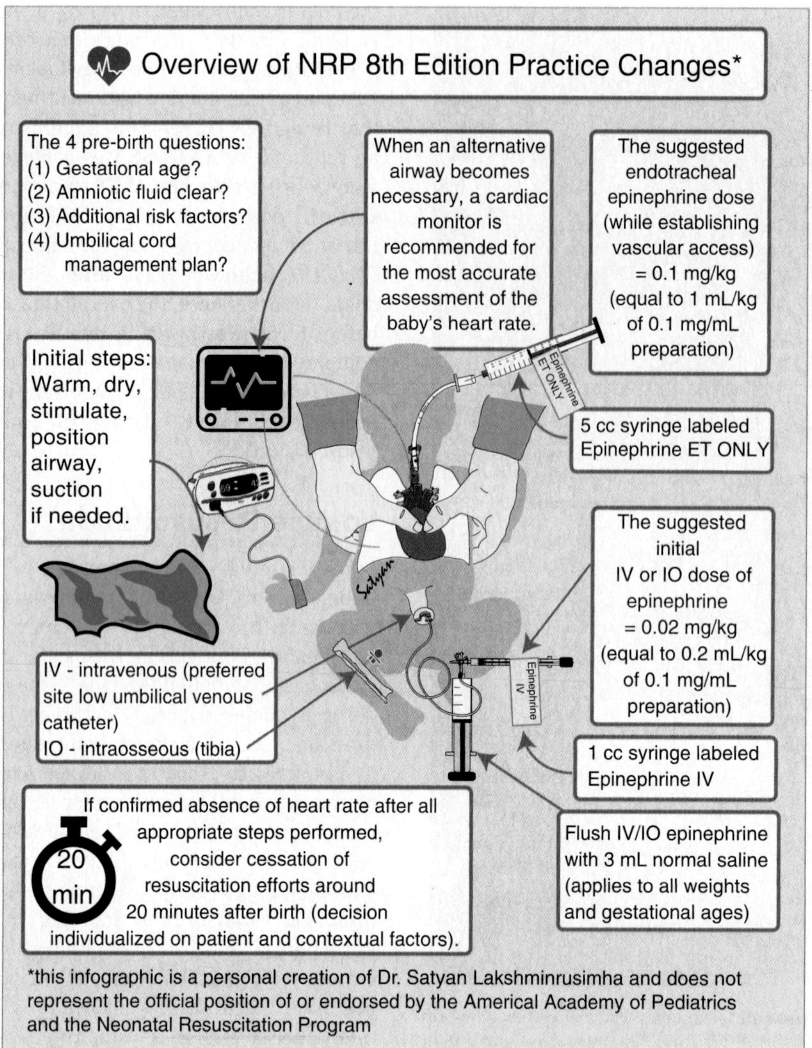

Fig. 8.10 Salient Changes in the 8th Edition of the *Textbook of Neonatal Resuscitation* Compared With Previous Editions. (Copyright Satyan Lakshminrusimha.)

care.[103] Video-assisted resuscitation has been shown to improve time to effective ventilation and use of corrective steps and to increase adherence to NRP guidelines in simulated resuscitation.[104] Telemedicine can also be used to assist in the performance of procedures needed during resuscitation and provide education to rural sites to better prepare them for advanced neonatal resuscitation.[105]

Postresuscitation Care (Fig. 8.11)

Neonates who have required significant resuscitation are at risk of developing complications and need support immediately after resuscitation. Infants with an Apgar score of <5 at 1 minute but who had recovered by 5 minutes after birth had a 5.8-fold increased risk of neonatal death and a 17-fold increased risk for cerebral palsy compared with infants with two normal Apgar scores at 1 and 5 minutes.[106] Therefore, it is recommended that newborns requiring significant resuscitation be moved to the neonatal intensive care unit for observation and postresuscitative care.[107] Additional complications that may occur in these infants during the postresuscitation period include the following.

Electrolyte Disturbances

Hyponatremia is a common finding in the asphyxiated neonate[108] and is thought to be due to an increased secretion of antidiuretic hormone and acute kidney injury in neonates with HIE leading to water retention and dilutional hyponatremia. Hyperkalemia secondary to metabolic acidosis or acute kidney injury is also common in infants with HIE.[108] Hypocalcemia can lead to cardiac dysfunction in asphyxiated newborns and can occur due to a sluggish response in parathyroid hormone (PTH) secretion to the postnatal fall in plasma calcium concentration.[109] Hypoglycemia has the potential to worsen brain injury in neonates with HIE. Routine monitoring of glucose and electrolytes and supplementation as needed is recommended.

Cardiovascular Monitoring

Heart rate, blood pressure, perfusion, and urine output should be monitored in the postresuscitative period. Volume replacement followed by inotropic support in infants who do not respond to volume may be used to provide cardiovascular support. For patients with sustained signs of cardiovascular compromise, an echocardiogram should be considered to rule out congenital heart disease and assess cardiac function.

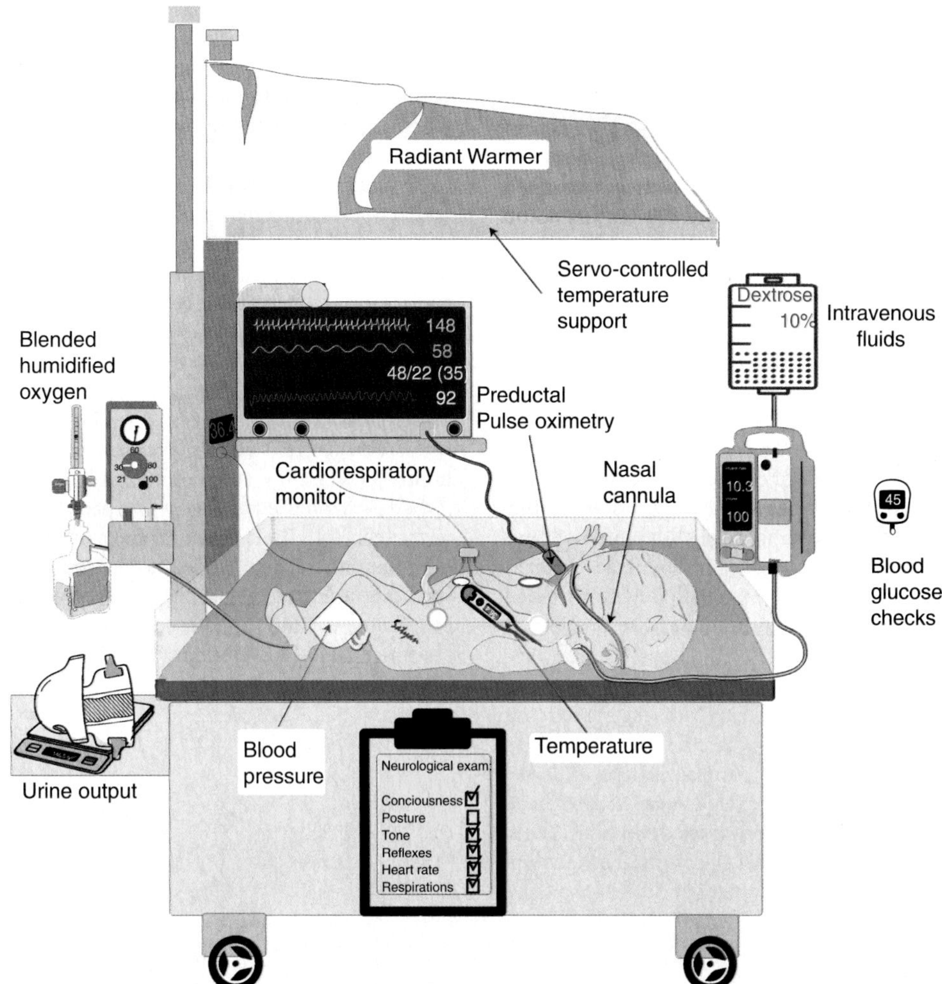

Fig. 8.11 Postresuscitation Management of a Newly Born Infant. After resuscitation (positive pressure ventilation or chest compressions) in the delivery room, abnormalities in various organ systems can occur. Hence close monitoring of temperature, respiratory status (including oxygenation), blood pressure, blood glucose, urine output, neurologic status, and hydration should be closely observed. (Copyright Satyan Lakshminrusimha.)

Temperature

Special attention must be taken to ensure that neonates are euthermic after resuscitation. Hypothermia in preterm infants has been associated with an increase in mortality and other morbidities (see the section on thermal management). Therapeutic hypothermia initiated within 6 hours of birth is the standard of care in infants with moderate to severe HIE.[110] Deep cooling (below 33°C)[111] and elevated temperature[112] are associated with adverse outcomes in neonates with HIE and should be avoided.

Respiratory Monitoring

Meconium aspiration syndrome and persistent pulmonary hypertension of the newborn (PPHN) are common among infants with HIE.[113] Avoiding acidosis and optimal ventilation and oxygenation are important in the postresuscitation period.

Neurologic Monitoring

The most common cause of neonatal seizures during the postresuscitation period is HIE, accounting for around 80% of all seizures.[114,115] Continuous electroencephalogram (EEG) monitoring is the best method of assessing for seizures, with a higher sensitivity and specificity than either brief conventional EEG or amplitude-integrated EEG monitoring.[116] Seizures are treated with the use of anticonvulsants.

Withholding Aggressive Resuscitation

Providing comfort care during delivery room resuscitations of extremely preterm infants involves complex ethical considerations. The American Academy of Pediatrics together with the American College of Obstetricians and Gynecologists define *periviable birth* as delivery occurring from 20 0/7 weeks to 25 6/7 weeks of gestation.[117] Due to the wide range of possible outcomes associated with periviable birth, the decision to resuscitate the neonate should involve collaboration between healthcare providers and the parents. Parents often struggle with the decision to resuscitate in hopes of survival or to withhold treatment to avoid suffering and potential long-term morbidities.[118–120] As such, prenatal counseling should be done as early as possible before preterm birth to allow parents time to discuss the presented options.

The primary goal of prenatal counseling is to provide parents with information that will aid their decision-making. Counseling should include not only expected outcomes for the infant but also a discussion of all available treatment options.[121] In general, there is a consensus that only comfort care should be offered to infants born at less than 22 weeks of gestation and that resuscitation should be offered for all infants born at or later than 25 weeks of gestation, leaving an area of ambiguity between 22 and 25 weeks of gestation within which recommendations vary.[89,121–123] When counseling parents, it is important to take an individualized approach. Multiple factors have been associated with an improvement in short-term and long-term outcomes of periviable infants, including (1) gestational age, (2) birth weight, (3) sex, (4) plurality, (5) use of antenatal corticosteroids, and (6) delivery at a center that has a large number of periviable births.[124]

The National Institute of Child Health and Human Development's Neonatal Research Network developed a tool to estimate outcomes for births between 22 and 25 weeks. This, in addition to other available estimators of neonatal outcomes, could be used to help relay outcomes to parents during counseling. Potential limitations of these tools are that the data are slightly outdated, and outcomes change with time; outcomes vary widely from center to center; and gestational age and estimated fetal weight estimates are not always accurate, especially in mothers who are late to receiving prenatal care.[125]

During consultation, it is useful to present the data on rates of survival and long-term neurodevelopmental disabilities separately, as the importance the parents give to these may be different. Coping with a minor disability may be difficult to handle for some families, whereas other families may be willing to adapt to a child with major disabilities.[123]

In addition to previable births, there are additional situations in which resuscitation may prolong life temporarily, prolong suffering, or result in a viable infant with major neurodevelopmental disabilities. In these cases, it may be acceptable to redirect toward comfort care. Specific examples include congenital abnormalities, genetic abnormalities, or marked disability noted in the postnatal period.

Finally, the choice of words matters. Providers must be sensitive toward the parents' ability to comprehend the situation, language preferences, cultural or religious considerations, and the family support structure. The use of visual aids and pamphlets may help improve counseling and parents' understanding of the situation.[126] Providers should consider and respect the wishes of parents who have been fully informed and have a good understanding of the information provided. When the decision is made to provide comfort care, the parents should be encouraged to spend time with the infant. Providing religious, psychosocial, and palliative care support may assist families at this difficult time.[121]

CHAPTER 9

Golden Hour and Thermoregulation

Erin E. Schofield, Lindy W. Winter

KEY POINTS

1. The first 60 minutes after birth constitutes a Golden Hour for a newborn infant, when appropriate clinical management can improve long-term outcomes.
2. The physiologic transition from intrauterine to extrauterine life is complex, and alterations in this transition can have lasting effects, particularly in premature infants.
3. After an antenatal consult, a delivery team should be assembled and briefed on maternal history, gestational age, and any prenatally known fetal diagnoses.
4. There is a need for timely and appropriate resuscitation, temperature control, and minimization of transcutaneous fluid losses in all infants.
5. Premature infants may need timely administration of surfactant, initiation of intravenous fluids, oxygen in appropriate concentrations, and other forms of respiratory support.

The "Golden Hour" is a well-defined term in adult trauma literature and has been adapted to the first hour of neonatal life. *The Golden Hour*, first published in the 1970s by R. Adams Cowley of the University of Maryland Medical Center, described use of evidence-based medicine to develop standardized protocols built around the initial hour of stabilization of the adult trauma patient (Table 9.1). These protocols led to a decrease in mortality and improvement in other outcomes.[1] In neonatology, Golden Hour terminology has been adapted to refer to the first 60 minutes of postnatal life. Evidence-based interventions and standardized protocols applied in the first hour of life (Table 9.2) have been shown to improve long-term outcomes in preterm infants.

The physiologic transition from intrauterine to extrauterine life is complex, and alterations in this transition can have lasting effects on the newborn, particularly the extremely low birth weight (ELBW) infant. Antenatal counseling, neonatal resuscitation, transportation of the ELBW infant to the neonatal intensive care unit (NICU), respiratory and cardiovascular support, attention to thermoregulation and glucose stability, and interventions to reduce intraventricular hemorrhage (IVH) are some but not all of the considerations when addressing the needs of the ELBW infant.

The Golden Hour can be implemented for either term or preterm neonates. When referring to the Golden Hour as it pertains to term neonates, there are three main goals as set forth by the World Health Organization and the United Nations Children's Fund (UNICEF). These goals include direct, immediate skin-to-skin contact between the mother and newborn, delayed cord clamping, and early initiation of breastfeeding where it is both medically appropriate and desired by the mother. Taken together, these interventions have decreased rates of hypothermia and hypoglycemia in the neonate and increased mother–child bonding.[2] Mothers who have been exposed to the Golden Hour protocol have decreased rates of postpartum anxiety and are more likely to continue to exclusively breastfeed.[3]

The Golden Hour of the Preterm or High-Risk Neonate

ELBW infants have high mortality and morbidity and are at risk for lifelong neurodevelopmental disabilities that range from subtle impairment to severe delays. In the preterm or critically ill neonate, Golden Hour protocols are more intensive and focus on many more facets of neonatal care.

A true Golden Hour protocol starts with prenatal counseling well before any planned delivery of a preterm or otherwise critically ill infant. The neonatal team should meet with the obstetric team to verify the estimated gestational age, estimated fetal weight, pregnancy complications, antenatal steroid administration, and comorbid diagnoses of any impending high-risk delivery. Based on this information, an antenatal consultation with parents should be performed to review the expected outcomes based on gestational age and comorbid diagnoses, expected length of the NICU stay, and potential interventions that may need to be performed to stabilize the infant. It is recommended that antenatal steroids be given for fetal lung maturation in infants of gestational ages 24 0/7 to 33 6/7 weeks, although institutional guidelines may vary and include lower gestational ages.[4]

In cases of periviability or expected poor prognosis, goals of care should be discussed with parents prior to delivery based on national and institutional guidelines. These goals may include conversations around providing comfort care in place of aggressive support. This decision needs to take into account regional guidelines, perceived accuracy of gestational age dating, presence of infection in the mother (such as chorioamnionitis), level of care available at the location of delivery, and personal and spiritual beliefs of the parents. Parents should be informed about the most accurate prognostic data on morbidity and mortality currently available, based on estimated gestational age, race, and sex of their infant. It is important that parents are given time to receive counseling and make decisions

Table 9.1 Trauma Golden Hour

Task	Time for Task, min	Total Time, min
Injury	0	0
On-scene response and assessment	10	10
On-scene emergency care	20	30
Extrication	10	40
Transportation	10	50
Emergency department stabilization	10	60
Surgical intervention by 60 min		

Table 9.2 Neonatal Golden Hour

Task	Time for Task, min	Total Time, min
Birth	0	0
Resuscitation	10	10
Transport	5	15
Lines	40	55
X-ray and intravenous fluids	5	60
Isolette closed by 60 min		

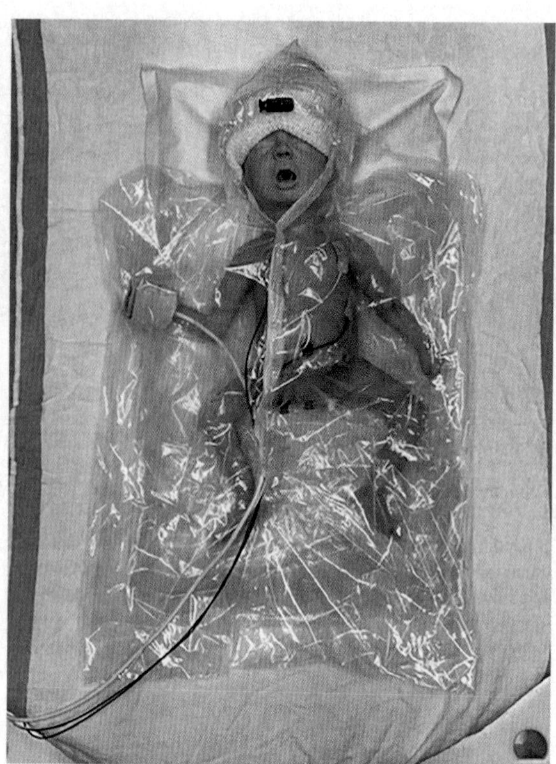

Fig. 9.1 Golden Hour Practices. The Golden Hour practices for clinical management of premature infants focus on timely and appropriate resuscitation, temperature control, minimization of transcutaneous fluid losses, timely administration of surfactant if indicated, early initiation of intravenous fluids containing dextrose and amino acids, and administration of oxygen only if or as needed and in appropriate concentrations to prevent hyperoxia-induced lung and eye injury.

regarding the management of their infant, which is why prenatal counseling is a vital component of Golden Hour management.

After the antenatal consultation is performed, a delivery team should be assembled. All team members should be briefed on maternal history, gestational age, and any prenatally known fetal diagnoses. The charge nurse and admitting nurse in the NICU should be included in this discussion and should inform the delivery team members of the bed spot to which the neonate will be admitted. The admitting team should have a prewarmed isolette, common medications and fluids available at bedside, and anticipated ventilatory support in the patient's room before arrival of the patient. Assignment of neonatal delivery team roles is especially important in a high-risk delivery. The team leader should be designated early and should assign specific roles to every team member attending the delivery. Before the delivery of the infant, all delivery room equipment should be checked and verified to be in appropriate working order, per Neonatal Resuscitation Program (NRP) guidelines. Adequate personnel and equipment should be on hand for deliveries with multiple gestations or known congenital anomalies.

Although the Golden Hour is, in name, focused only on the first hour of postnatal life, such protocols have lifelong benefits for at-risk infants. Implementation of Golden Hour practices has improved time to surfactant administration, early administration of dextrose and amino acids, rates of normothermia on admission to the NICU, odds of developing chronic lung disease, and odds of developing retinopathy of prematurity by providing a multifaceted protocol for care of the preterm neonate[5] (Fig. 9.1).

Delayed Cord Clamping

Preterm or high-risk newborns are at particularly high risk for anemia, both from prematurity and from iatrogenic losses. Delayed umbilical cord clamping (clamping of the cord 30 seconds to 3 minutes after birth) has been associated with a decreased need for postnatal blood transfusions, decreased IVH, and decreased rates of necrotizing enterocolitis.[6] The most current NRP 2015 guidelines acknowledge the benefit of delayed cord clamping but also acknowledge that there are inadequate studies on the safety of performing delayed cord clamping in a patient who requires resuscitation. For this reason, NRP recommends delaying cord clamping for 30 seconds after birth in only those term and preterm infants not requiring resuscitation at birth.[7]

Hypothermia

One of the main foci in the Golden Hour protocols is the prevention of hypothermia, defined as a temperature <36.5°C. Hypothermia is a dangerous condition in the newly born ELBW with a reported prevalence on admission estimated to be between 45% and 93%, depending on gestational age and birth weight of the infant.[8,9] Each degree of temperature drop is associated with a 28% increase in neonatal mortality, and temperature on admission to the NICU is a strong predictor for neonatal mortality.

Temperature regulation is most difficult in the initial first few minutes to hours after birth as a newly born infant transitions between in-utero and ex-utero environments where conduction, convection, and evaporative and radiative heat loss are much greater. Due to infants' relatively large body-to-surface area, heat losses due to these four mechanisms are increased, which makes infants uniquely susceptible to heat loss. Per NRP guidelines, the goal body temperature of the preterm neonate should be maintained between 36.5°C and 37.5°C.[7]

Hypothermia is associated with substantially increased morbidity and mortality,[10–13] including:

- Delayed adjustment to newborn circulation
- Hypoglycemia
- Metabolic acidosis
- Coagulopathy
- Oxygen dependency
- Intraventricular hemorrhage
- Late-onset sepsis
- Poor neurodevelopmental outcomes
- Death

Despite what is known about the risks of hypothermia, and strategies to combat it, hypothermia remains a common problem.

Strategies to prevent hypothermia include[14,15]:

- Prewarming the resuscitation table
- Prewarming and humidifying the isolette
- Maintaining the delivery room temperature between 25°C and 28°C
- Use of heated, humidified respiratory gases for resuscitation
- Use of a polyethylene wrap or food-grade plastic bag
- Use of an insulated head cap
- Exothermic heated mattresses (monitor closely for associated hyperthermia)
- Avoidance of drafts around the resuscitation area (no opening or closing of doors, no air vents, etc.)

In the delivery room, the radiant warmer, or isolette, that will be used for resuscitation should be prewarmed and positioned in an area that is as free from air drafts as possible. This means positioning the resuscitation area in the farthest point away from doors and air vents. Cardiorespiratory monitoring leads should be placed on the infant's skin upon arrival to the resuscitation area so that an insulated hat and polyethylene wrap can be immediately applied to the infant before any intentional drying has occurred. The wrap traps evaporative moisture losses between the infant's skin and the wrap, which creates humidity and further decreases evaporative water and heat losses. Once the wrap and hat are in place, they should not be removed. All resuscitative efforts can be performed through the thin film of the bag. Umbilical lines can also be placed with the polyethylene wrap in place, either by folding the edges of the wrap inward to surround the umbilical stump or by cutting a hole just large enough for the umbilical stump if the polyethylene covering is a continuous bag.

One member of the resuscitation team should be responsible for checking the body temperature of the newborn throughout the resuscitation. A transcutaneous temperature probe in servo control mode can be placed on the infant's abdomen per unit protocol, but this temperature should be periodically confirmed with axillary temperature readings. There are varying guidelines on when to remove the polyethylene wrap, but most sources agree that the infant should achieve and maintain normothermia for at least 1 hour prior to removal of the wrap or bag.

Respiratory Support in the Golden Hour

Initial respiratory support in the Golden Hour should focus on lung-protective ventilation strategies. The latest guidelines from the NRP should be followed, and pulse oximetry should be used as soon as possible in the delivery room.[7] For infants less than 35 weeks' gestation, a 21% to 30% fraction of inspired oxygen (Fio_2) should be used during resuscitation. In infants >35 weeks' gestation, a 21% Fio_2 should be used. The Fio_2 should be titrated to achieve optimum preductal saturations[7] (Table 9.3).

Table 9.3 Guidelines for Spo_2 Values in First 10 Minutes of Life[a]

Minute of Life	Spo_2, %
1	60–65
2	65–70
3	70–75
4	75–80
5	80–85
10	85–90

[a]Neonatal Resuscitation Program recommendations.
Spo_2, Oxygen saturation.

It is equally important for the resuscitation team to titrate the Fio_2 down as goal oxygen saturations are achieved so as to avoid injury resulting from hyperoxia. Preterm infants are at particularly high risk for oxidative stress, which contributes to the development of bronchopulmonary dysplasia, retinopathy of prematurity, necrotizing enterocolitis, and intraventricular hemorrhage.[16]

If an infant needs positive pressure ventilation in the delivery room, it is important to use the minimal amount of pressure necessary to affect an adequate increase in heart rate and oxygen saturation. In preterm infants requiring resuscitations, most institutions start at a peak inspiratory pressure of 20 cm H_2O and a positive end-expiratory pressure of 5 cm H_2O. Again, NRP guidelines should be followed, and the peak inspiratory pressure and positive end-expiratory pressure should be adjusted as necessary to achieve the targeted rise in heart rate. Early nasal continuous positive airway pressure (nCPAP) in the delivery room, as opposed to prophylactic early intubation and surfactant administration, has been shown to reduce the rate of future intubations in the delivery room and the NICU, reduce the rate of postnatal corticosteroid use, and lead to a shorter duration of mechanical ventilation.[17] When possible, early nCPAP should be initiated in the resuscitation of preterm infants. Compared with nCPAP, nasal intermittent positive pressure ventilation is more effective in decreasing rates of respiratory failure and the need for intubation in preterm infants with respiratory distress syndrome, but it can be harder to provide in the delivery room.[18] Exogenous surfactant replacement therapy should be administered for a persistent Fio_2 requirement >40% or per institutional guidelines.

Fluid Management and Prevention of Hypoglycemia During the Golden Hour

Hypoglycemia in the newborn is common, and even transient hypoglycemia can lead to lasting neurodevelopmental impairments. These effects are especially pronounced in preterm infants as opposed to term infants.[19,20] Preterm newborns are at high risk for hypoglycemia, particularly those who are growth restricted or large for gestational age or who have diabetic mothers. Like many other outcomes in the preterm neonate, the incidence of hypoglycemia is inversely related to gestational age.[21] The initial blood glucose level should be measured within the Golden Hour, because blood glucose levels reach a physiologic nadir within approximately 60 minutes of postnatal life in the absence of exogenous supplementation. Intravenous (IV) access should be established as soon as possible after birth in the preterm neonate, either with a peripheral IV or umbilical venous catheter, and parenteral fluids containing dextrose and amino acids should be administered at maintenance levels. Early administration of such fluid has been demonstrated to improve growth outcomes and decrease the incidence of hypoglycemia.[22] Obtaining stable intravenous access by 1 hour of life should be incorporated into any Golden Hour protocol.

Prevention of Sepsis in the Golden Hour

Neonatal sepsis is one of the most common causes of neonatal morbidity and mortality worldwide.[23] Adult and pediatric critical care medicine have instituted their own Golden Hour protocols around the administration of antibiotics in patients at high risk for sepsis. This has been shown to significantly decrease mortality from sepsis in these patients.[24,25] Risk factors for neonatal sepsis include prematurity, immunodeficiency, maternal Group B streptococcal colonization, and chorioamnionitis. Chorioamnionitis is a major risk factor for preterm birth and also independently increases the risk of early onset neonatal sepsis, development of cerebral palsy, and leukomalacia. Timely administration of appropriate antibiotics within the Golden Hour is critical in preventing early-onset sepsis and later sequelae of sepsis. Pharmacists should be included in the development of any Golden Hour protocol, because they can ensure that the NICU is stocked with the most common antibiotics used in the first days of a neonate's life. Having antibiotics, usually ampicillin and gentamicin, readily available for nurses to give negates the delay in having to order these medications from the pharmacy and have them approved prior to administration.

It is important to note that overtreatment with antibiotics is also associated with poor outcomes, so once blood cultures show no growth after 36 to 48 hours, antibiotics should be discontinued. If a blood culture becomes positive, antibiotic therapy should be tailored to the most appropriate regimen for the specific organism.[26]

Optimizing Outcomes by Minimizing Interventions

Neonatal intensive care is, by definition, intensive. It is our default, because intensive care practitioners want to know all that we can about our patients in order to help them. We need to balance our need for information with the potential harm that invasive procedures and laboratory tests can cause. Greater numbers of invasive (painful) procedures in neonates are associated with abnormal brain development.[27] Infants who undergo more painful or invasive procedures have reduced white matter and subcortical gray matter on magnetic resonance spectroscopic imaging.[28] These abnormalities in the white matter microstructure persist and are ultimately associated with a lower IQ in preterm neonates.[29]

Extremely preterm neonates typically have the highest rates of iatrogenic blood loss on the first day of life secondary to the routine laboratory studies done on admission to the NICU. These losses can be upward of 10 mL/kg, which is substantial considering that the average circulating red blood cell volume in a preterm neonate is just 90 to 100 mL/kg.[30] Throughout a NICU admission, iatrogenic phlebotomy losses are one of the key contributors to neonatal anemia.[31] Estimates for iatrogenic blood loss in the first 6 weeks of life in an ELBW infant range from 11 to 22 mL/kg/week, which represents 15% to 30% of circulating blood volume in an ELBW infant.[31–33] Of all red blood cell transfusions during the NICU admission of an ELBW infant, 44% are given during the first 2 weeks of life and 70% during the first month of life.[34]

The amount of blood drawn for laboratory tests in the NICU is directly correlated with the number of blood transfusions in preterm infants.[33,35–37] Therefore, as providers, we can decrease the number of blood transfusions given to patients and the degree of anemia by judiciously ordering laboratory studies. Golden Hour protocols should have guidelines for decreasing iatrogenic phlebotomy losses in neonates.

The initial "sticks" in the Golden Hour for laboratory blood draws can be reliably obtained from umbilical cord blood in the delivery room, provided that personnel have been properly trained in how to draw blood from the placenta via the umbilical cord. Multiple studies have demonstrated that laboratory tests such as complete blood cell count, blood culture, and blood type/antibody screens are equally reliable when drawn from the umbilical cord blood or directly from the infant.[38–44] Umbilical cord blood samples can still be used for neonatal laboratory studies even if delayed cord clamping is done after birth, because a substantial portion of fetal cells remains even after delayed cord clamping is completed. The placenta and umbilical cord are rich reservoirs of fetal blood cells and should not simply be discarded after birth. To further decrease laboratory blood draws and "sticks" upon admission to the NICU, noninvasive monitors such as transcutaneous or end-tidal CO_2 monitors should be considered.

Future Directions for the Golden Hour

Standardization of care in the initial resuscitation and the first hour of life of high-risk neonates has improved long-term mortality and neurodevelopmental, respiratory, and ophthalmologic outcomes. Even after a standardized resuscitation and after the first hour of life, neonates are still at high risk for developing other morbidities. It stands to reason that these morbidities could potentially be mitigated with further standardization of care past the Golden Hour. ELBW infants have a 30% to 40% overall risk of developing an IVH during their NICU stay, with 90% of these hemorrhages occurring during the first 72 hours of life. Some factors leading to increased IVH risk in ELBW infants are the following[45]:

- Capillary fragility
- Mechanical ventilation
- Sepsis
- Episodes of hypotension or hypertension
- Low Apgar scores
- Hypernatremia
- Hypothermia
- Early blood transfusions

Given these known risk factors, many centers have standardized multiple facets of neonatal care beyond the first 24 hours of life. One large academic medical center proposed a "Golden Week" for infants born at <28 weeks' gestation. The global aim was to build on the experience of other facilities and implement a standardized interdisciplinary approach to the care of ELBW infants as the foundation of quality improvement efforts to improve local clinical practice. The center extended the concepts of the Golden Hour care through the first week of life, building on protocol-driven, evidenced-based practice. Multiple quality outcomes encompassing all aspects of care were followed, including family-centered care, team performance, thermoregulation, respiratory management, neuroprotective strategies, fluid management, optimization of nutrition, and reduction of painful procedures and laboratory/radiologic testing. Checklists were implemented in an effort to move from provider-centered to team-centered management goals. The overarching goal was to improve morbidity and mortality in infants born at <28 weeks' gestation. Specific guidelines were created surrounding every aspect of neonatal care during the first week of life.

The Golden Week protocol built on Golden Hour guidelines and included such things as when patients should be intubated and given surfactant, what type of initial ventilator support should be used, and what lines should be placed. In this protocol, only experienced practitioners (attending MDs, fellows, and experienced nurse practitioners) were allowed to intubate and place umbilical lines in these high-risk infants. The purpose of this was not to exclude more inexperienced residents and nurse practitioners from the care of these patients but to improve efficiency in the delivery of care and reduce stress during the care of these most high-risk patients.

It was important to target specific outcomes for each organ system throughout the first week of life. Ventilator strategies were developed to keep the partial pressure of carbon dioxide and the pH in a defined range, with the ultimate goal of decreasing the severity of respiratory distress syndrome and the incidence of bronchopulmonary dysplasia. All infants admitted on continuous positive airway pressure or intubated were started on aminophylline or caffeine. Nutritional guidelines included early and aggressive enteral nutrition, with daily total fluid goals, serum sodium goals, and guidelines for total parenteral nutrition components. Adjustments to total fluid intake were made every 12 hours based on serum sodium goals and twice-daily weights. Strict calculation of total fluids received was performed every 12 hours, including total parenteral nutrition, other continuous drips, parenteral medication volumes, flush volumes, and feeds. Protocols were established for the use and duration of antibiotics for prevention of sepsis. Care was bundled to eliminate unnecessary touch and stimulation for these infants. In addition, indomethacin use was standardized as a method to reduce IVH.

Perhaps the largest practice change was the schedule of laboratory blood draws in this population. All admission lab samples were drawn off umbilical cord blood by obstetric staff who had been appropriately trained. Lab schedules were written so that there were only two planned lab draws per day. Physicians were not prohibited from obtaining additional lab samples outside of the protocol if the clinical status of the infant warranted them. Transcutaneous CO_2 monitors were used in every patient to decrease the frequency of blood draws or heel sticks for blood gas monitoring.

By implementing all of the strategies described above, the rate of severe IVH (grade 3–4) was reduced from 20.4% to 10.3%. The rate of combined death or severe IVH in the first week of life was reduced from 33% to 17%. Laboratory blood draws were decreased by 27%, and a 15% cost savings was effected. There was a 13% reduction in iatrogenic blood loss. These data are in the pre-publication stage, but the entire "Golden Week" protocol is expected to be made available to the public in the near future.

Although no single "Golden Hour" or "Golden Week" protocol has been demonstrated to be superior to others, standardization of care has been shown to improve clinical outcomes.[16] It is important for each institution to create protocols that standardize as many facets of care as possible. It is also important to continually educate all staff members on these protocols so that they are implemented with consistency. The importance of such protocols should be repeatedly stressed, because "buy in" from every team member involved in the care of these fragile neonates is essential. Protocols should be continually reviewed in multiple Plan-Do-Study-Act (PDSA) cycles and revised, as indicated, as part of ongoing quality improvement initiatives to allow individual institutions to fine tune Golden Hour strategies to best achieve local clinical outcomes.

FURTHER READING

Croop SEW, Thoyre SM, Aliaga S, McCaffrey MJ, Peter-Wohl S. The Golden Hour: a quality improvement initiative for extremely premature infants in the neonatal intensive care unit. *J Perinatol.* 2020;40:530–539.

Peleg B, Globus O, Granot M, et al. "Golden Hour" quality improvement intervention and short-term outcome among preterm infants. *J Perinatol.* 2019;39:387–392.

CHAPTER

10 Oxygen During Postnatal Stabilization

Maximo Vento, Ola D. Saugstad

KEY POINTS

1. There is a precisely controlled sequence of circulatory and respiratory changes at birth that leads to the establishment of adult-type circulation and airborne respiration.
2. Despite the well-established sequence of events, 1 in 10 infants, particularly those born before term, will require interventions to achieve an adequate postnatal adaptation.
3. Oxygen has been widely accepted as the most relevant drug for preterm resuscitation.
4. There is a need to achieve oxygen saturation between 80% and 85% within the first 5 minutes after birth in very preterm infants <32 weeks' gestation) independently of the initial fraction of inspired oxygen.
5. We need continued and critical appraisal of both the need for and the doses (concentrations) of oxygen administered during resuscitation.

Introduction

Fetal-to-neonatal transition in mammals is characterized by a precise sequence of circulatory and respiratory changes that contribute to the establishment of adult-type circulation and airborne respiration. As a consequence, there is an abrupt increase in the oxygen availability that fulfills the increased energy requirements of multicellular organisms.[1] Despite the exquisite physiologic arrangements that regulate this sequence of events, almost 10% of all newly born infants, and especially those born prematurely, require resuscitative interventions to achieve an adequate postnatal adaptation.[2] In the newborn period, resuscitation requires lung expansion, reducing pulmonary resistance, improving lung compliance, and achieving a functional residual capacity. All these changes improve alveolar capillary gas exchange and arterial blood oxygenation.[3]

The lungs, the thoracic cage, and respiratory muscles mature late in gestation.[4] Moreover, surfactant and the antioxidant enzymatic and nonenzymatic defenses, especially in males, are not readily available until the last weeks of gestation.[5] Hence preterm infants, especially very preterm infants with a gestational age (GA) below 32 weeks, frequently experience difficulties establishing effective respiration immediately after birth. Immaturity and surfactant deficiency lead to uneven lung ventilation with hyperventilated areas coexisting with atelectasis and the inability to establish a functional residual capacity. As a consequence, the premature baby is at increased risk of developing hypoxemia, hypercapnia, and increased work of breathing, which are characteristic of respiratory distress syndrome with hypoxemic respiratory failure. Therefore prenatal interventions such as the administration of antenatal steroids and postnatal resuscitation with positive pressure ventilation and oxygen supplementation constitute essential interventions necessary to overcome respiratory insufficiency.[6]

Oxygen has been widely accepted as the most relevant drug for preterm resuscitation. However, there are still important aspects regarding its use in the immediate postnatal period that have not yet been answered. It is necessary to address the optimal initial fraction of inspired oxygen (FiO_2), oxygen saturation (SpO_2) target ranges in the first minutes after birth, and how to titrate oxygen according to the infant's response. Of note, oxygen in excess leads to hyperoxemia and direct tissue damage secondary to oxidative stress, activation of proinflammatory and proapoptotic pathways, and other mechanisms.[5] At the other extreme, hypoxemia, especially when combined with bradycardia, significantly enhances the risk for intraventricular hemorrhage (IVH) and death. Both situations increase mortality and/or short- to long-term morbidities in survivors.[7]

The aim of the present chapter is to critically analyze the most relevant and recent literature concerning the use of oxygen in the delivery room (DR) to help neonatologists optimize the care management of preterm infants during postnatal stabilization.

Oxygen in Utero and During Fetal-to-Neonatal Transition

During late gestation, the arterial partial pressure of oxygen ranges between from 25 to 30 mm Hg in the fetus and 80 to 90 mm Hg in the mother. The oxygen gradient between the mother and fetus drives oxygen across the intervillous space of the placenta. The oxygen content in fetal blood is low during embryogenesis and progressively rises during fetogenesis, reaching a saturation plateau of 50% to 60% at approximately 14 to 20 weeks after conception. Thereafter, SpO_2 slowly decreases to values of 45% to 50% in the last trimester.[8] Oxygenated blood is redirected through circulatory shunts at the foramen ovale and ductus arteriosus to the lung, brain, and cardiac circulation. The brain and heart are extremely dependent on aerobic metabolism.[9] Immediately after birth, newly born infants initiate profound inspiratory movements, reaching negative pressures of as low as -40 to -50 cm H_2O that contribute to lung expansion and extrusion of lung fluid from the respiratory airways and alveoli to the interstitium. In addition, increased oxygen content causes vasodilatation of the lung vasculature, a drop in vascular resistance, closure of intracardiac and extracardiac shunting, and redirection of the ventricular output to the lungs.[7] The partial pressure of oxygen rises to 70 to 80 mm Hg in the first 5 to 10 minutes after birth, and arterial SpO_2, reflecting the percentage of hemoglobin that is saturated with oxygen, oscillates between 95% and 100% once fetal-to-neonatal transition is completed.[7]

Evolving Arterial Oxygen Saturation in the First Minutes After Birth

Dawson et al. merged databases from three research groups that included term and preterm newborn infants who did not need resuscitation or oxygen supplementation on stabilization (Fig. 10.1).[10] With these data, they assembled a graph of SpO_2 ranges with centiles for term and late preterm babies for the first 10 minutes after birth. Reference ranges for term infants have been adopted by international guidelines to establish target SpO_2 recommendations minute by minute. Thus recommended ranges for SpO_2 are 60% to 65% at 1 minute, 65% to 70% at 2 minutes, 70% to 75% at 3 minutes, 75% to 80% at 4 minutes, 80% to 85% at 5 minutes, and 85% to 95% at 10 minutes.[11] However, the reference ranges for preterm infants were based on a smaller population of 136 late preterm infants (33 6/7–36 6/7 weeks' gestation). The percentiles for preterm infants did not reflect the evolving SpO_2 in the first minutes after birth in very preterm infants ≤32 weeks' GA.[10] Vento et al.[12] retrieved the SpO_2 and heart rate (HR) minute by minute in very preterm infants ventilated with positive pressure and air, mimicking the real clinical situation in the DR. As shown in their nomogram, the results of the study by Vento et al. showed that very preterm infants on mask ventilation achieved higher SpO_2 values and stabilized significantly earlier than did preterm infants.[12]

Delaying cord clamping has been recommended by international guidelines in the past decade and is widely accepted as a routine intervention in the DR.[5,11,13] Delaying cord clamping contributes to the hemodynamic stabilization of the newborn infant by increasing the left ventricular preload and afterload, decreasing pulmonary vascular resistance, and facilitating pulmonary gas exchange.[14] Hence aerating the lungs and increasing pulmonary blood flow before umbilical cord clamping could avoid the reduction of cardiac preload and output caused by immediate cord clamping.[14] Based on these assumptions, several clinical studies have reported the feasibility of ventilating newborn infants with patent cord, although no improvement in outcomes has been yet reported.[15–18]

Recently, reference ranges for term infants born by vaginal delivery with cord patency delayed for more than 1 minute and no need for resuscitation or oxygen at birth have been constructed.[19] Minute-by-minute data for HR and SpO_2 were registered during the first 10 minutes after fetal expulsion. Significantly higher values for SpO_2 for the 10th, 50th, and 90th centiles, compared with the reference range of Dawson et al.[10] for the first 5 minutes, and for HR for the first 1 to 2 minutes after birth were reported.[19] Hence in healthy infants newly born by vaginal delivery and with cord clamping delayed for >60 seconds, a higher SpO_2 value and HR were achieved in the first 5 minutes after birth compared with term neonates born but with immediate cord clamping.[19]

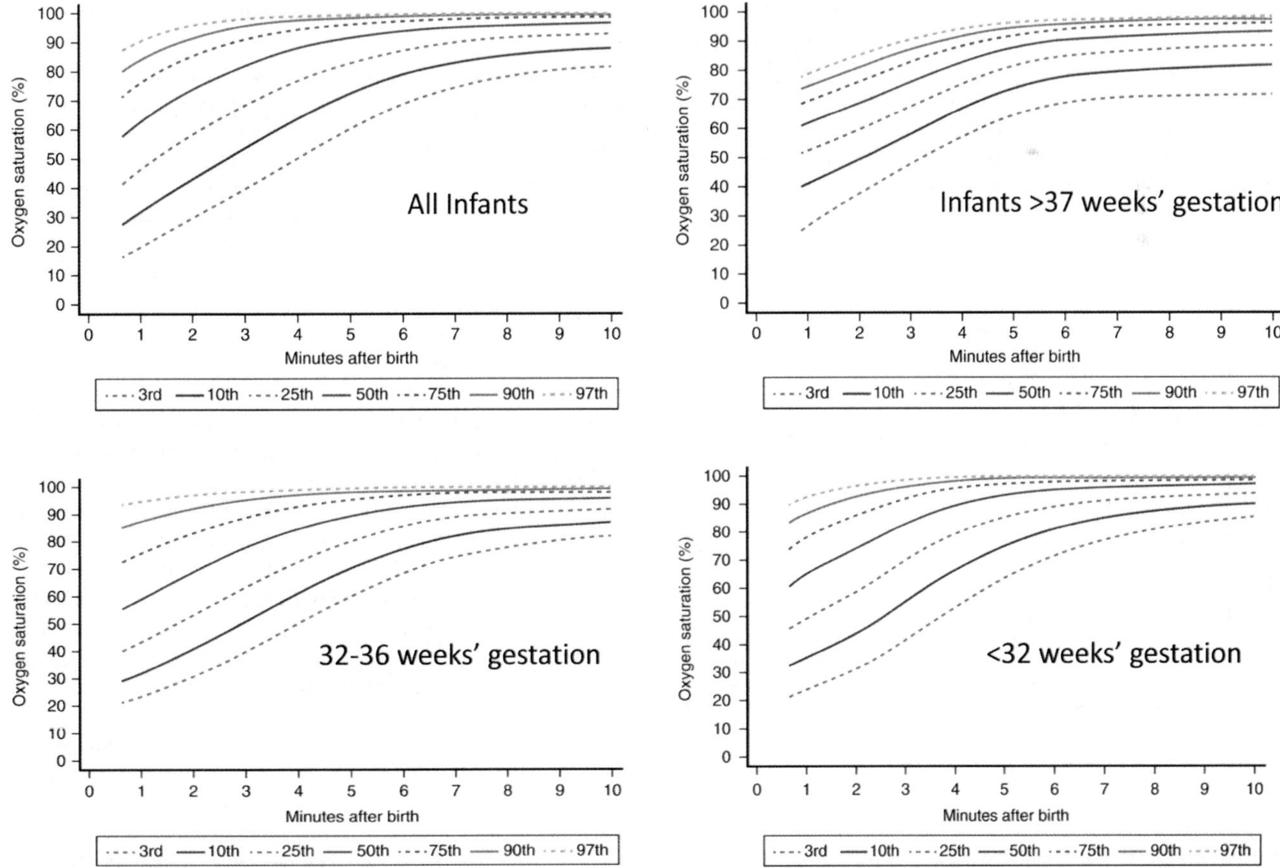

Fig. 10.1 Oxygen Saturation by Minutes After Birth. The 3rd, 10th, 25th, 50th, 75th, 90th, and 97th oxygen saturation percentiles, first for all infants and then in subgroups with decreasing gestational age. These infants did not receive any medical intervention. (Modified with permission from Vento. In: *Assisted Ventilation of the Neonate*. 16:153–161.)

Initial Fio_2 for Resuscitation in the Delivery Room

International guidelines established in 2015[11,13,20] strongly recommend initiating resuscitation of preterm infants born at <32 weeks' GA who have a low oxygen concentration (21%–30%; Fig. 10.2), although the evidence that supports this recommendation is of moderate quality. The recent 2019 European Consensus Guidelines on the Management of Respiratory Distress Syndrome[5] advocate the use of an Fio_2 of 0.21 to 0.30 as the initial gas admixture for preterm infants <28 weeks' gestation and 0.30 for babies 28 to 31 weeks' gestation. Oei et al.[21] launched an international survey that showed that the majority (77%) of neonatologists targeted Spo_2 between the 10th and 50th percentiles of the reference range by Dawson et al. for full-term infants[10] and would start with an Fio_2 of 0.3. Interestingly, most participants acknowledged a lack of sufficient evidence and recommended further research.[21] It could be hypothesized that the use of a lower initial Fio_2 would reduce the oxygen load and the oxidative stress on stabilization. Oxidative stress has been linked as a causative agent to a series of neonatal conditions including bronchopulmonary dysplasia (BPD), retinopathy of prematurity (ROP), necrotizing enterocolitis (NEC), and IVH, among others.[22,23] In two randomized controlled trials (RCTs), the initiation of resuscitation with a high initial Fio_2 (0.9 or 1.0) with subsequent titration resulted in increased oxidant stress and BPD incidence compared with starting with an Fio_2 of 0.21 or 0.30.[24,25] In contrast, when the difference between higher (≥0.60) and lower (≤0.30) initial Fio_2 was reduced, no differences in clinical outcomes or biomarkers of oxidative stress were found in two RCTs blinded for the air/oxygen blender.[26,27] In contrast, a nonblinded RCT performed in extremely premature infants (<28 weeks' gestation) raised concerns about the optimal strategy to supplement oxygen to extremely preterm infants. The TO2RPIDO study randomized infants <32 weeks' GA to air or 100% oxygen. The Spo_2 was targeted to 65% to 95% at 5 minutes and 85% to 95% at NICU admission.[28] A total of 287 infants with a mean GA of 28.9 weeks were included. In a nonprespecified post hoc analysis, infants <28 weeks' GA had an almost four-fold increase in mortality if initially started with air compared with 100% oxygen (risk ratio, 3.9; 95% CI, 1.1–13.4).[28] It should be underpinned that this study was underpowered to address this post hoc hypothesis reliably, and the trial was ceased per recommendation of the data and safety monitoring committee due to loss of equipoise for the use of 100% oxygen.[28] Furthermore, Oei et al.[29] performed a systematic review of the outcomes of infants born at ≤28 6/7 weeks' gestation randomized to resuscitation with a low (≤0.3) versus high (≥0.6) Fio_2 at delivery in eight RCTs that fulfilled these requirements. They did not find differences in the overall risk of death or other common preterm morbidities including BPD, NEC, ROP, PDA, or IVH after resuscitation was initiated at delivery in infants with lower versus higher Fio_2.[29] Additional evidence has been reported in two major systematic reviews and meta-analyses. Lui et al.[30] performed a Cochrane systematic review of 10 RCTs that included 914 infants. No significant impact was assessed on death at discharge or relevant neonatal conditions such as ROP, periventricular leukomalacia, IVH, NEC, BPD, PDA, or neurodevelopmental outcome in preterm infants born at ≤32 weeks' gestation with a lower (<0.4) or higher (≥0.4) initial Fio_2 titrated to target Spo_2.[30] Almost simultaneously, Welsford et al.,[31] in a systematic review and meta-analysis that included 10 RCTs and 4 cohort studies with a total of 5697 preterm infants born at <35 weeks' gestation, compared a higher (>50%) versus lower (<50%) initial Fio_2 for outcomes of resuscitation in the DR. This study also failed to show differences in short-term mortality, long-term mortality, neurodevelopmental impairment, or other relevant preterm morbidities in the neonatal period.[31] However, the authors pointed out that most of the subgroup of newborns of ≤32 weeks' gestation required oxygen supplementation on stabilization.[31]

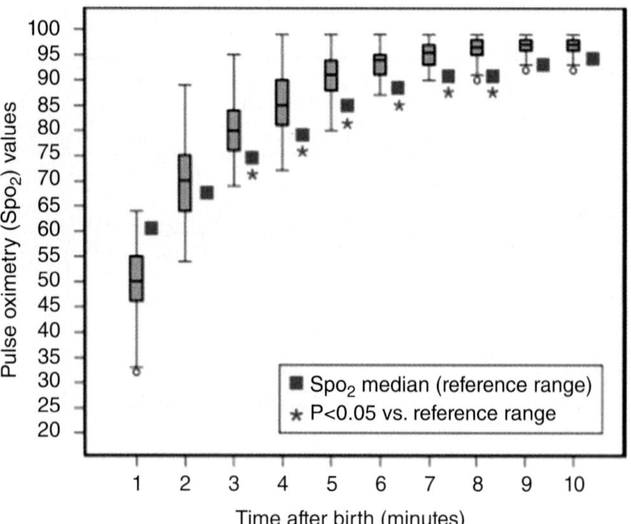

Fig. 10.2 Changes in Preductal Oxygen Saturations (Spo_2) After Birth. *Red squares* show the natural changes in Spo_2 in newborn infants born at a gestational age range of 25 to 42 weeks who did not receive any active resuscitation after birth. *Blue box-whisker plots* show the Spo_2 of preterm infants <32 weeks' gestation who received respiratory support immediately after birth with continuous positive airway pressure and air. (Modified with permission from Vento. In: *Fanaroff and Martin's Neonatal–Perinatal Medicine*, 33, 543–551.)

Higher Initial Fio_2: Critical Appraisal of Recent Evidence

Despite the results of both meta-analyses,[30,31] ongoing studies have approached the best option to stimulate respiration and achieve suitable Spo_2 values in the DR in preterm infants ≤28 weeks' gestation. Crawshaw et al.,[32] using phase contrast x-ray imaging, studied the effect of mask ventilation on glottis and epiglottis status and showed that immediately after birth, both remained predominantly closed, rendering intermittent positive pressure ventilation (IPPV) ineffective. Of note, after lung aeration, the larynx was predominantly open, allowing noninvasive ventilation to efficiently ventilate the lungs.[32] Hence in apneic preterm infants, noninvasive ventilation may be rendered inefficient because of the glottis remaining closed. However, tactile stimulation is a potent stimulator of spontaneous breathing and therefore should be routinely applied to avoid tracheal intubation.[33] Dekker et al.,[34] based on the inhibitory effect of hypoxia on spontaneous breathing, hypothesized that the use of a high Fio_2 would reduce the risk of hypoxia and increase the respiratory drive at birth. Preterm kittens were randomized to receive continuous positive airway pressure immediately after birth with either 21% or 100% oxygen. If apnea occurred, IPPV was applied with 21% or 100% to the 21% group and remained at 100% for kittens who started with 100%. Kittens receiving 21% oxygen had an unstable respiratory pattern compared with kittens on 100% oxygen. Apnea that required IPPV was significantly more frequent in kittens initially resuscitated with 21% oxygen, and recovery after apnea also showed a more unstable pattern of respiration in kittens on 21% oxygen. Thus initiating resuscitation with 100% oxygen contributed to a stable respiratory pattern and decreased the risk of apnea.[34] This group translated the results of their experiments into a small RCT in which preterm infants <30 weeks' gestation were initially ventilated with an FiO_2 of 0.3 (20 infants) versus 1.0 (24 infants).[35] The primary outcome was the minute volume of spontaneous breathing. Other clinical and oxidative stress parameters were also measured. Minute volumes, tidal volumes, and the mean inspiratory flow rate were significantly higher in the 100% oxygen group, and the duration of mask ventilation was significantly shorter. Oxygenation in the first 5 minutes was significantly higher and the duration of hypoxemia significantly shorter in infants in the 100% oxygen group. No differences in the oxidative stress marker were found. However, mortality and relevant morbidities in the neonatal period, such as BPD, IVH, NEC, or length of hospital stay, were not different between groups.[35] Despite the improvement in the immediate postnatal period, using 100% oxygen had no positive impact on clinical outcomes in the neonatal period. The beneficial effect of an initial ventilation with pure oxygen was limited to the stabilization period in the DR and did not influence longer-term clinical outcomes.

The aim should be to reach SpO_2 of 80% to 85% within 5 minutes of life. It has been shown that despite the initial FiO_2, there is little difference in the SpO_2 achieved in the first 2 to 3 minutes after birth. Moreover, reliable SpO_2 readings often are not achieved until this time elapses. Hence the chance to correctly adjust the FiO_2 to achieve an SpO_2 of 80% at 5 minutes is limited to a time span of 2 to 3 minutes. This is one of the strong arguments for starting with 100% oxygen, to reach targeted saturations and then titrate down. However, doing so only improves the infant's response in the first minutes, not the longer-term outcomes. In addition, there is a risk of unexpectedly prolonging hyperoxia, with inherent deleterious consequences. Very careful titration is necessary, starting with lower oxygen and increasing the FiO_2 rapidly if needed to avoid hypoxemia and its consequences.

To date, we still lack an SpO_2 reference range for very preterm infants, nor have we established saturation goals in the first minutes after birth. In the study by Dekker et al.[35] oxygen load was apparently lower in babies receiving less than higher initial FiO_2 in the first minutes after birth and titrating thereafter. However, there is no evidence supporting what is more detrimental—the oxygen load exposure or the peak concentration of oxygen. In this regard, the study by Dekker et al. measured 8-iso-prostaglandin F2α (8iPGF2α) at 1 and 24 hours after birth and did not find a significant increase.[35] Not all isoprostanes always reflect the presence of hyperoxic oxidative stress. In this regard, isofurans are the most reliable biomarkers to assess oxidative damage to lipids caused by hyperoxia.[36] Oxygen concentration differentially modulates the formation of isoprostanes and isofurans. As oxygen concentration increases, the formation of isofurans is favored, whereas the formation of isoprostanes becomes disfavored.[36] This could explain why, despite using 100% oxygen, the levels of isoprostanes did not increase as expected. However, the results of previous studies clearly correlate the use of higher oxygen concentrations with oxidative stress and increased incidence of associated conditions, especially BPD.[24,25] Oei et al.[37] analyzed data from 768 infants <32 weeks' GA who were enrolled in 8 RCTs and were initially resuscitated with a higher (≥0.6) or lower (≤0.3) initial FiO_2. Babies who, independent from the initial FiO_2, did not reach an SpO_2 of 80% within 5 minutes after birth had higher mortality, more severe IVH, and poorer neurodevelopmental outcomes compared with those who reached this level of oxygenation.[37]

These and other findings reflected in comprehensive updated reviews and meta-analyses should be taken into consideration before generalizing the use of a high initial FiO_2 in extremely preterm infants.[37] An infographic summarizing current evidence on initial FiO_2 for resuscitation of preterm infants is shown in Chapter 7.

Final Considerations

The key for this conundrum resides in the ability to achieve SpO_2 values between 80% and 85% within the first 5 minutes after birth in very preterm infants (<32 weeks' gestation) independently of the initial FiO_2, sex, or type of delivery. Reaching adequate oxygenation and avoiding episodes of bradycardia in the first 5 minutes after birth seems essential to enhance postnatal stability and avoid death or serious complications such as IVH.[38,39]

Based on the present evidence, consensus guidelines recommend initiating resuscitation of infants born at 28 to 31 weeks' gestation with an initial FiO_2 of 0.21 to 0.30, guiding oxygen titration up and down with the use of pulse oximetry, and aiming to achieve an SpO_2 of 80% to 85% and an HR >100 bpm within 5 minutes.[5,11,13,20]

CHAPTER 11 Respiratory Distress Syndrome

Kartikeya Makker, Colby L. Day-Richardson, Mark L. Hudak

KEY POINTS

1. **Respiratory distress syndrome (RDS) remains an important cause of morbidity and mortality in preterm infants.**
2. **The etiopathology of RDS involves structural immaturity and surfactant deficiency in the developing lung.**
3. **The diagnosis rests on the presence of characteristic clinical and radiographic features in premature infants.**
4. **Judicious use of antenatal steroids has reduced the frequency and severity of RDS.**
5. **The use of continuous positive airway pressure, technologically advanced neonatal ventilation, and the availability of surfactant preparations have changed the clinical outlook in this condition.**
6. **Heroic efforts by the neonatal community to conduct evidence-based testing of therapies have greatly advanced the science, sophistication, and outcomes of care.**

Introduction

Respiratory distress syndrome (RDS), formerly known as hyaline membrane disease (HMD) and more recently simply as surfactant deficiency, has been a topic of discussion in the medical community for over a century. The diagnosis of RDS is based on the summation of clinical observations, required respiratory support, and findings on chest radiographs rather than on a gold-standard single diagnostic criterion. HMD was first described in 1903 in the German literature by Hochheim, who detailed the presence of hyaline membranes at autopsy in the lung of an infant who had died of respiratory disease.[1] Over the next 50 years, multiple investigators proposed a variety of etiologies for HMD, including in utero inhalation of amniotic fluid.

In 1959, Avery and Mead authored a sentinel paper that compared the surface-tension-lowering abilities of extracts of minced lung from infants who had succumbed due to HMD and from infants without HMD who had died of other causes. They reported that the lung extracts of infants who died of HMD were not able to reduce surface tension on a modified surface-balance instrument, whereas lung extracts of infants who died of causes other than HMD were able to produce low surface tensions. Avery and Mead concluded that HMD was caused by a deficiency of a lung substance that prevents generalized atelectasis through its ability to reduce surface tension at the alveolar liquid-air interface.[2]

In 1959, clinicians and pathologists gathered informally and attempted to define necessary clinical criteria to diagnose HMD and to grade its severity. Some of the clinical criteria included prematurity, history of intrauterine distress, family history of respiratory distress, diabetes, birth weight, respiratory rate, work of breathing, cyanosis, temperature instability, and hypotonia. The group also discussed laboratory and radiographic and autopsy criteria for diagnosis.[3]

In 1963, President John F. Kennedy's son died of HMD at a gestational age of 34 weeks. This event accelerated a new focus on maternal and infant healthcare that the National Institutes of Health had initiated in 1962 with the creation of the National Institute of Child Health and Human Development.[1]

Research into mechanical ventilation, continuous positive airway pressure (CPAP), and eventually artificial surfactants expanded from the late 1960s into the 1980s. After years of failed attempts by the neonatology community to adapt adult techniques of mechanical ventilation to newborns, in 1971, Gregory and colleagues published a landmark study on the use of CPAP in infants with idiopathic RDS.[4] This simple technique represented the first major therapeutic advance that effectively targeted and ameliorated the underlying pathophysiology of RDS.

Unfortunately, clinical translation of Avery's observation of surfactant deficiency was delayed due to an imperfect understanding of the composition and physiologic function of natural surfactant. As a result, clinical trials that demonstrated no improvement in infants with HMD after tracheal instillation of phosphatidylcholine set back basic and clinical research on surfactant for nearly two decades. It was not until the late 1970s, when Fujiwara and colleagues showed efficacy of instillation of a bovine-derived surfactant in ameliorating lung disease in premature lambs, that interest in exogenous surfactant replacement therapy rekindled. Results from a series of in vitro studies that quantitated surface tension properties of artificial surfactants and animal studies that demonstrated efficacy of instilled artificial surfactants with respect to short-term improvements in pulmonary function led to small human trials in premature infants that replicated these effects. Subsequently, large randomized human clinical trials throughout the 1980s resulted in Food and Drug Administration (FDA) approval, in 1990 and 1991, of the first two exogenous surfactants for the prophylaxis and treatment of RDS.[1] Although surfactant replacement therapy of infants at risk for or who have established RDS significantly improved survival and reduced early respiratory morbidities such as pulmonary air leaks, the hopes of clinicians that this treatment would also translate into a reduction in the incidence of bronchopulmonary dysplasia (BPD) were soon dashed.

Pathophysiology

As with most pathologic processes in neonatology, a robust understanding of both normal in utero and abnormal ex utero development of the pulmonary airways and vascular bed is needed to understand the clinical features of RDS. Lung development begins early in

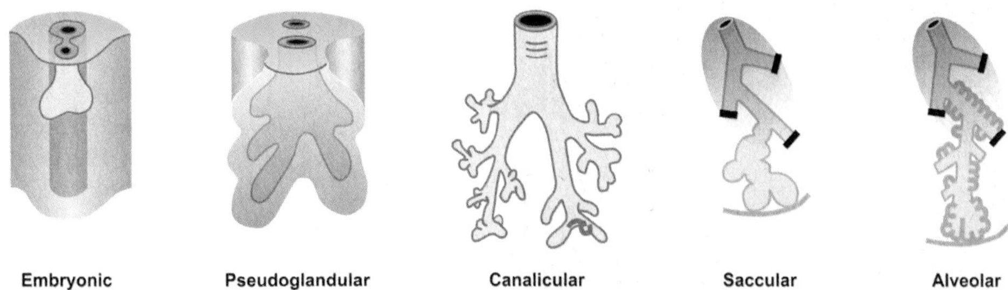

Fig. 11.1 Stages of Lung Development. There are 5 recognized stages of lung development: embryonic, pseudoglandular, canalicular, saccular, and alveolar. (Modified with permission from Sun and Mcculley. In: *Murray & Nadel's Textbook of Respiratory Medicine*. 2, 24–32.e3.)

gestation (as early as 3 weeks' gestation), and maturation progresses throughout the pregnancy, extending into childhood and potentially adolescence.[5–7] Respiratory tract development is divided into five stages, which perforce overlap but nonetheless represent different structural evolutions that occur under changing hormonal environments (Fig. 11.1). Depending at what point preterm birth exposes a neonate to unprogrammed treatment exposures and physiologic aberrations, subsequent disturbances of normal lung growth and development can have very different effects on long-term morbidity and mortality. The purpose of this chapter is not to provide a detailed description of embryology but instead to review the developmental biology briefly so that RDS and associated morbidities can be understood within the context of the embryologic background.

The first, or embryonic, stage of lung development occurs during the first 8 weeks of gestation. During this time, through complex interactions between transcription factors, growth factors, and surrounding mesenchyme, the early respiratory tract buds form from the developing foregut to create the trachea, the left and right main bronchi, and the bronchial buds (three on the right and two on the left) that will eventually become the lobes of the lungs.[6–8] The pulmonary vasculature bed also begins to form during the embryonic stage and continues to branch and mature in parallel with extension of the airway tree throughout gestation. By the end of the second, or pseudoglandular, stage at 17 weeks' gestation, branching of the large airways is completed.[7,9] The third or canalicular stage of lung development occurs between 16 and 26 weeks' gestation. Given current therapies, fetuses first become viable at 22 to 23 weeks' gestational age, in the middle of the canalicular stage. As might be expected, the formation of the first rudimentary gas exchange units occurs during this stage.[6] However, the total surface area for gas exchange is only a fraction of that of a term infant. In addition, surfactant production is minimal, with the result that most infants born at this developmental stage who are not treated with exogenous surfactant or supported very early after birth with positive distending pressure will manifest signs of RDS and be at risk to develop associated sequelae. During the saccular stage (24–38 weeks' gestation) and alveolar stage (36 weeks' gestation and beyond), expansion of acini, a dramatic increase in the surface area of the air-lung interface, maturation of surfactant production, and reduction in diffusion distance between the acinus and pulmonary capillaries combine to allow the lungs to replace the placenta as the organ of gas exchange.[7,9]

Diagnosis

The diagnosis of RDS depends on predisposing factors such as the degree of prematurity, the timing of onset, clinical conditions such as maternal diabetes, and the clinical and radiologic manifestations. The mainstay of diagnosis is radiography; findings such as low lung volumes, diffuse ground-glass haziness or a reticulogranular pattern, and air bronchograms are considered to be highly suggestive (Fig. 11.2). Exciting work on the possibility that modalities such as ultrasound and computerized

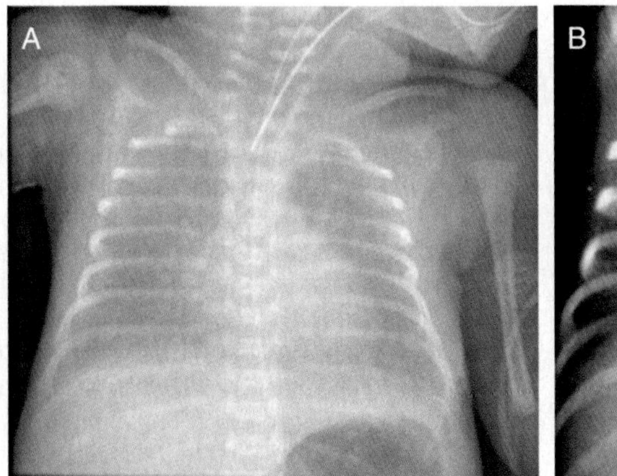

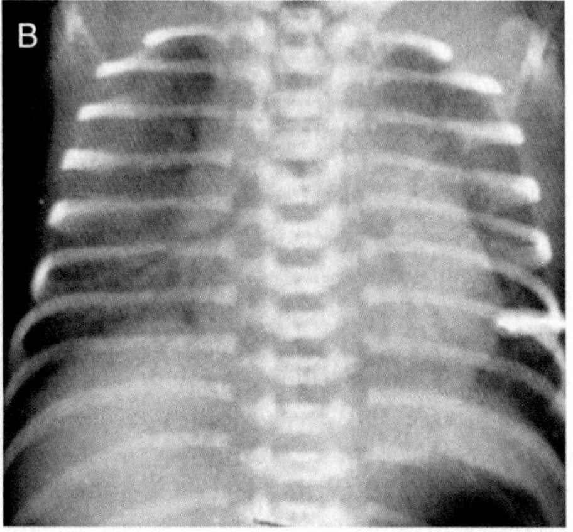

Fig. 11.2 Radiographs of Respiratory Distress Syndrome. (A) Premature infant born at 24 weeks' gestation. The radiograph shows low lung volumes, a diffuse ground-glass haziness, and some air bronchograms. (B) Large-for-gestational-age infant of a diabetic mother born at 34 weeks' gestation. There is a prominent reticulogranular pattern with air bronchograms. The haziness in the extremely premature infant reflects diffuse microatelectasis due to surfactant deficiency. The reticulogranular patten is usually caused by alveolar atelectasis, although there may be some component of pulmonary edema. The prominent air bronchograms represent aerated bronchioles superimposed on a background of nonaerated alveoli.

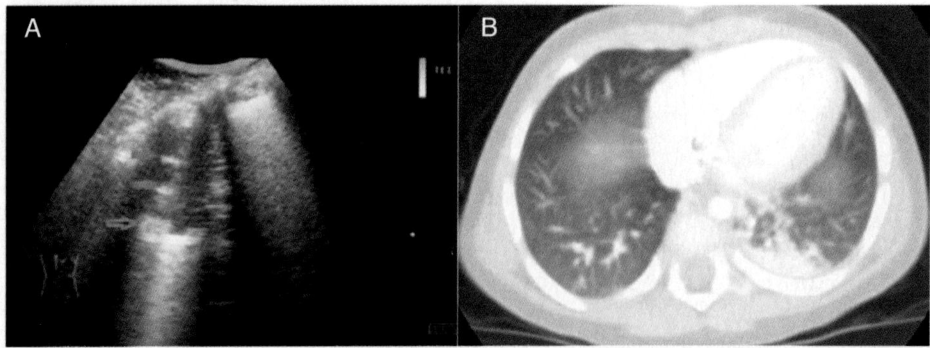

Fig. 11.3 Recent Advances in Lung Imaging Show Promise in the Assessment of Severity and in Progression of Respiratory Distress Syndrome. (A) Ultrasound of the lower left lobe with a convex probe (3.5–5 MHz) in an infant, showing hyperechoic spots and bands *(blue arrows)*. (B) A computed tomography scan shows a diffuse patten, although air bronchograms were not seen so readily. (Reproduced with permission from Quarato et al. *European J Radiol*. 2019;120:108664.)

tomography may help in the assessment of severity and/or recovery is also ongoing (Fig. 11.3).

Management

Early Interventions to Prevent RDS

In 2021, a gestational age of 22 to 23 weeks represented the earliest point in pregnancy at which preterm birth may result in a birth of an infant who survived to home discharge. However, many preterm infants who survive sustain significant respiratory and nonrespiratory morbidities. RDS is the hallmark respiratory morbidity of prematurity. Moreover, the treatment of RDS involves invasive procedures and intensive support that can lead to other complications. A major goal of prevention and early treatment strategies for RDS is to minimize other morbidities that may prolong recovery and affect the survival and long-term neurodevelopmental outcome. Although prevention or treatment of early RDS in the most premature infants does not by itself alter the likelihood of BPD, the totality of changes in the care of premature infants has altered the spectrum of anatomic, clinical, and physiologic manifestations of the "new BPD"—also referred to as chronic lung disease—among preterm survivors. Although beyond the scope of this chapter, continued focus on reducing the incidence and severity of BPD is critical because this condition can result in later infant mortality and often has long-term effects on subsequent respiratory health, neurodevelopment, and the quality of life of both the child and the family.

In this section, we will review several antenatal, delivery room, and early postnatal interventions with respect to their direct effect on the pathophysiology of RDS or their indirect effect as reflected by improved neonatal stabilization or via a reduction in the risk of later morbidity.

Antenatal Steroids

As more has been learned about the pathophysiology of RDS and the natural history of injury, repair, and development of the ventilated preterm lung, research has focused on the development of effective interventions that can reduce the severity of RDS. The most significant predisposing factor for RDS is premature birth. Administration of antenatal steroids in the setting of anticipated premature birth due to spontaneous labor or other maternal of fetal indication, for the purpose of accelerating the maturity of fetal lungs and other organs, remains the most effective antenatal therapy on behalf of the fetus. The benefit of antenatal steroids was first reported in 1969 by Liggins based on his observation that preterm lambs exposed to antenatal dexamethasone who normally would have succumbed to respiratory failure in fact had minimal respiratory dysfunction. The increase in lung inflation found on autopsy was likely due to accelerated production or secretion of surfactant.[10] Based on this seminal observation, Liggins and Howie performed a randomized controlled clinical trial in 1972 that investigated the effects of antenatal betamethasone administered to mothers with threatened preterm delivery on neonatal respiratory outcomes. Their initial study demonstrated a significant decrease in the incidence of RDS in infants whose mothers received antenatal betamethasone (9%) compared with infants whose mothers did not receive the steroids (25.8%); however, the authors noted that the difference was significant only among infants born at less than 32 weeks' gestational age and whose mothers had received treatment between 24 hours and 7 days prior to delivery.[11] Since the initial trials by Liggins and Howie, there have been many studies that have examined more focused issues related to the efficacy of antenatal corticosteroids and the potential risks of this therapy. A 2017 Cochrane Review of 30 individual studies comprising 7774 women and 8158 infants provided definitive evidence for the efficacy and safety of antenatal corticosteroids. This review also identified areas that require further study, including outcomes in countries with fewer resources, outcomes among infants in multiple-gestation pregnancies, and potential long-term adverse outcomes.[12]

The American College of Obstetricians and Gynecologists (ACOG) strongly recommends corticosteroid treatment for women between 24 0/7 and 36 6/7 weeks' gestation who are judged to be at risk of a preterm delivery within 7 days. The statement also advises consideration of corticosteroid treatment between 23 0/7 and 23 6/7 weeks' gestation, when active resuscitation is planned. This recommendation applies to multiple gestations and to pregnancies complicated by premature rupture of membranes. One additional "rescue" course of corticosteroids can be considered for women less than 34 0/7 weeks gestation who are at risk for preterm delivery within 7 days but who received their initial course of antenatal corticosteroids more than 14 days prior.[13] Some centers now offer antenatal steroid therapy in the 22nd week of gestation, based on increasing survival rates of infants born at 22 to 23 weeks' gestational age.

Delayed Cord Clamping

Until recently, clamping of the umbilical cord immediately after birth of an infant and prior to delivery of the placenta had been a routine obstetric practice. During the past two decades, multiple studies have revisited the optimal timing of cord clamping to elucidate potential benefits of delayed cord clamping (DCC) on short- and long-term outcomes of preterm and term infants. Two recent large meta-analyses of DCC in preterm infants reached different conclusions. Members of the International Liaison Committee on Resuscitation's Neonatal Life Support Task Force examined 42 randomized controlled studies of DCC and intact-cord milking (ICM) that included 5772 premature infants <34 weeks' gestational age. This analysis suggested at best a very modest survival benefit (risk ratio, 1.02) associated with either DCC or ICM, but the 95% confidence intervals for the risk ratios indicated there was no effect.[14] A second analysis reported by Canadian investigators included 56 studies that included 6852 preterm infants and found that both DCC and ICM were associated with significantly lower odds of intraventricular hemorrhage and a need for packed red cell transfusions.[15] DCC but not ICM was associated with lower odds of mortality. Nonetheless, neither study provided additional insight to alter a prior conclusion that the optimal duration of DCC is unknown.[16] In term infants, DCC increases blood hemoglobin levels after birth and iron stores during the first several months of life at the expense of a small increase in the percentage of infants who receive phototherapy to treat neonatal jaundice. Current ACOG guidelines from 2020 supported DCC for at least 30 to 60 seconds for vigorous term and preterm infants.[17]

Animal studies have suggested that resuscitation and assisted ventilation prior to cord clamping could assist with the cardiorespiratory transition at birth.[18,19] As a result, the feasibility, safety, and efficacy of resuscitation prior to cord clamping is under study.[20] A 2019 Cochrane Review concluded that data remain insufficient to provide guidance on the advisability of resuscitation prior to cord clamping.[16]

Oxygen Titration

Guidelines from the Neonatal Resuscitation Program (NRP) recommend resuscitation with 21% oxygen for infants greater than or equal to 35 weeks' gestational age and resuscitation with 21% to 30% oxygen for infants less than 35 weeks' gestational age. The NRP guidelines also provide recommended target peripheral oxygen saturations for newborns by minute after delivery to guide titration of supplemental oxygen. This focus on utilizing the lowest fraction of inspired oxygen (Fio_2) is based primarily on concerns that early high partial pressure of oxygen (Pao_2) levels increase the risk of severe retinopathy of prematurity; however, others have voiced concern that a 21% Fio_2 is insufficient for resuscitation of infants born at <28 weeks' gestational age.[21,22] A 2018 Cochrane Review also supports the need for further studies on the optimal Fio_2 at delivery.[23]

Respiratory Practices in the Delivery Room

Care for preterm infants immediately following birth has become more sophisticated during the past several decades with the advent of new pharmaceutical treatments and strategies of mechanical ventilation. A seminal 1987 report surveyed eight clinical centers to evaluate the incidence of chronic lung disease in preterm infants with birth weights between 700 and 1500 g. This report noted that one center, Columbia, reported a dramatically lower incidence of chronic lung disease among its preterm infants compared with all other centers. At the time, Columbia was the only center among the eight that initiated CPAP at birth, permitted partial pressure of carbon dioxide ($Paco_2$) levels as high as 60 torr (permissive hypercapnia), and eschewed muscle relaxants.[24] Since that controversial study, multiple other trials have compared the relative merit of CPAP to early intubation, especially in light of proposed benefits of early surfactant administration, including the COIN, SUPPORT, VON-DRM, CNRN, and CURPAP trials.[25-29] Together, these studies have shown that early CPAP reduces the need for intubation and decreases days of mechanical ventilation. However, these studies did not support that CPAP compared with early intubation significantly reduced the primary outcomes of survival and/or BPD. Others have interpreted these studies as supporting a practice that limits surfactant treatment to a rescue intervention for a select group of neonates rather than espousing routine prophylactic surfactant treatment of all high-risk neonates.[30] As a result, clinical practice has trended toward early use of noninvasive support directly after delivery rather than early intubation and surfactant treatment, although there are nuances in practice related to gestational age.

Postdelivery Care

Although the most clinically apparent effect of antenatal steroid therapy is a reduction in the incidence and/or severity of RDS due to accelerated fetal lung maturity, most postdelivery interventions and care guidelines aim to minimize other morbidities and other causes of mortality. With the increased emphasis on standardization of practice, the neonatology community has focused on choreographing care during the first "golden hour" of postnatal life. "Golden-hour" clinical protocols embrace a comprehensive bundle of practices that are supported in the evidence-based literature or that have some strong rationale based on expert consensus. This bundle best applies to the care of preterm infants who require some form of resuscitation following delivery.[31]

Postnatal Strategies to Treat Established RDS

Surfactant

The use of exogenous surfactant to prevent and treat RDS has been the standard of care for decades. Several surfactants, both synthetic and animal-derived, have reduced the incidence, severity, and some short-term respiratory morbidities associated with RDS. The composition of surfactant is increasingly better known (Fig. 11.4), and this has had exciting implications for both treatment and ongoing research focused on refining these products.

Types of Surfactants

First-Generation Synthetic Surfactants

In 1987, a multicenter trial of the synthetic surfactant pumactant (a 7:3 weight:weight ratio of the principal lung surfactant phospholipids dipalmitoylphosphatidylcholine [DPPC] and phosphatidylglycerol) demonstrated a significant reduction in mortality and respiratory support in very preterm infants even though this surfactant lacked surfactant proteins B (SP-B) and C (SP-C).[32] The development of alternate synthetic additives that were chosen to mimic the roles of SP-B and SP-C in achieving low surface tensions led to production of the first FDA-approved completely synthetic and protein-free surfactant, colfosceril palmitate (Exosurf), for the treatment of RDS in the United States. Several randomized clinical trials that tested Exosurf for the prevention and treatment of RDS showed significant reduction in neonatal and infant mortality as well as in pulmonary air leaks.[33] However, a 2001 meta-analysis established that treatment with these first-generation synthetic surfactants was associated with increased mortality and a greater risk of pneumothorax compared with treatment with animal-derived surfactants.[34] The inferiority of first-generation synthetic surfactants, as demonstrated in vitro via

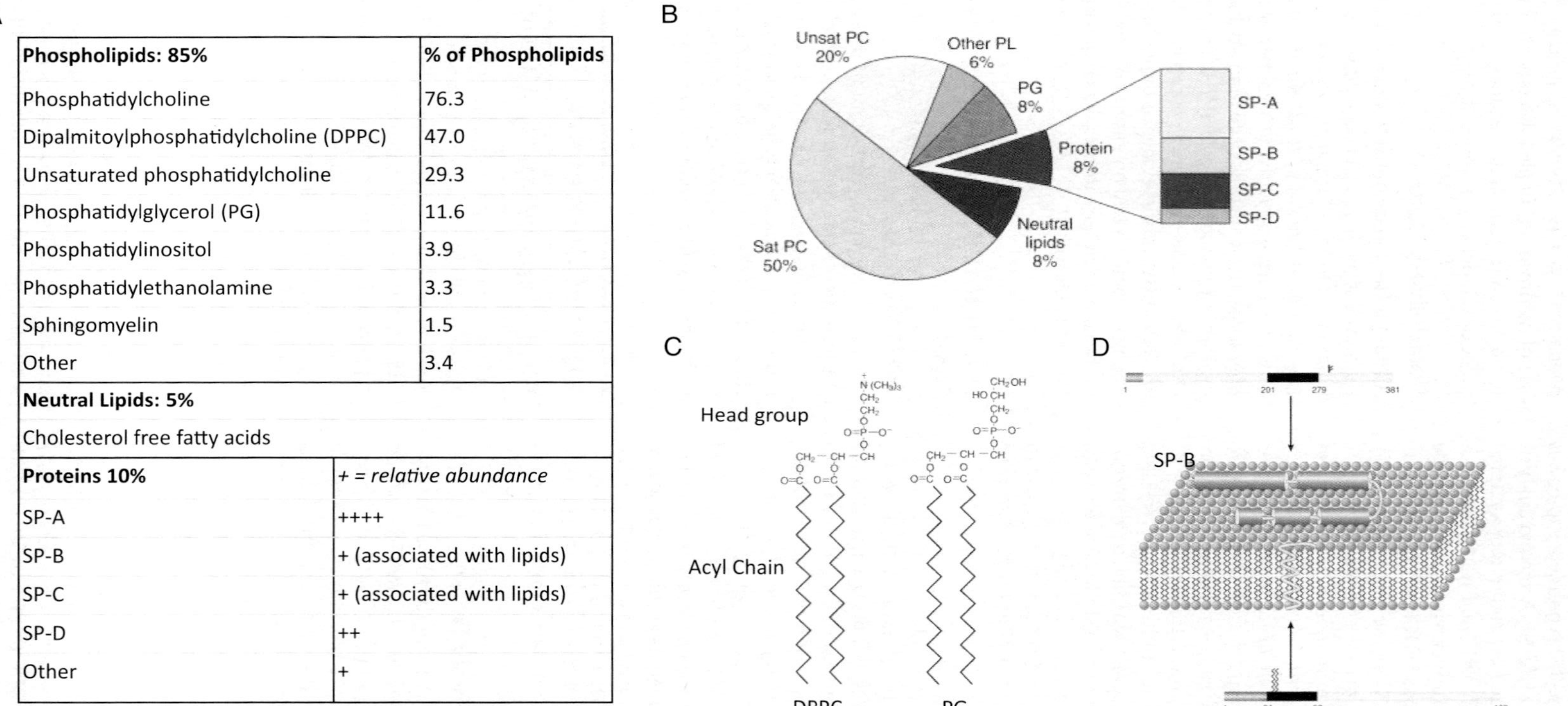

A

Phospholipids: 85%	% of Phospholipids
Phosphatidylcholine	76.3
Dipalmitoylphosphatidylcholine (DPPC)	47.0
Unsaturated phosphatidylcholine	29.3
Phosphatidylglycerol (PG)	11.6
Phosphatidylinositol	3.9
Phosphatidylethanolamine	3.3
Sphingomyelin	1.5
Other	3.4
Neutral Lipids: 5%	
Cholesterol free fatty acids	
Proteins 10%	*+ = relative abundance*
SP-A	++++
SP-B	+ (associated with lipids)
SP-C	+ (associated with lipids)
SP-D	++
Other	+

Fig. 11.4 Pulmonary Surfactant. (A) Details of chemical composition in a table. (B) Panoramic view with a pie-diagram. (C) Chemical structures of two important lipids, dipalmitoylphosphatidylcholine (DPPC) and phosphatidylglycerol (PG). (D) location of surfactant proteins B and C, which are most critical for surfactant function. (Reproduced with minor modifications and permissions from A [a] Zacharias et al. 3, 33–48.e9; [b], Sun and Mcculley. In: *Murray & Nadel's Textbook of Respiratory Medicine*. 2, 24–32.e3; B, Kingma and Jobe. In: *Kendig's Disorders of the Respiratory Tract in Children*, 5, 57–62.e2; and C, Whitsett. In: *Fetal and Neonatal Physiology*, 80, 798–808.e1.)

bubble surfactometry and in vivo in animal models of RDS, was principally owed to the lack of substances that reproduced the critical roles of SP-B and SP-C. Exosurf eventually fell into disfavor with neonatologists due to its slower mechanism of action and its lesser ability to protect against pulmonary air leaks compared with surfactants derived from animal sources that more closely mirrored the composition of natural surfactant.

Animal-Derived Surfactants

Preliminary proof-of-concept animal studies published in the 1970 showed that preterm rabbits treated with natural surfactant that contained both phospholipids and surfactant-associated proteins reduced the clinical severity of RDS.[35]

The first successful administration of exogenous surfactant to newborn infants with RDS was reported in 1980. An open-label trial of surfactant extract from bovine lungs (surfactant TA [Tokyo Akita]) improved mean respiratory parameters in 10 preterm infants.[36] Subsequently, large, randomized, placebo-controlled or surfactant-comparison trials for the prophylaxis and treatment of neonatal RDS led to FDA approval of several surfactants in the 1990s (Exosurf, 1990; beractant [Survanta], 1991; calfactant [Infasurf], 1998; and poractant alpha [Curosurf], 1999). These surfactants differ in source, mode of preparation, composition, in vitro profile of surface tension properties, and in vivo profile of onset, magnitude, and duration of physiologic effects in animal models of RDS.[37] Exosurf is a completely synthetic surfactant; Survanta and Infasurf are derived from an extract of minced cow lung and from a calf lung lavage, respectively; and Curosurf is derived from an extract of minced pig lung. Survanta requires addition of synthetic DPPC, tripalmitin, and palmitic acid to achieve acceptable surface-tension-lowering capabilities; Infasurf contains no additives; and Curosurf undergoes additional processing by liquid gel chromatography to concentrate polar phospholipids. Although Curosurf has higher concentrations of DPPC and SP-B than does Infasurf, Infasurf has a higher SP-B content as a percentage of phospholipids by weight that more closely approximates the composition of natural surfactant and may provide greater protection against natural proteins such as albumin and hemoglobin that can inhibit surfactant activity in vivo.[38] Poractant alpha exhibits the lowest viscosity of all four surfactants, which may provide advantages for less invasive surfactant treatment (LIST) techniques.

Two large studies compared Exosurf and Infasurf in the prophylaxis and treatment of RDS.[39,40] The prophylaxis study demonstrated that compared with Exosurf, Infasurf significantly reduced the incidence of RDS, the severity of early lung disease, the incidence of pulmonary air leak, and the rate of mortality due to RDS but did not improve long-term outcomes including the incidence of BPD or the rate of survival without BPD.[39] A parallel study of treatment of established RDS found that compared with Exosurf, treatment with Infasurf reduced the severity of lung disease and the incidence of pulmonary air leak without translation to a reduction in BPD or survival without BPD.[40]

Trials that compared Survanta and Infasurf did not demonstrate significant differences in long-term clinical outcomes or dosing-related complications. However, among infants treated for RDS, a subgroup of Infasurf-treated infants demonstrated greater clinical improvement as evidenced by a lower inspired oxygen concentration and mean airway pressure in the first 72 hours of life and a longer interval between doses compared with infants treated with Survanta.[41–43]

The first multicenter, placebo-controlled trial of Curosurf was reported in 1988. Among 146 infants, Curosurf significantly reduced neonatal mortality (from 51% to 31%), pneumothorax (from 35% to 18%), and pulmonary interstitial emphysema (PIE) (from 39% to 23%) and increased the PaO_2/FiO_2 ratio by nearly threefold.[44] A subsequent study demonstrated that retreatment with up to two additional doses of Curosurf within 24 hours of the initial dose led to lower ventilator requirements at 2 to 4 days after randomization compared with a single treatment.[45] Subsequent studies of Curosurf showed that early treatment produced more favorable results compared with later administration.[46–48]

Six randomized comparison trials of Curosurf and Survanta have been published to date.[49–54] These studies showed that Curosurf-treated infants demonstrated more rapid reductions in FiO_2 and mean airway pressure (MAP), less frequent repeat dosing, fewer days on mechanical ventilation, lower mortality among infants less than 32 weeks' gestational age, fewer air leaks, and increased survival without BPD compared with infants treated with Survanta. In a large retrospective study, Ramanathan et al. compared 14,173 infants treated with Curosurf, Infasurf, and Survanta and found significantly higher mortality rates in infants treated with Infasurf and Survanta compared with Curosurf-treated infants.[55] However, a larger retrospective study that evaluated comparative effectiveness between these three surfactants in 51,282 infants showed no differences in mortality.[56]

A systematic review and meta-analysis of five randomized controlled trials (RCTs) compared outcomes of 529 infants who received either Curosurf or Survanta treatment for established RDS. The incidence of oxygen dependence at a postmenstrual age of 36 weeks was similar in both groups. Infants treated with low-dose (100 mg/kg) or high-dose (200 mg/kg) Curosurf demonstrated statistically significant reductions in death, the need for repeat dosing, FiO_2 administration, and durations of treatment with mechanical ventilation and supplemental oxygen. Statistically fewer deaths occurred among Curosurf-treated compared with Survanta-treated infants. The need for repeat dosing was lower with high-dose but not with low-dose Curosurf.[57] Studies of other surfactant preparations have shown that use of a higher dose is associated with better clinical outcomes.[58–61] Use of a higher dose of Curosurf results in longer physiologic half-life, a lower oxygenation index, and less frequent repeat dosing.[62] Another meta-analysis concluded that compared with treatment with Survanta, treatment with Curosurf resulted in fewer complications associated with administration, reduced the need for repeat dosing, led to greater improvements in acute respiratory parameters, and reduced the risk of mortality.[63] In the most recent Cochrane reviews, significant differences in outcomes were noted when trials of beractant were compared with poractant alpha, including a significant increase in the risk of mortality prior to discharge, death, oxygen requirement at 36 weeks of postmenstrual age, patent ductus arteriosus (PDA) requiring treatment, and patients receiving more than one dose of surfactant in infants treated with beractant compared with poractant alpha.[64] The difference in these outcomes was observed only in the studies that employed the higher initial dose of Curosurf.

Second-Generation Synthetic Surfactants

Second-generation synthetic surfactants that incorporated compounds meant to reproduce in vivo functions of SP-B or SP-C offset some of the shortcomings of first-generation surfactants. The main attractions of these surfactants were the homogeneity of surfactant preparation and the elimination of any risk related to transmission of prion-mediated disease (mad cow disease or bovine spongiform encephalopathy that results in variant Creutzfeldt-Jakob disease in humans).[65,66]

The two second-generation synthetic surfactants that have undergone clinical trials are lusupultide (Venticute) and lucinactant (Surfaxin). Venticute contains recombinant SP-C, but it was not studied in neonates and was mainly used in clinical trials in adults with acute lung injury.[67] Surfaxin contains two phospholipids, a fatty acid, and a synthetic peptide that has surface-tension-lowering properties similar to that of SP-B, and it was approved for use by the FDA in 2012.[68]

Surfaxin was compared with Exosurf and Survanta in a trial that enrolled 1294 infants born before 33 weeks' gestational age.[69] Prophylactic Surfaxin (administered within 30 minutes of life) significantly decreased rates of RDS at 24 hours after birth and significantly reduced RDS-related mortality. Compared with Exosurf, Surfaxin also reduced the rate of BPD at 36 weeks' postmenstrual age. Compared with Survanta, Surfaxin reduced RDS-related and overall deaths but did not change other morbidities associated with prematurity. The Surfaxin Therapy Against RDS (STAR) study compared Surfaxin with Curosurf in preterm infants using a noninferiority trial design but was prematurely terminated due to slow recruitment.[70] These data collectively suggest that second-generation synthetic surfactants achieve outcomes comparable to those of first-generation animal-derived surfactants. However, the advantages of Surfaxin did not outweigh practical disadvantages (the need for large volumes, prewarming, and multiple doses), and the product was withdrawn from the market in 2015.

Third-Generation Synthetic Surfactants

In animal studies, third-generation synthetic surfactant has been shown to be superior compared with Infasurf.[71] In a study with preterm lambs, a synthetic surfactant containing both SP-B and SP-C analogs (CHF 5633) resisted inactivation better than Curosurf.[72] A phase 1 human clinical trial of synthetic surfactant CHF 5633 in RDS involved 40 preterm infants born at 27 to 34 weeks' gestational age (20 infants received 100 mg/kg and 20 received 200 mg/kg). Both doses were well tolerated and showed promising clinical efficacy.[73] Recently reported phase 2 multicenter double-blind randomized controlled clinical trials compared CHF 5633 (200 mg/kg dose with repeat doses of 100 mg/kg if indicated) with Curosurf for treatment of established RDS. The FiO_2 and the respiratory severity score (defined as $FiO_2 \times$ mean airway pressure) decreased from baseline at all time points assessed ($P < .001$), but there was no statistically significant difference between groups. Moreover, the use of rescue surfactant and the incidence of BPD and mortality at day 28 were similar in the two treatment groups. No immunogenicity was detected per the report, and the authors concluded that treatment with CHF 5633 demonstrated clinical efficacy and safety similar to that of Curosurf in the treatment of preterm neonates with moderate to severe RDS.[74]

Indications for Surfactant Administration

The American Academy of Pediatrics and the updated 2019 European Consensus Guidelines have recommended institution of nasal CPAP as the first treatment modality for an infant at risk for and demonstrating clinical signs of RDS, with deferment of intubations and surfactant administration until or unless the infant demonstrates apnea or develops severe disease.[75–77] These guidelines suggest that subsequent surfactant administration (persistent requirement of an FiO_2 >30%) may decrease mortality and morbidity in infants with RDS born before 30 weeks' gestational age. Multiple doses of surfactant using the INSURE procedure (intubate, administer surfactant, extubate) has also been successfully used and has not been shown to worsen outcome.[78]

The 2019 European Consensus Guidelines state that infants should be given natural surfactant, preferably as an early rescue treatment, if there is evidence of RDS ($FiO_2 > 0.30$ on CPAP pressure of at least 6 cm H_2O). They suggest administering higher doses of Curosurf (200 mg/kg) and support less invasive surfactant administration (LISA) as the preferred mode of administration in spontaneously breathing infants.[76]

Timing of Surfactant Administration

Prophylaxis Versus Rescue Surfactant

In an era where antenatal treatment with steroids is nearly universal, the strategy to treat with prophylactic surfactant compared with a strategy of immediate lung recruitment using nasal CPAP is associated with a greater risk of death or BPD (risk ratio [RR], 1.13; 95% confidence interval [CI], 1.02–1.25).[79] Hence, in infants who have the advantage of adequate antenatal steroid exposure and where the resuscitation team can achieve effective lung recruitment with nasal CPAP or noninvasive ventilation (NIV), surfactant therapy in the delivery room can be safely deferred.

Early Versus Delayed Rescue Surfactant

One clinical trial that compared the two strategies of early versus later threshold-based intratracheal surfactant treatment of preterm infants on nasal CPAP showed that early rescue treatment was associated with significantly less need for intubation and/or death before 7 days of life and lower mortality at hospital discharge.[80] A similar clinical trial a decade later demonstrated significantly less need for intubation as well as less a lower incidence of air leaks associated with early rescue treatment.[28] A decrease in the duration of mechanical ventilation is an important clinical outcome, especially when medical resources are limited, and it may result in less BPD in both developed and low-resource areas. However, the optimal timing for surfactant administration remains unclear, especially among infants treated with NIV.

Techniques of Surfactant Administration: INSURE, INSURE, and INRecSURE

Initially, surfactant administration occurred via prophylactic rapid bolus intratracheal instillation (to a fluid-rich lung in the delivery room) in infants at high risk for RDS or by slower infusion of multiple aliquots in infants with established RDS after endotracheal intubation. Prophylactic surfactant has fallen into disfavor because clinicians prefer to recruit surfactant-deficient lungs with early application of nasal CPAP and/or initiation of NIV support and to reserve surfactant treatment only for infants who exceed a prespecified threshold of respiratory support. The INSURE procedure originated in the early 1990s as an attempt to reduce the duration of an indwelling endotracheal tube.[81,82] This technique involves surfactant instillation after endotracheal tube intubation followed by rapid extubation after a brief period of mechanical ventilation. Leone et al. showed that the INSURE procedure resulted in a longer duration of improved oxygenation compared with rescue surfactant administration during invasive mechanical ventilation. In addition, premature infants treated with INSURE developed fewer respiratory comorbidities, including pneumothorax, BPD, and death or BPD.[83] A recent meta-analysis that included nine clinical trials and 1551 infants compared INSURE to CPAP alone. There were no statistically significant differences between early INSURE and CPAP alone for all outcomes, such as the combined outcome of BPD and/or death, BPD, death, air leaks, severe IVH, neurodevelopmental delay, or death and/or neurodevelopmental impairment.[84] The authors concluded that "currently, no evidence suggests that either early INSURE or CPAP alone is superior to the other." Although INSURE minimizes the duration of invasive ventilation, it may not represent the ideal method of surfactant administration because of (1) the need to administer opioid medication before intubation and (2) the not infrequent reluctance of providers to extubate promptly. Concerns that even a brief period of ventilation can initiate lung injury in a vulnerable preterm infant have led to the exploration of alternative surfactant administrations strategies to avoid tracheal intubation. This has led to use of the laryngeal mask airway (LMA) and special catheters such as feeding tubes for surfactant instillation and to the development of a modified INSURE (mINSURE) procedure.

A randomized trial of the LMA among preterm infants with RDS with a gestational age greater than 29 weeks and a birth weight greater than 1000 g found a decreased need to initiate mechanical ventilation in the LMA compared with the INSURE group.[85] The mINSURE procedure typically involves surfactant administration using a small tube (e.g., a feeding tube, an angiocatheter, or a specially made small-diameter catheter) while the baby is breathing spontaneously on nasal CPAP or nasal intermittent positive pressure ventilation (NIPPV), without using premedication. This technique, most commonly termed LISA[86,87] or minimally invasive surfactant treatment (MIST),[88,89] is currently being studied in many centers around the world. Investigators have used many other names for the mINSURE procedure, including avoidance of mechanical ventilation, surfactant without intubation, the Take Care method, Sonda Nasogastrica SURfactante Extubacion (SONSURE), Early CPAP and Large volume Modified InSure Technique (ECALMIST), and Minimally Invasive SURFactant administration (MISURF). Kanmaz compared surfactant administration in infants breathing spontaneously on CPAP using a 5F sterile flexible nasogastric tube (Take Care) with the INSURE procedure. The duration of CPAP and mechanical ventilation and the incidence of BPD were significantly shorter in the Take Care group compared with the INSURE group. With a decreased need for and duration of mechanical ventilation, infants in the Take Care group had a lower rate of BPD.[90] Use of the LISA technique in a single-center cohort of 224 infants born between 23 and 27 weeks' gestational age was associated with significantly higher survival rates and decreased incidences of total IVH, severe IVH, and cystic periventricular leukomalacia.[91] In a similar study, infants on CPAP who received surfactant replacement therapy via a thin catheter experienced a significantly lower rate of intubation and mechanical ventilation compared with infants treated using the INSURE procedure (19.2% versus 65%). In addition, the incidence of BPD was lower among infants who received surfactant via a catheter.[92] In a recent multicenter trial from the German neonatal network, use of the nonintubated surfactant application (NINSAPP) technique in 211 preterm infants born between 23 and 26 weeks' gestational age resulted in significantly higher combined survival without severe adverse events compared with administration of surfactant via an endotracheal tube to infants on mechanical ventilation.[93] In another study, MIST has been shown to result in a rapid and homogenous increase in end-expiratory lung volume and improved oxygenation.[94]

A systematic review and meta-analysis of six RCTs using mINSURE or LIST techniques to administer Curosurf in premature infants with RDS resulted in decreased risks of BPD (RR, 0.71 [0.52–0.99]; number needed to treat [NNT], 21), death or BPD (RR, 0.74 [0.58–0.94]; NNT, 15), early CPAP failure (RR, 0.67 [0.53–0.84]; NNT, 8), and invasive ventilation requirements (RR, 0.69 [0.53–0.88]; NNT, 6). Compared with INSURE, LIST decreased the risks of BPD and/or death (RR, 0.63 [0.44–0.92]; NNT, 11) and of early CPAP failure (RR, 0.71 [0.53–0.96]; NNT, 11).[95] In another meta-analysis, the use of the LISA technique reduced the composite outcome of death or BPD (RR, 0.75 [95% CI: 0.59–0.94]; P = .01) and BPD at 36 weeks' postmenstrual age among survivors (RR, 0.72 [0.53–0.97]; P = .03), the use of mechanical ventilation within 72 hours of birth (RR, 0.71 [0.53–0.96]; P = .02), and the use of mechanical ventilation at any time before hospital discharge (RR, 0.66 [0.47–0.93]; P = .02). There were no differences in total mortality and other neonatal morbidities.[96] A large, multinational, multicenter, randomized masked controlled trial (OPTIMIST TRIAL) in preterm infants born between 25 and 28 weeks' gestational age that compares surfactant delivery using a semirigid surfactant instillation catheter to sham treatment is currently underway.[97]

A 2021 report of a multicenter trial of 35 centers (involving 218 spontaneously breathing infants on nasal CPAP who met failure criteria) compared outcomes in infants randomized to INSURE versus a novel method of surfactant administration and rapid extubation after lung recruitment with high-frequency oscillation (INtubate-RECruit-SURfactant-Extubate: IN-REC-SUR-E). The use of mechanical ventilation during the first 72 hours of life was reduced in the IN-REC-SUR-E group (40%) compared with the IN-SUR-E group (54%; adjusted RR, 0.75; 95% CI, 0.57–0.98; P = .04; NNT, 7.2; CI, 3.7–135). Infants in the IN-REC-SUR-E group had nonsignificantly lower rates of mortality at discharge (19% in the IN-REC-SUR-E group versus 33% in the IN-SUR-E group), pneumothorax (4% versus 6%), and severe (grade 3 or 4) IVH (12% versus 15%). The authors speculated that the decreased use of mechanical ventilation in the first 72 hours may facilitate successful use of noninvasive respiratory support strategies.[98]

Some trials have studied even less invasive methods of surfactant administration by aerosolization, nebulization, or atomization. Actual or theoretical advantages of administering aerosolized surfactant include ease of administration, avoidance of hypoxemia, more homogenous distribution, less likelihood of airway complications, and less use of mechanical ventilation. In an open-label pilot study of aerosolized Surfaxin, the authors concluded that aerosolized surfactant could be safely given via CPAP as an alternative to surfactant administration via endotracheal tube.[99] Another study examined the feasibility of administering two doses of aerosolized Survanta (100 versus 200 mg phospholipid/kg) in infants on noninvasive respiratory support (high-flow nasal cannula [HFNC], nasal CPAP, and NIPPV) through short binasal prongs within 72 hours of birth.[100] Cummings et al. randomized infants with early RDS to aerosolized Infasurf or conventional therapy and found that aerosolized surfactant reduced the rate of intubation and mechanical ventilation by nearly 50% but did not affect respiratory or survival outcomes at 28 days.[101]

Other Respiratory Approaches

Caffeine Therapy

Many centers have adopted caffeine therapy as a standard practice in the management of premature infants. The typical loading dose of caffeine citrate is 20 mg/kg loading followed by a daily maintenance dose of 5 to 10 mg/kg. The Caffeine for Apnea of Prematurity (CAP) trial showed that caffeine was associated with earlier extubation and a reduced use of supplemental oxygen at 36 weeks' postmenstrual age. Most notably, neurodevelopmental follow-up through 18 to 21 months' corrected age showed significantly lower rates of cerebral palsy and cognitive delay in infants randomized to caffeine therapy.[102] The literature supports a strategy of early caffeine administration, before the onset of apnea of prematurity, to achieve maximum efficacy.[103–105]

Permissive Hypercapnia

Under the theoretical framework that the likelihood of BPD increases with longer exposures to supplemental oxygen and positive pressure ventilation, it was reasonable to test the hypothesis that use of ventilatory strategies that minimize volubarotrauma might reduce the incidence of BPD. One anticipated consequence of less aggressive mechanical ventilation is a higher $Paco_2$, referred to as permissive hypercapnia.

To date, no evidence supports greater efficacy for ventilation strategies that result in permissive hypercapnia. In fact, *post hoc* analysis of data from the SUPPORT trial showed an association between higher $Paco_2$ and a greater risk of death, intraventricular hemorrhage, BPD, and adverse neurodevelopmental outcome.[106] The Permissive Hypercapnia in Extremely Low Birthweight Infants (PHELBI) trial randomized ventilated preterm infants to two target Pco_2 levels for the first 14 days of ventilation, the higher arm reaching about 75 mm Hg and the lower arm about 60 mm Hg.[107] In this study, the primary outcome of death or BPD was the same in both groups. Moreover, the rates of mortality, intraventricular hemorrhage, and retinopathy of prematurity did not differ between groups. Results from these important trials highlight the need for further evaluation of ideal $Paco_2$ targets in preterm infants.

Postnatal Steroids

Lung inflammation is a characteristic finding in neonates who develop BPD. Strategies that reduce lung inflammation during the acute stage of RDS may potentially limit the time on mechanical ventilation and the incidence or severity of BPD. Dating back to the presurfactant study by Avery and colleagues, neonatologists have used postnatal steroids under diverse treatment protocols.[108] Enthusiasm for steroid use has waxed and waned over time, and it is fair to summarize that no consensus exists about an optimal treatment protocol. Although many studies showed that postnatal dexamethasone therapy improved short-term respiratory outcomes and decreased BPD, steroid treatment has declined dramatically after investigators identified an association with an increased risk of cerebral palsy.[109] However, BPD is also associated with death and adverse neurologic outcomes, and it is possible that infants who are at high risk of or have severe BPD might, on balance, benefit from steroid treatment.[110] A short course of low-dose dexamethasone (<0.2 mg/kg/day) is an option for infants who remain intubated, especially after 1 to 2 weeks.[111] Inhaled budesonide could be a viable alternative to systemic steroids. A large RCT of 863 infants showed that treatment with early (<24 hours after birth) inhaled budesonide significantly reduced the incidence of BPD (from 38% to 28%); however, a nonsignificant increase in mortality was also noted (16.9% versus 13.6%).[112]

Inhaled Nitric Oxide

Inhaled nitric oxide (iNO) achieves pulmonary vasodilatation and theoretically has anti-inflammatory effects. A meta-analysis of all clinical trials that have tested the hypothesis that iNO will decrease BPD or the combined outcome of mortality or BPD has concluded that neither routine prophylactic iNO initiation nor rescue therapy with iNO improves these outcomes. The state of the evidence is that that nitric oxide should not be used to treat preterm infants with RDS or later respiratory conditions that result in hypoxemia. Some evidence suggests that use of iNO in the premature infants with pulmonary hypoplasia and/or documented pulmonary hypertension, by extrapolation to studies in term neonates, may improve outcomes.[113]

Noninvasive Ventilation

NIV (e.g., modes of ventilation that do not require endotracheal intubation) is considered the preferred method of providing support to preterm infants with RDS. NIV modalities include CPAP devices, NIPPV, and humidified oxygen delivered by HFNC. Traditionally, noninvasive methods were used as a step-down from ventilation through an endotracheal tube, and initially, CPAP was the only method used. Further studies showed that initiation of CPAP immediately upon delivery followed by intubation and surfactant administration if needed was not inferior to strategies of routine intubation for stabilization or prophylactic surfactant administration.[85]

Many centers have adopted NIPPV as their primary mode of ventilatory support, using conventional ventilators to deliver peak inspiratory pressures.[114] NIPPV has been shown to reduce extubation failure, but it has not consistently been associated with a reduction in BPD. Studies in which NIPPV was most successful used synchronization of inspiratory pressure; however, delivering effective synchronization using flow sensors is challenging due to large leaks during CPAP, and it is unclear whether unsynchronized NIPPV is less effective.[115]

The use of heated humidified HFNC as an alternative to CPAP has increased in popularity as a respiratory support for newborn infants due to its relative ease of use and perceived improvement in patient comfort. A recent meta-analysis of 15 studies comparing HFNC with other modes of noninvasive respiratory support showed similar rates of efficacy for preventing treatment failure, death, and BPD. Additionally, following extubation, HFNC was reported to be associated with less nasal trauma and might be associated with reduced pneumothorax compared with nasal CPAP.[116] However, the role of HFNC as a first-line therapy for RDS has been studied in only a few trials, most of which have employed noninferiority designs. HFNC was used as the first-line mode of respiratory support in the delivery room in a small study that demonstrated feasibility,[117] but in a large multicenter clinical trial that compared HFNC with nasal CPAP as the initial support modality for preterm infants with respiratory distress, neonates managed with HFNC had a significantly higher rate of treatment failure than neonates whose care was managed with nasal CPAP (25.5% versus 13.3%).[118] Further studies are needed to evaluate the safety and efficacy of HFNC in subgroups of extremely preterm infants and to compare different HFNC devices.

In one noninferiority trial, a total of 316 infants were randomized either to HFNC (4–6 lpm) or CPAP/BiPAP (4–6 cm H_2O), and the initiation of mechanical ventilation within 72 hours from the beginning of respiratory support was examined as the primary outcome. Failure occurred in 10.8% versus 9.5% of neonates in the HFNC and CPAP groups, respectively (95% CI of risk difference, 6.0%–8.6% within the noninferiority margin; $P = .71$). The authors concluded that use of HFNC resulted in profile of safety and efficacy similar to that of the use of CPAP/ bilevel positive airway pressure (BiPAP) as the initial approach to managing preterm infants more than 28 weeks' gestational age with mild to moderate RDS.[119] In another recent and larger trial, 754 infants were randomized to either HFNC or CPAP in nontertiary intensive care nurseries. The primary outcome was a predefined treatment failure within 72 hours after randomization. Treatment failure occurred in 78 of 381 infants (20.5%) in the HFNC group and in 38 of 373 infants (10.2%) in the CPAP group (risk difference, 10.3 percentage points; 95% CI, 5.2–15.4).[120]

Mechanical Ventilation Strategies

Almost 50% of extremely preterm infants with RDS do not tolerate NIPPV and progress to intubation and mechanical ventilation.[121] Common to all mechanical ventilation strategies for RDS is the tenet of optimizing lung volumes for gas exchange without overdistending airways or alveolar units, thus avoiding volubarotrauma and hypocarbia. Hyperdistention increases the risk of air leaks such as pneumothorax and PIE. Using too low a mean airway pressure in an infant with RDS, on the other hand, will result in atelectasis that impairs gas exchange.

Pressure-limited, flow-cycled ventilation and volume-targeted ventilation are the most common modes used. Pressure-limited ventilation does not have any control over volume generated and potentially leads to excess tidal volumes, especially in the setting of rapid compliance change after surfactant administration in infants with RDS. Excessively high-tidal volumes expose the lung to volutrauma from overdistention, and the increased minute ventilation can cause hypocarbia that has been associated with certain types of brain injury.[122,123] In contrast, low-tidal volumes may cause uneven inflation of alveoli, resulting in hypercarbia and an agitated infant who must assume an increased work of breathing. A volume-targeted mode, on the other hand, delivers controlled tidal volumes and automatically will wean distending pressure as lung compliance improves. Compared with pressure-cycled ventilation, the volume-targeted ventilation may reduce the rate of death and/or BPD, the rate of intraventricular hemorrhage, and the duration of mechanical ventilation.[124,125]

When high pressures are needed to achieve adequate lung inflation, many clinicians use high-frequency oscillatory ventilation (HFOV) in preference to conventional mechanical ventilation. HFOV allows gas exchange at very low-tidal volumes delivered at very fast rates while optimal lung inflation is maintained using a continuous high distending pressure. A recently updated meta-analysis of RCTs that compared HFOV with conventional ventilation showed that use of elective HFOV compared with conventional ventilation resulted in a small reduction in the risk of BPD, but this evidence was weakened by the inconsistency of this effect across trials. In addition, infants managed with HFOV experienced a higher rate of acute air leak. Adverse effects on short-term neurologic outcomes have been reported in some studies, but these effects did not achieve overall significance. Most trials reporting long-term outcome have not identified any difference.[126]

Infants with air leaks, including PIE, can be effectively managed with the high-frequency jet ventilator (HFJV). The HFJV offers theoretical advantages compared with HFOV, including lower frequencies and higher expiratory times and the ability to "sigh" the lungs using a low rate of conventional breaths.

Irrespective of the choice of ventilator used, clinicians should be careful to avoid the extremes of hypocarbia and hypercarbia due to their association with an increased risk of BPD, periventricular leukomalacia, and intraventricular hemorrhage. Continuous end-tidal CO_2 monitoring can be helpful, especially during the first few days of ventilation. Weaning of pressure support should commence immediately upon establishment of effective gas exchange or improvement in lung compliance.

Nonrespiratory Strategies

Temperature Control

Maintaining body temperature between 36.5°C and 37.5°C during delivery room stabilization and NICU admission is extremely important for preterm infants. To facilitate achieving this goal, labor and delivery units should provide an environmental temperature greater than 25°C at the time of delivery of a preterm neonate. Initial stabilization of neonates less than 32 weeks' gestational age should be performed using a polyethylene bag under a radiant warmer.[127] Warming and humidification of gases required for stabilization are helpful in achieving normothermia.[128]

Following admission to the NICU, the premature neonate should be managed in servo-controlled incubators set at 36.5°C with high relative humidity to reduce insensible water losses.[129] For very premature infants, who have gelatinous skin and very high insensible water loss, a humidity of 70% to 80% is required initially, which can be reduced over time as the skin keratinizes and insensible losses decrease. Infants should be maintained in a thermal environment that maintains the core body temperature between 36.5°C and 37.5°C.

Fluid Management

Maintaining fluid balance can be challenging, because the most premature neonates initially can lose very high amounts of fluid per kilogram of body weight via evaporation through an immature skin barrier. One goal of fluid administration is to achieve a slightly negative balance to allow the reduction in extracellular fluid that occurs naturally after birth. Excessive fluid intake has been independently associated with higher rates of PDA, necrotizing enterocolitis, and BPD.[130]

Routine use of diuretics (particularly furosemide) in preterm infants with RDS should be avoided due to lack of demonstrated benefit.[131] Diuretic use often leads to electrolyte abnormalities, especially hyponatremia and hypokalemia, as well as hypochloremic alkalosis, which may elevate Pco_2 and result in higher ventilatory pressures.

Nutritional Management

Parenteral nutrition should be started immediately after admission to the NICU. Early initiation of amino acids leads to positive nitrogen balance,[132] decreases time to regain birth weight, and increases the rate of weight gain through discharge.[133] Minimal enteral nutrition with breast milk should be initiated as soon as possible. Breast milk is the preferred option for initiation of feeding; however, if unavailable, donor breast milk is a reasonable alternative to formula feeding and may reduce the risk of necrotizing enterocolitis.[134]

Judicious Use of Antibiotics

Traditionally, clinicians treat premature infants with RDS with antibiotics on the supposition that maternal infection is a cause of premature birth. More recent evidence has shown that routine prolonged antibiotic use without any evidence of infection may result in greater harm. Hence, antibiotics should be used more judiciously and discontinued promptly when there is no clear evidence of infection.[135–137] Neonatal treatment with antibiotics is not indicated when preterm delivery occurs for maternal or fetal indications without preterm labor or evidence of maternal infection.

Cardiovascular Management

In premature infants, blood pressure is lower in the first few hours of life and increases gradually during the first 24 hours of life.[138] Blood pressure varies with gestational age as well as chronologic age.[139] Hypotension in infants with RDS may result from hypovolemia, large left-to-right ductal shunts, or myocardial dysfunction.

Hypovolemia can be minimized by delaying cord clamping. When cautious volume expansion is unsuccessful, dopamine is more effective than dobutamine in increasing blood pressure and also may improve cerebral blood flow in hypotensive infants.[140] Epinephrine and hydrocortisone are typically used to treat refractory hypotension when other options have failed to optimize blood pressure and systemic perfusion.

PDA in very preterm infants with RDS can cause low blood pressure, poor systemic tissue perfusion, and pulmonary edema and may delay weaning from mechanical ventilation. Permissive tolerance of PDA in an infant without clear hemodynamic instability is an acceptable strategy if the infant is thriving, tolerating feeds, and requiring minimal respiratory support.[141]

Complications of Treatment

The routine use of antenatal steroid therapy and the avoidance of atelectasis with early initiation of positive pressure and/or surfactant administration has significantly reduced early pulmonary complications associated with RDS. Complications still occur related to the underlying nature of the disease or to therapeutic interventions such as placement of arterial catheters, the use of supplemental oxygen and positive pressure ventilation, and the use of endotracheal tubes.

Complications Due to Endotracheal Tubes

Adverse events related to intubation can occur in as many as 40% of neonates.[142] Displacement or misplacement of the endotracheal tube may occur on occasion. Inadvertent endotracheal tube positioning into a main stem bronchus (usually the right) is the most common occurrence and results in hyperinflation of the ventilated lung and atelectasis of the contralateral lung. The hyperinflation increases the risk of acute air leak. Other complications associated with prolonged intubation include subglottic stenosis and atelectasis after extubation.[143] Esophageal and pharyngeal perforations are rare and usually occur with devastating results in the most fragile and premature neonates.

Pulmonary Air Leaks

Pulmonary air leaks are common acute complications of RDS and occur with an incidence of approximately 6% in all low birth weight infants.[144] Air leaks result from the rupture of overdistended alveoli. These may occur during spontaneous breathing (in the era before ventilators, the incidence of pneumothorax was 25% in neonates with RDS) or in association with positive-pressure mechanical ventilation. Air may dissect toward the hilum, resulting in a pneumomediastinum, or more commonly into the pleural space, resulting in a pneumothorax.

Less commonly, air may dissect into the pericardial space, subcutaneous tissue, or peritoneal space to produce pneumopericardium, subcutaneous emphysema, or pneumoperitoneum, respectively. In the preterm infant, the more abundant and compliant perivascular connective tissue allows air to be trapped in the perivascular space, producing PIE.

The risk of pneumothorax increases with decreasing gestational age. Pneumothorax can also result from progressive lung overinflation as compliance improves after surfactant administration. Pneumothoraces can be managed by insertion of tubes or catheters connected to a negative pressure drainage system, and they usually resolve within days. On the other hand, intrapulmonary air leak (pulmonary interstitial emphysema) cannot be relieved by negative pressure drains and often takes more than 5 days to resolve.

Pneumothorax may occur spontaneously within the first few breaths, and if large, it will present with tachypnea, grunting, and retractions. In larger neonates who are more difficult to transilluminate, a chest radiograph may be required to differentiate it from RDS. Pneumothorax in a neonate on ventilatory support often presents acutely with an acute increase in heart rate, decrease in blood pressure due to cardiac tamponade, and sudden onset of hypoxemia and hypercapnia. Pneumothorax should always be suspected in neonates who have recently been treated with surfactant if they experience a sudden clinical deterioration after treatment.

A bronchopleural fistula is an abnormal acquired communication between the bronchial tree and pleural space. Clinically, this may present as a persistent air leak or as a failure of the lung to reinflate despite good chest tube drainage for greater than 24 hours. Neonates with a large fistula are difficult to ventilate (because most tidal volume is diverted through the fistula) and demonstrate persistent lung atelectasis and delayed weaning from mechanical ventilation.

Ventilator Management of Complications of RDS

Management of pneumothorax is based on the cause and severity of illness. Most often, pneumothoraces require continuous drainage and resolve within days. To minimize the likelihood of air leak, ventilatory parameters should be adjusted to maintain tidal volumes of 3 to 4 mL/kg and inspiratory times of approximately 0.3 seconds. A tension pneumothorax may be temporarily treated by needle aspiration but almost always requires subsequent chest tube placement due to a continuing large air leak. High frequency ventilation (HFV) is the preferred modality for management of persistent or refractory pneumothorax. Infants may be maintained on HFV until the pneumothorax resolves completely. Some infants may be able to be extubated to NIPPV.[145]

Infants with PIE are managed conservatively. The majority of these infants are extremely premature and already receiving significant ventilatory support. Most often these infants are transitioned to HFOV or HFJV. Lower peak pressures provided by HFV aid in decreasing ongoing air leak while promoting more rapid healing of distal airway injury.[146]

An HFJV is most frequently used when a neonate fails HFOV. This mode enhances ventilation at lower peak and mean airway pressures while maintaining a constant inspiratory time. One tradeoff in maintaining lower ventilatory pressures to facilitate resolution of PIE is a transient need for higher FiO_2 (0.5–0.75). Sigh breaths are not recommended for managing infants with air leaks. Unilateral PIE may be managed by positioning the infant with the affected side down to minimize lung aeration to that side. Some severe cases have responded to selective bronchial intubation.

Management strategies for bronchopleural fistula have included conservative measures such as the insertion of one or more large caliber chest tubes to accomplish more effective drainage and allow lung healing. In general, ventilatory pressures are scaled back, and higher levels of PCO_2 are tolerated.

Most air leaks will resolve spontaneously over a few days. Small tears or punctures usually heal quickly, whereas greater structural damage to the lung or a major bronchus may not heal with conservative management, particularly if high pressures are required for adequate gas exchange. Differential lung ventilation through double-lumen tubes has been used in some cases. For proximal leaks, fiberoptic bronchoscopy and direct application of sealants have been attempted with some success. Refractory cases have been managed surgically using thoracoplasty, lung resection/stapling, pleural abrasion/decortication, or other techniques.

Summary

During the past several decades, clinicians have translated many pharmacologic and device innovations to achieve improved early pulmonary outcomes and lower mortality of infants who have or are at risk for RDS. Unfortunately, the early hope that prevention or mitigation of lung disease caused by surfactant deficiency would lead to longer term improvements in respiratory outcomes such as BPD is unrequited. Increased success in the management of RDS has instead unmasked a much more complicated pathophysiology and biology of BPD. It is unlikely that any single new future therapy that will mimic the quantum improvement in early outcomes that surfactant achieved will soon be forthcoming. Continued progress in improving the survival and long-term respiratory and neurodevelopmental outcomes of extremely preterm infants will demand meticulous attention to continuous judicious respiratory management and to other nonrespiratory issues such as optimal management of the systemic circulation, enhanced nutritional therapy, and prevention of nosocomial infections.

CHAPTER 12 Invasive and Noninvasive Ventilation Strategies

Vikramaditya Dumpa, Vineet Bhandari

KEY POINTS

1. Endotracheal tube ventilation, also known as invasive ventilation, although life-saving, is associated with lung injury, especially in premature infants.
2. Volume-targeted ventilation is the preferred mode of invasive conventional mechanical ventilation.
3. High-frequency ventilation is recommended as a rescue mode in conditions not responsive to conventional mechanical ventilation.
4. Early nasal continuous positive airway pressure (NCPAP) and selective early surfactant use is beneficial over intubation and prophylactic surfactant administration in preterm infants at risk of respiratory distress syndrome.
5. Nasal intermittent positive pressure ventilation is preferred over NCPAP to prevent extubation failure in preterm infants.
6. There is not enough evidence to suggest the use of a high-flow nasal cannula as the primary respiratory support in preterm infants, although it is a reasonable alternative for postextubation support compared with NCPAP.
7. Short binasal prongs are preferred for the delivery of noninvasive respiratory support.
8. Noninvasive neurally adjusted ventilatory assist and nasal high-frequency ventilation are promising techniques on the horizon, but more trials are needed before recommending their routine use.

Introduction

Mechanical ventilation is perhaps the most significant life-saving intervention in neonatal medicine to date. Invasive ventilation refers to the ventilation of lungs through the endotracheal route. This is achieved by the use of either a conventional mechanical ventilator or in some circumstances a high-frequency ventilator. Although invasive mechanical ventilation definitely reduces neonatal mortality, there is some morbidity associated with its use. Newborn lungs, especially those of premature infants, are vulnerable to direct damage caused by ventilation, referred to as ventilator-induced lung injury (VILI). The mechanisms of VILI include damage caused by excessive stretch of the lung tissue from large gas volumes (volutrauma), by high airway pressures (barotrauma), by repeated alveolar collapse and reexpansion (atelectotrauma), and by release of inflammatory mediators from the injured alveolar epithelium (biotrauma).[1] Injury to the immature lung can disturb the normal postnatal lung development, potentially leading to bronchopulmonary dysplasia (BPD), and it can also have untoward effects on other organs such as the brain, resulting in poor neurodevelopment.[2] The recognition of these untoward effects sparked a renewed interest in noninvasive ventilation strategies. Noninvasive ventilation encompasses any form of ventilation delivered through the nares, and the established modes include nasal continuous positive airway pressure (NCPAP), nasal intermittent positive pressure ventilation (NIPPV), and high-flow nasal cannula (HFNC). Emerging techniques of noninvasive ventilation include neurally adjusted ventilatory assist (NIV-NAVA) and noninvasive high-frequency ventilation (NIHFV). The focus of this chapter is to discuss the various modalities of invasive and noninvasive ventilation and to review the evidence, or lack thereof, supporting their use in management of newborn respiratory disease.

Invasive Ventilation

Despite the recognition of the potential hazards of invasive mechanical ventilation, it remains an invaluable asset in the initial management of extremely preterm and critically ill infants. The goal of mechanical ventilation should be facilitation of adequate gas exchange with limitation of additional lung damage. Broadly, mechanical ventilation can be classified into two categories based on the tidal volumes delivered by the machine: (1) conventional mechanical ventilation (CMV), where volumes approximating physiologic tidal volumes are exchanged intermittently through a conventional ventilator, and (2) high-frequency ventilation (HFV), where low tidal volumes, at times less than the volume of the anatomic dead space, are exchanged at an extremely rapid rate through a high-frequency ventilator.

Conventional Mechanical Ventilation

There are multiple ventilator devices commercially available in the market, with each ventilator equipped to offer many different modes of ventilation. A thorough review of the devices, modes, and modalities of ventilation is beyond the scope of this chapter, and we chose to highlight the frequently used modes and modalities of mechanical ventilation and the rationale supporting their use in the next few paragraphs.

Modes of Ventilation

There are four main modes of CMV, depending on the manner in which the ventilator initiates and terminates the inspiratory phase of the respiratory cycle (e.g., based on time or on change in flow).

Intermittent Mandatory Ventilation

Intermittent mandatory ventilation (IMV) was the standard mode of ventilation used prior to the availability of synchronized ventilation. IMV is a time-cycled, pressure-controlled mode where the ventilator delivers a set number of mandatory inflations. Here, the operator sets the rate, peak inspiratory pressure (PIP), inspiratory time, positive end expiratory pressure (PEEP), and flow rate. The patient may breathe spontaneously between the mandatory breaths, and these spontaneous breaths are supported only by the PEEP, resulting sometimes in inadequate and unstable tidal volumes. Ventilator dyssynchrony is a major disadvantage of this mode, with potential consequences of gas trapping, air leaks, and intraventricular hemorrhage (IVH).[3,4] The mode is useful when the patient is completely apneic or is under heavy sedation, but it has largely been replaced by newer modes that can synchronize the inflations to the patient's respiratory efforts and can deliver mandatory breaths.

Synchronized Intermittent Mandatory Ventilation

In synchronized IMV (SIMV) (Fig. 12.1A), the inflations delivered by the ventilator are synchronized to the onset of spontaneous patient breaths or are delivered at a mandatory rate if the patient has inadequate or absent respiratory effort. The operator sets the rate, PIP or tidal volume (depending on whether the modality is pressure controlled or volume targeted, respectively), inspiratory time (if time cycled), PEEP, and flow rate. The spontaneous breaths are supported by the PEEP, so there can be a wide variation in tidal volumes, depending on the respiratory effort of the patient. The advantages include faster weaning from mechanical ventilation and reduced need for sedation/paralysis due to ventilator-synchrony.[5]

Assist Control

In assist control (AC) mode (see Fig. 12.1B), every spontaneous breath is supported (assist), and the ventilator provides a set number of inflations if the patient does not breathe (control). AC is time cycled and pressure controlled or volume controlled. The operator sets the control rate, PIP or tidal volume (depending on pressure controlled or volume targeted modality, respectively), inspiratory time, PEEP, and flow rate. The advantages include ventilator synchrony and uniform tidal volume delivery for each breath and improved work of breathing compared with SIMV. It is important to set a control rate just below the infant's spontaneous breath rate, because a high rate can make the patient not breathe spontaneously and a low rate can lead to excessive fluctuations in minute ventilation during periods of apnea. Weaning is done by reducing the PIP or tidal volume.

Pressure Support Ventilation

Pressure support ventilation (PSV) is a flow-cycled, pressure-controlled ventilation mode (see Fig. 12.1C) used in spontaneously breathing patients and is similar to AC in that every breath is supported but is flow-cycled. The operator sets the PEEP, the flow rate, and a pressure support level, which is the support delivered to spontaneous breaths in addition to the PEEP. With flow cycling, an inflation is terminated when inspiratory flow declines to a preset threshold, generally 5% to 15% of peak flow. This eliminates the need for unnecessary inflation time (inspiratory hold) if inspiration is completed early. This results in automatic adjustment of inspiratory time depending on the lung mechanics and leads to better ventilator–patient synchrony. However, because the inspiratory time is

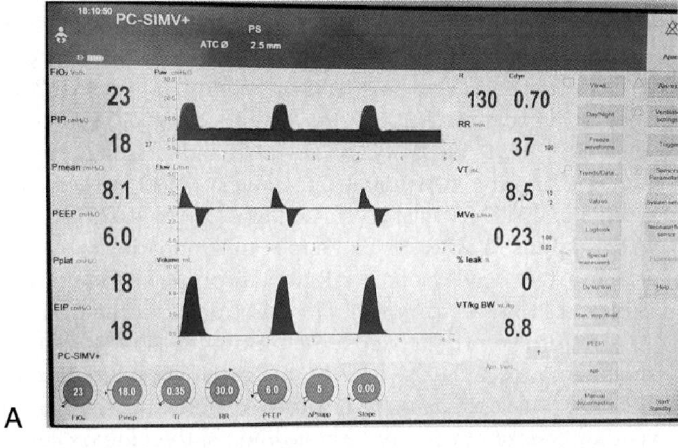

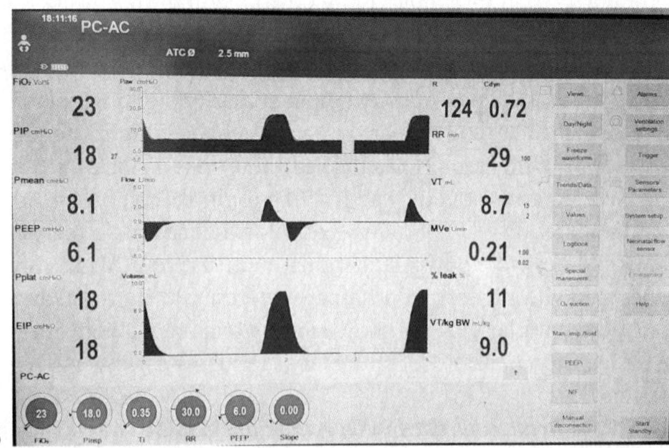

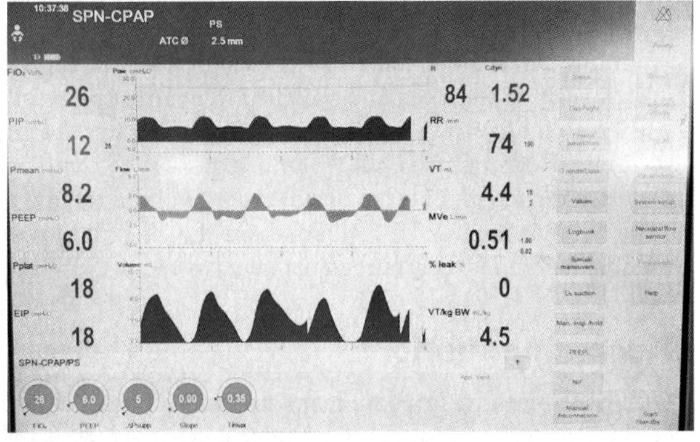

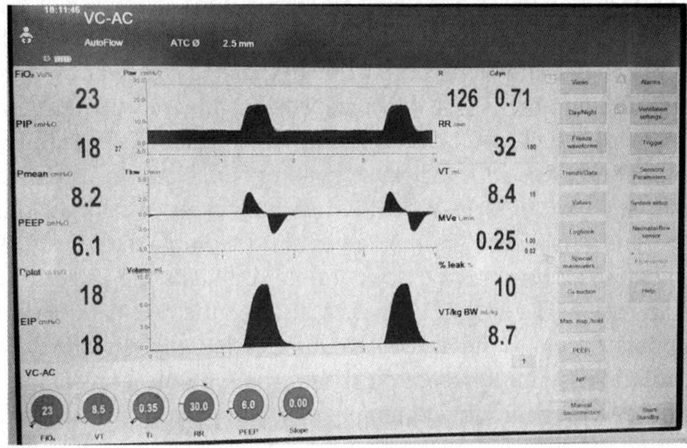

Fig. 12.1 Screenshots of Ventilator Modes. (A) Ventilator with pressure control-synchronized intermittent mandatory ventilation (PC-SIMV) mode. (B) Ventilator with pressure control–assist control (PC-AC) mode. (C) Ventilator with pressure support ventilation (PSV; spontaneous-continuous airway pressure support [SPN-CPAP/PS]) mode. (D) Ventilator with volume control–assist control (VC-AC) mode.

typically shorter, this might result in lower mean airway pressures, and hence adjusting the PEEP as necessary is important to prevent atelectasis. PSV can also be used along with SIMV, where the SIMV rate serves as the control and the spontaneous breaths are supported by the pressure support.

Modalities of Ventilation

The modality refers to the target or limit variable of the mechanical breath. There are two modalities of CMV: pressure targeted and volume targeted.

Pressure Targeted Ventilation

Ventilation where the operator targets the pressure while the volume delivered is dependent on the lung mechanics is termed *pressure targeted ventilation.* This modality of ventilation can be delivered using any of the above-mentioned modes. Time-cycled, pressure-limited (TCPL) ventilators were used extensively in the past to provide this modality of respiratory support.

Volume-Targeted Ventilation

In volume-targeted ventilation (VTV) (see Fig. 12.1D), the operator targets the volume, and the pressure delivered is dependent on the lung mechanics. Ever since the recognition that volutrauma, as opposed to barotrauma, is more injurious to the lung, there has been increased emphasis on the use of ventilation modalities that control the delivered tidal volume. Fluctuations in tidal volume can occur, with changes in lung mechanics leading to hyperventilation and excessive alveolar stretch on one hand and atelectasis and inadequate gas exchange on the other hand. Having control over the delivered tidal volume is therefore much more desirable than controlling the pressure. Despite the evidence of benefits of VTV over pressure-controlled (PC) ventilation, a survey of practicing neonatologists in the United States and Canada revealed that a majority of physicians still prefer to use PC ventilation.[6] In this survey, half of the responders cited a lack of understanding as the reason for not using VTV.[6] The use of uncuffed endotracheal tubes with resultant leak around the tube and the inability of the older ventilators to accurately measure the tidal volumes were potential barriers to the use of VTV for a long time. Most of the modern ventilators have the ability to measure exhaled tidal volume at the airway opening and have algorithms to calculate leak compensation, features that make the use of VTV more convenient.

The term *volume-controlled (VC) ventilation* is not to be used synonymously with *volume-targeted ventilation.* The VC mode, which is frequently used in adult and pediatric populations, involves delivery of a set tidal volume into the proximal end of the circuit, and the pressure changes in inverse proportion to the lung compliance. Here, the set tidal volume is not the same as the delivered tidal volume due to factors such as variable endotracheal tube (ETT) leak and compression of gas in the circuit, making it difficult to assess the desired tidal volumes. In VTV, the operator chooses a target tidal volume and a pressure limit. The ventilator compares the exhaled tidal volume of the previous inflation and adjusts the pressure to reach the set tidal volume. There is a limit on the pressure increase from one inflation to the next to avoid excessive tidal volume delivery. Inflation is also terminated if the tidal volume exceeds a set percentage above the target volume, as a safety feature. Thus, autoregulation of the inflation pressure occurs with changing lung compliance, and this results in automatic weaning without the need to manually adjust the settings based on blood gas measurements. This feature of VTV is termed the volume guarantee (VG) mode on Draeger ventilators (Draeger Medical, Lubeck, Germany) and the pressure-regulated volume control mode on Servo ventilators (Maquet, Solna, Sweden). Keszler[7] has discussed a detailed description of VTV and practical guidelines for its use in different disease conditions in a review article.

Evidence for Use of Different Modes and Modalities of Ventilation

Multiple studies on synchronized (patient-triggered) ventilation have shown beneficial effects of improved gas exchange and ventilation, consistent tidal volume delivery, and reduced breathing effort, stress, and blood pressure variability with use of synchronization.[8] However, a Cochrane meta-analysis of randomized clinical trials (RCTs) comparing synchronized (patient-triggered) to nonsynchronized CMV demonstrated no difference in outcomes of mortality, BPD, air leaks, or IVH but a benefit of shorter duration of ventilation with synchronization (mean difference [MD], −38.3 hours; 95% confidence interval [CI], −53.90 to −22.69).[5] The AC mode, compared with SIMV, was associated with a trend toward shorter duration of weaning in this meta-analysis (MD, −42.38 hours; 95% CI, −94.35 to 9.60).[5] In another meta-analysis of 20 RCTs with patients on 1 of 16 different ventilation modes, TCPL, high-frequency oscillatory ventilation (HFOV) mode, SIMV + VG mode, and VC ventilation mode were associated with lower mortality compared with the SIMV + PSV ventilation mode.[5,9] There is moderate-quality evidence from multiple RCTs to support the use of VTV in neonates. A Cochrane review of 20 RCTs comparing VTV with pressure-limited ventilation in infants concluded that use of VTV had resulted in decreased rates of death or BPD at 36 weeks' gestation (relative risk [RR], 0.73; 95% CI, 0.59–0.89), rates of pneumothorax (RR, 0.52; 95% CI, 0.31–0.87), mean days of mechanical ventilation (MD, 1.35 days; 95% CI, −0.86 to −1.83), rates of hypocarbia (RR, 0.49; 95% CI, 0.33–0.72), rates of grade 3 or 4 IVH (RR, 0.53; 95% CI, 0.37–0.77), and rates of the combined outcome of periventricular leukomalacia (PVL) with or without grade 3 or 4 IVH (typical RR, 0.47; 95% CI, 0.27–0.80).[10] A similar meta-analysis of 18 RCTs by Peng et al. comparing the outcomes of these two modes of ventilation in preterm infants showed reduced BPD, rates of hypocarbia, duration of mechanical ventilation, failure of primary mode of ventilation, grade 3 or 4 IVH, pneumothorax, and PVL with VTV but no difference in the outcome of death.[11] In a systematic review carried out to identify the optimal ventilation strategy in full-term newborns, the authors concluded that SIMV with a tidal volume of 6 mL/kg and a PEEP of 8 cm H_2O may be advantageous in full-term newborns.[12]

Infants must be weaned off invasive mechanical ventilation aggressively as tolerated and switched to noninvasive ventilation if needed to limit VILI. There are no RCTs comparing the efficacy of having a weaning protocol to limit exposure to ventilation and decrease the length of hospital stay.[13] Rather than relying on a protocol, clinicians must be vigilant about the changing dynamics of the lung and make constant adjustments as required.

Recommendations

For infants needing intubation and mechanical ventilation, there is enough evidence to suggest the use of volume-targeted ventilation modes. Synchronization of ventilation might be beneficial, with advantages of faster weaning and shorter duration of mechanical ventilation, but there is no evidence of long-term benefit. When pressure targeted ventilation is used, care should be taken to aim for adequate tidal volumes that prevent volutrauma.

High-Frequency Ventilation

HFV refers to any form of assisted ventilation in which small tidal volumes are delivered to the patient at extremely rapid rates. The advantages of HFV include the ability to deliver tidal volumes less than that of the anatomic dead space and to use low transpulmonary pressures that can result in decreased volutrauma and barotrauma compared with CMV. The small tidal volumes and attenuated pressure amplitudes at the level of the alveoli also enable the use of higher mean airway pressures, thus helping to maintain optimal lung volume without exacerbating lung injury. Another advantage is the ability to adequately and independently manage oxygenation and ventilation with HFV.

Gas transport in HFV occurs based on the mechanisms of convective flow, convection and diffusion, diffusive flow, high-frequency pendelluft, and laminar flow with Taylor-type dispersion.[14] The conventional linear relationship between minute ventilation, ventilator rate, and tidal volume does not apply in HFV. Small changes in tidal volumes bring about significant changes in ventilation. In fact, one of the primary risks of the use of HFV is the potential to cause hyperventilation leading to hypocarbia with subsequent cerebral injury, thus limiting its frequent use for respiratory insufficiency in neonates.[15]

The two most commonly used forms of HFV are high-frequency jet ventilation (HFJV) and HFOV. Although a variety of devices are approved to deliver HFV, the approved devices most commonly used in the United States are the Bunnell Life Pulse jet ventilator (Bunnell, Inc., Salt Lake City, Utah) and the CareFusion 3100A High Frequency Oscillatory Ventilator (CareFusion, San Diego, California).

High-Frequency Jet Ventilators

In the HFJV form of HFV, short pulses of pressurized gas are directly injected into the upper airway through the ETT at a rapid rate ranging from 240 to 660 pulses per minute. The gas volumes delivered are very small and even less than that of the anatomic dead space. The jet ventilator is used in conjunction with a conventional ventilator that provides PEEP and can be used to deliver sigh breaths if needed. The operator sets the PIP, rate, and inspiratory time on the jet ventilator and adjusts the PEEP on the CMV. Exhalation during HFJV is passive and results from the elastic recoil of the lungs. The inspiratory times are short (0.02–0.034 seconds) with prolonged expiratory times, making this ventilator very effective in the management of air leaks. Inhaled nitric oxide can be delivered with HFJV.

High-Frequency Oscillation

In HFOV, air is moved back and forth at the proximal ETT by a piston attached to a diaphragm at a rapid rate (typically 480–900 per minute). A constant mean airway pressure is set, which helps in alveolar recruitment and oxygenation. The amplitude of the oscillations around this mean airway pressure determines the tidal volumes delivered to the lungs and thus affects ventilation. The rapid rates make the inspiratory times very short. The operator sets the mean airway pressure, amplitude, frequency, and inspiratory time, which makes HFOV relatively easier to use than HFJV. Exhalation is an active process in HFOV, resulting from the negative pressure applied during expiration. The ability to recruit lung volume by controlling the mean airway pressure directly also makes HFOV an effective device to deliver inhaled nitric oxide.

Evidence for Use of HFV in Neonatal Respiratory Disease

Despite animal studies showing favorable outcomes with use of HFV compared with CMV, the beneficial effects were not consistently reproduced in human studies. There are no RCTs directly comparing outcomes in preterm infants who were on HFJV versus HFOV. Hence, there is no evidence to support one over the other as an elective or rescue mode in these infants.[16]

A Cochrane meta-analysis of 19 RCTs involving 4096 infants and comparing the elective use of HFOV versus CMV in preterm infants with respiratory distress syndrome (RDS) revealed no difference in mortality between the two groups. There was a reduction in chronic lung disease (CLD) at 36 to 37 weeks' postmenstrual age in the HFOV group (17 RCTs; N = 2786 infants; RR, 0.86; 95% CI, 0.78–0.96) but at the expense of an increase in the incidence of air leaks (13 RCTs; N = 2854; RR, 1.19; 95% CI, 1.05–1.34). Caution must be exercised in interpreting these data; there was significant heterogeneity between the groups, and this analysis was done on RCTs conducted over 25 years, with significant perinatal and neonatal practice changes during the period.[17,18] A systematic review by Bhuta et al. on rescue use of HFOV versus CMV in preterm infants included 1 RCT with 182 infants and it showed no significant difference in mortality or CLD but reduction in any new air leak (RR, 0.73; 95% CI, 0.55–0.96) with use of HFOV.[19] A Cochrane review of two RCTs (N = 199) comparing elective or rescue use of HFOV versus CMV in infants ≥35 weeks with pulmonary dysfunction did not show a difference in the studied outcomes, including mortality and CLD.[20] Another Cochrane review of three RCTs compared the elective use of HFJV versus CMV in preterm infants with RDS and found reduced CLD at 36 weeks in the HFJV group (two RCTs; N = 170; RR = 0.59; 95% CI, 0.35–0.99) with no difference in mortality.[21] Given no data on long-term pulmonary or neurodevelopmental outcomes from these trials, the authors did not recommend routine use of HFJV in preterm infants.[21] An RCT by Keszler et al. compared the rescue use of HFJV versus CMV (N = 166) in preterm infants with pulmonary interstitial emphysema and reported no difference in their studied outcomes including mortality and CLD.[22] A Cochrane review of the rescue use of HFJV in which only the trial by Keszler et al. met eligibility criteria concluded that there was not enough evidence to support routine use of HFJV as rescue therapy in preterm infants.[23] Table 12.1 summarizes the Cochrane reviews comparing HFV with CMV. It is important to remember that some of the above studies were done in the presurfactant era and before synchronized ventilation gained acceptance.

In summary, systematic reviews and meta-analyses suggest no clear benefit of using HFV (either HFJV or HFOV) as an elective or rescue mode for treatment of respiratory insufficiency in preterm and term neonates. Although HFV may theoretically seem to be lung-protective, there is not enough evidence to support its use to prevent air leaks. HFV has also been used with success in pulmonary hypoplasia,[24] but RCTs are not available to demonstrate this benefit. The VICI trial, comparing HFOV versus CMV as the initial ventilation strategy in patients with a prenatally diagnosed congenital diaphragmatic hernia, did not show any difference in BPD/death between the two groups, and infants randomized to the CMV group had shorter ventilation time and lesser need for extracorporeal membrane oxygenation.[25]

Table 12.1 Cochrane Systematic Reviews of RCTs Involving HFV Versus CMV and Outcomes of Mortality, CLD, and Air Leaks

Authors	Groups	Mode	RCTs/N	Criteria (GA, BW)	Mortality	CLD	Air Leaks
Cools et al.[17]	HFOV versus CMV	Elective	19/4096	Preterm and low BW (<36 weeks, 2 kg)	No difference	Reduced CLD at 36 weeks with HFOV (RR, 0.86; 95% CI, 0.78–0.96)	Increased with HFOV (RR, 1.19; 95% CI, 1.05–1.34)
Bhuta et al.[19]	HFOV versus CMV	Rescue	1/182	<35 weeks	No difference	No difference in IPPV at 30 days	Any new air leaks reduced with HFOV (RR, 0.73; 95% CI, 0.55–0.96)
Henderson-Smart et al.[20]	HFOV versus CMV	Elective or rescue	2/199	≥35 weeks	No difference	No difference	No difference
Bhuta et al.[21]	HFJV versus CMV	Elective	3/262	<35 weeks/ <2 kg	No difference	Reduced CLD at 36 weeks with HFJV (RR, 0.58; 95% CI, 0.34–0.98)	No difference
Rojas-Reyes et al.[23]	HFJV versus CMV	Rescue	1/166	<35 weeks/ <2 kg	No difference in overall mortality but decreased mortality with HFJV before crossover (RR, 0.66; 95% CI, 0.45–0.97)	No difference	No difference in new air leaks

BW, Birth weight; *CI*, confidence interval; *CLD*, chronic lung disease; *CMV*, conventional mechanical ventilation; *GA*, gestational age; *HFV*, high-frequency ventilation; *HFOV*, high-frequency oscillatory ventilation; *HFJV*, high-frequency jet ventilation; *IPPV*, intermittent positive pressure ventilation; *RCT*, randomized clinical trial; *RR*, relative risk.

Recommendations

There is not enough evidence suggesting use of HFV electively in the management of RDS in preterm neonates, but it can be trialed as a rescue therapy. We recommend use of HFV in established air leak syndromes, persistent pulmonary hypertension of the newborn, and pulmonary hypoplasia not responsive to CMV on a case-by-case basis.

Noninvasive Ventilation

Nasal Continuous Positive Airway Pressure

NCPAP is a form of respiratory assistance in which continuous distending pressure is delivered to the airway through nasal passages, which helps to maintain the lung end-expiratory volume. By maintaining adequate functional residual capacity in a spontaneously breathing infant and preventing atelectasis, NCPAP helps to decrease ventilation–perfusion mismatch and improves gas exchange and work of breathing. The NCPAP pressure is generated using a variety of devices and is delivered to the nasal airway opening via an interface. The operator sets the PEEP level, which typically ranges between 4 and 10 cm H_2O.

Depending on the technique used to control the gas flow to the patient, NCPAP systems are classified into constant-flow and variable-flow systems.

1. Constant-flow NCPAP systems, in which the gas is delivered at a set flow, include bubble NCPAP and ventilator NCPAP systems.
   a. In the bubble NCPAP system, inspiratory flow is provided from a blended gas source, whereas the expiratory side of the circuit is submersed in a water column. The depth of insertion into the water column can be adjusted, and it determines the level of NCPAP.
   b. In ventilator NCPAP, fresh gas is delivered into the inspiratory side of the circuit, and there is a pressure valve in the expiratory limb that can be adjusted to a desired level to deliver the pressure needed.
2. Variable-flow NCPAP is also known as fluidic NCPAP based on the fact that this system uses several fluidic principles of operation at the patient nasal interface. Here, gas is delivered at a varying flow rate, which generates the pressure during inspiration. There is an adaptive flip valve at the nasal interface that causes the flow of gas going toward the nares to flip around at the time of expiration and to leave the generator chamber via the expiratory limb. This phenomenon, termed the Coanda effect, minimizes exhalation against the flow of incoming gases and results in decreased work of breathing. Infant Flow (Cardinal Health, Dublin, Ohio), Arabella (Hamilton Medical, Reno, Nevada), and AirLife (Cardinal Health) are examples of variable flow NCPAP systems.

RCTs comparing the efficacy of different NCPAP delivery systems from the past few years are summarized in Table 12.2. Despite multiple RCTs,[26-33] there is lack of good evidence to suggest that any one CPAP system is superior to another for improving patient outcomes. The clinician's familiarity with a particular system and ability to respond to changes in the patient's disease process are more important factors than the benefits offered by any particular NCPAP system or device. However, bubble NCPAP has the advantage of cost-effectiveness and is an ideal NCPAP system for use in developing countries.

A variety of interfaces are used to deliver NCPAP. These include single prongs, short binasal prongs, nasal masks, long nasal prongs (also called nasopharyngeal prongs), and nasal ETTs. The long nasal prongs increase the work of breathing by increasing resistance compared with short prongs. Short binasal prongs have been shown in a Cochrane review to be superior to long nasopharyngeal prongs in preventing extubation failure and improving oxygenation.[34] There is very sparse literature on head-to-head comparisons between different interfaces. In a small crossover intervention study comparing two binasal prong interfaces in preterm infants with RDS requiring NCPAP, the RAM Cannula system (Neotech, Valencia, California) consistently delivered lower pharyngeal pressure than the set pressure when compared with Hudson prongs (Hudson RCI, Temecula,

Table 12.2 Randomized Clinical Trials Comparing Different NCPAP Delivery Devices in the Past Few Years

Authors	Eligibility	N	Groups	Outcomes
Mazmanyan et al.[30]	GA <37 weeks	125	Bubble CPAP versus flow driver	No difference in outcomes of duration of CPAP, supplemental O_2, ventilation, incidence of nasal injury, pneumothorax, and/or death
Tagare et al.[33]	GA <37 weeks	145	Bubble CPAP versus ventilator CPAP	CPAP failure less frequent in bubble CPAP
Agarwal et al.[32]	BW <1500 g	68	Bubble CPAP versus ventilator CPAP	No difference in outcome of CPAP failure
Bhatti et al.[31]	GA <34 weeks with RDS	170	Bubble CPAP versus jet CPAP (variable flow)	No difference in outcome of CPAP failure

BW, Birth weight; *CPAP*, continuous positive airway pressure; *GA*, gestational age; *NCPAP*, nasal continuous positive airway pressure; *RDS*, respiratory distress syndrome.

California) (mean pressure difference, −2.45 cm H_2O versus 0.4 cm H_2O).[35] An RCT of premature infants (n = 126) with RDS evaluating NIPPV failure on RAM cannula versus Hudson prongs showed a higher need for invasive ventilation (32.8% versus 9.6%; *P* = .002) and surfactant use (42.1% versus 19.3%; *P* = .007) in the RAM cannula group.[36]

Nasal Prongs Versus Nasal Mask

Nasal injury is a significant problem with use of nasal prongs. Nasal masks are gaining popularity as a means of decreasing or avoiding nasal injuries when delivering NCPAP. In an RCT (N = 175) by Bashir et al., NCPAP with a nasal mask significantly reduced nasal injury in comparison with nasal prongs alone and nasal prongs alternated with a nasal mask, with no difference in NCPAP failure rate.[37] In a meta-analysis of five RCTs, it was shown that use of nasal masks was associated with a decreased risk of NCPAP failure (four of the RCTs; n = 459; RR, 0.63; 95% CI, 0.45–0.88) and decreased incidence of moderate to severe nasal trauma (three of the RCTs; n = 275; RR, 0.41; 95% CI, 0.24–0.72) compared with binasal prongs.[38] In another recent meta-analysis of seven RCTs, use of a nasal mask for preterm infants requiring NCPAP was associated with a reduction in NCPAP failure (RR, 0.72; 95% CI, 0.53–0.97) and in the need for surfactant administration (RR, 0.78; 95% CI, 0.66–0.92) and a lower incidence of nasal injury (RR, 0.71; 95% CI, 0.59–0.85) and moderate to severe BPD (RR, 0.47; 95% CI, 0.23–0.95).[39] However, care should be exercised when interpreting the results, because the authors stated that the level of evidence was low to very low. The authors of the meta-analysis recommend use of nasal mask as a preferred interface in delivery of NCPAP/noninvasive respiratory support given the potential clinical benefit.

Evidence for Use of NCPAP as Primary Respiratory Support

Multiple large, multicenter RCTs have evaluated the efficacy of NCPAP in the early management of RDS. The CPAP or Intubation (COIN) trial was a large multinational RCT evaluating use of CPAP as primary respiratory support after delivery in extremely preterm infants. Six hundred and ten infants were randomized to CPAP versus intubation after birth. There was no difference in the outcome of BPD/death (odds ratio, 0.80; 95% CI, 0.58–1.12; *P* = .19), but infants in the CPAP group were exposed to lesser duration of ventilation. Although the incidence of pneumothorax was higher in the CPAP group (9% versus 3%; *P* < .001), it is important to note that these infants were started at a PEEP of 8 cm H_2O and had a threshold for intubation at a fraction of inspired oxygen of 0.6, both risk factors for development of air leaks.[40]

In the Surfactant Positive Airway Pressure and Pulse Oximetry Trial in Extremely Low Birth Weight Infants (SUPPORT trial), conducted by the National Institute of Child Health and Human Development Neonatal Research Network in 2010, 1316 infants across 16 US centers were randomized to NCPAP in the delivery room versus intubation and surfactant. There was no difference in the primary outcome of BPD/death (RR, 0.95; 95% CI, 0.85–1.05) between the groups. Infants in the NCPAP group spent fewer days on mechanical ventilation and had lesser need for postnatal corticosteroid therapy. There was no difference in other important outcomes such as air leaks, grade 3 or 4 IVH, or severe retinopathy of prematurity between the groups.[41] Post hoc analysis revealed that infants at 24 to 25 weeks' gestational age (GA) randomized to NCPAP had a lower death rate. Follow-up studies revealed that infants in the NCPAP group had less respiratory morbidity and no difference in death or neurologic impairment at 18 to 22 weeks.[42,43]

Another large trial conducted by the Vermont Oxford Network Study Group randomized 648 preterm infants across 27 centers to one of three arms: prophylactic surfactant followed by mechanical ventilation, intubate-surfactant-extubate, and NCPAP followed by surfactant if needed. There was no difference in BPD/death and other studied outcomes in the three groups. Infants in the NCPAP group needed less intubation and surfactant.[44] A Cochrane meta-analysis showed that early NCPAP use followed by selective surfactant if needed resulted in less BPD/death compared with use of prophylactic surfactant.[45]

Recommendation

There is enough evidence to conclude that early NCPAP and selective early surfactant use is beneficial over intubation and prophylactic surfactant administration in preterm infants at risk of RDS.[46]

Evidence for Use of NCPAP as Secondary Support After Extubation

A Cochrane meta-analysis of nine RCTs from 2003 comparing NCPAP with an oxygen hood/low-flow nasal cannula for postextubation support in preterm infants showed that use of NCPAP reduced the incidence of respiratory failure (RR, 0.62; 95% CI, 0.49–0.77).[47] Although it is desirable to extubate infants as early as feasible,[48,49] newer studies comparing the various modes of noninvasive ventilation suggest that NIPPV is a better alternative to NCPAP to reduce extubation failure (discussed in next section).

Nasal Intermittent Positive Pressure Ventilation

NIPPV is a form of noninvasive ventilatory assistance using a nasal interface to deliver intermittent peak inspiratory pressures above the PEEP. It is also referred to as noninvasive intermittent positive pressure ventilation or noninvasive intermittent mandatory ventilation. NIPPV is an intermediate approach between invasive ventilation with an ETT and noninvasive NCPAP. Although this technique was practiced as early as the 1970s, it went into disfavor in the 1980s after reports of increased gastrointestinal perforations with its use.[50] There was a renewed interest in its use after adequately powered RCTs using synchronized NIPPV (SNIPPV) showed efficacy without any major side effects, including a lack of intestinal perforations.[51,52] The mechanisms by which NIPPV and SNIPPV work include recruitment of the collapsed alveoli and stabilizing functional residual capacity, resulting in improved gas exchange, an increase in tidal and minute volumes, and a decrease in the work of breathing.[53-55] Other reported physiologic effects include improved stability of the chest wall, improved pulmonary mechanics, decreased flow resistance, and reduction in thoracoabdominal asynchrony.[56,57]

SNIPPV Versus NIPPV

NIPPV, if synchronized to the patient's respiratory efforts, is termed SNIPPV. In the past, SNIPPV was delivered using the Infant Star ventilator in the Star Sync mode (Infrasonics Inc., San Diego, California) with a Graseby capsule placed on the anterior abdominal wall to detect the patient's inspiratory efforts. This ventilator is no longer in production, but newer devices able to deliver SNIPPV are available. The Sophie ventilator (Fritz Stephan GmbH, Gackenbach, Germany) uses the Graseby capsule placed on the anterior abdominal wall, the GiULIA ventilator (Ginevri, Rome, Italy) uses a flow sensor at the airway opening, and NIV-NAVA uses a esophageal catheter to detect the electrical activity of the diaphragm for synchronization. Although there are no large RCTs evaluating outcomes of infants on SNIPPV versus NIPPV, small trials showed that SNIPPV has superior efficacy over NIPPV.[58,59]

NIPPV Versus BiPAP/SiPAP

Bilevel CPAP (BiPAP) or biphasic CPAP (such as Infant Flow SiPAP) is not to be confused with NIPPV. In BiPAP, variable flow is delivered to provide alternating high and low PEEP levels. The inspiratory times are much longer, with lower respiratory rates to allow spontaneous breathing. On the other hand, constant flow is delivered in NIPPV, with the PIP and PEEP levels being similar to those used in invasive ventilation with shorter inspiratory times. A subgroup analysis of a large multicenter RCT comparing outcomes of infants on NIPPV versus bilevel CPAP did not show a significant difference in the composite outcome of death and BPD or BPD alone, but morbidity was higher in the bilevel CPAP group.[60] It is important to recognize that these two modes of respiratory support are different and should not be referred to interchangeably.

Evidence for Use of NIPPV as Primary Respiratory Support

Ekhaguere et al. recently performed a pooled analysis of data from trials including those from a 2016 Cochrane meta-analysis comparing NIPPV to NCPAP (16 RCTs; N = 2014).[61] NIPPV, when used as a primary support, reduced respiratory failure compared with NCPAP (RR, 0.55; 95% CI, 0.46–0.65). It is worth noting that four RCTs included in this analysis compared BiPAP with CPAP. The Cochrane meta-analysis from 2016 had similar conclusions that early NIPPV is superior to NCPAP alone in decreasing respiratory failure and the need for intubation and ETT ventilation in preterm infants with RDS.[62]

Evidence for Use of NIPPV as Secondary Support After Extubation

In the analysis by Ekhaguere et al., which included 12 RCTs comparing use of NIPPV to NCPAP after extubation, it was noted that NIPPV significantly reduced the rate of postextubation failure (RR, 0.60; 95% CI, 0.45–0.81).[61] The Cochrane meta-analysis from 2017 had similar conclusions.[63]

Even though some RCTs comparing the use of NIPPV with NCPAP have shown a decreased incidence of BPD with NIPPV,[64-68] a meta-analysis from recent Cochrane reviews did not demonstrate a significant reduction in BPD with the use of NIPPV compared with CPAP.[62,63] A large, multicenter, pragmatic RCT conducted by Kirpalani et al. also showed no significant differences in BPD/death between the two groups.[69] In a recent RCT comparing NIPPV with NCPAP, the rate of BPD was not different in the two groups, but infants in the NIPPV group had a significantly shorter hospital stay (26.2 ± 17.4 days versus 38.4 ± 19.2 days; $P = .009$).[70]

Recommendations

There is strong evidence to recommend use of NIPPV as the preferred noninvasive mode to prevent postextubation failure. NIPPV may also be preferred for primary noninvasive respiratory support but does not decrease BPD/death. If an infant is intubated to administer surfactant, the infant should be extubated to NIPPV (Fig. 12.2).

High-Flow Nasal Canula

In this the HFNC method of noninvasive respiratory assistance, humidified air is delivered at flow rates generally ranging between 2 and 8 L/min through specialized nasal prongs. The mechanism of action of HFNC includes its ability to generate continuous distending pressure, helping to maintain functional residual capacity. It also helps in provision of gas flow sufficient to reduce inspiratory resistance and work of breathing, improves airway conductance, and reduces resistance through washout of the nasopharyngeal dead space.

The humidified flow decreases the adverse effects of dry air, such as nasal bleeding, thickened secretions, and obstruction of nasal passages. It is very difficult to measure the distending pressure achieved by HFNC. Any nasal cannula can be used to deliver HFNC, but two devices are in common use: Vapotherm 2000 (Vapotherm Inc., Stevensville, Maryland) and Optiflow Junior (Fisher & Paykel Healthcare, Auckland, New Zealand). The advantages of HFNC include the simple interface that makes it easy to maintain in place and fewer side effects such as nasal trauma, pneumothorax, etc.

Evidence for Use of HFNC as Primary Respiratory Support

HFNC is a less invasive form of noninvasive respiratory support compared with NCPAP but is considered to have similar efficacy in terms of using it as a primary mode of respiratory support. In a Cochrane review analyzing use of HFNC versus CPAP for primary respiratory support, it was found that there was no difference between HFNC and

A

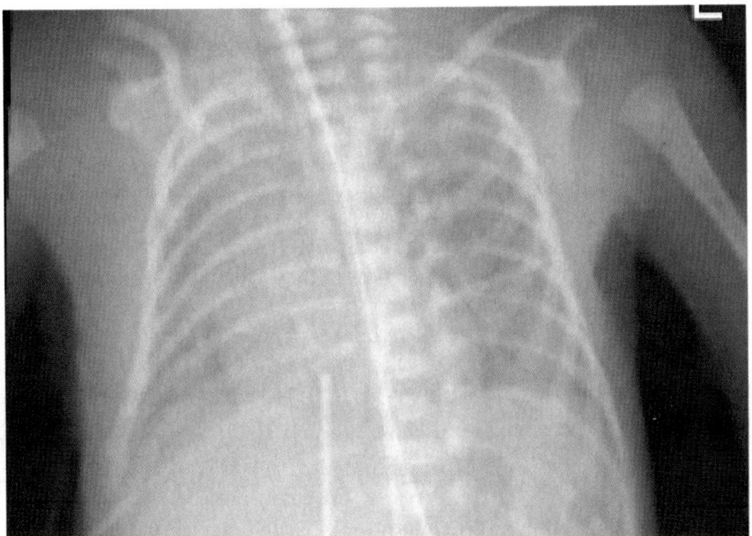

B

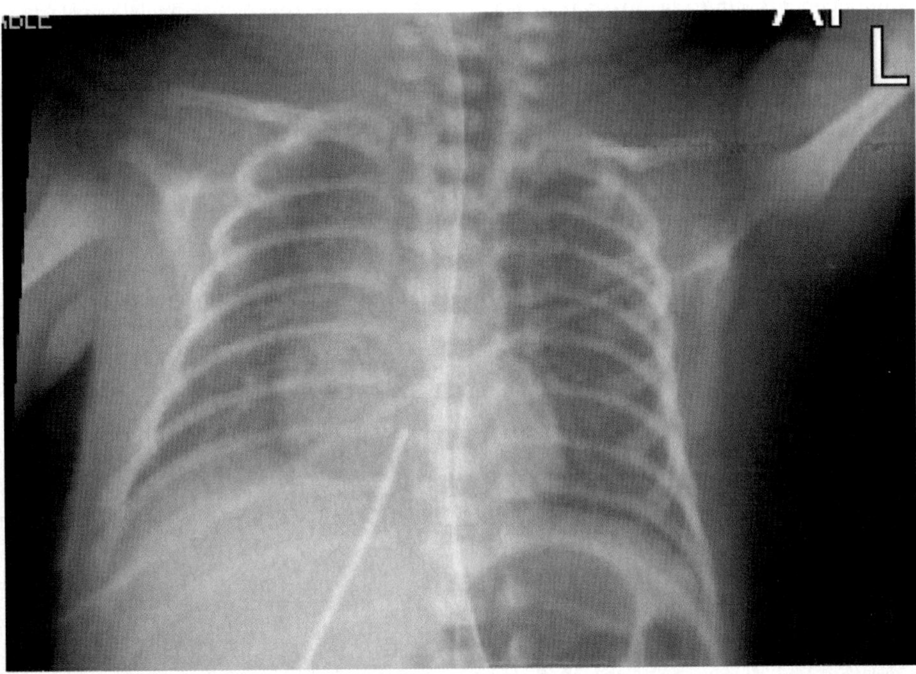

Fig. 12.2 Chest X-Rays of an Extremely Premature Infant With Respiratory Distress Syndrome, Taken on the Day of Birth. (A) Low lung volumes and hazy opacification of lung fields while on NCPAP (PEEP, 6 cm H_2O; Fio_2, 0.35). (B) Improved aeration of the lung fields when placed on NIPPV (PIP, 18 cm H_2O; PEEP, 5 cm H_2O; rate, 30 breaths per min; Ti, 0.45 sec; MAP, 11 cm H_2O; Fio_2, 0.28). *Fio_2,* Fraction of inspired oxygen; *MAP,* mean airway pressure; *NCPAP,* nasal continuous positive airway pressure; *NIPPV,* nasal intermittent positive pressure ventilation; *PEEP,* positive end expiratory pressure; *PIP,* peak inspiratory pressure; *Ti,* inspiratory time.

NCPAP groups.[71] Subsequent trials published after the Cochrane review, however, showed mixed results, and a pooled analysis of four additional trials along with the Cochrane review (total of seven RCTs; $N > 1500$) found that NCPAP is superior to HFNC in preventing respiratory failure (RR, 1.86; 95% CI, 1.46–2.37).[61] In another recent RCT comparing the use of NCPAP to HFNC in infants with GA >31 weeks, use of HFNC resulted in a higher rate of treatment failure than did NCPAP (20.5% versus 10.2%).[72] Use of HFNC compared with NIPPV for primary respiratory support did not show any significant differences in respiratory failure.[73,74] However, the study by Kugelman et al.[73] was a pilot RCT with a small number of patients (72) with a mean gestational age of approximately 32 weeks. The need for ETT was actually higher in the NIPPV group (34% versus 28%), but the difference was not significant. The other study, by Wang et al.,[74] had similar findings (i.e., no differences in studied outcomes, with a sample size of 89 very low birth weight infants).

Evidence for Use of HFNC as Secondary Support After Extubation

In terms of preventing postextubation failure, a Cochrane meta-analysis showed no additional risk of treatment failure or reintubation with use of HFNC compared with NCPAP.[71] Subsequent trials showed no difference between those modalities,[75,76] and one study[77] indicated higher failure rates with HFNC.

Recommendation

There is not enough evidence to suggest the use of HFNC as primary respiratory support in preterm infants, although it is a reasonable alternative for postextubation support compared with NCPAP. Minimal evidence exists to recommend use of HFNC in extremely preterm infants less than 28 weeks' gestation.[78]

Noninvasive High Frequency Ventilation

In NIHFV, high-frequency breaths are superimposed on constant positive airway pressure through a nasal interface. It is a relatively newer modality of respiratory support, mostly used in a few Canadian and European units currently. The presumed physiologic basis for its mechanism is thought to be similar to the benefit of invasive HFV, in which the low tidal volumes delivered at extremely rapid rates provide constant lung expansion and effectively eliminate CO_2.

A recent meta-analysis of eight RCTs (N = 463) comparing NIHFV with Bi-CPAP and NCPAP in preterm infants showed that NHFOV significantly removed CO_2 and reduced the risk of intubation (RR, 0.50; 95% CI, 0.36–0.70) compared with Bi-CPAP/NCPAP.[79] Another recently published RCT by Chen et al. comparing outcomes of infants extubated to NIHFV versus NCPAP had similar conclusions.[80] Ruegger et al. compared NIHFV with NCPAP in a randomized crossover trial and showed that NIHFV was associated with significantly reduced desaturations and bradycardia events but with increased oxygen requirements in preterm infants.[81]

Evidence for Use of NIHFV

Even though trials are showing promising results, a cautious approach to the use of NIHFV is warranted. Future large RCTs should focus on use in extremely preterm infants and the long-term safety effects before use of NIHFV can be routinely recommended.

Noninvasive Neurally Adjusted Ventilatory Assist

NAVA is a relatively new modality of respiratory support that can be provided invasively or noninvasively. The system uses the

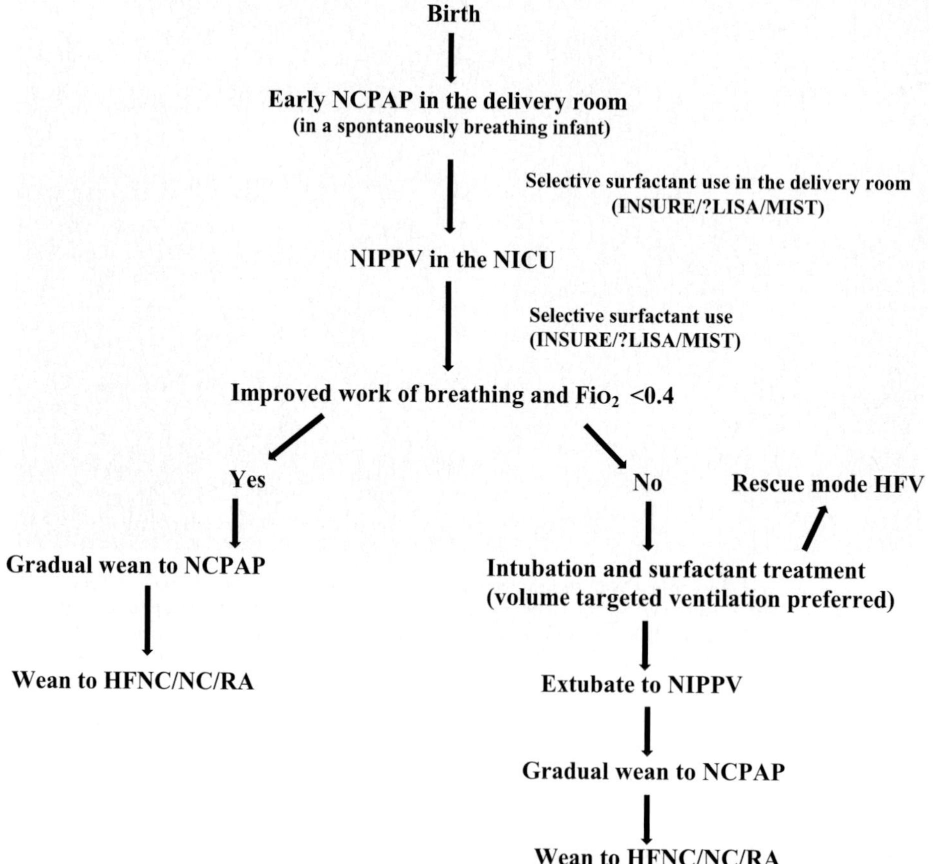

Fig. 12.3 Flow Diagram Showing a Suggested Approach in the Respiratory Management of an Extremely Premature Infant With Respiratory Distress Syndrome (RDS). *Fio_2*, Fraction of inspired oxygen; *HFNC,* high flow nasal cannula; *HFV,* high frequency ventilation; *INSURE,* intubate, surfactant, extubate; *LISA,* less invasive surfactant administration; *MIST,* minimally invasive surfactant therapy; *NC,* nasal cannula; *NCPAP,* nasal continuous positive airway pressure; *NICU,* neonatal intensive care unit; *NIPPV,* nasal intermittent positive airway pressure; *RA,* room air.

electrical activity of the diaphragm to deliver synchronized, pressure-controlled breaths and provides pressure support proportional to the patient's inspiratory efforts. This ability to synchronize with the patients' inspiratory efforts allows for decreased work of breathing, improved gas exchange, and earlier extubation.[82,83] Small RCTs have shown its efficacy, but large RCTs are needed before NIV-NAVA can be routinely recommended.[84,85]

Conclusions

There is no strong evidence for the basis behind many ventilation strategies applied in neonates. Many practices are driven by the clinician's experience, preferences, and available resources. There is good evidence to recommend use of NCPAP for delivery room stabilization of the preterm infant. NIPPV has been conclusively shown to be a better alternative to NCPAP to prevent extubation failure; it may also a preferred mode of primary respiratory support. HFNC seems to have lower efficacy compared with NCPAP as the primary mode of respiratory support. NHFOV and NIV-NAVA seem to be emerging promising techniques. VTV has been proven to be better than pressure-controlled ventilation, and there is not enough evidence to recommend use of HFV as primary support. Fig. 12.3 shows a suggested algorithm for initial respiratory management of a premature infant with RDS. Finally, it is worth remembering that good evidence behind the use of any strategy only supplements the clinician's knowledge of the pathophysiology and his or her familiarity with the device.

Section 2

CHAPTER

13 Pulmonary Hypertension of the Newborn

Praveen Chandrasekharan, Satyan Lakshminrusimha

KEY POINTS

1. Persistent pulmonary hypertension of the newborn (PPHN) represents continued high pulmonary vascular resistance (PVR) after birth resulting in extrapulmonary shunting of the blood from pulmonary to systemic circulation, leading to hypoxemia.
2. The disorder can be idiopathic or primary or could complicate respiratory, neurologic, and cardiovascular morbidities. Perinatal asphyxia with meconium aspiration syndrome or pneumonia can result in impaired lung recruitment, suboptimal oxygenation, and pulmonary vasoconstriction. Preterm neonates with severe respiratory distress syndrome could also have persistent high PVR after birth.
3. Pathophysiological mechanisms such as pulmonary vascular remodeling, abnormal pulmonary vascular reactivity, and pulmonary vascular hypoplasia can contribute to PPHN.
4. The molecular mechanisms of PPHN include abnormally high levels of pulmonary vasoconstrictors such as endothelin 1, leukotrienes, thromboxanes, and/or low levels of pulmonary vasodilators such as nitric oxide (NO) and prostacyclin.
5. Neonates with PPHN are often managed using positive pressure ventilation, oxygen to correct hypoxemia, surfactant replacement therapy, vasopressors to maintain systemic pressures, pulmonary vasodilators, and adequate sedation with minimal stimulation.
6. Regardless of treatment intervention, neonates with PPHN have 10% mortality along with poor pulmonary and neurodevelopmental outcomes. In neonates randomized to early inhaled NO with PPHN, 25% had impaired neurodevelopmental outcome and 22% had hearing impairment.

Introduction

Persistent pulmonary hypertension of the newborn (PPHN) is estimated to affect 1.9 per 1000 live births[1] and is characterized by a failure of transition from fetal to newborn circulation. PPHN is secondary to the persistence of high pulmonary vascular resistance (PVR), resulting in extrapulmonary shunting of the blood from pulmonary to systemic circulation and leading to hypoxemia. It is often secondary to respiratory disease, although occasionally, PPHN can present as primary or idiopathic, often associated with "black lungs" on a chest x-ray due to absence of lung disease and pulmonary oligemia. PPHN could complicate the course of a sick newborn infant, leading to respiratory, neurologic, and cardiovascular morbidities and mortality. Commonly identified in term infants, increasing evidence supports the presence of PPHN in preterm neonates.[2–4] Neonates with PPHN are often managed using positive pressure ventilation (PPV), oxygen to correct hypoxemia, surfactant replacement therapy, vasopressors to maintain systemic pressures, pulmonary vasodilators, and adequate sedation with minimal stimulation. According to the Extracorporeal Life Support Organization, 20% of neonates with PPHN required extracorporeal membrane support (ECMO),[5] although early surfactant and inhaled nitric oxide (iNO) can potentially further reduce the need for ECMO.[6] The focus of this chapter is to discuss the available evidence to guide management of PPHN.

Pathophysiology

Interference in the mechanism of transition during birth could lead to persistent elevation of pulmonary arterial pressures, leading to PPHN.[7] PPHN is characterized by labile systemic arterial hypoxemia secondary to elevated PVR in relation to systemic vascular resistance (SVR), with resultant right-to-left (pulmonary to systemic circulation) shunting through persistent fetal channels such as the ductus arteriosus and foramen ovale, bypassing the lungs (Fig. 13.1).

The transition from fetal to newborn circulation occurs at birth with aeration of the lungs, which drops PVR and increases blood flow to the lungs by 8- to 10-fold.[8,9] With clamping of the umbilical cord, there is an increase in SVR, increasing left ventricular afterload, and switching of the shunts at the foramen ovale and ductus arteriosus from right-to-left to left-to-right.

The following pathophysiological mechanisms can alter PVR and result in PPHN: pulmonary vascular remodeling, abnormal pulmonary vascular reactivity, and pulmonary vascular hypoplasia.

Pulmonary Vascular Remodeling

Idiopathic PPHN secondary to pulmonary vascular remodeling in the absence of lung pathology could present with histopathological features of smooth-muscle hypertrophy and extension of the muscular layer to more peripheral vasculature such as the preacinar arterioles. During fetal life, high pulmonary vascular pressures and resistance are maintained by humoral mediators such as endothelin 1, leukotrienes, and thromboxanes along with decreased levels of pulmonary vasodilators such as nitric oxide (NO) and prostacyclin (PGI_2).[8,10,11] NO exhibits its effect on pulmonary vasodilation by increasing cyclic guanosine monophosphate (cGMP) in the smooth muscles, which causes relaxation (Fig. 13.2). Higher endothelin 1 and lower cGMP could contribute to abnormal pulmonary vasculature, in turn contributing to the pathology.[12] Urea cycle defects leading to low levels of arginine, the precursor of NO, could contribute to PPHN.[13] Maternal ingestion of cyclooxygenase inhibitors such as aspirin during late pregnancy may be associated with ductal closure and lead to PPHN,[14] although this association has been recently questioned.[15] Maternal intake of selective serotonin reuptake inhibitors has also been

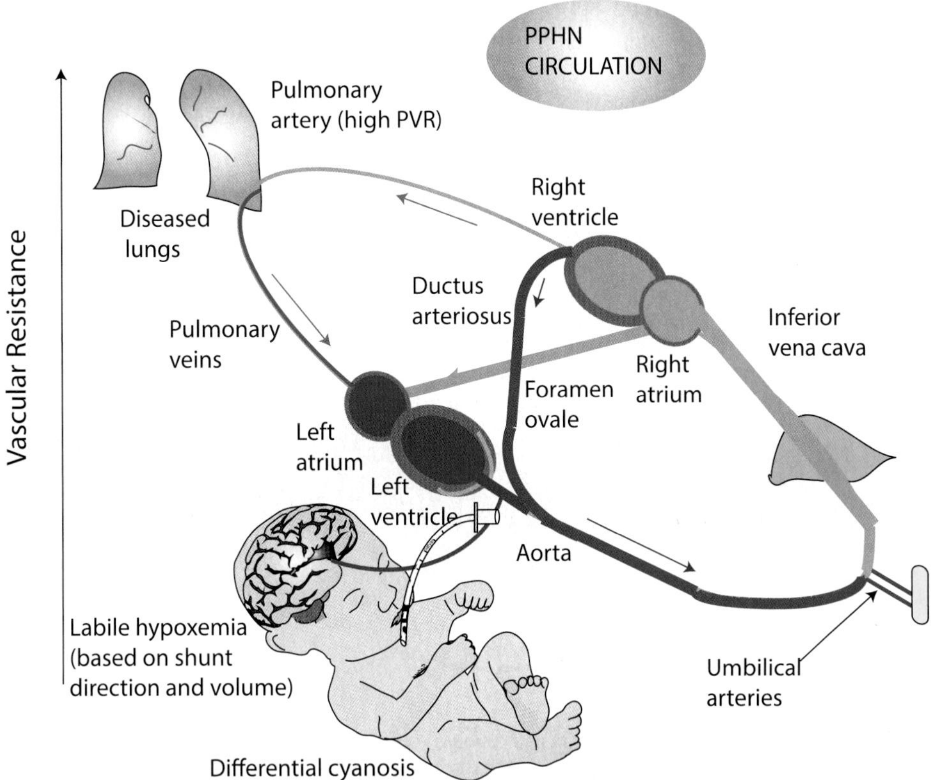

Fig. 13.1 Pathophysiology of Pulmonary Hypertension of the Newborn. The circulatory system in an infant with pulmonary hypertension of the newborn (PPHN) is shown with vascular resistance on the Y-axis. The pulmonary vascular resistance (PVR) is high in PPHN and is equal to or greater than systemic vascular resistance. As blood follows the path of least resistance, right-to-left shunts at the ductus arteriosus and foramen ovale result in cyanosis and hypoxemia. Labile hypoxemia is the hallmark of PPHN, because oxygenation varies based on shunt direction and volume. (Copyright Satyan Lakshminrusimha.)

associated with PPHN,[16] possibly due to pulmonary vasoconstrictive effects of serotonin.[17,18]

Abnormal Pulmonary Vasoconstriction

Optimal oxygenation leads to pulmonary vasodilation and also stimulates endogenous NO.[10] Failure to establish adequate lung recruitment as observed in asphyxia with meconium aspiration syndrome (MAS) or pneumonia could lead to suboptimal oxygenation and ventilation, in turn leading to pulmonary vasoconstriction. Preterm neonates with severe respiratory distress syndrome (RDS) and neonates delivered by cesarean section in the absence of labor could have persistent high PVR after birth. An imbalance between pulmonary vasodilators and constrictors can lead to PPHN with increased vascular reactivity, remodeling, and high PVR. Lung parenchymal diseases such as MAS, pneumonia, and RDS can trigger proinflammatory mediators that could stimulate endothelin and thromboxane, leading to pulmonary vasoconstriction.[19] Increased viscosity (such as severe polycythemia) can lead to pulmonary vascular obstruction and can elevate PVR (Fig. 13.3).

Pulmonary Vascular Hypoplasia

Disruption in the development of pulmonary vasculature reduces the cross-sectional area, leading to high PVR. Pulmonary hypoplasia can occur in conditions such as congenital diaphragmatic hernia (CDH), oligohydramnios secondary to prolonged rupture of membrane (PROM), Potter syndrome, and renal disease. The closure or restriction of ductus arteriosus in a fetus secondary to maternal ingestion of nonsteroidal anti-inflammatory drugs may be associated with pulmonary vascular hypoplasia and remodeling (see above).[15,16,20–22]

Pulmonary Venous Hypertension

Anatomic and functional abnormalities in the pulmonary venous system and left heart can lead to pulmonary venous hypertension. These conditions include pulmonary vein stenosis, left ventricular dysfunction, hypoplastic left heart syndrome, and mitral stenosis. These conditions may present with intractable PPHN with poor response to traditional inhaled pulmonary vasodilators such as NO (Fig. 13.4)

Clinical Conditions Presenting With PPHN

Based on a Neonatal Research Network study, the primary respiratory illnesses associated with PPHN in the order of descending frequency were MAS (41%), pneumonia (14%), RDS (13%), pneumonia and/or RDS (14%), CDH (10%), and pulmonary hypoplasia (4%).[23]

Meconium Aspiration Syndrome

A distressed fetus is at risk of exposure to meconium-stained amniotic fluid (MSAF), and approximately 5% to 10% of these newborns are at risk for MAS.[24] MAS presents as acute respiratory failure with the need for mechanical ventilation. The chemical pneumonitis and surfactant inactivation secondary to meconium aspiration result in impaired gas exchange. A combination of hypoxemia, hypercarbia, acidosis, and impaired pulmonary vascular transition contributes to

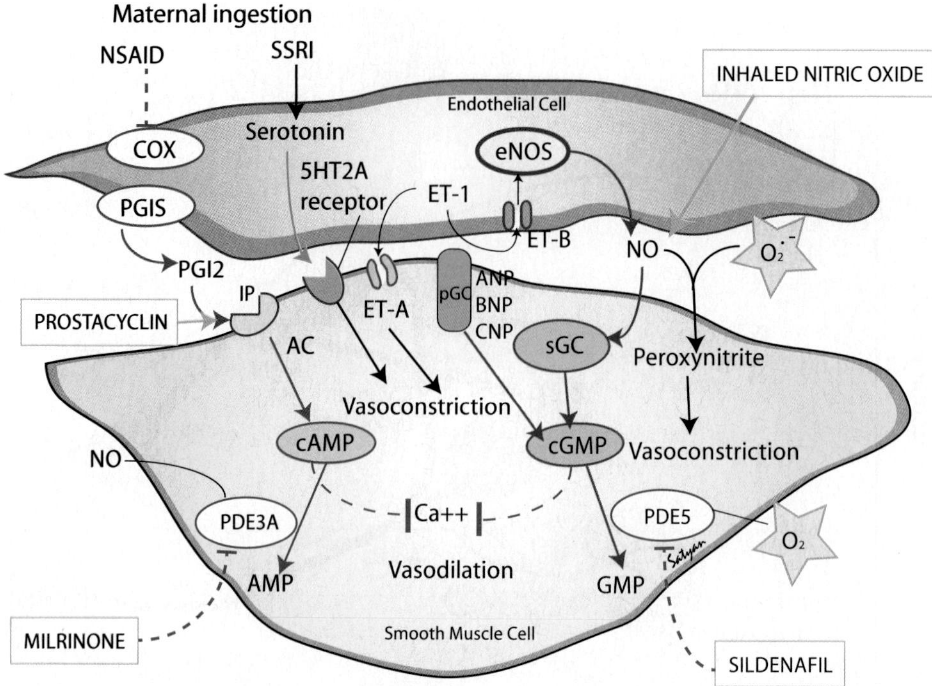

Fig. 13.2 Vasoactive Mediators in the Etiology and Management of Pulmonary Hypertension of the Newborn. The endothelial cell produces vasodilators such as nitric oxide (NO) from endothelial nitric oxide synthase (eNOS) and prostacyclin (PGI_2) from cyclooxygenase (COX) and prostacyclin synthase (PGIS). Nitric oxide stimulates soluble guanylyl cyclase (sGC) to produce cyclic guanosine monophosphate (cGMP). In addition, natriuretic peptides (atrial, brain, and C-type [ANP, BNP, and CNP]) stimulate particulate guanyl cyclase (pGC) to produce cGMP. Cyclic GMP mediates relaxation of the smooth-muscle cell, leading to pulmonary vasodilation. The enzyme phosphodiesterase 5 (PDE5) breaks down cGMP to inactive GMP. This enzyme is inhibited by sildenafil. Prostaglandins stimulate adenyl cyclase (AC) to release cyclic adenosine monophosphate (cAMP)—also a smooth-muscle relaxant. Cyclic AMP is broken down by the phosphodiesterase 3 (PDE3) enzyme, and this enzyme is inhibited by milrinone. Endothelin (ET) is a vasoconstrictor released by the endothelium and stimulates the endothelin A (ET-A) receptor to cause smooth-muscle contraction. *5HT2A*, 5-Hydroxy-tryptamine 2 A receptor; *ANP*, atrial natriuretic peptide; *BNP*, B-type natriuretic peptide; *CNP*, c type natriuretic peptide; *IP*, Prostaglandin or also known as prostacyclin I2 receptor; *NSAID,* Nonsteroidal anti-inflammatory drug; *SSRI,* selective serotonin reuptake inhibitor. (Copyright Satyan Lakshminrusimha.)

PPHN. The delivery room management of a newborn with MSAF has changed with the 2015 International Liaison Committee on Resuscitation recommendations based on available clinical and translational evidence.[25–30] The current recommendations as of 2015 are to initiate PPV in the nonvigorous neonate and not to perform routine endotracheal suctioning to minimize the interruptions in initiating resuscitative steps.[28] Although MAS is no longer the most common indication for neonatal respiratory ECMO, it continues to be a major contributor to PPHN (often associated with asphyxia) in low- and middle-income countries.

Pneumonia

Underlying parenchymal lung injury, along with elevated PVR, could lead to PPHN. These infants may or may not present with radiologic features of pneumonia. If pneumonia is associated with sepsis, it could lead to a drop in systemic pressures, which may further complicate PPHN.

Respiratory Distress Syndrome

RDS is a condition that primarily occurs in preterm neonates secondary to surfactant deficiency (93% of infants <28 weeks). Approximately 10% of late preterm neonates and 1% of term neonates could also have RDS. Newborns with RDS present with tachypnea, nasal flaring and grunting, intercostal retractions, and hypoxemia, presenting as cyanosis/color change secondary to intrapulmonary (ventilation–perfusion mismatch) and right-to-left extrapulmonary (across the ductus and foramen ovale) shunting. This condition is commonly managed with continuous positive airway pressure (CPAP), invasive mechanical ventilation with optimal mean airway pressure, and rescue surfactant therapy.

Congenital Diaphragmatic Hernia

Characterized by a defect in the diaphragm that leads to herniation of abdominal contents into the thorax, the incidence of congenital diaphragmatic hernia (CDH) ranges anywhere from 0.8 to 5 per 10,000 births.[31] Pulmonary hypoplasia, pulmonary vascular remodeling, and the associated PPHN are the major factors contributing to hypoxemia in CDH. An underdeveloped left ventricle and a hypertrophied right ventricle leading to biventricular dysfunction could further complicate the PPHN in these neonates.[32]

Pulmonary Hypoplasia

Besides CDH, pulmonary hypoplasia secondary to renal dysfunction, oligohydramnios, and/or skeletal abnormalities primarily affecting the thorax could be associated with PPHN.

Prematurity and PPHN

Traditionally a disease of term and late-preterm neonates, PPHN is increasingly diagnosed in extremely premature infants.[2,4,33] PPHN in preterm neonates has a biphasic presentation: early and late onset. Early-onset PPHN is associated with RDS and occurs within the first

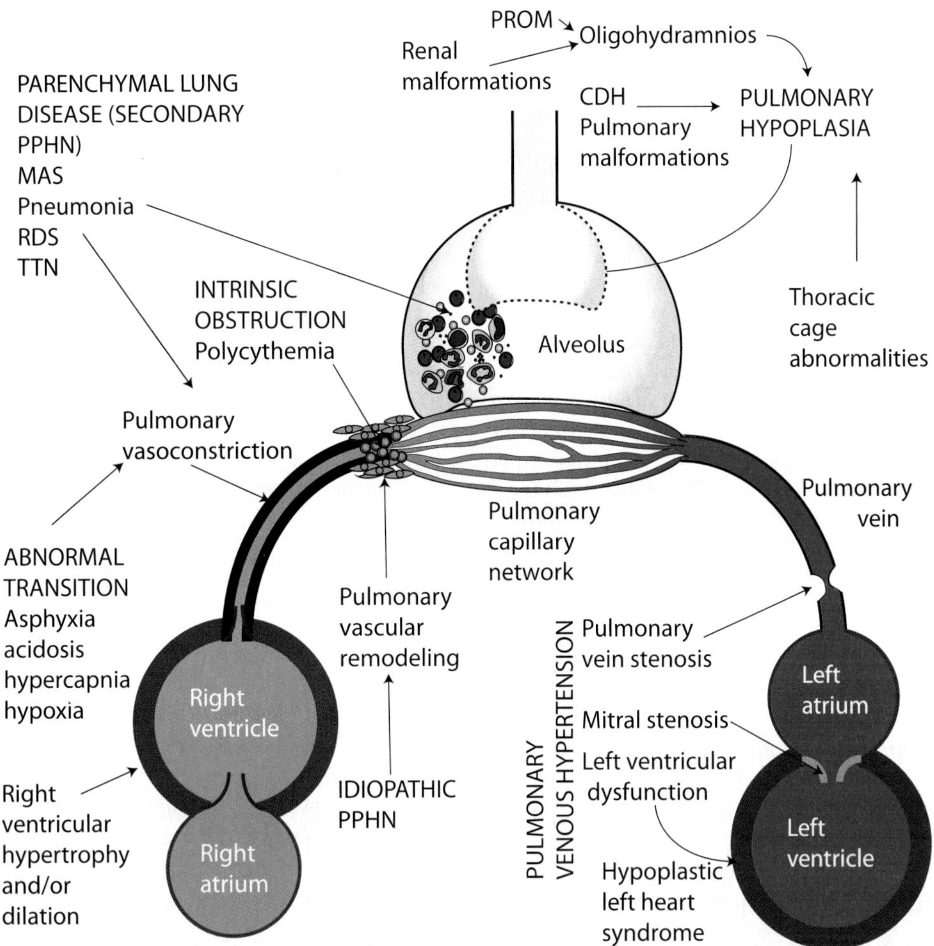

Fig. 13.3 Etiology of Pulmonary Hypertension of the Newborn. Important causes of pulmonary hypertension of the newborn (PPHN) include parenchymal lung disease (such as meconium aspiration syndrome [MAS], pneumonia, respiratory distress syndrome [RDS], and transient tachypnea of the newborn [TTN]) or abnormal transition (asphyxia). Idiopathic PPHN without parenchymal lung disease presents with a "black-lung" appearance on chest x-ray. Pulmonary hypoplasia and pulmonary venous hypertension often cause intractable pulmonary hypertension that may be resistant to conventional pulmonary vasodilators. *CDH,* Congenital diaphragmatic hernia; *PROM,* prolonged rupture of membrane. (Copyright Satyan Lakshminrusimha.)

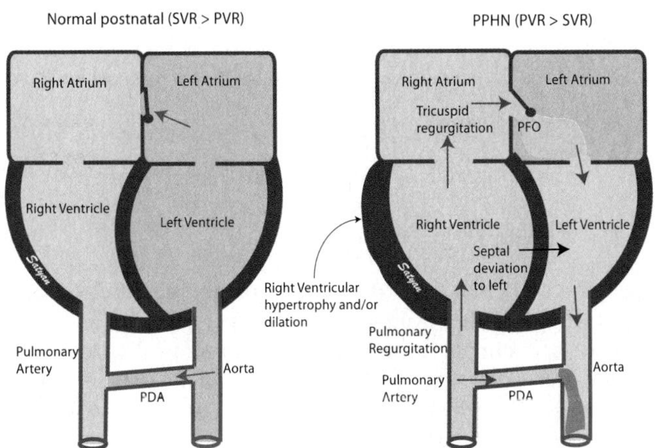

Fig. 13.4 Echocardiographic Features of Pulmonary Hypertension of the Newborn. A normal postnatal cardiac anatomy is compared with a pulmonary hypertension of the newborn (PPHN) heart with pulmonary vascular resistance (PVR) higher than systemic vascular resistance (SVR). High PVR leads to pulmonary regurgitation, tricuspid regurgitation, and deviation of the interventricular septum to the left. Right-to-left (or bidirectional) shunts at the patent foramen ovale (PFO) or patent ductus arteriosus (PDA) contribute to labile hypoxemia. (Copyright Satyan Lakshminrusimha.)

few weeks after birth. Although late-onset PPHN is often associated with bronchopulmonary dysplasia (BPD), there are preterm babies with echocardiographic evidence of PPHN without BPD reported.[34] Fetal growth restriction, premature PROM, oligohydramnios, and pulmonary hypoplasia are risk factors for PPHN in preterm neonates.[35,36] Preterm neonates who present with both acute and late-onset PPHN are at higher risk of mortality and morbidity.

Miscellaneous Causes

Other conditions such as alveolar capillary dysplasia and congenital surfactant deficiencies may present with PPHN requiring ECMO, and the disease process in these cases may not be reversible. Alveolar–capillary dysplasia with pulmonary vein misalignment could present beyond the neonatal age group and could pose a challenge to diagnose.[37]

Diagnostic Features

PPHN presents with clinical features, which could be evaluated further by blood gas analysis, imaging (x-ray of the chest), and echocardiography. Echocardiography is also required to rule out congenital heart defects (CHDs) and estimate the severity of PPHN.[38] Cardiac catheterizations are rarely performed to grade the degree and determine etiology of intractable PPHN.

Clinical Signs and Symptoms

The classic clinical feature is a newborn is labile hypoxemia with differential oxygen saturation (Spo_2), that is, higher Spo_2 in the right upper limb (preductal) compared with the lower-extremity Spo_2 (postductal), which fluctuates with or without the need for oxygen and PPV. PPHN often presents as acute hypoxic respiratory failure (HRF), usually requiring oxygen >50% while on PPV.

Prenatally diagnosed CDH and perinatal factors such as nonreassuring fetal heart tracing, birth asphyxia, meconium-stained amniotic fluid, PROM, and oligohydramnios should prompt a physician to have a high index of suspicion for PPHN. PPHN should also be considered if hypoxemia and the oxygen requirement are disproportionate to the lung pathology. Preductal and postductal saturations (Spo_2) should be monitored for labile hypoxemia and differential cyanosis (lower-limb Spo_2 is lower than the right-upper-limb Spo_2). The absence of an Spo_2 difference could occur in PPHN if the shunting occurs at the level of the foramen ovale. A chest exam may reveal a barrel chest in cases of MAS secondary to air trapping, with variable lung sounds on auscultation along with rales and rhonchi. Secondary to PPHN, the cardiac examination could reveal a loud second heart sound and a harsh systolic murmur best heard along the left sternal border secondary to tricuspid regurgitation.

Peripheral Saturations and the Utility of Blood Gas

Hypoxemia could also be secondary to heart defects, and it is important to differentiate PPHN from cyanotic CHD. A higher preductal-to-postductal saturation difference greater than 5% to 10% or an arterial oxygenation (Pao_2, in mm Hg) difference of greater than 10 to 20 mm Hg is suggestive of PPHN. In the absence of ductal shunting, both preductal and postductal saturations could remain low. In a condition such as coarctation of the aorta in the presence of ductus, differential cyanosis could be seen. In CHD, the low saturations persist despite oxygen supplementation, unlike in PPHN. In centers without immediate access to echocardiography or a cardiologist, the hyperoxia test could help differentiate CHD, PPHN, and lung disease causing hypoxemia.

Hyperoxia Test

Assessing a change in Pao_2 in arterial blood gas (ABG) before and after exposing a neonate to 100% supplemental oxygen could help differentiate PPHN from parenchymal lung disease and CHD. After exposing the neonate to 100% O_2, in a healthy neonate, the Pao_2 is usually >300 mm Hg. In a newborn with CHD, after a hyperoxia test, the Pao_2 is <100 mm Hg, and in a newborn with PPHN, it can be >100 mm Hg but is typically <150 mm Hg. In parenchymal lung disease, the Pao_2 could be between 150 and 300 mm Hg. A hyperoxia test is not a gold standard test and could be falsely negative or positive in cardiac lesions with high pulmonary blood flow. In the presence of easy access to echocardiography, a hyperoxia test should be avoided to limit oxygen toxicity and to avoid ductal closure and an excessive drop in PVR in the presence of ductal-dependent systemic circulation (such as hypoplastic left heart syndrome).

In the past, hyperventilation-induced alkalosis and hyperoxia were used to diagnose PPHN. Both oxygen and alkalosis induce pulmonary vasodilation and improve oxygenation in PPHN and could differentiate it from cyanotic CHD. However, respiratory alkalosis reduces cerebral blood flow and is associated with negative neurodevelopmental outcomes, and it should be avoided.

Severity of Hypoxemia in PPHN

Hypoxemia can be assessed by ventilator settings, ABG parameters, and oxygen saturations. The indices mentioned below can be used to assess severity and response to therapy in PPHN: the oxygenation index (OI); arterial oxygenation, the ratio of the partial pressure of oxygen in arterial blood (Pao_2) to the fraction of inspired oxygen (Fio_2) (P/F ratio); the A-a (alveolar-arterial) oxygen gradient; and the oxygen saturation index (OSI).

Oxygenation Index

The equation to calculate the OI is

$$Fio_2 * 100 * \left(\text{mean airway pressure } [\text{MAP}] \text{ in cm } H_2O\right) \div \left(Pao_2 \text{in mm Hg}\right).$$

Based on OI, HRF could be classified as

1. Mild (OI ≤ 15)
2. Moderate (OI > 15 and < 25)
3. Severe (OI 25–40)
4. Very severe (OI > 40)—an indication for ECMO

P/F Ratio

The severity of the P/F ratio, or the ratio of the Pao_2 to the Fio_2 in mm Hg, can be assessed as follows:

1. Mild: >200 to 300
2. Moderate: >100 to 200
3. Severe: 100

Alveolar-Arterial Gradient

The A-a gradient provides an estimate of the oxygen gradient between the alveolar and the arterial side. It is estimated as

$$\text{A-a gradient} = (Fio_2 *[\text{barometric pressure} - \text{water vapor pressure}] - [Paco_2/R] - Pao_2),$$

where $Paco_2$ in mm Hg is the arterial partial pressure of carbon dioxide and *R* is the respiratory quotient. *R* could be influenced by diet, for example, a neonate on intravenous dextrose (pure carbohydrate) may have an *R* of 1 and a neonate on a mixed diet may have an *R* of 0.8. The normal A-a gradient is usually less than 20 mm Hg.

Oxygen Saturation Index

The OSI is an alternate to the OI if access to ABG is not available. It is calculated using preductal Spo_2 instead of Pao_2:

$$OSI = Fio_2 * 100 * (MAP/Spo_2).$$

For an SpO_2 level of 75% to 99%, the OI is approximately twice the OSI.[39] Also, an OI derived from the OSI has been shown to have good agreement and be strongly predictive of clinically relevant OI cutoffs (in the range of 5 to 25).[40]

X-Ray Imaging of the Chest

Characteristic findings on chest x-ray could aide in the diagnosis of underlying lung pathology and management of PPHN.

- Dark lung fields—primary or idiopathic PPHN; these could also happen in pulmonic stenosis and pneumothorax
- Whiteout lung fields—severe RDS, pneumonia, collapse or atelectasis, or massive effusion (including chylothorax)
- Reticulo-granular pattern—RDS, pneumonia
- Patchy—pneumonia, MAS
- Fluffy pattern—MAS, hyperexpanded x-ray
- Bubbly—pulmonary interstitial emphysema
- Streaky pattern—transient tachypnea of the newborn

The appearance of the heart could also help in diagnosing CHD:

- Egg on a string appearance—transposition of great arteries
- Snowman appearance—total anomalous pulmonary venous return
- Boot-shaped heart—tetralogy of Fallot
- A figure three or reverse figure three—coarctation of the aorta

Optimal inflation of the lungs to functional residual capacity results in the lowest PVR. Adequately inflated lungs are usually indicated by eight to nine ribs expanded with a nonflattened diaphragm, as seen on an anterior-posterior view of a chest x-ray. In the presence of diaphragmatic hernia, eight-rib expansion on the contralateral side is considered to be optimal.

Echocardiography

Echocardiographic evidence of PPHN is of paramount importance to begin therapy and to assess response to therapy. Specific echocardiographic features help in the diagnosis of PPHN and estimation of pulmonary arterial pressure (PAP). A modified Bernoulli equation is used to estimate pressures from peak wave signals obtained from echocardiography. If a peak pulmonary regurgitation (PR) signal is obtained, the mean PAP (mPAP) can be approximated by the following Bernoulli equation: $mPAP = 4*(PR\ peak\ velocity)^2 + RAP$ (right atrial pressure).[41] Often, tricuspid regurgitation (TR jet) velocity is obtained, and the right ventricular systolic pressure (RVSP) is calculated as $4*(TR\ peak\ velocity)^2 + RAP$. The diagnosis of PPHN is based on the following echocardiographic findings in the absence of structural heart disease:

- RVSP higher than 30 to 40 mm Hg
- RVSP/systemic systolic blood pressure ratio higher than 0.5
- Cardiac shunt at the patent ductus arteriosus or patent foramen ovale level with bidirectional or right-to-left shunting
- Any degree of ventricular wall septal flattening
- Hypertrophied and dilated right ventricle
- Dilated right ventricle

Brain Natriuretic Peptide

Brain natriuretic peptide (BNP) is a biomarker that increases when there is left ventricular strain and dilation. Serial levels of BNP are more valuable to assess trends than is a single estimation. Serial BNP measurements along with echocardiography are performed to assess the severity of BPD-associated pulmonary hypertension in preterm neonates who require oxygen.[7]

Evidence-Based Management of PPHN

If available, the treatment recommendations are graded based on the class of recommendations (COR) and level of evidence (LOE) as recommended by the European Society of Cardiology and the American Heart Association and are adopted from recommendations by Abman et al.[38] and Hilgendorff et al.[7] A detailed description of the COR and LOE may be found in the executive summary by Hansmann et al.[42]

The goals of managing PPHN (Fig. 13.5) are to provide

- adequate oxygenation and ventilation support
- circulatory support by maintaining systemic blood pressure
- pulmonary vasodilator therapy to reduce pulmonary arterial pressures
- oxygenation, ventilation, and optimized gas exchange.

The care of a neonate with PPHN and HRF needs to be tailored based on the underlying disorder and the severity of the disease.

A newborn with PPHN or suspected PPHN is transferred to and cared for in a neonatal intensive care unit (NICU). In rare instances, PPHN could be detected in an infant with labile oxygen saturations but with preductal $SpO_2 > 90\%$ with minimal respiratory support and could be managed in a community hospital nursery with close follow-up. However, given the nature of the disease and risk of rapid progression, it is best to transfer these infants in a NICU. To minimize oxygen demand, infants are usually cared for in a neutral thermal environment (with the exception of infants with associated moderate to severe hypoxic-ischemic encephalopathy undergoing therapeutic hypothermia). The infant is placed on a cardiorespiratory monitor with preductal and postductal saturation monitoring. Systemic blood pressures are monitored invasively using an umbilical or peripheral arterial line or with an appropriate cuff if an arterial line is not available.

Supportive Care

Optimal temperature management, maintaining euglycemia, assessing the need for invasive ventilation, arterial line placement for access and blood draws, assessing the need for intravenous (IV) nutrition, minimal stimulation, and sedation should be considered for a newborn based on the degree of PPHN and the severity of hypoxemia.

When sepsis or pneumonia is suspected as the underlying cause, obtaining a blood culture and a complete blood count with differential and starting IV antibiotics is of prime importance.

In cases of birth asphyxia and hypoxic-ischemic encephalopathy for which the neonate is undergoing therapeutic hypothermia, PPHN could be associated with coagulopathy and hematologic and electrolyte abnormalities, which should be corrected.

Acidosis (pH of <7.25), both metabolic and respiratory, can worsen PVR and PPHN.[43] Correcting ventilator parameters and providing IV fluids (crystalloids and blood products if needed) is recommended to maintain perfusion, prevent lactic acidosis, and maintain pH in the normal range, whereas hyperventilation and alkali infusion are best avoided. A target pH of >7.25 with a lactate level of <5 mmol/L and with $PaCO_2$ in the range of 45 to 60 mm Hg is recommended (COR IIa and LOE B).[7]

Avoiding excessive stimulation and providing a comfortable environment is important for the management of PPHN, especially in intubated infants. Pain and agitation in an intubated neonate could lead to asynchrony of breathing and worsen gas exchange, aggravating hypoxia, hypercarbia, and respiratory acidosis. Catecholamine release with poor pain control could increase PVR and worsen PPHN. Infusion of opioids such as morphine and fentanyl provides comfort and pain relief and is often used in intubated neonates in the NICU along with rescue doses as needed. The role of paralytic drugs

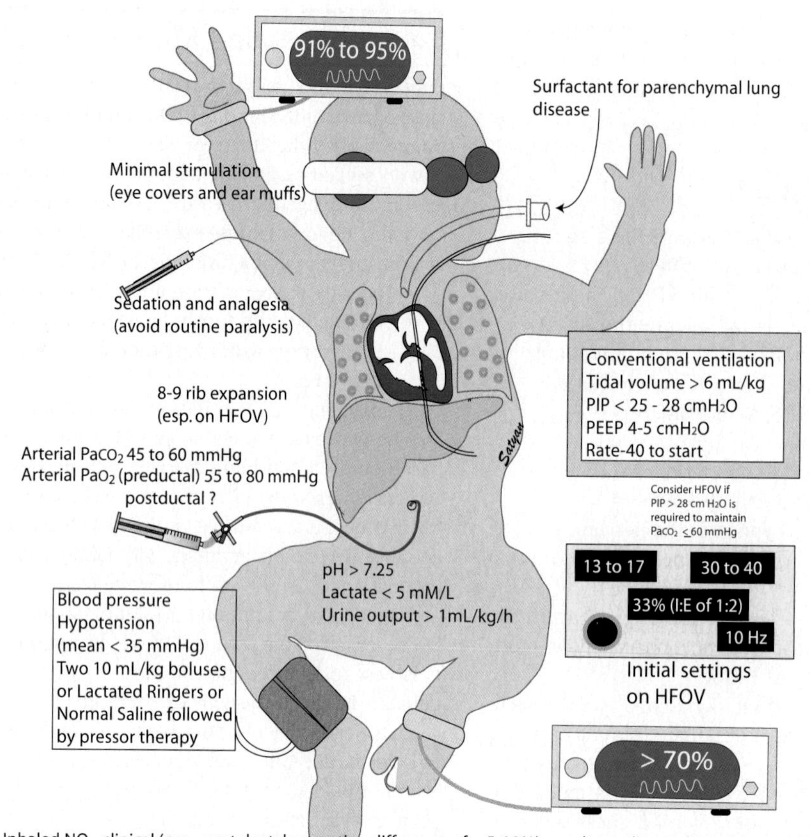

Fig. 13.5 Evidence-Based Management of Pulmonary Hypertension of the Newborn. Gentle ventilation (permissive hypercapnia with tolerable hypoxemia while avoiding hyperoxia and hypocapnia) along with lung recruitment is key to optimal management of pulmonary hypertension of the newborn. Systemic hemodynamics and pulmonary vasodilator therapy are also shown in the figure. *HFOV,* High-frequency oscillatory ventilation; *I:E,* inspiratory-to-expiratory time ratio; *OI,* oxygenation index; *Paco₂*, partial pressure of carbon dioxide; *PEEP,* positive end-expiratory pressure; *PIP,* peak inspiratory pressure. (Copyright Satyan Lakshminrusimha.)

remains controversial, and until further evidence is available, it is usually not recommended in managing PPHN.

Positive Pressure Ventilation and Types of Ventilation

The need for PPV and the mode of ventilation is decided based on underlying parenchymal lung disease and the extent of hypoxemia. Lung recruitment and maintaining functional residual capacity is essential to optimize gas exchange and can improve the efficacy of iNO therapy (COR I and LOE B).[38] With the advent of high-flow nasal cannula (HFNC), noninvasive ventilation is increasingly used in NICUs to manage PPHN.

Noninvasive Ventilation

In neonates with no lung disease, a noninvasive mode of ventilation that provides adequate positive end-expiratory pressure (PEEP) is often used. In idiopathic PPHN or black-lung PPHN, CPAP, HFNC, or noninvasive PPV could be used to recruit the lungs and avoid lung injury. High intrathoracic pressures could inhibit cardiac return and worsen PPHN and could be avoided by using the noninvasive mode of ventilation.

Invasive Mode of Ventilation

PPHN secondary to parenchymal lung disease associated with an inability to oxygenate (inspired oxygen requirement >60%) or ventilate ($Paco_2$ of >60 mm Hg with respiratory acidosis [pH < 7.25]) requires intubation and mechanical ventilation. Gentle ventilation strategies using low peak inspiratory pressures (PIPs) and/or a tidal volume (TV) with adequate PEEP will ensure optimal lung inflation and avoid atelectasis and overexpansion of the lung.

In cases of severe lung disease, such as MAS, high-frequency ventilators (HFVs) are used to provide higher MAPs to maintain lung inflation, avoid air leaks, and optimize oxygenation and ventilation. In cases where a PIP of >28 cm H_2O and/or a TV of >6 mL/kg is needed in a conventional ventilator, it is recommended that an HFV be used. Combination therapy of an HFV and iNO is more effective in severe PPHN associated with parenchymal lung disease, with a lower rate of mortality or ECMO compared with an HFV or iNO therapy alone.[44]

Intratracheal Surfactant Therapy (COR IIa and LOE B)

Rescue surfactant therapy in preterm and term infants with RDS may be beneficial. Surfactant inactivation could occur in parenchymal lung diseases such as MAS and pneumonia. Use of surfactant was shown to decrease the risk of mortality and/or the need for ECMO when used early before iNO therapy in HRF, but it did not have the same effect on idiopathic or black-lung PPHN.[6,45] Thus, surfactant therapy could be considered in parenchymal lung disease with PPHN.[38]

Oxygen Use and Saturation Targets

Pulmonary vascular transition occurs with an increase in arterial oxygenation at birth. Oxygen, a potent pulmonary vasodilator, is therapeutic in PPHN. Supplemental oxygen in conjunction with PPV to maintain optimal arterial oxygenation is essential. Brief exposure to 100% oxygen in transitioning animal models was shown to worsen pulmonary vascular contractility, reducing the subsequent response to iNO and increasing the risk of oxidative stress.[8,46,47] Targeting the preductal Spo_2 between 91% and 95% is optimal when PPHN is suspected or established (COR I and LOE A).[7] Intermittent desaturations and Spo_2 >97% should be avoided.[7]

Maintaining Systemic Pressures

It is important to maintain systemic pressures for gestational age in a neonate with PPHN. Ensuring adequate cardiac output and perfusion helps to maintain tissue oxygenation. Systemic hypotension worsens hypoxemia by increasing right-to-left shunting. The underlying cause of systemic hypotension should be addressed (Fig. 13.6). Sepsis should be treated adequately with antibiotics. If there is a volume deficit, a fluid bolus with crystalloid should be considered. The hematocrit level should be maintained between 40% and 45% to improve tissue oxygenation and maintain systemic blood pressure. Coagulopathy should be corrected with blood products. High intrathoracic pressures secondary to a high MAP should be addressed, especially if the neonate is on HFV. Excessive sedation using opioids could also drop systemic pressures and should be used cautiously. Once underlying causes have been addressed, if the infant remains hypotensive, vasopressors should be considered to maintain systemic pressures. Target blood pressures for the gestational age should be maintained (Table 13.1). Aiming for supraphysiological values to exceed estimated pulmonary arterial pressure by echocardiogram puts added stress on the right ventricle and should be avoided.

Vasopressors

Dopamine is the most commonly used vasopressor in the NICU, and its selective action in certain dose ranges remains unknown, especially in preterm neonates. Dopamine at higher doses of infusion could also

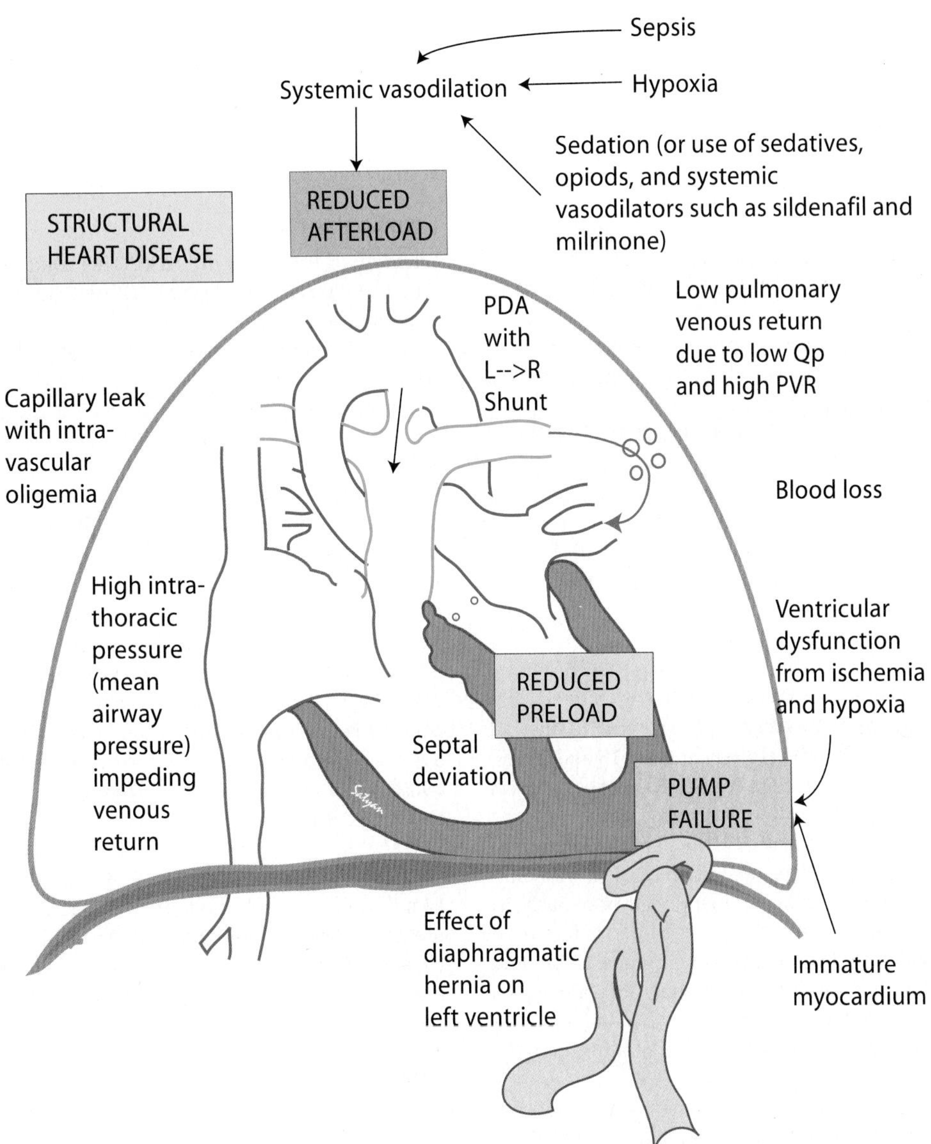

Fig. 13.6 Causes of Systemic Hypotension in Pulmonary Hypertension of the Newborn. Systemic hypotension in pulmonary hypertension of the newborn is common and is caused by the following pathogenic mechanisms: reduced afterload (due to sepsis or medications), reduced preload (due to high intrathoracic pressure from ventilators or septal deviation), and pump failure from hypoxia and ischemia (leading to systemic hypotension). *PDA*, Patent ductus arteriosus; *PVR*, pulmonary vascular resistance; *Qp*, pulmonary blood flow. (Copyright Satyan Lakshminrusimha.)

Table 13.1 Blood Pressure in Term Infants at Various Postnatal Ages[a]

Age	Systolic Blood Pressure	Mean Blood Pressure	Diastolic Blood Pressure
6–18 h	80 ± 13 (54)	57 ± 12 (33)	43 ± 10 (23)
18–30 h	83 ± 12 (59)	60 ± 11 (38)	46 ± 10 (26)
3 d ± 6 h	84 ± 14 (56)	60 ± 12 (36)	48 ± 13 (22)
7 d ± 1 d	91 ± 15 (61)	67 ± 13 (41)	52 ± 11 (30)

[a]The numbers in parentheses are the mean values minus two standard deviations and can be considered the lower limit of the normal range.

Based on Nascimento MC, Xavier CC, Goulart EM. Arterial blood pressure of term newborns during the first week of life. *Braz J Med Biol Res.* 2002;35:905–911.

constrict the pulmonary vasculature and increase the pulmonary pressure. Norepinephrine has been shown to increase systemic pressure and left ventricular output while decreasing the pulmonary–systemic ratio in neonates with PPHN and systemic hypotension.[48] Similarly, vasopressin may have some selectivity to systemic circulation and may be an optimal medication in PPHN. Hydrocortisone is used to treat systemic hypotension, especially if it is refractory to vasopressor therapy.[49] In clinical practice, steroids are also used in iNO-resistant PPHN and systemic hypotension, which may improve hemodynamic stability.

Pulmonary Vasodilator Therapy

Inhaled NO is indicated for the treatment of PPHN in neonates on a mechanical ventilator to improve oxygenation and reduce the need for ECMO (COR I and LOE A) if the OI is >25.[7,38] Endogenously, NO is produced in the endothelium and is an important regulator of pulmonary vascular tone.[50] Administered as an inhaled drug, iNO is a selective pulmonary vasodilator without a significant effect on systemic blood pressure. Ventilation–perfusion mismatch improves secondary to dilation of pulmonary vessels in the ventilated region of the lung (microselective effect of iNO).

Evidence from randomized controlled trials using iNO in PPHN includes the following:

- The Neonatal Inhaled Nitric Oxide study (NINOs) studied 235 late preterm and term infants; iNO therapy decreased the need for ECMO but did not affect mortality in severe HRF.[51]
- Davidson et al. evaluated 155 term infants with PPHN; early iNO improved oxygenation for 24 hours without sustained short-term adverse effects.[52]
- Clark et al. randomized 248 neonates after 34 weeks' gestation; iNO reduced the need for ECMO in neonates with PPHN.[53]
- Konduri et al. randomized 299 term and near-term infants and showed that initiation of iNO between an OI of 15 and 25 did not reduce mortality or the need for ECMO compared with initiation at an OI of >25.[54]

With echocardiographic evidence of PPHN and in the absence of CHD, iNO could be started at a dose of 20 ppm and its response assessed by a change in the P/F ratio, as mentioned previously. A dose >20 ppm is not recommended.

In the systemic circulation, iNO combines with hemoglobin and is converted to methemoglobin and nitrate, thus neutralizing its systemic effects. Methemoglobin is monitored at 2 hours and then at 8 hours after initiating iNO. Subsequently, it is monitored daily, and the preferred level is less than 5%.

Weaning from iNO therapy should be gradual because an abrupt decrease in dosing may lead to rebound hypertension.[55,56] There is no clear evidence to suggest a protocol to wean from iNO.[57] Many institutions decrease iNO by 5 ppm for a PaO_2 >60 mm Hg or a persistent O_2 of <60% every 4 hours until reaching 5 ppm, and subsequently by 1 ppm. This approach may safely avoid rebound PPHN.

iNO-Resistant PPHN

An inadequate or ill-sustained response to iNO could be due to poor lung recruitment, failure to optimize systemic hemodynamics (including the presence of LV dysfunction), excessive oxidative stress, or ineffectiveness of target enzymes. The first step is to optimize lung recruitment (COR I and LOE B). Subsequently, a repeat echocardiogram to assess pulmonary pressures and ventricular function and measures to optimize systemic circulation should be implemented. In infants with worsening hypoxemia, alternate pulmonary vasodilators and an assessment of the need for ECMO should be done. Cardiac conditions such as total anomalous pulmonary venous return, genetic conditions such as alveolo-capillary dysplasia, and congenital surfactant deficiency should also be considered.

Prostaglandins

Intravenous Prostaglandin E1 (PGE1) could be considered to maintain ductal patency in severe PPHN with no post-tricuspid unrestrictive shunt-like ventricular septal defect (COR IIa and LOE B). Ductal patency decreases right ventricular afterload, especially in neonates with CDH and PPHN.[58] Inhaled PGI_2 analogs could be considered in iNO-refractory PPHN with an OI >25 (COR IIb and LOE B).[38]

Sildenafil

Both oral and IV forms of sildenafil, a phosphodiesterase 5 inhibitor, are used in the treatment of PPHN.[59,60] In settings without access to iNO, sildenafil is the primary pulmonary vasodilator, and IV sildenafil could be considered for treatment of PPHN in a critically ill neonate refractory to iNO, especially if the OI is >25 (COR IIb and LOE B).[7] IV sildenafil has been shown to improve oxygenation even in neonates who were not exposed to iNO.[60] Oral sildenafil could be considered in BPD-associated pulmonary hypertension and PPHN, especially if iNO is not available (COR IIa and LOE B).[7] Systemic hypotension is a major side effect of using sildenafil and could affect the pulmonary/systemic pressure ratio, which could worsen PPHN.

Milrinone

IV milrinone is a phosphodiesterase 3 inhibitor that is reasonable to use in infants with PPHN and left ventricular (LV) dysfunction (COR IIa and LOE B).[38] It increases cyclic adenosine monophosphate in pulmonary, systemic, and cardiac muscle. Milrinone can also cause systemic hypotension and needs close monitoring of blood pressure.

Bosentan

Bosentan is an endothelin 1 receptor blocker and is used in adults with pulmonary hypertension. In a placebo-controlled exploratory trial involving 21 near-term and term neonates, bosentan did not improve oxygenation or improve outcomes.[61] However, it continues to be used for iNO-refractory PPHN, especially associated with CDH.

ECMO in Management of PPHN

ECMO is a lifesaving option available in select centers for neonates with severe PPHN who are >34 weeks with a weight of >2000 g and an OI >40 or A-a gradient of >600 after aggressive management for reversible lung disease.[7,38] ECMO is performed by cannulating large vessels, and the blood is run through an extracorporeal system that provides gas exchange and sustains life until there is improvement in pulmonary pressures. Venoarterial and venovenous ECMO are two types that are often used. Venovenous ECMO enhances pulmonary vasodilation by allowing oxygenated blood to flow through pulmonary circulation. Conditions such as CDH, MAS, and idiopathic PPHN constitute the majority of the respiratory illnesses in the neonatal age group that require ECMO.[62]

Special Scenarios

Preterm PPHN

Currently there is no evidence to support iNO therapy in preterm neonates with early PPHN. A consensus statement from the American Academy of Pediatrics and National Institutes of Health does not recommend using iNO in preterm neonates.[63,64] However, a recent expert recommendation from the American Thoracic Society suggests that selective use of iNO could be beneficial in preterm infants with severe hypoxemia secondary to PPHN physiology rather than parenchymal lung disease, especially with the antenatal risk factors of PROM and oligohydramnios.[65] Avoiding hypoxia by targeting an Spo_2 value in the low to mid-90s, maintaining systemic pressures, and using lung recruitment strategies are helpful in managing preterm PPHN. Inhaled NO therapy should not be used to prevent bronchopulmonary dysplasia.

Congenital Diaphragmatic Hernia

In neonates with CDH-associated PPHN, iNO did not reduce mortality or the need for ECMO.[66] Optimizing oxygenation/ventilation and improving systemic hemodynamics with supportive care is helpful in management. Lung-protective gentle ventilation is recommended in CDH management due to the presence of lung hypoplasia.

Outcomes in Neonates With PPHN

Regardless of treatment intervention, neonates with PPHN have 10% mortality along with poor pulmonary and neurodevelopmental outcomes.[23,67–70] In neonates randomized to early iNO with PPHN, 25% had impaired neurodevelopmental outcomes and 22% had hearing impairment.[67] Early-school-age follow-up at 5 to 10 years among 109 patients with PPHN enrolled in three trials showed that 24% had respiratory problems, 60% had abnormal chest x-rays, and 6.4% had some sensorineural hearing loss.[70] Also, full-scale intelligent quotient (IQ) evaluation showed that 9.2% of the patients had a score <70 and 7.4% had a score of 70 to 84. It is not clear if associated asphyxia, hypoxemia, and circulatory disturbances play a role in long-term outcomes of patients with PPHN. Multidisciplinary follow-up of neonates with PPHN is necessary to monitor outcomes and to provide appropriate support.

Conclusion

Decades of important research have led to management strategies centered around ventilation strategies to optimize oxygenation and ventilation, strategies to support systemic circulation, and pulmonary vasodilator therapy, which have resulted in improving survival rates from much lower than 50% to about 90%. Understanding underlying pathology is helpful in tailoring therapy for PPHN. Extensive research from both translational and clinical studies during the past two decades has focused on iNO as a treatment for PPHN. In term neonates with PPHN, iNO has been beneficial in reducing mortality and the need for ECMO. The management strategies for PPHN in neonates with CDH, acute PPHN in preterm neonates, and late BPD-associated pulmonary hypertension remain controversial. Alternate pulmonary vasodilator therapies, oxygen management strategies, and the role of genetic factors need further research. Quality-of-life outcomes in neonates with PPHN also warrant further evaluation.

Section 2

CHAPTER

14 Bronchopulmonary Dysplasia

Mireille Guillot, Bernard Thébaud

KEY POINTS

1. Minimally invasive surfactant therapy administered via a thin catheter is the most commonly studied less invasive surfactant administration strategy and has been shown to improve survival free of bronchopulmonary dysplasia (BPD).
2. Compared with continuous positive airway pressure, nasal intermittent positive pressure ventilation (NIPPV) is a useful method to avoid respiratory failure or intubation or extubation failure. However, NIPPV does not improve death or BPD.
3. Volume-targeted ventilation is superior to pressure-limited ventilation for short-term respiratory outcomes and for death or BPD.
4. Compared with an oxygen saturation target of 85% to 89%, a target of 91% to 95% decreases the risk of death and necrotizing enterocolitis without increasing blindness in extremely preterm infants.
5. The benefits and the risks of systemic postnatal steroids in neonates at high risk of BPD must be carefully evaluated by the clinician. The optimal dosage and duration of systemic corticosteroids are still under investigation.
6. Inhaled corticosteroids are not associated with a significant reduction in BPD and might increase mortality. Combined with surfactant administration, inhaled corticosteroids might be an attractive strategy to reduce BPD.
7. Intramuscular administration of vitamin A modestly reduces the incidence of BPD, but the concern by healthcare providers of repeated painful intramuscular administration has restricted its clinical use.
8. Caffeine reduces the incidence of BPD with some long-term mid–school-age neurodevelopmental benefits compared with placebo in extremely preterm infants.
9. Inhaled nitric oxide, diuretics, and bronchodilators have not shown effectiveness in reducing the risk of BPD.

Introduction

Bronchopulmonary dysplasia (BPD), a multifactorial disease affecting the normal sequence of lung growth, is one of the most frequent complications of prematurity. Approximately 40% of neonates born before 28 weeks' gestation are affected by BPD.[1] Despite improved neonatal intensive care unit therapies, the incidence of BPD has not significantly changed during the past two decades.[1,2] Survivors with BPD are at increased risk of adverse neurodevelopmental and pulmonary outcomes.[3–5] Consequently, BPD remains a major challenge for neonatologists, and it is a priority to improve the care of and optimize the outcomes for children with BPD.

BPD was originally described more than 50 years ago as a severe pulmonary disease occurring after treatment with mechanical ventilation and high levels of oxygen in preterm neonates.[6] The seminal report from Northway et al. in 1967 described a cohort of 32 preterm neonates born between 30 and 34 weeks' gestation, of whom only 4 survived.[6] Since this report, several changes in neonatal care have drastically improved the survival of preterm infants born at increasingly earlier stages of gestation. The originally described BPD disease, now coined "old" BPD (Fig. 14.1), has been replaced largely by "new" BPD, which affects predominantly extremely preterm infants (Table 14.1; Fig. 14.2).[7]

The etiology of BPD is multifactorial and results from the contribution of antenatal exposures and postnatal injuries, superimposed on an immature lung (Figs. 14.3 and 14.4).[8] The pathogenesis of "new" BPD is characterized by a highly immature lung (at the late canalicular and/or saccular stage of development) with abnormal alveoli and vascular development.[9,10] In the most severe cases, infants with BPD may develop pulmonary hypertension and pulmonary vascular disease.[11] Computerized tomography typically shows heterogeneously hyperlucent lungs owing to foci of air-trapping. Coarse interstitial markings can be seen (Fig. 14.5).

With evolving neonatal respiratory management and the increasing survival of preterm neonates during the past decades, several different definitions of BPD have emerged to better represent the population at risk.[12–15] In 1988, BPD was defined by the use of oxygen at 36 weeks' gestation.[14] In 2000, a more comprehensive definition was suggested and included a separate definition for infants born at <32 weeks' gestation versus at ≥ 32 weeks' gestation and for levels of severity (mild, moderate, and severe) based on the amount of oxygen provided and/or the need for respiratory support.[16] This definition was further changed to include an oxygen challenge test.[17] More recently, it was suggested that defining BPD only at 40 weeks' gestation might better predict pulmonary outcomes.[13] In practice, the definition of BPD as the need for supplemental oxygen beyond 36 weeks' gestation is the most commonly used.[12,14] Despite the best attempts at correctly defining BPD, the current definitions are simply based on the ventilation and/or oxygen treatment at a specific time point rather than including any pathophysiological or anatomic aspects of the disease.[12,18] The definition of BPD is an evolving concept, and it remains a challenge when used as an endpoint in evaluating preventive and therapeutic strategies.[18,19] Future definitions of BPD should attempt to include markers of severity of lung pathology or specific biomarkers that would potentially better standardize the disease and improve the prediction of long-term outcomes.[19–21]

This chapter's main focus is on strategies to prevent BPD, including recent respiratory support strategies and pharmacologic approaches (corticosteroids, vitamin A, caffeine, nitric oxide, diuretics, and bronchodilators). Unfortunately, none of these approaches has markedly decreased the incidence of BPD. New therapies, including stem cell–based therapies and insulinlike growth factor 1, are currently being studied and will be briefly discussed in this chapter.

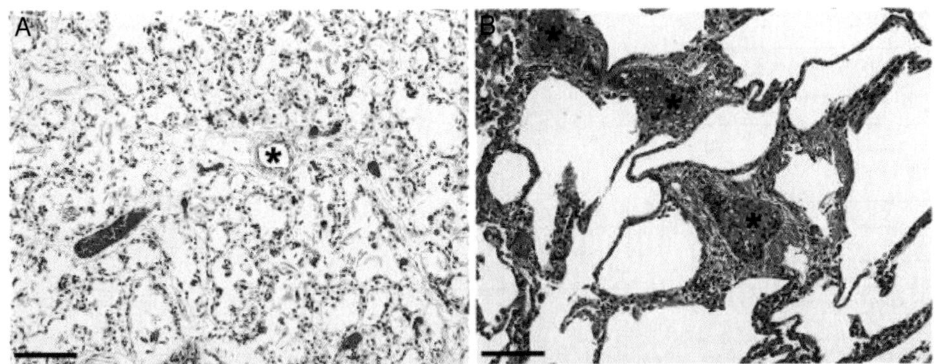

Fig. 14.1 Histopathological Changes Seen in Bronchopulmonary Dysplasia. Hematoxylin and eosin staining of tissue sections from (A) a term infant and (B) a patient of 55 weeks' corrected gestational age with bronchopulmonary dysplasia. Note severe alveolar simplification concomitant with medial wall thickening of pulmonary arteries in (B) compared with (A). Asterisks define pulmonary arteries. Scale bar = 10 μm. (Reproduced with permission from Christ LA, Sucre JM, Frank DB. Lung disease and pulmonary hypertension in the premature infant. *Prog Pediatr Cardiol*. 2019;54:101135.)

Table 14.1 Clinical and Pathologic Changes in Old and New BPD

Old BPD[a]	New BPD[b]
CLINICAL Stage 1: Acute respiratory distress syndrome. Stage 2: Opaque lung fields with air bronchograms due to patchy atelectasis alternating with emphysema. Lung volume normal to low. Pulmonary edema due to shunt across the ductus arteriosus. Stage 3: Small radiolucent fields and streaky densities with early hyperinflation. Stage 4: Hyperinflated lungs with generalized cystic areas.	CLINICAL Disorder of lung development in premature infants born at a gestational age <28 weeks and birth weight <1000 g with persistent respiratory insufficiency. Distinct stages not well-defined.
PATHOLOGY Fewer alveoli develop after birth. Many areas of the lung show inflammation and scarring. The size of alveoli varies with areas of atelectasis and hyperinflation. Strands containing hypertrophied peribronchial smooth muscle, fibroblasts, and dense fibrotic strands. Perimucosal fibrosis. Inflammation marked by newly infiltrated macrophages and resident histiocytes, many of which are enlarged with engulfed lipids (foam cells). Tortuous lymphatics. Altered microvascular development. Early changes of pulmonary hypertension can be seen with vessels showing medial hypertrophy and elastin-rich degenerative-regenerative lesions.	PATHOLOGY Overall fewer alveoli. Alveolar size varies with areas of atelectasis and hyperinflation. Altered microvascular development. Early changes of pulmonary hypertension can be seen with vessels showing medial hypertrophy and elastin-rich degenerative-regenerative lesions.

[a]Old BPD was seen in premature infants born at relatively later gestational ages who sustained lung injury related to barotrauma/volutrauma and infection; the most prominent histopathological changes were those of inflammation and scarring.

[b]New BPD most commonly occurs in extremely preterm infants born before 28 weeks gestational age, and the most prominent changes are those of inhibited alveolar development.

BPD, Bronchopulmonary dysplasia.

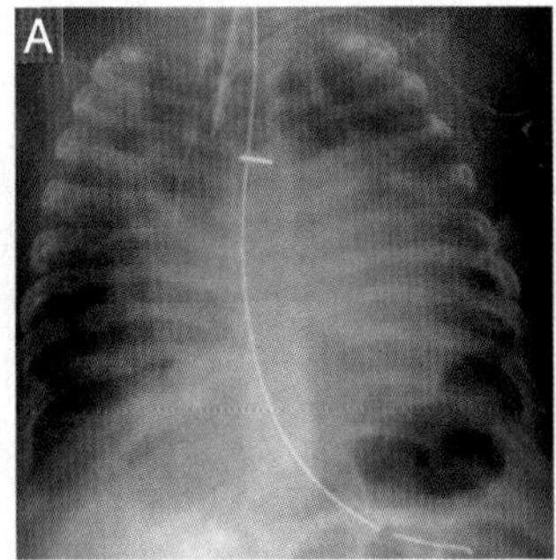

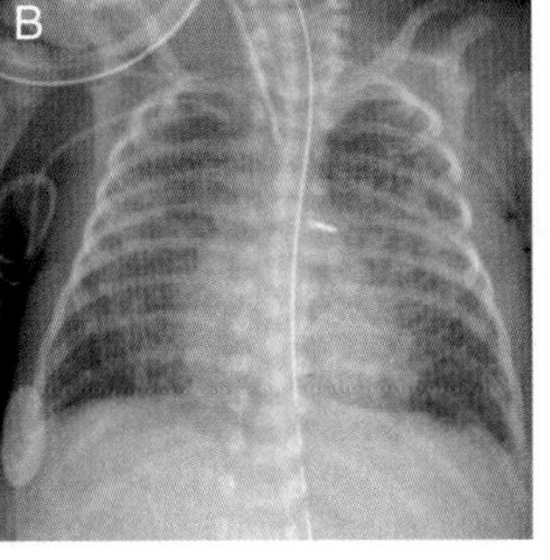

Fig. 14.2 Chest Radiographs. (A) Areas of hyperinflation and emphysema with adjacent dense areas of atelectasis. This picture is characteristic of "old" bronchopulmonary dysplasia. (B) "New" bronchopulmonary dysplasia, showing generalized homogeneous opacities with an interstitial pattern. (Reproduced with permission from Merrow AC, Hariharan SL. *Imaging in Pediatrics*. Philadelphia: Elsevier; 2018;56–57.)

Management

BPD is a multifactorial disease. Current approaches aim to use lung-protective c = ventilation strategies, combined with pharmacologic therapies to attenuate inflammation, promote lung repair, and stimulate respiratory drive.

Respiratory Support Strategies

Different ventilation strategies have been considered to prevent the development of lung injury and establishment of BPD. Table 14.2 summarizes recent respiratory support approaches studied in preterm infants.

Sustained Inflation

Preclinical studies have demonstrated that sustained inflation (SI) at the onset of neonatal resuscitation improves lung inflation

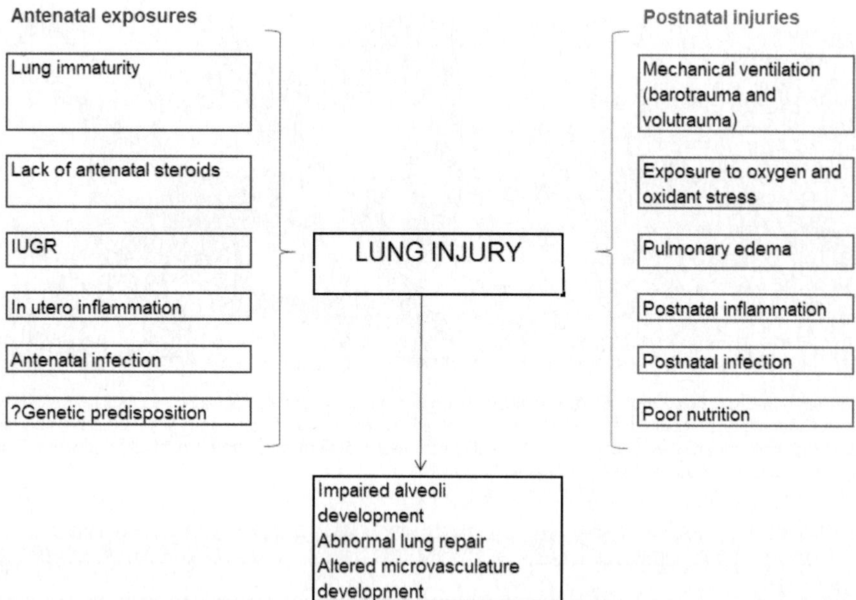

Fig. 14.3 Pathogenesis of Bronchopulmonary Dysplasia: Complex Interaction of Several Factors. *IUGR,* Intrauterine growth restriction.

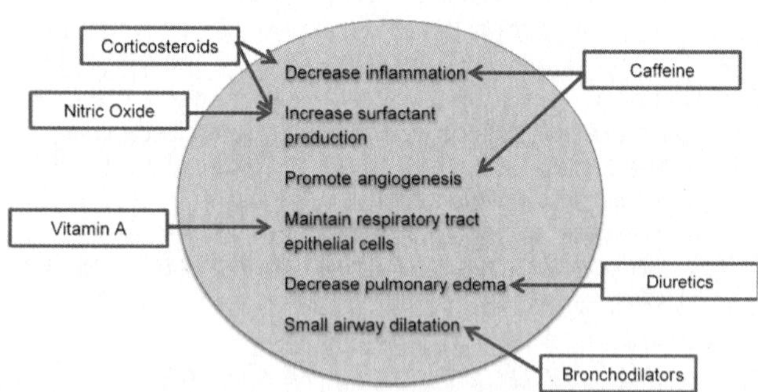

Fig. 14.4 Possible Mechanisms of Pharmacologic Approaches in Bronchopulmonary Dysplasia.

and produces a greater functional residual capacity without impairing the neonatal cardiovascular transition.[22,23] Subsequent to these studies, several randomized controlled trials (RCTs) compared SI to intermittent positive pressure ventilation (PPV) at the initiation of resuscitation.[24–26] Three meta-analysis compared the efficacy of SI immediately after birth versus intermittent PPV and showed no improvement in the rate of BPD and/or death.[24–26] One meta-analysis showed improvement in short-term respiratory outcomes of infants receiving SI, with a decrease in mechanical ventilation within 72 hours after birth.[25] The studies included in the three meta-analyses used heterogeneous SI strategies (one to multiple SIs, for 5 to 20 seconds, with variable positive inspiratory pressure) in a population of preterm infants of varied gestational age.

Recently a large multicenter RCT (SAIL trial), not included in the previous meta-analysis, reported on the effect of SI versus intermittent PPV in a cohort of extremely preterm infants.[27] The authors reported no difference in the outcome of death or BPD between the groups. However, the trial was stopped early due to increased mortality at less than 48 hours of life in infants receiving SI. Current evidence does not support the use of SI in the prevention of BPD and/or death.

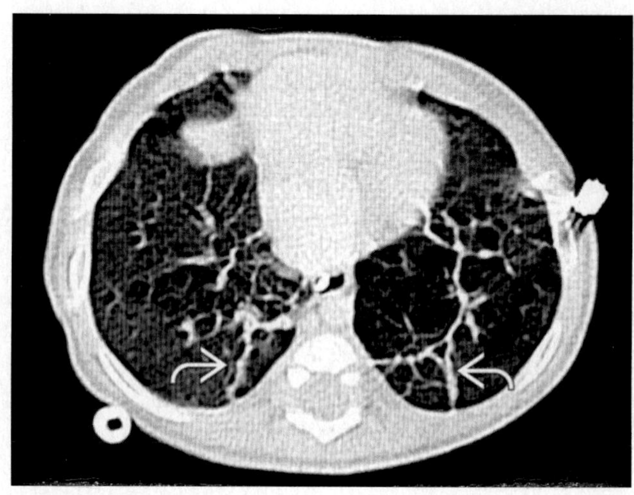

Fig. 14.5 Axial Chest Computed Tomography of an Infant With Bronchopulmonary Dysplasia. Heterogeneously hyperlucent lungs due to foci of air-trapping are shown. Coarse interstitial markings with parenchymal bands *(arrow)* are noted bilaterally. (Reproduced with permission from Merrow AC, Hariharan SL. *Imaging in Pediatrics*. Philadelphia: Elsevier; 2018;56–57.)

Surfactant

Based on a meta-analysis of studies comparing prophylactic versus selective administration of surfactant in very preterm neonates, the prophylactic use of surfactant is no longer recommended.[28] The meta-analysis included two studies designed to compare prophylactic surfactant treatment with early initiation of continuous positive airway pressure (CPAP) treatment and found an increased risk of BPD or death with the prophylactic administration of surfactant (2 trials; 1744 neonates; relative risk [RR], 1.12; 95% confidence interval [CI], 1.02–1.24).[28]

Surfactant administration traditionally involves intubation and mechanical ventilation. Exposure to mechanical ventilation is associated with risk of volutrauma, barotrauma, and inflammatory responses, known as important risk factors for the development of BPD. As such, new techniques to administer surfactant while avoiding prolonged ventilation have been developed.

Table 14.2 Recent Respiratory Support Strategies to Prevent Lung Injury

Approaches	Evidence
Sustained inflation	Three meta-analyses compared sustained inflation to intermittent PPV: no effect on BPD and/or death[24–26] One large RCT (SAIL trial): increased mortality at <48 h in infants receiving sustained inflation; no effect on BPD or death[27]
Surfactant	One meta-analysis compared prophylactic surfactant to routine stabilization on CPAP: reduction in BPD or death with early CPAP treatment[27a]
INSURE	Cochrane review compared INSURE to rescue surfactant: INSURE reduced mechanical ventilation and BPD[28] Meta-analysis compared early INSURE with CPAP alone: no effect on BPD and/or death[29]
MIST	One metanarrative review (10 studies—thin catheter administration evaluated in 6 studies): surfactant administration via thin catheter may be efficacious and safe[31] One systematic review comparing MIST to standard surfactant administration: MIST was associated with reduction in death or BPD[33] One systematic review comparing MIST to 6 other ventilation strategies: MIST was associated with the lowest likelihood of death or BPD[32]
NEWER VENTILATION STRATEGIES	
NIPPV	Cochrane review compared early NIPPV with early CPAP: NIPPV decreased respiratory failure and intubation; no effect on BPD[37] Cochrane review compared NIPPV with CPAP after extubation in preterm neonates: NIPPV decreased extubation failure; no effect on BPD or death[35] One RCT compared NIPPV with CPAP in infants aged <30 weeks: no effect on BPD or death[38]
Noninvasive HFV	One meta-analysis compared noninvasive HFV with CPAP: noninvasive HFV decreased intubation rate and improved CO_2 clearance[43]
Volume-targeted ventilation	Cochrane review compared volume-targeted ventilation to pressure-limited ventilation: volume-targeted decreased death or BPD[46]
Oxygen saturation target	One meta-analysis compared high (91%–95%) with low (85%–89%) Spo_2 target in extremely preterm infants: no difference in death or disability; higher risk of death in lower target Spo_2 group[49]

BPD, Bronchopulmonary dysplasia; *CPAP*, continuous positive airway pressure; *HFV*, high-frequency ventilation; *INSURE*, intubate, surfactant, extubate; *MIST*, minimally invasive surfactant therapy; *NIPPV*, nasal intermittent positive pressure ventilation; *PPV*, positive pressure ventilation; *RCT*, randomized controlled trial; Spo_2, oxygen saturation.

Intubate, Surfactant, Extubate

The intubate, surfactant, extubate (INSURE) approach involves intubation for early administration of surfactant followed by a brief period of mechanical ventilation and extubation to CPAP. A Cochrane review compared this approach to rescue administration of surfactant in preterm infants with respiratory distress syndrome and showed a decrease in mechanical ventilation and BPD.[29] A meta-analysis of 9 trials with a total of 1551 preterm infants compared early INSURE with CPAP alone.[30] The authors reported no benefits of early INSURE in the outcomes assessed, including BPD and/or death. However, the estimated RR favored early INSURE over CPAP alone (12% reduction in BPD and/or death; RR, 0.88; 95% CI, 0.76–1.02). Still, the need for premedication, the secondary effects, and the failure to extubate in a significant proportion of neonates led to the development of alternative techniques with noninvasive or minimally invasive administration of surfactant, with the goal to avoid intubation.[31]

Minimally Invasive Surfactant Administration

Several minimally invasive surfactant administration techniques (MIST) have been described, including administration via (1) a thin catheter, (2) aerosol or nebulization, (3) a laryngeal mask airway, and (4) the pharyngeal airway. A metanarrative review was conducted in 2014 to assess the safety and efficacy of these techniques.[32] It included 10 studies, 6 of which used a thin catheter for surfactant administration, which appears to be an efficacious and potentially safe technique. Other systematic reviews comparing different ventilation strategies also suggested that MIST with surfactant delivery via a thin catheter reduced the composite outcome of death or BPD at 36 weeks' gestation.[33,34]

Further RCTs of surfactant administration via less invasive methods are underway and will help clarify the short- and long-term benefits of this practice. These studies will also help identify the best technique, optimal patient selection, and adequate surfactant dosage.

Newer Ventilation Strategies

Newer noninvasive ventilation strategies have been developed to avoid endotracheal intubation and its associated complications.

Nasal Intermittent Positive Pressure Ventilation

Nasal intermittent positive pressure ventilation (NIPPV) has been studied extensively for a variety of neonatal disorders.[35–38] A Cochrane review compared the efficacy of early NIPPV versus early CPAP in preterm infants and showed that NIPPV was associated with a reduction in respiratory failure and intubation but no reduction in BPD.[38] Another Cochrane review compared NIPPV versus CPAP after extubation in preterm neonates.[36] The analysis showed that NIPPV decreased the incidence of extubation failure but had no significant effect on BPD or death. To our knowledge, only one RCT comparing NIPPV versus CPAP restricted enrollment to neonates born before 30 weeks' gestation and assessed BPD or death as the primary outcome.[39] In this large, multicenter study, there was no difference in the incidence of death or BPD among patients assigned to the NIPPV or CPAP group.

Noninvasive High-Frequency Ventilation

Noninvasive high-frequency ventilation (HFV) has been suggested as a gentler and highly efficacious mode of ventilation for CO_2 clearance.[40] Small observational studies previously showed potential benefits of noninvasive HFV over CPAP in preterm and term neonates.[41,42] Despite the limited evidence available, noninvasive HFV is already used clinically in some European neonatal intensive care units.[43] A meta-analysis including eight RCTs involving 463 patients evaluated the safety and efficacy of noninvasive HFV.[44] The authors showed that compared with nasal CPAP or biphasic nasal CPAP, noninvasive HFV was associated with a lower intubation rate (RR, 0.50; 95% CI, 0.36–0.70) and a more effective clearance of CO_2 (weighted mean difference, −4.61; 95% CI, −7.94 to −1.28). So far, available data are promising for the use of noninvasive HFV. However, larger trials with long-term safety data are required.

Volume-Targeted Ventilation

Mechanical ventilation remains an essential tool in the management of many preterm infants, especially those born before 29 weeks' gestation.[1,45] Newer modes of mechanical ventilation have been associated with better lung protection.[46] A volume-targeted ventilation strategy, in which a constant volume is delivered with each ventilator inflation, has been shown to be a safe and efficient approach.[47] A recent Cochrane review showed that this ventilation strategy, compared with pressure-limited ventilation, was associated with a decrease in death or BPD (RR, 0.73; 95% CI, 0.59–0.89).[47] Additionally, volume-targeted ventilation is associated with a decreased duration of mechanical ventilation and a reduction in pneumothorax, hypocapnia, and severe intraventricular hemorrhage.[47]

Several other ventilation strategies including high-frequency ventilation and patient-triggered ventilation have been evaluated but failed to show a difference in the risk of death or BPD.[48,49]

Oxygen Saturation Targets

The neonatal oxygen prospective meta-analysis (NeOProM) compared the impact of high (91%–95%) versus low (85%–89%) oxygen saturation (Spo_2) target ranges on death or major morbidities in extremely preterm infants.[50,51] The meta-analysis included 5 large, multicenter trials performed in different parts of the world (the United States, Australia, New Zealand, Canada, and the United Kingdom), which together enrolled 4965 infants. The authors showed no difference between the groups in death or disability at 18 to 24 months. However, although infants assigned to the group with lower target Spo_2 had a lower incidence of retinopathy of prematurity requiring treatment, they had a higher risk of death and necrotizing enterocolitis and no difference in blindness. The benefits also occurred in subgroups. Further studies could help determine whether the target should be modified according to postnatal ages,[52] but data are insufficient to make changes based on postnatal ages, because the benefits observed in these trials occurred with the same saturation targets across all postnatal ages. Pending better additional data, a target oxygen saturation of 90% to 95% might be safer.[53]

Pharmacologic Interventions

Several different medications have been investigated as potential therapies to prevent or treat BPD. These medications include corticosteroids, vitamin A, caffeine, inhaled nitric oxide, diuretics, and bronchodilators. As demonstrated in Fig. 14.4, these therapies target potential disease mechanisms related to lung injury and BPD.

Corticosteroids

Inflammation is known as an important mediator in the development of BPD.[54] The use of corticosteroids to reduce inflammation has been extensively investigated (Table 14.3).

Systemic Corticosteroids in the First 7 Days of Life

Several studies have assessed early dexamethasone treatment (≤7 days) in preterm neonates.[55,56] Although early dexamethasone reduced the

Table 14.3 Corticosteroids and Bronchopulmonary Dysplasia

	Recommendation
SYSTEMIC CORTICOSTEROIDS	
In the first 7 days of life	
Early dexamethasone	Not recommended Increase CP and combined outcome of death or CP[54,55]
Early low-dose hydrocortisone	To consider in selected population Increase survival without BPD[58,63] Risk of gastrointestinal perforation when used in association with indomethacin[63]
After 7 days of life	
Late corticosteroids	To consider in selected population Cochrane review: late corticosteroids (dexamethasone or hydrocortisone) associated with a reduction in BPD, with no difference in death or CP[64] Systematic review: in infants at higher risk of BPD, late corticosteroids associated with a reduction in death or CP[65,66]
Late hydrocortisone	Not recommended Multicenter RCT: 22-day course of hydrocortisone did not improve the composite outcome of death or BPD[68] Multicenter RCT: 10-day course of hydrocortisone between day 14 and 28 did not improve survival without BPD[68a]
INHALED CORTICOSTEROIDS	
Inhaled corticosteroids	Not recommended Cochrane review: inhaled steroids is not superior to systemic steroids for preventing BPD or death in ventilated preterm neonates, with similar neurodevelopmental outcomes[69]
Early inhaled corticosteroids	Not recommended Cochrane review to determine the impact of inhaled corticosteroids when initiated within the first 2 weeks of life: reduction in BPD or death, but questionable clinical relevance[70] Multicenter RCT on long-term outcomes of inhaled budesonide: higher mortality in neonates who received budesonide[71]
Combination of inhaled corticosteroids and surfactant	Not recommended; larger trials needed Meta-analysis (two studies) evaluating efficacy of budesonide-surfactant versus surfactant alone or no treatment: reduction in BPD in patients receiving budesonide with surfactant[72]

BPD, Bronchopulmonary dysplasia; *CP*, cerebral palsy; *RCT*, randomized controlled trial.

incidence of death or BPD (RR, 0.88; 95% CI, 0.83–0.93), it is associated with significant short-term side effects (hyperglycemia, hypertension, gastrointestinal hemorrhage, and gastrointestinal perforation).[56] Importantly, cerebral palsy was significantly more common in infants treated with dexamethasone (RR, 1.42; 95% CI, 1.06–1.91). Given the potential adverse effects of dexamethasone treatment in the first week of life, it is not recommended for the prevention of BPD.[56,57]

Because of the serious side effects associated with early dexamethasone treatment, researchers have investigated the role of low-dose hydrocortisone as an alternative. There is evidence that sicker preterm infants have relative adrenal insufficiency and therefore are unable to produce sufficient cortisol to control inflammation in case of critical illness.[58] Prophylaxis of early adrenal insufficiency with low-dose hydrocortisone to prevent BPD has been studied in five RCTs.[59–63] In 1999, Watterberg et al. first described the effect of early low-dose hydrocortisone in a randomized, placebo-controlled study of 40 mechanically ventilated extremely low birth weight infants.[60] These authors showed an increased likelihood of survival without BPD in patients treated with hydrocortisone. More recently, Baud et al. conducted a multicenter RCT (PREMILOC) including 523 neonates born at less than 28 weeks' gestation who received either low-dose hydrocortisone for 10 days or a placebo.[59] In this study, the authors showed a significant increase in survival without BPD in the hydrocortisone group (60% versus 51% in the placebo group; odds ratio [OR], 1.48; 95% CI, 1.02–2.16; number needed to treat [NNT], 12).[59] Similarly, an individual-patient-data meta-analysis that included 982 neonates showed that early low-dose hydrocortisone for 10 to 15 days improved survival without BPD at 36 weeks (OR, 1.45; 95% CI, 1.11–1.90).[64] Importantly, when hydrocortisone is given in association with indomethacin, there is an increased risk of spontaneous gastrointestinal perforation. Additionally, although neonates exposed to hydrocortisone were more likely to develop late-onset sepsis, there were no negative effects on mortality or neurodevelopmental outcomes at 2 years of age.[64]

In conclusion, based on the available evidence, low-dose hydrocortisone initiated early after birth appears safe when not associated with indomethacin and improves survival without BPD, without having a negative impact on early neurodevelopment assessed at 2 years of age. As suggested by Doyle et al. in a recent Cochrane review, longer-term neurodevelopmental follow-up is needed to assess effects of hydrocortisone on higher-order neurologic functions.[56] There is also a need to identify the patients who will benefit the most from this therapy. In its policy statement, reaffirmed in 2014, the American Academy of Pediatrics stated that early treatment with hydrocortisone may be beneficial in a selected population, but there is insufficient evidence to recommend its use for all neonates at risk of BPD.[57]

Systemic Corticosteroids After 7 Days of Life

In a Cochrane systematic review updated in 2017, Doyle et al. examined the effects of late (>7 days after birth) systemic postnatal corticosteroids for prevention of BPD in 1424 preterm neonates.[65] Infants treated with late systemic corticosteroids (dexamethasone or hydrocortisone) had less incidence of BPD at 36 weeks' gestation (RR, 0.77; 95% CI, 0.67–0.88). Benefits of late corticosteroids also included reductions in failure to extubate and to be discharged on home oxygen and less rescue corticosteroid treatment. Adverse effects included short-term side effects such as hyperglycemia and hypertension and an increase in severe retinopathy of prematurity (without increase in blindness). There was no difference in the combined outcome of death or cerebral palsy, although long-term developmental data were limited. Interestingly, a systematic review published in 2005 showed that in infants at higher risk of BPD, corticosteroid treatment was associated with a reduction in death or cerebral palsy.[66] In an updated analysis by the same authors with data from 20 RCTs, the same relationship was observed with greater statistical significance.[67] There is ongoing research to determine the ideal dose and duration of corticosteroid therapy. Marr et al. recently compared 42-day versus 9-day courses of dexamethasone in extremely preterm neonates at high risk of BPD.[68] The authors showed that the prolonged course of dexamethasone was associated with improved short-term outcomes and an increased rate of survival without handicap at 7 years old (75% of children in the 42-day group had intact survival at school age, versus 35% in the 9-day group; $P < .005$). Based on the available evidence, dexamethasone treatment may be considered in ventilator-dependent preterm infants at high risk of BPD.

Hydrocortisone has also been considered as an alternative to dexamethasone. A multicenter RCT (STOP-BPD) examined the effect of hydrocortisone initiated 7 to 14 days after birth on mortality or BPD among ventilated preterm neonates.[69] The 22-day course of hydrocortisone (with a starting dosage of 5 mg/kg/day, for a cumulative dose of 72.5 mg/kg) did not improve the composite outcome of death or BPD at 36 weeks' gestation (adjusted OR, 0.87; 95% CI, 0.54–1.38). More recently, a large multicenter RCT involving 800 infants born less than 30 weeks' gestation at high risk for BPD evaluated the efficacy of hydrocortisone initiated after 2 weeks of life on survival without BPD. In this trial, hydrocortisone, started between postnatal day 14 to 28, was given over a period of 10 days (with a starting dosage of 4 mg/kg/day). This intervention was not associated with an improvement in survival without BPD, nor with survival without neurodevelopmental impairment.

Inhaled Corticosteroids

Inhaled corticosteroids were investigated as a possibly safer alternative to systemic corticosteroids. Unfortunately, the data regarding their efficacy are not convincing, and there are concerns regarding associated increases in mortality.

A Cochrane review including three trials (431 participants) compared inhaled with systemic steroids and showed that inhaled steroids did not confer any significant advantages over systemic steroids.[70] Another Cochrane systematic review examined the effect of early (within the first 2 weeks) inhaled corticosteroids on BPD.[71] Ten trials were included (with a total of 1644 very low birth weight [VLBW] infants), and the authors reported a significant reduction in the incidence of BPD or death in neonates receiving inhaled steroids (RR, 0.86; 95% CI, 0.75–0.99). However, this benefit is of questionable clinical relevance because the NNT for an additional beneficial outcome was 17, with a 95% CI of 9 to infinity.[71] Importantly, a long-term follow-up study by Bassler et al.[72] was not included in the review. Bassler et al. reported on the 18 to 22–month outcomes of a cohort of 863 extremely preterm infants randomized to receive early (≤24 hours) inhaled budesonide or placebo. They showed a significantly higher mortality rate in the budesonide group (19.9%) versus the placebo group (14.5%) (RR, 1.37; 95% CI, 1.01–1.86).[72] Although inhaled steroids are associated with a reduction in BPD, the increased mortality reported in a large RCT of inhaled steroids for BPD prevention is worrisome. Thus inhaled steroids should not be routinely used in the care of preterm infants.

Inhaled corticosteroids administered in combination with surfactant has also been studied as a BPD prevention strategy. A meta-analysis of 2 studies including 381 VLBW infants with severe respiratory distress syndrome requiring mechanical ventilation with a high fraction of inspired oxygen reported a 43% reduction in the risk of BPD (RR, 0.57; 95% CI, 0.43–0.76; NNT, 5) with no difference in mortality.[73] The major limitation of these studies is the high incidence of BPD in the control group (50%).[74] The effect size in a cohort with lower incidence of BPD would likely be much lower. Larger trials are ongoing to determine the effect of budesonide-surfactant (NCT04019106, NCT02907593, NCT03275415, and NCT00883532).

Vitamin A

Vitamin A is an essential nutrient for lung development and for maintaining the integrity of the respiratory epithelium. As such, it has been examined as a potential way to prevent BPD. A meta-analysis showed that intramuscular administration of vitamin A in VLBW infants was associated with a modest reduction in the incidence of BPD (RR, 0.87 [95% CI, 0.77–0.99]; NNT, 11 [95% CI, 6–100]).[75] However, vitamin A is not routinely used in practice, mainly because it involves repeated intramuscular injections, a painful procedure, and because of limited access and a perception of limited efficacy. Additional research has focused on determining the optimal dose and route of administration.[76–78]

Caffeine

Caffeine is a methylxanthine widely used in neonatal care to prevent and treat apnea of prematurity. Caffeine acts by increasing minute ventilation, central sensitivity to CO_2, and respiratory muscle function.[79] The Caffeine for Apnea of Prematurity (CAP) trial showed that caffeine therapy, initiated in the first 10 days of life in VLBW neonates, was associated with a reduced risk of BPD (RR, 0.72; 95% CI, 0.58–0.89) and earlier discontinuation of positive airway ventilation and supplemental oxygen compared with placebo.[80] A recent study from the Canadian Neonatal Network showed that earlier initiation of caffeine (in the first 2 days after birth) had additional benefits because it was associated with a decreased risk of death or BPD (adjusted OR, 0.81; 95% CI, 0.67–0.98).[81] The 11-year follow-up study of the CAP trial showed that caffeine was safe, and although it did not improve functional outcomes, it was associated with a lower risk of motor impairment and improved visual-motor integration.[82,83] In summary, caffeine therapy for apnea of prematurity appears to be a safe and effective strategy to reduce the incidence of BPD in VLBW neonates.

Inhaled Nitric Oxide

Inhaled nitric oxide (iNO) is a pulmonary vasodilator currently used in term and near-term infants with pulmonary hypertension. Trials in preterm neonates were initiated after animal studies suggested that iNO could also have beneficial effects on lung injury and evolving BPD.[84–86]

Two published meta-analyses evaluated the impact of iNO in preterm infants on the rate of BPD and mortality.[87,88] First, Donohue et al. included 14 RCTs in their analysis and showed a small reduction in the composite outcome of death or BPD (RR, 0.93; 95% CI, 0.87–0.99) but no difference in death alone or BPD.[87] Second, a 2017 Cochrane review reported on 17 RCTs of iNO therapy in preterm infants, which were analyzed in three different categories based on their inclusion criteria.[88] Eight trials of early rescue treatment (iNO initiated before 3 days) showed no significant effect of iNO on BPD or mortality. Similarly, four studies using routine prophylactic use of iNO shortly after birth showed no benefit on BPD or mortality. Later treatment with iNO, used in infants at higher risk of BPD, also showed no significant reduction in BPD or death, but the effect size approached significance (RR, 0.92; 95% CI, 0.85–1.01).

A recent RCT from the Newborns Treated with Nitric Oxide Trial Group, not included in the two meta-analyses discussed in the previous paragraph, studied the impact of iNO on the rate of survival without BPD.[89] In a cohort of 451 preterm infants born before 30 weeks' gestation and requiring positive pressure ventilation support on postnatal day 5 to 14, infants were randomized to receive iNO or placebo for 24 days. The authors showed that iNO was not associated with improved survival without BPD or neurodevelopmental outcomes at 18 to 24 months.

In conclusion, current evidence does not support the use of iNO in preterm infants to improve survival without BPD.[90,91] Current investigations into detecting early pulmonary vascular disease in preterm infants may open new therapeutic avenues for iNO or other targeted approaches.[11]

Diuretics

Although diuretic therapy is frequently used to alleviate symptoms of BPD, there is only very limited evidence to support its use.[92–94] Most trials have shown that diuretics may improve short-term pulmonary outcomes.[94] However, there is no convincing evidence that the long-term use of diuretics (loop and thiazide diuretics) may improve important clinical outcomes such as BPD, duration of ventilation, or survival.[95,96]

Bronchodilators

There is very little evidence about the role of bronchodilators in preventing BPD.[97] One RCT studied inhaled salbutamol in ventilated preterm neonates and showed no effect on survival and/or BPD.[98] A posthoc analysis from the Neonatal European Study of Inhaled Steroids compared outcomes of preterm infants who received early bronchodilators versus no bronchodilators and showed no effect on BPD and/or death.[99] A systematic review investigating the role of bronchodilators in BPD concluded that there are insufficient data for a reliable assessment of this intervention.[100]

New Therapies

Stem Cell Therapies

Stem cell–based therapies are emerging as a potential therapeutic strategy for several neonatal diseases including brain injury and BPD. Evidence suggests that impaired function and/or loss of stem/progenitor cell populations contributes to abnormal organ development/repair.[101,102] Mesenchymal stromal cells (MSCs), originally identified as niche cells for hematopoietic stem cells in the bone marrow, have been investigated as a potential therapy for BPD in several preclinical studies.[103–106] A meta-analysis including 25 studies showed significant therapeutic benefits of MSCs in rodent models of BPD.[107] MSCs exert their effect via a paracrine mechanism, which may explain their pleiotropic therapeutic potential (antiinflammatory, antifibrotic, and antioxidative).[104]

Early-phase clinical trials investigating the feasibility and safety of MSC therapy for BPD are currently underway.[108–111] A phase 1 trial conducted in South Korea included nine ventilated preterm infants who received a single intratracheal administration of allogeneic, cord blood–derived MSCs.[112] The procedure was feasible and well tolerated, and the patients had no adverse effects on their growth, respiratory, or neurodevelopmental outcomes at 2 years.[112,113] A second phase 1 trial with a similar trial design, conducted with the same proprietary cell product in the United States in 12 preterm infants, confirmed feasibility and showed no short-term toxicity.[110] A phase 1 trial of a single intravenous administration of human amnion epithelial cells in six preterm, ventilator-dependent infants at 36 weeks' corrected age showed feasibility and absence of toxicity of this cell-based therapy approach.[111] Although stem cell–based therapies have entered the clinical arena based on promising preclinical data, much more needs to be learned about the biology of these putative repair cells. Further research is needed to determine the optimal cell product, source, dosage, route, and timing of administration.

Insulinlike Growth Factor 1

Insulinlike growth factor 1 (IGF-I) is an essential fetal growth factor that increases during gestation.[114] Preterm delivery is associated with a decrease in IGF-1 levels.[115] Low IGF-1 circulatory concentrations in extremely preterm infants have been associated with BPD, retinopathy of prematurity (ROP), poor weight gain, and abnormal brain growth.[115–118] A phase 2 RCT investigating the role of IGF-1 for the prevention of ROP did not demonstrate benefits in reducing severe ROP but found a decreased incidence of severe BPD, a secondary endpoint.[119] Another phase 2 trial assessing IGF-1 in the prevention of BPD is currently ongoing (NCT03253263).

Long-Term Outcomes

BPD is well recognized as a major risk factor for lifelong respiratory and neurologic impairment.[3–5] Survivors with BPD are described as having global dysfunction, affecting their motor, cognitive, language, and academic abilities.[120–123] Children with BPD also have worse respiratory function, an increased need for respiratory medications, and a higher rehospitalization rate in their first 2 years of life.[5,124]

Studies assessing respiratory function of adult survivors of BPD report more respiratory symptoms, impaired exercise capacity, and abnormal pulmonary function.[125–129] Emphysema, a lung disease characterized by the destruction of alveolar capillary units that is usually described in the aging population, is reported as one of the most common computed tomography findings in adult survivors of BPD.[129] Additionally, studies on adolescents and young adults born preterm have shown a significant increased risk for the development of pulmonary vascular disease and right ventricular dysfunction.[130] These limitations may contribute to the development of other chronic conditions known to be associated with prematurity, including obesity, hypertension, diabetes, and cardiovascular disease.[126]

The significant consequences of BPD underline the urgent need for transformative therapies and effective early intervention to prevent long-term complications.

Conclusion

Despite advances in neonatal care, BPD remains a frequent complication of extreme prematurity associated with mortality and long-term disability. Incremental progress has had only modest impact on the incidence of BPD as more and more extremely premature infants survive. Given the complexity of the pathophysiology of BPD, it is unlikely that a single therapy will substantially impact the disease. Instead, a combination of strategies targeting different disease mechanisms, both in the prenatal and postnatal periods, is more likely to be successful.

In parallel, there is a need to better understand normal lung development and the causal pathways involved in neonatal lung injury and the development of chronic lung disease in preterm infants. Disruptive new therapies such as stem cell–based approaches are currently being explored in preclinical studies and early clinical trials. Still, before implementing new therapies in the most fragile preterm population, several factors need to be considered, including solid preclinical evidence, well-designed clinical trials, and appropriate knowledge translation. Additionally, with the significant short- and long-term consequences of BPD, the impact of potential therapies should ideally be assessed longitudinally, with several years of respiratory and neurodevelopmental follow-up.

CHAPTER 15 Treatment of Apnea of Prematurity

Zeyar Htun, Richard J. Martin

KEY POINTS

1. There are three types of apnea: central, mixed, and obstructive. Mixed apnea is most common in longer episodes of apnea.
2. Apnea of prematurity is primarily due to the immaturity of respiratory and central nervous systems.
3. Direct interventions are first-line therapies that are evidence-based and include methylxanthine therapies, noninvasive respiratory supports, and/or invasive respiratory supports.
4. Indirect interventions are used in conjunction with direct interventions and can include environmental stimuli, the infant's positioning, and packed red blood cell transfusion for anemia.
5. More evidence-based management options seek to optimize neurorespiratory outcomes for preterm infants.

Introduction

Immaturity in respiratory control is of interest to scientists and clinicians alike. From a biologic perspective, it represents a unique link between the developing respiratory and central nervous systems. The resultant apnea precipitates repetitive oxygen desaturation and bradycardia, the longer-term consequences of which are uncertain. Nevertheless, the combination of immature respiratory control, an immature lung, and the resultant therapeutic ventilatory support predispose these infants to chronic respiratory morbidity. There is a need to optimize ventilatory support, both invasive and noninvasive, and provide safe pharmacotherapy that enhances respiratory neural output in this high-risk population of neonates. This is the primary focus of this chapter.

Pathophysiology

The multiple contributors to apnea of prematurity and resultant desaturation are summarized in Fig. 15.1. They comprise upregulation of brainstem-mediated inhibitory pathways, altered peripheral chemosensitivity, decreased central chemosensitivity, enhanced inhibition from upper airway afferents, and an unstable upper airway. Apnea is clearly more likely to elicit desaturation with the low functional residual capacity (and other abnormalities of lung function) that characterizes bronchopulmonary dysplasia (BPD) (see Fig. 15.1).

The neural circuitry that generates respiratory rhythm and governs inspiratory and expiratory motor patterns is distributed throughout the pons and medulla. The medulla contains a specialized region known as the pre-Bötzinger complex, which contains neurons that exhibit intrinsic pacemaker activity capable of producing rhythmic respiratory motor output without sensory feedback. Although a fundamental feature of this network is that it enables breathing to occur automatically, this systematic central rhythmicity may fail in preterm infants.[1–3]

Excitatory and inhibitory neurotransmitters and neuromodulators mediate the rhythmogenic synaptic communications between neurons of the medulla. Glutamate is the major neurotransmitter mediating excitatory synaptic input to brainstem respiratory neurons. Gamma-aminobutyric acid (GABA) and glycine are the two primary inhibitory neurotransmitters in the network. Interestingly, during late embryonic and early postnatal development, GABA can mediate *excitatory* neurotransmission secondary to changes in the chloride gradient across the membrane. It is unclear how this phenomenon relates to the inhibition of respiratory output and resultant apnea seen in preterm infants.[2] Neonatal rodent data suggest that caffeine, which is a nonselective adenosine receptor inhibitor, may block excitatory A_{2A} receptors at GABAergic neurons and so inhibit GABA output and contribute to the ability of caffeine to enhance respiratory drive.[3] Additionally, defects in the medullary serotonergic system likely contribute importantly to the pathogenesis of sudden infant death syndrome. For future advances in the pharmacotherapy of neonatal apnea, greater understanding of the maturation of these neurotransmitters/neuromodulators is imperative.

Responsiveness to CO_2 is the major chemical driver of respiratory neural output. This is apparent in fetal life, where breathing movements increase under hypercapnic conditions in animal models. As in later life, CO_2/hydrogen ion (H^+) responsiveness is predominantly based in the brainstem, although peripheral chemoreceptors contribute to the ventilatory response and respond more rapidly. The reduced ventilatory response to CO_2 in small preterm infants, especially those with apnea, is primarily the result of decreased central chemosensitivity; however, mechanical factors such as poor respiratory function and an unstable upper airway and/or chest wall may contribute.[4] It is difficult to distinguish the neural from mechanical factors that contribute to respiratory failure in this population, as highlighted in Fig. 15.2.

It has been known for many years that preterm infants respond to a decrease in inspired oxygen concentration with a transient increase in ventilation over approximately 1 minute, followed by a return to baseline or even depression of ventilation. The characteristic response to low oxygen in infants appears to result from initial peripheral chemoreceptor stimulation, followed by overriding depression of the respiratory center as a result of hypoxemia.[5] Such hypoxic respiratory depression may be useful in the hypoxic intrauterine environment where respiratory activity is only intermittent and not contributing to gas exchange. The nonsustained response to

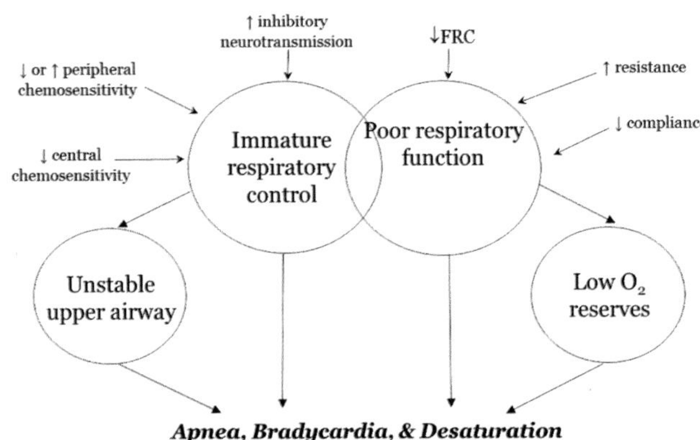

Fig. 15.1 Multiple factors contribute to both immature respiratory control and poor respiratory function and enhance vulnerability for development of intermittent hypoxic episodes. *FRC,* Functional residual capacity; ↑, increased; ↓, decreased.

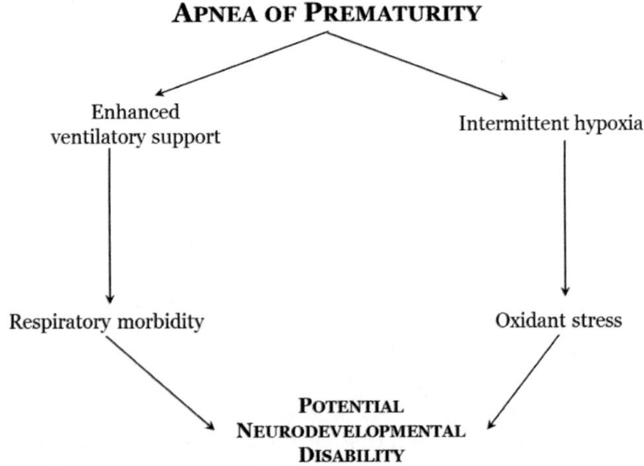

Fig. 15.2 Potential Pathways Whereby Apnea of Prematurity May Contribute to Adverse Neurodevelopmental Outcomes.

low inspired oxygen concentration may, however, be a disadvantage postnatally. It may play an important role in the origin of neonatal apnea and offers a physiologic rationale for the decrease in incidence of apnea observed when a slightly increased concentration of inspired oxygen is administered to apneic infants who have a low baseline oxygen saturation. Decreased peripheral chemoreceptor responsiveness to oxygen or central hypoxic depression of respiratory neural output may impair recovery from apnea. In contrast, excessive peripheral chemosensitivity has also been shown to compromise ventilatory stability and predispose to periodic breathing and even apnea in preterm infants.[2,6] Finally, inhibitory sensory inputs from the upper airway (larynx and pharynx) may be prominent in early postnatal life and serve a protective function yet precipitate potential clinically significant apnea.

Clinical Features and Evaluations

Apnea can be classified into central, obstructive, or mixed. Central apnea occurs from central nervous system immaturity, which causes decreased respiratory effort and an exaggerated response to laryngeal stimulation (a normal reflex that closes the airway as a protective measure). Obstructive apnea in premature infants is mostly due to position (the infant's neck is hyperflexed or hyperextended) in combination with low pharyngeal muscle tone preventing air flow through the pharynx. Mixed apnea is the most common cause of clinically significant apnea of prematurity, accounting for over 50% of the episodes. Mixed apnea in premature infants consists of central pauses secondary to the immature state of respiratory control and obstructive respiratory efforts secondary to decreased pharyngeal or laryngeal muscle tone.

Table 15.1 Widely Accepted Definition of Apnea of Prematurity

	Definition
Apnea of prematurity	Infants born at less than 37 weeks of gestation who have: Pause of breathing for more than 15–20 seconds *often with one or more of the following:* Oxygen desaturation (Spo_2 ≤80% for ≥4 seconds) Bradycardia (heart rate <100 or <2/3 of baseline for ≥4 seconds) Pallor/cyanosis

Moriette G, Lescure S, El Ayoubi M, Lopez E. *Arch Pediatr.* 2010;17(2):186–190.

Apnea of prematurity presents as cessation of breathing for longer than 20 seconds or a shorter duration if accompanied by bradycardia, oxygen desaturation, or cyanosis (Table 15.1). Incidence of apnea of prematurity is inversely related to gestational age.[7] The incidence is nearly 100% for infants born at or before 28 weeks' gestational age. At 30 weeks' gestational age the incidence decreases to approximately 80% and at 34 weeks' gestational age the incidence significantly decreases to 20%. Onset of apnea of prematurity is usually within the first week of life. The time period for resolution of apnea of prematurity is generally around 36 to 40 weeks' postconceptual age. Apneic spells typically stop by 37 weeks' postmenstrual age in 92% of infants and by 40 weeks' postmenstrual age in 98% of infants.[7] The time of resolution is also inversely related to gestational age. Infants born at <28 weeks' gestation may have recurrent apnea and bradycardia events that persist to or beyond 38 weeks' postconceptual age, whereas in infants born ≥28 weeks' gestational age, the time to resolution for recurrent apnea and bradycardia events is generally around 36 to 37 weeks' postmenstrual age.[8]

Although apnea in a premature infant can be physiologic, it can be a sign of change in clinical status of the preterm infant. Other etiologies should be considered if there is escalation in respiratory support or if apnea is associated with other clinical findings such as feeding intolerance or lethargy. If this is the case, the infant should be further evaluated for infectious etiologies (such as sepsis or bacteremia), central nervous system abnormalities (such as intracranial hemorrhage), anemia, genetic disorders, or metabolic disorders because all of these can contribute to apnea in both preterm and term infants.

More Evidence-Based (Direct) Management Approaches

Xanthines

Methylxanthine therapy consists of either caffeine or theophylline. Both therapies are known to be effective in treatment for apnea of prematurity. Caffeine is the most widely used xanthine therapy, constituting about 96% of all methylxanthines used in clinical practice, and is preferred over theophylline. Caffeine does not require drug-level monitoring because of its greater pharmacologic stability,

Table 15.2 Clinical Benefits and Challenges Associated With Caffeine Therapy

	Resolved	Unresolved
Early initiation	Starting caffeine within the first days appears optimal. Early use of caffeine as either treatment or prophylaxis can decrease time on mechanical ventilation.	Most studies are retrospective, case–control studies. A recent randomized controlled trial by Amaro et al.[17] questions initiation of caffeine prior to 3 days as expediting extubation.
Prolonged treatment	Median postmenstrual age where caffeine is discontinued or weaned approximates 34–36 weeks' postmenstrual age. There is an inverse relationship between gestational age and duration of cardiopulmonary events.	Optimal duration of therapy for infants who have severe BPD or prolonged mechanical ventilation. Uncertainty as to whether prolonged caffeine is beneficial in decreasing cardiopulmonary events and longer-term morbidity.
Dosage	No need to monitor serum caffeine levels. Higher doses of caffeine (both loading and maintenance) may decrease extubation failure and frequency of apnea.	Potential pro- and antiinflammatory effects of caffeine may depend on adenosine receptor subtype inhibition; this may relate to caffeine concentration.

BPD, Bronchopulmonary dysplasia.

longer half-life, and higher therapeutic index, in contrast to theophylline, which has a narrower therapeutic window requiring drug-level monitoring. Adverse effects for both caffeine and theophylline include tachycardia, cardiac dysrhythmias, emesis, and jitteriness, but important clinical side effects are uncommon.

Both xanthine therapies, caffeine and theophylline, increase respiratory neural output, which can have both central and peripheral effects. Centrally, due to increased inspiratory neuron response in the brainstem, there is enhanced CO_2 responsiveness, decreased hypoxic depression of breathing, and decreased periodic breathing. Peripherally, there may be a contribution from improved respiratory function. In addition to effects on the respiratory system and drive, xanthine therapies have been implicated to have antiinflammatory effects, shown in both hyperoxic exposure models and chorioamnionitis exposure models.[9,10]

Methylxanthine therapies are known to have two mechanisms of action: (1) nonselective adenosine receptor antagonist and (2) nonselective phosphodiesterase inhibitor. Due to xanthine having a molecular structure similar to that of adenosine, the primary mechanism of action is competitive antagonism of adenosine receptors. The two adenosine receptors that are primarily antagonized are A_1 and A_{2A}. Inhibition of A_1 receptors results in excitation of respiratory neural output because activation of A_1 leads to inhibition of adenylyl cyclase and some Ca^{2+} channels in the central nervous system. Inhibition of A_{2A} receptors decreases GABA release by the GABA ergic neurons in the medulla oblongata. GABA is a well-known inhibitor of respiratory neural output; therefore inhibition of A_{2A} results in decreased inhibition of respiratory neural output. In addition to respiratory neural output effects, antiinflammation properties can be promoted by xanthine therapies due to both nonspecific phosphodiesterase inhibition and antagonism of adenosine receptors.[11]

The current practice for treatment of apnea of prematurity with caffeine citrate is based on the doses used in the Caffeine for Apnea of Prematurity (CAP) Trial.[12] Caffeine citrate is approved by the US Food and Drug Administration with the recommended initial bolus dose of caffeine citrate (20 mg/kg) followed by maintenance dosing of 5 to 10 mg/kg/day. There have been multiple studies evaluating different dosing regimens, specifically with higher maintenance or loading doses. Similar findings were reported across multiple studies, showing that although the higher doses of caffeine were associated with decreased extubation failure and frequency of apnea, there was no difference in incidence of BPD, retinopathy of prematurity, and intraventricular hemorrhage.

Utilization of caffeine as either prophylaxis or treatment varies worldwide. The general trend in the past two decades has been a progression toward earlier initiation of caffeine (Table 15.2). Caffeine was initiated at a mean age of 10 days in 1997 versus 4 days in 2010.[13] In 2013, neonatal intensive care units (NICUs) from four different countries were surveyed and the result showed that 62% of the units used caffeine for prophylaxis.[14] Davis et al. studied the subgroups in the CAP Trial and noticed that use of caffeine before 3 days of life was associated with greater reduction of time on ventilation compared with caffeine initiated on or after 3 days of life.[15] A retrospective study by Lodha et al. suggested that early onset of treatment appears to be beneficial. In this study, neonates received caffeine within the first 2 days after birth (early group) or on or after the third day following birth (late group). The results showed early (prophylactic) caffeine use was associated with a reduction in the rates of death or bronchopulmonary dysplasia and patent ductus arteriosus.[16] However, a randomized, placebo-controlled trial by Amaro et al. testing early caffeine initiation versus placebo treatment raises caution with early use of caffeine in mechanically ventilated preterm infants until more efficacy and safety data become available. Amaro et al. found that early initiation of caffeine did not reduce the age of first successful extubation, but there was a nonsignificant trend toward higher mortality in the early caffeine group.[17] This implies that further randomized controlled studies are needed to identify the best time for initiating caffeine (see Table 15.2). Caffeine therapy is typically discontinued around 36 to 40 weeks' postmenstrual age because this is when apnea of prematurity generally resolves. For extremely premature infants or infants who have been mechanically ventilated for a prolonged period of time, apnea can persist past 36 weeks, and caffeine can be discontinued around 38 to 40 weeks' postmenstrual age.

Doxapram is a dose-dependent respiratory stimulant[18] that is administered intravenously. Due to its short half-life, it is administered as a continuous infusion with a dose range of 2 to 2.5 mg/kg/h to achieve safe and effective blood concentration levels.[18] The mechanism of action is initially on peripheral carotid and aortic chemoreceptors at lower dosage. As the dose is increased, the central respiratory centers in the medulla are stimulated. This leads to stimulation of the respiratory center in the brainstem, and the neurons here control the activity of the diaphragm, chest wall, and other respiratory accessory muscles. The overall effect is an increase in tidal volume and respiratory rate. However, doxapram may have adverse effects on cerebral blood flow. Utilizing cerebral Doppler ultrasonography, Dani et al. showed that doxapram induced an increase in cerebral oxygen consumption and a decrease in oxygen delivery.[19] In addition, doxapram can cause cardiac dysrhythmias. Overall, the efficacy and the safety profile of doxapram on premature infants have not been well studied. Before doxapram can be widely and routinely used, further trials should be performed.[20]

Respiratory Support

Nasal continuous positive airway pressure (CPAP) is a noninvasive form of respiratory support that is commonly used in preterm infants, provides safe and effective positive pressure at 4 to 7 cm H_2O, and is commonly used in conjunction with pharmacologic therapies such as methylxanthines. The positive pressure provides a constant distending pressure during both inhalation and exhalation for both upper and lower airways. When the upper airway is kept open, this reduces the risk of laryngeal or pharyngeal collapse, aiding in prevention of obstructive and mixed apnea. CPAP also increases functional residual capacity and improves oxygenation.[21]

High-flow nasal cannula (HFNC) and noninvasive positive pressure ventilation (NIPPV) are other forms of noninvasive respiratory support that can be used in conjunction with pharmacologic therapies and may avoid the need for invasive ventilation via endotracheal intubation. HFNC provides constant flow rather than intermittent inflation to enhance ventilation. However, pressure is not measured with the HFNC, and this raises a potential safety concern in very preterm infants. NIPPV is a noninvasive method of ventilation via nasal cannula that provides both peak inspiratory pressure and positive end expiratory pressure. Similar to CPAP, NIPPV is proposed to increase functional residual capacity. In addition, it can also increase mean airway pressure and increase tidal and minute volume. Therefore NIPPV may be a useful method of augmenting the beneficial effects of NCPAP in preterm infants with apnea that is frequent or severe.[22]

Neurally (EMG) adjusted ventilatory assistance (NAVA) can be used as either a noninvasive or invasive form of respiratory support. The support provided is similar to NIPPV except for the fact that NAVA utilizes a flow and neural sensor to synchronize its support with the infant's respiratory efforts. In comparison with NIPPV, synchronized nasal ventilation reduced breathing effort and resulted in better infant-ventilator interaction.[23] In a small, randomized crossover study, Gizzi et al. noted less incidence of desaturations, bradycardias, and central apnea episodes when infants were on flow-SNIPPV in comparison with when the infants were on NIPPV and NCPAP.[24] Similar results were also seen in a retrospective single-center study by Tabacaru et al., and NAVA was associated with a significant reduction in the number of isolated bradycardic events per day and overall bradycardia per day.[25]

For severe and/or refractory episodes of apnea that may or may not be accompanied with other clinical findings, endotracheal intubation and mechanical ventilation should be strongly considered. If an infant receives mechanical ventilation, the infant's spontaneous respiratory efforts should be encouraged by attempting to minimize ventilation settings. This can prevent further volu- or barotrauma in extremely preterm infants.

Therapeutic approaches should not primarily focus on apnea only. There has been increasing evidence that treatment of hypoxemia can secondarily prevent apnea. One speculation is due to the biphasic hypoxic ventilatory response of premature infants. This is composed of initial increased ventilation due to excitation by peripheral chemoreceptor activity and subsequent depression of ventilation by central chemoreceptors as discussed earlier.[26] Therefore although no studies have been performed yet, one possible way to decrease apneic episodes is to decrease the amount of hypoxemia exposure. Automated adjustment of FiO_2 increases the time that infants spend within the target SpO_2 range and a reduction in time of hyperoxemia and hypoxemia for infants on either noninvasive or invasive respiratory support.[27] In addition, the number of prolonged events with SpO_2 $<88\%$ was reduced with automated adjustments.[28]

Less Evidence-Based (Indirect) Management Approaches

Blood Transfusions

Blood transfusions may help reduce apnea events for a short period of time. Anemia in preterm infants can lead to decreased oxygen-carrying capacity, which may result in decreased oxygen delivery to the central nervous system, a decreased efferent output of the respiratory neuronal network, and an increase in apnea events.[29] Bell et al. performed a randomized trial comparing liberal versus restrictive guidelines for red blood cell transfusion. In this study, both groups showed decreases in apnea events after transfusions, and the infants who received more red blood cell transfusions had significantly less frequent apnea.[30] Zagol et al. demonstrated in very low birth weight infants that the probability of future apnea is inversely related to hematocrit in these infants, which provides further evidence that decreased oxygen-carrying capacity, rather than volume alone, may play a significant role in apnea of prematurity.[29] Although there are potential benefits to giving packed red blood cell transfusions, there can be potential complications from transfusions for preterm infants, such as intraventricular hemorrhage.

Management of Gastroesophageal Reflux

Gastroesophageal reflux (GER) is very common in preterm infants, with the incidence being about 22% for infants born at less than 34 weeks' gestational age.[31] Recent studies have shown that there is no strong association between GER and apnea of prematurity. Peter et al. utilized multiple intraluminal impedance techniques to investigate whether there is a temporal relationship between GER and apnea of prematurity and whether GER occurs predominantly before a cardiorespiratory event. They found that although both events were commonly occurring in their infant population of 30 weeks' median gestational age, the events did not seem to be temporally related.[32] Mousa et al. reinforced this finding with their study, also utilizing multichannel intraluminal impedance monitoring. They saw no difference between acid gastroesophageal reflux and nonacid gastroesophageal reflux in the frequency association with apnea.[33] Therefore GER is a common and physiologic occurrence in preterm infants, and there seems to be no strong association with apnea. Caution should be taken when initiating GER therapies because they can potentially increase the risk for sepsis or NEC in the preterm population.[34]

Infant Positioning

The American Academy of Pediatrics, since 1992, has recommended infants to be placed on their backs to reduce the risk of sudden infant death syndrome.[35] In the NICU, there are benefits to prone positioning for the preterm infant. Central apnea rates are decreased in the prone position compared with supine positioning.[36] Preterm infants also exhibit better oxygenation and improved functional residual capacity in prone positioning.[37–39] Therefore placing infants in the prone position can be beneficial and can help augment other therapeutic measures such as caffeine and CPAP. However, one must be aware that "back to sleep" is the recommended positioning for post-discharge NICU infants, and prone positioning should be avoided as discharge approaches.

Sensory Stimulation

Stimuli from the environment can be beneficial to preterm infants. Kangaroo care or skin-to-skin contact with the parents have been shown to have overall positive effects. Although no reduction in desaturation or in bradycardic or apneic events has been noted during kangaroo care, there is stability of these events during kangaroo care.[40] This should be highly encouraging to the medical staff to promote kangaroo care, because it has been shown to help modulate pain, improve sleep organization, and possibly improve neurodevelopmental outcomes.[41] Music therapy is another sensory stimulus that can benefit preterm infants. In utero, the infant is constantly exposed to the mother's voice, which plays a key role in the fetal development. However, the NICU environment may be insufficient in beneficial sensory exposure in comparison with the in utero environment. Music therapy has been shown to be beneficial to preterm infants.[42] Music therapy can have positive effects of stabilizing the heart rate and respiratory rate, increasing oxygen saturations, and modulating pain response.[43] When music therapy and kangaroo care are combined, there is a further decrease in heart rates and respiration and an increase in oxygen saturation.[42] Coinciding with music therapy, certain sounds or voices can be beneficial to cognitive development. Therefore preterm infants should be exposed to voices of family members, and the ambient noise levels in the NICU should be controlled so the infant can hear and discriminate human voices.[44]

Long-Term Outcomes

Multiple studies over several decades in preterm infants have shown an association between apnea of prematurity and morbidity. Unfortunately, it is very difficult to demonstrate a causal relationship. More recent data in neonatal models suggest that the accompanying desaturation and/or bradycardia may be the contributing factor(s) in initiating a pathologic cascade. Factors that can influence the initiation, duration, and severity of IH include baseline oxygen saturation, oxygen uptake from the alveoli, pulmonary oxygen stores, total blood oxygen carrying capacity, the slope of the hemoglobin oxygen dissociation curve, and metabolic oxygen consumption.[45] In extremely preterm infants, IH events are pervasive and transient during early postnatal life, with a relatively low incidence during the first week of life followed by a rapid increase during the second and third weeks and a plateau or decrease thereafter.[46] A significant challenge is that we are only beginning to understand the implications of patterns of IH events on morbidity.

Long-term recordings have now allowed for more reliable and detailed analyses of oxygen saturation patterns and morbidity. For instance, continuous pulse oximetry monitoring over the first 2 months of life revealed an association between severe retinopathy of prematurity and both a higher frequency and longer duration of IH events as well as a distinct timing between IH events.[47] A secondary analysis of infants enrolled in the Canadian Oxygen Trial has shown an association between increased time spent $<80\%$ during IH events and a greater probability of death or disability, cognitive or language delay, severe retinopathy of prematurity, and motor impairment at 18 months of age[48] that was limited to IH events of 1 minute or longer in duration. An association between bradycardia episodes and adverse outcomes could not be demonstrated.

In summary, the potential adverse consequences of apnea of prematurity are most likely associated with need for enhanced ventilatory support and compromised oxygenation (Fig. 15.3). Pathologic cascades such as greater prooxidant signaling may be initiated by specific high-risk patterns of IH and have both short-term and long-lasting effects, including sleep-disordered breathing, growth restriction, retinopathy of prematurity, neurodevelopmental impairment, and alterations in cardiovascular regulation.[49] Identification of high-risk patterns may provide insight on future intervention protocols in the NICU setting. The ongoing Pre-Vent Study, funded by the National Heart, Lung, and Blood Institute, seeks to characterize mechanisms of ventilatory control leading to postnatal respiratory morbidities.[50] This should lead to a more evidence-based approach to the management of apnea as a means of optimizing neurorespiratory outcomes in former preterm infants.

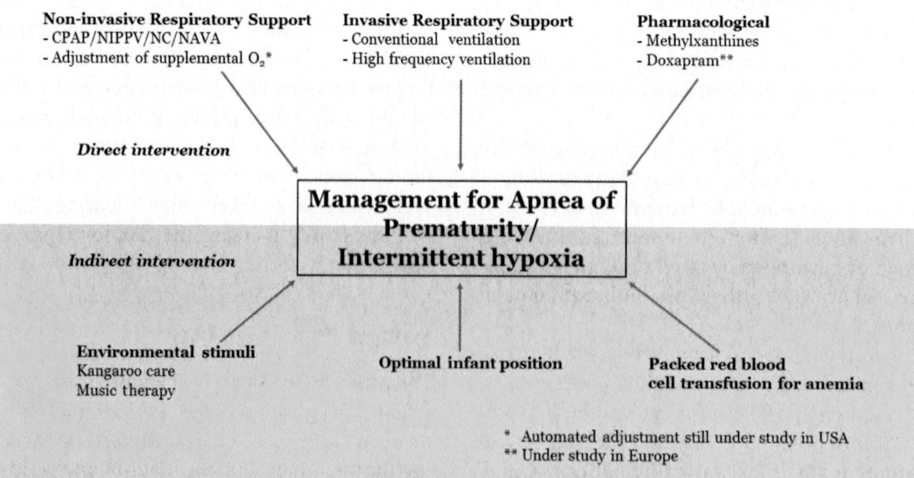

Fig. 15.3 Direct interventions have more evidence and are practiced more universally as first-line therapies for apnea of prematurity. Indirect interventions are less evidence-based. These are suggested to be used in conjunction with direct interventions to further augment management. *CPAP,* Continuous positive airway pressure; *NAVA,* neurally adjusted ventilatory assistance; *NC,* nasal cannula; *NIPPV,* noninvasive positive pressure ventilation.

SECTION 3

Feeding

OUTLINE

CHAPTER 16 Human Milk

Nitasha Bagga, Kei Lui, Arūnas Liubšys, Mohammad M. Rahman, Srijan Singh, Mimi L. Mynak, Akhil Maheshwari

KEY POINTS

1. The female breast develops with chronologic maturation, during pregnancy, and with major physiologic/endocrine changes in preparation for lactation after delivery.
2. Care providers need to begin preparing pregnant women for lactation during antenatal visits by providing information about the importance of breastfeeding and about early initiation of breastfeeding.
3. After birth, skin-to-skin contact, initiation of feeding within the first hour, positioning, identification of the infant's cues to start feedings, maintaining maternal-infant contact to promote bonding, and psychological support during the first hours can be helpful.
4. Maternal-infant bonding, maternal motivation, and successful establishment of breastfeeding are important to form the necessary feed-forward cycle for feeding.
5. For young mothers, education about posture, timing, and storage of milk and provision of information about the nutritional, immunologic, and other components is useful.
6. There is increasing information that shows the universal impact of encouraging maternal feeding on infant health and survival.

Introduction

The female breast progressively develops with chronologic maturation. This process is further accelerated during pregnancy, when major physiologic/endocrine changes prepare the breast tissue for lactation after delivery (Fig. 16.1). Hormones such as estrogen, progesterone, prolactin, and the placental lactogen augment proliferation and differentiation of the mammary glands (Table 16.1). The first milk, the colostrum, is rich in energy and immunologic factors to prepare the newborn infant for independent existence. Over the next few days, the colostrum "matures" with increased volume and changes in various constituents. Colostrum contains factors that can protect the newborn infant against infections and many metabolic disorders. Increasing information suggests that it may be protective in disorders such as sudden infant death syndrome, which we are still trying to understand.

Preparation of the Mother for Breastfeeding

The care providers need to prepare the mother-infant dyad for lactation.[1,2] The effort starts during the antenatal visits, where the mother must be informed about the importance of breastfeeding and motivated for early initiation and various techniques to breastfeed. Maternal-infant bonding, maternal motivation, and successful establishment of breastfeeding forms a feed-forward cycle (Fig. 16.2). Steps such as skin-to-skin contact (Fig. 16.3), breast crawl, initiation of feeding as early as within the first hour, correct positioning, identification of the infant's cues to start feedings, repeated opportunities for feedings, maintaining maternal-infant contact to promote bonding, monitoring for any difficulties in suckling, and psychological support during the first hours can be helpful.[3,4]

To encourage active feedings, keeping the baby awake with skin-to-skin contact and gentle, affectionate stroking may be helpful. Mothers may also find it helpful to have some support in recognizing when to switch sides.[5] The care providers can help the mother by ensuring adequate fluid intake. In this process, the fathers can contribute by arranging fluids of choice for the mother and by providing care to the baby when the mother begins to feel fatigued and needs rest.[6] After a few attempts, both parents begin to recognize when the baby settles between feeds.

The infant should have 5 to 7 wet nappies in 24 hours.[7] In the first few days, the stool color also changes from the darker meconium to a mustard-yellow appearance. It is not unusual for a baby to have 2 to 5 stools every day.[8] It is usually an instance of great joy for the parents when the baby gains weight for the first time after the first few days.

Information That We Have Found Useful to Encourage Mothers

Most mothers find information on the physiologic benefits of lactation (Fig. 16.4), healthy weight gain for the baby, and various nutritional and immunologic factors present in their milk to be very interesting and encouraging (Table 16.2).[9–11] Increasing information suggests that breast milk components, particularly specific types of fats, are ideal for the baby's intellectual development.[12] Mother's milk may also be protective against the risk of chronic disorders including allergic disorders such as eczema, and in the longer term, diabetes and hypertension.[13–16]

It is very comforting for the mother to know that her milk is all the nutrition the baby needs, including that needed to maintain hydration and to fulfill her/his needs for subcomponents of nutrition: proteins, fat, and carbohydrates.[17] There is no need for any supplements.[18]

Appropriate Postures for the Mother and Good Latch-On for the Baby

Information on the right posture should be provided, such as that the mother's back is straight and well-supported and the lap and feet are flat; the mother can use a pillow to support her back and arms

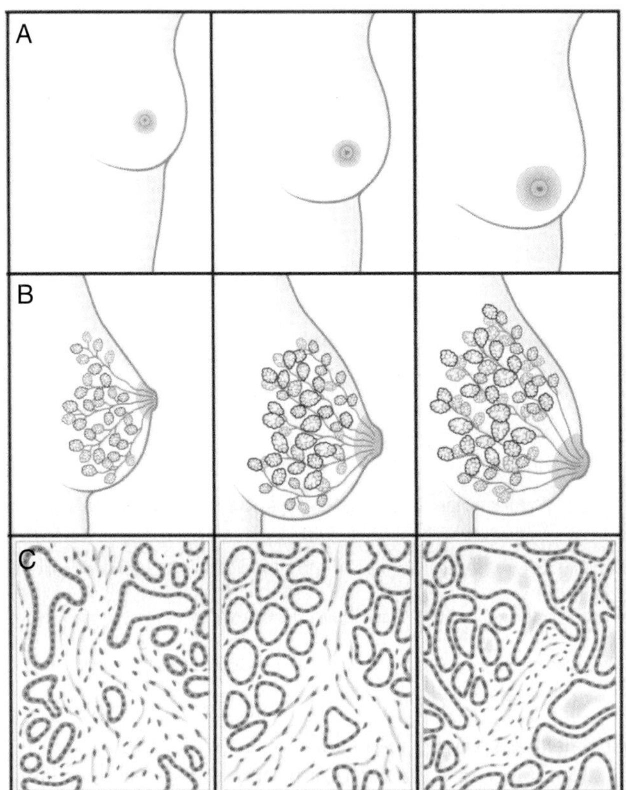

Fig. 16.1 Female Breast in Adulthood, Pregnancy, and During Lactation, With Corresponding Duct Structure and Tissue Cross-Sections. (A) Adult breast shows well-differentiated ductular and peripheral lobular-alveolar system. (B) Ductular sprouting and intensified peripheral lobular-alveolar development in pregnancy. Glandular luminal cells begin actively synthesizing milk fat and proteins near term; only small amounts are released into the lumen. (C) With postpartum withdrawal of luteal and placental sex steroids and placental lactogen, prolactin is able to induce full secretory activity of alveolar cells and release of milk into alveoli and smaller ducts. (From Lawrence RA, Lawrence RM. *Breastfeeding: A Guide for the Medical Profession.* 7th ed. St Louis, MO: Mosby; 2010:43. Modified with permission from Lawrence RM, Lawrence RA. The breast and the physiology of lactation. In: Creasy RK, Resnik R, Iams JD, eds. *Creasy and Resnik's Maternal-Fetal Medicine: Principles and Practice.* Philadelphia, PA: Saunders/Elsevier; 2009:11:161–180.e3.)

when she is raising baby to the level of her breasts.[19] Some mothers, particularly when fatigued, at night, or those who have had to undergo a cesarean section, may find feeding easier while lying down.[20] All these postures are shown in Fig. 16.5. The consideration of posture(s) may be particularly important when feeding premature/critically ill infants who may be physically too weak to feed adequately.[21,22]

The mother should try to hold the baby close to her, with her/his mouth facing the breast and close to the nipple and with the head, shoulders, and body in a straight line.[23] The baby should be able to latch on to the breast with the mouth wide open and the nipple pointing toward the roof of this mouth. Her/his chin should be touching the breast. If the mother can see the areola, less should be visible below the bottom lip than the top one (Fig. 16.6). When feeding premature infants, sometimes there may be a need to use devices such as nipple shields (Fig. 16.7).

The sucking pattern should be with long, deep sucks with pauses. Feeding should not be painful. If it is, the mother may need to adjust the position of the baby. It is good to involve fathers.[24] Most of the time, any discomfort felt by the mother is related to positioning while feeding or inadequate efforts to feed in terms of frequency. Babies differ in terms of their feeding patterns, and it may take a few days for the both the mothers and the baby to adjust. This is normal. The milk supply will also change to match the baby's needs. If the baby looks hungry, the mother may just try to feed more frequently, and her body will adjust accordingly. Some of the difficult situations that may make lactation difficult [25] and need supervision from a specialist are listed in Table 16.3.

Milk Expression

The mother may have to express milk using her hands or using a hand/electric pump (some of the equipment is shown in chapter 17 that is focused on milk storage).[26–28] The mother may also consider doing so if the breast feels too full and engorged.[29] Sometimes, there may also be a need to do so if she has to go back to work.[30] She should just wash her hands, and also wash all the containers, bottles, and pump pieces in soapy water before use. In geographic regions or countries with warmer climates, it may be useful to sterilize the equipment with steam; the equipment is easily available.[31]

To express milk, it may be easier to do so in quiet, private settings.[28,32] Some mothers find it easier to do so with a warm drink and with thoughts/pictures of the baby. Gently massaging the breast and rolling the nipples between the first finger and the thumb may help because it simulates the sensations that the baby would have provided during feeding. The nipple itself may be too sensitive, and it may be helpful to exert the pressure on the surrounding area. The milk may take a minute or two to flow. It may be useful to rotate the fingers around the nipple to ensure that all the sections can be emptied. After a few minutes, it may be easier to switch sides.

Some women find it more comfortable to use hand-held or electric breast pumps, particularly when the breasts are full. The pumps have a funnel that fits over the areola. These pumps may allow expressing milk from both sides at the same time and thus may add to the convenience. It may be useful to maintain a certain frequency, such as every 3 hours.

Milk Storage at Home

Milk can be stored at 2 to 4 degrees for up to 5 days.[33] In warmer climate areas, some hospitals recommend freezing the milk if the mother needs to store it for more than 24 hours.[34,35] When freezing for occasional use at home, a plastic container can be used, although many authorities are now beginning to consider using a glass container because of the concerns with potentially soluble toxins in some plastic vessels.[36] It may be useful to date and label each container.

Frozen milk should be thawed slowly by moving it to the refrigerator or to room temperature.[37] Once thawed, it should be used immediately if possible; if the milk does not get used, it may be better to discard it.[38] The use of a microwave to thaw milk is not recommended because of uneven heating, although there may not be major changes in the nutrient composition.[39] It is also undesirable if the milk has been stored in plastic containers for the reasons mentioned above.

Nutritional Components in Human Milk

The nutrient composition of human milk is dynamic and changes within a feeding, during the course of a day, and throughout

Table 16.1 Stages of Mammary Development

Developmental Stage	Hormonal Regulation	Local Factors	Description
Embryogenesis	—	Fat pad necessary for ductal extension	Epithelial bud develops in fetus at 18–19 weeks, extending short distance into mammary fat pad with blind ducts that become canalized; some milk secretion may be present at birth
Mammogenesis			Anatomic development
Puberty			
Before onset of menses	Estrogen, GH	IGF-I, hGF, TGF-β; others	Ductal extension into mammary fat pad; branching morphogenesis
After onset of menses	Estrogen, progesterone; PRL		Lobular development with formation of terminal duct lobular unit
Pregnancy	Progesterone, PRL, hPL	HER; others	Alveolus formation; partial cellular differentiation
Lactogenesis	Progesterone withdrawal, PRL, glucocorticoid	Not known	Onset of milk secretion Stage I: midpregnancy Stage II: parturition
Lactation	PRL, oxytocin	FIL	Ongoing milk secretion
Involution	PRL withdrawal	Milk stasis; FIL	Alveolar epithelium undergoes apoptosis and remodeling; gland reverts to prepregnant state

FIL, Feedback inhibition of lactation; *GH*, growth hormone; *HER*, heregulin; *hGF*, human growth factor; *hPL*, human placental lactogen; *IGF-I*, insulin-like growth factor I; *PRL*, prolactin; *TGF-β*, transforming growth factor-β.

Modified with permission and with minor modifications from Lawrence RM, Lawrence RA. The breast and the physiology of lactation. In: Creasy RK, Resnik R, Iams JD, eds. *Creasy and Resnik's Maternal-Fetal Medicine: Principles and Practice.* Philadelphia, PA: Saunders/Elsevier; 2009;11, 161–180.e3.

Originally from Neville MC. Mammary gland biology and lactation: a short course. Presented at: International Society for Research on Human Milk and Lactation annual meeting; October 1997; Plymouth, MA.

lactation and also differs between women.[17] Components of human milk have multiple nutritional and immunologic functions. A reference tabulation of the composition of human milk comparing term and preterm milk 1 week after delivery is given in Table 16.4. In the first few weeks after birth, milk from mothers who delivered prematurely contains more protein than does milk from those delivering at term, and the total protein content in both declines similarly to a plateau seen in "mature" milk. Milk protein content is not related to maternal diet but increases with maternal body mass index.[40]

Human milk contains more whey protein (70%) than casein (30%).[17] This differs from bovine milk (82% casein, 18% whey). Whey proteins remain in solution after acid precipitation, whereas caseins are less soluble in gastric acid. Whey proteins are more easily digested and emptied out of the stomach. The major whey protein in human milk is α-lactalbumin. Unlike caseins, whey contains less phenylalanine, tyrosine, and methionine but more taurine. The other whey proteins, namely lactoferrin, lysozyme, and secretory immunoglobulin A, also resist proteolytic digestion and provide mucosal immunity.

The lipid system of human milk is physiologically very important for the growing brain and eyes and for immunologic responses. Unlike the concentrations of protein and lactose, which are relatively constant during the day, fat content tends to be higher during the day and lower during the night.[41] The lipid system of human milk carries nearly half of all calories and is structured to be easily digested and absorbed.[42,43] Milk fat content and the feeling of breast fullness are related, and about 70% of the variance of fat content can be explained by the amount of

Fig. 16.2 Maternal-Infant Bonding, Successful Establishment of Maternal Feeding, and Breastfeeding: A Feed-Forward Cycle. (Image provided by Dr. Rachana Singh, USA; Global Newborn Society.)

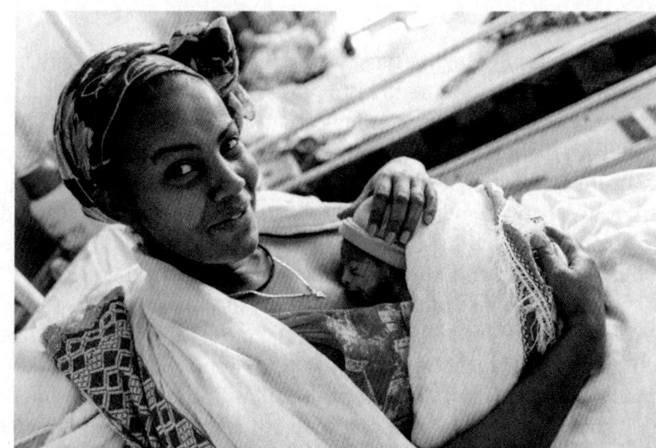

Fig. 16.3 Kangaroo Care. Kangaroo care was first introduced in Bogota, Colombia in 1979 because of inadequate resources to care for premature infants. This method of care has since been evaluated and found beneficial all over the world. Dressed only in a diaper, an infant is held skin to skin against the mother's chest between her breasts, snug inside the mother's clothing, often for hours. The father can do the same. Such care stabilizes breathing, heart rates, and temperatures. The infants show less uneasiness and spend more time either in a quiet, alert state or in deep sleep. These infants may show better weight gain and earlier discharge from the hospital. The mothers have also noted increased milk volume expression. (Dr. Misrak Tadesse, Wax and Gold, Inc.)

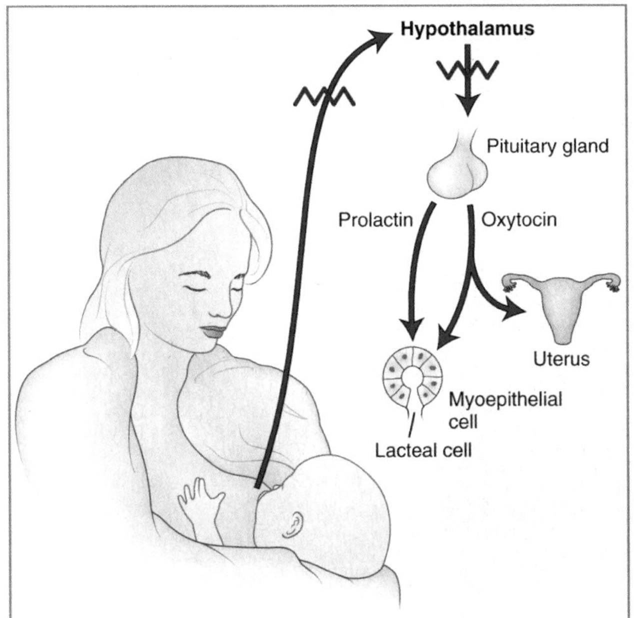

Fig. 16.4 The Let-Down (Ejection) Reflex Arc. When the infant suckles the breast, mechanoreceptors in the nipple and areola are stimulated, which sequentially stimulate the nerve pathways to the hypothalamus and the posterior pituitary gland and activate the release of prolactin and oxytocin. Prolactin is secreted by the anterior pituitary gland in response to suckling and promotes lactogenesis. Oxytocin stimulates myoepithelial cells in the breast to contract and eject milk from the alveolus and also promotes uterine recovery. Stress associated with pain or anxiety can inhibit the let-down reflex. Seeing or hearing the infant can stimulate the release of oxytocin but not prolactin. (Reproduced with permission and minor modifications from Lawrence and Lawrence. The Breast and the Physiology of Lactation. In: *Creasy and Resnik's Maternal-Fetal Medicine: Principles and Practice*, 11:161–180.e3.)

milk in the breast before and after feeding.[44] Neutral lipids include triglycerides, diacylglycerols, monoacylglycerols, and sterol esters, which contribute 98% (wt/wt) or more to the total fat in milk. Nearly 95% of these are contributed by fatty acids.[45] The fat content of milk varies with maternal diet and throughout the feed, with hindmilk (the last part of the feed) containing two to three times more fat than the initial milk (foremilk).[46] The essential fatty acids in human milk are derived from the maternal diet, either directly or after intermediate incorporation into a body storage pool. Diet and endogenous synthesis are the sources of milk long chain-polyunsaturated fatty acids, and for both steps, incorporation into storage pools is a possibility.

The lipid system in maternal milk is composed of an organized milk fat globule, bile salt–stimulated lipase, and a pattern of fatty acids marked by high palmitic acid (Cl6:0), which composes nearly 50%, and oleic acid (Cl6:1 ro9), which accounts for 12%. The linoleic (Cl8:2 ro6) and linolenic (C18:3 ro3) acids are also important.[47] Unlike the palmitate in most lipids, lipid system in maternal milk has a slight structural isomeric variation that facilitates the absorption of the monoglycerides released during digestion. Unlike bovine milk, human milk also contains large amounts of long chain-polyunsaturated fatty acids such as docosahexaenoic acid (C22:6 ro3) and arachidonic acid (C20:4 ro6), which are required for the developing brain and the infantile immune system.[48] These fatty acids are also important constituents of retinal and brain phospholipid membranes and are believed to be important for visual and neurodevelopmental outcomes.

The carbohydrates in human milk are an important source of lactose and oligosaccharides.[49] Unabsorbed lactose may promote a softer stool consistency, nonpathogenic fecal flora, and improved mineral absorption. Human milk oligosaccharides are bioactive carbohydrate polymers (also including glycoproteins) that promote mucosal immunity because they resemble specific bacterial antigen receptors and prevent bacterial attachment to the host mucosa.[50] Human milk oligosaccharides such as fucosylated glycans inhibit binding by *Hemophilus influenzae, Campylobacter jejuni,* and some viral agents.[51] Human milk oligosaccharides are also prebiotics that stimulate the growth of nonpathogenic bifidus bacteria.

The mineral composition of human milk is a subject of ongoing study.[52] Human milk has lower calcium and phosphorus concentrations than do other milks, but these are present in more bioavailable forms. Copper and zinc content appears adequate for nutritional needs. The concentration of iron, however, may not be adequate beyond 4 to 6 months, and oral iron supplement or iron-containing complementary feedings are indicated are needed beginning at about 6 months. Preterm and low birth weight infants should receive iron supplementation from birth.

Vitamin K concentrations in human milk are low, and all infants need one-time administration of vitamin K at birth.[52] Vitamin D concentrations in milk depend on maternal vitamin D status, and infants may need oral vitamin D supplementation.[53,54]

Table 16.2 Bioactive Factors Present in Human Milk
Immune factors
Growth factors
Hormones
Enzymes
Nucleotides
Vitamins
Lipids
Mucins

Nutritional Implications for the Premature Infant

Maternal milk is the preferred enteral feeding for premature infants, even though its nutritional contents may not always be adequate.[21,55–59] Preterm milk contains more protein than the milk from mothers who delivered at term, although it may still not meet the needs of all preterm infants. The fats are more easily digestible. The gastrointestinal advantages of human milk include faster gastric emptying, less feeding intolerance, and fewer days to full enteral feeds. When considered in addition to the immunologic benefits, these strengths are important.[21,55–59]

The concentrations of protein, sodium, and zinc decline throughout lactation and may not remain adequate for all infants. For very low birth weight (<1500 g) infants, human milk needs to be fortified for calories, protein, calcium, phosphate, and other micronutrients.[60,61] The use of an exclusive human milk diet, made with human milk–based fortifier, may be safer with a lower risk of necrotizing enterocolitis.[62]

Human milk fortifier is usually added once the premature infant begins to tolerate tube feedings, and its use is continued until the infant has achieved targeted oral feedings, a weight of 1800 g, or is close to being discharged from the hospital.[60,61] The importance of postdischarge multinutrient fortification is unclear, but many of these infants may benefit from individualized plans to consistently achieve a weight gain >20 g/day until the weight targets appropriate for the corrected age, linear growth of 0.5 cm/week, and an alkaline phosphatase level less than 450 IU/L have been achieved.[63]

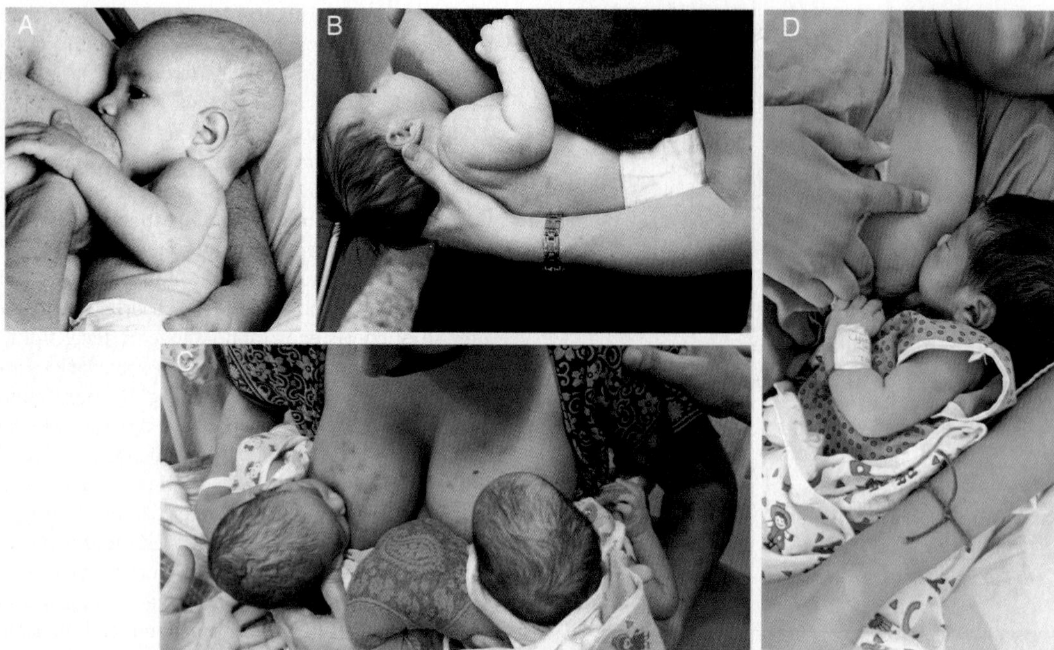

Fig. 16.5 Breastfeeding Positions. (A) Cradle position, the classic front hold. The baby's head is cradled near the mother's elbow, and her arm supports the infant along the back and neck. The mother and baby should be chest to chest. (B) Cross-cradle position. Another excellent position to use with young infants because it allows good visualization of the latch and provides firm head control of the neonate. The mother's hand is under the baby's neck. The baby's chin but not the nose is in the mother's breast. More of the areola is covered by the lower lip than by the upper lip, which is characteristic of a normal, asymmetrical latch. (C) Underarm position or Football hold. The mother tucks the baby close to her body. Useful for feeding twins. (D) Side-lying position. Suitable for mothers who have had a cesarean section, are tired, have a sore perineum, have a sleepy baby, and for nighttime feeding. The mother and baby are belly to belly, and the baby is held on the side by the mother's hand. (A, Image reproduced with permission and minor modifications from Newton ER and Stuebe AM. Lactation and Breastfeeding. In: *Gabbe's Obstetrics: Normal and Problem Pregnancies,* 25, 475-502.e3; B, Image reproduced with permission and minor modifications from Balest et al. Neonatology. In: *Zitelli and Davis' Atlas of Pediatric Physical Diagnosis*. 2:44–70. C and D, Images provided by Dr. Srijan Singh, Global Newborn Society.)

Immunologic Benefits

Human milk contains secretory IgA, lactoferrin, lysozyme, oligosaccharides, growth factors, and cellular components that protect the infant against known, frequently seen infections.[17] The mother may also form specific antibodies against any new antigens that may enter the shared environment and passes those on to the infant.[64]

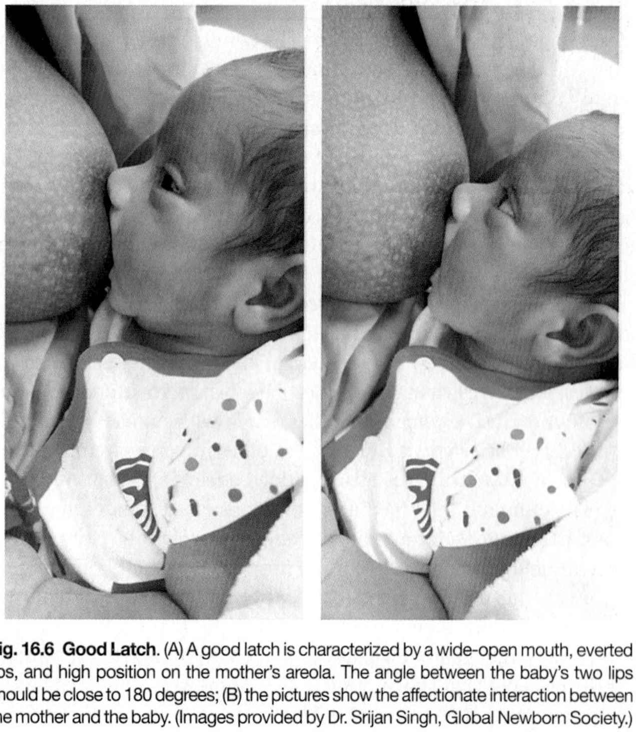

Fig. 16.6 Good Latch. (A) A good latch is characterized by a wide-open mouth, everted lips, and high position on the mother's areola. The angle between the baby's two lips should be close to 180 degrees; (B) the pictures show the affectionate interaction between the mother and the baby. (Images provided by Dr. Srijan Singh, Global Newborn Society.)

Neonatal Morbidity

Breastfed infants have a lower rate of respiratory and diarrheal illness and all-cause infection-related mortality.[65–67] Both mother's own and donor human milk reduce the risk of necrotizing enterocolitis, late-onset sepsis, retinopathy of prematurity, chronic lung disease, and the total length of hospital stay.[58] Breastfeeding also seems protective against sudden infant death syndrome.[68] Even though a direct mechanism is not known, the effect is strong and dose-dependent and does not appear to be only a marker for confounders such as passive smoking or demographic factors.[69]

Chronic Disorders

Breastfed infants likely have lower rates of dental caries, inflammatory bowel disorders, type 1 diabetes, and childhood leukemia.[70–73] The risk of allergic disorders seems somewhat conflicting, but meta-analysis shows reduced risk of asthma at age 5 to 18 years compared with infants who were never breastfed, or in comparison of more versus less breastfeeding, with no impact of stratification by family atopy. The risk of eczema seems lower before 2 years of age in infants who were exclusive breastfed for 3 to 4 months, but not after. Breastfeeding does not specifically reduce the risk of food allergies, although it appears to reduce the risk of generalized allergic disease before age 5 years.

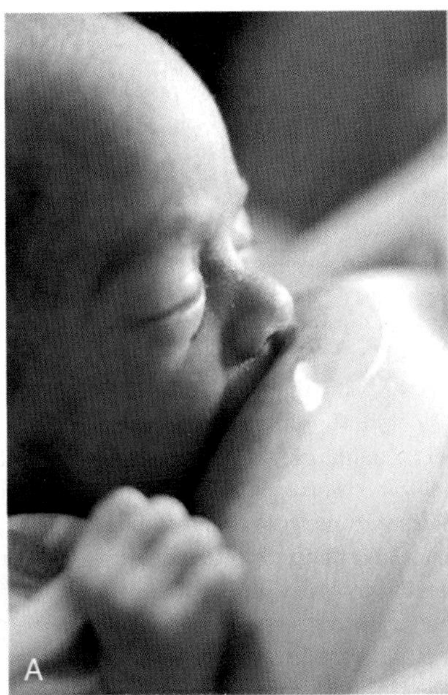

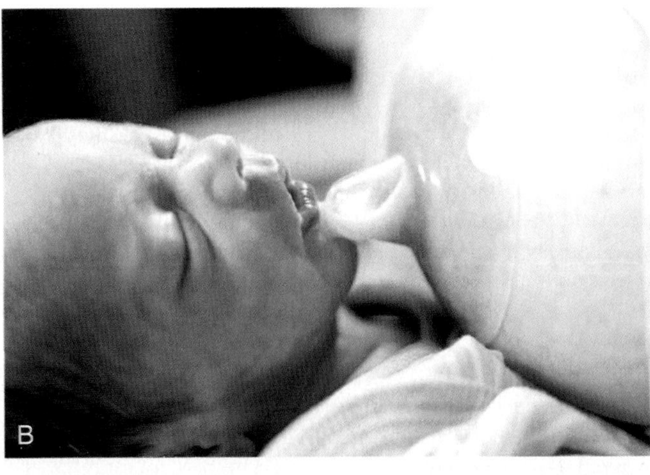

Fig. 16.7 Use of Nipple Shields. (A) A preterm infant breastfeeding with a nipple shield in place. Nipple shields can be used for preterm or term infants who have difficulty with latch for a variety of reasons, such as maternal flat or inverted nipples and engorgement. These are not intended for long-term use and should be used under the supervision of a person well trained in lactation support. (B) A preterm infant is full and satisfied after breastfeeding with a nipple shield in place. The nipple shield has multiple fenestrations, so the milk comes out as it does from the mother's nipple. (Reproduced with permission and minor modifications from Balest et al. Neonatology. In: *Zitelli and Davis' Atlas of Pediatric Physical Diagnosis*. 2:44–70.)

Obesity and Related Cardiovascular Changes

The exclusivity and duration of breastfeeding may reduce the risk of obesity and overweight in childhood and adulthood, which is noticeable both in individual studies an in meta-analysis (pooled odds ratio, 0.74; 95% confidence interval [CI], 0.70–0.78 points).[16,74] Suggested mechanisms include higher energy and protein/energy intake among formula-fed infants, leading to neonatal and hence childhood obesity, and endocrine differences that alter fat deposition patterns. Hormones in breast milk, including leptin, adiponectin, and ghrelin, also appear to regulate appetite, growth, fat deposition, and energy balance, which may alter the body composition.[75] Blood pressures and cholesterol levels in later life may also be impacted positively.[76]

Table 16.3 Difficulties in Lactation/Breastfeeding
Maternal chronic illness such as diabetes, cystic fibrosis, or sickle cell disease
Prior breast surgery
Obesity
Perinatal complications, cesarean section
Multiple births
Nipple injury, pain
Premature infants
Small-for-gestation infant
Large-for-gestation infant
Congenital anomalies in the infant, ranging from chromosomal errors to anatomic defects[a]
Infant with neurologic issues
Infants in the postoperative period for any reason
Infants recovering from birth asphyxia

[a]One important, frequently encountered difficulty is in feeding infants with cleft lip/palate. These infants should be evaluated on an individual basis, based on the size and location of the baby's clefts and the mother's wishes and previous experience with breastfeeding (Fig. 16.8). Most infants with cleft lip are able to generate at least some suction and may be able to feed successfully. Those with a cleft lip and palate may have difficulty generating enough suction. Some infants may be able to feed using a cup, spoon, or bottle, with the parents having to keep a close eye on the hydration and growth status of the infant. The families may be able to find some peer support from organizations such as Operation Smile. In some infants, modifications to breastfeeding positions may help.

Cognitive Ability

The evidence seems favorable but needs confirmation because of multiple confounders. A meta-analysis using strict study criteria noted breastfeeding promoted an average gain of 3.44 points (95% CI, 2.30–4.58 points) on intelligence testing in childhood.[12] When

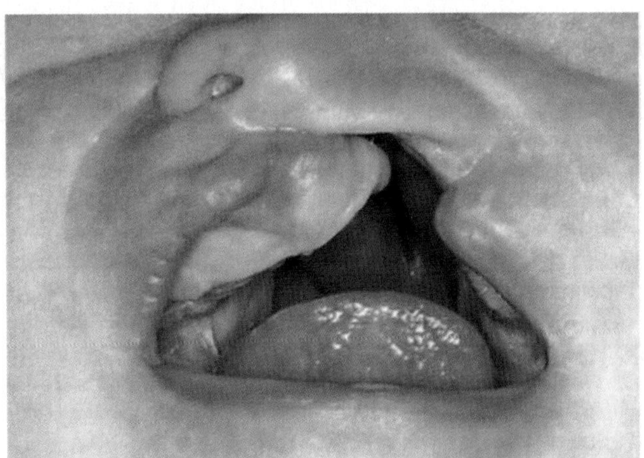

Fig. 16.8 Left Complete Unilateral Cleft of Lip, Alveolus, and Hard and Soft Palate. (Reproduced with permission and minor modifications from Elsevier Point of Care. Published January 19, 2018. From Goodacre T. Cleft lip and palate: current management. *Paediatr Child Health*. 2012;22[4]:160–168.)

only the highest-quality studies (n = 4; sample size >500; breastfeeding recall time <3 years; controlled for maternal intelligence) were examined, the gains were still significant (1.76 points; 95% CI, 0.25–3.26 points).

Studies show receipt of fortified human milk during hospitalization improves neurodevelopment among extremely low birth weight infants as measured during follow-up using the Bayley Scales of Infant Development II. The gains were particularly notable at 30 months; every 10 mL/kg/day increase in human milk increased the Mental Developmental Index score by 0.59 points, the Psychomotor Developmental Index score by 0.56 points, and the total behavior percentile score by 0.99 points.[77]

Benefits of Breastfeeding for Both the Mother and the Infant

Exclusive breastfeeding through 6 months of age has been noted to increase mother–infant bonding, possibly due to increased oxytocin levels, which are involved in the milk ejection reflex during nursing but are also an important neurotransmitter that directly affects maternal nurturing behaviors, and to mother–infant social interaction, gaze, vocalizations, and affectionate touch.[78] There are also important, known benefits to the mother, such as in protection against malignancies and cardiovascular disease.

Global Impact

Human milk feedings have positively affected preventive health interventions in childhood. The effects have been acknowledged in high-, middle-, and low-income countries with respect to infant nutrition, infant survival, gastrointestinal function, host defense, neurodevelopment, and psychological well-being.[79] The benefits of both exclusive or even partial breastfeeding are known.[80] However, health providers can elicit parents' perspectives about the challenges of exclusive breastfeeding and provide scientifically based guidance and personalized support, recognizing that any breast milk (including colostrum) gives a meaningful health benefit. The success of the United Nations Millennium Development Goals, with a reduction in the number of deaths of children younger than 5 years from 12.7 million per year in 1990 to 5.9 million per year in 2015, is multifactorial, but breastfeeding plays a large current and larger potential role (World Health Organization Media Centre, 2015).[80] Exclusive breastfeeding (0–5 months) is increasing by 1% annually in the Millennium Development Goals–tracked countries.[80] Each of the 2030 United Nations Sustainable Development Goals, for example, "Zero Hunger," can be linked to and supported by breastfeeding.[81]

Breastfeeding Goals

In the United States, the recognition of breastfeeding benefits grew during the 1970s, and rates more than doubled in the United States from 24.7% in 1971 to 59.7% in 1984.[82] The US Centers for Disease Control and Prevention began monitoring annual breastfeeding rates through the National Immunization Survey in 2001 and administered the first national survey of maternity practices related to breastfeeding, the Maternity Practices in Infant Nutrition and Care Survey, in 2007. The Healthy People 2020 infant feeding goals of >80% initiating breastfeeding postpartum, >14% breastfed within the first 48 hours, and >40% exclusively breastfeeding at 3 months were largely met in 2012.[83,84]

In 1992, the United Nations International Children's Emergency Fund and the World Health Organization (WHO) developed the Baby-Friendly Hospital Initiative (BFHI), an international program to promote breastfeeding-supportive policies for birthing hospitals.[85–87] The BFHI "10 steps" in combination with an "11th step," the WHO International Code of Marketing of Breastmilk Substitutes, which protects against free provision and advertising of breast milk substitutes (i.e., formula), effectively increased breastfeeding rates worldwide.[88] Adherence to these evidence-based maternity practices significantly increases the likelihood of mothers initiating breastfeeding, exclusively breastfeeding, and breastfeeding through 6 months. Possible expansion of a modified Ten Steps to Successful Breastfeeding program (Table 16.5) to neonatal intensive care units has been proposed, and state health departments have begun to create programs to support Ten Steps to Successful Breastfeeding practices (such as http://texastenstep.org/). The number of birthing hospitals designated as baby friendly (by Baby-Friendly USA Inc.) is increasing (Baby-Friendly, 2015).[89]

Association of women's, infants and children initiatives, including enhanced maternal food packages for breastfeeding mothers and peer counseling (Loving Support), hold promise, as do the Affordable Care Act mandates covering breastfeeding education and supplies and

Table 16.4 Nutrient Composition of Term and Preterm Milk

	Term (≥37 Weeks) Human Milk 1 Week After Birth	Preterm (28 Weeks) Human Milk 1 Week After Birth
Energy (kcal/dL)	**67±7**	**75±4**
Protein (g/dL)	**1.4±0.3**	**2.4±0.2**
Fat (g/dL)	3.9±0.3	4.1±0.6
Carbohydrates (g/dL)	6.2±0.4	7.5±0.4
Calcium (mmol/L)	5.4±0.3	6.5±0.2
Iron (mg/L)	**0.8±0.2**	**1.5±0.3**
Phosphate (mg)	1.9±0.2	2.1±0.3
Magnesium (mmol/L)	1.2±0.4	1.5±0.5
Sodium (mmol/L)	11±0.2	10±0.3
Potassium (mmol/L)	11±0.4	13±0.2
Chloride (mmol/L)	11±0.5	12±0.3

Our Own Data; Bolded Letters Indicate $P < .05$; N = 100.

Table 16.5 10 Steps to Successful Breastfeeding
Step 1: Have a written breastfeeding policy that is routinely communicated to all healthcare staff.
Step 2: Train all healthcare staff in the skills necessary to implement this policy.
Step 3: Inform all pregnant women about the benefits and management of breastfeeding.
Step 4: Help mothers initiate breastfeeding within 1 hour of birth.
Step 5: Show mothers how to breastfeed and how to maintain lactation even if they are separated from their infants.
Step 6: Give newborns no food or drink other than breast milk, unless medically indicated.
Step 7: Practice rooming-in: Allow mothers and infants to remain together 24 hours a day.
Step 8: Encourage breastfeeding on demand.
Step 9: Give no pacifiers or artificial nipples to breastfeeding infants.
Step 10: Foster the establishment of breastfeeding support groups, and refer mothers to them on their discharge from the hospital or birth center.

Table 16.6 Contraindications to Breastfeeding
Untreated active/miliary maternal tuberculosis
Active herpetic lesions on the breast (not vaginal)
Active varicella (chickenpox) lesions on the breast; can feed with expressed milk; infant should receive varicella immunoglobulin
Active human immunodeficiency virus (HIV) infection
Active human T-lymphotrophic virus (types 1 and 2) infection
Maternal use of illicit drugs is an absolute contraindication; can feed if drug-free and receiving methadone
Receiving cancer chemotherapy
Acute maternal illness with swine flu (H1N1 flu)
Infant with galactosemia; need consultation for other inborn errors

reasonable break time for "nonexempt" hourly employees to express milk.[90] Workday strategies that include feeding the infant directly from the breast appear more effective than pumping only. However, maternal employment outside the home, in general, is associated with decreased breastfeeding initiation and continuation. Public policy changes can increase national breastfeeding rates: provision of paid maternity leave for employed women increases breastfeeding exclusivity and duration, and longer maternity leaves are associated with increased breastfeeding initiation.[91] The United Nations International Labor Organization recommends 18 weeks of paid maternity leave, a "reasonable goal" that could push the United States closer to Healthy People breastfeeding targets.[92]

Prelacteal Feeding

In many countries, there is a practice of prelacteal feeding by offering foods and/or liquids other than milk before initiating breastfeeding.[93] Such feedings may include water, formula, honey, or thawed butter. If possible, these feedings should be gently discouraged because there is no need, and they could actually introduce exposure to contaminants/infectious agents.

Contraindications to Breastfeeding

There are very few true contraindications to breastfeeding (Table 16.6).[82,94] Mothers with fever or other minor illnesses should be permitted to breastfeed, because the infant has already been exposed to the infectious agent during the incubation period and will be able to benefit from the mother's immune factors that will be released in breast milk. Few maternal medications contraindicate breastfeeding; a list at the National Institutes of Health US National Library of Medicine Drugs and Lactation Database (https://www.ncbi.nlm.nih.gov/books/NBK501922/) is a useful resource. Mothers who have undergone breast reduction or breast implant surgery can breastfeed under supervision with a lactation specialist.

CHAPTER

17 Storage and Use of Human Milk in Neonatal Intensive Care Units

Nitasha Bagga, Kei Lui, Arūnas Liubšys, Mohammad M. Rahman, Mimi L. Mynak, Akhil Maheshwari

KEY POINTS

1. Human milk is an important source of nutrients, immunologic factors, and pre- and probiotic factors for preterm and critically ill infants for up to 6 months after birth.
2. Human milk has positive effects on enhanced maturation of vital organs such as the brain and gastrointestinal system and on immunity, and it is also known to protect at-risk infants against neonatal morbidities such as necrotizing enterocolitis, bronchopulmonary dysplasia, and retinopathy of prematurity.
3. Because mother's own milk is not always available for all critically ill infants, neonatal intensive care units (NICUs) have/are developing storage facilities for the storage, screening, processing, and careful use of human milk in ill infants.
4. In this chapter, we have summarized the information/guidelines for the development of physical infrastructure and human resources for milk storage units in NICUs.
5. There is a need for continued education of mothers about the importance of human milk and its storage, screening for infectious agents, and measures to improve safety of infant feeding with mother's own or stored donor milk.

Introduction

Human milk has a unique composition, and consequently, has unique bioactive properties that differ from milk from other mammals (Fig. 17.1). Breast milk not only meets complete nutritional needs of a newborn infant (Fig. 17.2) up to 6 months but also plays a vital role in development of the brain and immune system, and it has been constantly emphasized in literature. In-depth analyses show unique structural patterns in human milk-borne carbohydrates, which may have far-reaching effects and even after the patterns of gut microbial colonization extending into later infancy and beyond (Fig. 17.3). All these attributes make breastfeeding the single most cost-effective intervention to reduce infant mortality across the globe.[1] Although all newborn infants benefit from breast milk, not all are able to breastfeed at birth, which majorly includes preterm and low birth infants. The benefits of breast milk remain irreplaceable in preterm neonates. Prevention of prematurity-related morbidities such as necrotizing enterocolitis, bronchopulmonary dysplasia, and retinopathy of prematurity; better intestinal maturity; and improved neurodevelopmental outcomes are a few advantages.[2,3] Succinctly, the most vulnerable population of newborns is at the greatest risk of increased mortality and morbidity and is not able to receive the benefits of breast milk.[4] However, initiation and maintenance of mother's own milk (MOM) are of global concern in neonatal intensive care units (NICUs). The World Health Organization and European Society for Paediatric Gastroenterology, Hepatology, and Nutrition recommend pasteurized donor human milk as the next best option if MOM is not available.[5–7] This chapter outlines the basic requirements and principles for developing facilities in various NICUs for storage of MOM, and if possible, milk from mothers willing to share if there are volumes more than those needed for their own infants. For donated milk, a set of procedures needs to be developed similar to those used in larger milk banks to ensure safety from any infectious agents.

Definition

Human milk storage facilities in NICUs store, screen, process, and use human milk to feed the infants. These units promote, protect, and support breastfeeding by providing safe and appropriate storage to provide high-quality human milk to premature and critically ill infants. Such units also help prevent waste of this important resource during periods when the infant cannot be fed due to medical reasons.

Infrastructure of Human Milk Storage Units in NICUs[8]

The use and processing of human milk for use in the newborn infant units and NICUs is summarized in Fig. 17.4. In the following sections, we describe the structural and functional needs for developing a human milk storage unit in a hospital. We realize that the chapter is relatively weighted toward the policies and procedures needed for processing donated milk, but these details are needed to prevent infections and transmission of unknown toxins and to ensure safety when an infant is fed with donated milk. The procedures to ensure safety of using mothers' own and donated milk have been defined but need periodic reevaluation (Fig. 17.5).

Space

There are no standard guidelines or recommendations on the minimum or maximum space required for a milk bank, but it is considered to be approximately a 250-square-foot room, which accommodates milk bank equipment, a work area for technicians, and records storage. A breast milk expression room should be separate, which provides sufficient privacy to the mothers.

Equipment

Pasteurizer

To pasteurize milk, the Holder method is recommended (heat treatment of milk at 62.5°C for 30 minutes). It can be done by an automated pasteurizer or by the shaker–water bath (manual method), a less-expensive method that can be used in resource-limited settings. Another method of pasteurization is flash heat treatment (high

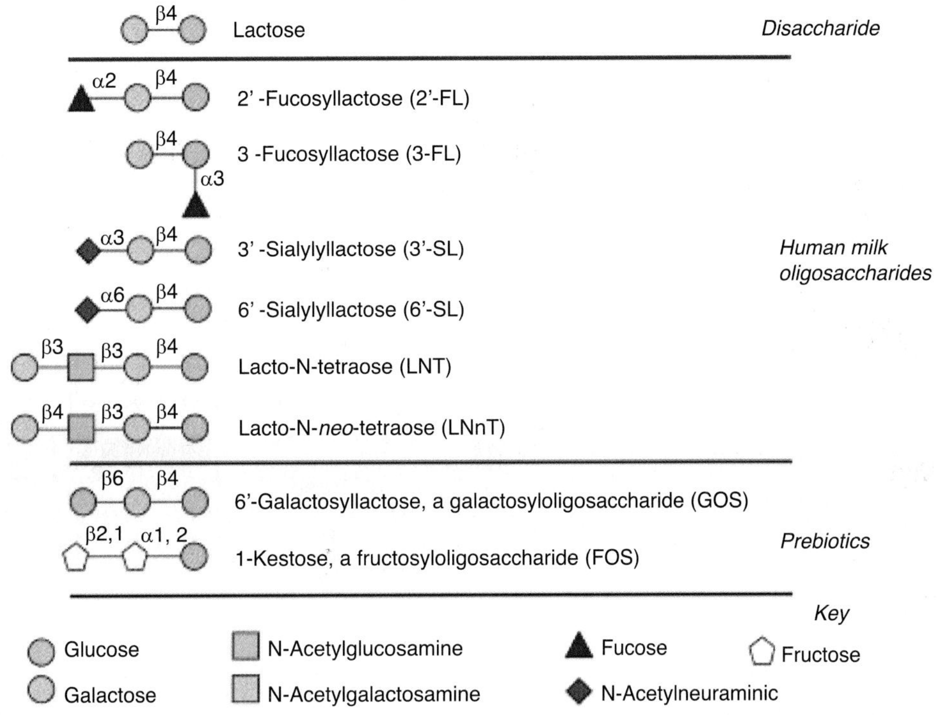

Fig. 17.1 Human milk carbohydrates show unique structural characteristics, which may impart important short- and long-term beneficial effects. *Upper row:* The disaccharide lactose, is the most abundant carbohydrate found in human milk and the core for human milk oligosaccharides. *Rows 2 to 7:* Selected examples of simple human milk oligosaccharide (hMOS) structures. Shown are two fucosylated structures (2′-FL and 3′-FL), two sialylated (acidic) structures (3′-SL and 6′-SL), and two precursor molecules without fucose or sialic acid. *Rows 8 to 9:* Two commercially available prebiotic carbohydrates are shown (fructo-oligosaccharide [FOS] and galacto-oligosaccharide [GOS]). (Morrow, Newburg, Human milk oligosaccharide. Gastroenterology and Nutrition: Neonatology Questions and Controversies, Chapter 4, 43–57.)

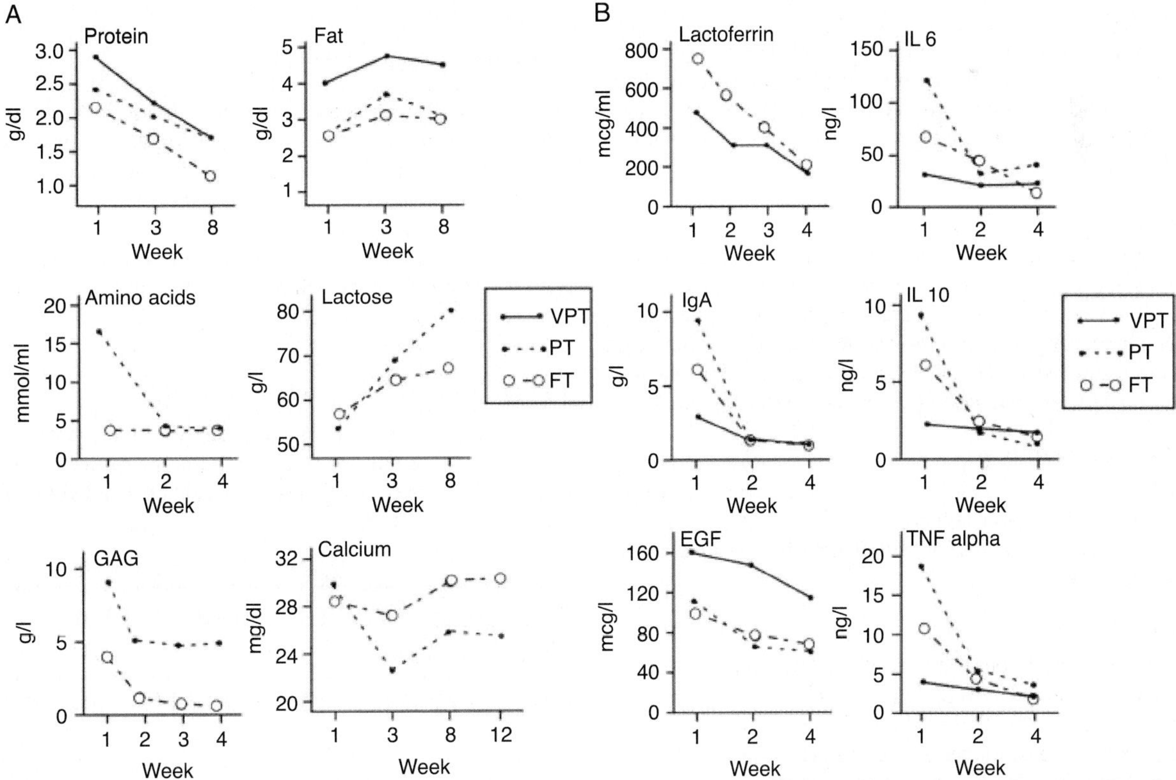

Fig. 17.2 Changes in Milk Composition Over Time in Term (FT, 37–41 Weeks), Preterm (PT, 30–36 Weeks), and Very Preterm (VPT, <28–30 Weeks) Infants. (A) Nutrients. (B) Bioactive molecules. *EGF,* Epidermal growth factor; *GAG,* glycosaminoglycans; *IgA,* immunoglobulin A; *IL 6,* interleukin 6; *IL 10,* interleukin 10; *TNF alpha,* tumor necrosis factor alpha. (Adapted from: Reproduced with permission and minor modifications from Underwood MA. Human milk for the premature infant. *Pediatric Pediatr Clin North Am.* 2013;60[1]:189–207.)

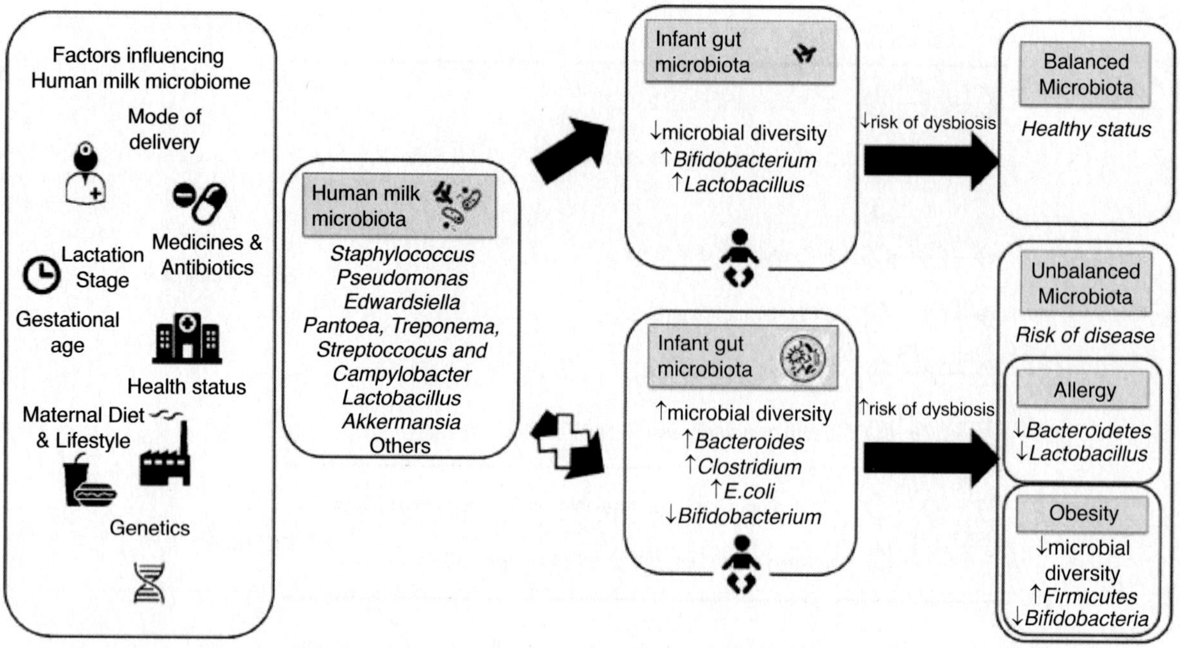

Fig. 17.3 Human Milk Microbiota Composition and Comparison Between Breastfeeding and Formula-Feeding Microbiota. Metagenome analysis of human milk shows that the human milk microbiota is mainly dominated by *Staphylococcus*, *Pseudomonas*, and *Edwardsiella*, but other groups are also represented in minor amounts. Breastfed and formula-fed infants have different bacterial populations, which seems to modulate the susceptibility of noncommunicable diseases such as allergy and/or obesity during infancy and/or in adult life. *E. coli*, *Escherichia coli*. (Adapted from: Reproduced with permission and minor modifications from Gomez-Gallego et al. The human milk microbiome and factors influencing its composition and activity. *Semin Fetal Neonatal Med*. 2016;21[6]:400–405.)

temperature, short time; 72°C for 16 seconds) or ultraviolet irradiation, which is not being used very commonly.

Deep Freezer

Milk is stored at −20°C in closely monitored refrigerators. A deep freezer with an automatic temperature display is desirable. For donated milk, two deep freezers are required, one to keep postpasteurized milk awaiting culture and another to keep culture-negative milk, ready for disbursement.

Refrigerator

A refrigerator is used when the collected milk cannot be used immediately and needs to be stored for 24 hours or longer. Donated milk should be pooled and pasteurized. Pasteurized milk is also kept in a refrigerator for thawing overnight before disbursement. Either two separate units should be used or clear demarcation should be present to prevent any confusion in usage of pre- and postpasteurization milk.

Hot Air Oven/Autoclave

Human milk storage units should have individual hot air ovens, autoclaves, or centralized sterile service departments to sterilize the containers used for milk expression, storage, pasteurization, and if needed, transport of milk.

Breast Milk Pump

Hospital-grade electrical breast pumps (Fig. 17.6) are preferred, as these are more comfortable, less painful, and can be used for expression of larger volumes. In resource-limited settings and for home expression, manual breast pumps are recommended. Cleaning and sterilization should be done as per the manufacturer's manual.

Storage and Expression Containers

The containers used to collect milk are made of polycarbonate, propylene, Pyrex, and food-grade stainless steel containers. Polythene milk bags can also be used for temporary purposes. The risk of spillage, contamination, and loss of lipids and fat is higher with milk bags.

Administrative Staff

Human milk storage units should have a dedicated director (a neonatologist/pediatrician for planning and implementing of services), a specifically assigned manager (for day-to-day running of the milk bank), and a team consisting of a lactation consultant, lactation nurses, a microbiologist, an infection control nurse, a biomedical engineer, and a milk bank attendant, and if needed/possible, personnel for transportation and collection of expressed milk from home or other centers.

Uninterrupted Power Supply

A dedicated, centralized source of uninterrupted power is recommended for any milk bank to run equipment, deep freezers, and refrigerators. There should also be a backup source of electricity in case of power failure.

Components and Process of a Human Milk Bank[9,10]

Encouraging Mothers and Recruitment of Donors

The goal of improving the feeding practices in any newborn infant unit or NICU is to encourage mothers to feed their infants. Any lactating mother who is healthy with extra expressed milk can also be recruited for donating milk for the milk bank. Such recruitment obviously has to be on a strictly voluntary basis. To

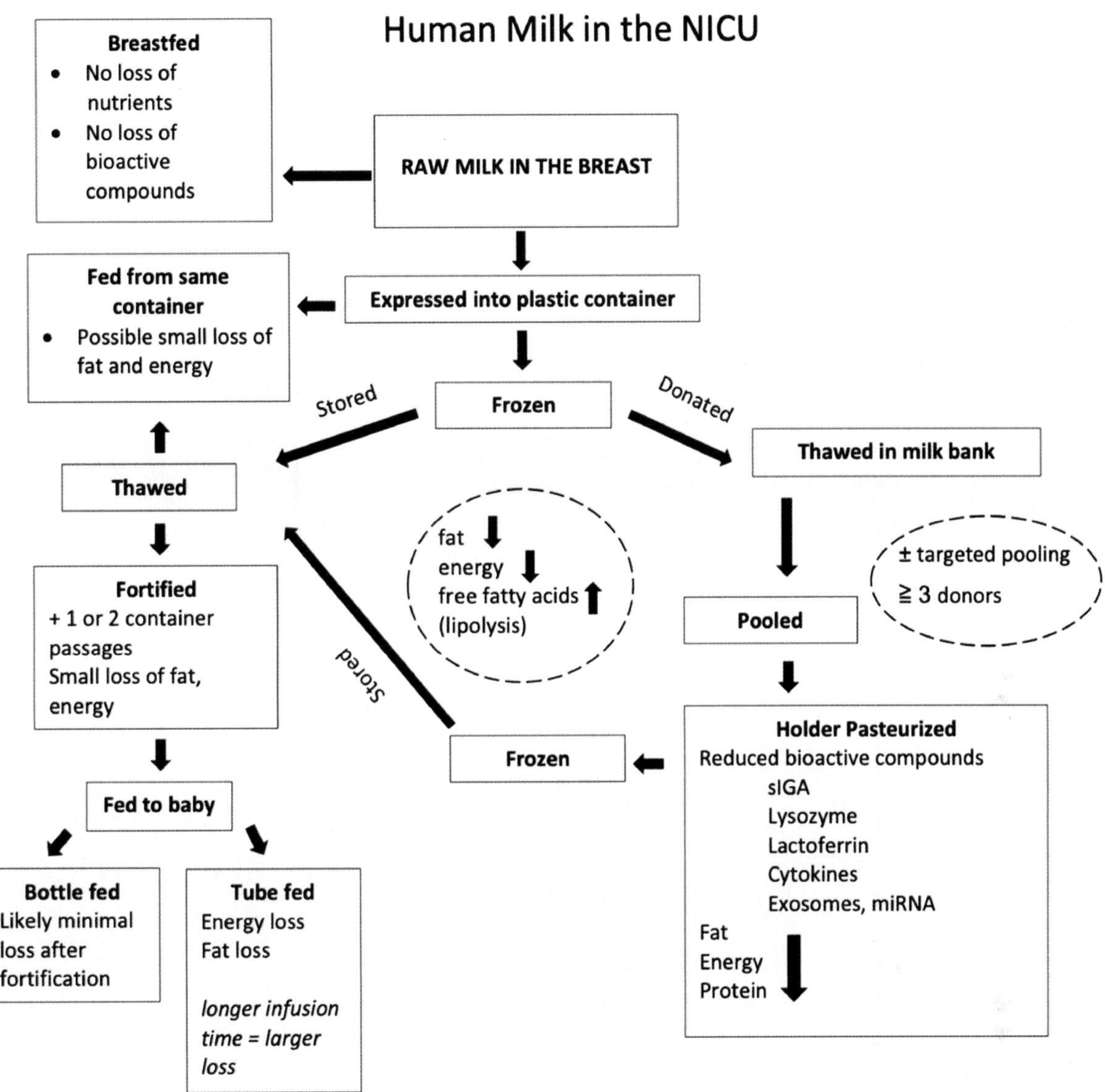

Fig. 17.4 Use and Processing of Mother's Own and Donor Milk for Use in Newborn Units and Neonatal Intensive Care Units (NICUs). The processing and storage of donor milk is known to cause some changes in the nutrient composition. (Adapted from: Reproduced with permission and with minor modifications from Colaizy T. Effects of milk banking procedures on nutritional and bioactive components of donor human milk. *Sem Perinat*. 2021;45:151382.)

reach mothers, a variety of communication methods can be used:

- Information leaflets to emphasize the importance of human milk feeding. These leaflets can include the importance of donation and eligibility criteria of the mothers and can be shared with mothers in maternity and postnatal wards, antenatal clinics, well-baby clinics, and other areas such as the milk expression rooms. Other media resources such as television and radio can also be used to reach a larger number of donors.
- A breastfeeding support team comprising obstetricians, pediatricians, nursing staff, and a lactation consultant should promote breastfeeding and counsel and motivate mothers for extra milk donation.
- Donors themselves can also encourage other donors for recruitment, and continual lactation support is important.

Donor Screening

Screening criteria must be tailored as per the local concerns and requirements (see Fig. 17.5), though all lactating mothers who are willing can donate milk, with minimum mandatory selection criteria as follows:

- Donor has enough milk after feeding her baby satisfactorily, and her baby is thriving and well.
- Donor is well as ascertained by history and physical examination.
- Donor's blood tests for HIV, VDRL, hepatitis B, and CMV are negative within 6 months of the current pregnancy or at the time of donor recruitment.
- Donor is not consuming any drugs such as antitubercular therapy, antipsychotics, chemotherapeutic agents, or any illicit drugs.

Informed written consent should be obtained from all the donor mothers so that the responsibility of maintaining the safety and quality of donor milk can be shared.

Milk Expression

Milk expression can be done by various methods at home, at the hospital, and at milk banks, with adequate precautions (see Fig. 17.6).

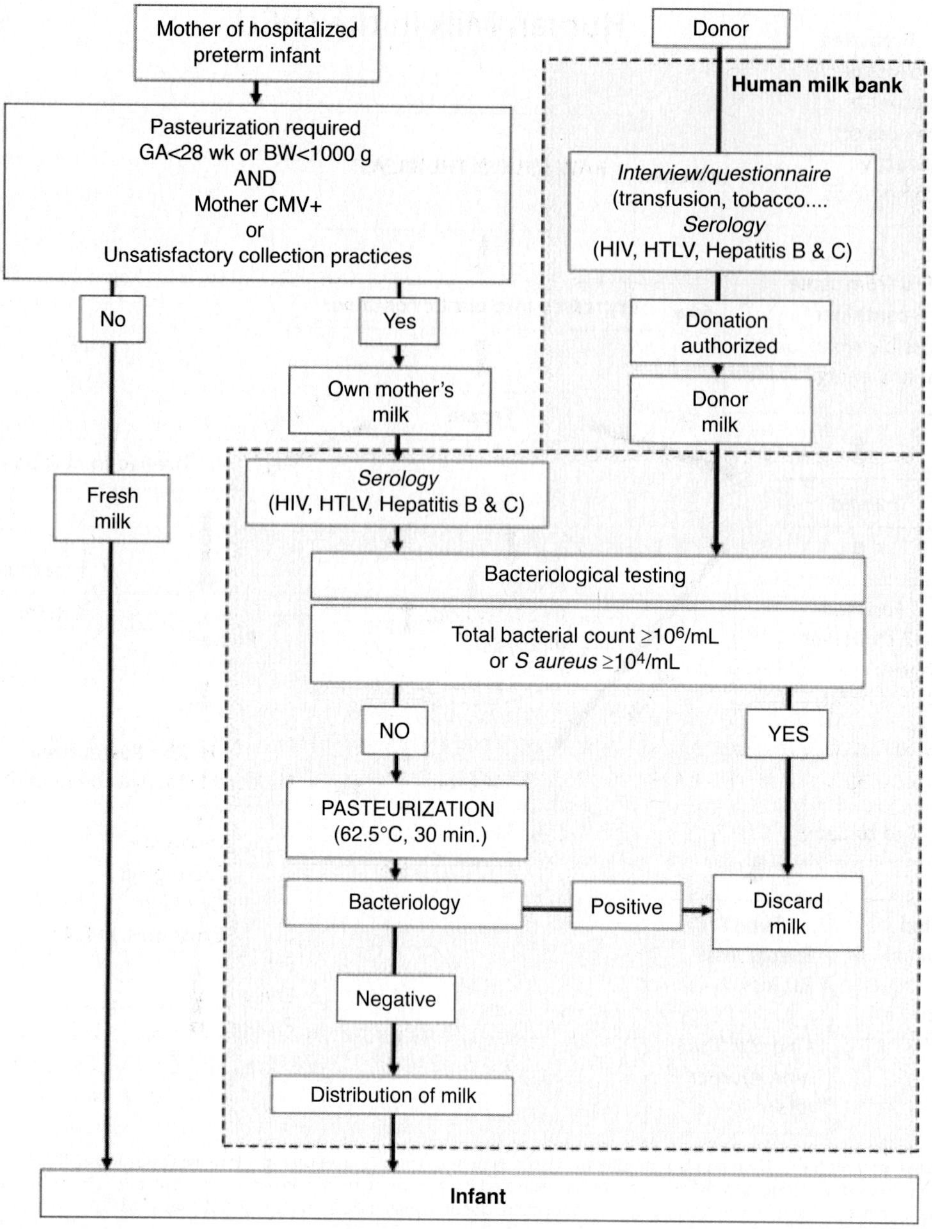

Fig. 17.5 Safety of Stored Maternal and Donor Milk. Banked human milk and feeding preterm infants with human milk. *BW,* Birth weight; *GA,* gestational age; *S aureus, Staphylococcus aureus*. (Adapted from: Reproduced with permission and minor modifications from Picaud J-C, Buffin R. Human milk—treatment and quality of banked human milk. *Clin Perinatol*. 2017;44:95–119.)

- Milk expressed either at home or at a hospital facility is stored in suitable containers, preferably plastic, glass, milk bags, or food-grade stainless steel. Frequency of milk expression in a single container should be labeled with date and time and the donor's identification.
- Educating donor mothers about appropriate techniques and equipment available for milk expression (manual and hospital-grade breast pumps) and proper cleaning methods of breast pumps should be a duty of the breastfeeding support team.

Increasing information shows that mother's own and donor milk may differ in the content of fat, protein, and lactose. However, very interestingly, these contents show considerable variation between individual mothers, seen both in mother's own and in donor milk (Fig. 17.7). When the plasma levels of key amino acids are compared with the levels seen in fetuses, the impact of different milk expression techniques on the levels seen in preterm infants becomes evident (Fig. 17.8). There are important differences in composition even between aliquots obtained by expression at different times in the same day. Similarly, different expression methods also affect the maternal prolactin levels, and consequently, the likelihood of the mother being able to continue producing enough milk for her infant. Further work is needed to understand the determinants of the composition and volumes of milk produced by a lactating mother.

Milk Handling

Risk of contamination is very high during all stages of milk handling (storage and transportation; see Figs. 17.4 and 17.5). Processing is important for donated milk.

- Donor milk expressed at home should be stored in a refrigerator immediately. Milk should not be stored more than 4 to

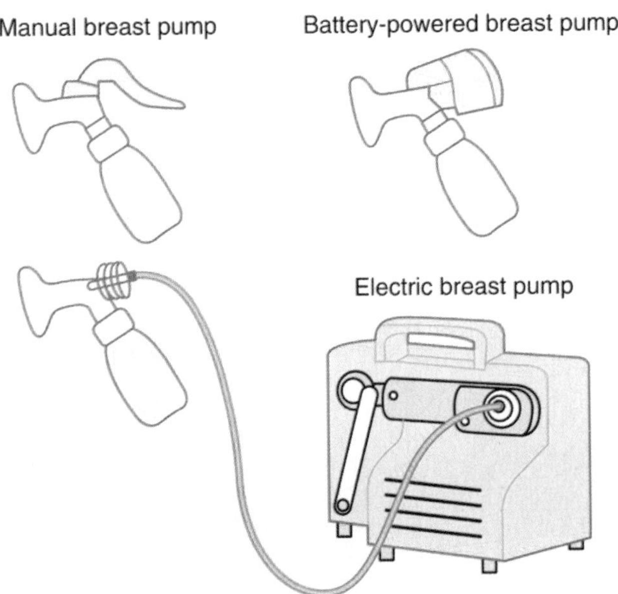

Fig. 17.6 The Collection and Storage of Human Milk and Human Milk Banking. (Adapted from: Reproduced from: US Food and Drug Administration. Types of breast pumps; 2018. https://www.fda.gov/medical-devices/breast-pumps/types-breast-pumps. Accessed December 26, 2019.)

6 hours at room temperature. The containers should be labeled appropriately with the name, time, and date of expression.

- If the milk is donated in a hospital or human milk bank (HMB), it should be kept in freezer at −20°C immediately unless it is to be used the same day.
- Milk must be stored in food-grade containers, labeled with an identification number and the time and date of collection/freezing.
- Transportation of milk should be done maintaining an appropriate freezing temperature to avoid bacterial contamination and degradation of milk. Insulated containers with ice packs can be used for transportation of milk from home or other healthcare facilities to the HMB.

Processing of Donated Milk

Processing of donated milk includes milk pooling and pasteurization.

- Once milk is expressed from multiple donors and transported to the HMB, pooling of milk is done. This helps in maintaining uniform and consistent nutrient content of milk.
- Pre- and postpasteurization screening for contamination should be considered either from each sample or from each batch of pooled milk. Milk that contains high counts (>100,000 colony forming units/mL) of any bacteria is discarded.
- After pooling, milk is kept in individual small bottles (100–130 mL, depending on the pasteurizer used). Pasteurization is a method to heat the milk to a certain temperature, which inactivates bacteria, viruses, and other pathogenic organisms but retains milk protective components such as proteins, vitamins, and antibodies. The method of pasteurization is decided by individual HMBs based on financial and staffing resources (see Fig. 17.4).

Allocation of Donated Milk

Every HMB should have a written policy for recipient prioritization and allocation of the donor human milk.

- Babies who are born prematurely, have a low birth weight, are diagnosed with necrotizing enterocolitis, have a feeding intolerance, have malabsorption syndromes, and/or require any gastrointestinal surgery should be given milk on a priority basis.
- If donor human milk is sufficient in quantity, it can be dispensed to babies with maternal lactation failure or ill health or after maternal death or adoption.
- Milk should be defrosted in the refrigerator and thawed before disbursement to the recipient.

Documentation

Every donated-milk storage unit should have an established system of records maintenance and documentation. This includes tracking of temperatures right from donor expression to transportation,

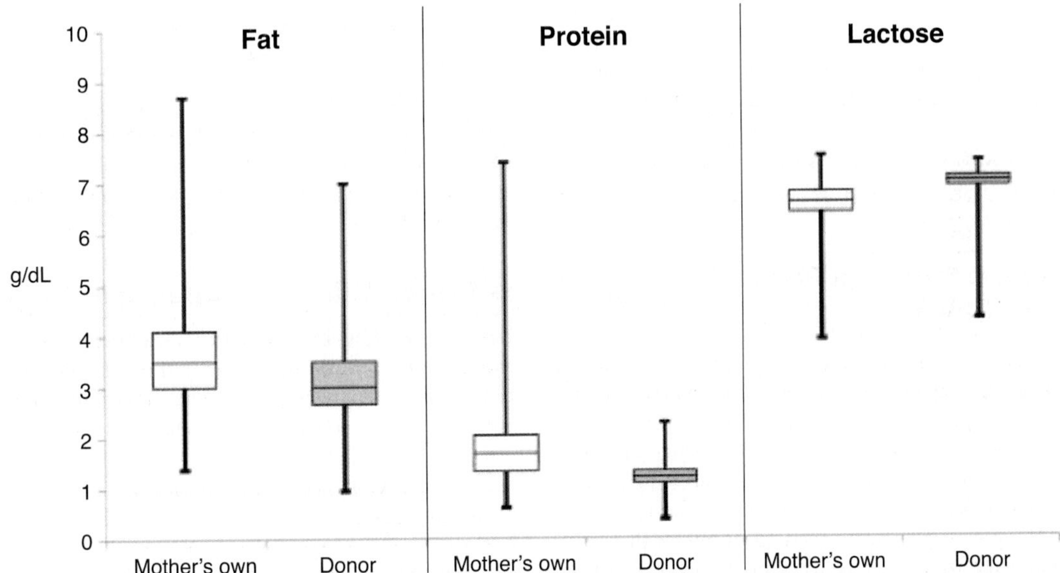

Fig. 17.7 Fat, Protein, and Lactose Content (Median, P25, P75, Minimum, and Maximum Values) Assessed by a Near Infrared Analyzer in Mothers' Own Milk (1350 Samples) and Donor Human Milk (860 Samples). (Adapted from: Reproduced after permission and minor modifications from Picaud J-C, Buffin R. Human milk—treatment and quality of banked human milk. *Clin Perinatol*. 2017;44:95–119.)

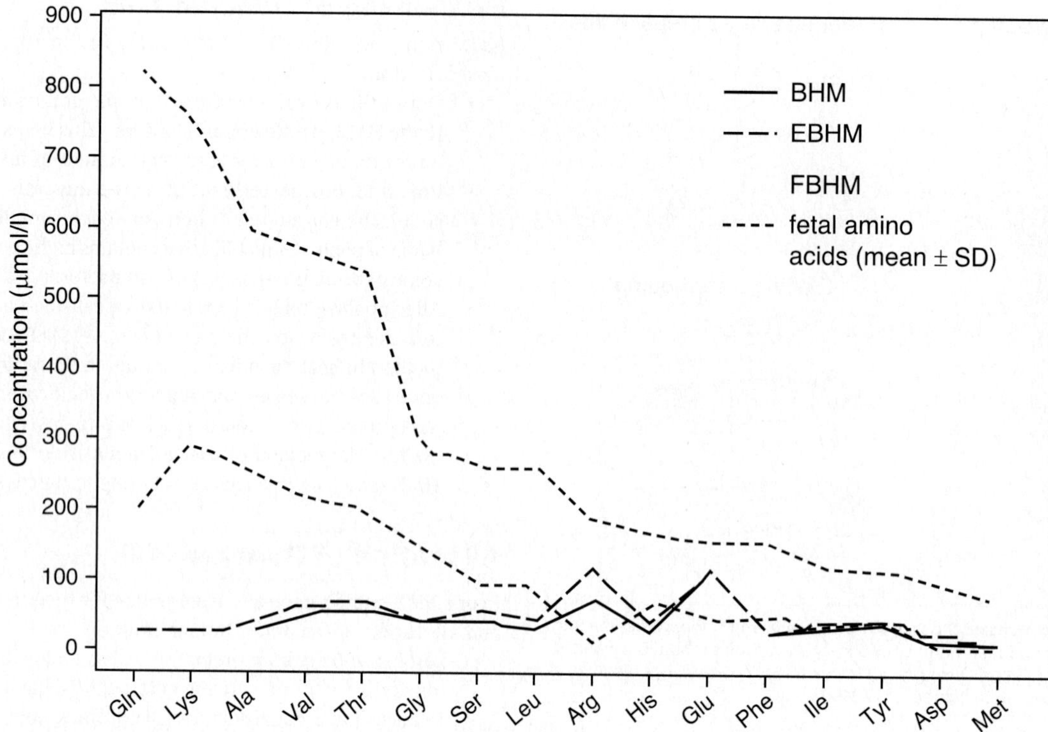

Fig. 17.8 Median Concentrations of Plasma Amino Acids in Preterm Infants Fed One of Three Milk Diets and Reference Values for Fetal Plasma Amino Acids. *BHM*, Banked human milk; *EBHM*, banked human milk evaporated to 70%; *FBHM*, banked human milk fortified with FM85. (Adapted from: Reproduced after permission and with minor modifications from dos Santos SC, et al. Plasma amino acids in preterm infants fed different human milk diets. *Clinical Nutrition ESPEN*. 2007;2.)

storage, and disbursement of milk. Date and time of expression, with donor identification and batch numbers of pooled milk, should be labeled. Prepasteurization and postpasteurization screening should be appropriately documented.

Staff Training

A breastfeeding support group comprising a pediatrician/neonatologist, lactation consultant, lactation nurse, infection control nurse, technical staff, and biomedical engineer should be formed and comprehensive training in various components of milk processing, infection control, equipment handling, and lactation counseling should be provided.

Myths and Doubts About Pasteurized Donor Human Milk[11]

Is Donor Human Milk at a Par With Mother's Own Milk?

Pasteurization of donor milk affects its antiinfective properties, cellular components, enzymes, growth factors, and some nutrients. Heat treatment also affects unsaturated fatty acids and pluripotent stem cells but retains some components such as oligosaccharides, which are heat resistant. High-temperature processing might lead to a decrease in antiinfective properties of milk but might not eradicate it. A meta-analysis by Chauhan et al.[12] comparing formula versus donor milk with regard to the incidence of necrotizing enterocolitis showed donor milk was significantly protective compared with formula. Narayan et al.,[13] in their prospective evaluation of antiinfective properties of donor human milk, showed a decreased protective effect of donor human milk compared with mother's own milk, but it was still significantly better than formula feeds (14.3% versus 10.5% versus 33% risk of infection). There is enough evidence in the literature to say that antiinfective properties and some other beneficial effects of donor human milk might not be at par with mother's own milk but it is the second best choice in the absence of mother's own milk. Also, once the donor milk is fortified appropriately, its nutrient component is equivalent to that of mother's own milk.

Is Donor Human Milk Safe for Preterm Neonates?

Because milk donated by multiple mothers is pooled and processed together, there is always a risk of transmission of many diseases that can spread through breast milk. The aggressive donor screening and screening of the milk pre- and postpasteurization essentially decreases the risk of transmission.

Is Donor Milk Cost-Effective?

Use of donor human milk not only decreases the incidence of necrotizing enterocolitis and sepsis in the preterm population but also reduces the hospital stay, and hence, it is considered to be the most cost-effective intervention while taking care of preterm babies.[14,15]

Summary

- Donor human milk is important for preterm, low birth weight, and sick neonates when mother's own milk is not available.
- Human milk storage units in hospitals and milk banks follow strict quality control procedures during donor recruitment, donor

screening, milk processing, and milk handling to ensure safety of donor milk.

- Adhering to the standard operating procedures of storage units in hospitals and milk banks, appropriate documentation and staff training are the key factors in sustenance of any human milk bank.
- There is a growing interest in storage units in hospitals and human milk banks worldwide, but human milk should be stored using strict safety guidelines.
- Human milk storage units in hospitals and milk banks play a pivotal role in catering pasteurized donor human milk to preterm infants, thereby decreasing their mortality and morbidity significantly. Donor human milk is highly recommended in the absence of mother's own milk.[16–18]
- Donor human milk is one the most important and cost-effective resources to improve infant health and survival.

CHAPTER 18 Possible Benefits and Risks of Using Probiotics in Neonates

Mohan Pammi, Monika S. Patil, Kristina Reber, Akhil Maheshwari

KEY POINTS

1. Probiotics are live microorganisms that, when consumed in adequate amounts by an adult host, are believed to and in many instances have been shown to confer health benefits.
2. The best-known probiotics belong to the genera *Bifidobacteria, Lactobacillus,* and *Saccharomyces.*
3. Extensive clinical evidence indicates that probiotics can reduce the risk of necrotizing enterocolitis (NEC) and late-onset sepsis in term and very low birth weight infants. Further work is needed to ensure safety in extremely low birth weight infants.
4. The baseline incidence of conditions such as NEC and other inflammatory conditions is an important consideration in deciding whether to initiate the administration of probiotics in a neonatal intensive care unit.
5. Several probiotics dampen inflammation by inhibiting TLR4 and TLR2 and by stimulating expression of antiinflammatory mediators. Several probiotics improve intestinal barrier function by strengthening the mucus layer and tight junctions between enterocytes. Many probiotics increase energy harvest by producing short-chain fatty acids, amino acids, vitamins, and secondary bile acids.
6. Many probiotics alter the intestinal microbiota by selectively competing for human milk oligosaccharides and by producing bacteriocins.

Probiotics are live microorganisms that, when consumed in adequate amounts, are believed to and in many instances have been shown to confer health benefits in adult hosts.[1] In older children, the gut microbiome is relatively stable and the addition of probiotics can potentiate intestinal homeostasis, nutrition, and mucosa immunity.[2] However, in neonates, particularly in the extremely low birth weight (ELBW) ones, early introduction of probiotics evokes debate. The proponents who advocate for the administration of probiotics emphasize that these agents could neutralize the dysbiosis associated with the acquisition of hospital-acquired gram-negative flora. Probiotics may not be natural, but neither are the nosocomial gram-negative bacilli. The opponents argue that the sequential appearance of gram-positive and gram-negative bacteria and anaerobes in the neonatal intestine at specific stages of development might have a natural rationale that we might not quite understand yet. They emphasize that the intention might be to promote health, but the safety of administering live bacteria in ELBW infants is not assured; recall that these bacteria may have caused sepsis-like illness in some infants.[3–6] The opponents question that the administration of live bacteria, even if apparently advantageous in mature adults and in many premature infants, could still be an underappreciated mistake in some that might not necessarily fix an earlier mistake that enabled the overgrowth of potentially harmful bacteria.

In neonatal intensive care units (NICUs), families now increasingly ask clinicians whether they should be adding probiotics to the feedings of their premature or critically ill infants, and if so, for help in choosing products. These questions create a dilemma, given that none of the currently available probiotic preparations are recognized as therapeutic agents. These are perceived as dietary supplements, and there is indeed some room for criticism of the scientific rigor and the "number needed to treat." Our neonatologists, pediatricians, and allied personnel long for guidance for these questions.

In this chapter, we have summarized the current information on the types of probiotics, available pharmaceutical preparations, effects, likely mechanism(s) of action, and evidence that favors and negates the impact of probiotics. Wherever possible, we provide evidence-based information to guide both clinicians and parents about the potentially protective effects of probiotics against necrotizing enterocolitis, sepsis, and other inflammatory conditions. In areas where sufficient evidence is available, we have tried to include information on the individual probiotic strains or combinations that may be effective and the clinical contexts that warrant further research. We have included a brief section on prebiotics and synbiotics, because those are perceived by many as potentially safer. The Grading of Recommendations Assessment, Development and Evaluation (GRADE) approach was used to assess the quality of evidence.[7]

Types of Probiotics

The International Scientific Association for Probiotics and Prebiotics defines probiotics as live microorganisms that confer a health benefit to the recipient when administered in adequate amounts. This definition does not include transplant of fecal microbiota or dead organisms. Many probiotic species are known and are commercially available (Table 18.1). Many probiotics have been accorded the GRAS (generally recognized as safe) status by the Food and Drug Administration (FDA) in the United States and have been safely used in food based either on a history of use before 1958 or on published scientific evidence, and they need not be approved by the FDA before being used.[8] Probiotics listed with GRAS status in the United States are listed in Table 18.1 (https://www.fda.gov/food/generally-recognized-safe-gras/microorganisms-microbial-derived-ingredients-used-food-partial-list).

The best studied probiotic species are *Bifidobacteria* and *Lactobacilli* (Fig. 18.1). A list of commercially available probiotic products can be easily found with a Google search using the search phrases "infant probiotics," "probiotics for infants," "commercially available infant probiotics," and "commercially available probiotics infant." The availability of specific products may differ by geographic region

Table 18.1 Probiotics[a] That Have Been Accorded GRAS Status in the United States
Bacillus coagulans GBI 30, 6086 (activated, inactivated, and spores)[b]
B. coagulans strain Unique IS2 spores preparation
B. coagulans SANK 70258 spore preparation
B. coagulans SBC37-01, spore preparation
B. coagulans SNZ1969 spore preparation
Bacteroides xylanisolvens strain DSM23964
Bifidobacterium animalis subsp. *lactis* strain Bf-6
Bifidobacterium breve M-16
Bifidobacterium lactis strain Bb12 and *Streptococcus thermophilus* strain Th4
Bifidobacterium longum BB536
B. animalis subsp. *lactis* strains Bf-6, HN019, Bi-07, B1-04, and B420
Carnobacterium maltaromaticum strain CB1 (viable and heat treated[a])
Lactobacillus acidophilus La-14
L. acidophilus, Lactobacillus lactis, and *Pediococcus acidilactici*
L. acidophilus NCFM
Lactobacillus casei subsp. *rhamnosus* strain GG
L. casei strain Shirota
Lactobacillus fermentum strain CECT5716
Lactobacillus plantarum strain 299v
Lactobacillus reuteri strain DSM 17938
L. reuteri strain NCIMB 30242
Lactobacillus rhamnosus strain HN001
L. rhamnosus strain HN001 produced in a milk-based medium
Propionibacterium freudenreichii ET-3, heat killed[a]
Saccharomyces cerevisiae strain ML01, carrying a gene encoding the malolactic enzyme from *Oenococcus oeni* and a gene encoding malate permease from *Schizosaccharomyces pombe*
S. cerevisiae strain P1Y0, a variant of *S. cerevisiae* parent strain UCD2034
Streptococcus salivarius K12

[a]The term "probiotic" is formally limited to live organisms.
[b]US Food and Drug Administration. GRAS notices. https://www.accessdata.fda.gov/scripts/fdcc/?set=GRASNotices.
GRAS, Generally recognized as safe.

and the variety used in trials and observational studies to date, and no product(s) can be specifically recommended yet (https://clinicaltrials.gov/ct2/show/NCT02472769; http://ibtherapeutics.com/the-phase-3-study-protocol-is-modified-after-ibts-meeting-with-the-fda/). Clinicians need to evaluate specific products for safety and efficacy.

Need for Standardization

A large number of probiotic preparations that are currently being marketed need more standardization. At least 30% of these formulations show discrepancies between the stated and actual number of viable organisms, the concentrations of the organisms, and/or the types of organisms compared with the product labeling. There is a need for a set of minimal manufacturing standards with clear guidelines for efficacy (Table 18.2).

In the United States, probiotics are classified as dietary supplements and are not subject to stringent regulatory processes, similar to therapeutic medicines.[10] The production of probiotics is required

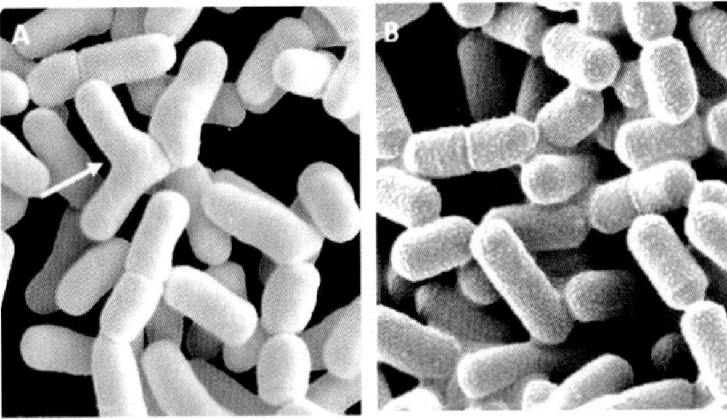

Fig. 18.1 Electron Microscopic Images. (A) *Bifidobacteria*. (B) *Lactobacilli*. Both are gram-positive, nonmotile, anaerobic or microaerophilic, non–spore forming bacteria. *Bifidobacteria* are so named because some show branching *(arrow)*. *Lactobacilli* have rough and smooth morphotypes[9]; this image shows a rough strain.

to comply with Good Manufacturing Practice guidelines but not with testing standards for quality or efficacy.[11] Similarly, in Europe, probiotics are regulated by the European Food Standards Agency at levels that are lower than those for medicines.[12] Lewis et al.[13] found that the contents of most bifidobacterial probiotic products differed from the ingredients list. Another observation is that most probiotic products contain a mixture of live bacteria with dead bacteria and their fragments. Hence the labeling information is not always accurate; dead bacteria and bacterial components can trigger immune responses. Many products may also contain contaminating pathogenic organisms, which is an important consideration in premature infants.[14] There has been one death from mucormycosis associated with a contaminated probiotic product,[15] and there have some reports of probiotic-associated sepsis.[3,5,6,16–18] There are some uncertainties as to which strain and dose is optimal in patients, owing to the heterogeneity in both clinical trials and implementation cohort studies.[19] Until high-quality pharmaceutical-grade probiotic preparations (single-dose packaging, stable strains, and cross-tested against contaminants) are available, consideration must be given to analyzing each new batch of probiotics to quantify probiotic organisms by polymerase chain reaction and microbiological techniques.

Van den Akker[20] identified 25 single-strain or combination products used in randomized clinical trials (RCTs) or studies that reported mortality, necrotizing enterocolitis (NEC), late-onset sepsis (LOS), or time to full enteral feeds. Three combination products reduced mortality, seven products (three single, four combination) reduced NEC, and two combination products reduced LOS. One combination product *(L. acidophilus, B. longum, B. bifidum, B. infantis)* used in two studies showed efficacy across all three outcomes. Earlier studies have compared single- and multiple-strain products, showing better results with multiple-strain products. It is not clear whether the effects are specific to strains, subspecies, species, or the genera.[21–23] Some observational studies and national databases with varying products still

Table 18.2 Concerns About Currently Marketed Probiotic Formulations
Inadequate labeling about taxonomic classification of microbial names
Inadequate information about numbers of viable probiotic organisms
Inadequate information on shelf life of products
Inadequate guidelines for storage conditions needed to maintain probiotic viability
Inadequate information on labeling about dosing or toxicity

show benefit,[23,24] suggesting that at least some of the clinical benefits are not likely to be strain specific.[25,26]

Although the current definition of probiotics emphasizes that the bacteria are alive when administered to the host, nonviable organisms may also elicit beneficial immune responses. The term "paraprobiotic" or "ghost probiotic" is used for intact but nonviable cells or cell extracts. *Bifidobacterium breve* M-16 V, currently available and used by some units, has demonstrated suppression of proinflammatory responses from a heat-killed form in a mouse model. A systematic review in 2017 identified 19 pediatric trials of "modified" probiotics, none targeted at NEC or LOS and only one in neonates (targeting atopic dermatitis), but showed no improvement in the safety profile compared with live probiotics. However, given the anxiety caused by the administration of live bacteria in preterm infants, this line of study merits further exploration.

Clinical Effects of Probiotics in Newborn Infants

Probiotic microbes have been historically identified as food stabilizers.[27] The microbial genera were associated with good health and have included *Lactobacillus, Bifidobacterium, Escherichia, Lactococcus, Streptococcus,* and *Saccharomyces.* These have shown resistance to gastric acid, bile acids, and intestinal enzymes.[28] In neonates, the earliest studies examined probiotics for prevention of NEC.[29] In one of these, all infants admitted to a NICU in Bogota, Colombia, were provided feedings supplemented with *Lactobacillus acidophilus* and *Bifidobacterium infantis* until discharge. Compared with historical controls, the incidence of NEC dropped from 6.6% to 3%. Since then, a large number of systematic reviews and randomized controlled studies have been completed to examine the impact of probiotics in neonates.

There are three possibilities regarding the future use of probiotics. Small clinical trials are currently being conducted, and there are believers and nonbelievers about potential benefit of these bacteria as a nutritional supplement. In one possibility, parents would be asked to make a choice, and the infants would be treated if the families agreed. In another possibility, probiotics would begin to be prepared with strict guidelines as a drug and be universally adopted as the standard of care. In the third, the products would still be prepared under strict oversight, and infants at high risk of conditions such as NEC or LOS would be treated. In this third possibility, infants in specific gestational age or birth weight ranges or those with high-risk conditions that are likely to benefit would continue to be identified and treated.

The outcomes of infants treated with probiotics may be reported with clinical end points such as all-cause mortality, chronic lung disease, NEC, LOS, retinopathy of prematurity, time to reach full feeds, and length of hospital stay. There may be some difficulty in separating these conditions, because infants with NEC may need respiratory support for longer periods and may be labeled as having chronic lung disease; may need central lines for parenteral nutrition, and consequently, may develop LOS; may need respiratory support with oxygen therapy that may increase the risk of retinopathy of prematurity; and with the higher severity of multisystem illness, may need a longer length of hospital stay and have a higher risk of mortality.

There is a need to evaluate composite outcomes such as all-cause mortality even in infants who develop NEC, because they are at risk of sepsis owing to the need for vascular catheters and also because of gastrointestinal injury and altered gut anatomy in the postoperative period. Many infants with secondary bacterial sepsis who remain culture-negative may be differentially labeled at various centers, and hence, this subgroup needs to be identified and evaluated. Table 18.3 shows a summary of the impact of probiotics in various clinical conditions.

Effect of Probiotics on Composite Outcomes Including NEC, LOS, and All-Cause Mortality

In Table 18.3, we show a summary of the studies by Deshmukh and Patole,[30] Chi et al.,[31] Morgan et al.,[32] Balasubramanian et al.,[33] Bi et al.,[34] Zhu et al.,[35] Deshpande et al.,[36] Dermyshi et al.,[37] Chang et al.,[38] and Olsen et al.[39] A large implementation cohort study in Germany used Infloran, a probiotic preparation of *L. acidophilus* and *Bifidobacterium bifidum*, and included more than 5000 infants.[40] Another cohort study of 3093 infants <29 weeks' gestation in Canada showed prophylactic probiotic supplementation to lower the risk of NEC (odds ratio [OR], 0.64; 95% confidence interval [CI], 0.41–0.99) and death (adjusted OR, 0.41; 95% CI, 0.26–0.63).[41] An earlier single-center cohort study in the United States and Canada had shown these formulations to be efficacious.[42] Other implementation cohort studies from France, Australia, and Switzerland have also reported decreased NEC after routine use of probiotics.[19] Additionally, the pooled treatment effects of probiotics on NEC, death, and LOS in observational studies are similar to those in clinical trials. These findings support the external validity of the pooled estimates of probiotic treatment effects from randomized trials and increase confidence in the findings from meta-analyses of randomized trials.[43]

Effect of Probiotics on the Risk of NEC

Data from the studies by Sharif et al.,[44] Liu et al.,[45] Jiao et al.,[46] Hagen et al.,[47] and Lau et al.[48] are summarized in Table 18.4. The table also shows the findings from the Probiotics in Preterm Infants (PiPS) trial,[49] which did not find a difference in the risk of NEC between the probiotic and the placebo group.

Most trials of probiotic supplementation have enrolled very low birth weight (VLBW) infants, but ELBW infants are underrepresented in many studies. A large German cohort study demonstrated beneficial effects of probiotics in ELBW infants. However, the subgroup analyses of the ProPrems trial did not find any significant differences in effects of probiotics on NEC between ELBW and other premature infants.[19] The use of probiotics in more mature populations to prevent NEC may substantially increase the number needed to treat (NNT) to prevent NEC, because the baseline incidence would be lower in this population.

The 2020 Cochrane Database of Systematic Reviews evaluated 56 trials with 10,812 infants.[44] Most trials were small (median sample size, 149), and there were concerns about the possibility of bias in about half of the trials. Trials varied by the formulation of the probiotics; most preparations contained *Bifidobacteria, Lactobacilli, Saccharomyces* species (spp.), and *Streptococcus* spp. alone or in combinations. Meta-analysis showed that probiotics may reduce the risk of NEC: relative risk [RR], 0.54; 95% CI, 0.45–0.65 (54 trials; 10,604 infants; $I^2 = 17\%$); risk difference [RD], −0.03; 95% CI, −0.04 to −0.02; NNT for an additional beneficial outcome (NNTB), 33; 95% CI, 25–50. Evidence was assessed as low certainty because of the limitations in trials design and the presence of funnel

Table 18.3 Effect of Probiotics on NEC, LOS, and All-Cause Mortality

Authors	Design	Outcomes	Studies, No.	Patients, No.	Outcome (Range)	Other Conclusions
Deshmukh and Patole	Systematic review of non-RCTs; routine probiotic supplementation (RPS)	NEC ≥stage II, LOS, all-cause mortality, and feeding intolerance	30	77,018	Less NEC (30 studies, n = 77,018; OR, 0.60; 95% CI, 0.50–0.73); less LOS (21 studies, n = 65,858; OR, 0.85; 95% CI, 0.74–0.97); less all-cause mortality (27 studies, n = 70,977; OR, 0.77; 95% CI, 0.68–0.88). In ELBW infants, RPS reduced NEC (4.5% versus 7.9%), but not LOS and mortality. Multistrain RPS was more effective than single-strain. One study reported nonfatal probiotic sepsis in three infants.	Moderate- to low-quality evidence indicating that RPS was associated with significantly reduced NEC ≥stage II, LOS, and all-cause mortality in neonates <37 weeks of gestation and NEC ≥stage II in ELBW neonates.
Chi et al.	Network meta-analysis	NEC, mortality	45	12,320		*Bifidobacterium* plus prebiotic had the highest probability of decreasing the mortality (surface under the cumulative ranking curve, 83.94%), and *Lactobacillus* plus prebiotic had the highest probability of having the lowest rate of NEC (surface under the cumulative ranking curve, 95.62%).
	Bifidobacterium plus *Lactobacillus*				NEC 0.47 (0.27–0.79); mortality 0.56 (0.34–0.84)	
	Lactobacillus plus prebiotic				NEC 0.06 (0.01–0.41)	
Morgan et al.	Network meta-analysis of RCTs	NEC, mortality	63	15,712		
	1 or more *Lactobacillus* spp. and 1 or more *Bifidobacterium* spp.				Combination of ≥1 *Lactobacillus* spp. and ≥1 *Bifidobacterium* spp. showed moderate- to high-quality evidence of reduced all-cause mortality (OR, 0.56; 95% CI, 0.39–0.80). *Bifidobacterium animalis* subsp. *lactis*, *Lactobacillus reuteri*, or *Lactobacillus rhamnosus* reduced severe NEC (OR 0.35 [95% CI, 0.20–0.59]; OR 0.31 [95% CI, 0.13–0.74]; OR, 0.55 [95% CI, 0.34–0.91]; and OR, 0.44 [95% CI, 0.21–0.90], respectively).	Moderate to high evidence for the superiority of combinations of 1 or more *Lactobacillus* spp. and 1 or more *Bifidobacterium* spp. versus single- and other multiple-strain probiotic treatments. The combinations of *Bacillus* spp. and *Enterococcus* spp. and 1 or more *Bifidobacterium* spp. and *Streptococcus salivarius* subsp. *thermophilus* might produce the largest reduction in the occurrence of NEC.
Balasubramanian et al.[33]	Systematic review of RCTs	Mortality, NEC, LOS	9	1514	Reduced risk of NEC ≥stage II (RR, 0.36; 95% CI 0.2–0.66), LOS in 7 studies (RR, 0.56; 95% CI, 0.45–0.71), and mortality in 8 RCTs (RR, 0.62; 95% CI, 0.41–0.95)	
Bi et al.[34]	Network meta-analysis	Prevention strategies	34	9161	Significant advantage of probiotic mixture and *Bifidobacterium* to prevent the incidence of NEC in preterm infants; a probiotic mixture showed effectiveness in reducing mortality in preterm infants.	The results showed that *Bifidobacteria* and a mixture of probiotics were effective; the other probiotic genera (*Saccharomyces, Bacillus, Lactobacilli*) failed to show an obvious effect to reduce the incidence of NEC, sepsis, and all-cause death.
Zhu et al.[35]	Meta-analysis of RCT	Mortality, NEC, sepsis	24	6155		
	Bifidobacterium groups				NEC (RR, 0.38; 95% CI, 0.25–0.58), mortality (RR, 0.74; 95% CI, 0.60–0.92)	No significant difference in the incidence of sepsis.

Continued

Table 18.3 Effect of Probiotics on NEC, LOS, and All-Cause Mortality—cont'd

Authors	Design	Outcomes	Studies, No.	Patients, No.	Outcome (Range)	Other Conclusions
Deshpande et al.	Meta-analysis of RCTs from 10 low- and middle-income countries	Mortality, NEC, LOS	23	4783	NEC ≥ stage II (RR, 0.46; 95% CI, 0.34–0.61), LOS (RR, 0.80; 95% CI, 0.71–0.91), and all-cause mortality (RR, 0.73; 95% CI, 0.59–0.90)	
Dermyshi et al.	Meta-analysis of 30 RCTs and 14 observational studies	Mortality, NEC, sepsis	44		Mortality: RCTs, RR, 0.77 (95% CI, 0.65–0.92), observational studies, RR, 0.71 (95% CI, 0.62–0.81); NEC: RCTs, RR, 0.57 (95% CI, 0.47–0.70), observational studies, RR, 0.51 (95% CI, 0.37–0.70)	A 12% reduction in the risk of sepsis in RCTs and a 19% reduction in observational studies.
Chang et al.	Fixed effects analysis	NEC, mortality	25	7345		
	Multiple strains				NEC: OR, 0.36 (95% CI, 0.24–0.53); mortality: OR, 0.58 (95% CI, 0.43–0.79)	
	Single strains				NEC: OR, 0.6; 95% CI, 0.36–1.0	No reduction in mortality with single strains
Olsen et al.	Meta-analysis	NEC, mortality, sepsis	12	10,800	NEC: RR, 0.55 (95% CI, 0.39–0.78); mortality: RR, 0.72 (95% CI, 0.61–0.85)	No significant reduction in sepsis
Samuels et al.	Cohort study using Infloran	NEC	1	5000	Surgical NEC: RR, 0.58; 95% CI, 0.37–0.91	
Singh et al.	Cohort study	NEC, mortality	1	3093	NEC: OR, 0.64 (95% CI, 0.41–0.99); mortality: OR, 0.41 (95% CI, 0.26–0.63)	

CI, Confidence interval; *ELBW*, extremely low birth weight; *LOS*, late-onset sepsis; *NEC*, necrotizing enterocolitis; *OR*, odds ratio; *RCT*, randomized clinical trial; *RR*, risk ratio; *spp.*, species; *subsp.*, subspecies.

Table 18.4 Effect of Probiotics on Risk of NEC

Authors	Design	Outcomes	Studies, No.	Patients, No.	Outcome (Range)	Other Conclusions
Sharif et al.	Meta-analysis	NEC, mortality, late onset infection	56	10,812	Total: NEC RR, 0.54; 95% CI, 0.45–0.65 (54 trials; 10,604 infants; I^2 = 17%) Trials with low risk of bias: NEC RR, 0.70; 95% CI, 0.55–0.89 (16 trials, 4597 infants; I^2 = 25%) Reduction in mortality (RR, 0.76; 95% CI, 0.65–0.89 (51 trials; 10,170 infants; I^2 = 0%) and late-onset infection (RR, 0.89; 95% CI, 0.82–0.97 (47 trials, 9762 infants; I^2 = 19%)	Probiotics may have little or no effect on severe neurodevelopmental impairment
Liu et al.	Meta-analysis	NEC, mortality, sepsis	23	4686	NEC RR, 0.34; 95% CI, 0.25–0.46 Mortality RR, 0.48; 95% CI, 0.36–0.64	No significant difference in the incidence of sepsis
Jiao et al.	Meta-analysis	NEC	16	4686		
	Mixture of *Bifidobacterium* and *Lactobacillus*				NEC RR, 0.34; 95% CI, 0.25–0.46	Single strain *Lactobacillus* or single strain *Bifidobacterium* did not show reduction in NEC
Hagen et al.	Meta-analysis	NEC	9			Some benefit in infants <34 weeks' GA with RR of 0.43 (95% CI, 0.21–0.87; P = .019) but not in neonates <28 weeks' GA
	Bifidobacterium lactis				NEC RR, 0.11; 95% CI, 0.03–0.47	
Lau et al.	Meta-analysis	NEC, mortality, sepsis	20	5982	NEC RR, 0.509; 95% CI 0.385–0.672 Mortality RR, 0.731; 95% CI, 0.577–0.926 Sepsis RR, 0.919; 95% CI 0.823–1.027	
Probiotics in Preterm Infants (PiPS) trial	RCT	NEC		1315		
	Bifidobacterium breve BBG-001 or placebo				No benefit in NEC, no harm	20% of infants in the placebo group were also colonized with the probiotic organism by 2 weeks of age and 49% by 36 weeks postmenstrual age, suggesting notable cross-contamination

CI, Confidence interval; *GA*, gestational age; *NEC*, necrotizing enterocolitis; *RCT*, randomized clinical trial; *RR*, relative risk.

plot asymmetry consistent with publication bias. Sensitivity meta-analysis of trials at low risk of bias showed a reduced risk of NEC: RR, 0.70; 95% CI, 0.55–0.89 (16 trials, 4597 infants; I^2 = 25%)); RD, −0.02; 95% CI; −0.03 to −0.01; NNTB, 50; 95% CI, 33–100. Meta-analyses showed that probiotics probably reduce mortality (RR, 0.76; 95% CI, 0.65–0.89 [51 trials, 10,170 infants; I^2 = 0%]; RD, −0.02; 95% CI, −0.02 to −0.01; NNTB, 50; 95% CI, 50–100), and late-onset invasive infection (RR, 0.89; 95% CI, 0.82–0.97; [47 trials, 9762 infants; I^2 = 19%]; RD, −0.02; 95% CI, −0.03 to −0.01; NNTB, 50; 95% CI 33–100). Sensitivity meta-analyses of 16 trials (4597 infants) at low risk of bias did not show an effect on mortality or infection. Meta-analysis showed that probiotics may have little or no effect on severe neurodevelopmental impairment (RR, 1.03; 95% CI, 0.84–1.26 (five trials, 1518 infants; I^2 = 0%). The certainty of this evidence is low because of design limitations.

Effect of Probiotics on the Risk of Late-Onset Sepsis and Other Conditions (Table 18.5)

Rao et al.[50] examined pooled results from 37 RCTs (N = 9416) of probiotics versus placebo/no probiotics using a fixed effects model. In meta-analysis, probiotics decreased the risk of LOS.

Qamer et al.[51] performed a systematic review of efficacy and safety of probiotics in the management of cow's milk protein allergy (CMPA). Primary outcomes were resolution of hematochezia and acquisition of tolerance to CMP, and the secondary outcomes included effects on allergic symptoms, growth, gut microbiota, and adverse effects. Ten RCTs (N = 845) were analyzed, but no significant benefits were seen. However, in confirmed CMPA, limited low-quality evidence showed that probiotics expedited the acquisition of tolerance to CMP at the end of 3 years.

Colic is defined as periods of inconsolable crying, fussing, or irritability that have no apparent cause and present in otherwise healthy infants. Simonson et al.[52] performed a systematic review and showed that oral administration of probiotics to breastfed infants with colic resulted in at least a 50% reduction in crying time compared with placebo. Ong et al.,[53] Sung et al.,[54] and Harb et al.[55] also showed benefit.

Probiotics seem to be efficacious in reducing the severity of neonatal hyperbilirubinemia. Deshmukh et al.[56] analyzed 9 RCTs (prophylactic: 6 trials, N = 1761; therapeutic: 3 trials, N = 279). Total serum bilirubin (TSB) was significantly reduced at 96 hours. Chen et al.[57] examined 13 RCTs involving 1067 neonates with jaundice in a meta-analysis and also noted efficacy.

In other gastrointestinal surgical conditions, probiotics may not be so effective. Rao et al.[58] examined two RCTs; the first was conducted in 24 neonates with gastroschisis, the second in 8 with various surgical conditions. Based on these data, the role of probiotics in neonates with gastrointestinal surgical conditions is still unclear and needs further study.

Effect of Probiotics on Fungal Infections

Hu et al.[59] examined 7 trials involving 1371 preterm neonates. Meta-analysis (fixed-effects model) showed that probiotic supplementation was associated with a lower risk of *Candida* colonization and invasive fungal sepsis. However, after excluding one study with a high baseline incidence of fungal sepsis, the effect of probiotics on invasive fungal sepsis became statistically insignificant. When using a random-effects model, the effect of probiotics remained favorable for *Candida* colonization but not for fungal sepsis.

Clinical Decision to Start Routine Probiotic Supplementation

The decision to start using probiotics in a NICU is a complex one (Table 18.6).[19] The proportion of infants receiving their mother's own or a banked human milk is important,[60] and therefore, promotion of human milk feeding should be the major focus of efforts to decrease NEC. Additionally, human milk contains oligosaccharides that can promote the growth of probiotic bacteria such as *B. infantis.*[61] Prebiotics can be useful in some instances, but further research is needed to determine the efficacy of prebiotics compared with live bacteria.[62] Some randomized trials have combined the use of prebiotics with probiotics,[63] but this strategy might still not adequately compensate for all the beneficial components of breast milk that may protect against NEC, including lowering gastric pH, enhancing intestinal motility, and decreasing epithelial permeability.[1,63]

At each center, the baseline incidence of NEC is an important consideration for making decisions about the routine use of probiotics. This incidence will provide an idea about the estimated NNT to prevent one case of NEC. The center will also need to consider the case-fatality and morbidity rates. As the baseline risks decrease, the NNT to prevent one case of NEC increases (Table 18.7).[19] This table is based on the incidence of NEC reported in the literature and estimates of treatment effect on NEC from Sawh et al.[64]

There are also several practical issues to consider. A team-based approach is important, including nursing leadership, pharmacy, infectious disease, and microbiology. Each stream of experts contributes to the program with expertise and infrastructure.[19] Some authors have suggested that local evaluation of bacterial species of probiotics is an important quality-control measure,[65] although such an approach for single-dose preparations may not always be feasible. The rationale for and approach to implementation should be documented.

Dosing and Duration

Most large trials have used 10^8 to 10^9 probiotic bacteria per dose because stool bacterial counts seem to plateau beyond these counts. Further work is needed to optimize these doses because the numbers of bacteria in stool may be more an indicator of transit than of ecological establishment. Existing studies have focused either on the prevention or on the correction of already established dysbiosis with *Enterobacteriaceae.* The time to initiate administration of probiotics is harder to decide until further data are available; determining the time to stop supplementation may be simpler when the risk of maturity-related complications related to dysbiosis, such as NEC, becomes lower.

Mechanisms of Probiotic Effects

Development of Microflora During the Neonatal Period

Vaginally delivered infants become colonized with microorganisms such as *Enterobacteriaceae, Bacteroides,* and *Parabacteroides* in the mother's vaginal tract, whereas those delivered by cesarean section become

Table 18.5 Effect of Probiotics on Other Risks

Authors	Design	Outcomes	Studies, No.	Patients, No.	Outcome (Range)	Other Conclusions
Rao et al.	Meta-analysis with fixed effects model	Late-onset sepsis	37	9416	RR, 0.86 (95% CI, 0.78–0.94)	
Qamer et al.	Systematic review	Cow's milk protein allergy	10	845	Probiotics expedited the acquisition of tolerance to cow's milk protein at the end of 3 years compared with placebo (RR, 1.47; 95% CI, 1.17–1.84)	Not associated with earlier resolution of hematochezia; no adverse events reported
Ong et al.	Systematic review	Infantile colic—minutes of crying	6	1886		
	Lactobacillus reuteri				Reduction of 44.3 minutes in daily crying with a random-effects model (95% CI, −66.6 to −21.9; $I^2 = 92\%$), favoring probiotics	No clear evidence that probiotics are more effective than placebo at preventing infantile colic
Sung et al.	Meta-analysis	Infantile colic—minutes of crying	4	345		
	L. reuteri DSM17938				Day 21 crying reduction of 25.4 (95% CI, −47.3 to −3.5) minutes	Intervention effects were dramatic in breastfed infants (number needed to treat for day 21 success, 2.6 [95% CI, 2.0–3.6]) but were insignificant in formula-fed infants
Harb et al.	Subgroup meta-analysis	Infantile colic—minutes of crying	6		Day 21: −55.8 (95% CI, −64.4 to −47.3) min/day of crying	
Deshmukh et al.	Meta-analysis	Hyperbilirubinemia—duration of phototherapy	9	279	Mean difference, −11.80 (95% CI, −17.47 to −6.13) TSB reduced at 96 h: mean difference, −1.74 (95% CI, −2.92 to −0.57) TSB reduced at 7 days: mean difference, −1.71 (95% CI, −2.25 to −1.17)	There were no probiotic-related adverse effects; limited low-quality evidence indicates that probiotic supplementation may reduce the duration of phototherapy in neonates with jaundice
Chen et al.	Meta-analysis of RCTs	Serum bilirubin, duration of phototherapy, need for hospitalization	12	1067	3 days: mean difference, −18.05 (95% CI, −25.51 to −10.58) 5 days: mean difference, -23.49 (95% CI, −32.80 to −14.18) 7 days: mean difference, −33.01 (95% CI, −37.31 to −28.70) Duration of phototherapy: mean difference, −0.64 (95% CI, −0.84 to −0.44) Hospitalization: mean difference, −2.68 (95% CI, −3.18 to −2.17)	
Rao et al.	Meta-analysis	Difference in microbiomes in gastroschisis patients	2	24	In one study, overall microbial communities were not significantly different between groups; in another study there were significantly more *Streptcoccaceae* in the fecal samples in the probiotic group and significantly more *Bifidobacteriaceae* in the no-probiotic group	The role of probiotics in neonates with gastrointestinal surgical conditions is still unclear and needs further study
Hu et al.	Meta-analysis	Candida colonization, invasive fungal sepsis	7	1371	Candida colonization: RR, 0.43 (95% CI, 0.27–0.67) Invasive fungal sepsis: RR, 0.64 (95% CI, 0.46–0.88)	

CI, Confidence interval; I^2, I-squared statistic (indicates treatment-effect heterogeneity across patient subgroups and populations); *RR*, relative risk; *TSB*, total serum bilirubin.

Table 18.6 Factors Important in Making Decisions About the Routine Use of Probiotics[19]

Support Starting Routine Probiotic Supplementation	Do Not Support Starting Routine Probiotic Supplementation
Preclinical and human data support biologic plausibility	No regulator-approved drug formulation (in US or UK)
Numerous RCTs enrolling >10,000 infants show consistent benefit (low heterogeneity) in decreasing the risk of NEC	Concerns regarding product quality and contamination
Large magnitude of effect on NEC in meta-analysis (decreases RR by approximately one-half); lower risk of late-onset sepsis and all-cause mortality	Well-conducted, multicenter trial (PiPS) showed no benefit on NEC (of note, relatively high rate of cross-colonization with probiotic strain in control arm)
Multiple implementation cohort studies support effectiveness of probiotic supplementation in routine practice	Uncertainty regarding optimal product/strain, including dose and duration of supplementation
Meta-analysis for subgroup of infants with birth weight <1000 g infants show no increased risks of sepsis	Limited long-term follow-up data (Two studies showed no evidence of harm; one showed a lower risk of deafness)
Low relative cost of supplementation	High NNT for centers with low NEC incidence
NEC remains a major cause of death in preterm infants.	Other opportunities (such as increasing human milk feeding) to decrease the risk of NEC

NEC, Necrotizing enterocolitis; *NNT*, number needed to treat; *RCT*, randomized clinical trial; *RR*, relative risk.

colonized with organisms such as *Staphylococci* and *Streptococci* from maternal skin and the oral cavity. However, exclusive breastfeeding in the first week can quickly introduce high levels of *Bifidobacteria* and *Lactobacillus.*[66] This pattern may not always remain intact in premature infants, who are more frequently delivered by cesarean section and get colonized with skin-related organisms.

Social structure and family interactions also play a role in the early-life microbiome. Breastfeeding may link the microbiome between mothers and infants, including transmission of probiotic-like organisms such as *Lactobacilli* and *Bifidobacteria*, and may protect against many infectious diseases and at least early onset of atopy. Family contacts can also increase the risk for acquisition of bacteria such as methicillin-resistant *Staphylococcus aureus*. There may be differences in the oral microbiota among infants for whom the parents did versus did not use pacifiers. In rural settings, microbiome sharing may extend to livestock, household surfaces, and household members.

Effects on Intestinal Inflammation

Toll-Like Receptor 4

Toll-like receptor (TLR) 4 is a membrane-spanning protein that binds lipopolysaccharide and activates immune responses. Low-level TLR4 stimulation may promote immune homeostasis and gut maturation *in utero*, but high-level stimulation with dysbiosis may trigger inflammation and NEC.[67–84] Neonatal enterocytes and leukocytes express higher levels of TLR4, MyD88, and NFκB than in adults.[75] Probiotic-conditioned media from *B. infantis* (ATCC 15697) and *L. acidophilus* (ATCC 53103) suppress inflammatory responses in tissue explants and rodent models.[85] *Lactobacillus reuteri* (DSM 17938 and ATCC PTA 4659) showed similar results.[86] In porcine peripheral blood monocytes, *L. acidophilus* suppressed lipopolysaccharide-induced inflammatory responses.[87] *Lactobacilli* and *Propiniobacteria* produce a surface-layer protein B (SlpB) that inhibits cytokine expression.[88]

Table 18.7 Estimates of Infant NNT to Prevent One Outcome of NEC

Baseline NEC Incidence, %	Absolute Risk Reduction, %	NNT (95% CI)
1.0	0.5	213 (172–294)
2.0	0.9	106 (86–147)
3.0	1.4	71 (57–98)
4.0	1.9	53 (43–74)
5.0	2.4	43 (34–59)
7.5	3.5	28 (23–39)
10.0	4.7	21 (17–29)
12.5	5.9	17 (14–24)
15.0	7.1	14 (11–20)
20.0	9.4	11 (9–15)

CI, Confidence interval; *NEC*, necrotizing enterocolitis; *NNT*, number needed to treat.

Toll-Like Receptor 2

Toll-like receptor 2 binds lipoteichoic acid on gram-positive bacteria.[89] Its expression is suppressed by conditioned media from *B. infantis* and *L. acidophilus.*[85] Both *Lactobacilli* and *Bifidobacteria* are gram-positive organisms and can stimulate TLR2.[90] In monocytes, *Lactobacillus paracasei* inhibited cytokine production.[91] Some *Lactobacillus* strains may activate macrophage expression of TLR2 and cytokine expression but eventually lead to increased phagocytosis and antibacterial activity.[92] *B. breve* MV-17 decreased the severity of rodent NEC.[42] A combination of probiotic microbes increased expression of TLR2 but not TLR3, TLR4, or TLR9, but the same combination attenuated the effect of other agonists.[93]

NLRP3 Inflammasomes

The nucleotide-binding oligomerization domain leucine-rich repeat-containing and pyrin domain-containing (NLRP)3 inflammasome is a cytosolic signaling receptor that activates several cytokines, leukotrienes, and prostaglandins.[94] The probiotic *Escherichia coli* Nissle 1917 suppresses inflammasome assembly.

Antiinflammatory Mediators

Probiotics can upregulate antiinflammatory cytokines and other mediators. Several *Bifidobacterium* and *Lactobacillus* strains increase IL-10 and TGF-β in several colitis models. Pili-like proteins in the outer membrane of *Akkermansia muciniphila* ATCC BAA-835 stimulate host production of IL-10 through both TLR2 and TLR4. In a rat model, *Bifidobacterium adolescentis* attenuated NEC, decreased expression of TLR4, and increased expression of toll interacting protein (TOLLIP) and single Ig IL-1-related receptor (SIGIRR), which block TLR4.

Adaptive Immunity

Probiotic *E. coli* and *Lactobacillus johnsonii* can restore T- and B-cells in the *lamina propria* that has been depleted by prolonged treatment with broad-spectrum antibiotics. These bacteria also increase the number of regulator T cells (T-regs) and activated dendritic cells. In mice, *B. breve* induced IL-10-producing T-regs, but *Lactobacillus casei* did not. *L. reuteri* DSM 17938 can reduce T-effector/memory activity and increase T-regs, which can reduce the severity of NEC-like intestinal injury. *Lactobacilli* and *Bifidobacteria* promote the maturation of the neonatal immune system and tone down its inflammatory responses by converting the prenatal T-helper 2 (Th2)-biased responses to more balanced patterns. *Lactobacilli* can prime monocyte-derived dendritic cells to drive the development of T-regs. These T-regs produce IL-10 to inhibit the proliferation of bystander T-cells. In addition, one study showed fewer Th2 cells in infants whose mothers had received perinatal probiotic supplementation.

Intestinal Permeability

Probiotic microbes strengthen epithelial junctions in immaturity and NEC. These bacteria also alter the mucus layer; there is an inner mucus layer that is normally composed of tightly linked mucins and an outer, more loosely linked layer that contains antimicrobial peptides and IgA. Commensal organisms such as *A. muciniphila* thrive in the outer mucus layer and use the host mucins as a food source. These increase mucin turnover but eventually thicken the mucus layer and improve the intestinal barrier. Other important probiotic microbes are *Bifidobacterium longum* GT15, *Escherichia faecalis* L3, and *Lactobacillus farciminis* CIP 103136. The mucus carbohydrate concentrations, which are likely altered by diet, change the adherence of bacteria such as *L. acidophilus* NCFM to mucus. *Lactobacillus rhamnosus* ATCC 53103 and *Lactobacillus plantarum* ATCC 10241 can also strengthen tight junction integrity.

Paneth Cells

Paneth cells are specialized epithelial cells in intestinal crypts that shape the intestinal microbiota and protect the neighboring intestinal stem cells by secreting a variety of antimicrobial peptides such as the defensins, lysozymes, C-type lectins, and cathelicidins. *B. bifidum* or *B. infantis* can attenuate NEC-like injury and suppress antimicrobial peptide expression.

Autophagy

Autophagy is a catabolic process of regulated destruction and recycling of lysosomal components. It plays an important role in the normal enterocyte life cycle but gets dysregulated in NEC upon exposure to invading pathogens. *L. reuteri* ZJ617, *L. rhamnosus* GG, *B. bifidum* ATCC29521, and some *E. coli* strains can reduce these changes.

Energy Regulation

Intestinal microbiota alter energy regulation in germ-free, obese, and malnutrition rodent models. Germ-free mice fed a high fat, high sugar diet do not become obese or develop fatty liver or insulin sensitivity, but lean mice gain weight and develop fatty liver even on a normal diet after fecal transplantation from obese mice. Some probiotics can prevent or treat obesity or malnutrition. Gut microbes can alter energy metabolism by processing of nondigestible fibers, production of short-chain fatty acids (SCFAs), and altered lipid metabolism.

Human Milk Oligosaccharides

Human intestinal cells lack the glycosidases to digest human milk oligosaccharides (HMOs). However, probiotic bacteria such as *Bifidobacteria* can digest these oligosaccharides. The addition of HMOs can also improve fat absorption and weight gain. *B. infantis* can degrade the full range of HMOs; four species are particularly important: *B. longum* subspecies *infantis*, *B. longum* subspecies *longum*, *B. bifidum*, and *B. breve*. Some probiotic microbes can also promote the digestion of plant fibers, potentially releasing monosaccharides and disaccharides that could serve as an energy source for the mother.

Short-Chain Fatty Acids

Many probiotic microorganisms such as *Bifidobacteria* and *Lactobacilli* produce SCFAs such as butyrate, propionate, and acetate, which can help maintain the epithelial barrier and the anerobic environment in the colon and stimulate the expansion of intestinal stem cells, Paneth cells, and goblet cells. Short-chain fatty acids may increase the resistance to gut mucosal injury. Administration of antibiotics can alter the microflora with decreased *Clostridia*, and increased facultative anaerobes (such as *Enterobacteriaceae*) can reduce SCFAs and increase the luminal oxygen to create a feed-forward loop for progressive alteration in the microflora.

Effects in Probiotics on Normal Turnover of Nutrients

Amino Acids

B. animalis subsp. *lactis* synthesizes the branched chain amino acids leucine, isoleucine, and valine, which play a role in skeletal muscle protein synthesis.

Vitamins

Many gut microbes produce vitamins that provide a nutritional benefit to the host. Thiamine, riboflavin, cobalamin, and biotin serve as cofactors to enzymes in the Krebs cycle and help produce energy. Niacin and pantothenic acid are also essential to energy generation in their roles as electron receptor and synthesis of coenzyme A, respectively. Vitamin K is not produced by probiotic microbes, but development of a Vitamin K–producing probiotic may have value.

Lipid Metabolism

Intestinal microbes can promote partial digestion of glycans that are normally not digestible, and although production of bacterial metabolites such as SCFAs and vitamins is strong, the impact of gut microbes on lipid metabolism remains uncertain. The role of lipids in diseases of premature infants remains understudied, and whether altering the microbiota will impact diseases other than NEC and sepsis remains unknown.

Effects in Probiotics on Intestinal Defense and Motility

Bacteriocins and Other Antimicrobial Molecules

Several probiotic bacteria may produce bacteriocins and other antimicrobial peptides, proteins, and lipoproteins to dominate a given anatomic niche. These toxins usually have a narrow spectrum and eliminate closely related competing species. These bacteriocin-producing probiotic bacteria may promote food safety. The bacteriocins discovered to date are categorized in several databases including BAGEL and BACTIBASE. These bacteriocins may also enhance gut mucosal permeability.

Intestinal Motility

Bifidobacteria can improve gut motility in the mature intestine. These effects are still being evaluated in infants. The impact of gut microbes on intestinal motility is complex, with effects on both the central and enteric nervous systems.

Biologic Plausibility for Effects of Probiotics in Preterm Infants

Preclinical and human data suggest several plausible mechanisms by which probiotics may protect preterm infants against NEC. The strongest clinical association of NEC is with prematurity. Fig. 18.2 shows a host-agent-environment model of strong associations with NEC and how probiotics may interrupt some of these factors. In a meta-analysis of 14 studies, infants who developed NEC showed low diversity of gut bacteria with abundance of *Proteobacteria* species and fewer *Firmicutes* and *Bacteroidetes* species. Probiotics could possibly protect the immature gut against inflammation and injury by several mechanisms: (1) suppressing inflammatory responses and activating cytoprotective mechanisms; (2) improving gut barrier function; (3) producing butyrate and other SCFAs, which protect colonocytes and lower the intestinal pH and oxygen tension; (4) reducing the dysbiosis and normalizing the ratio of *Firmicutes* versus *Enterobacteriaceae*; and (5) improving cellular immunity. Specific probiotic strains show some variation in impact.

The impact of probiotics on gut (and systemic) inflammation can be measured with biomarkers such as cytokines, enteral calprotectin, SCFAs, changes in the enteric microflora, and increased IgA expression. Data from the recently conducted MAGPIE (randomized comparison of magnesium sulfate with placebo for women with preeclampsia) and ELFIN (a multicenter randomized placebo-controlled trial of prophylactic enteral lactoferrin supplementation to prevent late-onset invasive infections in very preterm infants) studies compared stool microbiome, metabolome, host metabolomics, and biomarkers such as calprotectin. Such steps are needed to assess and refine probiotic mixtures for mechanisms and efficacy. Biobanks of stool and breast milk are needed to test theories and hypotheses. The understanding of the host/microbiome interaction may refine the processes used in tailored supplementation of banked or mother's own milk.

Efficacy of Individual Probiotic Strains

Many protective effects of human milk against NEC[60,95,96] may be mediated through its impact on probiotics, and consequently, on the whole gut microflora. In recent years, the role of probiotics in preventing NEC has been investigated through observational studies, RCTs, systematic reviews, and meta-analyses.[37,38,50,59,64,97–100] However, there is still a need for clinically meaningful recommendations.[101] Van den Akker et al.[102] performed a strain-specific network meta-analysis on probiotics' effects in preterm infants. More recently, the European Society of Pediatric Gastroenterology Hepatology and Nutrition (ESPGHAN) published a position paper in 2020[102] on the use of probiotic strains with proven efficacy and safety in preterm infants. There is still a need for information about possible confounding factors that might alter the perceived impact of probiotics.[98,101,103,104]

A recent network meta-analysis[32] examined the differential performance of multi- versus single-strain probiotics in reducing mortality and morbidity in preterm infants.[102] The overall network geometry was based on 13 treatment categories, assessed in 27 studies, versus the common comparator placebo, including 4173 patients. Four double-zero trials, including 378 infants, were initially excluded from the primary Bayesian meta-analysis.[105–107] In network meta-analyses, treatments are often ranked by the surface under the cumulative ranking curve (SUCRA). The authors used another comparison marker, which they defined as the P-score, that works without resampling. *Lactobacillus acidophilus* LB showed the highest SUCRA value, followed by *B. longum* BB536, *B. breve* M-16V, *L. reuteri* 17938, *B. lactis* Bb-12 OR B94, or combinations that were identified as potentially useful.[105–114] As known, human milk is protective against NEC but did not completely abrogate this disease.[105–109,111–128]

Among preterm infants who were not fed exclusively with human milk, *B. longum* 35,624 + *L. rhamnosus* GG were most effective; *B. longum* BB536, *L. reuteri* DSM17938, the multigenus probiotic group, *B. lactis* Bb-12 OR B94, and *L. rhamnosus* LGG ATTC 53103 also showed some efficacy. However, the ORs of *B. longum* 35,624 + *L. rhamnosus* GG, *L. rhamnosus* LGG ATTC 53103, the multigenus probiotic group, and *B. longum* BB536 showed wide credible-intervals. On the other hand, the ORs of *B. lactis* Bb-12 or B94, based on four trials[108,121,122,129] with 355 infants, and *L. reuteri* DSM17938, based on four RCTs[96,101,104,110,120,125,126] with 631 infants, indicate that these treatments reduced the risk of any-stage NEC in preterm infants

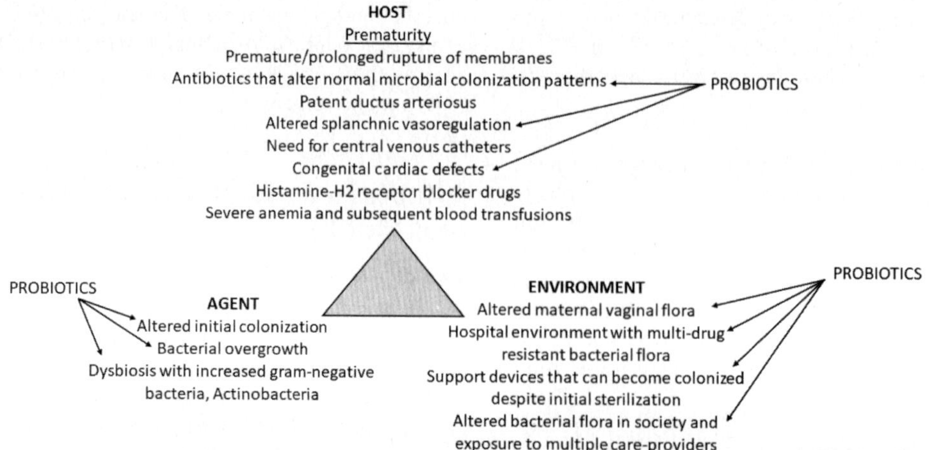

Fig. 18.2 Probiotics and Risk Factors Associated With Necrotizing Enterocolitis (NEC). Putative mechanisms *(arrows)* by which probiotics may alter or interrupt several risk factors associated with NEC.

nonexclusively fed human milk. Only *B. lactis* Bb-12 OR B94 showed a reliable reduction in the risk of stage ≥2 NEC.

A recent network meta-analysis focused on the differential performance of multistrain versus single-strain probiotics in reducing mortality and morbidity in preterm infants.[32] The results showed that combinations of one or more *Lactobacillus* spp. and one or more *Bifidobacterium* spp., *Bifidobacterium lactis* and *Lactobacillus reuteri*, may be more effective in *reducing* severe NEC.

Studies focused on probiotics need to evaluate both efficacy and safety. The ESPGHAN panel on probiotics and preterm infants has recently issued a conditional recommendation not to provide probiotic strains that produce D-lactate (i.e., *L. reuteri* DSM17938 or *L. acidophilus* NCO1748), because their potential risks or safety have not been adequately studied in preterm infants and remain uncertain. We need more information on the highest-risk infants, such as those with ELBW or intrauterine growth retardation.[105,117,124,130,131]

Follow-Up Studies

Infants treated with probiotics in trials need to be followed-up to confirm safety.[132] The 2018 strain-specific systematic review and network meta-analysis of probiotic use in preterm infants from ESPGHAN did not identify an optimal strain, dose, or combination of probiotics to reduce NEC.[102] Clinicians still do not have a choice but to use inadequately tested, potentially unsafe, and possibly ineffective treatments. There are fears about preterm babies being at risk from administration of live microbial products, and most evaluations are still limited to short-term follow-up. There are some individual case reports of bacteremia related to *Bifidobacteria* and *Lactobacilli.* A number of babies in these studies developed or had underlying intestinal pathology, and fortunately, the probiotics were sensitive to β-lactam antibiotics and there was no mortality from probiotic bacteremia. However, it is important to note that probiotics are fastidious anaerobes and are difficult to grow using standard culture media, so systemic infections may be underrecognized.

Probiotics may not primarily alter neurodevelopmental outcomes, except possibly as a positive secondary effect if these do prevent acute illnesses such as NEC or LOS. Akar et al.[133] published a randomized trial of 400 VLBW infants with follow-up of 249 infants at 18 to 24 months' corrected age. In this trial the use of *L. reuteri* had no effect on neurocognitive outcome assessed using the Bayley Scales of Infant and Toddler Development II. Follow-up programs in the Australasian ProPrems trial[134] also found no differences in neurodevelopmental impairment at a mean age of 30 months, although they did find a lower incidence of deafness among probiotic-treated children. They followed 1099 VLBW infants born at <32 weeks' gestation, who had been randomized to either receive a combination of *B. infantis, B. lactis,* and *Streptococcus thermophilus* or placebo. The trial reported a 54% reduction in the secondary outcome of NEC in probiotic-treated infants. At 2 to 5 years of age, the two groups showed no difference in survival free from major neurosensory impairment (281 [75.3%] vs. 271 [74.9%]; RR, 0.98; 95% CI, 0.76–1.26; $P = .88$). In another study, Chou and colleagues[135] evaluated 301 VLBW infants to study the probiotic combination of *B. infantis* and *L. acidophilus* versus placebo. Examination at age 3 years using the Bayley Scales of Infant and Toddler Development II showed no differences in mortality or neurodevelopmental impairment (45 of 153 [29.4%] vs. 49 of 148 [33.1%]; $P = .1$). Similarly, Sari et al.[136] followed up 242 VLBW infants born at <33 weeks' gestation to compare those who received *Lactobacillus sporogenes* versus placebo. They also found no difference in immediate neurodevelopmental outcomes (100 of 121 [82.6%] vs. 98 of 121 [81.0%]; $P = .92$). These similarities in early neurodevelopmental outcomes are reassuring, but cautious follow-up is still needed.[44,133,135,137]

Parental Perspectives

Parental awareness is increasing, but parents' perspectives are poorly reflected in the literature.[138–140] Parents are usually given positive information, which may not be fully representative. At our center, a survey of parents of infants identified dissatisfaction with the information provided, because they perceived NEC to be a "rare" disease. Most mothers (55%) did feel that probiotics were "safe" or "very safe," and 73% considered them to be "beneficial." Sixty-one percent felt that the information provided at the hospital and on the Internet could have some positive bias. Only 1.8% would use these supplements if research showed that there were permanent changes in the microbiota. There is a need to share information about the impact of probiotics on premature babies overall and in terms of NEC and LOS. We know that NEC and LOS are multifactorial disorders; thus a rate of "zero" is impossible. Written guidance supported by professionals developed in partnership with parents of infants with and without NEC would help.

Research Needs

Stating that there is further need for placebo-controlled trials receives strong and mixed opinions.[141] To make progress, future trials need appropriately calculated samples powered to address all NEC, LOS, and mortality; a high quality-control protocol; recording of underpinning mechanistic data (microbial taxa changes, establishment of the administered strain); an appropriately targeted ELBW infant population; an established dosing regimen; a rapid time frame (to prevent other practices changing); and refined recording tools.

Units using probiotics in current practice could study comparative effectiveness of strains or combination products, such that all infants would receive probiotics, but missing gaps in knowledge are filled and products and strategies optimized over time.[101] These units could compare the use of two prebiotic/probiotic combinations versus single-strain products. Randomization by baby or unit or opt-out randomization may be acceptable to parents. Group randomized trials needs a larger number of patients, but there are study designs that can help minimize these numbers. Group randomization by unit can help with cross-contamination issues but leaves other confounders.

Alternative Options With Prebiotics and Synbiotics: Quality and Safety

Prebiotics are nonviable substrates that are selectively used by host microorganisms and confer a health benefit to the host.[142] These include noncarbohydrates and can act outside the intestinal environment, such as in the skin or vagina.[143] Synbiotics are combinations of prebiotics and probiotics that are designed to have synergistic and/or additive effects benefiting the host. A well-resourced, randomized, double-blind, placebo-controlled field trial of synbiotic (*L. plantarum* plus the prebiotic fructo-oligosaccharide) administration to term or late-preterm infants in rural India reported reduction in combined sepsis and death (primary outcome) during the first 2 months of life.[144] These data are exciting and suggest a need for further study. Sestito et al.[145] reviewed the literature and noted that probiotics were effective in reducing the incidence of eczema in high-risk infants. The optimal prebiotic or strain of probiotic, dose, duration, and timing of intervention need study. A combined pre- and postnatal intervention may also be beneficial.

Yu et al.[146] examined the impact of probiotics, probiotics + fructo-oligosaccharides, pentoxifylline, arginine, and lactoferrin in preventing NEC in neonates. A total of 27 eligible studies with 4649 preterm infants were included in this network meta-analysis, and the efficacy and safety of five food additives were evaluated. Probiotic and arginine exhibited better preventive efficacy compared with placebo (OR, 0.50 [95% CI, 0.32–0.73] and OR, 0.30 [95% CI, 0.12–0.73], respectively). Only probiotics achieved a considerable decrease in the risk of mortality compared with placebo (OR, 0.68; 95% CI, 0.46–0.98). Patients with NEC receiving lactoferrin appeared to have a lower incidence of sepsis than those receiving placebo (OR, 0.13; 95% CI, 0.03–0.61) or probiotics (OR, 0.18; 95% CI, 0.03–0.83). Based on this network meta-analysis, probiotics had the potential to be the most preferable additive because they exhibited a significant superiority for NEC and mortality and a relatively balanced performance in safety.

Probiotics During Other Diseases Seen in Neonates and Young Infants

Studies show that the normal bacterial colonization on mucosal or skin surfaces becomes altered during many disease states. Some examples of this pathologic imbalance, dysbiosis, are provided in the following sections.

Unknown Effects of Probiotics in Premature Birth

Women in premature labor often show bacterial overgrowth and dysbiosis with *Gardnerella* spp. and *Lactobacillus crispatus*.[147] These findings are important because the amniotic cavity and the fetus are now known to be nonsterile before the rupture of membranes; low levels of *Enterobacteriaceae*, *Leuconostocaceae*, *Enterococcaceae*, and *Streptococcaceae* can be seen. However, the impact of antibiotic treatment of vaginosis before 22 weeks on preterm birth prior to 37 weeks is uncertain.[148] The role of probiotics needs to be clarified.

Probiotics and Atopy

Infants with atopic dermatitis carry more *Staphylococcus aureus* and *S. epidermidis* on the skin, whereas *Streptococcus* and *Corynebacterium* spp. may increase immediately preceding and during clinical improvement.[149] Administration of oral probiotics such as *Lactobacillus* spp. may decrease atopic dermatitis with an accompanying shift in the T-helper cell (Th1/Th2) balance.[150]

Probiotics and Neurobiological Functioning

The enteric microbiome can alter the gut-brain axis, particularly the hypothalamic-pituitary-adrenal system.[151] The tractus solitarius and the vagus nerve appear to mediate the enteral tract–brain connection.[152] *Bifidobacterium animalis* subsp. *lactis* can alter transcriptional profiles in individual cells, with a shift to increased carbohydrate fermentation to fatty acids.[153]

Conclusions

Current evidence suggests that probiotics reduce the risk of NEC, although the benefit in nosocomial sepsis may not be consistent. Despite evidence of efficacy in NEC, the acceptance of probiotics in routine neonatal intensive care has been variable. Some of the skepticism has philosophic roots, and many physicians and parents remain concerned about the short- and long-term safety of administering live bacteria in vulnerable newborn infants. Those with reservations have found strength in (1) lower or no efficacy in many large trials and meta-analyses; (2) difficulties in laboratory detection of probiotics, which are facultative anaerobes; and (3) increasing data that unlike in adults, bacterial colonization in the neonatal intestine passes through multiple phases, and altering these patterns may have unknown effects. The success of stringent quality-improvement efforts in lowering the incidence of NEC in infants weighing 1001 to 1500 g at birth has also enhanced the questions about risk-to-benefit ratios. There is a need to confirm the safety and benefit profile in ELBW infants, to refine the probiotic products with strict standards used for manufacturing pharmaceutical products, and to determine whether nonliving products such as prebiotics could be useful.

SECTION

4

Nutrition

OUTLINE

Section 4

CHAPTER

19 Enteral Nutrition

Allison Rohrer, Sarah N. Taylor

KEY POINTS

1. The benefits of enteral nutrition for the preterm infant extend beyond growth and encompass gastrointestinal development and gut inflammatory balance.
2. Preterm infant intake of mother's milk, including oral immune therapy, is associated with improved outcomes.
3. Pasteurized donor human milk is the preferred feeding supplement when mother's milk is contraindicated or unavailable and is associated with less necrotizing enterocolitis compared with formula.
4. Preterm infants tolerate initiation of enteral nutrition as early as the first postnatal day and most tolerate advancement of 30 mL/kg/day with no difference in long-term outcomes compared with infants with slower feed advancement.
5. Fortification of human milk with a multinutrient human milk fortifier is necessary to meet energy, protein, mineral, and micronutrient requirements and support growth.
6. Standardized fortification may not meet the needs of all infants due to variations in human milk composition. Modification of feeds should be individualized to support growth, especially for infants with higher energy and protein demands.
7. Exact protein needs are not well-defined; however, maintaining a protein intake of 3.5 to 4.3 g/kg/day with a minimum of 110 kcal/kg/day is recommended.
8. Sustaining mother's milk feeding with nutrient supplementation as needed to sustain adequate growth appears to be the best enteral nutrition practice to optimize neurodevelopment.
9. More research is needed to define the optimal diet of the very low birth weight infant at hospital discharge; however, supplementation of human milk with a multinutrient human milk fortifier for ≥50% of feedings until 52 weeks' postmenstrual age should be considered.

Introduction

Enteral nutrition delivery to preterm infants is evolving. Product options in preterm formula and human milk fortifier, availability of donor human milk, and improved methods to support maternal milk production have increased greatly in the past decade. Furthermore, the recognition that human milk feeding protects against necrotizing enterocolitis (NEC) has transformed the approach to preterm infant feeding from a belief that the infant must show that he is "safe" to be fed to a concept that feeding is protective, and therefore, initiation and continuation of feeding should be prioritized. Yet work is still needed in the design of methods to optimize nutrient delivery, including ways to minimize nutritional loss in human milk from the time of collection until the time the infant receives the feed. Furthermore, methods to protect preterm infants by extending the duration of mother's milk feeds, ensuring safe donor milk options, developing reliable probiotic options, and identifying the best enteral nutritional intake to optimize neurodevelopment should all be prioritized.

Preterm Infant Gastrointestinal Tract

When an infant is born preterm, the gastrointestinal tract must continue to develop outside the intrauterine environment, and while developing, it also must function to both absorb nutrients and block pathogens. At birth, the preterm infant gut is no longer exposed to amniotic fluid, which delivers 15% of fetal nutrition and provides growth-stimulating cytokines to the developing intestinal wall. Fortunately for the preterm infant, human milk and amniotic fluid share a cytokine profile that fosters maturation of the intestinal wall and immune system[1,2] (Table 19.1). Unlike the fetus who has minimal if any intestinal microbes, development of the preterm infant gastrointestinal system includes microbial colonization (Fig. 19.1). NEC occurs when the infant's intestinal barrier, antiinflammatory mediators, and commensal bacteria incline toward a proinflammatory process.

For the intestinal barrier, intestinal permeability is a marker of gut immaturity and is measured by the leakiness of the tight junctions between intestinal epithelial cells. Intestinal permeability is high at birth and is much higher in preterm infants compared with full-term infants.[3] Intestinal permeability decreases with postnatal age and decreases with intake of mother's milk in both full-term and preterm infants.[3–5] Intestinal permeability appears to be associated positively with intestinal microbial diversity, and one study demonstrated decreased permeability with a bifidobacterium supplement to cow's milk for preterm infants.[6,7]

Therefore, beyond providing adequate nutrition to achieve growth, gastrointestinal development and gut inflammatory balance are critical considerations in regard to enteral nutrition for a preterm infant. The type of feeding, timing of feed initiation, and speed of feed advancement not only are factors important for nutrient delivery but also have been studied extensively for their role in gut health. Additionally, consistency and accuracy in diagnosis of gut health and feeding tolerance is critical in safe enteral nutrition delivery. Refer to Fig. 19.2 for other nutritional limitations in the premature gastrointestinal tract.[8–12]

Human Milk Production and Delivery

Preterm infant health outcomes are optimized with intake of human milk. Unfortunately, efforts to ensure mothers can initiate and sustain lactation are not adequate for all mothers. Methods that have been shown to be beneficial are provided in Table 19.2.[13–16] Human milk feedings of mother's milk supplemented as needed with donor human milk are associated with significantly less NEC, less sepsis, and less severe retinopathy of prematurity. Benefit is seen in lower NEC and sepsis rates with exclusive human milk versus exclusive preterm formula, any human milk versus exclusive preterm formula, and higher versus lower human milk doses. For sepsis, the dose-dependent effect is observed in observational studies but not randomized-controlled trials. Meta-analysis also shows a potential decrease in severe retinopathy of prematurity. Evidence of a decrease in

Table 19.1 Growth-Stimulating and Immunomodulating Cytokines Found in the Fetal Intestine, Amniotic Fluid, and HUMAN Milk[1,2]

In fetal intestine, amniotic fluid, and human milk
• Erythopoietin • Granulocyte colony-stimulating factor • Interleukins -4, -7, -8, and -10 • Tissue necrotic factor–α • Epidermal growth factor • Transforming growth factors β and γ • Insulin-like growth factor I and II • Hyperglycemic-glycogenolytic factor
In amniotic fluid and human milk
• Interleukin-6 • Vascular endothelial growth factor

Adapted from Maheshwari A. Role of cytokines in human intestinal villous development. *Clin Perinatol.* 2004;31(1):143–155.

bronchopulmonary dysplasia is less certain.[17] Mechanisms by which human milk protects the infant from disease are shown in Fig. 19.3.[18]

Early Enteral Nutrition

Oral Immune Therapy With Mother's Milk

Oral immune therapy, or oral colostrum care, is when milk is placed on the infant's buccal mucosa. A Cochrane Review of six studies including 335 infants concluded that days to full enteral feeds were reduced, with a mean difference of −2.58 days (95% confidence interval [CI], −4.01 to −1.14) in the group that received oral colostrum care.[19] Evidence of potential immune benefit also has been demonstrated, with increased urinary lactoferrin and immunoglobulin A concentrations with oral immune therapy versus placebo.[20] Of note, the benefits of oral immune therapy are more apparent when the milk is delivered with a syringe versus a swab.[21]

Initiation of Feeds

Unless there is abdominal pathology or cardiovascular compromise, feeds should be initiated as early as the first postnatal hours and as late as 3 days. Meta-analysis results show no benefit to delaying feeds to 4 days or longer, including no decreased risk of NEC. Even though the meta-analysis demonstrates no benefit to introduction of feeds before 4 days, if early introduction leads to earlier attainment of full enteral nutrition, then central-line days and parenteral-nutrition days may be decreased, leading to less risk for infection, complications, and cost.[22] As to how early is too early to initiate feeds, no study has demonstrated an early time that is associated with morbidity. In a trial by the Abnormal Doppler Enteral Prescription Trial Collaborative Group that included infants born at less than 35 weeks with intrauterine growth restriction, outcomes were no different with initiation of feeds by 48 hours compared with after 48 hours in the whole group and in the subgroup of infants born at less than 29 weeks' postmenstrual age (PMA).[23] In regard to potential benefit with earlier feeding, intestinal permeability is

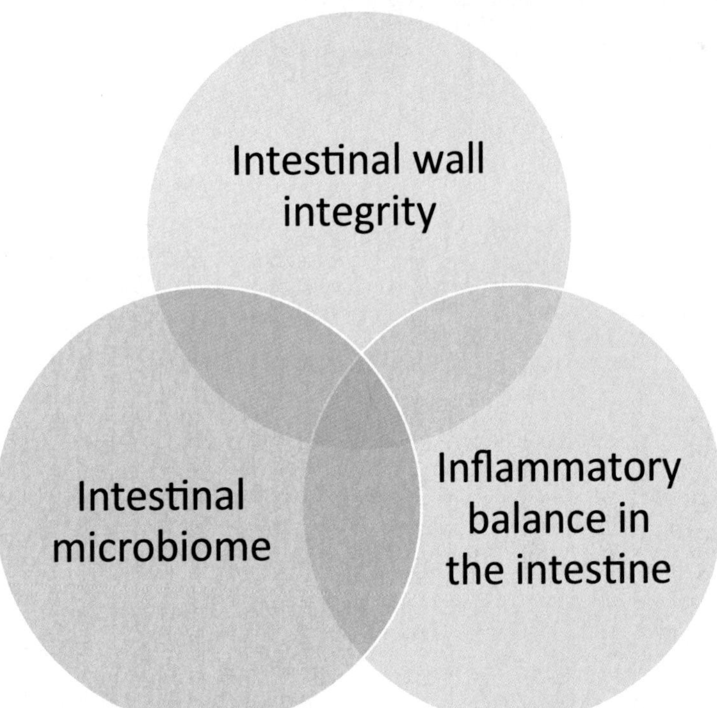

Fig. 19.1 Gastrointestinal Development Starts in the Fetal Environment and Continues Into Infancy. Although the primary function of the gastrointestinal tract is absorption of nutrients, the ability to avoid infection and inflammation also are critical functions. For the fetus, the development of the intestinal wall and antiinflammatory system of the gut is performed in a sterile or near-sterile environment. For the preterm infant, the development of the microbiome based on bacterial and antibiotic exposure affects both gut wall integrity and inflammatory balance. When this development is disrupted substantially, necrotizing enterocolitis occurs. Maheshwari A. Role of cytokines in human intestinal villous development. *Clin Perinatol.* 2004;31(1):143–155.

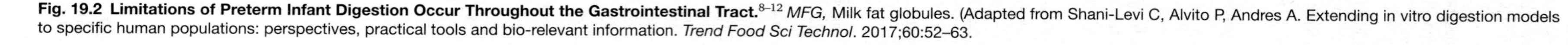

Mouth
• Preterm infants have limited oral phase with use of feeding tubes
• Unable to rely on activity of salivary amylase or lingual lipase
Small Intestine
Protein:
• Enterokinase activity occurs by 24 weeks gestation; activity is decreased in preterm infants
Carbohydrate:
• Lactase activity increases between 24 and 40 weeks gestation; activity is overall decreased in preterm infants
• Near-full activity of sucrase, maltase, and isomaltase
• Limited pancreatic amylase production begins 14-16 weeks gestation but does not reach adult levels until 2 years of age
Lipids:
• Preterm infants have low levels of pancreatic lipase and bile acids that contribute to inadequate or incomplete digestion of lipids
• Human Milk:
• Lipid digestion of MFG membrane appears to be independent of pancreatic enzymes
• Alkaline sphingomyelinase present at birth in preterm infant but activity undefined
• Bile-salt-stimulated lipase is activated in small intestine (absent in pasteurized donor milk or formula)
Stomach
• Delayed gastric emptying common
• Transient relaxation of Lower Esophageal Sphincter may contribute to gastroesophageal reflux
Protein:
• Preterm infants with limited gastric acid for protein denaturation
• Pepsinogen present in stomach by 17 to 18 weeks
Lipids:
• Gastric lipase present in early gestation although functional capacity not well defined
Colon
Carbohydrate:
• Undigested starches that pass into colon can be digested by microbes; production of short-chain fatty acids can be used as energy source

Fig. 19.2 Limitations of Preterm Infant Digestion Occur Throughout the Gastrointestinal Tract.[8–12] *MFG,* Milk fat globules. (Adapted from Shani-Levi C, Alvito P, Andres A. Extending in vitro digestion models to specific human populations: perspectives, practical tools and bio-relevant information. *Trend Food Sci Technol*. 2017;60:52–63.

Table 19.2 Evidence-Based Methods to Sustain Maternal Milk Production for Hospitalized Preterm Infants[13–16]

To Sustain Mother's Milk to 40 Weeks' Postmenstrual Age	To Have Adequate Milk Supply at Hospital Discharge
Express milk by 6 hours postbirth Perform kangaroo care Express milk at least 5 times per day	Pump both breasts simultaneously Produce 500 mL/day milk by postnatal day 10 Describe breast pumping as comfortable Have a NICU environment with: • Adequate staffing • Nurses with high level of lactation education • Nurse support of breastfeeding

NICU, Neonatal intensive care unit.

highest when an infant gut is not fed. Additionally, one study showed increased inflammatory markers in stool and increased inflammatory diseases such as bronchopulmonary dysplasia (BPD) and retinopathy of prematurity (ROP) with delaying feed initiation until after the third day.[24] Another study demonstrated tolerance when extremely low birth weight infants were fed at a median of 14 versus 33 hours and found less central-line-associated infections and less feeding intolerance and higher growth velocity in the cohort fed earlier.[25] A potential evidence-based guideline for feed initiation is provided in Table 19.3.

Enteral Feeding Selection

Human Milk

Human milk is the preferred feeding for nearly all infants, with numerous short and long-term advantages to the very low birth weight infant.[26] There are few contraindications to feeding mother's own milk (Table 19.4).[27] The use of marijuana during breastfeeding is one subject of debate, especially because lipid-rich milk is the ideal vector for cannabinoid metabolites. Unfortunately, long-term consequences due to exposure to human milk cannabinoids are not well described, and studies are confounded by use of other recreational substances like tobacco and alcohol.[28–30] The American Academy of Pediatrics (AAP) highlighted concern for neurodevelopment and growth sequelae with marijuana use during both pregnancy and lactation in a recently published report.[30] However, due to the lack of evidence, the guideline does not state that lactation is contraindicated for a mother who is using marijuana. Consequently, with the currently available information, mothers who are using marijuana should be educated regarding the potential consequences to their infant's growth and neurodevelopment and given appropriate social support and counseling, but after education, if the mother continues to provide her milk, she should be supported in her lactation.[30]

For most medications, the benefits of mother's milk for a preterm infant likely outweigh the potential harm of the medication. However, for some medications with minimal research, it is important to obtain the available drug information and discuss the risk benefits to develop a consensus among the interdisciplinary clinical care team and the family. Available resources are provided in Table 19.5.

It is important to note that the processes of pumping, storage, freezing, thawing, and preparing human milk feeds for neonatal intensive care unit (NICU) infants decrease concentrations of some nutritional and immunologic components of mother's milk. When providing mother's milk via tube, fat, vitamin C, vitamin B_6, carotenoids, calcium, and phosphorus are at risk for loss during tube feedings.[31] Therefore, attention to providing the freshest mother's

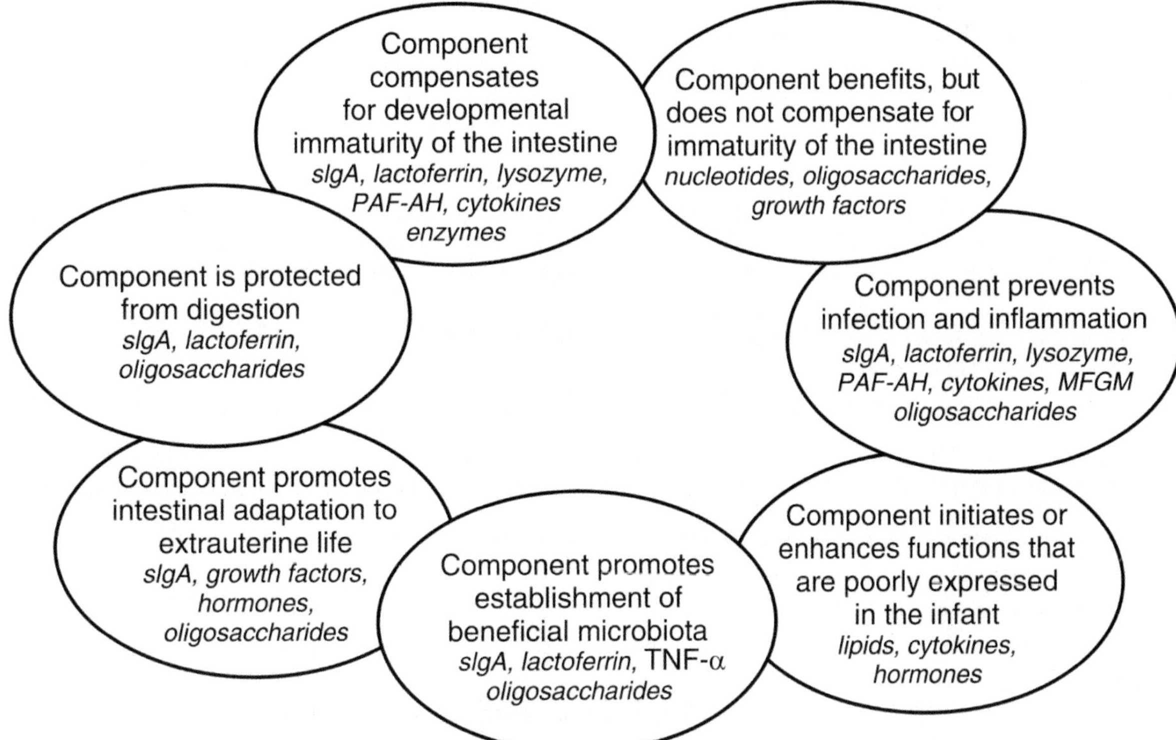

Fig. 19.3 Possible Beneficial Impact of Bioactive Agents Known to Be Present in Human Milk. *MFGM,* Milk fat globule membrane; *PAF-AH,* platelet-activating factor-acetylhydrolase; *sIgA,* secretory immunoglobulin; *TNF-α,* tumor necrosis factor-α. (Modified from Goldman AS. Modulation of the gastrointestinal tract of infants by human milk: Interface and interactions—an evolutionary perspective. *J Nutr.* 2000;130:426S.)

Table 19.3 Potential Evidence-Based Feed Initiation and Advancement Guideline for Infants ≥34 Weeks

	Feeding Volume	Feeding Type	
Days 1–3	Initiate feeds 12–25 mL/kg/day[a]	<1500 g or <32 Weeks	>1500 g and >32 Weeks
Days 2–4	Initiate feed advancement by 25 mL/kg/day	Mother's milk supplemented with donor human milk	Mother's milk supplemented with preterm formula
Days 3–12	Increase feed volume by 25 mL/kg/day to full volume, 120–160 mL/kg/day	Fortify with high-protein bovine-derived fortifier or human milk–derived fortifier at least at 100 mL/kg/day or as early as the first feed	Fortify with standard protein bovine-derived fortifier at least at 100 mL/kg/day or as early as the first feed; if formula feeding, start with 24 kcal/oz formula at first feed
Discharge	No less than 120 mL/kg/day when taking volumes ad libitum	If human milk–fed: Fortify with standard protein bovine-derived fortifier for ≥50% of feedings for up to 52 weeks' postmenstrual age If formula fed: Preterm-discharge formula until minimum of 40 weeks' corrected age; preterm formulas may be considered in some circumstances, i.e., severe growth restriction, metabolic bone disease	Provide preterm-discharge formula or supplement mother's milk with preterm-discharge formula until at least 40 weeks' corrected age
		Transition infants to either unfortified human milk/breastfeeding or to standard formula (for formula-fed infants) once the infant regains his or her birth percentile	

[a]Full-term breastfed infants: feed 10–15 mL/feed on day 1, 15–20 mL/feed on day 2, 20–25 mL/feed on day 3, and 25–30 mL/feed on day 4. Consider limiting to these volumes even in infants who weigh >3 kg.

milk in the shortest time benefits nutrition and immune-component delivery to the NICU infant.

Donor Human Milk

When mother's milk is not available, donor human milk is a feeding type associated with less NEC compared with formula feeding.[32] Current sources of donor human milk include raw milk, pasteurized milk (Holder or vat), and retort-sterilized milk. In a recent meta-analysis of 12 trials of donor human milk and preterm formula, all studies used pasteurized (Holder or vat) donor human milk except for one that used raw milk. No studies in this meta-analysis used retort-sterilized human milk. Three trials added bovine-derived milk fortifier to the donor milk, and one added human milk–derived milk fortifier. The meta-analysis results demonstrate significantly better weight, length, and head growth with formula compared with donor human milk. No difference in neurodevelopment was observed between infants fed formula or donor human milk. Formula-fed infants had a significantly higher risk of NEC (relative risk, 1.87; 95% CI, 1.23–2.85) with a number needed to treat of 33 preterm infants with donor milk to avoid one case of NEC.[32] The trials of donor human milk versus formula differ in their populations and duration of treatment, but many institutions and even state quality-improvement initiatives have chosen to provide donor human milk to the infants most at risk for NEC during the time that they are most at risk. A common standard is to provide donor human milk as a supplement to mother's milk for all hospitalized very low birth weight (<1500 g) and very preterm (<32 weeks' PMA) infants until they reach 34 weeks' PMA.

Although the benefit of donor human milk to prevent NEC is critical to preterm infant care, all donor human milk is lacking in some nutritional and immunologic factors compared with mother's milk. The lower values in donor human milk are due to differences in milk expressed for a preterm versus a full-term infant, the loss of nutritional and immunologic function with pasteurization or retort processing, and the loss of nutritional and immunologic concentrations during freezing, thawing, and container transfers that occur in donor milk processing. Preterm milk is higher in protein, sodium, and immune components (beta-defensin, secretory CD14 receptor,

Table 19.4 Contraindications to Mother's Milk Feeding[27]

When to substitute formula or donor milk for mother's milk
• Maternal HIV in developed countries (in low-resources countries without safe formula, exclusive breastfeeding may be recommended) • Maternal HTLV • Maternal Ebola virus • Maternal use of illicit street drugs (i.e., cocaine, methylamphetamines, PCP) except for narcotic-dependent mothers who are enrolled in a supervised program with no other contraindications • Maternal medications with known toxicity (radioactive agents, chemotherapy, cyclosporine, lithium, methotrexate)
When to temporarily substitute formula or donor milk for mother's milk
• Temporary use of maternal medications with known toxicity
When to not feed directly from the breast (but feeding mother's milk from bottle is acceptable)
• Maternal active tuberculosis • With maternal active herpes simplex virus (HSV) lesion on the breast, feed from unaffected breast or cover lesion completely
When to only feed formula (no human milk)
• Infants with galactosemia should only receive lactose-free formulas, i.e., soy formulas

HTLV, Human T-lymphotropic virus.

Table 19.5 Resources for Information on Safety of Medications for the Lactating Woman

Resource
LactMed https://www.ncbi.nlm.nih.gov/books/NBK501922/
Mother to Baby (a service of the nonprofit Organization of Teratology Information Specialists) https://mothertobaby.org/
InfantRisk Center (a service of Texas Tech University Health Sciences Center) http://www.infantrisk.com/categories/breastfeeding
CDC Breastfeeding and Special Circumstances: Vaccinations, Medications, & Drugs https://www.cdc.gov/breastfeeding/breastfeeding-special-circumstances/vaccinations-medications-drugs/prescription-medication-use.html
University of Rochester Medicine Breastfeeding Provider Resource Telephone Consultations for Healthcare Providers https://www.urmc.rochester.edu/breastfeeding/provider-resources.aspx

transforming growth factor–β 2, and potentially lysozyme) than is term milk.[33–36] In the pasteurization process for donor milk, live cells are killed and enzymes (such as lysozyme, alkaline phosphatase, amylase, and lipase) are inactivated. Additionally, immunoglobulins and water-soluble vitamins are reduced in the pasteurization process.[37]

Pathogen-free donor milk is available from nonprofit and for-profit milk banks with milk processed by Holder pasteurization, vat pasteurization, and retort processing for a shelf-stable milk. Other processes being investigated as methods to provide safe donor milk include high-pressure processing, high-temperature short-time pasteurization, UV irradiation, and (thermo-) ultrasonic processing.[38] Table 19.6 compares sources of human milk and implications on processing methods.[9,39–47]

Mothers should be educated on the dangers of informal milk sharing.[48] One group of investigators obtained and analyzed more than 100 samples of human milk from the Internet. The majority of samples were found to have evidence of dilution with bovine milk, high counts of bacterial growth, and evidence of mothers' use of nicotine and caffeine. Poor handling, storage, and shipping techniques were described.[49–51] Although fresh mother's milk that has never been frozen is the preferred source of feeding for the preterm infant, it is possible for human milk to have a bacterial or viral load that may be injurious to the infant.[50,52] One example is a mother with reactivated cytomegalovirus. Shedding of the virus can be detected in colostrum as early as 3 days. However, even though a preterm infant may become infected from cytomegalovirus in maternal milk, the benefit of fresh maternal milk appears to outweigh the risk of viral infection. The same cannot be said for informally shared donor milk. Therefore, shared donor milk even from a "trusted" source should not be provided to a hospitalized preterm infant. Institutions should have a policy that prohibits or at least requires parental informed consent for use of raw milk other than the mother's own, especially for the high-risk, immunocompromised infant.

Despite great efforts to obtain mother's milk as early as possible, when a mother is not directly breastfeeding, the ability to obtain milk drops via pump or hand expression may be difficult, especially in the early days. Therefore, a common question in preterm infant care is whether feeds should be started with donor human milk or formula or whether feed initiation should be delayed until mother's milk is available. The second question, then, is how long is it appropriate to wait for mother's milk? Unfortunately, evidence to answer these questions is lacking. Due to the apparent low toxicity of donor human milk, many institutions initiate donor human milk while awaiting mother's milk. When an infant does not "qualify" to receive donor human milk, and therefore, formula would be the initial feeding type, the practice is quite varied even within an institution. Until studies are performed to address these questions, no evidence-based recommendation is available. For the very low birth weight infant or very preterm infant, if a supplement to mother's milk is needed, donor human milk is the current standard of care until the infant is out of the PMA at which NEC risk is greatest. A common practice is to provide donor human milk to all infants born weighing <1500 g and/or at <32 weeks' PMA until they reach 34 weeks' PMA or until hospital discharge (whichever occurs first), but variations on this practice are widespread. Based on a Cochrane Review meta-analysis, the evidence-based goal with donor human milk is to provide it to preterm infants to decrease the risk of NEC.[32] Therefore, providing it to the infants most at risk for NEC during the time that they are most at risk for NEC is an evidence-based practice. The donor human milk provided to very preterm infants should be pasteurized donor milk.

Preterm Infant Formula

For neonatal units without access to donor milk or for larger premature infants who do not meet specific weight or gestation criteria to receive donor milk, preterm formula is recommended when mother's own milk is not available. Modest improvements of in-hospital growth are observed compared with standard formulas.[53] Preterm formulas are higher in protein, calcium, and phosphorus, contain a fat source that is predominantly medium-chain triglyceride-based, and have lactose and glucose polymers as their carbohydrate source to enhance digestion of calcium.[54] Ready-to-feed, 24-calories-per-ounce preterm formulas have an osmolality similar to that of breast milk (280–320 mOsm/kg water) and may be used from the start of the first feeding in the absence of human milk. Available preterm formulas are whey-predominant with varying amounts of protein, between 3.0 and 3.6 g per 100 calories. Higher-protein formulas may be best suited for the fluid-restricted infant in order to meet protein goals; however, providing >4 g/kg/day of protein long term in formula-fed infants has not been well-studied, and evidence is limited in terms of safety or neurodevelopmental outcomes.[55] Additionally, there is inconclusive evidence that use of a hydrolyzed protein formula for "easier digestion" affects the risk of NEC.[56] There are currently no protein hydrolysate or amino acid formulas within the US market that are designed to meet the nutritional requirements of preterm infants, and concern exists for nutrient bioavailability, especially with regard to protein, calcium, and phosphorus.

Advancement of Feeds

Preterm infants have small gastric size and slow motility; therefore the initial feeding volume is small, with the volume advanced over days. Historically, rapid advancement of feed volume appeared to be

Table 19.6 Comparison Sources of Human Milk[9,39–47]

Products (Distributors)	Processing Type and Description	Effects on Processing	Additional Information
MOM	Fresh milk preferred because changes to composition are observed with freezing	Freezing MOM ↓ concentration of lysozyme, secretory IgA, and lactoperoxidase Calorie and fat content decreases with freezing time; significant differences are observed at 90 days	Maximum recommendations for safe hold times: https://www.cdc.gov/breastfeeding/recommendations/handling_breastmilk.htm Average composition of human colostrum and mature breastmilk are available[47]
Pasteurized donor milk (Human Milk Banking Association of North America—includes the United States and Canada) https://www.hmbana.org/	Holder Pasteurization Initial freeze/thaw cycle, heated to 62.5°C during pasteurization process, then rapidly cooled to 4°C and stored frozen at −20°C or less Distributed to units frozen and must be thawed prior to being fed to infant Average of 2–6 mothers per batch	Eliminates bile salt–stimulated lipase ↓ Lactoferrin, IgA, IgM concentrations compared with MOM ↓ Lysozyme and secretory IgA activity compared with MOM, although retains significantly higher activity compared with retort sterilization	Must remain frozen and used within 48 hours of thawing/refrigeration Mothers are screened for health and drug/tobacco use and blood tested for bloodborne pathogens Mothers are not compensated for donation Milk is prioritized to preterm infants Labeling of calories and protein specific to individual milk banks and nutritional analysis may be used to target pool milk to obtain a minimum of 20 calories per ounce
PremieLact Prolact HM (Prolacta Bioscience) https://www.prolacta.com/	Vat Pasteurization Similar to Holder Pasteurization with two freeze/thaw cycles Milk is heated to 63°C for ≥30 minutes; additional details are proprietary Average of 250 mothers per batch	Fat and energy concentration significantly higher compared with the retort sterilization although not different compared with Holder Pasteurization	Must remain frozen and used within 48 hours of thawing/refrigeration Mothers are compensated for donation Donors are blood tested for bloodborne pathogens, and donated milk undergoes nucleic acids amplification testing for pathogenic viruses and bacteria Donor milk is DNA matched to the donor Donor milk is tested for microbes, adulteration, nicotine, and drugs of abuse Uniform caloric density with nutrition content provided on the product label; nutritional analysis via wet chemistry tests Guarantees a minimum of 20 calories/ounce and provides an average of 1.1 g protein per 100 mL
BENEFIT-18 BENEFIT-20 BENEFIT-24 (Medolac Laboratories, Boulder City, Nevada) https://www.medolac.com/	Retort Sterilization Initial freeze/thaw cycle, milk heated to 121°C for 5 minutes under pressure of 15 pounds per square inch; distributed in shelf-stable packaging	↓ Lysozyme and secretory IgA activity compared with MOM and Holder/Vat Pasteurization ↓ Protein, fat, immune-modulating proteins, and HMO function compared with Holder/Vat Pasteurization	Shelf-stable at room temperature for 3 years Commercially sterile and homogenized Can be refrigerated for 7 days after opening Mothers are compensated for donation Milk is tested for pathogens both before and after processing Uniform caloric density: Nutrition content provided and specific to each lot with minor variation between lots Refer to company-specific website for details; nutritional analysis via third-party analysis BENEFIT-24 is ultrafiltered and has increased amounts of key nutrients including 1.78 g protein per 100 mL and 24 calories/ounce
HDM Boost HDM Plus (Ni-Q) https://www.ni-q.com/	Proprietary Agitating Retort Process	No information available	Shelf-stable at room temperature for 12 months Commercially sterile and homogenized Donors are blood tested for bloodborne pathogens Donor milk is screened for alcohol and microbial contamination and is genetically tested to ensure donor matching Mothers are compensated for donation Uniform caloric density: nutrition content provided and specific to each lot, with minor variation between lots Refer to company specific website for details; nutritional analysis validated by a third party Calorically enhanced using a patent pending system: HDM Boost has a minimum of 1.5 g protein and per 100 mL and 24 calories/ounce HDM Plus has a minimum of 20 calories/ounce
Informally shared milk (includes any milk other than mother's own, i.e., milk from either the Internet or a known source)	None	No information available	Risks poor handling and inadequate temperature holding; thus no guarantee that milk is safe from harmful bacteria May be diluted with bovine milk or other nonhuman milk source No blood testing performed for transferrable diseases

HMO, Human milk oligosaccharides; *MOM*, mother's own milk.

associated with a higher risk of NEC. However, most but not all contemporary studies have disproved that association. Recent retrospective cohort studies have demonstrated a decrease in NEC with a slower feed initiation and advancement practice, but randomized, controlled trials show no benefit.[57–59] A 2014 Cochrane Review reported both no evidence of benefit for trophic or minimal volume feedings for a few days prior to feed advancement and no benefit to advancing less than 24 mL/kg/day.[22,60] The Speed of Increasing Milk Feeds Trial (SIFT) is a randomized, controlled trial of very low birth weight or very preterm infants randomized to receive feed volume advanced by 30 or 18 mL/kg/day increments. At 2 years of age, the two groups demonstrated no difference in outcomes including incidence of NEC and late-onset sepsis.[59] Although no benefit was demonstrated with feed advancement of 30 mL/kg/day, no detriment was observed either. With the risks and costs of parenteral nutrition, including both the compounding and the vascular access and also the difficulty of providing adequate nutrition, especially with the ever-recurring shortages of nutrients, the current evidence points to 30 mL/kg/day as an acceptable and potentially beneficial feed volume advancement strategy. In fact, the available evidence led the authors of one meta-analysis to recommend achieving full enteral nutrition within 7 days for infants born weighing 1 to 1.5 kg and within 14 days for infants born weighing <1 kg,[61] which is indeed feasible and has been established in clinical practice.[62]

Nutrition Requirements

Protein

Early and adequate protein intake is key to preventing accumulation of protein deficits in the preterm infant. Although studies have not identified the ideal protein requirement of the preterm infant, achieving a slightly higher enteral protein intake compared with parenteral intake is recommended due to incomplete and immature digestion and the biologic value of enteral protein sources. Older guidelines for protein were created on the basis of fetal accretion rates during gestation and have been adjusted over time. Current available evidence points to protein goals in the premature infant ranging from 3.3 to 4.3 g/kg/day. In randomized, controlled trials, higher protein intakes of 3.3 to 4.3 g/kg/day versus 2.8 to 3.7 g/kg/day are significantly associated with improved weight, height, and head circumference growth, but not consistently. This lack of consistent efficacy may be due to an overlap in protein delivery, as demonstrated by three studies defining protein intake of 3.6 to 3.7 g/kg/day as low protein. Additionally, the studies were also complicated by variation in maternal protein content.[63–69] One recent study did not show any growth benefit with higher protein fortification (3.7 g/kg/day vs. 4.3 g/kg/day) when milk protein content was confirmed with human milk analysis.[67] This suggests a saturation point or ceiling-effect of protein on growth in the preterm infant. Variation of growth is more likely contributed to an *energy* deficit when protein needs are met.

Calories

Energy needs of the premature infant are estimated based on several factors in addition to basal energy expenditure and requirements for growth and lean body mass deposition. Factors that are unique to the individual infant include levels of physical activity, temperature support, thermic effect of food, losses of energy in stool and urine, and clinical condition/disease state, that is sepsis or chronic lung disease. Exact energy requirements are difficult to identify based on the influence of protein on growth and the varying protein energy ratios in empirical studies. One group of studies that specifically identified the protein-to-energy ratio instead of protein or energy quantities alone identified a caloric intake of approximately 115 kcal/kg/day with a protein intake of 3.6 g/kg/day needed to achieve weight gain of 16 to 22 g/kg/day. A greater supply of energy, upwards of 150 kcal/kg, produced more body fat measured by triceps skinfold; however increasing protein above 4 g/kg/day did not increase gains in lean body mass.[70] Preterm infants do require a minimum of 110 kcal/kg/day to maintain fat deposition similar to the normally growing fetus. Adequate caloric intake is needed to maximize nitrogen retention with increase in protein delivery, as illustrated in Fig. 19.4.[71] Our recommendations for calories and protein are outlined in Table 19.7.[72] Enteral nutrient recommendations from different sources are compared in Table 19.8.[73–76]

Preterm Infant Enteral Nutrition Management

Human Milk Fortification

While maternal human milk is the gold standard for feeding preterm infants, it is unable to provide the appropriate combination of macro- and micronutrients or support growth when fed at typical volumes of 135 to 200 mL/kg. Therefore human milk fortification has become the standard of care for preterm infants to help promote short-term growth in the hospital.[77] A multinutrient human milk fortifier provides crucial nutrients including protein, essential fatty acids, calcium, phosphorus, vitamin D, zinc, and electrolytes and increases the caloric density of human milk. The combination of nutrients is critical to support growth of lean body mass and developing organs, including the lungs and rapidly growing brain. Commercial formula companies have improved human milk fortifiers during the past decades with regard to protein and nutrient content and currently market products that are available in both powder and liquid. Liquid is often preferred because it can be sterilized, but it is not universally accessible. The first liquid bovine human milk fortifier was acidified as a method to preserve nutrient composition while reducing heat treatment required to achieve sterility, although nonacidified preparations are now available. Nonacidified bovine human milk fortifiers are preferred because infants exhibit less metabolic acidosis, less feeding intolerance (emesis or gastric residuals), and improved growth compared with acidified bovine human milk fortifier.[78–81] One version of bovine fortifier has extensively hydrolyzed protein as the protein source to aid in digestion, although there was no difference in feeding intolerance compared with intact protein.[65] The amount of protein in bovine human milk fortifier varies both among and within manufacturer product lines (Table 19.9). The ideal amount of protein to add to human milk is unknown, though small improvements in weight gain are seen during hospital admission with fortifiers that provide an additional ≥1.4 g protein per 100 mL of human milk compared with moderate protein amounts (≥1–<1.4 g per 100 mL human milk).[82]

Prolacta Bioscience is a human milk bank that operates for profit and sells pasteurized human milk, exclusive human milk fortifiers, ready-to-feed human milk–based premature infant formula, and a human milk cream supplement. Exclusive human milk fortifier is concentrated, pasteurized donor human milk that is added to human milk to increase calorie and nutrient composition; however, exclusive human milk fortifiers tend to displace large quantities of the mother's own milk compared with bovine fortifiers and may be cost-prohibitive to some NICUs. Protein concentrations of exclusive human milk

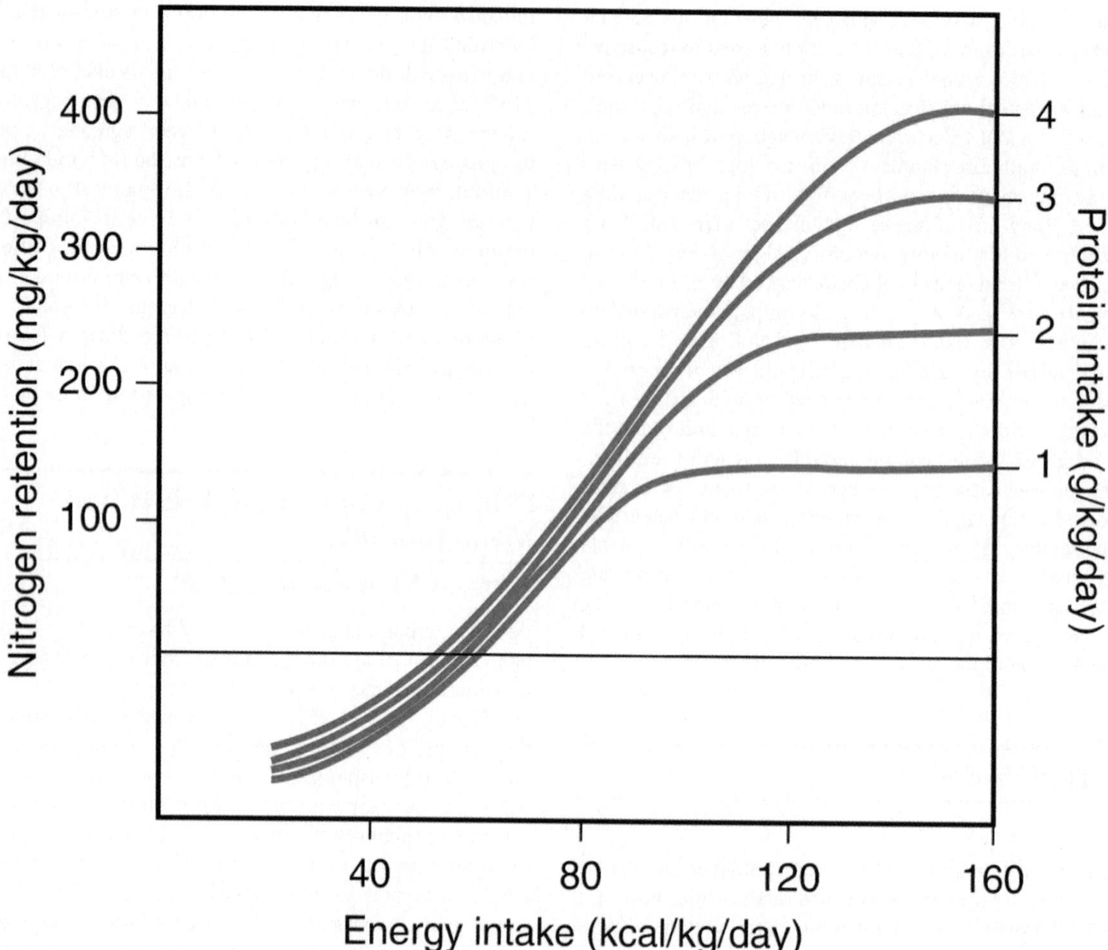

Fig. 19.4 Energy Intake and Protein Retention Based on Protein Intake in Low Birth Weight Infants. (From Senterre J, Rigo J. Protein requirements of premature and compromised infants. In: Xanthou M, ed. *New Aspects of Nutrition in Pregnancy, Infancy and Prematurity*. Amsterdam: Elsevier; 1997:109–115.)

fortifiers are not equivalent when compared with 24-calories-per-ounce bovine-fortified breast milk. Higher caloric concentrations of the exclusive human milk fortifier or volumes of feeding are usually needed to achieve protein goals, and caloric concentrations of up to 30 calories per ounce are available. There is limited evidence from a recent Cochrane Review that shows no reduction in risk of NEC (relative risk, 0.95; 95% CI, 0.2–4.54), feeding intolerance, or late-onset sepsis and no improvement in growth when using an exclusive human milk fortifier.[83] Specifically, the review included one randomized, controlled trial of 125 infants, which directly compared bovine and exclusive human milk fortifiers.[84] Previous randomized, controlled trials that demonstrated reduction of NEC and feeding intolerance with exclusive human milk fortifiers compared study arms that used preterm formula in infants weighing <1250 g and not the current standard of care of donor human milk as the milk base to which bovine fortifier was added.[85,86] Recently the NEC Society published results of a survey that highlighted confusion among both parents and providers with use of the term "human milk fortifier," because it applies to both bovine and pasteurized donor milk fortifiers. The authors call for a change in the labeling because using only the term "human milk fortifier" can be misleading. Although the addition of multinutrient fortifier is the standard of practice in most NICUs and often occurs automatically in unit protocols, providers should not withhold information about the type of fortifier that is being used.[87]

There is no evidence of exactly *when* to fortify human milk; however, there is a trend in favor of earlier fortification to optimize calorie, protein, and mineral provision during the period of transitioning off parenteral nutrition.[88] Published studies have indicated addition of human milk fortifier after attaining enteral volumes as low as 20 to 40 mL/kg/day and even as early as the first feed.[86,89,90] No studies evaluating earlier fortification have found benefit or harm.[86,89–92] One practice is to overlap fortification with parenteral nutrition to maintain at least 3 g/kg/day protein delivery. In general, as described in a 2016 Cochrane Review, feeding milk with multinutrient fortifier compared with milk without fortifier to preterm infants is associated with increased weight, length, and head

Table 19.7 Recommended Enteral Energy and Protein Intakes[72]

Age	Energy Goal (kcal/kg)	Protein Goal (g/kg)
Preterm <34 0/7 weeks	110–130	3.3–4.3[a]
Late preterm 34 0/7 to 36 6/7 weeks	120–135	3–3.2
Term ≥37 0/7 weeks	105–120	2–2.5

[a]Authors recommend slightly less protein compared with original text given limited data for higher protein intakes above 4.3 g/kg/day.

Adapted from Goldberg DL, Becker PJ, Brigham K, et al. Identifying malnutrition in preterm and neonatal populations: recommended indicators. *J Acad Nutr Diet.* 2018;118(9):1571–1582.

Table 19.8 Recommendations (per kg/day) of Select Nutrients for VLBW Infants When Fed Enterally[73–76]

Nutrient per kg	Koletzko, 2014[73]	ESPGHAN, 2010[74]	LSRO, 2002 (Formula-Fed Infants Only)[75]
Energy, kcal	110–130	110–130	100–141
Protein, g	3.5–4.5	4.0–4.5 (<1 kg) 3.5–4.0 (1–1.8 kg)	3.0–4.3
Lipids, g	4.8–6.6	4.8–6.6	5.3–6.8
Carbohydrate, g	11.6–13.2	11.6–13.2	11.5–15
Sodium, mg	69–115	69–115	46.8–75.6
Potassium, mg	78–195	66–132	72–192
Calcium, mg	120–200	120–140	148–222
Phosphorus, mg	60–140	60–90	98–131
Vitamin D, IU	400–1000 per day (from milk + supplement)	800–1,000 per day (milk to provide 100–350 per 100 kcal)	90–324
Vitamin A, mcg RE	400–1,100	400–1,000	245–456
Zinc, mg	1.4–2.5	1.1–2.0	1.32–1.8
Iron, mg	2–3	2–3	2–3.6
Iodine, mcg	10–55	11–55	7.2–42

ESPGHAN, European Society for Paediatric Gastroenterology Hepatology and Nutrition; *LSRO*, United States Life Science Research Office; *RE*, retinol equivalents; *VLBW*, very low birth weight.

Table 19.9 Nutrient Composition for Select Breast Milk and Formula Recipes for a 1-kg Infant Fed at Volumes of 150 mL/kg/day[a]

	20 kcal/oz	24 kcal/oz		25 kcal/oz	26 kcal/oz	27 kcal/oz		30 kcal/oz
Nutrients per kg	HM, Unfortified[b]	HM With Bovine Fortifier[c]	Preterm Formula[d] (High Protein Values in Parentheses)	HM[b] + Preterm Formula[e] (1:1)	HM + Human Milk–Derived Fortifier, +6 Calories/oz[f]	HM + Bovine Fortifier + MCT[g]	HM + Bovine Fortifier + Powder Formula[h]	Preterm Formula[e]
Calories, kcal	101	120	120	110	135	135	136	150
Protein,[i] g	2.1	3.5–4.8	3.7–4.1 (4–4.4)	3.3–3.5	4.0	3.5–4.8	3.9–4.7	4.6–5
Fat, g % DHA	5.8	5.9–7.8	6.2–6.6 0.25–0.34	6.7–8	8.3	7.8–9.2	6.8–7.1	8–10.1
Calcium, mg	38	169–203	201–219	144–156	181	169–203	200–226	251–274
Phosphorus, mg	20	93–116	110–122	78–86	99	93–116	112–128	137–152
Sodium, mEq	1.7	2.4–3	2.3–3.7	2.3–3.1	3.7	2.4–3	2.2–2.3	2.9–4.6
Potassium, mEq	2.3	3–4.5	3.1–4	3–3.6	3.75	3–4.5	4.8–4.9	3.8–5
Vitamin D, IU	3	177–254	183–360	116–227	6	177–254	187	228–450
Iron, mcg	0.2	0.7–2.4	2.2	1.2	0.1	0.7–2.3	0.9	2.7
Zinc, mcg	510	1558–1980	1826–1830	1395–1397	1407	1558–1980	1820–1890	2280–2283
% Mother's own milk	100	83–96	0	50	70	83–96	83–96	0

[a]Nutrients are expressed as a range of commercially available products.

[b]Preterm human milk. Values obtained from Pediatric Nutrition Product Guide 2017 (Abbott Nutrition, Columbus, Ohio), 162187/January 2017.

[c]Similac Human Milk Fortifier powder, Similac Human Milk Fortifier Concentrated Liquid, Similac Human Milk Fortifier Hydrolyzed Protein Concentrated Liquid (Abbott Nutrition, Columbus, Ohio); Enfamil Human Milk Fortifier Powder, Enfamil Human Milk Fortifier Acidified Liquid, Enfamil Human Milk Fortifier Liquid High Protein, Enfamil Human Milk Fortifier Liquid Standard Protein (Mead Johnson, Evansville, Indiana).

[d]Similac Special Care 24, Similac Special Care 24 High Protein (Abbott Nutrition, Columbus, Ohio); Enfamil Premature 24 Cal, Enfamil Premature 24 Cal HP (Mead Johnson, Evansville, Indiana).

[e]Similac Special Care 30 (Abbott Nutrition, Columbus, Ohio); Enfamil Premature 30 Cal (Mead Johnson, Evansville, Indiana).

[f]Prolacta Bioscience, Prolact+6 H²MF (Prolacta Bioscience, City of Industry, California).

[g]MCT = Medium Chain Triglycerides, MCT (Nestlé Health Science, Vevey, Switzerland), provides 115 calories and 14 g of fat per 15 mL. Values expressed dosing 2 mL/kg (provides an additional 3 kcal/oz when feeding 150 mL/kg/day of Human Milk with bovine fortifier[c]).

[h]Standard fortification (24 kcal/oz) Similac Human Milk Fortifier powder, Similac Human Milk Fortifier Concentrated Liquid, Similac Human Milk Fortifier Hydrolyzed Protein Concentrated Liquid + preterm discharge formula Similac Neosure (Abbott Nutrition, Columbus, Ohio).

[i]Protein values of human milk and fortified human milk analyzed with the base protein of 1.41 g/100 mL.

HM, Human milk.

circumference gain with no difference in neurodevelopment or NEC incidence.[77]

Cultural Considerations

Product selection is often dictated by unit-specific contracts and protocols, but cultural practices may exclude some infants from receiving specific products. There is a belief within Muslim communities that accepting donor human milk (or donor human milk fortifier) creates a kinship to the mother/infant who has donated, thereby generating concern for marrying with "milk siblings" later in life. For Muslim families living in Western countries, the European Council for Fatwa and Research has permitted preterm infants to receive donor human milk while in the NICU, citing that *kinship* specifically relates to *suckling* or nursing only from the breast.[93] Practices of Western milk banks and NICUs—pooling multiple donors, pasteurization, and fortification—all change the characteristics of donated breast milk, making it more permissible under Islamic Law.[94] Additionally, available preterm formulas and powdered fortifiers on the market are certified as kosher and halal; however, extensively hydrolyzed and acidified liquid bovine human milk fortifiers are not because pork enzymes are used in the hydrolysis process. Clinicians need to be conscientious of religious preferences when selecting enteral products. Providing parental education and adequate time for a family to discuss these medical interventions with their religious leaders may lead to accord in these decisions.

Individualized Fortification

Commercial bovine fortifier is typically added to maternal or donor milk to add 4 calories per ounce, otherwise known as standard fortification. Standard fortification assumes that human milk is uniform with regard to macronutrient content and energy density. However, the composition of human milk is known to vary depending on the length of gestation, stage of lactation, time of day, and even time within a feeding.[95–98] Most manufacturers provide nutrient analysis of prepared fortified human milk based on preterm human milk composition, which is higher in protein, fat, free amino acids, sodium, and zinc than is mature human milk in the first postnatal weeks.[99] Between postnatal weeks 1 and 2, preterm milk protein decreases from an average (±2 standard deviations) of 2.2 (0.3–4.1) g/100 mL to 1.5 (0.8–2.3) g/100 mL,[33] and the concentration of zinc follows a similar trend.[100–102] Assumed protein content provided with standard fortification is therefore overestimated compared with what the infant receives.[103] A recent study argues the need to consider the underlying nutrient variability of human milk with standardized fortification.[104] Using macronutrient analysis from their data set of banked human milk consisting of more than 400 individuals, addition of a commercial fortifier, which added 1.5 g protein/dL, was unable to meet target protein intakes of 4 g/kg/day in approximately 50% of mature milk samples if fed below volumes of 160 mL/kg/day. In response to the variation in maternal milk protein content and the individualized requirements for growth, two approaches have been described. "Adjustable fortification" allows clinicians to add protein in varying amounts based on basal urea nitrogen collected in routine labwork, whereas "targeted fortification" involves measuring exact quantities of protein, carbohydrate, and fat of human milk and supplementing with modular products.[105–109] Targeted fortification requires costly equipment, personnel, and time and is therefore not always feasible in clinical practice. Some studies are contradicting and have not shown any benefit with regard to weight gain,[67] and there is no consensus recommendation for frequency of analysis.[110] Several human milk analyzers are available to purchase for research, but only one is currently approved for clinical use (Miris Human Milk Analyzer, Miris, Uppsala, Sweden). Additionally, targeted fortification addresses only macronutrient variability, whereas the micronutrient content of human milk and donor human milk is equally variable. Maternal factors and diet influence quantities and composition of key nutrients such as fatty acids, fat-soluble vitamins, and carotenoids.[111] Although the most recent Cochrane Review suggests improvements in weight, length, and head circumference using adjustable or targeted fortification in comparison with standard fortification, further investigation is needed to identify the efficacy and efficiency of such interventions and to identify any benefit beyond short-term growth.[112] Future innovations in "lactoengineering" could potentially maximize the provision of human milk through use of a novel point-of-care, bedside device that passively concentrates human milk within a 2-hour time period.[113]

Probiotics

The intestinal microbiome plays a critical role in preterm infant health. Substantial high-grade evidence exists that multistrain, safe probiotic supplementation is associated with less NEC and less mortality in preterm infants.[114,115] Probiotics appear to be of most benefit when given in human milk or formula and include multiple strains. A few concerns remain regarding probiotic supplementation to preterm infants and account for why probiotics are not provided universally to preterm infants. These concerns include the potential for contamination. The manufacturing of probiotics is not a sterile procedure, and as a nutrient instead of a medication, probiotics are not held to the same federal requirements as a medication; contamination has led to infant death.[116] The lack of federal oversight also allows the potential for products to not contain the number or strains of bacteria advertised on the label, as was shown in a study of 16 samples in which only 1 matched its bifidobacterial label claim in all samples tested.[117] A third concern is that prebiotics may lead to cross-colonization of other infants in the NICU.[118,119] This may be beneficial but also may be of harm. Further investigation of this effect is warranted. A last consideration is that even when a safe multistrain product is available, the beneficial decrease in NEC and/or sepsis in some studies is reported for infants born more mature and larger (≥28 weeks' gestational age or ≥1000 g at birth).[120] Some NICU centers have a very low risk of NEC and/or sepsis in this population without the use of probiotics. Therefore the potential benefit may be small.

Vitamins, Minerals, and Osmolality

No method of standard fortification meets all the micronutrient requirements, and in some cases, excess amounts of certain nutrients are provided. Providing 1 mL of a commercial multivitamin product may supplement deficiencies but risks exceeding recommendations for both water- and fat-soluble vitamins.[121] Supplemental vitamin D is required when providing low volumes of fortified human milk in extremely small or fluid-restricted infants to ensure they receive 400 to 1000 IU/day.[76] Depending on the commercial fortifier, additional iron must be added separately to meet minimum requirements. Table 19.9 provides a comparison of select nutrients for the most commonly used products. Medications and nutritional supplements (including fortifiers) increase the osmolality of human milk.[122] In the 1970s, the AAP advised that the osmolality from milk and medication combined should not exceed 400 mOsm/L (450 mOsm/kg), based on little evidence that an increase in osmolality could lead to serious gastrointestinal events such as NEC. A recent systematic review identified no differences in feeding intolerance in the range of 300 to 500 mOsml/kg; however, large randomized controlled trials are needed to detect a difference in NEC.[123]

Preparation of Feeding

Fortified human milk and compounded formulas should be prepared in a dedicated, centralized room away from the bedside. Trained staff who are solely responsible for the preparation of human milk and formula can help ensure a safe, consistent, and accurate product. A decrease in nursing hours spent preparing infant feedings is observed when using a central milk-preparation room.[124] Moving the preparation of human milk away from the bedside allows more time for direct patient care and decreases risks of error.[125] Minimizing the handling of human milk is also key to prevent nutrient loss. From the time of human milk expression to the point at which it is fed to the baby, it is possible for milk to undergo up to a dozen steps including freezing, thawing, fortification, and container transfers into single-unit doses. Establishing a system to prevent milk misadministration is paramount. All institutions should have a policy to ensure the right milk is fed to the right baby, either by two-person verification or bar code scanning. Several professional organizations have resources available to outline best practices.[126,127]

Measures of Feeding Intolerance

Feeding intolerance in the preterm infant is poorly defined. Gastric residuals obtained prefeeding have historically been used as a measure of gastric emptying. Several studies including a randomized, controlled trial have not shown any increase in the incidence of NEC when gastric residuals are not routinely checked.[128–130] The practice of obtaining gastric residuals may delay feeding progression and increase the time taken to regain birth weight and achieve full feeds, thereby increasing parenteral nutrition days and potentially days of central access.[131] Therefore routine monitoring of gastric residuals is not recommended.

Unfortunately, other potential markers of feeding intolerance also have weaknesses. Abdominal girth is not a reliable measure of feed tolerance and has not been demonstrated in studies to be associated with clinical outcomes. Additionally, it may vary by 3.5 cm during one feeding cycle in a normal preterm infant.[132] Preterm infants have poor and sometimes retrograde motility, so emesis and even bilious emesis may only be markers of motility. Bloody emesis is more concerning as a sign of NEC and hematochezia. However, isolated bleeding due to gavage tube trauma or anal fissures may be the cause. With no definitive diagnosis for feeding intolerance, it is difficult to identify risk factors for it or outcomes associated with it. Other enteral feeding issues are outlined in Table 19.10.[128–130,133–142] Although NEC is the most feared and emergent gastrointestinal condition, there is no evidence that human milk fortification is associated with NEC.[77]

When to Modify Feeds

Given the evidence for positive neurodevelopmental outcomes associated with in-hospital growth, infants' weight should be measured daily and their feeding regimen adjusted to support growth goals. Several approaches to poor growth are outlined in Table 19.10. Few of the interventions have been described in the literature,[136–139,142] but they are common recommendations in clinical practices. High-calorie liquid preterm formula may be added as a supplement to unfortified human milk in place of a fortifier[139,140] or added directly to fortified maternal milk in varying amounts to increase the caloric density

Table 19.10 Common Enteral Feeding Issues in the Preterm Infant[128–130,133–142]

Enteral Feeding Problem	Recommendation

• Feeding intolerance
  • Abdominal distention
  • Emesis
  • Loose stools
	• Routine measurement of gastric residuals should be avoided[128–130]
	• Consider prolonging duration of bolus feeds with trial of continuous gastric feeds, if indicated
	• Shorter feeding interval (i.e., every 2 hours) may be considered
	• Minimize bacterial colonization of naso- or orogastric tubing
	  • Change feeding tubes at appropriate intervals
	  • Follow best-practice guidelines for the preparation and administration of human milk and formula

• Metabolic bone disease
  • Rickets
  • Fractures
	• Minimize prescription of diuretics and corticosteroid therapy
	• Maximize calcium and phosphorus provision with high-mineral human milk fortifier and preterm formula[133]
	• Provide 400–1000 IU/day vitamin D

• Bloody stools	• Routine testing for guaiac-positive stool is not recommended • Visible blood in stool warrants further investigation • Minimize bacterial colonization of human milk, formula, and naso- or orogastric tubing by following safe handling practices • If milk protein intolerance suspected, recommend milk protein elimination in maternal diet and use fortifier/formula that is a hydrolysate or amino acid–based
• Hypoglycemia	• Consider continuous feeds • Cornstarch is not an appropriate therapy for neonates

• Poor growth	• Provide enteral feeds via bolus with the shortest duration tolerated
	• Treat laboratory abnormalities, i.e., metabolic acidosis or hyponatremia, if present
	• Ensure protein goals of 3.5–4.3 g/kg/day are met
	• If meeting protein goals, increase caloric provision; consider increase in volume of feeds if infant is not fluid sensitive[142]
	• Other methods to increase the calories per ounce of human milk beyond standard fortification include:
	  • Additional lipid source: human milk cream, MCT oil[136–138]
	  • Addition of formula: transitional powdered formula, term liquid concentrate, preterm liquid formula[136,139,140]

• Oral aversion	• Focus on methods to prevent oral aversion:
	  • Encourage nonnutritive sucking
	  • Develop and follow a policy that utilizes cue-based, not volume-driven feeding
	• Recommend a multidisciplinary approach[134,135,141]

MCT, Medium-chain triglyceride.

beyond 24 calories per ounce. However, these methods do displace high volumes of human milk and may be discouraged in infants whose mothers are producing sufficient milk volumes to feed their infant.

Methods of Feeding

Preterm infants have limitations in their ability to orally feed and therefore commonly rely on gavage tubes for enteral nutrition. Gavage feeding for preterm infants is provided either to the stomach or small intestine. If feeding is transpyloric, the feeds cannot be bolused, but if feeding is gastric, the feeds may be bolused or extended over time and even given continuously. Although transpyloric or small-intestine feeding is sometimes the preferred method of feeding due to gastroesophageal reflux or feeding intolerance, this method of feeding has no demonstrated benefit, is associated with slower growth, and raises concerns about medication delivery to the small intestine instead of the stomach. Therefore, gastric gavage feeding is the evidence-based method to feed preterm infants who do not reliably feed orally. Additionally, feeding should be given by bolus, because increased duration of feeding leads to higher loss of nutrients in the feeding tube.

Oral feeding ability develops between 34 and 44 weeks' PMA in preterm infants and is negatively correlated with the degree of maturity. Additionally, respiratory, cardiovascular, or neurologic disease may delay oral feeding ability or endurance.[143] Recent research has focused on investigation of the best method to support infants who have a delay in oral feeding achievement. To continue hospitalization, to place a gastrostomy tube to facilitate discharge, or to discharge with a nasogastric tube are practices under review.[144,145] Infant outcomes, parental satisfaction, and cost are important considerations as these practices are compared.

Enteral Feeding Postdischarge

The World Health Organization and the AAP recommend exclusive breastfeeding for the first 6 months and continuation of breastfeeding for at least 12 months. Exclusive breastfeeding or feeding unfortified breast milk via bottle may not provide enough nutrition to support growth of the preterm infant, especially for those discharged from the hospital prior to term who have not yet developed the ability to regulate their volume to compensate for differences in energy density. It is difficult for mothers to sustain lactation throughout the duration of their infant's hospital stay; therefore care must be taken to support the mothers' decisions to feed the baby at breast while prescribing a nutrition regimen at discharge consisting mostly of human milk that also meets the needs of the rapidly growing infant. The situation is further complicated by accumulated nutrient deficits, medical comorbidities that may affect oral feedings, and individualized requirements to sustain current growth or meet needs for "catching up." Additional nutrients, provided as extra formula or fortifier, are typically provided via a bottle; however, cup or finger feeding is also described in the literature for infants who are exclusively breastfed.[146,147] One small study reported no differences in growth at 12 to 15 months in infants fed human milk complemented by two to three feeds per day of a 22 kcal/oz preterm discharge formula compared with infants fed only a diet of preterm discharge formula.[148] Only a few randomized controlled trials have evaluated growth with fortification of human milk after hospital discharge. One group of investigators found better weight, length, and head circumference growth in infants weighing <1250 g at birth, all maintained at 1 year, and better visual acuity at 9 months when the infant was provided with a commercial human milk fortifier for partial feedings from discharge to 52 weeks' corrected age.[146,149] Two other trials did not detect a difference in sustained growth at 1 year but used a different commercial fortifier at a much lower dose.[150] The AAP suggests that although fortification at discharge is now the standard of care, the duration and concentration should be individualized to maintain an appropriate growth trajectory.[76] Continuing multinutrient fortification for 12 weeks, or at least until 52 weeks' postterm equivalent age, are considerations in infants with appropriate growth and sufficient volumes of maternal milk.[146,149]

For exclusively formula-fed infants, a preterm-discharge formula containing more protein, calories, and minerals than a standard formula is commonly used (energy density approximately 73 vs. 67 kcal/100 mL). However, with available evidence, a Cochrane meta-analysis found no significant improvements in growth parameters or bone mineral content at 12 months' follow-up for infants who were fed preterm-discharge formulas compared with standard formula, and there was no difference in the Bayley Scales Mental or Psychomotor Development Index at 18 months postterm.[151] Thus there is limited evidence to support routine recommendation of preterm-discharge formulas. Infants fed preterm formula compared with standard formula also did not show any significant differences in weight, length, and head circumference up to 12 months, but differences appeared at 12 months for weight and at 18 months for head circumference. A large systematic review also supports the suggestion that providing a higher protein-energy ratio ≥2.5 to 3.0 at discharge seems to have a positive improvement in anthropometrics at 12 months; however, significant heterogeneity was observed among the studies included, and evidence is therefore limited.[152] Supplying extra energy and nutrients postdischarge has previously raised concern for the metabolic and cardiovascular health of preterm infants with risk of rapid "catch-up" growth; however, the potential for improved neurodevelopment may outweigh such risk and favors an optimal growth trajectory. Preterm formulas can provide excessive amounts of nutrients when taken ad libitum, specifically fat-soluble vitamins, calcium, and phosphorus, and clinicians should refer to product-specific guides for a safe weight limit, generally between 2.5 to 3.6 kg, to avoid toxicities.[153] If a preterm formula is indicated postdischarge, outpatient access may be limited by state contracts for the Special Supplemental Nutrition Program for Women, Infants, and Children (WIC), insurance coverage, or reliance on company-specific discharge programs. So far, meta-analyses and at least one other recent randomized, controlled control trial show no difference in neurodevelopmental outcomes with preterm or preterm-discharge formula feeding for preterm infants after hospital discharge compared with term formula.[151,154] However, infants discharged prior to term age and those with significant neurologic, respiratory, or cardiac disease are likely to need nutrient supplementation at discharge. Enriched feeds are needed until the infant has the maturity and endurance to "feed to grow." This occurs for most infants between 40 and 52 weeks' PMA. Infants with health limitations may need a longer duration of nutrient supplementation. Regardless of the feeding plan at the time discharge, ensuring parent education to prevent formula preparation and/or breast milk fortification errors is necessary given the high rate of mixing errors described.[155,156] A plan for early follow-up with a multidisciplinary team is also critical to address nutritional and other medical concerns in a timely manner.[155]

Long-Term Outcomes

Enteral nutrition practices are not only to optimize in-hospital outcomes such as avoiding NEC and demonstrating good head growth;

Table 19.11 In-Hospital and Prior to Term Corrected Age Nutrition and Growth Patterns Associated With Improved Neurodevelopmental Outcomes in Very Preterm, VLBW Infants[158–162,164–175]

Age at Evaluation	In-Hospital Growth Patterns Associated With Improved Neurodevelopment	In-Hospital Human Milk Intakes Associated With Improved Neurodevelopment
18–30 months	• Less decrease in weight *z*-score from birth to 36 weeks • Higher weight gain and head circumference gain from birth to hospital discharge • Highest quartile of weight gain velocity through hospitalization • Higher linear slopes of growth in weight, length, BMI, and head circumference from 1 week to term • Conserved head growth from birth to hospital discharge	• For every 10 mL/kg/day increase in breast milk
4–11 years	• Increasing SD scores for weight and head circumference from birth to discharge • Higher weight gain, length gain, and higher fat-free mass gain from birth to discharge	• More than 80% human milk feeds in first month • Human milk at the time of discharge • Greater than 50% of feeds as human milk in first 28 days • Duration of mother's milk feeding • Greater than 30% human milk in neonatal ward • Received human milk in neonatal ward
Adolescence/young adulthood	• Faster growth from birth to term age	• Higher percent of mother's milk during hospitalization

BMI, Body mass index; *VLBW*, very low birth weight.

the expectation would be that in-hospital enteral nutrition delivery would be associated with improvements in long-term outcomes. The most studied and arguably most important outcome is survival without moderate or severe neurodevelopmental delay. Meta-analysis of the evidence regarding neurodevelopmental outcomes has been performed in regard to several practices for preterm infant enteral feeding. No significant difference was demonstrated in a meta-analysis of the existing literature comparing preterm infant feeding of donor human milk versus formula, preterm infant feeding of fortified human milk versus unfortified milk, or preterm formula versus term formula for the preterm infant.[32,53,77] A meta-analysis also was performed measuring long-term neurodevelopment with preterm infant enteral intake of polyunsaturated fatty acids, with no significant improvement observed.[157] The SIFT study comparing slow versus rapid volume advancement of feeds has published 24-month outcomes, and the results showed no difference in survival without moderate or severe neurodevelopmental disability or secondary outcomes such as confirmed or suspected late-onset sepsis, NEC, and cerebral palsy.[59] In fact, only six factors associated with preterm infants' enteral nutrition were associated positively with neurodevelopment—weight gain, head growth, length growth, body mass index gain, and fat-free mass gain during hospitalization and mother's milk feeding.[158–172] Studies demonstrating neurodevelopmental outcomes associated with weight gain and head growth and associated with mother's milk feeding are shown in Table 19.11.[158–162,164–175] These associations of both mother's milk intake and growth trajectory with preterm infant neurodevelopment outcomes have been described by Rozé et al. as "the apparent breastfeeding paradox," because preterm infants receiving formula exhibit a higher growth velocity than do those receiving mother's milk.[167] Consequently, sustaining mother's milk feeding with nutrient supplementation as needed to sustain adequate growth appears to be the best enteral nutrition practice to optimize neurodevelopment. Other benefits of breastfeeding for full-term infants are provided in Table 19.12. Although not studied in preterm infants, until those studies are performed, preterm infants are assumed to obtain equal if not greater long-term benefit from breastfeeding.[26]

Table 19.12 Long-Term Outcomes With Breastfeeding Duration for Full-Term Infants[26]

Ever Breastfeeding 23% ↓ Otitis media 31% ↓ Inflammatory bowel disease 40% ↓ Type 2 diabetes mellitus 64% ↓ Gastrointestinal infections 72% ↓ Lower respiratory infections	>2 Months Breastfeeding 52% ↓ Celiac disease 3 Months Breastfeeding 26% ↓ Asthma w/o family history 40% ↓ Asthma with family history
>1 Month Breastfeeding 36% ↓ SIDS	>4 Months Breastfeeding 74% ↓ RSV bronchiolitis
Early cessation: Breastfeeding 4–6 months versus breastfeeding ≥6 months 1.95 × ↑ Recurrent otitis media 4.27 × ↑ Lower respiratory tract infection	

RSV, Respiratory syncytial virus; *SIDS*, sudden infant death syndrome.

Conclusion

In summary, enteral nutrition is by far the preferred method for nourishing the preterm infant. Using human milk for feeding and standardizing advancement of enteral nutrition practices can reduce the instances of NEC and achieve faster attainment of full feeds. This reduces the need for parenteral nutrition and its associated complications including central access and risk of infection, gut atrophy, and liver dysfunction; minimizing such complications and maximizing growth potential are favorable from a neurodevelopmental standpoint. At this time, an extensive literature review for enteral nutrition practices has revealed more questions than answers and calls for high-quality studies to assess the following: (1) protein and energy requirements in the preterm infant, specifically "high protein" fortification and formulas; (2) benefit versus cost of targeted fortification practices; (3) use of probiotics in the high-risk infant; and (4) an optimal feeding plan at discharge that provides adequate macro- and micronutrients to support the rapidly growing infant while minimizing risk of "overgrowth" and metabolic consequences.

CHAPTER 20 Parenteral Nutrition in Neonates

Stephanie M. Barr, Laura Cummings

KEY POINTS

1. Parenteral nutrition is a necessary component of the nutritional and medical management of the premature infant.
2. The fluid, macronutrient, and micronutrient requirements are unique to the premature infant due to their transition from the intrauterine to extrauterine environment, critically ill status, and lack of nutrient stores.
3. Understanding how to properly calculate a premature infant's parenteral nutrition requirements is critical to ensure adequacy of the administered solution. The increased risk of deficiency and toxicity in this population makes the accuracy of these calculations paramount.
4. It is necessary to consider product compatibilities, contamination, and availability when ordering parenteral nutrition.
5. Utilization of a multidisciplinary team is recommended for management of parenteral nutrition and its associated complications.

Indications for Parenteral Nutrition

If the gut works, use it is the characteristic recommendation of nutrition administration for the hospitalized patient. However, in the high-risk neonate there are many instances where the gut does *not* work, requiring utilization of parenteral nutrition (PN). Parenteral nutrition is a critical component of nutrition and medical intervention in the neonatal intensive care unit (NICU).

Appropriate initiation of PN is required to support appropriate growth in the acute and long-term stages of a premature infant's NICU course.[1,2] Early administration of a nutritionally complete PN solution promotes positive nitrogen balance,[3] reduces hyperglycemia,[3] and minimizes electrolyte and mineral imbalances associated with inadequate nutrient intake.[4]

Indications of initiation and length of parenteral nutrition use vary between institutions. Very premature infants (born at ≤32 weeks' gestation) and very low birth weight infants (born at ≤1500 g) require PN support due to complications of prematurity. Other indications of parenteral nutrition use are discussed in Table 20.1.

Initiation of "starter" or "early" parenteral nutrition within the first hours of life promotes an anabolic state and is a safe practice for very low birth weight infants.[5,6] Starter parenteral nutrition contains only dextrose, amino acids, and calcium; full parenteral nutrition should be initiated within the first 24 to 48 hours of life to meet the complete nutritional requirements of the premature infant. An example of parenteral nutrition composition progression can be seen in Table 20.2.

Nutrition Requirements in Parenteral Nutrition

Premature infants have unique nutrition requirements that necessitate specialized parenteral nutrition compositions. A summary of parenteral nutrition requirements from the most frequently cited references can be found in the following sections and in Tables 20.3, 20.4, 20.5, and 20.6.

Fluid

Fluid management is a challenging component of early-life neonatal care because requirements must be balanced with expected losses and rapidly changing serum electrolyte status. Weight loss is expected within the first 1 to 2 weeks of life due to the transition to the extrauterine environment and contraction of the extracellular fluid. As illustrated in Table 20.7, extracellular fluid volume increases with the degree of prematurity, resulting in greater expected weight loss after birth.[7,8]

Term infants typically experience 5% to 10% weight loss from birth weight in the first 7 to 10 days of life; preterm infants may experience up to 15% weight loss and may take up to 14 days to regain birth weight. More significant weight loss and a longer time to regain birth weight may be concerning for improper fluid and nutrition management.

Premature infants have increased fluid requirements due to elevated energy needs, high rates of insensible water loss, and immature renal function. Insensible water losses are caused from respiration and immature skin membranes but may be reduced with administration of antenatal steroids[9] and use of double-wall incubators.[10] Premature infants have an impaired ability to concentrate urine due to a reduced nephron count and immature tubular function causing decreased glomerular filtration; this puts them at an increased risk of dehydration and electrolyte abnormalities.[11]

Many disease states may necessitate modifications to fluid administration so as to not contribute to disease progression while preventing dehydration[12]; disease states include patent ductus arteriosus[13] and bronchopulmonary dysplasia.[14,15]

A gradual increase of fluid intake is recommended in preterm and term neonates after birth.[10] The smaller and more premature the infant, the higher the fluid requirements. An example of fluid progression in neonates is depicted in Table 20.8.

Energy

Energy requirements of preterm infants receiving parenteral nutrition are determined by the basal metabolic rate, growth requirements, and severity of illness. Meeting energy goals is necessary to meet

Table 20.1 Indications of Parenteral Nutrition Use

PREMATURITY	
Gestational age ≤32 weeks Birth weight ≤1500 g	Early introduction of PN is recommended for the proper nutritional management of premature infants. Early initiation of PN reduces time to regain birth weight, reduces weight loss after birth, and may improve total growth within the NICU stay.[2,104]
Umbilical arterial or venous catheter	The impact of umbilical catheters on intestinal perfusion has been disputed in the literature.[105] However, the practice of withholding enteral feedings while umbilical lines are present remains common due to the believed increased risk of necrotizing enterocolitis.[106]
ACQUIRED GASTROINTESTINAL DISEASES	
NEC	Following NEC diagnosis, PN is required to allow bowel rest and recovery during medical and/or surgical intervention.
SIP	Management of SIP necessitates cessation of the gastrointestinal tract use during medical and/or surgical management.
	Early postnatal dexamethasone[107] and maternal chorioamnionitis[108] have been associated with increased risk of SIP. The correlation of indomethacin administration and SIP occurrence has been debated in the literature.[109,110] Neonates with increased risk for SIP may have more conservative EN progression and thus may require more PN.
CONGENITAL GASTROINTESTINAL DISEASES	
Gastroschisis	Prior to and immediately following closure of the abdominal cavity necessitates use of PN. Progression to EN varies, but a standardized approach to EN advancement has been associated with improved outcomes.[111]
Omphalocele	Omphaloceles are often associated with other malformations, adding further complexity to this diagnosis. Use of PN is always indicated in this complex patient population.
Bowel obstruction Bowel atresia Hirschsprung disease	PN is required pre- and postoperatively to meet nutrition requirements for the high-risk neonate when it is not safe to provide enteral nutrition.
MALABSORPTION SYNDROMES	
SBS	PN is required in the management of infants with SBS. Length of time to wean from PN to EN is related to both small bowel length and percentage of expected bowel remaining based on gestational age. Gonzalez-Hernandez's model found that infants who lost 25%–50% of small bowel required an average of 1 year of PN; infants who lost 51%–75% small bowel required an average of 2 years of PN support.[112]
Cystic fibrosis with meconium ileus	A meconium ileus is frequently the first clinical manifestation of cystic fibrosis and occurs in about 20% of cases.[113] This diagnosis and presentation requires PN because infants are unable to receive EN prior to surgical intervention.
CONDITIONS OF HEMODYNAMIC INSTABILITY	
CHD	Concern for increased risk of NEC in patients with CHD due to mesenteric circulatory insufficiency may result in prolonged NPO periods with PN management in early life. A growing body of literature suggests that early enteral nutrition is safe in infants with CHD,[114,115] but use of PN in this patient population remains common.
PDA	Fluid restriction in management of PDAs often results in decreased energy and protein intake and may influence postnatal growth outcomes.[116] Use of nonsteroidal antiinflammatory drugs (e.g., indomethacin, ibuprofen) or requirement of surgical ligation may result in a patient being made NPO. Infants with large PDAs may have higher risk of necrotizing enterocolitis and feeding intolerance.[117]
Hypoxic ischemic encephalopathy	Due to critical illness and presumption of poor gut perfusion during therapeutic hypothermia, PN is required to meet the nutritional requirements of these infants. Although minimal enteral nutrition may be practiced during therapeutic hypothermia,[118,119] it is not sufficient to meet the nutrient requirements of this population.
ECMO	Use of ECMO in neonates with cardiac and respiratory failure requires PN to meet nutrient intake goals and avoid cumulative protein deficits.[120]
PPHN	Due to the severity of illness, PN is indicated in infants with PPHN. Providing appropriate PN to meet nutrition requirements of the critically ill infant is associated with lower mortality in this patient population.[121]
OTHER	
Chylothorax	Management of severe chylothorax often requires PN,[122] which allows for healing of the thoracic duct by preventing the formation of chylous fluid. Use of a midchain triglyceride-rich intravenous fat emulsion may be beneficial in PN management of chylothorax.[123]

CHD, Congenital heart disease; *ECMO*, extracorporeal membrane oxygenation therapy; *EN*, enteral nutrition; *NEC*, necrotizing enterocolitis; *NICU*, neonatal intensive care unit; *NPO*, nil per os; *PDA*, patent ductus arteriosus; *PN*, parenteral nutrition; *PPHN*, persistent pulmonary hypertension of the newborn; *SBS*, short bowel syndrome; *SIP*, spontaneous intestinal perforation.

Table 20.2 Parenteral Nutrition Composition Progression in the First Week of Life

	First Days of Life	Transition	Growth
Fluid (mL/kg)	80–120	100–140	140–160
Energy (kcal/kg)	45–55	60–85	90–120
Protein (g/kg)	1–2	2–3	3–4
Fat (g/kg)	0.5–2	1–2	2–3

Table 20.3 Energy and Macronutrient Recommendations

	ASPEN[124,125]		Koletzko[126]	ESPGHAN[19,24,35,127]	
	Preterm	Term	Preterm	Preterm	Term
ENERGY (KCAL/KG/DAY)					
Initial	—	—	60–80	45–55	Calculate needs using Schofield's equation
Goal	—	—	≥100	90–120	
Dextrose (mg/kg/min)					
Initial	6–8	6–8	—	4–8	2.5–5
Goal	10–14	10–14	—	8–10	5–10
Minimum	—	—	4	4	2.5
Maximum	14–18	14–18	7–12	12	12
Protein (g/kg/day)					
Initial	1–3	2.5–3	1.5–3	1.5	1
Goal	3–4	2.5–3	—	2.5–3.5	1–3
Maximum	3–4	—	4	3.5	3
SOY-BASED INTRAVENOUS LIPID EMULSION (G/KG/DAY)					
Initial	0.5–1	0.5–1	Start by DOL 2	Start by DOL 2	—
Goal	3	2.5–3	2–3	3–4 (pending type of lipid emulsion)	
Minimum	0.5–1 g/kg/day	0.5–1 g/kg/day	—	Minimum linoleic acid intake of 0.25 g/kg/day	Minimum linoleic acid intake of 0.1 g/kg/day
Maximum	Infusion rate of 0.15 g/kg/hour	Infusion rate of 0.15 g/kg/hour	—	4 g/kg/day	

ASPEN, American Society for Parenteral and Enteral Nutrition; *DOL*, day of life; *ESPGHAN*, European Society for Paediatric Gastroenterology. Hepatology and Nutrition.

Table 20.4 Macromineral Recommendations

	ASPEN[124,125]		Koletzko[126]	ESPGHAN[47,53]	
	Preterm	Term	Preterm	Preterm	Term
CALCIUM MEQ/KG/DAY (MMOL/KG/DAY)					
Initial	—	—	2 (1)	1.6–4 (0.8–2)	—
Goal	2–4 (1–2)	0.5–4 (0.25–2)	3.2–5 (1.6–2.5)	3.2–10 (1.6–3.5)	1–3 (0.8–1.5)
PHOSPHORUS (MMOL/KG/DAY)					
Initial	—	—	1	1–2	—
Goal	1–2	0.5–2	1.6–2.5	1.6–3.5	0.7–1.3
Calcium:phosphorus ratio	Use with caution in prescribing calcium and phosphorus related to compatibility		1–1.5 (mg)	0.8–1 (molar) in incomplete PN 1.3 (molar) in full PN	
MAGNESIUM MG/KG/DAY (MMOL/KG/DAY)					
Initial	—	—	0–3 (0–0.12)	2.5–5 (0.1–0.2)	—
Goal	3.6–6 (0.15–0.25)	3.6–6 (0.15–0.25)	7–10 (0.3–0.4)	5–7.5 (0.2–0.3)	2.4–5 (0.1–0.2)
IRON (MG/KG/DAY)					
Goal	—	—	0–0.25	0.2–0.25	0.05–0.1
				Should not be given in short-term PN (<3 weeks); enteral administration is preferential Max: 5 mg/day	

ASPEN, American Society for Parenteral and Enteral Nutrition; *ESPGHAN*, European Society for Paediatric Gastroenterology. Hepatology and Nutrition; *PN*, parenteral nutrition.

growth goals and improve clinical and developmental outcomes in neonates. Research has shown that meeting ideal nutrition administration in the first week of life is associated with improved growth and neurodevelopment in preterm infants.[2,16,17] Additionally, achieving energy intake goals in the first week of life may decrease the risk of adverse outcomes from critical illness in extremely low birth weight infants.[18] Excess energy administration may cause hyperglycemia, which may increase the risk of infection, impaired liver function, and long-term metabolic consequences and thus should be avoided.

Energy provided should promote appropriate, symmetric growth. A commonly used goal for weight gain is 17 to 20 g/kg/day.[19] A full discussion of growth goals and assessment can be found in the nutrition assessment chapter (Chapter 22).

Table 20.5 Vitamin Recommendations

	ASPEN[124,125]			ESPGHAN[54]	
	<1 kg	1–<3 kg	≥3 kg	Preterm	Term
Dose	1.5 mL	3.25 mL	5 mL		
Vitamin A	207 mcg	449 mcg	690 mcg	227–455 mcg/kg/day	150–300 mcg/kg/day
Vitamin D	120 IU	260 IU	400 IU	80–400 IU/kg/day	40–150 IU/kg/day
Vitamin E	2 mg	5 mg	7 mg	2.8–3.5 mg/kg/day	≤11 mg/day
				Monitor if receiving IV fat emulsions containing vitamin E. Max: 11 mg/day	
Vitamin K	60 mcg	130 mcg	200 mcg	10 mcg/kg/day	
Thiamine (B_1)	0.4 mg	0.8 mg	1.2 mg	0.35–0.5 mg/kg/day	
Riboflavin (B_2)	0.4 mg	0.9 mg	1.4 mg	0.15–0.2 mg/kg/day	
Niacin (B_3)	5 mg	11 mg	17 mg	4–6.8 mg/kg/day	
Pyridoxine (B_6)	0.3 mg	0.7 mg	1 mg	0.15–0.2 mg/kg/day	
Folate	42 mcg	91 mcg	140 mcg	56 mcg/kg/day	
Cobalamin (B_{12})	0.3 mcg	0.7 mcg	1 mcg	0.3 mcg/kg/day	
Biotin	6 mcg	13 mcg	20 mcg	5–8 mcg/kg/day	
Pantothenic acid	1.5 mg	3.3 mg	5 mg	2.5 mg/kg/day	
Vitamin C	24 mg	52 mg	80 mg	15–25 mg/kg/day	

ASPEN, American Society for Parenteral and Enteral Nutrition; *ESPGHAN*, European Society for Paediatric Gastroenterology, Hepatology and Nutrition; *IV*, intravenous.

Table 20.6 Trace Element Recommendations

	ASPEN[124,125]		Koletzko[126]	ESPGHAN[53]	
	Preterm	Term	Preterm	Preterm	Term
Zinc (mcg/kg/day)	400	250	400	400–500	250 (0–3 months) 100 (3–12 months)
				Max: 5 mg/day	
Copper (mcg/kg/day)	20	20	40	40	20
				Max: 0.5 mg/day	
Selenium (mcg/kg/day)	2	2	5–7	7	2–3
				Max: 100 mcg/day	
Manganese (mcg/kg/day)	1	1	1	Long term PN: ≤1 mcg/kg/day Max: 50 mcg/day	
Chromium (mcg/kg/day)	0.05–0.3	0.5	0.05–0.3	Addition to PN not required due to known PN contamination Max: 5 mcg/kg/day	
Molybdenum (mcg/kg/day)	—	—	0.25	1	0.25
				Max: 5 mcg/day	
Iodine (mcg/kg/day)	—	—	10	1–10	1

ASPEN, American Society for Parenteral and Enteral Nutrition; *ESPGHAN*, European Society for Paediatric Gastroenterology, Hepatology and Nutrition; *PN*, parenteral nutrition.

Table 20.7 Variation in Total Body Water Composition and Extracellular Fluid (ECF) Volume at Birth in Relation to Gestational Age and Body Weight (BW)[8]

Gestational Age (Weeks)	BW (g)	Total Body Water (%BW)	ECF Volume (%BW)
23–27	500–1000	85–90	60–70
28–32	1000–2000	82–85	50–60
36–40	>2500	71–76	~40

Macronutrients

Protein

Protein is required for growth in the preterm infant. Reaching protein goals in the first days of life may lessen hyperglycemia and reduce the need for insulin therapy.[20,21] Achieving protein goals in this critical window may also improve postnatal growth and neurodevelopmental outcomes in preterm infants.[22,23]

Protein requirements of parenterally fed infants are lower than those of infants receiving enteral nutrition due to the bypassing of

Table 20.8 Sample Fluid Progression (mL/kg/day)[a]

	DOL 1	DOL 2	DOL 3	DOL 4	DOL 5
Term neonate	60–80	80–100	100–120	120–140	140+
Preterm, BW >1500 g	80–100	100–120	120–140	140+	140+
Preterm, BW 1000–1500 g	100–120	120–140	140–160	140–160+	140–160+
Preterm, BW <1000 g	120	120–140	140–160	160–180	160–180

[a]Postnatal fluid requirements are highly dependent on treatment conditions and environmental factors. Certain clinical conditions may afford modifications of daily fluid intakes.
BW, Body weight; *DOL*, day of life.

Table 20.9 Amino Acid Solutions Available in the United States

STANDARD	
Aminosyn II	Hospira
Clinisol	Baxter
FreAmine III	B. Braun
Plenamine	B. Braun
Travasol	Baxter
PEDIATRIC/NEONATAL	
Premasol	Baxter
Aminosyn PF	Hospira
TrophAmine	B. Braun
LIVER DISEASE	
HepatAmine	B. Braun

intestinal uptake and utilization of amino acids. Protein administration should not exceed 4 g/kg/day, because exceedingly high protein has not been shown to be an effective therapy in improving any nutritional or clinical outcomes.

Preterm infants have altered metabolic requirements and have a higher need for conditionally essential amino acids including arginine, glycine, proline, tyrosine, cysteine, and glutamine.[24] Specialized amino acid solutions are used to meet preterm infants' parenteral needs (Table 20.9).

Carbohydrates

Dextrose (D-glucose) is the source of carbohydrate in parenteral nutrition and provides 3.4 calories per gram. Dextrose should be given at a level to meet energy needs while preventing excessive administration and hyperglycemia. Table 20.10 reviews dextrose and glucose infusion rate (GIR) recommendations and associated line requirements. Minimum GIRs have been estimated to ensure that organs that preferentially use glucose for energy (the brain, renal medulla, and erythrocytes) are able to receive a sufficient amount.

Excessive dextrose administration can cause hyperglycemia, which is associated with an increased risk of multiple morbidities including poor postnatal growth,[25] severe intraventricular hemorrhage,[26] increased need for respiratory support,[27] and poor neurologic outcomes.[28] Hyperglycemia is also associated with a higher rate of mortality among preterm infants.[28]

There may be a risk of long-term metabolic consequences of persistent hyperglycemia and high glucose infusion rate in the neonatal period. In pediatric studies, beta-cell dysfunction has been observed in children with prolonged hyperglycemia in the critically ill state.[29] Excess glucose administration causes lipogenesis and fat deposition; this may cause steatosis and impair liver function. This metabolic outcome may contribute to development of parenteral nutrition–related liver disease in the preterm infant.

Providing a balanced parenteral administration that meets carbohydrate, lipid, and amino acid goals helps minimize hyperglycemia and electrolyte abnormalities in preterm infants.[21,30]

Lipids

Lipids provide energy and essential fatty acids and aid in delivery of lipid-soluble vitamins. Infants receiving parenteral nutrition should receive 25% to 50% of nonprotein calories from a lipid source. Initiation of lipids in the first 2 days of life is believed to be safe and well tolerated in very low birth weight infants.[31,32] Additionally, early initiation of intravenous lipid emulsions has been shown to improve growth in the neonatal population and may reduce the incidence of retinopathy of prematurity.[33,34]

There is little research on the ideal dosing of intravenous lipid emulsions in the first days of life or in infants with sepsis or infection. In critically ill infants, monitoring of plasma triglycerides and adjustment of lipid infusion rates is recommended. An example of dosing of commonly discussed intravenous lipid emulsion products in the United States can be seen in Table 20.11.

Intralipid is a 20% lipid emulsion, is entirely soybean-oil based, and provides 10 calories per gram of fat. Intralipid is highly concentrated in essential fatty acids, thus allowing a minimum dose of 0.5–1 g/kg/day to meet essential fatty acid requirements. This product has historically been the only intravenous lipid emulsion product used in the neonatal population in the United States. Although Intralipid is effective in providing nonprotein calories and essential fatty acids, prolonged use is associated with negative clinical outcomes including increased oxidative stress, pulmonary vascular resistance, impaired pulmonary gas exchange, and increased rates of infection.[35]

Table 20.10 NICU Dextrose Administration

	%Dextrose	Glucose Infusion Rate	Line Requirements
First days of life	5%–10%	Minimum 4–8 mg/kg/min[127]	Peripheral
Maintenance PN	10%–12.5%	Target 8–10 mg/kg/min[127]	Peripheral
Increased dextrose requirements due to hypoglycemia/ energy requirements/fluid restrictions, etc.	13%–20%	Maximum 15 mg/kg/min[128]	Central

NICU, Neonatal intensive care unit; *PN*, parenteral nutrition.

Table 20.11 Example of Neonatal Intravenous Lipid Emulsion Dosing

	Composition	Minimum Dose to Meet EFA Requirements	Growing Preterm Infant	Growing Term Infant	Maximum Safe Dose
SMOFlipid (g/kg)	Soybean oil (30%)	2	2.5–3.5	2–3	4
	MCT oil (30%)				
	Olive oil (25%)				
	Fish oil (15%)				
Intralipid (g/kg)	Soybean oil	0.5–1	1.5–3		4
Omegaven (g/kg)	Fish oil	Not intended to meet EFA requirements	1		1
			0.5–0.75 in setting of hypertriglyceridemia		

Infusion rate should be <0.15 g/kg/hour
EFA, Essential fatty acid; *MCT*, medium chain triglyceride.

Omegaven is an entirely fish oil–based intravenous lipid emulsion that is approved for use in neonatal populations for treatment of parenteral nutrition associated cholestasis (PNAC), as diagnosed by a direct bilirubin level ≥2 mg/dL. Use of Omegaven is effective in reversing PNAC in neonates requiring prolonged parenteral nutrition administration.[36] Although Omegaven is an intravenous lipid emulsion, it is intended to be used for PNAC management and treatment; Omegaven does not contain sufficient essential fatty acids to meet the neonate's requirements.

SMOFlipid is a mixed oil lipid emulsion that has recently been approved for use in neonates in the United States by the Food and Drug Administration. SMOFlipid is a 20% lipid emulsion composed of 30% soybean oil, 30% midchain triglycerides, 25% olive oil, and 15% fish oil; and it provides 10 calories per gram of fat. Due to the decreased content of the essential fatty acid–rich soybean oil, a minimum dose of 2 g/kg/day is needed to avoid essential fatty acid deficiency.[37] Composite intravenous lipid emulsions such as SMOFlipid may have fewer proinflammatory components, thus causing less immune suppression, and a greater antioxidant effect than intravenous lipid emulsions composed of only soybean oil, such as Intralipid.[35] A reduction in phytosterol content in mixed-oil lipid emulsions has been proposed as a possible reasoning for the hepatoprotective effects of mixed-oil and soy lipid emulsions.[38] However, the reduction of cholestasis in preterm infants due to SMOFlipid use has been inconclusive in the neonatal population.[39–42] The medium chain triglyceride (MCT) content of SMOFlipid is beneficial because it has faster plasma clearance, more rapid oxidation, and less dependency on carnitine for beta oxidation. The increased vitamin E content in SMOFlipid may have antiinflammatory benefits but may require increased monitoring of serum alpha-tocopherol levels to prevent hypervitaminosis. Although further research must be completed to discern the full impact of SMOFlipid on neonates, there are significant potential benefits related to SMOFlipid use in this population, including reduction of PNAC, improved growth, reduction of retinopathy of prematurity, and reduction of bronchopulmonary dysplasia.[35,43] Infants with prolonged exposure to parenteral nutrition likely have the greatest potential to benefit from SMOFlipid administration.

All infants receiving intravenous lipid emulsions should have their triglyceride levels checked every 2 weeks. If the triglyceride level is >265 mg/dL, reduction of lipids may be considered.[32,35] For infants receiving SMOFlipid, testing of serum alpha tocopherol levels should be considered to monitor for hypervitaminosis due to increased vitamin E content in this product.

Electrolytes and Macrominerals

Sodium, Potassium, Magnesium, and Chloride

Administration of electrolytes (Na, Cl, and K) should be adjusted to maintain appropriate serum values on laboratory measurements and per the infant's clinical status. Fluctuation of fluid status in the first days of life often requires several changes to electrolyte supplementation. Example dosing of electrolytes can be viewed in Table 20.12. Chloride levels should be monitored to avoid iatrogenic metabolic acidosis. Potassium supplementation in early life should be closely monitored to avoid nonoliguric hyperkalemia.

While weaning off PN, serum sodium should be closely monitored to ensure adequate status with enteral supplementation provided as needed. Late-onset hyponatremia after discontinuing parenteral nutrition inhibits appropriate growth in preterm infants.[44]

Magnesium is an important cation that is required for DNA, RNA, and protein synthesis and plays a crucial role in bone matrix development. Neonates are at risk for hypermagnesemia in the first days of life if their mothers were treated with magnesium sulfate prior to delivery; this population may not immediately require supplementation parenterally.[45] If a neonate has hypermagnesemia at birth, magnesium should be added into the parenteral solution after neonatal serum levels have normalized.

Table 20.12 Usual Neonatal Ranges for Electrolytes[10,93]

Usual Pediatric Range	Neonates First DOL 1	Neonates	1 Month–1 Year
Sodium (mEq/kg)	0–2	2–5	3–4
Potassium (mEq/kg)	0–3	2–3	
Magnesium (mEq/kg) as sulfate	0–0.6	0.4–0.6	0.3–0.6
Chloride %anions as chloride	25%–50%	25%	

DOL, Day of life

Table 20.13 Factors Affecting Calcium and Phosphate Stability in Parenteral Nutrition

Factor Influencing Stability	Why Factor Influences Stability
Calcium and phosphate concentrations	Lower concentration is more soluble
pH of the total parenteral nutrition	Lower pH is more soluble
Dextrose and amino acids concentrations	Higher concentration is more soluble
Ratio of calcium to phosphate	The solubility is more sensitive to phosphate, so higher amounts of calcium can generally be added
Temperature	Lower temperatures are more soluble
Lipids	Obscures the ability to see precipitates
Cysteine	Increases the solubility
Calcium salt form	Calcium chloride is more likely to precipitate and is generally avoided in parenteral nutrition solutions; calcium gluconate should be used

Calcium and Phosphorus

Calcium and phosphate are essential minerals that play an important function in bone health and development. Phosphate plays a critical role in energy metabolism, whereas calcium is essential for muscle contractions.

The challenges of calcium and phosphate solubility in parenteral nutrition have been well studied, with numerous published solubility curves available for standard use of pediatric pharmacists.[46] Most commonly, the ideal ratio of calcium to phosphorus appears to be 1 mmol Ca to 1 mmol P (or 2 mEq Ca to 1 mmol P).[47] The percentage of amino acid in solution, inclusion of cysteine, pH, volume of PN, and temperature of the PN solution all increase the solubility of calcium and phosphorus in solution[48]; see Table 20.13 for further discussion of compatibility, and see Table 20.14 for example dosing of calcium and phosphorus with parenteral nutrition volume and amino acid content in mind.

Metabolic bone disease and serum calcium and phosphorus abnormalities can be common problems in the preterm infant. Inadequate and unbalanced parenteral nutrition administration in the first days of life may exacerbate these abnormalities. This "placental incompletely restored feeding syndrome" was first proposed by Bonsante et al. in 2013; they showed that excessive amino acid and energy administration without adequate mineral administration drove hypokalemia, hypophosphatemia, and hypercalcemia in preterm infants.[4] Neonatal refeeding syndrome may be prevented by introducing phosphorus at physiologic rates in the first 24 hours of life, rather than providing phosphate-free starter total parenteral nutrition (TPN) for the first few days of life.[49]

Prolonged use of parenteral nutrition puts neonates at an increased risk for metabolic bone disease of prematurity.[50] This is discussed in depth in the "Complications of Parenteral Nutrition" section of this chapter.

Iron

Iron plays a critical role in neurodevelopment and erythropoiesis. Iron deficiency in infancy can cause anemia and significant neurocognitive deficits later in life.[51,52] Enteral iron is nearly always the preferred method of administration, as parenterally administered iron bypasses the absorption regulation present in the gastrointestinal tract. When administered parenterally, there is a risk of iron overload because there is no mechanism for excretion or absorption regulation. Iron overload can increase oxidative stress and risk of infection. For patients on long-term parenteral nutrition, ferritin and hemoglobin should be monitored to assess iron status and avoid iron deficiency and toxicity.[53]

Vitamins

Vitamin supplementation in parenteral nutrition is largely driven by the commercial products available (described in Table 20.15). Daily parenteral nutrition doses of vitamins should be administered per Table 20.5. The use of these products in standard clinical practice meets current estimated requirements of the neonate due to prolonged use without detrimental effect.[54] Routine monitoring of serum vitamin levels is not necessary unless clinically indicated.

Trace Elements

Akin to vitamins, trace element supplementation is limited by the commercial products available (described in Table 20.16). The impact of individual trace element supplementation in the preterm neonate has been well studied.

Table 20.14 Example Calcium and Phosphorus Dosing Based on Parenteral Nutrition Volume and Amino Acid Content

	Parenteral Nutrition Volume				
	<50 mL/kg	50–74 mL/kg	75–100 mL/kg	≥100 mL/kg	Maximum Dose
Amino acid (g/kg/day)	0.5–1	2	3	3.5–4	4.5
Amino acid (%)	1–2%	2.7–4%	3–4%	3–4%	4%
Calcium (mEq/kg)	a	1.8	2.7	3	4
Phosphorus (mmol/kg)	a	0.8	1.3	1.5	2.5

[a]Only include calcium or phosphate when total parenteral nutrition volume is less than 50 mL/kg.

Table 20.15 Available Multivitamin (M.V.I.) Products in the United States

	Adult	Pediatric
	Infuvite (Per 10 mL) M.V.I. Adult (Per 10 mL)	Infuvite Pediatric (Per 5 mL) M.V.I. Pediatric (Per 5 mL)
Biotin	60 mcg	20 mcg
Dexpanthenol	15 mg	5 mg
Niacinamide	40 mg	17 mg
Folic acid	600 mcg	140 mcg
Vitamin A	3300 IU	2300 IU
Vitamin B_1	6 mg	1.2 mg
Vitamin B_2	3.6 mg	1.4 mg
Vitamin B_6	6 mg	1 mg
Vitamin B_{12}	5 mcg	1 mcg
Vitamin C	200 mg	80 mg
Vitamin D	200 IU	400 IU
Vitamin E	10 IU	7 IU
Vitamin K	150 mcg	200 mcg

Zinc

Zinc is a cofactor required for growth, cell differentiation, and metabolism of macronutrients. Premature infants have higher zinc requirements due to low body stores, increased endogenous losses, and increased rate of growth. Acute zinc deficiency may present as stunted growth, impaired immune function, or the classic perioral and/or perianal rash; prolonged, chronic zinc deficiency can result in renal and liver failure.[55] Infants with predicted significant zinc losses (e.g., high ostomy output) will require a greater level of parenteral zinc. Zinc toxicity in neonates and children has not been well studied, but a significant case report showed a fatal overdose in a premature infant who received a parenteral zinc dose 1000 times higher than typical.[56]

Copper

Copper is required for normal function of several physiologic enzymes within the body. Copper deficiency may present as neutropenia, iron deficiency and anemia, osteoporosis, or hair depigmentation, among other symptoms.[57,58] Copper is primarily excreted through bile; thus there is concern for inadequate clearance of excessive copper in premature infants due to their risk of biliary stasis.[59]

Copper excretion is reduced in cholestasis due to reduction of bile flow. Concern for hepatocellular injury due to copper accumulation in cholestasis has led to the common practice of removing copper from PN in cholestatic infants.[60,61] However, elimination of copper paired with low copper stores at birth and increased copper requirements may cause copper deficiencies in preterm infants with cholestasis.[57] Elimination of copper from PN in the setting of cholestasis is no longer advised.

Parenteral copper requirements for preterm infants have been estimated to be as high as 40 mcg/kg/day.[53,62] Conditions with excessive gastrointestinal losses result in higher copper requirements.[63] For example, infants with ostomies may have copper requirements that exceed those of other preterm or critically ill neonates, because a standard dose of copper may not prevent deficiency.[64] Copper status should be monitored in infants with cholestasis through plasma copper and ceruloplasmin levels, although it is important to note that these levels are increased in the setting of inflammation.[63]

Chromium

Chromium is involved in carbohydrate and lipid metabolism. Elevated serum chromium levels have been associated with decreased serum iron levels in children.[65] Chromium is believed to competitively inhibit iron binding to transferrin, thus interfering with iron metabolism and storage. Chromium is a known contaminant of parenteral nutrition solutions and may exceed ordered quantities in parenteral nutrition.[66] With estimations of 0.28 mcg additional chromium in neonatal parenteral nutrition solutions,[67] removal from standard PN composition should be considered.[53]

Table 20.16 Available Trace Element Products in the United States

		Zinc[a]	Copper[a]	Manganese[a]	Chromium[a]	Selenium[a]
STANDARD COMBINATION PRODUCTS						
Multitrace-4	Am Regent	1 mg	0.4 mg	100 mcg	4 mcg	
Multitrace-4 neonatal	Am Regent	1.4 mg	0.1 mg	25 mcg	0.85 mcg	
Multitrace-4 pediatric	Am Regent	1 mg	0.1 mg	25 mcg	1 mcg	
Multitrace-5	Am Regent	1 mg	0.4 mg	100 mcg	4 mcg	20 mcg
CONCENTRATED COMBINATION PRODUCTS						
Multitrace-4 concentrate	Am Regent	5 mg	1 mg	500 mcg	10 mcg	
Multitrace-5 concentrate	Am Regent	5 mg	1 mg	500 mcg	10 mcg	60 mcg
SINGLE ENTITY PRODUCTS						
Chromium	Pfizer				4 mcg	
Copper	Pfizer		0.4 mg			
Manganese sulfate	Am Regent Pfizer			100 mcg		
Selenious acid	Am Regent					60 mcg
Zinc sulfate	Am Regent	1 mg				
Zinc sulfate concentrate	Am Regent	5 mg				

[a]Dose per mL.

Selenium

Selenium is important for the body's immune function, thyroid hormone metabolism, and protection from oxidative stress and damage. Selenium is a component of active glutathione peroxidase, an enzyme that may protect against oxidative tissue damage in disease states such as bronchopulmonary dysplasia and retinopathy of prematurity. Appropriate supplementation of selenium in the preterm infant may reduce risk of both bronchopulmonary dysplasia and sepsis[68]; there is no evidence correlating selenium supplementation and the occurrence of retinopathy of prematurity.

Historical references have referred to 2 mcg/kg/day as appropriate supplementation levels of selenium in parenteral nutrition.[69] However, recent publications have suggested that 5 to 7 mcg/kg/day is a more appropriate dosage to achieve serum selenium levels in preterm infants comparable with those of healthy term infants.[53,70,71]

Selenium status is most commonly monitored by measuring plasma selenium levels, which should be done in infants on long-term parenteral nutrition and those with renal failure. While monitoring selenium, it is recommended to assess signs of a systemic inflammatory response syndrome, such as C-reactive protein, because inflammation decreases plasma selenium levels.

Carnitine

Carnitine is an important cofactor in beta-oxidation because it facilitates the transport of long-chain fatty acids as acyl carnitines into the inner mitochondrial matrix. Preterm infants are born with limited carnitine reserves, because accretion largely occurs during the third trimester. Infants on long-term total parenteral nutrition administration receiving L-carnitine supplementation have normalized serum carnitine levels and improved fatty acid oxidation.[72] L-carnitine supplementation may improve growth, but this finding is inconsistent in the literature.[73–75] Infants receiving an exclusive human milk diet are estimated to consume 2 to 5 mg/kg carnitine daily. Supplementation levels of L-carnitine in parenteral nutrition have been reported up to levels of 50 mg/kg/day in the literature. An ideal dose of supplemental L-carnitine has not been identified. Routine testing of serum carnitine levels is not recommended in preterm infants.

Iodine

Iodine is critical for brain development and thyroid function during infancy. Preterm infants have a higher iodine requirement due to minimal iodine and thyroid hormone stores. Maternal iodine deficiency is rising, partly due to many prenatal vitamins not containing iodine, putting mothers and their infants at greater risk for iodine deficiency.[76] Standard parenteral nutrition provides <1 mcg/kg/day of iodine.[77] Currently there is no parenteral source of supplemental iodine available for use in the NICU. The rate of iodine deficiency in preterm infants, specifically in preterm infants receiving prolonged parenteral nutrition, is not fully known, due to infrequent testing of iodine status. Urine iodine levels should be checked to monitor for iodine deficiency.[78,79] If deficiency is confirmed, enteral iodine may be given as potassium iodide, at a dose of 100 mcg/day once enteral feeds are established.

Manganese

Manganese is an essential trace element, playing a role in physiologic and neuronal functions and acting as a cofactor for several enzymes including pyruvate carboxylase. Enteral metabolism and absorption of manganese is well regulated by the gastrointestinal tract; however, the same regulation does not exist when manganese is administered parenterally. Long-term parenteral administration of manganese is a risk factor for direct hyperbilirubinemia and cholestasis.[78,80–82] Neurotoxicity has also been seen in excessive and prolonged manganese administration, because manganese can cross the blood–brain barrier, bind to catecholamine storage sites, and deplete central catecholamine stores. In instances of neurotoxicity, manganese deposits are visible in the basal ganglia in magnetic resonance imaging.[83] There has been no documentation of manganese deficiency in the published literature among adult, pediatric, or neonatal populations. Risk for deficiency is considered low, because manganese is a common contaminant of other trace minerals found in parenteral nutrition. This lack of evidence of deficiency in the neonatal population paired with the growing evidence of manganese toxicity suggests that it is not necessary to include manganese in parenteral nutrition administration.[84]

Aluminum

Aluminum is a known contaminant of parenteral nutrition solution additives, putting patients who require long-term parenteral nutrition at risk for toxicity.[85–88] Excessive exposure to aluminum has been associated with osteomalacia and impairment of parathyroid hormone secretion in adults.[89] In preterm infants dependent on parenteral nutrition, aluminum may play a role in slowed growth and decreased bone mass and density.[90] Aluminum can be found in cysteine, phosphorus, calcium, trace elements, and gluconate salts utilized in PN.[88,91] Calcium gluconate (in plastic vials), sodium phosphate, and sodium glycerophosphate are all potential calcium and phosphorus additives for parenteral nutrition that can be utilized to minimize aluminum exposure of the premature infant.[88]

Compatibilities in Parenteral Nutrition

Compatibility is important to consider during many steps of the parenteral nutrition process. Compatibilities of parenteral nutrition with medications is often a necessary consideration, particularly for the smallest premature infants who may have limited intravenous access. A list of Y-site compatibilities with references can be seen in Table 20.17. Compatibilities may vary based on a two-in-one administration (parenteral nutrition without lipids) or a three-in-one administration (parenteral nutrition combined with lipids). Some medications will have adverse effects on the intravenous lipid emulsion but be compatible with the two-in-one portion; in these instances, lipids should be administered via a separate line. For other medications, compatibility may be improved by lipids running through the same line.

When ordering the components, an important concern is the amount of calcium and phosphate included in the TPN. Many factors determine their solubility in solution (see Table 20.13). Final concentration of calcium and phosphate will be determined by the dose ordered and the final volume of the TPN. As the volume of TPN decreases, there may be a point where only calcium or phosphate can be added (see Table 20.14).

Once the product is prepared, temperature affects calcium/phosphate solubility. Contrary to expectations, increasing the temperature also increases the risk for precipitation. A TPN may form precipitates when removed from the refrigerator or when placed too close to a radiant warmer. Due to the risk of precipitate formation, it is important to infuse parenteral nutrition solutions with an inline filter. Per

Table 20.17 Y-Site Compatibility

	2 in 1 (No Lipids)	PN + Intralipid
Acetazolamide[129]	I	—
Acyclovir[129–131]	I	I
Alprostadil[132]	C	—
Amikacin[129–131,133,134]	C	I/var
Aminophylline[129–131]	I/var	C
Amphotericin B[130,131]	I	I
Ampicillin[129–131,134,135]	I/var	C
Ampicillin/sulbactam[130,131]	C	C
Aztreonam[130,131]	C	C
Bumetanide[130,131]	C	C
Caffeine[135,136]	C	—
Cefazolin[130,131,134,135]	I/var	C
Cefotetan[130,131]	C	C
Cefoxitin[130,131,134,135]	C	C
Ceftazidime[129–131]	C	C
Cefuroxime[130,131]	C	C
Chloramphenicol[134]	C	—
Chlorothiazide[129]	I	
Clindamycin[130,131,134–136]	C	C
Dexamethasone[129–131]	C	C
Digoxin[130,131,137]	C	C
Dobutamine[129–131]	C	C
Dopamine[129–131,137]	C	I/var
Enalaprilat[130,131,136]	C	C
Epinephrine[136]	C	—
Erythromycin[134,135]	C	C
Famotidine[130,131]	C	C
Fentanyl[129–131]	C	C
Fluconazole[130,131,136]	C	C
Ganciclovir[130,131]	I	I
Gentamicin[129–131,133–135]	C	C
Hydrocortisone[130,131,136]	C	C
Imipenem/cilastatin[130,131]	C	C
Insulin[130,131]	C	C
Levetiracetam[138]	—	C
Lorazepam[130,131]	C	I
Meropenem[131]	—	C
Methylprednisolone[130,131]	C	C
Metoclopramide[130,131,136]	I/var	C
Metronidazole[129–131]	C	C
Midazolam[130,131,136]	I/var	I
Milrinone[129]	C	—
Nafcillin[130,131,134]	C	C
Nitroglycerin[130,131]	C	C
Norepinephrine[130,137]	C	C
Octreotide[130,131]	C	C
Penicillin G potassium[129,134,135]	C	C
Phenobarbital[130,131,136]	I/var	I
Piperacillin/tazobactam[130,131]	C	C
Potassium chloride[130,131]	C	C
Ranitidine[129–131]	C	C
Rifampin[136]	I	—
Sodium nitroprusside[130,131]	C	C
Ticarcillin/clavulanate[130,131]	C	C
Tobramycin[129–131,133–135]	C	C
Vancomycin[129–131,134]	C	C
Zidovudine[129–131]	C	C

C, Compatible; *I*, incompatible; *I/var*, variable results in literature; —, no information found; *PN*, parenteral nutrition.

the American Society for Parenteral and Enteral Nutrition (ASPEN), a 0.22 micron or greater filter is used for two-in-one solutions and a 1.2 micron or greater filter is used for lipid-containing solutions.[92]

Osmolarity of the final solution is also an important consideration. The combination of multiple components quickly results in a hyperosmolar solution. Most guidelines recommend limiting the osmolarity of peripherally administered parenteral nutrition to ≤900 mOsm/L. When administration is combined with Intralipid, higher limits have been tolerated, but evidence is lacking.[92] Until a central line can be used, some components of the solution may need to be decreased (e.g., multivitamins, dextrose).

Practical Calculations for Parenteral Nutrition Administration

Glucose Infusion Rate

The GIR is the measure of administration of carbohydrates via intravenous nutrition and is reported in milligrams (of dextrose) per kilograms (of patient) per minute. GIR goals can be seen in Table 20.10.

$$\text{GIR} = \frac{\text{IV rate}\left(\frac{\text{mL}}{\text{hr}}\right) \times \text{dextrose concentration}\left(\frac{\text{g}}{\text{dL}}\right) \times 1000\frac{\text{mg}}{\text{g}}}{\text{weight (kg)} \times 60\frac{\text{min}}{\text{hr}} \times 100\frac{\text{mL}}{\text{dL}}}$$

Example: A 1.3-kg infant is receiving parenteral nutrition at 4.1 mL/hour with 14% dextrose.

$$\text{GIR} = \frac{4.1\frac{\text{mL}}{\text{hr}} \times 14\frac{\text{g}}{\text{dL}} \times 1000\frac{\text{mg}}{\text{g}}}{1.3\text{ kg} \times 60\frac{\text{min}}{\text{hr}} \times 100\frac{\text{mL}}{\text{dL}}} = \frac{57{,}400\frac{\text{mL*mg}}{\text{hr*dL}}}{7{,}800\frac{\text{kg*min*mL}}{\text{hr*dL}}}$$

$$= 7.36\text{ mg/kg/min}$$

Total Fluid, Energy, and Protein Administration

Example: A 0.75-kg infant is receiving parenteral nutrition at 2.6 mL/hour. The parenteral nutrition ordered is 11% dextrose, 3.2% amino acid, and 2.5 g/kg Intralipid.

Total Fluid

From parenteral nutrition:

$$2.6 \text{ mL/hour} \times 24 \text{ hours} = 62.4 \text{ mL/day}$$

$$62.4 \text{ mL/day} \div 0.75 \text{ kg} = 83.2 \text{ mL/kg/day}$$

From Intralipid:
There are 2 g fat per 10 mL Intralipid (or, 2 g/kg per 10 mL/kg).

$$\frac{2.5 \text{ g/kg}}{X} = \frac{2 \text{ g/kg}}{10 \text{ mL/kg}}$$

$$25 \frac{g^* \, mL}{kg^2} = 2X \frac{g}{kg}$$

$$12.5 \frac{ml}{kg} = X$$

Total fluid = 83.2 mL/kg + 12.5 mL/kg = 95.7 mL/kg ≅ 96 mL/kg

Total Protein

83.2 mL/kg from parenteral nutrition with 3.2% amino acid solution:

$$83.2 \text{ mL/kg} \times 0.032 \text{ g/mL} = 2.67 \text{ g/kg protein}$$

Total Energy

From protein:

2.67 g/kg protein × 4 kcal/g = 10.7 kcal/kg ≅ 11 kcal/kg from protein

From dextrose: note, dextrose, the d-isomer of glucose, provides 3.4 calories per gram.

83.2 mL/kg from parenteral nutrition with 11% dextrose

83.2 mL/kg × 0.11 g/mL = 9.15 g/kg dextrose

9.15 g/kg × 3.4 kcal/g = 31.1 kcal/kg ≅ 31 kcal/kg from dextrose

From fat: note, 20% intravenous lipid emulsions have 2 g fat/10 mL and provide 2 kcal/mL with calories from fat and glycerol. Thus calories can be calculated as 10 kcal/g.

2.5 g/kg Intralipid

2.5 g/kg × 10 kcal/g = 25 kcal/kg from fat

Total calories:

11 kcal/kg + 31 kcal/kg + 25 kcal/kg = 67 kcal/kg

Lipid Infusion Rate

Tolerance of intravenous lipid emulsion is the ability of the infant to hydrolyze the fat as assessed by serum triglyceride levels. Lipid infusion should not exceed 0.15 g/kg/hour.

Example: A 1.4-kg infant with an ordered dose of 2.5 g/kg/day Intralipid run over 18 hours.

$$2.5 \text{ g/kg} \div 18 \text{ hours} = 0.14 \text{ g/kg/hour}$$

Calories From Essential Fatty Acids

See Tables 20.18 and 20.19.

Table 20.18 Essential Fatty Acid Requirements for Term and Preterm Infants

	Linoleic (Omega-6)	Linolenic (Omega-3)
Institute of Medicine Adequate Intake for infants ages 0–6 months[139]	4.4 g/day	0.5 g/day
American Academy of Pediatrics recommendations for premature infants[140]	At least 3% of total energy	

Meeting the American Academy of Pediatrics' Recommended 3% of Calories From Linoleic Acid

Intralipid

Say we have a 1.0-kg infant receiving 100 kcal/kg/day from parenteral nutrition. This infant requires 3% of calories (or 3 kcal/kg, and in this case, 3 kcal) from linoleic acid to meet essential fatty acid requirements. We know that fat has 9 kcal/g and 50% of the fat in Intralipid is linoleic acid. Therefore,

1 g Intralipid = 9 kcal from fat = 4.5 kcal from linoleic acid

So we can determine:

$$3 \text{ kcal} = (X \text{ grams of fat} \times 9 \text{ kcal/g}) \times 0.5$$

$$X = 0.7 \text{ g Intralipid} = 0.7 \text{ g/kg Intralipid}$$

SMOFlipid

Say we have the same 1.0-kg infant receiving 100 kcal/kg/day from parenteral nutrition. This infant still requires 3% total calories from linoleic acid to meet essential fatty acid requirements. We know that fat has 9 kcal/g and 18% of the fat in SMOFlipid is linoleic acid. Therefore:

1 g SMOFlipid = 9 kcal from fat = 1.6 kcal from linoleic acid

So we can determine:

$$3 \text{ kcal} = (X \text{ grams of fat} \times 9 \text{ kcal/g}) \times 0.18$$

$$X = 1.9 \text{ g SMOFlipid} = 1.9 \text{ g/kg SMOFlipid}$$

Complications of Parenteral Nutrition

High-risk neonates requiring parenteral nutrition often experience a variety of metabolic complications related to immature processes and critical illness that require modification of parenteral nutrition. These may include electrolyte abnormalities, hypo- and hyperglycemia, acid–base disturbances, hypertriglyceridemia, and rises in blood urea nitrogen. Specific disease states related to prolonged parenteral nutrition administration are discussed below.

Metabolic Bone Disease

Preterm infants are at high risk for osteopenia of prematurity due to limited nutrient stores paired with an impaired ability to provide sufficient calcium and phosphorus. Approximately 80% of fetal accretion of calcium and phosphate occurs in the third trimester (Table 20.20), resulting in premature infants having low mineral stores at birth.[93] Parenteral nutrition is unable to meet the

Table 20.19 Composition of Intravenous Lipid Emulsion (ILE) Products

	Oil (%)				EFA Content (%)			
Product	Soy	MCT	Olive	Fish	Linoleic (Omega-6)	Linolenic (Omega-3)	g Fat Per 250 mL ILE	% EFA Per 250 mL ILE
Intralipid 20%	100%	—	—	—	50	9	50	59
SMOFlipid	30%	30%	25%	15%	18	2	50	20

EFA, Essential fatty acid; *MCT*, medium chain triglyceride.

Table 20.20 Calcium and Phosphorus Third Trimester Accretion Rates[126]

Average (maximum)	Calcium	Phosphorus
mmol/kg	2.5–3 (7.8)	1.6–2.1 (2.4)
mEq/kg	5–6 (15.6)	

intrauterine accretion rates of calcium and phosphorus of the premature infant, thus putting this population at higher risk for metabolic bone disease.

Parenteral administration of calcium and phosphorus is limited by their solubility in solution. The presence of aluminum as a contaminant in parenteral nutrition solution is a long-term risk factor for reduced bone mineral density and stunted bone growth of former premature infants.[94] Additionally, many commonly used medications (e.g., loop diuretics, corticosteroids) are deleterious to bone health.

Early initiation of phosphorus-containing parenteral nutrition helps prevent prolonged early-life hypophosphatemia and reduce hypercalcinemia.[4,49,95] ASPEN recommends use of parenteral nutrition containing high doses of calcium and phosphorus to minimize risk of metabolic bone disease.[50] However, there is no clear evidence of an improvement in bone health in the long term with this type of intervention.[96]

Cholestasis

Intestinal failure–associated liver disease (IFALD) is used to describe liver disease occurring due to the medical and surgical management of intestinal failure, which was previously described as PNAC or parenteral nutrition–associated liver disease. The pathogenesis of IFALD is multifactorial and includes intestinal and biliary stasis, poor enterohepatic circulation, immature bile secretion from the liver, and the immature liver's sensitivity to lipid peroxidation.[97]

The best treatment for IFALD is to initiate enteral nutrition as soon as medically appropriate. When this is not feasible, modifications to parenteral nutrition administration may be indicated. Ensuring appropriate rather than excessive administration of energy and nitrogen should be done to prevent fatty liver deposition.[97] It is no longer recommended that copper be removed from parenteral nutrition in the setting of cholestasis due to the risk of cholestasis. Use of a fish oil–based lipid emulsion has been proven an effective and approved treatment for IFALD.[36,98]

Contamination of Parenteral Nutrition Components

The contamination of parenteral nutrition products by trace elements is a well-documented issue with potential for toxicity risks. Aluminum,[85–88] chromium,[66,67] and manganese[67] are the most concerning contaminants, and their inclusion in standard parenteral nutrition orders should be reconsidered.[53,67] Multitrace element packages are problematic because neonatal/pediatric solutions provide potentially toxic amounts of manganese and chromium.[99] The risk of trace-element toxicity should be considered when creating parenteral nutrition plans, particularly for long-term parenteral nutrition–dependent patients.

Parenteral Nutrition Shortages and Clinical Deficiencies

Premature infants' lack of nutrient stores and potential for long-term parenteral nutrition use puts them at a unique risk for significant nutrient deficiencies. Thiamine deficiency presenting with severe lactic acidosis was seen in a preterm infant born at 28 weeks post menstrual age was born in a Turkish hospital, who received parenteral nutrition lacking the vitamin.[100] Essential fatty acid deficiency has been described in infants receiving inadequately dosed SMOFlipid intravenous fat emulsions.[37] Appropriate composition of parenteral nutrition solution is vital to prevent significant nutrient deficiencies.

As intravenous nutrient shortages are occurring with greater frequency, NICUs need to modify their approach to parenteral nutrition to prevent severe deficiencies.

What to do about shortages?

- Stay informed. ASPEN: http://www.nutritioncare.org/public-policy/product-shortages/
- Implement strategies early
- Search for alternate suppliers/products
- Change to enteral nutrition/supplements
- Limit use to the most vulnerable populations
- Observe patients for resultant clinical deficiencies
- Be aware of increased risk for errors with alternate procedures
- Restart use when reliable supply has returned

Transition to Enteral Nutrition

Transitioning off parenteral nutrition is often a unit-specific practice, with few guidelines on the best recommended approach. Balancing the minimizing of parenteral nutrition–associated complications such as central line–associated bloodstream infections, cholestasis, or metabolic bone disease with determining how quickly to advance enteral nutrition is a clinical challenge.

The potential for nutrient deficits in the transition phase has been increasingly documented in the literature.[101,102] Fig. 20.1 depicts examples of calorie and protein deficits that can be seen in this transition period. Efforts to reduce transitional nutrition discrepancies improve growth in premature infants.[102] Strategies to maximize nutrition in this period include:

- Creating a transition nutrition guideline to ensure minimum nutrient requirements are met[103]
- Utilizing concentrated parenteral nutrition
- Continuing full parenteral nutrition, rather than solutions containing dextrose and electrolyte only, until enteral nutrition alone can meet nutrient requirements
- Initiation of earlier human milk fortification.

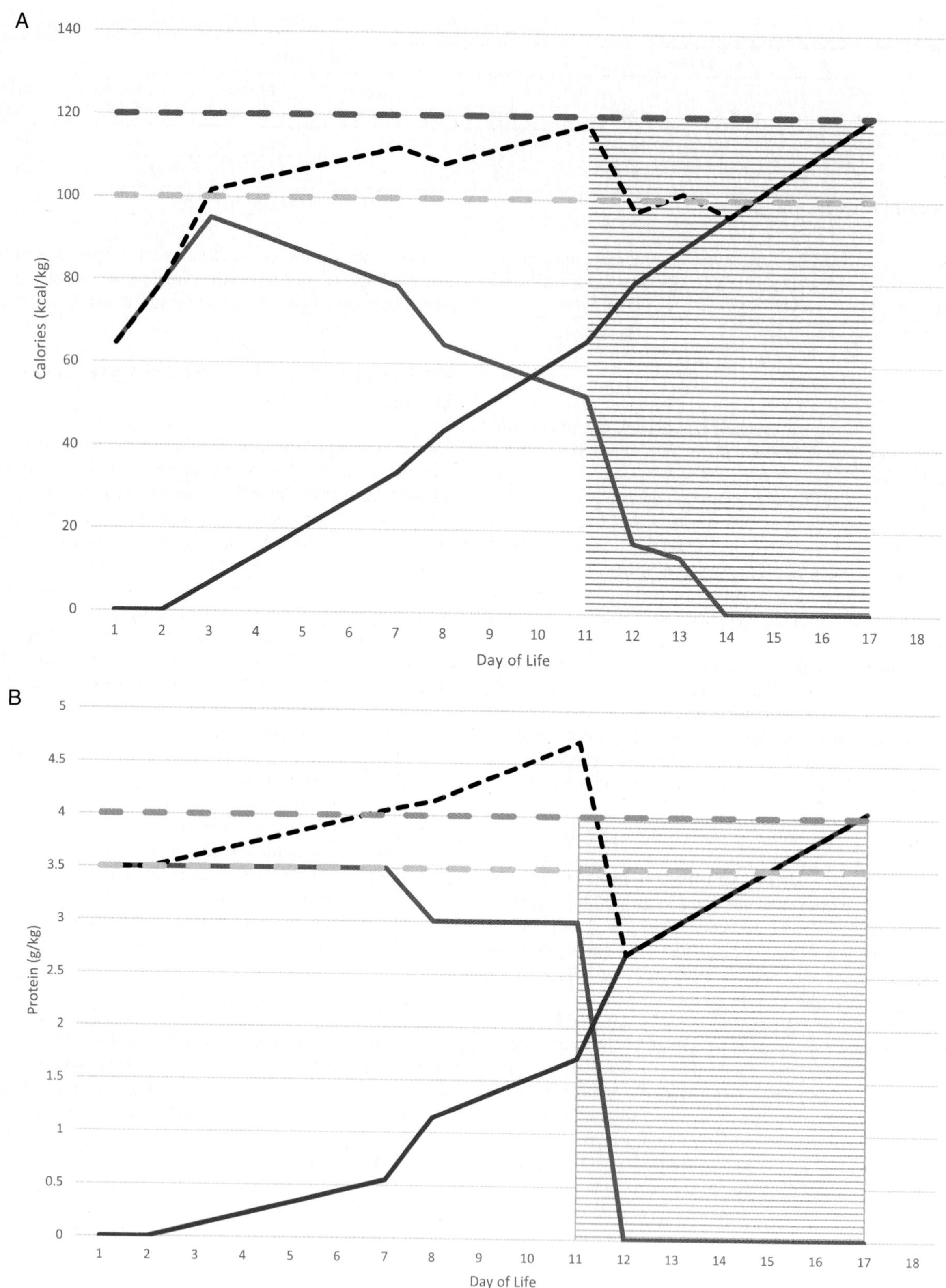

Fig. 20.1 Discrepancies in (A) Calories, (B) Protein, and (C) Calcium Administration When Transitioning From Parenteral to Enteral Nutrition. This depicts a typical example of a premature infant progressing from parenteral to enteral nutrition. This infant starts on parenteral nutrition with D10%, AA 3.5 g/kg, and IVFE 2 g/kg, increases to D12%, AA 3.5g/kg, and 3 g/kg IVFE on DOL 3. Enteral nutrition starts on DOL 3 and is advanced 10 mL/kg/day. Enteral feeds of expressed breast milk (EBM) at half fortification (1 packet human milk fortifier to 50 mL EBM) starts at 60 mL/kg and full fortification at 100 mL/kg. Parenteral nutrition is replaced with D10% when enteral feeds reach 100 mL/kg and all IV nutrition is discontinued when enteral nutrition reaches 120 mL/kg. The gray-shaded portion of the graph depicts the nutrient deficit that occurs over 4 days when parenteral nutrition is stopped prematurely. The calcium figure shows a parenteral nutrition goal that is significantly different than the enteral goal; the parenteral calcium goal reflects the chemical limitations of fitting calcium in the parenteral nutrition solution, and the enteral goal depicts the premature neonate's true calcium requirement. The necessity of human milk fortifier is clear for calcium requirements to be met. Unit guidelines should account for the transition nutrition phase to prevent nutrient deficits. *AA,* Amino acid; *D,* dextrose; *DOL,* day of life; *IVFE,* intravenous fat emulsion. (©Stephanie Merlino Barr.)

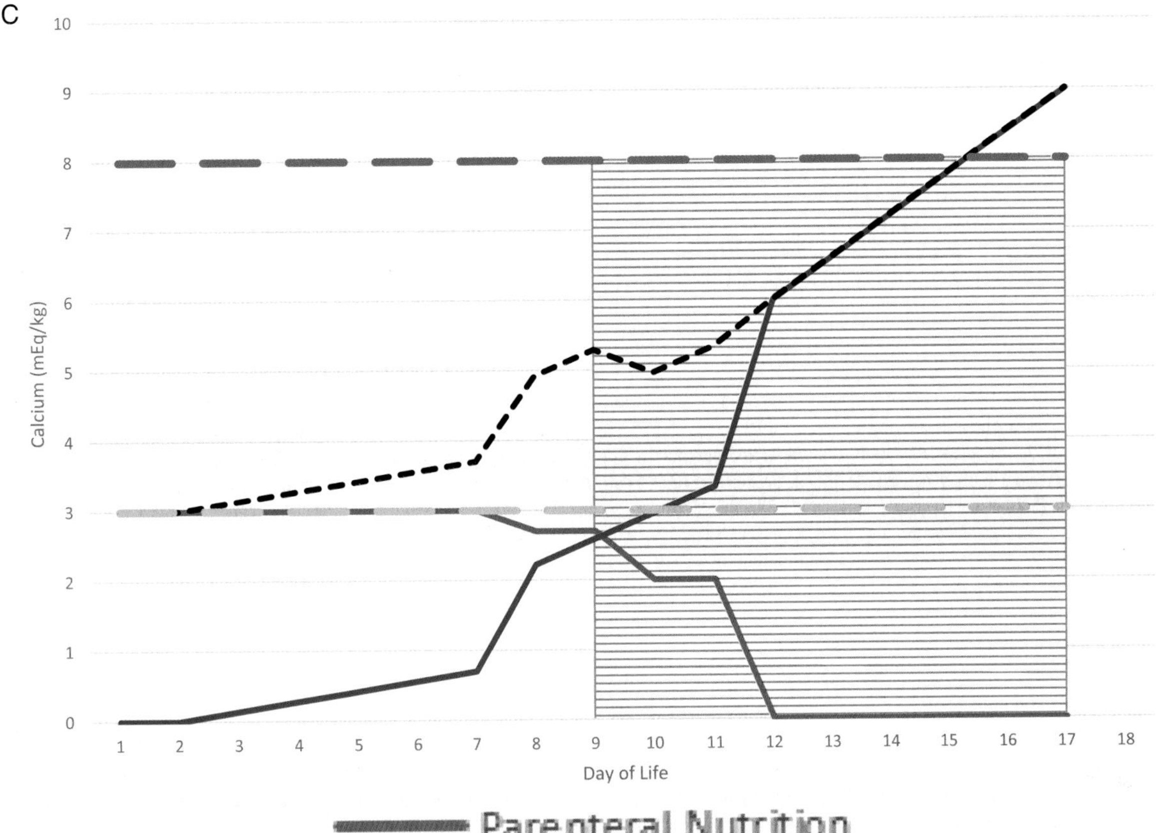

Fig. 20.1 Continued

CHAPTER

21 Nutrition in Short Bowel Syndrome

Muralidhar H. Premkumar, Alvaro Dendi, Akhil Maheshwari

KEY POINTS

1. Intestinal failure (IF) is defined as the loss of functional gut mass to levels below those needed for digestion and absorption of fluid and nutrients required to support adequate nutrition and growth.
2. Short bowel syndrome (SBS) is a subtype of IF that occurs due to the anatomic loss of a part of the intestines.
3. Gastroschisis and necrotizing enterocolitis (NEC) are the most frequently seen congenital and acquired causes of IF in neonates and young infants.
4. Loss of specific parts of the intestine may predispose an infant to various nutritional deficiencies.
5. SBS from surgical resection of the intestine may show phasic adaptive recovery: an initial acute period of intestinal dysfunction, subacute recovery over several weeks, and then a chronic phase of consolidation over months to years depending on the extent of the loss.
6. Many infants with IF require parenteral nutrition for long periods and are consequently at risk of cholestasis and liver failure.
7. In many patients, specific nutritional supplements such as dietary fiber, lipid preparations such as fish oil, probiotics; and motility-altering agents may be helpful.

Introduction

Intestinal failure (IF) is defined as the reduction of functional gut mass to levels below those needed for digestion and absorption of fluid and nutrients at levels adequate for nutrition and growth, resulting in prolonged dependence on parenteral nutrition.[1,2] It can result from either anatomic or functional loss of the intestines (Table 21.1). The term "short bowel syndrome" (SBS) refers to a specific subtype of IF that results from the anatomic loss of absorptive and digestive surface of the intestines.[2–4] IF can also result from mucosal dysfunction due to various congenital and acquired enteropathies and from gastrointestinal dysmotility states.

Congenital IF is associated most frequently with gastroschisis, which accounts for about 15% of all cases of IF and SBS in infants (Pediatric Intestinal Failure Consortium study).[5] In the same study, necrotizing enterocolitis (NEC) was noted to be the most frequent postnatal cause, accounting for 26% of IF in infants (Fig. 21.1).[5] These data are not surprising, because NEC still has a fairly high incidence; in a study from 820 centers in the United States, NEC occurred in 7.6% of all very low birth weight (VLBW) infants.[6] In another study conducted by the Neonatal Research Network of the National Institute for Child Health and Human Development (NICHD), NEC caused 96% of all IF and SBS in VLBW infants.[5] The increasing prevalence of SBS is likely related to improved survival of extremely premature infants with severe NEC and other gastrointestinal conditions.[6,7] The NICHD network has reported the incidence of SBS to be 7 per 1000 VLBW infants and 11 per 1000 extremely low birth weight infants.[8] SBS is also an important cause of infant morbidity and mortality in other countries; the Canadian Collaborative Study Group reported an overall incidence of 0.25 cases of SBS per all 1000 live births, increasing to 3.5 per 1000 in preterm infants.[9]

Development of the Gastrointestinal System and Relevance to Short Bowel Syndrome

The human gut develops from an infolding of the endodermal layer of the embryo, beginning at about 2 to 3 weeks after conception. All three germ layers are involved: the endoderm, the mesoderm, and the ectoderm. Many endodermal cells differentiate into gut epithelium and associated glands; mesoderm contributes to the *lamina propria, muscularis mucosa, muscularis externa,* and the blood vessels; and the ectoderm gives rise to the gut neuronal network in the submucosal and myenteric plexuses. The longitudinal growth of the small intestines can be described in three phases: an initial linear phase, a second and more accelerated phase between 20 and 40 weeks of gestation, and then a second phase of linear growth during infancy. The small intestines grow from about 2 to 20 cm between the 7th and 14th weeks of gestation and then double in length from 20 to 40 weeks.[10] The mean length of the small intestines at 20 weeks is 125 cm, and this increases to 275 cm at full term.[11] The cylindrical growth, both linear and circumferential, occurs secondary to binary fission or duplication of intestinal crypts and is most prominent in the submucosa. The surface area of the intestinal mucosa increases with the formation of mucosal folds of Kerckring, deepening of the

Table 21.1 Causes of Intestinal Failure

Anatomic Loss of Function: Reduced Absorptive Area (Short Bowel Syndrome)
- Congenital
  - Gastroschisis
  - Intestinal atresia
  - Midgut volvulus
- Acquired
  - Necrotizing enterocolitis
  - Midgut volvulus
  - Vascular thrombosis
  - Spontaneous intestinal perforation
  - Intussusception

Mucosal Dysfunction: Inefficient Mucosal Surface
- Congenital enteropathy
  - Microvillus inclusion disease
  - Intestinal epithelial dysplasia
- Postinfectious diarrhea

Neuromuscular Dysfunction: Motility Disorders
- Extensive Hirschsprung disease
- Chronic intestinal pseudoobstructions

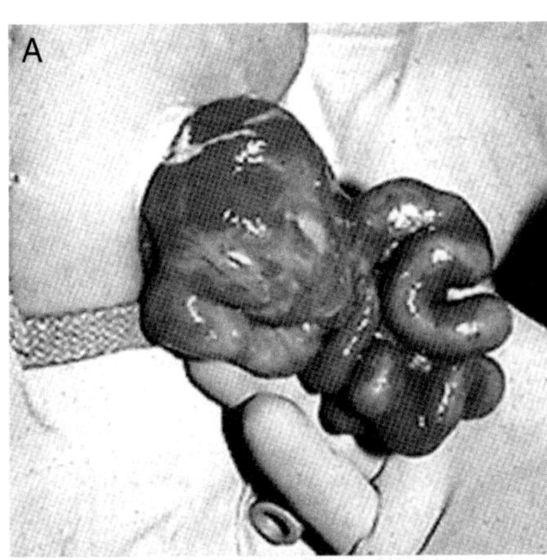

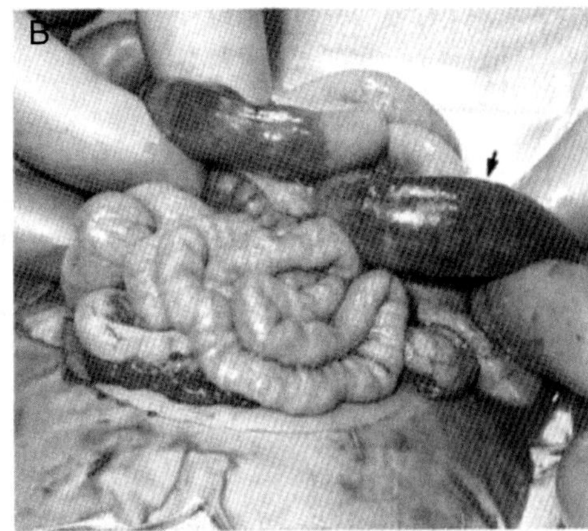

Fig. 21.1 Common Causes of SBS in Infants. (A) Gastroschisis with marked inflammatory peel. Reproduced with permission and minor modifications from Gastroschisis. Elsevier Point of Care. Updated May 27, 2021. (B) Clearly defined segments of necrotizing enterocolitis–affected bowel, seen during laparotomy. (Reproduced with permission and after modifications from Thakkar HS, Lakhoo K. The surgical management of necrotizing enterocolitis [NEC]. *Early Human Development*. 2016;97:25–28.)

crypts, and the development of microvilli in the brush border. This mucosal and submucosal growth increases the absorptive area of the intestines by more than 600 times. Finger-shaped villi with apical microvilli can be seen as early as the 14 weeks' gestation, and this development continues during early infancy.[10,12] This "reserve" ability of the small intestines to grow in structure and function in the second half of gestation provides some adaptability to the loss of some length secondary to disease and/or surgical resection.

Nutritional Challenges in Short Bowel Syndrome

The signs and symptoms of SBS are defined by the loss of function of specific parts of the gastrointestinal tract.[3] The direct impact of SBS is attributed to the loss of the digestive and absorptive surface of the mucosal ultrastructure and/or shortened length of the intestine. The transit of the food may also be reduced, and the resulting feeding intolerance (emesis) may reduce its contact period with the mucosa, thus impairing digestion and absorption. The loss of specific parts of the gastrointestinal tract, which have evolved to absorb different nutrients, may also predispose the infant to various nutritional deficiencies. Fig. 21.2 summarizes these data.

The stomach is resected less frequently, but the disturbances to gastric physiology can lead to several signs and symptoms seen in SBS. The stomach primarily receives the ingested food, initiates digestion, and transfers the food in a series of well-coordinated movements between the fundus-body and the pylorus-antrum. Gastric hypersecretion is a state of increased gastric secretions often noted with resection of the terminal ileum. The terminal ileum secretes a hormone called peptide YY, which slows down the motility and secretion of the stomach and the duodenum.[13,14] After resection of the ileum, this negative feedback look is lost, leading to states of hypergastrinemia and hypermotility. Incoordination between different parts of the stomach can lead to gastroparesis, impairing the ability to transfer gastric content to the duodenum, leading to increased gastrointestinal output.

Pancreatic enzymes are detected as early as 15 weeks' gestation, but the ontogeny of pancreatic exocrine function is slower compared with the anatomic development of the gut. The pancreatic exocrine function is fairly mature beyond 20 to 25 weeks but then plateaus to continue to develop through early infancy.[15] In SBS, the loss of pancreatic function leads to exocrine pancreas insufficiency and subsequent malabsorption of nutrients. Pancreatic amylase in the duodenum resumes the digestion of complex carbohydrates initiated by salivary amylase in the mouth. Thereafter, brush border hydrolases found on the enterocytes, such as lactase, maltase, and sucrase, continue the disintegration of disaccharides into monosaccharides and facilitate their absorption into the bloodstream via hexose transporters such as SGLUT-1 and GLUT5. Intestinal lactase activity is low between 14 and 20 weeks' gestation before reaching a high level at term. Although human milk is high in lactose concentration, VLBW infants tolerate human milk very well. This is probably aided by the colonic salvage pathways that convert unabsorbed lactose into short-chain fatty acids, which are then absorbed and used for energy production. In fact, early feeding promotes increased intestinal lactase in preterm infants. Many other effects of SBS may not be directly related to the loss of digestion and absorption of nutrients. Examples include intestinal failure–associated liver disease (IFALD), cholelithiasis, bloodstream infections, metabolic bone disease, oral aversion, and long-term growth failure with neurodevelopmental delays.

Intestinal Adaptation/Rehabilitation

The events and recovery of intestinal functions after the sentinel event resulting in IF can be broadly categorized into three stages (Fig. 21.3):

1. Acute phase, seen immediately after a surgical event, lasting between a few days to weeks. The acute phase is characterized by postoperative ileus and consequent high outputs either through the gastric tube or the gastrostomy. Consequent to high gastrointestinal outputs, this is accompanied by fluid and electrolyte losses and acid–base imbalance.
2. Subacute phase, spanning several weeks. The intestinal function gradually returns; the previously high gastrointestinal output decreases with less severe fluid and electrolyte disturbances. During this period, enteral nutrition is initiated and advanced on a foundation of a stable parenteral nutritional regimen. This phase is significant for linear and circumferential growth and the adaptation of previously retained sections of the intestines. This process facilitates feed tolerance, enabling the advancement of enteral nutrition and weaning of parenteral nutrition.
3. Chronic consolidation phase, spanning several months to years depending on the extent of the loss.

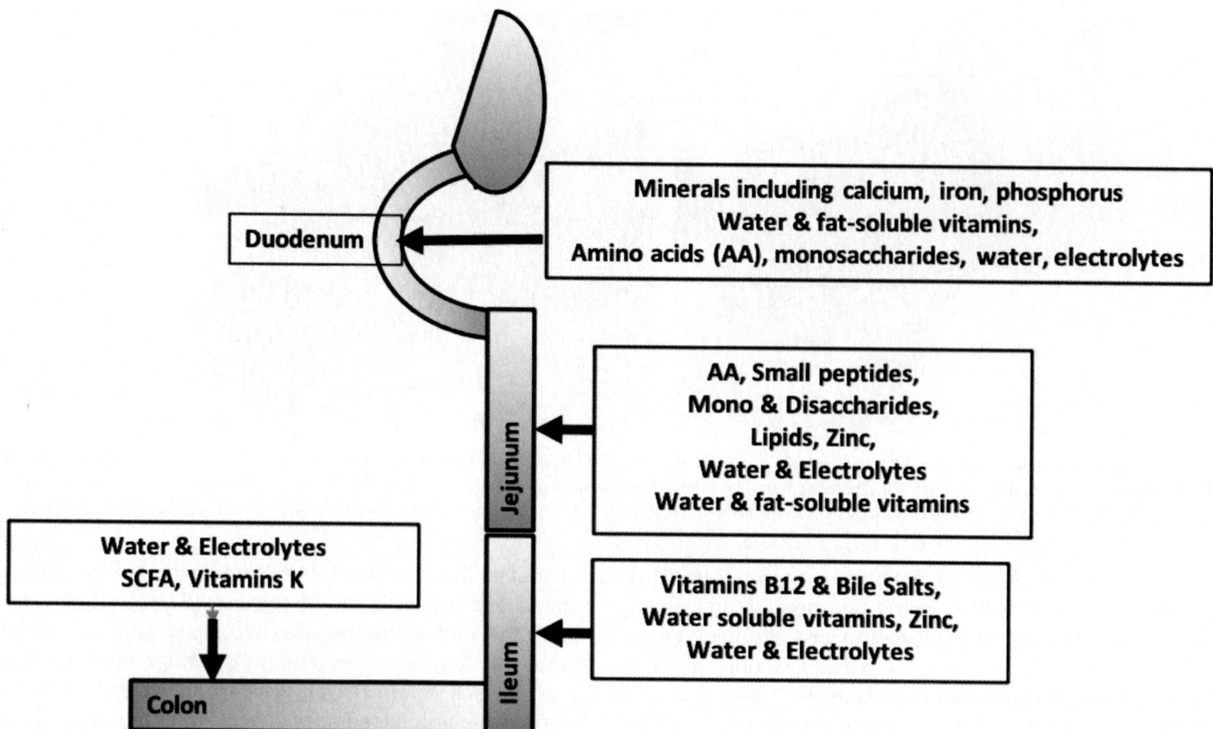

Fig. 21.2 Absorption of Various Nutrients in Specific Parts of the Gastrointestinal Tract. The duodenum is involved primarily in the absorption of monosaccharides, whereas both monosaccharides and disaccharides are absorbed in the jejunum. Both the duodenum and jejunum are the primary sites of protein digestion and absorption of amino acids and peptides. The jejunum also participates in fat absorption, along with the absorption of water and fat-soluble vitamins. The primary site for absorption of minerals such as iron, calcium, and phosphorus is the duodenum, whereas the jejunum is the primary site for zinc absorption. The ileum is the main site of the absorption of vitamin B_{12} and bile salts. Apart from these functions, the ileum and jejunum also participate in water and electrolyte absorption. The colon is a major site for absorption of water and electrolytes and partakes in "carbohydrate salvage," where the colonic microflora ferment the undigested carbohydrate residues, generating short-chain fatty acids. These short-chain fatty acids serve as additional caloric sources and stimulate water and sodium absorption.

All stages show progressive intestinal adaptation, marked by a series of anatomic and physiologic changes that begin as early as 48 hours after surgery and continue throughout rehabilitation.[16,17] During this process, compensatory changes are observed in the mucosa and muscular layers of the intestines. Changes in the mucosal cytoarchitecture involve lengthening of villi, deepening of crypts, and enterocyte proliferation resulting in expansion of the subluminal mucosal surface, increasing the surface area by many times. This process results in increased enterocyte per villus and is achieved by increasing mucosal DNA and RNA content. This process of intestinal adaptation is mediated by gastrointestinal hormones such as growth hormone, insulin-like growth factor, glucagon-like peptides, peptide YY, and neurotensin. This process of intestinal adaptation is further enhanced by exposure of the intestinal mucosa to enteral feeds, which prompts the release of hormonal mediators mentioned above, facilitating a trophic effect. The extent of intestinal adaptation varies with the anatomic site of the gastrointestinal tract; studies suggest that the capacity for anatomic and function adaptation is highest in the ileum and limited in the jejunum.[18] The process of intestinal adaptation provides the host with the anatomic and physiologic machinery required to improve the function of the residual bowel. As the intestinal adaptation progresses, it results in the gradual return of the function of the residual bowel, restoring the capacity to digest and absorb fluids, electrolytes, and nutrients.

Goals of Intestinal Rehabilitation

The goals of intestinal rehabilitation are listed sequentially in the order of appearance in Table 21.2. Enteral autonomy is often mentioned as the final goal in the process of intestinal rehabilitation. Enteral autonomy is defined as a clinical state in which the demands for adequate nutrition are met entirely by enteral feeds with complete independence from parenteral nutrition. However, the ultimate goal should be to promote and achieve appropriate developmental milestones with the best-tolerated combination of enteral and parenteral nutrition while striving toward enteral autonomy. There is wide variability in the definition of enteral autonomy, with different durations of independence from parenteral nutrition used as criteria. Short-term definitions have included achievement of feeds of 130 mL/kg/day with freedom from parenteral nutrition for a period as short as 48 hours.[19,20] However, long-term definitions in which independence from parenteral nutrition for over 3 to 12 months with appropriate growth parameters offer a more meaningful definition of enteral autonomy.[21–23] The latter is a better definition because it stands the test of a more significant duration of time and incorporates goals of growth and development. Although the parenteral nutrition–free period of 12 months is more stringent, it is reported that a period of 3 months free from parenteral nutrition captures most instances of enteral autonomy without any relapses.[22]

Nutritional Strategies in Short Bowel Syndrome

Replacement of Fluid and Electrolyte Losses

Fluid and electrolyte losses are a significant concern in the acute phase after intestinal surgery. The most common cause of gastric

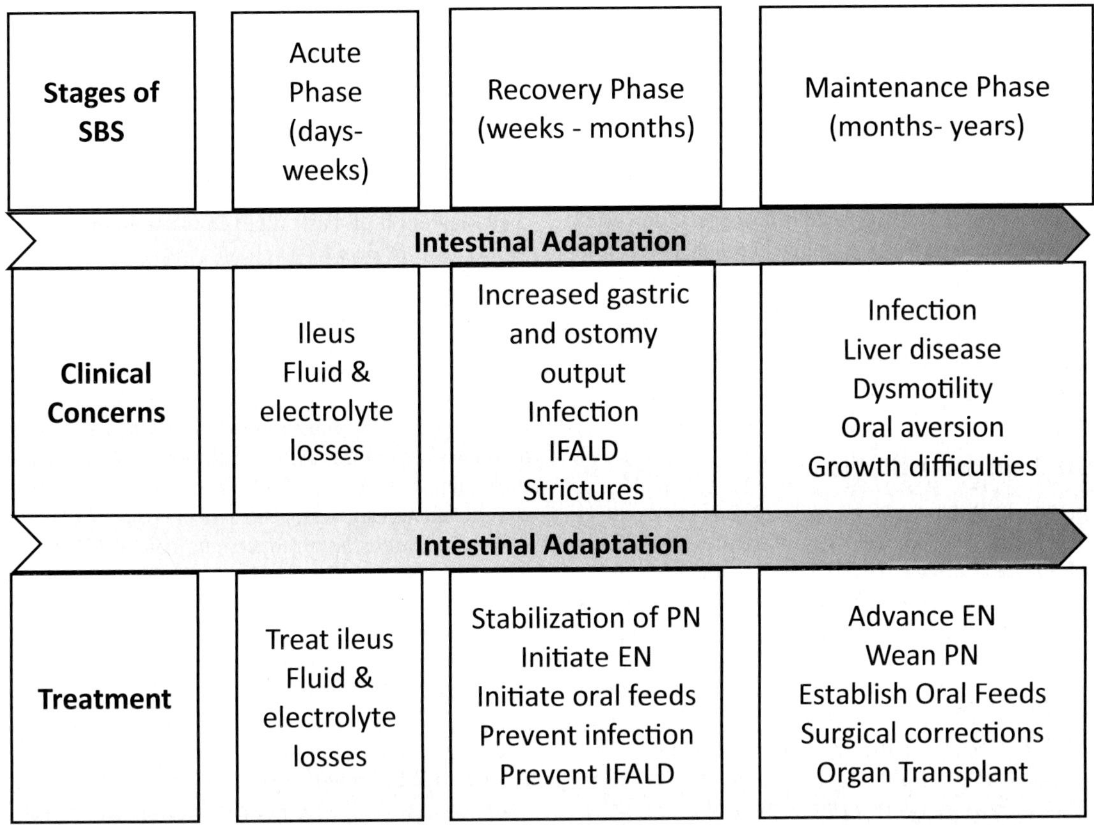

Stages of SBS
Acute Phase (days-weeks)
Recovery Phase (weeks - months)
Maintenance Phase (months- years)
Intestinal Adaptation
Clinical Concerns
Ileus
Fluid & electrolyte losses
Increased gastric and ostomy output
Infection
IFALD
Strictures
Infection
Liver disease
Dysmotility
Oral aversion
Growth difficulties
Intestinal Adaptation
Treatment
Treat ileus
Fluid & electrolyte losses
Stabilization of PN
Initiate EN
Initiate oral feeds
Prevent infection
Prevent IFALD
Advance EN
Wean PN
Establish Oral Feeds
Surgical corrections
Organ Transplant

Fig. 21.3 Stages of Recovery, Clinical Concerns, and Management of Short Bowel Syndrome. *EN,* Enteral nutrition; *IFALD,* intestinal failure–associated liver disease; *PN,* parenteral nutrition; *SBS,* short bowel syndrome.

losses is postoperative ileus. As the ileus resolves over days to weeks, the gastric secretions decrease. As the acute phase transitions to the subacute phase, gastric secretions through the gastric tube or gastrostomy can still be a concern even after the ileus has resolved. In these situations, the cause for increased gastric output is either due to gastroparesis or gastric hypersecretion. Gastroparesis is treated symptomatically with promotility medications. The most commonly used promotility medication is erythromycin. Erythromycin acts on the motilin receptors by promoting the type 3 migrating motor complexes, propagating the luminal content down the intestines. Gastric hypersecretion is often due to the loss of the inhibitory loop from the terminal ileum transmitted through peptide YY.[14,24] H2 blockers and proton pump inhibitors are of some benefit in treating gastric hypersecretion.[25–27]

The fluid losses from the gastrointestinal tract should be closely monitored because they are a source of dehydration and electrolyte derangements. Small-volume fluid losses equal to or slightly greater than physiologic secretions do not require any intervention. The volume of output greater than accounted by the normal physiologic secretions are replaced either half or full volume (0.5 or 1 mL 0.9% normal saline replacement for every 1 mL of gastrointestinal output). Volumes greater than 20 to 30 mL/kg/day are replaced with 0.9% normal saline either in half or full volume. Volumes greater than 40 mL/kg/day can cause fluid and electrolyte imbalance; hence such volumes are repleted at frequent intervals and full volume with close monitoring of fluid and electrolyte status.

Table 21.2 Goals of Intestinal Rehabilitation

- Support nutritional needs
  - Replace nutrients based on gastrointestinal losses
  - Meet nutritional needs with parenteral and enteral nutrition
  - Prevent nutrient deficiencies
- Avoid complications
  - Parenteral nutrition–related cholestasis, bloodstream infections, metabolic bone disease
- The transition from parenteral nutrition to all enteral nutrition
- Transition to all oral feeds
- Promote appropriate developmental milestones

Parenteral Nutrition

Parenteral nutrition forms an essential mode of nutrition delivery from the time of diagnosis of SBS until enteral autonomy is achieved. During the acute and subacute phases, parenteral nutrition is the mainstay of nutrient delivery. For the recommended goals for energy and protein delivered through parenteral nutrition, please refer to Chapter 25 on Parenteral Nutrition. The goal for calories ranges from 90 to 110 calories/kg/day depending on the age and maturity of the infant, the nutritional state, and the metabolic demands. This goal can be achieved with a combination of glucose, proteins, and lipids delivery. A glucose infusion rate of 11 to 12 mg/kg/min is regularly reached; In situations where calories originating from lipids are restricted, the glucose infusion rate is increased to a rate as high as 14 mg/kg/min.[28] Proteins are delivered at 3.2 to 4 g/kg/day in preterm infants and at a lower delivery rate of 2 to 3 g/kg/day in term infants, based on the nutritional demands.

Deficiencies of micronutrients in infants with SBS are common but underreported.[29,30] In a retrospective study of 178 children with IF, deficiencies of multiple micronutrients were noted during the transition from parenteral nutrition to enteral nutrition and after enteral autonomy.[29] Iron was the most common micronutrient deficiency, with 84% and 37% of children with IF having iron deficiency and iron deficiency anemia, respectively. In the United States, parenteral nutrition solutions are usually devoid of iron due to issues with compatibility and anaphylaxis. For this reason, iron is often supplemented as 25 to 50 mg/month as a separate intravenous infusion.[31] Infants with an ostomy are at an increased risk for deficiencies of zinc and copper due to losses from the ostomy. Extra supplementation with zinc and copper is made to offset the losses from the ostomy (100–150 μg/kg/day of zinc; 10–15 μg/kg/day of copper). However, because copper and manganese are excreted through bile, these micronutrients are retained in cholestatic states. In presence of cholestasis, the delivery of copper and manganese should be restricted to prevent the toxicities. Periodic biochemical measurements of these micronutrients in infants with SBS will help deliver appropriate amounts.

Intravenous Lipid Emulsions

Lipids are integral building blocks of the cell wall and play a crucial role in retinal and brain development. As a nutrient source, lipids are a calorie-rich source and act as a vehicle for fat-soluble vitamins and essential fatty acids. IFALD is a multifactorial complication noted in SBS. It is diagnosed by increased blood levels of conjugated bilirubin (≥2 mg/dL) and transaminases and may affect 22% to 30% of all infants on long-term parenteral nutrition.[32–34] There is a strong association between the use of 100% soybean oil–based lipid emulsion and IFALD,[28,35] possibly due to the high content of n-6 fatty acids that have a proinflammatory profile. Stigmasterol, a phytosterol present in soybean oil–based lipid emulsion, antagonizes the hepatoprotective farnesoid X receptor and causes hepatocyte damage.[36] Based on these concerns, efforts have focused on reducing the administration of soybean oil–based lipids to prevent IFALD.[35,37,38] This lipid-limiting technique has involved the use of lower doses (1–1.5 g/kg daily or just twice a week) of 100% soybean oil–based lipid emulsions.[39] However, randomized controlled trials showed only a modest clinical impact and actually increased the frequency of essential fatty acid deficiency with this strategy.[40,41] Newer-generation lipid emulsions have been formulated to mitigate the proinflammatory profile of n-6 fatty acids and to augment the antiinflammatory profile of n-3 fatty acids. This led to the emergence of fourth-generation lipid emulsions, namely multi-oil-based and 100% fish oil–based lipid emulsions. The multi-oil-based lipid emulsions contain soybean oil, medium-chain triglyceride oil (coconut oil), olive oil, and fish oil in proportions of 30:30:25:15, respectively. The newer-generation lipid emulsions, compared with 100% soybean oil–based lipid emulsion, have a higher antiinflammatory profile due to n-3 content, higher antioxidant activity due to greater content of vitamin E, and lower levels of the hepatotoxic phytosterol. Because of the improved antiinflammatory profile, the fourth-generation lipid emulsions have become a major strategy in both prevention and treatment of IFALD. The use of 100% fish oil–based lipid emulsions has been shown to be effective in treating IFALD in several retrospective and prospective cohort studies.[42–44] In a pair-matched analysis, infants with cholestasis who received 100% fish oil–based emulsion, in comparison with 100% soybean oil–based emulsion, showed higher rates of resolution of cholestasis (65% versus 16%) and lower rates of liver transplantation (4% versus 12%). The sole randomized controlled trial comparing 100% soybean oil–based lipid emulsion versus 100% fish oil–based lipid emulsion was inconclusive due to early termination after parental refusal to participate in the study.[45] A recent meta-analysis showed multi-oil-based lipid emulsions to have only a modest effect on prevention and treatment of IFALD.[46,47] A meta-analysis conducted by the European Society for Paediatric Gastroenterology Hepatology and Nutrition suggested that multi-oil-based lipid emulsions may be beneficial to infants with prolonged exposure to lipid emulsion. Infants who received multi-oil-based lipid emulsions for >4 weeks had decreased levels of conjugated bilirubin.[48] Although the quality of evidence to support the use of newer-generation lipid emulsions is of very low quality, the use of 100% fish oil–based lipid emulsion in the treatment of and the use of multi-oil-based lipid emulsion in the prevention of IFALD should be considered.

Enteral Nutrition

Because intestinal adaptation begins within 48 hours, enteral feeding should be commenced as soon as the postoperative ileus resolves. Enteral feeding promotes intestinal adaptation and improves feed tolerance, facilitating earlier achievement of enteral autonomy. Early introduction of enteral feeding reduces the number of days with central venous catheters, decreases the risk of catheter-related bloodstream infections, and reduces the risk of IFALD. Apart from the early introduction of feeds, there is little consensus on the choice of initial feeds (breast milk versus formula feeds), route of feeds (oral versus enteric drip), or continuous versus bolus feeds. There is a serious limitation in data to make confident recommendations; most of our current information is from observational studies.

If available, the first choice of initial feeds in infants with SBS is breast milk. Human breast milk contains many protective and trophic factors, which offer numerous benefits, including effects on digestion, immunity, and the development of a healthy gut microbiome.[49] Factors such as α_1-antitrypsin and β-casein in the breast milk aid in the process of nutrient digestion and absorption and facilitate enterocyte proliferation and growth. Despite its content of lactose, relatively low content of medium-chain triglycerides, and complex proteins, breast milk is well tolerated in infants with SBS.

There are no randomized controlled trials comparing the outcomes between breast milk and formula in infants with SBS. If there are concerns for persistent feeding intolerance, protein allergy, or increased risk of NEC, hydrolyzed protein or amino acid–based formula can be used. In a retrospective study involving 32 patients with SBS, those who received either breast milk or amino acid–based formula had shorter durations of parenteral nutrition.[50] Medium-chain triglycerides do not require emulsification and esterification; these are converted to free fatty acids and can be directly transported to the liver by portal circulation, even in states of pancreatic deficiency.[51] For this reason, formulas high in medium-chain triglycerides are often preferred. However, long-chain triglycerides in the diet are also important as sources of the essential fatty acids linoleic and α-linolenic acid. In animal studies, long-chain triglycerides demonstrate more trophic effects with better mucosal hyperplasia compared with medium-chain triglycerides.[52]

Continuous enteral feeds are achieved by either nasogastric or orogastric tube feeding, feeding gastrostomy, or jejunal tube feeding. Continuous feeds thoroughly saturate the luminal receptors and optimize the transporters, thereby promoting better digestion and absorption. Small-volume feeds provided continuously is often the strategy when feeds are introduced after recovery from postoperative ileus. However, the downsides include loss of calories to adherence of fats to the tubing,[53,54] loss of appetite, and alterations in gastrointestinal motility due to the absence of type 3 migrating motor complexes seen during fasting states. The advantages of bolus feeds include better gut motility and adaptation and better amino acid and insulin levels after the feed. Transpyloric feeds are tried in the presence of concerns for emesis and gastric distension due to gastric hypomotility.

In general, in the initial states of SBS, feedings are initiated as continuous enteral feeds at a rate of 0.5 to 1 mL/hour or 5 to 10 mL/kg/day. As tolerance to feeds is demonstrated, feeds are advanced once in 2 to 4 days by increasing the infusion rate while closely monitoring the stoma or stool output. Feed advancement is continued even if stoma or stool output of 20 to 30 mL/kg/day is noted as long as adequate weight gain and electrolyte balance are maintained. If the stool output is more than 30 mL/kg/day, feed advancement should be held, or feeds should be decreased until an improvement in stool output is noted. As one approaches the volumes of full feeds, fortification of milk should be considered to meet the growth demands.

Oral feeds should be attempted in smaller quantities when the infant shows appropriate behavioral cues. Early introduction of oral feeding facilitates the development of safe suck-swallow cycle skills and decreases the likelihood of oral aversion. Oral feeding may stimulate gall bladder contractions and release of luminal and pancreatic hormones, which promote digestion and gastrointestinal motility. Provision of parenteral nutrition during the night and bolus tube feeds during the daytime facilitates the development of oral feeding skills.[55] For recommended energy and protein goals for complete enteral nutrition, please refer to Chapter 26 on Enteral Nutrition.

Although enteral autonomy is the ultimate goal, this should not be achieved at the expense of appropriate growth. Parenteral nutrition should be increased, resumed, or extended to augment growth when the expected growth requirements are not satisfied, even if enteral feeds are well tolerated. The goals of nutritional support in infants with SBS should meet the appropriate growth parameters as measured by weight, head circumference, and height.

Nonnutritional Strategies in the Management of Short Bowel Syndrome

Mucous Fistula Refeeding

In infants with SBS after resection of the intestines, two conduits or ostomies are often created, namely a proximal stoma and a distal mucus fistula. Mucus fistula refeeding is the practice of collecting proximal ostomy effluent and reinfusing it into the distal mucous fistula to mimic the normal physiologic intestinal flow, digestion, and absorption. In infants with ostomies, the likelihood of achieving sustained enteral autonomy without mucous fistula refeeding is very challenging and hence low.[20] The process of mucous fistula refeeding exposes the otherwise unused portion of the intestines and colon distal to the mucous fistula to enteral feeds. This exposure of the distal intestine to stoma effluent stimulates and sustains the process of intestinal adaptation. There is emerging evidence suggesting that mucous fistula refeeding provides several advantages to the patient with IF. Mucous fistula refeeding improves the absorptive capacity of the distal bowel for nutrition, with related notable effects including an increase in weight gain, decreased electrolyte imbalance, decreased dependence on parenteral nutrition, and lower peak conjugated bilirubin levels.[56–58] Although mucous fistula refeeding has emerged as the standard of care in infants with IF and ostomy, more research is required to better define the short and long-term outcomes associated with mucous fistula refeeding.

Cycling of Parenteral Nutrition

Once a steady metabolic state has been stabilized with a combination of parenteral and enteral nutrition in infants with SBS, cycling of parenteral nutrition should be initiated.[59] Cycling parenteral nutrition has several benefits. It has been shown to decrease the risk of hyperglycemia, hyperinsulinemia, hepatic steatosis, and IFALD.[55] In a retrospective study involving 107 infants with gastroschisis, cycling of parenteral nutrition was associated with reduced incidence of cholestasis at 25 and 50 days.[60] However, the evidence to support the cycling of parenteral nutrition in the prevention of IFALD is weak. In a randomized clinical trial, VLBW infants who received cycling of parenteral nutrition did not demonstrate a reduction in IFALD.[61] Importantly, cycling of parenteral nutrition during the day releases the infant from being tethered to the parenteral nutrition pole, improving mobility and physical activity, thus promoting neurodevelopment. Cycling of parenteral nutrition should be instituted before discharge from the hospital and continued at home.

Multidisciplinary Care

Multidisciplinary care of infants with SBS in a tertiary center has been shown to improve the chances of achieving enteral autonomy.[21,50,62] Multidisciplinary care brings together expertise from various specialties such as neonatology, surgery, gastroenterology, nursing, nutrition, pharmacy, and family support. Standardization of feeding regimens, medical therapies, surgical techniques, and nursing has improved survival and decreased morbidity. In a study conducted in Canada, the outcomes from two different eras, before and after instituting multidisciplinary care, were compared. In the latter epoch, feeding protocols were standardized, prophylactic antibiotics were used, lipid was minimized, and the use of newer lipid emulsions were introduced. The era of multidisciplinary care was associated with improved outcomes, including decreased mortality, higher rates of achievement of enteral autonomy, and shorter durations of parenteral nutrition.[62]

Medications

Advancement and tolerance of enteral feeds are often hampered by complications of SBS such as slow motility, hypermotility, hypergastrinemia, and small intestinal bacterial overgrowth. Treatment of these conditions with medications can alleviate the symptoms associated with these complications and improve the tolerance to enteral feeds. Gastroparesis and hypomotility of the small intestines have been treated with promotility agents. Erythromycin and amoxicillin-clavulanate are motilin agonists, which act on the motilin receptors in the upper gastrointestinal tract and stimulate gastric and intestinal motility.[63,64] Studies of erythromycin in infants with SBS are limited. Erythromycin failed to show significant benefits in patients with gastroschisis compared with placebo in the only randomized controlled trial.[63] Amoxicillin-clavulanate acts on the duodenum and jejunum and is a better prokinetic medication than erythromycin. Although there are very few studies of amoxicillin-clavulanate in infants with an intact gastrointestinal system,[65] there are no studies in infants with SBS. Antidopaminergic medications such as domperidone and metoclopramide and serotoninergic agents such as cisapride are avoided in infants due to their unfavorable side effects, including tardive dyskinesia and cardiac arrhythmia, respectively.[66,67] Opioid medications used as antidiarrheal agents include loperamide and diphenoxylate, to treat hypermotility in infants with SBS. Small intestinal bacterial overgrowth is a common complication of short bowel syndrome associated with decreased transit times, seen in hypomotility and blind intestinal loops. Antibacterial agents such as metronidazole, amoxicillin-clavulanate, and trimethoprim-sulfamethoxazole are often used to treat small intestinal bacterial overgrowth. The GLP-2 analog teduglutide is a modulator that increases the enterocyte mass by the expansion of mucosa by crypt cell growth and reduction in enterocyte apoptosis. In a 12-week-long open-label study, infants and children who received teduglutide showed a reduction in parenteral nutrition volume and an increase in tolerated enteral feed volume with no serious adverse effects.[68] The use of teduglutide in children less than a year old with SBS has not been studied.

Dietary Fibers

Dietary fibers act as absorbents and are of two varieties: insoluble and soluble. Both these forms work by osmotically absorbing water, slowing transit, and improving stool consistency.[69] Examples of dietary fiber include substances such as guar gum and pectin. When dietary fiber reaches the colon in an undigested form, it is acted on by the intestinal bacteria–liberating short-chain fatty acids, which serve as metabolic fuel to the enterocytes in the colon, supporting their proliferation and growth. The use of dietary fibers in children with SBS has demonstrated a reduction in stool output, increased gastrointestinal transit time, and increased positive nitrogen balance.[70]

Enteral Fish Oil and Lipid Supplements

Enteral lipid preparations are obtained from various sources, including plant oil, fish oil, or synthetic preparations. The benefits of enteral lipid supplementation include enhancing nutrient absorption, improving intestinal motility, promoting mucosal growth, and reducing IFALD. In experimental models of SBS, enteral fish oil supplementation improved absorption of total fat and individual fatty acids and increased the DNA content of enterocyte.[71,72] Enteral lipid also enhances the level of the hormone peptide YY that slows motility, lengthening the transit time and resulting in increased mucosal contact with the nutrients. The use of enteral lipid in infants with SBS is promising and deserves more research.

Probiotics

Probiotics are live microorganisms that, when administered in adequate amounts, confer a health benefit on the host. The data on probiotics in children with SBS dependent on parenteral nutrition are limited. The altered gut permeability and dysmotility in SBS increase the risks for bacterial translocation and subsequent bacteremia with the use of probiotics. The use of probiotics in animal models of SBS has demonstrated an increase in villus length, crypt depth, and increase in enterocyte count in the jejunum but not the ileum.[73] *Saccharomyces boulardii* in rat models of SBS has been demonstrated to reduce bacterial translocation along with having trophic effects on the mucosa.[74] The data regarding the use of probiotics in infants with SBS are restricted to observation studies and case reports. Although laboratory studies suggest potential benefits, observations of bacteremia in infants with SBS treated with probiotics raise serious concerns. In one account, two patients with SBS and cholestasis developed *Lactobacillus* bacteremia during supplementation with *Lactobacillus rhamnosus* GG.[75] In another case series, four patients with SBS and a central venous catheter developed *S. boulardii* fungemia.[76] These patients were receiving *S. boulardii* as a nutritional supplement to treat diarrhea. In a systematic review on the use of probiotics in infants with SBS, the authors highlighted the absence of randomized controlled trials of the use of probiotics in infants with SBS.[77] The authors further reported that the benefits of probiotics in infants and children with SBS were inconsistent. Apart from the aforementioned adverse effects of *Lactobacillus* bacteremia, the authors also reported concerns for lactic acidosis. In light of the yet unproven benefits and reported concerns of bacteremia, they concluded that the current data were insufficient to support the use of probiotics in infants and children with SBS. Until evidence for safety and efficacy emerges, the use of probiotics in infants with SBS should perhaps be restricted to closely monitored research protocols.

Predictors of Successful Outcomes

Although the survival of infants with SBS has improved dramatically, the morbidity continues to be high.[21–23] In a study of infants with neonatal-onset SBS, the overall survival at last follow-up exceeded 95%, and nearly 85% of infants achieved enteral autonomy.[22] However, in infants with ultra-SBS, the achievement of enteral autonomy can be challenging and delayed. In infants with a residual bowel length <31 cm, only 50% achieved enteral autonomy at the last follow-up of 44 months. Also, in those infants with <31 cm residual bowel length, it took a median of 585 days to achieve enteral autonomy. Patient variables associated with improved outcomes include a longer length of the residual bowel, presence of ileocecal valve and colon, fewer infections, and use of breast milk or elemental formula.[21,22,50,78]

Future Directions

The advances in the past two decades in the nutritional management of SBS have improved the outcomes tremendously. The survival is high, and the rates of intestinal and liver transplants are low. This vast improvement in outcomes is widely attributed to the multidisciplinary care in highly specialized centers, wide use of newer-generation lipid emulsions, and better infection-control bundles. Although the mortality is low, morbidity is still high, stressing the need for improvements in the care of infants with SBS. Because residual bowel length is a crucial variable on the outcomes of infants with SBS, advances in surgical techniques resulting in retaining longer bowel lengths are needed. Although newer-generation lipid emulsions have vastly improved the outcomes of infants with SBS, the search for the ideal intravenous lipid emulsions is not over. Current development of the newer generation of lipid emulsions includes further depletion of phytosterols, enhancing antioxidant properties, and optimizing the n-3:n-6 ratio. The hope is to generate a lipid emulsion with the optimal balance of fatty acids, readily metabolized, with a reduced oxidative stress and antiinflammatory profile promoting a better long-term neurodevelopmental outcome. The use of intestinal growth modulators such as GLP-2 has not been adequately studied, particularly in infancy, and can improve outcomes significantly. The use of probiotics in animal models with SBS is promising and deserves further study in closely monitored trials in infants with SBS. The beneficial effect of probiotics observed in preventing NEC and the benefits noted in animal models of SBS raises the possibility of similarly improved infant outcomes. Finally, there is an urgent need to address the lack of an evidence base for the current practices of intestinal rehabilitation. The current treatment strategies are mainly experience-based rather than evidence-based. In particular, with the increasing availability of donor breast milk and evolving technologies with lacto-engineering, there is an urgent need to determine the best choice of enteral feeding in infants with SBS. Studies that promote the development of evidence-based therapeutic approaches are needed.

CHAPTER

22 Neonatal Nutrition Assessment

Kera M. McNelis, Tanis R. Fenton

KEY POINTS

1. All infants should be classified at birth with the use of appropriate anthropometric measurement techniques to determine risk status for complications such as hypoglycemia or catabolism. Growth charts and tools to determine *z*-scores are readily available and should be used.
2. Hospitalized infants are at higher risk for growth impairment, so patterns on a growth chart and growth velocity throughout hospitalization should be routinely monitored as part of standard clinical care.
3. A nutrition-focused physical examination includes anthropometric assessments, vital signs, and careful assessment for any evidence of nutritional deficiencies.
4. Controversy exists regarding frequency and timing of biochemical monitoring for common complications of prematurity, such as metabolic bone disease and cholestasis. Clinicians should consider adopting a standardized approach that incorporates expert opinion when evidence is lacking.
5. All high-risk infants should have daily assessment of nutrient intake.
6. A registered dietitian should be part of the healthcare team to assess neonatal growth and nutrient intakes.

Introduction

Growth is a normal state for infants and an indicator of wellness. All infants deserve personalized nutritional care that will promote growth and a healthy start to life. Nutritional assessment based on growth history; biochemical, clinical, and physical parameters; and nutritional intake can allow the clinician to determine which infants are not growing well and/or have not achieved adequate nutrition.

Preterm and critically ill infants need focused growth monitoring, because nutrient needs are not based on the cues from the infant but have to be estimated and delivered by the medical team. In this chapter, we seek to describe clinically available tools and the highest-quality evidence available to assess neonatal nutritional status. Further information on parenteral and enteral nutrition is included in separate chapters focused on nutrition requirements.

Classification of the Newborn

Newborn assessment and anthropometric classification at the time of delivery reflect intrauterine growth and allow identification of infants who are at higher nutrition risk. Many of these small- and large-for-gestational age (SGA and LGA) infants are also at risk of early metabolic complications such as hypoglycemia in the first days of life. SGA infants often have low glycogen stores, whereas many LGA infants may be at risk of abnormal glucose levels due to maladaptation to higher glucose loads from uncontrolled maternal diabetes.[1] Symptoms of hypoglycemia include jitteriness, poor feeding, tachypnea, floppy tone, and even seizures. In subsequent days, these early metabolic abnormalities may resolve, but multiple studies have shown these infants to also be at risk of abnormal growth trajectories (Chapter 19, 20).

Birth Weight Classification

- Per Centers for Disease Control and Prevention 2019 data, about 8.3% of all infants have a birth weight of less than 2500 g and are categorized as low birth weight (LBW).[2,3] Those born with a birth weight of less than 1500 g are identified as very low birth weight (VLBW) infants, which is about 1.4% of all infants.[3] Less than 1% of infants are born with a weight of less than 1000 g and are categorized as extremely low birth weight (ELBW).[3]
- Birth weight may reflect the adequacy of nutritional stores, such as those of protein, fat, iron, calcium, phosphorus, and other important nutrients.
- Higher gestational age reflects maturity with better ability to tolerate fluctuations in biochemical levels of various nutrients. Adjusting age for prematurity assists in setting expectations for developmental achievements.
- Premature birth is the most common cause of low birth weight. We have nutritional guidelines for VLBW, preterm infants that aim to meet the metabolic and growth needs and achieve growth rates similar to those in utero.[4,5]
- Besides prematurity, another important cause of low birth weight is fetal or intrauterine growth restriction (IUGR). At any gestation, infants may be classified as SGA (birth weight < the 10th percentile), appropriate for gestational age (AGA), or LGA (birth weight > the 90th percentile). Based on these definitions, 20% of the population is expected to have a birth weight outside the AGA category. Not all infants who meet criteria to be labeled SGA or LGA are medically compromised, nor have they suffered from an obvious intrauterine insult that may explain their abnormal growth. Some conditions are definitely more frequent in the LGA and SGA categories, but it is important to understand that these definitions are statistical and somewhat arbitrary, and therefore, not everyone in these categories has ongoing pathology. Many of these infants have weights that are normal, healthy metrics for their genetic profiles. In some infants, IUGR may also be due to maternal factors that did not support in utero growth at their genetic potential. These infants also may not have intrinsic abnormalities.
- Newer technologies can often allow the identification of the cause for IUGR. Many fetuses are growth restricted because of compromised fetal blood flow; the Doppler waveform of blood flow in

the umbilical vessels can provide useful information.[6,7] Similarly, magnetic resonance imaging of whole-body fetal adipose tissue can also provide useful information to aid assessment of fetal growth and placental sufficiency.[8]

Features of Fetal Growth Restriction

- Can be identified via prenatal ultrasound or by physical exam at birth
- Thin, wasted appearance on prenatal imaging and after birth[9]
- Deficiency of subcutaneous tissue and muscle, noted in the cheeks, neck and chin, arms, back, buttocks, legs, and trunk
- Cranial sutures may be widened, and the umbilical cord may be thin and lacking in Wharton's jelly
- Dysmorphic features could indicate a congenital syndrome

One scoring system is the Clinical Assessment of Nutritional Status (CANS) (Fig. 22.1).[10] The intent of this exam is to distinguish a term infant who suffered from fetal malnutrition from an infant who is simply physiologically small for gestational age.[11] This malnutrition might result in altered body composition and impaired neurodevelopmental potential. The signs of malnutrition include:

- Hair: silky versus straight
- "Staring" or flag sign
- Reduced buccal fat in the cheeks
- Sharply defined thin chin or fat double chin
- A thin, clearly evident neck with loose, wrinkled skin
- "Accordion" pleating of the skin of arms and legs with loose, easily lifted skin over major joints
- Loss of subcutaneous fat on the back with skin easily lifted
- Minimal fat and wrinkled skin over abdomen
- Buttocks with deep folds

This CANS simple scoring system was developed for term infants and is intended to be used in the first 48 hours of life.[12,13] Some researchers then applied the CANSCORE to preterm infants. They found that maternal hypertension and preeclampsia, oligohydramnios, disturbed umbilical artery Doppler flow, neonatal hypoglycemia, polycythemia, feeding intolerance, and necrotizing enterocolitis were all associated with what was described as fetal malnutrition.[14] Interestingly, not all of the infants who were identified as having had fetal malnutrition were classified as SGA based on anthropometrics. We clearly need ways for more accurate identification of the predisposing factors and validation of the CANSCORE for preterm infants.

LGA infants can be born to constitutionally tall parents or to mothers with uncontrolled diabetes or obesity.[15,16] Infants of diabetic mothers may have increased adiposity resulting from storage of the fat generated from the conversion of high glucose supply from the hyperglycemic mothers. These fat stores may be visually obvious to the examiner and can also be objectively identified by measuring body composition, using indices such as an elevated weight, mid-upper arm circumference, and/or triceps skinfold thickness in the absence of an elevated length and head circumference.[17] During the early neonatal period, infants of diabetic mothers are important to identify because they are at higher risk for hypoglycemia, hypocalcemia, polycythemia, and congenital malformations.

Anthropometric and Growth Assessment

Growth Charts

Infant growth charts have been developed to provide normative growth references for monitoring an infant's postnatal growth. Even though this information is not diagnostic, the data do help differentiate infants who are growing well from those who need more support and/or additional follow-up assessments. Several growth charts exist, each of which have strengths and limitations (Table 22.1). Broadly, these growth charts show normative data of serial anthropometric measurements of fetuses at the time of their birth (intrauterine chart) or preterm infants (postnatal charts). Because the ideal preterm infant growth is not yet defined, many expert groups recommend that the growth of preterm infants should mimic that of the fetus, as seen in intrauterine growth charts.[4] Fetal growth slows down in late pregnancy for two reasons—the space limitations of the in-utero environment and slowing from the peak growth at about 34 weeks, which is displayed on intrauterine growth charts as a flattening after about 36 weeks. Preterm infants do not always slow their growth as much as their fetal counterparts at the same gestational age and can demonstrate some catch-up growth at this age.[18,19]

Most infants usually lose some weight after birth due to changes in total body water and in nutrient supply, which transfers their growth chart position to lower percentiles. Hence, at any age after the day of birth, weight less than the 10th percentile should not be used to define size for gestational age and categorize infant growth.[19]

Growth Velocity

A goal weight gain of 15 to 20 grams/kilogram/day (g/kg/day) after the postnatal weight loss and up to 36 weeks' postmenstrual age (Fig. 22.2) is required to maintain intrauterine growth rates, as recommended to support optimal neurodevelopmental outcomes for premature infants.[20–22]

For the growth of head circumference, estimates from fetal and postnatal growth rates show an increase of approximately 1 to 1.3 centimeters per week (cm/week) until 30 weeks, which then decreases to about 0.4 cm/week by 40 weeks (see Fig. 22.2).[22] For growth measured in length, estimates from fetal and postnatal growth rates are a velocity of approximately 1.2 to 1.4 cm/week to 34 weeks, decreasing to about 0.8 cm/week by 40 weeks.

After 36 weeks' corrected age, the expected weight gain slows to less than 15 g/kg/day. It can be useful to change at this point to grams per day and aim for 20 to 40 g/day until 2 months' corrected age.[22] Using a growth chart to examine the patterns of weight, head, and length growth from birth adds to the perspective of understanding the growth history, which assists in assessing an infant's weight in relation to their length and head size and in setting expectations for the future. The typical growth pattern of preterm infants is to lose weight in the first days of life, which places them lower on growth chart percentiles. Not all infants lose weight after birth, and losing no weight may occur more frequently among SGA infants. Head growth seems to be the priority for growth in the first weeks and months of life to gradually catch up to the population average as represented by the intrauterine and Fenton growth charts' median. Weight catch up generally occurs after term age.

The goal for infants to grow at intrauterine rates applies well to weight gain, because many infants gain weight approximately parallel to the curves on growth charts. Length growth seems to have a lower priority for preterm infants in their first months, because length gain is usually slower than intrauterine rates until after term age. It is important to consider parental size, because parents with short stature are not likely to have the tallest children.[15] Small size at birth may also be due at least in part to socioeconomic disadvantages and thus may identify parents who need additional support.[23]

If preterm infants are plotted on growth charts without correcting for their preterm birth, their size will appear inappropriately

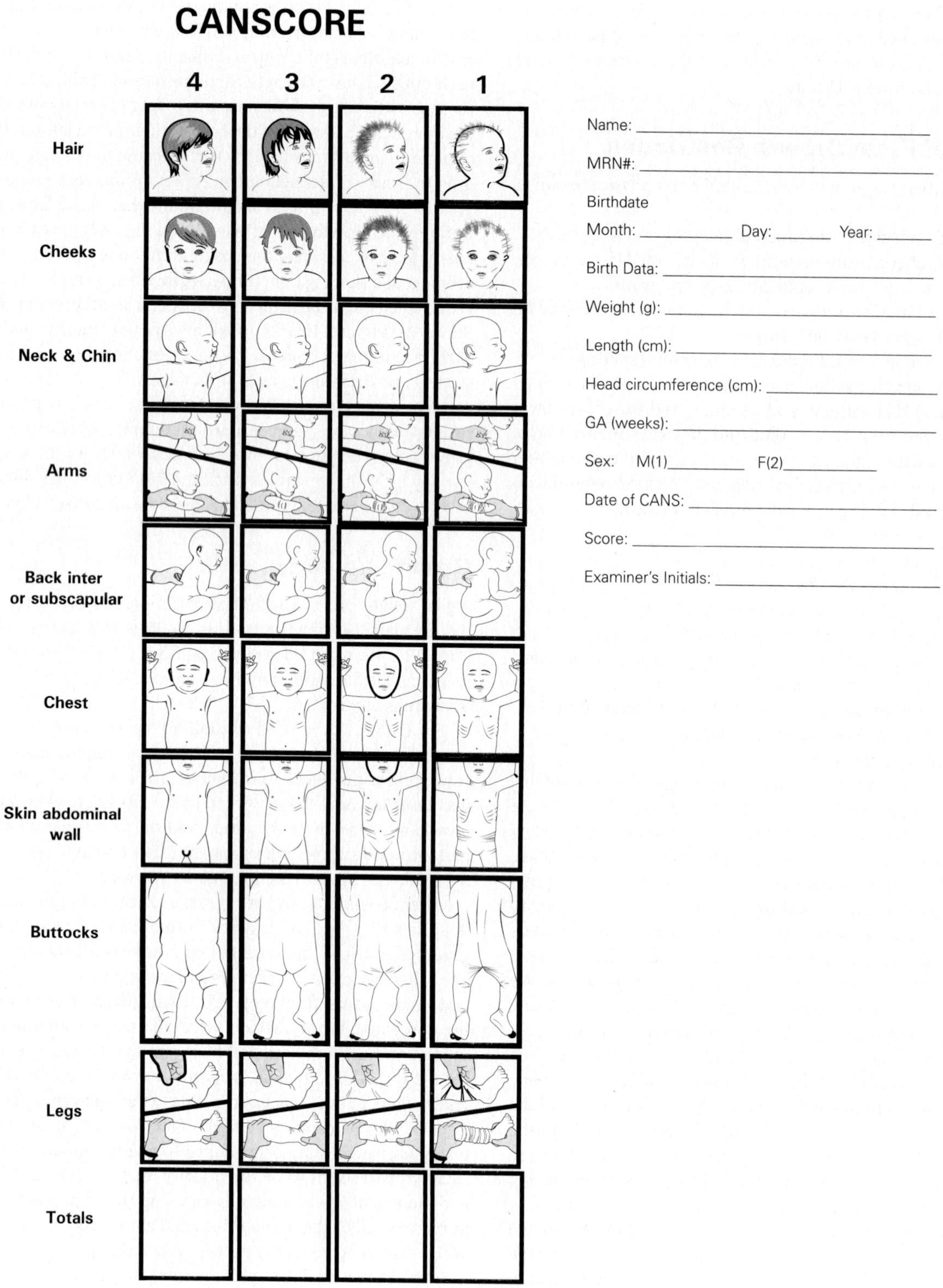

CANSCORE

4 3 2 1

Hair

Cheeks

Neck & Chin

Arms

Back inter or subscapular

Chest

Skin abdominal wall

Buttocks

Legs

Totals

Name: ____________________

MRN#: ____________________

Birthdate

Month: ________ Day: ______ Year: ______

Birth Data: ____________________

Weight (g): ____________________

Length (cm): ____________________

Head circumference (cm): ____________________

GA (weeks): ____________________

Sex: M(1)________ F(2)________

Date of CANS: ____________________

Score: ____________________

Examiner's Initials: ____________________

Fig. 22.1 Clinical Assessment of Nutritional Status (CANS), a Scoring Tool for Fetal Malnutrition. This tool was developed for term newborns and should be used with physical exam findings in the first 48 hours of life. Infants with scores less than or equal to 24 have clinical evidence of fetal malnutrition. *GA*, Gestational age. (Adapted from Metcoff J. Clinical assessment of nutritional status at birth. *Pediatr Clin North Am*. 1994;41[5]:875-891.)

small on a growth chart. For example, a 25-weeks' gestational age female infant with a birth weight of 700 g is at the median on a Fenton preterm growth chart, which reveals this as a normal weight. If this same infant was inappropriately plotted at birth on the World Health Organization (WHO) Growth Standard as a term infant, she appears to have an extremely low birth weight. In the case of a preterm, VLBW infant, it is necessary to continue to adjust for an infant's early birth throughout the first 3 years of life to accurately assess size.[24] Therefore it is very important to correct for prematurity when an infant is transitioned to growth charts that begin at term/40 weeks' gestational age, such as the WHO Growth Standard.

Table 22.1 Comparison of Infant Growth Charts

Growth Curve	Intrauterine Growth or Postnatal Growth	Population (Including #)	Strengths	Limitations	Access
Fenton 2013	Intrauterine combined with term postnatal growth	Represents 3,986,456 preterm births from developed countries (Germany, United States, Italy, Australia, Scotland, Canada)	Harmonized with the WHO Growth Standard Produced using meta-analysis; age is actual age instead of completed weeks; largest sample size Use for classifying infants <36 weeks: SGA/AGA/LGA status, for older gestational age use the 6-country meta-analysis	Should not be used to assign size for gestational age at birth after 37 weeks; use the WHO Growth Standard for these infants; the 6-country meta-analysis can be used for gestational ages 22–42 weeks	PDFs, *z*-score/percentile calculators, apps, and growth chart curve data for noncommercial use available at www.ucalgary.ca/fenton/
Olsen 2010	Intrauterine	Represents 257,855 preterm births from 33 US states who survived to discharge	Useful for assessment of size for gestational age at birth for American infants May be used for classifying infants <36 weeks: SGA/AGA/LGA status	Limited use as a growth chart after 36 weeks because fetal growth slows in late pregnancy	https://downloads.aap.org/DOSP/20200Is-enCurveUpdated.pdf
INTERGROWTH-21st	Postnatal growth	Represents 224 singleton preterm births (mean gestational age, 35.5 weeks) from antenatally enrolled mothers of low-risk birth with early prenatal care in 8 worldwide locations (Brazil, Italy, Oman, United Kingdom, United States, China, India, Kenya)	More specific for EUGR Harmonizes with WHO	Small sample size at low gestational ages; not data informed <33 weeks Overestimates SGA because growth-restricted infants were excluded	PDFs and apps available at https://intergrowth21.tghn.org
WHO 2006	Postnatal growth for term infants and for preterm infants after term corrected age	8,440 healthy breastfed infants from diverse ethnic backgrounds	Selected children from communities in which economics were not likely to interfere with growth Longitudinal measures to 2 years of age; *z*-score charts also available Use for growth monitoring of term infants and preterm infants after term postmenstrual age (using age adjusted for prematurity) Use for classifying infants GA 37 weeks+: SGA/AGA/LGA status	It is appropriate to use these charts to assign size for gestational age at birth for infants 37+ weeks	https://www.who.int/childgrowth/standards/en/

AGA, Appropriate for gestational age; *EUGR*, extrauterine growth restriction; *GA*, gestational age; *LGA*, large for gestational age; *SGA*, small for gestational age; *WHO*, World Health Organization.

The American Academy of Pediatrics recommends that the phrase "corrected gestational age" be used until up to 3 years of chronologic age for infants who are born prematurely.[25] It recommends that corrected gestational age be "calculated by subtracting the number of weeks born before 40 weeks of gestation from the chronological age. Therefore, a 24-month-old, former 28-week gestational age infant has a corrected age of 21 months according to the following equation: 24 months − [(40 weeks − 28 weeks) × 1 month/4 weeks]."

In the NICU, it is important to assess growth patterns from birth by examining the patterns of weight, length, and head circumference together. Short-term assessments have high variability due to fluid fluctuations.[20] Caution should be used when interpreting weight gain of an infant with fluid accumulation, such as infants with lymphatic malformations, hydrops fetalis, cardiac lesions, renal anomalies, or hydrocephalus, because weight will be elevated by the excess fluid. Likewise, after diuretics are started, an infant is likely to temporarily fail to meet weight gain goals due to fluid weight loss. Irremovable equipment such as respiratory support and drainage tubes may hinder precise measurements. Monitoring weight gain over a 5- to 7-day period instead of daily weight gain improves the understanding of growth velocity.[20]

To calculate growth velocity, the Average 2-point method is the most accurate calculation (see Fig. 22.3 for an example) because the Early 1-point method overestimates weight gain, especially for time periods greater than 1 week.[21] Although growth charts reflect cross-sectional fetal growth, many preterm infants achieve similar growth rates after the postnatal weight loss phase.[18,26]

The best practice is to monitor length and head circumference weekly and to use this information along with weight changes to make anthropometric assessments. Recumbent length is best

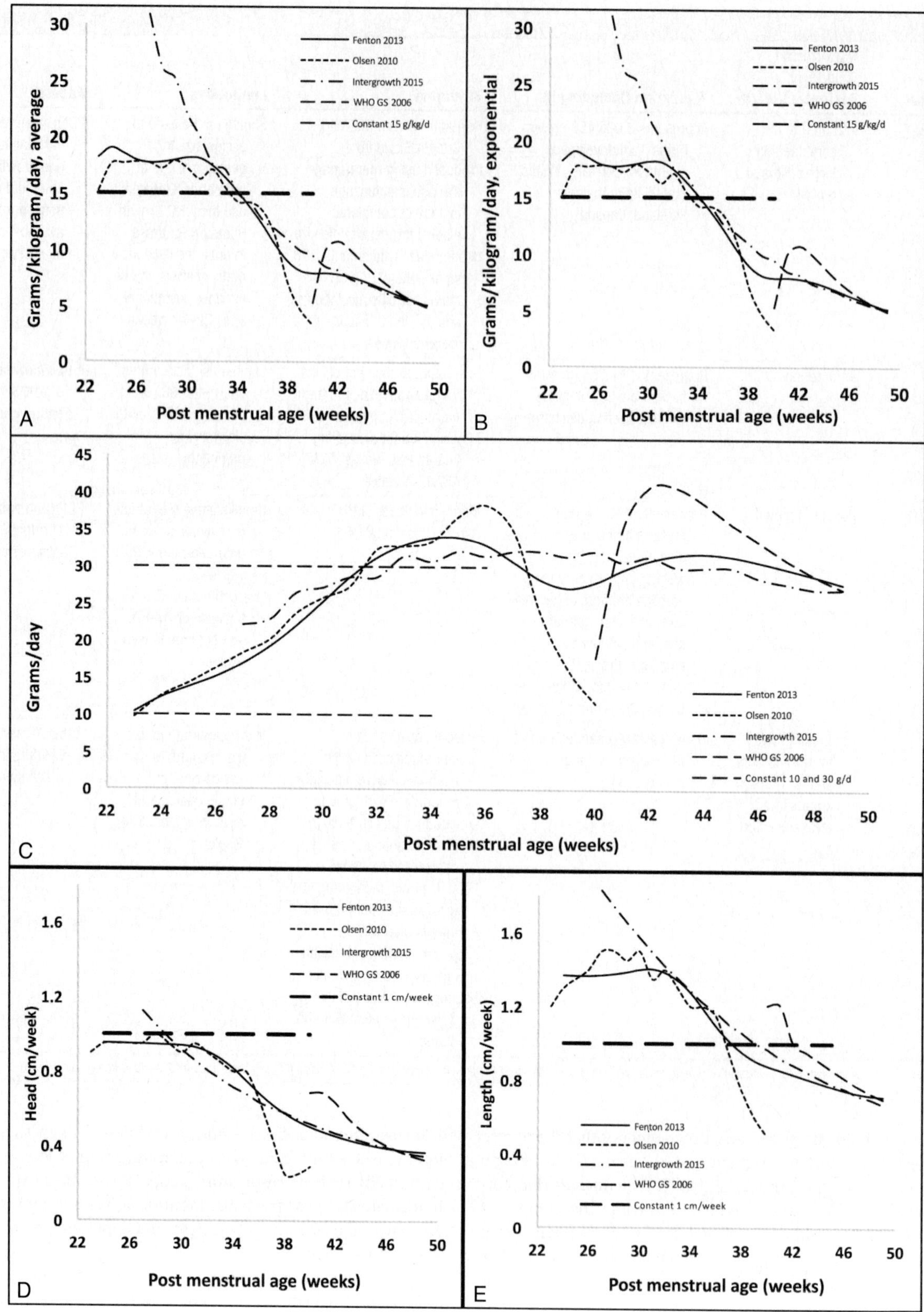

Fig. 22.2 Growth in weight (as grams/kilogram/day [A: average method as defined in Fig. 22.3, B: exponential method] and C: grams/day), D: length, and E: head circumference (in centimeters per week) as reflected by commonly used growth charts for preterm infants from 22 to 50 weeks' postmenstrual age. (Reprinted with authors' permission from Fenton TR et al. *J Peds*. 2018.)

Average weight gain,
grams/kilogram/day =

$$\frac{\dfrac{(w2-w1)}{((w1+w2)\div 2)\div 1000}}{\text{Number of days}}$$

Example:

DOL 7: weight 1500 g = w1

DOL 14: weight 1700 g = w2

$$\frac{\dfrac{(1700-1500)}{((1500+1700)\div 2)\div 1000}}{7}$$

Average weight gain = 17.9 grams/kilograms/daily

Fig. 22.3 Two-Point Method for Average Weight Gain. *DOL*, Day of life; *w1*, week 1; *w2*, week 2.

measured with use of a solid length board and two examiners. One person holds the infant's head against the fixed headboard while the other person gently extends the infant's legs and places the footboard at the flat feet. For an infant who is too unstable for this measurement, a nonstretchable tape measure can provide a length estimate,[27,28] but it is better to use a length board whenever possible.

Head circumference (occipitofrontal circumference) is measured with a nonstretchable tape measure around the widest part of the infant's head. The tape measure will cross the infant's skull over the frontal bones, along the parietal bones, and over the occipital bones. The head circumference should be measured at delivery but also after 24 hours of life or later in infants who experienced labor, as the skull shape will normalize and soft-tissue swelling and molding will resolve. Length and head circumference should be measured to the nearest one decimal place (e.g., 25.3 cm) and plotted weekly through hospitalization.

Using *Z*-Scores to Describe Growth Rates

Z-scores define the size of an infant compared with a growth chart at a specific age, in terms of how many standard deviations the infant's measure is above (positive values) or below (negative values) the median of the growth chart (Fig. 22.4). By examining two or more *z*-scores for an infant's anthropometric measurements, the changes in the *z*-scores reflect whether the infant is maintaining the growth velocity reflected in the growth chart over that time period. As with any anthropometric measurements, *z*-score fluctuations are normal and expected. Do not expect an infant to maintain *z*-scores identical to previous measures. As with weight gain monitoring, *z*-score changes should be assessed over at least 5- to 7-day periods instead of shorter time periods.

If an infant is not maintaining their weight, length, and/or head circumference *z*-scores after the postnatal weight loss phase in their first week of life, they may be finding their genetic potential, or their growth may be limited by insufficient nutrition or morbidities. When an infant is not maintaining their *z*-score(s), ensure that nutrition is adequate and not limiting. See Table 22.2. Many genetic and environmental factors contribute to an infant's size, which can be indicated at least in part by parental size. The birth *z*-score is not an appropriate weight gain goal, as the postnatal weight loss that most babies experience after birth lowers the magnitude of their *z*-score goals. Instead, use the *z*-score at day 7 as the starting value for comparisons, but do not expect that *z*-scores will be perfectly maintained, because growth fluctuations are normal.

Z-SCORES

- Standardized for age relative to a growth reference
- Specify size relative to growth charts

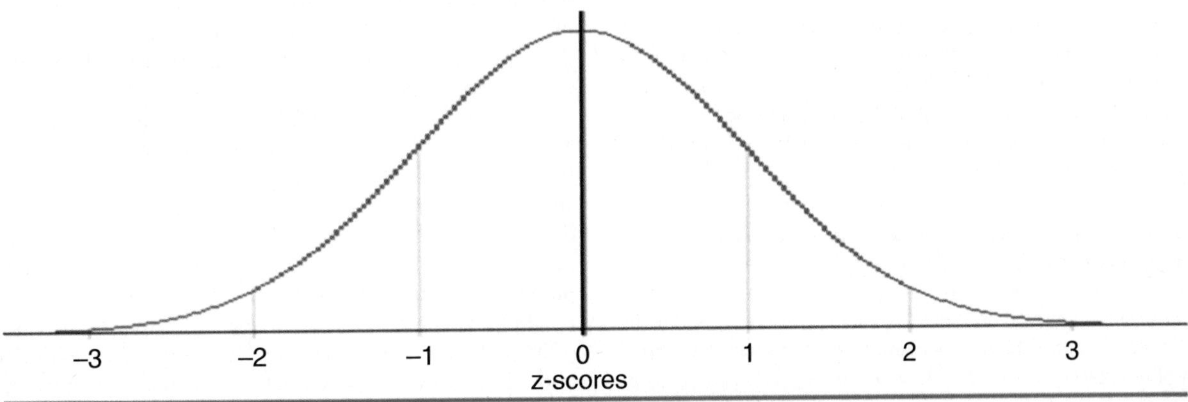

Fig. 22.4 Illustration of *Z*-Score Frequency Distribution of a Population.

Table 22.2 Reasons for Growth Rates Less Than Intrauterine Rates (as Reflected by Fenton or Olsen Growth Charts)

Problem	Solution
Inadequate intakes due to inadequate nutrition provision[68,69] or intolerance(s)	Refer to dietitian Optimize nutrient intakes
Human milk has variable composition	Refer to dietitian Assess milk for true protein and energy content Increase fortification of inadequate nutrients
Previous fluid overload	Examine growth patterns from birth, consider past and present fluid status
Excess weight at birth due to poorly controlled maternal diabetes or excess fluid (e.g., hydrops)	Reassess expectations; when infants have excess weight gain from poorly controlled diabetes, they are likely to have slower subsequent weight gain velocity as they follow their genetic potential for growth
Time period of assessment is too short, which can under- or overestimate growth	Assess growth by looking at the patterns of weight, length, and head growth on a growth chart; avoid calculating weight gain velocity over periods shorter than 5–7 days[20]

Precise weight gain goals can be found by using the website https://www.PediTools.org,[29] but caution is needed when applying these precise numerical goals because individual patient growth is somewhat variable day to day and week to week. Whether estimating precise weight gain goals is superior to examining growth patterns on a growth chart has not been validated. One concern with using these precise weight gain goals is that infants are not likely to achieve any specific numerical growth velocity goals, so using numerical z-score values could lead to excess concern.

Body Mass Index

Body mass index (BMI) is a common measurement for older pediatric and adult populations, and there is increasing interest in using it in infancy (Fig. 22.5). One large cohort study found that infants 4 to 6 months of age with a BMI > the 85th percentile had a higher risk of developing childhood obesity.[30] However, these findings could be due to a few study patients with extreme BMIs, because sensitivity for identifying at-risk infants was only 33%. This study did not account for gestational age or history of prematurity.

In older age groups, such as adults, BMI is primarily used to identify high body fat in older populations. A detailed magnetic resonance imaging study in average preterm infants of former 28 weeks' gestational age found that both BMI and weight at hospital discharge were strongly associated with total body fat (*r*, 0.95 and 0.89, respectively), whereas waist circumference was not associated with body fat (*r*, 0.28).[31]

BMI, and other similar indexes such as the ponderal index, do not discriminate between fat and lean tissue.[32] The use of these indices in preterm infants could incorrectly assume that an infant has high body fat if her lean body mass is higher than average or when length growth lags behind weight gain. For this reason, preterm infant nutrition should not be restricted if a preterm infant's BMI is elevated. Care is needed in the first years of life because any error in age will provide the incorrect BMI reference interval. BMI should not be used with stunted infants or those with restricted length, because these infants are not represented in the reference intervals.

Body Composition Modalities

Direct measurements can be limited by resource availability and technical challenges.[33] Table 22.3 summarizes the strengths and limitations of each of these methods. Publication of normative body composition growth charts allows for comparison of preterm and term infants' measures.[34] Caution is needed when using body composition measurements in care, because validated techniques to alter care based on these measurements have not been developed. Nutrition should not be provided outside of recommended intake levels (above or below the recommendations) in the neonatal intensive care unit (NICU) even if body composition measures exceed or are below reference intervals. It is not yet known if low lean mass of growing preterm infants can be improved with dietary changes, especially those with morbidities, SGA, or previous nutritional intolerance.

When direct measurement is unavailable, there are validated equations to predict body fat in infants over 2000 g.[35,36]

$$\text{Neonatal fat mass (kg)} = (\text{Body weight [kg]} \times 0.39055) + (\text{Flank skin fold [mm]} \times 0.0453) - (\text{Length [cm]} \times 0.03237) + 0.54657$$

$$\text{Neonatal body fat percentage} = \text{Fat mass (kg)}/\text{Body weight (kg)} \times 100$$

Evidence of Healthy Body Composition

Body composition measurement provides additional information that may assist the nutritional assessment over anthropometric measurement alone; however, validated methods to use this information have not been established. Body fat provides insulation to aid in temperature stability and is an important alternative substrate for the glucose-dependent brain while early oral feeding is established. In a study of term infants, low fat mass and low body fat percentage had greater predictive value than low birth weight percentile for neonatal morbidities including hypothermia, poor feeding, and extended length of stay,[37] suggesting that body composition data may assist differentiating infants with fetal growth restriction from small, healthy infants better than weight percentiles do. Body composition may provide more information to aid assessments and may reflect the infant's medical and nutritional history rather than provide guidance to change care.

The body composition of former preterm infants at term-corrected gestational age is different than the body composition of equivalent term counterparts. Former preterm infants have less lean tissue but similar fat mass at term-corrected gestational age, resulting in a different proportionality, including a higher proportion of body fat.[38–40] Researchers have expressed great concern that this higher proportion of body fat is a concern for later body composition, but it should be noted that term infants also increase their proportion of body fat in the first months of life[40] (Figs. 22.6 and 22.7). Lean body mass growth is an indication of protein accretion as well as organ and brain growth. Higher lean body mass gain among preterm infants during NICU hospitalization is associated with higher

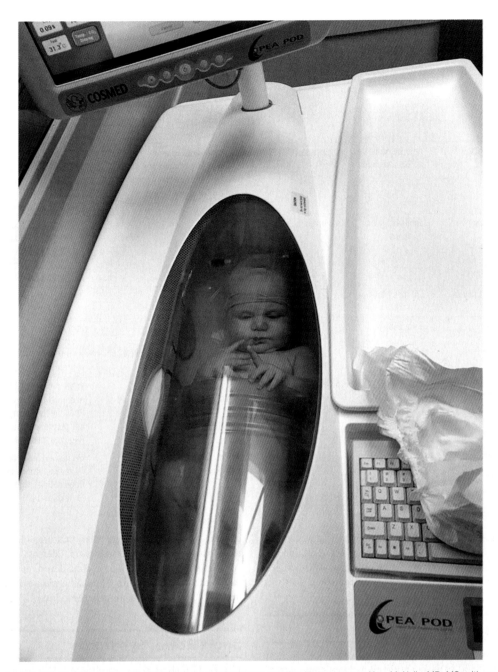

Fig. 22.5 Measuring Infant Body Composition Via Air Displacement Plethysmography. (Photo courtesy Kera McNelis, MD, MS, with parents' permission.)

neuronal processing speed and superior neurodevelopment.[41,42] Postnatal fat accretion, which occurs at an earlier postmenstrual age in preterm infants (i.e., before 40 weeks' postmenstrual age) compared with term infants (i.e., after 40 weeks' postmenstrual age), has been suggested to be a normal postnatal development for all infants.[43]

Biochemical Assessment

Biochemical laboratory testing can add additional information to a nutritional assessment (Table 22.4). Judicious testing can augment clinical decision making regarding nutritional provision as long as the risks of additional blood loss and challenges interpreting the results do not outweigh the benefits. Besides costs, iatrogenic blood loss can be an important contributor to neonatal anemia. An infant's circulating blood volume is between 80 and 100 mL/kg, so every lab draw of 1 mL represents up to 1% of an ELBW infant's blood volume. Micro laboratory techniques are needed to use smaller blood samples than are used for adults. Infants receiving parenteral nutrition should have their intolerance evaluated using laboratory monitoring, whereas stable premature infants receiving full enteral feedings should rarely need a lab draw. Infants with short bowel syndrome and chronic compromise of nutrient absorption will need ongoing lab testing.[44]

A final consideration for monitoring is increasing the frequency of tests in times of restricted nutrient delivery, such as during an injectable-product shortage. Clinicians can stay abreast of the current shortages by accessing the Food and Drug Administration's website.[45] The American Society for Parenteral and Enteral Nutrition provides clinical guidance about parenteral nutrition product shortages.[46] Restricted dose delivery of micronutrients has been associated with adverse outcomes,

Table 22.3 Body Composition Measurement: Comparing the Different Modalities

Method	Parameters	Strengths	Limitations
Air displacement plethysmography	Body fat percentage, fat mass, fat free mass	Quick test Designed for longitudinal, repeated measurements Easy interpretation Growth charts available[34] Safe, noninvasive	Requires machine Only tests infants breathing room air
Magnetic resonance imaging[70–74]	Adipose tissue volume, fat mass, and fat-free mass	Safe, noninvasive Assesses regional distribution of adipose tissue, not only volume	Expensive Expert interpretation required Patient must be able to go to scanner and must be still Requires technician and machine
Isotope (deuterium) dilution[75,76]	Total body water, fat-free mass, fat mass	Accurate Noninvasive	Requires mass spectrometry Expert interpretation required Requires technician and machine 2–4-hour completion time Hydration status will affect results
Bioelectrical impedance analysis	Fat mass, fat-free mass	Quick test Safe, noninvasive	Poor individual accuracy
Skin fold thickness	Total body fat	Safe, noninvasive Quick test Can be measured regardless of clinical status	Poor accuracy, especially for preterm infants who have low subcutaneous fat[77]
Dual energy x-ray absorptiometry	Bone mineral density, fat-free mass, fat mass	Accurate for bone mineral density Quick test	Patient must be able to go to scanner and must be still Radiation exposure Inaccurate fat measure Requires machine and technician
Mid-upper arm circumference		Quick test Safe, noninvasive	Limited evidence does not support its use for preterm infants[78,79] Does not discriminate between fat and lean tissue[80]

so careful monitoring and prioritization of the restricted products during times of shortage is essential.[47–49] NICU patients should be among the highest priority groups during shortages due to their critical illness, lack of physiologic reserve, and smaller total dosages required.

Clinical Assessment

Daily nutritional clinical assessment of the hospitalized infant includes monitoring of vital signs, quantification of input and output, and calculation of the nutrient content of enteral and parenteral provision, compared with recommended intakes. The relevance of vital signs to nutritional status is displayed in Table 22.5. Daily nutritional calculation from the provision of enteral feeds requires knowing the nutrient content of the human milk, human milk fortifier, commercially available infant formulas, and nutritional supplements provided; please refer to the chapter on enteral nutrition (Chapter 19). Necessary calculations for parenteral nutrition are discussed in the Parenteral Nutrition chapter (Chapter 20).

All hospitalized infants should have careful monitoring of fluid intake and output to aid assessment of volume status. Fluid intakes include parenteral and enteral nutrition and fluid intake from medications, intravenous lines, and intravenous flushes. Care should be taken to monitor the actual daily intakes of the infant and not the prescribed volume, because there may be considerable differences. Output includes urine, stool, gastrointestinal losses (emesis and discarded residuals), and insensible (skin) losses and also includes drainage from any drainage tubes or stoma (Table 22.6). Insensible fluid losses from skin, open abdominal defects, respiration, and third-space fluid shifts should all be considered, even if it is not possible to assign numerical values. Humidification of respiratory equipment and isolettes may mitigate insensible losses.

Short Bowel Syndrome

Infants with short bowel syndrome and intestinal failure represent a challenging patient population that requires particular care.[50] Determining the remaining bowel length for infants who undergo a surgical intestinal resection is an important step in nutritional assessment.[51] Remaining intestinal length is one of the critical predictors of outcome for infants with short bowel syndrome and is a predictor of parenteral nutrition dependence, growth restriction, and dysbiosis.[52,53] A study by Struijs et al. developed a predictive model using height and a reference table of preresection small bowel length and colon length per postmenstrual age.[51]

Preresection small bowel length (SBL) can be predicted with the equation:

$$\ln(\mathrm{SBL}) = 6.741 - 80.409 / \mathrm{height}$$

Preresection colon length (CL) can be predicted using the equation:

$$\mathrm{CL} = 0.111 \times \mathrm{height}^{1.521}$$

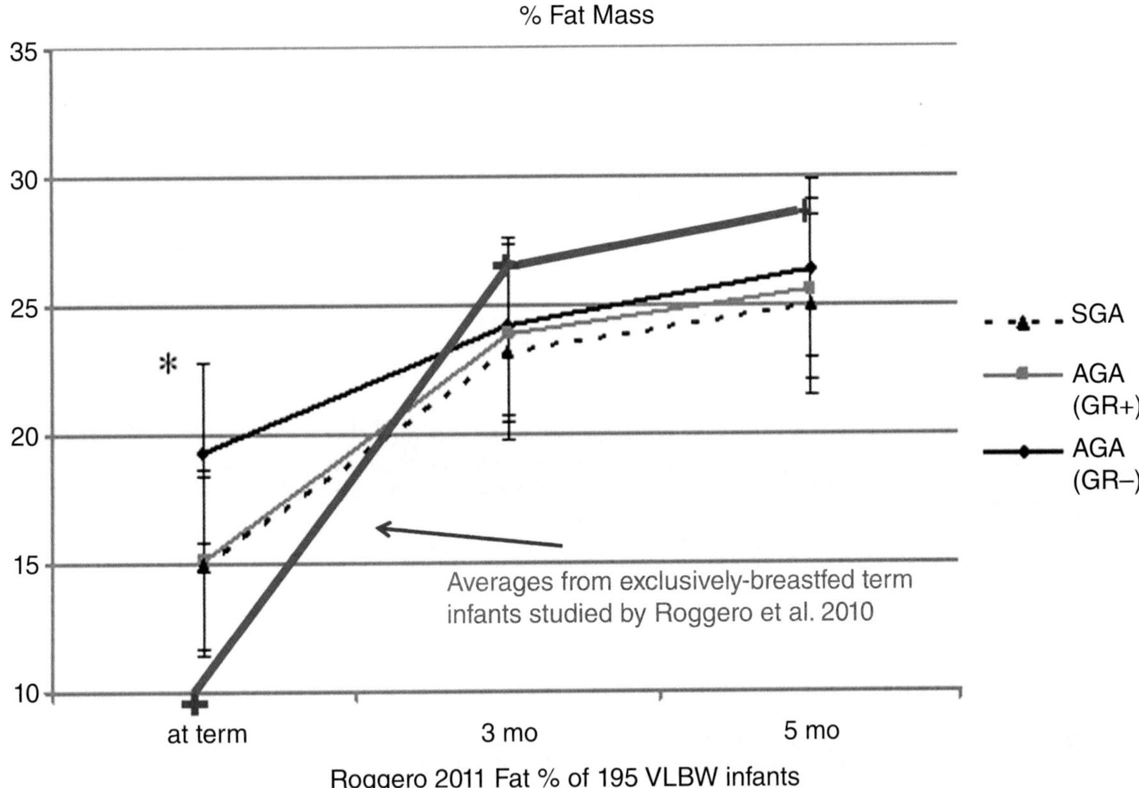

Fig. 22.6 Healthy Growth Entails Proportionate Deposition of Lean and Fat Mass. Both preterm and term infants increase their proportion of body fat after birth, preterm infants at an earlier postmenstrual age than term infants. When the percent body fat begins to level off, term infants on average have a higher percent body fat than do preterm infants. This means that the concern about percent body fat in preterm infants at term is not necessary and that gains in percent body fat are a normal postnatal event. *AGA*, Appropriate for gestational age; *GR*, growth restriction; *SGA*, small for gestational age; *VLBW*, very low birth weight. (Data supported by the conclusions in: [1] Roggero P et al. Rapid recovery of fat mass in small for gestational age preterm infants after term. *PLoS One*. 2011;6[1]:e14489–e14489; [2] Roggero P et al. Quality of growth in exclusively breast-fed infants in the first six months of life: an Italian study. *Pediatr Res*. 2010;68[6]:542–544; and [3] Griffin IJ, Cooke RJ. Development of whole body adiposity in preterm infants. *Early Hum Dev*. 2012;88[suppl 1]:S19–S24.)

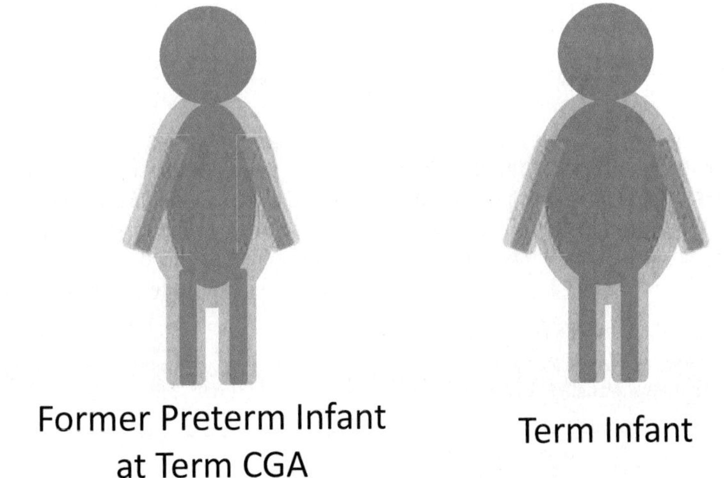

Fig. 22.7 Relative Proportion of Fat and Lean Mass Between Preterm Infants and Term Infants at Term-Corrected Gestational Age (CGA). In this figure, *yellow* represents fat, and *blue* represents lean mass. Preterm infants have a higher body fat percentage at term-corrected gestational age than do their term peers, but this is primarily due to lower lean mass deposition and not increased fat mass.

Table 22.4 Indications and Limitations of Common Nutritional Biochemical Tests

Lab Test	Common Clinical Indications	Reasons to Consider Limiting Testing	Society Guidelines and Expert Opinions
Serum glucose	Prematurity, postoperatively, fetal growth restriction and SGA, infant of diabetic mother, polycythemia, LGA, HIE, congenital syndromes, midline malformations[1]	Mixed evidence regarding neurodevelopmental outcomes of asymptomatic infants with low plasma glucose[81] Transitional hypoglycemia is common and frequently resolves within 48 hours of birth[82]	American Academy of Pediatrics, 2011[1] Pediatric Endocrine Society, 2015[83] American Society for Parenteral and Enteral Nutrition, 2012[84]
Serum electrolytes	Parenteral nutrition, diuretics, renal disease, impaired wound healing, preterm infant renal sodium wasting	Serum sodium is limited; surrogate of total body sodium content	European Society of Pediatric Gastroenterology, Hepatology, and Nutrition; and the European Society for Clinical Nutrition and Metabolism, 2005[85]
Blood urea nitrogen	Evaluate nitrogen status	BUN concentration is not a marker of amino-acid intolerance[86,87] because it is highly associated with renal function[88] Higher protein intake improves growth in preterm infants[88] Growth at approximate intrauterine rates, with deposition of lean tissue, is a better assessment of nitrogen status	
Urine sodium[89,90]	Preterm kidneys, renal sodium, wasting growth, faltering due to inadequate sodium intakes, malabsorption, post–bowel resection[90]	No consensus on the interpretation of urinary sodium values Commonly used medications (diuretics, aminoglycosides, caffeine, steroids) have natriuretic effects	Bischoff et al., 2016[91]
Iron studies	Refractory anemia (anemia despite appropriate iron supplementation) Long-term parenteral nutrition or delays in beginning enteral iron, large quantity of blood testing	Anemia is the final state of iron depletion Ferritin may not differentiate between iron overload and inflammation[92]	ESPGHAN/ESPEN/ESPR/CSPEN, 2018[93] Biomarkers of nutrition for development, 2018[92] Georgieff, 2017[94]
Liver function tests, including direct bilirubin	Long-term parenteral nutrition, cholestasis, short bowel syndrome[95]		American Pediatric Surgical Association Outcomes and Clinical Trials Committee, 2012[96]
Alkaline phosphatase and phosphate	Screen for inadequate phosphate intake and for metabolic bone disease of prematurity[97]	Controversial values May normalize over time given sufficient mineral intakes[61]	Backström et al., 2000[98] Faerk et al., 2002[99] Fenton et al., 2011[97]

BUN, Blood urea nitrogen; *HIE,* hypoxic-ischemic encephalopathy; *LGA,* large for gestational age; *SGA,* small for gestational age.

See Table 22.7 for the reference small bowel length. Best practice includes calculating predicted small bowel length for each patient by age, weight, and length and then either using the average value from these three equations or excluding an outlier.

It is helpful when surgical reports describe the amount and location of any intestinal loss during surgery. In addition to postsurgery bowel length, other prognostic factors include sustained cholestasis and absence of the ileocecal valve.[44] It is of great importance to understand the function of the remaining bowel to assess which

Table 22.5 Relevance of Vital Signs to Nutritional Status

Vital Sign	
Respiratory rate	Normal range: 40–60 breaths/min Tachypnea is a contraindication for oral feeding Apnea (pause in breathing >20 seconds) and bradypnea may delay oral feeding ability[100]
Heart rate	Normal range: 100–180 beats/min Tachycardia may be due to crying, pain, or dehydration Bradycardia may present during sleep or suggest instability
Blood pressure	Varies by gestational age[101] Hypertension defined as systolic or diastolic blood pressure that exceeds 95th percentile for postmenstrual age Hypotension may be sign of severe dehydration

Table 22.6 Pediatric Gastrointestinal Electrolyte losses

	Sodium (mEq/L)	Potassium (mEq/L)	Chloride (mEq/L)	Bicarbonate (mEq/L)
Gastric	140	15	155	
Ileostomy	80–140	15	115	40
Colostomy	50–80	10–30	40	20–25
Secretory	60–120			
Diarrhea	30–40	10–80	10–110	30
Normal stool	5	10	10	

Modified and reprinted with authors' permission from Wessel JJ. Short bowel syndrome. In: Groh-Wargo S, Thompson M, Cox JH, eds. *Nutritional Care of High Risk Newborns.* Chicago, IL: Precept Press; 2000:469.

nutrients are likely to have compromised absorption. The jejunum has less ability to take over the function of the ileum, because the ileum has specific sites for absorption and greater capacity for adaptation. Table 22.8 describes the nutrients absorbed by each section of bowel.

Bronchopulmonary Dysplasia

Many extremely preterm and very preterm infants will develop bronchopulmonary dysplasia (BPD), a chronic lung disease of prematurity. Below are some considerations for assessing the nutritional status of infants with BPD:

- Birth weight and gestational age are the most predictive of risk of developing BPD.[54] BPD's etiology is due to immaturity of a premature infant's lungs at birth (insufficiency of surfactants that lower surface tension to allow the lungs to expand and contract easily) followed by chronic damage
- Specific evidence-based recommendations for established BPD do not exist, but expert recommendations are to focus on adequate nutrition provision and avoid fluid overload[55,56]
- Barriers to achieving adequate growth can include inadequate respiratory support, inflammation, limited fluid and inadequate nutrition provision, stress, and infection[57]
- Zinc supplementation may improve growth in ELBW infants who are at risk for BPD[58]
- Nutritional management of patients with BPD is critical; therefore registered dietitians represent a key member of a multidisciplinary care team[59]
- With the benefits of a multidisciplinary care team, patients with BPD may achieve a "progrowth" state: improved growth, improved respiratory status, unimpaired neurodevelopment, and respiratory progress[57]

Table 22.7 Calculating Percent of Remaining Bowel

	Mean (cm)	Standard Error
Postconception Age		
24–26 weeks	70.0	6.3
27–29 weeks	100.0	6.5
30–32 weeks	117.3	6.9
33–35 weeks	120.8	8.8
36–38 weeks	142.6	12.0
39–40 weeks	157.4	11.2
0–6 months	239.2	18.3
7–12 months	283.9	20.9
13–18 months	271.8	25.1
19–24 months	345.5	18.2
25–36 months	339.6	16.9
37–48 months	366.7	37.0
49–60 months	423.9	5.9
Weight at Surgery (g)		
500–999	83.1	9.2
1000–1499	109.9	6.6
1500–1999	120.1	4.6
2000–2999	143.6	8.0
3000–4999	236.5	23.8
5000–7999	260.3	14.1
8000–9999	300.1	22.0
10,000–12,999	319.6	16.4
13,000–15,999	355.0	19.2
16,000–19,999	407.0	13.2
Length at Surgery (cm)		
30–39	97.4	6.0
40–49	129.0	5.6
50–59	205.9	21.6
60–74	272.0	11.1
75–89	308.5	16.5
90–99	382.5	15.2
100–120	396.4	15.3

Percent of remaining bowel = remaining length measured by surgeon/preresection predicted bowel length.

Predicted mean small bowel length per infant age, weight, or length.

Table reprinted with authors' permission from Struijs MC et al. *J Peds Surg.* 2009.

Metabolic Bone Disease

There is a lack of consensus for screening and radiographic diagnosis of metabolic bone disease in premature infants. Risk factors associated both with development of osteopenia and spontaneous fractures include smaller birth weight, earlier gestation, severity of lung disease, duration of parenteral nutrition, and use of certain medications such as diuretics and systemic steroids.[60] Preterm infants are at risk of metabolic bone disease due to low body stores of the bone minerals calcium and phosphorus at birth, missing the high fetal accretion of late pregnancy, limited solubility of these minerals in parenteral nutrition, limited absorption from enteral feedings, low mineral content of some feedings (e.g., unfortified human milk or formulas designed for term infants, such as protein hydrolysate formulas), and some medications.

The best approach to metabolic bone disease is to prevent its occurrence by providing calcium and phosphorus close to maximum solubility in parenteral nutrition, fortifying human milk with these minerals, and using preterm formulas when formula feeding.[4] Assessment practices for metabolic bone disease vary widely. Biochemical markers that have been studied include calcium, phosphorus, alkaline phosphatase, parathyroid hormone, tubular reabsorption phosphate,

Table 22.8 Nutrients by Section of Bowel Where Predominantly Absorbed

Bowel	Nutrient
Duodenum/jejunum	Fats Sugars Peptides/amino acids Folate Calcium Water-soluble vitamins
Duodenum/proximal jejunum	Iron
Jejunum/proximal ileum	Lactose
Distal ileum	Bile salts Vitamin B_{12}
Colon	Water, sodium, potassium, and minor amounts of energy from unabsorbed nutrients, fiber, and oligosaccharides

osteocalcin, urine calcium, and urine phosphate.[61] A recent survey of American neonatologists found that half of them used x-rays for workup[62] even though x-rays lack sensitivity and specificity for diagnosing metabolic bone disease. Dual-energy x-ray absorptiometry is the gold standard for bone mineral density testing, but limitations to widespread use include movement artifacts, the length of the test, radiation exposure, costs, and limited availability of equipment. Metabolic bone disease may be noticed incidentally on routine x-rays, but a dedicated wrist x-ray film can be used in conjunction with alkaline phosphatase levels to grade the severity of disease.[63]

Nutrition-Focused Physical Exam

Fluid status is readily assessed on physical exam. An infant with hypovolemia can have some or all of these findings: dry mucous membranes, sunken fontanel, poor skin turgor, lack of tears, and tachycardia. Severe dehydration presents with delayed capillary refill, hypotension, and altered activity. Fluid overload can present with excessive weight gain and edema, which may be especially noticeable around the eyes or in the genitals.

As discussed previously, having lower than expected body fat could increase the risk of morbidities. The skin, the largest organ of the body, can have many features relevant to an infant's nutritional status. Pallor, defined as unusual lightness of the skin or mucous membranes, can indicate anemia or poor perfusion. This may be more challenging to appreciate on dark skin and may only be appreciated in the nailbeds and palpebral conjunctivae. Central cyanosis may indicate diminished perfusion, including poor gut perfusion. Flaky-paint dermatitis can be a sign of protein deficiency. Essential fatty acid deficiency, which is rare, can present with generalized scaly dermatitis. Other rashes or compromised skin integrity are indicative of specific nutrient deficiencies; see Table 22.9. Handbooks that include photographs of examination findings are available.[64]

Respiratory compensation for metabolic acidosis can present as tachypnea. Lactic acidosis can result from impaired tissue perfusion or oxygenation or, rarely, thiamine deficiency, among other causes. Increased work of breathing will indicate a higher metabolic demand for energy. Sufficient nutrition is needed to support growth of respiratory musculature.

Surgical wounds require special consideration. Surgery can induce a metabolic stress response to enable tissue repair, but this can lead to increased catabolism. Deficiency of protein or micronutrients can impair wound healing.[65] There is suggestive evidence that vitamins A and E, selenium, and copper aid in wound healing, whereas vitamin C, zinc, and protein are critical for this function; it is not known whether requirements are elevated beyond usual infant intakes. Thompson et al. created a consensus and evidence-informed clinical pathway for delayed wound healing based on nonpediatric studies, and they recommended assessing and intervening for vitamin C, zinc, and protein deficiency.[66] Additional supplementation of these nutrients may obviate the need for testing levels. The primary medical team should obtain a consultation from a dietitian for all infants with delayed wound healing or wound dehiscence to formally assess and optimize the provision of these nutrients.

Table 22.9 Micronutrient Deficiencies and Physical Exam Findings

Nutrient	Functions	Risks of Deficiency	Signs of Deficiency
Essential fatty acids	Growth of neural tissues, cellular functions	Inadequate provision, intestinal failure,[102] chylothorax	Dermatitis; scaly, dry skin; poor wound healing
Vitamin B_{12}[103,104]	Cofactor for numerous enzymes	Stomach and ileal resection Breastfed infant of deficient mother, vegan mother	Hypotonia, inflamed mucous membranes, pallor (due to megaloblastic anemia)
Zinc[50]	Cofactor for numerous enzymes	Intestinal resection, insufficient parenteral delivery, SGA[105]	Dermatitis; scaly, dry skin; poor wound healing; poor growth[106]
Vitamin A	Development of retina, GI tract, brain, immune systems	Premature infants, insufficient parenteral delivery	Scaly, dry skin; dry corneas; poor wound healing
Copper[107]	Free radical scavenger, metabolic processes	Serious illness,[108] administration of Cu-free PN, malabsorption (GI) disorders	Impaired wound healing, skeletal demineralization
Iodine	Component of thyroid hormones	Fetal iodine deficiency, prematurity, insufficient delivery (including environmental exposure)	Hypothyroidism leading to cretinism, goiter, slower growth
Iron	Major component of heme proteins	Premature infants, excessive blood loss	Pallor, pale sclerae, neurodevelopment
Folate	Cofactor for enzymes involved in DNA and RNA biosynthesis	Intestinal resection (duodenum)	Pallor, pale sclerae, anemia
Selenium	Free radical scavenger	Prematurity, administration of Se-free PN	Abnormal fingernail beds, skin depigmentation, alopecia

GI, Gastrointestinal; *PN*, parenteral nutrition; *SGA*, small for gestational age.

Table 22.10 Primary Indicators of Neonatal Malnutrition

Indicator	Mild Malnutrition	Moderate Malnutrition	Severe Malnutrition	Use of Indicator
Primary Indicators Requiring 1 Indicator				
Decline in weight-for-age *z*-score	Decline of 0.8–1.2 standard deviations	Decline of >1.2–2 standard deviations	Decline of >2 standard deviations	Not appropriate for first 2 weeks of life
Weight gain velocity	<75% of expected rate of weight gain to maintain growth rate	<50% of expected rate of weight gain to maintain growth rate	<25% of expected rate of weight gain to maintain growth rate	Not appropriate for first 2 weeks of life
Nutrient intake	>3–5 consecutive days of protein/energy intake <75% of estimated needs	>5–7 consecutive days of protein/energy intake <75% of estimated needs	<25% of expected rate of weight gain to maintain growth rate >7 consecutive days of protein/energy intake <75% of estimated needs	Preferred indicator during first 2 weeks of life
Primary Indicators Requiring 2 or More Indicators				
Days to regain birth weight	15–18	19–21	>21	Use in conjunction with nutrient intake
Linear growth velocity	<75% of expected rate of linear gain to maintain expected growth rate	<50% of expected rate of linear growth to maintain expected growth rate	<25% of expected rate of linear gain to maintain expected growth rate	Not appropriate for first 2 weeks of life May be deferred in critically ill, unstable infants
Decline in length-for-age *z*-score	Decline of 0.8–1.2 standard deviations	Decline of >1.2–2 standard deviations	Decline of >2 standard deviations	Not appropriate for first 2 weeks of life May be deferred in critically ill, unstable infants Use in conjunction with another indicator when accurate length measurement is available

Modified and reprinted with permission from Goldberg DL et al. *J Acad Nutri Diet.* 2018.

Diagnosing Malnutrition in the Newborn

Malnutrition may be apparent in early life (signifying restricted fetal growth) or may develop through the neonatal course. Please refer to the previous section, "Classification of the Newborn." Premature infants are at higher risk for malnutrition than their term counterparts due to lower body stores at birth and higher nutrient requirements to match fetal accretion. If nutrient delivery is compromised by feeding intolerance, difficulties with absorption or metabolism, and/or morbidities, infants can be at increased risk of malnutrition. To diagnose newborn malnutrition, indicators have been suggested by Goldberg et al. that apply to both preterm and term infants.[67] These primary malnutrition indicators include a decline in weight-for-age *z*-score of >0.8 standard deviations after the first 2 weeks of life, diminished weight gain velocity <75% of expected, and/or insufficient protein and/or energy intake. Given the physiologic weight loss that most babies experience after birth, the birth *z*-score is not an appropriate growth goal. Other indicators of malnutrition that require more than the indicator to be present include delayed regaining of birth weight, diminished linear growth velocity, and decline in length-for-age *z*-score (Table 22.10).

Conclusion

Patients requiring neonatal intensive care have exceptional and specific needs, and a careful assessment of their nutritional status is part of the best-practice care. Nutritional provision is hardly a "one size fits all" proposition for a newborn, because preterm infants have very high nutritional needs, and their size at birth and neonatal morbidities can increase risks of malnutrition.[4] A full nutrition assessment, including classification, anthropometric measurements, a focused physical examination, and assessment of nutrient intake should be completed on all hospitalized infants and those with chronic disease. Select patients will also benefit from additional assessments such as biochemical monitoring, body composition measurement, or estimation of bowel length. A multidisciplinary team approach, using tools supported by the latest evidence, improves outcomes for high-risk newborns.

SECTION

5 Endocrine Disorders

OUTLINE

CHAPTER 23

Neonatal Hypoglycemia

Winnie Sigal, Diva D. De Leon

KEY POINTS

1. Hypoglycemia is frequently seen in premature and critically ill term infants.
2. Neonates are at risk of hypoglycemia in the early neonatal period because of the abrupt interruption of maternal glucose transfer to the baby at birth, imposing a need for independent regulation of plasma glucose concentrations by adjusting insulin secretion and mobilizing counterregulatory responses.
3. Many neonates experience a transitional period of lower glucose concentrations soon after birth because of lower thresholds for glucose-stimulated insulin secretion during the perinatal period.
4. The clinical manifestations of neonatal hypoglycemia can be nonspecific, ranging from fussiness, hypothermia, apnea, and lethargy to seizure activity. A high index of suspicion is needed.
5. The Pediatric Endocrine Society guidelines identify that neonatal hypoglycemia can occur due to a variety of causes, each of which requires careful evaluation. Persistent neonatal hypoglycemia can cause long-term morbidity and requires a high index of suspicion and tailored management.

Introduction

Normal brain function depends on a continuous supply of glucose, the principal metabolic fuel of the human brain, from the bloodstream. Low plasma glucose concentrations, and as a consequence, low brain glucose availability result in cerebral energy failure, neuronal death, and irreversible brain damage. The developing brain is particularly vulnerable to the deleterious effects of hypoglycemia, as demonstrated by the high frequency of neurodevelopmental deficits in children with congenital hypoglycemia disorders.[1–3] Thus it is critically important to screen, identify, and treat neonates with persistent hypoglycemia.

During fetal development, facilitated diffusion of glucose from the maternal circulation to the fetal circulation guarantees an appropriate supply of glucose to the fetus. The abrupt interruption of maternal glucose transfer to the baby at delivery imposes a need for the newborn infant to independently control plasma glucose concentrations by adjusting insulin secretion and mobilizing counterregulatory responses. These "fasting systems" are intact and functional in the newborn period and provide defense against hypoglycemia when working properly. The "fasting systems" include hepatic glycogenolysis, hepatic gluconeogenesis, and fatty acid oxidation. These processes are all coordinated by endocrine counterregulatory hormones; insulin suppresses these processes whereas glucagon, cortisol, epinephrine, and growth hormone are stimulating.[4] Fasting adaptation's essential function is to maintain the brain's fuel supply. The redundancy in hormonal signaling provides for additional layers of security to prevent hypoglycemia. Hepatic glycogenolysis provides energy for only a few hours; beyond that, hepatic gluconeogenesis provides glucose for energy requirements. During extended fasting, lipolysis and fatty acid oxidation mobilize fatty acids and generate ketones as an alternative fuel source for the brain. Hypoglycemia beyond the immediate newborn period is often a consequence of a defect in fasting adaptation.

It is essential to identify neonates with hypoglycemic disorders prior to newborn hospital discharge, because there is a high risk of long-term morbidity. Specifically, persistent and repeated episodes of hypoglycemia in the neonatal period lead to irreversible brain injury and developmental disabilities.[1–3] In addition to prompt stabilization, early identification of the precise etiology of hypoglycemia allows for tailored interventions to minimize hypoglycemic events and ultimately improve long-term outcomes.

In this chapter, we will review the evaluation and management of neonates with persistent hypoglycemia with a special emphasis on hyperinsulinism (HI), the most common cause of persistent hypoglycemia in neonates and infants.

Transitional Neonatal Hypoglycemia

There is a transitional period immediately after birth when mean plasma glucose concentrations fall in normal newborn infants from 70 to 80 mg/dL (close to maternal glucose values) to 55 to 60 mg/dL.[5,6] There is evidence that suggests that this transitional period of lower glucose concentrations in normal newborns is explained by a lower threshold for glucose-stimulated insulin secretion and thus should be considered as "transitional neonatal hyperinsulinism." This includes observations that during the period that plasma glucose is low in normal newborns, lipolysis and ketogenesis are suppressed and liver glycogen reserves are maintained, as shown by the large glycemic responses elicited by administration of glucagon or epinephrine.[7] An important feature of transitional neonatal hypoglycemia in normal newborns is that the hypoglycemia progressively improves over the first few days of life and the plasma glucose concentration reaches the normal range for older infants and children by the third to fourth day of life.[6–8] Additionally, the plasma glucose concentration in transitional hypoglycemia is impressively stable and relatively unaffected by initial feeds, which has been demonstrated in multiple studies.[7,9,10] Of prime importance, however, is that transitional neonatal hypoglycemia is self-limited, and in the absence of other factors, the hypoglycemia should resolve within the first 3 days of life as the threshold for glucose-stimulated insulin secretion rises and fasting adaptation mechanisms become fully functional.[7]

The process of beta cell maturation after birth may be impacted by perinatal factors resulting in a prolongation of this state of hyperinsulinism. This is a specific entity known as perinatal stress-induced hyperinsulinism, a distinct form of hyperinsulinism that spontaneously resolves within the first few weeks of life, although it sometimes persists for a few months. Perinatal factors associated with perinatal stress-induced hyperinsulinism include birth asphyxia, maternal preeclampsia, prematurity, intrauterine growth retardation, and other peripartum stress.[11–13] Up to 50% of neonates in these at-risk categories may be affected.[14] Hyperinsulinism secondary to perinatal stress can be as severe as the genetic permanent forms and is also associated with a high risk for neurodevelopmental deficits.[15]

In 2015, the Pediatric Endocrine Society (PES) published recommendations for evaluation and management of neonatal hypoglycemia.[16] The purpose of this publication was to provide guidance beyond the immediate stabilization period. The PES recommendations highlight the importance of differentiating transitional neonatal hypoglycemia from persistent hypoglycemia disorders, because failure to identify these at-risk neonates can lead to devastating consequences from repeated and prolonged episodes of hypoglycemia and resultant brain damage. The recommendations also emphasize the need for evaluation to determine the underlying etiology of persistent hypoglycemia in order to provide tailored treatment to optimize patient care and minimize long-term morbidity.

Screening Neonates at Risk for Hypoglycemia

Symptoms of hypoglycemia are well defined in older individuals; however, they may be difficult to discern in a neonate.[17] Adult guidelines highlight the utility of Whipple's triad to verify hypoglycemia: symptoms consistent with hypoglycemia, documented low plasma glucose during symptoms, and resolution of symptoms with normalization of plasma glucose.[4,16] These criteria cannot be applied to neonates. Thus a high index of suspicion is needed, in addition to repeated plasma glucose measurements in neonates at risk, to recognize and confirm neonatal hypoglycemia and to prevent adverse consequences. In a neonate, hypoglycemia may present as a wide range of clinical manifestations including fussiness, hypothermia, apnea, lethargy, and seizure activity.

Neonates that should be screened for hypoglycemia include those with symptoms suggestive of hypoglycemia and those with risk factors for either transient or prolonged hypoglycemia. Risk factors include prematurity, low birth weight, small or large for gestational age, infants of diabetic mothers, suspected infection, maternal medications such as beta blockers, exposure to perinatal stressors, midline congenital defects, and a family history of hypoglycemia disorders (Table 23.1).

Plasma glucose concentrations should be assessed using a laboratory-based method.[18] Although point-of-care glucose meters provide a rapid and convenient method to measure plasma glucose at the bedside, one should be aware that there is a limitation in accuracy, with an error margin in the setting of hypoglycemia of up to ±15 mg/dL. Thus it is important to confirm the presence of hypoglycemia using a lab-based assay prior to embarking on further evaluation. Furthermore, it should be noted that whole-blood glucose values are approximately 15% lower than plasma glucose concentrations, and additionally, a delay in sample processing can result in further reduction of glucose up to 6 mg/dL/hour due to red blood cell glycolysis.[19]

Neonates at Risk for Persistent Hypoglycemia and Indications for Evaluation

The PES hypoglycemia guidelines identify four categories of neonates at high risk of persistent hypoglycemia that require evaluation (see Table 23.1): (1) neonates with severe hypoglycemia (i.e., those requiring intravenous dextrose and those with an episode of symptomatic hypoglycemia), (2) neonates unable to maintain plasma glucose >60 mg/dL by the third day of life, (3) neonates with family history of a genetic form of hypoglycemia, and (4) neonates with a congenital syndrome known to be associated with hypoglycemia (Beckwith-Wiedemann syndrome, panhypopituitarism).[16]

Given the confounder of transitional neonatal hypoglycemia in the immediate postnatal period, diagnostic evaluation should be deferred until at least the third day of life.[16] Failure to perform a diagnostic fast prior to hospital discharge greatly increases the risk of delaying definitive diagnosis and treatment and thus increases the likelihood of neurologic sequelae.

Table 23.1 Screening and Evaluation of Neonates at Risk of Hypoglycemia

A. Neonates at Increased Risk of Hypoglycemia Who Require Screening

1. Symptoms of hypoglycemia
2. Perinatal stress
   - Birth asphyxia
   - Fetal distress
   - Prematurity
   - Intrauterine growth restriction/small for gestational age
   - Meconium aspiration syndrome
   - Maternal preeclampsia/eclampsia
3. Large for gestational age
4. Premature or postmature delivery
5. Infant of diabetic mother
6. Family history of genetic form of hypoglycemia
7. Congenital syndromes associated with hypoglycemia (e.g., Beckwith-Wiedemann syndrome), congenital anomalies (e.g., midline facial malformations, microphallus)

B. Neonates in Whom a Persistent Hypoglycemia Disorder Should Be Excluded Before Discharge

1. Neonates with severe hypoglycemia (e.g., episode of symptomatic hypoglycemia, hypoglycemia that requires intravenous dextrose)
2. Inability to consistently maintain plasma glucose >50 mg/dL during first 48 hours of life or >60 mg/dL after 48 hours of life
3. Family history of a genetic form of hypoglycemia
4. Congenital syndromes associated with hypoglycemia (e.g., Beckwith-Wiedemann syndrome, congenital hypopituitarism)

Initial Treatment and Stabilization

Once neonatal hypoglycemia is recognized, the first step is to stabilize the patient. In neonates with suspected congenital hypoglycemia disorders, effort should be made to maintain plasma glucose greater than or equal to 70 mg/dL to minimize repercussions of prolonged hypoglycemia. This can be done with an intravenous bolus of dextrose-containing fluids, typically 2 mL/kg of 10% dextrose solution, followed by starting a glucose infusion rate and gradually up-titrating to meet requirements to maintain a plasma glucose of 70 mg/dL. Per the PES guidelines,[16] for infants without a suspected congenital hypoglycemia disorder, plasma glucose should be maintained above 50 mg/dL in the first 48 hours of life and above 60 mg/dL beyond the first 48 hours of life. The decision to have a lower glucose target for infants without a suspected congenital hypoglycemia disorder was made to balance the risk of transient hypoglycemia with the risk of intervention.[16] If an infant is requiring an intravenous glucose infusion to maintain normoglycemia beyond 48 hours of life, a formal evaluation for a hypoglycemia disorder in consultation with a pediatric endocrinologist is indicated.

There is no role for glucocorticoid therapy to treat neonatal hypoglycemia, and as such, it should be avoided. Glucocorticoids are ineffective at treating hypoglycemia unless the hypoglycemia is due to adrenal insufficiency, and they can have harmful side effects including iatrogenic adrenal suppression.

Evaluation of Persistent Hypoglycemia: The Diagnostic Fast

The purpose of pursuing a diagnostic evaluation is to identify the underlying mechanism of the hypoglycemia and subsequently provide tailored treatment. A thorough history should be conducted including pregnancy, birth, and family history. Close attention should be paid to clues on the physical examination that may suggest a particular diagnosis—for example, facial midline defects such as cleft lip or palate and micropenis are suggestive of hypopituitarism, whereas omphalocele, hemihypertrophy, and macroglossia are consistent with Beckwith-Wiedemann syndrome. A carefully monitored diagnostic fast should be conducted in order to obtain a blood specimen, or critical sample, at the time of hypoglycemia. Alternatively, the sample can be obtained opportunistically if a spontaneous episode of hypoglycemia is captured. This is not a "safety fast" (performed to ensure that a patient with a known hypoglycemia disorder can fast long enough to be safely discharged home) but a "diagnostic fast" for a neonate who has been determined to have persistent hypoglycemia and in whom a cause is being investigated; a pediatric endocrinologist should be involved at this point if possible.

The critical sample measures alternative fuels and counterregulatory hormones and should be obtained when the plasma glucose is 50 mg/dL or below in order to prevent false positive results. Alternatively, the fast can be stopped if the β-hydroxybutyrate is >2.5 mmol/L. During a diagnostic fast, feeds are held and glucose support is slowly withdrawn (if necessary) while closely monitoring glucose levels. Once the glucose reaches 50 mg/dL or lower, it should be confirmed using a laboratory-based assay, and once confirmed, the critical sample is obtained. A complete critical sample measures glucose, β-hydroxybutyrate, free fatty acids, insulin, C-peptide, cortisol, growth hormone, lactate, ammonia, bicarbonate, insulin-like growth factor binding protein 1, acylcarnitine profile, total and free carnitine, and urine organic acids. If a complete critical sample is unable to be obtained, at minimum one should obtain plasma glucose, bicarbonate, β-hydroxybutyrate, lactate, and free fatty acids at the time of hypoglycemia, because these alone can provide significant metabolic clues to the underlying diagnosis[16] (Fig. 23.1).

Subsequently, a glucagon stimulation test is performed by administering 1 mg glucagon and measuring plasma glucose every 10 minutes for 40 minutes. The glucagon stimulation test is a crucial step if hyperinsulinism is suspected, as a rise in plasma glucose greater than 30 mg/dL in response to glucagon stimulation is highly suggestive of hyperinsulinism. If the plasma glucose does not increase by 20 mg/dL in the first 20 minutes, however, the test should be concluded and the infant should be fed. Of note, the test should be terminated early if the infant becomes symptomatic.

The most common causes of neonatal hypoglycemia and their relative frequency are summarized in Fig. 23.2. Hyperinsulinism is the most common cause of persistent neonatal hypoglycemia. Other rare causes of neonatal hypoglycemia include hypopituitarism, fatty acid oxidation defects, gluconeogenesis defects, and glycogenoses. Neonatal hypopituitarism presents with a similar biochemical profile to hyperinsulinism in the neonatal period with hypoketotic hypoglycemia, whereas in older infants and children, hypoglycemia due to growth hormone and cortisol deficiency is associated with elevated ketones. Patients with midline craniofacial abnormalities such as septo-optic dysplasia are at increased risk. Growth hormone deficiency is the most common pituitary hormone deficiency, with an estimated prevalence of 1 in 4000 to 1 in 10,000 neonates.[20] Fatty acid oxidation defects, if not detected on the newborn screen, often present with hypoketotic hypoglycemia in infancy after fasting. Medium-chain acyl-CoA dehydrogenase (MCAD) deficiency is the most common fatty acid oxidation defect, with an incidence of 1 in 15,700 neonates.[21] Gluconeogenesis defects are characterized by hypoglycemia associated with lactic acidosis. Most glycogenoses do not present in the neonatal period, with the exception of glycogen storage disease type I (GSD I),

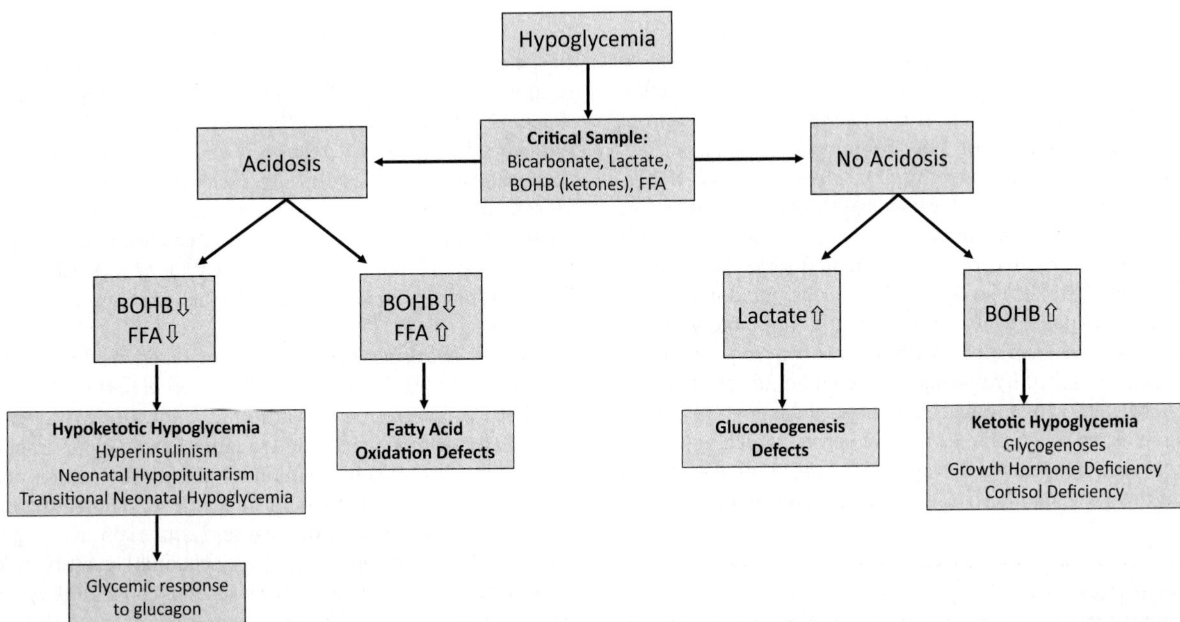

Fig. 23.1 Differential Diagnosis Based on the Critical Sample. This algorithm outlines how the characteristic biomarkers obtained in a critical sample are useful in determining the underlying cause of neonatal hypoglycemia. *BOHB*, Betahydroxybutyrate; *FFA*, free fatty acids.

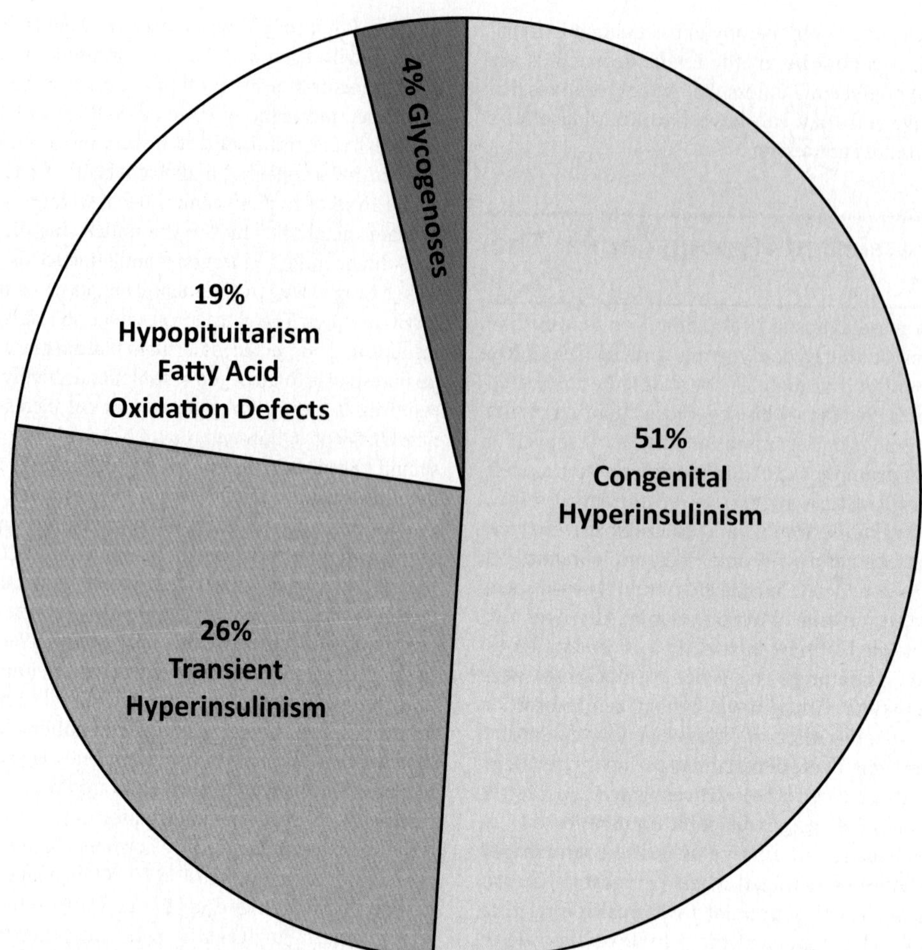

Fig. 23.2 Relative Frequency of Hypoglycemia Disorders in Neonates Evaluated at the Children's Hospital of Philadelphia. Of note, the relative frequencies of congenital and transient hyperinsulinism (HI) displayed come from data collected at a major HI referral center, which may skew the results toward congenital HI. Nonetheless, the point of emphasis is that HI is the most common cause of hypoglycemia in the neonate.

which presents with severe hypoglycemia and lactic acidosis because it impairs both glycogenolysis and gluconeogenesis. GSD I is exceedingly rare, with an estimated incidence of 1 in 100,000 live births.

In a review of 156 neonates with persistent hypoglycemia at CHOP over a 5-year period, more than 75% of neonatal hypoglycemia disorders were attributable to hyperinsulinism (see Fig. 23.2). Hyperinsulinism can be transient and secondary to perinatal factors or permanent due to monogenic mutations affecting the regulation of insulin secretion. The estimated incidence of monogenic (congenital) HI in the United States is 1 in 50,000 live births,[22] and hyperinsulinism due to perinatal stress (transient) is quite common, affecting up to 50% of at-risk neonates[14] with a conservatively estimated incidence of 1 in 12,000 live births.[13,23,24] Of note, the relative frequencies of congenital and transient HI displayed in Fig. 23.2 come from data collected at a major HI referral center, which may skew the results toward congenital HI. Nonetheless, the point of emphasis is that HI is the most common cause of hypoglycemia in the neonate.

Hyperinsulinism

Hyperinsulinism is the most common cause of persistent hypoglycemia in neonates.[25] The biochemical profile of hyperinsulinism includes detectable insulin and C-peptide, suppressed β-hydroxybutyrate and free fatty acids, and an inappropriate positive response to glucagon (Table 23.2). Laboratory assays are not always able to detect an elevated insulin level due to the limitations of the assays with the threshold of detection,[26,27] so obtaining other supportive diagnostic data is imperative. Because neonatal hypopituitarism can closely resemble hyperinsulinism, growth hormone and cortisol assays should be obtained, and if values are insufficient, further provocative simulation testing to assess for central growth hormone and adrenal insufficiency should be pursued if deficiency is suspected.

Hyperinsulinism is caused by dysregulated insulin secretion from the pancreatic β-cells and can be the result of perinatal factors (perinatal stress–induced HI), syndromic (as in Beckwith-Wiedemann syndrome), or monogenic, due to mutations in genes important for the regulation of insulin secretion.[28] The most common and severe type of congenital hyperinsulinism is due to inactivating mutations in *ABCC8* or *KCNJ11*, which cause dysfunction in the pancreatic β-cell ATP-sensitive potassium (K_{ATP}) channel, resulting in dysregulated insulin secretion.[29–31] Other causes of congenital hyperinsulinism are mutations in genes encoding different proteins involved in insulin secretion from the β-cells, including activating mutations in glutamate dehydrogenase *(GLUD1)* and glucokinase *(GCK)*. In

Table 23.2 Diagnostic Criteria for Hyperinsulinism[27]

Diagnostic Criteria (When Plasma Glucose Is <50 mg/dL)	Sensitivity (%)	Specificity (%)
Hypoketonemia (plasma β-hydroxybutyrate <1.8 mmol/L)	100	100
Hypofattyacidemia (plasma free fatty acids <1.7 mmol/L)	86.9	100
Hyperinsulinemia (detectable plasma insulin)[a]	82.2	100
Inappropriate glycemic response to glucagon, 1 mg IV (delta glucose ≥30 mg/dL)	88	100
SUPPORTIVE PARAMETERS		
C-peptide ≥0.5 ng/Ml	89	100
Suppressed IGFBP-1 (≤110 ng/mL)	85	96.6

[a]Please note that newer, more sensitive insulin assays may result in higher sensitivity.

IGFBP-1, Insulin-like growth factor binding protein 1; *IV*, intravenous.

Ferrara C, Patel P, Becker S, et al. Biomarkers of insulin for the diagnosis of hyperinsulinemic hypoglycemia in infants and children. *J Pediatr.* 2016;168:212–219.[27]

addition to monogenic forms of congenital HI, hyperinsulinism is associated with certain syndromes, most notably Beckwith-Wiedemann syndrome. In contrast to genetic congenital etiologies, hyperinsulinism can also be transient, occurring as a result of perinatal stressors. This distinct form of transient HI, known as perinatal stress–induced HI, typically responds to treatment with diazoxide and spontaneously resolves within the first few months of life.[5] Hyperinsulinism due to perinatal stress is quite common, affecting up to 50% of at-risk neonates exposed to perinatal stressors.[4] Perinatal stress–induced hyperinsulinism is often perceived as less severe than permanent congenital HI, but children with perinatal stress–induced hyperinsulinism are also at risk for severe hypoglycemia and long-term neurologic sequelae.[5,15]

Treatment

Once a diagnosis of hyperinsulinism is established, the short-term goal should be to maintain plasma glucose greater than 70 mg/dL. This can be accomplished with an intravenous glucose infusion. If high glucose infusion rates are required to maintain normoglycemia, central access should be obtained in order to administer fluids with a higher dextrose concentration and thus minimize fluid overload. In severe cases, a glucagon infusion can be employed, which will temporarily decrease the glucose requirement.[32]

There are limited available medical treatments for hyperinsulinism (Table 23.3). Diazoxide is the only drug approved by the Food and Drug Administration for the treatment of hyperinsulinism. Diazoxide opens the K_{ATP} channel and thereby inhibits insulin secretion.[33,34] Side effects include hypertrichosis (prevalence, 26%–30%), fluid retention (prevalence, 5.5%–16%), pulmonary hypertension (prevalence, 2.4%–4.8%), bone marrow suppression (prevalence, 15%), and hyperuricemia (prevalence, 5%).[35,36] To avoid fluid retention, all patients should be started on chlorothiazide at the start of diazoxide treatment, typically at twice the dose of diazoxide, rather than wait for symptoms to occur to begin treatment. Concurrent initiation of chlorothiazide decreases risk of fluid overload and secondary respiratory effects. The PES therapeutic committee has recently published practice guidelines for dosing and monitoring for adverse events in infants treated with diazoxide, which includes tailoring the dose according to the suspected type of hyperinsulinism, i.e., transient versus permanent; a comprehensive evaluation of cardiopulmonary health; and consideration of a baseline echocardiogram.[37] Determining diazoxide responsiveness should be done expeditiously once a diagnosis of hyperinsulinism is established, because the response indicates which infants require a more specialized evaluation. It takes up to 5 days for diazoxide to reach a steady state, and waiting to assess for improved fasting tolerance is recommended, with titration to maximum diazoxide dosing of 15 mg/kg/day, divided twice daily as necessary. Not all forms of

Table 23.3 Medical Treatments for Hyperinsulinism

Treatment	Dose	Route	Mechanism of Action	Side Effects	Monitoring	Notes
Diazoxide	5–15 mg/kg/day divided twice daily	Oral (only suspension available in the United States)	Activates the β-cell K_{ATP} channels	Fluid retention Hypertrichosis Bone marrow suppression Appetite suppression Pulmonary hypertension	Electrolytes CBC with differential Echocardiogram	Concomitant use of diuretics decreases fluid retention
Octreotide	10–20 mcg/kg/day (every 6 hours)	Subcutaneous injection	Somatostatin analog; inhibits insulin release	Elevated liver enzymes Diarrhea Gall stones Growth failure Hypothyroidism Necrotizing enterocolitis	Liver function Growth factors Thyroid function RUQ ultrasound	Use in infants >8 weeks due to risk of necrotizing enterocolitis
Glucagon	1 mg/24 h	Continuous infusion	Promotes glycogenolysis and gluconeogenesis	Nausea Rash	Frequent glucose monitoring	Used as temporary measure Lowers GIR requirement and associated risk of fluid overload
Continuous dextrose	Up to 10 mg/kg/min	Enteral—via gastrostomy tube	Increased glucose intake	Risk of hypoglycemia if infusion is interrupted	Frequent glucose monitoring	Requires use of an infusion pump

CBC, Complete blood cell count; K_{ATP}, ATP-sensitive potassium.

hyperinsulinism are diazoxide responsive, and given the side-effect profile, discontinuation of diazoxide is recommended if there is minimal or no response. If a neonate with hyperinsulinism is found to be diazoxide unresponsive, the patient should be transferred to a congenital hyperinsulinism center for further specialized intervention.

Somatostatin analogs are second-line agents used for treatment of hyperinsulinism, due to their insulin inhibitory effects.[38] Octreotide is most commonly used, although treatment failure is not uncommon due to tachyphylaxis. Unfortunately, necrotizing enterocolitis is a concerning known treatment risk, and thus use in neonates is limited.[39] Other side effects of somatostatin analogs include transaminitis, gallstones, hypothyroidism, poor growth, and diarrhea.[40] Glucagon can be used as a short-term agent via continuous infusion of 1 mg per day in infants requiring surgery, to decrease dextrose requirement and thus lessen fluid burden.[32] As a general rule, using feeds to maintain glycemic control is not recommended, because this increases risk for future feeding difficulties, such as oral aversions, and excessive weight gain from overnutrition.[41]

Genetic testing helps identify the specific cause of HI and is particularly helpful in guiding the management of diazoxide-unresponsive cases. The most common and severe type of congenital hyperinsulinism is due to mutations in *ABCC8* or *KCNJ11*, which cause dysfunction in the pancreatic β-cell K_{ATP} channel, resulting in dysregulated insulin secretion.[29,30] There are two distinct histologic forms of K_{ATP} HI. The disease may be focal, affecting only a localized area of the pancreas. Focal disease is caused by paternally inherited recessive mutations in *ABCC8* or *KCNJ11*, in combination with somatic loss of heterozygosity of the 11p15 chromosomal region and compensation via uniparental disomy.[42,43] Alternatively, diffuse hyperinsulinism, in which all the pancreatic β-cells are affected, is most often caused by biallelic recessive mutations in the K_{ATP} genes.

Long-term tailored management should begin with expedited genetic testing for *ABCC8* and *KCNJ11* mutations, with reflex testing to the expanded genetic hyperinsulinism panel. Genetic testing including parent-of-origin analysis is highly efficient at predicting focal disease, because the positive predictive value of a single recessive paternally inherited *ABCC8* or *KCNJ11* mutation for focal hyperinsulinism is 94%.[31] Genetic testing should be sent shortly after diagnosis, because results will provide prognostic information and impact disease-management decisions.

Surgical Management

If focal disease is suspected based on identification of the specific genetic inheritance pattern associated with the focal histologic phenotype, then surgical management via excision of the affected lesion should be pursued, because it would likely be curative. A review of 500 surgically managed hyperinsulinism cases at the Children's Hospital of Philadelphia demonstrated that 97% of patients with focal hyperinsulinism were cured after surgical resection of the lesion.[44] Patients with suspected focal hyperinsulinism should undergo a specialized PET imaging technique using an ^{18}Fluoro-L-3,4-dihydroxyphenylalanine (^{18}F-DOPA) tracer, which is taken up by neuroendocrine tissue, to confirm and localize a focal lesion prior to surgical resection.[45] While surgical management is often curative for focal lesions, in diffuse hyperinsulinism, surgical management is employed when medical therapy alone is insufficient at maintaining normoglycemia. In these cases, a near-total pancreatectomy is performed, which is often only palliative and results in continued hyperinsulinism disease, Lthough less severe and thus medically manageable. These patients should also undergo gastrostomy tube placement at the time of pancreatectomy, given the high likelihood of a continuous dextrose requirement to manage residual hypoglycemia.[46] Unfortunately, a near-total pancreatectomy has long-term

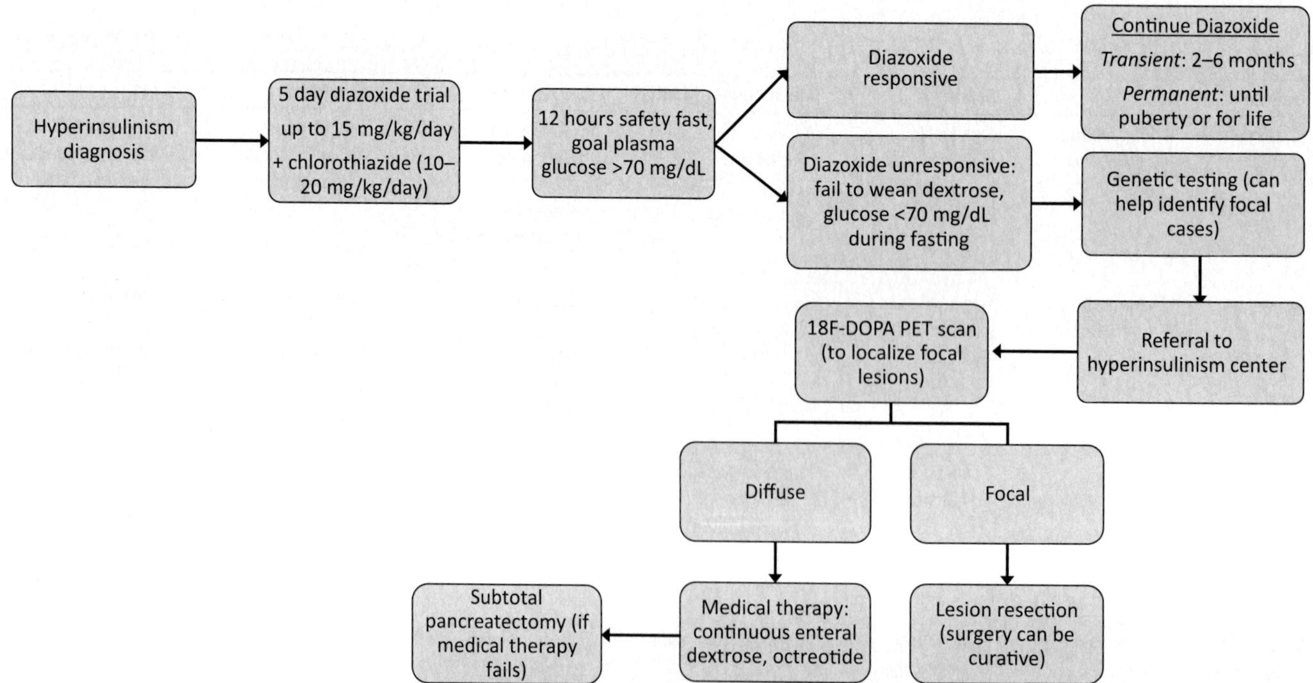

Fig. 23.3 Hyperinsulinism Management Algorithm. This algorithm outlines the general treatment approach to a patient with a diagnosis of hyperinsulinism. Treatment begins with a trial of diazoxide followed by genetic testing and specialized imaging at a congenital hyperinsulinism center if the patient is diazoxide unresponsive.

consequences of its own, including an almost guaranteed risk of diabetes later in life.[24] If indicated, surgical management via pancreatectomy should be pursued at a specialized hyperinsulinism center. Fig. 23.3 outlines the management approach to the neonate with hyperinsulinism.

Conclusion

Persistent neonatal hypoglycemia is an important cause of long-term morbidity, and thus persistent hypoglycemia disorders should be distinguished from transitional neonatal hypoglycemia. Providers must maintain a high index of suspicion for an underlying hypoglycemia disorder, particularly if hypoglycemia persists beyond the first 2 to 3 days of life or if an infant has risk factors for a hypoglycemia disorder. In the initial days of life, management should be directed toward maintaining glucose stability, and further evaluation with a diagnostic fast should be deferred until after the period of transitional neonatal hypoglycemia is over. Furthermore, failure to adequately assess for an etiology of hypoglycemia and provide a treatment plan prior to discharge home can have lasting consequences due to hypoglycemia-mediated neurologic injury.

CHAPTER

24 Infants of Diabetic Mothers

Vinayak Mishra, Kei Lui, Robert L. Schelonka, Akhil Maheshwari, Rajesh Jain

KEY POINTS

1. Diabetes in pregnant women can be visualized in two distinct subsets: 1% to 2% of women have pregestational disease, whereas 6% to 9% develop diabetes during pregnancy.
2. In mothers with pregestational or early-onset diabetes, placental vasculopathy may cause growth restriction, altered organogenesis, and congenital anomalies.
3. In mothers with gestational diabetes, the fetuses tend to become large for date, show a wide range of metabolic changes, and may be predisposed to short- and long-term complications.
4. The most frequently seen metabolic complications in infants of diabetic mothers (IDMs) are hypoglycemia, hypocalcemia, and hypomagnesemia.
5. Respiratory and cardiovascular complications contribute importantly to neonatal morbidity and mortality, especially in preterm neonates.
6. IDMs have a two- to four-fold increase in the risk of congenital malformations compared with the general population. These malformations are seen most frequently in the cardiovascular, neurologic, renal, gastrointestinal, and skeletal systems.

Infants born to mothers with diabetes mellitus (DM) in pregnancy are predisposed to short- and long-term complications.[1] The extent of these complications depends on the type of diabetes (pregestational or gestational); onset and duration of glucose intolerance; severity of diabetes (degree of glucose intolerance, presence of complications); and therapeutic control. This chapter will review the epidemiology of maternal diabetes, pathophysiology of complications, clinical features, management, and prognosis in affected infants.

Epidemiology

In 2019, an estimated 20 million women experienced hyperglycemia during pregnancy. This accounted for nearly 16% of all live births in the world.[2] Diabetes noted during pregnancy may have already been there as a pregestational disease, referring to type 1 or type 2 DM diagnosed before pregnancy, or it may get diagnosed during pregnancy and then be labeled as gestational diabetes mellitus (GDM). The overall incidence of pregestational diabetes is about 1% to 2%, and that of GDM is about 6% to 9%.[3]

The global incidence of diabetes during pregnancy is rising. In the United States the prevalence of pregestational diabetes increased by 37% and that of GDM by 56% during the period 2000 to 2010.[3] The most important risk factors for maternal diabetes are maternal age ≥35 years, urban residence, and low socioeconomic status.[4,5] Prevalence varies by race and ethnicity; Black women have higher rates of pregestational diabetes, whereas Asian women are more susceptible to GDM. Latinas are at higher risk of both pregestational diabetes and GDM.[6] Obesity, family history of diabetes, high parity, and older age at first birth increase the risk of gestational diabetes.[3]

Pathophysiology

Because maternal plasma glucose can cross the placenta by facilitated diffusion, maternal hyperglycemia leads to fetal hyperglycemia. Early-onset placental vasculopathy may cause growth restriction and may alter organogenesis (diabetic embryopathy) with recognizable patterns of congenital anomalies.[1] Poorly controlled GDM and hyperglycemia can cause macrosomia (Fig. 24.1).

The metabolic changes in infants of diabetic mothers (IDMs) are summarized in Fig. 24.2. In the second trimester, the fetal pancreas responds to the rise in glucose levels by producing insulin, leading to fetal hyperinsulinemia. Fetal hyperglycemia and hyperinsulinemia drive the multisystemic pathology present in IDMs.[7] Elevated fetal insulin levels, upregulated glucose transporters, and increased intracellular glucose concentrations can enhance mitochondrial oxidative phosphorylation. The resulting increase in the production of reactive oxygen species can contribute to diabetic embryopathy. Chronically upregulated fetal metabolic rate and oxygen consumption lead to relative hypoxemia, which in turn elevate proangiogenic factors such as leptin, vascular endothelial growth factor, fibroblast growth factor 2, and matrix metalloproteinases (MMPs) such as MMP14 and MMP15, which lead to altered tissue histoarchitecture and epigenetic changes.

IDMs experience several types of metabolic stress, including in the oxidative, nitrosative, endoplasmic reticulum (unfolded protein response), and hexosamine pathways.[8] Smith et al.[9] demonstrated that insulin impedes the cortisol-induced synthesis of phosphatidylcholine (an essential substrate for surfactant production) by type II alveolar pneumocytes. Hyperinsulinemia has also been shown to suppress the structural maturation of the fetal lung. Together, all these changes predispose IDMs to respiratory distress syndrome even at peri-term gestational ages. IDMs also have an excessive accumulation of liver glycogen, cardiac and skeletal muscles, adipose tissue, and other tissues. Fetal hyperglycemia and hyperinsulinemia accelerate glycogenesis, lipogenesis, and protein synthesis.[7] The cellular effects include hypertrophy and hyperplasia of the pancreatic islets of Langerhans, myocardial hypertrophy, and increased cytoplasm in hepatocytes.[7]

IDMs are at a higher risk of hypoxia and ischemia at peri- and intrapartum stages than are infants of nondiabetic mothers. Fetal hypoxemia raises erythropoietin levels, which can stimulate erythroid progenitor growth that is already activated by hyperinsulinemia. These two phenomena can lead to polycythemia and consequently to neonatal hyperviscosity syndrome.[8,9] Many fetal regions have

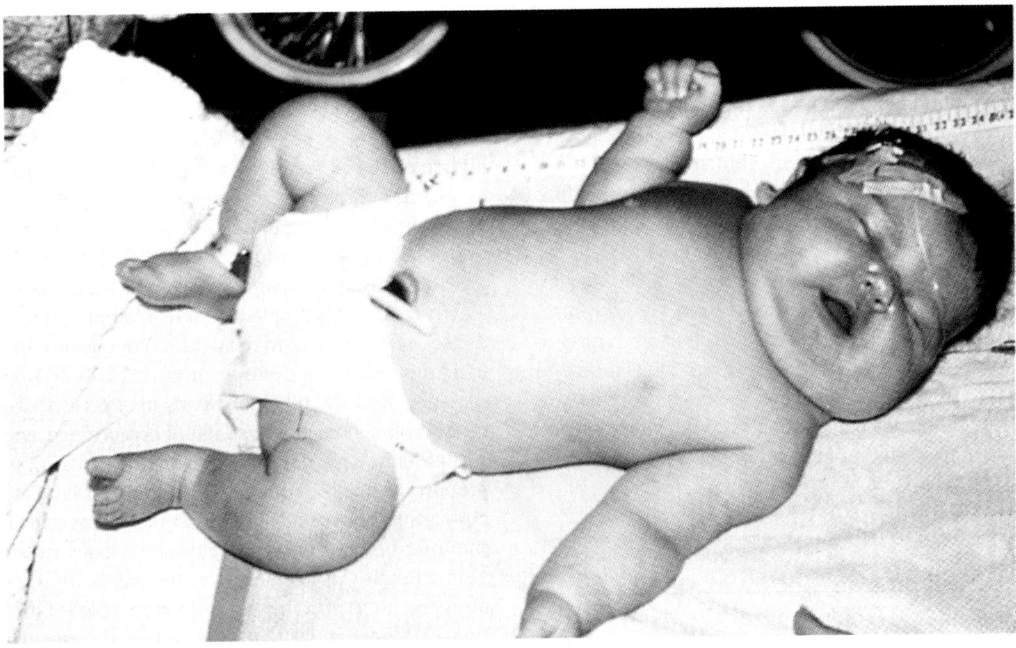

Fig. 24.1 Large-for-Gestation Term Infant of a Mother With Gestational Diabetes. The infant weighed 5 kg. (Reproduced with approval and minor modifications from Balest et al. *Zitelli and Davis' Atlas of Pediatric Physical Diagnosis*. 2018.)

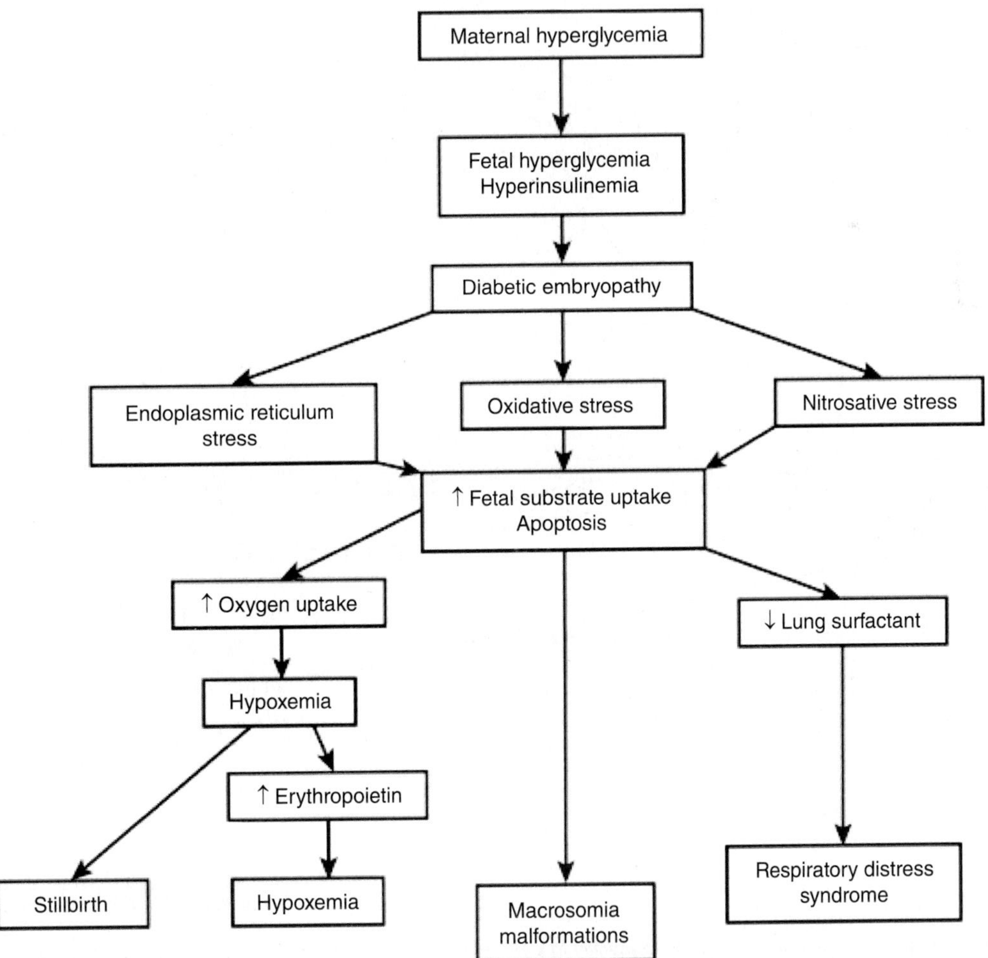

Fig. 24.2 Flow Diagram of Pathogenic Events That Result in Fetal and Neonatal Morbidity in Infants of Diabetic Mothers. (Reproduced with approval and minor modifications from Garg and Devaskar. Disorders of carbohydrate metabolism in the neonate. In: *Fanaroff and Martin's Neonatal-Perinatal Medicine*. 86:1584–1610.)

concomitant tissue hypoxia due to increased glycation of hemoglobin and low concentrations of 2,3-diphosphoglycerate, which increase erythropoietin expression and red blood cell (RBC) production. Some premature infants develop polycythemia, and the larger RBC mass and turnover may increase the bilirubin loads to exceed the capacity of the developing liver and cause hyperbilirubinemia.[10]

In the fetal metabolic environment, even small changes can induce epigenetic modifications with altered gene expression and phenotypic changes (Fig. 24.3).[11,12] The risk of diabetic embryopathy increases with prolonged fetal exposure to maternal hyperglycemia.[1,13,14] Insulin binds to the type I insulin-like growth factor receptor to induce intracellular phosphorylation pathways, which activate cellular growth-promoting factors.[13] In IDMs, myocardial hypertrophy leads to cardiomegaly with asymmetric, disproportionate septal hypertrophy.[15,16] There is also widespread cellular apoptosis with altered genetics and epigenetic systems, resulting in dysmorphogenesis.[17]

Clinical Features

Fetal Effects

A brief summary of clinical manifestations is provided in Table 24.1.

Diabetic mothers experience preterm delivery and unexplained intrauterine demise more often than mothers who do not have diabetes.[1,18] The risks are particularly high with pregestational diabetes.[1] In GDM, the odds of congenital anomalies are slightly higher than in the general population (odds ratio, 1.1–1.3) and increase with higher maternal fasting blood glucose or body mass index.[19,20]

Macrosomia with birth weights >4000 g may be seen in up to 25% to 45% of infants born to mothers with pregestational diabetes and 15% to 20% of those born to mothers with GDM.[1,21–24] Many IDMs show greater adiposity compared with infants born to nondiabetic mothers.[25] Macrosomic IDMs frequently show altered growth with higher chest-to-head and shoulder-to-head ratios compared with infants of nondiabetic mothers[21,26] and are at increased risk of a birth injury such as shoulder dystocia, brachial plexus injury, clavicular or humeral fractures, cephalohematoma, subdural hemorrhage, and facial palsy.[27–29]

Epidemiologic data show a recent encouraging downtrend in the proportion of macrosomic IDMs from 9.1% to 7% of the newborn population between 1990 and 2005.[30] However, these figures need cautious evaluation because these changes in birth weights could also originate in prematurity, increased multiple births, or early obstetric intervention with induction of labor and/or cesarean sections. Mothers with type 1 DM and good medical care (HbA_{1c} ≤7%) still have a 50% increased risk for fetal macrosomia (>90th

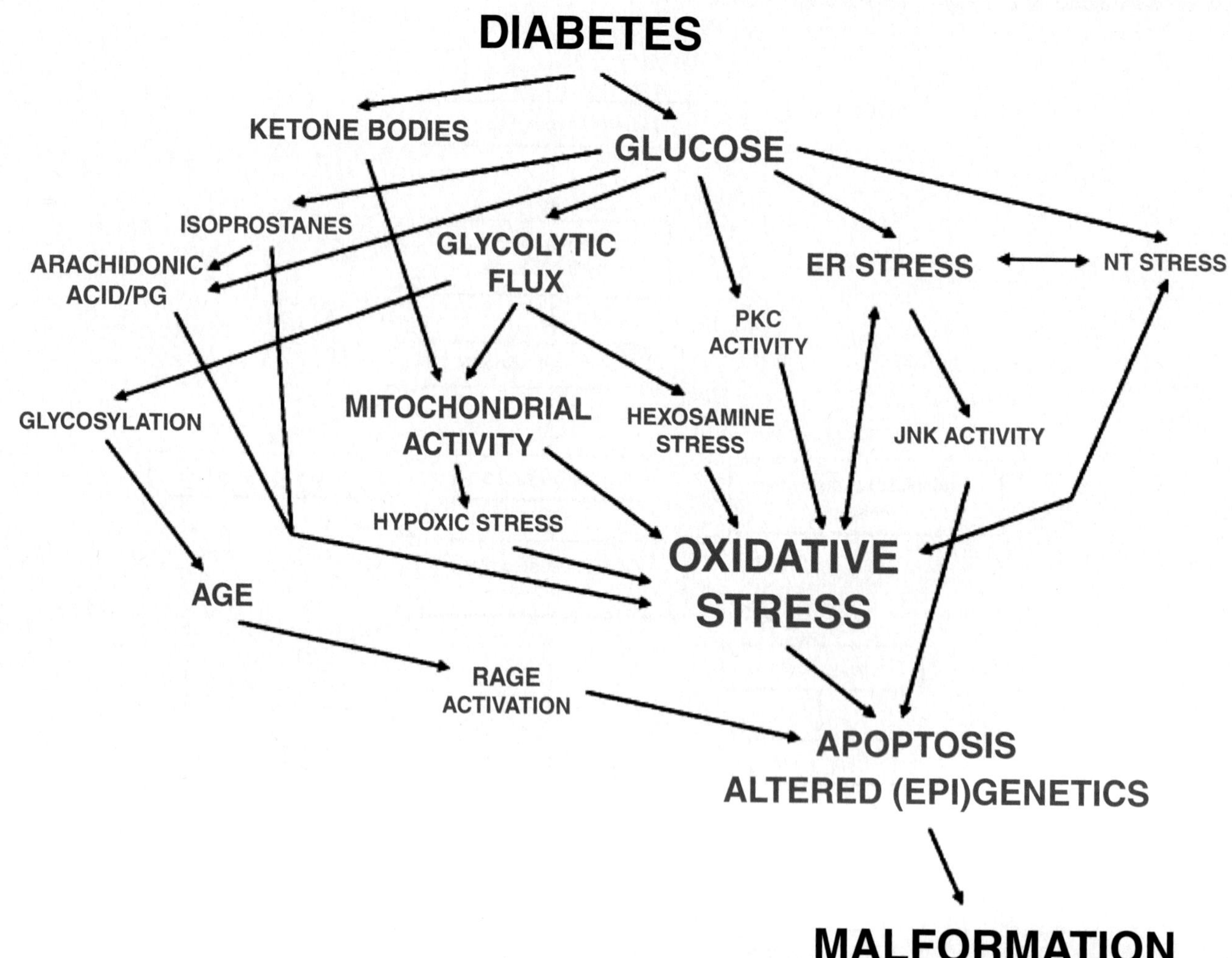

Fig. 24.3 Schematic Outline of the Development of Diabetic Embryopathy. *Blue* indicates increased activity/amount and *red* indicates decreased or disturbed activity/amount of compounds or processes. Note that more interactions between the items are likely to be present than those denoted here and that the putative importance of genetic predisposition is not included. *ER*, Endoplasmic reticulum; *JNK*, c-Jun N-terminal kinase. *PG*, prostaglandin; *PKC*, protein kinase C. (Reproduced with approval and minor modifications from Eriksson UJ, Wentzel P. The status of diabetic embryopathy. *Ups J Med Sci*. 2016;121:96–112.)

Table 24.1 Clinical Manifestations Frequently Seen in Infants of Diabetic Mothers

- Fetal/perinatal deaths (18–28 per 1000 births, compared with 4.5 per 1000 in nondiabetic mothers).
- Large for date/macrosomia (birth weights ≥90th percentile in 40%–60% of type 1 diabetic pregnancies, 30%–55% of type 2 diabetic pregnancies, and 10%–20% of pregnancies complicated by gestational diabetes. For infants born to nondiabetic mothers, macrosomia (birth weight ≥4000 g) is seen in 7%–8% and LGA in 8%–14% infants.
- Birth trauma with shoulder dystocia, brachial plexus injury, clavicular or humeral fractures, cephalohematoma, subdural hemorrhage, and facial palsy. Cesarean deliveries in 50%.
- Metabolic problems such as hypoglycemia (25%–50%, compared with 5% in nondiabetic), hypocalcemia (4%–40%), and hypomagnesemia (up to 40%, mostly asymptomatic).
- Polycythemia.
- Transient tachypnea of the newborn, surfactant deficiency/respiratory distress syndrome, persistent pulmonary hypertension (5%–40%, compared with 3% in nondiabetic mothers).
- Hyperbilirubinemia (10%–25%).
- Abdominal visceromegaly.
- Asymmetric septal hypertrophy of the heart (30%–40% of IDMs show cardiac changes on imaging, but only approximately 5% of infants will manifest symptoms), heart failure.
- Renal vein thrombosis.
- Small left colon.
- Congenital anomalies, caudal regression syndrome.

IDMs, Infants of diabetic mothers; *LGA*, large for gestational age.

percentile) and a 33% greater chance of having a very large for gestational age neonate (>97th percentile) compared with the general population.[31] Glycemic control in midpregnancy could be one of the most important determinants of abnormal growth.[32]

About 5% to 10% of IDMs may be small for date with birth weights below the 10th percentile.[33,34] These infants may be born to mothers with longstanding diabetes who may have notable placental vascular changes on ultrasound/histopathology.[35,36] There is a strong correlation between fetal intrauterine growth restriction and the severity of maternal changes of type 1 DM and preeclampsia.[37] In these pregestational diabetic mothers, microvascular complications such as retinopathy increase the risk of small-for-gestational-age (SGA) birth.[36] Excessive glycemic control may also increase the risk, possibly due to decreased fetal nutrition.[37] Conversely, a few cohort studies have shown that diabetes during pregnancy reduces the risk of SGA.[38,39] Coexisting conditions such as preeclampsia, markers of prolonged diabetes such as retinopathy, and the control of diabetes during pregnancy are important for the determination of risk to the fetus.[40] Further studies are also needed to determine the anthropometric measures of adiposity and skeletal growth.[41]

Recent efforts include evaluating 3-dimensional ultrasound to predict fetal weight based on the estimation of subcutaneous tissue in limbs.[42] The amniotic fluid volume also seems to be related to fetal weight.[43] These measurements can be performed with high accuracy. However, further work is needed to assess the impact of these studies on maternal management of diabetes during pregnancy and fetal/neonatal outcomes.[44]

Peripartum Effects

Birth asphyxia occurs more frequently in IDMs due to obstetric complications such as failure to progress, shoulder dystocia, and fetal diabetic cardiomyopathy.[27,45,46] Mimouni et al.[46] showed that maternal nephropathy, maternal hyperglycemia before delivery, and premature births were associated with the rate of birth asphyxia.

Neonatal Effects

Metabolic

The common metabolic complications in IDMs are hypoglycemia, hypocalcemia, and hypomagnesemia.[47] Neonatal hypoglycemia commonly presents in the first few hours of birth.[48] It occurs due to the cut-off of maternal glucose transfer in a state of persistent hyperinsulinemia.[49] Macrosomic neonates, preterm neonates, and SGA neonates have greater risk of developing hypoglycemia.[50,51] Hypocalcemia in IDMs may present as jitteriness, lethargy, apnea, tachypnea, or seizures between 24 and 72 hours of birth.[18]

Cardiorespiratory

Respiratory and cardiovascular complications contribute importantly to neonatal morbidity and mortality, especially in preterm neonates.[52] Respiratory complications including respiratory distress syndrome due to prematurity, relatively immature structure of the developing lung, surfactant deficiency, patent ductus arteriosus, and transient tachypnea of the newborn (Fig. 24.4) predispose the infant to neonatal hypoxia.[8,16,52–57] IDMs are vulnerable to transient hypertrophic cardiomyopathy, characterized by left ventricular outflow obstruction due to disproportionate thickening of the interventricular septum and reduced left ventricular size (Fig. 24.5).[16,57–59] Way et al.[60] showed that symptomatic infants recovered within 2 to 4 weeks and echocardiographic findings of septal hypertrophy resolved within 2 to 12 months.

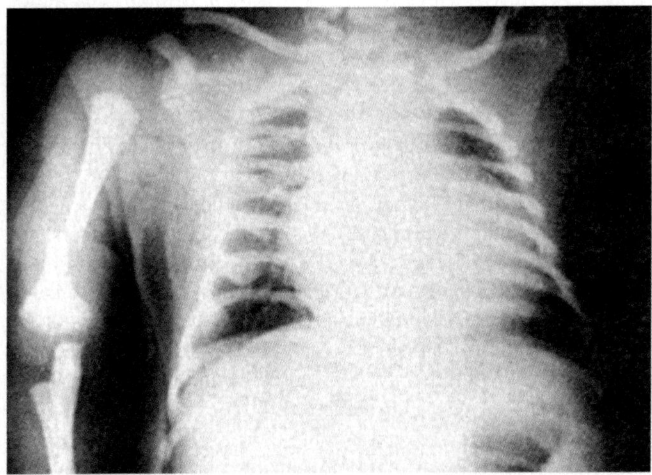

Fig. 24.4 Chest Radiograph of a Vaginally Delivered, Full-Term Infant (4.7 kg) of a Diabetic Mother. The infant had cardiomegaly, hepatomegaly, congested lung fields, and fractures of the right humerus and left clavicle. (Reproduced with approval and minor modifications from Garg and Devaskar. Disorders of carbohydrate metabolism in the neonate. In: *Fanaroff and Martin's Neonatal-Perinatal Medicine*, 86:1584–1610.)

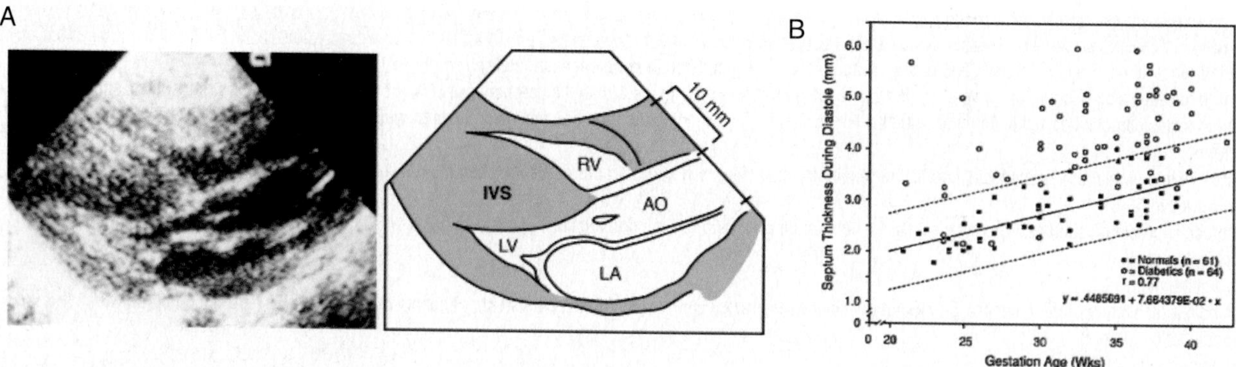

Fig. 24.5 Maternal Diabetes Is Associated With Increased Thickness of the Ventricular Septal Thickness. (A) Parasternal long-axis view of a 2-dimensional echocardiogram of an infant of a mother with diabetes. There is asymmetric hypertrophy of the interventricular septum (IVS), which is at least two times as thick as the posterior wall of the left ventricle (LV). (B) Correlation between septal thickness during diastole and gestational age. *AO*, Aorta; *LA*, left atrium; *RV*, right ventricle. (A, Reproduced with approval and minor modifications from Park and Salamat. Primary Myocardial Disease. In: *Park's Pediatric Cardiology for Practitioners*. 18:248–263. B, Reproduced with approval and minor modifications from Weindling. Offspring of diabetic pregnancy: short-term outcomes. *Seminars in Fetal and Neonatal Medicine*. 2009;14[2]:111–118.)

Transient hypertrophic cardiomyopathy is usually a benign condition that does not require pharmacologic treatment in most cases.[60,61]

Hematologic

IDMs can have higher hematocrit values owing to the chronic fetal hypoxemia and consequently raised erythropoietin; these changes can set up a feed-forward cycle.[62] Many IDMs develop polycythemia, defined as a central venous hematocrit above 65%. This higher incidence of polycythemia in IDMs has been noted in several studies.[18,63] Polycythemia could predispose infants to neonatal hyperviscosity syndrome, which involves ischemia and infarction of major organs due to blood vessel obstruction by sludging.[64] Renal vein thrombosis is a significant complication of hyperviscosity syndrome in IDMs (Fig. 24.6).[65,66]

Another consequence of chronic fetal hypoxemia is the shunting of iron into the expanding erythrocyte mass, which can cause low iron stores in many organ systems to be notable during the third trimester and at birth.[67] The breakdown of excess RBCs could possibly restore the iron stores, so iron supplementation therapy is not recommended. As mentioned above, the increased RBC breakdown can cause hyperbilirubinemia in IDMs.[18] The risk of pathologic jaundice in IDMs may also be augmented by other factors such as prematurity and total RBC mass with macrosomia.[68]

Congenital Malformations

IDMs have a two- to four-fold increase in the risk of congenital malformations over the generally presumed 3% risk in the general population.[69,70] The mechanisms underlying the increased incidence of congenital malformations in IDMs are incompletely understood but are likely multifactorial (see Fig. 24.3). The risk of major malformations is higher; the Atlanta Birth Defects Case-Control Study reported a risk of major malformation in 2.3% of live births in the general population and a relative risk of 5.2 (95% confidence interval [CI], 2.1–13.2) in mothers who required insulin during pregnancy and up to 7.9 (1.9–33.5) in mothers with type 1 DM.[71]

In the Baltimore-Washington Infant Study, the strongest associations were noted between maternal diabetes and cardiovascular malformations, particularly with double-outlet right ventricle anomalies (odds ratio [OR], 21.33; 99.5% CI: 3.34–136.26) and truncus arteriosus (OR, 12.81; 1.43–114.64).[72] The relative risk for major cardiovascular malformation is 12.9 (95% CI, 4.8–34.6) in mothers who require insulin during pregnancy, with an absolute risk of 6.1% of live births. Many studies show increased incidence of pulmonary atresia, transposition of the great vessels, ventricular septal defects, coarctation of the aorta, and patent ductus arteriosus in neonates ≥2500 g.[73]

Maternal diabetes is also increased with fetal neurologic anomalies (Fig. 24.7) such as neural tube defects, anencephaly, microcephaly, holoprosencephaly, hydrocephalus, and spina bifida.[73] Caudal regression syndrome, a rare anomaly in terms of the overall

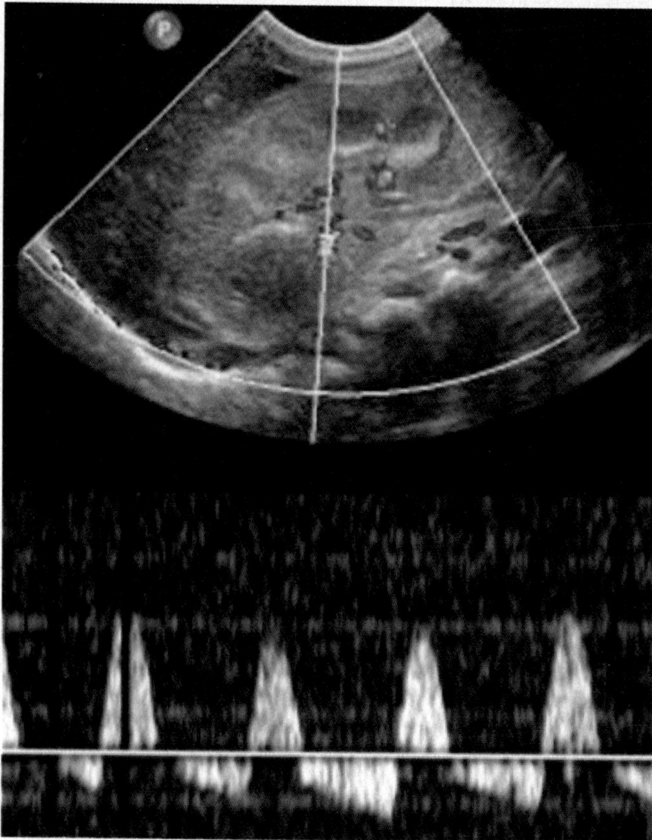

Fig. 24.6 Renal Vein Thrombosis. Longitudinal sonogram of this 2-day-old infant shows an enlarged, echogenic kidney. A highly resistive patter of intrarenal arterial flow is present with reversal of diastolic blood flow. (Reproduced with approval and minor modifications from Wells et al. Vascular conditions. In: *Caffey's Pediatric Diagnostic Imaging*, 2019.)

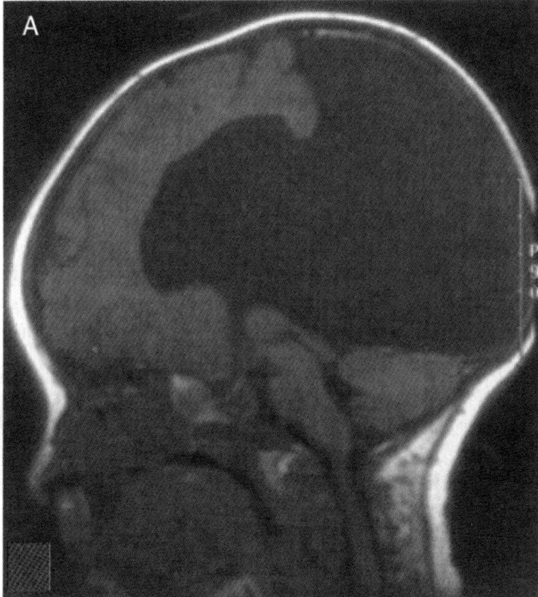

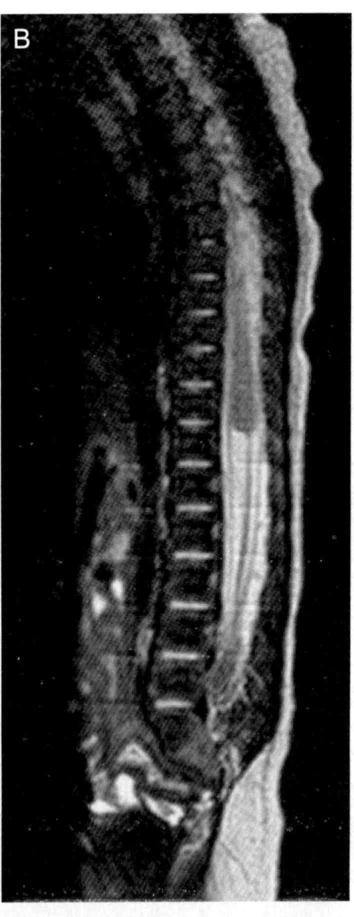

Fig. 24.7 Neurologic Abnormalities in IDMs. (A) Holoprosencephaly. Midsagittal, T1-weighted magnetic resonance imaging (MRI) of a child with alobar holoprosencephaly shows a pancake of brain anteriorly, with the single, midline ventricle leading into a large, dorsal cyst. The corpus callosum is absent. (B) Caudal regression syndrome. One-week-old neonate with caudal regression syndrome and absence of sacral segments. The cord ends at the level of T11, with a club-shaped distal cord. (A, Reproduced with approval and minor modifications from Sarnat et al. Neuroembryology. In: *Youmans and Winn Neurological Surgery*. 46:e286–e312. B, Reproduced with approval and minor modifications from Gilbert. MR imaging of the neonatal musculoskeletal system. In: *Magnetic Resonance Imaging Clinics of North America*. 2011;19:841–858; ix.)

incidence, is seen with a 200 times higher frequency in IDMs than in the general population.[74–76] It is defined by agenesis or dysgenesis of variable parts of the sacrococcygeal and/or lumbar spine and can be associated with anomalies in other systems.[77] It can be diagnosed by ultrasound as early as in the first trimester of pregnancy.[78,79] Gastrointestinal anomalies include duodenal atresia, imperforate anus, anorectal atresia, and small left colon syndrome.[76] Genitourinary defects include ureteral duplication, renal agenesis, and hydronephrosis; skeletal defects include sacral agenesis and hemivertebrae.[80,81]

Management

The management of IDMs is primarily preventive and depends on appropriate antenatal care and neonatal care. Antenatal care of women with GDM or pregestational diabetes should include strict diabetes control, frequent biophysical profile assessment, routine ultrasonography to assess fetal maturity and detect anomalies, and delivery planning in a hospital where operative delivery and neonatal resuscitation provisions are available.

IDMs should be cautiously and frequently monitored after birth and evaluated for congenital anomalies. If the infant does not require resuscitation or transfer to the neonatal intensive care unit, the infant should be handed over to the mother for early initiation of breastfeeding. Early establishment of skin-to-skin contact and breastfeeding within 30 minutes of birth is essential. The newborn should be monitored for hypoglycemia and its clinical features such as jitteriness, lethargy, floppiness, central cyanosis, apnea, poor feeding, and seizures. Glucose monitoring to detect hypoglycemia should be performed soon after the first breastfeeding and continued at regular intervals for the first 24 hours of postnatal age (details in the chapter on neonatal hypoglycemia). Many infants also have polycythemia and need to be evaluated and treated with intravenous fluids. If seen to be jittery or as having seizures, calcium levels may have to be checked and treated.

The management of neonatal hypoglycemia is a stepwise process depending on the plasma glucose levels and clinical features. If there are hypoglycemic signs or symptoms, aggressive treatment with parenteral glucose should be started immediately, whereas if there are no hypoglycemic clinical features, oral feeds should be encouraged first.[82,83] Buccal dextrose gel is a simple and inexpensive treatment that could be used along with milk feeding for asymptomatic neonates.[84] In rare cases of refractory hypoglycemia, when the blood glucose stays below 50 mg/dL despite maximum parenteral glucose infusion, glucagon administration should be considered.[85] Glucocorticoids, diazoxide, and octreotide are other treatment options in refractory cases of neonatal hypoglycemia.[86]

Many IDMs with asymmetric cardiac septal hypertrophy show an enlarged cardiac silhouette on chest radiography.[87] On clinical examination, there may be altered peripheral perfusion and/or hypotension. Echocardiography may show characteristic features: there may be hypertrophy of the right ventricular anterior wall and left ventricular posterior wall with a thickness of ≥5 mm.[88] The septum is considered hypertrophic if it is ≥6 mm.[88] A septal-to-left-ventricle posterior wall thickness of ≥1.3 is also a useful parameter.[89] Cardiac magnetic resonance imaging can be utilized as a complimentary tool to characterize the myocardium and assess viability. In autopsy studies, the ventricular muscle fibers show hypertrophy; there is some subendocardial patchy necrosis, interstitial edema, and a mononuclear inflammatory infiltrate.[90]

The treatment of asymmetric cardiac septal hypertrophy in IDMs is largely supportive with close monitoring. If symptomatic, some infants may respond to intravenous fluids. In some, enteral propranolol (typically 1 mg/kg every 8 hours) may be useful. Inhibition of the angiotensin-converting enzyme could be useful. If the infant has heart failure, specific treatment may be needed with expert consultation.[91] Fortunately, most signs of outflow obstruction tend to resolve by 3 to 6 months of age.[92]

Several other neonatal congenital anomalies seen in IDMs need treatment. Unfortunately, the therapeutic options available in many are limited to supportive measures, and once clinical stability is attained, to surgical measures. We intentionally have not covered those issues because the frequencies of these conditions are fortunately low and consultations with specific subspecialties would be needed.

Prognosis

IDMs are genetically susceptible to developing DM later in life.[81] There is a 65% lifelong risk of type 1 DM in identical twins.[93] The lifelong risk for obesity and impaired glucose metabolism is higher in IDMs than in infants of nondiabetic mothers. Pettitt et al.[94] showed a 45% prevalence of non-insulin-dependent diabetes mellitus (NIDDM) in offspring of Pima Indian women with NIDDM, 8.6% in offspring of women with GDM, and 1.4% in offspring of nondiabetic pregnant women.

Fetal hyperinsulinemia increases lipogenesis and adipose tissue development, which augments the lifetime risk of obesity.[25] Mughal et al.[95] found that offspring of mothers with type 1 diabetes have higher body mass index, body fat, linear length, and bone dimensions than do offspring of nondiabetic mothers. Sobngwi et al.[96] demonstrated that IDMs have an increased risk of impaired glucose tolerance and defective insulin secretory response irrespective of family history of type 2 DM.

There are several reports of poor neurodevelopmental outcomes in IDMs; however, the evidence is limited and of poor quality.[97] A systematic review by Adane et al.[98] reported that diabetes during pregnancy is related to poor cognitive development in the offspring. Bytoft et al.[99] showed poorer cognitive outcomes in adolescent offspring of women with type 1 diabetes compared with age-matched controls. Neurodevelopmental impairment in IDMs could be attributed to prematurity, neonatal hypoglycemia, hypoxia-ischemia episodes, and poor diabetes control during pregnancy.[100]

Conclusion

Optimal management of IDMs requires a coordinated and multidisciplinary approach from obstetric, perinatal, and neonatal healthcare teams to reduce the risk of perinatal asphyxia, stillbirths, congenital anomalies, and early neonatal complications. A careful and vigilant approach to managing adverse neonatal outcomes such as hypoglycemia could reduce the risk for long-term neurodevelopmental or cognitive impairment.

CHAPTER 25

Evidence-Based Neonatology: Neonatal Pituitary Hormone Deficiencies

Lauryn Choleva, Mabel Yau, Christopher J. Romero

KEY POINTS

1. Congenital pituitary hormone deficiencies can be caused by maldevelopment of central brain structures, acute injury, and pituitary gene mutation.
2. The anterior pituitary is composed of four distinct cell types that produce five different hormones.
3. Understanding the role of each of these hormones allows more timely diagnosis of pituitary hormone deficiencies.
4. Treatment is typically replacement of missing hormones and can be safely accomplished, allowing children to grow and develop properly.

Introduction

The diagnosis of pituitary hormone deficiency or congenital hypopituitarism in the neonate can often be a challenge to the provider. Patients may present either extremely ill in an intensive care setting or apparently healthy in the newborn nursery or pediatric office without apparent signs or symptoms suggesting deficiency. The provider, therefore, requires adequate knowledge of the multiple roles of the pituitary, symptoms of pituitary hormone deficiency, and/or select phenotypes that may suggest a risk for pituitary abnormalities.

The development of the pituitary gland is a complex process that is achieved through an orchestrated expression of transcription factors and signaling molecules. The pituitary gland is composed of an anterior lobe (adenohypophysis) and a posterior lobe (neurohypophysis) (Fig. 25.1). The adenohypophysis contains five distinct cell types that produce six different hormones. These include somatotrophs, which produce growth hormone (GH); thyrotrophs, which produce thyroid stimulating hormone (TSH); lactotrophs, which produce prolactin; corticotrophs, which produce adrenocorticotrophic hormone (ACTH); and gonadotrophs, which produce both luteinizing hormone (LH) and follicle-stimulating hormone (FSH). The neurohypophysis does not contain hormone-producing cells but instead is a reservoir for both antidiuretic hormone and oxytocin. These hormones are produced in cells in the paraventricular and supraoptic nuclei of the hypothalamus; they are then transported to the posterior pituitary within the axons of these cells, which form the posterior pituitary.

The true incidence of congenital hypopituitarism is not entirely clear, but reports have cited estimates of 1 in 3500 to 1 in 10,000 or even less in patients diagnosed with a single or multiple hormone deficiencies.[1,2] Congenital hypopituitarism may occur as an isolated disorder, although in some cases, pituitary disease can occur as part of a syndrome. In addition, breech delivery or perinatal insult may be associated with idiopathic hypopituitarism.[3,4] Once one or more deficiencies are established, hormone replacement is typically successful in bringing levels to normal and providing a means for continuation of normal growth and development.

This chapter will focus on reviewing the presenting signs and symptoms of pituitary hormone deficiency, diagnostic tools used to assess deficiencies, and the treatment required. Given the complexity of pituitary disease and the fact that single or multiple hormone deficiencies can occur, we will present each hormone deficiency individually for clarity. The provider must understand, however, that an evaluation of the pituitary should involve diagnostic measures to assess the function of as many of the cell types as possible simultaneously in order to guide the provider with appropriate treatments. This also helps with counseling the parents. By helping the provider to better understand each deficiency, early recognition and an appropriate diagnosis will expedite treatment that can ultimately prevent comorbidities and mortality associated with congenital hypopituitarism.

Genetics of Pituitary Disease

Congenital pituitary disease, whether it originates from a structural abnormality, an isolated hormone deficiency, or both, often has a genetic basis. Alternatively, perinatal stress such as ischemia could presumably injure the pituitary or impact its development without an underlying genetic abnormality. Despite advances in genetic screening, however, identifying a precise etiology of pituitary disease remains a challenge. The identification of specific genetic mutations leading to hypopituitarism continues to be a rare occurrence, with reports citing less than 5% of cases.[5] Nevertheless, our understanding of pituitary development has expanded tremendously over the past several decades. We now recognize that pituitary development is a complex, temporally regulated cascade of events orchestrated through the expression of various transcription factors and signaling molecules.[6–9]

Given the complexity of pituitary development and the numerous genes associated with pituitary hormone deficiency, this chapter will not discuss the topic in detail. The clinician should be aware, however, that improvement in genetic technology has enabled easier access and affordable options for studies such as whole exome sequencing.[10,11] Some research centers have also developed panels to screen for various genetic mutations involved in pituitary development and function. Currently, however, there are limited resources for pituitary genetic screening to be done commercially.

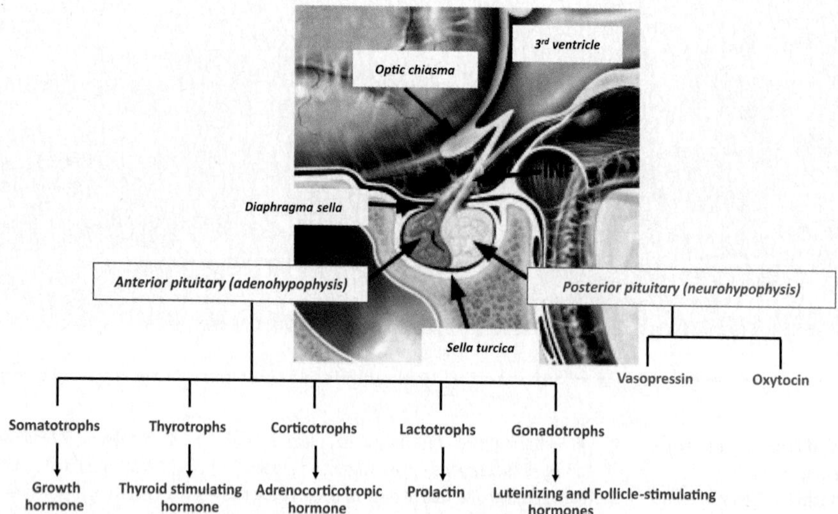

Fig. 25.1 The Pituitary Gland and Its Cell Types. The pituitary gland is composed of two main lobes, an anterior (adenohypophysis) and a posterior (neurohypophysis). The anterior lobe houses five cell types that produce six different hormones, and these hormones activate downstream glands. The posterior lobe stores two hormones, vasopressin and oxytocin, that are produced and transported from the paraventricular and supraoptic nuclei of the hypothalamus. Genetic mutations, maldevelopment, or injury can lead to dysfunction of one or several of these cell types, leading to congenital hypopituitarism. (The figure was drawn using an image, after permission, of the pituitary and surrounding structures from Chapman et al. Neuroimaging of the pituitary gland. In: *Radiologic Clinics of North America*. 2020;58:1115–1133.)

Syndromes Associated With Pituitary Deficiency

Various syndromes have been associated with a risk for pituitary hormone deficiency. In addition, given the location of the pituitary gland, an infant noted to have midline defects such as cleft lip, cleft palate, and holoprosencephaly should be considered for evaluation for pituitary hormone deficiencies.[12] Abnormal pituitary magnetic resonance imaging (MRI) findings, such as seen in pituitary stalk interruption syndrome, should alert the provider to screen for pituitary dysfunction.[13] In cases of isolated GH deficiency (GHD), some have commented on the utility of pituitary MRI findings.[14]

One particular phenotype the clinician should recognize is septo-optic dysplasia. A diagnosis is made by identifying two of the following: pituitary hypoplasia/hormone deficiency, midline forebrain defects (e.g., absence of the septum pellucidum), and optic nerve hypoplasia. A clinical clue to optic nerve hypoplasia is an infant who presents with nystagmus along with symptoms suggesting pituitary hormone deficiency. This condition may also present with other neurologic manifestations such as schizencephaly, which may be a risk for the development of seizures. Although mutations in several transcription factors known to be important in pituitary development have been implicated as the etiology, such as *HESX1*, the identification of a genetic mutation is rare.[15,16] Table 25.1 summarizes several possible clinical syndromes or phenotypes that may be diagnosed in the newborn period and have been associated with pituitary disease. Although a genetic etiology is not always identified nor is pituitary dysfunction diagnosed, the clinician should have high suspicion for possible pituitary hormone deficiency in these patients.

Growth Hormone Deficiency

GH is a polypeptide produced by somatotrophs in the anterior pituitary. Its mode of action is both anabolic and mitogenic with a primary role in growth during childhood. These actions are mediated through insulin-like growth factors (IGFs), of which peripheral and hepatic IGF-1 is the most important in growth. GH is secreted in a pulsatile pattern under the control of two hypothalamic antagonistic hormones, growth hormone–releasing hormone and somatotropin release-inhibiting factor (also known as somatostatin).

In contrast to later in life, neonates demonstrate a nonpulsatile secretion pattern of GH such that serum levels are often detectable. It may be several months before an infant develops the pulsatile pattern of GH secretion characteristic of later life. This physiologic pattern provides some convenience when attempting to test the GH axis in neonates.

Infants with GHD do not typically present with below-average length at birth, although some have argued that in those with severe GHD there may be abnormal growth as an infant.[17] In part, this is because maternal factors play a more vital role in gestational growth. In addition, the GH receptor is poorly expressed in the infant, explaining why infants with GHD may not be easily detected at birth. These receptors may take up to 6 months to become functional and typically it may be several years until growth deceleration is detected. Therefore size and growth may not be a sign suggesting GHD in neonates and infants. However, GH also has a metabolic role as a counterregulatory hormone for glycemic control. Hypoglycemia is a common symptom in infants with GHD. This is in contrast with older children and adults, where isolated GHD rarely causes hypoglycemia. Hypoglycemia is also a symptom of cortisol deficiency; therefore hypoglycemia in the neonate should prompt a suspicion for pituitary hormone deficiency. This presentation leads to the request of a critical sample that can often be helpful in documenting pituitary dysfunction (Fig. 25.2).

In both the intensive care unit and newborn nursery, the definition of hypoglycemia varies depending on the day of life and can sometimes be controversial. The Pediatric Endocrine Society recently published data helping to better define expectations of glycemic control in term infants given the known risks for complications of neurodevelopment among infants with chronic hypoglycemia.[18,19] Strict definitions of hypoglycemia become challenging when prematurity and illness complicate the medical picture. These

Table 25.1 Syndromes/Clinical Phenotypes Associated With Congenital Hypopituitarism[a]

Diagnosis	Gene(s) Defect	Clinical Description
Axenfeld-Rieger syndrome	*PTX2*	Ocular anterior compartment abnormalities, craniofacial abnormalities, cardiac defects, variable anterior pituitary hormone deficiencies
Central hypothyroidism/macroorchidism	*IGSF-1*	X-linked syndrome of central hypothyroidism delayed puberty despite testicular enlargement, GH, and PRL deficiencies
CHARGE syndrome	*CHD7*	Eye coloboma, heart defects, choanal atresia, retardation of growth, hypogonadism, ear abnormalities, may also be MPHD
DAVID (deficient anterior pituitary with variable immune deficiency)	*NFKB2*	Anterior pituitary hormone deficiency and common variable immunodeficiency—hypogammaglobulinemia, ACTH deficiency is less common
Eye development abnormalities (microphthalmia, anophthalmia, optic nerve maldevelopment)	*PAX6, OTX2, RAX*	Abnormalities in eye or optic nerve development associated with isolated or MPHD, anterior pituitary hypoplasia
Holoprosencephaly	*SHH, GLI2*	Cephalic disorder where forebrain fails to develop two hemispheres, severe midline defects, polydactyly, MPHD
Moebius syndrome	Usually unknown; reported genes: *PLXND1, REV3L, TUBB3*	Neurologic disorder with weakness/paralysis of cranial nerves, pituitary hormone deficiencies (GH, ACTH, LH/FSH), hypoplastic optic disc
Pallister-Hall syndrome	*GLI3*	Hypothalamic hamartoma, polydactyly, bifid epiglottis
Pituitary stalk interruption syndrome	*HESX1, LHX4, OTX2, SOX3, PROKR2*	Pituitary stalk, ectopic posterior pituitary gland, hypoplastic anterior pituitary, IGHD, MPHD
Septo-optic dysplasia	*HESX1, SOX2, SOX3, OTX2, FGFR1*	Complex midline brain defects (absent septum pellucidum/corpus callosum, optic nerve dysplasia, MPHD

[a]Listed are various syndromes or clinical phenotypes that are associated with congenital hypopituitarism. Some of these have gene defects associated with the diagnosis, although quite often a genetic etiology may not be available. Pituitary hormone deficiency(s) may also not be detectable at the time of diagnosis or may develop over time. Therefore the clinician should be vigilant to consider evaluating pituitary function. In addition, future follow-up to ensure appropriate growth and development is recommended given the risk of pituitary disease.

ACTH, Adrenocorticotrophic hormone; *CHARGE*, Coloboma, Heart defects, Atresia choanae, Retardation of mental and somatic development, Growth retardation/Genital abnormalities, and Ear abnormalities; *FSH*, follicle-stimulating hormone; *GH*, growth hormone; *IGHD*, isolated Growth hormone deficiency; *LH*, luteinizing hormone; *MPHD*, multiple pituitary hormone deficiency; *PRL*, prolactin.

recommendations state that blood glucose levels should be >50 mg/dL in the first 48 hours of life and >60 mg/dL afterward.[18] The clinician should be aware that if neonatal hypoglycemia is detected, an evaluation for possible GHD should be considered, along with the other causes of neonatal hypoglycemia. Fig. 25.2 delineates the investigations to diagnose the etiology of hypoglycemia.

Phenotypically, another associated finding with severe GHD in a male infant is micropenis. A stretched penile length that measures more than 2.5 SD below the mean should raise suspicion for either

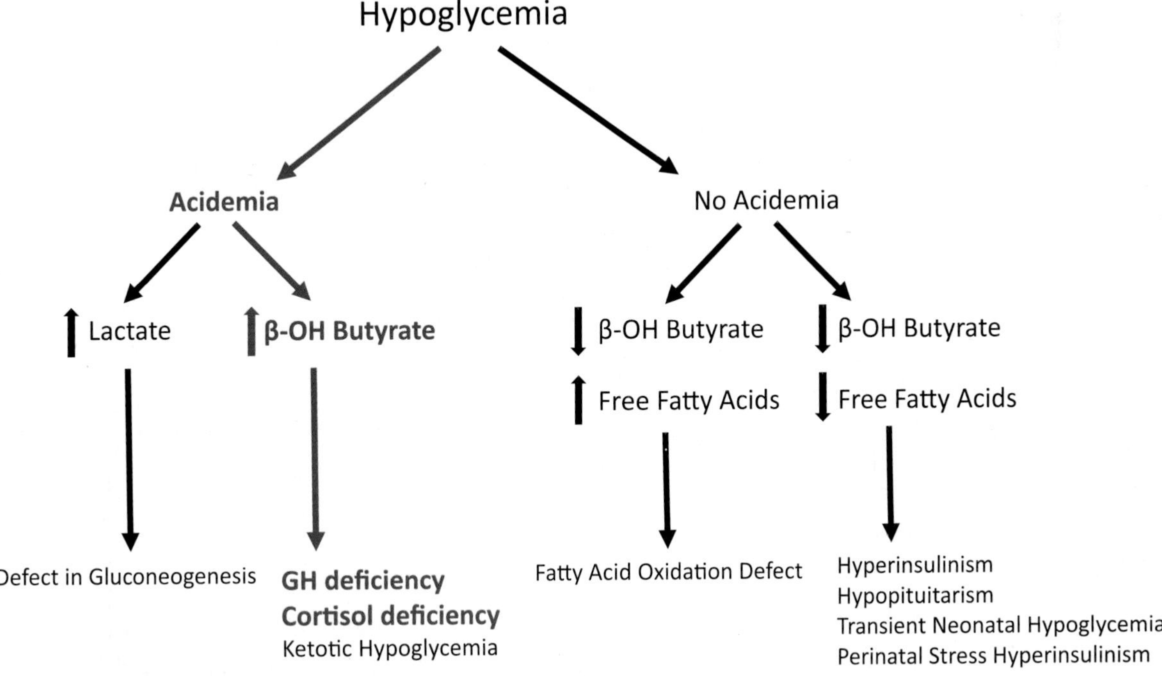

Fig. 25.2 Clinical Suspicion and Evaluation of a Hypoglycemic Infant for Hypopituitarism. At a time of hypoglycemia, serum measurement of the pituitary counter-regulatory hormones, growth hormone and cortisol (boldfaced *red*) can help identify the diagnosis or raise suspicion for pituitary hormone deficiencies. When evaluating the cause of hypoglycemia, the clinician should be mindful that several diagnoses can place a patient at risk for hypoglycemia, as shown in the figure. *GH*, Growth hormone. (Revised from reference 18.)

GHD or gonadotropin deficiency. In addition, prolonged conjugated hyperbilirubinemia has also been noted in infants with GHD.[20–22]

Diagnosis of GHD

An accurate diagnosis of GHD continues to be a clinical challenge in infants. Classically, stimulation tests that utilize provocative agents to recreate a GH pulse are used in an attempt to assess whether a child can appropriately produce GH. These stimulation tests are not standardized and many pose the risk of adverse effects, especially in younger patients. Furthermore, there is low specificity and reproducibility with the currently available pharmacologic agents used during testing (including clonidine, arginine, levodopa, and glucagon). Fig. 25.3 shows a simplified algorithm for such considerations.

In the neonate, however, guidelines suggest a diagnosis can be made without GH provocative testing. There is increased GH production in the first few days of life and/or at times hypoglycemia, providing an opportunity to more accurately detect levels.[23,24] These levels can range from 20 to 50 ng/mL in the first few weeks of life and then gradually decline. Therefore a measured GH level less than

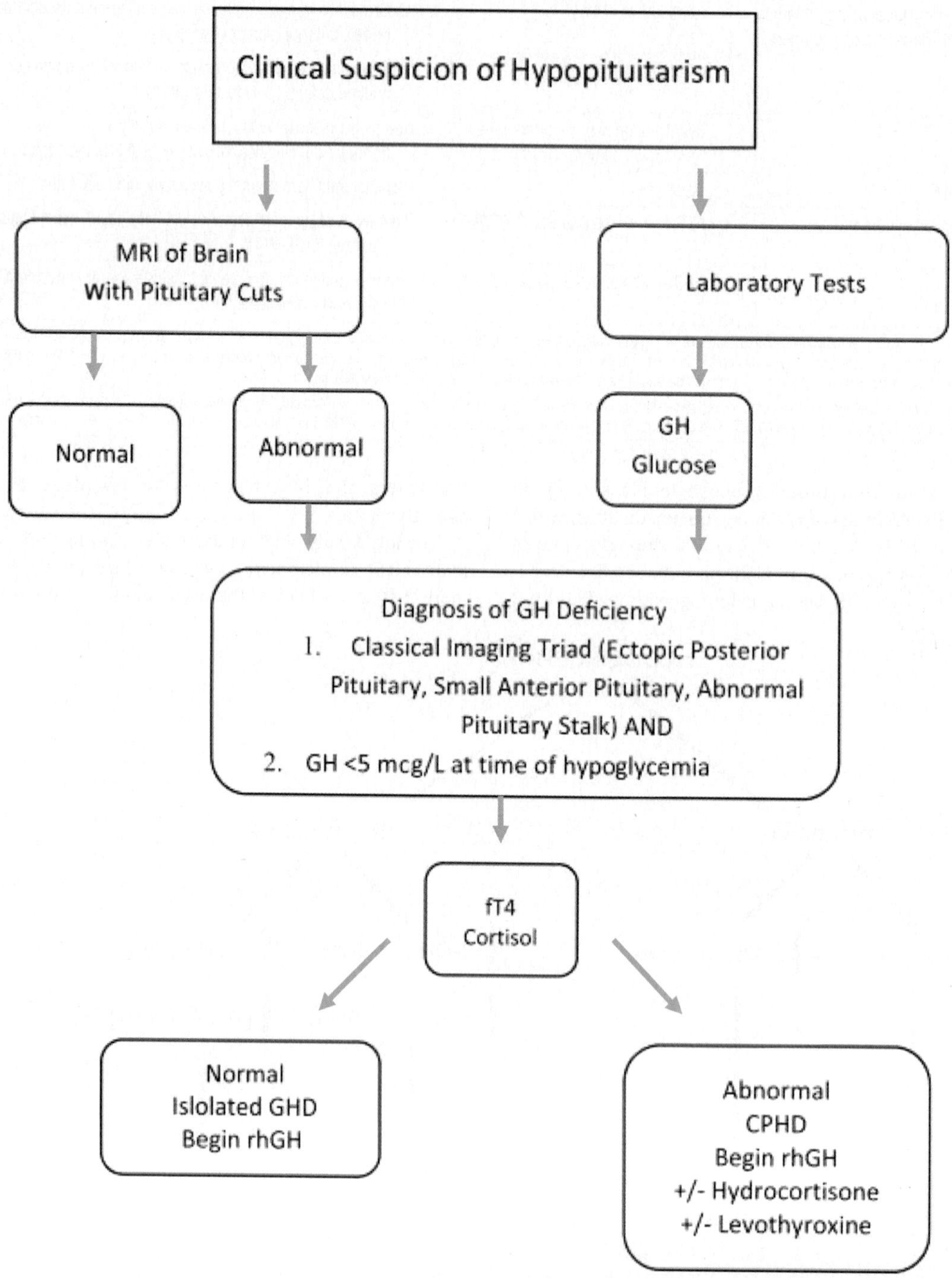

Fig. 25.3 Simplified Algorithm Demonstrating an Evaluation Strategy for Children With Suspected Hypopituitarism. Although not an absolute requisite, anatomic pituitary gland malformations should increase suspicion for possible hormone deficiencies. The provider should also be aware that repeat testing is sometimes necessary if clinical symptoms occur even after initial workup. *CPHD*, Combined pituitary hormone deficiency; *GH*, growth hormone; *GHD*, GH deficiency; *rhGH*, recombinant human growth hormone. (Reproduced, after permissions and modifications, from Parks. Clinical suspicion of hypopituitarism. In: Congenital Hypopituitarism. *Clin Perinatol*. 2018;45:75–91.)

10 ng/mL would be considered diagnostic for GHD. However, by day 15, reports suggest the mean falls to 5.5 ± 3.7 ng/mL.[25] More recently, research efforts are being made to determine whether dried blood spots, similar to newborn screening, can be used to diagnosis deficiency.[26] Results are reported as a possible alternative option for testing GH levels but have not yet been validated.

Diagnostic imaging with MRI of the pituitary can sometimes assist to confirm the risk for pituitary hormone dysfunction if an anatomic abnormality is identified (Fig. 25.4). This can include abnormalities such as anterior pituitary hypoplasia, ectopic posterior pituitary, interrupted pituitary stalk, or absence of the corpus callosum. The ability to accurately image a neonate or infant, however, may be limited and require the risk of sedation. Therefore the authors do not feel imaging is absolutely necessary at first for diagnosis. These patients may also have been diagnosed with another pituitary hormone deficiency, therefore already signifying a risk for other hormone deficiencies.

Treatment

Replacement with recombinant growth hormone therapy is the standard of treatment for infants diagnosed with deficiency. Guidelines for growth hormone treatment established by the Pediatric Endocrine Society state that an initial GH dose should be 0.16 to 0.24 mg/kg/week or 22 to 35 mcg/kg/day.[27] Some manufacturers have recommended higher doses up to 0.3 mg/kg/week in prepubertal children, but the provider should recognize that a decision to treat an infant with recombinant growth hormone is in part dictated by preventing ongoing hypoglycemia and not just to promote normal growth; the higher doses are generally not required to alleviate hypoglycemia.

Central Hypothyroidism

Clinical Presentation

The classical signs of central hypothyroidism are typically absent in the neonate and diagnosis is usually made biochemically. The measurement of low free T4 concentrations with a low or inappropriately normal TSH concentration are diagnostic of central hypothyroidism.[28] Prolonged untreated congenital hypothyroidism, however, can also lead to a high prevalence of complications including hypoglycemia, jaundice, seizures, feeding difficulties, and temperature instability.[26,29,30] Even without signs suggesting hypothyroidism, if there is clinical suspicion for pituitary dysfunction, thyroid levels should be checked.

The concentrations of triiodothyronine (T3) and thyroxine (T4) are maintained in a stable range by feedback mechanisms mediated by thyrotropin releasing hormone (TRH), which is synthesized in the paraventricular nucleus of the hypothalamus as a prohormone. Central hypothyroidism occurs due to a lack of stimulation of the thyroid gland TSH. The etiology of central hypothyroidism may be caused by a mutation in several genes involved in the development of the pituitary gland, including *POU1F1*, *PROP1*, and *HESX1*. Mutations in these genes have been linked to the development of multiple pituitary hormone deficiencies, including hypothyroidism.[30] In addition, mutations of the TRH receptor, the TSH β-subunit, and the immunoglobulin superfamily factor 1 have all been identified as possible genetic causes of central hypothyroidism.[31]

Diagnosis

Central hypothyroidism is diagnosed in patients who have a low free T4 based on the assay and age-specific reported reference ranges with a low, normal, or slightly elevated TSH (no higher than twice the upper limit of the reference range). Because there is typically no significant elevation in TSH seen in patients with congenital central hypothyroidism, these patients may be missed by newborn screening programs that are designed to detect congenital hypothyroidism by TSH elevation. It is also important to note that these laboratory findings can also be seen in infants who are critically ill. The use of the TRH-stimulation test as an adjunct test for diagnosis of central hypothyroidism is controversial and is not currently available in the United States. The TRH stimulation test involves measuring TSH at baseline and then at 20 and 60 minutes after

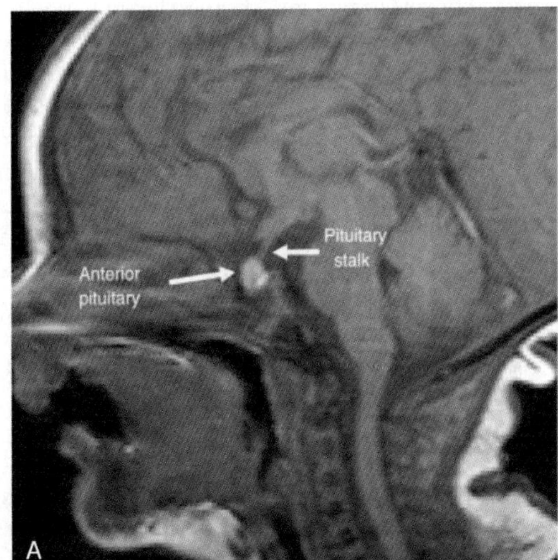

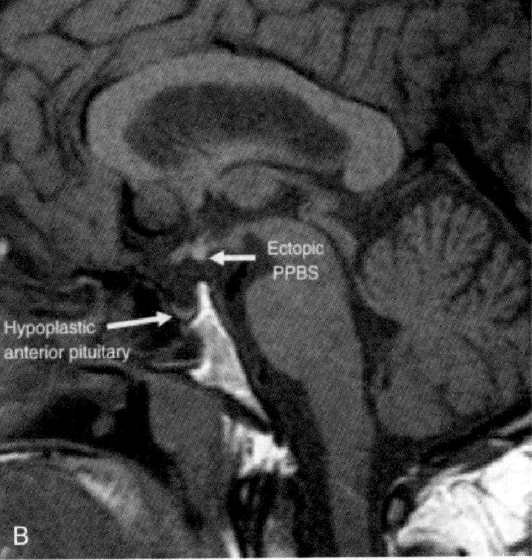

Fig. 25.4 Magnetic Resonance (MR) Imaging. (A) MR scan of an infant brain (1 month old). The anterior pituitary has a relatively bright appearance in early life on T1-weighted images. (B) MR scan of baby with pituitary hormone deficiency. *PPBS*, Posterior pituitary bright spot. (Reproduced after permission and minor modifications from Jane et al. *Rennie and Roberton's Textbook of Neonatology*. 2012:849–926.)

administration of 7 mcg/kg (up to a maximum of 200 mcg) of intravenous (IV) TRH. In patients without pituitary dysfunction, the administration of TRH causes a rise in serum TSH concentration that peaks at 20 minutes and is followed by a decrease in TSH levels at 60 minutes.[32]

Treatment

Treatment of congenital hypothyroidism is by replacement with synthetic levothyroxine. Although T3 is the biologically active hormone, T4 has a longer half-life and is converted in peripheral tissues to T3. Treatment is started with 10 to 12 mcg/kg/day of oral levothyroxine with the goal of a free T4 in the upper half of the reference range for age.[29] Measurement of free T4 is used to assess the adequacy of replacement therapy and should be monitored every 2 to 4 weeks initially. Serum TSH levels are not useful for monitoring adequacy of therapy in patients with central hypothyroidism and are typically suppressed in patients on treatment. It is important that cortisol deficiency be assessed prior to the initiation of thyroid hormone replacement. Rapid correction of thyroid hormone deficiency has been linked to the development of an adrenal crisis via acceleration of cortisol metabolism in patients with cortisol deficiency. In neonates and infants, cortisol levels can typically be checked any time of day or, more appropriately, during a stressful event to assess the cortisol axis (see section on adrenal insufficiency for more details). It is recommended that oral treatment with levothyroxine be given on an empty stomach. The ingestion of products containing soy, calcium, and/or iron can impair the bioavailability of levothyroxine and should not be administered concurrently. Compounded solutions of levothyroxine are not recommended because they do not provide reliable dosing.[33] In patients who require parenteral dosing, it is recommended to give 50% of the oral dose intravenously once daily, with careful monitoring of serum free T4 levels. Thyroid hormone plays an integral role in normal growth and development. Even mild abnormalities in thyroid function may disrupt normal neurocognitive development.[34] Rapid initiation of treatment, within the first 2 weeks of life, in patients with hypothyroidism results in normal body composition, motor function, and IQ.[34]

Gonadotropin Deficiency

Puberty is an important developmental process that provides the means for both sexual maturation and accelerated growth later in childhood. It is marked by a reawakening of the hypothalamic-pituitary-gonadal axis through the increased pulsatility of gonadotropin-releasing hormone (GnRH) targeting the gonadotrophs in the pituitary. It is an axis that is initially active during fetal life and is suppressed at the time of birth but then reactivated in the first months of life.[35] Subsequently, the axis becomes quiescent during most of childhood. Therefore making a diagnosis of gonadotropin deficiency is difficult after the neonatal period. The occurrence of congenital hypogonadotropic hypogonadism is rare in isolation but is associated with congenital hypopituitarism. The etiology has been identified as either deficiency of GnRH or gonadotroph function but also GnRH receptor function. Much research has been devoted to identifying genetic causes of hypogonadism leading to any of the mentioned abnormalities.[36,37] The complications of this condition are absent or incomplete puberty and infertility. In addition, given the importance of sex hormones in potentiating growth during puberty, there is risk for a patient to not obtain his/her expected optimum final adult height.

Diagnosis

Infants will typically experience a "minipuberty" postnatally, which represents a reactivation of the axis leading to a rise in gonadotropins. Therefore, in addition to detection of gonadotroph activity within 48 hours of birth (before the axis is suppressed after birth), there is also the opportunity to assess the axis between 4 and 8 weeks after birth.[38,39] This increase in gonadotropins and sex steroid levels occurs in both sexes. It has been suggested that detection during this time is very reliable and possibly more accurate than dynamic tests performed later in childhood.[40] LH levels predominate in boys and then decline, whereas FSH levels in girls remain elevated for several years in childhood. Because Sertoli cells do not express the androgen receptor in infancy, the testes do not mature despite almost pubertal levels of testosterone.

In the male infant, the measurement of serum LH, FSH, and total testosterone during these critical periods can assist in diagnosis. In addition, the measurement of levels of inhibin B, which is a glycoprotein member of the transforming growth factor (TGF) superfamily and secreted by the Sertoli cells, can be utilized as an indicator of Sertoli cell function. It is secreted soon after birth and is found to increase until about 4 to12 months of age. In cases of hypogonadotropic hypogonadism, the plasma concentration of inhibin B remains low.[41,42] Anti-Müllerian hormone (AMH) is another glycoprotein member of the TGFβ family noted to be detectable in cord blood of males but not females. These levels also rise rapidly in the first month of life and then peak by 6 months.[43,44] Therefore, both inhibin B and AMH can be clinically useful in determining Sertoli cell function and assist in the diagnosis of hypogonadism. In girls, one can detect elevated gonadotropin levels, which do result in increased ovarian follicular development and a rise in estradiol levels; this has been studied in preterm and term infants.[45,46] This rise can at times lead to palpable breast tissue during the minipuberty.

The phenotype of congenital hypogonadism is a spectrum, and in cases of severe deficiency, males can present with cryptorchidism and/or micropenis. In some cases of partial GnRH deficiency, however, there may not be abnormal genitalia findings on examination. Phenotypically, GnRH deficiency does not have clear signs. As with concerns of pituitary dysfunction in hypopituitarism, findings of midline defects should raise suspicion. One etiology of isolated hypogonadotropic hypogonadism is Kallmann syndrome, which is a condition of GnRH deficiency. GnRh neurons actually populate outside the central nervous system in the olfactory placode and migrate to the hypothalamus. In Kallmann syndrome this migration does not occur, and clinically, a patient may also be born with anosmia. This finding, of course, cannot be assessed in a newborn. Interestingly, recent literature demonstrates there may be some genetic overlap between patients with isolated hypogonadotropism and other pituitary hormone disease.[47] Such findings further demonstrate the wide phenotypic spectrum of pituitary dysfunction.

Treatment

In most cases, there is no necessity for treatment during infancy. The exception may be with male infants presenting with micropenis and/or cryptorchidism. The use of androgen therapy, such as testosterone, has been utilized to increase penile size; however, it is not clear if this addresses appropriate adult penile size.[48,49] Studies have also looked at the use of recombinant human LH and FSH to stimulate testosterone production and improve penile size.[42,50,51] Despite promising results in these studies, formal randomized trials are needed to affirm the utility and safety in infants. In addition, some have advocated for the use of human chorionic gonadotropin that also leads to increased serum testosterone to facilitate descent of testes in cases of cryptorchidism.[52–54] There is concern that untreated cryptorchidism may contribute to an increased risk of male infertility and testicular malignancy. Surgery (orchidopexy), however, remains the treatment of choice.

By establishing the diagnosis of hypogonadotropic hypogonadism in the infant, the timing of hormone replacement therapy at the age of puberty can be optimized and the uncertainties and delay in making a definitive diagnosis avoided.

Adrenal Insufficiency

Clinical Presentation

Adrenal insufficiency in neonates can present with shock, hypoglycemia, and apnea in the first few days of life or can develop more insidiously over several weeks and present with poor feeding, vomiting, and failure to thrive. Electrolyte abnormalities are not commonly seen with central adrenal insufficiency because the renin-angiotensin-aldosterone axis remains intact.[55] The characteristic hyperpigmentation associated with primary adrenal insufficiency is not seen in patients with central adrenal insufficiency.

Diagnosis

The variability in criteria used to diagnosis adrenal insufficiency has made interpretation of results challenging. The greatest controversy has been defining the threshold cortisol concentration for the adrenal stress response to be deemed acceptable and below which a patient should be considered to have adrenal insufficiency and be treated.

Although an early morning cortisol represents the peak in humans, the cortisol diurnal variation is yet to be established in neonates so that a random level can be obtained.

The standard ACTH stimulation test is performed using IV or intramuscular (IM) synthetic ACTH (cosyntropin) at a dose of 15 mcg/kg in infants, 125 mcg/dose in younger children (<2 years of age), or 250 mcg/dose in older children (>2 years of age) with measurements of cortisol levels at baseline, at 30 minutes and at 60 minutes following the administration of ACTH. Historically, a cortisol level of less than 5 mcg/dL during a period of stress and the failure of cortisol to rise to more than 18 mcg/dL 30 minutes after IV cosyntropin is consistent with adrenal insufficiency and should be treated appropriately with replacement hydrocortisone.[56] A study in London reported a low sensitivity (60%) of the stimulated cortisol level.[57] Current assays, however, that utilize highly specific liquid chromatography/mass spectroscopy and newer immunoassays suggest the threshold for stimulated cortisol levels to diagnose adrenal insufficiency may be lower. These studies report that cutoffs for normal stimulated cortisol levels using such assays are approximately 12.7 mcg/dL to 17.5 mcg/dL with a sensitivity and specificity above 90%.[58,59] Clinical presentation and repeat measurements of physiologic cortisol secretion may be required to confirm the diagnosis. Like GHD, the diagnosis of adrenal insufficiency can be made without stimulation testing in the setting of hypoglycemia.[55]

As with most endocrine/metabolic disorders, obtaining a blood sample prior to the initiation of treatment is critical, because interpretation of laboratory data after the onset of treatment can be misleading and may delay diagnosis.

Treatment

Patients with adrenal insufficiency should be treated with daily maintenance hydrocortisone (5–10 mg/m^2/day). Hydrocortisone is the drug of choice because it represents the major glucocorticoid secreted physiologically by the adrenal glands. The goal of maintenance therapy in children is to treat the adrenal insufficiency while ensuring normal growth velocity and minimizing the side effects associated with long-term glucocorticoid treatment.[56]

In non–life-threatening periods of illness or physiologic stress, the corticosteroid dose should be increased to 30 to 50 mg/m^2/day for the duration of that period, divided into 3 to 4 daily doses. Each family should be given injection kits of hydrocortisone, that is, Solu-Cortef, for emergency use, and all family members should be trained in its intramuscular administration. The injectable dose of hydrocortisone in an emergency is 50 mg/m^2 and approximately 25 mg for infants. In the event of a surgical procedure, 30 to 50 mg/m^2/dose of hydrocortisone is needed, with 25 to 100 mg hydrocortisone IM/IV administered to infants before and during a surgical procedure, followed by high doses of hydrocortisone during the first 24 to 48 postoperative hours. The dose can then be tapered over the following days to resume the patient's normal preoperative schedule.

Posterior Pituitary Hormone Deficiencies

Anterior pituitary hormones are more common than posterior hormone deficiencies. However, deficiency of the posterior pituitary antidiuretic hormone can pose a great risk to an infant's health. We review below deficiencies of antidiuretic hormone (also known as vasopressin).

Diabetes Insipidus

Presentation and Diagnosis

Central diabetes insipidus (DI) is caused by a deficiency in antidiuretic hormone secretion by the posterior pituitary gland, resulting in increased urine production and intravascular volume depletion. Patients with DI usually present with classic symptoms of polyuria and polydipsia. These symptoms can be associated with nausea, vomiting, and weight loss due to dehydration. Urine output usually exceeds 2 L/m^2/day (150 mg/kg/day in neonates). Hypernatremia (serum sodium >145 mEq/L) in the setting of a net negative fluid balance or low urine specific gravity is suggestive of DI. A serum osmolality greater than 300 mOsm/L, with urine osmolality less than 300 mOsm/L, establishes a diagnosis of DI.[60]

A water deprivation test may be performed under close medical supervision to confirm the diagnosis but poses some challenges in neonates and infants. The test challenges the body's ability to conserve water and concentrate urine. It is often a long test to administer (it may exceed 20 hours in older children), which is not feasible in a neonate. If at any time during the test the serum osmolality exceeds 300 mOsm/L while the urine osmolality is less than 600 mOsm/L, DI is confirmed.[60]

Treatment

In older children and adults with an intact thirst mechanism, fluid balance can often be maintained with free access to water and

1-deamino-8-D-arginine vasopressin (DDAVP) administered via several routes. This includes IV, intranasal, or an enteral route in subacute conditions.

Treatment of DI in neonates poses a challenge, because patients are dependent on caregivers and fluid intake includes breast milk and/or formula for nutrition. DDAVP has been used in the treatment of neonates with DI, but an increased risk of water intoxication and hyponatremia has been reported. These patients are at risk of severe hyponatremia if they receive both excessive amounts of fluids and DDAVP treatment. Furthermore, patients with DI and persistent adipsia were reported to have increased frequency of hyper- and hyponatremia compared with patients with an intact thirst mechanism.[61] There is debate on the best administration modality of DDAVP to allow for fine titration of dosing. Subcutaneous administration of diluted DDAVP, oral ingestion of the intranasal formulation of DDAVP, and oral administration of desmopressin lyophilisate have all been proposed. In some mild cases in neonates, however, sufficient fluid intake can balance increased urine output.[60,62] Daily monitoring of fluid input and output in addition to weight should be performed to monitor for fluid overload and prevent hyponatremia. Diabetes insipidus can also be treated with increased free water intake along with diuretics such as thiazides and amiloride.[60] Given the complexity of DI treatment, close follow-up with pediatric endocrinology and accurate monitoring of fluid intake and output by caregivers can ensure favorable outcomes.

Conclusion

The pituitary gland is a complex gland that is responsible for the production of multiple hormones essential for proper growth, development, and physiologic homeostasis. Although a deficiency in one or more of these hormones has long-term negative effects, the newborn can also present with acute biochemical abnormalities. Understanding how pituitary dysfunction can present and what may pose an infant to be at risk for deficiency can avoid any delay in diagnosis.

As genetic causes for pituitary hormone deficiency become better defined, genetic screenings will provide easy and efficient means to identify babies born at risk for pituitary dysfunction. This could potentially avoid the need for risky testing such as the critical sample during provoked hypoglycemia and provide replacement hormones in a timelier manner. In all at-risk cases, providers should consult with a pediatric endocrinologist, especially because patients diagnosed with pituitary dysfunction will require long-term care. This includes appropriate education, counseling, and treatment to ensure normal growth and development.

Section 5

Neonatal Thyroid Disease

CHAPTER 26

Andrew J. Bauer

KEY POINTS

1. Thyroid hormone signaling is required for both normal fetal and pediatric development.
2. The identification of genes critical for thyroid gland development and migration and thyroid hormone metabolism, transport, and receptor function has revealed that derangement of local thyroid hormone signaling can impact development, even in the absence of primary thyroid disease.
3. The goal of thyroid hormone replacement in neonates is to optimize normal growth and development.
4. For many neonates, levothyroxine (LT4) replacement is anticipated to be lifelong; however, there is potential to discontinue LT4 in patients with transient congenital hypothyroidism.
5. In neonates with hyperthyroidism, there is a risk of acute morbidity and mortality as well as some evidence to suggest the potential for long-term adverse neurocognitive outcomes.
6. Further clinical research is needed to better understand the long-term consequences of fetal and neonatal hypothyroxinemia, as well as thyrotoxicosis, to better understand the potential benefits and risks of treatment.

Introduction

The incidence of congenital hypothyroidism (CH) is reported to be between 1 in 2000 and 1 in 4000 births, with the higher incidence associated with lowering of the thyroid-stimulating hormone (TSH) diagnostic level for diagnosis.[1] The most common inheritable cause of primary CH is failure of normal thyroid gland development (dysgenesis) or failure of a eutopic thyroid gland (a gland located in its usual position, anterior to the second to fourth tracheal rings) to produce thyroid hormone normally (dyshormonogenesis). Thyroid dysgenesis accounts for approximately 85% of permanent CH, and thyroid ectopy is the most common cause of dysgenesis, with the ectopic thyroid tissue located anywhere along the path of migration, from the foramen cecum in the base of the tongue to the thyroid bed.[2] The identified transcription factors critical for thyroid gland formation include *NKX2-1*, *FOXE1*, and *PAX8*; for thyroid folliculogenesis, *NKX2-1* and *PAX8*; and for migration, *FOXE1* and *CDCA8*/Borealin.[3,4] Several of these transcription factors are also involved in nonthyroid related organogenesis. As an example, expression of *NKX2-1* is critical in the development and function of interneurons in the central nervous system, surfactant producing cells in the lungs, and expression of thyroid peroxidase and thyroglobulin. Mutations in *NKX2-1* are associated with brain-lung-thyroid syndrome, characterized by hereditary chorea, respiratory distress syndrome, and congenital hypothyroidism secondary to thyroid dysgenesis.[2] Tables 26.1 and 26.2 review the genetic alterations and phenotypes for thyroid gland dysgenesis (Table 26.1a) and dyshormonogenesis (Table 26.1b).

Congenital central hypothyroidism is rare, with an incidence between 1 in 16,000 and 1 in 20,000.[5] Because transcription factors regulate expression of multiple pituitary cell types, multiple pituitary hormone deficiencies are present in about 75% of infants with congenital central hypothyroidism (Table 26.1c).[6]

Lastly, several extrinsic factors can cause hypothyroidism in neonates. Iodine deficiency remains the most common cause of neonatal hypothyroidism worldwide. Preterm infants are at increased risk of iodine-related thyroid dysfunction; iodine deficiency–associated hypothyroidism can occur due to low iodine content of preterm infant formulas and parenteral nutrition.[7] Iodine excess can also cause hypothyroidism secondary to iodine-induced decreased synthesis of thyroid peroxidase, leading to decreased organification of iodine and production of thyroid hormone (called the Wolff-Chaikoff effect).[8] The most common sources of excess iodine are exposure to topical iodine-based antiseptics,[9] exposure to high content iodine medications such as amiodarone,[10] radiographic contrast agents,[11,12] or high maternal dietary intake of iodine that is passed through breast milk.[13] Other extrinsic causes include transplacental passage of antithyroid medications used to treat hyperthyroidism (methimazole, carbimazole, or propylthiouracil), transfer of maternal immunoglobulin G antibodies that block activation of the TSH receptor,[14] and many additional medications that can alter thyroid hormone levels (see Table 26.2).[15,16]

Neonatal thyrotoxicosis (hyperthyroidism) is less common than congenital hypothyroidism; however, it can lead to significant morbidity and mortality if not promptly recognized and adequately treated. The majority of cases are transient, secondary to transplacental passage of maternal thyroid-stimulating immunoglobulin (maternal Graves disease, [GD]); however, neonatal hyperthyroidism can also occur secondary to activating mutations in the TSH receptor or activating mutations in the alpha subunit of stimulatory G proteins *(GNAS)* in McCune-Albright syndrome.[17]

Pathophysiology

Hypothyroidism

Normal embryonic development requires the coordinated action of thyroid hormones. In mammals, these iodothyronine hormones (T3 and T4) are derived from both maternal and fetal sources and regulate the proliferation, differentiation, and apoptosis of developing tissues in a temporally and anatomically precise manner. During most of gestation, extracellular concentrations of active thyroid hormones in the fetus are low (compared with maternal serum) and the local action of thyroid hormones is regulated by the dynamic expression of cellular thyroid hormone transporters, metabolizing enzymes, and nuclear receptors.

During the first trimester, maternal T4 production increases by approximately 20% under stimulation of placental human chorionic

Table 26.1a Genes and Phenotype Associated With Thyroid Dysgenesis

Gene (OMIM)	Name	Thyroid Phenotype	Additional Features
NKX2-1 (600635)	NK2 homeobox 1 or thyroid transcription factor 1	Thyroid hypoplasia, hemiagenesis, or athyreosis	Brain-lung-thyroid syndrome; benign hereditary chorea, infant respiratory distress syndrome (surfactant deficiency)
PAX8 (167415)	Paired box 8	Thyroid hypoplasia, ectopy, or athyreosis	Urogenital tract abnormalities
FOXE1 (602617)	Forkhead box protein E1 or thyroid transcription factor 2	Thyroid hypoplasia or athyreosis	Bamforth-Lazarus syndrome; cleft palate, choanal atresia, bifid epiglottis, and spiky hair
TSHR (603372)	Thyroid stimulating hormone receptor	Thyroid hypoplasia	None
HHEX (604420)	Hematopoietically expressed homeobox	Thyroid hypoplasia and ectopy	None

OMIM, Online Mendelian Inheritance in Man.

Table 26.1b Genes and Phenotype Associated With Thyroid Dyshormonogenesis

Gene (OMIM)	Name	Mode of Inheritance	Phenotype
TSHR (603372)	Thyroid stimulating hormone receptor	AD	TSH resistance with elevated TSH and T4 in the normal range
SLC5A5 (601843)	NIS: sodium-iodide symporter	AR	Absent or low iodide uptake on scintigraphy with elevated serum Tg; variable hypothyroidism and goiter
SLC26A4 (605646)	Pendrin: anion transporter	AR	High level of uptake on scintigraphy with positive perchlorate discharge test and elevated serum Tg; sensorineural hearing loss with enlarged vestibular aqueduct hypothyroidism and goiter
DUOX1/DUOX2 (606758/606759)	Dual oxidase 1 and 2	AR or AD	High level of uptake on scintigraphy with positive perchlorate discharge test and elevated serum Tg; transient or permanent hypothyroidism and goiter
DUOXA2 (612772)	Dual oxidase associated protein	AR	High level of uptake on scintigraphy with positive perchlorate discharge test and elevated serum Tg; transient or permanent hypothyroidism and goiter
TPO (606765)	Thyroid peroxidase	AR	High level of uptake on scintigraphy with positive perchlorate discharge test and elevated serum Tg; severe hypothyroidism and goiter
Tg (188450)	Thyroglobulin	AR	Positive uptake on thyroid scintigraphy and low to undetectable serum Tg; variable hypothyroidism and goiter
IYD/DEHAL1 (612025)	Iodotyrosine dehalogenase	AR	Positive uptake on thyroid scintigraphy and elevated serum Tg; variable hypothyroidism and goiter
GNAS (139320)	Alpha subunit of the stimulatory guanine nucleotide-binding G-protein	Imprinted gene	Hypothyroidism with partial TSH resistance

AD, Autosomal dominant; *AR,* autosomal recessive; *NIH,* Na-I-Symporter; *OMIM,* Online Mendelian Inheritance in Man; *Tg,* thyroglobulin; *TSH,* thyroid stimulating hormone.

Table 26.1c Genes and Phenotype Associated With Central Hypothyroidism and Defects in Thyroid Hormone Metabolism

Level of Defect	Gene(s) Involved (Primary Mode[s] of Inheritance)	Phenotype
CONGENITAL CENTRAL HYPOTHYROIDISM		
Isolated central hypothyroidism[a]	*TRHR* (AR); *TSHB* (AR) *IGSF1* (X-linked)	Central hypothyroidism (low T4, normal or low TSH)
THYROID HORMONE CELL MEMBRANE TRANSPORT DEFECT		
Allan-Herndon-Dudley syndrome	*SLC16A2* (X-linked)	Abnormal serum thyroid tests (high T3, low T4, low rT3, normal or high TSH); low body mass index, central hypotonia, spastic quadriplegia, mental retardation, speech delay
THYROID HORMONE METABOLISM DEFECT		
SBP2 defect	*SECISBP2* (AR)	Abnormal serum thyroid tests (high T4 and rT3, low T3, normal or high TSH); growth retardation, delayed bone maturation, developmental delay
THYROID HORMONE ACTION DEFECT		
RTHα	*THRA* (AD)	Abnormal serum thyroid tests (low T4 to T3 ratio); impaired cognition, short lower limbs, delayed bone/dental development, macrocephaly, constipation
RTHβ	*THRB* (AD)	Abnormal serum thyroid tests (high T4, nonsuppressed TSH); goiter, attention deficit hyperactivity disorder, tachycardia

[a]Central hypothyroidism may also develop as a component of combined pituitary deficiency from *HESX1, LHX3, LHX4, SOX3, PROP-1,* or *POU1FI* mutations.

AD, Autosomal dominant; *AR,* autosomal recessive; *rT3,* reverse T3; *TSH,* thyroid stimulating hormone.

Table 26.2 Drugs That Alter Thyroid Hormone Levels

Level of Alteration	Medications
Decreased TSH secretion	Glucocorticoids Dopamine Octreotide
Decreased T3 and T4 secretion	Iodide Amiodarone Lithium
Decreased T4 absorption	Aluminum hydroxide Omeprazole (proton pump inhibitors) Ferrous sulfate
Displacement of T3 and T4 from binding proteins	Furosemide Heparin
Increased hepatic metabolism	Phenobarbital Phenytoin Carbamazepine

TSH, Thyroid stimulating hormone.

gonadotropin. Maternal T4 then crosses the placenta to augment fetal organogenesis and development after conversion to T3 by type 2 deiodination within fetal tissues.[18] During the second trimester, concentrations of thyroid hormone in fetal serum rise, and in the early third trimester (25 weeks), the fetal pituitary response to thyroid-releasing hormone (TRH) develops, as well as maturation of the negative feedback control of pituitary TSH from T3 and T4. After delivery the infant begins transitioning to an adult pattern of thyroid hormone metabolism over the ensuing 2 to 4 weeks.[18–20] This transition may be altered by the gestational age at the time of delivery, illness, exogenous medications administered to the mother or infant, abnormal development of the hypothalamic-pituitary-thyroid axis, or disorders of thyroid hormone production and/or metabolism.

Thyroid hormone deficiency has a negative impact on fetal development. In humans, this is most significantly illustrated by the permanent neurocognitive injury associated with combined maternal and fetal thyroid deficiency due to either profound, untreated maternal autoimmune hypothyroidism (Hashimoto thyroiditis) or severe maternal iodine deficiency.[21,22] In other settings, where at least one thyroid axis is intact, thyroid hormones from either maternal or fetal secretion can function as a protective homeostatic mechanism for the fetus. As an example, in complete fetal athyreosis, maternal thyroid hormone alone is sufficient to support normal fetal development as is illustrated by the normal growth and intellectual outcome of athyreotic children who receive adequate levothyroxine treatment from birth.[18,19] The effective transplacental transfer of maternal thyroid hormone in this setting has been directly documented in humans by the demonstration of T4 and T3 in the serum of infants with complete organification defects or athyreosis prior to treatment.[23]

In contrast to the protection afforded by maternal thyroid hormones, fetal compensation for the converse pathophysiology of maternal hypothyroidism appears to be incomplete. In pregnant women who have associated maternal hypothyroxinemia, offspring have decreased intellectual outcome even in the presence of normal fetal thyroid gland development and function.[24,25] The risk is greatest in the first trimester when the fetal thyroid is developing and does not have secretory capacity.[18] This is the rationale for current recommendations to monitor thyroid status frequently upon the diagnosis of pregnancy in women with preexisting hypothyroidism.[21] However, even in the unfortunate occurrence of untreated, overt maternal hypothyroidism discovered late in pregnancy (second or third trimester), aggressive thyroid hormone replacement therapy to achieve a maternal TSH <3 μU/mL may result in infants without significant cognitive delay.[26]

At birth, the neonate rapidly shifts to postnatal thyroid physiology. Thyroid secretion is acutely stimulated, with a rapid peak in TSH (as high as 60–80 μU/mL) approximately 30 to 60 minutes after delivery, followed by elevations in T4 and a decrease in reverse T3 levels (the neonatal surge).[27] The TSH surge is transient, decreasing to around 20 μU/mL at 24 hours, with a continued, gradual decline over the first week.[28] Subsequent to the TSH surge, there is an increase in T4 levels, which peak about 3 days after delivery.[29,30] For the majority of healthy, term infants, the serum concentration of TSH approximates adult levels within 2 weeks.[29] Serum T3 levels increase more slowly than T4 up to approximately 3 months of age, when both T3 and T4 begin to decrease toward adult levels.[20]

The above transition from fetal to neonatal thyroid physiology is altered in prematurely born infants. Neonates born before 28 weeks' gestation often exhibit a blunted TSH and T4 surge, followed by a period of prolonged hypothyroxinemia (total T4) with inappropriately normal or low serum TSH concentrations.[31] A major contributor of the fall in T4 is loss of transplacental maternal T4 and iodine secondary to early parturition. Due to immaturity of the hypothalamic-pituitary-thyroid (HPT) axis, serum TSH does not increase in response to the low T3 and T4 and may remain "inappropriately" low for 2 to 3 months until the HPT axis begins to mature.[32]

This pattern of altered HPT tone is called *transient hypothyroxinemia of prematurity* and the etiology is multifactorial, reflecting persistence of the fetal thyroid hormone metabolic state (low T3 and T4 with elevated reverse T3 [rT3]), reduced maternal transfer of iodine and T4, and a lack of response of the neonatal HPT axis feedback loop to low T3 and T4 levels, which begins to mature at approximately 30 weeks adjusted gestational age. Nonthyroidal illness syndrome, the suppression of thyroid function that occurs in patients of all ages during critical illness, is often confounded by administration of drugs or agents known to suppress TSH release (dopamine, glucocorticoids) and/or production and secretion of T3 and T4, including iodine-containing antiseptics, amiodarone,[33] and iodine-containing radiologic contrast agents.[12] The overlap between the severity of illness and common therapies used in the ICU setting complicates the interpretation of the thyroid axis laboratory values and may prolong the period of HPT axis maturation.[19,34–36] In nonthyroidal illness syndrome, T3 and the reverse T3 (rT3) levels correlate with severity of illness and mortality, respectively, T3 negatively and rT3 positively.[37]

The severity of the transient hypothyroxinemia correlates with increased morbidity and decreased survival.[38–40] Although some studies have shown an association between the severity of this hypothyroxinemia and later intellectual outcome, none have demonstrated a consistent benefit of levothyroxine treatment.[41–44] Consequently, controversy exists regarding the appropriateness of treatment, and more research is needed to address this.

While the HPT axis matures, preterm infants display a delayed elevation in TSH (dTSH).[45] The increase in TSH may be modest (between 5 and 15 μU/mL) or more significant (>25 μU/mL), and it typically occurs between 2 weeks and 6 months of age, with a mean of 30 days.[28] T4 levels are also low and decrease to a nadir 2 to 3 weeks after delivery, with lower levels correlating with the degree of prematurity and birth weight.[40,45,46] Although the majority of infants who develop dTSH have a normal thyroid on imaging and ultimately recover normal thyroid function, up to 25% have

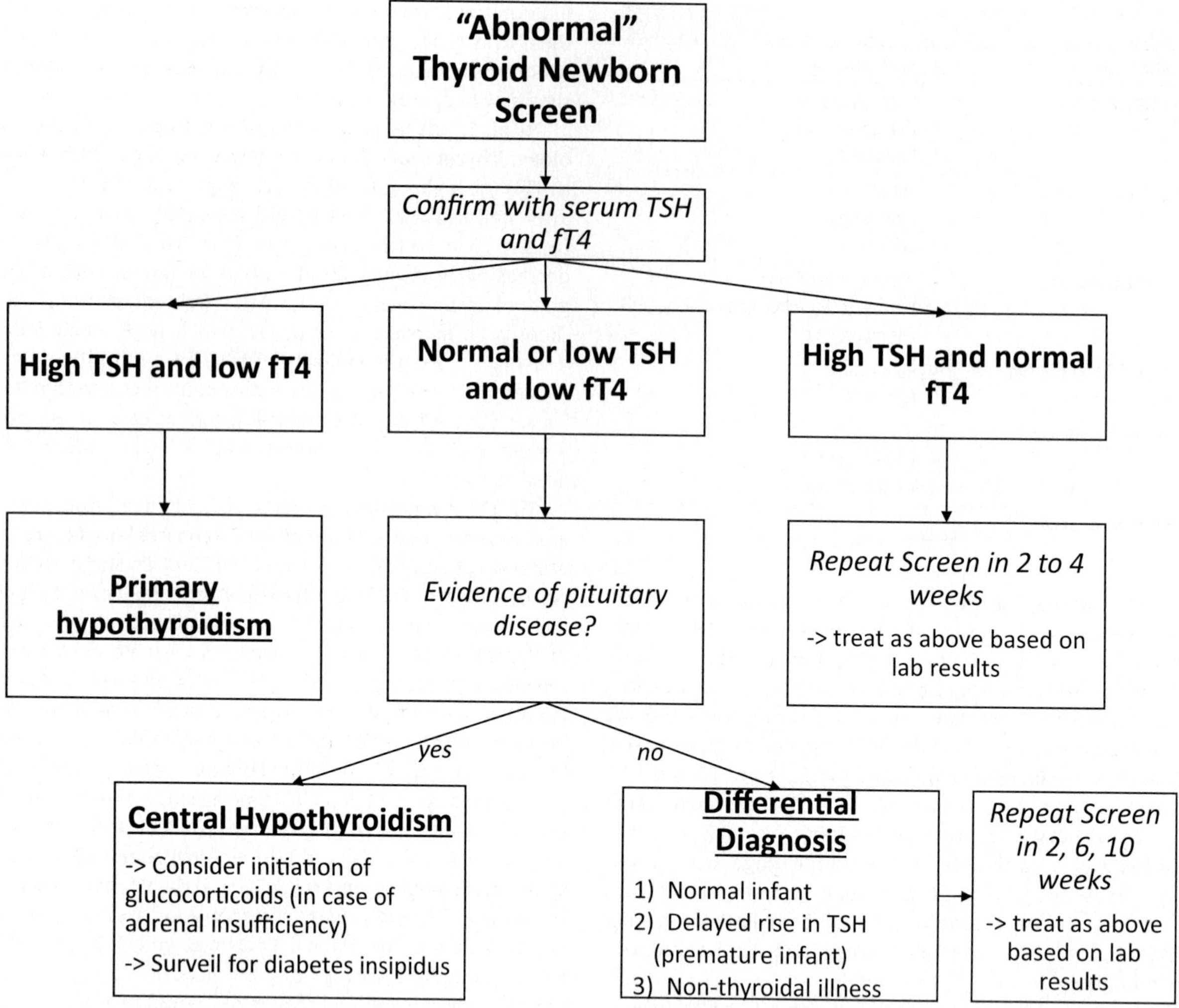

Fig. 26.1 Screening Algorithm for Newborns With Potential Congenital Hypothyroidism. *TSH*, Thyroid-stimulating hormone.

permanent hypothyroidism.[35,47] Fig. 26.1 reviews an algorithm for screening infants with potential congenital hypothyroidism.

Hyperthyroidism

Neonates of mothers with GD are at increased risk for neonatal GD, but hypothyroidism can also occur. There are two types of TSH-receptor (TSHR) antibodies (TRAbs): TSHR-stimulating immunoglobulins, which cause overproduction of thyroid hormone (hyperthyroidism), and TSH-receptor inhibitory (blocking) immunoglobulins, which can cause hypothyroidism. Fetal thyroid hormone synthesis begins at approximately 10 to 12 weeks' gestation, and the fetal TSH receptor starts responding to stimulation, including stimulation by thyroid-stimulating immunoglobulins, during the second trimester.[48] TRAbs, which belong to the immunoglobulin G class, freely cross the placenta, similar to iodine, thyroxine (T4), and antithyroid drugs (ATDs) the mother may be taking for the treatment of GD. The balance of stimulatory and inhibitory TRAbs, as well as ATD dose, influence the thyroid status in the fetus and neonate, and the fluctuation of maternal antithyroid antibody titers may result in different risks to the fetus or neonate.[49] In cases of transient neonatal GD, maternal TRAbs typically clear from the infant's circulation by 4 to 6 months of age, with resultant resolution of hyperthyroidism.[48]

As mentioned in the introduction, neonatal hyperthyroidism can also occur secondary to activating mutations in the TSH receptor or activating mutations in the alpha subunit of stimulatory G proteins *(GNAS)* in McCune-Albright syndrome.[17] This form of hyperthyroidism is permanent. Long-term antithyroid medical therapy is indicated until the child is old enough to safely complete definitive therapy to convert to hypothyroidism. Thyroidectomy is the treatment of choice, with some patients requiring radioactive iodine even after thyroidectomy if residual tissue is associated with persistent or recurrent hyperthyroidism.[50–52]

Clinical Features

Fetuses of euthyroid women are protected from the effects of hypothyroidism by placental transfer of maternal thyroid hormone and because they commonly have some functioning thyroid tissue. Prenatal treatment of CH may be considered in rare cases of dyshormonogenesis that present with a large fetal goiter, which can cause polyhydramnios and airway compromise that may obstruct breathing after birth.[53] The pattern and timing of dyshormonogenesis-associated goiter may vary based on the genetic etiology. Mutations in *TG*,[54] *TPO*,[55] and *DUOXA2*[56] have been reported as etiologies of fetal goiter.

Infants with severe congenital hypothyroidism may present with hypothermia, bradycardia, poor feeding, hypotonia, large fontanelles, myxedema, macroglossia, and umbilical hernia. This presentation is most common when both fetal and maternal hypothyroidism are present, as in iodine deficiency or untreated maternal hypothyroidism. However, many neonates manifest few or no symptoms even with significant hypothyroidism, making clinical diagnosis difficult in this age group. Implementation of universal newborn screening has nearly eradicated severe intellectual impairment due to CH in areas where screening is practiced, but CH remains a leading cause of preventable intellectual impairment in areas without newborn screening programs.

Signs of hyperthyroidism can be detected in the fetus, and if present, are highly predictive of neonatal hyperthyroidism. Particularly in cases where maternal GD is poorly controlled, features concerning for fetal hyperthyroidism include fetal tachycardia (heart rate >160 beats/min), thyroid enlargement (goiter; fetal neck circumference >95%), intrauterine growth retardation, polyhydramnios or oligohydramnios, advanced bone age, craniosynostosis with microcephaly, and hydrops.[57,58] Polyhydramnios is typically associated with a goiter with resultant esophageal and/or tracheal obstruction. Fetal bone age is assessed at the distal femur as the distal femoral epiphysis becomes detectable at about 32 weeks' gestation.[59] An advanced bone age is present if the femoral epiphysis is present prior to the 31st gestational week. For fetuses with severe thyrotoxicosis, there is an increased risk for premature delivery, and at the extreme, fetal death may occur.[48]

After delivery, a newborn may present with tachycardia, irritability with tremors, poor feeding, sweating, and difficulty sleeping secondary to thyrotoxicosis. Newborns may also have an emaciated appearance, proptosis with stare, and a goiter. Premature closure of cranial sutures (craniosynostosis) may be noted in severely affected infants. Other signs of neonatal hyperthyroidism, which may be confused with infection/sepsis, include thrombocytopenia, hepatosplenomegaly, and jaundice.[60] Fulminant liver failure and pulmonary hypertension secondary to neonatal hyperthyroidism may also be features of thyrotoxicosis.[61–64]

Evaluation

Screening protocols vary but generally begin with measurement of TSH and/or T4 in a dried blood spot collected from the infant within a few days after delivery. The initial sample generally should be obtained at least 24 hours after delivery to avoid false-positive results due to the physiologic TSH surge.[65,66] Prompt diagnosis and treatment of CH is critical to optimize developmental outcome, so any abnormal newborn screen result should prompt immediate confirmation of TSH and free T4 concentrations in a serum sample.[67] If a repeat newborn screen is obtained after the first few days of life, whether to confirm an abnormal result or as standard practice in all or selected newborns, gestational age– and postnatal age–specific reference ranges must be used to avoid misinterpreting an elevated TSH as normal in the context of the higher TSH reference range that is applicable only to the first few days after birth.[1]

In preterm infants, the timing of thyroid hormone testing should be adjusted to surveil over the time required for HPT axis maturation and acute illness. In an effort to avoid missing appropriate treatment, serial thyroid hormone monitoring should be implemented. A standardized monitoring schedule should be considered, with two examples including testing at (1) 48 hours, 2 weeks, 6 weeks, 10 weeks, or until the infant is >1500 g,[68] or (2) 72 to 120 hours, 1 week, 2 weeks, 4 weeks, and at term-corrected gestational age (see Fig. 26.1).[47] There is no consensus on criteria for initiation of thyroid hormone replacement therapy, but treatment should be considered if the TSH is >10 μU/mL with a low T4.[28] Levothyroxine (LT4) replacement should also be considered if the TSH is persistently between 5 and 10 μU/mL or if the TSH is >5 μU/mL with an upward trend on serially repeated thyroid function testing.

Determining the etiology of CH via radiologic imaging rarely alters initial management but may provide insight into prognosis. Ultrasound or thyroid scintigraphy (using ^{99}mTc or ^{123}I) can be used to assess the presence or absence of a normally located thyroid gland.[69] Although hypothyroidism due to dysgenesis is usually permanent, about 35% of patients with a eutopic thyroid gland have transient disease and will not require lifelong therapy.[70,71]

Neonates considered to be at high risk for development of thyrotoxicosis include (1) infants born to mothers with GD, especially if the maternal TRAb level is greater than twice the upper limit of normal; (2) infants in whom intrauterine surveillance revealed fetal signs of hyperthyroidism; and (3) infants with a known family history of genetic causes of congenital hyperthyroidism including activating mutations in the TSH receptor. If possible, TRAbs should be measured in cord blood of infants at high risk for neonatal hyperthyroidism, because there is a strong correlation between maternal and neonatal TRAb levels. Cord blood TSH and free thyroxine (fT4) are less helpful in predicting the onset of neonatal hyperthyroidism. Maternal ATDs are usually metabolized and excreted by 5 days of life. Unless symptoms of hyperthyroidism develop earlier, thyroid function studies (TSH and fT4) should be sent between 3 and 5 days of life, when biochemical hyperthyroidism typically develops in neonates with hyperthyroidism secondary to maternal GD. Onset of signs and symptoms of thyrotoxicosis may be delayed for several days, either from the effect of maternal ATDs or due to a coexistent effect of blocking antibodies. Thyroid function studies should therefore be sent again at 10 to 14 days of life, as studies have shown that most cases of neonatal GD present within the first 2 weeks of life.[72] However, there have been case reports of overt thyrotoxicosis secondary to neonatal GD occurring as late as 45 days of life.[73] After 2 weeks of age, infants with no clinical or biochemical hyperthyroidism should continue close monthly follow-up with their primary care providers. Algorithms summarizing the evaluation and management of neonatal hyperthyroidism are available.[17,72]

Management

Hypothyroidism

In newborns whose screening whole blood TSH is ≥40 mIU/L, LT4 should be initiated as soon as the confirmatory serum sample is obtained, without awaiting the results. In infants with screening TSH <40 mIU/L, LT4 should be initiated if the confirmatory serum TSH is >20 mIU/L or between 6 and 20 mIU/L with a low free T4 concentration (see Fig. 26.1).[67] The management of infants with mild TSH elevation (serum TSH 6–20 mIU/L) and normal free T4 levels is controversial. Although such patients are frequently identified by more stringent newborn screening thresholds, the neurodevelopmental risks posed by untreated mild disease remain uncertain.[74–77] Although there is a lack of consensus, if the TSH remains in the 6 to 20 mIU/L, beyond 21 days in a healthy, term neonate, LT4 replacement may be initiated with reevaluation for the need of continued therapy at 2 to 3 years of life.[78]

The initial dose of LT4 for CH is 10 to 15 micrograms (μg)/kg daily. For the majority of term infants, the typical starting dose is 37.5 mcg/day of LT4. For infants with marked elevation in TSH, >100 mIU/L, 50 mcg/day may be considered as a starting dose[79,80] with close follow-up and dose reduction to avoid overtreatment that may be associated with altered neurodevelopmental outcome.[81,82] Serum thyroid function testing is monitored every 1 to 2 weeks until normal, and then every 1 to 2 months during the first year of life and every 2 to 4 months during the 2nd and 3rd year of life with LT4.[69] The target parameter for LT4 treatment is normalization of

TSH within the first weeks of initiation of therapy.[80,83] LT4 dose is adjusted to maintain the serum TSH in the midnormal range and the serum free T4 in the mid- to upper half of the normal range. A subgroup of infants with CH displays variable degrees of thyroid hormone resistance with persistently elevated TSH levels despite high-normal or frankly elevated free T4 concentrations.[84] For these patients, the addition of LT3 to LT4 therapy can facilitate normalization of the TSH, but whether this improves outcomes is unknown.[85] To initiate combined therapy, the LT4 dose is typically decreased by 10% to 20% with addition of liothyronine (LT3) between 0.3 and 0.66 μg/kg/day, with the minimal reliable dose of 2.5 μg/day (1/2 tab) based on the smallest available tablet size (5 μg).[85]

In patients with suspected transient CH, based on the presence of a normal-appearing, eutopic thyroid gland on ultrasound and an initial borderline elevated TSH between 6 and 20 mIU/L, an LT4 dose of <1.7 μg/kg/day at 1 year of life or <1.45 μg/kg/day, without a need for an increase in LT4 dose despite normal growth and development, is associated with a high likelihood of normal thyroid function after discontinuation of LT4 supplementation.[53,71,86] LT4 doses >4.9 μg/kg/day or >4.7 μg/kg/day at 12 months or 24 months, respectively, are associated with an increased likelihood for permanent hypothyroidism.[86] A trial off of LT4 is typically delayed until the child is 2 to 3 years of age, when the risk of potential hypothyroidism-related neurocognitive development is lower.[78]

In central hypothyroidism, the TSH is low or inappropriately normal despite low T4 levels, secondary to abnormalities in the hypothalamus (thyrotropin-releasing hormone, TRH) or pituitary gland (TSH). The goal of treatment in central hypothyroidism, in which, by definition, serum TSH does not reflect systemic thyroid status, is to maintain the serum free T4 level in the upper half of the reference range.[87] However, before initiation of thyroid hormone replacement therapy in patients with suspected central hypothyroidism, assessment of the other anterior pituitary hormone axes must be completed to avoid inducing adrenal insufficiency secondary to thyroid hormone–associated increased clearance of cortisol.

LT4 tablets should be crushed, suspended in a small volume of water, breast milk, or non–soy-based infant formula, and administered via a syringe or teaspoon (not in a bottle). LT4 should not be administered with multivitamins containing calcium or iron. Limited data suggest that brand-name LT4 may be superior to generic in children with severe congenital hypothyroidism but not in those with equally severe acquired hypothyroidism.[67,88] Compounded LT4 solutions do not provide reliable dosing and should not be used.[89] Tirosint-SOL is a stable liquid form of levothyroxine that is available in Europe and the United States with reported unaltered absorption when administered with milk (and other breakfast beverages, in adults).[90] With the potential of improved absorption, optimal dosing of liquid LT4 preparations in neonates may differ compared with tablet formulations.[91,92] In patients that cannot tolerate LT4 by mouth or by nasogastric or gastrostomy tube, intravenous levothyroxine may be administered with a dose reduction of 25% based on a 70% to 80% absorption rate of oral levothyroxine in healthy subjects (thyroid hormone is absorbed in the jejunum and ileum).[87]

Prenatal treatment of CH may be considered in rare cases of dyshormonogenesis that present with a large fetal goiter, which can cause polyhydramnios as well as airway compromise that may obstruct breathing after birth. Intraamniotic injection of LT4 may help decrease fetal goiter size to prevent these complications. Although there is no consensus on intraamniotic LT4 dose or schedule, several reports have employed 150 to 500 μg/dose (or 10 μg/kg estimated fetal weight) every 2 weeks, with adjusted frequency based on fetal goiter response.[19,93,94] Intrauterine demise and need for intubation at birth are potential complications in such cases.[54]

Hyperthyroidism

In cases of suspected neonatal GD with biochemical hyperthyroidism, antithyroid drugs, (methimazole (MMI), and others) should be started

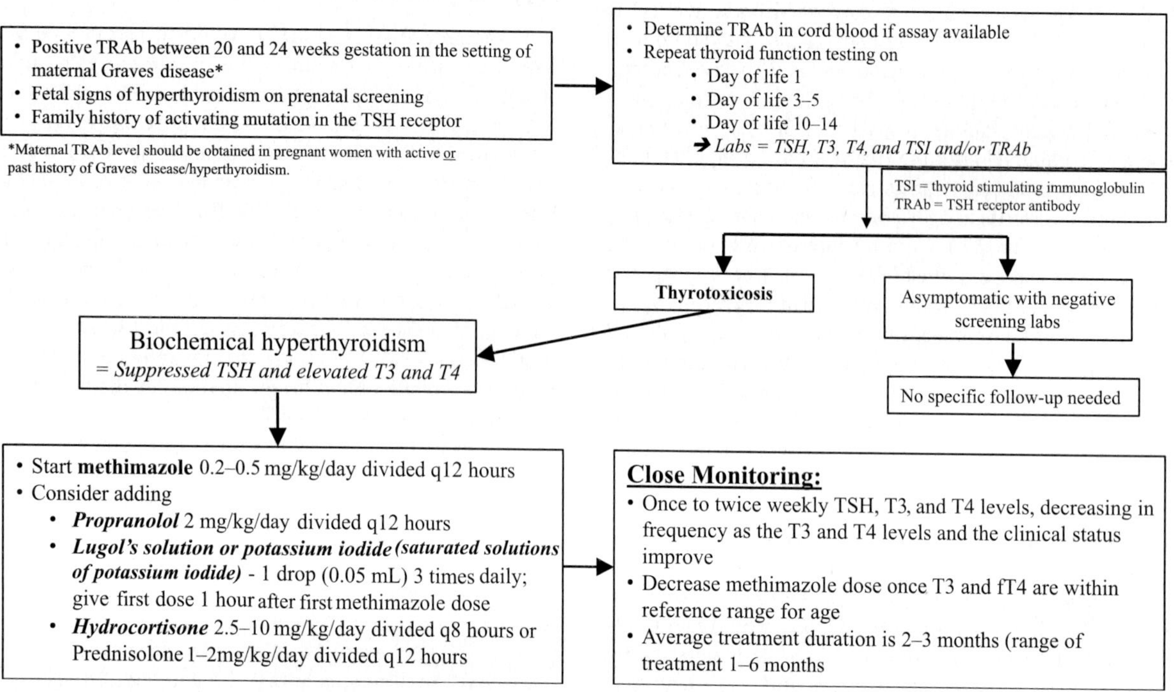

Fig. 26.2 Screening and Treatment Algorithm for Newborns at Risk for Neonatal Thyrotoxicosis. *TSH*, Thyroid-stimulating hormone.

at a dose of 0.2 to 0.5 mg/kg/day.[17] Propranolol should be added at a dose of 2 mg/kg/day for signs of sympathetic hyperactivity including tachycardia and hypertension. Propylthiouracil (PTU) is not recommended in neonates and throughout childhood due to the increased risk for hepatotoxicity.[95] In severe cases with hemodynamic compromise, Lugol's solution or potassium iodide may be given. Glucocorticoids may also be beneficial in the short term (Fig. 26.2). Because neonatal hyperthyroidism is more often transient and resolves with clearance of maternal TRAbs from the circulation, thyroid function tests should be monitored every 1 to 2 weeks after initiation of treatment to ensure appropriate MMI dose titration.[72]

In cases of nonautoimmune neonatal hyperthyroidism (activating mutations of the TSH receptor or McCune-Albright syndrome), MMI should be used for treatment similarly to cases of neonatal GD. Definitive therapy including thyroidectomy and/or radioiodine ablation will ultimately be required but can be delayed for months to years if the baby is responsive to medical therapy.[96,97]

Current guidelines note that breastfeeding is safe for mothers on antithyroid medications at moderate doses of MMI (20–30 mg/day) and PTU (less than 300 mg/day).[98] Infants of mothers with GD who are breastfeeding should have periodic thyroid function screening to ensure they have not developed hypothyroidism.[99]

Conclusion

Abundant basic and clinical research demonstrates that thyroid hormone signaling is required for both fetal and pediatric development. The identification of genes critical for thyroid hormone metabolism, transport, and receptor function has revealed that derangement of local thyroid hormone signaling can impact development, even in the absence of primary thyroid disease.

The goal of thyroid hormone replacement in neonates is to optimize normal growth and development and reduce or eliminate hypothyroidism-related signs and symptoms. For many neonates, LT4 replacement is anticipated to be lifelong; however, there is potential to discontinue LT4 in patients with transient congenital hypothyroidism[100,101] and drug-induced hypothyroidism (amiodarone[33] and others).

In neonates with hyperthyroidism, there are known short-term consequences of acute illness, a risk of craniosynostosis, and some evidence to suggest the potential for long-term adverse neurocognitive outcomes.[102,103]

Further clinical research is needed to understand the consequences of fetal and neonatal hypothyroxinemia and thyrotoxicosis, especially for preterm and/or critically ill infants, to better understand the potential benefits and risks of treatment.

CHAPTER

27 Hypothalamic-Pituitary-Adrenal Axis in Neonates

David W. Cooke, Yasmin Akhtar

KEY POINTS

1. Normal hypothalamic-pituitary-adrenal (HPA) axis production of cortisol and a normal renin-angiotensin-aldosterone axis are needed for the normal regulation of volume status, blood pressure, and serum sodium, potassium and glucose levels in the neonate. Disorders of these axes can be life-threatening.
2. Cortisol deficiency can be due to a disorder of the adrenal gland itself or to impaired ACTH secretion from the pituitary gland.
3. Mineralocorticoid deficiency can result from deficient production of aldosterone from the adrenal gland or from impaired mineralocorticoid signaling.
4. A disorder of sex development, resulting in virilization of a 46,XX fetus or undervirilization of a 46,XY fetus, may indicate an underlying disorder of adrenal steroid synthesis.
5. Transient, relative glucocorticoid deficiency can occur in all newborns in the transition to extrauterine life. This may be exacerbated in the premature infant due to immaturity of the HPA axis and as a consequence of critical illness.

Introduction

The adrenal glands sit on top of the upper pole of each kidney. The inner adrenal medulla produces catecholamines, predominantly epinephrine, which protect against hypotension and hypoglycemia. There are no significant disorders of the adrenal medulla during infancy. The adrenal cortex produces steroid hormones: aldosterone (a mineralocorticoid); cortisol (a glucocorticoid); and androgens, predominantly dehydroepiandrosterone (DHEA) and dehydroepiandrosterone sulfate (DHEAS). Mineralocorticoid action regulates the body's fluid volume and serum potassium level, whereas glucocorticoids have a wide range of actions, including controlling the immune response and protecting against hypoglycemia and hypotension. The role of glucocorticoids to protect against hypoglycemia and hypotension are particularly important during times of stress, when healthy individuals will increase cortisol secretion by as much as 10-fold. Neonatal disorders of the adrenal cortex include those that result in deficiency of mineralocorticoid and glucocorticoid action and those that cause excessive mineralocorticoid and androgen action.

Embryology and Development of the HPA Axis

The cells of the adrenal cortex are of mesodermal origin whereas the cells of the adrenal medulla are from the neuroectoderm. Adreno-gonadal progenitor cells appear around the 4th week of gestation, and these cells give rise to steroidogenic cells of the gonads and adrenal cortex around the 7th to 8th weeks of gestation. The complete hypothalamic-pituitary-adrenal (HPA) axis is established by 20 weeks of gestation.[1] The fetal adrenal cortex (Fig. 27.1A) consists of a relatively small outer definitive zone and a larger fetal zone. At about midgestation, a transitional zone develops between the definitive and fetal zones. During fetal life, the fetal zone produces large amounts of DHEA and DHEAS, which serve as precursors for placental estrogen production. The definitive zone of the fetal adrenal can produce glucocorticoid and mineralocorticoid. The role of the transitional zone is unclear, although it may be a site of fetal cortisol synthesis. Fetal adrenal glands grow through the third trimester. At birth, they are the same size as adult adrenal glands, that is, they are very large relative to body size. After birth the fetal zone involutes and disappears by about 6 to 12 months of age, with a concomitant decrease in the size of the infant adrenal gland. After birth, while the fetal zone is involuting, the definitive zone slowly enlarges and ultimately forms the three distinct zones of the fully developed adrenal cortex (Fig. 27.1B): the outer zona glomerulosa, which produces aldosterone; the middle zona fasciculata, which produces cortisol; and the inner zona reticularis, which produces DHEA, DHEAS, and androstenedione. The glomerulosa and fasciculata zones are not fully differentiated until about 3 years of age, whereas the zona reticularis does not begin to differentiate until after 3 years of age and is not fully developed until 15 years of age.[2]

Steroid hormones are produced using cholesterol as the precursor. Although the adrenal gland can make cholesterol *de novo* from acetate, most of the cholesterol for postnatal steroid synthesis comes from plasma low-density lipoprotein from dietary cholesterol. The synthetic pathway of adrenal steroid synthesis is shown in Fig. 27.2. The expression of a subset of the enzymes in the synthetic pathway results in temporal and zone-specific expression of the steroid hormones. Note that although the postnatal adrenal gland makes little or no testosterone, there is evidence that the fetal adrenal gland can synthesize testosterone through the expression of 17β-hydroxysteroid dehydrogenase 5 (17βHSD5). In virilizing forms of congenital adrenal hyperplasia, this adrenal testosterone production can be significant and contributes to the virilization of female fetuses.

In the first half of gestation, maternal cortisol crosses the placenta, inhibiting the fetal HPA axis (Fig. 27.3A). However, starting at midgestation and increasing through the last trimester, there is increased expression of placental 11β-hydroxysteroid dehydrogenase type 2 (11βHSD2), whose activity converts cortisol to the inactive cortisone (Fig. 27.3B). This limits exposure of the fetus to maternal glucocorticoid, decreasing the negative feedback effect on the fetal HPA axis and resulting in an increase in fetal ACTH production.[3,4] Although all the enzymes necessary for the synthesis of cortisol are expressed in the developing adrenal gland very early in gestation,

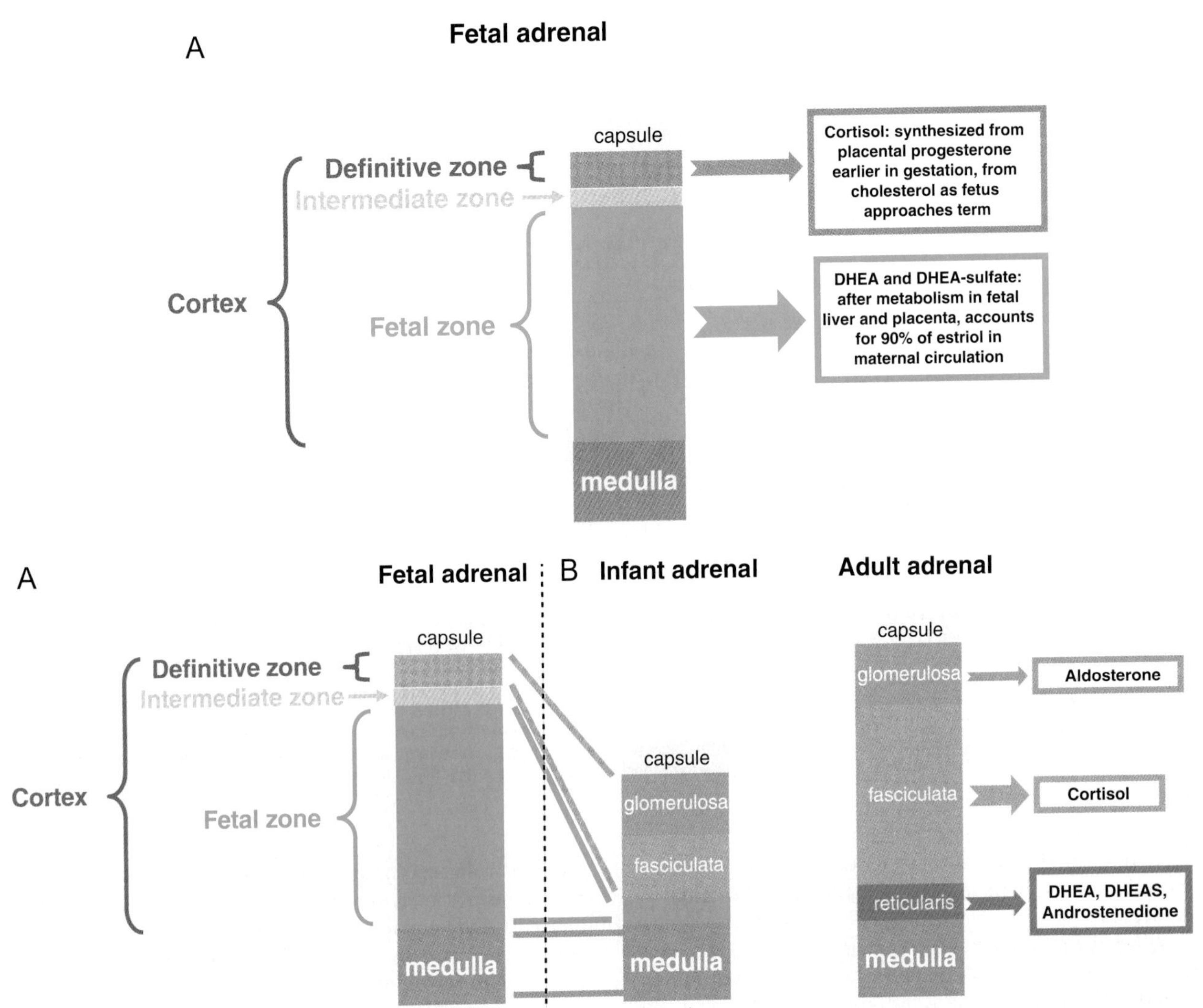

Fig. 27.1 Development of the Adrenal Cortex. (A) In later gestation, the fetal adrenal cortex consists of a large fetal zone and a small outer definitive zone, with an intermediate zone between the two. The fetal zone makes large amounts of dehydroepiandrosterone sulfate (DHEAS), and dehydroepiandrosterone (DHEA). The DHEAS and DHEA are metabolized by the fetal liver and the placenta to estriol. The definitive zone produces cortisol, initially from placental progesterone, but as 3βHSD2 expression increases as the fetus approaches term, the cortisol can be produced from cholesterol, as it will be after birth. (B) At term, the fetal adrenal glands are approximately the same size as the adult adrenal glands. After birth, the fetal zone involutes (as does the intermediate zone). The definitive zone differentiates into the outer aldosterone-producing zona glomerulosa and the cortisol-producing zona fasciculata. Throughout childhood, the adrenal cortex grows and the zona reticularis develops between the zona fasciculate and the medulla.

by 14 weeks of gestation, 3β-hydroxysteroid dehydrogenase 2 (3βHSD2) is no longer expressed. Until expression of 3βHSD2 returns in the definitive zone (and possibly the intermediate zone) later in gestation, the fetal adrenal cannot synthesize cortisol from cholesterol. This lack of 3βHSD2 expression drives the production of DHEA and DHEAS by the fetal zone. Prior to expression of 3βHSD2 later in gestation, the fetal adrenal can synthesize cholesterol, but it does so by utilizing placental progesterone as the substrate. It is not until after 30 weeks' gestation that the fetal adrenal typically produces cortisol *de novo* from cholesterol. Thus infants born at less than 27 to 30 weeks' gestational age may have more impairment in the HPA axis than infants born at a later gestational age. For infants born after 27 weeks' gestational age, serum cortisol levels over the first week of life change in response to illness, with infants who are ill showing a rise in serum cortisol and well infants having a decline in serum cortisol. In contrast, serum cortisol levels decrease in infants born prior to 27 weeks' gestational age, whether they are ill or well.[5] This transient adrenal insufficiency of prematurity seems to be limited to the first 2 weeks of life.[3] A final unique aspect of the fetal HPA axis is that the placenta produces corticotropin releasing hormone (CRH), with the production increasing through the end of gestation (see Fig. 27.3C). At that time, fetal ACTH is stimulated by the high circulating levels of placental CRH, with suppression of fetal hypothalamic CRH.

Although the enzymes necessary for the production of aldosterone are present in the fetus, mineralocorticoid production is only required postnatally.

Clinical Features of Adrenal Insufficiency

The presentation of neonates and infants with disorders of the adrenal gland and the HPA axis depends on which class of adrenal hormone production is disrupted. If there is impairment of mineralocorticoid signaling, the infant may present with acute life-threatening dehydration and hyponatremia and hyperkalemia. Mineralocorticoid deficiency can also present in infancy with a subacute or chronic presentation of failure to thrive.

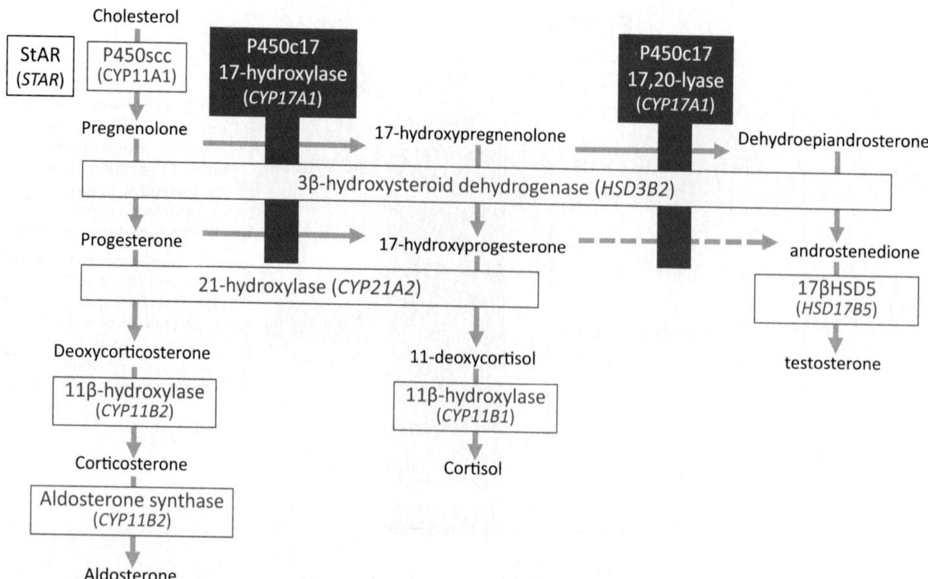

Fig. 27.2 Adrenal Steroidogenic Pathway. Biosynthetic pathway of the adrenal steroids aldosterone, cortisol, dehydroepiandrosterone (DHEA), and androstenedione. Enzyme reactions are shown in filled and open red boxes, with gene names indicated in parentheses. Synthesis of pregnenolone from cholesterol requires the steroidogenic acute regulatory protein (StAR) to transport cholesterol into the mitochondria where side chain cleavage enzyme (P450scc) catalyzes the reaction. P450c17 has both 17-hydroxylase and 17,20-lyase activity. P450c17 only very inefficiently catalyzes the synthesis of androstenedione from 17-hydroxyprogesterone; most androstenedione is produced by the action of 3β-hydroxysteroid dehydrogenase (3βHSD2) on DHEA. Until late in gestation, the fetal adrenal expresses very little 3βHSD23 so that the major steroid product is DHEA. Cortisol can be synthesized in the fetal adrenals before the expression of 3βHSD2 by utilizing placental progesterone as the initial substrate. Aldosterone synthase (the product of the *CYP11B2* gene) has 11β-hydroxylase activity to convert deoxycorticosterone to corticosterone and 18-hydroxylase and 18-methyl oxidase activities to convert corticosterone to aldosterone. Although the adrenal glands do not produce large amounts of testosterone, there is 17β-hydroxysteroid dehydrogenase expression (17βHSD5) to allow for some synthesis of testosterone. In males, the vast majority of testosterone synthesis occurs in the testis through the action of 17βHSD3.

Glucocorticoid deficiency can present with hypotension and hypoglycemia; the hypotension is compounded by the dehydration that occurs with mineralocorticoid deficiency if that is also present. When the adrenal insufficiency is due to hypopituitarism, there is glucocorticoid deficiency, but there is not mineralocorticoid deficiency, because aldosterone production is under control of the renin-angiotensin system, not ACTH. Disorders of adrenal androgen production can result in a disorder of sexual development, presenting as ambiguous genitalia in the newborn.

Causes of Adrenal Insufficiency

Primary adrenal insufficiency refers to disorders of the adrenal cortex, whereas central adrenal insufficiency refers to glucocorticoid deficiency as a result of impaired ACTH secretion. Depending on the underlying cause, primary adrenal insufficiency can result in mineralocorticoid deficiency in addition to glucocorticoid deficiency. The main causes of adrenal insufficiency in the neonate are listed in Table 27.1. Primary adrenal insufficiency can occur because of underdevelopment of the adrenal gland or impaired function of the adrenal gland.

Disorders of Adrenal Gland Development

X-linked adrenal hypoplasia congenita (AHC) is caused by mutation of the *NROB1* gene encoding DAX1 on chromosome Xp21.[6] AHC may be caused by a specific mutation of DAX1 but can also be part of a contiguous gene syndrome along with glycerol kinase deficiency and Duchenne muscular dystrophy.[7] In the most common form the definitive zone of the fetal adrenal gland does not develop. Half of the boys present with salt loss and glucocorticoid insufficiency early in infancy and the rest with adrenal insufficiency throughout childhood. AHC is also associated with hypogonadotropic hypogonadism because DAX1 is involved in pituitary gonadotrope development. Heterozygous mutations in steroidogenic factor 1(SF1, coded for by *NR5A1*) result in complete or partial gonadal dysgenesis, resulting in ambiguous genitalia or a female phenotype in 46,XY infants. There have been rare reports of individuals with *NR5A1* mutations also having primary adrenal failure (in at least one case due to a homozygous *NR5A1* mutation), although in most patients with heterozygous *NR5A1* mutations, adrenal steroidogenesis appears normal.[8] IMAGe syndrome (intrauterine growth retardation, metaphyseal dysplasia, adrenal hypoplasia, and genitourinary anomalies) and MIRAGE syndrome (myelodysplasia, infection, restriction of growth, adrenal hypoplasia, genital phenotypes, and enteropathy) are also associated primary adrenal insufficiency from impaired adrenal gland development. IMAGe syndrome is due to a dominant missense mutation of the *CDKN1C* gene on the maternal allele (*CDKN1C* is paternally imprinted). This gene encodes the tumor suppressor P57KIP2. Different mutations in this gene cause Beckwith-Wiedemann syndrome. MIRAGE syndrome is caused by heterozygous missense mutations in the *SAMD9* gene.

Familial glucocorticoid deficiency (also called hereditary unresponsiveness to ACTH) is an autosomal recessive condition of impaired cortisol synthesis caused by mutations in a number of genes including *MC2R* (which codes for the ACTH receptor), *MRAP* (melanocortin receptor accessory protein gene), *MCM4*, *TXNRD2*, and *NNT*. Classically, these patients do not have mineralocorticoid deficiency, although mineralocorticoid deficiency has been described in patients with mutations in *NNT*.[9] The first symptoms of familial glucocorticoid deficiency typically occur in early

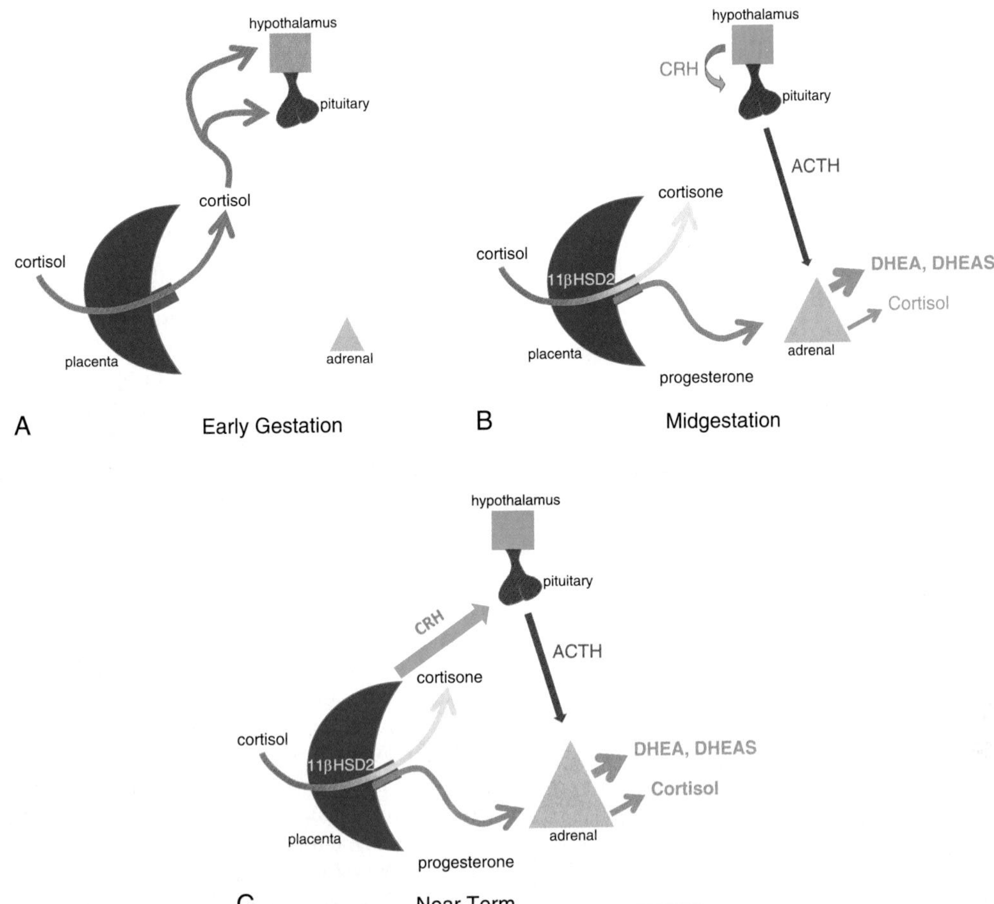

Fig. 27.3 Adrenal Cortex Function Through Gestation. (A) Early in gestation, maternal hydrocortisone crosses the placenta to the fetus, without inactivation. This cortisol suppresses corticotropin releasing hormone (CRH) production in the hypothalamus and adrenocorticotropic hormone (ACTH) production in the pituitary. (B) By midgestation, placental expression of 11βHSD2 has increased, so that cortisol is converted into inactive cortisone. Without suppression from maternal cortisol, the fetal hypothalamus produces CRH, which stimulates the fetal pituitary to secrete ACTH, which stimulates the fetal adrenal gland to grow and synthesize steroid hormones. Because of the lack of expression of 3βHSD2, cortisol cannot be synthesized *de novo* from cholesterol, and the majority of the steroid produced is dehydroepiandrosterone (DHEA) and dehydroepiandrosterone sulfate (DHEAS). A small amount of cortisol can be made using placental progesterone as the initial substrate. (C) As term approaches, the placenta produces increasing amounts of CRH. This high level of circulating CRH in the fetus becomes the stimulator of fetal pituitary ACTH secretion, with fetal hypothalamic CRH secretion being suppressed. Development of the definitive zone of the fetal adrenal gland, which expresses 3βHSD2, progresses as the fetus approaches term, allowing *de novo* synthesis of cortisol from cholesterol.

infancy and include recurrent hypoglycemia, failure to thrive, or an adrenal crisis precipitated by an illness. The patients often are hyperpigmented at presentation due to the effects of an elevated ACTH level.

Impaired Adrenal Gland Function

A number of metabolic disorders affecting steroid hormone synthesis result in adrenal insufficiency—in some cases affecting just glucocorticoid production, in others affecting both glucocorticoid and mineralocorticoid production. Congenital adrenal hyperplasia, which impairs the synthesis of cortisol from cholesterol, is the most common metabolic disorder causing adrenal insufficiency. Smith-Lemli-Opitz syndrome impairs adrenal function due to a defect in cholesterol synthesis.

Congenital Adrenal Hyperplasia

Congenital adrenal hyperplasia (CAH) is a family of autosomal recessive diseases caused by mutations in the enzymes that are necessary for the production of cortisol (see chapter 27 for further details on these disorders). The impaired fetal production of cortisol results in a rise in ACTH, driving adrenal gland hyperplasia and the overproduction of adrenal steroids that are not dependent on the mutated enzyme. Depending on the type of CAH, this can result in an infant being born with ambiguous genitalia due to virilization of the 46,XX fetus or to undervirilization of the 46,XY fetus. When the infant is not born with ambiguous genitalia (or when the ambiguous genitalia are not recognized, as in the severely virilized 46,XX infant with 21-hydroxylase deficiency who is mistaken for a male without ambiguous genitalia), the infant is at risk of presenting with an acute adrenal crisis with hypotension and hypoglycemia from cortisol deficiency, along with dehydration, hyponatremia, and hyperkalemia if mineralocorticoid deficiency is also present. In part because infants are born in a relatively volume-expanded state, the presentation with a salt-wasting adrenal crisis (from combined glucocorticoid and mineralocorticoid deficiency) classically occurs in the second week of life, although it can occur both earlier and later.

Virilization of the 46,XX fetus with CAH occurs due to the overproduction of DHEA and (in some forms of CAH) androstenedione. These adrenal androgens are converted into testosterone and dihydrotestosterone either in the adrenal gland (due to the expression

Table 27.1 Major Causes of Adrenal Insufficiency in the Neonatal and Infant Period

- Primary adrenal insufficiency
  - Disorders of adrenal gland development
    - Adrenal hypoplasia congenital (AHC): DAX1 mutation
      - Isolated DAX1 mutation
      - Xp21 continuous gene deletion
    - Mutations of SF1
    - IMAGe syndrome
    - MIRAGE syndrome
  - Impaired adrenal gland function
    - Isolated glucocorticoid deficiency
      - Familial glucocorticoid deficiency
    - Metabolic disorders
      - Congenital adrenal hyperplasia
        - 21-Hydroxylase deficiency
        - 11-Hydroxylase deficiency
        - 3BHSD-deficiency
        - 17-Hydroxylase deficiency
        - Congenital lipoid adrenal hyperplasia
          - StAR deficiency
          - P450SCC deficiency
        - P450 Oxidoreductase Deficiency (Antler-Bixley Syndrome)
      - Smith-Lemli-Opitz Syndrome
  - Adrenal hemorrhage
- Disorders of the renin-angiotensin-aldosterone axis
  - Aldosterone synthase deficiency
  - Pseudohypoaldosteronism (PHA)
    - Autosomal dominant PHA, *NR3C2* mutations
    - Autosomal recessive, systemic PHA, ENaC mutations
    - Secondary to renal disease
- Central adrenal insufficiency
  - Hypopituitarism
    - Developmental
    - Postinjury
  - Suppression of HPA axis from exogenous glucocorticoid treatment
    - Treatment of the infant
    - Maternal treatment during gestation
  - Relative adrenal insufficiency
    - Illness-associated
    - Immaturity of the HPA axis

3BHSD, 3-β-hydroxysteroid dehydrogenase; *HPA,* hypothalamic-pituitary-adrenal; *IMAGe,* intrauterine growth retardation, metaphyseal dysplasia, adrenal hypoplasia, and genitourinary anomalies; *MIRAGE,* myelodysplasia, infection, restriction of growth, adrenal hypoplasia, genital phenotypes, and enteropathy; *StAR,* steroidogenic acute regulatory protein.

of 17βHSD5 in the fetal adrenal[10] or outside the adrenal gland due the peripheral expression of 3βHDS1, 17βHSD5, and 5α-reductase). CAH due to deficiency of 21-hydroxylase causes over 90% of CAH. The presentation of 21-hydroxylase deficiency depends on the degree of enzyme deficiency. The mildest form (attenuated or nonclassic) presents in adolescent females with hirsutism and menstrual irregularity. With greater enzyme deficiency (simple virilizing form), 46,XX newborns will present with ambiguous genitalia at birth, and 46,XY children will present as a boy with peripheral precocious puberty in later infancy or early childhood. The most severe form (salt-wasting CAH) will present with ambiguous genitalia in the 46,XX infant, with the virilization sometimes severe enough to appear as a male with bilateral undescended testes. 46,XY infants with salt-wasting 21-hydroxylase deficiency are born with normal male genitalia, presenting with a salt-wasting adrenal crisis in the first week or two of life. Other, rarer forms of CAH that can virilize the 46,XX fetus are those due to mutations in 3βHSD2 (*3BHSD2* gene) and 11-β-hydroxylase (*CYP11B1* gene). Mutations that result in severe deficiency of 3βHSD2 activity will lead to a risk of a salt-wasting crisis, just as in 21-hydroxylase deficiency. In the 46,XY infant, 11-β-hydroxylase deficiency presents with peripheral precocious puberty. Although this enzyme defect impairs the production of aldosterone, there is overproduction of deoxycorticosterone, which, at the high concentrations achieved, activates the mineralocorticoid receptor. Although these infants can have a salt-wasting crisis in infancy, it is less common than in 21-hydroxylase deficiency. These infants are, however, at risk of having an adrenal crisis from glucocorticoid deficiency, such as during an intercurrent illness or other stress. The unregulated activation of the mineralocorticoid receptor by deoxycorticosterone leads to hypertension in these individuals, although this generally does not occur until after the neonatal period.

Some of the same enzymes that produce cortisol from cholesterol in the adrenal gland are needed to produce testosterone in the testis. Therefore some forms of CAH also impair testosterone production in the 46,XY fetus. Because a high fetal concentration of dihydrotestosterone, derived from a high concentration of testosterone, is needed for the development of normal male genitalia, these forms of CAH result in ambiguous genitalia in the 46,XY fetus. The forms of CAH that result in undervirilization of the 46,XY fetus are those due to mutations in *3BHSD2* and mutations that impair the 17-hydroxylase activity of *CYP17A1*. Note that *3BHSD2* CAH can cause ambiguous genitalia in both the 46,XX and 46,XY fetus: the overproduction of DHEA in the adrenal virilizes the 46,XX fetus, and the impaired testosterone production in the testis results in undervirilization of the 46,XY fetus. *CYP17A1* CAH will not virilize the 46,XX fetus (because there is no overproduction of adrenal DHEA) and also does not put infants at risk of a salt-wasting crisis (because aldosterone synthesis is not impaired.)

Another form of CAH that both virilizes the 46,XX fetus and results in undervirilization of the 46,XY fetus is that due to mutations in P450 oxidoreductase (POR). POR transfers electrons to all microsomal cytochrome P450 enzymes, including P450c17, P450c21, and P450aro; impairing 17-hydroxylase, 17,20-lyase, 21-hydroxylase, and aromatase activities in steroid synthesis (aromatase converts androgens to estrogens).[11] Presumably related to impairment of other P450 enzymes, these patients have the Antley-Bixler skeletal malformation syndrome (ABS), which includes craniosynostosis, brachycephaly, radio-ulnar or radio-humeral synostosis, femoral bowing, midface hypoplasia, and choanal atresia. ABS can also be caused by heterozygous gain-of-function mutations of fibroblast growth factor receptor 2 (in this case, ABS is not associated with abnormal steroid synthesis). POR deficiency does not impair aldosterone production, and glucocorticoid deficiency is variable but is generally mild, with normal baseline cortisol levels but subnormal cortisol levels after ACTH stimulation. Because of impaired placental aromatization of fetal androgens to estrogens, there can be virilization of the mother of a fetus with POR deficiency.

Disorders of Cholesterol Metabolism

Smith-Lemli-Opitz (SLO) syndrome is an autosomal recessive defect in cholesterol biosynthesis due to mutations in the steroid delta-7 reductase gene, *DHCR7*. Features include microcephaly, developmental delay, proximal thumbs, syndactyly of of the second and third toes, cardiac abnormalities, and undervirilized genitalia in 46,XY infants (due to impaired in utero production of dihydrotestosterone). Low serum cholesterol with elevated 7-dehydrocholesterol and 8-dehydrocholesterol and decreased steroid delta 7 reductase activity are found in these patients, with genetic analysis of *DHCR7* confirming the diagnosis. In addition to adrenal insufficiency, SLO patients may also have hypoparathyroidism, hypothyroidism, and immunodeficiency.[12] Most patients with SLO have normal-sized adrenal glands, although adrenal hyperplasia has been reported. Milder forms of SLO may not have adrenal insufficiency. In more severe forms of SLO, it is possible that cholesterol deficiency and accumulation of 7DHC and other oxysterols alter the cell membrane and cell membrane rigidity. This leads to absence or malformation of vesicles needed for endocrine and exocrine functioning.[13] One study showed that adrenal function was preserved in patients with mild or moderate SLO treated with dietary cholesterol supplementation.[14]

Other metabolic disorders, including peroxisomal disorders such as Zellweger syndrome, and mitochondrial disorders such as Kearns-Sayre syndrome can have adrenal insufficiency as part of their features. However, the adrenal insufficiency may not be present in infancy, and the other aspects of these diseases predominate.

Adrenal Hemorrhage

Because the neonatal adrenals are large and highly vascular, they are at risk of developing adrenal hemorrhage. In most cases, this is asymptomatic. However, adrenal hemorrhage can also present with marked jaundice, anemia, or a large flank mass. Adrenal insufficiency rarely occurs from adrenal hemorrhage, perhaps only 1% to 2% of the time,[15] in large part because it is only bilateral about 10% of the time. When bilateral adrenal hemorrhage causes adrenal insufficiency, there will be both glucocorticoid and mineralocorticoid deficiency. Risk factors for the development of adrenal hemorrhage include asphyxia, sepsis, coagulation disorders, traumatic deliveries, and perinatal injuries.[16]

Isolated Disorders of Mineralocorticoid Signaling

Aldosterone synthase deficiency is caused by mutations of the *CYP11B2* gene that produces the aldosterone synthase enzyme p450C11aldo. These infants present in the first weeks of life with nausea, vomiting, and feeding problems with failure to thrive. Laboratory investigation reveals metabolic acidosis, hyponatremia, hyperkalemia, and a high renin level, with a low or inappropriately normal level of aldosterone.[17]

Aldosterone resistance (pseudohypoaldosteronism [PHA]) can present similar to aldosterone deficiency (nausea, vomiting, failure to thrive, hyponatremia, and hyperkalemia) but with an elevated serum aldosterone level.[18] There are two congenital forms for this. Heterozygous mutations in the *NR3C2* gene coding for the mineralocorticoid receptor cause aldosterone resistance that typically has resolution of a need for salt supplementation by 18 to 24 months of age. Mutations in the genes encoding the epithelial sodium channel subunits (*SCNN1A*, *SCNN1B*, and *SCNN1G*) cause an autosomal recessive form of PHA that results in a more systemic disorder that includes significant pulmonary and skin disease. This systemic form does not ameliorate with age. Transient PHA is secondary to renal disease, including pyelonephritis and obstructive uropathy.

Central adrenal insufficiency, resulting in deficient ACTH secretion from the pituitary, may be due to developmental hypopituitarism, hypopituitarism from perinatal central nervous system (CNS) injury, or from temporary impairment of ACTH secretion. Central adrenal insufficiency impacts glucocorticoid synthesis, but mineralocorticoid function is normal.

Hypopituitarism

Hypopituitarism as a cause of adrenal insufficiency is discussed in detail in Chapter 27. Neonates with hypopituitarism may present with direct hyperbilirubinemia or hypoglycemia from the hormone deficiency and with midline defects such as cleft palate or an absent septum pellucidum, which point to a risk for hypopituitarism.

Suppression From Exogenous Glucocorticoid

Prolonged use of systemic or inhaled glucocorticoids can suppress ACTH secretion, which results in atrophy of the adrenal cortex. Both of these issues take time to resolve after withdrawal of exogenous glucocorticoid treatment, and until they do, the patient will have a form of central adrenal insufficiency (the renin-angiotensin-aldosterone axis is not affected). The risk of adrenal suppression in infants appears to be the same as that in older children and adults: if there is use of supraphysiologic doses of systemic glucocorticoid for more than 2 weeks, this places the infant at risk of adrenal suppression.[19] The data on how much inhaled corticosteroids can suppress the HPA axis in infants are incomplete. One study found that 21 days of inhaled beclomethasone (starting at an expected delivered dose of 40 mcg/kg/day) in infants born at a mean gestational age of 26.2 to 26.4 weeks resulted in lower baseline serum cortisol levels but no difference in cortisol levels after an ACTH stimulation test.[20] In older children, moderate or higher doses of inhaled corticosteroids result in a risk of adrenal suppression.[21,22]

Maternal use of glucocorticoids can cause adrenal suppression in the newborn if the glucocorticoid is not inactivated by placental 11βHSD2 and the treatment extends until close to the time of delivery. Thus, this will occur with maternal treatment with dexamethasone or betamethasone or with extremely high doses of other glucocorticoids that then overwhelm the capacity of placental 11βHSD2. Because placental 11βHSD2 expression is low early in gestation, maternal glucocorticoid treatment can more easily result in suppression of the HPA axis of infants born extremely prematurely. Although the effect of a particular maternal glucocorticoid regimen is difficult to predict, recovery of the infant HPA axis typically occurs within about 2 weeks after birth. However, some studies have shown a decreased HPA axis response to painful stress for up to 4 months after birth.[23]

Relative Adrenal Insufficiency

Relative adrenal insufficiency refers to the inability of a patient to generate sufficient cortisol needed during a state of physiologic stress in the absence of a permanent, underlying disorder of the HPA axis. This has been best described in critically ill adults but also occurs in critically ill neonates. The mechanism for this critical illness–associated relative adrenal insufficiency includes cytokine-induced suppression of ACTH and cortisol synthesis and possibly decreased adrenal gland perfusion.[24] Additionally, in the first week of life the HPA axis may be relatively sluggish in responding to stress due at least in part to the fact that the fetal hypothalamic production of corticotropin releasing factor is quiescent because of the large amount of corticotropin releasing factor produced by the placenta at the end of gestation,[24] which can induce a lag in the recovery of the infant's production of hypothalamic CRH after birth. In premature infants, there may also be transient adrenal insufficiency due to immaturity of the HPA axis. As discussed previously, the 3βHSD2 that is necessary for synthesis of cortisol from cholesterol is not fully expressed until after about 30 weeks' gestation, although the increase in 3βHSD2 expression can be accelerated by premature birth. Nonetheless, with premature birth, the progesterone source that is utilized for fetal cortisol synthesis is cut off, potentially further impairing the capacity for cortisol synthesis of premature newborns. For all of these reasons, clinicians must be cautious about attributing adrenal insufficiency in infants to a permanent disorder. One challenge when evaluating for relative adrenal insufficiency is the difficulty in quantitating the physiologic stress. Because cortisol levels increase with stress, it is not surprising that higher cortisol levels may be a marker for increased morbidity and mortality as in a study by Rameshbabu et al., where basal serum cortisol levels at 24 to 36 hours of life were significantly higher in preterm infants (< 30 weeks' gestational age or < 1250 g birth weight) who died or developed vasopressor refractory hypotension.[25]

Studies have attempted to correlate cortisol levels, either baseline or ACTH-stimulated levels, with outcomes in premature infants. These have given conflicting results. Some have found that higher cortisol concentrations correlate with an increase in short-term adverse outcomes, suggesting the higher cortisol concentrations are a marker for disease severity.[26,27] Other studies have found that lower levels correlate with worse outcomes, raising the possibility of adrenal insufficiency as a potential contributor to worse outcomes. However, a number of other studies found no correlation of cortisol levels with clinical outcome.[27,28]

Evaluation

Evaluation of primary or central adrenal insufficiency involves testing the adrenal axis. If the concern is for primary adrenal insufficiency, both mineralocorticoid and glucocorticoid insufficiency are expected. In older children, there is a circadian variation in serum cortisol levels through the day. Neonates do not initially have this circadian variation. Although some studies have demonstrated circadian variation as early as the first few days of life, the classic circadian variation of peak serum cortisol concentration in the early morning and a nadir at midnight typically develops starting around 2 months of age, becoming fully established in most infants by about 9 months of age.[29] Therefore, in neonates, time of day generally does not matter when measuring basal cortisol levels. A baseline cortisol level above 10 mcg/dL (285 nmol/L) is generally a good indication of a normal HPA axis.[30] Baseline cortisol levels below 10 mcg/dL do not always indicate adrenal insufficiency, however, and in some situations (such as a critically ill infant), a level above 10 mcg/dL may not exclude adrenal insufficiency. When primary adrenal insufficiency is being evaluated, a serum ACTH level should be measured with the serum cortisol, because the combination of an ACTH concentration more than twice the upper limit of the reference range with a cortisol concentration less than 5 mcg/dL is diagnostic. In situations where the baseline cortisol level does not give a definitive answer, ACTH stimulation testing may need to be performed to further evaluate for adrenal insufficiency. This testing can be used to evaluate for both primary and central adrenal insufficiency, with the important caveat that it will miss the diagnosis of acute (< 2–4 weeks) central adrenal insufficiency (as might occur after a CNS injury) because a positive result in the case of central adrenal insufficiency relies on the atrophy of the adrenal gland that occurs in the absence of normal ACTH stimulation. The standard ACTH stimulation test uses 250 mcg of synthetic ACTH in adults, with the equivalent dose for infants being 15 mcg/kg.[31] The low-dose ACTH stimulation test uses a 1-mcg dose of ACTH in adults (0.1 mcg/kg or 1 mg/m^2 in infants) and is proposed to have a higher sensitivity for central adrenal insufficiency. There is significant risk of false positives with the low-dose test, particularly in settings were the testing is not done frequently. The 2016 Endocrine Society Clinical Practice Guidelines recommend the standard-dose ACTH stimulation test over the low-dose test until more evidence demonstrates superiority of the low dose-test.[31] In the past, a peak cortisol value more than 18 mcg/dL (500 nmol/L) made adrenal insufficiency unlikely. However, newer cortisol assays, including liquid chromatography-tandem mass spectrometry (LC-MS/MS) and newer, highly specific immunoassays, result in lower cortisol results than the assays that were used to define the 18 mcg/dL threshold. Although specific validation of the proper threshold to define adrenal insufficiency in infants using these newer assays has not been performed, a threshold of 12.5 to 14.5 mcg/dL (350–400 nmol/L) is more appropriate, because this is the level that corresponds to the 18 mcg/dL on the older assays.[32]

Blood electrolytes should be obtained to identify hyponatremia and hyperkalemia when primary adrenal insufficiency is suspected. Hyponatremia (but not hyperkalemia) can also occur with isolated glucocorticoid deficiency (as in central adrenal insufficiency), although in this case it is due to impaired water excretion rather than the sodium loss that occurs with mineralocorticoid deficiency.

If cortisol deficiency is being evaluated because of hypoglycemia, a serum cortisol level should be obtained at the time of hypoglycemia (when the serum glucose concentration is less than 50 mg/dL or 2.8 mmol/L) to look for the appropriate counterregulatory response with a rise in cortisol to above the same threshold considered normal on the ACTH stimulation test. Because hyperinsulinism is a common cause of neonatal hypoglycemia, and in this case, the hypoglycemia can develop so quickly that the serum cortisol has not yet increased at the time the hypoglycemia is detected, a subsequent serum cortisol level 30 minutes after the detection of the hypoglycemia should be measured.

To evaluate for CAH, the appropriate steroid precursors proximate to the enzyme deficiency are measured (e.g., 17-hydroxyprogesterone in 21-hydroxylase deficiency).

If there is concern about adrenal hemorrhage, imaging with abdominal ultrasound can be obtained but is not necessary to diagnose primary adrenal insufficiency. Similarly, if adrenal insufficiency from hypopituitarism is suspected, magnetic resonance imaging of the hypothalamus and pituitary should be obtained.

Management

Treatment of adrenal insufficiency consists of replacing the missing cortisol and/or aldosterone (Table 27.2). The usual daily requirement for cortisol is 6 to 8 mg/m^2/day. Hydrocortisone is preferred for replacement therapy over synthetic glucocorticoids because the risk of side effects from overtreatment is substantial when synthetic glucocorticoids are used. In congenital adrenal hyperplasia, a slightly

Table 27.2 Hydrocortisone Doses for Adrenal Insufficiency

Daily dose:
• 6–8 mg/m²/day hydrocortisone
Stress dose:
• 25–50 mg/m²/day
Critical illness:
• 50–100 mg/m²/day
Perioperative coverage:
• 25 mg/m² hydrocortisone IV on call to the operating room
• 50 mg/m² hydrocortisone IV given as an infusion over the course of the surgery
• 50 mg/m²/day hydrocortisone IV given over the subsequent 24 hours

IV, Intravenous.

higher dose than the usual 6 to 8 mg/m²/day dose may be needed because the goal of treatment is to lower adrenal androgen production in addition to replacing the cortisol deficiency. Oral bioavailability of hydrocortisone is close to 100%, so the same dose may be used for both oral and parenteral delivery.

At times of illness and medical stress, higher amounts of cortisol are made in individuals with a normal HPA axis, and this higher requirement is needed in patients with adrenal insufficiency in order to avoid an adrenal crisis. 25 to 40 mg/m²/day of hydrocortisone is an appropriate stress dose with illness, with the higher dose allowing for the possibility of impaired absorption when using an enteral dose. For critical illness, a stress dose of 100 mg/m²/day is appropriate. For the stress of surgery, a typical regimen is outlined in Table 27.2.

The half-life of cortisol is increased in the newborn, particularly in very preterm infants, in whom the half-life may be twice as long as in adults. Therefore hydrocortisone may be dosed every 12 hours in premature infants, changing to every 6 to 8 hours in late-preterm and term infants.[33]

When adrenal insufficiency is being considered in an acute situation, such as in vasopressor refractory hypotension, an appropriate course is to measure a serum cortisol concentration and to treat with 1 mg/kg of intravenous (IV) hydrocortisone. If there is a response, with an improvement in the blood pressure after 2 to 6 hours, this can be followed by 0.5 mg/kg of IV hydrocortisone every 12 hours (equivalent to about 8–10 mg/m²/day.) If the initial cortisol level suggests normal adrenal function (e.g., a level above 15–20 mcg/dL, or 400–550 nmol/L), discontinuation of the hydrocortisone could be considered.[34]

For mineralocorticoid deficiency, 0.1 to 0.2 mg of fludrocortisone is given to newborns, given either daily or dosed every 12 hours. Fludrocortisone is not available in a parenteral formulation, so if a patient is unable to take oral fludrocortisone, hydrocortisone should be given at the higher stress dose, because this higher dose of hydrocortisone will supply the desired mineralocorticoid activity. Because of the low sodium content of an infant diet, additional sodium supplementation is generally needed, at a dose of 1 to 2 g/day of NaCl. For patients with PHA, treatment is with salt supplementation at a dose of 3 to 20 mEq/kg/day.

The treatment of SLO syndrome is primarily dietary cholesterol supplementation. The estimated daily synthetic need for cholesterol during infancy is 30 to 40 mg/kg/day. The goal is to provide sufficient dietary cholesterol to downregulate endogenous sterol synthesis and limit *de novo* production of 7DHC. When children with SLO syndrome are hospitalized for surgery or acute medical problems and cholesterol cannot be given enterally, cholesterol in the form of low-density lipoprotein containing fresh frozen plasma can be beneficial in the treatment of acute infections and poor wound healing.[35] Although dietary changes are the primary management, there have been studies looking at treatment with HMG-COA reductase inhibitors (such as simvastatin) for the management of SLO syndrome.[36]

CHAPTER

28 Disorders of Neonatal Mineral Metabolism and Metabolic Bone Disease

Andrew C. Calabria, Sarah A. Coggins

KEY POINTS

1. Disorders of mineral homeostasis in the neonatal period are often exaggerated responses to the normal physiologic transition. Parathyroid hormone (PTH) is the principal regulator of postnatal calcium metabolism, with vitamin D and its metabolites involved in the regulation of serum calcium levels.
2. Neonatal hypercalcemia is uncommon and often asymptomatic; calcium concentrations need to be interpreted based on age-related norms, which are higher in neonates, and in concert with serum phosphorus and PTH levels.
3. Hypocalcemia is common in the neonatal intensive care unit and is transient in most infants; congenital hypoparathyroidism should be considered in the setting of prolonged hypocalcemia.
4. Metabolic bone disease of prematurity (MBD) results from interrupted maternal–fetal mineral transfer during the third trimester and is exacerbated by inadequate postnatal nutritional mineral intake and pharmacologic exposures.
5. No single biochemical marker is sufficient for diagnosis of MBD, but common screening approaches include measurements of alkaline phosphatase, PTH, calcium, phosphorus, and 25-hydroxyvitamin D (25(OH)D).
6. Prevention and treatment of MBD are often the same and include nutritional optimization, targeted enteral calcium and phosphorus supplementation, limiting bone active medications, and physical therapy interventions.
7. MBD slowly self-resolves over time, although long-term follow-up in former preterm infants suggests negative impacts on overall growth and bone mineralization in childhood and adulthood.

Background

Neonatal calcium and phosphorus metabolism are influenced by fetal and maternal factors and are postnatally controlled by complex parathyroid-renal hormonal interactions. Homeostasis of calcium and phosphorus is critical for physiologic stability (with roles in signal transduction, neurotransmitter release, and muscle contraction) and for postnatal growth and skeletal development. Preterm infants are at particular risk for disordered mineral metabolism, resulting from interrupted maternal–fetal mineral transfer in the third trimester and exacerbated by inadequate postnatal mineral intake in the setting of rapid growth. Metabolic bone disease (MBD), or osteopenia of prematurity, primarily occurs in very low birth weight (VLBW) infants with birth weight <1500 g, although extremely low birth weight (ELBW) infants <1000 g are disproportionately affected. MBD rates were as high as 50% among ELBWs in the 1980s,[1] although with advancements in overall neonatal care, MBD rates have declined, and 10% to 40% of ELBW infants are affected in more contemporary reports.[2,3] In this chapter, we review fetal and postnatal mineral physiology and discuss disorders of neonatal mineral metabolism, including calcium derangements and metabolic bone disease of prematurity.

Fetal Bone Development

Fetal bone mineralization primarily occurs during the third trimester and is reliant on active transport of calcium and phosphorus across the placenta. Eighty percent of total gestational calcium accretion occurs during the third trimester, during which time the fetus is supplied (approximately 120–150 mg/kg/day of calcium),[4] with phosphorus accretion of approximately half that amount (70 mg/kg/day).[5] It is thus unsurprising that perinatal conditions of decreased placental efficiency (preeclampsia, intrauterine growth restriction) in preterm infants are associated with MBD postnatally. Rapid fetal bone length growth in the third trimester (about 1.2 cm/week) is supported by these nutrients as well as bone remodeling via mechanical forces between the fetal skeleton and the uterine wall.[6]

The fetus exists in a state of relative hypercalcemia, which is mediated by the calcium-sensing receptor (CaSR) and suppresses fetal parathyroid hormone (PTH). In addition to promoting fetal bone mineralization, fetal hypercalcemia may also buffer the physiologic drop in serum calcium that occurs after birth.[4] Calcium binding to albumin is dependent on pH—as the neonate initiates breathing, the serum pH rises, albumin is increasingly able to bind calcium, and the free ionized calcium level falls. Active ATP-mediated transport of minerals from mother to fetus appears to be primarily mediated by elevations in fetal PTH-related peptide (PTHrP). Fetal calcitonin is also elevated and enhances bone mineral absorption; PTH and calcitriol are suppressed.[4,5,7] PTHrP is expressed in the placenta and is instrumental in regulation of active placental calcium transport from mother to fetus as well as in modulating chondrocyte differentiation and osteoblast development.[4] However, PTHrP is not routinely measured in clinical practice because it is transiently present in serum, technically difficult to assay, and challenging to interpret given the lack of reference ranges for age.

The role of vitamin D in placental mineral transport is unclear; 25(OH)D crosses the placenta, but calcitriol does not. Fetal calcitriol levels are less than half of maternal levels,[4] and some authorities assert that maternal 25(OH)D levels do not significantly influence fetal bone development.[8] However, lower maternal 25(OH)D levels at 34 weeks' gestation were associated with greater femoral metaphyseal cross-sectional area and femoral splaying at both 19 and 34 weeks' gestation.[9] Maternal vitamin D status does correlate with neonatal serum vitamin D levels postnatally,[10] and additional evidence suggests that maternal 25(OH)D status influences later bone mineralization. Higher maternal serum 25(OH)D levels in late gestation were associated with increased bone area and bone mineral content as measured by dual energy x-ray absorptiometry (DXA) in female infants at 2 weeks of life.[11] Lower maternal 25(OH)D stores in the third trimester have been associated with lower bone mineral content in offspring at 9 years of age.[12]

The mechanisms for placental phosphorus transfer are less understood, but they also appear to be governed by PTHrP-mediated active transport. Phosphorus is also essential for fetal bone development; it mediates apoptosis of chondrocytes and is subsequently incorporated into newly formed osteoid matrix.[4]

Postnatal Mineral and Hormone Physiology

Upon umbilical cord clamping, previously high rates of placental-fetal mineral transfer abruptly cease. In the first 12 to 24 hours of life, both serum total and ionized calcium concentrations drop by 20% to 30% (with deeper nadirs in preterm than term infants),[5] while serum phosphorus concentrations rise, both returning to normal values within the first few days of life.[4] In the neonate, calcium is almost entirely (99%) located in bone matrix, where it is complexed to phosphorus. In the remaining 1% of circulating calcium, 50% is ionized and biologically active, 40% is protein-bound (mostly to albumin) and biologically inactive, and the remainder is complexed to organic and inorganic acids.[5,13] Phosphorus is primarily (85%) stored in the skeleton, with the remainder circulating in the serum either in ionized form (55%), complexed to cations (35%), or protein-bound (10%).[5]

Postnatal control of calcium and phosphorus metabolism is governed primarily by PTH, calcitonin, and vitamin D (Fig. 28.1). PTH is the primary hormone governing calcium homeostasis after birth. Suppressed in the fetus due to relative hypercalcemia, PTH is secreted by the parathyroid gland in the setting of hypocalcemia and induced two- to five-fold in both preterm and term infants after the postnatal calcium drop.[5] Although an acute increase in PTH has anabolic effects on the neonatal skeleton and promotes bone formation,[14] prolonged elevation in PTH promotes osteoclast proliferation and differentiation, leading to bone resorption and release of calcium and phosphorus. In the kidney, PTH promotes calcium reabsorption and phosphorus excretion at the distal convoluted tubule and stimulates production of calcitriol in the proximal tubule by activation of renal 1-hydroxylase.[13] Calcitonin is produced by parafollicular cells of the thyroid gland and acts in opposition to PTH, decreasing serum calcium by inhibition of osteoclasts and increasing renal excretion of calcium and phosphate.

Vitamin D is either ingested or synthesized in skin after UV exposure. In the neonatal intensive care unit (NICU), vitamin D comes almost exclusively from dietary intake. It is first hydroxylated to 25(OH)D in the liver, and given its long half-life, 25(OH)D is most reflective of overall vitamin D status. PTH mediates hydroxylation of 25(OH)D in the kidney, to produce 1,25(OH)$_2$D (calcitriol). Calcitriol has multiple effects via binding of the vitamin D receptor, including increased intestinal absorption of calcium and phosphorus, promotion of bone formation by mineralization of osteoid, and negative feedback over PTH via transcriptional downregulation. Calcitriol levels are low at birth but increase to adult levels in the first day of life.[5] Postnatal mineral and hormone kinetics change rapidly in the first several postnatal days and are summarized in Fig. 28.2.

Hypercalcemia

Hypercalcemia is far less common than hypocalcemia in the neonatal and infantile periods. Interpretation of an elevated serum total calcium level with suspected hypercalcemia requires measurement of the either the ionized calcium level or determination of the serum albumin concentration, with appropriate adjustment of the serum calcium level if the albumin level is abnormal. The effects of acid-base status must be considered as well, with acidosis resulting in decreased calcium binding to albumin and an increase in the ionized calcium, whereas alkalosis increases protein binding of calcium and a decrease in ionized calcium. In addition, the reference range for neonates is higher than at other ages, with the upper limit of normal at 11.3 mg/dL.[15] Initial biochemical testing must also include

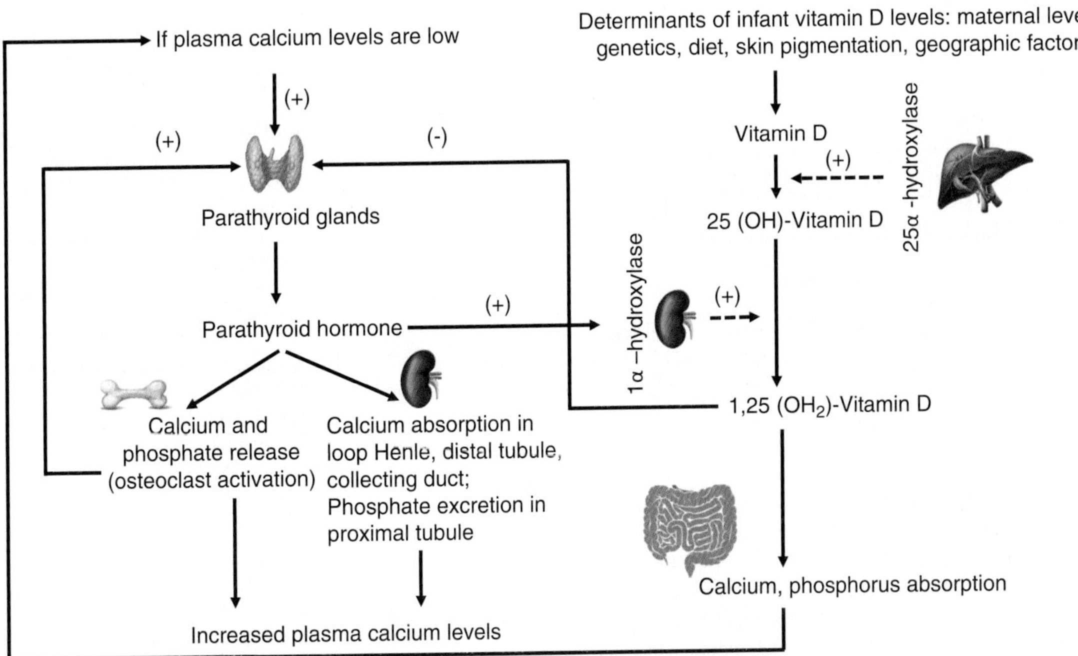

Fig. 28.1 Physiology of Calcium and Metabolism Regulation. (Modified from Montaner Ramón A. Risk factors of bone mineral metabolic disorders. *Semin Fetal Neonatal Med.* 2020;25[1]:101068. doi:10.1016/j.siny.2019.101068.)

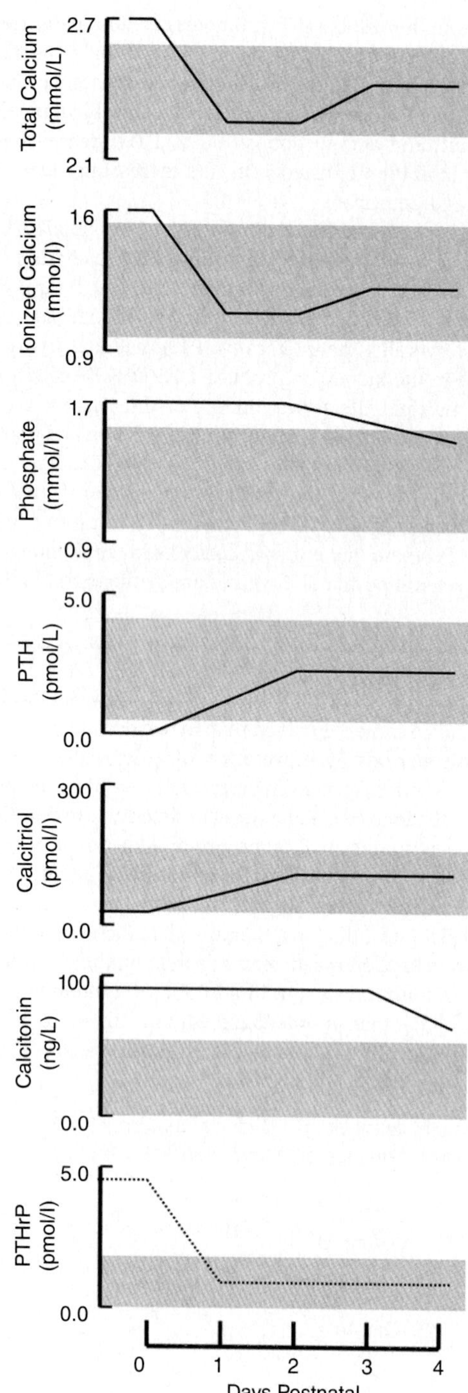

Fig. 28.2 Mineral and Hormone Levels Over the First Four Postnatal Days. Shaded areas denote normal values in adults. (Reproduced from Ryan BA, Kovacs CS. Calciotropic and phosphotropic hormones in fetal and neonatal bone development. *Semin Neonatal Fetal Med.* 2020;25[1]:101062.)

determination of the serum phosphorus level, because hypophosphatemia can cause hypercalcemia, particularly in premature or low birth weight infants who receive inadequate dietary phosphorus.

Symptoms of hypercalcemia are highly variable and depend on the age of the patient, the degree of hypercalcemia, and the clinical disorder. For cases of mild to moderate hypercalcemia, usually up to 13 mg/dL, patients may be without symptoms or with nonspecific symptoms such as anorexia, feeding intolerance, irritability, or constipation. Chronic hypercalcemia can present as failure to thrive, but the vague nature of symptoms can lead to delayed diagnosis and increase the risk for morbidity and mortality. Hypercalcemia can also lead to shortened ST segment and heart block, polyuria secondary to renal resistance to vasopressin leading to nephrogenic diabetes insipidus with associated dehydration, and hypertension due to the direct vasoconstriction from elevated serum calcium levels. Renal complications such as hematuria, nephrocalcinosis, and nephrolithiasis can be early manifestations of hypercalcemia. Severe hypercalcemia can directly affect the nervous system, leading to lethargy and seizures, with rare progression to coma.

The differential diagnosis of neonatal hypercalcemia can be broadly divided into PTH-dependent and independent causes (Table 28.1). Iatrogenic causes of hypercalcemia can be seen with hypophosphatemia, excessive administration of calcium and/or vitamin D, and the use of thiazide diuretics, which lead to decreased urinary calcium excretion.

PTH-Dependent Hypercalcemia

Neonatal hyperparathyroidism is characterized by high serum calcium levels with inappropriately elevated PTH levels, with low

Table 28.1 Differential Diagnosis for Neonatal Hypercalcemia and Hypocalcemia

Category	Differential Diagnoses
NEONATAL HYPERCALCEMIA	
Iatrogenic	Hypophosphatemia Vitamin D excess Excessive calcium supplementation Thiazide diuretics
PTH-dependent	Maternal hypocalcemia/transient neonatal hyperparathyroidism Inactivating mutations of the calcium-sensing receptor • Familial hypocalciuric hypercalcemia (OMIM #145980) • Neonatal severe hyperparathyroidism (OMIM #239200) Jansen's metaphyseal chondrodysplasia (OMIM #156400)
PTH-independent	Subcutaneous fat necrosis Williams syndrome (OMIM#194050) Idiopathic infantile hypercalcemia/CYP24A1 mutations (OMIM #143880) Inborn errors of metabolism (e.g., lactase deficiency) Hypophosphatasia Endocrine causes (adrenal insufficiency, thyrotoxicosis)
NEONATAL HYPOCALCEMIA	
Early onset (days 1–4)	Infant of diabetic mother Perinatal asphyxia Preeclampsia Prematurity Maternal hyperparathyroidism
Late onset (days 5–10)	Vitamin D deficiency Dietary phosphate load (e.g., cow's milk formula) Hypomagnesemia Transient PTH resistance Transient hypoparathyroidism Congenital hypoparathyroidism (see Table 28.2)

OMIM, Online Mendelian Inheritance in Man; *PTH*, parathyroid hormone.

levels of serum phosphorus, normal or elevated alkaline phosphatase (ALP) levels, and relative hypocalciuria.

Neonatal transient primary hyperparathyroidism can occur in response to low in utero maternal calcium concentrations. This more commonly occurs in lower birth weight infants but otherwise comes without clinical signs. Thorough investigation of the infant's mother will disclose previously known but inadequately treated hypoparathyroidism or clinically unsuspected hypocalcemia.[16] Decreased calcium transport from the hypocalcemic mother to the fetus leads to fetal hypocalcemia, with secondary increased secretion of fetal PTH, stimulating mobilization of calcium from the fetal skeleton and causing bone demineralization and subperiosteal resorption. This hyperfunction of the developing parathyroid glands may persist after birth, resulting in postnatal hyperparathyroidism with resulting transient moderate hypercalcemia. Postnatally, the skeleton avidly takes up calcium, and the bone lesions heal spontaneously within 4 to 6 months. Careful management of the plasma calcium concentration in hypoparathyroid women during pregnancy will prevent the development of functional hyperparathyroidism in the fetus.

Neonatal Severe Hyperparathyroidism and Familial Hypocalciuric Hypercalcemia

Inactivating mutations of the CaSR result in altered calcium sensing with inappropriate PTH production with respect to the serum calcium level. Hypercalcemia results from this altered set point, with higher calcium levels required to suppress PTH release, resulting in higher serum calcium levels. Most cases of neonatal severe hyperparathyroidism (NSHPT) and familial hypocalciuric hypercalcemia (FHH) are homozygous and heterozygous manifestations, respectively, of the same genetic defect in the *CASR* gene at 3q13.3–21 that inactivates the CaSR.[17,18] Despite this relationship, the clinical presentations of NSHPT and FHH are distinct. NSHPT is a severe and life-threatening disorder and usually presents in the first week of life. It likely begins in the fetal period, as suggested by the finding of generalized skeletal demineralization and localized erosions at the ends of long bones and subperiosteal resorption along the shafts of tubular bones. Parathyroid glands are enlarged and biochemical findings include markedly elevated serums levels of PTH and 1,25$(OH)_2$D, low-to-normal serum phosphorus, normal-to-high serum magnesium, elevated ALP, and inappropriately normal or low urinary calcium excretion. A family history of NSHPT or FHH in a sibling can provide strong confirmation of the diagnosis. Genetic testing is available for evaluation of *CASR* gene mutations and the less common *AP2S1* and *GNA11* gene mutations, which can cause NSHPT/FHH in some families.[19] By contrast, FHH is characterized by a relatively benign course and is generally asymptomatic despite mild-to-moderate hypercalcemia. It is most commonly discovered as an incidental finding or during the evaluation of relatives of patients with hypercalcemia. The hypercalcemia may be present at birth, or the diagnosis may be made during infancy and childhood. Circulating levels of PTH are normal or high-normal, but in the presence of hypercalcemia, they are inappropriately high, reflecting the higher set point of the parathyroid calciostat.

The treatment of hypercalcemia depends on the severity of the presentation. Hypercalcemia seen in newborns exposed to maternal hypocalcemia is often mild, transient, and self-limiting and responds to conservative management. Most patients with FHH lack symptoms and treatment is not required. By contrast, cases of severe hypercalcemia such as with life-threatening hypercalcemia of NSHPT require more aggressive treatments. In NSHPT, traditional management has involved subtotal parathyroidectomy, but appropriate medical treatments can preclude the need for surgical intervention in select cases. Initial therapies include maintenance of adequate hydration and avoiding excessive vitamin D and calcium. Intravenous isotonic fluids are the primary treatment for hypercalcemia, with the goal of increasing the urinary excretion of sodium because sodium and calcium clearance are closely linked during osmotic diuresis. Loop diuretics such as furosemide have traditionally been used to enhance calciuresis once hydration has been optimized. However, such agents must be used with caution because they may induce dehydration, which can actually worsen hypercalcemia through reduction in the glomerular filtration rate. In cases of NSHPT, hypercalcemia is often life-threatening and requires urgent medical intervention. Glucocorticoids are ineffective in the treatment of NSHPT-associated hypercalcemia. Calcitonin (2-4 U/kg every 6–12 hours) can be given by subcutaneous injection and can directly reduce osteoclastic bone resorption and lower serum calcium levels. However, calcitonin typically only works for a short time because tachyphylaxis develops quite rapidly. Nitrogen-containing bisphosphonates (e.g., pamidronate 0.5–1.5 mg/kg/dose × 3 days, zoledronic acid 0.015–0.05 mg/kg/dose), are analogs of inorganic pyrophosphate that adsorb to the hydroxyapatite matrix and can provide a more sustained inhibition of bone resorption and effectively lower serum and urinary calcium in NSHPT.[20] Calcimimetics such as cinacalcet could be potential therapeutic options in NSHPT because they increase CaSR sensitivity to calcium and can lower serum calcium levels. Although a trial of cinacalcet may be considered in infants with severe hypercalcemia related to *CASR* mutations, this approach must be pursued with caution because only limited information is available regarding its safety and efficacy in children with primary hyperparathyroidism.

PTH-Independent Hypercalcemia

Subcutaneous fat necrosis is common in neonates with complicated deliveries and may lead to hypercalcemia within days or weeks of birth. Affected infants often have a history of birth asphyxia and may have the added risk factor of receiving hypothermia treatments after asphyxia. Subcutaneous fat necrosis usually presents as reddish or purple subcutaneous nodules at sites of pressure such as the back, buttocks, and thighs or in areas of direct trauma that occur during a difficult birth process, such as forceps or vacuum extraction. Hypercalcemia results from excess circulating 1,25$(OH)_2$D levels produced by macrophages present within the granulomatous reaction to the necrotic fat. The hypercalcemia is compounded by calcium release from fat tissues and possibly from increased prostaglandin E activity, as well the expression of ectopic 1-α-hydroxylase activity that is not regulated by PTH, calcium, phosphorus, or 1,25$(OH)_2$D.[21] Hypercalcemia may persist for several weeks, and infants should receive a low calcium, reduced vitamin D diet until serum calcium levels normalize. Traditional management has involved isotonic intravenous fluids, loop diuretics, and glucocorticoids, but other therapies may be required in refractory cases. Glucocorticoids, most commonly prednisone at a dose of 1 to 2 mg/kg/day, may be effective in lowering serum calcium levels and decreasing inflammation of the fat necrosis but come with risk of adrenal suppression. Calcitonin can be used but requires multiple daily injections, and tachyphylaxis can develop. Bisphosphonates, either pamidronate or zoledronic acid, can be used for long-term management of hypercalcemia and should be strongly considered in refractory cases.

Williams syndrome (WS) is a sporadic multisystem disorder characterized by dysmorphic facies, cardiovascular disease (most commonly supravalvular aortic stenosis), “cocktail party” personality despite intellectual disability, and hypercalcemia in 15% to 45% of cases, although hypercalciuria may be more common.[22] WS has been associated with microdeletions of 7q11.13 and likely represents a contiguous gene deletion that typically includes the gene for elastin *(ELN)*, found in connective tissue of many organs. Hemizygosity of the *ELN* gene likely accounts for some of the features, such as cardiac defects and some of facial characteristics, but cannot explain the hypercalcemia. The majority of cases of WS are detected through a chromosomal microarray or fluorescent in situ hybridization of lymphocytes using a probe for *ELN*. Hypercalcemia typically occurs during infancy and usually resolves between 2 and 4 years of age. PTH is most commonly suppressed, and hypercalciuria may be seen even in children who do not have hypercalcemia. Nephrocalcinosis and soft-tissue calcifications may be seen in WS. Patients typically show exaggerated responses to pharmacologic doses of vitamin D and blunted calcitonin responses to calcium loading.[23,24] Elevated plasma concentrations of calcitriol have been reported in some patients despite low or normal circulating PTH levels.[25] Overall, studies have failed to show any consistent abnormality in vitamin D metabolism to explain the mechanism of hypercalcemia in WS.

Of note, some children with hypercalcemia have similar disturbances in vitamin D sensitivity but lack other phenotypic features of WS and do not have a 7q11.13 deletion. Termed “idiopathic infantile hypercalcemia” (IIH), biallelic loss-of-function mutations of *CYP24A1*, which encodes the key degradative enzyme in vitamin D catabolism, have been identified. These mutations likely account for the increased vitamin D sensitivity. With defective catabolic activity, elevated 25(OH)D and 1,25$(OH)_2$D are accompanied by hypercalcemia and hypercalciuria. The hypercalcemia in IIH usually resolves within the first few years of life, but persistent hypercalciuria is common. Inactivating mutations of *CYP24A1* have been increasingly identified in older children and adults with nephrocalcinosis and recurrent nephrolithiasis and present a long-term risk for chronic kidney disease.[26] 24,25$(OH)_2$D levels can be measured by certain commercial laboratories, with increased 25(OH)D/24,25$(OH)_2$D supporting the diagnosis of reduced *CYP24A1* activity. Genetic analysis of *CYP24A1* can confirm the diagnosis.

Treatment of hypercalcemia in WS and IIH includes a low calcium diet with elimination of vitamin D. Bisphosphonate therapy could also be considered in cases refractory to initial therapies of severe hypercalcemia. Case reports suggest rifampin, a powerful inducer of CYP3A4, with a dose of 10 mg/kg/day, can restore vitamin D homeostasis in individuals with *CYP24A1* mutations through an alternative pathway for vitamin D and can lead to inactivation of vitamin D metabolites.[27] Other options such as CYP27B1 inhibitors fluconazole and ketoconazole have also been used but have less desirable safety profiles.

Hypocalcemia

Neonatal hypocalcemia is the most typical form of hypocalcemia encountered by the pediatrician and is particularly common in the NICU. A fall of total calcium (adjusted for albumin) below 7.5 mg/dL or of ionized calcium below 4 mg/dL (1 mmol/L) is considered hypocalcemia in newborns, whereas in infants 3 months of age or younger, it is defined as total serum calcium less than 8.8 mg/dL or ionized calcium less than 4.9 mg/dL (1.22 mmol/L).

Infants with hypocalcemia will often lack specific signs or symptoms and may only be identified by lab studies. Potential symptoms can include neuromuscular irritability, which may manifest as myoclonic jerks, twitching, exaggerated startle responses, and seizures. Apnea, cyanosis, tachypnea, vomiting, laryngospasm, or heart failure may also be seen. Marked reduction in ionized calcium levels can lead to Q-Tc prolongation on electrocardiogram. Particular attention should be paid to high-risk infants such as preterm infants and infants of diabetic mothers. Different causes of neonatal hypocalcemia can be grouped according to the time of onset.

Early Neonatal Hypocalcemia

Early neonatal hypocalcemia occurs within the first 4 days of birth and represents an exaggeration of the physiologic fall in plasma calcium that occurs during the first 24 to 48 hours of life. Early neonatal hypocalcemia is thought to result from insufficient release of PTH from immature parathyroid glands or inadequate responsiveness of the renal tubules to PTH. An exaggerated rise in calcitonin secretion in premature infants may also contribute. Perinatal stress (e.g., difficult delivery), respiratory distress, prematurity, low birth weight, hypoglycemia, and maternal diabetes mellitus are common associated findings. Hypomagnesemia has been especially noted in infants of diabetic mothers but is typically mild and transient and is unlikely to play a prominent role in pathophysiology of neonatal hypocalcemia in these infants. Transient neonatal hypoparathyroidism may occur in infants exposed to maternal hypercalcemia in utero, as intrauterine hypercalcemia suppresses fetal parathyroid activity and leads to delayed responsiveness of parathyroid glands to postnatal hypocalcemia.

Late Neonatal Hypocalcemia

Late neonatal hypocalcemia typically occurs from days 5 to 10 after birth and is considered to be a manifestation of relative resistance of the immature kidney to PTH.[28] This leads to renal retention of phosphorus and hypocalcemia, with biochemical features that strongly resemble those of pseudohypoparathyroidism, albeit without the defects in the *GNAS* gene that characterize genetic forms of pseudohypoparathyroidism. The high phosphorus content of cow’s milk and many infant formulas can reduce intestinal calcium absorption. In addition, many infants are unable to excrete the high phosphate load and develop hyperphosphatemia, which in turn directly reduces serum calcium levels. PTH resistance also inhibits renal production of 1,25$(OH)_2$D, further reducing intestinal calcium absorption. Because human milk (HM) is low in phosphorus, breast-fed infants rarely develop late hypocalcemia. Neonatal vitamin D deficiency can also present with late onset hypocalcemia, especially in preterm infants (<28 weeks) and infants born to mothers with poor vitamin D status. Because neonatal vitamin D stores are exclusively derived from maternal stores in utero, hypocalcemia occurs after the first few days when intestinal absorption of calcium becomes dependent on vitamin D. Hypomagnesemia is a rare cause of late onset hypocalcemia because it causes resistance to PTH and impairs PTH secretion.

In most infants, neonatal hypocalcemia is transient and calcium levels normalize within a few weeks. Genetic causes of parathyroid dysfunction (i.e., congenital hypoparathyroidism) are more likely to underlie hypocalcemia and hyperphosphatemia that persist beyond 1 month of age. Depending on the severity of the defect in parathyroid development or function, hypoparathyroidism may present in the newborn period, may be transient or permanent, or may not manifest until the child is older. Causes of congenital hypoparathyroidism can be divided into defects that impair formation of the parathyroid glands or those that interfere with normal function of the parathyroid glands. In both cases, PTH levels will be inappropriately low in the context of hypocalcemia and hyperphosphatemia, with elevated fractional excretion of urinary calcium.

Advances in molecular genetic testing have led to the identification of a growing number of genes that are associated with hypoparathyroidism (Table 28.2). One of the best-known examples is the DiGeorge sequence (DGS), a common developmental field defect that includes cardiovascular malformations, hypoparathyroidism, thymic hypoplasia, and characteristic facial (e.g., low-set posteriorly rotated ears, short palpebral fissures, shortened philtrum) and palatal (submucous or overt cleft palate) dysmorphism as major clinical features. Hemizygous microdeletions within chromosome 22q11.21–23 are the most common cause of DGS and account for about 85% of cases. Hypoparathyroidism is present in up to 60% of patients with DGS but is highly variable and can range from severe, early-onset hypocalcemia with neonatal seizures to mild asymptomatic hypocalcemia that is only discovered later in childhood or even adulthood. Hypoparathyroidism is more common in DGS during the neonatal/infantile period, especially among those with congenital heart disease and receiving concomitant loop diuretics. Hypocalcemia may resolve during childhood, even in some children as young as 1 year of age, but hypoparathyroidism is often latent and can be unmasked during times of stress (e.g., surgery or severe illness), presumably due to insufficient parathyroid reserve. Hypoparathyroidism can be a component of the CHARGE (Coloboma, Heart defects, Atresia choanae, Restricted growth and development, Genital hypoplasia, and Ear anomalies/deafness) syndrome. More than 75% of CHARGE cases are due to heterozygous loss-of-function mutations in the coding region of the *CHD7* gene at chromosome 8q12.2. There is significant clinical overlap with DGS because both conditions display hypoparathyroidism, cardiac anomalies, cleft palate, renal anomalies, ear abnormalities/deafness, and developmental delay. In fact, hypoparathyroidism may be more common in newborns with CHARGE syndrome compared with newborns with DGS.

Hypocalcemia Management

The management of neonatal hypocalcemia depends on its presentation, which can vary from an asymptomatic biochemical finding to a life-threatening condition. Symptomatic hypocalcemia should be treated with IV calcium, preferably as 10% calcium gluconate administered as 100 to 200 mg/kg (1 to 2 mL/kg), with 9.4 mg elemental calcium per ml, given over 10 minutes. Additional boluses given every 4 to 6 hours may be required within several hours of initial therapy, but caution must be taken to avoid extravasation of IV calcium because it can cause severe soft-tissue necrosis. If prolonged IV calcium is required, IV calcium can be given as a continuous infusion (1–3 mg/kg/hour elemental calcium), best given with central access.

To maintain normal calcium levels, oral calcium (50–100 mg/kg/day) should be given, most commonly available as calcium carbonate suspension (40% elemental). Vitamin D should be provided at standard doses of 400 U/day (10 mcg), with higher doses in infants with vitamin D deficiency. In cases of refractory hypocalcemia or with suspected permanent hypoparathyroidism, calcitriol should be used (0.025–0.05 mcg/kg/day). Formula-fed infants with late-onset neonatal hypocalcemia and hyperphosphatemia benefit from additional calcium to increase the calcium:phosphorus ratio up to 3:1 or 4:1. Low-phosphate formulas such as Similac PM 60/40 or breast milk are preferred. For symptomatic patients requiring IV calcium, IV calcium can usually be weaned and/or discontinued within 48 hours, once oral therapy becomes effective. For cases of suspected transient hypocalcemia, calcium and/or calcitriol can be weaned over time. If unable to wean supplementation, a permanent cause should be considered. Patients

Table 28.2 Genetic Disorders Associated With Hypoparathyroidism

Disease	Gene	Locus	OMIM[a]	Associated Comorbidities
DISORDERS OF PARATHYROID GLAND FORMATION				
Isolated parathyroid aplasia	*GCM2* *SOX3*	6p23–24 Xq-26–27	*603716 *307700	
DiGeorge sequence Type 1 Type 2	 *TBX1* *NEBL*	 22q11.21–q11.23 10p13	 #188400 %601362	Thymic hypoplasia with immunodeficiency, cardiac defects, cleft palate, dysmorphic facies
CHARGE syndrome	*CHD7* *SEMA3E*	8q12.2 7q21.11	#214800 #214800	Cardiac defects, cleft palate, renal anomalies, ear abnormalities/deafness, developmental delay
Hypoparathyroidism, deafness, renal dysplasia	*GATA3*	10p14–15	#146255	Deafness and renal dysplasia
Hypoparathyroidism, retardation, dysmorphism (Sanjad-Sakati syndrome)	*TBCE*	1q42–43	#241410	Growth retardation, developmental delay, dysmorphic facies
Kenny-Caffey syndrome Type 1 Type 2	 TBCE FAM111A	 1q42–43 11q12.1	 #244460 #127000	Short stature, medullary stenosis, dysmorphic facies; type 1 with developmental delay and type 2 with normal intelligence
Smith-Lemli-Opitz syndrome	DHCR7	11q13.4	#270400	Microcephaly, abnormal male genital development, renal dysplasia, syndactyly, adrenal insufficiency, developmental delay
DISORDERS OF PARATHYROID HORMONE SYNTHESIS OR SECRETION				
PTH gene mutations	*PTH*	11p15.3-p15.1	*168450	
Autosomal dominant hypocalcemia Type 1 Type 2	 *CASR* *GNA11*	 3q13.3–q21.1 19p13.3	 #601198 #615361	Milder phenotype, may not present until second decade Hypercalciuria Short stature; no hypercalciuria

[a]OMIM indexing guide: * is a gene description, # is a phenotype with known molecular basis, and % is a phenotypic description or locus with unknown molecular basis.

OMIM, Online Mendelian Inheritance in Man; *PTH,* parathyroid hormone.

with hypoparathyroidism typically require calcium and calcitriol, especially during times of stress.

Biochemical Changes in Metabolic Bone Disease of Prematurity

There is no consensus clinical definition for MBD, but most experts consider it a condition of decreased bone mineralization, as demonstrated by biochemical data (elevated serum ALP, hypophosphatemia, secondary elevation in serum PTH), and/or radiographic evidence of demineralization or rickets.[7,29,30] These clinical signs typically develop within the first 6 to 16 weeks of life,[29] and in the long term, poor bone mineralization may contribute to fractures, respiratory compromise, and poor growth.

MBD develops in preterm infants secondary to deficient mineral intake with secondary bone resorption. The majority of VLBW infants require initial parenteral nutrition (PN) until enteral feeds can be advanced. Due to precipitation issues in PN, calcium and phosphorus intake is limited and does not compare to the equivalent high mineral accretion at the corresponding gestational age (GA) in-utero. Hypophosphatemia (with or without urinary phosphorus wasting) is the earliest biochemical finding, occurring within the first 7 to 14 days of life.[31,32] Phosphorus deficiency suppresses PTH secretion, limiting urinary phosphate wasting, but directly stimulates increased $1,25(OH)_2D$ concentrations that promote intestinal phosphorus reabsorption (and as a by-product, increase calcium reabsorption and can lead to secondary hypercalcemia, hypercalciuria, and nephrocalcinosis). ALP, present in osteoblasts, increases physiologically in the first several weeks of life as bone is formed. Although the degree of hyperphosphatasia does not appear to correlate with severity of demineralization, persistently elevated ALP after 6 weeks of life is suggestive of increased risk for osteopenia and MBD.[29]

Isolated serum calcium levels are generally unreliable markers of calcium stores and risk for MBD. Although some infants with primary hypophosphatemia may exhibit normal or elevated serum calcium secondary to PTH-mediated reabsorption, other infants may develop MBD in the setting of low total body calcium (i.e., premature infants on calcium-wasting loop diuretics with secondary hyperparathyroidism).[29] Hypophosphatemia and hypercalciuria were seen in VLBW infants fed unfortified breast milk, suggesting that there is inadequate mineral content in HM and that supplemental dietary intake of phosphorus is required for calcium retention in preterm infants.[33]

The differential diagnosis for osteopenia and/or fractures in a neonate is limited, and in addition to MBD, it includes genetic bone disorders and nonaccidental trauma. Skeletal hypomineralization noted during fetal life or immediately after birth is concerning for congenital or genetic underlying etiologies (Table 28.3).

Risk Factors for Metabolic Bone Disease

Infants born prematurely (<28 weeks' GA) and/or with VLBW (<1500 g) are at highest risk for MBD, taking into account the loss of in-utero mineral accretion. Postnatal pharmacologic exposures can place additive risk. Neonates receiving chronic loop diuretics are at risk for excessive calcium excretion and secondary hyperparathyroidism. Caffeine can interfere with bone marrow progenitor differentiation and induce urinary calcium wasting.[34–36] Glucocorticoids promote apoptosis of osteoblasts and osteocytes while disproportionately stimulating osteoclast differentiation.[37] Phenobarbital induces cytochrome P450 3A4 enzymes, which can contribute to hypocalcemia by hastening vitamin D degradation.[38] Long-term exposure to unfractionated heparin and prostaglandin have been associated with osteopenia and periosteal changes with increased bone resorption, respectively.[39–41]

Infants unable to tolerate enteral nutrition fortified with additional macronutrients and minerals are at risk for MBD, particularly those with intestinal failure (e.g., necrotizing enterocolitis) requiring prolonged PN (>4 weeks). Copper deficiency may occur in VLBW infants due to suboptimal nutrition[42] and causes bone demineralization very similar to that seen in MBD (putatively related to deficient copper cofactors required for bone matrix production). Risk factors for copper deficiency and MBD overlap (long-term PN dependence, malabsorption, short gut syndrome), although copper deficiency is additionally distinguished by factors such as neutropenia, anemia, and edema.[42,43] Additionally, VLBW infants fed either HM or preterm formula are known to develop serum zinc nadirs at 4 to 8 weeks postpartum.[44] Animal data suggest that zinc regulates osteoclastic bone resorption, either via direct local effect or by indirect effect mediated by osteoblasts.[45]

Biochemical Screening for MBD

No consensus guidelines exist regarding optimal timing of and screening algorithms for diagnosis of MBD. Preterm infants with MBD risk

Table 28.3 Differential Diagnosis for Osteopenia or Fractures in the Neonate

Disorder	Etiology	Characteristics
GENETIC BONE DISORDERS		
Osteogenesis imperfecta	Collagen I gene mutations and inadequate production of osteoid matrix	Severe osteoporosis, decreased bone density and mineralization, and multiple fractures
Hypophosphatasia	Loss-of-function mutations in the tissue-nonspecific isoenzyme of alkaline phosphatase	Very low serum alkaline phosphatase, hypercalcemia, slender "gracile" ribs with thoracic insufficiency, and associated pulmonary hypoplasia, complete demineralization, and fractures[84]
Neonatal severe primary hyperparathyroidism	Inactivating mutations of the calcium-sensing receptor	Marked hypercalcemia, elevated PTH, severe bone demineralization, fractures
TRAUMA		
Birth trauma	In context of appropriate delivery history; shoulder dystocia and/or instrument-assisted delivery commonly reported	Noted at birth; clavicular fractures most common[85–87]; fractures of the humerus,[88] femur,[89] and skull[90] also reported
Nonaccidental trauma		Diagnosis of exclusion

PTH, Parathyroid hormone.

factors should be screened. Given the low incidence of radiographic MBD among preterm infants >1500 g, there are minimal data to support screening in this group unless additional risk factors for bone disease exist (long-term PN, pharmacologic exposures, etc.).[8] Most experts recommend beginning testing between 4 to 6 weeks of life because neither radiographic rickets nor elevations in ALP manifest prior to 4 weeks of life, regardless of GA.[7,8,29] There are no official society recommendations guiding the composition of initial screening labs, although survey data of US level III NICUs suggests some homogeneity in initial lab testing (including ALP, serum phosphorus, and serum calcium).[46] Multiple groups have echoed this finding in recommendations to begin MBD screening algorithms with initial testing of serum calcium, serum phosphorus, ALP, and tubular reabsorption of phosphate (TRP),[7,29] with some advocating additional use of PTH and 25(OH) vitamin D[30,47] (Table 28.4). Once screening is initiated, repeat monitoring every 1 to 2 weeks is suggested (Fig. 28.3).

ALP is useful as a marker of overall bone remodeling, with higher values associated with MBD in preterm infants. There are four human ALP isoenzymes, although the tissue nonspecific form (present in liver, kidney, and bone) is most commonly measured clinically. The bone isoform predominates (up to 90% of total ALP) in both preterm and term infants[48,49] and correlates strongly with total ALP.[50] Both total and bone-specific ALP increase physiologically in the first several weeks of life, peaking at approximately 600 U/L by 6 weeks of life, though preterm infants fed with mineral-enriched formulas had lower peak ALP than those not receiving supplemented formula.[48] Measurement of the bone-specific isoform can be useful if the etiology of hyperphosphatasia is unclear (particularly if concurrent liver disease is present); however, measurement of the bone isoform does not improve diagnosis in routine MBD screening.[50] There is no defined cutoff value for MBD diagnosis, with varying studies identifying values of ALP above 500 to 900 IU/L as associated with MBD.[2,3,50,51] Backström et al.[50] demonstrated that total ALP greater than 900 IU/L had 88% sensitivity and 71% specificity for low bone mineral density (BMD), and the best screening performance was seen when combined with serum phosphorus less than 1.8 mmol (5.5 mg/dL), with a sensitivity of 100% and specificity of 70%.

Despite the association of elevated ALP and MBD, the correlation of elevated ALP and low bone mineralization is controversial. Among a cohort of ELBW infants,[2] ALP elevation was common, but ALP was not significantly different among infants with radiographic rickets vs osteopenia alone. Serial ALP measurements in preterm infants were not correlated with whole-body BMD as measured by DXA at term[52]; DXA measurements of regional BMD have shown limited[50] or no[53] correlation of ALP and BMD. Concurrent glucocorticoid use also impairs interpretation because steroids suppress ALP by inhibiting bone formation, and thus low ALP levels may be falsely reassuring.

Serum calcium and phosphorus are routinely screened. Infants with serum phosphorus levels below 5.5 mg/dL (1.8 mmol) are at increased risk for osteopenia and rickets.[54] This cutoff comes from a 1993 British study of 24 VLBW infants, 6 of whom (25%) developed severe radiographic rickets; of note, these infants received enteral feeds with mineral content far below that of current recommendations. Isolated serum calcium is an unreliable marker of total body calcium stores, given the ability for compensatory action of PTH to maintain normocalcemia in MBD.

TRP is useful for determining the degree of phosphate wasting in premature infants and is calculated with time-correlated phosphorus and creatinine in serum and urine with the following equation: TRP = (1 − [UPhos/UCr × SCr/SPhos] × 100).[29] Normal TRP in premature infants ranges from 78% to 91%; very high TRP (above 95%) suggests almost complete renal phosphate reabsorption secondary to insufficient intake. Renal phosphate losses are exaggerated in the most preterm infants (<28 weeks), whose renal phosphate excretion threshold is lower than in infants with moderate prematurity, and thus they have the potential for excessive excretion even if total body phosphorus is low.[7]

PTH can be elevated in MBD secondary to hypocalcemia and can be associated with hypophosphatemia due to urinary losses. Prolonged PTH elevation and osteoclast stimulation can cause pathologic bone resorption. A small pilot study in VLBW infants suggests a physiologic reference range for PTH in preterm infants (9.4–66 pg/mL; 1–7 pmol/L), similar to that of adults.[55] Rustico et al.[29] suggested that screening PTH levels >100 pg/mL should raise clinical concern for elevated risk of MBD. PTH may have value as an earlier biochemical marker for MBD; among preterm infants <1250 g screened for MBD at 3 weeks of life, Moreira et al.[56] found higher specificity and sensitivity of PTH (at maximal diagnostic accuracy of 180 pg/mL) of 71% and 88%, respectively, compared with ALP (at 660 U/L) with sensitivity of 29% and specificity of 93%. PTH and TRP may be useful in elucidating underlying mineral deficiencies; a low TRP with high PTH suggests underlying calcium deficiency whereas a high TRP with low or normal PTH suggests phosphorus deficiency. Of note, PTH may also be elevated in infants with chronic kidney disease and must be interpreted with caution in that population.

Vitamin D levels can be less frequently monitored unless certain conditions are present that may exacerbate deficiency, such as short bowel syndrome with malabsorption, phenobarbital therapy

Table 28.4 Screening Biochemical Markers in MBD

	Level of Interest	Key Points
ALP	>600 IU/L or trending up[2,48–51]	Total ALP isoform usually sufficient; can send bone-specific isoform if liver disease present
PTH	>100 pg/mL	Suggested reference range in preterm neonates: 9.4–66 pg/mL (1–7 pmol/L)[37]
Serum calcium	<8.5 or >10.5 mg/dL (<2.12 or >2.62 mmol/L)[54,91]	Isolated measurements of serum Ca are unreliable for estimation of total body Ca; levels often normal in MBD
Serum phosphorus	<5.5 mg/dL (1.8 mmol/L), although typically worse if <4 mg/dL[54]	Lower levels increase risk for osteopenia and rickets
TRP	>95% in setting of low phosphorus[49]	Normal range 78%–91% in preterm infants; high TRP denotes low urinary phosphorus wasting and may suggest need for supplementation
25(OH) vitamin D	<20 ng/mL denotes deficiency 20–30 ng/mL suggests insufficiency	Vitamin D levels usually normal in MBD

ALP, Alkaline phosphatase; *MBD,* metabolic bone disease of prematurity; *PTH,* parathyroid hormone; *TRP,* tubular reabsorption of phosphate.

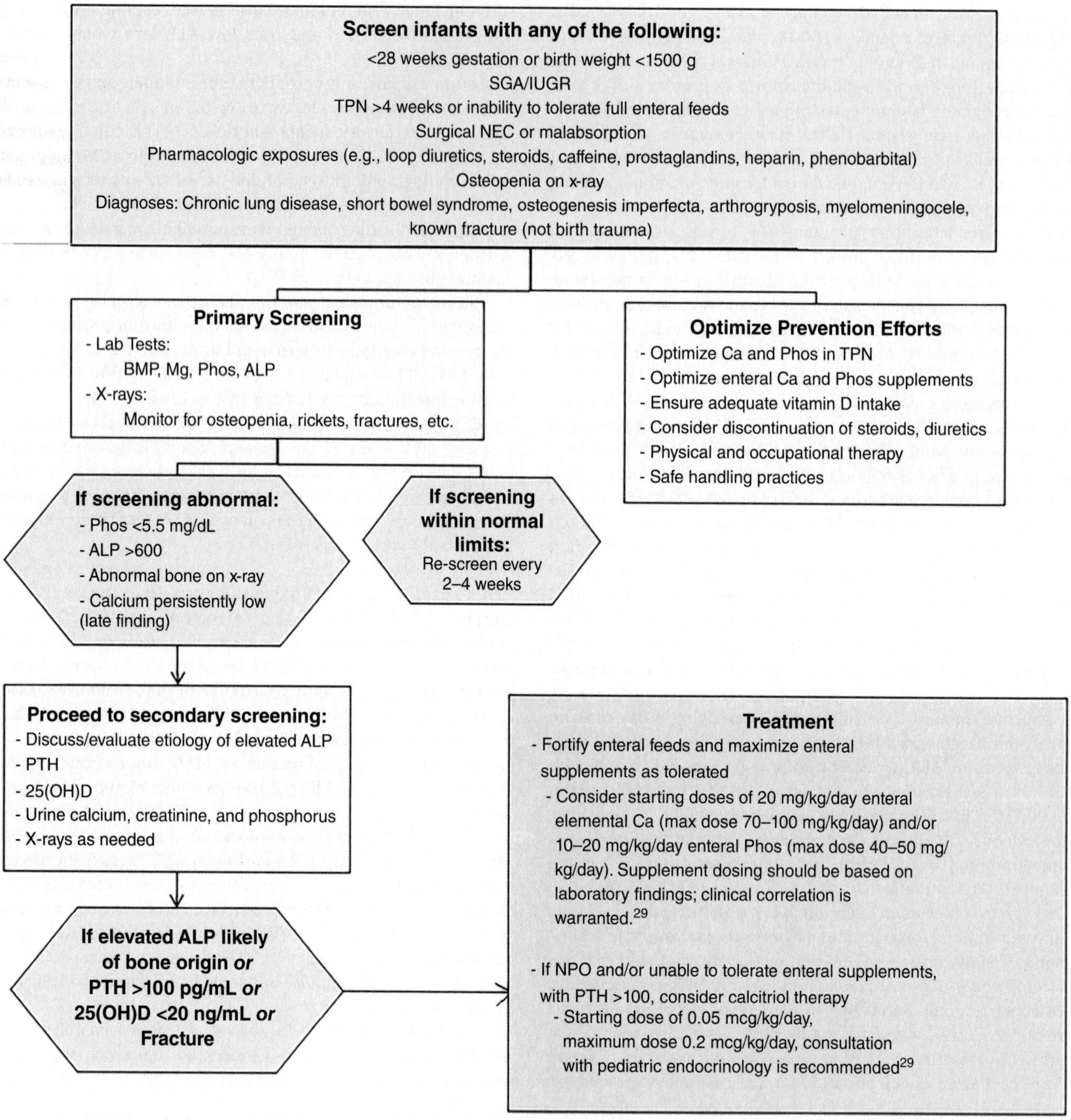

Screen infants with any of the following:
<28 weeks gestation or birth weight <1500 g
SGA/IUGR
TPN >4 weeks or inability to tolerate full enteral feeds
Surgical NEC or malabsorption
Pharmacologic exposures (e.g., loop diuretics, steroids, caffeine, prostaglandins, heparin, phenobarbital)
Osteopenia on x-ray
Diagnoses: Chronic lung disease, short bowel syndrome, osteogenesis imperfecta, arthrogryposis, myelomeningocele, known fracture (not birth trauma)

Primary Screening
- Lab Tests:
  BMP, Mg, Phos, ALP
- X-rays:
  Monitor for osteopenia, rickets, fractures, etc.

Optimize Prevention Efforts
- Optimize Ca and Phos in TPN
- Optimize enteral Ca and Phos supplements
- Ensure adequate vitamin D intake
- Consider discontinuation of steroids, diuretics
- Physical and occupational therapy
- Safe handling practices

If screening abnormal:
- Phos <5.5 mg/dL
- ALP >600
- Abnormal bone on x-ray
- Calcium persistently low (late finding)

If screening within normal limits:
Re-screen every 2–4 weeks

Proceed to secondary screening:
- Discuss/evaluate etiology of elevated ALP
- PTH
- 25(OH)D
- Urine calcium, creatinine, and phosphorus
- X-rays as needed

If elevated ALP likely of bone origin *or* PTH >100 pg/mL *or* 25(OH)D <20 ng/mL *or* Fracture

Treatment
- Fortify enteral feeds and maximize enteral supplements as tolerated
  - Consider starting doses of 20 mg/kg/day enteral elemental Ca (max dose 70–100 mg/kg/day) and/or 10–20 mg/kg/day enteral Phos (max dose 40–50 mg/kg/day). Supplement dosing should be based on laboratory findings; clinical correlation is warranted.[29]
- If NPO and/or unable to tolerate enteral supplements, with PTH >100, consider calcitriol therapy
  - Starting dose of 0.05 mcg/kg/day, maximum dose 0.2 mcg/kg/day, consultation with pediatric endocrinology is recommended[29]

Fig. 28.3 Proposed Algorithm for Surveillance, Screening, and Treatment of Metabolic Bone Disease in Preterm Infants.

(promotes increased catabolism via induction of cytochrome P450 3A4 enzymes), and increased risk of vitamin D intoxication (daily vitamin D intake >1000 U, often due to concurrent use of fortified breast milk/preterm formula and/or vitamin supplements).[29] Maternal vitamin D deficiency appears to influence development of neonatal vitamin D deficiency, but the degree to which GA influences neonatal vitamin D levels is unclear.[8,29,57] 25(OH)D (and not 1,25$(OH)_2$D) is most reflective of total body vitamin D stores and should be used for screening purposes.[8] Levels below 20 ng/mL indicate vitamin D deficiency.[29] However, 25(OH)D levels do not appear to differ between preterm infants with and without rickets or fractures.[57]

Role of Radiographic Screening for MBD

There is no consensus on the role of radiographs in screening and diagnosis of MBD. Classic radiographic findings of MBD include demineralization (particularly in long bone metaphyses) and thinning of bones (osteopenia) and can occasionally show rickets (frayed metaphyses, rachitic rosary) and fractures. Radiographic evidence of osteopenia or rickets typically appears later than biochemical changes, and it is estimated that bone must undergo significant (20%–40%) demineralization before osteopenia is apparent.[58] In the early 1980s, a three-stage grading system for radiographic rickets in preterm infants was developed based on signs of cortical thinning, rickets, and/or fractures,[59] but despite attempts to standardize interpretation of radiographs, this remains a subjective endeavor that ultimately reflects impressions of radiographic and clinical evolution over time.

Fractures are most commonly seen incidentally on radiographs obtained in the course of routine clinical care; when identified, additional long bone imaging should be undertaken to evaluate for occult fractures. Fracture rates vary per study, all with relatively small sample sizes. A 1987 report of 48 ELBW infants with wrist radiographs revealed that 21% had osteopenia, 54% had radiologic rickets, and 17% had spontaneous fractures.[1] In a more contemporary cohort of 230 ELBW infants published in 2014, 71 (31%) developed radiographic MBD, and of those infants, 24 (33%) had spontaneous fractures.[3]

Given the limitations of plain radiographs, DXA and ultrasonography have gained interest as potential screening tools, although they are currently primarily used for research purposes. DXA employs quick, low-dose ionizing radiation to measure calcium content and calculate BMD.[60] DXA appears to be the most accurate noninvasive method for evaluation of BMD in adults and children and may be particularly useful in infants because its accuracy is unaffected by GA or body length.[61] However, use is limited by the lack of established reference values for premature infants and of established cutoff BMD values for diagnosis of MBD. Potential limitations of DXA may include cost, portability for use in small and/or ill neonates, and two-dimensional measurement (and thus estimation) of BMD.[62] Quantitative ultrasound is also under investigation as a potential tool for estimation of neonatal bone mineral status (measured at standard anatomic locations, i.e., forearm or tibia), with benefits including common availability, portability, and lack of ionizing radiation. However, reference ranges for ultrasound parameters are undefined, and challenges exist in standardizing data from different anatomic sites and ultrasound machines.[62]

Prevention of MBD

Mitigating risk of MBD requires avoidance of established risk factors, along with optimization of nutrition and mineral intake. Minimizing prolonged loop diuretic, glucocorticoid, and/or caffeine therapy may limit mineral wasting and bone resorption, but benefits of these medications for treating other chronic sequelae of prematurity must be weighed with their risks in potentiating MBD.

Nutritional interventions for prevention of MBD focus on provision of calcium and phosphorus to simulate in-utero bone accretion rates. Full enteral feeds are preferred because PN limits optimal calcium and phosphorus delivery due to solubility and precipitation issues. Fortification of enteral feeds (either HM or formula) is essential to provide adequate calcium and phosphorus content for premature infants. The Ca:P ratio is 2:1 in HM and 1.7:1 to 1.8:1 in preterm formulas (mg:mg), which accounts for increased mineral bioavailability and higher phosphorus absorption from HM compared with formula. Various sources have identified optimal enteral Ca:P ratios (mg:mg) in formulas ranging from 1.5:1 to 1.7:1[8,63] to 1.6:1 to 1.8:1.[64] Evidence suggests that slightly lower Ca:P ratios in formula best mimic in-utero mineral accretion ratios, with the higher 2:1 ratio providing insufficient phosphorus without significantly increased calcium accretion.[64] HM and preterm formula fortified to 24 kcal/oz at a volume of 160 mL/kg/day provides 180 to 220 mg/kg calcium and 100 to 130 mg/kg phosphorus as well as 200 to 400 IU vitamin D per day, reaching daily mineral content goals for premature infants. In contrast, unfortified breast milk at 20 kcal/oz provides only 37 mg/kg calcium and 21 mg/kg phosphorus, or about 20% of total daily mineral requirements.[8] Infants with a birth weight <1800 g should receive fortified HM or formula (this recommendation is made based on weight rather than GA, given that infants who are small for gestational age [SGA] also have low bone mineral content).[65] Clinicians may consider defortification of breast milk or conversion to transitional formula at around 36 weeks' corrected GA or 2000 g, although this decision ultimately depends on growth. Continuation of highly fortified preterm formula in an infant weighing greater than 3000 g has raised concerns for potential overdosing of nutrients, particularly of vitamin A.

PN is a clearly identified risk factor for MBD in preterm infants. Based on available evidence, the American Society for Parenteral and Enteral Nutrition (ASPEN) recommends PN prescriptions with high-dose calcium and phosphorus.[66] The European Society for Pediatric Gastroenterology, Hepatology and Nutrition (ESPGHAN) recommends that premature infants on PN receive calcium at 64 to 140 mg/kg/day (1.6–3.5 mmol/kg/day) and phosphorus at 50 to 108 mg/kg/day (1.6–3.5 mmol/kg/day) at a Ca:P mass ratio of 1.7:1.[67] Pelegano et al.[68] investigated mineral retention at various Ca:P ratios (1.3:1, 1.7:1, and 2:1) and determined that the 1.7:1 Ca:P ratio in PN provided superior retention of calcium and phosphorus while minimizing phosphaturia. Aggressive provision of amino acids in PN in the first week of life is important for promotion of rapid growth and avoidance of early nitrogen deficit, but at high levels (mean intake >2 g/kg/day) has been associated with hypophosphatemia (likely due to concomitant phosphorus consumption in ATP and nucleic acids).[69] Long-term exposure to aluminum-containing components in PN[67] has been associated with reduced bone mineralization, potentially by aluminum accumulation and interference at sites of new bone formation.[66] Hip bone mineral content at adolescence in former preterm infants was significantly lower (8%) among individuals with neonatal aluminum intake above the median.[70]

Initially, intestinal calcium and phosphate absorption appears to occur in a vitamin D–independent fashion in preterm infants. Vitamin D comes to play a crucial role in mineral absorption, but it is unclear when this shift occurs.[5,7] Optimal dosage is of some controversy, with the American Academy of Pediatrics recommending 200 to 400 IU/day for infants <1500 g and 400 IU/day when infants reach full enteral feeds or >1500 g.[8] European guidelines recommend intake of 800 to 1000 IU/day, although they do not specifically address vitamin D provision at these levels in ELBW infants.[71] Koo et al. randomized 62 VLBW infants to either 200, 400, or 600 IU/day of vitamin D for 3 to 4 weeks with no difference in outcomes, including serum vitamin D levels and growth parameters.[72] Backström et al.[73] randomized 39 infants (<33 weeks' GA) to receive either 200 IU/kg/day (up to 400 IU) or 960 IU/day until 3 months of life, with no significant differences between groups in serum vitamin D concentration or bone mineral content at 3 and 6 months' corrected age. Finally, Tung et al.[74] retrospectively examined serum vitamin D levels among 152 infants receiving protocolized supplementation of 400 IU/day vitamin D. Not only was there no association between vitamin D intake and serum 25(OH)D levels, but both insufficient (<20 ng/mL, 5.9% of infants) and excessive (>100 ng/mL, 8.6% of infants) serum vitamin D levels persisted among this cohort.

Aside from nutritional optimization, physical therapy has been implemented as a strategy to promote bone mineralization. In utero, skeletal loading forces are acquired via fetal movements against the uterine wall. A systematic review studying the effects of daily physical therapy in preterm infants concluded that some data suggested short-term weight gain, linear growth, and bone mineralization benefits. However, long-term effects were unclear and data were insufficient to recommend standard implementation of physical therapy programs for preterm infants.[75]

Treatment of MBD

Mineral supplementation should be initiated based on biochemical findings consistent with MBD. Low serum phosphorus levels, with adjunctive high TRP with low/normal PTH, suggests phosphorus deficiency with compensatory attempts at renal absorption. Phosphorus deficiency should be treated when serum levels fall below 4 mg/dL (some consider treating if levels are below 5.5 mg/dL if elevated ALP is also present). Potassium phosphate is the supplement of choice, at a starting dose of 10 to 20 mg/kg/day and maximal dose of 40 to 50 mg/kg/day; preterm infants are generally prescribed the intravenous formulation of potassium phosphate for enteral use given the lack of oral formulations of other phosphorus salts.[8,29]

Calcium supplementation is also often required for treatment of MBD. Serum calcium levels can be normal or high even in the setting of bone resorption in neonates, and deficiency is suggested by secondary elevations in PTH with low TRP. Enteral supplement options include calcium glubionate and calcium carbonate, with a recommended starting dose of 20 mg/kg/day of elemental calcium and the upper limit of the dosing range at 70 mg/kg/day,[8] although in our experience some infants require even higher doses (up to 150 mg/kg/day) to normalize biochemical data. When initiating mineral supplementation, one should ensure that overall mineral intake continues to target the goal 2:1 Ca:P ratio in enteral intake, but some children require altered Ca:P ratios to normalize their biochemical markers.

Proper supplement administration is critical for ideal absorption. Calcium and phosphorus supplements should not be coadministered because they will precipitate with one another. Furthermore, calcium and phosphorus supplements should not be given concurrently with enteral feeds because they will precipitate with phosphorus or calcium (respectively) within the milk or formula.[30] Discontinuation of mineral supplements may be considered once serum levels normalize and ALP is steadily trending down below 500 IU/L.

In a subset of patients who develop secondary hyperparathyroidism while on PN, with inability to tolerate enteral supplements, calcitriol ($1,25[OH]_2D$) therapy may be of use. Calcitriol can be given either enterally or intravenously at equivalent dosing (starting at 0.05 mcg/kg/day, up to 0.2 mcg/kg/day).[29,76] Rustico et al.[76] retrospectively studied 32 premature infants who received calcitriol for MBD treatment, diagnosed by osteopenia on x-rays and PTH >100 pg/mL. After calcitriol therapy (median duration 207 days at median dose 0.08 mg/kg/day), these infants had significantly decreased PTH and increased calcium, phosphorus, and TRP, with only three infants developing hypercalcemia (which resolved after dose reduction).

Postdischarge Management

Preterm infants remain at risk for growth failure postdischarge. They are often converted from preterm formula to 22 kcal/oz transitional fortification of HM or formula at a weight of approximately 2000 g or prior to discharge. ASPEN guidelines do not clearly define how long fortification should be continued postdischarge[66]; ESPGHAN recommends continuation of fortified HM or formula until at least 40 weeks' corrected age, and possibly up to 52 weeks' corrected age if growth is suboptimal.[77] With increasing volumes of fortified feeds (and minerals therein) taken as infants age, ongoing mineral supplementation may be unnecessary.[8,78] If a former VLBW infant is exclusively breastfeeding at discharge, a serum ALP should be checked 2 to 4 weeks postdischarge, with mineral supplementation considered if ALP >800 to 1000 IU/L.[8] Infants who are discharged on mineral supplementation for established MBD should continue to have laboratory monitoring (serum calcium, phosphorus, ALP, PTH) every 2 to 4 weeks.[29]

Long-Term Outlook for Growth and Bone Mineralization

MBD appears to self-resolve slowly with time, although there are limited long-term data on bone mineralization outcomes, particularly in the most preterm infants. Long-term follow-up of a large cohort of preterm infants born in the 1980s (mean GA of 31 weeks) demonstrated persistent effects on long-term linear growth, with peak ALP >1200 IU associated with significantly shorter height at age 9 to 12 years.[79] SGA preterm infants may have additive risk of growth stunting.[80] Although preterm infants do demonstrate catch-up bone mineralization (as measured by DXA) by 9 to 10 years of life,[81,82] VLBW adults have lower BMD and 2.4-fold increased odds of osteopenia/osteoporosis, compared with term SGA and appropriate for gestational age (AGA) controls.[83]

However, results of these follow-up studies must be taken in the context of the current state of neonatal care. Cohorts of VLBW infants followed in the 1980s, or even in the early 2000s, are likely to be intrinsically different than their contemporaries. With increasing resuscitation of infants at the limits of viability (22–24 weeks' gestation), the proportion of ELBW infants surviving to NICU discharge (and at highest risk for MBD) is likely to increase. Ongoing research is needed to inform development of consensus guidelines for MBD screening and treatment and to oversee long-term follow-up of preterm neonates.

Conclusion

Neonates (particularly preterm infants) are at risk for disorders of mineral metabolism, related to dramatic shifts in mineral physiology during the transition from fetal to extrauterine life. Metabolic bone disease is an important complication of prematurity that results from loss of transplacental mineral accretion in the third trimester and requires diligence in laboratory monitoring and nutritional optimization to promote long-term bone health and improve growth potential.

CHAPTER 29

Disorders of Sex Development for Neonatologists

John Fuqua

KEY POINTS

1. Disorders of sex development (DSD) is an umbrella term referring to the large collection of conditions in which establishment of chromosomal, gonadal, or anatomic sex development is atypical.
2. Estimates of the prevalence of DSD vary widely, but it is likely 1 in 5000 to 6000 in the general population.
3. The genetic regulation of sex determination and differentiation involves a complex cascade of transcription factors beginning with the SRY gene and its major target, SOX9.
4. Current nomenclature for DSD is mechanistically based and includes categories of 46,XX DSD, 46,XY DSD, and sex chromosome DSD. Within these categories, individual diagnoses are specified based on their genetic, enzymatic, or receptor defect.
5. The evaluation and management of an infant with DSD should be overseen by a multidisciplinary DSD team.
6. Using panels of targeted genes permits a genetic diagnosis in about 20% to 40% of infants with DSD, with higher diagnostic rates in cases of 46,XY DSD.
7. The most common identifiable cause of DSD is congenital adrenal hyperplasia due to 21-hydroxylase deficiency.
8. When assigning a gender to an infant with DSD, the overarching goal is to make an assignment that will match the individual's gender identity.
9. Although there is a paucity of data to inform the gender assignment decision, there is sufficient information for some of the more common or well-defined conditions.

Definition

Disorders of sex development (DSD) was coined in 2005 as an umbrella term referring to the large collection of conditions in which establishment of chromosomal, gonadal, or anatomic sex development is atypical.[1] Many, but not all, individuals included in the DSD rubric have genital ambiguity at birth. The term is controversial among those affected, and some have called for it to be changed to differences of sex development or abolished entirely. Nevertheless, it remains in widespread use as an overarching term encompassing conditions leading to over- or undermasculinization of a fetus.

Epidemiology

Congenital malformations of the genitalia, including isolated cryptorchidism and mild hypospadias, occur in approximately 1 in 200 to 300 live born infants,[2] but these conditions usually do not constitute DSD. Estimates of the prevalence of DSD range widely, depending on the definition and which specific disorders are included. A reasonable estimate is 1 in 5000 to 6000, although some have placed the number as high as 2%.[3,4] Although chromosomal disorders such as Turner and Klinefelter syndromes may be included in the spectrum of DSD, the most common cause of genital ambiguity is congenital adrenal hyperplasia (CAH), the vast majority of which is caused by deficiency of the 21-hydroxylase enzyme. CAH is estimated to occur in 1 in 14,000 to 15,000 live births.[5]

Embryology

In order to understand the pathophysiology and the medical evaluation of the infant with a DSD, a firm grasp of normal embryology is critical.

Embryology of the Gonadal Ridge

At approximately 5 weeks of gestation in the human embryo, the gonadal ridge appears on the surface of each mesonephros (primitive kidney). The gonadal ridge is morphologically undifferentiated in both 46,XX and 46,XY embryos, hence it is frequently termed the bipotential gonad (Fig. 29.1). Germ cells arise from the wall of the yolk sac and migrate toward the undifferentiated gonad, arriving at 5 to 6 weeks' gestation.[6]

Embryology of the Testis

The earliest morphologic changes specific to the testis occur at about 6 weeks of gestation.[7] At this time, Sertoli cells begin to differentiate within the primitive sex cords.[8] The Sertoli cells cluster around the germ cells as the primitive sex cords develop into the seminiferous tubules. The appearance of Sertoli cells is generally recognized to be the first sign that the gonad will become a testis. Approximately 1 week after Sertoli cells appear, Leydig cells differentiate from the mesenchyme between the primitive sex cords and become functional soon after their appearance.

Embryology of the Ovary

In the absence of testis determination, ovarian determination occurs. The earliest sign that the bipotential gonad will become an ovary occurs at approximately 7 weeks' gestation, when the cortical cords form. Germ cells become incorporated into these cords and enter prophase I of meiosis at approximately 10 weeks' gestation. The cortical cords subsequently break up into clusters of cells surrounding each germ cell, forming ovarian follicles. The precursors of the follicular cells are of the same lineage as the Sertoli cells of the testis.[9]

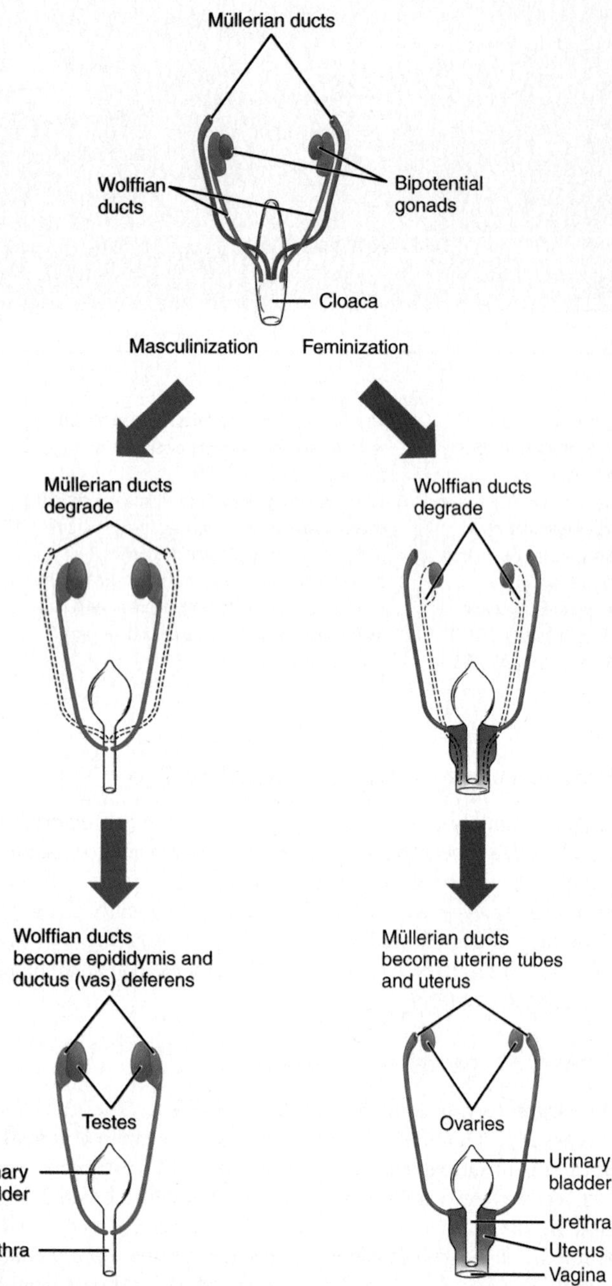

Fig. 29.1 Formation of Bipotential Gonads, Wolffian Ducts, and Müllerian Ducts. After testis determination, testosterone and anti-Müllerian hormone are produced, leading to masculinization of the internal genitalia, with involution of the Müllerian ducts. The Wolffian ducts proliferate, resulting in the formation of the epididymis, vas deferens, and seminal vesicles. In the absence of testis determination, the Wolffian ducts degenerate and the Müllerian ducts form the fallopian tubes, uterus, and posterior vagina. (Courtesy OpenStax College, https://commons.wikimedia.org/wiki/File:2915_Sexual_Differentation-02.jpg.)

Endocrinology of the Fetal Testis

Sertoli cells produce anti-Müllerian hormone (AMH), beginning at 7 weeks' gestation.[10] AMH acts to disrupt development of the Müllerian ducts (see below). At 8 weeks' gestation, the fetal testis starts to produce testosterone. Leydig cells require stimulation by human chorionic gonadotropin (hCG) to produce testosterone in appropriate amounts. The effects of hCG are mediated via the luteinizing hormone (LH)/CG receptor on the Leydig cell. Pituitary LH is not initially required for testosterone production, and indeed, it is not secreted from the pituitary until 11.5 weeks' gestation.[11] In response to hCG, the first of a series of enzymatic steps resulting in testosterone synthesis occurs (Fig. 29.2). Secreted testosterone subsequently diffuses into target cells, where it may act directly or be enzymatically converted by 5α-reductase to the more potent androgen, dihydrotestosterone (DHT). Placental aromatase serves the important role of protecting the mother from virilization due to placental transfer of fetal androgens. Conversely, aromatase also protects XX fetuses from the masculinizing effects of placentally transferred maternal androgens.

Embryology of the Internal Ducts and External Genitalia

By 6 weeks of gestation, all embryos possess two sets of ducts (see Fig. 29.1). The Wolffian ducts, precursors of the male system, originate as the excretory ducts of the mesonephros.[8] The Müllerian ducts, precursors of the female system, form lateral to the Wolffian ducts at 6 weeks of gestation. The Müllerian ducts meet in the midline to form the uterine canal.

In the XY fetus, testis determination occurs, and AMH secretion begins. In the presence of AMH, the Müllerian ducts involute. The timing of this is critical, because the ducts become insensitive to the effects of AMH after 8 weeks of gestation.[12] Testosterone leads the Wolffian ducts to differentiate into the epididymis, vas deferens, and seminal vesicles.

In the XX fetus, no testosterone or AMH is produced early in gestation. The Wolffian ducts regress if they are not exposed to androgen by 10 weeks of gestation. In the absence of AMH exposure early in gestation, the Müllerian ducts proliferate. The superior portion of the Müllerian ducts eventually differentiates into the fallopian tube, whereas the uterine canal differentiates into the uterus, cervix, and upper third of the vagina.[13]

The external genitalia of a 46,XY embryo prior to 8 weeks of gestation cannot be distinguished from those of an XX embryo. Bilateral ridges of tissue known as the urethral folds meet anteriorly to form the genital tubercle. The labioscrotal folds develop lateral to the urethral folds. Under the influence of androgen, the genital tubercle elongates to form the phallus. The urethral folds begin to fuse, starting posteriorly and moving anteriorly along the ventral surface of the phallus to form the penile urethra. The labioscrotal folds increase in size and fuse in the midline to form the scrotum. The differentiation of the external genitalia in the male is complete by 12 to 13 weeks gestation. If androgen secretion is delayed past this time, development of the external genitalia cannot be completed, even in the face of normal androgen levels. Masculinization of the external genitalia in XY fetuses occurs under the influence of DHT.

In the XX embryo, few changes occur in the appearance of the external genitalia after 6 weeks' gestation. The genital tubercle enlarges slightly to form the clitoris, whereas the urethral folds form the labia minora and the labioscrotal folds develop into the labia majora.

Genetic Regulation of Sex Determination and Sex Development

Sex determination refers to the path by which the bipotential gonad forms either a testis or ovary, whereas sex development includes the subsequent formation of internal and external genital structures. These processes are mediated by a complex network of genes required

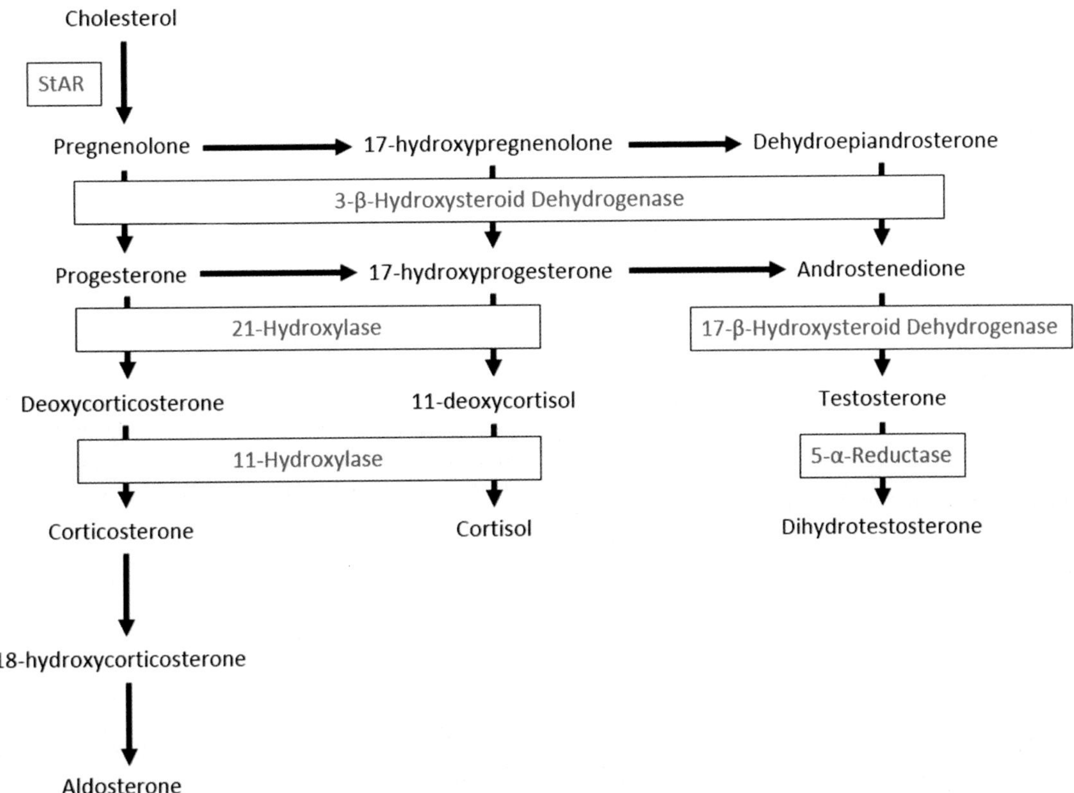

Fig. 29.2 Biosynthesis of Aldosterone, Cortisol, Testosterone, and Dihydrotestosterone. Abnormalities in StAR, 3β-hydroxysteroid dehydrogenase, 21-hydroxylase, 11-hydroxylase, and 17α-hydroxylase/17,20 lyase (not shown) lead to forms of congenital adrenal hyperplasia (CAH). Mutations in the genes encoding 17β-hydroxysteroid dehydrogenase type 3 and 5α-reductase interfere with androgen synthesis and are not forms of CAH. *StAR,* Steroidogenic acute regulatory protein.

for formation and maintenance of the gonadal ridge/bipotential gonad and testis or ovarian determination, which require a fine balance between genetic factors. This has been described as "a story of opposing forces and crucial alliances but, although the winning team takes all, its rule can be surprisingly tenuous."[14,15] Although in many cases the specific genes and their interactions in humans are known, much of our understanding comes from mouse models.

Normal formation of the gonadal ridge is critical for both testis and ovarian determination. Although much of the genetic regulation remains unknown, the WT1 gene is a critical component of this mechanism. WT1 activates the NR5A1 gene, which produces a protein known as steroidogenic factor 1 (SF-1). Both WT1 and SF-1 proteins are critical for activation of NR0B1, producing the DAX-1 protein. Maintenance of the gonadal ridge prior to testis determination requires a balance of this genetic interaction, likely involving additional genetic inputs.[14]

Beginning at 6 weeks of gestation, SRY expression commences in the XY fetus. Initiation of SRY expression likely involves input from GATA4 and its cofactor FOG2, which upregulate SRY expression. WT1 appears to stabilize SRY mRNA. The MAPK pathway also appears to have a role in SRY regulation.[16]

The major target of SRY appears to be SOX9. In turn, SOX9 activates a cascade of genetic events comprising dozens of genes leading to formation of a functioning testis. This activation of SOX9 is enhanced by SF-1, which also serves to activate AMH expression.[17] Interestingly, SF-1 is also critical for expression of a number of genes encoding steroidogenic enzymes and for genetic control of gonadotropin releasing hormone, LH, and FSH. While SOX9 is the mediator of SRY's role in sex determination, abnormal overexpression of other SOX genes may mimic SOX9 action, leading to testis development in an XX individual.[18]

An alternative genetic cascade exists for ovarian determination, although it is less well understood than that for the testis. WNT4 gene expression promotes ovarian differentiation, and abnormalities of WNT4 and altered WNT4 activity in response to RSPO1 mutation may interrupt ovarian development.[14] Genetic variants in NR5A1 encoding SF-1 may interfere with the WNT pathway and normal ovarian development.[19] FOXL2 is another gene that plays a role in ovarian function by suppressing SOX9 activity, thus maintaining ovarian differentiation.[20]

Nomenclature and Etiologies of Disorders of Sex Development

Historical terminology for DSD were fraught with controversy, as many people considered the terms to be pejorative. The nomenclature was revised at a consensus conference held in Chicago in 2005.[1] Although this nomenclature has also proved to be controversial in some quarters, it remains the standard. The new terminology has replaced categories such as "pseudohermaphroditism" and "hermaphroditism" with more mechanistically oriented language such as "sex chromosome DSD," "46,XY DSD," and "46,XX DSD."[1] Within these categories, individual diagnoses are specified based on their genetic, enzymatic, or receptor defect.

46,XX Disorders of Sex Development

This category includes conditions in which a 46,XX fetus is exposed to inappropriately high concentrations of androgens (Table 29.1). The source of these androgens may include aberrantly formed

Table 29.1 Etiologies of Disorders of Sex Development

I. 46,XX DSD
A. Virilizing congenital adrenal hyperplasia[a]
1. 21-hydroxylase deficiency
2. 11β-hydroxylase deficiency
3. 3β-hydroxysteroid dehydrogenase deficiency
B. 46,XX testicular DSD
C. 46,XX ovotesticular DSD
D. Maternal androgen exposure
E. Fetal aromatase deficiency
F. 46,XX gonadal dysgenesis
II. 46,XY DSD
A. 46,XY gonadal dysgenesis
1. Complete gonadal dysgenesis (Swyer syndrome)
2. Partial gonadal dysgenesis
B. 46,XY ovotesticular DSD
C. Leydig cell hypoplasia
D. Defective testosterone biosynthesis
1. Feminizing congenital adrenal hyperplasia
a. StAR deficiency (lipoid adrenal hyperplasia)
b. 3β-hydroxysteroid dehydrogenase deficiency
c. 17α-hydroxylase/17,20 lyase deficiency
2. 17β-hydroxysteroid dehydrogenase deficiency
E. 5α-reductase deficiency
F. Androgen insensitivity syndrome
1. Complete androgen insensitivity syndrome
2. Partial androgen insensitivity syndrome
G. Persistent Müllerian duct syndrome
III. Sex chromosome DSD
A. 45,X/46,XY mosaicism
B. Turner syndrome[a]
C. Klinefelter syndrome[a]
IV. Other abnormalities of sexual differentiation
A. Syndromes of multiple congenital anomalies

[a]Not considered as a disorder of sex development by some groups.

testicular tissue, excessive adrenal or placental androgen production, or exogenous exposure. A subcategory includes isolated abnormal ovarian development.

Congenital Adrenal Hyperplasia

CAH accounts for the majority of cases of masculinization of female infants. CAH is caused by a group of autosomal recessive disorders of adrenal steroidogenesis in which there is deficient activity of one of the enzymes necessary for the production of cortisol (see Fig. 29.2). Cortisol deficiency increases production of ACTH, leading to adrenal hyperplasia and overproduction of adrenal androgens. Virilizing CAH may be caused by 21-hydroxylase deficiency, 11β-hydroxylase deficiency, or 3β-hydroxysteroid dehydrogenase deficiency (3β HSD).

21-Hydroxylase deficiency accounts for more than 90% of CAH and is the most important diagnosis to consider in an infant with genital ambiguity. Based on newborn screening studies, the classical form of the disease occurs in 1 in 10,000 to 15,000 live births.[21] In the classical form there is masculinization, with or without salt-wasting. The salt-wasting form accounts for 75%, whereas the simple-virilizing form accounts for approximately 25% of cases.[5] Diagnosis is supported by increased baseline and adrenocorticotrophic hormone (ACTH)-stimulated 17-hydroxyprogesterone and androstenedione and increased serum androgens and may be confirmed by genetic testing. Prenatal diagnosis is available via molecular analysis of the CYP21A2 gene.

11β-Hydroxylase deficiency accounts for about 5% of cases of CAH. Although salt-wasting may occur in the newborn period, it is less common than in 21-hydroxylase deficiency. In later infancy and childhood, hypertension may occur due to accumulation of 11-deoxycorticosterone and its metabolites.[22]

3β-Hydroxysteroid dehydrogenase deficiency is the least common form of CAH. Clinical presentation is usually that of mild clitoromegaly due to accumulation of dehydroepiandrosterone (DHEA) and its peripheral conversion to testosterone via the type I 3βHSD enzyme, with salt-wasting.[23]

46,XX Testicular DSD

46,XX testicular DSD is a condition in which testicular tissue develops in the presence of a 46,XX karyotype. Although 80% of affected individuals have Y-chromosome sequences translocated to the X chromosome, the remaining 20% do not have any identifiable translocations.[24] In the absence of SRY translocation, other genes have been implicated, including SOX9,[25] NR5A1,[19] WT1,[26] and NR0B1,[27] all genes involved in the early stages of gonadal ridge and testis formation. Clinical presentation is variable, with most having normal male genitalia, but 10% to 15% exhibit some form of genital ambiguity or hypospadias.

Ovotesticular DSD

Ovotesticular DSD refers to the presence of both testicular tissue with seminiferous tubules and ovarian tissue with ovarian follicles in the same individual. Patients may have a 46,XX, 46,XY, or mosaic karyotype. In a review of 228 cases, 46,XX was the most common karyotype (70.6%), chromosomal mosaicism was the second most common karyotype (20.2%), and 7% had a 46,XY karyotype.[28] There may be various combinations of ovaries, testes, and ovotestes, but most common is an ovary and an ovotestis. Genitalia are almost always ambiguous. The genetics of this condition are incompletely understood, but there is overlap with the causes of 46,XX testicular DSD.[29] Diagnosis is made by biopsy of the gonads and examination of external and internal genitalia.

Exposure to Maternal Androgens

Masculinization of female external genitalia has occurred after exposure to endogenous or ingested maternal androgens during pregnancy.[30,31] This may occur due to ingestion of androgenic progestational compounds, maternal androgen-secreting tumors, or maternal CAH. Placental aromatase activity protects fetuses against typical concentrations of maternal androgens, but it may be insufficient to prevent masculinization in pathologic situations.

Aromatase Deficiency

Placental aromatase deficiency may lead to an accumulation of maternal and fetal androgens, such as DHEA, which are then converted to androstenedione and testosterone by placental 3βHSD and 17βHSD enzymes. Virilization of both the infant and the mother is usually seen in this extremely rare condition. Biochemically, testosterone and androstenedione levels are elevated whereas estrogen levels are very low or undetectable.

Gonadal Dysgenesis

46,XX gonadal dysgenesis occurs when ovarian development does not proceed normally and is characterized by streak gonads with normal internal and external female genitalia, delayed puberty with poorly developed secondary sex characteristics, and primary amenorrhea.[8] Although these girls have streak gonads, similar to those with Turner syndrome, they lack the phenotypic features of Turner syndrome. The genetic etiology of 46,XX gonadal dysgenesis is heterogeneous but may be due to mutations in the FSH receptor and in genes related to ovarian maintenance.[32]

46,XY Disorders of Sex Development

This category includes conditions in which a 46,XY fetus experiences insufficient androgen effect for normal masculinization. This may result from abnormal testicular formation, androgen biosynthetic deficits, or receptor abnormalities. A subcategory includes the isolated persistence of Müllerian structures.

Gonadal Dysgenesis

Gonadal dysgenesis in 46,XY individuals may be complete or partial. In 46,XY complete gonadal dysgenesis (Swyer syndrome) there is defective testis determination. This leads to streak gonads without germ cells, persistence of Müllerian structures, absence of Wolffian structures, and female external genitalia.[33] Patients with 46,XY complete gonadal dysgenesis thus have normal female genitalia, delayed puberty with poorly developed secondary sex characteristics, and primary amenorrhea.[33]

46,XY partial gonadal dysgenesis is defined by incomplete testis determination with varying degrees of dysgenesis. Patients usually present with ambiguous genitalia at birth and have a mixture of Wolffian and Müllerian duct structures due to deficient testosterone and AMH production.[33]

The etiology of 46,XY gonadal dysgenesis has been attributed to mutations in SRY, specific SRY-related genes, and many others, although a genetic diagnosis is currently made in only about 40% of cases.[34,35] Gonadal tumors occur in approximately 25% to 30% of patients with 46,XY gonadal dysgenesis, and arrangements should be made for the removal of gonadal tissue when the diagnosis is made.[36]

46,XY Ovotesticular DSD

As discussed in the section on 46,XX DSD, ovotesticular DSD indicates that an individual carries both testicular and ovarian tissue. Although 46,XX is the most common karyotype, 7% have a 46,XY complement.[28] Genitalia are almost always ambiguous. Ovarian tissue and female sex organs can function normally, because pregnancies have occurred; however, seminiferous tubules are often atrophic and spermatogenesis is extremely rare. Gonadal tumors occur in approximately 10% of patients with 46,XY or 46,XX/46,XY ovotesticular DSD.[36]

Leydig Cell Hypoplasia

Leydig cell hypoplasia is due to an abnormal LH/CG receptor causing unresponsiveness to LH and hCG. This results in insufficient production of testosterone and incomplete or absent differentiation of male external genitalia. Affected patients have 46,XY karyotypes with phenotypes varying from normal female external genitalia to hypospadias and undescended testes.[37] Müllerian structures are not present. Levels of testosterone and its biochemical precursors are low or undetectable, LH levels are elevated, and there is no steroid hormone response to hCG stimulation testing.

Abnormal Androgen Biosynthesis

Deficiencies of enzymes involved in the biosynthesis of testosterone and DHT are all associated with abnormal differentiation of male genitalia. However, AMH production from the otherwise normal testes leads to involution of Müllerian structures with absence of a uterus, fallopian tubes, and vagina.

StAR Protein Deficiency

Steroidogenic acute regulatory protein (StAR) facilitates the movement of cholesterol to the inner mitochondrial membrane to be available to many of the steroidogenic enzymes. 46,XY patients with StAR deficiency (lipoid congenital adrenal hyperplasia) present with ambiguous or female genitalia. Both 46,XY and 46,XX infants develop hyponatremia and hyperkalemia due to aldosterone deficiency.[38]

Cytochrome P450c17 (17α-Hydroxylase/17,20 Lyase) Deficiency

Mutations of the gene encoding this multifunctional enzyme impair steroid formation in the adrenals and gonads, leading to incomplete masculinization of 46,XY infants with ambiguous or female genitalia. Depending on the specific gene mutation and the affected enzymatic activity, some patients will have feminizing CAH.[39] Salt-wasting is not present, and some affected patients may be hypertensive.

3β-Hydroxysteroid Dehydrogenase Deficiency

Complete absence of 3βHSD results in aldosterone, cortisol and testosterone deficiency. The clinical manifestations of 3βHSD deficiency in XY infants vary from female external genitalia with salt-wasting crises if there is complete deficiency to ambiguous genitalia without salt-wasting if there is partial deficiency.[8]

17β-Hydroxysteroid Dehydrogenase-3 Deficiency

17β-Hydroxysteroid dehydrogenase-type 3 (17βHSD-3) is responsible for the conversion of androstenedione to testosterone in the testis. Mutations in the gene for the type 3 isozyme cause undermasculinization of male genitalia due to inadequate testosterone levels in utero.[40] The diagnosis is suggested by an increased androstenedione/testosterone ratio and elevated LH level.

5α-Reductase Deficiency

5α-Reductase deficiency due to mutations in the SRD5A2 gene impairs the conversion of testosterone to DHT, the more potent androgen, leading to undermasculinization and ambiguous or female-appearing external genitalia, because normal differentiation of the external genitalia is dependent on DHT.[41] Laboratory data indicating this diagnosis include normal to increased testosterone and LH levels, low levels of DHT, and an increased ratio of testosterone to DHT.

Androgen Insensitivity Syndrome

Mutations of the androgen receptor result in complete or partial insensitivity to androgens (testosterone and DHT) and abnormal male sexual differentiation. Hundreds of specific mutations have been described, causing complete or partial androgen insensitivity syndrome (AIS) depending on the resulting function of the receptor.

Patients with complete AIS have normal female external genitalia at birth. Müllerian structures are absent due to normal testicular AMH secretion. Unless there is a family history of AIS, discordant prenatal gender testing, or palpable testes or inguinal masses in infancy, the diagnosis is usually not made until the patient presents with primary amenorrhea in adolescence. In contrast, partial AIS may present with a variety of phenotypes. A classification system for partial AIS has been developed consisting of seven grades ranging from normal male phenotype (grade I) to normal female phenotype without pubic or axillary hair (grade VII).[42] At puberty, increased androgen levels may lead to some maturation of the genitalia, anabolic growth, and spermatogenesis in individuals with partial AIS; however, the degree of virilization at puberty is variable.[43] Laboratory investigations in newborns with AIS reveal normal male testosterone and AMH concentrations. LH may be normal or elevated.

Persistent Müllerian Duct Syndrome

A defect of either the gene encoding AMH or its receptor leads to insufficient production or action of AMH. Affected individuals have normally masculinized genitalia, well-developed but bilaterally undescended testes, normal male internal genitalia, and a uterus and fallopian tubes.[44] Otherwise, there are no obvious phenotypic features, and affected infants are detected when undergoing evaluation or surgical repair of an inguinal hernia or undescended testes. With AMH gene defects, serum AMH levels are low; conversely, with receptor defects, AMH levels are elevated.

Sex Chromosome Disorder of Sex Development

This DSD category includes conditions in which the complement of sex chromosomes is abnormal. Although Turner syndrome (45,X and variants), and Klinefelter syndrome (47,XXY and variants) are sometimes included in this grouping because of abnormal gonadal development, individuals with these conditions have otherwise normal reproductive anatomy and will not be discussed in this chapter.

45,X/46,XY Karyotypes

45,X/46,XY mosaic karyotypes may lead to gonadal dysgenesis or an ovotesticular DSD. The term "mixed gonadal dysgenesis" is used to refer to individuals with a dysgenetic gonad on one side with a normal testis on the other. 45,X/46,XY individuals may have male, female, or ambiguous genitalia depending on the degree of testis differentiation. However, in a series reported by Chang et al., 95% of 92 prenatally diagnosed patients with 45,X/46,XY mosaicism had normal male genitalia.[45] This patient population also carries a 15% to 20% risk of gonadal tumors,[36] and prophylactic gonadectomy should be considered in selected cases.

Syndromes and Multiple Congenital Anomalies

There are several known syndromes of multiple congenital anomalies that are associated with ambiguous genitalia or abnormal sex development. This section is not meant to be all-inclusive but only to briefly outline some of these anomalies.

Renal and genital anomalies often are related. Denys-Drash syndrome, caused by a mutation in WT1, is associated with 46,XY gonadal dysgenesis and genital ambiguity, progressive renal failure, and Wilms tumor.[46] Also caused by a mutation in WT1, Frasier syndrome is associated with 46,XY karyotype, streak gonads, female external genitalia, progressive glomerulopathy, and gonadoblastoma.[47] Smith-Lemli-Opitz syndrome is characterized by mental retardation, hypotonia, facial dysmorphisms, limb anomalies including syndactyly, and upper and lower genitourinary tract anomalies including hypospadias, cleft scrotum, and cryptorchidism.[48] Syndromes of multiple congenital anomalies that feature renal anomalies, such as VACTERL[49] and CHARGE[50] syndromes, are also associated with abnormal sexual differentiation. Some chromosomal deletion syndromes, including 4p-, 11q-, and 13 q-, are associated with hypospadias and cryptorchidism.

Evaluation of the Infant With a Disorder of Sex Development

The evaluation of an infant with abnormal sexual differentiation or ambiguous genitalia is an endocrinological emergency. The initial contact with the family must be established in a timely yet sensitive and confidential manner. The complex medical work-up required for diagnosis must be well coordinated with rapid initiation of appropriate consultation including endocrinology, urology, genetics, neonatology, and social work/clergy/patient support. Large medical centers often have multidisciplinary DSD teams. Various algorithms have been proposed to guide the evaluation of infants with DSDs. Fig. 29.3 shows an approach to the evaluation based initially on the infant's anatomy and karyotype, with further testing to focus on specific disorders. Other algorithms incorporate genetic testing in addition to anatomic and biochemical features.[51]

History

The family and pregnancy histories should be obtained as soon as possible. Family history of other affected infants, deaths in early infancy, or infertility may be significant. Pregnancy history of exposures (drugs, chemicals, or androgens) or of virilization during pregnancy is important to establish.

Physical Examination

A careful and objective physical examination must be performed (Fig. 29.4). Dysmorphic features or evidence of other anomalies should be noted. Midline structures, face, thorax, abdomen, limbs, anus, and spine should be carefully inspected. The abdomen should be carefully palpated for masses. The presence or absence of palpable gonads in the scrotum or inguinal canal is important to note. The genitalia should be examined in a careful, objective manner, with specific attention to phallic size and structure, location of the urethral meatus, visualization of a vaginal orifice or posterior labial fusion, presence of pigmentation and rugation of the labioscrotal folds, and the placement of the anus. It is important to note whether the genitalia are symmetric.[52]

Diagnostic Studies

Imaging studies are very helpful in evaluating the internal genital structures and the kidneys. A pelvic ultrasound should be obtained in an urgent manner in a patient undergoing work-up for ambiguous genitalia and awaiting sex assignment. A genitogram may be useful in evaluating the urethra and the presence of structures such as a urogenital sinus or vagina. These imaging studies will help document the presence of a uterus or other Müllerian structures, the lack of which indicates AMH secretion from testicular tissue. Direct cystoscopy by a pediatric urologist may also help define the anatomy and has largely replaced genitograms.

Laboratory studies should include a rapid karyotype sent to a reliable laboratory as soon as possible. Electrolytes are important to

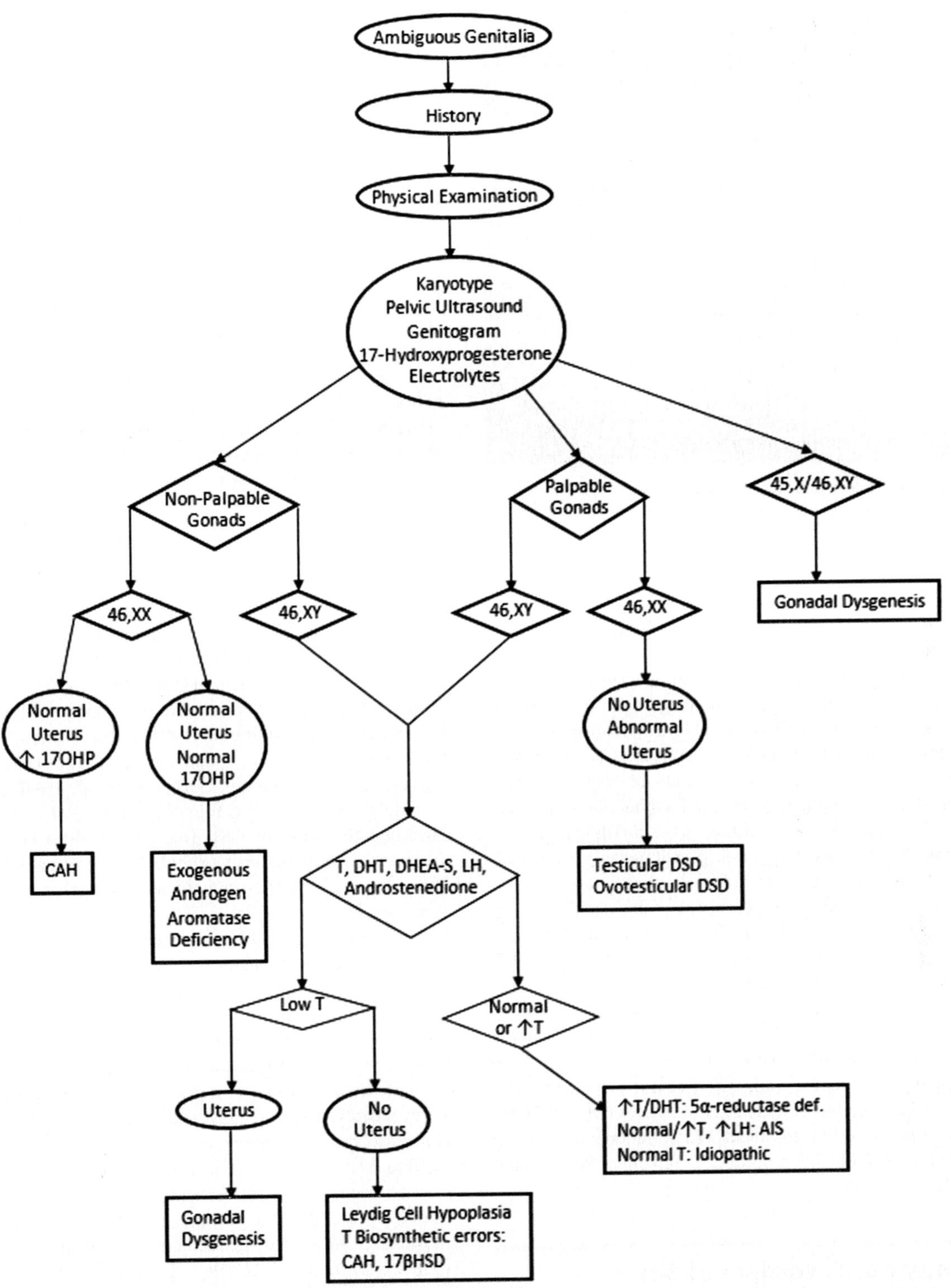

Fig. 29.3 Algorithm for the Diagnosis of Disorders of Sex Development Based on Karyotype and the Presence/Absence of Palpable Gonads. *17βHSD,* 17β-Hydroxysteroid dehydrogenase; *17OHP,* 17-hydroxyprogesterone; *AIS,* androgen insensitivity syndrome; *CAH,* congenital adrenal hyperplasia; *DHEA-S,* dehydroepiandrosterone sulfate; *DHT,* dihydrotestosterone; *DSD,* disorder of sex development; *LH,* luteinizing hormone; *T,* testosterone.

obtain after 24 hours of life, looking for salt-wasting as evidence of adrenal insufficiency. Because 21-hydroxylase deficiency CAH is the most frequent cause of DSD, a 17-hydroxyprogesterone level is indicated. If gonads are palpable, the infant is more likely to have a 46,XY karyotype, and additional adrenal and testicular hormones including DHEA, androstenedione, testosterone, and DHT are indicated for diagnosis. ACTH stimulation testing is useful if adrenal hormone levels are borderline or nondiagnostic.[53] Other useful diagnostic studies include measurement of gonadotropin levels and AMH. AMH levels can be used to indicate the presence of testes and Sertoli cell function.[54] hCG stimulation testing is useful to evaluate Leydig cell function and 5α-reductase activity.[53] When the above evaluation fails to indicate a diagnosis, gonadal dysgenesis and ovotesticular DSD should be considered. These two diagnoses are dependent on

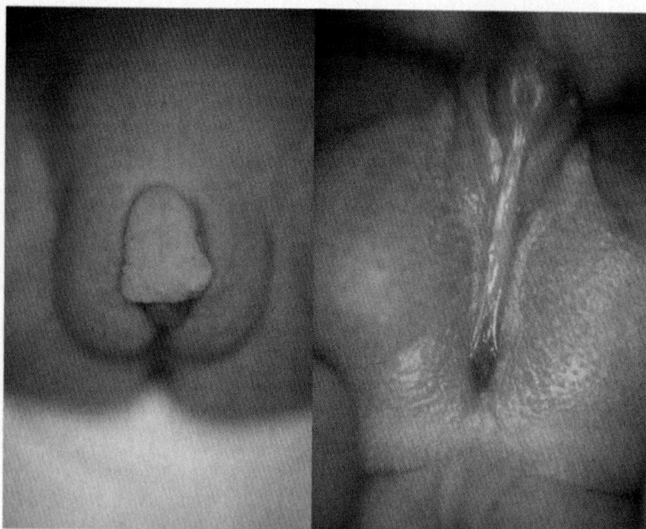

Fig. 29.4 Genitalia of an Infant With 45,X/46,XY Mosaicism. The left panel shows an enlarged phallic structure with mildly rugated labioscrotal folds. The right panel shows the same infant with the phallus lifted to demonstrate chordee, posterior labial fusion, and a single urogenital orifice located on the perineum.

histologic examination of gonadal tissue, hence surgical exploration may be necessary.[52]

If the anatomic and biochemical evaluation suggests a specific etiology, genetic testing may be confirmatory, such as mutational screening/sequencing of the CYP21B gene for 21-hydroxylase deficiency CAH or the androgen receptor gene for partial AIS. However, the genetic evaluation of 46,XX or 46,XY, gonadal dysgenesis, ovotesticular DSD, 46,XX testicular DSD, or an idiopathic DSD is difficult. In these cases, large panels comprising dozens of potential candidate genes are available. Use of existing panels permits a genetic diagnosis in about 20% to 40% of cases, with higher diagnostic rates in cases of 46,XY DSD.[55] Chromosomal microarrays may be useful for identifying copy number variants, particularly in cases of syndromic gonadal dysgenesis, where diagnostic rates are 20% to 30%.[56] Although whole exome sequencing approaches show promise, they remain imperfect, in part due to difficulty determining the significance of variant sequences. One study identified pathologic or likely pathologic variants in 25% of patients with a 46,XY DSD using whole exome sequencing.[57] Microarrays and whole exome sequencing offer the advantage of being able to identify novel genes not previously known to play roles in sex development. Whole genome sequencing is now being applied to the diagnosis of DSD and offers the potential to increase diagnostic accuracy.

Management of Disorders of Sex Development in the Neonatal Period

It has become standard practice for larger institutions to use a team-based approach to the diagnosis and treatment of infants born with DSDs. Such teams usually comprise neonatologists, endocrinologists, urologists, and clinical psychologists but may also include medical geneticists, radiologists, chaplains, and nursing.[58] The need for a team approach was laid out in the 2005 Chicago consensus meeting and was reinforced in more recent publications.[59] The role of the multidisciplinary team includes education and support for families as well as diagnosis and development of treatment plans. Continuing education of team members is critical as diagnostic techniques steadily improve and standard practices evolve. Family involvement, education, psychosocial support, and counseling is critical for a successful outcome. Parents should play the major decisional role regarding gender assignment, with input from the multidisciplinary team.

The most common identifiable cause of DSD is congenital adrenal hyperplasia due to 21-hydroxylase deficiency. Early diagnosis of this condition is critical, because approximately 75% of newborns with classic CAH have the salt-wasting form due to insufficient aldosterone secretion. This leads to progressive hyponatremia and hyperkalemia with volume loss, hypotension, and shock. The accompanying glucocorticoid deficiency compounds the hypotension and may also result in hypoglycemia. Babies with the simple virilizing form of CAH do not present with salt loss, but in the first week after birth this group cannot be easily distinguished from those with salt loss. The electrolyte abnormalities may develop within the first 1 to 2 weeks after birth, potentially before results of diagnostic studies have been received. Hence, careful monitoring of electrolytes and glucose is advisable until a CAH diagnosis is excluded. Male infants with salt-losing CAH have no obvious anatomic abnormalities but will develop similar electrolyte and hemodynamic problems. Fortunately, routine newborn screening often identifies boys with CAH before clinical illness is apparent. A special case is the phenotypic male infant with bilaterally nonpalpable testes. Such infants may be genetic females with severe virilization and are at high risk for salt-losing crises. Because premature infants and sick newborns normally have higher levels of 17-hydroxyprogesterone than healthy term infants, they may have falsely positive CAH newborn screens. False positive rates on newborn screens may be reduced by stratifying infants based on gestational age and/or birth weight and in one report ranged from 0.03% to 0.5% of normal infants.[60] Although testing protocols are designed to minimize false negative tests, this does occur, with recently reported false negative rates of 1.5% to 15.7%. Thus a negative newborn screen does not necessarily exclude CAH, particularly if the clinical picture is consistent. Fortunately, most missed cases have the simple virilizing form.[60]

If there is a high index of suspicion for CAH, glucocorticoid and mineralocorticoid treatment may be started, but only after diagnostic laboratory studies have been drawn. Typical laboratory findings include a significantly elevated serum 17-hydroxyprogesterone (usually >5000 ng/dL) and elevated androstenedione and testosterone levels. Initial treatment in newborns consists of hydrocortisone 25 mg divided into 3 doses if given enterally or into 4 doses if given intravenously. The dose may be decreased if the baby is doing well clinically. Typical maintenance hydrocortisone doses are in the range of 10 to 20 mg/m^2 body surface area per day. Other glucocorticoids may be used, but hydrocortisone is recommended for long-term therapy. Mineralocorticoid replacement is required in babies with salt-losing CAH and often recommended in those with the simple virilizing form. This is usually administered enterally as fludrocortisone, 0.1 to 0.2 mg daily. High doses of hydrocortisone provide adequate mineralocorticoid activity. Thus fludrocortisone may not be required during stress dose hydrocortisone therapy. Oral salt supplementation is also recommended, usually in the range of 3 to 6 mEq/kg/day.

The assignment of gender to a newborn with a DSD is a major decision that is often a source of significant distress for parents. The overarching goal is to assign a sex of rearing that will match the individual's gender identity. Unfortunately, very little is known about biologic and psychosocial influences of gender identity. Interestingly, the most predictive factor for gender identity in a person with a DSD is the sex of rearing.[61] That being said, prenatal and perhaps postnatal androgen exposure does appear to influence the development of male gender identity.

There is a paucity of data to inform the gender assignment decision, in part related to the relative rarity of some of the diagnoses subsumed under the DSD nosology and in part related to biologic variation. We do have sufficient information for some of the more common or well-defined conditions.[62] Of infants with a 46,XY DSD, those without genital masculinization generally have a female gender identity as adults. Specifically, girls with complete androgen insensitivity syndrome (CAIS) and 46,XY complete gonadal dysgenesis (Swyer syndrome) nearly universally identify as female.[62] Babies with these conditions are phenotypically female and usually would only be identified if there were prenatal gender testing or if inguinal masses were noted in the case of CAIS. In girls with CAH, although male gender role behavior patterns are common, 95% percent of 46,XX infants with CAH who are raised as female have a female gender identity as adults, and babies in this category should be assigned female in the absence of other factors. However, it is estimated that 5% of these infants will experience gender dysphoria by adulthood.[63]

In 46,XY DSD conditions other than CAIS and Swyer syndrome, gender assignment is more problematic. Compared with the normal population, individuals with 46,XY DSD have a much higher prevalence of gender dysphoria. One study of a clinic population showed a 15% rate of dissatisfaction with assigned gender.[64] In another study of a larger population of adults with DSD, 3.3% had changed genders.[61] Most studies confirm that the most reliable predictor of adult gender identity is the assigned gender at birth.[61,62] Two 46,XY DSD conditions that deserve special mention are 5α-reductase and 17β-hydroxysteroid dehydrogenase deficiencies. Both conditions are related to a block in the biosynthesis of androgen and are associated with a more consistent male gender identity than other 46,XY DSDs. Of persons raised in the female gender, 56% to 63% of those with 5α-reductase deficiency and 39% to 64% of those with 17β-hydroxysteroid dehydrogenase changed to the male gender, usually in adolescence or young adulthood.[65]

Conclusion

DSD refers to a group of uncommon conditions leading to abnormal genital development. An understanding of the differential diagnosis and pathophysiology requires familiarity with the developmental biology of the reproductive system. The approach to diagnosis includes a careful assessment of historical and physical features as well as imaging, laboratory, and genetic testing. Working together with family, multidisciplinary DSD teams can effectively determine a diagnosis and recommend appropriate treatment. Gender assignment is a critical decision that may be clear cut but is often difficult.

SECTION

6 Infections

OUTLINE

CHAPTER 30

Early-Onset Sepsis

Karen M. Puopolo

KEY POINTS

1. Early-onset sepsis (EOS) is defined by blood and/or cerebrospinal fluid culture-confirmed infection occurring 0 to 6 days after birth.
2. Incidence is highest among preterm infants, particularly those born with low gestational ages and with birth weight <1500 g.
3. Pathogenesis commonly involves ascending colonization of the uterine compartment with maternal flora, with subsequent colonization of the fetus and transition to invasive infection in utero or in the hours and days after birth
4. Risk factors include low gestational age, duration of rupture of membranes, colonization with high-risk organisms such as group B *Streptococcus* (GBS), and evidence of maternal intraamniotic infection, such as intrapartum maternal fever.
5. The most common causative organisms are GBS and *Escherichia coli.*
6. Newborns with EOS may be well-appearing at birth, but ~90% have signs of infection within 24 hours after birth.
7. Ampicillin and gentamicin are currently the recommended choice for empiric antimicrobial therapy. Broader-spectrum therapy should be considered for critically ill newborns at highest risk of EOS, until culture results are known.

Introduction

Early-onset sepsis (EOS) among term infants is a low-incidence but potentially fatal complication of birth. Among preterm, particularly low-gestation, very low birth weight (VLBW, birth weight <1500 g) and extremely low birth weight (ELBW, birth weight <1000 g) infants, EOS is more common and a significant contributor to morbidity and mortality. EOS is defined by isolation of a pathogenic species from blood or cerebrospinal fluid (CSF) culture in the first week after birth. Among continuously hospitalized, primarily preterm infants, EOS diagnosis is limited to infection occurring ≤72 hours after birth. For these infants, risk factors for infection and microbiology of infection both transition away from the perinatal period to reflect nosocomial factors around this time frame. Among term infants, EOS diagnosis is most commonly made at <48 hours after birth; for example, 95% of EOS caused by group B *Streptococcus* (GBS) occurs at <48 hours of age.[1] Rarely, otherwise healthy infants may be discharged from the birth hospital and develop EOS in the first week after birth.[2] Bacteria are the primary cause of EOS; fungal species are very occasionally isolated.[3,4]

Epidemiology

The incidence of EOS is inversely related to gestational age at birth. National surveillance conducted by the Centers for Disease Control and Prevention (CDC) demonstrates that overall US national incidence was constant from 2005 to 2014 at 0.7 to 0.8 cases/1000 live births.[3] Among infants born at ≥37 weeks' gestation, the incidence is approximately 0.5 cases/1000 live births.[3–5] In contrast, prospective surveillance among centers participating in the Eunice Kennedy Shriver National Institute of Child Health and Human Development Neonatal Research Network (NRN) from 2015 to 2017 found an incidence of 18.5 cases/1000 live births occurring at 22 to 28 weeks gestation and 6.2/1000 among those born at 29 to 33 weeks' gestation.[4] This study observed an incidence of 13.9 cases/1000 live birth among VLBW infants.

Pathophysiology

The pathogenesis of EOS begins with invasion of the intraamniotic compartment with bacterial species from maternal sources. The pathologic processes of EOS were described in seminal papers by Benirschke and Blanc, who described the "amniotic infection syndrome" as the cause of congenital bacterial sepsis and pneumonia, contrasting this entity with the transplacental, hematogeneous origin of congenital viral infection.[6,7] Rarely, pathogenic bacteria infecting the maternal bloodstream may cause EOS via the transplacental route. The classic example is EOS caused by *Listeria monocytogenes,* a foodborne pathogen with placental tropism that can cause fetal infection via the maternal bloodstream.[8] Most commonly, EOS pathogenesis begins by ascending colonization via the cervix into the uterine compartment with bacteria normally resident in the maternal gastrointestinal and genitourinary colonizing flora. Transition from fetal colonization to invasive infection via membranous surfaces then occurs, either in utero or after birth. Fetal infection may also occur in utero by aspiration of infected amniotic fluid. This pathogenesis primarily proceeds during labor and is promoted by membrane rupture but rarely can occur before the onset of labor.

Risk Factors

Factors that promote or reflect intraamniotic infection (IAI) may be used to assess risk of EOS. Preterm birth and low birth weight are strong risk factors for infection: IAI infection is a significant cause of preterm birth itself,[9,10] and the preterm infant is immunologically more vulnerable to bacterial infection compared with those born at term gestation.[11] Neonatal immune defenses derive primarily from innate immune responses including transplacentally acquired, maternally derived antibody.[11] Effective immune response to the majority of organisms causing EOS require neutrophil and complement-mediated defense mechanisms that are poorly developed among preterm infants. Preterm infants are also relatively deficient in maternally derived antibodies, which are primarily transferred from mother to fetus late in the third trimester. At the other end of the gestational age spectrum, postterm infants born after 41 weeks' completed gestation are also at slightly higher (~1.6-fold) risk of EOS compared with those born at 37 to 40 weeks' gestation.[5] The etiology of increased risk associated with postterm birth is unclear, but changes in the integrity of the amniotic membranes and cervical mucosa as well as placental senescence may contribute to decreased barrier defenses to infection.

Multiple intrapartum characteristics are also predictive of EOS. Duration of rupture of membranes (ROM) is a risk factor for EOS among term and late preterm infants,[5] as longer ROM promotes ascending colonization and infection of the uterine and fetal compartments. Preterm, prelabor rupture of membranes (PPROM) is associated with increased risk of EOS among preterm infants, but the exact relationship between duration of PPROM and infection is modified by the administration of latency antibiotics and obstetric management. Signs of maternal IAI (previously referred to as clinical chorioamnionitis) are strong predictors of neonatal infection. These signs include maternal intrapartum fever, maternal tachycardia, and uterine tenderness, all of which are reasonably sensitive for but lack specificity for predicting EOS. The American College of Obstetricians and Gynecologists (ACOG) provides guidance for the definitive and suspected diagnosis of maternal IAI.[12] The diagnosis of IAI is confirmed by amniotic fluid culture, gram stain and/or biochemical analysis consistent with infection, and placental histopathology consistent with infection and inflammation. Amniotic fluid-based diagnostic information is usually obtained when assessing a pregnant woman who presents with preterm labor and is less relevant to women laboring at term, for whom definitive evidence of IAI is more often obtained by placental histopathology. Suspected IAI is diagnosed in the laboring woman when a maternal intrapartum temperature ≥39.0°C occurs alone or a maternal temperature in the 38.0°C to 38.9°C range occurs when maternal leukocytosis, purulent cervical drainage, or fetal tachycardia is present. Isolated maternal fever is defined as the occurrence of a maternal intrapartum temperature ≥39.0°C alone or a persistent maternal temperature in the 38.0°C to 38.9°C range without additional clinical risk factors. The ACOG recommends the administration of maternal intrapartum antibiotics for confirmed or suspected IAI, as well as for isolated intrapartum maternal fever, due to the risks to both the pregnant woman and the fetus from progressive IAI, if indeed present.

Maternal vaginal-rectal colonization with GBS is a predictor for GBS-specific EOS.[13] Vertical transmission of GBS from mother to fetus and newborn is almost exclusively the source of neonatal early-onset GBS disease, in contrast to late-onset neonatal GBS disease, which may be due to either vertical or horizontal maternal transmission or horizontal transmission from nonmaternal caregivers and household sources. The risk posed by maternal GBS colonization is significantly reduced by administration of intrapartum antibiotic prophylaxis to laboring GBS-colonized mothers.[13,14] The widespread implementation of recommended practices for maternal antenatal culture-based screening for GBS colonization and appropriate administration of IAP has been associated with a nearly 10-fold decline in the incidence of GBS-specific EOS in the United States.[1]

Higher rates of both EOS and GBS-specific EOS have been found among infants born to US mothers of Black race compared with those who identify as of white non-Hispanic background.[13] Obstetric practices such as the frequency of vaginal exams during labor and the use of invasive fetal monitoring have been associated with increased risk of GBS-specific EOS in some observational studies. These findings are confounded by their associations with other factors such as length of labor, ROM, and preterm delivery and are therefore difficult to interpret. Current ACOG guidance for prevention of perinatal GBS disease states that such procedures should be performed as clinically indicated and notes that GBS IAP will likely minimize the impact of these factors.[14]

Microbiology

EOS is associated with organisms vertically acquired from the maternal gastrointestinal and genitourinary tract. The distribution of organisms causing EOS in surveillance or cohort studies conducted by the CDC,[3] NRN,[4] and within the Pediatrix Medical Group–affiliated neonatal intensive care units (NICUs)[15] is shown in Table 30.1 and Fig. 30.1. Gram-positive organisms compose 50% to 70% of all infections. Fungal infections were reported in the NRN surveillance, composing 1% to 2% of all infections and occurring exclusively among preterm infants. Despite use of targeted IAP, GBS is the most common organism isolated in EOS case infants born at ≥37 weeks' gestation, whereas *Escherichia coli* is the predominant organism isolated among those born at <37 weeks' gestation. The differential between these two most common causes of EOS is greater with decreasing gestational age: among those born at 22 to 28 weeks' gestation, the rate of *E. coli* disease is 120-fold higher than among those born at ≥37 weeks' gestation (12 cases/1000 among low-gestation versus 0.10 cases/1000 among term infants).[4]

Table 30.1 Organisms Causing Early-Onset Sepsis

Organism, n (% Total)	CDC[2] n = 1484	NRN[3] n = 235	Pediatrix[4] n = 1178
GRAM-POSITIVE			
Group B *Streptococcus*	532 (35.8)	70 (29.8)	473 (40.2)
Streptococcus viridans	280 (18.9)	7 (3.0)	—
Enterococcus	46 (3.1)	13 (5.5)	63 (5.3)
Group D *Streptococcus*/ *Streptococcus bovis*	21 (1.4)	6 (2.6)	—
Listeria spp.	19 (1.3)	2 (0.9)	4 (0.3)
Streptococcus pneumoniae	14 (0.9)	3 (1.3)	11 (0.9)
Staphylococcus aureus	52 (3.5)	3 (1.3)	23 (2.0)
Group A *Streptococcus*	—	9 (3.8)	1 (0.1)
CONS	—	2 (0.9)	18 (1.5)
Other gram-positive cocci	—	5 (2.1)	208 (17.7)
GRAM-NEGATIVE			
E. coli	368 (24.8)	83 (35.3)	145 (12.3)
Hemophilus influenzae	67 (4.5)	9 (3.8)	23 (2.0)
Klebsiella spp.	14 (0.9)	7 (3.0)	7 (0.6)
Citrobacter spp.	—	1 (0.4)	3 (0.3)
Enterobacter spp.	—	1 (0.4)	4 (0.3)
Pseudomonas spp.	—	1 (0.4)	2 (0.2)
Other gram-negative rods	—	5 (2.1)	43 (3.7)
Other			
Candida spp.	—	4 (1.7)	1 (0.1)
Other/unknown[a]	71 (4.8)	4 (1.7)	149 (12.6)

Individual organisms listed if identified in >1 study.

[a]Other/unknown category refers to (1) any species for which <10 isolates were identified (CDC), (2) polymicrobial infections (NRN), or (3) isolates not identified by name in the database (Pediatrix).

CDC, Centers for Disease Control and Prevention; *CONS*, coagulase-negative staphylococci; *NRN*, Neonatal Research Network; *spp.*, species.

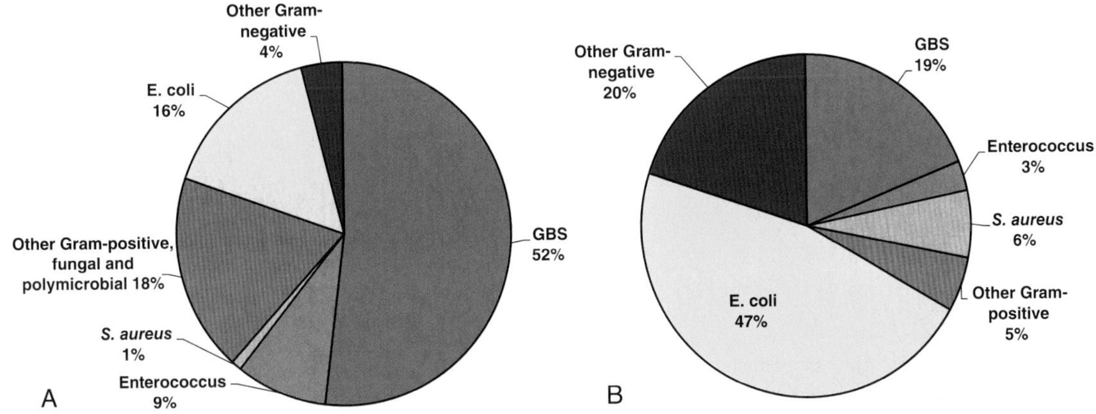

Fig. 30.1 Distribution of Early-Onset Sepsis Organisms. (A) Term infants. and (B) Preterm infants. (A, Adapted from Stoll BJ, Puopolo KM, Hansen NI, et al. Early-onset neonatal sepsis 2015 to 2017, the rise of escherichia coli, and the need for novel prevention strategies. *JAMA Pediatr*. 2020;174(7):e200593; B, Adapted from Puopolo KM, Draper D, Wi S, et al. Estimating the probability of neonatal early-onset infection on the basis of maternal risk factors. *Pediatrics*. 2011;128(5):e1155–e1163.)

Clinical Features

The signs of EOS among newborns are often nonspecific and may be especially difficult to distinguish from transitional instability that may occur among term infants and from cardiorespiratory immaturity commonly displayed among preterm infants. Vital sign instability is often present, including tachycardia, tachypnea, and temperature instability. Respiratory signs may range from mild tachypnea, with or without a requirement for supplemental oxygen, to profound respiratory failure due to pneumonitis, surfactant deficiency, and/or pulmonary hypertension with persistent fetal circulation. Cardiovascular systemic symptoms range from poor perfusion and metabolic acidosis to hypotension, tachycardia and cardiac dysfunction. Severe sepsis may be complicated by hypoxic-ischemic encephalopathy with or without meningitis. Septic shock may evolve to multisystem organ failure with oliguria, liver dysfunction including coagulopathy, bone marrow suppression with leukopenia, neutropenia, and thrombocytopenia. Approximately 50% to 70% of infants with EOS will present with signs of illness at the time of birth and the majority will present by 24 hours of age.[2,16] However, a small proportion of term infants can present after 24 hours of age, particularly those ultimately determined to be infected with GBS, despite negative maternal antenatal screening results and no significant intrapartum risk factors for EOS. Such cases may represent infants born to mothers who screened falsely negative for GBS or whose colonization status changed during the period between screening and delivery.[16]

Risk Assessment

Term and near-term infants should be considered separately from preterm infants. Among term infants (defined as those born ≥35 0/7 weeks' gestation), the pathogenesis of EOS most commonly develops during the course of labor. Given the relatively low incidence of EOS among term infants (approximately 1/2000 live births), the goal of risk assessment is to determine which newborns are at *high* enough risk to *warrant* EOS evaluation and empiric antibiotic therapy. In contrast, the majority of infants born preterm are born due to spontaneous preterm labor with or without preterm ROM, meaning that infection may be both a cause and a complication of preterm birth. Further, the baseline risk is as high as 1/50 live births for infants born at <29 weeks' gestation—meaning that the goal of EOS risk assessment among preterm infants is to determine which infants are at *low* enough risk to be *spared* initiation of empiric antibiotics.

EOS Risk Assessment Among Infants Born at ≥35 0/7 Weeks' Gestation

There are three basic approaches that can be taken to determine empiric antibiotic administration for EOS risk among term and late preterm infants. Each approach has advantages and limitations; centers can assess their local resources and their view of the risk/benefit balance of empiric antibiotic therapies to determine the approach best suited to their local care structure. Table 30.2 outlines the three approaches currently recommended by the American Academy of Pediatrics (AAP)[17] and summarizes the primary advantages and limitations of each. The *categorical approach* uses dichotomous cutoff values for risk factors, assigning risk on the basis of the presence or absence of specific risk factors, and recommends laboratory evaluation and empiric therapy be administered when the risk factor is present. This approach was recommended in GBS perinatal prevention guidance from 1996 to 2010 and widely applied to the evaluation of newborns for all microbial causes of EOS. The categorical approach to EOS risk assessment was not prospectively evaluated prior to recommendation, but retrospective studies among infants born at ≥35 to 36 weeks' gestation demonstrate that implementation results in 5% to 12% of infants treated with empiric antibiotics.[2,5,18] Multivariate prediction models have been developed that utilize specific risk factors for EOS and account for use of intrapartum antibiotics and the evolving clinical condition of the newborn over the first 6 to 12 hours after birth. These models provide estimated risk of EOS for the individual infant and have been formulated as a web-based "*Neonatal Early-Onset Sepsis Calculator*" (https://neonatalsepsiscalculator.kaiserpermanente.org). Prospective implementation studies in large birth cohorts demonstrate that this approach can reduce the rate of EOS evaluation and empiric antibiotic administration without safety concerns.[2] Depending on the thresholds used for specific clinical actions, empiric antibiotic rates of 2.6% to 3.7% have been reported among infants born at ≥35 to 36 weeks' gestational age using the sepsis risk calculator.[2,19] The final recommended approach to EOS evaluation relies on the use of serial *observation only* among infants categorized as at risk for EOS. Centers that have studied this approach have utilized it by first categorizing infants as at risk

Table 30.2 EOS Risk Assessment Among Infants Born ≥35 0/7 Weeks' Gestation

	Categorical Approach	Neonatal Early-Onset Sepsis Calculator[a]	Observation Only
Risk factors considered	• Signs of newborn clinical illness • Maternal intrapartum temperature ≥100.4°F (≥38°C) • Inadequate IAP in a GBS-colonized mother	• GA at birth • Highest maternal intrapartum temperature • Duration of ROM • Maternal GBS status • Type and duration of intrapartum antibiotic • Infant clinical status over the first 6–12 hours of age	• Signs of newborn clinical illness • Maternal intrapartum temperature ≥100.4°F (≥38°C) • Inadequate IAP in a GBS-colonized mother
Infant clinical status	Determination of what constitutes "signs of newborn clinical illness" is left to local center determination	Guidance on content and duration of vital signs and specifics of clinical status provided to determine whether infant is well-appearing, equivocal, or clinically ill	Determination of what constitutes "signs of newborn clinical illness" is left to local center determination

Recommended clinical actions	• Blood culture and empiric antibiotics recommended for infants:
	  ○ with clinical illness
	  ○ born to mothers with intrapartum temperature ≥38°C/100.4°F
	• Clinical observation for 24–36 hours in the birth hospital for infants born to mothers with inadequate GBS IAP
		Recommended actions are provided based on final risk estimate at birth and the risk estimate adjusted for clinical condition.	• Blood culture and empiric antibiotics recommended for infants with clinical illness
			• At-risk infants who appear well at birth should have serial, structured clinical assessments from birth through 36–48 hours of age and undergo EOS evaluation if signs of illness develop

Advantages	• Familiar • Multiple retrospective studies available	• Prospectively validated in large cohorts • Individualized management • Overall lower use of empiric antibiotics compared with categorical approach	Overall lower use of empiric antibiotics compared with categorical and (possibly) multivariate approach
Limitations	• Poor discrimination within risk categories • Higher use of empiric antibiotics compared with multivariate and observation-only approaches	• Requires structures for risk calculation • Require process for enhanced newborn observation at some levels of estimated risk	• Validation in small cohorts where risk was primarily determined by obstetric diagnosis of chorioamnionitis • Requires structures for serial newborn observation and development of rules for evaluation and empiric treatment

[a]Neonatal Early-Onset Sepsis Calculator found at: https://neonatalsepsiscalculator.kaiserpermanente.org/.

EOS, Early-onset sepsis; *GA*, gestational age; *GBS*, group B *Streptococcus*; *IAP*, intrapartum antibiotic prophylaxis; *ROM*, rupture of membranes.

based on categorical criteria such as the obstetric diagnosis of chorioamnionitis. Infant who are clinically ill at birth are provided empiric antibiotic treatment and those who are well-appearing undergo serial, structured physical assessments for 24 to 36 hours after birth. A single center in the United States has reported on the use of this approach among infants born to mothers diagnosed with chorioamnionitis, which the center had previously universally treated with empiric antibiotics. Depending on the criteria set for illness and the environment used for serial observation, the use of empiric antibiotic administration declined from 100% to 10% to 20% among initially well-appearing infants flagged for observation.[20,21]

EOS Risk Assessment Among Infants Born at ≤34 6/7 Weeks' Gestation

The comparatively high rate of EOS among preterm infants compared with term infants and the high rates of sepsis-associated mortality among preterm infants has resulted in near-universal use of empiric antibiotic administration among these infants. In a study of more than 40,000 preterm infants cared for in 297 centers across the United States from 2009 to 2015, 78.6% of VLBW and 87% of ELBW infants were treated with empiric antibiotics for risk of EOS. Prolonged administration of antibiotics for proven or presumed infection occurred in 20% to 40% of VLBW and ELBW infants, respectively, rates that are roughly 10-fold higher than the incidence of EOS in this population.[22] AAP management guidance[23] now recommends that clinicians focus on delivery characteristics of preterm infants to identify those who are low risk for EOS and may be spared antibiotic initiation (Fig. 30.2). This guidance is based on evidence from studies of both VLBW and ELBW populations that demonstrate the markedly lower risk of EOS among preterm infants born for maternal health indications (primarily preeclampsia) or fetal indications (primarily growth restriction) when there is no additional concern for IAI. When such infants are born by cesarean section in the absence of labor or attempts to induce labor, with ROM at delivery, they are not subject to factors that promote the pathogenesis of EOS and are at very low to no risk of EOS, regardless of their clinical condition at birth.[24,25] Although an ELBW infant born to a woman with clinical concern for IAI and with evidence of histologic chorioamnionitis on placental pathology may have a risk of EOS as high as 1/20, the risk among infants born by cesarean section, without labor or ROM prior to delivery for maternal preeclampsia, may be close to zero.[25] One center reported on the impact of using this approach to EOS risk assessment in a study of 918 VLBW infants admitted to the NICU over an 11-year period. With use of the algorithm in Fig. 30.2, overall empiric antibiotic use declined from 81% to 59% among all VLBW infants and from 95% to 66% among all ELBW infants. The decline was attributed to the use of antibiotics among VLBW

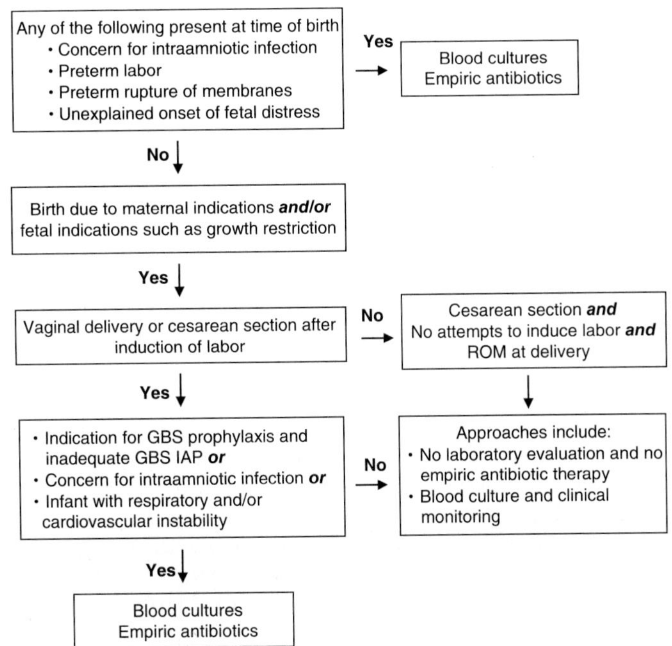

Fig. 30.2 Early-Onset Sepsis Risk Assessment Among Infants Born ≤34 6/7 Weeks' Gestation. *GBS*, Group B *Streptococcus*; *IAI*, intraamniotic infection.

infants categorized as low-risk; empiric antibiotic use declined from 62% to 13%.[26] No safety issues were associated with use of the low-risk algorithm over the study period.

Diagnostic Evaluation

Blood and Cerebrospinal Fluid Cultures

The diagnosis of EOS is made by a culture of a pathogenic species from blood and/or CSF. Although meningitis is most often a metastatic complication of bacteremia, meningitis can very rarely occur in isolation. CDC surveillance identified 1277 cases of GBS EOS occurring in the United States from 2005 to 2016; CSF was the only source of bacterial isolation in 11 (0.1%) of these cases.[1] The optimal approach to diagnosis of EOS includes blood and CSF culture prior to administration of empiric antibiotics; however, if not done previously, CSF analysis and culture should be performed when bacteremia is identified. Urine culture is not indicated for EOS diagnosis, and culture of tracheal or gastric secretions or skin surfaces will not distinguish colonization from infection. Appropriate blood culture technique can minimize concerns about the sensitivity of blood culture to detect bacteremia. Standard pediatric blood culture bottles should be inoculated with a minimum of 1 mL of blood to optimize organism recovery. The use of both aerobic and anaerobic culture bottles can optimize isolation of strict anaerobic species, particularly among preterm infants. One site that routinely obtained both aerobic and anaerobic cultures among VLBW infants reported that 17% of isolates were strict anaerobes, primarily *Bacteroides* species.[24] Obtaining two blood cultures may optimize recovery of potentially low-level bacteremia. Modern blood culture systems use automated, continuous detection technologies with identification of a positive culture within 24 hours for most clinically relevant bacterial pathogens. Time-to-positivity (TTP) data for neonatal EOS cultures collected from multiple sites over a 20-year period found that the median TTP was 21.0 hours (interquartile range [IQR], 17.1–25.3 hours), with 68% of bacterial pathogens isolated by 24 hours, 94% by 36 hours, and 97% by 48 hours of incubation.[27] Neither gestational age (term versus preterm), organism gram stain (gram-positive versus gram-negative), nor the administration of maternal intrapartum antibiotics significantly impacted TTP.

Complete Blood Count

Multiple studies have evaluated the utility of the complete blood cell count (CBC) for EOS diagnosis using test characteristics such as sensitivity, specificity, and positive and negative predictive value. These test characteristics are impacted by the incidence of disease; because of the relatively low incidence of EOS, the optimal test characteristic for evaluation of laboratory test performance is the likelihood ratio (LR). The test is also impacted by a variety of factors other than infection: gestational age at birth, sex, in utero growth restriction, mode of delivery, time (in hours) after birth, and maternal pregnancy complications such as preeclampsia and diabetes all can impact some component of the CBC. Two large studies addressed the performance of the white blood cell (WBC) count, immature/total neutrophil ratio (I/T), and absolute neutrophil count (ANC) in predicting culture-confirmed EOS using large multicenter data sets.[28,29] Both studies found that values obtained at <1 hour of age were associated with low likelihood ratios, meaning that the results did not significantly modify the prior probability of EOS. Values obtained at >4 hours of age were more predictive; extreme values (total WBC count <5000/μL; I/T >0.3; ANC <2000/μL in one study and WBC count <1000/μL, ANC <100/μL, and I/T >0.5 in the other) were associated with the highest likelihood ratios but very low sensitivities. A WBC count >20,000/μL and platelet counts were not associated with EOS in either study. The I/T squared (I/T divided by the ANC) performs better than any of the more traditional tests and is independent of age in hours but also had modest sensitivity and specificity.[30] Overall, no component of the CBC has adequate sensitivity to be used alone as a screen to make decisions regarding antibiotic initiation for EOS.

Inflammatory biomarkers such as C-reactive protein (CRP) and procalcitonin (PCT) have been studied for use in determining risk of EOS, both as single screening values and as serial assessments. CRP is an acute-phase reactant synthesized by the liver in response to interleukin 6 release from immune cells. CRP levels do rise during bacterial infection, but CRP will also rise in the setting of common perinatal noninfectious conditions. Elevated CRP has been associated with respiratory conditions including transient tachypnea of the newborn and meconium aspiration and with birth-associated tissue damage such as bruising and cephalohematoma, as well as with iatrogenic tissue damage such as with placement of a chest tube for pneumothorax.[31] The sensitivity of CRP at the time of EOS evaluation is particularly poor; in one series of 1002 EOS evaluations, CRP levels performed at the time sepsis evaluation had a 35% sensitivity for EOS, with a positive predictive value of 6.7% and a positive LR of 3.5.[32] In this study, three serial CRP levels obtained over the 48 hours after EOS evaluation together had increased sensitivity for EOS, but the positive predictive value (5.2%) and LR (3) declined. The poor performance of CRP at the time of EOS evaluation means that this laboratory test should not be used alone to determine empiric antibiotic therapy for EOS, particularly among the lowest-risk term infants, for whom an LR of 3 to 4 will not substantially increase the estimated risk of infection. PCT is an inflammatory mediator that is produced both by the liver and directly by WBCs and rises in response to bacterial infection faster than CRP. However, PCT rises normally in the hours after birth, and specific normative ranges by age in hours and by gestational age at birth are needed to optimally interpret PCT, limiting its use for evaluating the risk of EOS. Like CRP, PCT levels also rise in response to noninfectious perinatal conditions. Interleukin 6 itself and other cytokines such as soluble interleukin

2 receptor, interleukin 8, and tumor necrosis factor as well as inflammatory cell adhesion molecules have been studied as predictive markers of EOS. None have demonstrated sufficient sensitivity and specificity and none are currently in clinical use.[17,33] Other tests including advanced molecular-based methods for identification of infectious organisms are emerging, such as polymerase-chain reaction and microarray techniques. Advantages include small sample volume, quick turnaround time, and improved sensitivity and specificity. However, such techniques are currently limited by cost, inability to distinguish between colonization and true infection, inability to distinguish bacterial DNA from live bacteria, and lack of antimicrobial susceptibility testing.

Empiric Therapy

Empiric therapy for EOS should target the most common microbial isolates identified in national surveillance studies (GBS and *E. coli*). GBS remain universally susceptible to ampicillin, and although *E. coli* isolates are increasingly resistant to ampicillin, most remain sensitive to gentamicin.[1,3] Resistance to both ampicillin and gentamicin was, however, reported in 10% of EOS cases caused by *E. coli* in recent reports.[3,34,35] Less common causes of EOS, such as *Staphylococcus aureus* and ESBL gram-negative species, may not be susceptible to the combination of ampicillin and gentamicin. Enterococci and *Listeria monocytogenes* are not susceptible to cephalosporin antibiotics. With these considerations, AAP guidance recommends the primary use of ampicillin and gentamicin; the addition of a broader-spectrum antibiotic to this combination may be considered among VLBW infants at highest risk of EOS and for critically ill term newborns until culture results are known.[17,23] If blood cultures are sterile, empiric antibiotic therapies should be discontinued in most cases. If blood cultures identify an organism, definitive therapy should follow recommended durations of treatment for that organism, using the most narrow-spectrum antibiotic indicated by organism susceptibility results.

CHAPTER 31

Late-Onset Sepsis

Dustin D. Flannery, Karen M. Puopolo

KEY POINTS

1. Late-onset sepsis in the neonatal intensive care unit is defined by culture-confirmed infection ≥72 hours after birth.
2. Incidence is highest among preterm infants.
3. The pathophysiology involves colonization with perinatally and/or hospital-acquired organisms, with transition to invasive infection promoted by hospital devices and immature mucosa.
4. Risk factors include prematurity, presence of a central venous catheter, prolonged parenteral nutrition, and lack of breast milk feeding.
5. The most common causative organisms are coagulase-negative *Staphylococci* and *Staphlycoccus aureus.*
6. Clinical manifestations are nonspecific and often difficult to distinguish from instability characteristic of prematurity.
7. Identification of a pathogenic organism by culture of a normally sterile bodily fluid, primarily blood or cerebrospinal fluid, is currently the gold standard for diagnosis.
8. The choice of empiric antimicrobial therapy should be based on local microbiology and antibiotic susceptibility patterns, and targeted therapy should be narrowed based upon the isolate susceptibility profile and clinical response.

Introduction

Late-onset sepsis (LOS) is an important contributor to morbidity and mortality among both term (≥37 weeks' gestational age [GA]) and preterm (<37 weeks' GA) newborn infants. LOS is defined by isolation of a pathogenic species from a normally sterile body fluid. Among preterm infants, LOS is most commonly defined by isolation from blood or cerebrospinal fluid (CSF) culture. Infection confined to the urinary tract, joints, or bones may also occur as part of LOS with specific organisms. Bacteria, fungi (primarily *Candida* species), and viruses (herpes simplex virus, cytomegalovirus) may cause LOS. A consensus, physiology-based definition for neonatal sepsis does not currently exist.[1] LOS is also defined based on the timing of the infection relative to birth. Among continuously hospitalized infants cared for in the neonatal intensive care unit (NICU), LOS is defined as occurring in infants ≥72 hours or 3 days after birth. Risk factors for infection and organisms causing infection rapidly change from those reflecting perinatal risk and perinatally acquired flora to those reflecting nosocomial risk factors and hospital-acquired flora. In contrast, among infants discharged home from the birth hospital in the first week after birth, LOS is defined as occurring in infants 7 to 90 days of age. This chapter will focus on bacterial and fungal LOS among primarily preterm infants cared for in the NICU.

Epidemiology

The incidence of LOS is inversely related to the degree of maturity (GA and birth weight [BW]) and varies across populations.[2–4] Up to 40% of very preterm infants (<28 weeks' GA) admitted to the NICU have at least one episode of LOS, compared with 30% of moderately preterm infants (28–32 weeks' GA) and 17% of late preterm and term infants (≥33 weeks GA).[5–8] The peak incidence of LOS is between the 10th and 22nd postnatal day.[3,5] The incidence of LOS has increased over time, likely related to improved survival of extremely preterm infants with prolonged hospitalization and intensive care.[9]

Pathophysiology

The pathogenesis of gram-positive LOS, particularly that due to coagulase-negative *Staphylococci* (CONS) and *Staphylococcus aureus*, is often related to adherence and proliferation of bacteria on indwelling plastic medical devices, whereas gram-negative LOS often occurs by transmission from healthcare workers and contamination of catheters, parenteral solutions, or enteral formulas.[7,10] Intestinal, nasal mucosal, and skin colonization with invasive pathogens may also promote LOS both in the presence and absence of invasive medical devices.[11,12]

Risk Factors

Multiple studies provide evidence for both nonmodifiable and modifiable risk factors for LOS. Nonmodifiable risk factors include lower GA and lower BW.[7,8,13] Among preterm infants, some studies suggest small-for-GA infants may be at increased risk for LOS, particularly CONS infection.[8,14] Potentially modifiable risk factors for LOS include prolonged parenteral nutrition, presence of a central venous catheter (CVC), and breast milk feeding.[6–9,13,15,16] The decreased risk of LOS with breast milk is likely attributable to the complex immunomodulatory and antiinfective components of breast milk; more rapid achievement of full enteral feeds and decreased exposure to parenteral nutrition time and CVCs; and potentially to differences in constitution of the infant gut microbiome.[17] Multiple studies identify presence and duration of a CVC as a risk factor for LOS.[18–20] This may be due to entrance of commensal skin organisms into the catheter track or contamination of the catheter hub.[6,19] Mechanical ventilation and bladder catheterization also increase the risk of LOS. There is conflicting evidence for the role of early antibiotic administration on subsequent risk of all-cause LOS, fungal LOS, and comorbidities associated with LOS, such as necrotizing enterocolitis (NEC).[6,9,21–24] Racial disparity has been observed in LOS caused by group B *Streptococcus* (GBS), with maternal black race a significant risk factor.[25] Additional specific risk factors for fungal LOS due to *Candida albicans* include treatment with cephalosporin antibiotics, steroids, intralipids, and gastric acid suppressing medications.[26–28]

Microbiology

LOS is primarily (but not exclusively) associated with organisms acquired from the environment after birth (Fig. 31.1).[29] In a cohort of preterm infants born with BW <1000 g and GA <29 weeks from the Neonatal Research Network during 2000 to 2011, the majority of LOS was caused by gram-positive bacteria (73%).[2] Gram-negative bacteria caused 17% of LOS, and fungal organisms caused 7%.[2] CONS were isolated in 55% of the LOS cases.[2] Other reports confirm that CONS are the most frequent blood culture isolates associated with neonatal LOS.[3,30] CONS are common commensal organisms that colonize human skin and mucosal membranes and can adhere to indwelling catheters and plastic medical devices in susceptible patients, forming multilayered biofilms.[30,31] CONS are also common blood culture contaminants in NICU patients, and determining true infection can be challenging.[32] Other gram-positive bacteria causing LOS include *S. aureus*, *Enterococci*, and GBS, whereas *Escherichia coli*, *Klebsiella*, *Pseudomonas*, *Enterobacter*, and *Serratia* species are among the most common gram-negative LOS isolates.[2,3,7] The majority of fungal LOS is caused by *Candida* species, primarily *C. albicans* and *Candida parapsilosis*.[2,3,7] Although less common, viral infections can mimic bacterial LOS among preterm infants, and appropriate contextual consideration should be given to etiologies such as herpes simplex virus, seasonal respiratory viruses such as respiratory syncytial virus, and influenza, as well as cytomegalovirus among preterm infants fed their mother's own breast milk. The prevalence of causative organisms may vary widely based on geographic region.[4,9,33–39]

Clinical Features

The signs and symptoms of LOS among newborns are often nonspecific and may be especially difficult to distinguish from physiologic instability characteristic of preterm infants. Respiratory decline from established baseline, feeding intolerance, and increased apnea are among the most common reasons for LOS evaluation. In a prospective cohort study of preterm infants with suspected infection, delayed capillary refill and gray skin were specifically associated with LOS.[40] Infants may also present with hypothermia or hyperthermia (although temperature can be normal during isolette care), decreased activity, and tachycardia. Late signs may include cyanosis and/or hypotension; oliguria or anuria may be the first indication of significant hypotension. Jaundice may be a presenting symptom, particularly for urinary tract infection (UTI).[41] Irritability and fontanelle bulging may accompany central nervous system infection.[10] The combination of hyperglycemia and thrombocytopenia is a common feature of infants with fungal LOS.[42]

Evaluation

Cultures

The diagnosis of LOS is made by culture of a pathogenic species from blood and/or CSF. Although meningitis is often a metastatic complication of bacteremia, late-onset meningitis can occur in isolation among preterm infants.[43] Site-specific infection may occur without bacteremia: UTI, pneumonitis, and cellulitis may be diagnosed by site-specific culture (urine, tracheal fluid, drainage fluid). The optimal approach to diagnosis of late-onset infection includes blood and CSF culture prior to administration of empiric antibiotics. Urine culture should be obtained in older infants (especially those without CVCs), and site-specific cultures and radiographic studies should be obtained as clinically indicated. Appropriate blood culture technique can minimize concerns about the sensitivity of blood culture to detect bacteremia.[44] Standard pediatric blood culture bottles should be

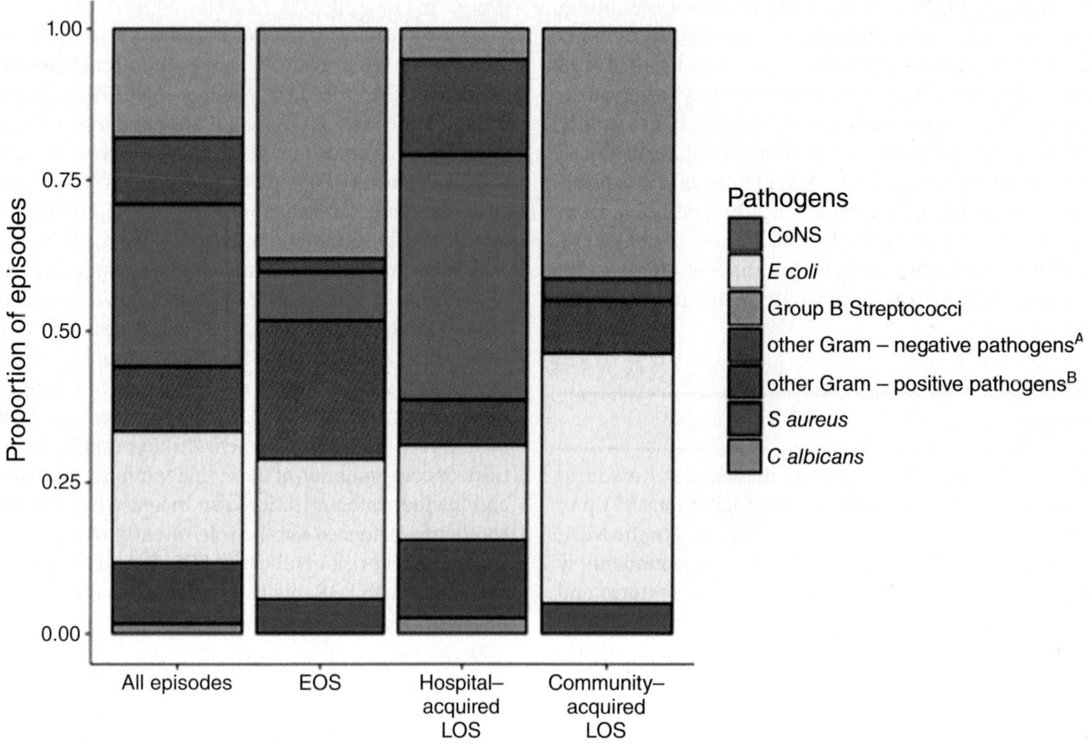

Fig. 31.1 Pathogens in Neonatal Sepsis. Episodes were stratified by early-onset, hospital-acquired late-onset, and community-acquired late-onset sepsis.

inoculated with a minimum of 1 mL of blood to optimize organism recovery.[45] When there is concern for gastrointestinal infection, the use of both aerobic and anaerobic culture bottles can optimize isolation of strict anaerobic species.[46] Obtaining two blood cultures from separate sites, especially when a central line is present, aids in determination of contamination versus true infection.[47] Modern blood culture systems use automated, continuous detection technologies with identification of a positive culture within 24 hours for most clinically relevant bacterial pathogens.[48] Time-to-positivity data for neonatal cultures in one study suggest that 95% of bacterial and 84% of fungal pathogens are detected within 48 hours of incubation.[49] Another study found that 71% of positive blood cultures were detected by 24 hours; CONS were detected after a mean of 21.7 hours.[50] When bacteremia is identified, CSF analysis and culture should be performed if not done previously. Empiric antibiotic therapy should be adjusted as needed in response to isolate susceptibility data, using the narrowest spectrum of appropriate therapy. Repeat blood cultures (and CSF cultures, when meningitis is present) should be obtained to document sterility in response to therapy. Persistent bacteremia (>2–3 positive cultures on appropriate antimicrobial therapy) should prompt investigation for a site-specific complication such as venous thrombosis, abscess, osteomyelitis, or other organ-specific infection.

Inflammatory Markers

Multiple studies have evaluated the efficacy and utility of the complete blood cell count (CBC) for LOS diagnosis. Overall, the CBC and its components have poor predictive value, and no CBC index possesses adequate sensitivity to reliably rule out LOS.[29,51] Serial normal CBC values may, however, provide reassurance that LOS is not present. Inflammatory biomarkers may also be used, such as C-reactive protein (CRP), procalcitonin, and interleukin 6.[52] CRP is an acute-phase reactant synthesized by the liver and reflects tissue damage, infection (bacterial, fungal, or viral), necrosis, or general inflammation. Sensitivity of CRP may be low during the early stages of infection, and elevation is nonspecific to LOS and may be related to other causes. These issues limit its utility, although serial levels may be of higher yield.[10,52] CBC and CRP may be of most predictive value in the individual infant if the clinician is able to compare baseline values with those obtained at the moment of clinical concern. Procalcitonin, an acute-phase reactant produced by hepatocytes and macrophages, has shown promise given its specificity for bacterial infections among neonates, early rise in levels during infection, and quick reduction in response to appropriate therapy, but wide variation in levels across uninfected infants has limited its use.[29,52] Interleukin 6 is a cytokine released in response to exposure to bacterial endotoxins and demonstrates an ability for early detection given its rise in the very early stage of infection, but thus far it has limited use in clinical care due to its very short half-life.[29,52] Other biomarkers and cytokine profiles have been studied to improve the diagnostic accuracy of LOS, but none are currently routinely used by neonatal providers.[29,53]

Other Tests

Advanced molecular-based methods for identification of infectious organisms are emerging, including polymerase-chain reaction and microarray techniques.[54] Advantages include small sample volume, quick turnaround time, and improved sensitivity and specificity. However, such techniques are currently limited by cost, inability to distinguish between colonization and true infection, inability to distinguish bacterial DNA from live bacteria, and lack of antimicrobial susceptibility testing.[20] Heart rate characteristic variability has been studied in LOS prediction, both in isolation and in combination with laboratory tests and/or other physiologic data.[55–57] Decreased heart rate variability and transient decelerations related to inflammation may indicate a high risk of LOS.[20] Although one trial demonstrated decreased mortality in very preterm infants with displayed heart rate characteristics, the mechanism of decreased mortality was unclear.[57] Available monitors are currently limited by a lack of specificity for LOS, meaning that frequent abnormal values may prompt additional evaluations for infection and create alarm fatigue among clinicians.

Prevention

Primary prevention of LOS should focus on the sources of infection. Nosocomial LOS is largely due to central-line–associated bloodstream infections (CLABSIs). Guidelines promoting strict hand-hygiene practices, barrier precautions, skin antiseptics, optimized daily care practices, management of infused fluids and infusion sets, and prompt removal of CVCs have been shown to reduce the incidence of LOS.[58–61] Centers should develop local CVC care guidelines informed by best practice. Optimizing feeding strategies and interventions to reduce the need for CVCs may also contribute to CLABSI prevention. Secondary bloodstream infections can result from organ-specific diseases such as NEC, UTI, pneumonia, or cellulitis. Prevention of secondary LOS should focus on strategies to reduce the incidence of the primary condition. The risk of some conditions (e.g., NEC and UTI) may be impacted by specific practices such as breast milk feeding for NEC and minimal indwelling bladder catheters for UTI, but neither of these conditions is entirely preventable among preterm infants. There are no currently known approaches to the prevention of GBS-specific LOS. Probiotics have been studied as a potential means of preventing LOS by populating the intestinal microbiota with low-virulence organisms that normally constitute the microbiome of healthy term infants. Trials of probiotic supplementation for the prevention of LOS have inconsistent results, and in meta-analyses, the intervention was not shown to decrease the incidence of the disease.[62,63] Lactoferrin supplementation has also been studied for the prevention of LOS; a review of six randomized controlled trials suggests that the intervention decreases LOS without adverse effects but found the current evidence quality is low.[64] A recent randomized controlled trial of lactoferrin supplementation among 2203 infants born at <32 weeks' gestation found no impact on LOS.[65] Fluconazole prophylaxis reduces the incidence of invasive candidiasis among extremely low BW infants.[66] Centers with high rates of *Candida* colonization/infection should consider empiric therapy for such infants. Among centers with a relatively low burden of *Candida* infection, evidence does not support universal, BW based administration of fluconazole prophylaxis, although such centers may opt to administer targeted prophylaxis to extremely low BW infants (<1000 g) at highest risk, such as those receiving prolonged antibiotic therapy.[67] National surveillance on incidence rates can indirectly reduce LOS by providing contemporary data to facilitate interhospital comparison, benchmarking, and continuous improvement efforts.[68]

Empiric Therapy

Empiric therapy should be based on local center data informing the most commonly isolated organisms and antibiotic susceptibility patterns among LOS cases. Typical regimens should include coverage for gram-positive and gram-negative bacteria, although there is a lack of clinical consensus on the most appropriate regimen.[32] Vancomycin is often used for gram-positive coverage because the majority of CONS are not susceptible to penicillinase-resistant β-lactams, and vancomycin provides coverage for methicillin-resistant *S. aureus* (MRSA) and ampicillin-resistant *Enterococci*. Empiric vancomycin prescription may not always be necessary, however, given that LOS with CONS has low virulence and is rarely fatal.[69] Empiric use of penicillinase-resistant β-lactam antibiotics such as oxacillin or nafcillin may be appropriate in centers with low rates of MRSA infection, particularly if the center also utilizes prospective screening for MRSA colonization.[70] Empiric gram-negative therapy typically includes an aminoglycoside such as gentamicin, amikacin, or tobramycin. Alternative gram-negative coverage options may include a cephalosporin, although emergence of colonization and infections with cephalosporin-resistant gram-negative organisms has been reported in units that routinely use these medications.[32,71] Amphotericin B should be used when empiric antifungal therapy is indicated. When blood cultures are sterile, antimicrobials should be discontinued after 36 to 48 hours based on local time-to-positivity data unless additional diagnoses (e.g., NEC) are present. Persistent symptoms in the face of sterile cultures and empiric broad-spectrum antibiotic therapy should prompt additional investigations such as renal and brain imaging for signs of focal fungal infection, cytomegalovirus testing among preterm infants fed their mother's own milk, and respiratory viral testing among infants with respiratory symptoms and/or decline.

Table 31.1 Pathogen-Specific Therapy[80]

Organism	Antimicrobial Regimen
Coagulase-negative *Staphylococci*	Vancomycin
Methicillin-susceptible *Staphylococcus aureus*	Staphylococcal penicillin (nafcillin or oxacillin)
Methicillin-resistant *Staphylococcus aureus*	Vancomycin
Enterococcus	• Ampicillin and gentamicin • Ampicillin-nonsusceptible: vancomycin and gentamicin
Group B *Streptococcus*	Penicillin; ampicillin is an acceptable alternative
Escherichia coli[a]	• Ampicillin • Ampicillin-resistant: aminoglycoside or cephalosporin • ESBL: meropenem, or cefepime, or amikacin
Other gram-negative bacilli[a]	• Antipseudomonal penicillin, or cephalosporin, ± aminoglycoside • ESBL: meropenem, or cefepime, or amikacin • Carbapenemase: seek infectious diseases consultation
Candida species[b]	• Amphotericin • Fluconazole

[a]Infectious disease specialist consultation is strongly recommended in cases of gram-negative meningitis and all cases of ESBL or carbapenemase-producing gram-negative infections.

[b]Amphotericin deoxycholate is recommended unless renal infection can be ruled out. Fluconazole should only be used for systemic infection if isolate susceptibility data are available.

ESBL, Extended-spectrum beta-lactamase.

Targeted Therapy

The duration of therapy for infants with culture-confirmed bacterial LOS is typically 10 days after documenting sterile cultures but may vary from 7 to 21 days depending on the pathogen, type of infection, and time to culture clearance. Longer treatment duration is appropriate for a site-specific infection such as meningitis, septic arthritis, or osteomyelitis, and longer treatment may also be indicated for fungal infection. Once a pathogen is identified, antimicrobial therapy should be narrowed based upon the susceptibility profile. Antimicrobial therapies for the most common causative organisms of LOS are shown in Table 31.1. Repeat blood cultures should be obtained every 1 to 2 days until sterility is achieved. When persistent bacteremia occurs (generally defined as >2 positive cultures on appropriate therapy), an isolated source of infection (abscess, septic thrombus, septic arthritis, osteomyelitis, or endocarditis) should be considered and appropriate imaging obtained. Consultation with infectious disease specialists is recommended for cases involving prolonged bacteremia, meningitis, or organ-specific fungal infection.

Adjunctive Therapy

Supportive care includes maintaining adequate oxygenation, ventilation, and intravascular volume, with close attention blood glucose levels, acid-base status, and serum electrolytes. Infants with severe sepsis or septic shock may require escalated respiratory support, volume resuscitation, and/or vasopressor medications. There is no clear consensus on when CVCs should be removed in the setting of culture-confirmed LOS, and practice varies.[32] Considerations include the clinical stability of the infant, pathogen virulence, duration of bacteremia, suspicion for contaminant versus true infection, and ability to obtain alternative access.[72] When CVCs are removed promptly, infants experience fewer infection-related complications.[72] Delayed removal of CVCs is associated with increased infection-attributable morbidity and mortality among infants infected with *Candida* species.[28] Multiple trials of adjunctive intravenous immune globulin have not demonstrated clinical benefit for infants with sepsis.[73,74]

Long-Term Outcomes

Preterm infants with LOS are two to three times more likely to die than gestational-age-matched infants.[75,76] Infection-related mortality is lower for otherwise healthy term infants.[77,78] Among preterm infants, mortality is also related to the infecting organism, with the highest death rates attributed to gram-negative and fungal infections and the lowest infection-attributable mortality among infants infected with CONS.[75–77] Most mortality related to LOS caused by gram-negative bacteria occurs within 72 hours of the blood culture, and LOS caused by multidrug-resistant strains are associated with increased mortality compared with nonresistant strains.[77,79] Preterm infants who survive after LOS are at increased risk for a prolonged NICU length of stay, NEC, bronchopulmonary dysplasia, and neurodevelopmental impairment.[5,7,75,76] Fungal LOS carries a particularly poor prognosis among survivors, with higher incidence of cerebral palsy and neurodevelopmental impairment compared with bacterial LOS.[26]

CHAPTER 32

Neonatal Herpes Simplex Virus Infections

Yahya Ethawi, Steven Garzon, Thierry A.G.M. Huisman, Suresh Boppana, Akhil Maheshwari

KEY POINTS

1. Neonatal herpes simplex virus (HSV) infections can cause potentially devastating infections in newborn infants.
2. HSV has a double-stranded linear DNA genome and is seen in two variants, HSV-type 1 and HSV-type 2.
3. Neonatal HSV infections occur in three patterns: prenatal, perinatal, and postnatal. Perinatal infections are most common and are associated with serious morbidity and mortality.
4. HSV infections can be confirmed by isolating the virus in enhanced viral culture, detecting herpes DNA in polymerase chain reactions, detecting herpes antigens by rapid direct fluorescent antibody tests, and enzyme immunoassays.
5. Acyclovir is the recommended antiviral agent for treatment of all types of HSV disease. The duration of acyclovir therapy depends on the type of infection and the response of neonatal HSV.
6. The outcome of HSV infection of neonates depends on clinical types. HSV infection is life-lasting, even with appropriate treatment. Neonatal central nervous system infection is an important cause of neurodevelopmental delay. The disseminated disease is most serious and may cause mortality in up to 30% of infected infants.

Background

Neonatal herpes simplex virus (HSV) can cause potentially devastating infection in newborn infants. These infections have been noted in about 0.2% of all neonatal intensive care admissions and account for 0.6% of neonatal mortality in the United States. Infected infants need prolonged monitoring and treatment, and with a high incidence of long-term morbidity, they frequently need considerable healthcare resources.[1–4]

Virus

HSV has a double-stranded linear DNA genome of 150,000 base pairs that encode more than 80 polypeptides. The nucleocapsid is composed of 162 capsomeres arranged in a 20-faced polyhedron, which is covered by a lipid tegument containing polyamines (Fig. 32.1).[1] There are two variants, HSV-type 1 and HSV-type 2, but the two share several homologous DNA sequences and encoded glycoproteins, suggesting evolution from a common ancestor virus.[1] Acute infections have a cytolytic effect, but the virus may also persist lifelong in an intracellular latent state that is not susceptible to antiviral agents.

Epidemiology

Neonatal HSV infections are seen in 3 to 30 per 100,000 live births.[5–10] In the United States about 1500 cases are reported per year[11]; the incidence of neonatal HSV disease has a direct relationship with the prevalence of HSV-type 2 genital infections in the general population. There are some concerns that the incidence of central nervous system (CNS) and disseminated HSV infections may have increased since the year 2000.[1,12,13] Early testing and empiric treatment for HSV infections should be considered in all ill febrile neonates, and this approach may improve the survival rate and reduce the long-term sequelae.

There are three patterns of neonatal (<3 months of age) HSV disease[5–8,11]:

1. Prenatal, seen in 1 in 250,000 infants;
2. Perinatal, seen in 1 in 3200 to 10,000 live births and associated with serious morbidity and mortality; and
3. Postnatal, seen in about 1 in 100,000 live births.

Neonatal HSV infections account for 1.2% of all emergency room admissions in the United States. Studies show three patterns of neonatal HSV disease: localized to the skin, eyes, and mouth (SEM) in approximately 40%; to the CNS in 30%; and disseminated infection in 30%.[14] These infections are seen most often between 7 and 14 days after birth, and the frequency declines in the second month after birth.

Clinical Manifestation

The clinical manifestations of neonatal HSV infections may vary depending on the timing of infection. Both HSV-type 1 and HSV-type 2 may cause any of these three patterns, although HSV-type 2 infections may have poorer outcomes.[1,13,15,16]

Prenatal infections account for 1% to 2% of all neonatal HSV disease. Some infants show only residua of past disease with cutaneous scarring, eye involvement, and CNS features such as microcephaly or hydranencephaly.[21–24] Others may show active infection, ranging from just a few skin vesicles to severe pneumonitis or disseminated disease with fatal multisystem organ failure.[21,22]

Prenatal or congenital HSV infections result from maternal viremia and transplacental acquisition or ascending infections through the membranes that are either ruptured or may be intact but with altered permeability. The histopathological changes may be limited to placental infarcts, plasma cell deciduitis, and lymphoplasmacytic villitis or may clearly extend to the fetus with necrotizing, calcifying funisitis. Severe cases show hydrops fetalis and fetal death. HSV can often be cultured from the placenta or identified using molecular techniques, such as polymerase chain reaction

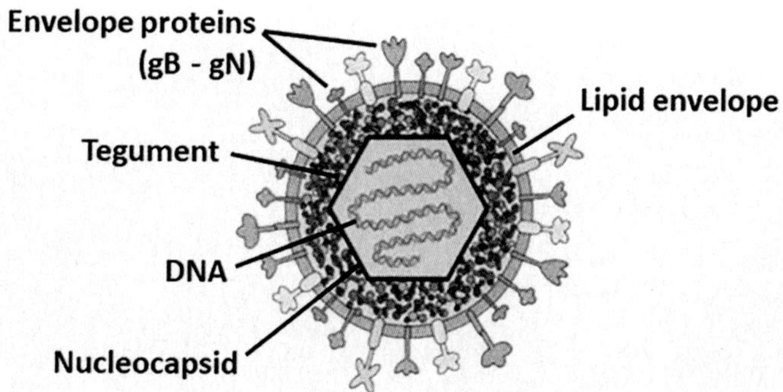

Fig. 32.1 Schematic Figure Showing the Structure of a Herpes Simplex Virus. There is a lipid envelope studded with proteins, a protective tegument, and a protein nucleocapsid shell, all of which enclose a central DNA core.

(PCR), immunohistochemistry, or in-situ hybridization. A high index of suspicion is needed.[20]

Perinatal infections account for nearly 85% of all neonatal HSV infections.[11] The virus may be transmitted to the infant during delivery from visible or unnoticed lesions in the maternal genital tract. It can enter the baby's body via the oral or genital mucosa, conjunctiva, or breaches in the skin; move into the sensory nerve endings; and then be transported retrograde via the axons to the dorsal root ganglia.[1]

The risk of perinatal infections increases with[13]:

- Primary (versus recurrent) maternal infection
- Low maternal immunity to HSV
- Prolonged rupture of membranes
- Use of fetal scalp monitors
- Mode of delivery (higher risk in vaginal versus cesarean section delivery)

Ascending infections frequently follow prolonged rupture of membranes, but an intact amniotic membrane may not be protective in all cases. Neonatal HSV infections have even been documented after cesarean delivery in women with intact membranes.[23,24]

Perinatal infections may be difficult to diagnose because there may not be a recorded maternal history of HSV infection.[25] Maternal fever is a risk factor, but it is not very useful because of its frequent occurrence during labor.[15,25–29] In infected neonates, the initial manifestations may be vague, such as variability in temperature, respiratory difficulties, jaundice, feeding problems, and lethargy.[1,29] However, these symptoms can quickly progress to hypotension, disseminated intravascular coagulation, and multisystem organ failure. Perinatal HSV infections are seen in three patterns: SEM, CNS, and disseminated disease.

Skin, Eye, and Mouth Disease

SEM disease constitutes approximately 40% of neonatal HSV infections.[10,11] Many infants may recover just from these localized lesions, whereas others may progress to develop CNS involvement or disseminated disease. SEM disease can present in the first 2 to 8 weeks after birth.[30] The vesicular lesions are often seen clustered on an erythematous base, and many coalesce,[1] making the distinction between HSV and bacterial skin infection difficult in many cases. These are seen most frequently on the presenting parts during labor and those of localized trauma such as that caused by scalp monitors. However, in infants with disseminated disease, skin vesicles may be seen in any part(s) of the body.

Eye infections are frequently asymptomatic at onset. Early signs may include watery eyes, crying from possible eye pain, and conjunctival erythema with or without vesicles in the periorbital area. The keratoconjunctivitis of neonatal HSV infections may lead to cataracts and chorioretinitis, causing permanent vision problems.[1,17]

Oropharyngeal disease may also be asymptomatic in its early stages and may begin as localized ulcerative lesions in the mouth, palate, and on the tongue. Distinction must be made between HSV infection and local trauma or other viral infections such as enterovirus.

Infants suspected to have SEM disease can have herpes viremia and subclinical multiorgan involvement in the liver, lungs, kidneys, cardiovascular system, and/or the CNS. These infants should be evaluated and managed as having early disseminated disease. With prompt treatment, many of these infants with early dissemination may have a good prognosis.

CNS Disease

About 30% of infants with HSV disease have isolated CNS involvement.[11,30] This CNS infection may result either from retrograde extension from the nasopharynx and olfactory nerves or via hematogenous spread. HSV meningoencephalitis typically manifests between 7 and 21 days after birth but can be delayed up to the second month.[30] CNS involvement may or may not be associated with SEM (skin lesions are seen in 60%–70% of patients) and/or disseminated disease.[11]

Early CNS disease is often asymptomatic, but clinical features such as irritability, tremors, lethargy, poor feeding, fluctuation of temperature, focal or generalized seizures, and bulging anterior fontanel can be seen with disease progression.[16,31,32] Cerebrospinal fluid (CSF) analysis may be inconclusive in early phases of the disease, but as the disease progresses, there may be mononuclear cell pleocytosis, moderately low glucose levels, and elevation in protein concentrations. The presence of red blood cells is not common.[25] Infants with CNS disease need to be evaluated and treated promptly with a high index of suspicion, because in the absence of noticeable skin lesions, it may be hard to distinguish CNS disease from other causes of neonatal sepsis or meningitis.[11,12] In many infants, there may be a need for empiric acyclovir therapy until the results of HSV DNA, PCR, and other CSF studies are available.[33,34]

Brain neuroimaging such as computed tomography (CT) and magnetic resonance imaging (MRI) may be normal at disease onset, but abnormalities such as parenchymal brain edema or attenuation, hemorrhage, or destructive lesions start appearing within a few hours (Fig. 32.2).[1,31] Although not specific, electroencephalographic abnormalities are often seen early in the course of CNS infection, with focal or multifocal periodic epileptiform discharges and frank seizure activity.[1,35]

Disseminated Disease

Approximately 30% of patients present with disseminated disease that presents with sepsis-like features and multisystem organ failure.[1,11,29,30,36] These infants may have lesions in the skin and mucous membranes (vesicles, seen in 60%–80% of patients),[11] meningoencephalitis (60%–75%),[30] hepatitis (40%),[37] lung infection (pneumonia, hemorrhagic pneumonitis, pleural effusions, and respiratory failure [40%]),[38] myocarditis and/or cardiac failure (25%), adrenal dysfunction with hypotension (70%), renal failure (70%), gastrointestinal tract abnormalities with necrotizing enterocolitis-like lesions (30%), hematologic abnormalities (thrombocytopenia, neutropenia [30%]), and disseminated intravascular coagulation (30%). Fever is seen in 60% to 70% of patients, but critically ill infants with multisystem organ failure may frequently have hypothermia.[1,29,39] Without

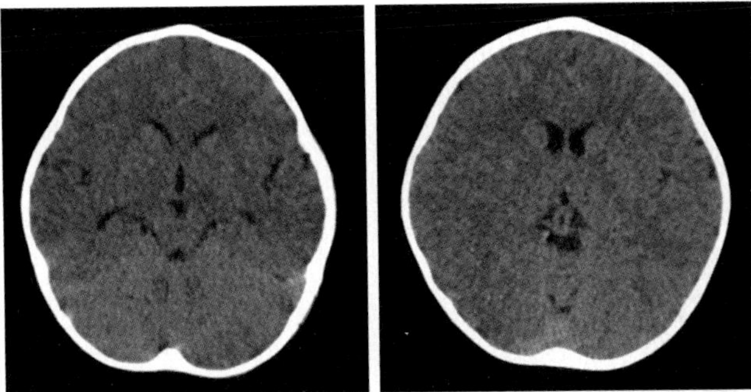

CT scan on day of onset was normal

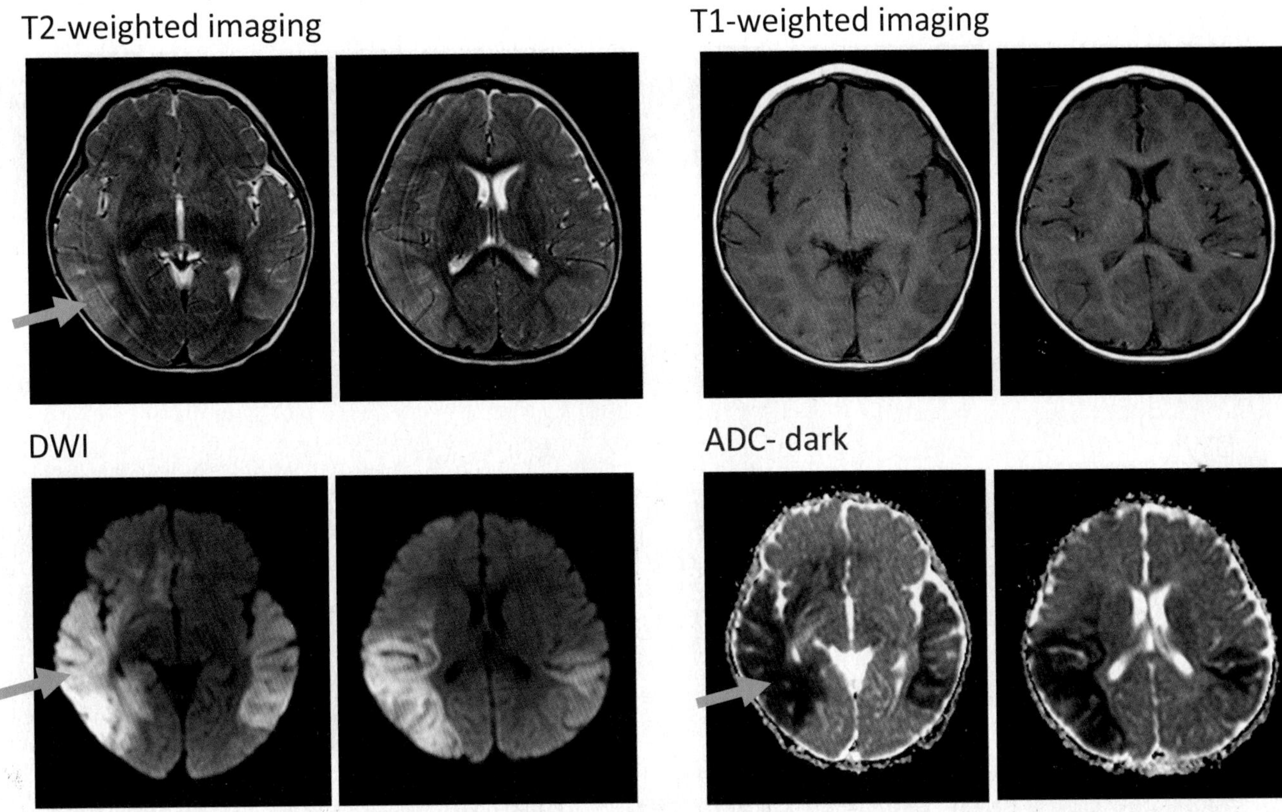

Fig. 32.2 Central Nervous System Imaging From an Infant With Herpes Simplex Virus Encephalitis. (A) On the day of disease onset, (1) noncontrast computed tomography (CT) appeared normal, but (2) magnetic resonance imaging (MRI) showed restricted diffusion in bilateral temporoparietal lobes, suggesting cytotoxic edema *(blue arrows)*. T2- and T1-weighted images showed signal changes and mild edema *(blue arrows)*. (B) Three days later, (1) noncontrast CT showed bilateral temporoparietal lobe hypodensities *(arrow)*, and (2) MRI showed worsening of cytotoxic edema *(blue arrows)*. Postcontrast images showed subtle meningovascular enhancement *(white arrows)*. These changes were prominent in diffusion-weighted (DW) and apparent diffusion coefficient (ADC) images. (C) One month after disease onset, MRI showed resolving cytotoxic edema, but there was global volume loss and gyriform enhancement *(arrow)*. (D) Three months later, there was extensive cystic encephalomalacia *(blue arrows)*. DW MRI and ADC maps show signal changes based on diffusion of water molecules in cells. Failure of normal diffusion across cell membranes and consequent cytotoxic edema (restricted diffusion), such as in encephalitis and stroke, is hyperintense on DW imaging and hypointense on ADC maps. T2-weighted images show edema and inflammation as hyperintense signals. T1-weighted images are useful for morphologic assessment but are relatively insensitive to detect pathology, particularly in early disease. Encephalomalacia looks hypointense on T1 images.

treatment, 80% of infants with disseminated HSV infections may die due to extensive organ damage.[3,25,28,40]

Diagnosis

Neonatal HSV disease is a clinically challenging problem because it starts with subtle, nonspecific manifestations that may mimic bacterial sepsis or other viral diseases such as those due to enteroviruses. A history of perinatal exposure in mothers with active genital lesions is helpful but frequently not present. A recent study matched 149 infants ≤60 days of age with 1340 control infants, all of whom were evaluated for infection, including CSF analysis.[41] Age, preterm birth, a history of seizure activity at home, ill appearance, abnormal temperature, vesicular rash, thrombocytopenia, neutropenia, and CSF pleocytosis were all significantly associated with HSV infection.

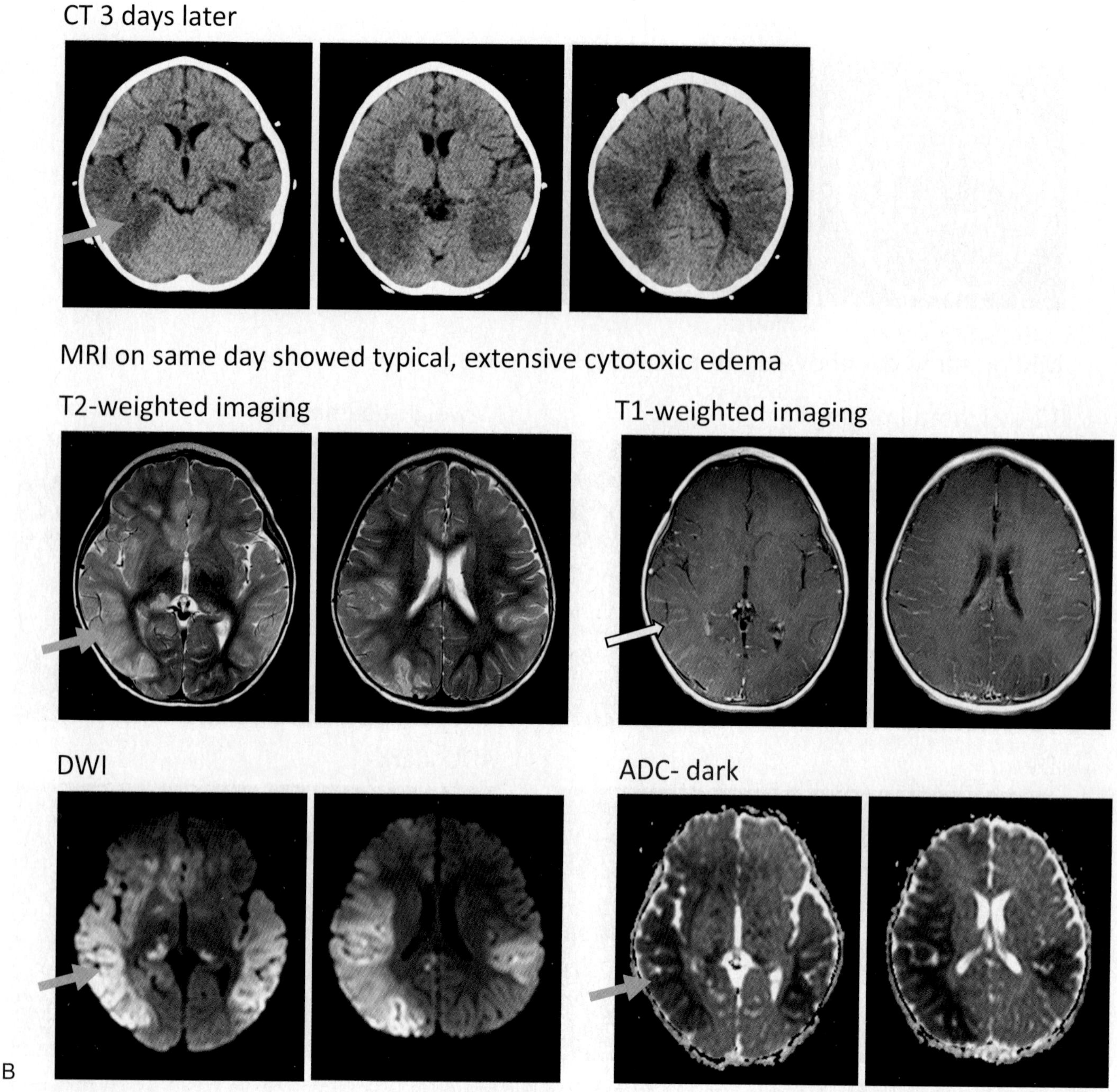

CT 3 days later

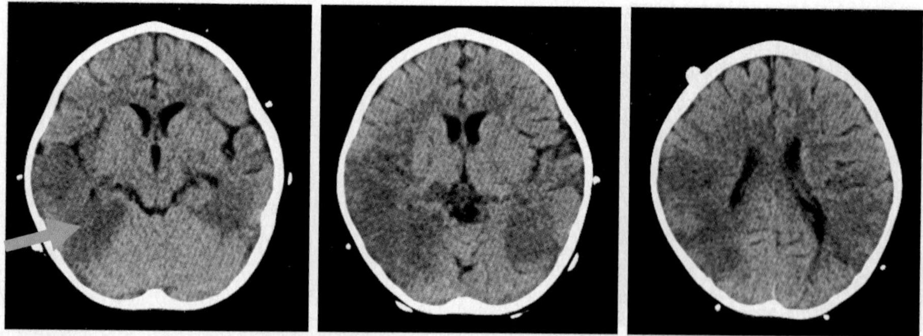

MRI on same day showed typical, extensive cytotoxic edema

T2-weighted imaging

T1-weighted imaging

DWI

ADC- dark

B

Fig. 32.2 Cont'd

The study authors proposed a scoring mechanism based on these factors, to aid in HSV clinical decision-making.

HSV infections can be confirmed by isolating the virus in enhanced viral culture, detecting herpes DNA in PCR, or detecting herpes antigens by rapid direct fluorescent antibody tests[42,43] and enzyme immunoassays.[43,44] Direct fluorescent antibody is specific but not as sensitive.[44] Generally, the serology is not of help in the diagnosis of neonatal herpes infection at the time of presentation. For culture, surface swabs from the conjunctivae, mouth, nasopharynx, and rectum are used.[30] Viral cultures may be positive in >90% cases.[1,30] If obtained 12 to 24 hours after birth, positive cultures indicate ongoing viral replication and not contamination from intrapartum exposure. Specimens from fresh vesicular lesions usually are positive within 24 hours of incubation, whereas CSF or other site specimens may need few days. Negative viral cultures after 10 days of incubation are usually considered negative.

If skin or mucous membrane lesions are present, swabs/scrapings can be obtained for cultures, PCR, or direct immunofluorescence (may not be as sensitive). HSV PCR assays of the skin and mucosal specimens are accepted alternatives.[16,30] All infants suspected of having an HSV infection should undergo a lumbar puncture and CSF analysis by PCR. Cultures are useful but may not be as sensitive as PCR.[36,45–51] Blood and plasma may be used for culture and/or PCR but are not as sensitive (positive in about 85% of cases). However, the detection of herpes DNA in the blood or plasma of neonatal disseminated HSV disease confirms the diagnosis and provides the opportunity for starting acyclovir early in the course of the disease.[49,52,53] Detection of >7 log10 copies per mL suggests increased

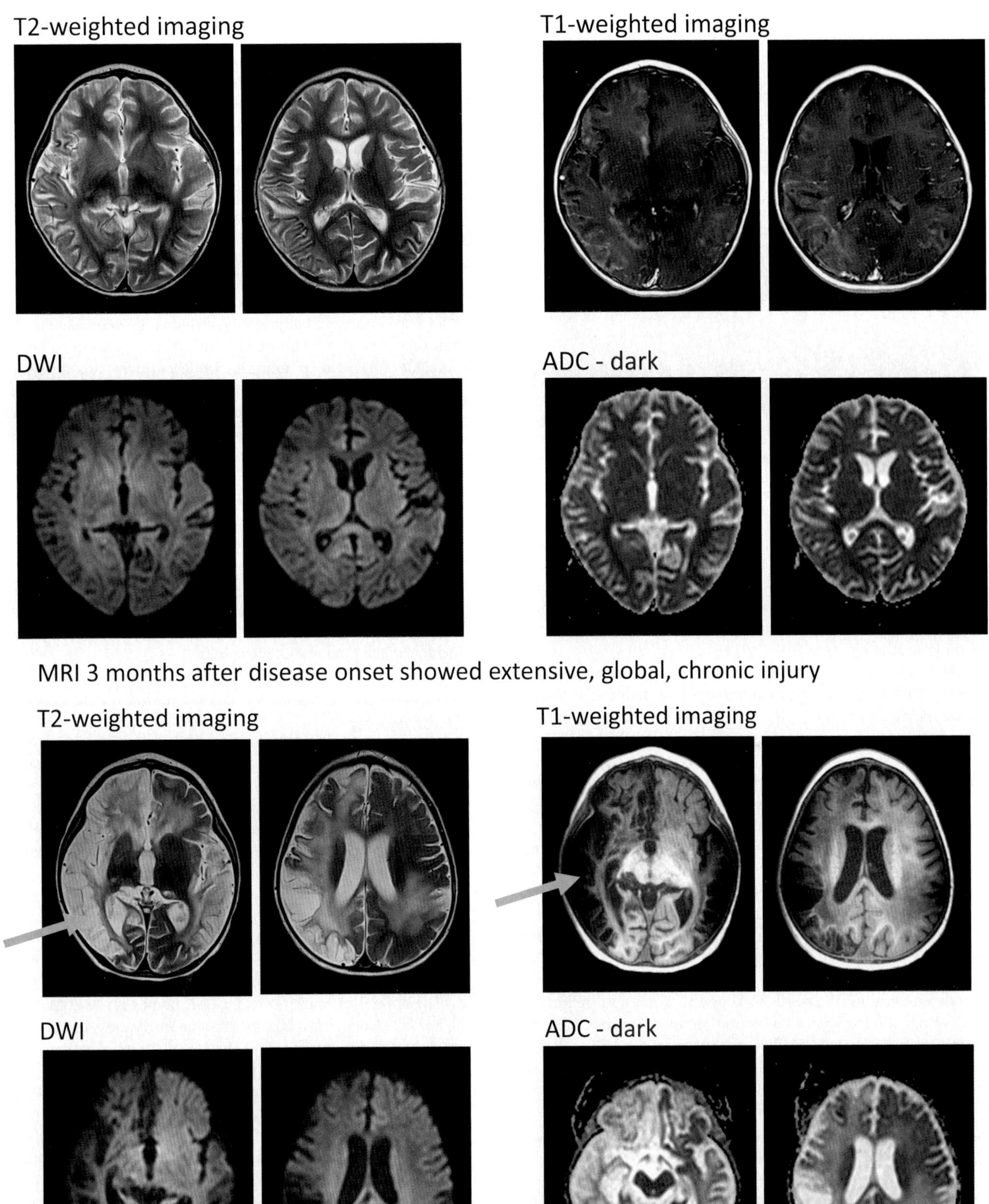

Fig. 32.2 Cont'd

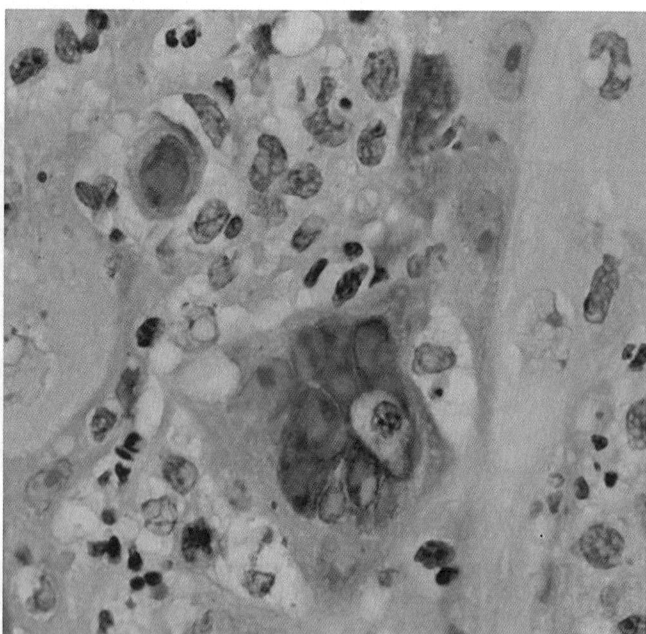

Fig. 32.3 High Magnification (1000×) of Cells With Herpes Simplex Virus Infection. Cells show multinucleation, nuclear modeling, and chromatin margination giving the typical ground-glass appearance. In the upper left quadrant, another infected cell is seen. Neutrophils are usually present due to ulceration of the lesions.

risk of mortality.[53] Specimens such as tracheal aspirates in intubated infants, peritoneal fluid in neonates undergoing peritoneal drainage, or laparotomy for other reasons can also be used for viral culture and PCR. Suspicious skin lesions can also be evaluated by biopsy and histopathology (see Fig. 32.2).

All infants with HSV disease should undergo neuroimaging with MRI or CT.[30] MRI is generally more sensitive than CT.[1,31] Neuroimaging may be normal early in the course of the disease, but as the disease progresses, parenchymal brain edema or abnormal attenuation, hemorrhage, or destructive lesions become evident.[1,31] The classic destructive lesions may be multifocal, with involvement limited to the temporal lobe or extended to the brainstem or cerebellum (Fig. 32.3).[31,35] Prenatal ultrasound may be useful; it may show damage in the fetal brain. However, postnatal ultrasound is not so accurate for estimating the extent of CNS disease. Infants with CNS HSV disease should undergo electroencephalography, particularly if there are seizures, abnormal movements, or abnormal CSF. The most common findings are focal or multifocal periodic or quasiperiodic epileptiform discharges.[1,25,30,31,40]

All infants with HSV disease should undergo standard laboratory tests to determine the need for supportive therapy. Infants with respiratory signs may need chest radiography. Primary HSV pneumonia or disseminated HSV disease may be seen as bilateral, diffuse lesions. Those with HSV hepatitis and acute liver failure may show ascites and hepatomegaly on ultrasound.

Management and Prevention

Acyclovir is the recommended antiviral agent for treatment of all types of HSV disease.[54–57] A virus-specific thymidine kinase converts acyclovir to acyclovir monophosphate, and other cellular enzymes then convert it to acyclovir triphosphate. This triphosphate form inhibits viral replication.[54–64] The recommended dose of acyclovir for all types of neonatal herpes is 60 mg/kg/day intravenously, divided every 8 hours.[55] The dose should be adjusted for abnormal renal function.[25,55] The duration of acyclovir therapy depends on the type and response of neonatal HSV.[54,55,57,58] SEM disease needs to be treated for a minimum of 14 days. CNS and disseminated diseases should be treated for a minimum of 21 days. The CSF should be reevaluated prior to cessation of treatment to ensure that HSV is no longer detectable by PCR.[54,58,65–69] If the test is positive, then the treatment should be continued and CSF herpes PCR repeated weekly until negative.[54,65,70]

If started early in HSV disease, acyclovir improves survival and outcome.[55,56,71] Early introduction of acyclovir may prevent 50% to 60% of SEM disease from progression to CNS and disseminated herpes.[72] In disseminated disease, acyclovir has reduced 1-year mortality from 85% to 29%.[27,55,56,65,73] The mortality in CNS disease has dropped from 50% to 4%.[55,56,65] Unfortunately, the improvement in neurodevelopment is not certain.[55,56,65,73]

Acyclovir is generally well tolerated.[55,58,65] Some infants may show mild renal injury, and others may develop dose-dependent reversible neutropenia.[58,65,74,75] The neutropenia does not seem to affect the outcome. Acyclovir is definitely preferred over vidarabine, which has more systemic toxicity and also brings logistical difficulties with the need for a 12-hour infusion dosing schedule.[56] If intravenous acyclovir is not available, ganciclovir (6 mg/kg/12 hours) can be used.[76–78] Another option is foscarnet at a dose of 60 mg/kg/12 hours. To treat eye disease, a topical ophthalmic solution such as 1% trifluridine, 0.1% idoxuridine (iododeoxyuridine), or 0.15% ganciclovir can be used.[54,58,65,69]

The use of orally administered acyclovir after neonatal HSV infection for at least 6 months after birth is recommended to suppress recurrent outbreaks in infancy. Such treatment has been demonstrated to improve neurodevelopmental outcomes, with higher average development scores at 1 year of age[74] without affecting the incidence and degree of neutropenia.[79]

Outcomes

The outcome of HSV infection of neonates depends on clinical types. HSV infection is life-lasting, even with appropriate treatment. All types of neonatal HSV infection may recur even despite oral suppressive therapy. Eye assessment and follow-up by an ophthalmologist for up to 12 months are recommended. Later-onset recurrences beyond 12 months have been documented.[80,81]

Neonatal CNS infection is associated with significant survival with neurodevelopmental delay.[79] Neonatal SEM disease has good outcomes, with $<2\%$ of infants treated per recommended protocols having any developmental delay.[54,55,57,65,74,75,82,83] Ocular involvement may increase the risk of vision loss and needs close follow-up.[58,65]

The annual mortality rate for CNS herpes is 4%.[55] Mortality is higher in infants with a history of prematurity, seizures, and altered sensorium at presentation.[65,82,84] In this subgroup of patients, 30% of survivors may have normal neurologic development.[55,65,73]

The annual mortality rate for disseminated disease is approximately 30%.[55,65,82,85] Most survivors may have normal or near normal neurologic development,[55,65,73] but as many as one-quarter may have developmental delay, hemiparesis, persistent seizures, microcephaly, or blindness.[65,85–87]

Vaccine

There are no licensed, effective vaccines available. A candidate HSV-type 2 gD subunit vaccine is in phase 3 clinical trials.[58,88]

Management of the Asymptomatic Exposed Infant

The optimal management of an asymptomatic patient exposed to maternal herpes infection at delivery with documented maternal virologic testing or active genital lesions has not been assessed in controlled trials.[57,69] Recommendations for evaluation of asymptomatic, exposed newborns are made by the American Academy of Pediatrics.[89] The risk of transmission is 25% to 60% higher in infants delivered vaginally or more than 4 hours after rupture of membranes to mothers with active genital lesions.[54,69,90,91] The risk is lower in infants born by cesarean section.[54,69,90,91]

Conclusions

A full evaluation is needed for all neonates with suspected or proven herpes infection to assess the degree of organ involvement and exclude other causes of the clinical situation. Pending definitive diagnosis, empiric therapy for neonatal HSV may be warranted. Acyclovir is the medication of choice for the treatment of all types of neonatal herpes disease. The duration of intravenous acyclovir treatment should be based on clinical situations and response to therapy from a minimum of 14 days for SEM to a minimum of 21 days for CNS and disseminated types. Ocular involvement needs eye drops and evaluation by specialists.

CHAPTER

33 Postnatal Cytomegalovirus Infection Among Preterm Infants

Sagori Mukhopadhyay, Kristin Weimer

KEY POINTS

1. Cytomegalovirus (CMV) infection is acquired in the postnatal period primarily from mother's milk feeding.
2. Postnatal CMV (pCMV) infection is usually asymptomatic in healthy term infants. Among very low birth weight (VLBW, birth weight <1500 g) infants, infection occurs in ~6.5% and is associated with a sepsis-like syndrome in ~1% but is rarely fatal.
3. Symptomatic pCMV infection is associated with lower gestation, younger age at acquisition, and an increased number of preexisting comorbid conditions.
4. VLBW pCMV infection has been variably associated with increased risk of chronic lung disease, retinopathy of prematurity, hearing loss, and neurodevelopmental impairment.
5. There are no standard recommendations for use of antiviral therapies for pCMV infection.
6. Prevention of pCMV transmission from mother to preterm infant is an area of ongoing research that has focused on methods to inactivate the virus in milk. The risks and benefits of such approaches remain unclear.

Introduction

Human cytomegalovirus (CMV) is a double-stranded DNA virus of the beta-herpes family. Primary infection with CMV commonly occurs via mucosa, but transmission can also occur after a transfusion or transplant or *in utero.* Like other herpes viruses, CMV persists after primary infection, predominantly by residing in myeloid cells where the virus does not replicate and avoids elimination by the host immune system.[1] During times of altered immune function, such as immunosuppression for transplant therapy, the virus can reactivate, proliferate with multiorgan involvement, and cause substantial morbidity and mortality.[2] In neonates, both congenital CMV infection (cCMV) and postnatally acquired CMV infection (pCMV) occur almost exclusively among infants born to CMV-infected mothers. cCMV may occur in the newborn due to primary maternal infection during pregnancy or with reactivation of a latent maternal infection, with resulting transplacental or intrapartum transmission.[3] In contrast, pCMV is primarily acquired via breast milk feeding. A majority of lactating women with latent CMV infection (positive for CMV-specific immunoglobulin G [IgG] serum antibodies) experience viral reactivation with secretion of CMV in breast milk.[4] This reactivation is localized in mammary tissue without consistent maternal viremia.[5] Although vertical CMV transmission during pregnancy can be devastating for the immune-naïve fetus, primary infection from breast milk in the postnatal period is largely asymptomatic among both term and preterm infants.[6] Preterm and very-low birth weight (VLBW, birth weight <1500 g) infants, however, may manifest acute illness after pCMV, with symptoms ranging from isolated laboratory abnormalities to acute clinical decompensation.[4,7–9] In the following, we will address neonatal CMV infection, with an emphasis on pCMV among preterm, VLBW infants.

Viral Pathogenesis

CMV entry into host cells is driven by interactions between glycoprotein complexes present on the outermost lipid envelope of the virus and host receptors (Fig. 33.1).[10,11] Once intracellular, a tightly regulated sequence of immediate early, early, and late gene expression occurs. Viral effects on the host cell can include a variety of outcomes including lysis, immune evasion, immune activation, and an altered cellular environment, depending on the type of cell, stage of development (especially important in fetal infection), and the immune state of the host.[11] Mechanisms of CMV persistence and immune evasion involve a multipronged approach by viral gene products against each arm of human immune defense. The virus produces cytokines that mimic host interleukin 10 and suppress inflammation; interferes with immune action requiring major histocompatibility complex I and II presentation; slows cell apoptosis; encodes microRNAs that alter cell cycle regulation; and produces a chemokine that is thought to allow dissemination of the virus in the body.[1,11] CMV establishes latency in specific hematopoietic cell lines, establishing life-long persistence.

Disease Pathogenesis

Despite a robust host immune response and tropism for a variety of organ systems, CMV infection is clinically asymptomatic in most immunocompetent hosts. Symptomatic clinical illness among transplant recipients and cCMV infants is associated with high viral load.[12] Although viral load may have a predictive role in cCMV sequelae and is used for decision-making in transplant settings,[10,13–15] the relationship between viral load and pCMV clinical disease among preterm infants remains unclear.[16,17] CMV viral replication causes cell lysis and immune-mediated injury that together create a clinical picture similar to bacterial sepsis with multiorgan involvement. Among solid-organ transplant recipients, CMV reactivation/infection appears to cause an additional "indirect effect," resulting in increased secondary infection, decreased graft survival, and increased mortality[12] that are reduced by CMV prophylaxis.[2] Latent infection among immunocompetent hosts may also alter the baseline immune state by active engagement of mechanisms required to maintain latency. In a study of 210 twins, discordant CMV carriage in monozygotic

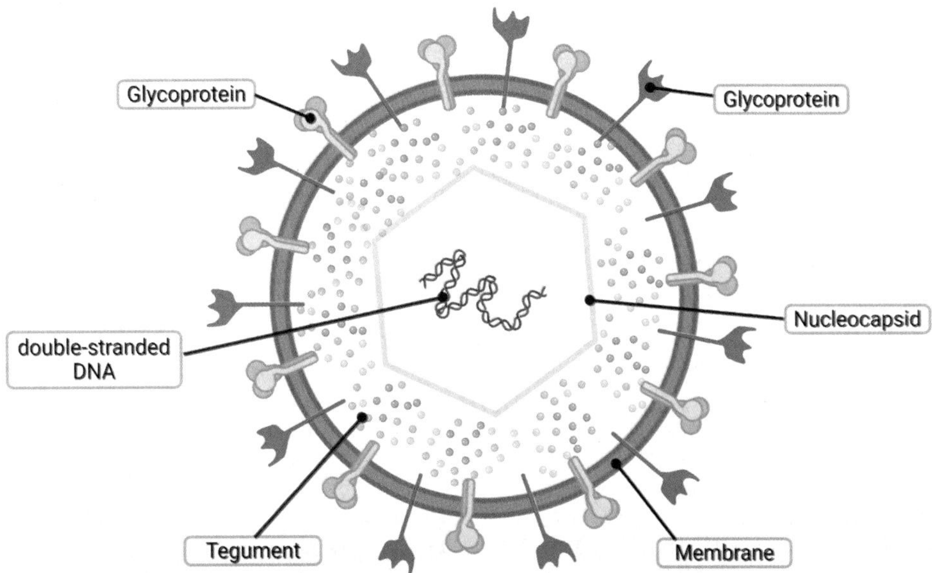

Fig. 33.1 Illustration of Cytomegalovirus (CMV) Structure. (Figure made in collaboration with Biorender.com.)

twins altered 50% of immune markers.[18] Latent CMV infection has been associated with altered cardiovascular health outcomes, attributed to this altered immune state.[19]

Perinatal Epidemiology

A multicenter study of 34,989 primarily term-born infants in 7 US hospitals (2008–09) reported a 0.5% incidence of cCMV infection.[20] A single-center study conducted from 1993 to 2008 among 4594 VLBW infants found cCMV in a similar proportion (0.39%).[21] The incidence of pCMV among preterm infants has varied in different reports. Using blood or urine CMV polymerase chain reaction (PCR) screening of VLBW infants at regular intervals from birth to 90 days, a study set in the United States found that pCMV occurred in 33/381 (8.7%) among those fed breast milk from CMV-positive mothers; no pCMV occurred among infants who were not fed mother's milk.[22] In a study conducted in Germany, VLBW infants were tested biweekly with urine CMV PCR testing until hospital discharge and then again at 3 to 6 months of age.[4] Of the 78 CMV-positive mothers and their 92 infants, CMV acquisition was reported in 21/92 infants (23%) while in the hospital and an additional 12/92 (13%) after discharge, for a total of 36% with pCMV. Differences in duration of follow-up, amount of breast milk ingested, and use of fresh or frozen milk may all account for the difference in transmission rates observed in these studies. Estimated seroprevalence for CMV in United States among women 20 to 49 years of age is 61.3% (95% confidence interval [CI], 58.9%–63.6%).[23] In a meta-analysis of 17 pCMV studies, annual pCMV incidence was estimated to be 2800 VLBW infants (6.5%; 95% CI, 3.7%–10.9%), with 1500 symptomatic cases (3.4%; 95% CI, 1.7%–5.8%) and 600 manifesting sepsis-like syndrome (1.4%; 95% CI, 0.7%–2.4%).[24] Estimations using frozen-thawed breast milk showed lower transmission rates but similar rates of symptomatic disease and sepsis-like presentation.[24]

Preterm pCMV

With the use of leuko-reduced and irradiated blood products, CMV transmission via mother's milk is the primary cause of pCMV.[22] High rates of viral DNA detection in breast milk have been reported across diverse racial/ethnic cohorts in multiple studies: 70% (Italy), 76% (United States), >80% (Sweden), 87% (Japan), 94% (Taiwan), and 95% (Netherlands).[5,17,25–28] CMV is detected in breast milk as early at 3 days to as late as 1 month postpartum.[4] Viral transmission is low when breast milk contains viral DNA alone (<10%) but approaches 50% when infectious virus is also present.[4] In all prospective studies, rates of infection are many-fold higher than rates of symptomatic disease.[4,22,29,30] Table 33.1 lists risk factors for transmission and symptomatic presentation.

Clinical Features of CMV Infection

Symptomatic congenital infection has a wide spectrum of presentation, from isolated hearing deficit to multisystem organ involvement and severe neurologic deficits, with severity of injury related to fetal age at acquisition.[31] A detailed discussion of the prevention, diagnosis and treatment of cCMV can be found in the review by Rawlinson et al.[31] Term and preterm infants commonly acquire pCMV from breast milk feeding without signs of infection.[6] In preterm infants the immature immune system, combined with a lack of maternally derived CMV antibody, contribute to the risk for symptomatic disease. Both direct viral damage and immune dysregulation may result in end organ injury.[32,33] Although there is an accepted causal link for manifestations such as bone marrow suppression (with evidence for direct tissue invasion, prevention with prophylaxis, and reversal with treatment),[2,8] causation is more difficult to establish with preterm outcomes that have a multifactorial pathogenesis, such as chronic lung disease, necrotizing enterocolitis (NEC), or childhood neurologic sequelae.[26,30,34–38] Attribution of clinical symptoms to pCMV is limited by the small number of cases in prospective studies (Table 33.2).[22,30,36,37,39,40] and variation in case definition and ascertainment bias for symptomatic infants.[7,32,34,41] Severe sepsis-like illness can occur, particularly among extremely low birth weight infants. Isolated thrombocytopenia, respiratory decompensation, and colitis are commonly reported signs in symptomatic pCMV cases among VLBW infants.[7,41] CMV-associated enteritis can present as atypical NEC,[42] and CMV-specific antigens and DNA have been identified in resected

Table 33.1 Predictors of Postnatal CMV Acquisition in Infants

Characteristic Associated With Transmission	Study Design
Maternal serostatus positive for CMV[4,22]	Prospective screening
Early detection of viral DNA in both the whey and cell components of breast milk[4]	Prospective screening
Higher (and earlier) breast milk viral load[26,70]	Prospective screening
Detection of virus that could be cultured (versus detection of viral DNA only)[4]	Prospective screening
Prolonged secretion of virus in milk[17]	Prospective screening
Exposure to greater volume of mother's milk[22,39,71,72]	Prospective screening
CMV genotype differentially associated with severely symptomatic cases[73,74]	Prospective screening and cross-sectional
Milk lactoferrin and maternal CMV IgG levels not shown to impact transmission[26,70,71]	Prospective screening
Milk IgG avidity associated with decreased transmission[75]	Prospective case study
Lower gestational age, birth weight, and preterm rupture of membrane[22,29,71]	Prospective screening
Characteristics Associated With Symptomatic Disease	
Lower birth weight, gestational age, and early acquisition[29]	Prospective screening
Higher preexisting morbidity[7,41]	Retrospective case study
Glucocorticoid use; hypothesized to reduce the viral load threshold for symptomatic disease[10,76,77]	Prospective, case-control, and post hoc analyses in adult and neonatal populations

CMV, Cytomegalovirus; *IgG*, immunoglobulin G.

intestinal specimens in NEC cases[33,43]; however, latent CMV can be enriched at sites of inflammation, complicating attribution.[12] In a post hoc analysis of a prospective screening study, NEC (≥ stage II) was significantly related to pCMV (adjusted hazard ratio, 8.45; 95% CI, 1.83–38.9).[26] In contrast, a study addressing the impact of pasteurizing mother's milk found decreased pCMV transmission after pasteurization but a trend toward higher incidence of NEC.[44] Longer-term outcomes associated with pCMV infection in preterm infants are summarized in Tables 33.3 and 33.4.

Diagnostic Testing

Maternal serum testing for CMV IgM and IgG can determine maternal serostatus and identify infants at risk for CMV infection. Urine testing is considered the standard for diagnosing neonatal CMV. Infants with cCMV continue to shed virus in urine for months to years after birth; pCMV can only be rigorously diagnosed if testing at < 14 to 21 days of age rules out cCMV. Nucleic acid testing (NAT) with PCR-based amplification has replaced traditional viral culture and shell vial assays (which detect early antigen expression) as the standard for urine CMV detection in many centers. cCMV detection with saliva NAT in term infants has a high sensitivity and specificity, whereas NAT from dried blood spots lacks sensitivity.[20,45,46] Saliva PCR is less sensitive than urine as a screening tool for pCMV among preterm infants, likely because of lower viral loads and a small volume of saliva.[47] NAT can detect CMV in a variety of clinical specimens including blood, cerebrospinal fluid, tracheal aspirate specimens, and bronchoalveolar lavage fluid. Quantitative NAT in blood is common for determining acute and ongoing viral replication and is used to monitor viral load in the management of transplant patients. There is no standardized recommendation for the use of viral load measurements in pCMV management. Immunofluorescent staining can be used to detect CMV in pathology tissue specimens.

The risks and benefits of universal screening for cCMV are currently a source of considerable debate in the United States. The primary benefit is anticipated to be more accurate identification of otherwise well-appearing term newborns at risk for CMV-mediated hearing loss. Among preterm infants, routine cCMV screening would offer the additional advantage of increased accuracy in diagnosis of pCMV.[45,48,49] The distinction has implications for ancillary testing and management, as outlined below. Testing for pCMV should be considered whenever there is clinical concern for late-onset sepsis or unexplained onset of thrombocytopenia among preterm infants fed mother's own unpasteurized breast milk.

Disease Management

Supportive management is central to care for preterm infants with symptomatic pCMV. Such infants may need an increase in cardiorespiratory support, transfusions, and periods of bowel rest to allow recovery.[7,8,41,42] Ganciclovir (administered intravenously [IV]) and its prodrug valganciclovir (administered per oral) are nucleoside analog DNA polymerase inhibitors that preferentially bind to CMV DNA (versus human DNA), inhibit CMV replication, and are the antiviral therapy of choice for CMV infection. Drug toxicity occurs in hematopoietic cells, where neutropenia is the most common side effect and has been associated with secondary infection in transplant patients.[2,50] The drug is not labeled for use in neonates or for the indication of cCMV or pCMV. Data for neonatal use comes from cCMV trials.[51,52] A trial of 109 infants with cCMV reported improved hearing and cognitive outcomes after 6 months of valganciclovir treatment compared with 6 weeks.[52] Approximately 20% of subjects had significant neutropenia in the first 6 weeks of treatment, and treatment had to be interrupted in three subjects; however, there was no difference in neutropenia between the two treatment groups from 7 weeks to 6 months. Mild transaminitis occurred less frequently.

Experience with antiviral therapy in preterm infants for pCMV is limited to case reports. Neither safety nor efficacy has been rigorously established, but no serious long-term effects of ganciclovir or valganciclovir therapy have been reported despite many years of off-label neonatal treatment. There are several case studies of infants with severe pCMV disease that report clinical improvement after antiviral therapy and an apparent shortening of disease course.[7,8,53,54] Although pCMV infection is rarely associated with mortality,[32,40] it is possible that pCMV-associated mortality is underreported due to lack of disease recognition. At this point, antiviral therapy for pCMV should be decided on an individual basis, accounting for severity of illness and evidence for systemic disease. One approach to diagnosing and managing pCMV cases is shown in Fig. 33.2. Consultation with pediatric infectious diseases experts and risk/benefit discussions with parents are both recommended. Unlike cCMV, antiviral therapy for pCMV is administered with a goal of resolving acute symptoms rather than prolonged viral suppression, and a shorter course of 2 to 3 weeks based on symptom resolution and viral load has been suggested.[55,56] If congenital infection cannot be ruled out and symptomatic disease is present, treatment for presumptive congenital infection may be considered. Current recommended treatment dosing follows that established for cCMV treatment ganciclovir 6 mg/kg IV q12 hours or valganciclovir 16 mg/kg PO q12 hours. Monitoring includes

Table 33.2 Acute Clinical Presentation Attributed to Postnatal CMV Infection Among Preterm Infants in Prospective Screening Studies

Study Symptomatic/ All Cases	GA Range, wk	Low Platelets	Low Neutrophils	Transaminitis or Cholestasis	GI Abnormality	Respiratory SLS	Mean Age at CMV Detection, Days (Range)	Mean Days at Symptoms (Range)	Mean Days From CMV Detection to Symptoms (Range)
Hamprecht et al.[4,a] 16/33	24–31	5	14	5	—	4	58.4 (29–120)	58 (22–118)	0.7 days (−14 to 7)
Mussi-Pinhata et al.[78] 1/21	28	1	1	1	—	—	49	63	14
Doctor et al.[39] 1/4	23	—	—	1	—	1	57	47	−10
Miron et al.[79,a] 3/4	27–29	—	—	3	—	1	32 (28–42)	NR	NA
Lee et al.[80,a] 1/2	24	1	—	1	1	—	37	37	0
Omarsdottir et al.[28] 1/2	24	—	—	1	—	—	34	34	0
Omarsdottir et al.[67] 2/5	26	—	—	2	—	—	51 (50–52)	51 (50–52)	0
Pilar et al.[81] 4/13	24–27	—	—	—	1	3	48 (15–88)	NR	NA
Patel et al.[26,b] 6/33	24–29	—	—	—	6	—	34 (12–66)	29 (19–60)	−5 (−47 to 28)
Total, No. (%)	—	**7 (20)**	**15 (43)**	**14 (40)**	**8 (23)**	**9 (26)**	—	—	—

[a]Each study had one child with petechiae and one with hepatospleenomegaly.

[b]Only reported GI manifestations.

CMV, Cytomegalovirus; *GA*, gestational age; *GI*, gastrointestinal; *NA*, not available; *NR*, not reported; *SLS*, sepsis lile syndrome; *WK*, weeks.

Table 33.3 Association of Postnatal CMV With Hospital Outcomes for Preterm Infants

Study Number of CMV Cases (n)	Description of Results Associated With Postnatal CMV Acquisition
BRONCHOPULMONARY DYSPLASIA (BPD)	
Kelly et al.[34] n = 303	Retrospective matched study of infants with and without pCMV (pCMV cases, n = 303) Relative risk for BPD: 1.33 (1.19–1.50) Relative risk for death/BPD: 1.21 (1.10–1.32)
Mukhopadhyay et al.[41] n = 19	Retrospective cohort study of symptomatic pCMV cases Adjusted odds ratio for BPD: 4.0 (1.3–12.4)
Prosch et al.[82] n = 12	Prospective screening study; included congenital infection (n = 2) CMV prevalence in BPD cases 7/24 (29%) versus 5/42 (12%) in infants without BPD (p not significant)
Patel et al.[26] n = 33	Prospective screening study; included symptomatic and asymptomatic infections Adjusted relative risk, mild BPD, 1.00 (0.69–1.46); moderate/severe BPD, 1.02 (0.57–1.80)
Martins-Celini et al.[71] n = 24	Prospective screening study; included symptomatic and asymptomatic infections Adjusted relative risk, 1.46 (0.82–2.55)
RETINOPATHY OF PREMATURITY (STAGE 2 OR 3)	
Martins-Celini et al.[71] n = 24	Prospective screening study; includes symptomatic and asymptomatic infections Adjusted relative risk, 2.51 (1.07–5.91)
Patel et al.[26] n = 33	Prospective screening study; includes symptomatic and asymptomatic infections Adjusted relative risk, stage 2: 0.85 (0.34–2.09); stage 3: 0.73 (0.10–5.21)
HEARING LOSS	
Weimer et al.[83] n = 273	Retrospective matched study of infants with and without pCMV (pCMV cases, n = 273) Relative risk for failed hearing screen: 1.80 (1.14–2.85)
Nijman et al.[9] n = 84	Prospective screening at term-corrected age; includes symptomatic (n = 6) and asymptomatic infants No case of sensorineural hearing loss at 1 year of age

CMV, Cytomegalovirus; *pCMV,* postnatal cytomegalovirus.

Table 33.4 Long-Term Neurologic Outcomes of Postnatal CMV Infection

Study Design (Reference)	n	Follow-Up Age	Measure	Finding
Prospective[17]	42 infants/ 6 infected	6 months	—	No difference
Prospective matched[84]	14 infected/ 41 uninfected VLBW	12–24 months	Bayley-II (MDI <70 or PDI <70) Gross motor quotient/Infant international battery	No significant differences
Prospective matched[85]	82 infants/ 21 infected	Term equivalent	MRI, Griffiths' Mental Developmental Scales at 16 months	Reduced fractional anisotropy of occipital region
Prospective matched[86,a]	44 infants/ 22 infected	2–4.5 years	Essential developmental milestones (<10th percentile for age) and structured neurologic exam for identifying cerebral palsy	No difference
Prospective matched[87,a]	41 infants/ 20 infected	7–8 years	Cog-Kaufman Assessment Battery for Children; Surveillance of Cerebral Palsy in Europe; Neuromotor function: Movement Assessment Battery for Children	Both cognitive and motor delay (manual dexterity and ball skills)
Prospective matched[88,a]	84 infants/ 42 infected	>4 years	Cog-Kaufman Assessment Battery for Children; Surveillance of Cerebral Palsy in Europe	Cognitive delay (simultaneous processing scale); no motor delay
Prospective matched[36]	71 infants/ 34 infected/ 37 term controls	12–15 years	Functional MRI	Increased activation in hippocampal and anterior cingulate regions
Prospective matched[37]	42 infants/ 19 infected/ 24 term controls	11–16 years	Cog-Wechsler Intelligence Scale	Cognitive delay

[a]Includes overlapping case and control preterm infants, from a single center in Germany.

CMV, Cytomegalovirus; *MDI,* mental development index; *MRI,* magnetic resonance imaging; *PDI,* psychomotor development index; *VLBW,* very low birth weight.

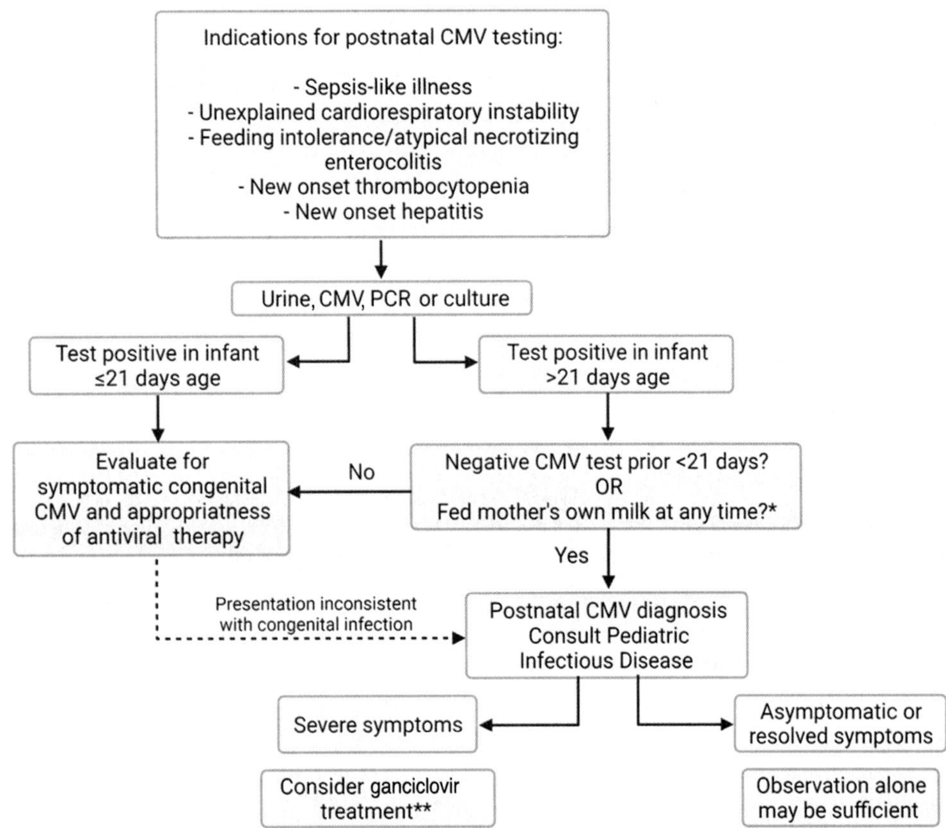
Indications for postnatal CMV testing:
- Sepsis-like illness
- Unexplained cardiorespiratory instability
- Feeding intolerance/atypical necrotizing enterocolitis
- New onset thrombocytopenia
- New onset hepatitis
Urine, CMV, PCR or culture
Test positive in infant ≤21 days age
Test positive in infant >21 days age
Evaluate for symptomatic congenital CMV and appropriatness of antiviral therapy
No
Negative CMV test prior <21 days? OR Fed mother's own milk at any time?*
Yes
Presentation inconsistent with congenital infection
Postnatal CMV diagnosis Consult Pediatric Infectious Disease
Severe symptoms
Asymptomatic or resolved symptoms
Consider ganciclovir treatment**
Observation alone may be sufficient
*Among infants never fed breastmilk, the probability of postnatally acquired CMV is low but may rarely occur via other modalities. For example, transfusion of non-irradiated or non-leukoreduced blood may transmit CMV.
**Ganciclovir 6 mg/kg IV q12 hours; valganciclovir 16 mg/kg PO q12 hours. Monitor weekly complete blood counts and liver function tests.

Fig. 33.2 Approach to pCMV Diagnosis and Management. *CMV*, Cytomegalovirus; *pCMV*, postnatal cytomegalovirus. (Flowchart made in collaboration with Biorender.com.)

weekly complete blood counts and liver function tests. Viral blood load may be followed to assess response. An eye exam to rule out retinitis, head imaging, and a hearing screen should be considered before discharge, especially if cCMV cannot be ruled out.

Infection Prevention

Preventive approaches to cCMV focus on prevention of primary infection in pregnant women by minimizing contact with saliva/urine from young children. Routine serologic testing of pregnant women is only recommended if ultrasound findings consistent with fetal CMV infection are observed. Trials of administering CMV-specific immunoglobulin to pregnant women to prevent cCMV have thus far been unsuccessful.[57]

With the development of reliable methods to prevent CMV transmission from transfused blood products, pCMV prevention efforts have focused on reducing exposure from breast milk. Donor milk banks generally use Holder pasteurization (62.5°C for 30 minutes), which inactivates and eliminates infectivity of the majority of bacteria and viruses, including CMV.[58] Treatment of mother's own milk is not routine in the United States due to concerns that such treatment reduces many of the nutrients and immune components in breast milk.[59–61] In addition, most neonatal intensive care units do not have the necessary equipment available for Holder pasteurization. One study demonstrated that short-term pasteurization (62.5°C for 5 seconds) significantly reduced pCMV transmission but did not eliminate it.[62] Another study evaluated ultraviolet-C irradiation (254 nm) of breast milk, which inactivates many bacteria while preserving immune components.[63] Although full CMV replication was inhibited, there was still evidence of viral transcription.[64] A small study eliminated CMV after microwaving at 750 W for 30 seconds, but such treatment impacts immune and nutrient components.[65,66] Finally, freeze-thawing breast milk prior to feeding may reduce viral load but does not eliminate infectivity.[24,60,67]

Consensus regarding strategies to address CMV transmission through breast milk is lacking. The American Academy of Pediatrics does not make any recommendations for treatment of breast milk to prevent pCMV acquisition, while the other guidelines in several European countries recommend strategies including Holder pasteurization of all milk until 34 weeks' gestational age.[44,68,69]

CHAPTER 34 Congenital Syphilis

Alvaro Dendi, Helena Sobrero, María Mattos Castellano, Akhil Maheshwari

KEY POINTS

1. Congenital syphilis is a global public health problem, particularly in the Americas where its incidence appears to be rising.
2. At birth 90% of infants are asymptomatic, the remaining 10% present a wide variety of symptoms from mild to lethal.
3. To confirm the presence of spirochete may be challenging, diagnosis will usually be based on maternal syphilis history, treponemal and non treponemal test performed (maternal and newborn's) and the presence of symptoms.
4. Patients will be treated with aqueous/procaine penicillin if congenital syphilis is proven or probable. Possible disease may be treated with a single dose of benzathine penicillin. This might also be the case if infection is less likely.
5. Follow up is paramount to ensure infants do not develop long term complications. Follow up will consist of periodical physical examination and non treponemal serologic test.
6. Prevention is key in diminishing the burden of congenital syphilis. Screening during pregnancy is recommended. Epidemiological surveillance through notifications systems remains a cornerstone to tackle this problematic.

Introduction

Congenital syphilis is the infection of a fetus and newborn infant caused by *Treponema pallidum*, a bacterium from the family *Spirochaetaceae.* The infection was described for the first time in Europe during the 15th century by Gaspar Torella.[1] In the Americas, the infection might have been brought by Europeans during colonization. *T. pallidum* was first identified in 1905 by Fritz Schaudinn, a zoologist, and Erich Hoffmann, a dermatologist. Penicillin was tested and proven to be an effective bactericidal agent against *T. pallidum* by John Mahoney, Richard Arnold, and A.D. Harris in 1943, and these findings provided an effective treatment for this infection.[2]

Syphilis is seen all over the world, particularly in urban areas. The reservoir of *Treponema* is exclusively human, and it is transmitted by body fluids or lesions that contain high concentrations of spirochetes, leading to a systemic and chronic infection.[3] Despite all the medical advances and the availability of an effective, affordable, and universally available treatment, congenital syphilis continues to cause considerable morbidity and mortality worldwide and is seen to evolve into various stages in patients with age (Fig. 34.1A). The consequences are particularly dire in infected pregnant women and newborn infants. Congenital syphilis remains a globally relevant public health problem.

Epidemiology

A large number of new cases of syphilis continue to be diagnosed each year. In 2016, 5.6 million new cases were diagnosed. The burden of congenital syphilis was estimated to be 473 per 100.000 births.[4–6] The incidence of syphilis showed some improvement during the period from 2007 to 2016, but it has plateaued since then. The number of new patients may be diminishing worldwide, but the incidence seems to be rising in the Americas. In the United States, the Centers for Disease Control and Prevention (CDC) has reported an increased number of new cases since the year 2000. The frequency of new cases has increased from 11.2 to 39.7 per 100,000 inhabitants, particularly in the western parts of the United States.[7,8] Syphilis is seen less frequently in women than in men, but the rate of new infections has increased by 178.6% during the period from 2015 to 2019. The prevalence is higher among women aged 20 to 39 and in African American, Latino, and Native American individuals living in the United States, Alaska, or the Pacific Islands.[7,8] The frequency of congenital syphilis has also increased during this period (see Fig. 34.1B).

In 2017, most parts of Latin America and the Caribbean region had reported advances in prevention of congenital syphilis; 15 out of the 17 countries in these regions reported virtual elimination of vertically transmitted syphilis (incidence <0.5 new cases per 1000 newborn infants per year). However, most of these advances have since been lost with a resurgence in the past few years. The largest rise in case load has been noted in Brazil.[9] Studies suggest that inadequate treatment of infected mothers is an important factor. Lack of proper prenatal care, difficulties in timely diagnosis of the infection, and clinical evidence of maternal infection despite proper treatment were also found to be fundamental to determining obstetric results.[10]

Pathogenesis

T. pallidum is a helical-shaped bacterium in the family *Spirochaetaceae,* subspecies *pallidum* (Fig. 34.2). These bacteria are host-dependent and can survive only in the human body, not freely in the environment. The unique adaptations in the outer membrane help circumvent clearance by the patient's immune system and facilitate prolonged subclinical/low-grade infections.[11,12]

After infection in the mother, the transmission to the fetus occurs most frequently during the incubation phase and in the primary stage of infection, when bacteremia is more frequent. Most infants get infected across the placenta *in utero. T. pallidum* has been detected in placental tissue as early as 9 to 10 weeks of gestation,[13] although the risk of infection increases with advancing gestation.[14,15] Some infants get infected during labor after exposure to the mother's body fluids or to lesions in the birth canal that contain high concentrations of these spirochetes, which can penetrate the fetal mucous membranes or skin.[12,16,17]

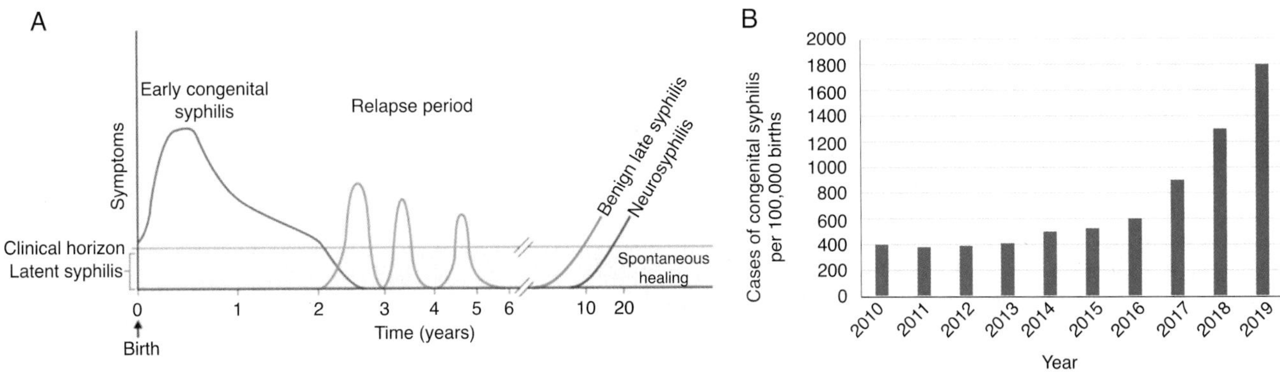

Fig. 34.1 Congenital Syphilis. (A) Time course for clinical manifestations of congenital syphilis. (B) Increasing incidence of congenital syphilis in the past few years. (Data in [A] modified permission from Stary and Stary. *Dermatology*. 82:1447–1469; Histogram in [B] based on data reported by Centers for Disease Control and Prevention, Sexually Transmitted Disease Surveillance 2019, Dos Santos et al. *PLoS One*. 2020;15[4]:e0231029; and Kojima and Klausner. *Current Epidemiology Reports*; 2018;5:24–38.)

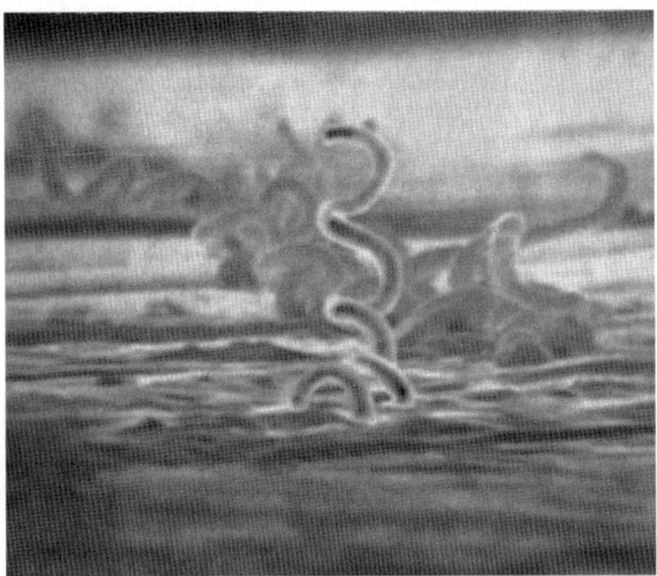

Fig. 34.2 Electron Micrograph of *Treponema pallidum* on Cultures of Cotton-Tail Rabbit Epithelium Cells, Displaying the Characteristic Helical Structure of Treponemes. (Reproduced with permission from Kollmann et al. In: *Remington and Klein's Infectious Diseases of the Fetus and Newborn Infant*, 16, 512–543.)

After a highly variable incubation period of 9 to 90 days, the primary stage of congenital syphilis begins. During this stage, the characteristic lesion, known as a chancre or a hallmark ulcer, appears. The chancre is a painless, indurated ulcer that develops at the site of inoculation in the genital region, anus, or oral cavity and is usually associated with locally enlarged lymph nodes.[16–18] The chancre then usually disappears spontaneously in a few days. Once inside the host, the microorganisms proliferate locally and are then disseminated extensively via the lymphatic and blood vessels.

The secondary stage begins 4 to 10 weeks later, when the spirochete can be detected in high concentrations in blood and infected tissues. The hematogenous dissemination and infiltration of various tissues can explain the variable clinical presentation, such as with fever; maculopapular nonpruritic lesions *(syphilitic roseola)* on the skin, including the palms and soles; papular lesions known as *condyloma lata*; alopecia; and hepatosplenomegaly. Generalized infections may also present with anorexia, irritability or lethargy, myalgia, arthritis, and/or generalized lymphadenopathies.[16–18] This stage usually resolves spontaneously in 1 to 6 months and is followed by a latent period, which is usually asymptomatic. However, recurrent symptomatic episodes of bacteremia may continue to occur. There may be an early latent stage in the first 12 months after the primary infection and a late latent stage that occurs after 12 months.[16–19]

About 30% to 50% of untreated patients develop a tertiary stage that might be seen in a period extending up to 30 years after the primary infection. This stage may involve multiple organs and show diverse presentations including cardiac valvulitis, aortitis with aortic aneurysms, meningitis, cerebrovascular accidents, neurosyphilis, or cutaneous granulations that have been described as gummas due to a gum-like or rubbery consistency.[16–18]

Clinical Features

Fetal *Treponema* infections are frequently associated with adverse outcomes. Up to 21% of pregnancies end in miscarriages, 9% in stillbirths, and 6% in preterm deliveries. Intrauterine growth restriction and nonimmune hydrops fetalis (Fig. 34.3) are seen frequently. Multiple prenatal findings may be observed in 31% of affected fetuses, particularly hepatomegaly (seen in 80% of affected pregnancies). Increased blood flow in the middle cerebral artery is seen in one-third of all infected fetuses. The placenta is enlarged with inflammation and edema in 27%. In some fetuses, cardiomegaly, pericardial effusion, splenomegaly, and bone alterations are also seen. Unfortunately, prenatal ultrasonography is not a sensitive method to detect these changes.[20,21]

The infected placenta may appear edematous and pale. Microscopically, a typical triad of enlarged, hypercellular villi, proliferative vascular changes, and acute or chronic villitis is seen. The decidua may show leukocytosis and erythroblastosis, particularly in stillbirths.[22,23] The umbilical cord is normal in most cases, but some may show necrotizing funisitis with nonspecific inflammatory changes.[24]

At birth, more than 90% of infants are asymptomatic. About 10% present with a wide variety and severity of symptoms ranging from mild nonspecific constitutional signs to lethal hydrops (Box 34.1 and Fig. 34.4).[14,25,26] Mucocutaneous lesions on the palms and soles (syphilitic pemphigus), genitourinary areas, and hepato- and/or splenomegaly are frequently seen.[16,25,26] The hepatosplenomegaly is likely caused by both inflammation and extramedullary hematopoiesis. In a study conducted by Lago et al. in 2013, hepatomegaly and

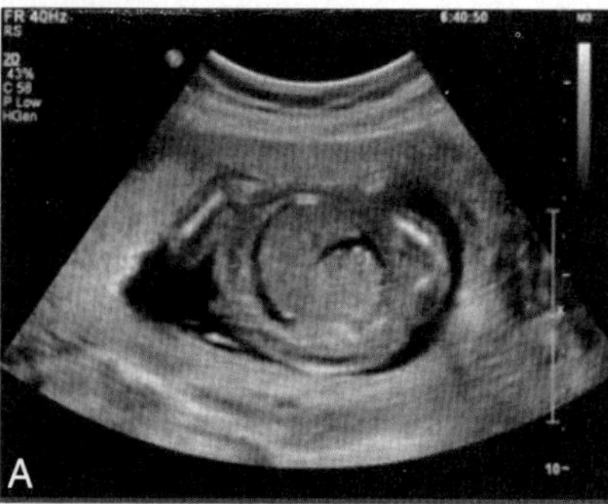

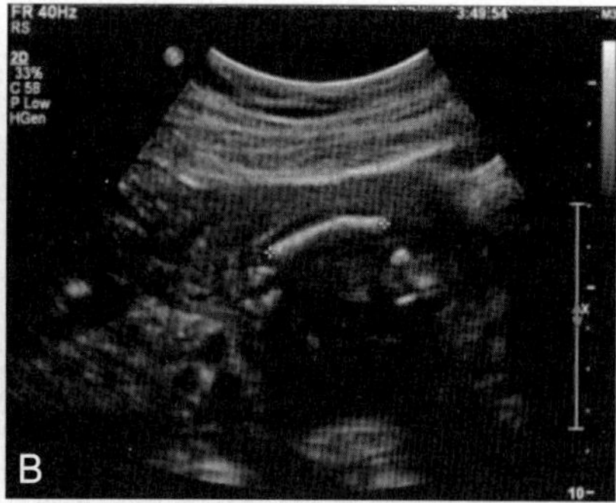

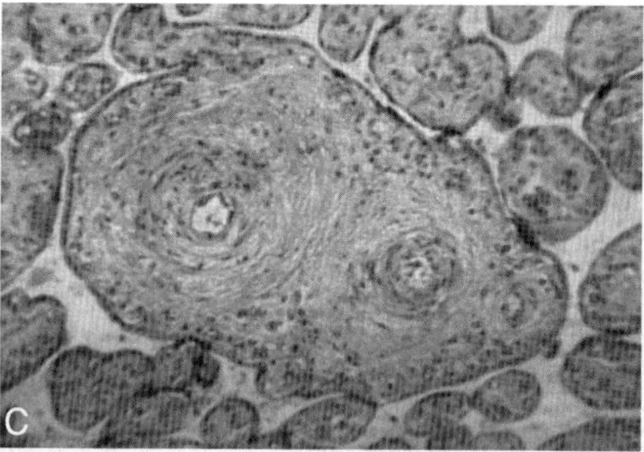

Fig. 34.3 Prenatal Ultrasound Shows Changes of Congenital Syphilis. (A) Nonimmune hydrops fetalis with mild ascites and epidermal edema. (B) Osseous abnormalities in long bones. (C) Cytoarchitectural changes seen in the placenta in congenital syphilis. Chorionic villi are enlarged and contain dense laminated connective tissue, and the capillaries distributed throughout the villi are compressed by this connective tissue proliferation. (From Johnson et al. Congenital syphilis. In: *Obstetric Imaging: Fetal Diagnosis and Care*. 2018.)

■ Box 34.1 Diagnosis of Congenital Syphilis

Clinical findings

- Prematurity
- Small for gestational age
- Fever
- Nasal discharge ("sniffles")
- Maculopapular rash, syphilitic pemphigus, wart-like lesions in genital areas (condyloma lata), perioral or perianal fissures
- Hepatosplenomegaly
- Lymphadenopathy
- Thrombocytopenia
- Nonimmune fetal hydrops
- Bone pain, and consequently, decreased limb movement ("pseudoparalysis of Parrot")
- Encephalitis, cranial nerve palsies, seizures
- Uveitis, chorioretinitis
- Myocarditis
- Pneumonia
- Ileitis, necrotizing enterocolitis, malabsorption
- Nephritis

Laboratory findings

- Nonhemolytic anemia, leukocytosis/leukopenia, thrombocytopenia
- Abnormal liver function
- CSF shows reactive VDRL, pleocytosis, increased protein levels

Radiologic findings

- Metaphyseal lucent bands in long bones
- Symmetric destruction of the medial portion of the proximal tibial metaphysis (Weber sign)
- Diaphyseal periostitis

CSF, Cerebrospinal fluid; *VDRL*, Venereal Disease Research Laboratory.

splenomegaly were seen in 71% and 60%, respectively, of infected infants.[27]

Infections in the bone marrow may explain the hematopoietic insufficiency and consequent anemia, thrombocytopenia, and leukopenia. Other frequently seen laboratory findings may include elevated direct and indirect bilirubin levels and hepatic enzymes.[25–28] Coagulation disorders may be caused by a deficiency of vitamin K–dependent clotting factors.

Radiologic changes are seen in long bones in 90% of symptomatic and 20% of asymptomatic patients.[29] Bilateral periostitis, cortical demineralization, and osteochondritis are seen frequently. Many cases may show lucent metaphyseal bands reflecting periostitis and demineralization.[30,31] Subepiphysial fractures or subluxation may cause the infant to avoid painful limb movements, a condition that is known as "pseudoparalysis of Parrot."[29,32]

Cerebrospinal fluid (CSF) abnormalities, particularly pleocytosis (sensitivity 38%, specificity 88%) and elevated protein levels, can be seen in up to 60% of patients.[25,26] The Venereal Disease Research Laboratory (VDRL) test has high specificity and should be performed to diagnose neurosyphilis. The findings do need cautious evaluation because a few patients may have false positive results due to passive antibody passage from the plasma.[26] Clinical signs of central nervous system (CNS) involvement are seen in 25% of patients, including seizures, cranial nerve palsies, or signs of meningits.[28] Other organs such as the pancreas, heart, and kidneys can also be affected in some cases.

Late congenital syphilis is caused by long-lasting infections and inflammation. The Hutchinson triad, which includes interstitial keratitis, neurosensory hearing loss, and dental anomalies, is well described. Bone deformities such as saddle nose, high-arched palate, bony prominence of the jaw and forehead, short upper jawbone, and saber-shaped tibia have been described. Rhagades, linear scar lines at the angle of the mouth, may also be present. CNS compromise is frequently observed in these patients, including severe neurodevelopmental delay, hydrocephalus, optic nerve atrophy, and cranial nerve paralysis.[16,26,33]

Diagnosis

The diagnosis of congenital syphilis in newborn infants can be challenging. Direct visualization under dark field microscopy would provide the best possible confirmation, but this technique is not used very frequently because of its complexity. In infants with suggestive maternal history, the diagnosis is based on maternal antibody titers, history of treatment, the newborn's physical examination, and the newborn's antibody levels (Fig. 34.5).[19,34] The polymerase chain reaction assay to detect genetic material from *T. pallidum* can be very useful.

The diagnostic techniques can be classified into direct identification tests, serologic treponemal tests, and serologic nontreponemal tests. Tissue samples from the placenta, amniotic fluid, umbilical cord, mucocutaneous lesions, or eventually necropsy may be used for diagnostic purposes.[26] To test newborn infants, blood samples should be collected from peripheral venipuncture, not the umbilical cord, which have higher false-positive and false-negative results.[9] Dark field microscopy is an important method for direct visualization of the spirochete but is technically difficult. The

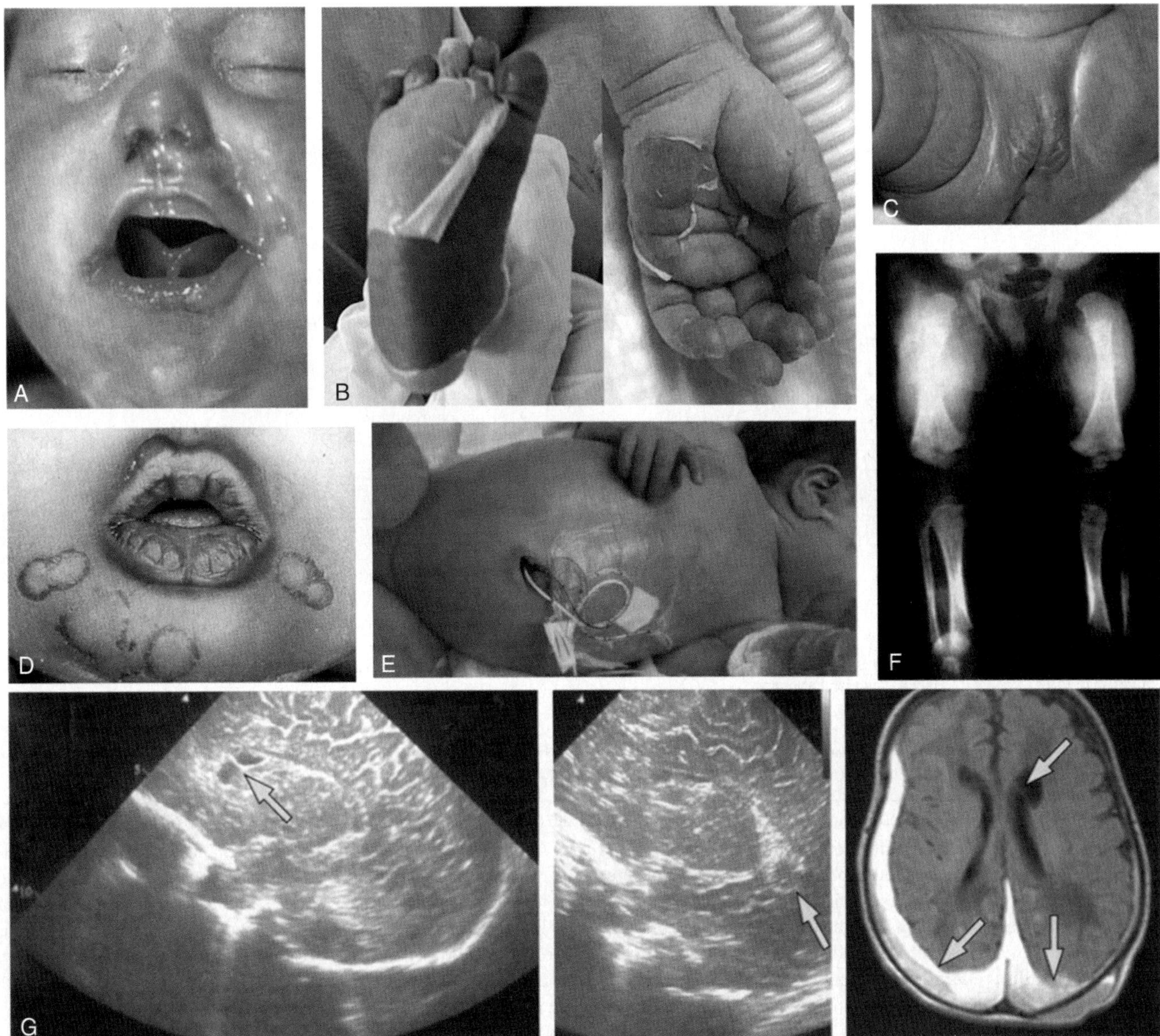

Fig. 34.4 Physical Signs in Early Congenital Syphilis. (A) Sniffles. (B) Palmoplantar syphilitic pemphigus. (C) Characteristic skin lesions in genital and perianal areas. (D) Perioral papules, ulcerous lesions, and labial fissures. (E) Hepatomegaly. (F) Radiographs show bilateral demineralization and destruction of the proximal medial tibial metaphysis (Wimberger sign). (G) Cranial ultrasound shows cystic lesions in the periventricular areas. (Images taken at the Newborn Unit, Pereira Rossell Hospital, Montevideo, Uruguay. The following images have been reproduces with permission. Image [D] is from Radolf et al. In: *Mandell, Douglas, and Bennett's Principles and Practice of Infectious Diseases*, 237, 2865–2892.e7; image [E] from Kollmann et al. *Remington and Klein's Infectious Diseases of the Fetus and Newborn Infant*, 16, 512–543; [G] Silva et al. *Lancet Infect Dis*. 2012;12:816–816.)

presence of the spirochete can also be confirmed by direct immunofluorescence, silver staining, or polymerase chain reaction.[35–39] Other methods for clinical evaluation and serial follow-up are the VDRL and rapid plasma reagin (RPR) tests, which provide quantitative measurements of nonspecific antibody responses during syphilis infections. The concentrations of these two reagins increase with increasing infection and decrease in patients responding to treatment, becoming nondetectable when the patients are completely cured. There are some differences between the two tests; RPR may be more sensitive than VDRL.[34] It may also be preferable to use kits from a single manufacturer for serial tests to eliminate the variability from zero-errors. Finally, positive results need cautious interpretation up to 15 months of age because of the possibility of passive passage of maternal antibodies (Box 34.1).

Specific tests for *Treponema* serology are the fluorescent treponemal antibody absorption test, particle agglutination test, chemiluminescence immunoassay, and treponemal enzyme immunoassay. These tests are used to confirm the results of a positive nontreponemal test. Treponemal tests remain positive during a patient's entire lifetime and are not suitable for interpreting infection activity or response to treatment. These tests are highly specific, particularly the treponemal enzyme immunoassay and chemiluminescence immunoassay.[40–42]

The diagnosis of neurosyphilis can be challenging. As mentioned above, most patients with CNS involvement are asymptomatic but have abnormalities in CSF examination. Nontreponemal serologic tests may be helpful, but the possibility of passive passage of antibodies from plasma to CSF needs to be considered. VDRL is preferred to RPR when testing CSF.[38,43]

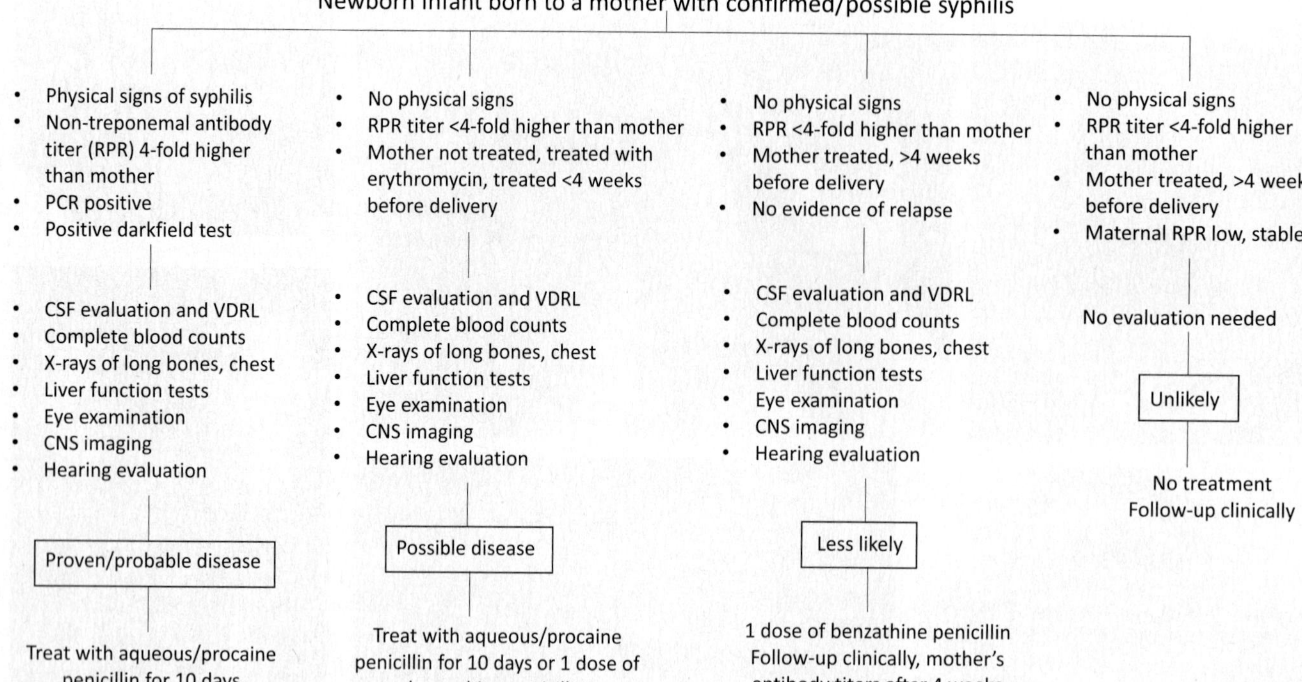

Fig. 34.5 Evaluation of a Newborn Infant Born to a Mother With Confirmed/Possible Syphilis. *CSF,* Cerebrospinal fluid; *CNS,* central nervous system; *RPR,* rapid plasma reagin; *VDRL,* Venereal Disease Research Laboratory.

Treatment

Penicillin is the only antibiotic with proven efficacy to treat maternal syphilis and prevent congenital infection by treating the fetus *in utero.*[44,45] Pregnant women should be treated with benzathine penicillin, and the number of doses will depend on the stage of infection.[19] In primary, secondary, and early latent stages, treatment should consist of two doses of 2.4 million international units of benzathine penicillin, separated by a week. When maternal syphilis is in a late latent stage or of unknown origin, treatment should consist of three weekly doses of 2.4 million international units of benzathine penicillin. The last dose should be administered at least 28 days before delivery.[44] Alternative antimicrobial treatments such as amoxicillin or some cephalosporins require more data and are currently not recommended.[46–56] At this time, recommendations state that mothers allergic to penicillin should undergo desensitization.

Newborn infants need to be treated according to the risk of infection and according to protocols presented in Fig. 34.5. The recommended treatment protocols include crystalline penicillin G, 50,000 international units (IU) per kg per dose, during a 10-day period, given every 12 hours during the first 7 days of life and in 8-hour intervals thereafter.[19] An alternate treatment regimen in lower-risk patients recommends a single dose of benzathine penicillin 50,000 IU/kg.[57–61] Ceftriaxone may be used if the mother is allergic to penicillin or if crystalline penicillin G or benzathine penicillin are not available. However, these patients will need careful follow-up.[62–64] The Jarisch-Herxheimer reaction is an acute infrequent pathologic response to penicillin treatment, which may affect the pregnant mother and cause preterm labor. It may cause a severe reaction in the fetus/newborn infant. These infants will require intensive are to support vital functions until recovery.[65,66]

Follow-Up

Affected newborn infants should be closely followed up every 2 to 3 months, with a physical examination and a nontreponemal serologic test. With adequate treatment, most infants do not develop long-term complications. Titers should decrease consistently in treated infants and should be checked repeatedly until the levels drop to one-fourth of the original or turn negative. If the titers increase during follow-up, particularly if by four-fold at any time, or if the patient remains positive with stable titers after 12 to 18 months, the patient should be treated again with a new course of penicillin. Patients who presented with a positive VDRL test in CSF should undergo a new lumbar puncture at 6 months of age; if the VDRL persists as positive, or if there is no change in CSF laboratory findings, the patient should receive a second course of treatment.[19]

Prevention

Syphilis prevention strategies have proven to be cost-effective. The US Preventive Services Task Force recommended universal screening of all pregnant women at their first contact with the healthcare system. Women with risk factors were recommended to be screened for a second time during the third trimester and then again at the time of delivery. These screenings may be performed with a nontreponemal serologic test (conventional diagnostic approach) but could also use a treponemal serologic test. If there are conflicting results, a treponema pallidum haemagglutination (TPHA) test should be used to confirm.[67–70] All positive tests should be recorded in a notification system, particularly for more vulnerable populations. Most countries in the American region have notification guidelines in order to register syphilis cases and develop healthcare policies. In the United States, syphilis cases should be reported to the CDC's National Notifiable Disease Surveillance System.

CHAPTER 35

Invasive Fungal Infections in the NICU: *Candida*, Aspergillosis, and Mucormycosis

David A. Kaufman, Namrita J. Odackal, Hillary B. Liken

KEY POINTS

1. Fungal infections including invasive *Candida* infections and molds (aspergillosis and mucormycosis) are devastating infections most commonly complicating extreme preterm infants due to their underdeveloped immune system combined with the need for intensive care and any neonate with complex gastrointestinal disease.
2. Dermatologic findings of candidiasis and molds are critical to their prompt diagnosis and correct empiric antifungal selection.
   - Congenital cutaneous candidiasis is an invasive infection that requires prompt recognition and evaluation as well as systemic treatment for 14 days. Dermatologic findings of congenital cutaneous candidiasis commonly involve skin desquamation and maculopapular, hypopigmented, and/or erythematous rashes.
   - Cutaneous aspergillosis presents as erythematous indurated papules or white plaques that progress to ulceration and white-gray-yellow coloration or exudates. They can evolve into target lesions with a white-yellow ring with an erythematous interior and exterior ring. Voriconazole or echinocandins are first-line therapy for aspergillosis infections.
   - Mucormycosis presents as an erythematous to purple papule with a central ulceration or induration that evolves into a black eschar, usually in a skin area that has been covered, injured, or in a pressure area such as the back. Amphotericin is the first-line therapy for mucormycosis.
3. Major risk factors for invasive *Candida* infections include extreme prematurity during the time period the infant requires intravenous access, gastrointestinal immaturity, dysmotility, injury, or disease and exposure to broad spectrum antibiotics, acid suppression medications, and postnatal steroids.
4. The highest-risk patients for invasive *Candida* infections are infants less than 1000 g at birth or 28 weeks' gestation until they no longer require intravenous access, due to their high mortality and risk of neurodevelopmental impairments from infection. Preventative measures including targeted antifungal prophylaxis have lowered the incidence in this group significantly, approaching zero.
5. *Candida* pathogenesis involves exposure, adherence, and colonization, followed by infection and commonly organ involvement. All infected infants need screening for end organ dissemination.
6. Cultures are critical for diagnosis of invasive *Candida* infections and should include blood, urine, and cerebrospinal fluid at the time of presentation. Additionally, peritoneal cultures should be obtained in any infant bowel perforation or necrotizing enterocolitis requiring laparotomy or drainage.
7. Survival and infection-related outcomes are improved with central venous catheter removal for candidemia, prompt antifungal dosing for all infected patients, and empiric therapy in high-risk patients.
8. Amphotericin B is the optimal choice for systemic treatment of invasive *Candida* infection due to *Candida* susceptibility patterns and cost. Fluconazole should not be the first choice until speciation and susceptibilities are known, because several *Candida* species are resistant to fluconazole. Additionally, if fluconazole is used for prophylaxis, a different antifungal should be selected to minimize emergence of resistance.

Introduction

Fungal pathogenesis involves exposure, adherence, colonization, and ultimately infection. Measures can be applied for each of these four aspects to prevent infections and improve outcomes in those infected. Invasive *Candida* infections (ICIs) in the neonatal intensive care unit (NICU) most commonly include bloodstream and urinary tract infections, meningitis, peritonitis, and congenital cutaneous candidiasis, whereas mold infections more often present as cutaneous lesions or complicate necrotizing enterocolitis (NEC). NICU patients are at increased risk for invasive fungal infections due to their developing immune system and need for intensive care including catheters and tubes that breach important protective barriers (Figs. 35.1 and 35.2). Furthermore, molds take advantage of skin that has been covered, in dependent areas, and at the site of any skin injury or complicated NEC.

Extremely preterm infants represent the highest-risk patients in the NICU, and incidence is inversely proportional with gestational age (Fig. 35.3). Many studies demonstrate rates of ICI >10% in infants less than 25 weeks' gestation and decreasing to around 5% in infants 27 weeks' gestation.[2–4] The highest risk patients are infants <1000 g or <28 weeks' gestation, in whom the incidence is significant and infection is associated with high mortality and neurodevelopmental impairment. Mold infections are less common but are increasing as we care for more infants at the lowest gestational ages.

Targeted antifungal prophylaxis in high-risk patients is the most effective prevention measure for ICI and has been critically studied in randomized controlled trials. For the entire NICU, a prevention bundle should include (1) targeted antifungal prophylaxis in high-risk patients <1000 g or <28 weeks' gestation during their high-risk period while they have intravenous access (A-I evidence, *Strong Recommendation*); (2) central line associated

The Level of Evidence used in this chapter is the US Public Health Service Grading System for ranking recommendations in clinical guidelines[1]: Strength of recommendation and levels of evidence. A: good evidence; B: moderate evidence; C: poor evidence. I: at least one randomized clinical trial; II: at least one well-designed but nonrandomized trial; III: expert opinions based on experience or limited clinical reports.

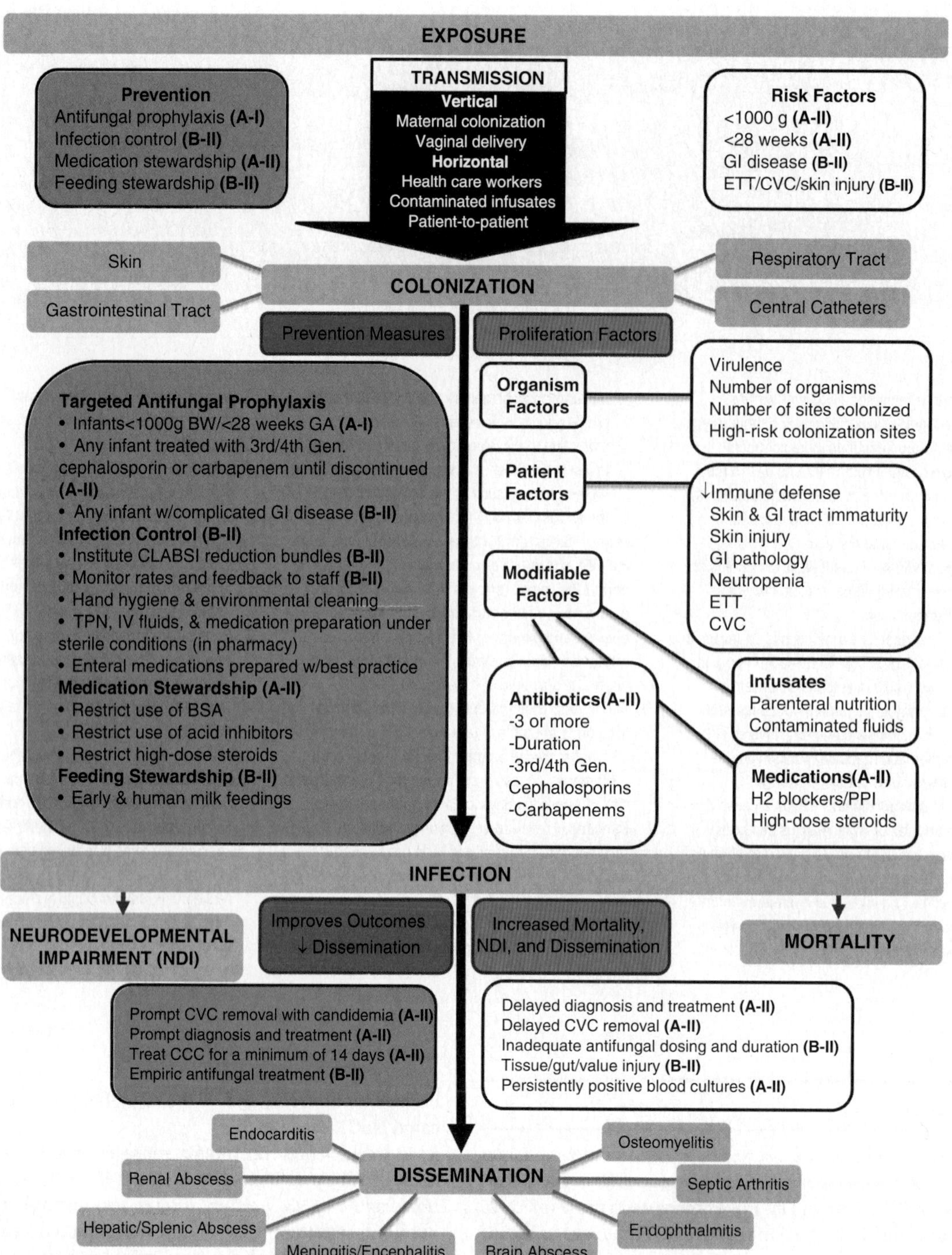

Fig. 35.1 Pathophysiology of Invasive *Candida* Infections: Exposure, Colonization, Infection, and Dissemination. High-risk colonization sites include the central venous catheter, endotracheal tube, and urine. *BSA*, Broad spectrum antibiotics; *BW*, body weight; *CCC*, congenital cutaneous candidiasis; *CLABSI*, central line-associated bloodstream infection; *CVC*, central venous catheter; *ETT*, endotracheal tube; *GA*, gestational age; *Gen*, generation; *GI*, gastrointestinal; *PPI*, proton pump inhibitor; *TPN*, total parenteral nutrition; *IV*, intravenous.

bloodstream infection (CLABSI) preventative practices (A-II, *Strong Recommendation*); (3) antibiotic, medication, and feeding stewardship (A-II, *Strong Recommendation*); and (4) infection control.

Infectious morbidity and mortality can be improved by (1) starting the appropriate antifungal agent and dose (A-II, *Strong Recommendation*); (2) prompt central venous catheter removal when candidemia is present (A-II, *Strong Recommendation*); (3) prompt recognition of dermatologic findings of invasive cutaneous fungal infections, evaluation, and systemic treatment for 14 days (A-II, *Strong Recommendation*); (4) end organ dissemination (EOD) screening and treatment (A-II, *Strong Recommendation*); (5) empiric antifungal therapy in high-risk patients when there is a high suspicion for fungal infection (A-II, *Strong Recommendation*); and (6) antenatal treatment of vaginal candidiasis (B-II, *Weak Recommendation*).

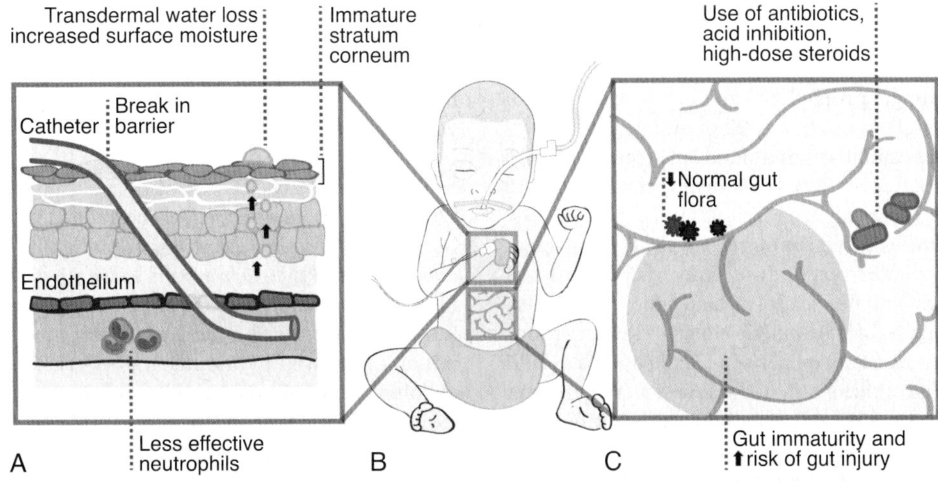

Fig. 35.2 Risk Factors for Invasive *Candida* Infections in Intubated Preterm Infant. (A) Effects of immature skin and neutrophil function, skin injury or puncture, as well as a central venous catheter. (B) Presence of an endotracheal tube. (C) Gastrointestinal tract predisposing factors of immaturity, dysmotility, dysbiosis, medications, mucosal disruption, and potential gut disease. *PPI,* Proton-pump inhibitor.

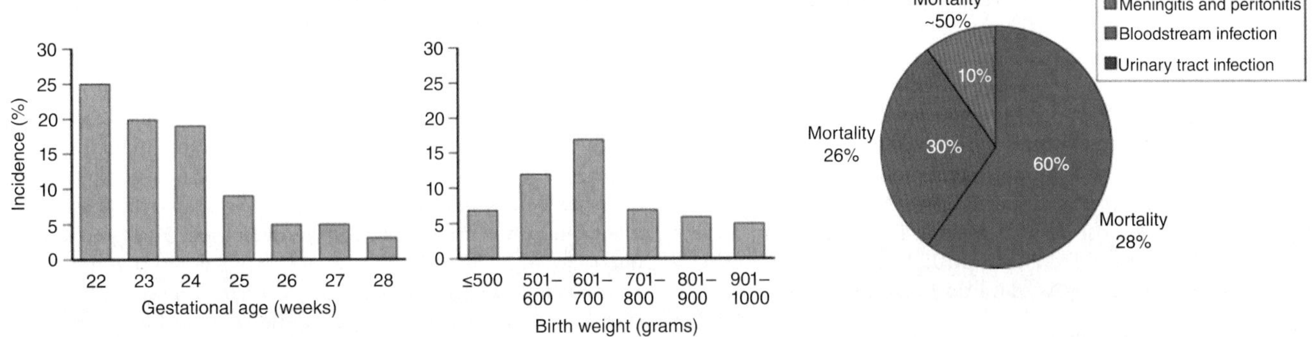

Fig. 35.3 *(Left)* Incidence of invasive *Candida* infection (ICI) by gestational age and birth weight groups in infants less than 1000 g birth weight not receiving antifungal prophylaxis. Gestational age has a linear relationship to ICI compared with birth weight and aids in defining the highest-risk patients. *(Right)* Distribution of type of ICI and their associated mortality. Note similar mortality for bloodstream infection (BSI) and urinary tract infection (UTI). Data from 137 infections in 1515 infants less than 1000 g from 19 centers of the NICHD Neonatal Research Network. (From Fungal and protozoal infections of the neonate. Kaufman and Manzoni. *Fanaroff and Martin's Neonatal-Perinatal Medicine*. 49:809–843.)

Candida

Epidemiology and Case Definition

ICI is defined as the presence of *Candida* species in a body fluid or tissue sample and includes bloodstream infections (BSIs), urinary tract infections (UTIs), peritonitis, meningitis, congenital (or diffuse) cutaneous candidiasis, and any infection of otherwise sterile tissue such as bones and joints.[2,4–7] These invasive infections are diagnosed based on a positive culture of blood, urine, cerebrospinal fluid (CSF), peritoneal fluid, or tissue. For congenital cutaneous candidiasis, diagnosis requires a diffuse rash with identification of *Candida* or yeast from the skin, placenta, or umbilical cord.[5] These ICIs can disseminate directly or hematogenously. They can lead to end organ abscesses due to multiple adhesive factors of *Candida* and damage the heart, kidneys, brain, liver, spleen, bone, and joints (see Fig. 35.1).

The majority of ICIs in the NICU are due to *Candida albicans* (~50%), followed by *C. parapsilosis* (30%–40%) and to a lesser degree *C. glabrata.* Infections due to *Candida tropicalis, C. lusitaniae, C. krusei, C. guilliermondii,* and other species occur less frequently. *C. albicans* is the most pathogenic of the *Candida* species, with mortality rates two to three times higher compared with nonalbicans candidemia.[8]

Extremely preterm infants represent the highest-risk patients in the NICU, and incidence is inversely proportional with gestational age.[4,9] There is variation in rates of ICI in NICUs as well as the incidence reported in the literature due to the factors listed in Table 35.1.

Table 35.1 Factors Affecting Variation in ICI in the NICU	
Reporting bias	• Most studies report only candidemia and/or meningitis, missing important data on UTIs and peritonitis • 40% of ICIs are not *Candida* BSIs
Resuscitation gestational age cutoff	• NICUs that do not resuscitate infants <24 or <25 weeks' GA will have lower rates than NICUs caring for these patients
Surgical and complex gastrointestinal diseases	• Centers caring for infants with NEC, gastroschisis, and other complex gastrointestinal diseases will have higher rates[1]
Targeted antifungal prophylaxis	• Centers using antifungal prophylaxis will have the lowest rates (nearly eliminating these infections), even in the highest-risk patients of the lowest gestational ages (<26 weeks) and birth weights (<750 g)

BSI, Bloodstream infection; *GA,* gestational age; *ICI,* invasive *Candida* infection; *NEC,* necrotizing enterocolitis; *NICU,* neonatal intensive care unit; *UTI,* urinary tract infection.

Risk Factors (See Fig. 35.1)

Prematurity

In the absence of antifungal prophylaxis, the incidence of ICIs in extremely low birth weight (ELBW; <1000 g) infants, not including congenital cutaneous candidiasis, is around 10% (see Fig. 35.3).[4] The incidence decreases from >20% at 23 weeks' gestation to 3% at 28 weeks' gestation. The incidence of 5% in infants of 27 weeks' gestation marks a potential cutoff for targeted antifungal prophylaxis in the first weeks after birth while other risk factors are present (central venous catheter, endotracheal tube, antibiotics, and/or parenteral nutrition).[4,10] Although bloodstream infections account for the majority of ICIs in ELBWs, *Candida* UTIs would increase the incidence an additional 3% to 4%, and meningitis and peritonitis (complicating any bowel perforation) an additional 1% to 2%.[9,11–16] The average candidemia rates are much lower in larger infants (1.32%, 0.36%, and 0.29% for birth weights of 1001–1500, 1501–2500, and >2500 g, respectively).[17]

Medications

Proliferation is favorable under certain conditions such as when antibiotics are used, as they eradicate competitive flora; when H2 blockers and proton pump inhibitors are used, because they decrease stomach acidity, which is an important defense against *Candida*; or when postnatal steroid exposure impairs granulocyte function. Longer antibiotic duration or exposure to multiple antibiotics, particularly third- and fourth-generation cephalosporins or carbapenems, are associated with increasing risk for ICI.[4,18,19] Dexamethasone and high-dose hydrocortisone (>1 mg/kg/day) are associated with increased incidence of ICI, but physiologic dosing of hydrocortisone (≤1 mg/kg/day) does not appear to increase risk.[20–22]

Catheters, Tubes, and Feedings

Central venous catheters, endotracheal tubes, and certain feeding practices increase the risk of ICI. Risk of ICI is decreased by receiving an early as well as an all human milk diet, because it is shown to lower rates of NEC and its associated ICI rate of 10%. While increased amounts of fresh expressed human milk are associated with fewer bacterial infections, studies have not demonstrated a decrease in ICI.[23]

Gastrointestinal Pathology and Abdominal Surgery

Gastrointestinal pathology is associated with an increased risk for candidemia and/or *Candida* peritonitis in patients with NEC, bowel perforation, gastroschisis, Hirschsprung disease, omphalocele, intestinal atresia, or tracheoesophageal fistula.[10,24,25]

Pathophysiology (See Fig. 35.1)

Candida pathogenesis involves exposure, followed by colonization, infection, and dissemination.

Exposure

As discussed above, prematurity is the greatest risk factor for ICI. This is due to these infants' underdeveloped immune system and immature and often breached (by central catheters and endotracheal tubes) defense barriers including the skin and the gastrointestinal and respiratory tracts (see Fig. 35.2). *Candida* species are potential opportunistic pathogens for preterm infants because they are naturally present on the skin, oral, and gastrointestinal mucosa, primarily as saprophytes. *Candida* species can also lead to infections if the host is exposed to a large number of organisms (at birth or with poor infection control) and after colonization when risk factors allow *Candida* to proliferate easily or barriers are compromised (e.g., skin breakdown, NEC, or the presence of an endotracheal tube or intravenous catheter).

Colonization

Colonization rates are inversely correlated with gestational age and birth weight, similar to infection. In the first weeks of life, >50% of ELBW and 25% to 50% of very low birth weight (VLBW; <1500 g) infants may become colonized, as compared with 5% to 10% of full-term infants.[2] Skin and gastrointestinal colonization occurs initially, followed by the respiratory tract.[26] Approximately 25% of colonized VLBW infants will progress to infection; risk is influenced by the number and location of colonized sites.[27] Colonization of multiple sites or colonization at a single high-risk site (endotracheal tube, urine, catheter tips, drains, and surgical devices) is associated with higher ICI risk than colonization at a single low-risk site.[9,28–31]

Infection and Dissemination

At the time of presentation, *Candida* often has already disseminated to other tissues, organs, or body fluids and formed microabscesses. This is due to adherence properties of *Candida*, its slow growth prior to clinical signs and symptoms, and the patient's immunocompromised state. Additionally, central vascular catheters can cause local trauma to valvular, endocardial, or endothelial tissue, followed by a thrombus to which yeast can adhere. More rapid diagnosis, treatment, and prevention of ICIs have decreased EOD, but it still is important to screen for EOD. Among infants with ICI, the incidence of concomitant endocarditis is around 5%, kidney abscesses 5%, central nervous system (CNS) abscesses 4%, and endophthalmitis 3%.[32] EOD is higher in ELBW infants and any infant with candidemia lasting >5 days.[33–35]

Clinical Features, Management, and Treatment

Congenital Cutaneous Candidiasis

Diagnosis of congenital cutaneous candidiasis (CCC) involves the presence of a diffuse CCC rash of major skin areas of the body, extremities, face or scalp, and/or funisitis, presenting in the first week (≤7 days), with identification of *Candida* species or yeast from (1) skin or mucous membranes cultures, (2) placenta staining or cultures, or (3) umbilical cord staining or cultures. CCC is usually present at birth but can emerge during the first week of life.[5] Dermatologic findings include desquamation alone (scaling, peeling, flaking, or exfoliation); maculopapular, papulopustular, and erythematous rashes; or a combination of these skin manifestations (Fig. 35.4).[5] CCC is an invasive infection that can occur with or without dissemination. There is a high burden of yeast with invasion into the dermis, which brings *Candida* close to the dermal vasculature. Therefore preterm and term infants need to be treated promptly at the time of rash presentation with systemic antifungal therapy and for a minimum of 14 days (A-II, *Strong Recommendation*). Delaying systemic treatment, solitary use of topical therapy (nystatin), and treating for <10 days is associated with *Candida* dissemination to the bloodstream.[5]

In evaluating a diffuse CCC rash in the first-week life, aerobic skin cultures for both fungal and bacterial organisms need to be

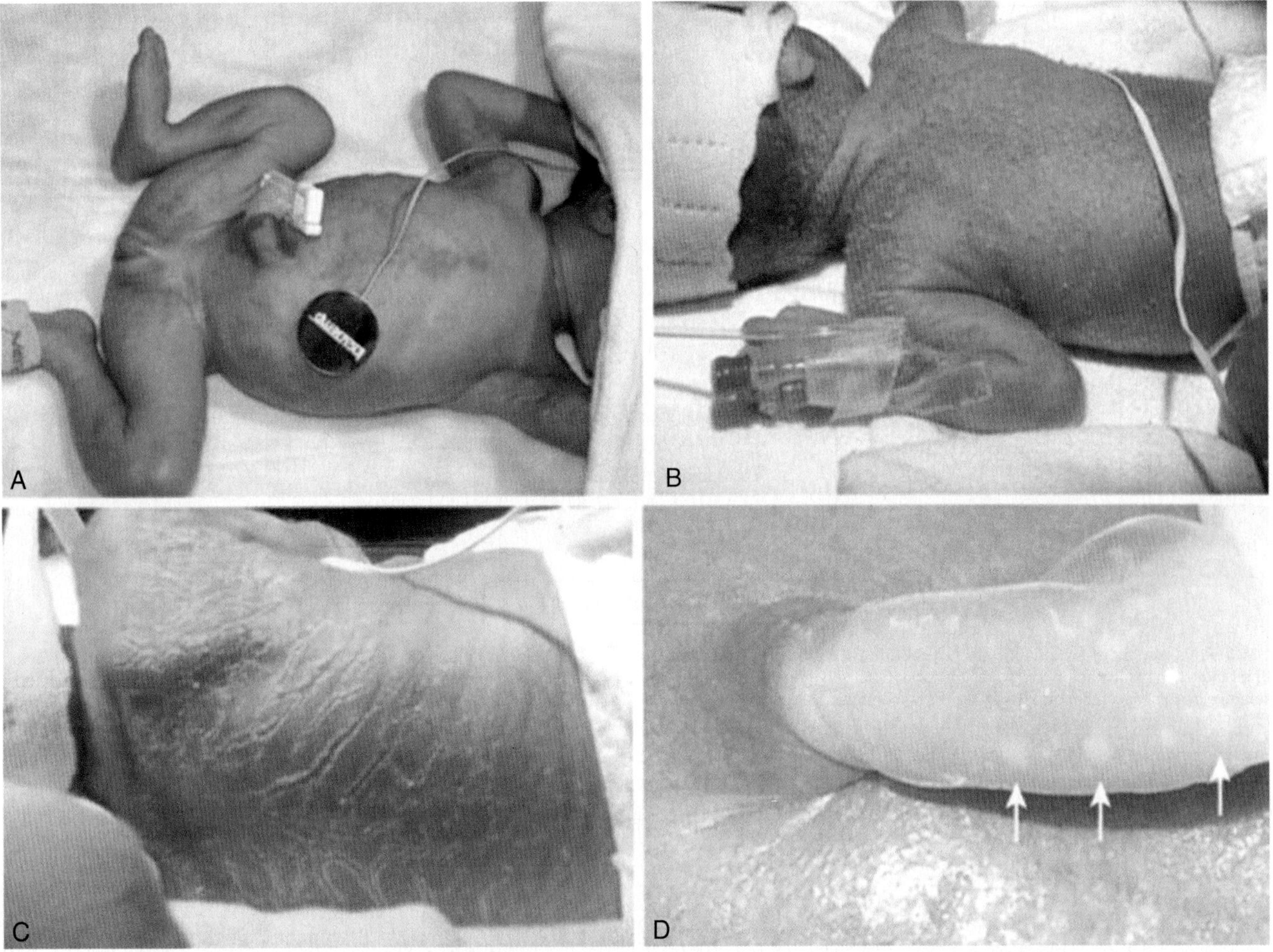

Fig. 35.4 Congenital Cutaneous Candidiasis. (A) Macular papular rash. (B) Dry, flaky rash. (C) Dry, cracking scaly rash. (D) White plaques of the umbilical cord. (From: Fungal and protozoal infections of the neonate. Kaufman and Manzoni. *Fanaroff and Martin's Neonatal-Perinatal Medicine*, 49, 809–843.)

obtained to identify the source of infection. Specific fungal staining and aerobic culture of the umbilical cord and placenta also aid in the diagnosis. Additionally, blood culture, urine culture if older than 48 hours, and CSF (if no rash on the back is present) should be performed. Lumbar puncture should not be performed or deferred if there is cutaneous involvement on the back due to risk of invasion into the dermis and of introducing *Candida* into the CSF. Differential diagnosis includes staphylococcal as well as other bacterial and fungal skin infections. In certain cases when the rash appearance could be due to bacterial or fungal pathogens, empiric staphylococcal and fungal empiric coverage should be initiated pending culture results. Cutaneous (or mucocutaneous) candidiasis presents as a diffuse rash with similar skin manifestations as CCC, but it occurs later, at age ≥8 days.[2]

Candidemia

Signs and symptoms of *Candida* bloodstream infections are similar to bacteremia, with candidemia having some unique patterns related to thrombocytopenia. In VLBW infants, candidemia has greater decrease (>50%), lower initial platelet counts, lower platelet nadirs, and a greater duration of thrombocytopenia compared with gram-positive sepsis (Fig. 35.5).[36]

Candidemia may be associated with disseminated EOD (see Fig. 35.1).[32] Initial screening for dissemination should include an echocardiogram, renal ultrasound, cranial ultrasound or magnetic resonance imaging (MRI), and ophthalmologic exam (Fig. 35.6) (A-II, *Strong Recommendation*). If there has been significant bowel pathology such as NEC or a focal bowel perforation, a complete abdominal ultrasound should be performed to rule out peritoneal abscesses. Hepatic abscesses are common if at any time a central venous catheter was positioned below the diaphragm in the liver. This could be performed within a few days of diagnosis of candidemia. Reevaluation for EOD should occur with candidemia that persists for >7 days.[34]

Studies in the era prior to antifungal prophylaxis have demonstrated candidemia complicating ~10% of cases of NEC due to *Candida* translocation or bowel perforation. Evaluation of the gastrointestinal tract by culture of the rectum, stool, or oral flora in patients with a diagnosis of stage II NEC or greater for the presence of *Candida* species or yeast should be performed, and if isolated, the addition of systemic antifungal therapy in addition to antibacterial treatment of NEC should be considered (Fig. 35.7).[25] This may not be needed if patients have been on antifungal prophylaxis since birth.

Prolonged positivity of blood cultures occurs with candidemia with a median of 3 days even in the absence of EOD.[3] Candidemia should be given time to clear with systemic antifungals with documentation of blood clearance >72 hours into treatment and

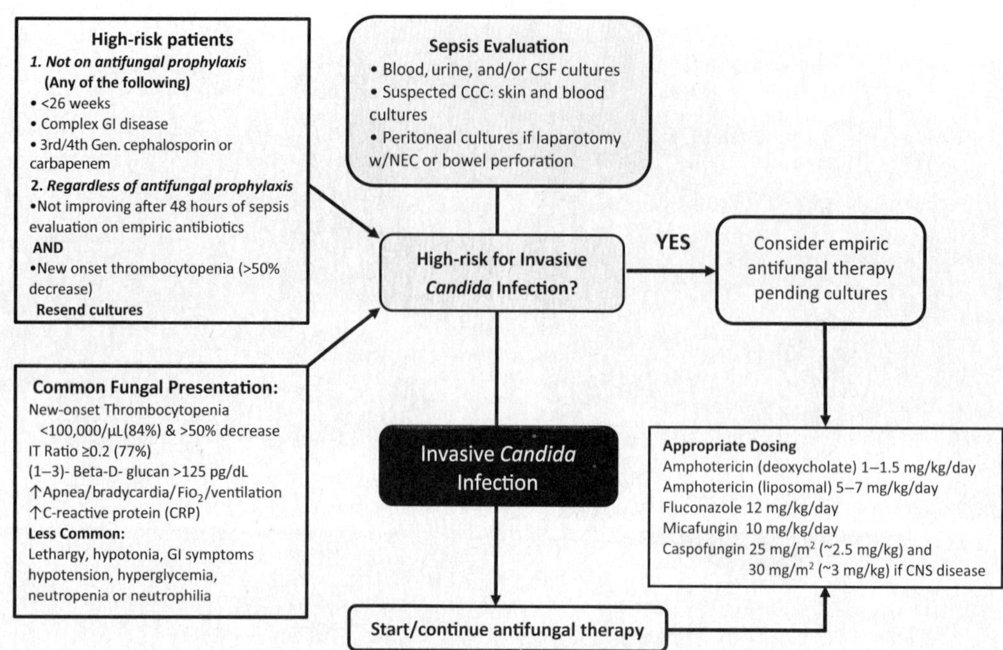

Fig. 35.5 Presentation of Invasive *Candida* Infections, Empiric and Treatment Therapy. Consider empiric antifungal therapy in sepsis evaluations in high-risk patients or when there is high suspicion for fungal infection. *CCC,* Congenital cutaneous candidiasis; *GI,* gastrointestinal; *IT ratio*, immature neutrophils (band cells + myelocytes + metamyelocytes) to total neutrophils ratio; *NEC*, necrotizing enterocolitis.

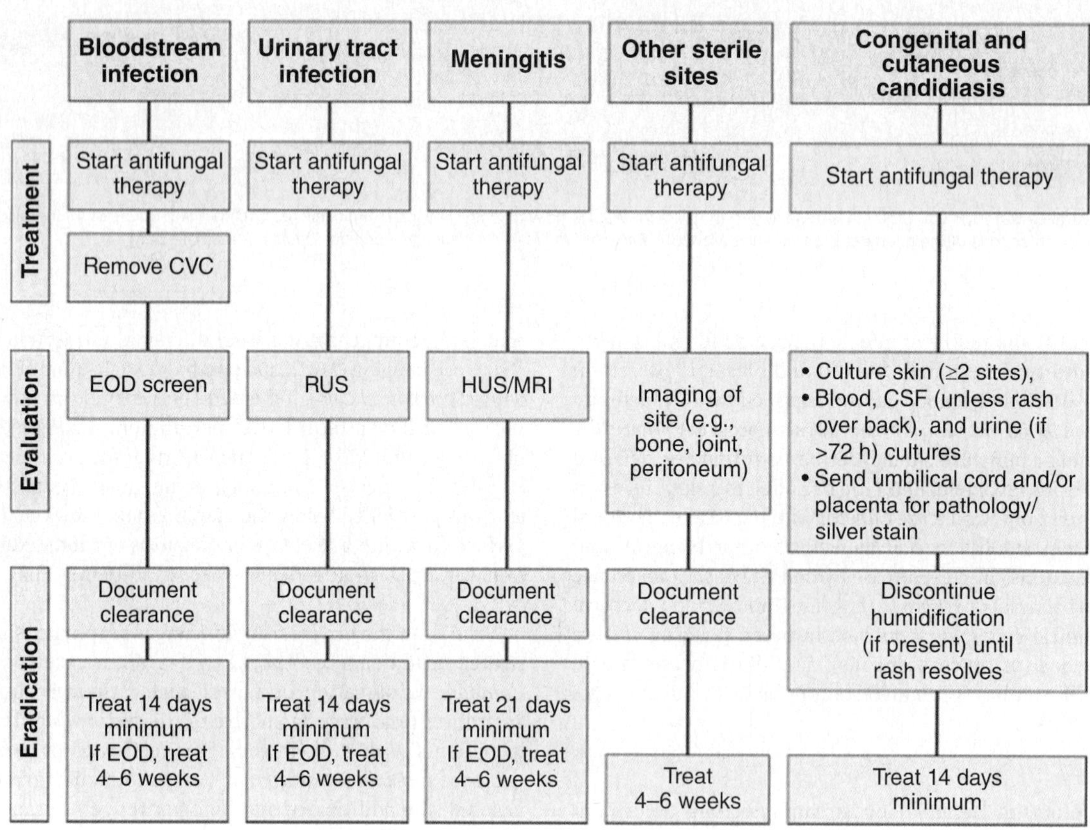

Fig. 35.6 Algorithm for Evaluation and Treatment of Invasive *Candida* Infections in Neonates. Combination therapy with a second antifungal is recommended based on susceptibilities for meningitis, persistent candidemia greater than 7 days, or end organ dissemination (EOD) (fluconazole is most commonly selected due to water solubility and cerebrospinal fluid penetration). See Fig. 35.5 for antifungal dosing. Repeat cerebrospinal fluid culture should be obtained near the end of therapy to ensure sterility. EOD screening: Initial EOD screening should be performed at presentation or after 5 to 7 days of appropriate antifungal treatment and repeated if candidemia persists after 7 days of antifungal therapy. EOD screen with candidemia includes surveillance for cardiac, renal, eye, and brain involvement. If bowel disease such as necrotizing enterocolitis or focal bowel perforation is present or previously occurred, a complete abdominal ultrasound for abscess should be performed. For UTI and meningitis, focal EOD screening can be performed. *CSF*, Cerebrospinal fluid; *CVC*, central venous catheter; *HUS*, head ultrasound; *ICI*, invasive *Candida* infection; *MRI*, magnetic resonance imaging; *RUS*, renal ultrasound; *UTI*, urinary tract infection. (From Fungal and protozoal infections of the neonate. Kaufman and Manzoni. *Fanaroff and Martin's Neonatal-Perinatal Medicine*, 49,809–843.)

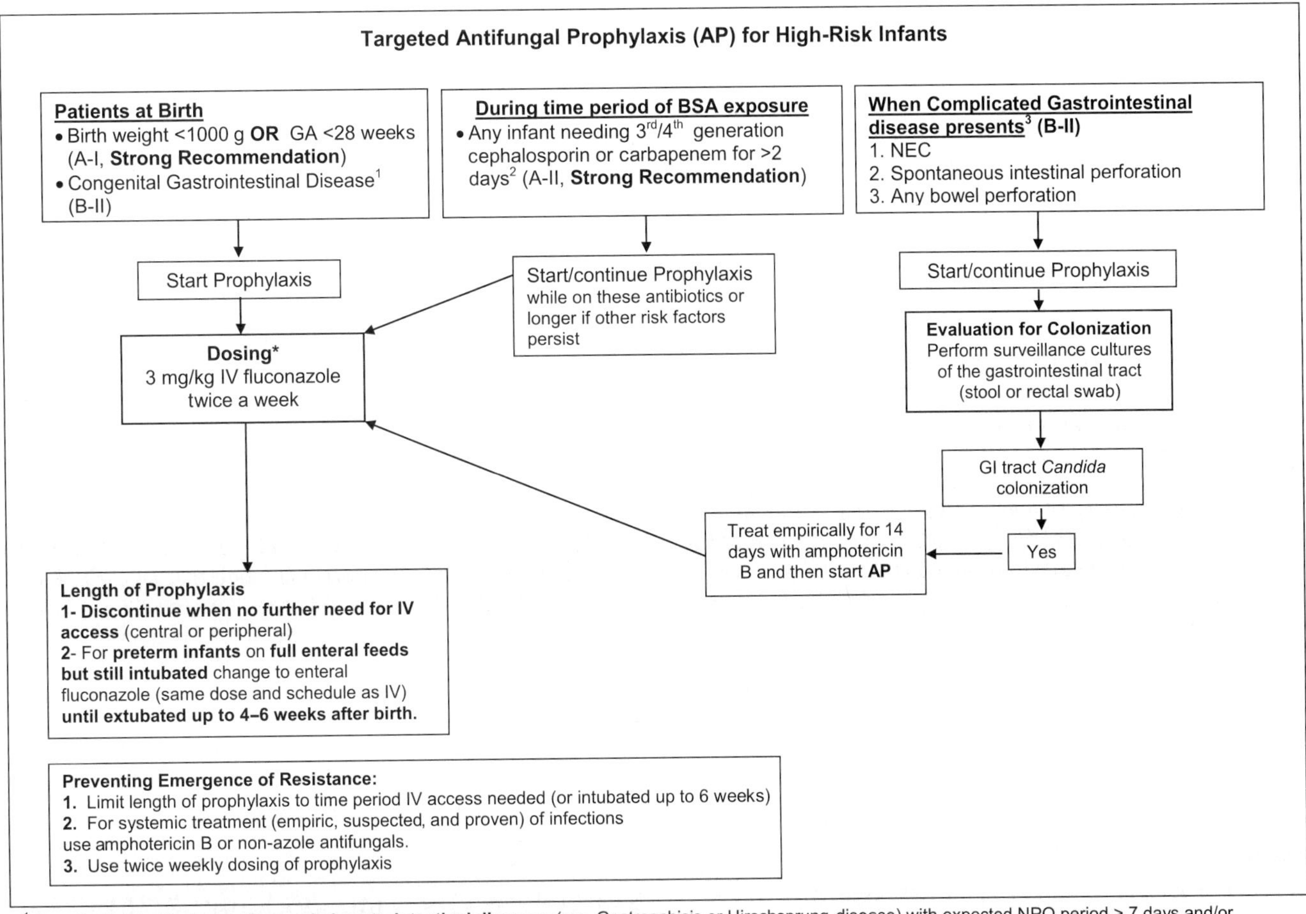

[1] **Acquired complicated or Congenital gastrointestinal diseases** (e.g. Gastroschisis or Hirschsprung disease) with expected NPO period > 7 days and/or need for prolonged antibiotics use > 7 days. Start AP upon presentation or day of birth and continue until no longer a need for IV access (B-II Evidence).

[2] **Treatment of infection requiring Broad spectrum antibiotics (BSAs)=3rd or 4th generation cephalosporins or carbapenems**. Cover with AP while the patient is receiving these antibiotics (A-II Evidence).

[3] For any bowel perforation with or without NEC, if laparotomy performed send aerobic cultures to evaluate for fungal peritonitis and treat 4-6 weeks if present.

Dosing Notes: First dose on day of birth, then twice a week (e.g., Tuesdays, Fridays, at 10AM)

Fig. 35.7 Targeted Antifungal Prophylaxis for High-Risk Neonates. *GA*, Gestational age; *NEC*, necrotizing enterocolitis; *NPO*, nil per os (no oral feedings).

documenting two or more negative cultures. However, with persistent candidemia greater than 5 days, four key areas should be explored, as summarized in Table 35.2.

Urinary Tract Infection

Late-onset sepsis evaluations should include a urine culture obtained via sterile catheterization because *Candida* UTIs and sepsis have similar presentations (A-II, *Strong Recommendation*). *Candida* UTIs often occur in the absence of candidemia, emphasizing the need to obtain urine cultures. An elevated creatinine level without clear etiology may be another sign of a UTI. In the absence of antifungal prophylaxis, candiduria can occur in up to 2.4% of VLBW and 6% of ELBW infants.[2,9]

UTIs are most commonly defined as growth of ≥10,000 CFU/mL from a sterile catheterization or ≥1000 CFU/mL for bladder aspiration. Some experts consider the presence of any *Candida* in

Table 35.2 Management of Persistent Candidemia >7 Days

Does the patient still have a central venous catheter?	• If yes, remove or replace at another site if central access is critical to maintain.
Is antifungal dosing appropriate?	• If not, adjust dosing with the assistance of a pediatric infectious disease specialist and/or pharmacist. • Consider adding a second antifungal until candidemia clears.
Is there end organ dissemination (EOD)?	Rescreen. If candidemia persists after >7 days, EOD is even more likely, and the initial screen should be repeated and expanded to include: (1) ultrasound of the location of the tip of any current or previous central catheter for an infected thrombus. (2) complete abdominal ultrasound if there is a history of NEC or bowel perforation for abscesses (laparotomy is sometimes considered if clinical suspicion is high). (3) draining of abscesses that are amenable to drainage.
What is the absolute neutrophil count?	• If neutropenia is present with candidemia or another invasive Candida infection while on appropriate antifungal therapy for >2 days, correction of neutropenia with granulocyte colony-stimulating factor should be given.

the urine as infection and risk for adverse outcomes.[4] Others consider a urine culture with lower CFUs representative of colonization at a high-risk site needing preemptive treatment.[30] Renal ultrasonography is warranted for all *Candida* UTIs to evaluate for abscess formation (A-II, *Strong Recommendation*). Abscess formation may occur with candiduria via an ascending infection or dissemination to the kidneys with candidemia. Prompt and appropriate antifungal therapy with candiduria decreases the risk for this dissemination. Renal imaging should be performed at presentation and repeated in cases with persistent candiduria or candidemia of 7 or more days.

Central Nervous System Infection

Meningitis, meningoencephalitis, or abscess formation may complicate candidemia or occur separately. Studies have found that about 50% of meningitis cases occur in the absence of candidemia.[3,37] Lumbar puncture at the time of sepsis evaluation prior to the initiation of antifungal therapy is important because CSF cell counts and chemistries may not be abnormal, especially in preterm infants.[38] If lumbar puncture is unable to be performed at the time of presentation, it is important to obtain it as soon as possible in cases of candidemia or CNS disease and presumptively treat for at least 21 days. If meningitis is present, a repeat lumbar puncture should be performed after several days or near the end of 21 days of treatment to document clearance in case antifungal therapy needs to be extended. Neuroimaging (MRI best, followed by ultrasound) is needed to evaluate for abscess formation in cases of candidemia, meningitis, or infections with CNS symptoms.

Peritonitis

An ICI can complicate patients presenting with stage III NEC or focal bowel perforation.[16,39,40] If exploratory laparotomy or drains are placed, cultures should be obtained to determine what organisms may be present (B-II, *Strong Recommendation*).[16] Peritonitis may initially present with or without erythema as part of abdominal symptomatology. Identification of pathogens in the peritoneal cavity is critical to appropriate management of bowel perforation, peritonitis, and preventing potential abscess formation.[16] *Candida* species are the predominant organism causing peritonitis in 44% of focal bowel perforation and in 15% of perforated NEC cases.[16] Although radiographs can identify "free air" indicating a bowel perforation, complex fluid collections on ultrasound may indicate perforation or abscess formation. Some cases of perforation or abscess formation may be missed, and exploratory laparotomy may be needed if clinically indicated. Abscesses amenable to removal should be drained (B-II, *Strong Recommendation*).

Pneumonia

Pneumonia remains a difficult diagnosis in ventilated neonates with chronic lung disease, because radiologic findings of infection versus atelectasis, fluid, or scarring are often similar. Respiratory colonization is a high-risk site for infection, especially in intubated ELBW patients.[9,31] Preemptive treatment has been shown to prevent dissemination when *Candida* is detected in a tracheal aspirate by culture, polymerase chain reaction (PCR), or *Candida* mannan antigen in infants <1000 g or ≤ 28 weeks.[41,42]

Osteoarticular Infection

If an infant with candidemia also has signs of septic arthritis or osteomyelitis (swelling, immobility, erythema), a clinical diagnosis of osteoarticular infection can be made. Joint aspiration may be needed for diagnosis in the absence of candidemia. Evaluation with MRI or bone scan may help define the extent of involvement but cannot be used to rule out joint or bone involvement in neonates in the face of clinical symptoms. Treatment should be for 4 to 6 weeks.

Endocarditis or Infected Vascular Thrombi

Candida endocarditis or infected vascular thrombi are the most common complication of candidemia and associated with higher mortality than candidemia alone.[34,35] A second antifungal should be added if candidemia persists. When antifungal therapy alone is unsuccessful in resolution of the endocarditis or thrombus, thrombolytic or anticoagulation therapy has been used in some cases, depending on the infant's gestational age and associated conditions.

Endophthalmitis

Endophthalmitis presents most commonly as an intraocular dissemination from candidemia but also could be a rare complication of retinopathy of prematurity surgery, or local trauma.[35] Endophthalmitis progresses from a chorioretinal lesion that breaks free in the vitreous body. Fundoscopy reveals one or more yellow-white, elevated lesions in the posterior retina or vitreous body, generally appearing as a white fluffy ball. The clear cell-free vitreous body can also become hazy due to an influx of inflammatory cells. Even in absence of visible retinal abscesses or chorioretinitis, *Candida* sepsis increases the risk for severe retinopathy of prematurity, and screening for retinal pathology is recommended even if not indicated by gestational age or birth weight criteria.

Evaluation (See Figs. 35.5 and 35.6)

Cultures

Cultures of blood, urine, CSF, or other sterile body fluids remain the best method for diagnosing ICIs. For infection evaluations, blood, urine (if age >48 hours), and CSF cultures should be obtained and are critical to making a prompt diagnosis. When laparotomy is performed in cases of stage III NEC or focal bowel perforation, peritoneal cultures should always be obtained.[16] *Candida* will grow on regular media; fungal-specific cultures are not required. For infants with an ICI, $>50\%$ of cultures will be positive by 36 hours and 97% by 72 hours.[43] Prophylactic antifungal therapy does not affect fungal detection or time to positivity.[43]

Non–Culture Based Methods

Fungal cell wall polysaccharides such as 1,3-beta-D-glucan (BDG) and mannan as well as PCR and can be extremely useful identifying high-risk patients who would benefit from early empiric antifungal therapy while awaiting culture results, detecting nonbloodstream infections, or following the response to antifungal therapy. However, they are not better than cultures in identifying true infections at this time. Levels are less helpful in diagnosing infection and are not reliable, especially in infants receiving transfusions, but they can be used to follow a patient's response to treatment because they decrease significantly in response to antifungals.[44–46] BDG levels may help guide decisions to send cultures or start empiric antifungal therapy pending culture results.

The cutoff for BDG is higher (>125 pg/mL) for neonates than adults (>80 pg/mL) due to the effect of fungal colonization, other infections, and transfusions. Median BDG levels in infants with ICI are 364 pg/mL (interquartile range [IQR], 131–976) versus 89 pg/mL (IQR, 30–127) in noninfected neonates.[45,46] Caution should be used if there have been red blood cell or fresh frozen plasma transfusions, because BDG levels can be significantly high afterward for weeks (170 pg/mL; IQR, 65–317); caution should also be used in those who are or were recently infected with coagulase-negative *Staphylocuccus* (CoNS) (116 pg/mL; IQR, 46–128).[45,46]

PCR to identify 18S ribosomal RNA (rRNA) in preterm infants can detect candidemia as well as nonbloodstream infections including *Candida* peritonitis, candiduria, previous candidal infections, and endotracheal colonization.[47] Similar to adjunctive tests, the question of whether PCR is detecting infection or only colonization has not been critically studied in neonates. Finally, another method that may help with the decision to start early empiric therapy is direct fluorescent assay of the buffy coat.[48] This test is a fluorescent stain that binds to structures containing cellulose and chitin, yielding results in 1 to 2 hours.

Management

Antifungal Treatment

Antifungal dosing and duration are outlined in Figs. 35.5 and 35.6. An ICI (BSI, UTI, CCC) in the absence of dissemination should be treated for a minimum of 14 days, meningitis for 21 days, and EOD and abscesses for 4 to 6 weeks.[49,50] Once culture results are positive, prompt appropriate antifungal dosing needs to be initiated (A-II, *Strong Recommendation*). Most experts would recommend adding a second antifungal in the cases of CNS disease.

Amphotericin B deoxycholate (AmBd) is the optimal first choice for treatment because it has similar efficacy to other agents, low cost, and a favorable susceptibility pattern, because many nonalbicans species may be resistant to azoles and echinocandins (A-II, *Strong Recommendation*). Studies have demonstrated similar efficacy and safety of AmBd compared with AmB lipid preparations or echinocandins (micafungin).[51,52]

Central Venous Catheter Removal

Immediate central catheter removal[3] with candidemia is critical for clearance, decreasing risk for EOD, and improving survival and neurodevelopmental (A-II, *Strong Recommendation*).[53]

Empiric Treatment (See Fig. 35.5)

In high-risk patients with suspected ICI, empiric antifungal therapy on the day cultures are sent improves survival and neurodevelopmental outcomes (B-II).[53,54] Fig. 35.5 outlines risk factors and clinical presentations that may prompt the addition of empiric antifungal therapy to empiric antibiotics in certain sepsis evaluations.

Preemptive Treatment

Several studies have demonstrated that when high-risk sites are colonized (e.g., the respiratory tract), infants <1000 g or <28 weeks' gestation benefit from treatment. Studies have used endotracheal positive *Candida* cultures or mannan levels ≥0.5 ng/mL to decide on preemptive treatment and significantly decreased ICI (B-II).[41,42]

Neutropenia

Neutrophils are one of the most important components in the innate immune system's initial response to *Candida* infections, both through direct phagocytosis and other neutrophil functions. If neutropenia is present while on appropriate antifungal therapy for >2 days and central venous catheters have been removed, granulocyte colony-stimulating factor should be given (see Table 35.2).

Prevention (See Fig. 35.7)

Antifungal Prophylaxis

Targeted prophylaxis in extremely preterm infants (<1000 g or <28 weeks) during the period when they require intravenous access focuses on high-risk patients and individualizes each patient to receive prophylaxis during their high-risk period based on individual risk factors (A-II, *Strong Recommendation*). Linking the duration of prophylaxis to intravenous access correlates to the time period preterm infants are likely to have risks for ICI, such as significant immune immaturity, central catheters, parenteral nutrition, antibiotic exposure, and lack of enteral feedings. Targeting prophylaxis to individual patients' risk factors limits exposure to the patient as well as fungi, which helps limit toxicity, costs, and the emergence of fungal resistance.

For antifungal prophylaxis, the recommendation is intravenous fluconazole, starting shortly after birth at a dose of 3 mg/kg, twice a week until intravenous access no longer is required for care.[9,15,27,49] This dosage and duration of chemoprophylaxis has not been associated with emergence of fluconazole-resistant *Candida* species. Administering fluconazole prophylaxis twice weekly on the same days (e.g., Tuesdays and Fridays) and at the same times (e.g., 10:00 a.m.) reduces pharmacy costs and time and may limit medication errors. Additionally, if antifungal prophylaxis is used, a different antifungal (amphotericin B or another non-azole) should be used for empiric therapy.

High-risk infants >1000 g in the NICU include infants with NEC, gastroschisis, and those with gram-negative infections being treated with third/fourth-generation cephalosporins or carbapenems.[4,19,24]

Infection Control Measures

Prevention can begin in utero in pregnancies complicated by preterm labor or prolonged rupture of membranes; screening and treatment of vaginal candidiasis may be beneficial in preventing *Candida* colonization and subsequent infection in the newborn.[55] After delivery, standard NICU infection control, including hand hygiene, environmental cleaning during each shift, family education, and pharmacy preparation and handling of all infusions and medications, remains a critical part of prevention.[56] The use of medications that increase the risk for ICI (third/fourth-generation cephalosporins, carbapenems, gastric acid inhibitors, and postnatal steroids) should be monitored with stewardship and guidelines and avoided when possible. Feeding protocols and promoting use of human milk feedings are associated with a decreased incidence of NEC and therefore fewer ICIs that can complicate NEC. Finally, standardized protocols for insertion and management of central venous catheters, attention to sterile practices, hub and dressing care, and closed medication delivery systems have been shown to decrease CLABSIs, including those due to *Candida* (A-II, *Strong Recommendation*).[57,58] A "bundled approach" including antifungal prophylaxis as part of CLABSI prevention is associated with near elimination of ICIs.

Long-Term Outcomes

Mortality and Morbidity

Mortality after any type of ICI is approximately 25% to 30% among ELBW infants (Fig. 35.3). All-cause mortality rates are similar for candidemia (28%) and candiduria (26%) and increase to >50% for other sterile sites (meningitis and peritonitis) or if multiple sites are involved (blood, urine, and/or CSF).[4] Attributable mortality—the difference in mortality between ICI-infected and noninfected

Cutaneous Fungal Infections in Neonates	*Candidiasis* (*Candida albicans, C. parapsilosis*)	Aspergillosis (*Aspergillus fumigatus*)	Mucormycosis (*Rhizopus* and *Mucor* species)
Presentation	Desquamation (scaling, peeling, flaking or exfoliation), maculopapular, papulopustular, hypopigmented and erythematous rashes	Dry white powdery rashes Yellow crusted lesions Yellow ulceration areas Dark scab-like lesions Evolves into target lesions	Initially begins as erythema, sometimes with central ulceration or induration, progressing to necrosis leading to a black eschar Occurs at a skin area that has been covered, injured or in a pressure area such as the back
Evaluation	Culture (aerobic or fungal)	Culture (aerobic or fungal) or biopsy	Fungal culture or biopsy
Diagnosis	Yeast cells and pseudohyphae can be found with Gram, calcofluor white, or fluorescent antibody stains or in a 10%–20% KOH prep	Dichotomously branched and septate hyphae, identified by microscopic examination of 10% KOH wet prep or of Gomori methenamine-silver nitrate stain	Broad non-septate or, rarely, pauciseptate hyphae that become twisted and ribbon-like and branch at right angles from the parent hyphae. Pauci-septate (few septa) differentiates from aspergillosis
Treatment-start empirically when rash/lesions present	Amphotericin B and other susceptible antifungals	Voriconazole, echinocandins	Amphotericin B and surgical debridement if indicated
Dermatological findings	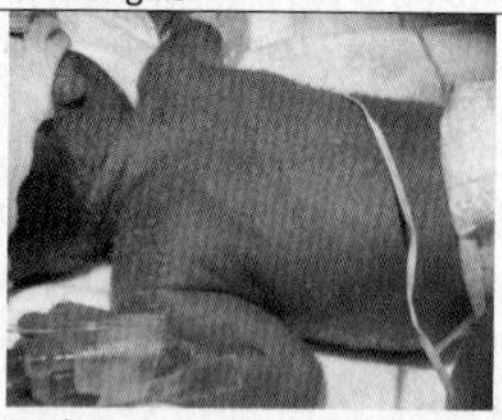 Back	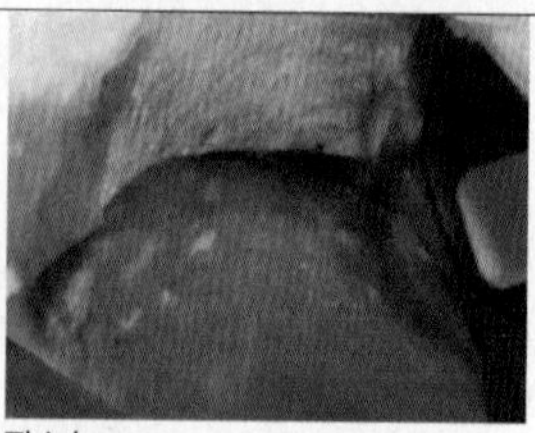 Thigh	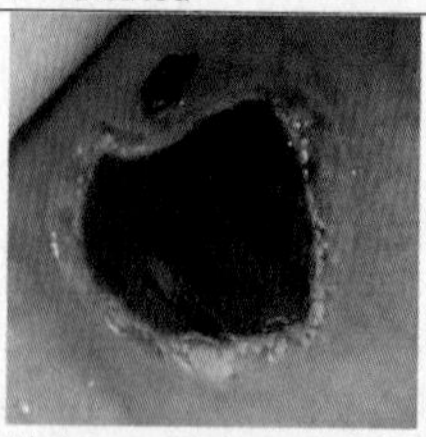 Abdomen next to umbilicus (area was discovered when hydrocolloid dressing was removed)[4]
	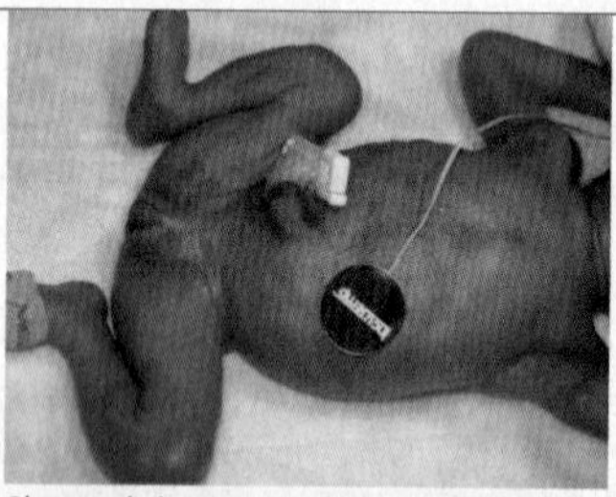 Chest, abdomen, and perineal area	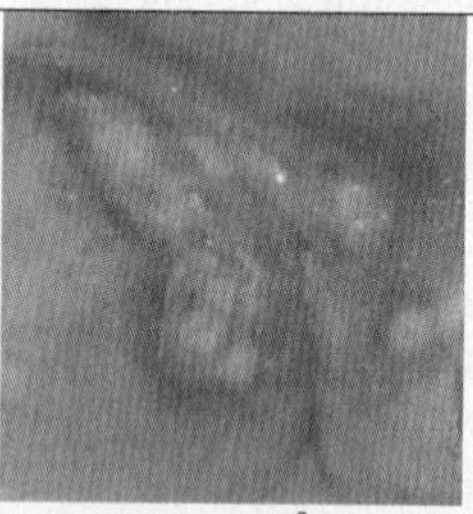 Leg and groin area[2]	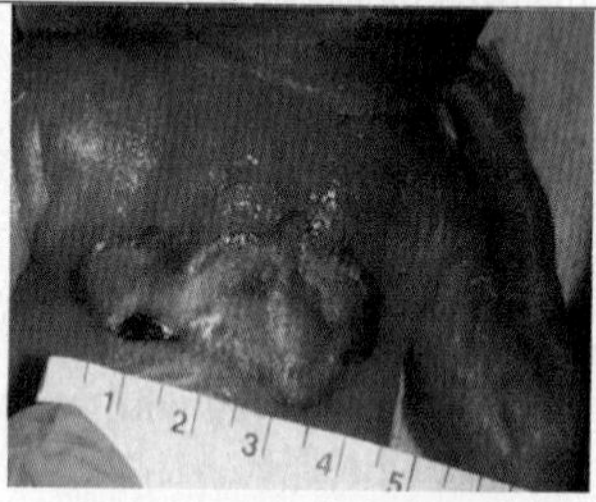 Back[5]
	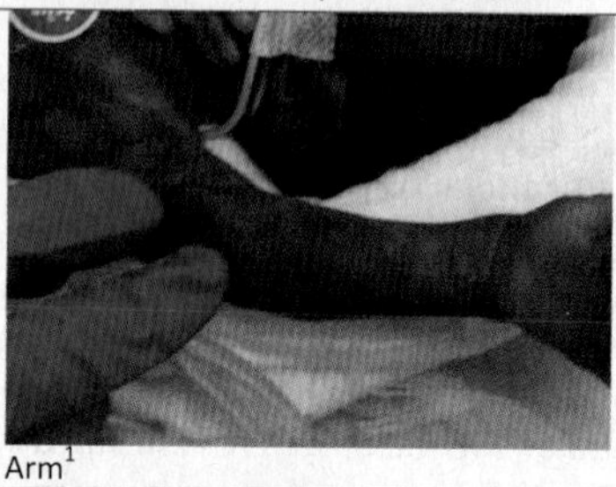 Arm[1]	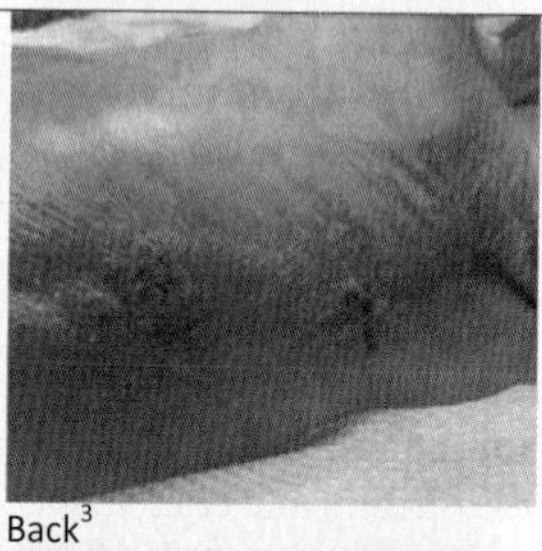 Back[3]	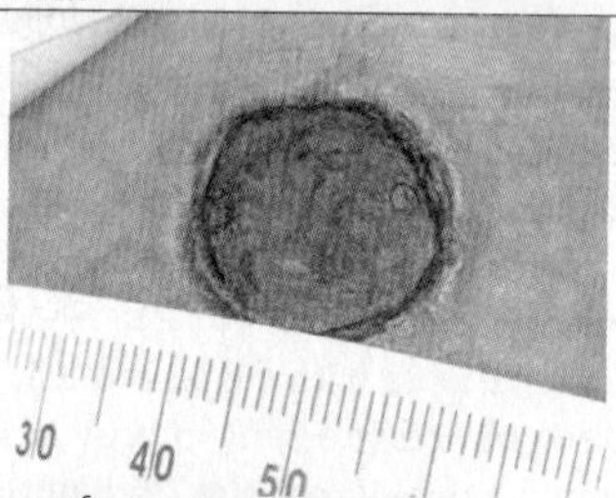 Back[6]
	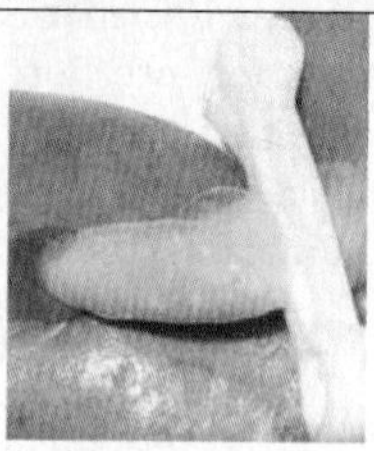 Funisitis	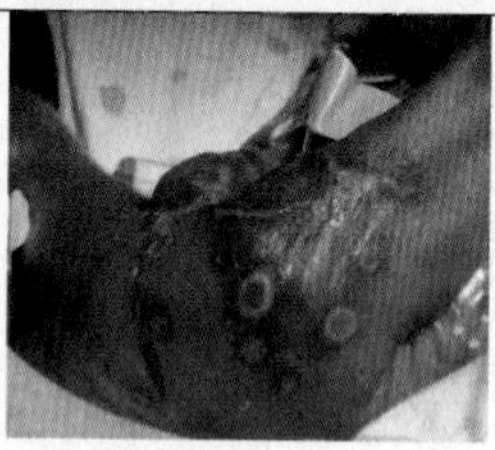 Leg and perineal area	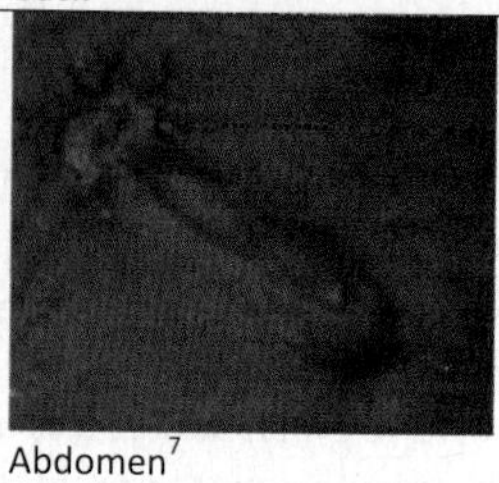 Abdomen[7]

1. Photo with permission (Neiman E, 2017)
2. Photo with permission (Rogdo B, 2014)
3. Photo with permission (Nakra NA, 2019)
4. Photo with permission (Murphy J, 2018)
5. Photo Courtesy of Joshua Attridge.
6. Photo with permission (Lowe CD, 2017)
7. Photo with permission (Gupta A, 2010)

Fig. 35.8 Cutaneous Fungal Infections.

infants—is 20% in ELBWs. In contrast, infants >1000 g with ICI have a much lower mortality risk of 2% compared with 0.4% in uninfected infants.[59] Survival is improved in candidemia cases with prompt removal of a central venous catheter, prompt empiric antifungal therapy, and in centers using antifungal prophylaxis.[3,53,60]

Survivors of ICI are at increased risk for morbidity. Even with prompt treatment, neurodevelopmental impairment or delay exceeds 50% for both candidemia and *Candida* meningitis.[3] Compared with uninfected, age-matched controls, candidemia in infants is associated with a 3-fold and candiduria a 2.5-fold increased risk for neurodevelopmental impairment.[7]

Aspergillosis and Mucormycosis

Aspergillosis and mucormycosis are caused by filamentous fungi or molds, and although uncommon, they occur and cause severe infections in extremely preterm infants.

Aspergillosis presents in neonates most commonly as a cutaneous infection and rarely as pulmonary or disseminated disease. Voriconazole as a first-line agent would be indicated in neonatal aspergillosis cases. The cutaneous manifestations are shown in Fig. 35.8.

Infections maybe the result of environmental contamination such as dust from hospital construction or faulty cleaning practices that can carry spores that may settle in wounds or be inhaled. This makes the extremely preterm infant at risk due to their diminished macrophage chemotaxis and phagocytosis, which are the major host defenses against aspergillosis. Prevention includes regular cleaning of the ventilation systems in the NICU to avoid buildup of dust contaminated with spores, as well as appropriate containment of dust during any work performed in the NICU, hospital renovation, and construction.

Mucormycosis initially presents as a black eschar at the site of local trauma, a covered area, or the back.[61] Skin lesions often begin as an erythematous to purple papule with central ulceration and an erythematous halo; they become necrotic, developing into an eschar that also can have an erythematous halo. They often progress to necrotizing soft-tissue infections. Extreme prematurity, neutropenia, and exposure to postnatal steroids are major patient risk factors. Mucormycosis may also complicate an intravenous catheter infiltrate. These fungi may contaminate adhesive tape, monitor leads, and wooden tongue blades used for splints in the NICU.

Early diagnosis and prompt therapy with amphotericin B are needed to prevent ulceration, necrosis, and rapid fatal dissemination in the majority of cases. Surgical debridement is sometimes needed, but studies show resolution of cutaneous cases with or without surgical debridement. A high degree of suspicion is needed. Fungal culture with Sabouraud and potato dextrose agar media positivity has improved in recent years to ~80%. Tissue biopsy may be needed to diagnose the right-angle, branched, nonseptated hyphae. Mortality from the infection without prompt diagnosis and treatment was reported as 61% (11 of 18) of infants in one small study.[62]

Although rare, gastrointestinal mucormycosis may occur in NICU infants and has a similar presentation as NEC (it may or may not have pneumatosis intestinalis).[63] It should be suspected if a patient, often with neutropenia, does not respond to medical NEC treatment and needs surgery. Gastrointestinal mucormycosis may also complicate NEC. Tissue biopsy and resection are needed for diagnosis and management in addition to at least 21 days of amphotericin B.

Malassezia and *Trichosporon* Infections

Malassezia furfur and *M. pachydermatis* are not highly virulent but have been associated with nosocomial infections in preterm infants. *M. furfur* is an obligatory lipophilic yeast and saprophyte that can colonize the skin, gastrointestinal tract, and intralipid solutions of NICU patients as well as lipid hand lotions and can be spread from patient to patient via hands of healthcare workers or family members. Bloodstream infection with *M. furfur* is more common in extremely preterm infants. Treatment involves antifungal treatment with discontinuation of intralipid infusion and/or removal of central vascular catheters. Amphotericin B should be used for treatment until a clinical response and negative blood culture are documented. However, in preterm infants with significant symptomatology and documented *M. furfur* fungemia, treatment with systemic antifungal therapy is warranted. *M. pachydermatis* invasive infections have also been described in neonates, including an outbreak that may point to infection control strategies. *M. pachydermatis* infections should prompt infection control measures and potential screening because the source may be other infants, healthcare workers, and dogs.

Trichosporon infections can occur in outbreaks and have high mortality in ELBW infants if not detected and treated. They are susceptible to amphotericin.

SECTION

7 Cardiac Defects and Dysfunction

OUTLINE

CHAPTER

Congenital Heart Defects 36

Diana Vargas Chaves, Shazia Bhombal
Ganga Krishnamurthy

KEY POINTS

1. Congenital heart disease (CHDs) are seen in 6 to 10 per 1000 live births. These include structural defects of the heart, of the great vessels, or both.
2. During the newborn period, the most important presenting features of CHD are central cyanosis, decreased perfusion to the body, and tachypnea. Cardiac murmurs are frequently heard but have a low sensitivity (44%) and low positive predictive value (54%).
3. The most useful screening methods to detect CHD include prenatal ultrasound, routine newborn physical examination, and pulse oximetry screening of newborns.
4. Three types of CHD can present soon after birth, including d-transposition of great arteries with intact ventricular septum and a restrictive foramen ovale, hypoplastic left heart syndrome with an intact atrial septum, and total anomalous venous connections with obstruction.

Overview

Congenital heart disease (CHD) is the most common birth defect. Recent incidence estimates for CHD range from 6 to 10 per 1000 live births.[1] One out of every four neonates with CHD has *critical CHD*, that is, a defect that requires either a surgical or transcatheter procedure within the first year of life.[2] These lesions can be broadly viewed as structural defects of the heart, of the great vessels, or of both.[3] Another way to classify these lesions could be based on the presence or absence of ventricular inflow/outflow abnormalities (Table 36.1). Defects range from relatively simple lesions, which neither cause clinical symptoms nor require therapy, to complex life-threatening lesions, which require emergent intervention in the neonatal period.[3,4]

Current screening methods to detect CHD include prenatal ultrasound, routine newborn physical examination, and pulse oximetry screening of newborns.[3–5] Although prenatal diagnosis of CHD is increasing, a significant proportion of babies are not diagnosed as having CHD before birth.[6,7] Postnatal diagnosis of CHD in the delivery room or newborn nursery is possible only if symptoms and signs of CHD manifest during the hospital stay or if there is a universal screening protocol using pulse oximetry.[3,5] Left-sided obstructive lesions such as coarctation of aorta are more likely to be diagnosed in babies after discharge from the nursery,[5,8] whereas those who have cyanotic CHD are more likely to be identified while still in the nursery.[9] Many neonates with serious CHD do not exhibit clinical manifestations of the underlying heart disease before discharge from the nursery.[10]

Clinical Features

Although a cardiac murmur is often considered the most common presenting sign of CHD, murmurs have a low sensitivity (44%) and low positive predictive value (54%) in the newborn period.[11] Rather, the three major presenting features of CHD in the newborn period are *central cyanosis, decreased perfusion to the body*, and *tachypnea*.[3] The predominant clinical manifestation depends on the type of CHD. Timing and severity of clinical presentation of CHD can vary depending on the nature of the defect.

Central Cyanosis

When cyanosis is restricted to the periphery, that is, in the nail beds or extremities, it is called peripheral cyanosis, a common and often

Table 36.1 Classification of Congenital Heart Defects Based on the Presence (or Absence) of Ventricular Inflow or Outflow Abnormalities

Defect	Description
WITH VENTRICULAR INFLOW OR OUTFLOW ABNORMALITY	
Tricuspid valve stenosis or atresia	Stenosis or atresia of tricuspid valve
Ebstein anomaly	Inferior displacement of tricuspid valve
Pulmonary atresia with intact ventricular septum	Atresia of pulmonary valve
Pulmonary stenosis	Subvalvar, valvar, or supravalvar obstruction to pulmonary blood flow
Tetralogy of Fallot with pulmonary stenosis or atresia	Anterior malalignment of conal septum leading to variable degree of obstruction to pulmonary blood flow, overriding aorta, VSD, and right ventricular hypertrophy
WITHOUT RIGHT VENTRICULAR INFLOW OR OUTFLOW ABNORMALITY	
Transposition of great arteries	Aorta arises from right ventricle, and pulmonary artery arises from left ventricle (ventriculoarterial discordance)
Truncus arteriosus	Single arterial trunk arises from ventricles, with variable origins of pulmonary arteries from trunk
Totally anomalous pulmonary venous connection with obstruction	Abnormal connection of all pulmonary veins to systemic venous system

VSD, Ventricular septal defect.

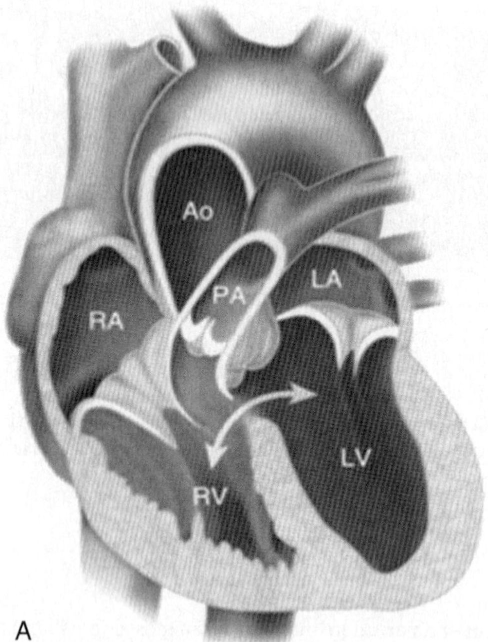

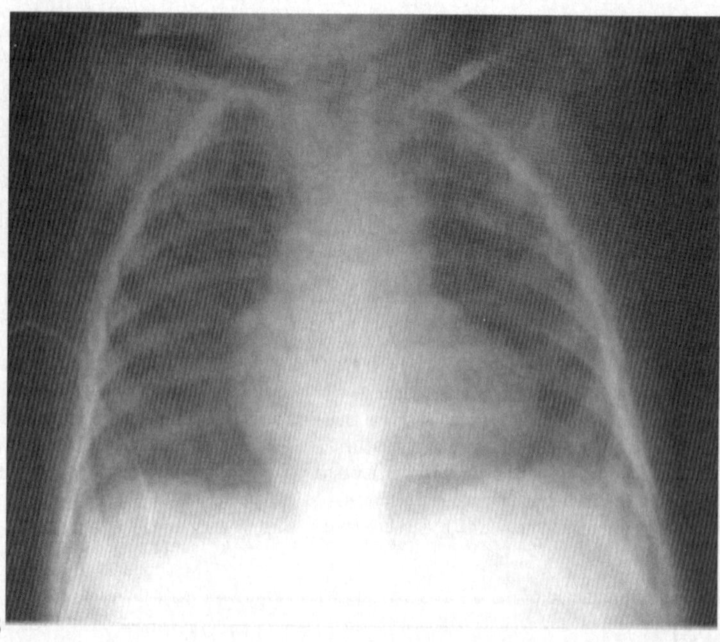

Fig. 36.1 Tetralogy of Fallot (TOF). (A) Schematic shows a large VSD with an enlarged aorta (Ao) overriding the defect. There is a notable valvular pulmonic stenosis and compensatory right ventricular (RV) hypertrophy. (B) Chest radiograph of a 3-month-old infant with TOF shows a boot-shaped heart. *LA,* Left atrium; *LV,* left ventricle; *PA,* pulmonary artery; *RA,* right atrium; *RV,* right ventricle; *VSD,* ventricular septal defect.

innocuous condition in newborns. Peripheral cyanosis should be differentiated from central cyanosis, a more ominous sign. Unlike peripheral cyanosis, central cyanosis is indicative of *hypoxemia.*[3]

In patients with CHD, shunting of systemic venous blood into the arterial circuit causes arterial hypoxemia and central cyanosis. Examples of lesions likely to present with central cyanosis include those that involve restriction of blood flow into the lungs, such as pulmonary stenosis, pulmonary atresia, and tetralogy of Fallot (TOF) with pulmonary stenosis (Fig. 36.1).[3] Typically, these defects are diagnosed when constriction of the ductus arteriosus causes further decrease in pulmonary blood flow. Congenital heart defects without restriction to pulmonary blood flow but characterized by the presence of desaturated blood in the aorta may also present with central cyanosis. These include dextro-transposition of the great arteries (d-TGA) (Fig. 36.2) and truncus arteriosus (Fig. 36.3).[3] Table 36.1 lists congenital heart defects, which commonly present with central cyanosis.

Cyanosis can also be seen in other types of CHD that may cause hypoxemia and systemic hemoglobin oxygen desaturation.[3] In the differential diagnosis, diseases involving lung parenchyma or the

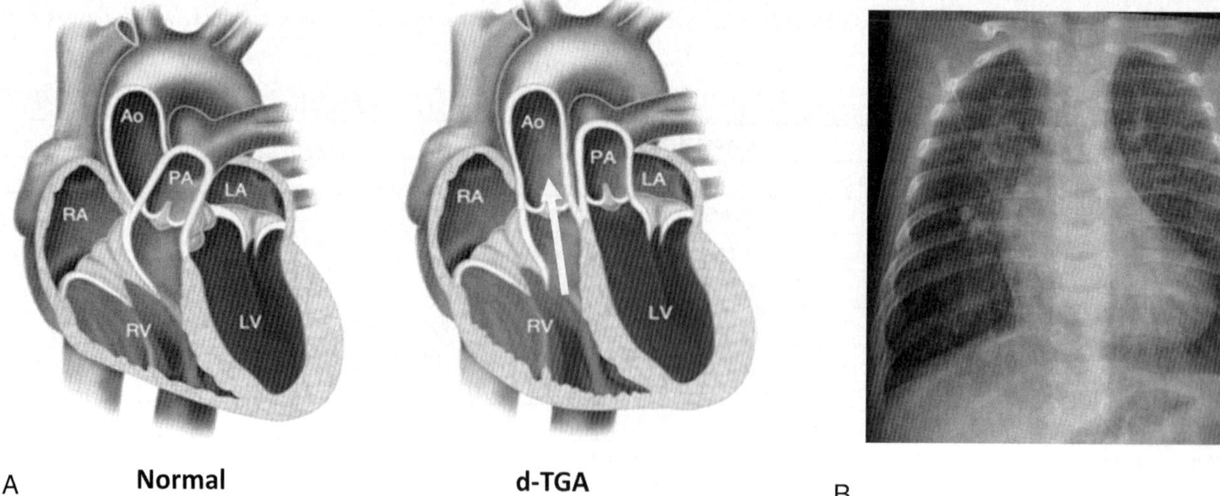

Fig. 36.2 (A) Anatomy of a normal heart and in complete d-transposition of the great arteries (d-TGA). With d-TGA, the aorta arises from the RV *(arrow)*, and the PA arises from the LV. Before corrective surgery, delivery of oxygenated blood to the systemic circulation depends on intracardiac shunting via an atrial septal defect or a ventricular septal defect. (B) Chest radiograph of an infant with d-TGA showing the egg-on-string appearance. *Ao,* Aorta; *LA,* left atrium; *LV,* left ventricle; *PA,* pulmonary artery; *RA,* right atrium; *RV,* right ventricle. (This figure was modified and reproduced with permission from Otto. *Textbook of Clinical Echocardiography*, 17, 473–506.)

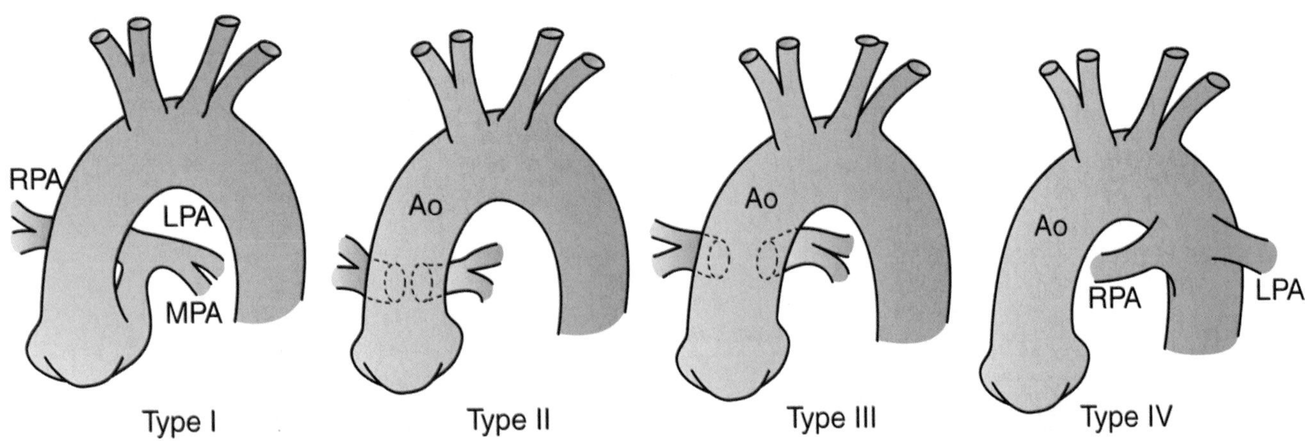

Fig. 36.3 Truncus Arteriosus (Collett-Edwards Classification). Type I: common main PA with subsequent origins of the branch PAs; Type II: branch PAs arise closely, but separately, from the truncus; Type III: branch pulmonary arteries widely separated in origin on the truncus; Type IV: no pulmonary arterial branch arises from the common trunk. This defect is now recognized as a form of pulmonary atresia with ventricular septal defect. *Ao,* Aorta; *LPA,* left pulmonary artery; *MPA,* main pulmonary artery; *RPA,* right pulmonary artery. (This figure was modified and reproduced with permission from Well and Fraser. In: *Sabiston Textbook of Surgery*, chap 59, 1641–1678.)

pleural space, such as a pleural effusion or pneumothorax, may affect gas exchange and oxygenation. In patients with these conditions, other clinical features suggestive of respiratory disease, such as nasal flaring, grunting, dyspnea, and hypercarbia, often accompany cyanosis. Neonates born with congenital neurologic, muscular, or neuromuscular conditions may present with cyanosis and hypercarbia caused by hypopnea. In neonates with cyanotic CHD, cyanosis is often the *sole* clinical feature. The *absence* of respiratory distress and hypercarbia in a cyanotic newborn should raise a strong suspicion of CHD.

On several occasions, infants with cyanotic heart disease may not *appear* cyanotic.[9] A critical amount of deoxyhemoglobin must be present in the capillary microcirculation for cyanosis to be apparent. Detection of cyanosis may be difficult if deoxy-hemoglobin is less than 3 to 5 g/dL or in babies with darkly pigmented skin. For this reason, serious cyanotic CHD often goes unrecognized unless measurement of oxygen saturation by pulse oximetry is performed.

Decreased Perfusion to the Body

Lesions that involve obstruction to blood flow from the left side of the heart present with decreased systemic perfusion (Table 36.2).[3,12] These defects range in severity from obstruction limited to the aortic isthmus, such as coarctation of the aorta (Fig. 36.4), to those causing severe hypoplasia of the left-sided structures of the heart, such as hypoplastic left heart syndrome (HLHS; Fig. 36.5).[3,12] Despite the obstruction, systemic blood flow is maintained before birth through a patent *ductus arteriosus* (PDA). In infants with critical left-sided obstructive lesions, signs of compromised systemic perfusion become evident with ductal constriction in the first few days after birth. Pulses become diminished, perfusion worsens, and capillary refill time increases. Metabolic acidosis ensues, and rapid progression into circulatory failure leads to severe end organ ischemia and death. It is not unusual for babies with left-sided obstructive lesions to manifest these symptoms after discharge from the nursery. The initial symptoms caused by left-sided heart obstruction are subtle but often progress rapidly. These patients may initially present to the pediatrician's office with mild tachypnea, difficulty or frequent interruptions in feeding, diaphoresis, and poor weight gain. Critical left-sided heart obstruction must be suspected when the infant presents in extremis to the emergency department.[3,13]

Table 36.2 Congenital Heart Defect Lesions That Involve Obstruction to Blood Flow From the Left Side of the Heart Present With Decreased Systemic Perfusion

Defect	Description
Aortic valve stenosis or atresia	Stenosis or atresia of aortic valve
Hypoplasia of aortic arch	Varying degrees of underdevelopment of ascending aorta, transverse arch, or both
Interruption of aortic arch	Complete separation or interruption of aortic arch; blood supply distal to interruption is via ductus arteriosus
Coarctation of aorta	Narrowing of aorta, usually at isthmus in juxta ductal region
Hypoplastic left heart syndrome	Underdevelopment of entire left-sided structures of heart

Tachypnea

Infants with heart lesions characterized by excessive pulmonary blood flow present with increased work of breathing.[3] Lesions can range from defects of the atrial or ventricular septum, or both, to abnormal communications at the venous or great artery level (Table 36.3).

Abnormal communication between the pulmonary and systemic circuit allows left-to-right shunting of blood and an increase in pulmonary blood flow.[3] Because the pulmonary vascular resistance is still elevated, symptoms of the underlying heart defect are usually not present at birth.[3,14] As the resistance in the pulmonary vascular circuit declines, left-to-right shunting of blood increases and symptoms emerge. Clinical manifestations usually appear at 4 to 6 weeks of life, when the low pulmonary vascular resistance and physiologic anemia of infancy contribute to increased left-to-right shunt. Earlier presentation is likely in preterm infants or those with multiple defects or if communication is at the arterial level (e.g., truncus arteriosus or aortopulmonary window). Newborns with isolated atrial septal defects (ASDs) do not usually exhibit symptoms in the neonatal period or even in infancy; diagnosis of an ASD is often missed unless an echocardiogram is obtained for evaluation of a murmur.

Increased blood flow into the pulmonary vascular bed and interstitial edema decrease lung compliance and cause an increase in work

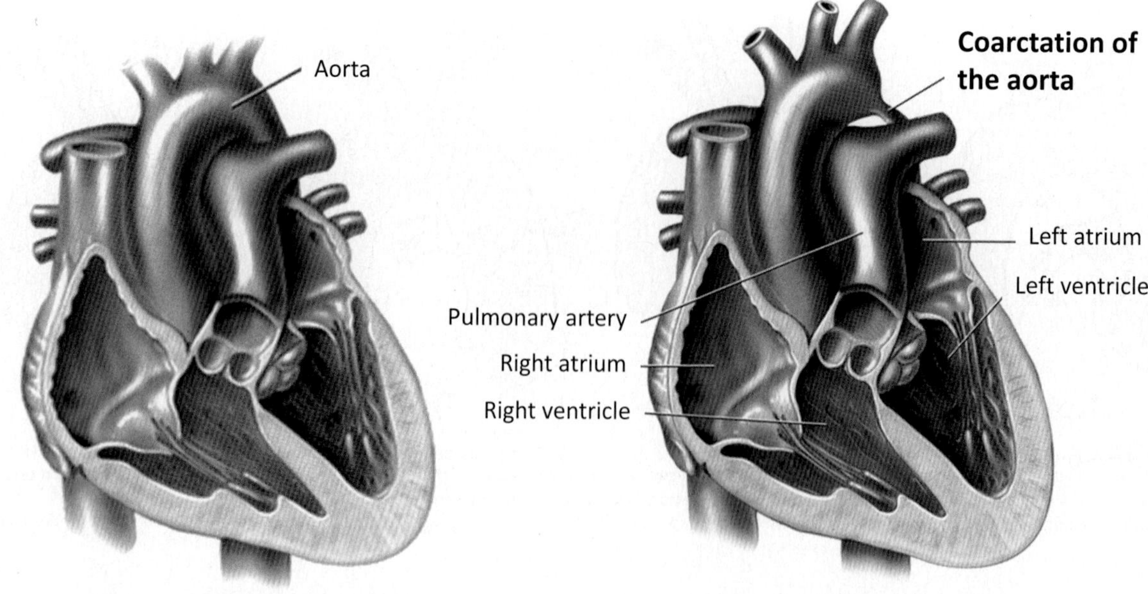

Fig. 36.4 Anatomy of a Normal Heart *(Left)* and With Coarctation of the Aorta *(Right)*.

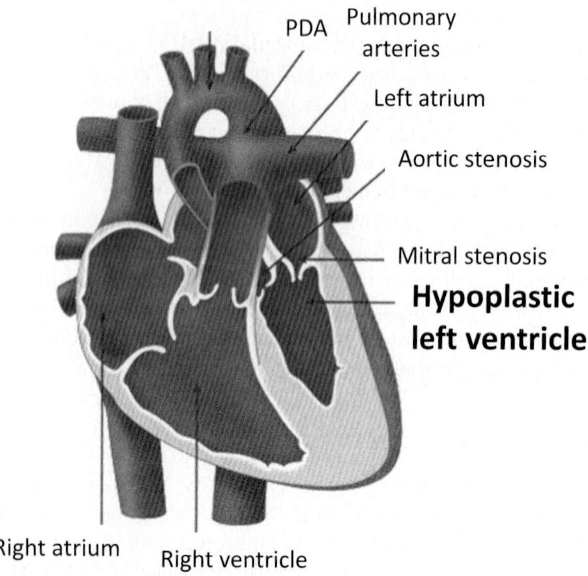

Fig. 36.5 Anatomy of Hypoplastic Left Heart Syndrome.

Table 36.3 Congenital Heart Defect Lesions Can Range From Defects of the Atrial or Ventricular Septum, or Both, to Abnormal Communications at the Venous or Great Artery Level

Defect	Description
Ventricular septal defect	Single or multiple defects in ventricular septum
Atrial septal defect	Single or multiple defects in atrial septum
Common atrioventricular canal	Defects of atrial and ventricular septa, along with a common atrioventricular valve
Patent ductus arteriosus	Pathologic patency of ductus arteriosus
Aortopulmonary window	Defect between aorta and main pulmonary artery
Truncus arteriosus	Single arterial trunk arises from ventricles, with variable origins of pulmonary arteries from trunk
Transposition of great arteries with ventricular septal defect	Aorta arises from right ventricle, and pulmonary artery arises from left ventricle (ventriculoarterial discordance); one or many defects in ventricular septum may also be present
Unobstructed total or partial anomalous pulmonary venous connection	Abnormal connection of some or all pulmonary veins to systemic venous system

of breathing. Babies with large left-to-right shunts exhibit tachypnea, easy fatigability during feeding, and diaphoresis.[3,14] Decreased oral intake and increased respiratory effort lead to poor weight gain and failure to thrive. Cyanosis is usually absent, unless there is a concomitant mixture of desaturated blood escaping into the arterial circuit, such as with unobstructed total anomalous pulmonary venous connection (TAPVC; Fig. 36.6) or truncus arteriosus.[3,15] In patients with these lesions, oxygen saturation levels measured by pulse oximetry are lower than usual. Clinical manifestations of large left-to-right shunts are usually not apparent at birth or prior to discharge from the nursery. These symptoms are often first reported to the pediatrician during routine office visits in the first 2 months of life.

Respiratory symptoms caused by a left-to-right shunt should be differentiated from those caused by primary lung disease. Underlying CHD should be suspected when symptoms described above are present, if there is an active precordium or a murmur on examination, or if cardiomegaly with prominent pulmonary vascular markings is noted on a chest radiograph.

Timing of Presentation

The age when symptoms or signs of CHD appear varies.[3] It can range from immediate and life-threatening presentation at birth to subtle symptoms of heart failure several weeks after birth.

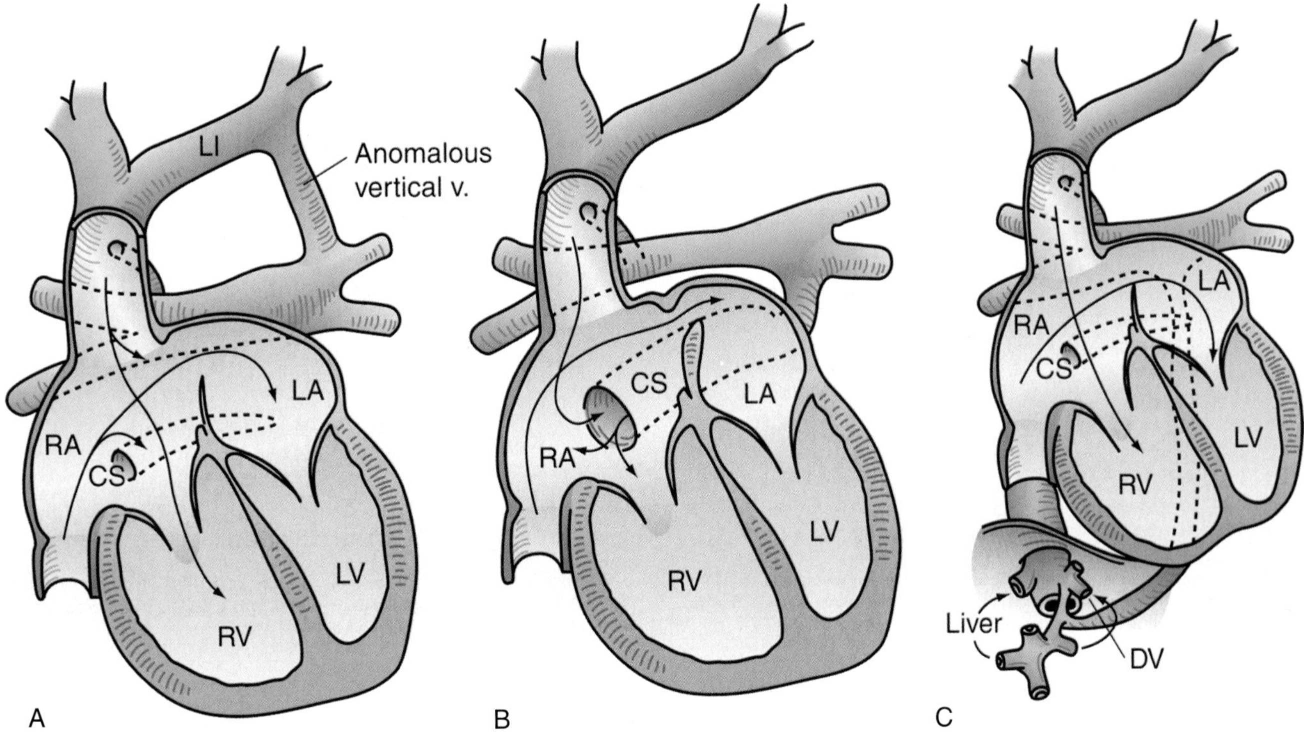

Fig. 36.6 Types of Total Anomalous Pulmonary Venous Connection (TAPVC). (A) Supracardiac type with a vertical vein joining the left innominate (LI) vein. (B) Intracardiac, connected to the coronary sinus (CS). (C) Infracardiac type with drainage through the diaphragm via an inferior connecting vein. *DV*, Ductus venosus; *LA*, left atrium; *LV*, left ventricle; *RA*, right atrium; *RV*, right ventricle. (This figure was modified and reproduced with permission from Hammon JW Jr, Bender HW Jr. Anomalous venous connections: pulmonary and systemic.)

Immediate and Life-Threatening

Three types of CHD can present soon after birth.[3] These lesions include d-TGA *with intact ventricular septum and a restrictive foramen ovale*, HLHS (with mitral atresia) *with intact or restrictive atrial septum*, and total anomalous pulmonary venous connection (TAPVC) *with obstruction*.[16–18] Babies with d-TGA, intact ventricular septum, and a restrictive foramen ovale are profoundly hypoxemic and cyanotic in the first minutes to hours after birth. Babies with HLHS and intact or restrictive foramen ovale have severe cyanosis, respiratory distress, and signs of low cardiac output that are evident within minutes after birth. Survival depends on urgent creation of an atrial-level communication by interventional cardiologists. This procedure can be performed only in cardiac centers; hence, early diagnosis and transfer are critical to survival. Babies with obstructed TAPVC present with profound cyanosis and respiratory distress within the first day of life. Temporary medical stabilization is possible, but very difficult, and urgent surgical repair is necessary for survival.

Symptoms in the Nursery

Lesions likely to be diagnosed in the nursery are those that usually present with cyanosis or murmur in the first couple days of life. Cyanotic lesions, including those with restriction to blood flow into or out of the right ventricle (see Table 36.1), are likely to be diagnosed in the nursery, as are d-TGA with intact ventricular septum and TAPVC with obstruction. Pathologic murmurs that present soon after birth are usually caused by turbulent flow across ventricular septal defects (VSDs) or stenotic semilunar valves, for example, aortic or pulmonary valvar stenosis. Often, the tricuspid regurgitation murmur of Ebstein anomaly (Fig. 36.7) may be recognized in the first few days of life. In absent pulmonary valve syndrome, turbulent antegrade and retrograde flow across a functionally incompetent pulmonary valve creates a to-and-fro murmur.

First 1 to 2 Weeks of Life

Lesions dependent on the ductus arteriosus for pulmonary or systemic blood flow usually present in the first week of life, either before discharge from the nursery or soon thereafter. Ductal-dependent systemic lesions, that is, left-sided obstructive lesions, are likely to present after discharge from the nursery. The more severe the lesion, the earlier the presentation, for example, HLHS is likely to present earlier than isolated juxta ductal coarctation of aorta.[3,13,17]

At 4 to 6 Weeks of Life

Most lesions causing significant left-to-right shunts present at this age, often with subtle earlier signs of mild tachypnea and feeding difficulties.

History and Physical Examination

History

Babies with critical CHD who present soon after birth have a very brief and benign perinatal history.[3] The *absence* of important clinical information that would allow the entertainment of an alternative diagnosis is a notable feature of CHD. For example, babies with severely obstructed TAPVC present with respiratory distress and cyanosis in the first 24 hours of life. However, there is usually no history of prematurity to suggest surfactant deficiency, no premature rupture of membranes or history of chorioamnionitis to suggest sepsis or pneumonia, or no meconium-stained amniotic fluid to suggest meconium aspiration. Hence, the *absence* of critical key historical information makes the diagnosis of CHD more likely.

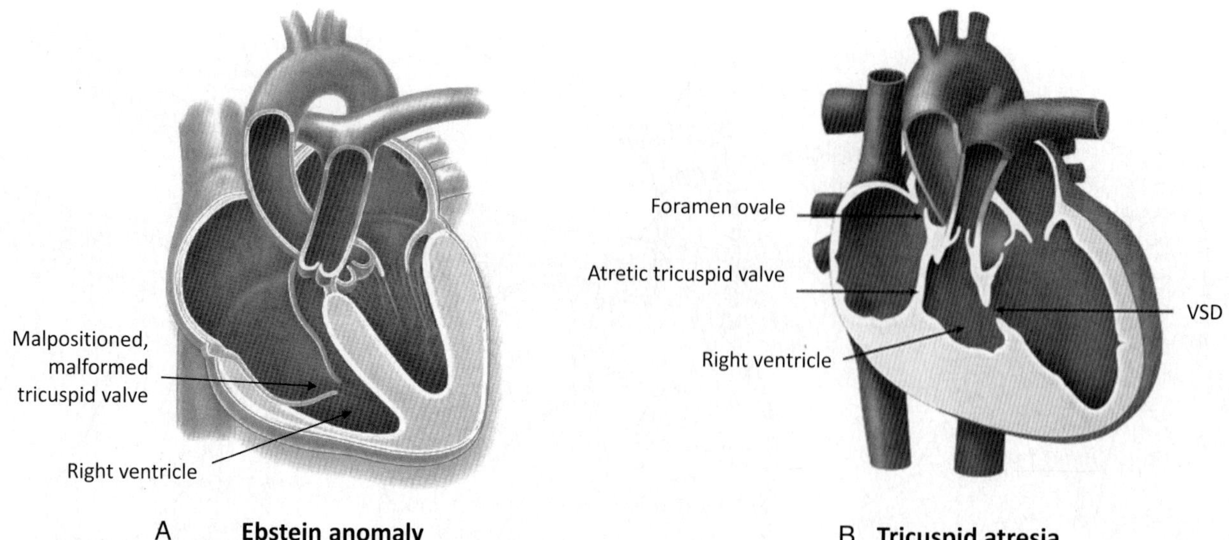

Fig. 36.7 Tricuspid Valve Anomalies. (A) Ebstein anomaly, where an apically displaced tricuspid valve is associated with atrialization of the right ventricle (located on the atrial side of the tricuspid valve). The functional right ventricle is small. (B) Tricuspid atresia. *VSD,* Ventricular septal defect. (Part A was modified and reproduced with permission from Lange and Cigarroa. *Conn's Current Therapy*. 2021; 107–112; part B was reproduced after modifications from Well and Fraser. In: *Sabiston Textbook of Surgery*. 2022; 1641–1678.)

Maternal history of CHD or diabetes increases the risk of CHD in the fetus. Maternal exposure to teratogenic drugs (e.g., lithium, phenylhydantoin, and alcohol) and viral infections (e.g., rubella) increases the risk of CHD in the fetus.[19–22] History of CHD in a sibling or other members of the family increases the risk of CHD in the fetus by several fold over the general population.[23]

Babies with cyanotic CHD usually present with cyanosis or cyanotic spells. Lesions, which cause obstruction to pulmonary blood flow or poor mixing, often present during the initial hospital stay in the nursery. Cyanosis in these patients may not be noticed at birth because the ductus arteriosus is still patent. Parents or physicians may initially note transient cyanosis during crying. As the ductus arteriosus begins to close, cyanosis becomes more apparent and persistent. Most important, despite cyanosis, a history of respiratory distress is usually not elicited.

Parents of babies with left-sided obstructive lesions may report tachypnea, irritability, and progressive difficulty in feeding. Symptoms emerge as systemic blood flow becomes compromised with closure of the ductus arteriosus. These newborns usually present after nursery discharge, typically within the first 2 weeks of life. As circulatory failure ensues, patients may present to the emergency department in extremis.[3,13]

Babies with large left-to-right shunts manifest symptoms of heart failure, that is, rapid respirations, diaphoresis, and feeding difficulties. These symptoms are subtle at first, usually appearing by 4 to 6 weeks of age, and worsen over time.[3]

Physical Examination

Anthropometric Measurements

Weight, height, and head circumference should be measured. A small head circumference is noted in some types of CHD, for example, HLHS.[24] In babies with congestive heart failure who are several weeks of age, comparison of current weight to birth weight may uncover inadequate interim growth.

Vital Signs

Tachycardia (within-reference-range heart rate: 120–160 beats/min at rest) in babies with CHD may be reflective of depressed ventricular function. An increased respiratory rate (within-reference-range: 20–60 breaths/min) may be caused by pulmonary edema, excessive pulmonary blood flow, or metabolic acidosis. Blood pressure should be measured in all four extremities; normally, the measured blood pressure in the lower extremities is a little higher than that measured in the upper extremities. A blood pressure gradient of greater than 10 to 20 mm Hg between the right arm and lower extremities may indicate coarctation of aorta or interruption of the aortic arch. Preductal and postductal hemoglobin oxygen saturation, measured with pulse oximetry, is critical in the evaluation of a neonate for CHD. A pulse oximetry sensor placed on the right hand of a neonate with a presumed left aortic arch and normal branching pattern of the head vessels measures preductal hemoglobin oxygen saturation; a sensor on either leg measures postductal oxygen saturation. A pulse oximetry sensor on the left hand is not an accurate reflection of preductal oxygen saturation, as the origin of the left subclavian artery is close to the region at which the ductus arteriosus connects to the aorta. By 15 to 20 minutes of life, babies with a structurally normal heart and good transition to extrauterine life have similar values for preductal and postductal hemoglobin oxygen saturation (>95%). Ideally, preductal and postductal hemoglobin oxygen saturation values should be recorded simultaneously. Low (<95%) preductal or postductal oxygen saturation may be suggestive of cyanotic CHD. Postductal oxygen saturation may be lower than the preductal oxygen saturation (differential cyanosis) in babies whose pulmonary vascular resistance is elevated, and shunting across the PDA is predominantly right to left. Differential cyanosis is also noted in neonates with critical coarctation of aorta or interrupted aortic arch in which the right ventricle provides flow into the descending aorta via the ductus arteriosus. Reverse differential cyanosis occurs when postductal saturation is *higher* than preductal saturation. Causes of reverse differential cyanosis include d-TGA with pulmonary hypertension or d-TGA with coarctation of aorta. In patients with d-TGA, blood with "high" oxygen tension enters the pulmonary artery from the left ventricle and is shunted into the descending aorta in the face of elevated pulmonary vascular resistance or the presence of either coarctation or interruption of aorta.

General Examination

Congenital heart disease often has an underlying genetic etiology with a recognizable pattern of physical features. Babies with Down syndrome have typical craniofacial features and are at high risk of having CHD.[25] Similarly, babies with a 22q11 deletion are at risk for conotruncal malformations, for example, truncus arteriosus or TOF, and have characteristic facies.[26]

Central cyanosis is best recognized in the buccal mucosa and tongue.[3] Central cyanosis is difficult to detect in babies with a within-range hemoglobin level unless systemic saturation is less than 80% to 85%. Cool extremities, feeble pulses, mottled skin, and prolonged capillary refill time indicate poor cardiac output and decreased systemic perfusion. Peripheral pulses are globally diminished when ventricular function is depressed. Disparity in pulses and blood pressure between the upper and lower extremities suggests coarctation of aorta with decreased flow in the descending aorta.

Cardiovascular Examination

The site of precordial activity should be noted. Dextrocardia should be suspected if the precordial impulse or activity is noted in the right hemithorax rather than the left. Parasternal impulse, rather than an apical impulse, is normal in neonates and signifies right ventricular dominance. A prominent parasternal impulse is noted with right ventricular pressure overload (right ventricular outflow tract obstructive lesions, pulmonary hypertension, and d-TGA). A diminished parasternal impulse is noted in right ventricular inflow obstruction, for example, tricuspid atresia or tricuspid stenosis with hypoplasia of the right ventricle. Left ventricular volume overload in left-to-right shunts (large VSD) causes a hyperdynamic apical impulse.

Auscultation of the heart includes evaluation of the heart rate and rhythm, heart sounds, and murmurs. S_1 is caused by closure of the atrioventricular valves. Abnormalities of S_1 are rarely appreciated in newborns. Split S_1 may be seen in newborns with Ebstein anomaly. S_2 reflects closure of both semilunar valves. Soon after birth, when pulmonary vascular resistance is still elevated, closure of both aortic and pulmonary valves occurs almost simultaneously. Hence, a single S_2 is commonly heard. As pulmonary vascular resistance falls, the pulmonary valve closes after the aortic valve and a split S_2 becomes apparent. A rapid heart rate makes it difficult to appreciate physiologic splitting of S_2 in newborns. Fixed splitting of S_2 in newborns is heard when pulmonary blood flow is excessive, as in unobstructed total or partial anomalous pulmonary venous connection. Wide, fixed splitting of S_2 occurs with ASDs but is not typically heard in the newborn period. A split S_2 is also appreciated when there is right ventricular obstruction or conduction delay. A single S_2 is appreciated when there is only one semilunar valve, as in pulmonary or aortic atresia or truncus arteriosus. Quality of the S_2 should also be assessed. An accentuated S_2 component reflects increased vascular resistance distal to the corresponding semilunar valve. A loud P_2 is heard in patients with pulmonary hypertension, while a soft P_2 may suggest pulmonary stenosis. S_3 and S_4 reflect abnormal ventricular filling dynamics. Stenosis of semilunar valves, a bicuspid aortic valve, or a dysplastic truncal valve in patients with truncus arteriosus may produce additional sounds or ejection clicks. A midsystolic click is sometimes appreciated in patients with Ebstein anomaly or with mitral valve prolapse.

Murmurs are often associated with structural abnormalities of the heart. Often, murmurs are innocent and bear little clinical significance. It may be difficult for the inexperienced physician to distinguish innocent from pathologic murmurs. A systematic approach to evaluation may assist in identifying an underlying anatomic malformation causing the cardiac murmur. Intensity, quality, location, radiation, duration, and timing of the murmur should be assessed. Murmurs can occur during systole, during diastole, or continuously during the entire cardiac cycle. Timing and duration of murmurs during the different phases of systole or diastole should be noted. A harsh murmur of at least grade 3 intensity, best heard in the lower-left sternal border and occupying the whole duration of systole, is likely to be secondary to a VSD. A harsh grade 3/4 intensity murmur with a crescendo-decrescendo configuration, best heard in the upper-right sternal border and radiating to the carotids, may relate to stenosis of the aortic valve. A murmur heard continuously across systole and diastole and best appreciated in the upper-left sternal border (or midclavicular region) is probably caused by a large PDA. Innocent murmurs are softer, occur in systole, and have no accompanying symptoms. *The absence of murmur does not rule out CHD.*

Pulmonary Examination

Respiratory rate and respiratory effort, quality of breath sounds, and the presence of adventitious sounds should be assessed. Babies with significant left-to-right shunts and increased pulmonary blood flow are tachypneic and show an increased respiratory effort. Most babies with cyanotic CHD exhibit normal respiratory activity, despite low oxygen saturation. *Normal* findings on respiratory examination in the presence of cyanosis *strongly* suggest CHD.

Abdominal Examination

Location and size of the liver should be assessed. A left-sided liver is present in situs inversus, and a midline liver is often noted in heterotaxy syndrome.[27] Hepatomegaly suggests hepatic congestion and right ventricular dysfunction or volume overload. Neonates with hepatic arteriovenous malformation and high-output heart failure may have a bruit over the liver.

Evaluation

Chest Radiograph

Position and contour of the cardiovascular silhouette on chest radiographs are informative.[28] Dextrocardia and presence of a right-sided stomach bubble or midline liver may indicate complex CHD, including heterotaxy syndrome.[27,28] Presence or absence of thymic shadow and sidedness of the aortic arch should be assessed. An absent thymic shadow may suggest 22q11 deletion syndrome and raises the possibility of conotruncal malformation. Characteristic radiographic features are noted in some types of CHD, for example, boot-shaped heart in TOF and "egg on string" appearance in d-TGA. Prominence of pulmonary vasculature indicates excessive pulmonary blood flow; relatively oligemic lung fields suggest paucity of blood flow to the lungs. Pulmonary venous congestion and pulmonary edema with a normal heart size are noted in newborns with TAPVC with obstruction.

Electrocardiogram

A 12-lead electrocardiogram (ECG) often reveals characteristic ECG findings in some types of CHD. However, normal ECG findings do *not* rule out presence of a serious underlying CHD.

Hyperoxia Test

A hyperoxia test is helpful to differentiate hypoxemia caused by structural heart disease from that caused by lung disease.[29] An arterial blood gas value is obtained at baseline and after exposure to 100% oxygen for at least 15 minutes. In babies with structural heart disease,

PaO_2 remains less than 100 mm Hg after exposure to 100% oxygen. Babies with lung disease will typically have an increase in PaO_2 to greater than 150 mm Hg but may not if intrapulmonary shunting is significant.

Echocardiography

An immediate cardiology consultation should be requested when CHD is suspected. Echocardiography is often the only definitive procedure required to confirm a diagnosis of structural heart disease.[30,31]

Blood Tests

Baseline blood work includes complete blood cell count to help rule out concurrent infection, serum chemistry to assess for electrolyte and renal function abnormalities, and an arterial blood gas with lactate level to assess gas exchange and the presence or absence of lactic acidosis.

Screening for CHD

Many neonates with serious CHD do not exhibit clinical manifestations of the underlying heart disease before discharge from the nursery.[31,32] More than 50% of newborns with CHD can have normal neonatal physical examination findings at the time of initial discharge from the hospital.[33] Many congenital heart defects do not produce visible central cyanosis, despite hypoxemia. Screening by pulse oximetry provides an opportunity to detect clinically silent hypoxemia in patients with critical CHD (Class IIb, Evidence Level C).[5,29,32] The US Department of Health and Human Services has recommended that all newborns be screened for critical CHD using pulse oximetry prior to discharge from the newborn nursery.[34] This recommendation has been endorsed by the American Academy of Pediatrics.[35] Pulse oximetry has now been included in the Recommended Uniform Screening Panel for newborns across several states in the United States.[35] Primary targets for newborn screening by pulse oximetry are HLHS, pulmonary atresia with intact ventricular septum, d-TGA, truncus arteriosus, tricuspid atresia, TOF, and TAPVC. Screening by pulse oximetry is highly specific for detection of critical CHD (>99%) and has moderate sensitivity (70%). The false-positive rate is very low (0.035%) when screening is done after 24 hours of age. Pulse oximetry may not detect *all* critical CHD, particularly lesions with obstruction to systemic blood flow.[5]

Critical CHD may escape detection at all three stages, that is, on prenatal ultrasound, routine neonatal examination in the nursery, and screening pulse oximetry. Patients in whom a diagnosis of CHD is missed may present in the pediatrician's office or emergency department. A high index of suspicion along with prompt and timely recognition of babies with critical CHD improves prognosis.[3,5,32]

Management

Airway, breathing, and circulation must be assessed in patients with cardiorespiratory symptoms. In patients presenting with severe hypoxia and increased respiratory effort, intubation and mechanical ventilation may assist in improving gas exchange. Circulation cannot be reestablished without a PDA in patients with ductal-dependent lesions. Prostaglandin E_1 (PGE_1) infusion can reopen a closing ductus arteriosus and must be initiated as soon as ductal-dependent CHD is suspected. It is not necessary to wait for an echocardiogram for confirmatory evidence prior to initiating a PGE_1 infusion except in cases of TAPVC, in which PGE_1 infusion has the potential of increasing pulmonary edema, thereby worsening oxygenation. Reopening the ductus arteriosus will improve oxygen saturation in patients with ductal-dependent pulmonary circulation, and systemic perfusion will improve in patients with ductal-dependent systemic circulation after initiating PGE_1 infusion. Correction of hypovolemia and initiation of cardiotonic infusions to enhance inotropy may be required for patients presenting in cardiogenic shock (Class IIb, Evidence Level C). Metabolic derangements, including hypoglycemia and hypocalcemia, should be corrected. Early transfer to a cardiac center is important.

Long-Term Considerations

Surgical or transcatheter therapy is available for almost all types of CHD. Survival for neonates born with CHD has improved in recent years, with more than 90% surviving to discharge from the hospital after surgery.[36] Long-term prognosis for newborns with CHD depends on several factors including severity of the heart defect and the presence of genetic anomalies.[37] Babies born with the most severe heart defects (e.g., HLHS) and with associated serious chromosomal malformations have significantly worse neurodevelopmental outcomes compared with babies with simpler heart defects.[38,39]

CHAPTER 37

Cardiac Defects—Anatomy and Physiology

Rune Toms, Rachana Singh

KEY POINTS

1. Congenital heart diseases (CHDs) are an important cause of morbidity and mortality in young infants. These malformations account for approximately 300,000 deaths yearly.
2. Cardiac septal defects are the most common type of anomalies. Ventricular septal defects (VSDs) are seen most frequently, in 5 to 50 per 1000 live births. Atrial septal defects (ASDs) also common and account for 8% to 10% of all congenital heart defects.
3. Atrioventricular canal (AVC) defects are commonly associated with Trisomy 21 and heterotaxy, although patients with normal chromosomes can also show AVC defects.
4. Tetralogy of Fallot is the most frequently seen cyanotic heart defect; it is characterized by pulmonic valve stenosis, VSD, overriding aorta, and right ventricular hypertrophy. Transposition of the great arteries is another important cyanotic defect.
5. Aortic stenosis and interrupted arch are important anomalies in the left outflow tract. With improved cardiac imaging, many infants with hypoplastic left heart syndrome are now being recognized prenatally and being treated with timely, appropriate intensive care services.
6. Further work is needed to determine the predisposing molecular defects that increase the risk of congenital cardiac defects. There is room for improvements in cardiovascular support and management. However, some of most complex defects have limited therapeutic options and need cardiac transplantation.

Congenital heart diseases (CHDs) are an important cause of morbidity and mortality in the neonatal period and beyond. Despite major advances in the medical and surgical treatment, CHDs pose a significant global health and economic burden and account for approximately 300,000 deaths yearly. In this chapter, we have focused on the prevalence, anatomic details, and pathophysiology of the most frequently seen congenital cardiac diseases (defects).

Septal Defects

Atrial Septal Defects

Prevalence

Atrial septal defects (ASDs) account for 8% to 10% of all congenital heart defects and are about twice as common in females as in males.[1,2] With the advent of echocardiography and increasing access to healthcare, the prevalence has increased over time, especially with increasing age of the patient population.[3]

Embryology and Anatomy

The septation of the atrium begins during the fourth week of life when the septum primum grows inferiorly in the direction of the endocardial cushion.[4] The failure of septum primum attachment and fusion with the endocardial cushion leaves an opening called the ostium primum. Additionally, in the mid to superior portion of the septum primum, tissue reabsorption occurs, creating an opening called the ostium secundum opening. These result in two defects in the septum primum: (1) the ostium primum, located inferiorly in the septum just above the endocardial cushion, and (2) the ostium secundum, located superiorly and in the center of the septum.[5,6] To the right of the septum primum, due to an anterosuperior folding of the atrium, a second septum grows inferiorly, named the septum secundum.[5,6] This septum consists of a superior and inferior limb. The inferior limb of the septum secundum grows inferiorly and completes the septation of the lower part of the septum by fusing with the endocardial cushion closing the ostium primum. The superior limb of the septum secundum has a more muscular ridge and covers the ostium secundum incompletely. This incomplete covering of the foramen secundum and adhesion by the septum secundum results in the fetal communication between the right and left atrium called the *foramen ovale.*[7,8] The superior ridge of the *foramen ovale* is called the limbus of *fossa ovalis* and is the inferior ridge of the superior *septum secundum.*

Secundum ASD is the most common form of ASD, accounting for 75% of all ASDs, followed by primum ASD, accounting for 20% of all ASDs.[9] Less common types of ASD are sinus venosus and coronary sinus ASDs.[9] Fig. 37.1 shows schematic figures of various types of ASDs.

Although most ASDs occur sporadically, a mother with an ASD has an 8% to 10% chance of having a child with ASD. Inherited mutations in genes encoding cardiac transcription factors and sarcomeric proteins have been reported as an underlying cause for familial recurrence of nonsyndromic CHD in humans, in particular cardiac septal defects.[10] Holt-Oram syndrome, an autosomal dominant syndrome that is a result of a *TBX5* mutation, is the most common syndrome associated with an ASD.[11] Holt-Oram syndrome is characterized by varying degrees of thumb hypoplasia, absent metacarpals, and radius. Heterozygous mutation in the *NKX2.5/CSX* transcription factor is associated with familial cases of ASD.[10,12] This *NKX2.5* mutation is also associated with first-degree heart block, which may progress to complete heart block. Therefore all babies with ASD should have a baseline electrocardiogram to evaluate for heart block. A dominantly inherited form of ASD is found with a missense mutation in an alpha-myosin heavy chain locus on chromosome 14q12.[13] This myosin heavy chain protein is a structural protein found in high concentrations during atrial septation.

Patent Foramen Ovale

The patent foramen ovale (PFO) is a normal anatomic communication in the atrial septum that allows oxygenated blood to flow from the placenta via the ductus venosus through the PFO to the left atrium

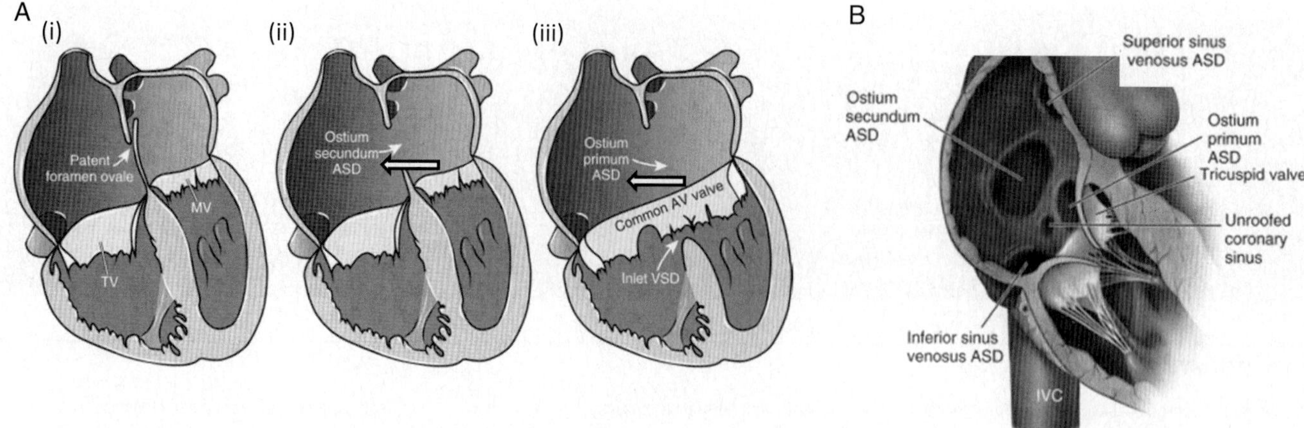

Fig. 37.1 (A) Schematic of atrial level shunts. (i) Patent foramen ovale; (ii) ostium secundum atrial septal defect (ASD); (iii) ostium primum ASD with a common atrioventricular (AV) valve and associated inlet ventricular septal defect (VSD). (B) Right atrial view of the interatrial septum demonstrating the location of different types of ASD. *Ao*, Aorta; *IVC*, inferior vena cava; *MV*, mitral valve; *SVC*, superior vena cava; *TV*, tricuspid valve. (Reproduced with permission and minor modifications from Lin J, Aboulhosn JA: Congenital shunts. In: Otto CM, ed. *The Practice of Clinical Echocardiography*, 5th ed. Philadelphia: Elsevier; 2017:881–883, Fig. 44.2–44.3.)

(LA) during fetal life. The septum primum and the septum secundum are developed normally. The foramen ovale is anatomically located in the fossa ovalis.[14] Immediately after birth, with an increase in pulmonary venous return to the LA and lowering of the pulmonary vascular resistance (PVR), the pressure in the LA exceeds that of the right atrium (RA), resulting in the septum primum being pushed toward the septum secundum and closing the PFO like a flap, leading to functional closure of the PFO. Over time the septum primum adheres to the superior limbus of the septum secundum, causing permanent anatomic closure of the PFO.

Secundum ASD

A secundum defect is a defect of the septum primum within the fossa ovalis, with a normally developed septum secundum.[6] The defect size may vary from a few millimeters to 2 to 3 cm, with significant defects resulting from an almost complete absence of the septum primum.

In infants, secundum defects less than 5 mm in size have an 80% to 90% chance of closing spontaneously. The chance of spontaneous closure decreases with age, and defects in children older than 5 years are more likely to increase in size.[15]

Primum ASD

A primum ASD results from the septum primum failing to attach to the endocardial cushion and results in a defect located just above the atrioventricular valves anterior and inferior to the fossa ovalis.

Sinus Venosus Defect

A sinus venosus defect is a defect between the posterior-superior wall of the RA and one or both of the right pulmonary veins.[16] This defect results in a left-to-right shunt from the right pulmonary vein to the RA. Physiologically, this left-to-right shunt is similar to the left-to-right shunting over an ASD. However, anatomically, a sinus venosus defect is not an ASD because there is no direct shunting over the atrial septum from the LA to the RA.

Coronary Sinus Defect

A coronary sinus defect results from "unroofing" of the coronary sinus, which wraps posteriorly around the heart, creating a channel for left atrial blood to enter the coronary sinus and empty into the RA.[17]

Pathophysiology

Fig. 37.2 shows a brief summary of the pathophysiology of ASDs. A defect in the atrial septum allows for mixing of oxygenated and deoxygenated blood. The maximum shunt across the atrial septum occurs mainly during diastole when both atrioventricular valves are open, with the atria emptying into the ventricles. The compliance of the ventricles in turn will mainly determine the degree of shunting across the ASD. In a neonate, the right ventricle (RV) is more active, dominant, and muscular compared with the left ventricle (LV) because it has been functioning primarily as the systemic ventricle in utero, working against a relatively high PVR. As the PVR naturally falls with postnatal transition, the RV becomes less muscular with improved compliance. This results in an increase in left (systemic) to right (pulmonary) shunting postnatally during this expected transition. Thus the atrial-level shunting can be used indirectly as a marker for both RV and LV compliance in critically ill neonates. By comparing the flow pattern of the atrial-level shunt, one can assess changes in ventricular compliance.[6]

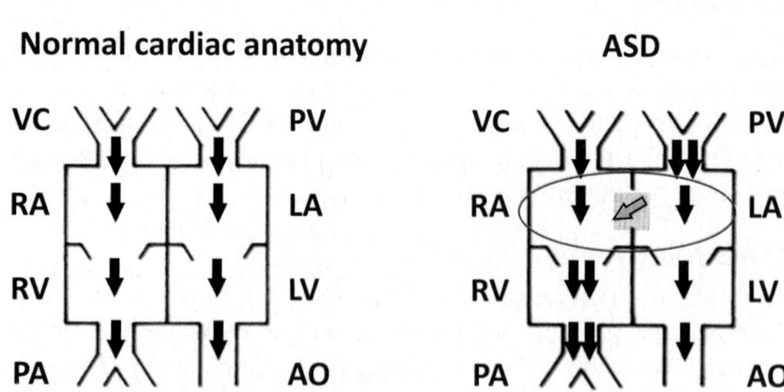

Fig. 37.2 Pathophysiology of Atrial Septal Defects (ASDs). Some of the pulmonary venous blood entering the left atrium (LA) flows left-to-right (L→R) through the ASD into the right atrium (RA) and right ventricle (RV). The degree of L→R shunting is determined by the compliance of the "downstream" RV. L→R shunting is low in neonates with poor RV compliance. It increases once the pulmonary vascular resistance (PVR) drops and the RV compliance improves. Most shunting occurs in diastole and during expiration. Most ASDs do not become symptomatic in neonates. Symptoms related to ASDs are usually related to long-standing large L→R shunting, which cause volume overloading in the RV. Patients with ASDs are at risk for paradoxical embolism. The second heart sound (S2) and its variations with respiration are lost because of increased RV volume. This is heard as wide, fixed splitting of S2 on auscultation. Increased blood flow through the tricuspid valve causes a systolic ejection murmur.

Ventricular Septal Defects

Prevalence

Ventricular septal defects (VSDs) are the most common type of congenital heart disease diagnosed in neonates and infants. The incidence of VSDs ranges between 5 and 50 per 1000 live births.[1]

Embryology and Anatomy

The ventricular septum anatomically separates the RV and LV. The RV comprises cardiomyocytes that originate from the secondary heart field and require the transcription factor Hand2 to develop. The LV develops from cardiomyocytes originating from the primary heart field, requiring the transcription factor Hand1 to develop.[18]

The ventricular septum develops between days 27 and 37. Septation occurs as a result of three mechanisms: (1) Tissues from opposite ends expand and grow toward each other and ultimately fuse; (2) one end of a cavity grows actively toward the opposite side of the lumen; and (3) the two expanding portions of one end of the heart merge, creating a wall. However, this mechanism will never lead to full septation of the cavity. VSD is commonly seen in trisomy 13, 18, and 21 and Holt-Oram syndrome (*TBX5* mutation). There is an association between maternal marijuana and cocaine use, as well as paternal exposure to paint stripping, and VSD in the offspring. There are several ways in which the anatomic locations of VSDs are classified and named. This chapter will use the most common clinical division of inlet, outlet, perimembranous, and apical trabecular (muscular) VSDs.

Based on location, VSDs are classified into 4 subtypes (Fig. 37.3):

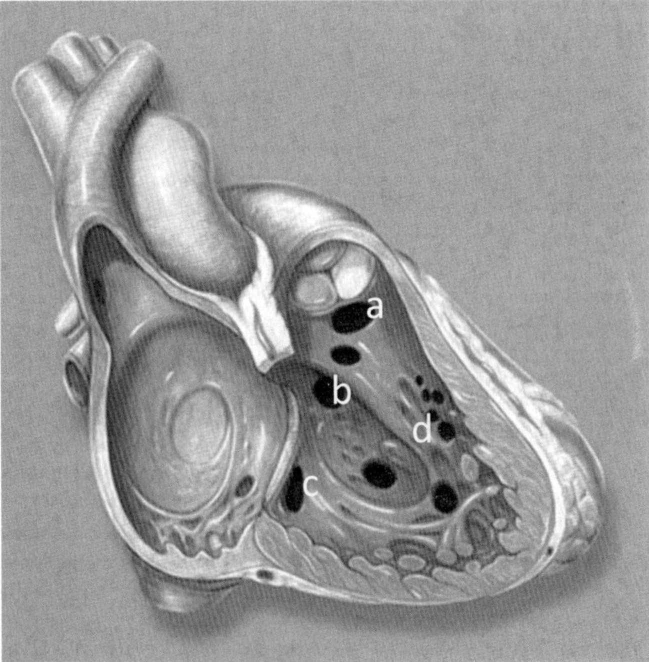

Fig. 37.3 Ventricular Septal Defect (VSD). VSDs classified based on location: (a) outlet; (b) perimembranous; (c) inlet; and (d) muscular. (Lynch PJ, illustrator; Jaffe CC, cardiologist; Yale University Center for Advanced Instructional Media Medical Illustrations by Patrick Lynch, generated for multimedia teaching projects by the Yale University School of Medicine, Center for Advanced Instructional Media, 1987–2000. Lynch PJ, http://patricklynch.net; http://commons.wikimedia.org/wiki/File:Heart_right_vsd.jpg. From Steppan and Maxwell. Congenital heart disease. In: *Stoelting's Anesthesia and Co-Existing Disease*, chap 7, 129–149.)

Perimembranous VSDs

Perimembranous VSDs are sometimes also referred to as central VSDs and are located in the membranous part of the ventricular septum. Many of these defects touch the fibrous continuity region between the anterior mitral valve and the aortic valve. Often these VSDs can be restrictive because they are partially covered by accessory tricuspid valve (TV) tissue. Complications in the form of aortic valve regurgitation can occur if the right or noncoronary cusp prolapses into the VSD. In anticipation of surgery, it is always important to know where the conduction system runs in relation to the defect. In perimembranous VSD, the bundle of His passes just behind and below the VSD (along the posterior-inferior margins of the VSD).[19]

Outlet VSDs

Outlet VSDs are located in the outflow portion of the tripartite RV and are associated with an absence or hypoplasia of the conal septum. The conal septum is a muscular structure that surrounds the pulmonary artery (PA) and defines the right ventricular outflow tract (RVOT). Because these defects are associated with the muscular conal septum, lack of and hypoplasia of that muscular septum changes the relative position between the PA, septum, and aorta. Therefore outlet VSDs are also referred to as malalignment VSDs, where anterior malalignment is seen in tetralogy of Fallot (TOF) and posterior malalignment is seen in interrupted aortic arch (IAA).[20]

Inlet VSDs

Inlet VSDs are posteriorly located just below the atrioventricular valves. These are the types of VSDs seen in atrioventricular canal defects.[20]

Muscular VSDs

Muscular VSDs are located within the muscular ventricular septum and have muscular borders all around. Their location often classifies them within the muscular septum and in relation to the moderator band. Midseptal VSDs are posterior to the septal band, anterior VSDs are anterior to the septal band, and the inferior muscular VSDs are deep in the septum close to the diaphragmatic surface.

Pathophysiology

The hemodynamic effect of the VSD is determined by the size of the defect and the relative resistance of the pulmonary versus the systemic hemodynamic systems (Fig. 37.4).

Large VSDs

In the immediate neonatal period, the PVR is relatively high and limits the degree of left-to-right flow over a large nonrestrictive VSD. However, as the PVR physiologically decreases during the first several days of life, the left-to-right shunt progressively increases. This increase in blood shunting from left to right circulation results in more blood going to the pulmonary vascular bed and an increase in the blood volume coming back to the left side of the heart from the lungs. The pulmonary pressures can approximate systemic levels secondary to pulmonary overcirculation. The increased pulmonary venous return subsequently results in left ventricular hypertrophy, an adaptive measure to increase output and decrease ventricular wall tension. This left ventricular hypertrophy lowers the LV compliance and increases the left ventricular end-diastolic pressure (LVEDP). The decrease in LV compliance and increase in LVEDP results in left atrial dilatation and left atrial and pulmonary venous hypertension. Untreated, this will over time result in an increase in the hydrostatic pressure in the pulmonary capillary bed and the

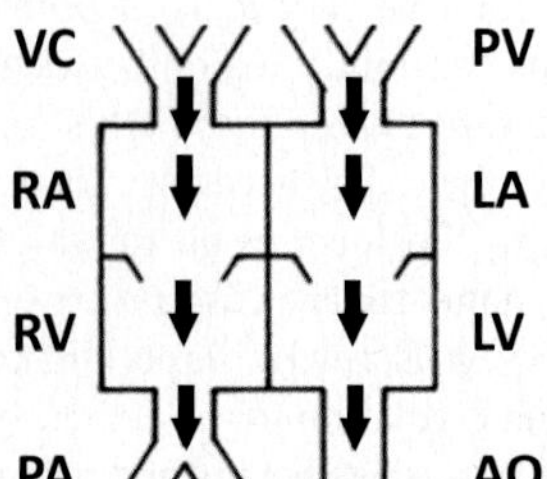

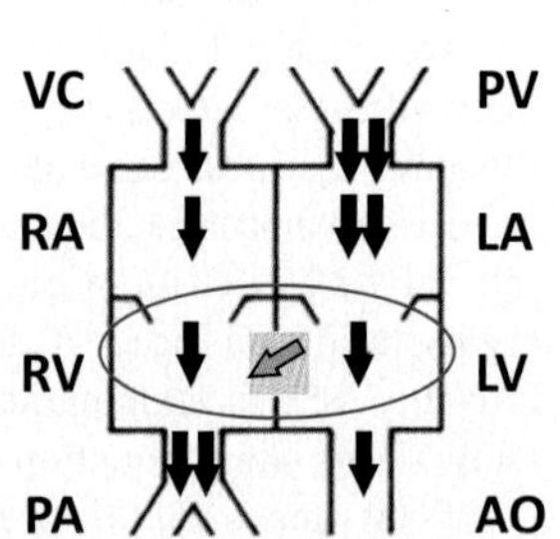

Fig. 37.4 Pathophysiology of Ventricular Septal Defects (VSDs). In patients with a VSD, left ventricle (LV) contraction ejects some blood into the aorta and some is shunted left-to-right (L→R) across the VSD into the right ventricle (RV) and pulmonary artery *(blue arrow)*. Severity of L→R shunting is determined by (a) the size of the VSD; and (b) difference in resistance in the pulmonary and systemic vascular circulation. LV hypertrophy occurs to compensate for decreased wall tension and increased output. The hypertrophied LV has decreased compliance and increased end-diastolic pressures. Neonates with VSDs develop symptoms when the pulmonary vascular resistance (PVR) drops with increased L→R shunting and RV/pulmonary blood flow. As pulmonary blood flow increases, the systemic blood flow can become compromised. Increased pulmonary venous return can cause left atrial (LA) pressures, LA dilatation, pulmonary venous congestion, and pulmonary edema.

development of neonatal heart failure symptoms by the accumulation of pulmonary interstitial fluid.

Small VSDs

Small VSDs usually have restrictive pressures and limit the left-to-right shunting once the PVR drops in the neonatal period. The left-to-right volume load is much less, and the compensatory mechanisms described for large VSDs do not typically develop. The pulmonary vascular flow and the pulmonary vascular pressures remain low, and the risk of developing pulmonary vascular disease in turn is lower. There is, of course, a clinical spectrum of VSDs between the pathophysiology of a large nonrestrictive VSD and a small restrictive VSD. Therefore every VSD warrants close monitoring of clinical status and follow-up. The hemodynamic assessment of VSDs can be challenging in preterm infants and neonates with other morbidities, requiring extended hospitalization and prolonged ventilation. Notable long-term complications after VSD repair may include double chamber RV, subaortic membrane resulting in left ventricular outflow tract (LVOT) stenosis, and aortic insufficiency secondary to valve prolapse.

Atrioventricular Canal Defects

Prevalence

Atrioventricular canal (AVC) defects are commonly associated with trisomy 21 and heterotaxy. Patients with normal chromosomes can also develop AVC defects, but it is 1000 times more common in neonates with trisomy 21, with about 50% of all patients with AVC defects having trisomy 21.[21–23] In patients with heterotaxy syndrome, the AVC defect association is mostly with right atrial isomerism and asplenia rather than left atrial isomerism and polysplenia.[24] AVC defects can also be seen with higher prevalence in patients with Ellis–Van Creveld syndrome.

Embryology and Anatomy

In the embryonic heart, one valve connects the atrium to the ventricle, which is called the common atrioventricular (AV) valve. This one common valve is divided by muscle tissues that grow toward each other on opposite sides of the common AV valve. This muscle tissue is called the endocardial cushion. Under normal development, the endocardial cushion divides the common AV valve into the left-sided mitral and right-sided TVs. Failure of the endocardial cushions to grow toward each other and fuse to form the AV septum results in one common AV connection. It is believed to be a defect in a cell adhesion molecule that results in the failure of the endocardial cushion to approximate and ultimately fuse to divide the common AV valve.[25] The common AVC defect classically consists of a primum ASD, an inlet VSD, and a common AV valve consisting of five leaflets.

In a normal heart, the AV septum and the hinge points of the AV valves make it such that the mitral valve is always superior to the TV, which defines the AV septum. With a failure to form the AV septum, the left-sided AV valve is displaced downward, placing the right and left sides on the same level. Having the right and left AV valves on the same level is a pathognomonic finding of an AVC defect. Another feature specific to AVC defects is an elongated LVOT. This characteristic shape of the LVOT in AVC defects is often called a "gooseneck" deformity.[25] The elongated LVOT is why a late complication of AVC repair is progressive subaortic stenosis. Fig. 37.5 shows the anatomic abnormalities in AV canal defects.

Classifications of the AV Canal

Complete AV Canal

The complete form of AV canal has an atrial-level defect and an intraventricular defect. Typically, the entire membranous septum is deficient, resulting in shunting at both an atrial and ventricular level. There is also just one common AV valve with five leaflets. It has one anterior and posterior bridging leaflet extending the entire length of the valve. There are two lateral leaflets and one right-sided anterior leaflet, which represent what would have been the anterior tricuspid leaflet.

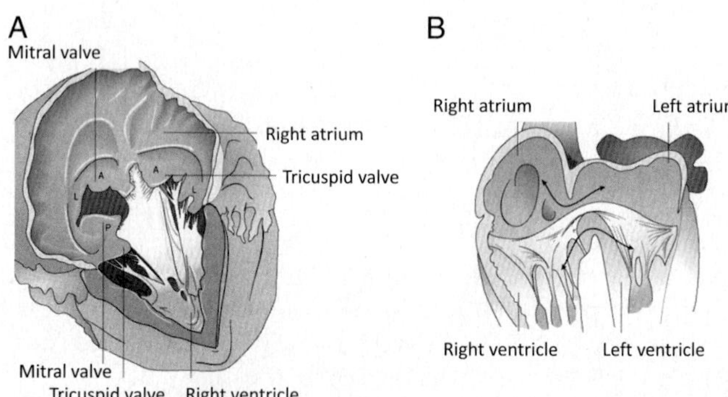

Fig. 37.5 Atrioventricular (AV) Septal Defects (Also Termed as AV Canal Defects). (A) The most frequently seen form of complete AV septal defects (Rastelli type A; details in Fig. 37.6) is classified according to (a) the division of the anterior bridging leaflet; and (b) attachment to the septum. The current interpretations emphasize the left-sided portion of anterior leaflet as the anterior bridging leaflet. The right-sided portion is described as the "true" anterior tricuspid leaflet. (B) Schematic 4-chamber view of a complete atrioventricular septal defect, showing common valve and atrial and ventricular communications. *A,* Two anterior leaflets of the mitral valve (MV) and tricuspid valve (TV) portions of leaflets; *L,* the two lateral leaflets corresponding to posterior mitral valve (MV) and tricuspid valve (TV); *P,* posterior bridging leaflet; *RA,* right atrium; *RV,* right ventricle. (A, Redrawn from Porter CJ, et al. Atrioventricular septal defects. In: Emmanouilides GC, Riemenschneider TA, Allen HD, Gutgesell HP, eds. *Moss and Adams Heart Disease in Infants, Children, and Adolescents: Including the Fetus and Young Adult.* Baltimore: Williams & Wilkins; 1995; B, From Castaneda AR et al., eds. Atrioventricular canal defect. In: *Cardiac Surgery of the Neonate and Infant.* Philadelphia: Saunders; 1994; From Andropoulos and Gottlieb. Congenital heart disease. In: *Anesthesia and Uncommon Diseases*, chap 3, 75–136.)

Intermediate AV Canal

There is a division of the right- and left-sided AV valves but a large primum ASD, and a significant VSD component persists.

Transitional AV Canal

A transitional AV canal is the formation of left- and right-sided AV valves with a large primum ASD but a small VSD component.

Partial AV Canal

A partial AV canal has division of the right and left AV valves and no VSD component, just a primum ASD. Anatomically, the right and left AV valves are not normal in the intermediate, transitional, and partial canals. They are on the same level, and there is a variable degree of tissue connecting the anterior and posterior bridging leaflets.

The Rastelli classification is based on how and mostly where the anterior bridging leaflet is attached and where it divides between the left superior leaflet and the right superior leaflet (Fig. 37.6).[24]

Type A: The anterior bridging leaflet is divided at the level of the ventricular septum and has chordal attachments to the septum. This is the most common form of AV valve in AVC defects and is primarily found in patients with trisomy 21.

Type B: The anterior bridging leaflet is not divided at the level of the ventricular septum and continues over to the RV, where it is attached with chordae to a papillary muscle located on the right side of the septum. This is the least common form of AVC defect.

Type C: The anterior bridging leaflet extends over into the RV, is not attached to the ventricular septum, and is attached to chordae extending to papillary muscles located on the free wall of the RV. This type of AV valve is most commonly found in TOF and AVC defects.

The pathophysiology of AV canal defects is summarized in Fig. 37.7. A panoramic view of left-to-right shunting lesions is shown in Fig. 37.8.

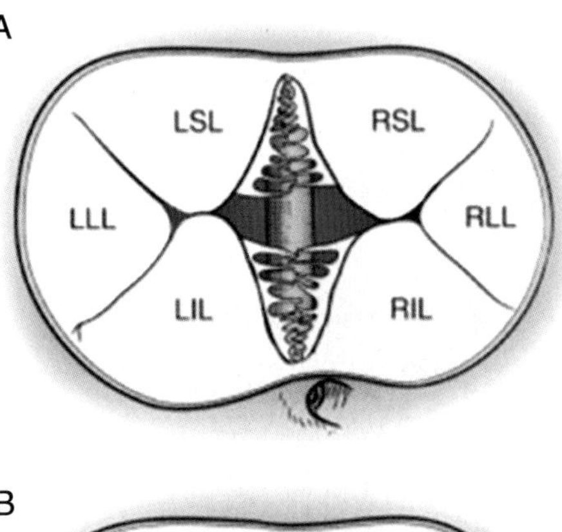

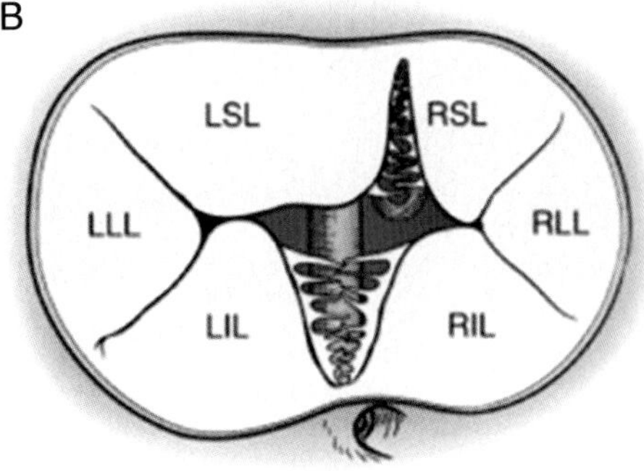

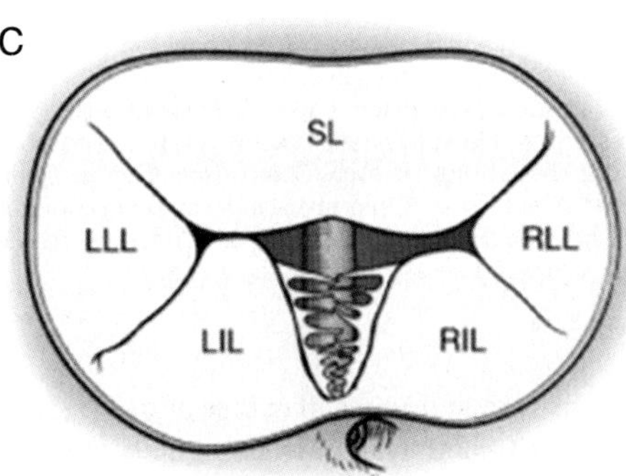

Fig. 37.6 Rastelli Classification of Complete AVSDs. (A) Type A has an SBL that is divided and attached to the crest of the ventricular septum. (B) Type B has straddling chordae from the left SBL to the RV papillary muscles. (C) Type C is a free-floating SBL that is not divided or attached to the crest. *AVSD,* Atrioventricular septal defect; *LIL,* left inferior leaflet; *LLL,* left lateral leaflet; *LSL,* left superior leaflet; *RIL,* right inferior leaflet; *RLL,* right lateral leaflet; *RSL,* right superior leaflet; *RV,* right ventricle; *SL or SBL,* superior bridging leaflet. (From Jacobs JP, Burke RP, Quintessenza JA, et al. Congenital Heart Surgery Nomenclature and Database Project: atrioventricular canal defect. *Ann Thorac Surg.* 2000;69[4 suppl]:S36-S43, with permission; and from Sassalos et al. Atrioventricular septal defects. In: *Critical Heart Disease in Infants and Children*, 50, 606–614.e2.)

Outflow Septation and Conal Defects

Tetralogy of Fallot

TOF is historically defined by its four distinct findings: pulmonic valve (PV) stenosis, VSD, overriding aorta, and right ventricular hypertrophy. These characteristics of TOF are all a result of the unique VSD found in TOF alone. Therefore the four features result from a single primary defect (sometimes referred to as monology of Fallot)—the anterior malalignment cono-ventricular VSD. This malalignment of the conal septum results in a wide communication between the RV and LV.

The RVOT obstruction seen in TOF is highly variable in both its severity and location. The obstruction is frequently found at many levels, starting from the superior muscular lip of the VSD to the narrow subvalvar infundibular region, with a frequently thickened, often bicuspid and stenotic pulmonary valve and supravalvar stenosis being common. Various degrees of anatomic abnormalities resulting in stenosis of the pulmonary vasculature tree are frequently present.[26] This multilevel obstruction to pulmonary blood flow is very characteristic of TOF.

Figs. 37.9 and 37.10 show a typical and a simplified version of the anatomy of TOF lesions, respectively. Fig. 37.11 highlight the pathophysiology of these anomalies, and the changes seen during cyanotic spells.

The clinical spectrum of TOF based on anatomy can be very broad, from VSD with almost no RVOT obstruction or PV stenosis to variable degrees of pulmonary valve stenosis. Occasionally, PV can be so stenotic that the pulmonary circulation may become dependent on systemic to pulmonary blood flow over the ductus. The takeoff of the left pulmonary artery is often stenotic because it has a variable degree of ductal tissue that can result in narrowing and anatomic distortion. TOF is commonly associated with a right aortic arch, meaning the arch crosses the right bronchus in 25% of cases, often with mirror image branching. The first branch is the left-sided brachiocephalic artery, which divides into the left subclavian and left carotid arteries. Approximately 7% of patients with

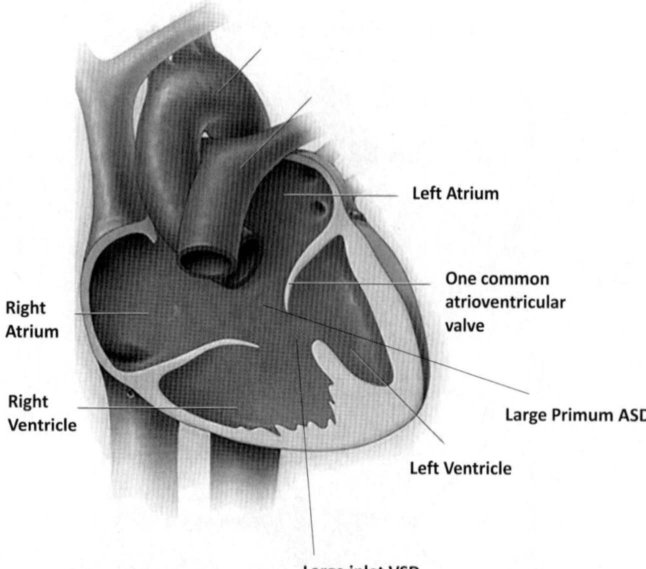

Fig. 37.7 Atrioventricular (AV) Canal Defects and Inlet ventricular septal defects (VSDs). AV canal defects are characterized by a primum atrial septal defect and consequent large left-to-right shunt. There is: right sided volume overload and right atrium (RA)/right ventriculum (RV) dilatation. Increased volume flows through the right side AV valve to the RV. Inlet VSDs are large left-to-right shunts. The flow increases as the pulmonary vascular resistance (PVR) drops. The lesions are notable for: increased pulmonary venous return. Left-sided AV valve regurgitation associated with increased left atrial pressures, volume overload, pulmonary venous congestion, and resulting pulmonary edema. Increased pulmonary blood flow (pulmonary-to-systemic blood flow ratios of 2–4:1) result in decreased systemic perfusion and decreased oxygen delivery. Compensatory left ventricular (LV) hypertrophy. Increased LV end-diastolic pressures and worsening compliance increase the left-to-right atrial level shunting. RV dilatation can further impede LV and RV function as well as exacerbate any AV valve regurgitation.

TOF will have abnormal origin and course of the coronary arteries. The coronary artery anatomy must be thoroughly understood before surgery to minimize the risk of damage to the coronary arteries, especially because 4% of patients may have a left anterior descending artery originating from the right coronary artery, which in turn crosses the RVOT in the exact area where a transannular patch may be placed.

Because TOF with pulmonary atresia has no anterograde blood flow through the RVOT, its only source of pulmonary blood flow is through major aortopulmonary collaterals (MAPCAS) or a patent ductus arteriosus (PDA). The right and left pulmonary arteries can be confluent or nonconfluent if the collateral feeds a confluent main pulmonary artery, the "seagull" sign classic when contrast is injected in the aorta or collateral. MAPCAS are structured and function more like systemic arteries compared with pulmonary arteries; they are frequently stenotic and can be reactive. MAPCAS refers to multiple collaterals feeding the pulmonary tree and one single systemic artery feeding a pulmonary segment leading to a unifocal blood supply.

Transposition of the Great Arteries

Prevalence

The prevalence of dextro-transposition of the great arteries (D-TGA) is 4.7 per 10,000 live births and accounts for 3% of all congenital heart disease and 20% of cyanotic heart disease.[27] It is more common in males and is generally not associated with any specific chromosomal anomalies or syndromes. It is associated with heterotaxy—in particular, right isomerism. D-TGA has also been associated with infant of a diabetic mother (IDM), maternal use of vitamin A and ibuprofen, and exposure to organic solvents and pesticides.

The pathogenesis of D-TGA results from failure of the conal tissue below the pulmonary valve to develop and failure of the conal tissue below the aortic valve to regress. This results in failure to position the pulmonary valve anteriorly and committed to the RV as it migrates during the RV and RVOT muscle growth. The most commonly associated cardiac lesion in D-TGA is a VSD. D-TGAs are frequently characterized as either with an intact ventricular septum (IVS) or with a VSD. Most D-TGAs will not have a VSD and have a normal aortic arch. A D-TGA with an accompanying VSD is at risk of having various degrees of LVOT obstruction, often associated with a malalignment VSD, pulmonary valve stenosis, septal hypertrophy, subpulmonary membrane, or accessory mitral valve tissue.[28] The anatomical changes in D-TGA are shown in Fig. 37.12.

The coronary arteries in D-TGA originate from the anteriorly positioned aorta and the sinuses facing the pulmonary valve. There are several described variations of the coronary arteries in D-TGA. The most common coronary artery pattern is the left anterior descending artery from the left-facing sinus giving rise to the left circumflex and the right coronary artery originating from the right-facing sinus. The next most common pattern is the circumflex coming off the right coronary artery (RCA) with an otherwise normal anatomic path.[29]

A Note on the Conus

The conus is a muscular structure that in embryology surrounds the base of the truncus. The conus plays an essential role in the septation of the RVOT, and the structure continues to embed the base of the PA and involutes around the aorta.[29] In doing so, it moves the PA anteriorly and slightly to the left of the aorta. The involution of the conal tissue around the aorta allows for the anterior leaflet of the mitral valve and the aorta to be in fibrous continuation. The conus is mainly associated with the RV. Therefore the more conal tissue is located below the great vessel, the more likely that great vessel will be associated with the RV. Congenital heart diseases that result from developmental problems with the conus are TOF, double outlet right ventricle (DORV), truncus with IAA, and D-TGA. In TOF, the conus is mainly associated with the RA; with DORV, there is a variable conus under both the PA and the aorta. There is conal tissue between the aorta and mitral valve. In D-TGA, there is no conus associated with the aorta, and there is no conus under the PA.

Malalignment refers to the position of the outflow septum in relation to the rest of the muscular septum. Anterior malignment means that the superiorly located outflow tract is shifted in an anterior (and often superior) position. The terminology here is essential as the anterior malalignment VSD is uniquely associated with TOF and DORV, whereas a posterior malalignment VSD is associated with an IAA.

Double Outlet Right Ventricle

Prevalence

DORV is usually not associated with any specific genetic anomalies and accounts for less than 1% to 3% of congenital heart defects. Obler et al.[30] reported that a large number of genes have been associated with DORV in both humans and animal models. The different anatomic subtypes seen in specific etiologies suggest several distinct pathogenetic mechanisms for DORV, including impairment of neural crest derivative migration and impairment of normal cardiac situs and looping. The large number of genes associated with DORV in both humans and animal models and the different anatomic subtypes

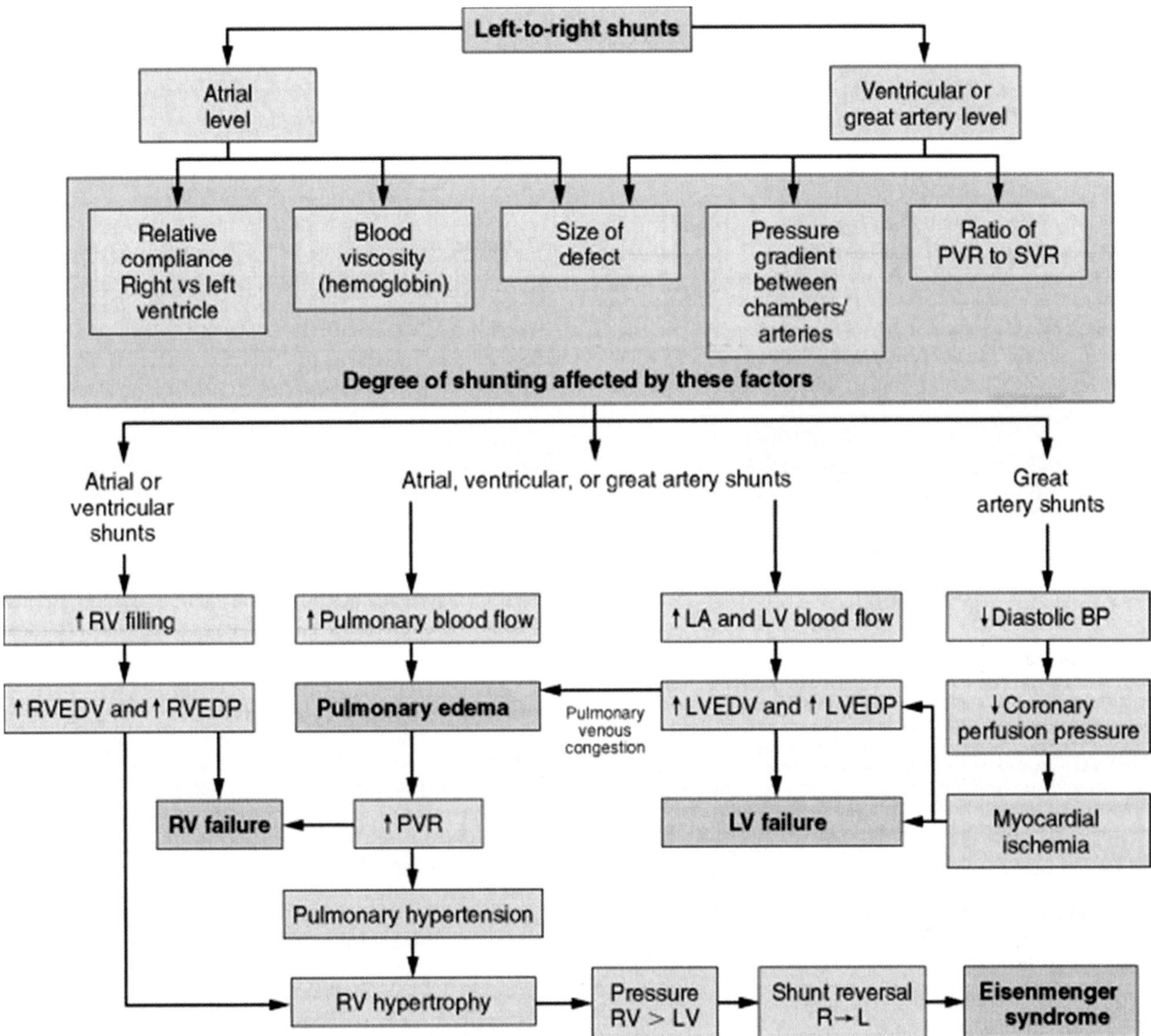

Fig. 37.8 Pathophysiology of Left-to-Right Shunting Lesions. Flow diagram depicts factors that affect left-to-right shunting at atrial, ventricular, and great artery level and pathophysiology produced by these shunts. A large shunt will result in left ventricular (LV) failure, right ventricular (RV) failure, and pulmonary edema. Increased pulmonary blood flow and pulmonary artery pressures lead to pulmonary hypertension and eventually Eisenmenger syndrome. These final common outcomes are highlighted in bold. *BP,* Blood pressure; *LA,* left atrial; *LVEDP,* left ventricular end-diastolic pressure; *LVEDV,* left ventricular end-diastolic volume; *PVR,* pulmonary vascular resistance; *R→L,* right to left; *RVEDP,* right ventricular end-diastolic pressure; *RVEDV,* right ventricular end-diastolic volume; *SVR,* systemic vascular resistance. (Data from Walker SG: Anesthesia for left-to-right shunt lesions. In Andropoulos DB, et al, editors: Anesthesia for congenital heart disease, ed 2, Oxford, UK, 2010, Wiley-Blackwell.)

seen in specific etiologies indicate the likelihood of several distinct pathogenetic mechanisms for DORV, including impairment of neural crest derivative migration and impairment of normal cardiac situs and looping.

DORV tends to be described by one of two definitions. One definition is that both the great arteries are 50% or more committed to the RV. The PA will need to be committed to the RV 50% or more than in TOF-like anatomy. Another frequently used definition based on echocardiography is that there is conal tissue located between the aorta and the anterior leaflet of the mitral valve, lacking the classic fibrous continuation. DORV, thus, is a conotruncal defect where the location of the great arteries in relation to each other defines the type of DORV and the physiology. The location of the great arteries depends on the location of the conus as the conus moves its associated great artery anteriorly and superiorly. DORV anatomy can range from anatomy and physiology similar to TOF, where there will be a subaortic VSD, to anatomy and physiology of a TGA where the VSD will likely be in a subaortic location. The VSD is located in the conoventricular septum stretching from the membranous septum into the upper part of the muscular ventricular septum. Pulmonary valve or subvalvular pulmonary stenosis is found in 50% of patients with DORV, and 25% of DORV hearts will have a secundum ASD. The anatomical changes characteristic of DORV are shown in Fig. 37.13.

Truncus Arteriosus

Truncus arteriosus is the resulting failure of the conus and neural crest cell migration to septate the truncus into the aorta and the main pulmonary artery. This results in a single artery leaving, giving

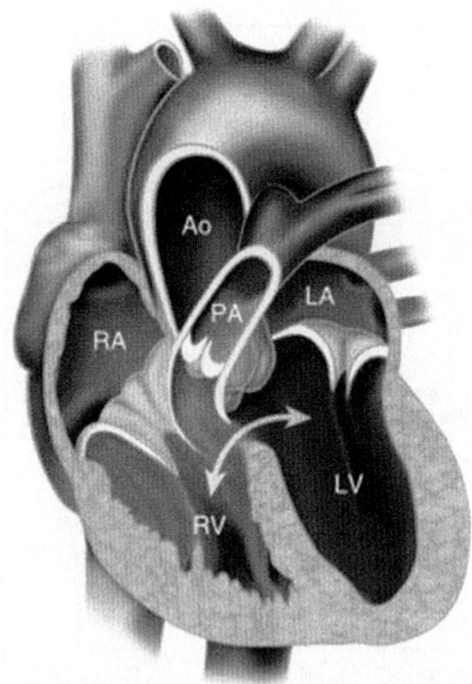

Fig. 37.9 Tetralogy of Fallot (TOF). TOF includes a large anterior malalignment ventricular septal defect (VSD), obstruction of the right ventricular outflow tract (RVOT), right ventricular hypertrophy, and an aorta that overrides the left and right ventricles. The degree of the RVOT obstruction determines the severity of right-to-left (R→L) shunting of blood across the VSD *(arrow)*. TOF with mild/no RVOT obstruction and a large VSD can develop pulmonary overcirculation similar to a VSD. TOF with some degree of RVOT obstruction and a large VSD may not have a large increase in pulmonary circulation and is less symptomatic. The severity of RVOT may increase with postnatal age with increasing hypertrophy of the outflow tract muscle tissue. Infants with mild/no RVOT may not need surgery during the neonatal period. Surgery is needed in infants with decreasing saturations, increasing RVOT obstruction, and TOF spells. (Reproduced with permission and minor modifications from Otto CM, *Textbook of Clinical Echocardiography*, 17, 473–506.)

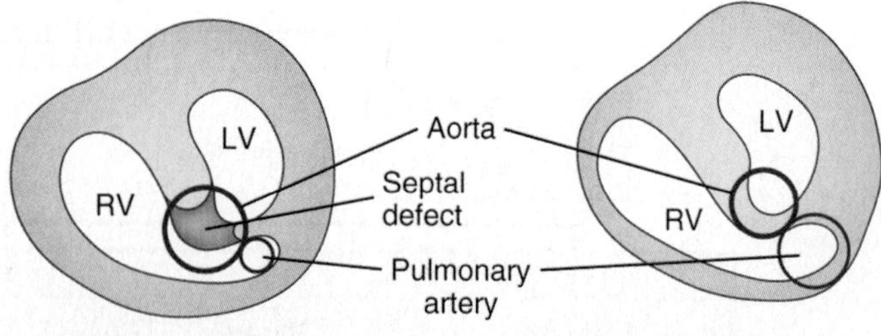

Fig. 37.10 Tetralogy of Fallot Anatomy (TOF). Image of the cross section of a TOF heart seen from above. The *red circles* show location of the pulmonary and aortic valves in TOF *(left)* as compared to that in a normal heart *(right)*. Note the relative location of the ventricular septal defect, the aorta (which overrides the defect), the pulmonary stenosis, and the right ventricular hypertrophy. This image highlights the convoluted geometry of the RVOT in TOF, showing its location as just below the potential subvalvar and valvar stenoses. *LV,* Left ventricle; *RV,* right ventricle; *RVOT,* right ventricular outflow tract; *VSD,* ventricular septal defect. (CONGENITAL MALFORMATIONS OF THE HEART, VOLUME II: SPECIFIC MALFORMATIONS, SECOND EDITION by Helen B. Taussig, Cambridge, Mass.: Harvard University Press, Copyright © 1947, 1960 by the Commonwealth Fun Used by permission. All rights reserved.)

rise to the coronary arteries, the aortic arch with head and neck vessels, and the pulmonary arteries.[31]

Prevalence

Truncus arteriosus is seen with an annual incidence of 7 per 100,000 live births, and although it accounts for less than 1% of all congenital heart lesions, it accounts for 4% of critical congenital heart defects.[32]

The anatomical changes in tricuspid atresia (TA) are shown in Fig. 37.14; the lesions are classified based on the anatomy of the origin of the pulmonary arteries off the TA.[33,34]

Type 1: Type 1 is the most common type of truncus, accounting for approximately 50%. A short main pulmonary trunk comes off the truncus, giving rise to the left and right pulmonary arteries.

Type 2: The second most common form of truncus, type 2 accounts for approximately 40%. There is no main pulmonary trunk, and the right and left pulmonary arteries arise directly from the truncus. In type 2, they arise adjacent to each other.

Type 3: Type 3 accounts for approximately 10% of truncus. It is anatomically very similar to type 2, but the right and left pulmonary arteries arise at variable distances and locations from each other.

The truncal valve is the TV in approximately 40% of cases but can be either quadricuspid or bicuspid 30% of the time. Truncal valve insufficiency adds to the complexity of the disease. The VSD in truncus is typically nonrestrictive and represents a defect in the infundibular outflow septum. Truncus can be associated with hypoplastic aortic arch and 20% of cases with IAA.

Aortopulmonary Window

Prevalence

Aortopulmonary window is rare, accounting for 0.1% of congenital heart defects, and is twice as frequent in males compared with females. It can be seen in association with other forms of congenital heart disease, especially IAA.[35]

Normal cardiac anatomy

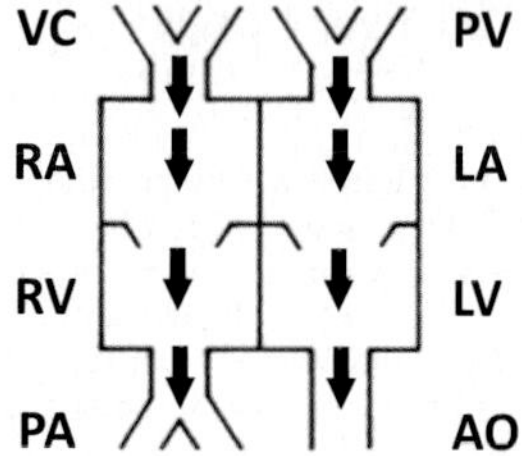

TOF

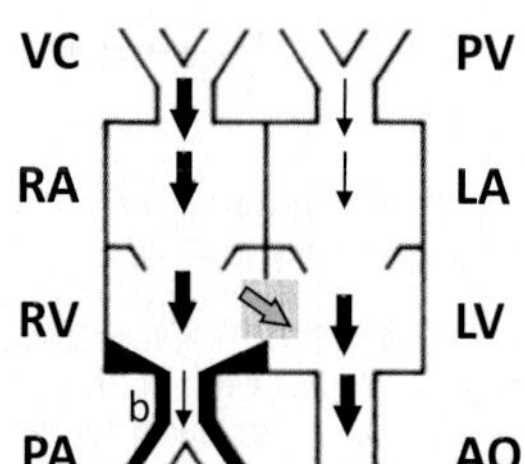

The blue arrow on the pink background shows R→L shunt across the malalignment VSD

The RV shows structural infundibular stenosis with RVOT (a). Crying can further increase PVR due to vascular spasm (b).

Fig. 37.11 Pathophysiology of Tetralogy of Fallot (TOF) and Cyanotic Spells. Infants with TOF with severe, multilevel right ventricular outflow tract tend to have tenuous pulmonary blood flow. Crying can increase the tissue oxygen demand, and at the same time, increase the pulmonary vascular resistance (PVR). Increased PVR worsens the R→L shunting across the VSD and reduces the pulmonary blood flow. The resulting hypoxemia, decreased tissue oxygen delivery, and metabolic acidosis lead to a feed-forward loop with increased PVR, tightening of the infundibular stenosis, and anterior displacement of the pulmonary valve, all of which further accentuate the R→L shunting with reduced pulmonary blood flow. With increasing postnatal age, the muscle hypertrophy reduces RV compliance with poor diastolic filling and more R→L shunting.

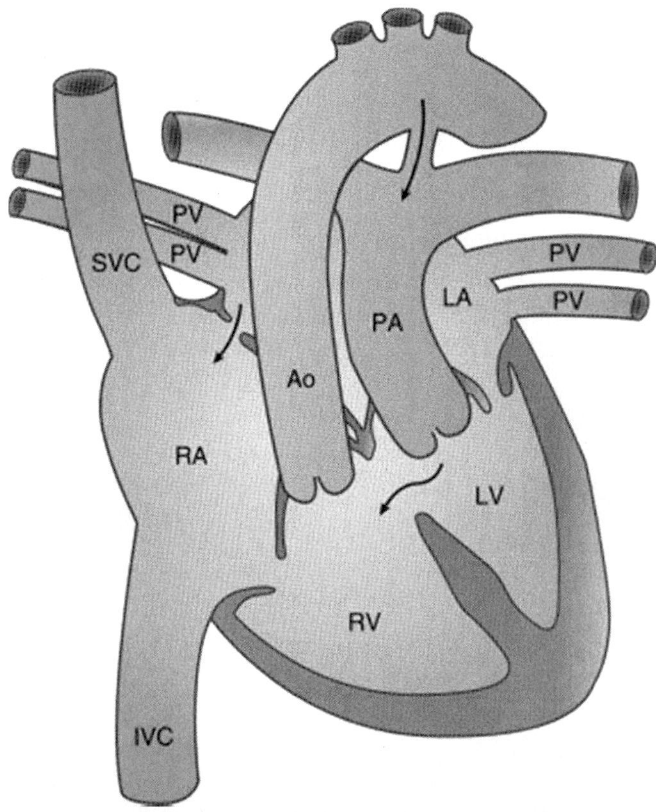

Fig. 37.12 Transposition of the Great Arteries (D-TGA). The right ventricle (RV) and left ventricle (LV) are connected in parallel to each other, creating independent circulations, with the aorta (Ao) arising from the RV and the pulmonary artery (PA) arising from the LV. The clinical presentation depends on mixing of blood between the two circulations through an ASD, VSD, or PDA. Consistent mixing of the blood only occurs at the level of the atrial septum; therefore, in cases of restrictive ASD, a balloon atrial septostomy is indicated prior to an arterial switch operation to ensure adequate mixing. Some centers will do a balloon atrial septostomy in all neonates with D-TGA to ensure atrial-level mixing, because the atrial communication can become restrictive over time. *ASD,* Atrial septal defect; *IVC,* inferior vena cava; *LA,* left atrium; *PDA,* patent ductus arteriosus; *PV,* pulmonary vein; *RA,* right atrium; *SVC,* superior vena cava; *VSD,* ventricular septal defect. (From Steppan and Maxwell. Congenital heart disease. In: *Stoelting's Anesthesia and Co-Existing Disease*, chap 7, 129–149.)

Aortopulmonary window results in the failure of complete septation of the truncus into the aorta and the PA. Depending on the area of communication, aortopulmonary windows are divided into three types by the Mori classification[36]:

Type 1: Very proximal defect just above the semilunar valves.
Type 2: Distal defect involving the PA bifurcation with almost an unroofing of the superior right side of the main PA.
Type 3: A significant defect that extends just superiorly of the aortic and pulmonary valve up to the bifurcation of the main pulmonary artery.

A Note on the Classification of the Aortic Arch

Terminology regarding the aortic arch: The ascending aorta is the ascending distance from the aortic valve to the brachiocephalic artery, the proximal transverse arch is the region between the brachiocephalic and the common carotid artery, and the distal transverse arch is the region between the common carotid artery and the area immediately distal to the left subclavian artery and the ductus or the ligamentum arteriosus. Distal to the ductus or ligamentum arteriosus is the descending aorta. A normal aortic arch is a left-sided arch, defined by the first artery that leaves the aorta and divides in two or the brachiocephalic artery. Another reliable clinical way of defining a left arch is on a simple AP chest x-ray to see if the aortic arch loops over the left bronchus. A schematic diagram of the aortic arch is shown in Fig. 37.15.

Interrupted Aortic Arch

Three variations of IAA have been described, and the pathogenesis seems to be different in each (Fig. 37.16).[37] The types of IAA are classified by the location at which the aorta is interrupted. DiGeorge syndrome is associated with a type B IAA, so 50% of patients with IAA type B will have DiGeorge syndrome.

Type A: The aortic arch is interrupted at the isthmus level or after the left subclavian artery and proximal to the ductus.
Type B: The aortic arch is interrupted between the common carotid artery and the left subclavian artery. This type of IAA is associated with a posteriorly aligned VSD, subaortic stenosis, and bicuspid aortic valve.
Type C: The aortic arch is interrupted between the brachiocephalic artery and the common carotid artery.

Outflow Tract Pathology

Isolated Pulmonary Valve Stenosis

Prevalence

Isolated congenital pulmonary valvular stenosis (PS) is a relatively common abnormality accounting for 7% to 12% of all congenital cardiac abnormalities.[38,39]

In isolated PS the PA leaflets can be identified, but there are variable degrees of separation. The PV is often dome-shaped, and the degree of stenosis depends on how much the valve opens. The aortic and pulmonary valve formation depends on the neural crest cell migration to fully septate the truncus and ultimately develop the leaflets. Noonan syndrome is associated with PS because signaling pathways influencing the valve formation are influenced by *PTPN11*.[40] The pulmonary valves in Noonan syndrome tend to be more dysplastic and thickened compared with nonsyndromic PS. Secondary to the PS, the RVOT can become hypertrophied and result in some degree of outflow tract obstruction. Often a poststenotic pulmonary arterial dilatation can be seen, and this is a good prognostic sign.

Critical pulmonary stenosis decreases RV flow during development because of significant PS resulting in a hypoplastic RV. This results in an increase in the right-to-left atrial shunting in the fetal circulation. Critical pulmonary stenosis will result in a cyanotic neonate with ductal-dependent pulmonary blood flow. The gold standard for classifying the degree of pulmonary valve stenosis is directly measuring the RV pressure and the pressure gradient across the valve. Pulmonary valve stenosis is divided into mild (gradient 35–40 mm Hg), moderate (gradient 40–60 mm Hg), and severe (gradient 60–70 mm Hg) stenosis.

Pulmonary Atresia With Intact Ventricular Septum

In pulmonary atresia with an IVS, the RVOT is atretic by a thick atretic PV or a longer segment muscular atresia with no associated

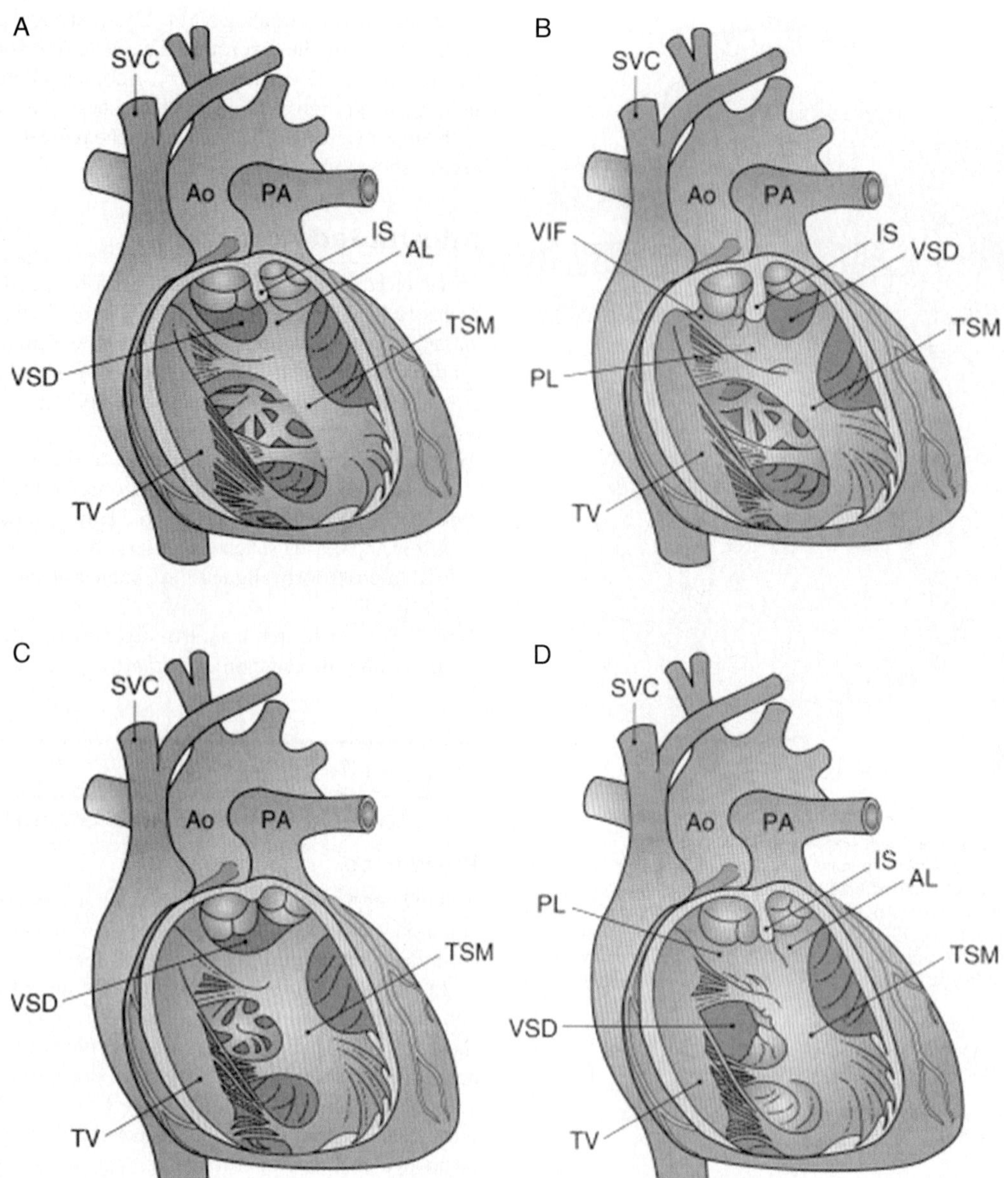

Fig. 37.13 Double Outlet Right Ventricle (DORV). DORV is a conotruncal defect in which both the great arteries are more than 50% committed to the right ventricle and there is conal tissue separating the anterior leaflet of the mitral valve and the aorta. The spectrum of DORV is determined by the conus and its effect on the rotation of the great arteries. In greater than 90% of cases the position of the VSD is the same, located in the perimembranous area. (A) DORV with subaortic VSD (about 70% of cases). The IS is attached to the anterior limb of the TSM. (B) DORV with subpulmonary VSD accounts for about 20% of cases. The IS is attached to the PL of the TSM. (C) DORV with doubly committed VSD. Absent or virtually absent IS. (D) DORV with remote VSD. Here the VSD is in the inlet portion of the septum; remote VSDs also occur as muscular VSDs unrelated to either great vessel. *AL,* Anterior limb of TSM; *Ao,* aorta; *IS,* infundibular septum; *PA,* pulmonary artery; *PL,* posterior limb; *SVC,* superior vena cava; *TSM,* trabeculae septomarginalis; *TV,* tricuspid valve; *VIF,* ventricular infundibular fold (same as the conus); *VSD,* ventricular septal defect. (Reproduced with permission and after minor modifications from Gu et al. Double-outlet right ventricle. In: *Diagnosis and Management of Adult Congenital Heart Disease*, 54, 553–561.)

VSD. Depending on the atrial-level communication, RV compliance, and the TV anatomy and function, the RA can be mildly to significantly dilated because there is no outflow from the RV. In cases where the heart is significantly dilated, this could result in developmental problems of the lung and, to some degree, lung hypoplasia because the dilated heart functions as a space-occupying lesion within the chest. The pulmonary blood flow is usually provided by the PDA alone. There is much variation in the degree to which the RV is developed. In cases where the RV has developed, the characteristic tri-partite RV cavity can be found with a well-developed RVOT but with a thickened, atretic PV. The three leaflets of the semilunar valve can often be defined, but they are completely fused. In cases where the infundibulum has a longer segment muscular atresia, the RV and PV tend to be very poorly formed.

The TV also displays various degrees of stenosis and regurgitation. In general, the smaller and more underdeveloped and dysplastic the RV, the more dysplastic with abnormal chordae and stenotic the TV will be. In patients with a more developed RV, the TV tends to be more dilated, still dysplastic, and frequently with significant regurgitation. Some of the dysplastic TV seen in pulmonary atresia with IVS may have a dilated annulus and be downward displaced, similar to Ebstein anomaly. With both RV inflow and outflow pathology in pulmonary atresia with IVS, the Congenital Heart Surgeons' Society suggests using the *z*-score of the TV annulus to characterize because this correlates with the RV cavity.[41]

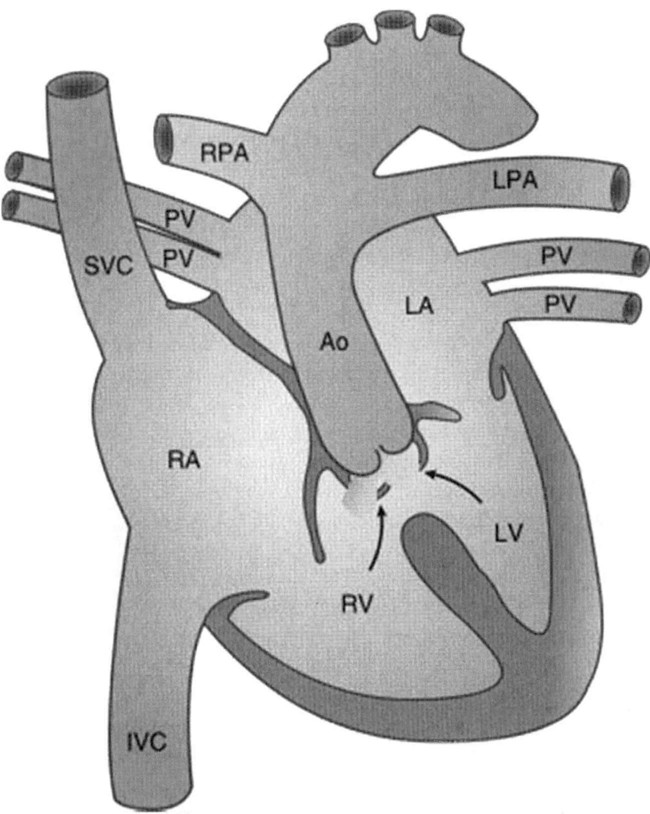

Fig. 37.14 Truncus Arteriosus. In patients with truncus arteriosus, a single vessel arises from the heart, overrides the left ventricle (LV) and right ventricle (RV), and gives rise to the aorta and pulmonary arteries. *Ao*, Aorta; *IVC*, inferior vena cava; *LA*, left atrium; *LPA*, left pulmonary artery; *PV*, pulmonary vein; *RA*, right atrium; *RPA*, right pulmonary artery; *SVC*, superior vena cava. (From Steppan and Maxwell. Congenital heart disease. In: *Stoelting's Anesthesia and Co-Existing Disease*, chap 7, 129–149.)

Aortic Stenosis

As a broader term, LVOT obstruction includes subvalvular stenosis, valvular stenosis, and supravalvular stenosis.

Subvalvular aortic stenosis refers to outflow obstruction below the aortic valve and is divided into membranous and fibromuscular origin. Membranous subvalvular stenosis is the most common type and accounts for the majority of subvalvular aortic stenosis. The stenosis is a result of a thin fibrous membrane immediately below the aortic valve. Fibromuscular subvalvular stenosis is characterized by a much thicker ridge located lower in the LVOT. Both types of subvalvular aortic stenosis develop over time secondary to abnormal flow patterns resulting from CHD and surgery resulting in damage of the endothelium in the LVOT.

Valvular aortic stenosis is the most common type and is a result of abnormal aortic valve tissue and bicuspid aortic valve. Bicuspid aortic valve is the most common congenital heart disease and results from partial to complete fusion of two valve cusps; in 80% of cases, it is the fusion of the right and left coronary cusps. Poststenotic dilatation of the ascending aorta is commonly observed in both bicuspid aortic valve and aortic stenosis. The severity of aortic valve stenosis is based on cardiac catheterization measurements of the pressure gradient over the stenotic valve and are graded as mild stenosis when there is a mean gradient of <25 mm Hg; moderate stenosis with a mean gradient of 25 to 40 mm Hg; and severe aortic stenosis with a mean gradient of >40 mm Hg.

Supravalvular aortic stenosis is a result of the narrowing just above the sinuses of Valsalva in the proximal ascending aorta. Supravalvular stenosis is often an inherited disorder secondary to a defect in the *ELN* gene located on chromosome 7q11.3. Disorders in the

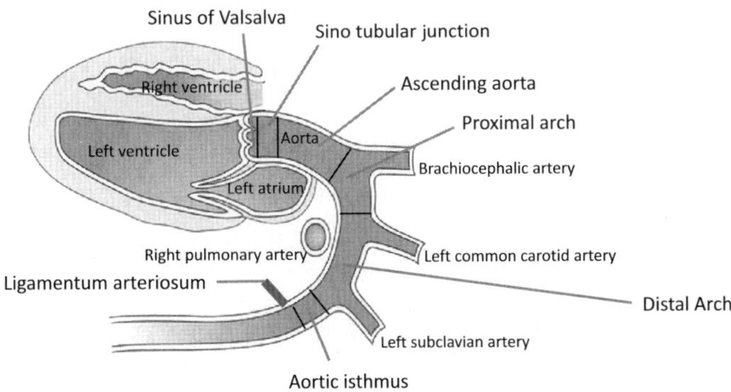

Fig. 37.15 Aortic Arch. Schematic diagram of fetal aortic arch, sagittal view. The aortic arch crosses over the right pulmonary artery. The isthmus is the section after the left subclavian artery and ends at the level of the ligamentum arteriosum. The figure shows the brachiocephalic artery, aortic isthmus, left atrium, left common carotid artery, left subclavian artery, left ventricle, and right ventricle (Courtesy Irving R. Tessler, MD. Reproduced with permission and after minor modifications from Sklansky. Fetal cardiac malformations and arrhythmias: detection, diagnosis, management, and prognosis. In: *Creasy and Resnik's Maternal-Fetal Medicine: Principles and Practice*, 25, 348–392.e5.)

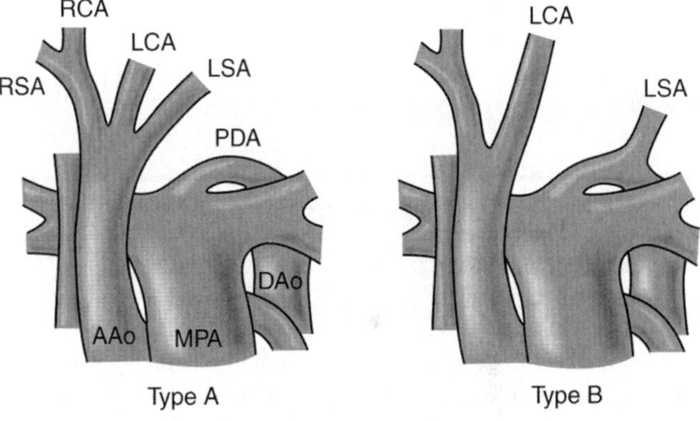

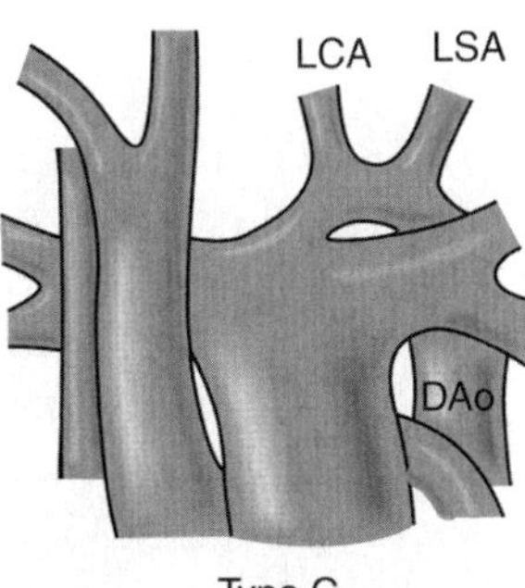

Fig. 37.16 Classification of Interrupted Aortic Arch. Type A: Interruption after the left subclavian artery and before the ductus arteriosus or ligamentum arteriosum. Type B: Interruption between the common carotid artery and the left subclavian artery. Type C: Interruption between the brachiocephalic artery and the common carotid artery. *AAo*, Ascending aorta; *DAo*, descending aorta; *LCA*, left common carotid artery; *LSA*, left subclavian artery; *MPA*, main pulmonary artery; *PDA*, patent ductus arteriosus; *RCA*, right common carotid artery; *RSA*, right subclavian artery. (Adapted from Monro JL. Interruption of aortic arch. In: Stark J, de Leval M, eds. *Surgery for Congenital Heart Defects*. 2nd ed. Philadelphia, PA: Saunders; 1994:299; reproduced with permission and after minor modifications from Weil and Fraser. Congenital heart disease. In: *Sabiston Textbook of Surgery*, chapter 59, 1641–1678.)

ELN gene potentially affect all arteries, but the aorta tends to be the most impacted. Often referred to as ELN arteriopathy, the aorta can be affected along its entire course. Patients with supravalvular stenosis are at high risk for stenosis at the origin of the coronary artery, most often the left coronary artery.

Coarctation of the Aorta

Prevalence

The prevalence of coarctation of aorta (CoA) is 5% to 8% among children with CHD, either as an isolated defect or in association with other CHDs.[42,43] CoA is commonly associated with Turner syndrome and the *Notch1* gene. Patients with Turner syndrome are not only at risk of neonatal CoA but are at risk of developing CoA later in life. Up to 5% of female patients with CoA will have Turner syndrome.

The area of the dorsal aorta between the fourth and sixth aortic arch is called the isthmus. The isthmus is the smallest part of the arch in an embryo, likely because it only carries 10% of the combined ventricular output, making it about 80% of the ascending aorta size. The pathogenesis behind CoA is that ductal tissue is located in the aortic arch, just distal to the isthmus and proximal descending aorta, where the sixth arch and fourth arch connect. When this ductal tissue contracts similarly to the ductus, the arch narrows and results in a CoA.

The neonatal presentation of CoA results in relatively acute compromise of systemic perfusion with high afterload, shock, LV wall stress, and LV dilatation. Later in life, coarctation can present with hypertension, and 20% of patients with coarctation will have berry aneurysms.[44]

Arch Anomalies and Ductus Arteriosus

Aortic Arch Anomalies

Embryonic Pharyngeal Arch Arteries

The thoracic, head, and neck vessels develop from the six aortic arches. The embryo has a right and left parallel system that consists of one truncus arteriosus, one aortic sac, two dorsal aortas, and six aortic arches. These blood vessels are shown in Fig. 37.17.[45]

Truncus Arteriosus: This is the most proximal part of the ascending aorta and pulmonary trunk. As embryonic differentiation progresses it gets divided into the pulmonary valve and the aortic valve.

Dorsal Arch: The right dorsal arch becomes part of the right subclavian artery, whereas the left dorsal arch becomes the descending and abdominal aorta.

Aortic Sac: The aortic sac forms the ascending aorta and right brachiocephalic trunk.

First and Second Arch: Both involute and disappear.

Third Arch: The third aortic arch becomes the right and internal carotid arteries.

Fourth Arch: The left fourth aortic arch becomes part of the aortic arch, whereas the right aortic arch becomes part of the right subclavian artery.

Fifth Arch: The fifth arch plays no significant role in main vessel development

Sixth Arch: The right sixth arch becomes the right pulmonary artery, and the left sixth arch becomes the PDA and the left pulmonary artery.

Types of Abnormal Arch and Vessel Constellations

The most frequently seen arch anomalies are summarized in Fig. 37.18.

Left Arch

Left aortic arch with an aberrant right (retroesophageal) subclavian: normal left arch with an aberrant retroesophageal right subclavian. This does not result in a tracheal ring, and patients can have mild swallowing dysfunction. This is the most common arch anomaly.

Aberrant right subclavian with diverticulum of Kommerell: normal left arch with a right retroesophageal diverticulum of Kommerell connected to the left pulmonary artery via the ligamentum arteriosus.

Right Arch

Right aortic arch with aberrant left (retroesophageal) subclavian: abnormal right aortic arch with an aberrant retroesophageal left subclavian artery. Patients are usually asymptomatic.

Right aortic arch with aberrant left subclavian with diverticulum of Kommerell: abnormal right arch with a left retroesophageal

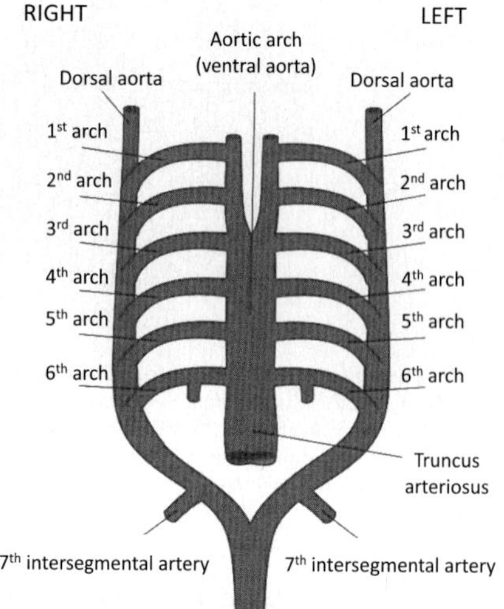

Truncus arteriosus = Proximal ascending aorta
1st and 2nd arch = Dissolve
3rd arch = Left and right common and internal carotid arteries
4th arch = Right part of right subclavian
Left part of aortic arch
5th arch = Does not exist in humans (controversial)
6th arch = Right becomes the right pulmonary artery
Left becomes the left pulmonary artery

Fig. 37.17 Schematic Diagram of the Embryonic Pharyngeal Arch Arteries. These details are important to understand the development of the aortic arch.

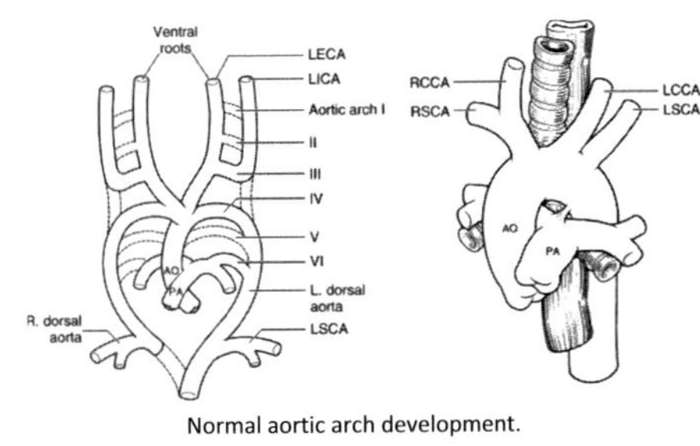

Normal aortic arch development.

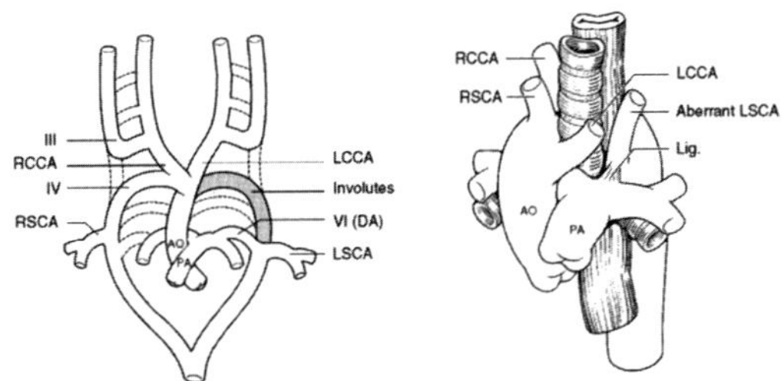

A right aortic arch with aberrant left subclavian and retroesophageal left ligamentum arteriosum.

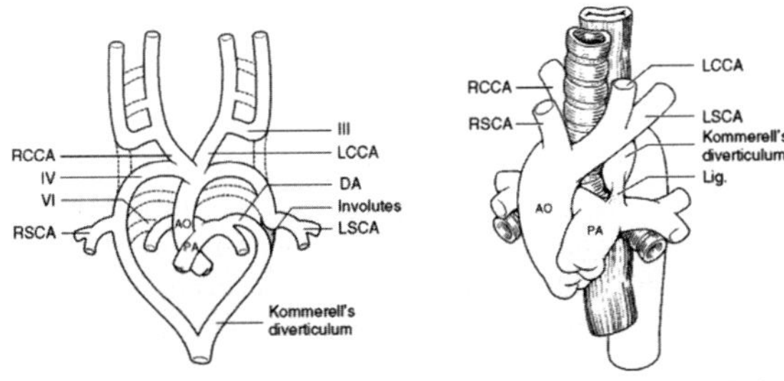

Formation of a right aortic arch with mirror image branching and retroesophageal left ligamentum arteriosum.

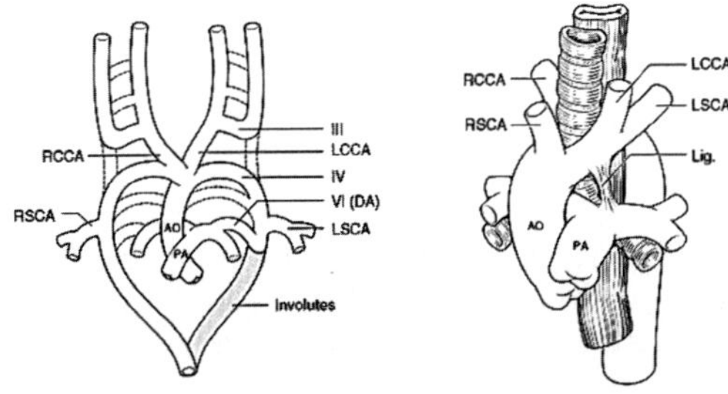

A right aortic arch with mirror imaging branching and left ligamentum arteriosum, which does not form a vascular ring.

Fig. 37.18 Most Frequently Seen Abnormalities of the Aortic Arch. *AO,* Aorta; *DA,* ductus arteriosum; *LCCA,* left common carotid artery; *LECA,* left external carotid artery; *LICA,* left internal carotid artery; *Lig.,* ligamentum arteriosum; *LSCA,* left subclavian artery; *PA,* pulmonary artery; *RCCA,* right common carotid artery; *RSCA,* right subclavian artery. (From Ohye RG, Wild LC, Mutabagani K, Bove EL. Vascular rings and slings. In: Franco KL, Putman JB, eds. *Advanced Therapy in Thoracic Surgery*. Hamilton, Ontario, BC: Decker; 2004; and Ohye and Hirsch. Congenital heart disease and anomalies of the great vessels. In: *Pediatric Surgery*, chap 127, 1647–1671.)

diverticulum of Kommerell connecting to the left pulmonary artery via the ligamentum arteriosus.

Right aortic arch with retroesophageal left brachiocephalic (innominate) artery: abnormal right arch with a retroesophageal left brachiocephalic (innominate) artery.

Right aortic arch with mirror image branching: abnormal right arch with the right subclavian artery and right carotid coming off the right arch and a proximal left innominate artery anterior to the trachea giving rise to the left subclavian and the left carotid artery. This arch anomaly is primarily seen in patients with TOF and truncus.

Double Aortic Arch

This results from the persistence of both the right and left aortic arch resulting in an ascending aorta dividing in a right and left arch encircling the esophagus and trachea completely. Fig. 37.19 shows a double aortic arch compressing the trachea.

Normal
Double aortic arch
Esophagus
Trachea
Aorta

Fig. 37.19 Double Aortic Arch. The image shows mechanical obstruction of the trachea secondary to a double aortic arch (http://www.nlm.nih.gov/medlineplus/ency/article/007316.htm). (From Steppan and Maxwell. Congenital heart disease. In: *Stoelting's Anesthesia and Co-Existing Disease*, chap 7, 129–149.)

Pulmonary Artery Sling

The main pulmonary artery bifurcates typically just before the trachea and gives rise to the left pulmonary artery. In a pulmonary artery sling, the main pulmonary artery bifurcates to the right of the trachea, and the left pulmonary artery travels behind the trachea and in front of the esophagus. Pulmonary slings tend to result in early symptoms of expiratory stridor and respiratory distress. Fig. 37.20 shows a pulmonary artery sling.

Persistent Ductus Arteriosus

Prevalence

Overall, symptomatic PDA accounts for up to 10% of congenital heart disease. There is an inverse relationship between gestational age and PDA, with up to 70% of infants of extremely low gestational

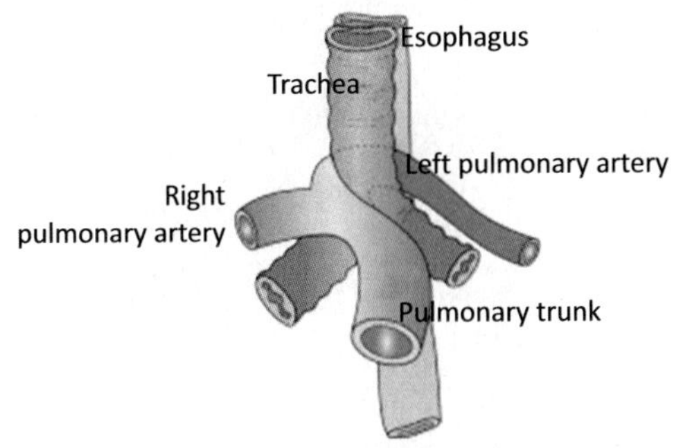

Fig. 37.20 Pulmonary Artery Sling. Pulmonary Vascular Sling. There is an anomalous origin of the left pulmonary artery from the right encircling the trachea. (Reproduced with permission and after minor modifications from Quail et al. Vascular rings, pulmonary slings, and other vascular abnormalities. *Diagnosis and Management of Adult Congenital Heart Disease*, 42, 429–439.)

age having a PDA. A PDA is seen more frequently in term neonates with following genetic syndromes: trisomy 21, Holt-Oram syndrome, Carpenter syndrome, incontinentia pigmenti, and Char syndrome. Congenital rubella syndrome is also associated with a PDA, which is secondary to the proliferation of the internal elastin layer, mimicking a premature ductus's anatomy. Such a ductus has a low likelihood of closing spontaneously.

In fetal life, the ductus is a necessary structure that allows communication between the PA and the aorta. The PDA is established during the sixth week of gestation and develops from the sixth branchial arch. Fig. 37.21 shows the anatomy of the ductus arteriosus.

Fetal Ductus

The ductus plays an essential role in the fetal circulation, where it allows for the more deoxygenated blood from the head and neck vessels of the fetus to be pumped from the RV via the main pulmonary artery directly into the descending aorta toward the two umbilical arteries to the placenta for gas exchange. The fetal right-to-left shunting results from high pulmonary arterial pressures, low systemic pressures, placental pressures, and a fully open ductus with the same caliber as the aortic arch. The ductus takes off at the very proximal part of the left pulmonary artery. Its entry into the aorta marks the end of the isthmus and the most proximal part of the descending aorta.

The ductus is structured like an artery with a tunica intima consisting of the endothelium and the internal elastin layer; tunica media with smooth muscle; and tunica externa with the external elastin layer. All arterial oxygen reaches the tunica media via a network of the vessel walls' own supply, called the vasa private, and through the diffusion of oxygen directly from the lumen. Arteries thinner than 0.5 mm generally have no vasa privata in the smooth muscle zone of tunica media because they are thin enough for oxygen to diffuse from the vessel lumen or the vasa privata located only in the tunica externa.

Two significant factors contribute to keeping the ductus wide open during fetal life:

1. Prostaglandins. Prostaglandins, both prostaglandin E2 and prostacyclin (PGI2), are produced in the placenta. Additionally, prostaglandins are also produced in the wall of the PDA and function as local vasodilators, keeping the smooth muscle within the wall of the ductus relaxed. This results in an increased concentration of prostaglandins in the fetus and a very localized increase in prostaglandins in the arterial ductus.
2. Low oxygen concentration. The blood that passes through the ductus in the fetus has particularly low oxygen concentration because it is mainly the deoxygenated blood from the head and neck vessels. These low oxygen concentrations support the patency of the ductus as it prevents the smooth muscle in the ductus from contracting.

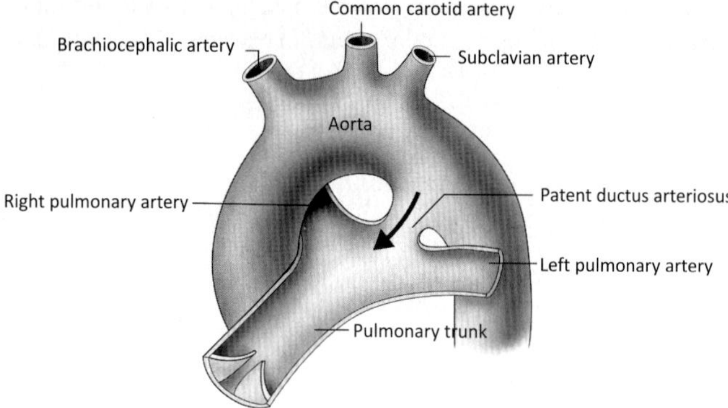

Fig. 37.21 Anatomy of a Patent Ductus Arteriosus. Blood from the aorta shunts across the ductus arteriosus into the pulmonary artery *(arrow)*. The degree of left to right shunting depends on the resistance in the ductus (diameter and length) and the pressure gradient between the systemic and pulmonary circulation. (Reproduced with minor modifications from Perloff JK, ed. *Clinical Recognition of Congenital Heart Disease*. 4th ed. Philadelphia: WB Saunders; 1994:510.)

Physiologic functional closure of the ductus arteriosus starts once the newborn infant takes the first breath. This immediately lowers the PVR significantly by opening the alveoli and the surface of the entire pulmonary vascular bed. The second step is removing the low-resistance large vascular surface area of the placenta once the umbilical cord is clamped. This again results in increased systemic vascular resistance and changes the direction of the blood flow from systemic to pulmonary flow. This provides oxygen-rich arterial blood to pass through the ductus, causing vasoconstriction of the smooth muscle in the tunica media. Removal of the placenta also removes a source of prostaglandin and significantly lowers the concentration of circulating prostaglandins, resulting in smooth muscle contraction in the tunica media. Smooth muscle contraction of the tunica media results in significant thickening of the vessel wall, resulting in an immediate effect of flow restriction and functional closure of the ductus. This significant thickening of the ductus vessel wall makes the previously thin avascular zone of 0.5 mm depending on oxygen diffusion from the vascular lumen increase to more than 1 cm in distance. This results in ischemia beyond the 0.5-mm diffusion length, resulting in circumferential cell death of smooth muscles in the tunica media and starting the complete anatomic closure and transformation into the ligamentum arteriosus.

Ductus in Preterm Neonates

The ductus in preterm neonates often fails to close despite the effects of lower circulating prostaglandins and higher oxygen content in the blood, resulting in some constriction and thickening of the ductus. The vessel wall of the ductus in a preterm infant is, on average, only 0.2 mm. It may thicken to approximately 0.6 mm; however, this is not enough to create a significant avascular zone, and local hypoxia and ischemia lead to cell death. Therefore the ductus is at risk of remaining patent in preterm neonates. Additionally, Fan et al. described the PDA maturation pathway in their rabbit model and demonstrated that patency of the preterm ductus is maintained by high levels of PGE1, prostaglandin E2 (PGE2), which binds the prostaglandin E2 receptor 4 (EP4) receptors under conditions of hypoxia as opposed to the term ductus, where the EP3 receptor levels are higher and exposure to PGE2 causes vasoconstriction under normoxic conditions.[46] Once functional closure of the ductus occurs, anatomic closure follows with intraluminal remodeling in response to hypoxemic conditions. Hence, delayed ductal closure in term infants is primarily related to structural alterations, whereas the lack of spontaneous closure in preterm infants is due to immaturity.[47] Some of the pathophysiological factors changes associated with persistent patency of the ductus arteriosus are highlighted in Fig. 37.22.

Inflow Tract Anomalies

Tricuspid Atresia

Prevalence

TA is seen in 1 per 10,000 births, making it one of the more common congenital cyanotic heart lesions.[48] The pathogenesis of TA is unknown; however, 7% of TA patients will have 22q11 microdeletion. It is also seen associated with trisomy 13, 18, and 21.

TA is defined by complete agenesis of the TV and lacks any communication between the RA and the RV. The floor of the RA in the

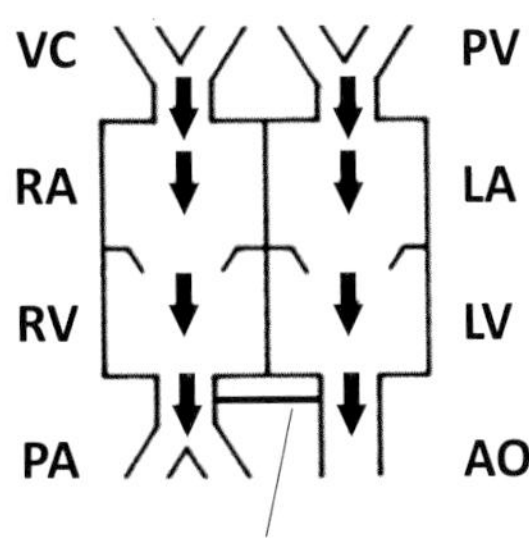

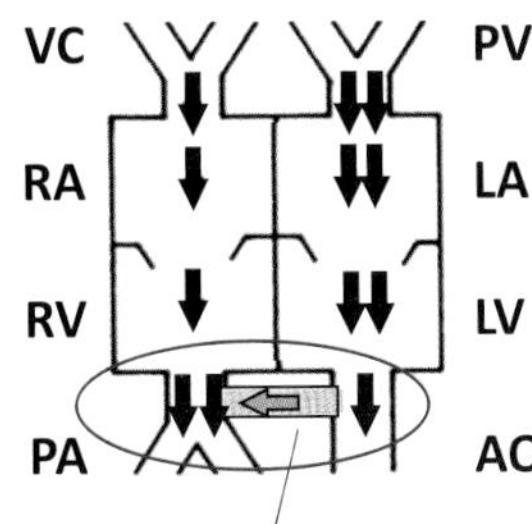

Fig. 37.22 Pathophysiology of Patent Ductus Arteriosus (PDA). In infants with a nonrestrictive PDA, pulmonary arterial (PA) pressures resemble the aortic pressures. Right ventricle (RV) diastolic function deteriorates when it has to pump against systemic-like PA pressures and because of geometric changes in the ventricular septum due to left ventricular (LV) overload. Large left-to-right (L→R) shunts can increase pulmonary blood flows to levels as high as twice those of the systemic circulation. Increased pulmonary blood flows result in pulmonary edema, increased pulmonary venous return, left atrial (LA) dilatation, and LV volumes.

area where the TV should have been tends to show a little tissue ridge, referred to as the fibromuscular ledge. The pathogenesis of TA is unknown. The anatomy of the underdeveloped RV is such that unless there is PA, only the outflow portion of the RV is developed. The size of the RV cavity is primarily dependent on the size of the associated VSD. Because there is no inflow from the RA to the RV, an ASD allows for blood to flow from the RA to the LA. For that reason, there tends to be a well-developed, nonrestrictive ASD in TA. TA is classified based on the size of the VSD, degree of PS, and whether the great vessels usually are related or transposed. Up to one-third of TA will have transposed great vessels, especially in cases with no pulmonary valve stenosis. In TA with TGA, there is an increased risk of having left-sided outflow tract obstruction in the form of subaortic stenosis and coarctation. The systemic circulation may, in such cases, be ductal dependent. The VSD seen in TA can be classified as a muscular VSD and tends to become smaller and more restrictive.

Ebstein Anomaly

Prevalence

The inheritance of Ebstein anomaly is sporadic and is not associated with a specific syndrome or gene. It occurs in about 1% of all cases of CHD.[49]

Ebstein anomaly is a complex congenital heart disease that affects the TV, the RV morphology, and RV function. Adherence of the TV leaflets to the RV myocardium results in an inferiorly displaced TV annulus. This is a result of the TV hinge points being displaced downward into the RV. In normal cardiac development, the leaflets of the TV are developed by a process known as delamination. Delamination refers to the cavity-forming layer of the myocardium separating from the rest of the myocardium, starting from the apex and delaminating in a proximal direction toward the AV junction, becoming the TV leaflets and chordea.[50] Ebstein anomaly results from a failure of the delamination process leading to an arrest in the formation of the TV leaflets, which never become unattached from the RV myocardium. Delamination starts in the apex and progresses proximally toward the AV junction, resulting in various degrees to which the RV is impacted depending on the stage of the delamination process. Because the delamination process involves the myocardium, variable degrees of cardiomyopathy are associated with Ebstein anomaly. This cardiomyopathy can also involve the LV. The TV in Ebstein anomaly is not only displaced toward the apex but tends to have significant coaptation failure resulting in severe TV regurgitation. Some of the anatomic features of Ebstein anomaly are shown in Fig. 37.23.

Secondary to marked cardiomegaly, the fetus with Ebstein anomaly may have lung hypoplasia secondary to prevention of lung expansion and growth. Fetal hydrops is not uncommon in Ebstein anomaly secondary to severe TV regurgitation, RA hypertension, and a very volume-overloaded heart. In cases where the TV regurgitation is severe, patients may have functional pulmonary atresia where the RV does not generate enough force to open an otherwise normal pulmonary valve because it all goes retrograde as tricuspid regurgitation into the RA. Postnatally this results in ductal-dependent pulmonary circulation. Pulmonary valve regurgitation can further complicate this pathophysiology, where a circular shunt can develop. This is a situation where the systemic to pulmonary shunt over the ductus does not perfuse the pulmonary arteries but escapes as pulmonary regurgitation into the RV and back via the highly abnormal and regurgitant TV to the RA and right to left to the LA mixes with the PV blood and back out via the LV to the systemic circulation without being able to oxygenate. The presence of pulmonary valve regurgitation in Ebstein anomaly is a risk factor for poor outcomes.

Single Ventricles

Single ventricle physiology is defined as one ventricle pumping blood, both to the systemic circulation and the pulmonary circulation. Anatomically and embryologically, there is always some remnant of an underdeveloped ventricle. Anatomically, the CHDs presenting with single ventricle physiology are TA, hypoplastic left heart syndrome (HLHS), some unbalanced AV canals, and a group of CHDs referred to as univentricular AV connections or simply as a univentricular heart.

Univentricular AV connections are described based on the atrial to ventricular connection, the dominant ventricle, the hypoplastic ventricle, and finally by the relationship of the great arteries.

Double Inlet Left Ventricle

Double inlet LV is the most common form of univentricular AV connection. Often, the great vessels are transposed, the aorta comes

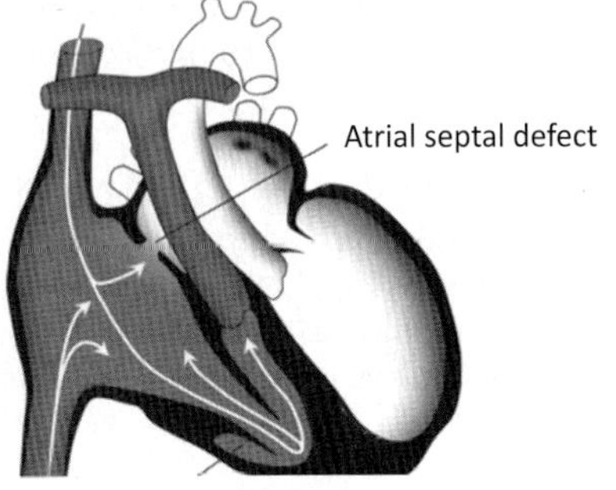

Fig. 37.23 Schematic Depiction of Ebstein Anomaly. This patient had an associated atrial septal defect (ASD), which is seen in (1/3) of these patients. The *white lines with arrows* represent the pathway of venous blood returning to the heart. (Reproduced with minor modifications from Cardiovascular Disease. In: Vidovich, Mladen I. *Chestnut's Obstetric Anesthesia*. Published January 1, 2020. Pages 987–1032.)

off a very hypoplastic RV, there is a VSD, and the pulmonary arteries are normally developed.

Hypoplastic Left Heart Syndrome

Prevalence

HLHS is a congenital heart disease characterized by underdeveloped to absent left-sided heart structures, frequently resulting in a single functioning RV. The prevalence of HLHS is close to 3% of all congenital heart disease. The incidence is about 2.1 per 10,000 live births. The clinical and surgical management of HLHS has evolved over the past 20 years, and now survival is between 80% and 90% after the first neonatal surgical palliation.[51]

A genetic predisposition has not been defined. However, first-degree relatives of patients with HLHS tend to have some degree of left-sided pathology from bicuspid aortic valve, mitral stenosis, or LVOT obstruction. Patients with Turner syndrome and duplication of the short arm of chromosome 12 are at increased risk of HLHS. Patients with HLHS frequently have other noncardiac anomalies and genetic syndromes. The pathogenesis of HLHS is progressive during embryology and is believed to be secondary to decreased blood flow via the foramen ovale via the LA to the LV in fetal life. The decrease in LV blood flow reduces LV volume, cardiac output, and wall stress needed for optimal growth of the LV, resulting in an underdeveloped, rudimentary abnormal hypoplastic LV. HLHS incorporates left-sided pathology to various degrees and is frequently defined by whether mitral and aortic valve stenosis or atresia is present. The various constellations and relative percentages of all HLHS are (1) aortic stenosis/mitral stenosis (AA/MA): 25%; (2) aortic atresia/mitral atresia (AA/MA): 50%; and (3) aortic atresia/mitral stenosis (AA/MS): 25%. The anatomical changes seen with HLHS are summarized in Fig. 37.24.

The ascending aorta usually is extremely hypoplastic, with a diameter frequently less than 3 mm. Most patients with HLHS also have CoA. The coronary arteries still arise from the base of the aorta, and perfusion in severe aortic stenosis (AS) and aortic atresia (AA) is achieved by retrograde flow down the ascending aorta to the coronary arteries. The coronary arteries in HLHS tend to be of standard caliber with a normal course. The LV anatomy ranges from barely having a lumen to a small, noncompliant LV cavity, frequently with endocardial fibroelastosis, to a small but more cavity-forming LV.

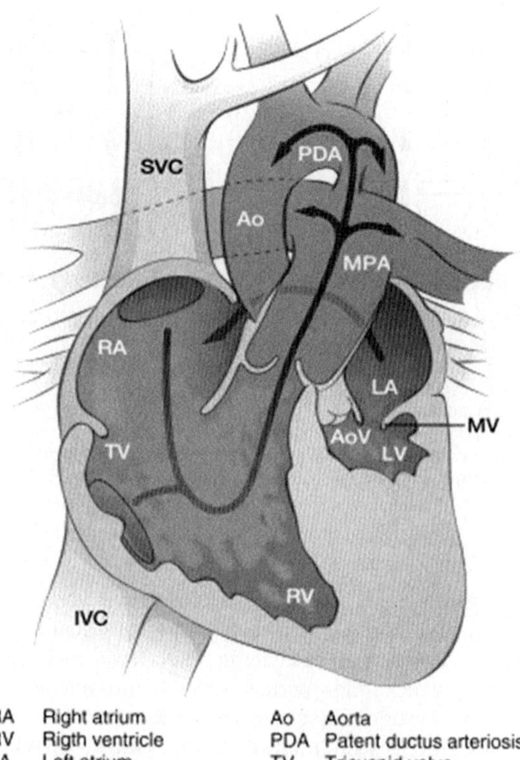

RA	Right atrium	Ao	Aorta
RV	Rigth ventricle	PDA	Patent ductus arteriosis
LA	Left atrium	TV	Tricuspid valve
LV	Left ventrticle	MV	Mitral valve
SVC	Superior vena cava	PV	Pulmonary valve
IVC	Inferior vena cava	AoV	Aortic valve
MPA	Main pulmomary artery		

Fig. 37.24 Hypoplastic Left Heart Syndrome. Hypoplastic left heart (MS/AS): Hypoplastic ascending aorta; small stenotic aortic valve; often there are abnormal attachments of the chordea such as parachute—valve where the chordae are attached only to one papillary muscle; underdeveloped, hypertensive LV (https://www.cdc.gov/ncbddd/heartdefects/hlhs.html). (From Steppan and Maxwell. Congenital heart disease. In: *Stoelting's Anesthesia and Co-Existing Disease*, chap 7, 129–149.)

A Note on Hemodynamics and Single Ventricle Pathophysiology

In order to understand the physiology and pathophysiology of a single ventricle heart, a few classic hemodynamic terms need to be defined.

Oxygen Consumption (VO_2)

Oxygen consumption is how much oxygen the body is using and needs to maintain metabolic equilibrium, and it varies based on certain states. Oxygen consumption increases with illness, fever, and exercise. Baseline oxygen consumption in a neonate is between 10 and 14 mL O_2/kg.

Oxygen Capacity

The amount of oxygen that can be bound by hemoglobin (Hgb) in the blood is calculated by using formula = Hgb × 1.36.

Oxygen Content

The amount of dissolved oxygen in the blood and the oxygen bound to hemoglobin (oxygen capacity).

Oxygen Delivery (DO_2)

Oxygen delivery describes how well the body uses the blood and heart to deliver oxygen to the tissue to meet the oxygen consumption ultimately.

Arterial-Venous Oxygen Saturation Difference

Comparing the oxygen saturation in the arterial end of the circulation with the venous side gives a measure of the degree of oxygen extracted by the tissue. The oxygen extraction indirectly provides information on whether oxygen delivery is sufficient for the body's oxygen demand. As a rule of thumb, oxygen extraction of greater than 45% suggests that the oxygen delivery is not sufficient, often due to reduced stroke volume in heart failure or decreased systemic blood flow (Qs).

The underlying challenge with single ventricle physiology is the inability to compensate for low mixed venous saturations secondary to increased oxygen extraction. In a four-chamber heart, the pulmonary venous return will have an oxygen saturation in the high 90s (assuming normal lungs) even if the mixed venous saturations are very low. In a single ventricle heart, the low mixed venous saturation is seen in high oxygen extraction, and a low oxygen delivery state will mix with the oxygenated blood returning from the lungs and lower the oxygen content of the mixed blood leaving the heart, further reducing the oxygen delivery as the arterial oxygen content is reduced. A single ventricle can never quite compensate for

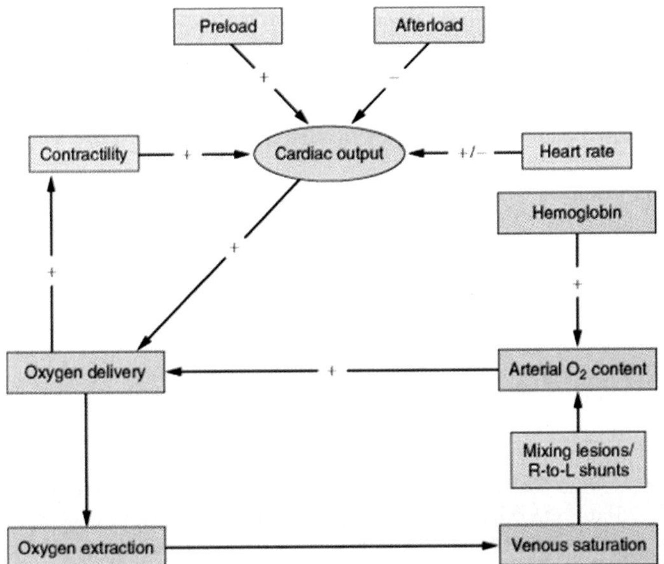

Fig. 37.25 Cardiac Output and Oxygen Delivery Determinants of Cardiac Output and Oxygen Delivery in Congenital Heart Disease. (Data from Andropoulos DB. Hemodynamic management. In: Andropoulos DB et al., eds. *Anesthesia for Congenital Heart Disease*. 2nd ed. Oxford, UK: Wiley-Blackwell; 2010; and from Andropoulos and Gottlieb. Congenital heart disease. In: *Anesthesia and Uncommon Diseases*, chap 3, 75–136.)

increased oxygen extraction. The relationship between the cardiac output and oxygen delivery is summarized in Fig. 37.25.

Cardiac Output

The cardiac output (CO) places a numerical value on how well the heart is functioning as a pump. Cardiac output can be described as the stroke volume (SV) multiplied by heart rate, ultimately describing how much blood leaves the heart in a minute.

It can also be described as the amount of blood flow (Q) leaving the ventricle. In a normal heart without shunts, the CO of the RV is the same as the CO of the LV, or the blood flow leaving for the lungs (Qp) from the RV is the same as the blood flow leaving for the systemic circulation (Qs) from the LV. In single ventricle physiology, one ventricle pumps blood both to the pulmonary circulation and the systemic circulation. Depending on anatomic obstructions and/or relative resistance between the pulmonary and systemic circulation, flow to one circulation may be greater than the other. This can result in an unbalanced blood flow; for example, a newborn with TA, normally related great vessels, restrictive VSD and pulmonary valve stenosis, and relatively high postnatal PVR will have anatomic and physiologic limitations to pulmonary blood flow, resulting in decreased Qp and an increase in Qs. This will be a cyanotic neonate with strong peripheral pulses and good systemic blood pressures.

In another example, a 2-week-old neonate with HLHS, on PGE for PDA patency, gets cold and develops some degree of vasoconstriction resulting in a slight increase in the systemic vascular resistance and then receives oxygen, which dramatically lowers the PVR, resulting in pulmonary overcirculation (Qp) and a decrease in the systemic circulation (Qs). This results in a less cyanotic infant with signs of systemic shock, poor peripheral perfusion, and pulses. This is why understanding and estimating the pulmonary blood flow (Qp) ratio to the systemic blood flow (Qs) is essential; the Qp:Qs is important in understanding and managing patients with single ventricle physiology.

Under normal circumstances in a healthy individual, the amount of oxygen extracted or consumed by the body is equal to the amount of oxygen taken up in the lungs. This physiologic fact sets the stage for calculating the blood flow (or cardiac output) using the Fick principle. Blood flow is proportional to the oxygen content of the blood before and after a capillary bed. This is true for both the pulmonary vascular bed (Qp) and the systemic vascular bed (Qs). The Fick principle states that the amount of blood flow is proportional to oxygen consumption (VO_2) divided by the change in oxygen content across the capillary bed (A-VO_2 difference).

$$Q = CO = \frac{VO_2}{\text{A-}VO_2\,\text{Difference}}$$

$$Q_{\text{systemic}} = \frac{VO_2}{(\text{Ao Sat} - \text{MV Sat}) \times (\text{Hgb} \times 1.36 + \text{dissolved } O_2) \times 10}$$

$$Q_{\text{Pulmonary}} = \frac{VO_2}{(\text{PV Sat} - \text{Pa Sat}) \times (\text{Hgb } \times 1.36 + \text{dissolved } O_2) \times 10}$$

In a normal heart without a shunt, the Q = Qp = Qs because pulmonary venous saturation is the same as systemic arterial saturation and the pulmonary arterial saturation is the same as the mixed venous saturation. This sets the basis for being able to calculate the Qp:Qs. Because Qp should be the same as Qs, mathematically that can be stated as follows:

$$\frac{VO_2}{(\text{Ao Sat} - \text{MV Sat}) \times (\text{Hgb} \times 1.36 + \text{dissolved } O_2) \times 10} = \frac{VO_2}{(\text{PV Sat} - \text{Pa Sat}) \times (\text{Hgb } \times 1.36 + \text{dissolved } O_2) \times 10}$$

With multiple cancellation maneuvers the above formula can be simplified as

$$\text{Qp: Qs} = \frac{\text{Ao MV}}{\text{PV} - \text{PA}}$$

A Qp:Qs of 1 is normal or balanced in a single ventricle, less than 1 reflects decreased pulmonary blood flow, and greater than 1 means too much pulmonary blood flow.

Abnormal Venous Connections

Anomalies of Systemic Venous Connections

During cardiac development, there exists an almost symmetric left and right venous system in the fetus, which ultimately develops to make systemic venous structures only run on the right side of the body in the form of the superior and inferior vena cava (IVC). The venous drainage from the left side of the body needs to connect with this right-sided system. It makes this through four connections: the common iliac vein, the left renal vein, the left azygous vein, and the left brachiocephalic (innominate) vein. Anomalies related to the systemic venous return are often a result of involution of the left-sided fetal venous system.

Anomalies of the Superior Vena Cava

Failure of the left anterior and common cardinal veins to involute results in a persistent left superior vena cava (SVC) and no innominate vein. The left SVC drains into the coronary sinus in up to 90% of cases, where some will have a partial or complete unroofed coronary sinus resulting in drainage both into the LA and the RA. Bilateral SVCs are frequently associated with other congenital heart disease, including heterotaxy with asplenia (right atrial isomerism), TOF, complete AVC, and mitral atresia.

Retroaortic Innominate Vein

The left innominate vein has an abnormal course and runs behind the ascending aorta instead of anterior to it and joins the right aspect of the innominate vein and drains into a right-sided SVC.

Anomalies of the Inferior Vena Cava

Interruption of the Inferior Vena Cava

Absence of the IVC is an anatomic constellation. The hepatic segment of the IVC is absent; the venous return travels via the azygous vein into a right- or left-sided SVC. This is associated with heterotaxy and polysplenia with left atrial isomerism in up to 90% of cases.

Bilateral Inferior Vena Cava

Bilateral infrarenal vena cava can be seen in up to 30% in right atrial isomerism and asplenia syndrome.

Total Anomalous Pulmonary Venous Return

In a normal heart, there are four pulmonary veins that connect to the back of the LA. The pulmonary veins are the most posterior structure of the heart in the mediastinum. The pulmonary veins start forming at the end of the fourth week, and the rudimentary capillary system of the pulmonary mesenchyme all join in one common pulmonary vein initially that drains into the common atrium. A tissue structure called the mesenchymal protrusion extends from the roof of the LA as atrial septation begins and surrounds the pulmonary ridge, where the common pulmonary vein enters the left side of the still common atrium. The mesenchymal protrusion now separates the common pulmonary vein into four veins and orifices and ensures that the pulmonary veins remain a left atrial structure. Total anomalous pulmonary venous return (TAPVR) is believed to be a failure of the dorsal mesenchymal protrusion in committing the pulmonary veins to the LA and splitting them in four. This failure leads to all lung segments draining into a common PV, often called a bridging or vertical vein, which is not committed to the LA and can drain into the RA, coronary sinus, or a systemic vein.

There are four types of total anomalous pulmonary venous return, classified by where the pulmonary vein travels:

1. Supra cardiac TAPVR: All pulmonary veins combine to make a vertical vein that drains into the superior vena cava and, ultimately, the RA.
2. Cardiac TAPVR: In this form of TAPVR, all the pulmonary veins drain into the coronary sinus or directly into the RA.
3. Infracardiac TAPVR: All pulmonary veins drain directly to the IVC or deliver through the hepatic veins or portal veins to the RA.
4. Mixed-type TAPVR: This type of TAPVR may have any combination of supra, cardiac, or infracardiac type features.

The pulmonary venous blood flow in TAPVR can become obstructed at various areas along the course of the common pulmonary vein confluence. Infracardiac TAPVR has the highest risk of becoming obstructed at the level where the common pulmonary vein enters the diaphragm or within the liver. Cardiac TAPVR can develop obstruction at the level where the common pulmonary vein enters the coronary sinus. Supracardiac TAPVR can have obstructed flow at the level where the vertical vein travels between the left bronchus and the main to left pulmonary artery.

CHAPTER 38

Medical and Surgical Management of Critical Congenital Heart Disease

David M. Kwiatkowski

KEY POINTS

1. The natural history of congenital heart diseases (CHDs) varies tremendously. Some critical CHDs become symptomatic and require therapeutic intervention in the neonatal period.
2. Patients with CHDs that result in inadequate pulmonary blood flow typically demonstrate cyanosis within minutes of life that does not improve with the administration of oxygen. Many of these patients need treatment with a prostaglandin infusion (PGE1) while awaiting confirmation of CHD.
3. Infants with transposition of the great arteries with dextro-transposition of the great arteries (dTGA), tricuspid atresia, pulmonary atresia, critical pulmonary valve stenosis, total anomalous pulmonary venous return, or Ebstein anomaly may present with cyanosis soon after birth.
4. Patients with hypoplastic left heart syndrome, coarctation of the aorta, or critical aortic valve stenosis have inadequate systemic blood flow and typically present with poor pulses, poor perfusion, or cardiogenic shock.
5. Neonates with a surgical aortopulmonary shunt, patent ductus arteriosus, unrepaired aortopulmonary window or truncus arteriosus can develop pulmonary overcirculation.
6. Patients with dTGA sometimes do not have sufficient mixing of the blood from the two cardiac sides. Many of these infants require balloon septostomy to promote mixing.
7. Myocardial disease can present with either systolic or diastolic dysfunction.

The natural history of congenital heart disease varies tremendously, because some lesions will self-resolve or go unnoticed throughout a full lifetime, whereas other lesions cause patients to present in extremis at a very young age. Congenital heart disease that requires medical or surgical intervention in the neonatal period for survival or prevention of end organ compromise is often referred to as critical congenital heart disease (CCHD) and is the focus of this chapter. The management of CCHD in neonates has great variability but centers on several core tenets of cardiovascular function, maintaining (1) adequate systemic blood flow, (2) adequate but not excessive pulmonary blood flow, and (3) adequate return of oxygenated pulmonary blood flow. This chapter will discuss the evaluation and early management of patients with one of four common problems, including inadequate pulmonary blood flow, inadequate systemic blood flow, inadequate obligate intracardiac shunting, and abnormal myocardial function (Fig. 38.1). Although different types of CCHD vary tremendously, a focus on these three basic tenets of cardiovascular function guides management in all described lesions.

It is not uncommon for a woman carrying a fetus with CCHD to have a full, seemingly uncomplicated pregnancy, yet for that infant to be critically ill shortly after birth. Fetal-placental circulation provides the means for adequate oxygen and nutrient delivery for the limited metabolic demands, even in many of the most severe cardiac lesions. Earlier prenatal diagnosis with fetal imaging allows the time for thoughtful planning of postnatal management[1] and allows families time to begin learning about and coping with a new diagnosis. Multiple studies have demonstrated the benefit to allowing a full pregnancy for fetuses with CCHD, without early induction of birth.[2–4] Although organ perfusion and oxygenation is intact throughout pregnancy, the heart may continue maldevelopment. In several specific cardiac lesions, such as critical aortic stenosis, pulmonary atresia with intact ventricular septum (PA/IVS), and hypoplastic left heart syndrome (HLHS) with intact atrial septum, some centers advocate for fetal intervention to palliate a cardiac lesion and halt further sequelae.[5] However, these interventions remain novel with yet unestablished safety, efficacy, and optimal patient selection.

At the time of birth, the umbilical cord is clamped and placental flow is removed from circulation, causing systemic vascular resistance to abruptly rise and the supply of oxygenated blood to cease. With the first breaths, alveolar beds begin to open and the lungs are exposed to higher oxygen content, prompting pulmonary vascular resistance to begin to fall. In normal physiology these changes are accompanied by closure of the ductus venosus due to lack in placental flow, an increase in pulmonary venous return and functional closure of the foramen ovale, and beginning of closure of the ductus arteriosus.

Patients with critical anatomic or physiologic cardiac abnormalities often develop signs and symptoms during this transitional period (Fig. 38.2) and may develop cardiogenic shock due to an inability to supply the body with adequate oxygenated blood for metabolic demands. This can be due to inadequate pulmonary blood flow, inadequate systemic blood flow, inadequate intracardiac mixing, or inadequate cardiac myocardial performance. Although these issues can individually be the subject of a textbook, this chapter serves as a brief review of common issues associated with the evaluation and management for common physiologies with references to further discussion (Fig. 38.3).

Inadequate Pulmonary Blood Flow

Patients with CHD that results in inadequate pulmonary blood flow (e.g., tricuspid atresia, pulmonary atresia, critical pulmonary valve stenosis, etc.) typically demonstrate cyanosis within minutes of life and have a low oxygen tension that does not improve with the administration of oxygen. After confirmation of cardiac disease or while awaiting confirmation, initiation of a prostaglandin infusion (PGE1) to maintain patency of the ductus arteriosus often allows clinical

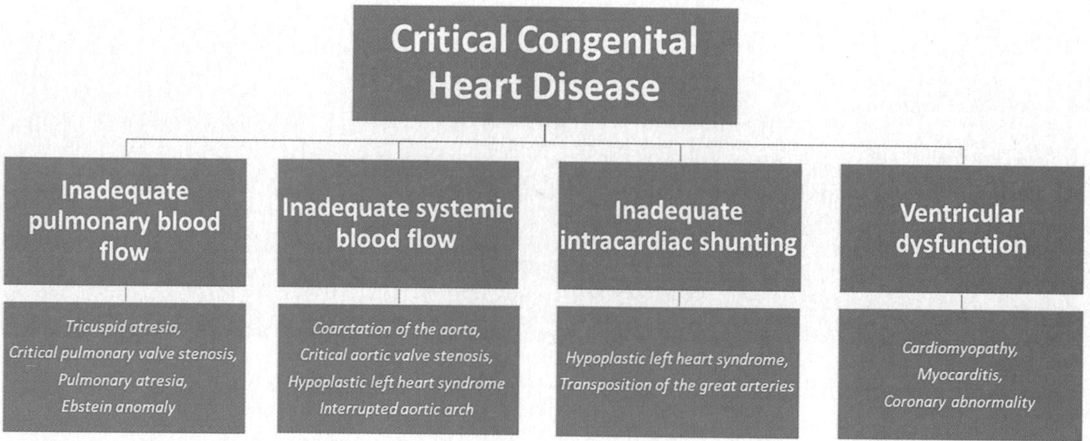

Fig. 38.1 Critical congenital heart diseases (defects) can be broadly classified into four categories, including those with inadequate pulmonary blood flow, inadequate systemic blood flow, inadequate intracardiac shunting, and ventricular dysfunction.

stability to gather information for surgical planning. Meanwhile, initial patient management must address pulmonary etiologies of hypoxia and ensure adequate airway, respiratory drive, and lung expansion. These aspects must be addressed as appropriate. In the majority of patients with CHD that results in inadequate pulmonary blood flow, patency of the ductus arteriosus and basic respiratory care is sufficient to maintain adequate oxygen carrying delivery while awaiting surgical intervention. There are specific cardiac lesions that require special considerations, some of which are detailed below.

Total anomalous pulmonary venous return is a disease in which the pulmonary veins connect to a confluence that drains to the right atria through abnormal supracardiac, infracardiac, or intracardiac connections. In some patients, particularly those with infracardiac and supracardiac drainage, the pulmonary venous drainage may be obstructed by external compression or narrow vessels in its course back to the heart (Fig. 38.4). All patients with total anomalous pulmonary venous return have some degree of cyanosis due to mixing of oxygenated and deoxygenated blood; however, patients with even minor obstruction may develop pulmonary edema and worse oxygen saturations. If the obstruction is more significant infants may develop elevated pulmonary artery pressures resulting in profound cyanosis from right-to-left shunting at the patent ductus arteriosus (PDA) or low cardiac output if a PDA is not present. Although the role of PGE1 is debated in this lesion, it can be detrimental if ductal patency results in greater left-to-right shunting and worsening pulmonary edema. These patients should be intubated and given high concentrations of oxygen as necessary to maintain adequate oxygen saturations; however, the only true treatment for obstructed pulmonary venous drainage is prompt surgical intervention. Obstructed pulmonary veins remain one of the few neonatal cardiac surgical emergencies. Unobstructed pulmonary venous drainage is often treated with diuretics in the neonatal period and repaired at a few weeks of age; however, results suggest that morbidity is decreased with earlier repair.[6]

	Inadequate pulmonary blood flow	Inadequate systemic blood flow	Inadequate intracardiac shunts	Ventricular dysfunction
Example lesions	Tricuspid atresia Critical pulmonary valve stenosis Pulmonary valve atresia Ebstein anomaly	Severe coarctation of the aorta Critical aortic valve stenosis Hypoplastic left heart syndrome Interrupted aortic arch	Hypoplastic left heart syndrome Transposition of the great arteries	Cardiomyopathy Myocarditis Coronary abnormality
Prostaglandin necessary	Often	Yes	Yes	No
Clinical signs and symptoms	Profound cyanosis Tachypnea Increased work of breathing Decreased lung markings on chest x-ray	Poor pulses Cool dusky extremities Tachypnea Lactic acidosis Low urine output	Variable- Profound cyanosis poor pulses Cool dusky extremities Tachypnea Lactic acidosis Low urine output Increased lung markings on chest x-ray	Poor pulses Cool dusky extremities Tachypnea Lactic acidosis Low urine output
Timing of Intervention	Depending on the lesion. Most patients are stable receiving prostaglandin while planning surgery within the first 2 weeks of life. Some lesions, such as tricuspid atresia or Ebstein anomaly, may not require neonatal surgery	Depending on the lesion. Critical aortic valve stenosis should have an intervention emergently, while many other lesions are often stable receiving prostaglandin while planning surgery within the first 2 weeks of life	Variable depending on amount of shunt present. Creation of a shunt is potentially emergent, within minutes to hours of life	Variable depending on severity. May need pharmacologic or mechanical circulatory support emergently

Fig. 38.2 Clinical presentation and management typically needed for the four categories of critical congenital heart diseases (defects) described in Fig. 38.1.

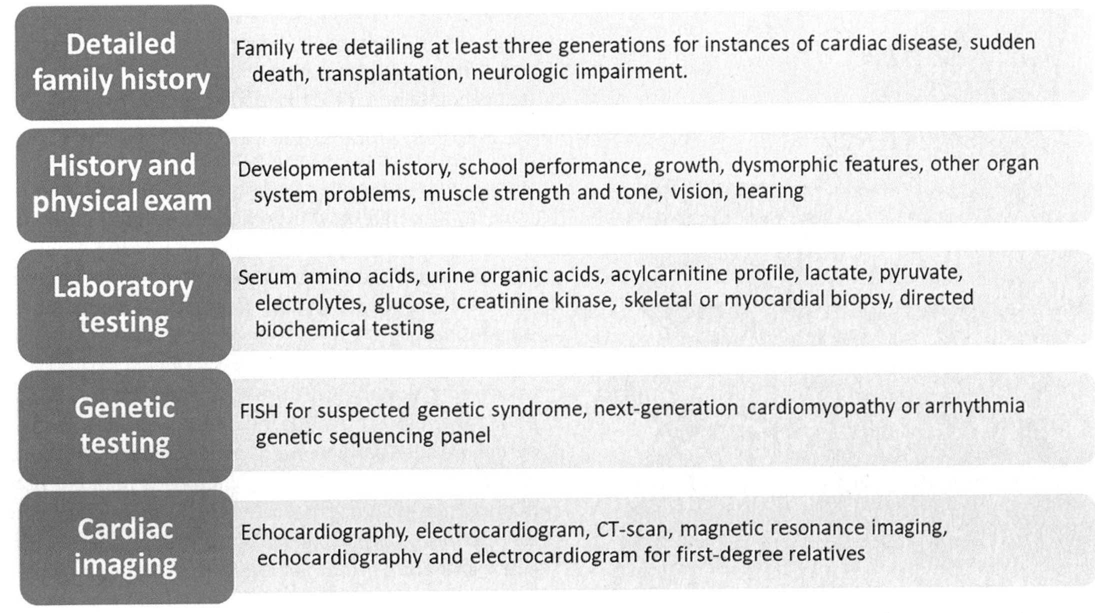

Detailed family history
Family tree detailing at least three generations for instances of cardiac disease, sudden death, transplantation, neurologic impairment.
History and physical exam
Developmental history, school performance, growth, dysmorphic features, other organ system problems, muscle strength and tone, vision, hearing
Laboratory testing
Serum amino acids, urine organic acids, acylcarnitine profile, lactate, pyruvate, electrolytes, glucose, creatinine kinase, skeletal or myocardial biopsy, directed biochemical testing
Genetic testing
FISH for suspected genetic syndrome, next-generation cardiomyopathy or arrhythmia genetic sequencing panel
Cardiac imaging
Echocardiography, electrocardiogram, CT-scan, magnetic resonance imaging, echocardiography and electrocardiogram for first-degree relatives

Fig. 38.3 Clinical Evaluation Needed for Infants With Congenital Heart Diseases (Defects). *CK*, Creatine kinase; *CT*, computed tomography; *FISH*, fluorescence in situ hybridization.

Ebstein anomaly is a heterogenous disease caused by a failure of normal development of the tricuspid valve in utero, causing tricuspid valve insufficiency and a decrease in the function cavity size of the right ventricle (Fig. 38.5). Although mild forms of the disease may result in a long asymptomatic life, more severe subtypes may result in patients with inadequate pulmonary blood flow and potentially functional or structural pulmonary atresia if the right ventricle is unable to generate antegrade blood flow. These patients will present with hydrops fetalis or postnatal cyanosis and potentially cardiogenic shock. Given the poor outcomes associated with neonatal repair, surgery is only indicated in patients who have cyanosis, overt heart failure, or poor cardiac output causing inadequate organ perfusion. Neonatal intervention is typically only performed in patients who fail to wean from PGE1 or have an unacceptably low oxygen saturation after weaning. Overall, this represents a minority of patients with Ebstein malformation. There are several approaches to neonatal intervention, all of which have less than optimal outcomes. Although many patients are able to have a biventricular repair, neonatal surgical interventions are commonly performed in patients who will have a functionally single ventricle physiology and are focused on creation of adequate yet controlled pulmonary blood flow either through a surgical systemic to pulmonary shunt or placement of a stent in the ductus arteriosus. These patients often have poor cardiac output due to ventricular-ventricular interactions, in which the large right ventricle (RV) compresses the left ventricle (LV). Management of this complication remain controversial and include surgical reduction and potentially oversewing of the tricuspid valve.[7] Neonates with anatomic pulmonary stenosis or atresia but reasonable RV function may rarely benefit from a balloon valvuloplasty as initial palliation. However, this procedure is likely to cause pulmonary

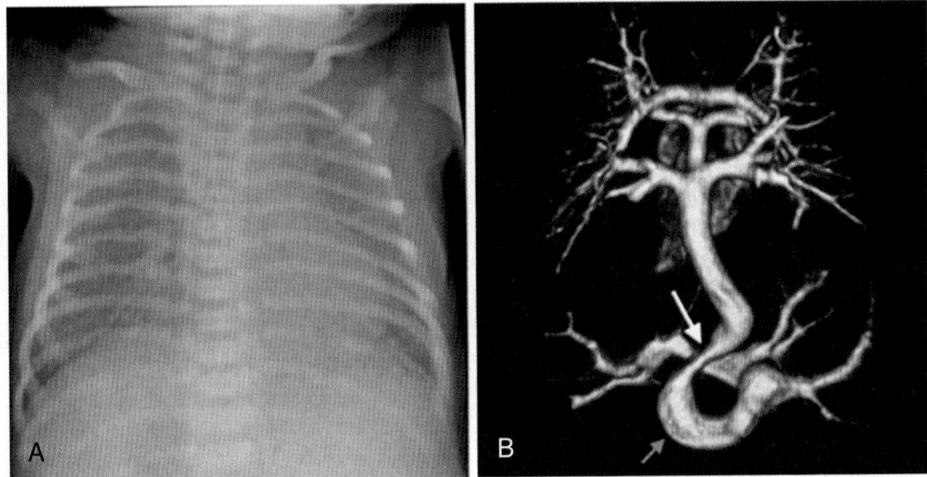

Fig. 38.4 Infracardiac Total Anomalous Pulmonary Venous Drainage. (A) Anterior-posterior chest x-ray in newborn infant presenting with cyanosis and respiratory distress showing pulmonary edema. (B) Volume-rendered 3-D reconstruction of magnetic resonance angiography showing total anomalous infracardiac drainage of the pulmonary veins in the same patient. Note the narrowing of the veins as they pass through the diaphragm *(white arrow)* before draining into the portal vein *(blue arrow)*. (Reproduced with permission and after minor modifications from Quail et al. Congenital heart disease: general principles and imaging. *Grainger & Allison's Diagnostic Radiology*, 13:289–314.)

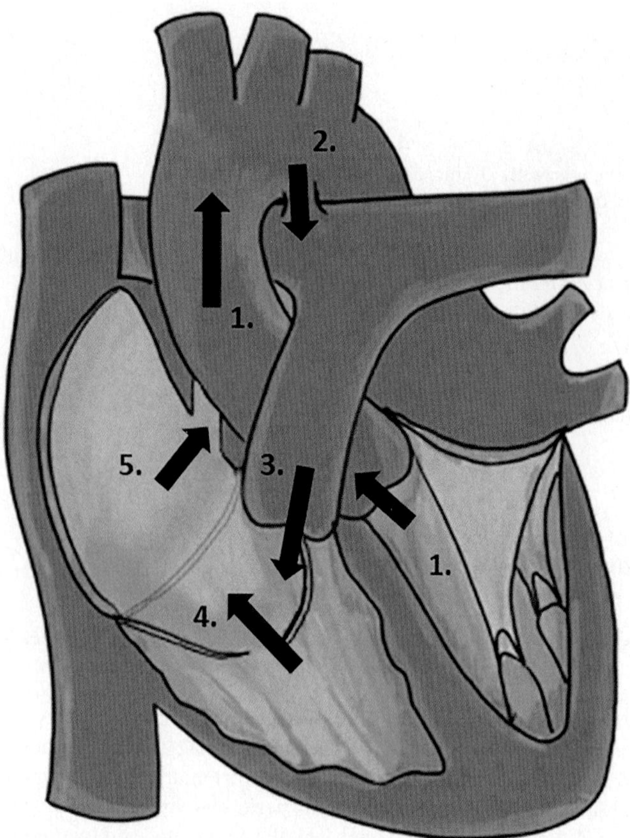

Fig. 38.5 The "Circular Shunt" of Ebstein Anomaly. (1) Blood is ejected from the left ventricle into the aorta. (2) Blood goes from the aorta to the pulmonary artery through the PDA. (3) Blood goes backward from the pulmonary artery to the right ventricle through the insufficient pulmonary valve. (4) Due to poor right ventricular function, blood regurgitates across the insufficient Ebsteinoid tricuspid valve. (5) Blood goes across the atrial septal defect and back into the left ventricle. (Charitha D. Reddy MD.)

insufficiency and is subject to the particular risk of the creation of a "circular shunt" in patients with significant tricuspid regurgitation (Fig. 38.5). In the "circular shunt," blood will flow from the aorta to the pulmonary artery via the PDA, enter the RV through the insufficient pulmonary valve, enter the right atria due to the tricuspid regurgitation, then cross the ASD and exit the left heart only to again cross the PDA. This ineffective circulation is poorly tolerated, and closure of the PDA is often performed in the same catheterization procedure.

Patients with PA/IVS have wide variability in their management and outcomes. After maintenance of a PDA is ensured with PGE1 administration, an echocardiogram is obtained to evaluate tricuspid valve effective orifice size and whether the right ventricle is of adequate size and function for an eventual biventricular repair. Patients with hypoplastic tricuspid valves commonly form coronary sinusoids, and those with more severe disease may rely upon these sinusoids for coronary circulation, a physiology termed right ventricular dependent coronary circulation. Many centers perform cardiac catheterization on all neonates with PA/IVS to define coronary anatomy and to determine coronary dependence. Catheterization data along with echocardiographic description of the tricuspid valve and right ventricle size, function, and morphology are often adequate to determine the initial course of management, which can include PDA stent or percutaneous pulmonary valvuloplasty in the catheterization lab, biventricular surgical repair, surgical aortopulmonary shunt, or primary listing for transplantation. The most classic management algorithm is based on a study that recommends biventricular repair in patients with a tricuspid valve *z*-score greater than -3.[8] However, many centers favor a biventricular repair even for patients with smaller tricuspid valves.[9,10] Some centers advocate creation of a patent right ventricular outflow tract in all patients who do not have right ventricular dependent coronary circulation, because decompressing the RV may be beneficial to encourage ventricular growth and prevent hypertensive RV cavities and the associated negative ventricular-ventricular interactions.[11]

Pulmonary valve stenosis is considered "critical" when maintenance of a ductus arteriosus is necessary to maintain adequate pulmonary blood flow. After diagnosis is confirmed with echocardiography, these patients are typically referred to the cardiac catheterization laboratory for transcutaneous pulmonary valve balloon dilation. Surgical approach to critical pulmonary valve stenosis is reserved for complex (particularly sub- or supravalvar) lesions or when catheterization has failed to relieve obstruction. Although balloon or surgical dilation is often effective at removing the valve gradient, the patient will often remain cyanotic due to hypertrophy of the right ventricle and right-to-left shunting at the atrial level. This may prompt use of prostaglandin to maintain ductal patency while waiting for the ventricular hypertrophy to regress. However, preservation of ductal patency causes the pulmonary artery to remain at systemic level pressure and may delay regression of hypertrophy. Judicious use of prostaglandin infusions to maintain oxygen saturations greater than 75% is certainly reasonable. In patients who have prolonged desaturation, it is reasonable to consider stenting of the PDA or surgical placement of a systemic-to-pulmonary shunt. In patients with severe infundibular hypertrophy, relief of valvar stenosis may create dynamic right ventricular outflow obstruction.[12] Dynamic infundibular hypertrophy may be treated with fluid administration, sedation, and beta blockade and rarely requires surgical myomectomy.

An important scenario in which neonates may have inadequate pulmonary blood flow is when there is a source of shunting (either intracardiac or at a PDA) with severe elevation of pulmonary vascular resistance. In the neonatal population, there are a multitude of etiologies for this physiology. Initiation of medications to decrease the pulmonary vascular resistance (PVR) should be considered in patients with right-to-left shunting before shunts are removed due to the potential of precipitating right ventricular failure or inadequate cardiac output. This topic is more thoroughly discussed elsewhere in this text.

Inadequate Systemic Blood Flow

Patients with CHD that result in inadequate systemic blood flow (e.g., hypoplastic left heart syndrome, coarctation of the aorta, critical aortic valve stenosis, etc.) typically present with poor pulses, poor perfusion, or cardiogenic shock, commonly when the ductus arteriosus closes. Similar to other discussed lesions, many of these diseases are well stabilized with the administration of prostaglandin while undergoing further evaluation and surgical planning. Delayed diagnosis of some of these lesions may result in increased afterload on the left ventricle, which might cause ventricular dysfunction. In these patients, use of inotropic or vasoactive medications and resuscitative therapies might be necessary before surgical intervention

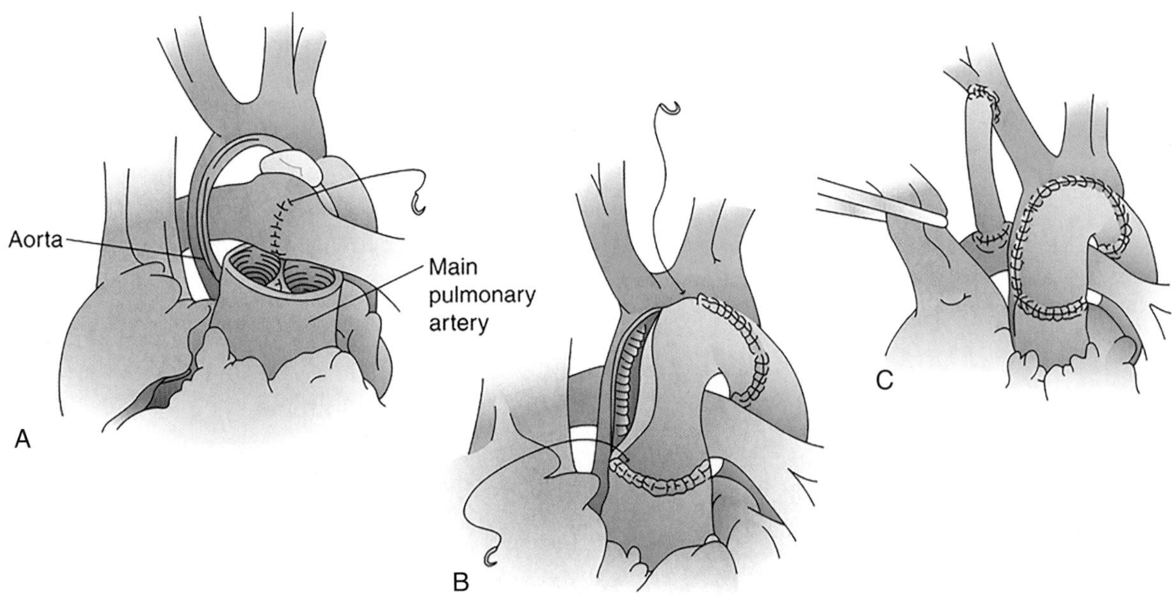

Fig. 38.6 Norwood Procedure for First-Stage Palliation of Hypoplastic Left Heart Syndrome. (A) The main pulmonary artery is divided proximal to the bifurcation, the ductus arteriosus is ligated and divided, and the aortic arch is opened from the level of the transected main pulmonary artery to a point distal to the ductal insertion in the descending aorta. (B) A segment of homograft is cut to an appropriate size and shape. This is sutured into place, creating an unobstructed outflow from the right ventricle to the pulmonary artery and aorta. (C) A polytetrafluoroethylene tube graft is placed from the innominate artery to the right pulmonary artery. The atrial septectomy is done while the patient is under circulatory arrest. (Reproduced with permission and after minor modifications from Well and Fraser. Congenital heart disease. In: *Sabiston Textbook of Surgery*, chapter 59, 1641–1678.)

can be pursued. Although the initial approach to lesions that cause inadequate systemic blood flow is often similar, there are lesions that require special considerations in their evaluation and management, some of which are discussed below.

Hypoplastic left heart syndrome is the most common cyanotic heart disease that would present with inadequate systemic blood flow in the absence of intervention. Patients with suspicion of HLHS should be started on a PGE1 infusion, and this should be continued through the ultimate palliation. Preoperative evaluation is often limited to echocardiography; however, many centers will refer patients with mitral valve stenosis and aortic atresia to cardiac catheterization to assess for the development of LV-dependent coronary circulation, a potential risk factor for poor outcome.[12a] The knowledge of this association may be beneficial for preoperative counseling, surgical planning, and management of hemodynamics and as a factor in the consideration of pursuing cardiac transplantation. Ideally, surgery for patients with HLHS will be performed within 5 to 7 days of birth. Because normal transitional changes cause a decrease in pulmonary vascular resistance, patients with HLHS are prone to pulmonary overcirculation and may develop hemodynamics that are difficult to medically manage without emergent surgery (Fig. 38.6). There remains variation in the surgical intervention for HLHS with centers performing either a Norwood with an aortopulmonary shunt, a Norwood with a right ventricle to pulmonary conduit, or a hybrid-Norwood procedure (PDA stent, atrial septostomy, and bilateral pulmonary artery band placement). Although outcomes have improved in all of these palliative procedures, morbidity and mortality remain disproportionately high compared with other CHD.

Critical aortic valve stenosis is defined as the presence of a normal-sized mitral valve and left ventricle with aortic valve stenosis that requires maintenance of a ductus arteriosus for adequate cardiac output. After diagnosis with echocardiography, these patients are emergently referred to the cardiac catheterization laboratory for percutaneous valve dilation (Fig. 38.7). Delays in intervention can be associated with left ventricular dysfunction, even with the administration of PGE1. Patients with critical aortic stenosis can be managed with either a biventricular or single ventricle palliation, with consideration toward the mitral valve size, left ventricular size, fibroelastosis of the ventricle, and systolic function.[13,14] Although there is often a push to obtain biventricular circulation,[15] borderline cases may have better outcomes with a single ventricular palliation.

Fetal echocardiography is notoriously poor at diagnosing coarctation or interruption of the aortic arch because these diseases often are not evident until the PDA closes. Therefore a high index of suspicion is necessary (Fig. 38.8) for any fetal echocardiogram that demonstrates hypoplasia of the aorta or left-sided cardiac structures or for interruption of the aorta in patients with associated abnormalities of posterior-malalignment ventricular septal defect (VSD), aortopulmonary (AP) window, or truncus arteriosus. Postnatal echocardiogram, physical exam, and monitoring for metabolic derangement as the PDA closes is necessary in patients at high risk for coarctation. For patients with hypoplastic left heart syndrome or interruption of the aorta, symptoms may develop even before the PDA has closed. It is important to remember that the PDA closes first at the pulmonary artery and last at the aorta and ductal ampulla; therefore a closed duct with dilated ductal ampulla may still develop coarctation as that region constricts. Furthermore, a moderate coarctation may not demonstrate any signs or symptoms initially but may lead to ventricular dysfunction that will demonstrate symptoms weeks later. After diagnosis of a severe coarctation or interruption of the aorta, awaiting surgical repair on PGE1 is almost always indicated. In the case of a late diagnosis of aortic arch obstruction in an infant presenting in shock, initial management includes PGE1 to open the duct in conjunction. In patients

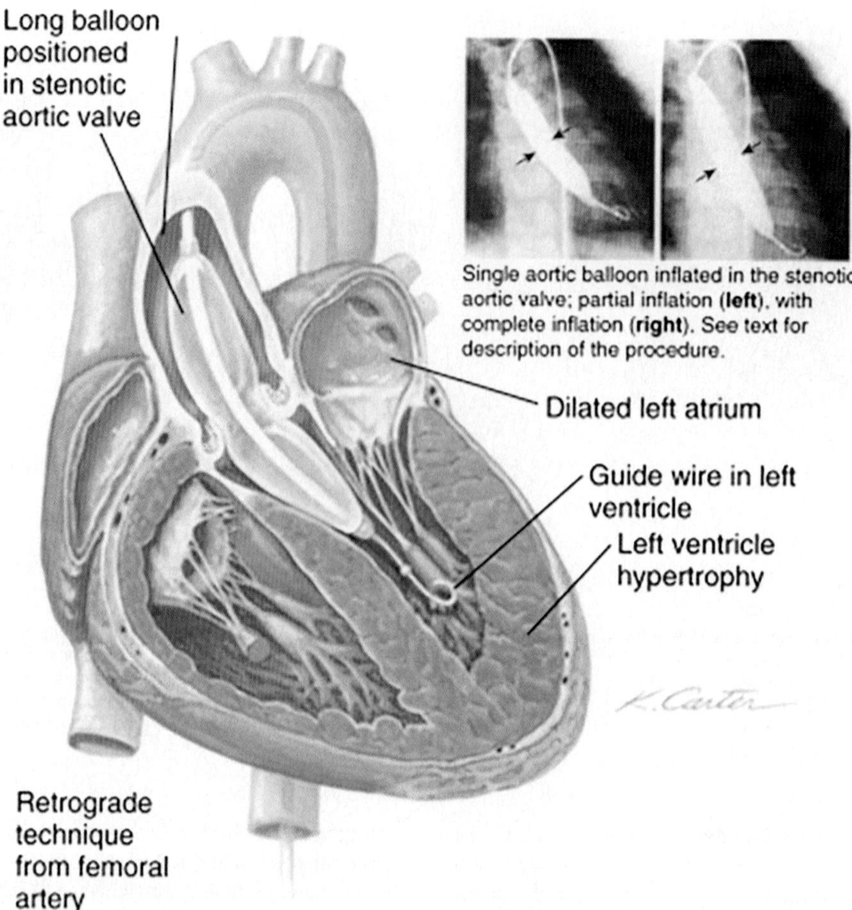

Fig. 38.7 Percutaneous Dilatation of Critical Aortic Valve Stenosis. A balloon catheter can be advanced across the aortic valve via the femoral vein, across the patent foramen ovale, through the left atrium, and antegrade out the aortic valve. Under both echocardiographic and angiographic guidance, the properly sized balloon can be inflated to dilate a stenotic aortic valve. (Reproduced with permission and after minor modifications from Alsoufi et al. Left ventricular outflow tract obstruction. In: *Critical Heart Disease in Infants and Children*, 51, 615–631.e3.)

with ventricular dysfunction, this should be done in conjunction with inotropic medications to support left ventricular function and cardiac output because the vasodilatory effects of PGE1 and re-creation of a left-to-right shunt may cause low cardiac output. Several days of medical management may be beneficial for the recovery of end organ function before surgical repair. If the duct does not reopen or cardiac function is deemed too poor to survive surgical intervention, some have advocated for the consideration of percutaneous aortic stent placement to allow organ recovery before definitive repair.[16,17]

Neonates with a surgical aortopulmonary shunt or PDA for pulmonary blood flow and patients with an unrepaired aortopulmonary window or truncus arteriosus are particularly vulnerable to the development of "pulmonary overcirculation." This term describes a physiology in which pulmonary blood flow is uncontrolled to the extent that systemic circulation becomes inadequate. This is most commonly due to an oversized aortopulmonary communication in conjunction with low pulmonary vascular resistance. Pulmonary overcirculation can lead to necrotizing enterocolitis, renal dysfunction, or other end organ failure. Although medication and ventilatory maneuvers to balance the blood flow to the body and lungs are often employed,[17a] mechanisms to increase total cardiac output is often more effective.[18] Ultimately, surgical manipulation of the aortopulmonary shunt or the underlying cardiac defect is the best way to manage severe or persistent pulmonary overcirculation. The term *pulmonary overcirculation* is commonly and erroneously also used to describe patients with pulmonary edema or respiratory symptoms due to excessive pulmonary blood flow. Patients with excessive blood flow but adequate cardiac output can often be managed with diuretic medication and medications to reduce systemic vascular resistance. This physiology is common in diseases with single ventricle physiology without pulmonary outflow obstruction or other large left-to-right shunts. In patients with persistent excessive pulmonary blood flow or congestive heart failure, it may be necessary to repair the underlying lesion or palliate with a pulmonary artery band placement.

Inadequate Intracardiac Shunts

Patients with CHD that result in inadequate intracardiac shunting may present with cyanosis or low cardiac output in a lesion that otherwise would be stable with the administration of PGE1 and adequate ventilation. Although many cyanotic heart lesions and single ventricle physiologies rely on intracardiac shunting for adequate delivery of oxygenated blood, there are particular lesions that commonly are affected by restrictive intracardiac shunts. The two most common cardiac pathologies that may need urgent diagnosis and management of inadequate intracardiac shunting include

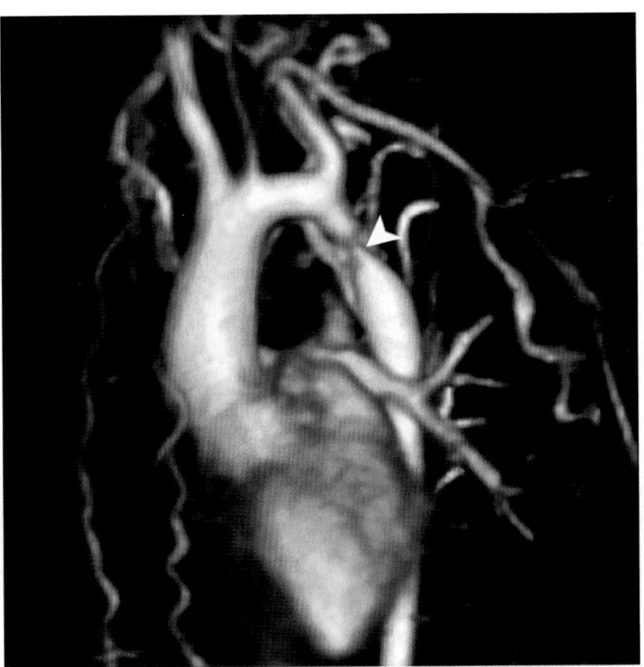

Fig. 38.8 Prenatal echocardiography is poor at diagnosing coarctation of the aorta (*arrowhead* seen here in volume-rendered 3-D reconstruction of magnetic resonance angiography showing a tight coarctation *arrowhead*) and multiple enlarged collateral vessels. (Reproduced with permission and after minor modifications from Grant and Griffin. Congenital heart disease. In: *Grainger & Allison's Diagnostic Radiology Essentials*, 2.1, 144–165.)

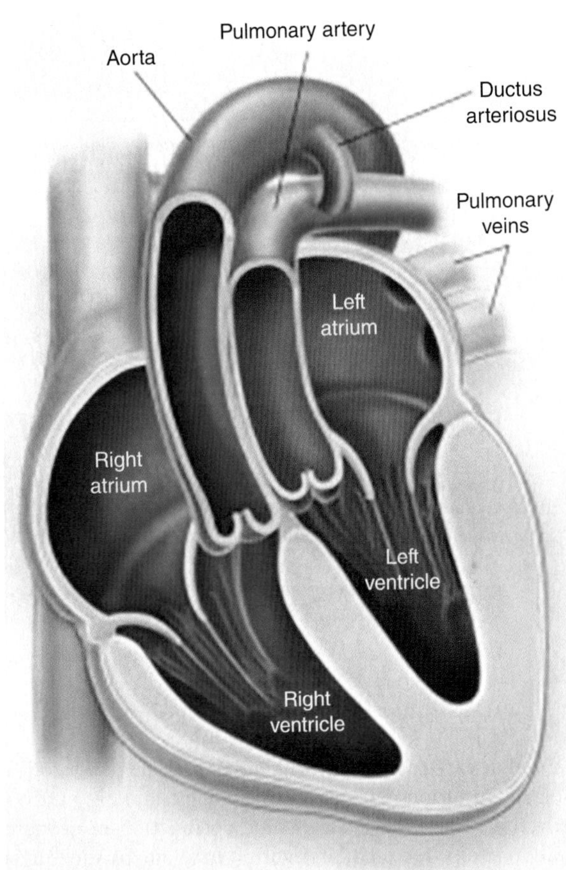

Fig. 38.9 Dextro-Transposition of the Great Arteries The atria and ventricles are in their usual position, but the aorta arises anteriorly from the right ventricle (RV) and the pulmonary artery (PA) arises posteriorly from the left ventricle (LV). (Reproduced with permission and after minor modifications from Haeffele and Lui. Dextro-Transposition of the Great Arteries. From: *Cardiology Clinics*, 2015-11-01, Volume 33, Issue 4, Pages 543-558.)

transposition of the great arteries and hypoplastic left heart syndrome (or its variants).

Patients with transposition of the great arteries (dTGA) have systemic and pulmonary circulations in parallel, such that deoxygenated blood is returned to the right atria, then is ejected from the right ventricle to the body while oxygenated blood is ejected from the left ventricle to the lungs (Fig. 38.9). Neonates with dTGA rely on atrial-level mixing to get oxygenated blood to their body. Although infants may also have bidirectional shunting at the PDA and at times VSD, these shunts are less effective at bringing oxygenated blood but are more effective at increasing pulmonary blood flow, which will potentiate the atrial level shunt. Infants who are born with a restrictive or intact atrial septum will demonstrate profound cyanosis not responsive to oxygen or mechanical ventilation and require intervention to allow improved mixing, most commonly with an urgent or emergent percutaneous balloon atrial septostomy. Although this commonly performed procedure is often without complication, vascular injury is possible and there has been shown a higher incidence of stroke in patients undergoing a septostomy. In patients with a small atrial communication that allows marginally adequate intracardiac shunting, one potential strategy is to continue a PGE1 infusion to maintain patency of the ductus arteriosus. This encourages increased pulmonary blood and greater atrial-level mixing. This technique to improve systemic oxygenation has the risk of creating worsening pulmonary edema and therefore is best tolerated when a prompt surgical plan has been made, ideally in the first 3 to 5 days of life.

Patients with HLHS or similar variants with severe hypoplasia of left-sided cardiac structures rely on atrial-level shunting of oxygenated blood to the right side of the heart to be ejected. A fetus that has an inadequate communication may develop left atrial hypertension, pulmonary arteriolar muscle hypertrophy, pulmonary lymphangiectasia, and pulmonary venous abnormalities. Some of these infants will develop hydrops fetalis, while others will have a seemingly uncomplicated pregnancy. A neonate with severe atrial restriction may present with cardiogenic shock and metabolic acidosis shortly after birth and need emergent resuscitation and creation of an intraatrial communication.[1] Given hypoplasia of left-sided structures, these infants commonly have a hypoplastic left atria with a thickened atrial septum, making creation of an atrial communication technically difficult with high incidence of adverse events. These patients typically need an atrial stent placement or atrial septectomy to maintain adequate communication. Given the technical challenges involved in the procedure and the rapid deterioration of these patients, some have strategized for patients to be delivered with cesarean section in the cardiac catheterization laboratory for immediate intervention. Despite many adaptations in this intervention, the outcomes for a patient with HLHS and a restrictive septum are universally poor, largely due to chronic issues with pulmonary lymphangiectasia, pulmonary artery hypertension, and pulmonary vein stenosis.

Ventricular Dysfunction

There is a subset of patients who have a structurally normal heart yet have inadequate cardiac output due to myocardial dysfunction.

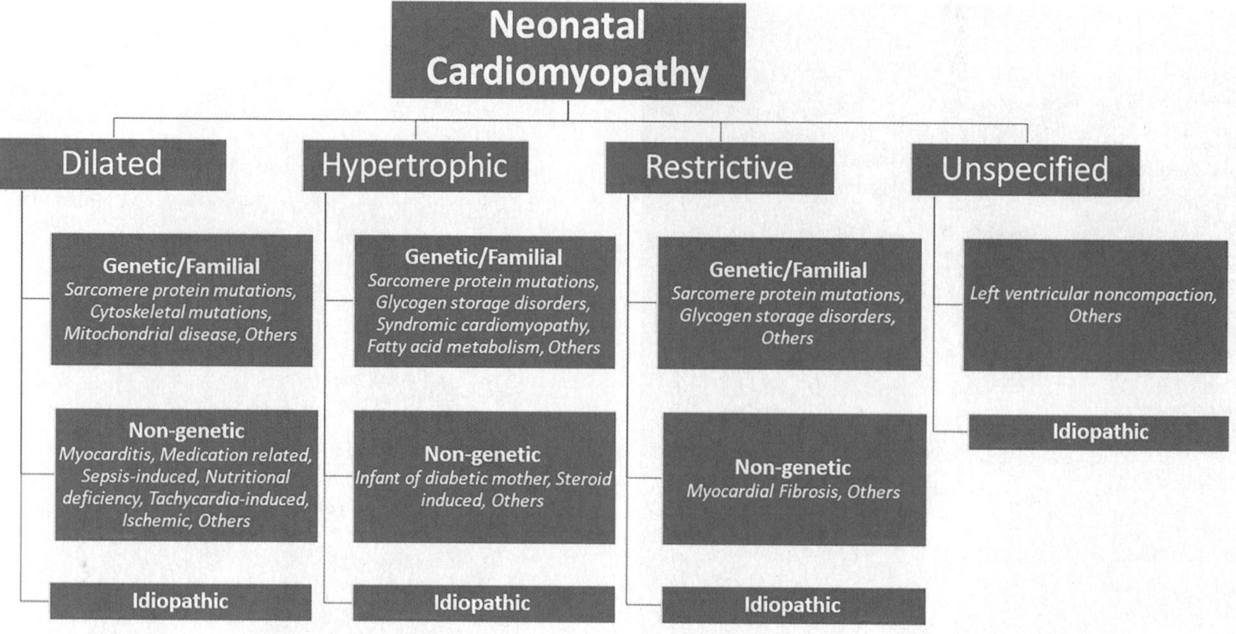

Fig. 38.10 Neonatal Cardiomyopathy Can Be Viewed in Four Broad Categories.

Myocardial disease can present with either systolic or diastolic dysfunction and in various phenotypes, including dilated, hypertrophic, or restrictive. The etiology of systolic dysfunction in neonates is generally one of three broad categories: cardiomyopathy, myocarditis, or coronary abnormality.

Thorough evaluation is necessary to determine the etiology of ventricular dysfunction. Clarification of the underlying cause may aid in prognostication but more importantly must exclude a reversible etiology. Echocardiography is helpful to establish cardiac structure and function but alone is often inadequate to determine the mechanism of dysfunction. For example, echocardiography has notoriously been poor at the identification of anomalous left coronary artery from the pulmonary artery and is unable to differentiate between myocarditis and cardiomyopathy as the etiology for dilated cardiomyopathy (Fig. 38.10). Laboratory studies may demonstrate a metabolic etiology of cardiomyopathy that may benefit from modified medical management. Diagnostic tools necessary for elucidation vary by patient but often include laboratory testing (Fig. 38.3), advanced imaging modalities, and potentially cardiac catheterization.

The medical management of neonates with a dilated cardiomyopathy is focused on interventions that ensure maximal cardiac output while ideally decreasing cardiac work. Although inotropic medications such as dopamine and epinephrine may be effective at increasing contractility and total cardiac output, they do so at the cost of increasing myocardial work and have been associated with arrhythmia, apoptosis, and increased myocardial oxygen demand. One of many maladaptive responses to low cardiac output is increased blood pressure via the increase in systemic vascular resistance through the renin-angiotensin system. Therefore, when blood pressure is adequate, the use of medications that decrease blood pressure may allow increased cardiac output while also decreasing myocardial oxygen demand. Diuresis may be necessary to decrease the symptoms associated with dilated cardiomyopathy and may improve heart failure exacerbations.

Neonates with hypertrophic cardiomyopathy have a range of presentations, from benign outflow tract murmurs to hydrops fetalis or cardiogenic shock. Hypertrophic cardiomyopathy may exist in isolation or in conjunction with other congenital heart disease.[19] Any patient with echo findings of hypertrophic myocardium needs evaluation of potential metabolic, mitochondrial, or genetic abnormalities for direction of management and prognostication. In addition to laboratory studies, skin or muscle biopsy may also be helpful for diagnosis,[20] and a genetics or cardiogenomics consultation is often of value. Diagnosis of neonatal hypertropic cardiomyopathy related to LEOPARD syndrome, Noonan syndrome, or Pompe disease may portend a more severe or progressive phenotype,[20–23] and evaluation for neonatal transplantation may be considered. Unlike dilated phenotypes, patients with hypertrophic cardiomyopathy often have hypercontractile myocardium, and inotropic medications are not clinically indicated. Medical management has not been demonstrated to change outcomes but may be employed to improve symptoms.[24] Beta blockade medications may decrease myocardial tone, allow for more time for ventricular filling, and prevent arrhythmia, all of which might aid adequate cardiac output and therefore are used as first-line therapy.

Although supportive medical management is typically the only treatment provided for neonates with impaired ventricular function, the use of mechanical circulatory support is occasionally necessary. The use of extracorporeal membrane oxygenation (ECMO) in infants is covered elsewhere in this text; however, it is important to review specific consideration for patients requiring mechanical circulatory support for inadequate cardiac output. The use of ECMO in neonates for cardiac indications is rising and now composes more than one-third of all neonatal ECMO.[25] The most common setting for neonatal cardiac ECMO is after cardiac surgery, most commonly in patients with single ventricle physiology. However, an important indication remains primary cardiomyopathy or myocarditis. Importantly, more than half of neonates who require ECMO for cardiomyopathy or myocarditis survive to discharge.[25] Neonates with fulminant myocarditis have the longest mean duration of ECMO; however, they have among the highest survival rates. ECMO is not suitable as a bridge to cardiac transplantation due to high rates of adverse events and posttransplant mortality, and this indication has almost completely been replaced with use of a ventricular assist device.[26,27] The increase in use of ventricular assist devices among neonates has led to a decrease in wait-list mortality with improving morbidity and has been described in increasingly small infants.[27]

Conclusion

As demonstrated through this brief review, neonates with critical congenital heart disease have a multitude of problems that present with several different pathophysiologies. Although initiation of a PGE1 infusion typically stabilizes most neonatal heart disease, there are special considerations that become evident after the initial diagnosis becomes evident. With good neonatal care, thoughtful cardiology consultation, and skilled neonatal cardiac surgery, optimal patient outcomes can be achieved. Most of these patients need cautious, meticulous follow-up care.

Section 7

CHAPTER

39 Neonatal Arrhythmia and Conduction Abnormalities

Shazia Bhombal, Megan L. Ringle, Yaniv Bar-Cohen

KEY POINTS

1. The normal cardiac electrical signal travels from the atria to the ventricles through a conduction system comprised of the sinus node, atrioventricular (AV) node, His bundle, and Purkinje system.
2. The AV node normally regulates the electrical action potentials from the atria to the ventricles. In some instances, the electrical signal bypasses the decremental AV node via an accessory pathway. AV block is a disturbance in conduction between the atrial depolarization and the ventricular response and may occur anywhere along the AV node–His bundle system.
3. Long QT syndrome (LQTS) refers to an abnormality in ventricular repolarization and is associated with syncope and sudden death.
4. Arrhythmias are relatively common in the neonatal period and can range from benign premature atrial contractions to wide-complex ventricular tachycardia (VT). Atrial arrythmias include the supraventricular tachycardias, which may be tolerated in the short term but can cause cardiovascular compromise over longer periods. Atrial flutter is a rapid atrial tachycardia due to a reentrant circuit revolving around the tricuspid valve.
5. Wide complex tachycardias from ventricular loci are uncommon in neonates. Rapid polymorphic VT or ventricular fibrillation can be seen in patients with channelopathies such as LQTS.

Normal Atrioventricular Conduction

In normal sinus rhythm, the electrical signal travels from the atria to the ventricles through the conduction system, comprising the sinus node (SA node), atrioventricular (AV) node, His bundle, and Purkinje system (Fig. 39.1). After the electrical signal reaches the end of the Purkinje system conduction, depolarization of the ventricle is completed through cell-to-cell activation from ventricular myocyte to ventricular myocyte. The cells then must complete repolarization prior to the next heart beat and activation. Pathology along any portion of the electrical conduction pathway will lead to varied conduction defects.

The role of the AV node is to conduct electrical action potentials from the atria to the ventricles. The AV node has decremental properties and therefore slows the electrical impulse from the atria to the ventricles. By causing a delay between the atrial contraction and the ventricular conduction, this decremental property of the AV node allows for enhanced ventricular filling due to ventricular contraction following the atrial kick. Abnormal signal conduction along the AV node can lead to relatively benign presentations such as first-degree AV block or pathologic defects such as third-degree heart block. Alternatively, in instances when atrial to ventricular conduction can bypass the decremental AV node, such as with accessory pathways, a short PR interval results and alters the sequence of ventricular activation (this is a feature of Wolff-Parkinson-White [WPW] syndrome).

Atrioventricular Block

AV block is a disturbance in conduction between the atrial depolarization and the ventricular response and may occur anywhere along the AV node–His bundle system. In adults, the most common etiology for AV conduction delay is not related to structural disease but rather to progressive fibrosis.[1] In neonates, congenital heart block is defined as the presence of AV conduction system disease in any form diagnosed prior to 29 days of life, with an incidence of 1 in 22,000 live births.[2] When diagnosed postnatally, congenital heart disease is associated with approximately one-third of AV conduction delays; however, when diagnosed prenatally, approximately one-half have congenital heart disease, most commonly left atrial isomerism and L-transposition of the great vessels.[2] When fetuses with congenital heart block have structurally normal hearts, a majority had exposure to maternal autoantibodies.[3]

AV block is designated as one of three degrees (first, second, and third), with nomenclature also including the ratio of atrial to ventricular contractions (1:1, 2:1, 3:2, etc.). Because the block occurs below the sinus node, the PP interval stays constant and can be marched out through any of the AV blocks, although the PR interval may change.

First-Degree Atrioventricular Block

First-degree AV block is defined as a delay between atrial and ventricular conduction and is most commonly due to delays through the AV node (although slow intraatrial conduction can also be responsible[4]). In first-degree AV block, the PR interval is prolonged beyond the upper limits of normal for the patient's age and heart rate, but a 1:1 atrial to ventricular contraction ratio is maintained. The PR interval includes (1) the time required for depolarization of the atrial myocardium from the start of the atrial contraction to its reaching the AV node (sometimes denoted as the PA interval, from onset of the P wave to the A wave on the His bundle electrocardiogram [ECG]), (2) the delay of conduction in the AV node (AH interval; the time interval between the onset of the atrial signal and the onset of the His bundle signal in His catheter recording), and (3) conduction

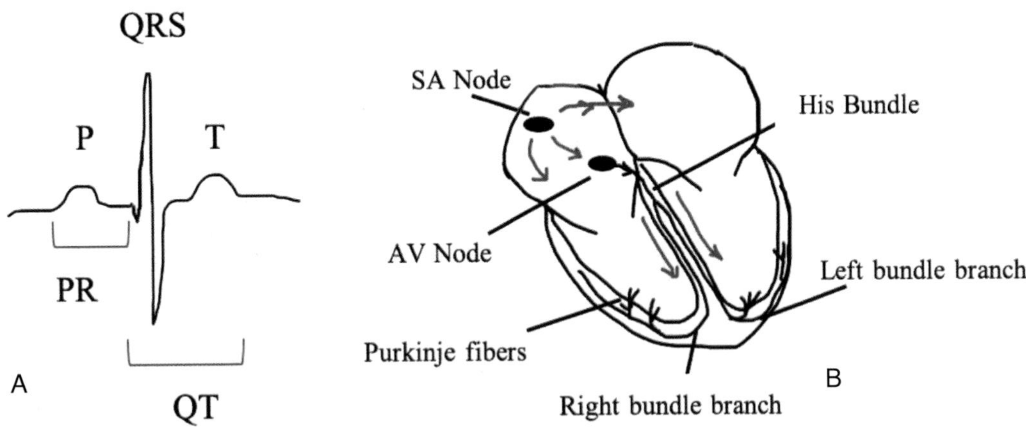

Fig. 39.1 (A) The electrical signal initiates from the sinus node leading to atrial depolarization (P wave), pauses due to the decremental conduction of the AV node (PR interval), and then rapidly depolarizes the ventricle through the His-Purkinje system. As the ventricular myocytes depolarize, they create the QRS complex and immediately begin repolarizing, ultimately completing repolarization with the end of the T wave (QT interval). (B) Electrical signal from the SA node to the decremental AV node, to the His bundle, and to the right and left bundle branches to the Purkinje fibers. *AV*, Atrioventricular.

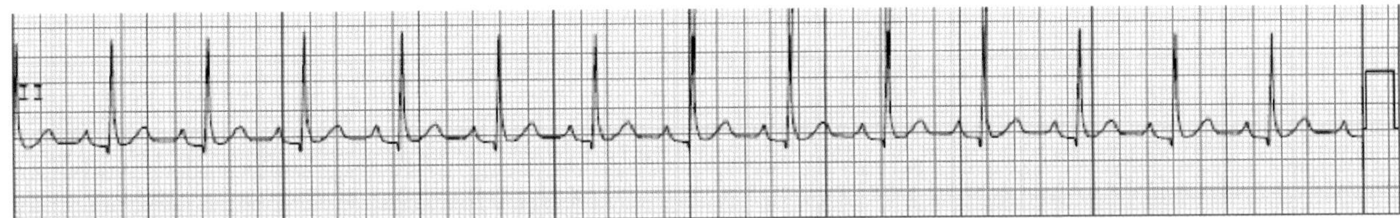

Fig. 39.2 First-Degree Block With Sinus Rhythm (PR Interval Measures Approximately 200 ms).

through the bundle of His until the time of onset of ventricular depolarization (HV interval) (Fig. 39.2). First-degree AV block can be seen in otherwise healthy young individuals and in athletes, which is generally due to increased vagal tone. Other less frequently implicated causes include congenital heart disease, infectious and inflammatory conditions, and drugs (such as digoxin or beta blockers). In the absence of heart disease, a prolonged PR interval does not typically progress to further degrees of block or produce hemodynamic instability; intervention is therefore not generally required.[4,5] A congenital prolonged PR interval does not typically progress to higher-grade block in neonatal life. In a cohort of 32 fetuses with exposure to maternal autoantibodies that can lead to heart block, eight developed first-degree AV block in utero. All had resolved by the first month of life without intervention in pre- and postnatal life.[5a]

Second-Degree Atrioventricular Block

Second-degree AV block is defined by interruption in conduction, typically within the AV node, where some, but not all, P waves result in a QRS, thus resulting in dropping of one or more ventricular beats. Second-degree AV block is usually divided into two patterns, Mobitz type I (Wenckebach) and Mobitz type II. For the purpose of this chapter, Mobitz type I and Wenckebach will be used interchangeably.

Mobitz Type I (Wenckebach)

In Mobitz type I, the PR interval becomes gradually prolonged from beat to beat as the AV node progressively fatigues until one QRS complex is dropped[4] (Fig. 39.3). Most examples of Wenckebach AV block in neonates demonstrate a narrow QRS, are asymptomatic, do not require intervention, and are related to medications or maternal connective tissue disease.[6,7] Wenckebach is generally related to abnormalities within the AV node and is manifested as prolonging PR intervals due to the ability of the AV node to decrement (prolonged conduction).

Mobitz Type II (Hay Phenomenon)

Mobitz type II AV block is a far rarer cause of second-degree block in neonates and generally occurs as a result of block in the distal conducting pathway below the AV node. Mobitz type II block presents with intermittent dropped ventricular beats without any prior prolongation of the PR interval and can rapidly progress to complete AV block (Fig. 39.4). In addition, because a junctional escape rhythm cannot conduct to the ventricles during severe Mobitz II block, very slow (if any) escape rates can be seen with progressive Mobitz II block. Mobitz type II block therefore has a more ominous prognosis, and permanent pacemaker placement is often recommended. Causes of Mobitz type II include myocarditis, cardiomyopathies, widespread sclerodegenerative conduction disease, myocardial infarction, congenital heart disease, and cardiac surgery.[4,5,8]

In the setting of 2:1 AV conduction, differentiating Mobitz I from Mobitz II conduction can be difficult. A prolonged PR during 2:1 conduction suggests Mobitz I block, but with a normal PR interval, either is possible. An additional consideration in the neonatal (and fetal) period is that 2:1 AV block can be a manifestation of long QT syndrome (LQTS) (where a prolonged repolarization period does not allow conduction through the ventricle when the next signal appears). As a result, LQTS (whether congenital or acquired) should be considered when 2:1 AV block is seen in the neonate.

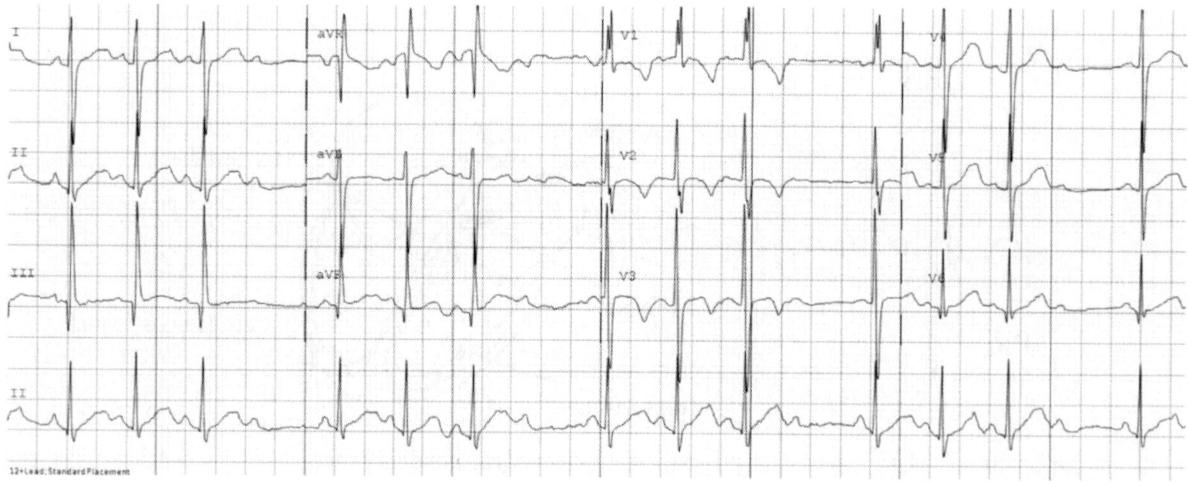

Fig. 39.3 Second-Degree Atrioventricular Block, Type I Wenckebach, With Small Prolongations of the PR Intervals Occurring Prior to a Dropped QRS.

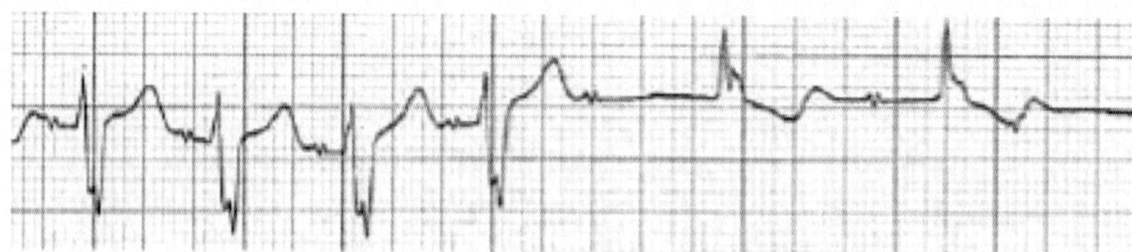

Fig. 39.4 Second-Degree Mobitz II Atrioventricular Block. A normal PR is seen followed by complete heart block with a wider-complex (ventricular) escape rhythm.

Complete Atrioventricular Block

In complete heart block (CHB), also referred to as third-degree AV block, the atrial and ventricular activations are entirely independent of each other (Fig. 39.5). Atrial impulses are not conducted to the ventricles through the AV conduction system, and the ventricles depolarize in response to a subsidiary intrinsic pacemaker, usually resulting in a slow escape rate. As with the previously discussed AV blocks, the P waves are regular, with regular PP intervals, and with an atrial rate usually comparable to the normal heart rate for age. The QRS complexes are also usually very regular but at a much slower rate than the P wave rate. A narrow QRS complex indicates that the subsidiary pacemaker (escape rhythm) is junctional and originates above the bifurcation of the bundle of His. Alternatively, a wide-complex escape rate suggests that the subsidiary pacemaker originates in the ventricular muscle (see Fig. 39.4). Most cases of congenital CHB have a narrow QRS complex and typically have a higher escape rate than is seen with wide-complex escape; these narrow-complex escape rates can vary in response to physiologic conditions.[5] During slow escape rates, cardiac output can be maintained by augmenting a slow heart rate with a stronger myocardial contractile force, a long diastolic filling time, and an increased end-diastolic volume resulting in an increased stroke volume.[9–11]

CHB can be divided into congenital and noncongenital forms as well as immune and nonimmune forms. The most common cause of congenital immune CHB is exposure to maternal autoantibodies. Nonimmune congenital forms of CHB are usually associated with structural heart disease such as left atrial isomerism, complete AV canal defects, and congenitally corrected transposition of the great arteries (accounting for approximately 14%–42% of cases of congenital CHB).[12] Noncongenital forms of CHB are usually due to AV node injury during congenital heart disease surgery; other forms of noncongenital CHB are extremely rare in the neonatal period.

Heart block affects an estimated 2% to 5% of infants born to primigravid women with anti-Ro/SSA and anti-La/SSB antibodies, and the risk is as high as 15% to 20% in women who have had a previously affected newborn.[13,14] CHB can result in significant morbidity, and mortality rates of up to approximately 20% have been reported, with the following factors associated with increased mortality: diagnosis in fetal life (particularly <20 weeks' gestation), presence of fetal hydrops, delivery prior to 33 weeks' gestation, ventricular rate <50 bpm, and decreased LV function.[13,15,16] Anti-Ro/SSA and/or anti-La/SSB bind to fetal cardiac tissue and cause an immune-mediated injury to the AV node and its surrounding tissue. Although most signs and symptoms in neonatal lupus are transient and disappear as the maternal antibodies fade within the first 6 months of life, congenital heart block is caused by fibrous replacement of the AV node and is frequently permanent, especially when third-degree AV block is present. In addition to congenital heart block, antibody-mediated cardiomyopathy may occur with neonatal lupus, with cardiac failure due to cardiomyopathy a leading cause of early death.[17] A majority of patients with congenital CHB require a permanent pacemaker before adulthood, with one study reporting an epicardial pacemaker approach in the majority of patients at a median of 10 days after birth.[15] Permanent pacing is a Class I indication for the symptomatic individual with congenital complete AV block or the infant with a resting heart rate of <55 bpm, or <70 bpm if associated with congenital heart disease.[18]

Standardized therapy for congenital CHB in utero is lacking. In patients with congenital CHB and normally structured hearts, early access to pacing wires immediately after birth is associated with improved survival.[19] Once in-utero CHB develops, it is generally irreversible, with goals of fetal therapy to halt advance to higher degrees of block and reduce clinical compromise and

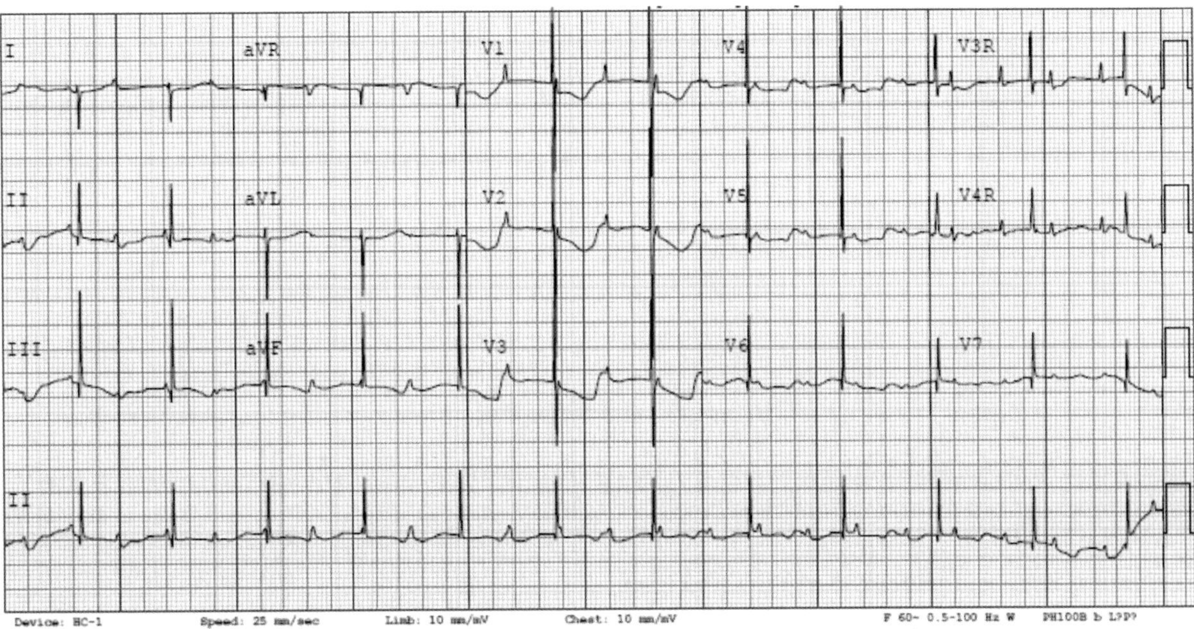

Fig. 39.5 Complete Third-Degree Heart Block With Atrial Rate Nearly Twice the Ventricular Rate.

development of hydrops.[12] Although there is no standardized management due to lack of definitive efficacy, antenatal medical therapies that have been utilized include steroids to mitigate the inflammatory response, plasmapheresis and intravenous immunoglobulin (IVIG) to reduce autoimmune antibodies, and beta-sympathomimetics to increase heart rate and augment cardiac output.[12,19] Studies have demonstrated mixed benefit to providing steroids to mothers with fetuses in CHB, and with the risks to mother and fetus of steroid administration, such as risk of maternal diabetes and risk of postnatal neurodevelopmental delay, there remains no generalized recommendation for steroid administration in utero for CHB.[12,15,19]

Intraventricular Conduction Delays

From the AV node, the electrical signal conducts through the His–Purkinje system into left and right bundle branches. Intraventricular conduction delays can occur anywhere along this path (Fig. 39.6). Whereas the right bundle branch remains as one, the left bundle divides into the left anterior and posterior fascicles to activate different portions of the ventricle. In adults, fascicular blocks are most commonly associated with coronary artery disease.[20] These are uncommon in the pediatric population, although younger patients may demonstrate hemiblocks in the setting of cardiac surgical repairs such as ventricular septal defect closure.[20]

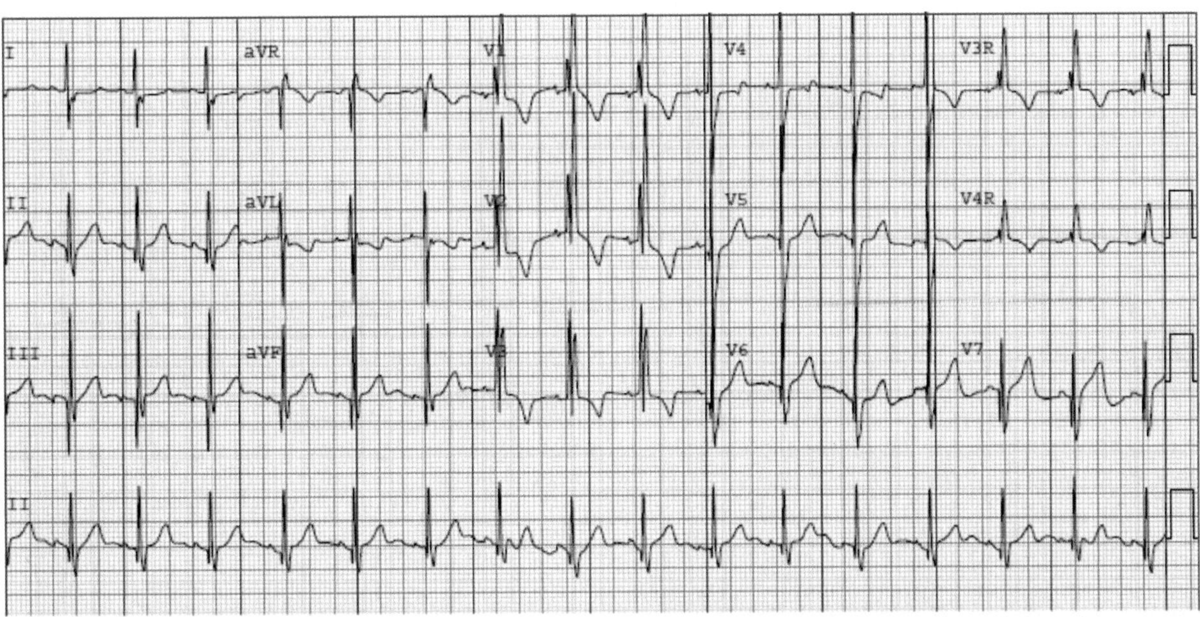

Fig. 39.6 Right Bundle Branch Block. Note the widened QRS and RSR′ morphology in right precordial leads (e.g., V_1).

Table 39.1 Sample of Congenital LQTS Genes and Associations, Including Triggers for Events

LQTS Type	Gene	Channel	Frequency	Findings
LQTS 1	*KCNQ1*	Potassium	40%–55%	Triggered by exercise (swimming), stress Homozygous in Jervell and Lange-Nielsen syndrome type 1
LQTS 2	*KCNH2*	Potassium	30%–45%	Triggered by auditory stimulation (e.g., alarm clock) or emotional stress
LQTS 3	*SNC5A*	Sodium	5%–10%	Triggered by sleep
LQTS 5	*KCNE1*	Potassium	Rare	Homozygous in Jervell and Lange-Nielsen syndrome type 2
LQTS 7	*KCNJ2*	Potassium	Rare	Andersen-Tawil syndrome: muscle weakness and facial dysmorphism
LQTS 8	*CACNA1C*	Calcium	Rare	Timothy syndrome: hand/foot, facial, and neurodevelopmental anomalies

(Adapted from Mizusawa Y, Horie M, Wilde AA. Genetic and clinical advances in congenital long QT syndrome. *Circ J.* 2014;78:2827–2833; Schwartz PJ, Crotti L, Insolia R. Long-QT syndrome. *Circ Arrhythm Electrophysiol.* 2012;5:868–877.)

Long QT Syndrome

LQTS refers to an abnormality in ventricular repolarization and is associated with syncope and sudden death. LQTS occurs when the ionic current leading to ventricular repolarization is affected by abnormalities in potassium channel, sodium channel, or sometimes calcium channel function that prolong the action potential and result in a prolonged QT interval on the ECG.[21] The incidence of LQTS is estimated to be approximately 1 in 2000, and approximately 10% of sudden infant death syndrome (SIDS) cases are found to have a genetic mutation associated with LQTS.[22,23] There is a strong genetic association in LQTS, but making a diagnosis is at times challenging. In one large screening study, 90% of infants with QTc intervals of greater than 470 ms had genetic testing and 43% had disease-causing LQTS mutations identified, of which approximately 94% were inherited from a parent.[22] There are multiple types of LQTS; however, the most common are LQTS 1 to 3, which compose approximately 90% of all genotyped LQTS (Table 39.1).[24]

Cardiac events such as syncope, cardiac arrest, or sudden cardiac death can occur in approximately one-third of patients with LQTS. Symptoms in LQTS manifest due to development of Torsades de Pointes, a ventricular tachycardia (VT) that can degenerate into ventricular fibrillation.[24] Undiagnosed, symptomatic LQTS results in death in up to 20% of patients in their first year and 50% by 10 years.[25] In patients with genotyped LQTS, approximately 50% do not have symptoms and up to 30% do not manifest LTQS on ECG.[25] If symptoms occur, 90% occur by 40 years of age, with 50% having their first event as a teenager.[21] Beta blockers have long been used as primary therapy for LQTS, including in infancy, and decrease the incidence of cardiac events. However, for patients with a history of cardiac events or other symptoms in the first year of life, those who demonstrate 2:1 AV block in the setting of LQTS (Fig. 39.7), or patients with Jervell or Lange-Nielsen syndromes, additional strategies are often necessary, such as placement of pacemakers, implantable cardioverter defibrillators, and/or left cardiac sympathetic denervation.[21,25] Implantable

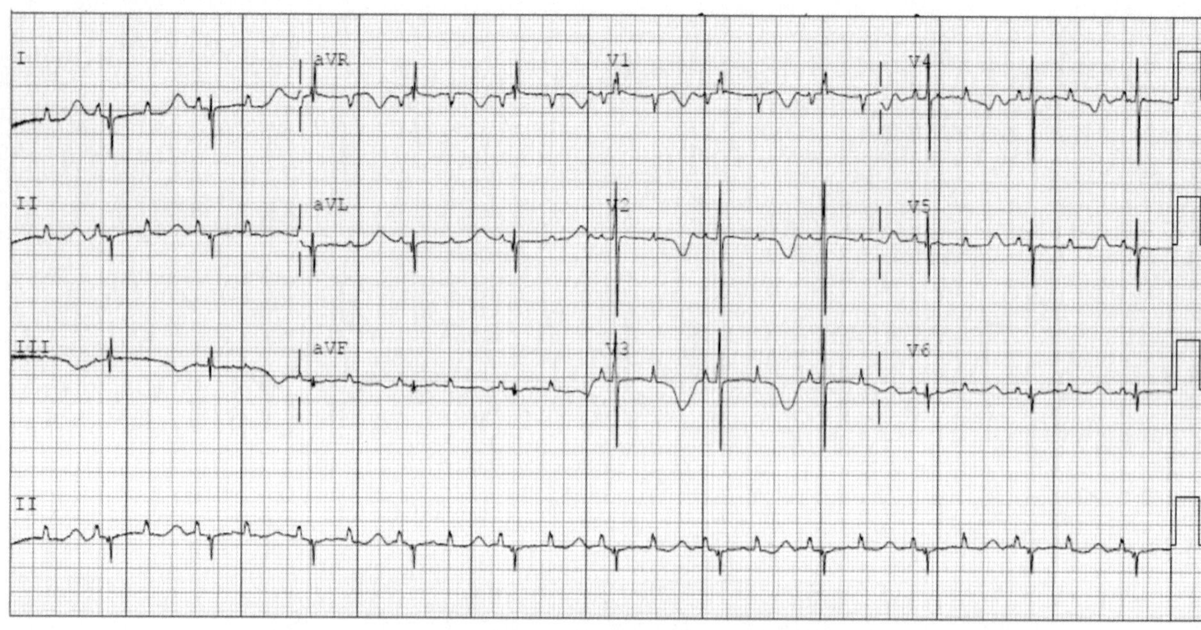

Fig. 39.7 Long QT Syndrome With 2:1 Atrioventricular Block.

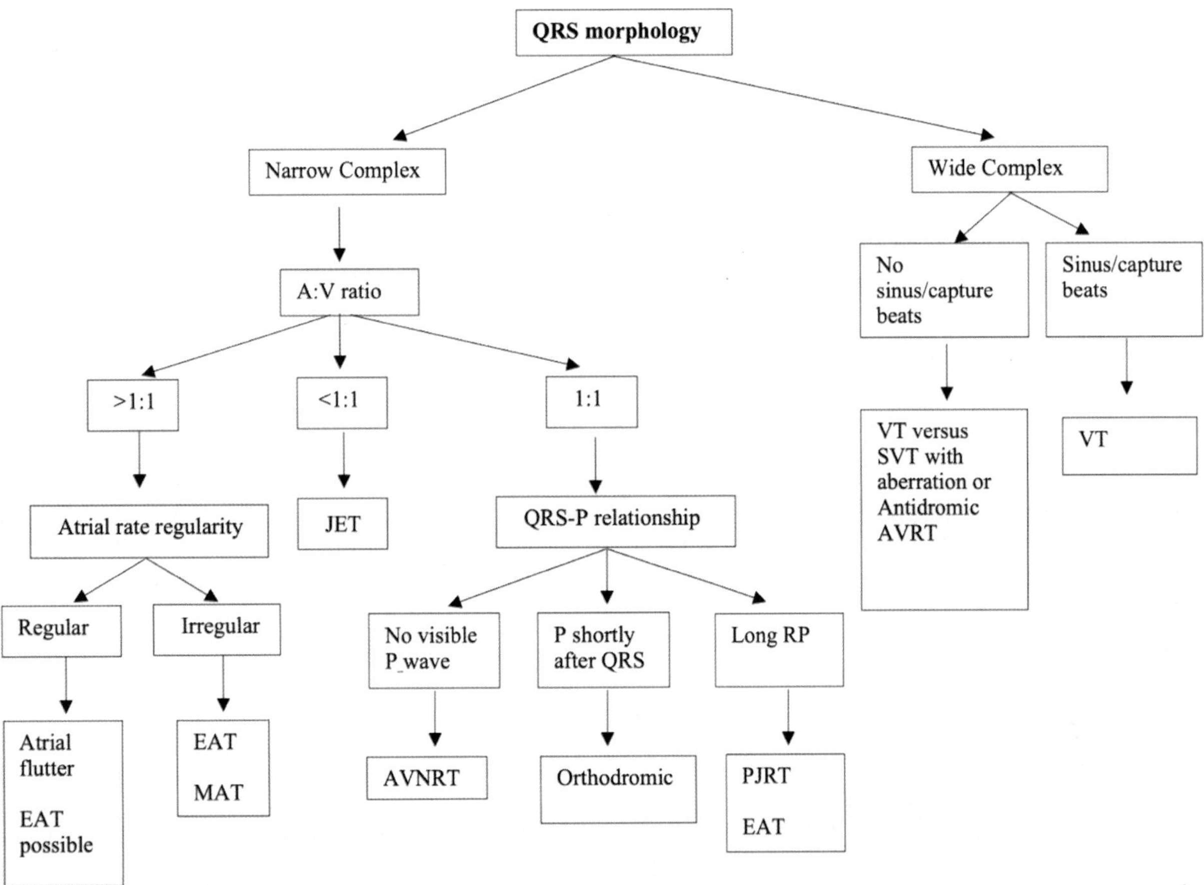

Fig. 39.8 Algorithm for Categorizing Tachyarrhythmias. *AVNRT,* Atrioventricular nodal reentry tachycardia; *AVRT,* atrioventricular reentry tachycardia; *EAT,* ectopic atrial tachycardia; *JET,* junctional ectopic tachycardia; *MAT,* multifocal atrial tachycardia; *PJRT,* permanent junctional reciprocating tachycardia; *SVT,* supraventricular tachycardia; *VT,* ventricular tachycardia. (Adapted from Kothari DS. Neonatal tachycardias: an update. *Arch Dis Child Fetal Neonatal Ed.* 2006;91:F136–F144).

cardioverter defibrillator placement is recommended if patients have a history of cardiac arrest (class 1) and may be useful in patients on beta blockers with syncopal events (class II).[26] Infants with LQTS and third-degree AV block or 2:1 AV block have a high mortality rate, and permanent pacemaker placement may be necessary.[18,27] Although 2:1 AV block in LQTS has been traditionally viewed as portending a very poor prognosis, one entire cohort survived to follow-up (earliest at 15 months).[28] Notably, all patients had early initiation of beta blockers, and 92% had a cardiac rhythm device placed.

Tachyarrhythmias

Arrhythmias are relatively common in the neonatal period. They can range from benign premature atrial contractions (PACs) to malignant wide-complex VT. Supraventricular tachycardia (SVT) is a particularly important arrhythmia in neonatal care and refers to tachycardia arising from above the ventricle, including atrioventricular tachycardia (AVRT), atrioventricular nodal reentrant tachycardia (AVNRT), atrial flutter, ectopic atrial tachycardia (EAT), and multifocal atrial tachycardia (MAT). SVT has an incidence of approximately 1 in 250 to 1 in 1000 children, with AVRT the most common pathologic tachycardia in the neonate.[29]

When assessing tachyarrhythmias, differentiating wide complex from narrow complex followed by other cues from the ECG can narrow the differential diagnosis and allow for tailoring of management (Fig. 39.8). Reviewing inpatient telemetry monitoring may be particularly important for diagnosing SVT, because gradual rate increases are far more suggestive of sinus tachycardia versus abrupt increases more commonly associated with SVT.

Premature Contractions/ Extrasystolic Beats

PACs are the most common benign arrhythmia in the neonatal population, with one study demonstrating this finding on 51% of ECGs in normal newborns.[30] PACs result in a P wave occurring prior to when the next sinus beat would have occurred. Depending on the timing of the PAC in relation to the last sinus beat and on the patient's AV conduction properties, the PAC can generally result in one of three scenarios: (1) the PAC can conduct normally through the AV node and His–Purkinje system and result in a normal-complex QRS, (2) the PAC can block through the AV conduction system and result in no ventricular contraction (no QRS), or (3) the PAC can conduct through the AV node but aberrate (due to part of the His–Purkinje system still being in its refractory period from the last sinus beat) and therefore result in a wider QRS than the normal-complex QRS. At times, PACs can come in repeating patterns, such as atrial bigeminy (an alternating pattern of the normally conducted signal followed by a premature atrial beat) or atrial trigeminy (a repeating pattern

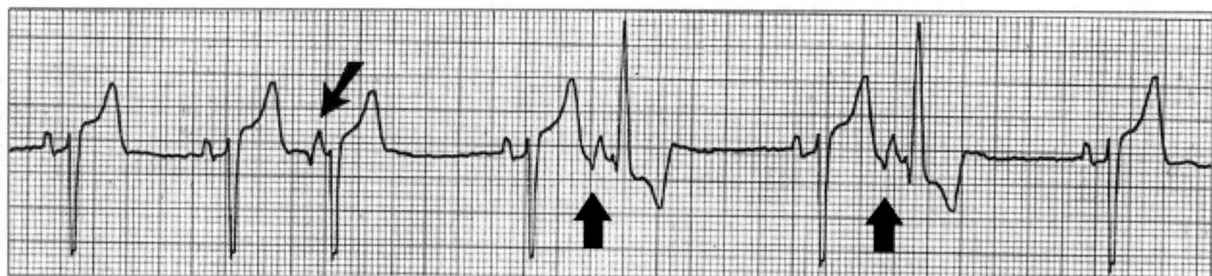

Fig. 39.9 Atrial Bigeminy. With the first premature atrial contraction *(narrow arrow)*, conduction through the AV node with a narrow-complex QRS is seen. With the subsequent premature atrial contractions *(wide arrows)*, aberration results in a wider QRS.

of two normally conducted signals followed by a premature atrial beat) (Fig. 39.9).

Premature ventricular contractions (PVCs) are less common than PACs; however, 18% of newborns were found to have benign isolated PVCs on a Holter monitor within the first 24 hours of life.[30] In a small study of neonates with frequent PVCs and no underlying structural heart disease, resolution occurred in the first few months of life.[31]

Supraventricular Tachycardia

SVT in the neonatal period is often well tolerated in the short term but can result in severe cardiovascular compromise (especially if not identified for potentially days prior to presentation). SVT can be categorized as reentrant (most commonly due to AVRT) or result from abnormal automacity (such as in EAT). Generally, SVT is associated with a narrow-complex QRS. However, if the His–Purkinje system is still in its refractory period at the time of the next fast heart beat, the QRS may widen, characterizing the tachycardia as SVT with aberration. The most common SVT subtype in neonates is atrioventricular reentrant tachycardia (AVRT), with orthodromic reciprocating tachycardia (ORT) being the most common type of AVRT. The next most common is atrial flutter, with other forms of SVT fairly uncommon. Differentiating the type of SVT is imperative, because response to therapy differs depending on the subtype (Fig. 39.10). As such, obtaining an ECG with rhythm strip before, during, and after intervention can be integral to making a diagnosis.

Atrioventricular Reentrant Tachycardia

AVRT occurs due to accessory pathways that allow conduction from ventricles to atria (or atria to ventricles) outside of the normal AV node. These accessory pathways are located along the AV groove and disrupt the usual fibrous continuity of the AV valves that separate the atria and ventricles. Forms of AVRT include ORT, antidromic

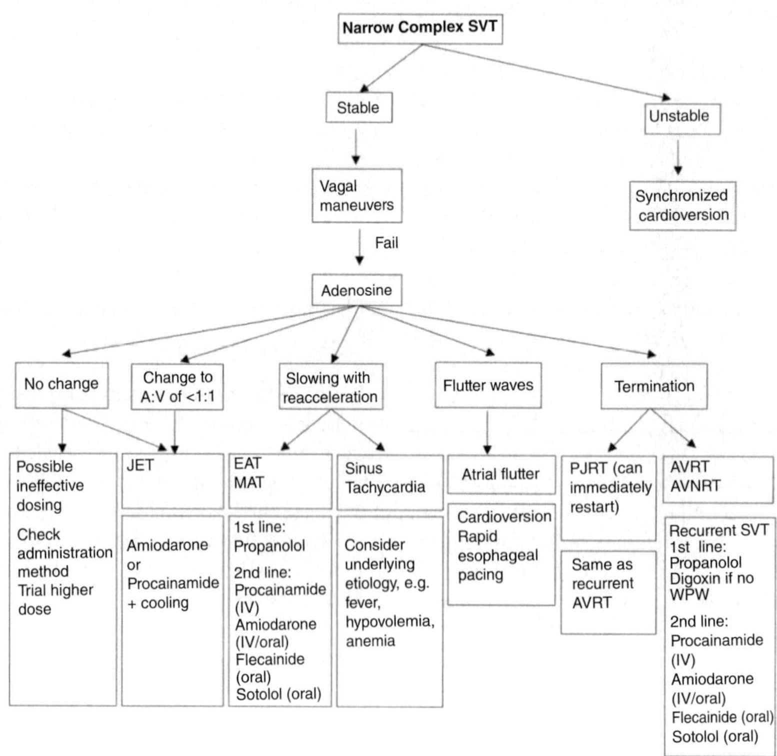

Fig. 39.10 Management of Tachyarrhythmias. *AVNRT,* Atrioventricular nodal reentry tachycardia; *AVRT,* atrioventricular reentry tachycardia; *EAT,* ectopic atrial tachycardia; *JET,* junctional ectopic tachycardia; *MAT,* multifocal atrial tachycardia; *PJRT,* permanent junctional reciprocating tachycardia; *SVT,* supraventricular tachycardia; *VT,* ventricular tachycardia.

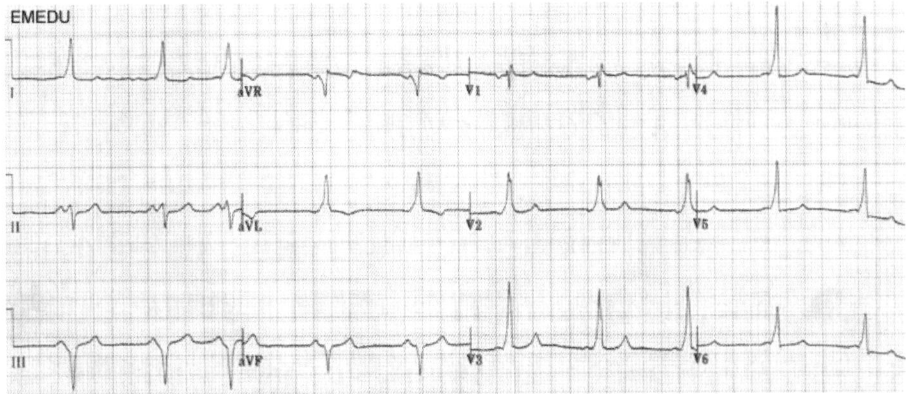

Fig. 39.11 ECG During Sinus Rhythm on a Patient With Wolff-Parkinson-White Syndrome. *Arrow* points to the delta wave (upslurring at the start of the QRS).

reentrant tachycardia (ART), and permanent junctional reciprocating tachycardia (PJRT).

Orthodromic Reentrant Tachycardia

Accessory pathways can manifest as WPW syndrome when antegrade conduction through the accessory pathway (from atria to ventricles) causes the QRS to prolong during sinus rhythm. In WPW syndrome, a short PR interval is seen and demonstrates the ability of the electrical conduction to travel from the atria to the ventricle while bypassing the decremental AV node (which otherwise slows conduction). A delta wave with a wider QRS is also seen due to the early activation of the ventricle and as the ventricle more slowly depolarizes through cell-to-cell mediated activation outside of the His–Purkinje system (Fig. 39.11). Most commonly, the tachycardia that occurs in the setting of WPW syndrome is due to retrograde conduction through the accessory pathway (from ventricles to atria). This form of AVRT is called ORT, where the electrical signal travels antegrade through the AV node to the His–Purkinje system (causing a narrow QRS), then back to the atria through the accessory pathway. WPW syndrome is typically associated with a normally structured heart, although it can occur in patients with congenital heart disease, most commonly Ebstein anomaly.[32] ORT can also occur in the setting of a concealed accessory pathway where there is no antegrade conduction possible through the accessory pathway, and the ECG during sinus rhythm does not demonstrate a delta wave (i.e., no WPW syndrome).

Antidromic Reentrant Tachycardia

Rarely, tachycardia propagates in reverse, causing another form of AVRT called ART. In ART, the electric circuit travels antegrade through the accessory pathway (causing a wider QRS) and retrograde through the AV node. Although ART is possible in WPW patients, it is considered extremely rare and is sometimes associated with a slowly conducting accessory pathway called a Mahaim fiber.

Permanent Junctional Reciprocating Tachycardia

PJRT is a form of AVRT that can affect the neonatal population, occurring in approximately 1% of neonatal SVT, and is typically an isolated finding with no associated congenital heart disease. PJRT characteristically manifests as a relatively slow AVRT (approximately 200 bpm) compared with what is typically seen with SVT from concealed accessory pathways. This is due to the slow (and decremental) retrograde conduction in PJRT accessory pathways, resulting in long ventricular atrial conduction times and slower tachycardia cycle lengths. ECG findings include a 1:1 tachyarrhythmia with a long RP interval. Although adenosine is effective in stopping the slow circuit and returning to sinus rhythm, this response is sometime short-lived, with recurrences often occurring immediately after terminations. As a result, PJRT can at times be very difficult to control.[33] Spontaneous resolution is unlikely, and if persistent, PJRT can lead to tachycardia-induced cardiomyopathy. PJRT often requires transcatheter radiofrequency ablation, sometimes early in life if antiarrhythmic medications are not sufficient.[34]

AVRT Management

The initial management for AVRT is vagal maneuvers followed by adenosine, both of which can slow or stop the conduction at the AV node and thus break the circuit. Recurrent episodes are often managed with propranolol or digoxin as first-line oral antiarrhythmic medications (although digoxin is contraindicated in patients with WPW syndrome due to potential effects on antegrade conduction, increasing the risk for ventricular fibrillation). A multicenter randomized controlled study of digoxin versus propranolol in infants with AVRT (excluding patients with WPW syndrome) or AVNRT did not demonstrate a difference in effectiveness between the two medications.[29] At times, stronger agents are required for management, including intravenous (IV) medications such as procainamide (sodium channel blocker), amiodarone (potassium channel blocker), or sotalol (beta receptor and potassium channel blocker) and second-line oral agents such as flecainide (sodium channel blocker), amiodarone, and sotalol. The accessory pathway and episodes of SVT can resolve in many patients with AVRT by 1 year of age.[6,29] Although patients with SVT are often on medication for control through the first year of life, a majority in the study were arrhythmia-free by 4 months of age.[29] Further studies are needed to elucidate optimal duration of therapy for neonatal SVT.

Atrial Flutter

Atrial flutter is due to a reentrant circuit revolving around the tricuspid valve that causes a rapid atrial tachycardia. Atrial flutter can initiate in fetal life and result in fetal hydrops. Atrial flutter can have variable conduction, with 2:1, 3:1, or 4:1 block referring to the ratio of atrial to ventricular contractions (Fig. 39.12). Because the AV node is not involved in the pathway, blocking the AV node with adenosine will be diagnostic by unmasking the flutter waves but will not terminate the arrhythmia. Rapid atrial overdrive pacing (often accomplished via placement of an esophageal pacing catheter) or

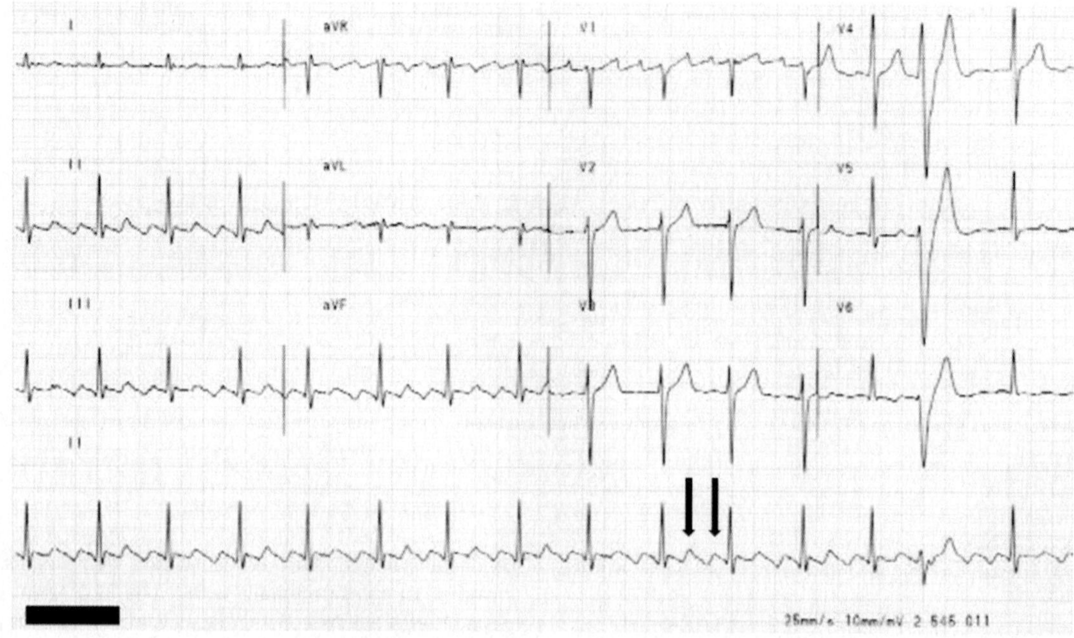

Fig. 39.12 Neonatal Atrial Flutter. *Arrows* denote typical "saw tooth" pattern flutter waves.

direct current (DC) cardioversion is generally required to stop atrial flutter, most commonly with no further medical management needed because recurrences outside of the early neonatal period are rare.[35]

AV Nodal Reentrant Tachycardia

AVNRT is due to a reentrant circuit involving a slow pathway and fast pathway of conduction into the AV node. AVNRT is extremely rare in the neonatal population, and when it occurs, it involves a similar management strategy to AVRT with vagal maneuvers/adenosine initially used to break the circuit.

Ectopic Atrial Tachycardia

EAT results in a narrow-complex (and sometimes irregular) tachycardia that originates from an ectopic focus within the atria. Unlike many neonatal SVTs that are due to a reentrant mechanism, EAT is typically due to an abnormality of automaticity resulting in rapid atrial depolarizations. In addition, because the etiology of EAT is usually related to abnormal automaticity, rate variability is often seen in the atrial tachycardia (Fig. 39.13). Due to the lack of a reentrant mechanism as the etiology, EAT generally does not terminate with adenosine or DC cardioversion. Cardiac dysfunction from tachycardia-induced cardiomyopathy can result if EAT is not controlled, and antiarrhythmic medications are often similar to those used for AVRT (despite EAT's usually being due to automaticity instead of reentry). EAT can resolve within the first year of life.

Multifocal Atrial Tachycardia

Multifocal atrial tachycardia (MAT, also known as chaotic atrial tachycardia) manifests as multiple ectopic foci within the atria initiating the cardiac rhythm and results in rapid and varied P wave morphologies. As with EAT, prolonged, uncontrolled MAT can lead to cardiac dysfunction. MAT can be very difficult to control medically, with potential need for multiple antiarrhythmic medications.

Management of Supraventricular Tachycardia

Although SVT is a fairly common diagnosis, it can be challenging to recognize and difficult to control, with as many as 50% of infants presenting with cardiomyopathy as a result of unrecognized and incessant SVT.[29] In a patient presenting with SVT, performing a 12-lead ECG prior to intervention can be paramount, because it may provide information regarding underlying etiology. Adenosine administration, which blocks the AV node, may terminate the tachycardia or uncover an underlying atrial flutter. In a hemodynamically unstable patient, synchronized cardioversion is appropriate to administer (see Fig. 39.10). In cases with acute, refractory SVT, amiodarone and procainamide have been utilized with success, with one study demonstrating procainamide was more efficacious than amiodarone (71% improvement/arrhythmia control with procainamide compared with 34% with amiodarone).[36] Even with resolution from an initial arrhythmia episode, with the high morbidity with neonatal SVT, many pediatric cardiologists and electrophysiologists elect to initiate preventive therapy in patients presenting with SVT.[37] Medical management options start with the common first-line therapies of beta

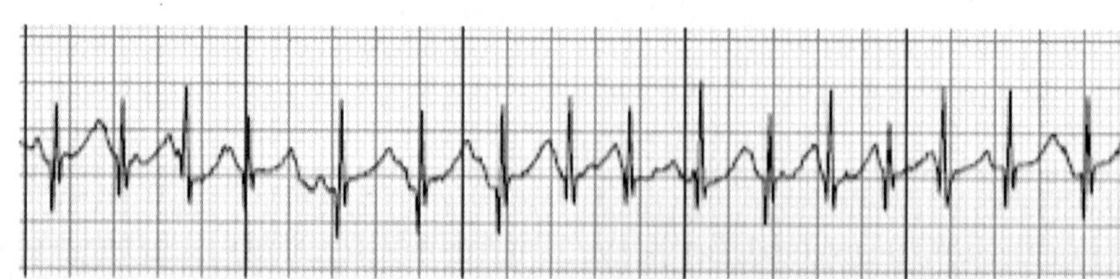

Fig. 39.13 Ectopic Atrial Tachycardia With Irregular P Waves Seen (Often Buried in the Preceding T-Waves).

blockers (e.g., propranolol) or digoxin (in non-WPW cases). Although calcium channel blockers (such as verapamil) can be used in older patients without WPW syndrome, these are contraindicated in infants due to their low calcium reserves and reports of hemodynamic collapse.[38] In more difficult cases, IV infusions of amiodarone (potassium channel blocker), procainamide (sodium channel blocker), esmolol (beta-blocker), and sotalol (beta receptor and potassium channel blocker) can be used. Additionally, second-line oral agents can be imperative for discharging patients home and include flecainide (sodium channel blocker), amiodarone (potassium channel blocker), and sotolol (beta receptor and potassium channel blocker).

In older children and adolescents, catheter ablation procedures are often utilized to eliminate the arrhythmia substrates. These procedures are typically performed on an outpatient basis and are usually considered elective and generally safe in the older child. In infants, however, these procedures carry significantly higher risks and are generally only considered when antiarrhythmic medications have failed.[39] The desire to avoid these procedures in very young patients is also due to the possibility for many tachyarrhythmia substates (such as accessory pathways and EAT) to resolve during infancy.

Junctional Ectopic Tachycardia

Although usually considered a form of SVT, the treatment of junctional ectopic tachycardia (JET) is often very different from the management of SVT described above. Similar to EAT and MAT, JET is due to abnormal automaticity (originating from the AV node instead of the atrial muscle). This arrhythmia is rarely seen in neonates except in the immediate postoperative period after repair of congenital heart disease. IV amiodarone or procainamide (with cooling) are often used, but this arrhythmia almost always resolves within days of the cardiac surgery. There is a rare nonpostoperative subtype (also known as congenital JET) that can occur in neonates and has high morbidity and mortality. Options for management include medical management (including amiodarone) and rarely transcatheter cryoablation.[40]

Ventricular Tachycardia

Wide-complex tachycardia resulting from VT is very rare in the neonatal population. Rapid polymorphic VT or ventricular fibrillation can be seen in patients with channelopathies such as LQTS. In addition to LQTS, etiologies of VT in neonates include other hereditary cardiomyopathies, cardiac tumors, myocarditis, congenital heart disease (especially after surgical repair), and electrolyte abnormalities (especially hypokalemia).[41] Rhabdomyomas are the most common type of cardiac tumor in the pediatric population (60%), with approximately 40% diagnosed in fetuses and with most located within the ventricular myocardium. Over 80% of rhabdomyomas are associated with tuberous sclerosis or a family history. Arrhythmia, most commonly VT, occurs in about one-third of these patients.[42] Antiarrhythmic medications such as propranolol may be utilized for rhythm control as the tumor regresses, with incessant cases potentially benefitting from tumor resection (especially in nonrhabdomyomas).

VT can occur in a neonate due to myocarditis, with patients presenting as critically ill and with myocardial depression. Medical management with amiodarone is beneficial in approximately 50% of cases, with extracorporeal membrane oxygenation sometimes required while managing the arrhythmia.[43] Finally, myocardial infarction, although extremely uncommon in neonates, should be on the differential diagnosis in a neonate presenting with VT.[43]

Overall, VT is much less common than SVT in neonates. One potential source of confusion is that SVT can present as wide-complex tachycardia due to aberration (when portions of the His–Purkinje system are in their refractory period and the result is slower ventricular activation). These tachycardias can be confused with VT. Sinus capture and fusion beats are unique to VT and can help elucidate a diagnosis. Capture beats represent sinus beats that are able to conduct through the AV node and lead to narrow complex beats during VT, whereas fusion beats are similar but change the QRS morphology due to fusion of a narrow complex sinus beat with the wide-complex arrhythmia.[44] If the infant is stable, adenosine may be considered to potentially terminate the tachycardia and differentiate VT from an aberrated SVT. However, if the infant is unstable, cardioversion is the appropriate management, and emergent therapy should not be delayed due to diagnostic exercises.

Summary

The synchronized cardiac cycle relies on a sequence of electrical events from the initial sinus node depolarization to the coordinated contraction of the ventricles. Failure can occur at a number of sites along these pathways, and although often benign, some arrhythmias can be life-threatening if not treated adequately. An understanding of the conduction pathways and their potential failings can therefore be mandatory for determining the correct arrhythmia diagnosis and the optimal management strategies. Whenever possible, an ECG should be obtained before, during, and after an intervention because this can make or confirm a diagnosis. In some cases, such as with neonatal atrial flutter, once an intervention is successful, no further management is needed. In others, such as accessory-pathway–mediated SVT, medications are necessary to prevent recurrences. A majority of neonatal arrhythmia resolves within the first year of life, and although it is a cause of high anxiety for parents, in many patients with arrhythmia, it is well-controlled and has good outcomes.

CHAPTER

40 Pulmonary Hypertension in Chronic Lung Disease

Megan L. Ringle, Gabriel Altit

KEY POINTS

1. Pulmonary hypertension (PH) in young infants is defined as a resting mean pulmonary artery pressure (mPAP) ≥20 mm Hg.
2. The mPAP at birth resembles the systemic blood pressure and then drops to infrasystemic levels over the first few days. However, many infants develop pathologic structural/functional changes in the pulmonary circulation due to lung injury and develop PH.
3. Prematurity-related bronchopulmonary dysplasia (BPD) is a leading cause of PH in infants. With improvements in our ability to salvage ever more premature infants, the histomorphology of BPD has changed from one appearing as altered healing and scarring in the "old BPD" to that of oversimplification of the lung structure in "new BPD," but the rates of PH continue to be high.
4. Imaging techniques such as echocardiography and continuous-wave Doppler with various exponents and cardiac catheterization for dye-enhanced radiography can help estimate the severity of PH.
5. Guidelines are available for clinical management, including for the enhancement of general care, oxygen supplementation, treatment with inhaled nitric oxide, and pharmacotherapy.

Introduction

Pulmonary hypertension (PH) is a state of "abnormally high pressures" in the pulmonary artery and is defined in neonates and young children as a resting mean pulmonary artery pressure (mPAP) ≥20 mm Hg. These pressure thresholds were originally defined for a postnatal age beyond 3 months after birth but are now being increasingly extrapolated to younger infants.[1–4] At the neonatal stage, pulmonary arterial pressure is often expressed relative to the systemic blood pressure.[5] As such, during the progressive fall of pulmonary vascular resistance, although the pulmonary pressure may be isosystemic in the immediate postnatal life (first days), it should shortly become infrasystemic after birth.[6] In many of these patients, the pathologic structural/functional changes in the pulmonary circulation are related to the developmental stage at which lung injury occurs.[7] In addition, the timing of injury, as in prior to or after birth, and consequent exposures to fluid, air, and the microbiome are also important determinants of whether these changes are most prominent in lung structure, metabolism, and/or the gas exchange.[8] One of the leading causes of PH in young infants is prematurity-related bronchopulmonary dysplasia (BPD) and related "chronic lung disease" with persistent needs for oxygen.[5,9–12] In the following sections, we describe the pathophysiology, clinical features, evaluation, and management of BPD-related PH.

Infants who develop PH in a setting of BPD do so despite the application of preventive strategies such as antenatal steroid use, surfactant administration, and noninvasive and gentle ventilation. BPD-related PH affects nearly one-third of very low birth weight infants; many survivors need long-term respiratory support and have poor neurodevelopmental outcomes and overall higher morbidity and mortality.[9,13–18] Most of these patients develop extensive changes in pulmonary arteries, veins, and capillaries.[5,11,19–21] An important difficulty in understanding the pathophysiology of BPD, and consequently, in the development of effective therapeutic strategies has been the lack of a clear definition of the disease. There are some concerns that the variability of the clinical course and outcomes or the histopathology in tissue specimens obtained from those with lethal disease actually indicate the disease to be a conglomeration of multiple forms of chronic lung injury, and the clinical definitions may be an oversimplification of the complexity of injury to the developing lung. Some of these subgroups may be related different genetic backgrounds, perinatal events, hyperoxia-related cellular injury, infections, altered healing after barotraumatic injury, and multiple other hitherto unknown causes. In the context of BPD, severe PH has been defined as being two-thirds systemic or more, advocated as a threshold of concern in that population frequently evaluated below 3 months.[5] Defining BPD is still shrouded in controversy.

Pathophysiology

BPD can be thought of as the classic "old BPD" with fibroproliferative changes of the pulmonary parenchyma in infants who require long-term ventilation and the "new BPD" seen in the most premature, extremely low birth weight infants.[22–24] The old BPD was seen from late 1968 to the 1980s with (1) altered pulmonary healing after severe respiratory distress syndrome (RDS); (2) hyperoxia-induced lung injury superimposed on severe RDS; or (3) a combination of tissue injury secondary to hyperoxia, healing RDS, barotrauma, and poor bronchial drainage and stasis of secretions following endotracheal intubation.[22,24]

The evolution of "new BPD" was rooted in the survival of more premature infants.

As the field of neonatology advanced, ventilatory management was gradually modified with acceptance of the lowest possible oxygen concentrations and gentle, noninvasive ventilation for the shortest durations that were adequate. Furthermore, advances in technology/management strategies in neonatal care, such as the use of exogenous surfactant, and in obstetric care, such as the administration of antenatal steroids, has improved survival in ever more premature infants with increasingly immature lungs.

The pathophysiology of "new BPD" in extremely preterm infants has been associated with multiple, concomitant risk factors related to pulmonary immaturity, ventilation-related lung injury, and altered tissue healing during the subsequent weeks to months.[25,26] The alveolar stage of lung development in humans extends from 36 weeks' gestation to 18 months after birth, but most of the alveolarization occurs within 5 to 6 months after term birth.[26] These infants with "new" BPD show two prominent changes: (1) hyperinflation with fewer, large-sized alveoli, with restricted septation and an overall reduction in alveolar surface area;[26–28] and (2) paucity and abnormal development of the pulmonary microvasculature. Unlike classic BPD, the airways usually remain free of epithelial metaplasia, smooth-muscle hypertrophy, and fibrosis but show increased elastic tissue.[26] There is focal inflammation.[26,29,30] Animal models of chorioamnionitis induced by the administration of *Escherichia coli* or *Ureaplasma* show altered lung maturation, increased angiogenesis, and inflammation similar to the changes seen in "new" BPD.[31–33]

The prominent vascular changes in new BPD have been a focus of intense investigation. BPD has been associated with decreased expression of vascular endothelial growth factor (VEGF) and the angiopoietin receptor Tie-2, and consequently, altered angiogenesis and endothelial cell proliferation of endothelial cells.[9,34] Decreased endothelial proliferation and development of the pulmonary vascular bed results in a smaller gas exchange surface area, which results in hypoxic vasoconstriction and impaired pulmonary blood flow. VEGF is known to promote angiogenesis and vasculogenesis and acts via nitric oxide (NO) production to promote the normal postnatal reduction in pulmonary vascular resistance.[9,35,36] Over time, these vascular changes contribute to pulmonary arterial vasoreactivity and cause structural remodeling with intimal hyperplasia and muscularization in the pulmonary vasculature. Preterm infants with severe BPD show abnormal intrapulmonary arteriovenous anastomoses, which may promote the shunting of deoxygenated blood into the pulmonary veins.[5,8,11,12,20,21,37–39] These vascular abnormalities tend to persist for longer periods in infants with severe BPD and may contribute to hypoxemia with secondary vasoconstriction and vascular remodeling.[9,36,40–42] Areas of ventilation-perfusion mismatch, abnormal airway architecture, inflammatory responses, subclinical infections, or oxidative stress may also contribute to BPD lesions. Many of these infants also have pulmonary hypertension and venous disease.[10]

Evaluation

Advanced BPD and associated PH frequently lead to right ventricular (RV) failure. These infants also remain susceptible to secondary events such as viral or bacterial pulmonary infections and associated changes in pulmonary blood flow. RV failure usually manifests with dyspnea, hypoxemia, and poor growth. Physical examination may show tachycardia and/or increased work of breathing. Some infants may have a systolic ejection murmur related to tricuspid regurgitation. RV afterload and RV dilation can cause loss of valvular coaptation.

Echocardiography is useful for screening of PH and evaluation of cardiac anatomy and function. The assessment of secondary changes is reliable at pulmonary pressures ≥40 mm Hg, although echocardiography does not allow direct estimation of pulmonary vascular resistance and may miss pulmonary venous drainage anomalies. In the presence of shunts, echocardiography may still detect but not always decipher the underlying cause of high pulmonary pressures. Current guidelines recommend use of echocardiography for screening of PH at 36 weeks' postmenstrual age in extreme premature newborns (<29 weeks of gestational age at birth).[5,8] Table 40.1 outlines recommendations regarding the evaluation and management of BPD-PH and is largely based on guidelines established by the American Heart

Table 40.1 Summary of Guidelines Regarding Evaluation and Management of Premature Newborns With or at Risk of Pulmonary Hypertension[a]

Team	A multidisciplinary team (NICU, PICU, Cardiology, Pulmonology, ENT, Nutrition, Occupational Therapy, Developmental Medicine/Neonatal Follow-up, Respiratory Therapy, Nursing) should be involved in the care of infants with BPD-PH. Infants with BPD-PH should have inpatient and outpatient follow-up with the multidisciplinary PH team and at intervals of 3–4 months (or earlier). Echocardiography, biomarkers, hemodynamic studies, and sleep studies should be done at follow-up, when indicated, and depending on the clinical progression and severity of underlying disease.
Screening	Echocardiography should be considered for screening of PH in a premature infant if: 1. there is severe hypoxemic respiratory failure after birth thought to be consistent with acute PH (i.e., persistent pulmonary hypertension of the newborn), despite optimal pulmonary management; 2. invasive mechanical ventilation is needed at day 7 of postnatal life, because early indicators of PH may be associated with a later adverse BPD profile; 3. significant and sustained respiratory support is required at any age, especially if there are recurrent events of hypoxemia; and 4. BPD is diagnosed (36 weeks' PMA); one may also consider screening if there is no formal BPD diagnosis but there is respiratory deterioration after 36 weeks' PMA.
Echocardiography	Echocardiography done for PH screening in the context of prematurity should be as complete as possible and include at least: 1. full anatomic evaluation, with special attention to the evaluation of shunts, structural abnormalities, pulmonary veins, and valvular stenosis/regurgitation; 2. assessment of ventricular (right and left) dimensions, hypertrophy, and systolic and diastolic performance; 3. estimation of pulmonary pressures (tricuspid regurgitant jet, pulmonary insufficiency jet, ductal flow); 4. assessment of septal configuration at the peak of systole at the midpapillary area (indicator of increased RV afterload relative to the LV afterload in the context of normal cardiac anatomy) and diastole (indicator of RV volume overload when flat)—consider measurement of septal deformation using the left ventricular peak-systolic eccentricity index; 5. documentation of the systemic blood pressure at the time of the screening (to compare the estimated pulmonary pressures relative to the systemic pressures).
BNP/NT-pro-BNP	When evaluation is consistent or suspicious for PH, consider baseline and serial measurements of brain natriuretic peptide (BNP) or NT-pro-BNP as a marker of ventricular overload—values do not replace other mean of screening or diagnosis modalities (such as: echocardiography or cardiac catheterization study).

Continued

Table 40.1 Summary of Guidelines Regarding Evaluation and Management of Premature Newborns With or at Risk of Pulmonary Hypertension[a]—*cont'd*

Other evaluations	Infants with a diagnosis/suspicion of underlying PH should have exhaustive evaluation for comorbidities that may impact an underlying lung condition, prior to the initiation of pulmonary arterial hypertension (PAH)-targeted medications. Investigations should include: 1. Evaluation for sustained hypoxemia 2. Evaluation for aspiration (consider evaluation by a swallowing specialist and videofluoroscopic swallowing study) 3. Evaluation for pathologic gastroesophageal reflux disease 4. Evaluation for structural airway disease (ENT) 5. Evaluation of pulmonary artery and vein stenosis 6. Evaluation of left-sided disease, such as ventricular diastolic dysfunction, mitral regurgitation, mitral stenosis, and aortic stenosis 7. Evaluation for aorto-pulmonary collaterals 8. Depending on clinical scenario and evolution, consider other rare etiology of pulmonary hypertension (infectious, genetic, thromboembolic, etc.)
Cardiac catheterization	Cardiac catheterization should be considered in selected cases, such as: 1. to confirm echocardiographic suspicion of PH, evaluate for disease severity and for contributions of shunt lesions (atrial septal defect, ventricular septal defect, or patent ductus arteriosus—when present), and address them by closure if appropriate; evaluate for the contribution of left-sided disease, if present, such as presence of pulmonary vein stenosis or LV dysfunction; evaluate for possibility of aorto-pulmonary collaterals; 2. to define need for addition of combination pharmacotherapy, especially if there is a need for systemic prostanoid therapy; 3. prior to the introduction of another pharmacologic agent (PAH-targeted therapy), in the setting of deterioration and echocardiography evidence of worsening PH or altered ventricular function.
Oxygen supplementation	Supplemental oxygen therapy should be administered to avoid episodic or sustained hypoxemia to achieve oxygen saturations between 92% and 95% in those with established BPD-PH.
iNO	Inhaled nitric oxide (iNO) should be considered in the context of an acute PH crisis and to be weaned after stabilization. The use of sildenafil may be helpful in the weaning of iNO.
PAH-targeted therapy	PAH-targeted therapy may be considered in those with BPD-PH after optimal management of their underlying pulmonary/cardiac condition. Pharmacologic treatment should be considered in those with evidence of high pulmonary vascular resistance and RV functional impairment, not related to left-sided heart disease (or pulmonary venous disease). The use of these medications is, for the majority, off-label and should be used with caution. Initiation or adjustment of PAH-targeted pharmacotherapy should be made based on disease severity, tolerance to effects (availability/cost/route of administration), and in conjunction with a specialist with expertise in PH.
Infection prevention	When eligible (according to vaccine product), ensure exhaustive and adequate protection with vaccination of the infant with BPD-PH and its entourage (respiratory syncytial virus prophylaxis, pneumococcal vaccination, influenza vaccination, SARS-CoV-2 vaccine [for the family and caregivers]). Crowds should be avoided, and caregivers should be taught appropriate infection prevention strategies (such as hands hygiene) to avoid flare-ups in the context of respiratory infections.
Parental/caregiver teaching	Training to recognize signs of respiratory distress or cardiac decompensation: diaphoresis, retraction, work of breathing, cyanosis, abnormal neurologic status. Caregivers should receive training regarding basic maneuvers for cardio-pulmonary resuscitation.
Traveling/altitude	Experts should be consulted if the family/caregivers consider traveling by plane (or moving to a higher-altitude area). The infant with BPD-PH may need a fit-to-travel assessment with, possibly, a hypoxic challenge test.

[a]Largely based on guidelines by American Heart Association/American Thoracic Society[6] and Pediatric Pulmonary Hypertension Network.[7]
BNP, Brain-type natriuretic peptide; *BPD,* bronchopulmonary dysplasia; *ENT,* Otorhinolaryngology; *iNO,* inhaled nitrous oxide; *LV,* left ventricle; *NICU,* neonatal intensive care unit; *NT-pro-BNP,* N-terminal pro-BNP; *PICU,* pediatric intensive care unit; *NT-pro-BNP,* N-terminal pro-BNP; *PAH,* pulmonary arterial hypertension; *PH,* pulmonary hypertension; *PMA,* postmenstrual age; *RV,* right ventricle.

Association/American Thoracic Society and the Pediatric Pulmonary Hypertension Network (PPHNet).[5,8]

The most reliable modality to assess pulmonary pressure and pulmonary vascular resistance is cardiac catheterization, but it is used less frequently in young infants because it is a relatively risky, invasive procedure. Catheterization can help exclude the possibility of left-sided cardiac anomalies. The procedure can also help assess the pulmonary vascular reactivity to pulmonary vasodilators. Unlike echocardiography, which can detect secondary changes seen at pulmonary pressures ≥ 40 mm Hg, cardiac catheterization can reliably detect mean pulmonary arterial pressures >20 mm Hg.[4,8,9]

In the absence of structural cardiac anomalies, systolic RV pressure may resemble systolic pulmonary arterial pressure (sPAP). Echocardiography can help estimate RV pressures through measurement of the peak tricuspid regurgitation (TR) jet velocity. Continuous-wave Doppler of the TR jet estimates the peak gradient between the systolic RV pressure and the right atrial (RA) pressure (Fig. 40.1). The modified Bernoulli equation ($4 \times \text{velocity}^2$) converts the velocity to a pressure gradient.[43,44] The sPAP is estimated by adding the presumed RA pressure of 5 to 10 mm Hg.[43,44] In the presence of a large ventricular septal defect (VSD) or large patent ductus arteriosus (PDA), the RV compartment is exposed to the systemic pressures during systole. Thus by definition, the TR jet may yield to systolic pressure in the absence of abnormal pulmonary vascular resistance. Similarly, newborns with pulmonary valvular stenosis or pulmonary arterial stenosis may have increased RV pressure (and TR jet) in the absence of increased pulmonary vascular resistances. Notably, TR jet may not be seen in all newborns; a reliable TR jet envelope may be seen only in about 61% of pediatric echocardiographic scans. There may also be erroneous estimations of the RV pressures due to increased angles of insonation (beam nonparallel to the regurgitant jet) and the absence of a complete Doppler envelope.[45]

In infants with mild pulmonary valve insufficiency (PI), echocardiography can help estimate the diastolic pulmonary arterial pressure (Fig. 40.2). Indeed, the continuous-wave Doppler of the PI can help estimate the gradient between the peak diastolic pressure in the main pulmonary artery and the RV. A similar approach may be used to estimate sPAP in the context of a restrictive PDA (Fig. 40.3) or a restrictive VSD (in the absence of left-sided inflow or outflow tract congenital anomalies). Indeed, the pressure gradient through the PDA/VSD may inform on the gradient between the systemic and pulmonary compartment. Comparisons of the estimated pulmonary arterial pressures to the corresponding

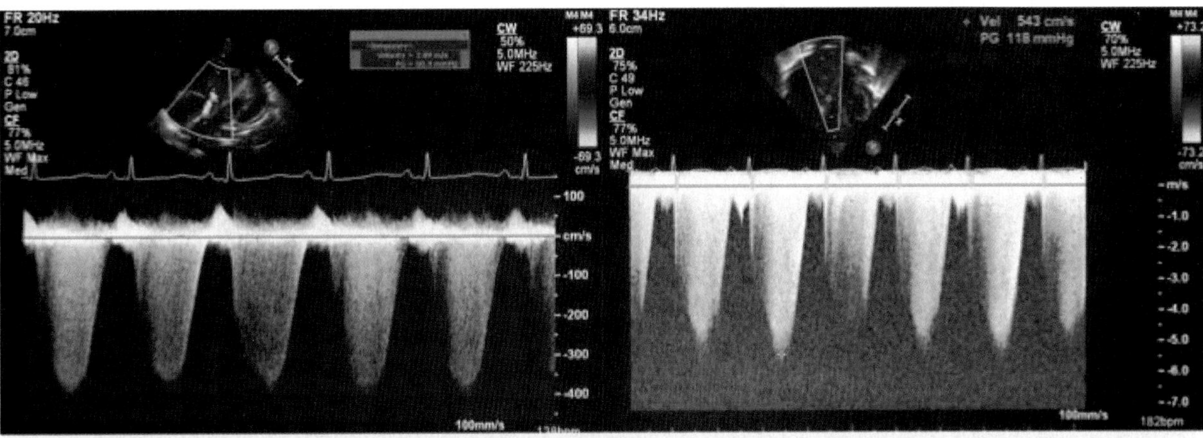

Fig. 40.1 Tricuspid Regurgitant Jet Velocity. Tricuspid regurgitation jet (TRJ) velocity by continuous-wave Doppler. The TRJ may be evaluated in various views (first panel, parasternal long axis view; second panel, apical four-chamber view). The TRJ, when a full envelope is obtained, it informs on the right ventricular to right atrial pressure gradient using the modified Bernoulli equation. In the context of normal cardiac anatomy, TRJ may estimate systolic pulmonary arterial pressure by adding the assumed right atrial pressure (usually 5 mm Hg unless there is RV diastolic dysfunction) to the RV-RA gradient. *RA,* Right atrium; *RV,* right ventricle.

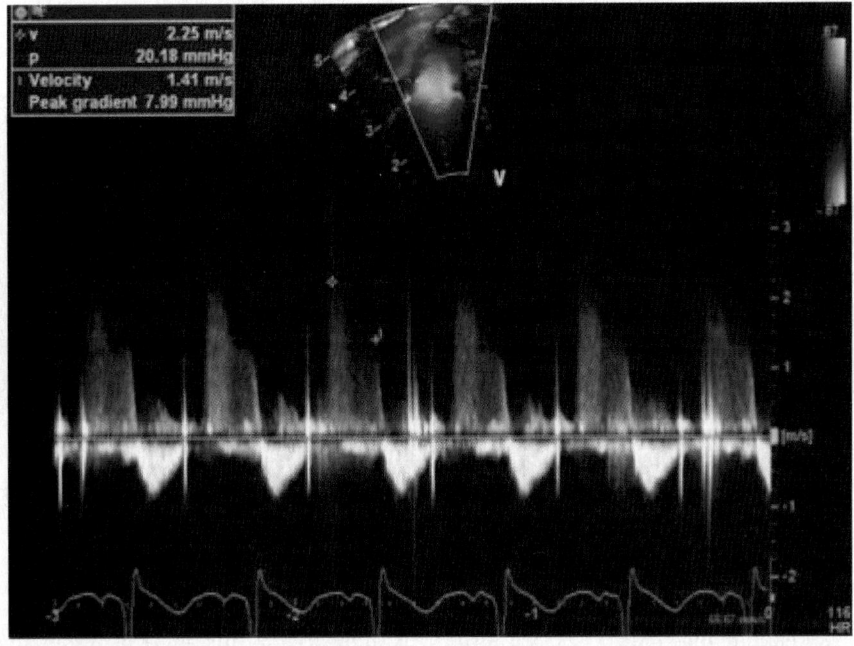

Fig. 40.2 Pulmonary Insufficiency Jet Velocities. Pulmonary insufficiency (PI) by continuous-wave Doppler. The modified Bernoulli equation may be used to estimate the pulmonary artery to RV gradient. The peak PI velocity informs on the mean pulmonary artery pressure, and the end PI velocity informs on the diastolic pulmonary artery pressure (adding the estimated end-diastolic RV pressure of about 5 mm Hg). *RV,* Right ventricle.

systemic arterial pressures measured using invasive or noninvasive techniques can be helpful; such estimations can allow the classification of PH into infra-, iso-, and suprasystemic pulmonary pressures. The shunting direction through the ductus arteriosus also informs about the relationship between the pulmonary and systemic compartment. One may need to put this into context, because systemic hypotension may be associated with bidirectional or right to left shunting. Similarly, the direction of blood flow assessed by color Doppler at the level of an interatrial communication informs about the end-diastolic pressures of the respective ventricles. A bidirectional or right-to-left atrial shunt may be associated with poor RV compliance in the context of pulmonary hypertension.[46] The right and left ventricle (LV) share muscular fibers and a septum. The septal curvature is assessed in the parasternal short axis view at the peak of systole at the papillary muscle level.[43,47] The RV-LV cross-talk may be disturbed in the context of increased RV afterload, leading to septal flattening (isosystemic pulmonary pressures) or bowing into the LV cavity (suprasystemic pulmonary pressures; Fig. 40.4). In the context of pulmonary hypertension but infrasystemic pulmonary pressures, a round LV is found and can miss an underlying pathologic process, making it an imprecise indicator. In order to quantify septal distortion, some have used the left ventricular eccentricity index (LVEI).[12,48–51] The LVEI is measured at the end of systole from the parasternal short-axis view at the papillary muscle level. It is the ratio of the LV diameter parallel to the septum to the diameter perpendicular to the septum (with a round LV providing a ratio close to 1.0). Abnormal LVEI in the context of PH has been described when >1.23.[12,52]

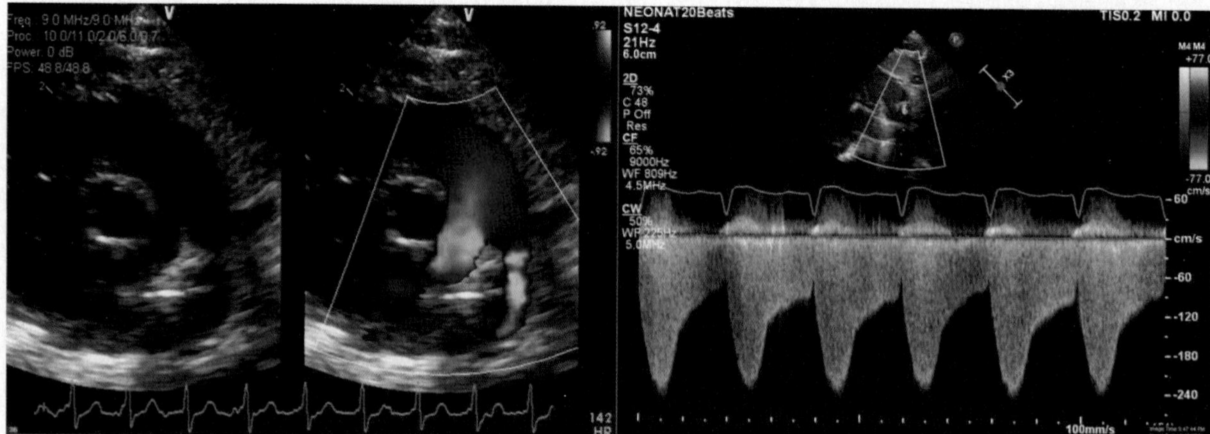

Fig. 40.3 Patent Ductus Arteriosus. Patent ductus arteriosus (PDA) visualized in the upper left parasternal short axis view. The color box indicates that the flow is right to left, indicating that there is suprasystemic pulmonary pressure. The continuous-wave Doppler informs on the velocity gradient between the pulmonary and aortic end. Because of the PDA tubular nature, the Bernoulli equation may underestimate the velocity gradient.

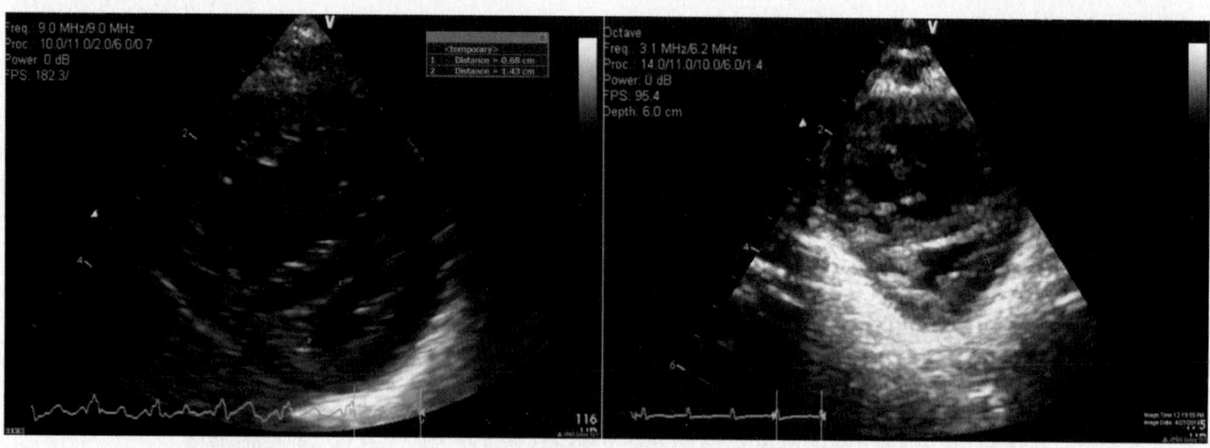

Fig. 40.4 Septal Configuration. The two panels indicate that there is RV overload with bowing of the interventricular septum. The LV eccentricity index (LV-EI; first panel) may be used to quantify the degree of septal deformation. The LV-EI should be measured at the peak of systole. The LV-EI represents the ratio between the largest measurement of the LV parallel to the septum and the largest measurement perpendicular to the septum (a perfect circle giving a ratio of 1). A flat septum at the peak of systole indicates that the pulmonary arterial pressure is estimated to be at least two-thirds systemic. When the septum is bowing into the LV cavity (as is the case in these two panels), one may suspect that there is suprasystemic pulmonary pressure. *LV*, Left ventricle; *RV*, right ventricle.

An acceleration time to RV ejection time ratio >0.3 measured from the pulsed-wave Doppler envelope of the RV outflow tract, at the tip of the pulmonary valve, has been associated with increased pulmonary artery pressure in infants with BPD.[9,12,53–56] Pulmonary artery acceleration time is the time to reach the peak of stroke distance within the main pulmonary artery. It is influenced by underlying RV performance, heart rate, and cardiac output.[39,53,57] With increasing RV afterload, the stroke distance profile changes toward a more triangular shape from a smooth, curved pattern.[58] Acceleration time is normalized to the heart rate by using the RV ejection time.

Although imprecise, other indirect indicators of pulmonary hypertension should be sought during echocardiography, such as RV hypertrophy or dilation, RA enlargement, pulmonary artery enlargement, hepatic veins dilation, or retrograde flow in the inferior vena cava. A ratio of the RV/LV longitudinal measure (perpendicular to the septum) in the parasternal short axis view at the papillary muscle level can also be used to quantify degree of RV dilation.[58] A ratio greater than 1.0 has been associated with pulmonary hypertension in the pediatric population.[12,50,58] This measure is influenced by the angle of insonation and is highly operator dependent.

In the context of BPD-PH, RV function should be quantified. RV contraction follows a longitudinal displacement of the inflow toward the outflow tract, a bulging of the septum toward the cavity, and a contraction of the free wall toward the septum. The RV geometry is complex, and assessment of systolic function by 2D echocardiography is usually limited to the use of tricuspid annular plane systolic excursion (TAPSE), fractional area change (FAC), and the use of tissue Doppler imaging (TDI) velocities (or myocardial performance index derived from TDI). Indeed, both markers have been described as predictors of mortality in the BPD-PH population.[12] TAPSE is measured by M-mode in the apical-4-chamber view with the line of interrogation passing through the apex of the RV and the lateral tricuspid valve attachment. It measures the longitudinal displacement of the tricuspid valve during systole. FAC is calculated in the apical-4-chamber view by the formula (RV diastolic area—RV systolic area)/RV diastolic area. Finally, TDI allows for the evaluation of systolic and diastolic myocardial velocities. TDI also allows for the calculation of the RV myocardial perfusion index (or Tei), a combined index of systolic and diastolic performance.[59] The RV myocardial perfusion index has been described has abnormal in the context of pediatric and neonatal PH.[37,60] Jain et al. have published normative values for RV function in term newborns.[61] Furthermore, normative data for TAPSE,[61–63] FAC,[64] and TDI velocities[61,65–70] are available in the newborn population at various gestational ages.

In infants with BPD, the presence of left-sided disease (mitral regurgitation, mitral stenosis, LV systolic or diastolic dysfunction, and LV outflow tract anomalies) and of pulmonary vein stenosis can be informative. Pulmonary vein stenosis is suspected on echocardiography/pulsed-wave Doppler of the pulmonary veins at their ostia, with monophasic Doppler flow profiles with a mean gradient >4 mm Hg.[71] Computed tomography scans can also be helpful for evaluation of pulmonary veins in the context of BPD-PH.[5]

Recent guidelines have also advocated for the evaluation of biomarkers such as the brain-type natriuretic peptide (BNP) or the *N*-terminal pro-BNP (NT-pro-BNP), which may be increased in the context of RV dysfunction.[5,9] BNP is a peptide released by cardiomyocytes secondary to stretch (during dilatation of cardiac structures),[72,73] and NT-pro-BNP is its inactive fragment.[73] Infants with PH frequently show elevated levels of these biomarkers.[74–76] Having said that, these markers may be more helpful for follow-up of disease progression, rather than to establish diagnosis. Vigilance in interpreting these markers is important, because newborns with BPD may have concomitant systemic hypertension and LV hypertrophy, which may also be associated with an increase in BNP/NT-proBNP.

Management

Using a nationwide database in the United States, Stroustrup and Trasande reported the incidence and resource use of infants with BPD. They found that the incidence of BPD decreased by 4.3% per year for 1993 to 2006. There was an increase in the use of noninvasive ventilation, but with it came an increase in the cost and length of hospitalization.[28,77] In recent years, BPD has remained stable (or even increased) according to the National Institute of Child Health and Development (NICHD) reports.[78,79] Furthermore, advances in neonatology have led to an increase in survival at the extremes of prematurity (22–24 weeks' gestational age) and birth weight (severe intrauterine growth restriction), possibly explaining the stability in BPD rates. Major predictors of BPD include early gestational age at birth and mechanical ventilation on day seven.[80] Furthermore, fetal growth restriction in infants born in the range of 23 to 27 weeks' gestation leads to increased risk of developing BPD.[28,81] Risk factors for PH in the context of BPD include extreme prematurity, oligohydramnios (associated with pulmonary hypoplasia), intrauterine growth restriction, prolonged mechanical ventilation, maternal preeclampsia and hypertension, and protracted oxygen supplementation.[9,11,12,82] Infants with BPD who have PH have a higher incidence of comorbidities, including retinopathy of prematurity, gastroesophageal reflux, pulmonary aspiration, airway anomalies, and dependence on technology (gastrostomy, gavage, tracheostomy, home oxygen).[11,12]

General Care

General management principles for care include maintenance of normal homeostasis with optimization of normal temperature, electrolytes, and intravascular volume.[83] The presence of acidosis may promote pulmonary vasoconstriction. However, intentional alkalosis should also be avoided, because it can worsen vascular tone, intracellular acidosis, reactivity, and permeability edema and can cause cerebral vasoconstriction.[83,84] Systemic blood pressure should be maintained at normal levels according to postmenstrual age.[85] Care should be taken to optimize lung recruitment and functional residual capacity. Impaired gas exchange results in hypoxemic vasoconstriction and eventually structural remodeling of the vasculature. Bronchospasm, airway obstruction, and tracheobronchomalacia should be identified and treated.[36] Surfactant administration in the immediate postnatal period can be beneficial in cases of deficiency (respiratory distress syndrome [RDS]) or inactivation (sepsis, meconium aspiration) and helps to improve oxygenation, reduce air leak, and reduce the need for extracorporeal membrane oxygenation in infants with meconium aspiration and other parenchymal lung diseases.[83,86] Gastroesophageal reflux and aspiration also warrant treatment.[36] Careful attention is needed to nutrition, including to specific components such as the total protein intake and vitamin A.

Oxygen Supplementation

Vento et al. evaluated resuscitation in preterm infants <28 weeks' gestation using 30% or 90% fraction of inspired oxygen and found that resuscitation with 30% caused less oxidative stress and inflammation, fewer days of supplemental oxygen, fewer days of mechanical ventilation, and a reduced risk of BPD than in the infants resuscitated with 90%.[31,87] In the BPD phase, monitoring with oximetry may allow detection of repetitive hypoxic events that may be prevented with oxygen supplementation titrated to obtain appropriate saturations. Repetitive desaturation may be associated with further vascular remodeling and worsening of pulmonary hypertension.[8,88] Despite many trials confirming the deleterious effects of hyperoxia on the lung, none have clearly demonstrated the most appropriate oxygen saturations to target in the premature neonate. The determination of appropriate oxygen targets is also complicated by the use of supplemental oxygen for conditions other than hypoxemia, such as apnea, bradycardia, desaturations during feedings, high work of breathing with suboptimal growth, and the variability in target oxygen saturations in infants with BPD.[10,89]

The PPHNet released guidelines in 2017 for the evaluation and management of pulmonary hypertension in children with BPD. The PPHNet recommends supplemental oxygen should be used to avoid episodic or sustained hypoxemia with the goal of maintaining oxygen saturations between 92% and 95% in patients with established BPD and PH. Even mild degrees of oxygen desaturations can markedly elevate pulmonary artery pressures in infants with BPD and related PH.[5,90–95] Overzealous use of high levels of oxygen beyond the recommended range may theoretically contribute to airway inflammation and should be avoided.[5,8,96,97]

Inhaled Nitric Oxide

In the setting of acute PH (persistent pulmonary hypertension of the newborn [PPHN]) in the term and near-term infant, inhaled nitric oxide (iNO) remains the first-line therapy.[98] In the context of prematurity, the use of iNO for acute pulmonary hypertension may lead to a rapid drop of pulmonary vascular resistance and steal effect via the ductus toward the pulmonary vascular compartment. This may theoretically increase the risk of intraventricular hemorrhage due to diastolic blood flow steal. Inhaled NO has been used in premature infants with acute PH in the setting of oligohydramnios and pulmonary hypoplasia.[99] Otherwise, data are lacking regarding the use of iNO in preterm infants.[100] Inhaled NO is a potent vasodilator and has strengths such as direct delivery to the pulmonary microvasculature and its rapid onset of action.[36,101] The vasodilatory effects of iNO are most pronounced in the well-ventilated lung regions, resulting in decreased ventilation-perfusion (V/Q) mismatch.[36] The mechanism of action involves guanylyl cyclase activation leading to production of cyclic guanosine monophosphate (cGMP) and subsequent smooth-muscle relaxation.[102–105] Despite its impact in the treatment of infants and children with pulmonary hypertension and experimental findings in animal models that suggest enhanced lung growth and reduced lung inflammation, the impact in neonates for the prevention or treatment of BPD remains uncertain.

The PPHNet recommends iNO use in an acute PH crisis. Infants with BPD can have worsening of PH or acute elevations in pulmonary artery pressure secondary to viral infections with parenchymal inflammation or hypoxia that trigger sudden lability in their saturations with profound desaturations and hypotension.[5] Inhaled NO at 10 to 20 ppm may be considered during acute crises and should be carefully weaned after stabilization.[5,90,106] Weaning strategies vary and usually involve rapid weaning to a dose of 3 to 5 ppm, followed by a gradual reduction to cessation.[5]

The National Institutes of Health Consensus Development statement regarding iNO therapy for premature infants examined several trials and meta-analyses evaluating the use of iNO in the preterm population and found that among those requiring oxygen at 36 weeks' postmenstrual age, treatment with iNO in the neonatal period does not reduce the occurrence or severity of BPD.[107] Clinical trials of iNO therapy for the prevention of BPD have shown little benefit, and it remains indicated only in the setting of PH.[36,108]

Pharmacotherapy

Pulmonary hypertension in the context of BPD is a multifactorial disease, including a fixed component (decreased pulmonary vascular territory), heterogenous vasculature (with varying degrees of vascular wall anomalies), abnormal vascular constriction, disturbed venous drainage, and intrapulmonary shunting. Whether the use of pulmonary vasodilator therapy affects survival in the BPD-PH population is unknown. Also, these therapies have not been studied in the context of BPD-PH, and it is unknown if an earlier administration may impact outcomes (positively or negatively). For the initiation of any pharmacotherapy, the PPHNet recommends that pharmacotherapy be considered for infants with BPD and sustained PH after optimal treatment of underlying respiratory and cardiac disease and that pharmacotherapy should be initiated in patients with significantly elevated pulmonary vascular resistance and RV impairment not related to left heart disease or pulmonary vein stenosis.[5,8] Despite an absence of evidence in this population, initiation of therapy is often considered in newborns with iso- to suprasystemic PH and RV failure. Decisions regarding selection, initiation, and modification of PH-specific therapy should be made based on disease severity, drug tolerance, and consultation with a PH specialist. Once a medication is initiated, close clinical monitoring with serial echocardiography and NT-pro-BNP levels are recommended by the PPHNet experts, along with clinical assessment to define the response to therapy and the need for combination therapy.[5]

Phosphodiesterase Inhibitors

Phosphodiesterases (PDEs) hydrolyze and inactivate cGMP and cyclic adenosine monophosphate (cAMP), regulate intracellular calcium concentrations, and minimize pulmonary vasoconstriction[109] structural remodeling.[36]

Sildenafil, a PDE5 inhibitor, is easily administered and is well tolerated but may be associated with systemic hypotension. PDE5 is highly expressed in the lungs and is a critical controller of NO-mediated vasodilation.[109,110] It is often used in BPD-associated PH, although its efficacy in young infants still needs to be proven conclusively. Small, retrospective studies have suggested accelerated recovery of PH with improved RV function and reduced mortality,[109,111–115] and supportive data demonstrate efficacy in the treatment of PPHN.[5,8] There have been some reports of dose-increased mortality in PH secondary to congenital heart disease.[36,111,112,116] The US Food and Drug Administration (FDA) issued a warning statement about higher mortality in children taking high doses of sildenafil for PH.[116-118] Clarifications from the FDA acknowledge that there may be risk-benefit profiles in which sildenafil may be acceptable for certain pediatric patients. It is not approved for use in neonates, and the STARTS-2 study, which triggered this controversy, did not enroll any infant under the age of 1 year.[118,119] Currently, sildenafil continues to be used in neonates as an acute adjuvant to iNO in iNO-resistant PPHN or to facilitate weaning of iNO, as an acute primary treatment of PPHN where iNO is unavailable or contraindicated, and in chronic primary treatment of pulmonary hypertension in conditions such as BPD and congenital diaphragmatic hernia.[118] Side effects to consider when using sildenafil include hypotension, ventilation-perfusion mismatch, irritability (headache), bronchospasm, nasal stuffiness, fever, and rarely, priapism.[5,109,111,120]

Milrinone, a phosphodiesterase-3 inhibitor, increases cAMP levels in the arterial smooth-muscle cells and the myocardium, resulting in decreased pulmonary vascular resistance and increased cardiac contractility. It also has systemic vasodilatory effects, reduces afterload, and has the potential for improved cardiac function. It may be considered in patients with PH associated with ventricular dysfunction.[109] Animal studies suggest that milrinone may reduce pulmonary artery pressure and may act synergistically with inhaled prostanoids[83,121] and additively with iNO.[83,122,123] Case reports suggest milrinone may prevent rebound PH after discontinuation of iNO and that it may enhance pulmonary vasodilation in infants with PPHN is refractory to iNO.[83,124,125] There may be some adverse effects such as systemic hypotension and reduced myocardial perfusion. It may promote V/Q mismatch because it may be being unselective for pulmonary vascular territories that are underventilated. It may also be arrhythmogenic and needs to be used very cautiously in patients with renal dysfunction.[5,109] Finally, there is some inconvenience because it needs to be administered intravenously.

Endothelin 1 Receptor Antagonists

Endothelin 1 acts via two G protein–coupled receptors: ET_A, which promotes smooth-muscle cell proliferation and vasoconstriction; and ET_B, which promotes proliferation and vasoconstriction and mediates vasodilation by release of NO and prostacyclin (PGI_2) from endothelial cells.[36,126–129] Bosentan is the most commonly used agent and has nonselective antagonist properties to both ET_A and ET_B. Bosentan has been shown to improve PH in the newborn with PPHN and in adults.[36,109,130,131] Treatment may improve oxygenation, echocardiographic parameters, and hemodynamics as noted upon cardiac catheterization. Bosentan monotherapy or in combination with sildenafil could improve pulmonary hypertension in patients with chronic lung disease.[132] There are some case reports of bosentan to have allowed weaning prostacyclin therapy for the treatment of BPD-associated PH.[133] Common side effects of bosentan include liver dysfunction during viral infections, V/Q mismatch, hypotension, and anemia.

Rarely, edema and airway issues may occur.[5,109] Ambrisentan is an ET_A receptor antagonist that is approved for adults with PH but lacks data in the pediatric population.[36,109,126]

Prostacyclins

Prostacyclins are metabolites of arachidonic acid that are produced by the vascular epithelium; these stimulate adenylate cyclase to produce cAMP, which results in smooth-muscle relaxation via reduction in the intracellular calcium concentrations. PH is associated with decreased synthesis of prostacyclin, reduced expression of its receptor, and increased synthesis of the vasoconstrictor prostanoid thromboxane A_2, and hence there is sound scientific basis for such treatment.[109,121,134]

Epoprostenol

Epoprostenol has a short half-life and requires continuous infusions, but it can show considerable improvement in PH.[109,135,136] There are sporadic case reports of epoprostenol use in infants with BPD, but rigorous data and the safety profile continue to be sparse.[137] A recent retrospective Canadian study of infants with PPHN <28 days showed that epoprostenol improved oxygenation index after 12 hours of treatment. There was improvement in echocardiographic markers, but many infants showed a rebound deterioration after cessation of the nebulization.[138] Neonates (<30 days) may show a more consistent response to epoprostenol than older children; there was improved oxygenation index and echocardiographic evidence of decreased right-sided pressures and/or improved RV function for 20% of patients.[139] There were some adverse effects, including hypotension, platelet dysfunction, V/Q mismatch, feeding intolerance, and a risk of rebound PH following cessation of therapy. In addition, the need for a central line added to the risk.[5,109]

Iloprost

Iloprost is a prostacyclin analog with a half-life of 20 to 30 minutes, delivered via inhalation with fewer systemic side effects.[109,140] Iloprost has been shown to improve oxygenation in infants with PPHN[141–143] and BPD-associated PH.[144,145] Potential side effects include bronchospasm, hypotension, ventilator tube crystallization and clogging, and pulmonary hemorrhage.[5,109]

Treprostinil

A longer-acting prostacyclin analog, treprostinil can be administered via inhalation or by an intravenous/subcutaneous route. Subcutaneous administration was appealing for infants treated with home vasodilatory therapy.[109,146,147] There is a need for further research to confirm efficacy and safety in this population.[148] The adverse effects of treprostinil resembled that of epoprostenol, but with a longer half-life, the risk of rebound pulmonary hypertension may be minimized.[5,109]

Glucocorticoids

Many preclinical and clinical studies advocate a role for glucocorticoid use in restoring normal pulmonary vascular function.[118,149,150] Hydrocortisone use has been postulated as a safer drug than dexamethasone to use for the prevention of BPD and with an improved safety profile for long-term neurodevelopmental outcomes.[151–153] Historically, dexamethasone was considered the drug of choice for preventing and treating BPD and decreased mortality.[151,154,155] However, dexamethasone was found to carry a high risk for adverse neurodevelopmental outcomes including cerebral palsy and developmental delay in newborns exposed to early administration and higher dosages than the regimen used for the DART protocol.[151,154–157] Hydrocortisone seems to be a promising avenue, but more data are needed.

The French multicenter, randomized controlled Premiloc study utilizing prophylactic low-dose hydrocortisone concluded that survival without BPD was reduced in extremely low birth weight infants.[158] However, most newborns were still managed with intubation, administration of surfactant, and use of invasive mechanical ventilation. The effect(s) of prophylactic hydrocortisone in premature newborns managed with noninvasive ventilation since birth or in those born at 22 to 23 weeks remain unknown.[159] In a recently published meta-analysis of hydrocortisone use in the preterm population, early initiation of systemic hydrocortisone was noted to be modestly effective for prevention of BPD in preterm infants.[151] No conclusions were drawn regarding the use of late hydrocortisone use or its effects on the pulmonary circulation.[151,160]

Conclusion

Although medical advances in the care of preterm infants have improved survival, BPD and subsequent development of pulmonary hypertension remain a significant morbidity in these patients. We still need a specific definition for BPD and standardized protocols for evaluation and management of pulmonary hypertension.

Section 7

CHAPTER

41 Hemodynamic Assessment and Management of a Critically Ill Infant

Tai-Wei Wu, Shahab Noori

KEY POINTS

1. Shock is a clinical condition marked by poor tissue perfusion resulting in inadequate oxygen delivery and tissue hypoxia.
2. Neonates with shock have hypotension or poor tissue perfusion, and there are important surrogate markers such as prolonged capillary refill time, low urine output, and lactic acidosis.
3. Early neonatal hypotension seems to increase the risk of brain injury and intraventricular hemorrhage.
4. Current models of the circulatory system show the laws of fluid dynamics to be valid with a strong relationship between blood pressure, blood flow, and calculated/measured values of the cardiac output. The systemic vascular resistance can also be assessed.
5. The impact of the preload, cardiac contractility, and afterload on cardiac output has been discussed.

Introduction

A healthy circulatory system delivers oxygen and nutrients to meet metabolic demands of the tissue and end organs. Shock is a clinical condition characterized by poor tissue perfusion resulting in inadequate oxygen delivery and tissue hypoxia. When cellular metabolic needs are unmet for a prolonged period of time, mitochondrial dysfunction, energy failure, cell death, and organ failure may ensue. Similar to pediatric and adult patients, shock in neonates can be categorized by its pathophysiological state (vasodilatory, cardiogenic, or hypovolemic shock) or severity (compensated, uncompensated, or irreversible shock). Unique to the newborn, the timing of shock (immediate postnatal or posttransitional period) may provide clues to the underlying etiology. In the immediate transitional period, newborns face the challenges of adjusting to abrupt alterations in systemic and pulmonary vascular resistance influenced by events such as timing of umbilical cord clamping and lung aeration. This is further complicated by underlying risks such as sepsis, asphyxia, or immature myocardium in preterm infants.[1] After the transitional period, infection and necrotizing enterocolitis are among the most common causes of shock.

Neonatal shock is most readily recognized in the clinical setting by hypotension or poor tissue perfusion indicated by surrogate measures such as prolonged capillary refill time, low urine output, lactic acidosis, etc. For the sake of practicality, the gestational age of the preterm infant is commonly used as the lower limit of "acceptable" blood pressure range. This notion is derived from population studies of preterm infants of varying gestational and postnatal ages and recommendations from the Joint Working Group of the British Association of Perinatal Medicine.[2–4] As demonstrated in Fig. 41.1, mean blood pressure increases accordingly with gestational and postnatal age. The incidence of neonatal hypotension varies widely depending on the definition of hypotension and gestational age of the population studied. Because the cutoff for normal blood pressure range is elusive, studies have instead investigated the use of antihypotensive medication as an indirect measure for neonatal hypotension. Accordingly, the incidence of vasopressor-inotrope use within first 24 hours ranged from 4% to 39% in very low birth weight infants among 6 units in a regional observational study,[5] 4.4% to 38% among 34 hospitals using a resource utilization national database, and 55% among infants born at 23 to 26 6/7 weeks' gestational age within a research network.[6]

In relation to outcome, numerous studies have found an association between early neonatal hypotension in preterm infants and intraventricular hemorrhage (IVH)[2,7,8] or adverse neurodevelopmental outcomes at a later age.[9,10] On the other hand, several studies have not found such association between early hypotension and poor neurologic outcome.[11,12] Furthermore, the mere presence of an association without shedding light on possible causation provides little guidance for the clinician managing these patients. The relationship between hypotension and subsequent brain injury is supported by a limited amount of data. For example, hypotensive preterm infants who respond to vasopressors/inotropes with normalization of blood pressure have been reported to have a similar rate of IVH as normotensive preterm infants[13] and a lower risk of IVH compared with nonresponders.[14] As part of a national prospective population-based cohort study of extremely preterm infants, 119 infants with untreated hypotension (mean blood pressure [BP] < gestational age [GA]) were matched with 119 infants who were treatment for isolated hypotension in the first 3 days of life.[15] The treated group had a higher rate of survival without severe morbidity and a lower rate of severe IVH and cerebral injury. There was even a stronger association between treatment and a better outcome when hypotension was defined as mean blood pressure < GA minus 5. This dose-effect relationship strengthens the possibility for causality between hypotension and brain injury in extremely preterm infants. However, even if hypotension contributes to development of poor outcomes, given the ambiguity regarding the blood pressure threshold below which organ perfusion is compromised and, more importantly, organ damage occurs, it is clear that monitoring blood pressure alone is not enough in assessing adequacy of circulatory function. Because other clinical (capillary refill time, core-peripheral temperature difference, heart rate, urine output) and laboratory (lactate, base deficit) markers of circulatory compromise have low sensitivity/specificity or lag in terms of manifestation, further monitoring technology is needed. In this chapter, we will review hemodynamics and discuss several tools that can enhance clinicians' ability to assess adequacy of cardiovascular function and guide management.

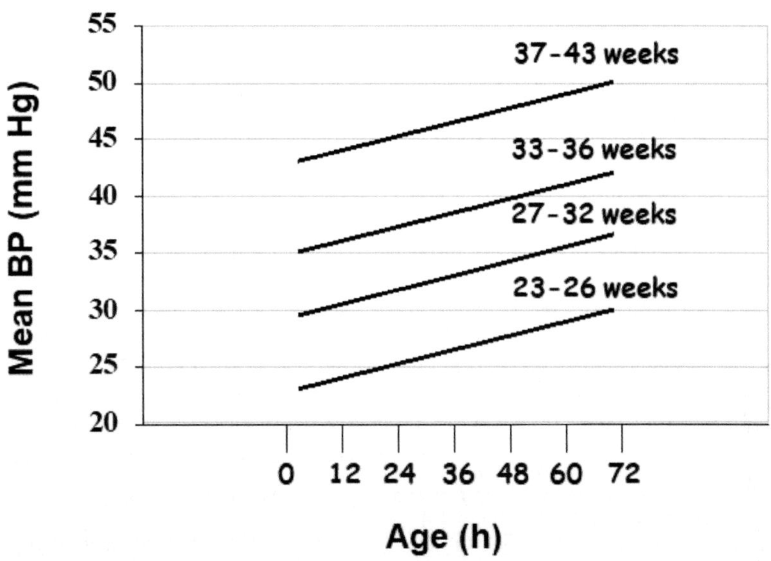

Fig. 41.1 An Example of Statistically Defined Normal Blood Pressure Values. The lines represent the lower limit of the 80% confidence interval of mean blood pressure in neonates during the first 3 postnatal days. (Modified from Nuntnarumit et al. Blood pressure measurements in the newborn. *Clin Perinatol.* 1999;26:981–996, x.)

Fluid Dynamics: Understanding the Relationship Between Pressure and Flow

The circulatory system as a whole can be better understood by applying Ohm's law of electricity to fluid dynamics, which grossly explains the relationship between blood pressure and blood flow:

$$\Delta P(\text{Pressure}) = \text{Q}(\text{flow}) \times (\text{resistance})$$

Further applying the principle to cardiovascular physiology:

$$\text{Mean blood pressure} - \text{Right atrial pressure} \\ = \text{Cardiac output} \times \text{Systemic vascular resistance}$$

From the above equation, it can be appreciated that blood pressure is a *dependent* hemodynamic variable resulting from the product of cardiac output (CO) and systemic vascular resistance (SVR). Unlike blood pressure, the two other major parameters (CO and SVR) are not routinely measured in the neonatal intensive care setting. Therefore circulatory compromise or shock may exist (and be subclinical or compensated) despite having a "normal" blood pressure. For example, in the setting of myocardial dysfunction, CO and overall systemic blood flow are reduced. Neuronal and hormonal signals mediate vasoconstriction at the level of the arteriole and increase SVR in response to decreased perfusion pressure and blood flow. The compromised hemodynamic state can remain clinically undetectable by way of this compensatory mechanism that acts to maintain blood pressure. The concept is illustrated in Fig. 41.2, which further explains why the use of abnormal blood pressure as a sole indicator for hemodynamic instability may not provide the full hemodynamic picture. Furthermore, the "normal" cutoff range may vary between individuals and even in the same individual in different pathologic states.

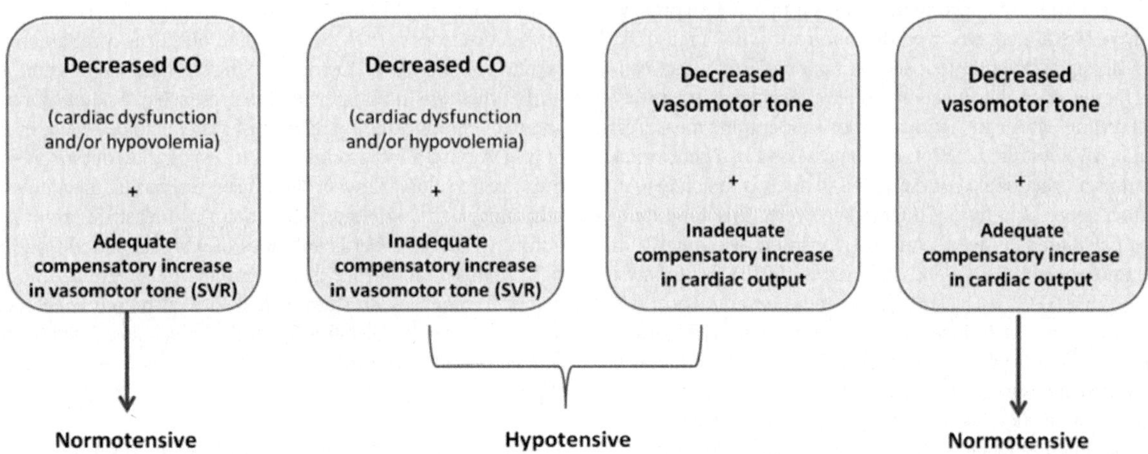

Fig. 41.2 Pathophysiology of Neonatal Cardiovascular Compromise in Primary Myocardial Dysfunction and Primary Abnormal Vascular Tone Regulation With or Without Compensation by the Unaffected Other Variable. This figure illustrates why blood pressure can remain in the "normal" range when there is appropriate compensatory increase in either vasomotor tone or cardiac output. In the hypotensive scenarios, the compensatory mechanisms have been exhausted. *CO,* Cardiac output. (From Wu T, Noori S, Seri I. Neonatal hypotension. In: Polin R, Yoder M, eds. *Workbook in Practical Neonatology*. 5th ed. Philadelphia: Elsevier; 2014:230–243.)

Determinants of Cardiac Output

Cardiac output is an important hemodynamic parameter that is not routinely measured or monitored in the neonatal intensive care setting. Cardiac output (measured in milliliters per minute) is the product of the volume of blood that the left ventricle ejects (stroke volume [SV]) multiplied heart rate, CO = SV × HR. The following sections briefly explain determinants of SV (preload, contractility, afterload) because this may aid the clinician in arriving at the etiology of the low cardiac output and administering appropriate treatment.

Echocardiography is the quintessential and most convenient bedside tool for the evaluation of cardiac dysfunction. The following section will include various echocardiographic indices that may guide the bedside clinician in developing treatment strategies to improve cardiac output and systemic blood flow.

Preload

Preload is best described as the amount of stretch of cardiac muscle fiber before myocardial contraction occurs. An optimal amount of stretch is necessary for the subsequent ejection force. The Frank-Starling law describes this length-tension relationship, when stretching of muscle fibers to a certain point increases actin-myosin cross bridges and calcium release from sarcoplasmic reticulum and improves SV. Physiologically, the volume of blood or pressure within the ventricles prior to contraction dictates the degree of stretch of the ventricular myocardial fibers. Factors affecting preload include but are not limited to blood volume, venous return, intrathoracic pressure, and systolic and diastolic function of the heart. On echocardiography, a few surrogate measures of preload have been proposed: left atrium to aortic root ratio, end-diastolic left ventricular internal diameter (LVIDD), and inferior vena cava diameter and collapsibility. LVIDD is the most commonly used index for preload assessment.[16] Inferior vena cava diameter and collapsibility have not been validated in the neonatal population. The commonly seen description of "underfilled" heart as a qualitative measure of inadequate preload in echocardiography reports is a testament to the difficulty of objectively estimating preload.

Contractility

Contractility or cardiac inotropy, regulated mainly by adrenergic activation and vagal inhibition, is a measure of intrinsic contractile strength in the form of myocardial fiber shortening. For example, when preload and afterload are fixed, increases in cardiac inotropy will increase SV. However, physiologically, both preload and afterload will affect contractility, and therefore, cardiac function is often evaluated in its entirety in the clinical setting using conventional echocardiographic measures. Left ventricular (LV) systolic function can be assessed by echocardiographic measures of fractional shortening (FS), which is the change in myocardial fiber shortening during the cardiac cycle. This commonly used index is calculated by measuring the LV internal diameter in M-mode at end-diastole (LIVDD) and end-systole (LVIDS) as follows: FS = (LVIDD − LVIDS)/LVIDD. Because the measurements are in a two-dimensional plane, FS assumes uniform movement and normal geometry of the left ventricle, which may not be true in pathologic conditions. As such, measuring area changes by tracing the ventricular endocardium in systole and diastole may be a more accurate representation of systolic function when septal flattening or myocardial dyskinesis is present. Newer modalities such as tissue Doppler and speckle tracking can give a better assessment of myocardial segmental function, but due to their complexity and time-consuming nature, their application in clinical settings is currently limited. Another limitation of FS is load-dependency, which means it can be affected by other factors that alter preload and afterload. Load-independent contractility can be assessed invasively by cardiac catheterization; however, echocardiographic measures such as the stress-velocity index and strain rate may be good surrogates for true contractility. A detailed description of load-independent indices is beyond the scope of this chapter.

Afterload

Afterload can be described as the force that the myocardial fibers must overcome to eject blood out of the ventricles during systole. This "load" is quantified as LV wall stress and follows the law of Laplace (P ∝ Thickness × Tension/Radius), which describes the relationship of pressure, radius, and tension within a sphere. Applying this law, wall stress (tension in the equation) is directly related to LV diameter and pressure and inversely related to wall thickness:

$$\text{Wall Stress} \propto \text{Pressure} \times \text{Radius} / \text{Wall thickness}$$

For example, in dilated cardiomyopathy, the ventricles are dilated with thin walls (↑ radius; ↓ wall thickness), which increases wall stress and afterload (Fig. 41.3). In the same regard, when an infant is hypotensive and the LV is already stretched from fluid boluses, further volume resuscitation can decrease wall thickness, increase LV diameter, and ultimately worsen cardiac output by increasing the afterload. Because the determinants (ventricular pressure, radius, and thickness) change throughout the cardiac cycle, wall stress changes as well. Clinically, wall stress at the end systole best represents afterload. Two determinants of wall stress can be measured by way of echocardiography—LV internal diameter and wall thickness (LV posterior wall). The third determinant, ventricular pressure, can be estimated using mean arterial blood pressure because it has been found to correlate well with end systolic LV pressure.[17] Lastly, it is important to note that SVR does not equate to afterload.[18] SVR is one of the determinants of blood pressure and contributes to LV cavity pressure. In this manner, it contributes to afterload but should not be confused to be synonymous with afterload. SVR is explained in more detail below.

Cardiac Output

As mentioned earlier, the interaction among preload, afterload, and contractility defines the SV, which together with heart rate determines cardiac output. When there are no intracardiac shunts or a patent ductus arteriosus (PDA), LV cardiac output is a reliable measure of systemic blood flow. However, in the neonatal population, especially during the transitional period, the presence of a patent foramen ovale and PDA complicates assessment of systemic blood flow. In the setting of a PDA with a left-to-right shunt, LV cardiac output overestimates the systemic blood flow. In such cases, estimating the amount of blood returning to the right side of the heart by measuring right ventricular output would be a better measure of systemic blood flow. However, right ventricular output is also inaccurate in the setting of a large patent foramen ovale shunt. Therefore, although echocardiography provides a wealth of hemodynamic information, much attention is needed in understanding the limitations of various indices in different clinical situations.

Assessment of Cardiac Output by Impedance Cardiometry

Echocardiography enables bedside visualization and assessment of cardiac function and output but is also operator-dependent and

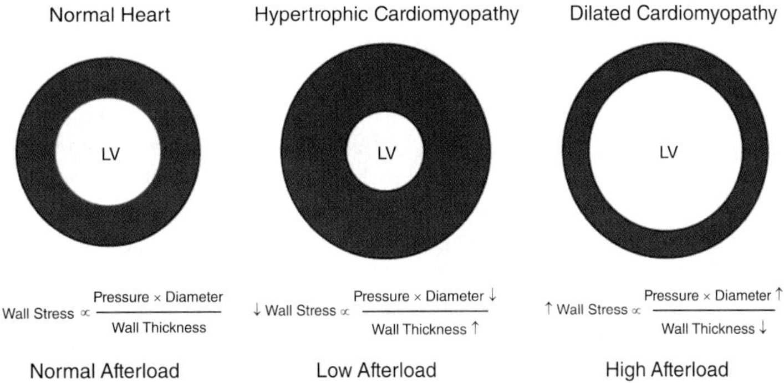

Fig. 41.3 End-Systolic Wall Stress Is Considered a Good Measure of the Afterload. Left ventricular (LV) wall stress is directly related to LV diameter and LV pressure (which in turn is related to systemic blood pressure) and inversely proportional to LV wall thickness. In hypertrophic cardiomyopathy the afterload is very low, promoting a hyperdynamic state, whereas in the case of dilated cardiomyopathy the afterload is very high, further compromising systolic function. (From Noori S, Wu T. Myocardial dysfunction, heart failure and shock. In: Siassi B, Noori S, Wong P, Acherman R, eds. *Practical Neonatal Echocardiography*. McGraw-Hill; 2019.)

requires prior training, experience, and in-depth understanding of developmental cardiovascular physiology.[19] Another means of noninvasive real-time cardiac output evaluation is impedance cardiometry. Estimation of SV and CO by impedance cardiometry is based on changes in bioimpedance induced by blood flow movement through the aorta during the cardiac cycle. In concept, prior to opening of the aortic valve, the red blood cells within the aorta assume a random orientation, which contributes to an increase in bioimpedance. The thoracic bioimpedance, measured by placement of electrodes, changes when cardiac contraction propels red blood cells forward through the aorta. This is thought to be due to a change in orientation of red blood cells from random to parallel, a property of disc-shaped blood cells moving in the direction of fluid flow. In this instance the parallel and organized orientation of red blood cells allows for decreased impedances (or higher conductivity). Because the above conductivity signal is altered due to pulsatile blood flow generated by heart contraction, the waveform can be recorded and analyzed. The rate and timing of changes in conductivity signal are used to estimate flow velocity and ejection time. In summary, impedance cardiometry utilizes the changing orientation of the red blood cells throughout the cardiac cycle to mathematically calculate blood flow velocity and flow time and ultimately arrive at a SV and CO value.

Several studies have tested the accuracy and precision of impedance cardiometry in adults and children by comparisons with the "gold standard" measures of CO: from direct Fick,[20] thermodilution,[21,22] or cardiac MRI.[23–25] These studies have found mixed results, with some reporting clinically acceptable accuracy and precision and others reporting poor accuracy and precision compared with the "gold standard" method. In the neonatal population, a study using AESCULON (Cardiotronic, La Jolla, California, USA) in the first two postnatal days found good accuracy but poor precision in estimating cardiac output compared with echocardiography.[26] Because echocardiography has its own limitations in estimating cardiac output, the authors concluded that impedance cardiometry has a clinically acceptable percentage error. In another study using NICOM (Cheetah Medical, Massachusetts, USA), the authors consistently found lower CO compared with echocardiography, suggesting a systemic bias perhaps owing to use of the algorithms derived from adults.[27] In a study of cardiac output in preterm infants, AESCULON had an acceptable agreement with echocardiography in infants without any respiratory support but poor agreement in preterm infants on mechanical ventilation, especially high-frequency ventilation.[28] Most studies of impedance cardiometry have reported no effect of PDA on estimating CO, but some investigators have found PDA to reduce agreement with echocardiography,[29] especially with CO >280 mL/kg/min.[30] Thus far, no studies have evaluated the utility of impedance cardiometry in neonatal shock.

In summary, impedance cardiometry appears to have a percentage error of about 30%, which may be considered borderline acceptable for clinical application. However, there may be a greater utility of impedance cardiometry in trending changes in CO rather than its absolute value.[31,32] Although accurate measurements of CO may not be feasible with impedance cardiometry, its noninvasive nature, ease of application, and ability to trend CO changes by continuous monitoring may still hold value in the assessment of neonatal hemodynamics.

Determinants of Systemic Vascular Resistance

The vascular system in general and arterioles in particular generate resistance to flow. Through hormonal, neuronal, and local factors, the vascular tone of arterioles is modulated to regulate blood flow to various tissue beds. These changes in arteriolar vascular tone determine SVR.

SVR cannot be measured, but with the knowledge of cardiac output and blood pressure, it can be calculated by rearranging Ohm's law: SVR = (mean arterial blood pressure − right atrial pressure)/CO. SVR is a measure of resistance in the entire circulatory system, which is a culmination of varying degrees of vascular tone within different organs. In states of decreased systemic blood flow, selective vasoconstriction in the nonvital organs shunts blood preferentially to vital organs such as the brain, adrenal glands, and heart. The overall increase in SVR may be adequate in maintaining organ perfusion pressure despite a compromised CO, manifesting as compensated shock that can be overlooked clinically in the setting of stable blood pressures. An abnormal systemic vascular response in systemic inflammatory diseases can present as vasodilatory shock. On clinical exam, the infant may present with warm extremities, rapid capillary refill time, and bounding pulses. Neonatal sepsis is one of the most common etiologies underlying vasodilatory shock. In addition, adrenal insufficiency, severe cases of necrotizing enterocolitis, significant perturbance of K_{ATP} channels, or vasoparalysis from vasomotor cell death associated with severe asphyxia can lead to low SVR and severe hypotension unresponsive to vasopressors and fluid resuscitation.

Pathophysiology of Shock

Combining the above determinants of cardiac output and SVR, a pathophysiology map can be constructed. From Fig. 41.4, hemodynamic assessment of the hypotensive newborn can be broken down to quantifiable parameters that aid the clinician in developing an individualized and pathophysiology-based approach to treatment of neonatal shock.

Role of Near-Infrared Spectroscopy in Neonatal Shock

In addition to assessment of hemodynamics at the macrocirculation level, monitoring end organ tissue oxygenation provides us with arguably even more important information regarding adequacy of the circulatory function. Indeed, if the critical blood pressure is elusive and individualized, the ability to continuously assess tissue oxygenation might provide insight about the critical oxygen delivery point. This is the threshold where oxygen utilization is delivery-dependent in the tissue[33] and any further reduction of organ blood flow induces an oxygen debt.

Light in the near-infrared wavelength (600–900 nm) has better tissue penetrance than visible light. Differences in optical absorption properties of oxyhemoglobin and deoxyhemoglobin in this spectrum allow near-infrared spectroscopy (NIRS) to quantify different absorbance and derive regional tissue oxygenation. The proportion of oxygenated hemoglobin to total hemoglobin (total hemoglobin = oxyhemoglobin + deoxyhemoglobin) is the regional oxygen saturation (rSO_2). In contrast to pulse oximetry, which removes nonpulsatile signals (venous and capillary light absorption), NIRS does not negate nonpulsatile signals and captures the mixture of arterial, venous, and capillary oxygenation. The distribution of signals from the vascular compartments is generally estimated to be 20% arterial, 75% venous, and 5% capillary,[34] which can be variable among individuals, organs examined, or physiologic conditions. For practical purposes, the signal is composed mainly of venous (75%) and partly arterial (25%) oxygenation.

The simple application of an NIRS sensor for assessment of end organ blood flow is appealing but dependent on stability of various factors: arterial oxygen saturation, organ blood volume, hematocrit, distribution in various vascular compartments, and metabolism. When the above factors are unchanged or stable, rSO_2 can then be trended and used as a surrogate for regional tissue blood flow. In the absence of data on the critical threshold for organ injury, the main goals of continuous organ blood flow monitoring are mainly two-fold: to identify state of compensated shock and to monitor response to intervention. Referring to the physiologic principle that nonvital organs (muscles, gastrointestinal tract, kidneys) shunt blood toward vital organs (heart, brain, adrenals) in circulatory compromise, some have proposed the use of the peripheral to cerebral oxygenation ratio as a method of early detection of blood centralization or impending circulatory compromise.[31,35,36] Because absolute rSO_2 values may not be comparable across individuals and NIRS devices, some have proposed the use of relative or percent decrease from baseline as an indication for further assessment or treatment.[37] One small, randomized study tested if early detection of microcirculation compromise by NIRS together with prompt treatment reduces the burden of hypotension (defined as mean blood pressure below gestational age) and found a nonsignificant reduction.[37] Another large, randomized clinical trial (Safeguarding the Brain of Our Smallest Infants-SafeboosC phase II) investigated

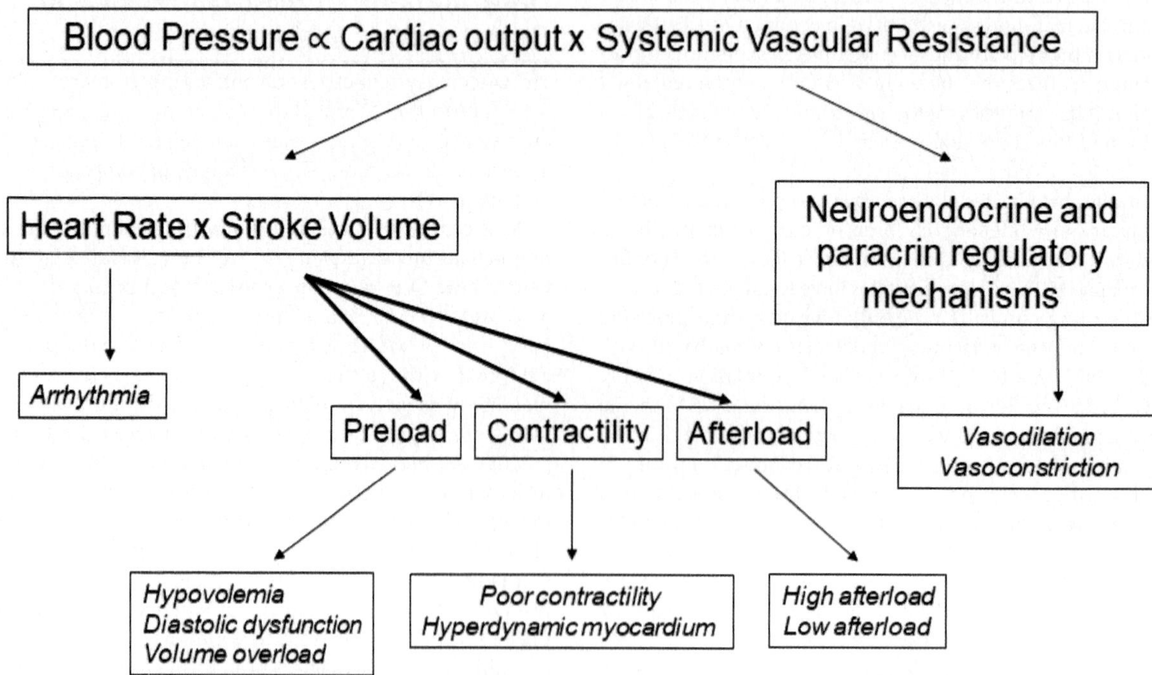

Fig. 41.4 Blood Pressure Is the Product of the Interaction Between Cardiac Output and Systemic Vascular Resistance. Assessment of each component of this interaction is important and useful in identifying the underlying cause of cardiovascular compromise. (From Noori S, Seri I. Hypotension. In: Stevenson DK, Cohen RS, Sunshine P, eds. *Neonatology: Clinical Practice and Procedure*. McGraw-Hill; 2015.)

the implementation of standard treatment guidelines in combination with rSO_2 cutoff thresholds (<55% or >85%) versus treatment as usual.[38] With the standardized protocol and implementation of rSO_2 monitoring, cerebral hypoxia or hyperoxia burden was reduced by 58%,[39] but there were no differences in early markers of brain injury[40] nor 2-year-old neurodevelopmental outcome.[41]

The use of NIRS in monitoring end organ perfusion is no doubt an important arm of hemodynamic assessment in sick infants. However, its current value in routine clinical surveillance is unclear.

SECTION

8 Jaundice, Blood Disorders, and Transfusions

OUTLINE

CHAPTER 42

A Practical Guide to Evaluating and Treating Severe Neonatal Indirect Hyperbilirubinemia

Timothy M. Bahr

KEY POINTS

1. We still need a universally accepted definition of severe hyperbilirubinemia; no particular thresholds of unconjugated or total bilirubin levels have been definitively associated with acute or chronic bilirubin encephalopathy.
2. Several measurements can be useful for the assessment of hemolysis, such as those of end-tidal carbon monoxide, blood levels of analytes such as carboxyhemoglobin and haptoglobin, reticulocyte percent and number, cell-free hemoglobin, and hemoglobinuria.
3. Hemolytic causes of hyperbilirubinemia include alloimmune hemolytic diseases. Nonimmune negative hemolytic disease can arise in red blood cell (RBC) enzymopathies, RBC membrane disorders, and globin disorders.
4. Phototherapy is the standard of care for all cases of hyperbilirubinemia. In severe hyperbilirubinemia, exchange transfusion may also be indicated. Efforts are ongoing to evaluate whether intravenous immunoglobins, metalloporphyrins, and phenobarbital might be useful in specific conditions.

Overview

There is no universal definition of severe hyperbilirubinemia because no threshold of laboratory values has been definitively associated with acute or chronic bilirubin encephalopathy. Some groups have suggested that the unconjugated fraction of bilirubin alone can cross the blood-brain barrier and cause bilirubin encephalopathy, and therefore only the unconjugated bilirubin fraction should be considered when evaluating a neonate for treatment of hyperbilirubinemia. Others have suggested that it is the unconjugated bilirubin, not bound to plasma proteins (e.g., albumin), that is more robustly associated with bilirubin encephalopathy.[1,2] Because none of these hypotheses have been upheld with uncontroversial evidence, we utilize the total serum bilirubin measurement in our evaluation of neonatal hyperbilirubinemia.[3]

Understanding the evaluation and treatment of severe neonatal indirect hyperbilirubinemia is simplified by understanding the fundamental steps in heme metabolism and bilirubin conjugation and excretion (Fig. 42.1). These crucial steps include (1) red blood cell (RBC) lysis or death, (2) the conversion of heme into biliverdin by heme oxygenase, and (3) the intrahepatic conjugation or glucuronidation of bilirubin by uridine diphosphate (UDP) glucuronosyl transferase (UGT1A1). In the most simple terms, hyperbilirubinemia is the result of either (1) excessive bilirubin production, (2) decreased bilirubin metabolism or elimination, or (3) a combination of the two. Aberrations in these crucial steps result in any of these broad etiologies.

This chapter will explore both well-established and innovative approaches to the evaluation and treatment of severe hyperbilirubinemia. Ultimately, the goal of evaluation and treatment of severe hyperbilirubinemia is to prevent bilirubin-induced neurologic dysfunction.

Determining Causes of Severe Hyperbilirubinemia

Determining the cause of severe indirect hyperbilirubinemia can have implications on immediate and long-term management of infants. Historically, our ability to identify the cause of severe hyperbilirubinemia has been poor. In the US voluntary Kernicterus Registry, conducted in the 1990s by Drs. Bhutani and Johnson, no clear explanation for the hyperbilirubinemia was identified in 55% of the 125 patients in the registry.[3] Christensen et al. reported similar findings retrospectively in the Intermountain Healthcare system in the Western United States, where among 302,399 live births, 32 neonates had a total serum bilirubin >30 mg/dL. Of these 32, only 11 (65.6%) had an explanation found for their extreme hyperbilirubinemia and the remaining patients were listed as having "idiopathic" jaundice.[4]

Subsequently, in a pilot registry in the state of Utah, Christensen successfully identified the cause of hyperbilirubinemia in all cases of acute bilirubin encephalopathy between 2009 and 2018 (seven cases). Two cases were caused by immune-mediated hemolysis. The remaining five had genetic mutations causing increased bilirubin production through hemolytic mechanisms. Two of these five patients also had a genetic mutation retarding bilirubin conjugation (Gilbert syndrome).[5] This study, although small, illustrated the growing availability and value of genetic sequencing in seeking the diagnosis of Coombs-negative hemolytic jaundice (and even nonhemolytic jaundice). At least two laboratories in the United States offer next-generation sequencing panels designed to diagnose genetic causes of severe hyperbilirubinemia: ARUP Laboratories (Salt Lake City, Utah) and Mayo Clinic Laboratories (Rochester, Minnesota). Although these panels are labeled "hereditary hemolytic anemia" panels, they both also include genes involved in bilirubin transport, conjugation, and excretion. Due to cost, we reserve these panels for more severe cases when a narrower differential diagnosis does not lead us to a more directed approach to diagnosis.

Our general approach to evaluating severe hyperbilirubinemia is to first determine whether hemolysis (increased bilirubin production) is a contributing factor, keeping in mind that the presence of hemolysis does not exclude coinheritance of mutations that slow bilirubin elimination. In fact, it is our experience that cases where increased bilirubin production and retarded bilirubin elimination are *both* present result in the most severe hyperbilirubinemia.[5] Determining

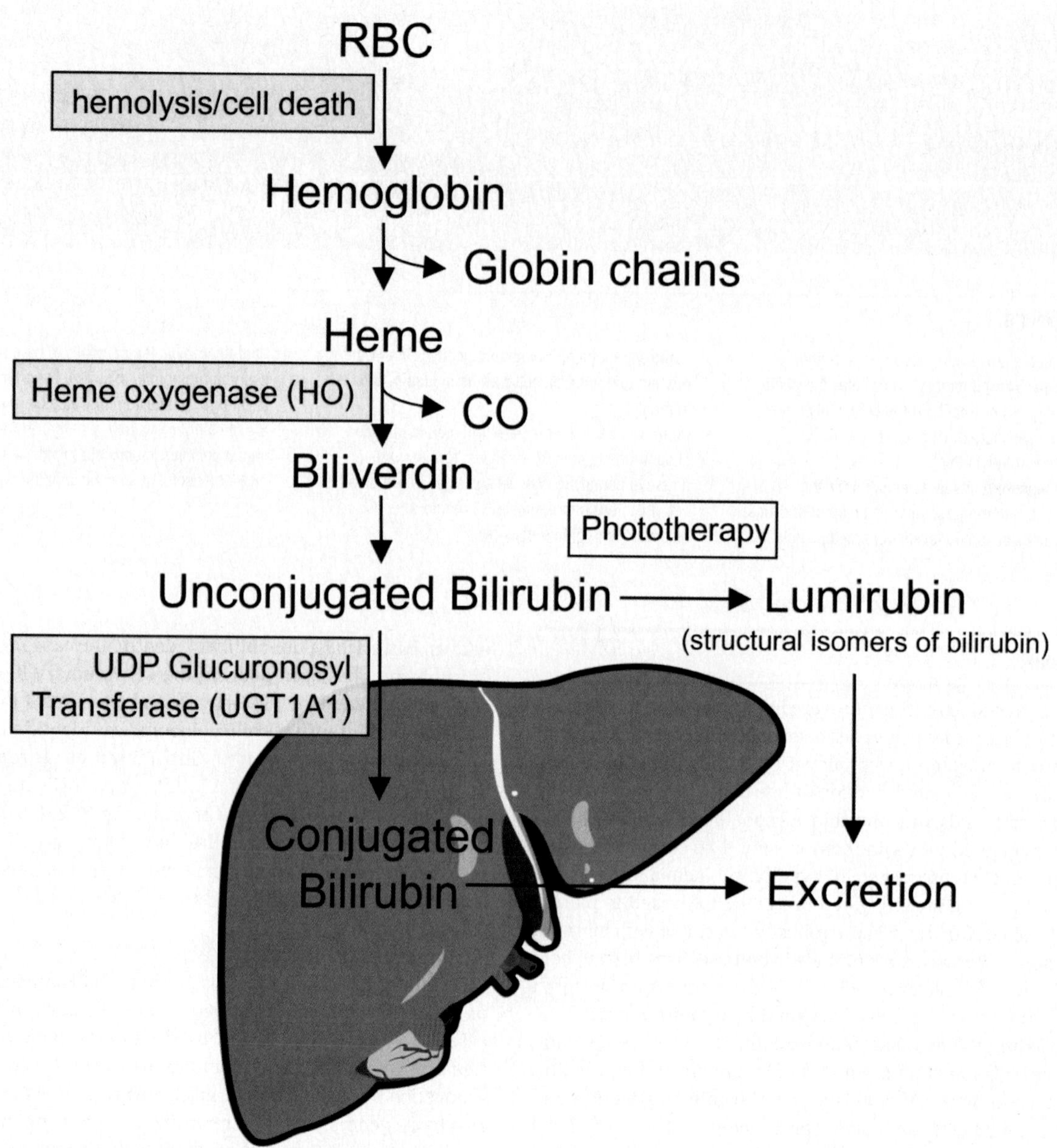

Fig. 42.1 Steps in Heme Metabolism and Bilirubin Conjugation and Excretion. *CO,* Carbon monoxide; *HO,* heme oxygenase; *RBC,* red blood cell.

whether the rate of bilirubin production is significantly increased will then help refine the differential diagnosis and guide the approach to the patient (Fig. 42.2). Here, we will first discuss tools used to differentiate hemolytic from nonhemolytic jaundice. Then we will discuss the most common hemolytic and nonhemolytic causes of severe hyperbilirubinemia.

Assessing for Hemolysis

End-Tidal Carbon Monoxide (ETCO)

Elevated carbon monoxide levels in neonates with erythroblastosis fetalis was first described in the 1971 by Jeffrey Maisels in the laboratory of David Nathan.[6] Carbon monoxide (CO) is generated in equimolar amounts to bilirubin as heme is metabolized to bilirubin.[7] Thus ETCOc (end-tidal carbon monoxide [CO] "corrected," which is end-tidal CO minus ambient CO) in exhaled breath can be used to quantify the hemolytic rate.[8] For many years, measurements of CO in the blood were only available by gas chromatography, and devices to measure CO in the breath did not exist. Portable devices are now available to obtain an accurate measurement of the ETCO noninvasively, at the patient's bedside, in less than 2 to 3 minutes. A wealth of literature supports the use of ETCOc measurement devices to quantify the rate of hemolysis in a patient and therefore identify patients with hyperbilirubinemia for whom increased hemolysis is a contributing factor.[8–11] Of the techniques described here, we consider ETCOc determinations to be the most helpful because they are sensitive and accurate, require little time, and require no phlebotomy. Based on a publication by Christensen et al. in 2015, we

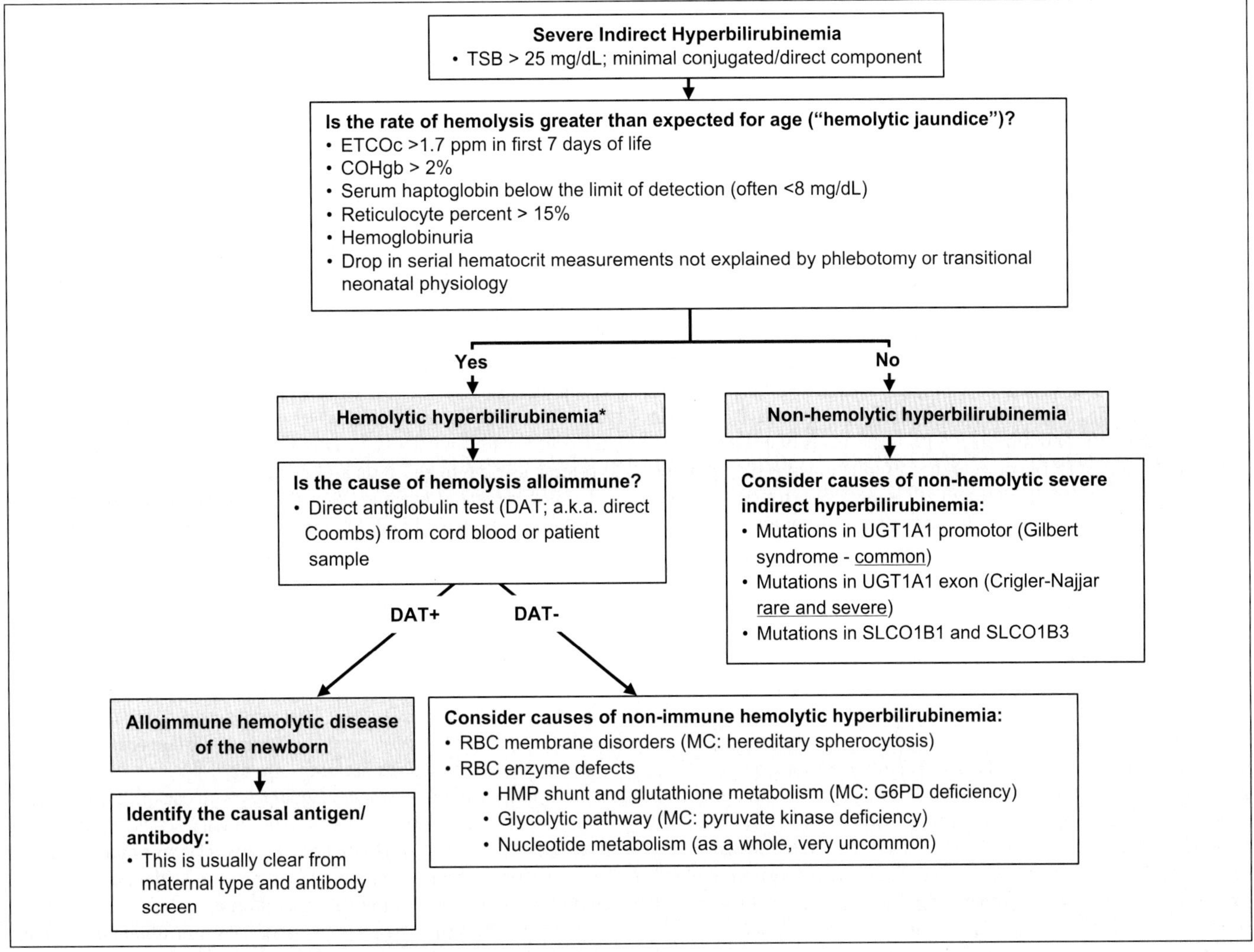

Fig. 42.2 Approach for Diagnostic Evaluation of Neonatal Hyperbilirubinemia. *COHgb*, Carboxyhemoglobin; *ETCOc*, End-tidal carbon monoxide "corrected" (end-tidal CO minus ambient CO); *HMP*, Hexose monophosphate; *MC*, Most common; *TSB*, total serum bilirubin.

consider an ETCOc measurement >1.7 ppm in a term newborn in the first week of life to be consistent with hemolysis.[9] Beyond 1 week, ETCOc determinations >1.0 ppm should raise concern for hemolysis.

Blood Carboxyhemoglobin

Carboxyhemoglobin levels can be measured directly in the blood and have utility to detect increased hemolysis similar to the ETCOc measurement.[12] Carboxyhemoglobin values are often obtained from a blood gas by cooximetry and are reported as a percentage of hemoglobin "saturated" with CO. The upper limit in the newborn has been reported between 1.5% and 2.0%.[13] Although this measure is not sensitive, it seems to be specific when elevated above 2.0%.

Serum Haptoglobin Concentration

Haptoglobin is a protein synthesized by the liver that is used to scavenge and recycle free hemoglobin. Once plasma hemoglobin is bound to haptoglobin in a haptoglobin-hemoglobin complex, it is rapidly cleared from the circulation. Therefore depletion of serum haptoglobin can be a sign of excess cell-free hemoglobin resulting from hemolysis.[13] However, haptoglobin levels are normally lower in the newborn than in a child or adult. Therefore the validity of the serum haptoglobin concentration as a marker of hemolysis is variable.[14] We judge that in a neonate, a serum haptoglobin level that is falling or is below the lower limit of detection is consistent with hemolysis.

Reticulocyte Percentage and Number

Reticulocytosis is the physiologic response to hypoxia due to anemia. At the time of delivery, the newborn is exposed to a relative hyperoxic environment that suppresses erythropoietin production and results in a decrease in red cell production and decreased reticulocyte production. Therefore the reference interval for reticulocyte percentage or number in the newborn is highly dependent on postnatal age. Because anemia may not be a result of ongoing RBC destruction, reticulocytosis is not specific for hemolysis. A reticulocyte percentage >15% can support the diagnosis of hemolysis but could also arise several days after severe hemorrhage. The immature reticulocyte fraction, reported as a percentage, is an automated reticulocyte parameter that quantifies the proportion of reticulocytes that have a particularly high RNA fraction by flow cytometry. It provides an early and sensitive index of marrow erythropoietic activity and therefore may be even more sensitive than standard reticulocyte measurements.[15] Immature reticulocyte fraction values greater than 7% at birth or >3% after 24 hours of life are consistent with a diagnosis of hemolysis.[13]

Hemoglobinuria

Cell-free hemoglobin should be uncommon in the healthy newborn. Therefore, trace hemoglobinuria or greater is evidence of hemolysis.[13]

Hemolytic Causes of Hyperbilirubinemia

Alloimmune Hemolytic Diseases of the Newborn

The primary differentiation to be made when determining causes of hemolytic hyperbilirubinemia is whether or not the process is immune-mediated (see Fig. 42.2). Historically, there has been significant emphasis placed on alloimmune-mediated hemolysis as the primary cause of severe neonatal hyperbilirubinemia (hemolytic disease of the fetus and newborn [HDFN]). This is likely due to the mortality burden of HFDN prior to the introduction of Rh(D) immune globulin (RhIg) in 1968. Although alloimmunity remains a serious and common cause of hyperbilirubinemia, its frequency in North America and Europe has decreased dramatically.

Some hospitals in the United States and Canada perform a blood type and antibody screen on all newborns born to mothers with blood type O. In the case of a mother who has a positive antibody screen, significant concern for the welfare of the fetus and newborn is warranted. The 2004 American Academy of Pediatrics guidelines, though, state that if the maternal blood group is O (+), it is an option to test the cord blood for the infant's blood type and to perform a direct antiglobulin test (DAT), *but it is not a requirement to do so* provided there is appropriate surveillance.[16] Recent studies by our group and others support eliminating routine blood typing and DAT in neonates born to blood group O (+) mothers in the absence of a positive antibody screen.[17–19] We found that neonates who were blood group A or B and born to mothers of group O (+) (and thus were at some risk for ABO hemolytic disease) did not have a higher incidence of severe neonatal hyperbilirubinemia than did neonates of blood group O who were born to group O (+) mothers (and thus were at no risk for ABO hemolytic disease). We found more in-hospital phototherapy use among babies born to group O mothers compared with mothers of other blood groups. We suggested that this supports our theory that universal bilirubin screening of neonates in the birth hospital identifies those who need phototherapy, including those with significant ABO hemolytic disease, and that this obviates their need for routine blood type testing and DAT.[8]

Because alloimmune HDFN is well-covered in other texts, this chapter will focus on DAT-negative causes of hemolysis in the newborn.[20]

Nonimmune (DAT-Negative) Hemolytic Disease of the Newborn

There are many causes of increased RBC breakdown, and therefore increased bilirubin production, that are not due to alloimmunity. All of those described here have a genetic etiology that results in a shortened RBC life span and are called hereditary hemolytic anemias. They can be subdivided into the following groups: (1) RBC enzymopathies, (2) RBC membrane disorders, and (3) globin disorders. Here, we will further subdivide RBC enzymopathies into (1) enzymes involved in the hexose monophosphate (HMP) shunt and glutathione metabolism, (2) enzymes involved in the glycolytic pathway, and (3) enzymes involved in nucleotide metabolism.

RBC Enzymopathies—HMP Shunt and Glutathione Metabolism

The unifying characteristic of defects in the HMP shunt and glutathione synthesis and metabolism is the inability of the RBC to withstand oxidative stress. Therefore the phenotype of red cell morphologies observed in these disorders is similar. Glucose-6-phosphate dehydrogenase (G6PD) deficiency accounts for a vast majority of cases attributed to RBC enzymopathies in the HMP shunt.

Glucose-6-Phosphate Dehydrogenase Deficiency

G6PD is an enzyme in the HMP shunt pathway responsible for the oxidation of glucose-6-phosphate to 6-phosphogluconate, at the same time reducing NADP to NADPH. The HMP shunt results in the production of glutathione, an important antioxidant in RBCs. Inability to maintain adequate glutathione levels, especially as newborns transition to an oxygen-rich *ex-utero* environment at birth or encounter other oxidative stress, results in denatured and dysfunctional proteins leading to cell lysis and death.

G6PD is located within q28 of the X chromosome and therefore is inherited in an X-linked dominant fashion. Symptomatic patients are almost exclusively male, but female carriers with unfavorable lyonization can also be affected. It is the most common enzymatic disorder of RBCs and affects 400 million people worldwide.[21–23] The geographic distribution G6PD deficiency prevalence is highly correlated with regions in which malaria was once endemic, leading to the hypothesis that G6PD deficiency may have conferred an advantage against malaria infection. Different genetic variants result in varying degrees of disease severity. Disease variants are named for and usually coincide with patients' ethnicities.

The peripheral blood smear of a patient who has G6PD may reveal eccentrocytes, also known as "bite" or "blister" cells, which result from splenic removal of Heinz bodies. Special stains can reveal the presence Heinz bodies, which are collections of denatured globin chains often attached to the RBC membrane.

When G6PD is the suspected cause of hyperbilirubinemia, a quantitative enzyme measurement assay is the preferred initial screening test. This test is available at many reference laboratories. Values less than 10.0 U/g hemoglobin (Hgb) are concerning for G6PD deficiency. The quantitative enzyme assay is sufficient to confirm the diagnosis for G6PD. If the patient's clinical course is consistent with the suspected variant based on ethnicity, further genetic sequencing is likely unnecessary. If the patient has refractory hyperbilirubinemia or anemia not expected based on ethnicity, then genetic sequencing may be indicated. Newborn physicians and hematologists should counsel parents of newborns with G6PD deficiency regarding drugs and foods to avoid prior to discharge. Our group schedules each child with uncomplicated G6PD deficiency in the hematology clinic between 2 and 3 months of life to recheck a complete blood cell count and provide additional counseling.

Glutathione Reductase Deficiency and Glutathione Synthetase Deficiency

Both glutathione reductase deficiency and glutathione synthetase deficiency are very rare diseases. Both result in increased RBC susceptibility to oxidative stress and present with phenotypes similar to G6PD deficiency.

RBC Enzymopathies—Glycolytic Pathway

The primary purpose of the glycolytic pathway, also known as the Embden-Meyerhof pathway, is the oxygen-independent production of energy. Enzymatic defects in this pathway result in common RBC morphologies suggestive of inadequate energy production.

Pyruvate Kinase Deficiency

Pyruvate kinase (PK) is responsible for the conversion of phosphoenolpyruvate to pyruvate with concomitant phosphorylation of adenosine diphosphate to adenosine triphosphate. PK deficiency is rare, with a prevalence estimated at <51 cases per million population. It has a worldwide distribution, but it is more common among people of northern European ancestry. Despite being rare, PK deficiency is the most common enzymopathy in the glycolytic pathway, and some have suggested that PK deficiency is the second most common hereditary variety of Coombs-negative, nonspherocytic hemolytic disease in the United States.[24]

The *PKLR* gene located on chromosome 1q22 encodes both the liver and RBC isozymes.[25] PK deficiency follows an autosomal recessive inheritance pattern (often compound heterozygosity), and as such, heterozygous carriers of *PKLR* mutations are asymptomatic. More than 260 different *PKLR* mutations have been described and associated with hemolytic anemias, most of which are single-nucleotide missense mutations.[26]

Newborns with PK deficiency present with severe hyperbilirubinemia that can be difficult to control with phototherapy.[24] Although the severity of symptoms and chronic anemia vary greatly, the disease is lifelong and may result in a need for chronic transfusions.

Other enzyme deficiencies of the glycolytic pathway have been described in case reports but are rare. Those described include aldolase, phosphofructokinase, phosphoglycerate kinase, glucose phosphate isomerase, hexokinase, and triosephosphate isomerase.

RBC Enzymopathies—Disorders of Nucleotide Metabolism

There are two main types of 5′-nucleotidases found in erythrocytes. They are known as P5′N1 and P5′N2. Defects resulting in hemolytic anemia have only been described in P5′N1 (NT5C3A).[27,28] The nucleotides of normal red cells consist largely of purine derivatives, with very low levels of pyrimidine nucleotides. P5′N1 deficiency results in accumulation of pyrimidines because it converts pyrimidine nucleoside monophosphates into cytidine and uridine, which can diffuse across the cell membrane. Excessive pyrimidines are thought to have toxic effects on RBCs. Their accumulation and subsequent intracellular persistence of ribosomes/RNA results in basophilic stippling. Although this finding is sensitive for P5′N1 deficiency, it is clearly not specific for this condition. It is also seen in lead poisoning, sideroblastic anemia, and certain hemoglobinopathies.[29,30]

More than 25 different mutations have been identified in NT5C3A. The majority of patients with P5′N1 deficiency are homozygous for a single mutation and the remainder are compound heterozygotes. The clinical manifestations of P5′N1 deficiency are lifelong mild-to-moderate hemolytic anemia accompanied by jaundice and splenomegaly.[28]

Assaying for the presence of pyrimidine nucleotides serves as a surrogate marker for P5′N1 deficiency and is available at a few reference laboratories including the Mayo Clinic. Alternatively, the *NT5C3A* gene is included as part of the hereditary hemolytic anemia gene panels available at the Mayo Clinic and ARUP laboratories.

RBC Membrane Disorders

Disorders due to RBC membrane structural protein defects include hereditary spherocytosis (HS), hereditary elliptocytosis, and hereditary pyropoikilocytosis. The structural proteins involved in these disorders are closely related.

Hereditary Spherocytosis

HS is a disorder characterized by defects in RBC membrane proteins resulting in a loss of RBC membrane surface area and thus sphere-shaped, hyperdense, poorly deformable RBCs. The cells have a shortened life span, which causes a hemolytic anemia found worldwide in individuals from all races and ethnicities. HS is the most common inherited hemolytic anemia in people with Northern European ancestry, with an estimated incidence of 1 per 1000 to 1 per 3000 births.[25,31] Seventy-five percent of cases are inherited in an autosomal dominant manner and the remaining are inherited in an autosomal recessive manner or are from a *de novo* mutation. The most commonly mutated gene associated with HS in the Northern European population is *ANK1* (40%–65%). Other genes where mutations cause HS include *SPTA1*, *SPTB*, *SLC4A1*, and *EPB42*.

The practitioner should consider HS when a neonate has Coombs-negative jaundice, anemia, and microcytosis. Christensen and Henry in 2010 also showed that an mean corpuscular hemoglobin concentration (MCHC) >36 g/dL in newborns with a total serum bilirubin >20 mg/dL is both sensitive and specific for HS.[32] In a subsequent publication by Christensen, the author estimated the ratio of mean corpuscular hemoglobin concentration to mean corpuscular volume (MCHC/MCV) >0.36 to be 97% sensitive and >99% specific for HS.[33]

The traditional diagnostic test for HS has been osmotic fragility. However, more recently it has been shown that the diagnostic criteria for HS used in adults and older children are unreliable in newborn infants because in both preterm and term infants, RBC membranes have an increased osmotic resistance. A relatively new diagnostic test for HS, eosin-5-maleimide flow cytometry, quantifies the erythrocyte membrane band 3 complex using an eosin-5-maleimide dye flow cytometric analysis.[34,35] A reduction in band 3 complex is consistent with HS. Therefore the test is commonly referred to as "band 3 reduction" at reference laboratories that offer it. This test performs well in neonates even in the first days of life.[36,37] If the patient has no family history of HS or the causal mutation is unknown, sequencing the genes that can cause HS is indicated. Different mutations result in a variety of disease severities. Identifying the causal mutation can also aid in identification of the inheritance pattern and reproductive risk for the proband.

Nonhemolytic Causes of Indirect Hyperbilirubinemia

Most known nonhemolytic causes of indirect hyperbilirubinemia are due to either (1) impaired uptake into the hepatocyte or (2) impaired conjugation of the unconjugated bilirubin molecule, with the latter being much more common.

SLCO1B1 and SLCO1B3

Solute carrier organic anion transporter family members 1B1 and 1B3 (SLCO1B1 and SLCO1B3) encode proteins expressed on the hepatic cell membrane that facilitate the transport of bilirubin into the hepatocyte.

Gilbert Syndrome

Both Gilbert syndrome and Crigler-Najjar syndrome are caused by inadequate glucuronidation (conjugation) of bilirubin by UDP-glucuronosyltransferase *(UGT1A1)*. Gilbert syndrome is typically caused by genetic variants in the promotor region of *UGT1A1*. Therefore, in contrast to patients with Crigler-Najjar syndrome, patients with Gilbert syndrome produce UDP-glucuronosyltransferase enzymes that have normal function but are decreased in amount. The normal sequence of the TATAA element within the promoter of *UGT1A1* is A(TA)6TAA, or simply (TA)6. The most common variant is a longer version of the TATAA sequence A(TA)7TAA, known as *UGT1A1*28*, that reduces the production of UDP-glucuronosyltransferase due to decreased affinity of transcription factors to the promotor region. Traditional thought is that Gilbert syndrome manifests only in people who are homozygous for the variant promoter. As a result, its inheritance is most consistent with an autosomal recessive trait. However, heterozygotes for the Gilbert genotype also have a partially decreased UGT1A1 enzyme level. We observed moderate to severe hyperbilirubinemia in *UGT1A1*28* heterozygotes when combined with another mildly hemolytic etiology (e.g., anti-A alloimmunization or heterozygosity for allele alpha-LELY in *SPTA1*). Epidemiologic studies of Gilbert syndrome (specifically, TA[7]) in Caucasian populations estimate a prevalence between 9.8% and 16%. Other alleles such as TA(5) and TA(8) are found in Caucasian populations but with much lower prevalence. These alleles can also result in decreased *UGT1A1* expression, resulting in bilirubin levels above normal. Because of the high prevalence of *UGT1A1* promoter polymorphisms, we find it that it is a common contributor to hyperbilirubinemia—often in combination with other bilirubin production or elimination aberrations.

Crigler-Najjar Syndrome

Crigler-Najjar can be divided into two types. Type I is characterized by absent uridine diphosphate glucuronosyltransferase (UGT) activity and little or no conjugated bilirubin. This results in early-onset, severe, lifelong indirect hyperbilirubinemia and is caused by a subset of mutations within *UGT1A1* coding regions that result in essentially no functional UGT enzyme. Type II is characterized by varying degrees of decreased enzyme activity that are caused by less deleterious mutations in the coding regions of *UGT1A1*. Children with Crigler-Najjar Type I and those with persistent hyperbilirubinemia due to Crigler-Najjar Type II should be referred to a transplant hepatology center for evaluation and management.

In 2020, Straus and colleagues published their experience in caring for 28 children with Crigler-Najjar Type I over 30 years.[38] Seventeen required liver transplantation. Prior to liver transplantation, neonates are phototherapy-dependent and require 15 to 20 hours per day on phototherapy.

Treatment of Severe Hyperbilirubinemia

Phototherapy is the standard of care for nearly all cases of hyperbilirubinemia. In cases of severe hyperbilirubinemia, especially those with signs of acute bilirubin encephalopathy, exchange transfusion may also be indicated. This section will briefly review evidence for or against less common therapies with unproven efficacy.

Intravenous Immunoglobulin

Because of the risks associated with exchange transfusions, intravenous immunoglobulin (IVIg) has been suggested as an alternative to avoid exchange transfusion. IVIg may reduce the rate of hemolysis by blocking the Fc receptors on macrophages that are thought to mediate destruction of RBCs coated with anti-D antibodies. The 2018 Cochrane Review (systematic review and meta-analysis) by Zwiers et al. examines the most relevant literature regarding IVIg for the treatment of alloimmune hemolytic disease of the newborn.[39] That review identifies the only two published studies with sufficiently low risk of bias to assess the efficacy of the therapy: a 2011 study by Smits-Wintjens et al. conducted in the Netherlands[40] and a 2013 study by Santos et al. conducted in Brazil.[41] Both of those trials conclusively found no benefit of IVIg in reducing the need for and number of exchange transfusions in cases of Rh hemolytic disease. The authors of the Cochrane Review state that the seven other studies included in their analysis were observational and had a high risk of bias. Our group has concluded that the Netherlands and Brazil studies were sufficient to show that IVIg has little or no benefit in the treatment of alloimmune hemolytic disease of the newborn, and children with hyperbilirubinemia not controlled by phototherapy should be transferred to a center that is able to perform an exchange transfusion.

Metalloporphyrins

Currently, the only means available to reduce the hemolytic rate in neonates with severe hemolytic jaundice is to perform a double-volume exchange transfusion, removing hemolyzing erythrocytes and replacing them with donor adult erythrocytes. Metalloporphyrins are potent inhibitors of heme oxygenase, the rate-limiting enzyme in the production of bilirubin from heme. Two metalloporphyrins have been studied to assess their ability to decrease the risk of hyperbilirubinemia. Tin mesoporphyrin has been tested in animals and humans and has shown promising results. Zinc protoporphyrin has been studied in only animals. Unfortunately, these drugs are not approved for use in the United States and have not been produced for clinical use.

Phenobarbital

Phenobarbital can induce UGT activity and can promote conjugation of bilirubin to its water-soluble form. We reserve the use of phenobarbital for neonates with genetically proven Crigler-Najjar Type II (or strong suspicion of the disease, awaiting confirmation). Neonates with Crigler-Najjar Type I do not respond to phenobarbital therapy and this lack of response can be used to differentiate Type I from Type II.

CHAPTER 43

Neonatal Anemia

Robert D. Christensen

KEY POINTS

1. Anemia is an abnormal, and an unhealthy, reduction in the blood hemoglobin concentration or the hematocrit. There are limitations in our current definitions of anemia, which are based on "reference intervals" constructed from clinically obtained laboratory tests, not from tests performed on healthy volunteers.
2. Erythropoietin is the main physiologic regulator of red blood cell (RBC) production.
3. Neonatal RBCs frequently show morphologic features of immaturity such as anisocytosis, poikilocytosis, and macrocytosis. Some nucleated erythrocytes may also be seen.
4. The combination of shortened RBC survival, decreased production, and growth-related expansion of the blood volume is responsible for a progressive decrease of hemoglobin concentrations in early infancy.
5. Neonates with anemia should be evaluated for losses due to hemorrhage or hemolysis and for possible hyporegenerative etiologies. In growing premature infants, anemia of prematurity is an important cause of hyporegenerative anemia beyond 4 weeks after birth.

Introduction

Anemia is an abnormal, and an unhealthy, reduction in the blood hemoglobin concentration or the hematocrit.[1] These two laboratory tests (hemoglobin and hematocrit) are somewhat similar in that each assesses the capacity of a subject's blood to deliver oxygen to that subject's tissues. It should be recognized, however, that neither measurement directly quantifies oxygen delivery or assesses whether the tissue's oxygen needs are indeed being met. In fact, very often in neonatal medicine, poor oxygen delivery to tissues is not the result of anemia at all but is due to respiratory, or sometimes cardiac, disease. Consequently, a practical definition of anemia, in neonatal medicine, focuses on quantifying an erythrocyte *number*, not on the physiologic concept of inadequate oxygen delivery. Specifically, by convention, the *number* that defines anemia in a neonate is a blood hemoglobin concentration or a hematocrit that falls below the 5th percentile of the appropriate reference interval.[2] The "appropriate" reference interval is one that accounts for the gestational age and the postnatal age of the neonate. This is because gestational age and postnatal age both profoundly affect where the hemoglobin concentration or hematocrit "should be." This chapter reviews the reference interval–based definition and pathogenesis of neonatal anemia and provides practical approaches for diagnosing the exact cause of this condition when the cause is not obvious.

Fetal and Neonatal Erythropoiesis

Erythropoietin (Epo) is the main physiologic regulator of red blood cell production.[3] However, it has additional biologic roles, some of which are particularly relevant during fetal and neonatal development. For instance, Epo is an important constituent of amniotic fluid, typically in concentrations of 25 to 40 mU/mL. A normal human fetus swallows 200 to 300 mL of amniotic fluid/kg/day and thus swallows 10 to 15 U of Epo/kg/day.[4,5] Epo does not cross the human placenta, and the source of the Epo in amniotic fluid is not the maternal circulation. In the second and third trimesters, amniotic fluid is largely derived from fetal urine, with minor constituents from fetal tracheal effluent and the placenta and fetal membranes. However, Epo in amniotic fluid is not derived from fetal urine. Fetal kidneys produce little Epo before delivery, and the first-voided urine of neonates generally has no detectable Epo.[6] Studies using *in situ* hybridization and immunohistochemistry indicate that the source of Epo in amniotic fluid is largely maternal, from mesenchymal and endothelial cells in the deciduae and amnion.[4]

Colostrum and breast milk contain biologically active Epo in concentrations of 10 to 20 mU/mL.[7–9] Epo levels in milk do not correlate with Epo levels in the mother's blood. In fact, during the first weeks of lactation, the mother's serum Epo concentrations decrease, whereas her milk Epo concentrations increase, reaching the highest concentrations in women breastfeeding for a year or more. The source of Epo in breast milk is mammary gland epithelium.[10] Epo in human amniotic fluid, colostrum, and breast milk is relatively protected from proteolytic digestion in the fetal and neonatal gastrointestinal tract. However, rather than being absorbed from the gastrointestinal tract into the blood, the Epo swallowed by the fetus and neonate binds to Epo receptors on the luminal surface of villous enterocytes, where it serves as an intestinal growth and development factor. Experimental animals artificially fed formulas devoid of Epo have retarded villous development, a condition that can be remedied by enteral recombinant Epo and blocked by anti-Epo antibody.[11]

Cells in the developing central nervous system produce Epo, which is present in relatively high concentrations in fetal cerebrospinal fluid (CSF).[12–16] In fact, the highest concentrations of Epo in the CSF are in the most premature neonates, and by several years of age, CSF Epo concentrations are typically <1 mU/mL.[15] Epo receptors are expressed on human fetal neurons,[12,14] and at least small quantities of recombinant Epo administered intravenously cross the blood-brain barrier and appear in the CSF.[17] Epo is a natural neuroprotectant.[18–22] Its production increases rapidly in the brain during hypoxia, and when Epo binds to receptors on neurons, antiapoptotic activity is induced. The clinical utility of recombinant Epo as a neuroprotectant is a topic of ongoing studies.

The liver is the primary site of fetal Epo production. The kidneys produce only about 5% of the total Epo during midgestation. The mechanisms regulating the switch in Epo production from the liver to the kidneys are not completely known but may involve developmental expression of transcription activators such as hypoxia inducible factor and hepatic nuclear factor 4[23,24] or developmental methylation of promoter and enhancer regions. The switch might involve the GATA transcription factors, particularly GATA-2 and GATA-3, which are negative regulators of Epo gene transcription.

Identifying Anemia Using Reference Intervals

"Reference intervals" are generally used to interpret laboratory tests in neonatology in place of "normal ranges."[2] The difference is that reference intervals are constructed from clinically obtained laboratory tests, not from tests performed on healthy volunteers. In order to approximate a normal range, the laboratory tests included in a reference interval data set are only those from neonatal patients who have minimal pathology or pathology not thought to be related to the test under consideration. For instance, reference intervals for the hematocrit of neonates exclude data from neonates with clinical issues known to affect the hematocrit, such as erythrocyte transfusions, hemolytic disease, hemorrhage, or reduction transfusion. Reference intervals for hematocrit on the day of birth, according to gestational age of the neonate, are shown in Fig. 43.1A.[25] Before 28 weeks' gestation, anemia is defined by a hematocrit below 30%. At term, anemia is defined by a hematocrit below 42%. Clearly, the hematocrit should increase gradually during the period from 23 weeks to term. Thus the definition of anemia, at birth, requires knowledge of the gestational age. Fig. 43.1B gives the same information for blood hemoglobin concentration on the day of birth. The same basic pattern is seen as in Fig. 43.1A.

In the days and weeks after birth, the hematocrit and hemoglobin gradually decrease. Fig. 43.2 demonstrates the reference interval for decreasing hematocrit (A) and hemoglobin (B) of term neonates ($\geq$35 weeks) and the hematocrit (C) and hemoglobin (D) of preterm neonates ($<$35 weeks).[25]

Circulating erythrocytes in the fetus have features reminiscent of "stress erythropoiesis" in adults. These features include anisocytosis, poikilocytosis, macrocytosis, and the presence of nucleated erythrocytes. Marrow cellularity in the fetus is relatively high. Erythroid precursors account for 30% to 65% and myeloid cells for 45% to 75% of nucleated marrow cells at birth.[26] The myeloid to erythroid ratio at birth is approximately 1.5:1. Marrow cellularity decreases after birth, attaining a density that is normal for adults by 1 to 3 months. Initially, this decrease in cellularity results from a rapid decline in red cell production. At 1 week of age, erythroid elements account for only 8% to 12% of nucleated cells, and the myeloid to erythroid ratio exceeds 6:1. The normal adult proportion of myeloid to erythroid precursors is not established until the third month. Both the percentage and absolute number of lymphocytes increase during the first 2 months, so that by 3 months of age, they constitute nearly 50% of marrow nucleated cells. Differential counts of bone marrow aspirates from preterm infants are similar to those of term infants.[27]

In newborn infants the hemoglobin (Hb) concentration and hematocrit of capillary blood are 5% to 10% higher than those of venous blood.[1] The difference between capillary and venous values is greatest at birth but disappears by 3 months of age. The discrepancy is greatest in preterm infants and in those with hypotension, hypovolemia, and acidosis.[28,29]

Reticulocytes at birth are approximately 5% of erythrocytes, with a range of 4% to 7%.[1,27] Reticulocytes remain elevated for the first 1 to 3 days, typically dropping abruptly to 0% to 1% by day 7. Nucleated red cells are seen regularly on blood smears during the first day of life, constituting about 0.1% of the red cell population (500 normoblasts/mm^3)[30] but are not common in the circulation after the first 3 days unless intermittent or chronic hypoxia is present.[31–33]

Red cell morphology is characterized by macrocytosis and poikilocytosis. Target cells and stomatocytes are prominent. Similarly, a high proportion of siderocytes (3.2% vs. the normal adult mean of 0.1%) is seen.[34]

Measuring the circulating red blood cell (RBC) volume in a fetus or neonate is difficult. Mock et al. used a nonradioactive method, based on *in vivo* dilution of biotinylated RBCs enumerated by flow cytometry, to estimate the correlation between hematocrit and circulating RBC volume in infants $<$1300 g and found that venous hematocrit values correlated highly with the circulating erythrocyte volume (r, 0.907; $P<.0001$).[35,36]

Neonates have a shorter red cell survival than do children and adults. The life span of red cells from term infants is estimated to be 60 to 80 days using the ^{51}Cr method and 45 to 70 days using methods involving ^{59}Fe.[37] Fetal studies using [^{14}C] cyanate-labeled red cells in sheep revealed an average red cell life span of 64 ± 6 days.[38] The mean red cell life span increases linearly from 35 to 107 days as the fetal age increases from 97 days (midgestation) to 136 days (term).

Neonatal red cells transfused into adults have a short survival,[39] indicating that factors intrinsic to the newborn red cell are responsible. This conclusion gains further support from a demonstration that adult red cells survive normally in newborn recipients. The life span frequency function is not parametrically distributed, in that most cells are destroyed before the mean survival is reached. Shortened red cell survival corresponds with erythropoietic rates at birth that are three to five times greater than those of normal adults.

The abrupt transition from the relative hypoxia of the uterus to an oxygen-rich environment profoundly alters erythropoiesis. During the first 2 months of life, the infant experiences both the highest and lowest Hb concentrations occurring at any time in development. Epo levels at birth are usually well above the normal adult range and fall markedly in the immediate postnatal period.[40] By 24 hours, the Epo value is below the normal adult range, where it remains throughout the first month of life. The decrease in Epo level is followed by a decline in the number of bone marrow precursors[41] and a decrease in the reticulocyte count.

The combination of shortened RBC survival, decreased production, and growth-related expansion of the blood volume is responsible for a progressive fall of the Hb concentration to a mean of approximately 11 g/dL at 2 months of age.[1] The lower reference interval for infants of this age is approximately 9 g/dL. This nadir is called *physiologic anemia*, in that it is not associated with apparent distress and is not prevented with nutritional supplements. Stabilization of the Hb concentration is heralded by an increase in reticulocytes at 4 to 8 weeks. Thereafter, the Hb concentration rises to a mean level of 12.5 g/dL, where it remains throughout infancy and early childhood.[1]

At term, the placenta and umbilical cord contain 75 to 125 mL of blood (30–40 mL/kg), or approximately one-fourth to one-third of the fetal blood volume.[42] Linderkamp et al. compared postnatal alterations in blood viscosity, hematocrit, plasma viscosity, red cell aggregation, and red cell deformability in the first 5 days of postnatal life in full-term neonates with early (less than 10 seconds) and late (3 minutes) cord clamping.[42] The residual placental blood volume decreased from 52 ± 8 mL/kg of neonatal body weight after early cord clamping to 15 ± 4 mL/kg after clamping. The neonatal blood volume was 50% higher in the late cord-clamped infants.

Additional placental transfer of blood to preterm infants occurs by delayed clamping of the umbilical cord. Transfer of about 10 to 15 mL/k

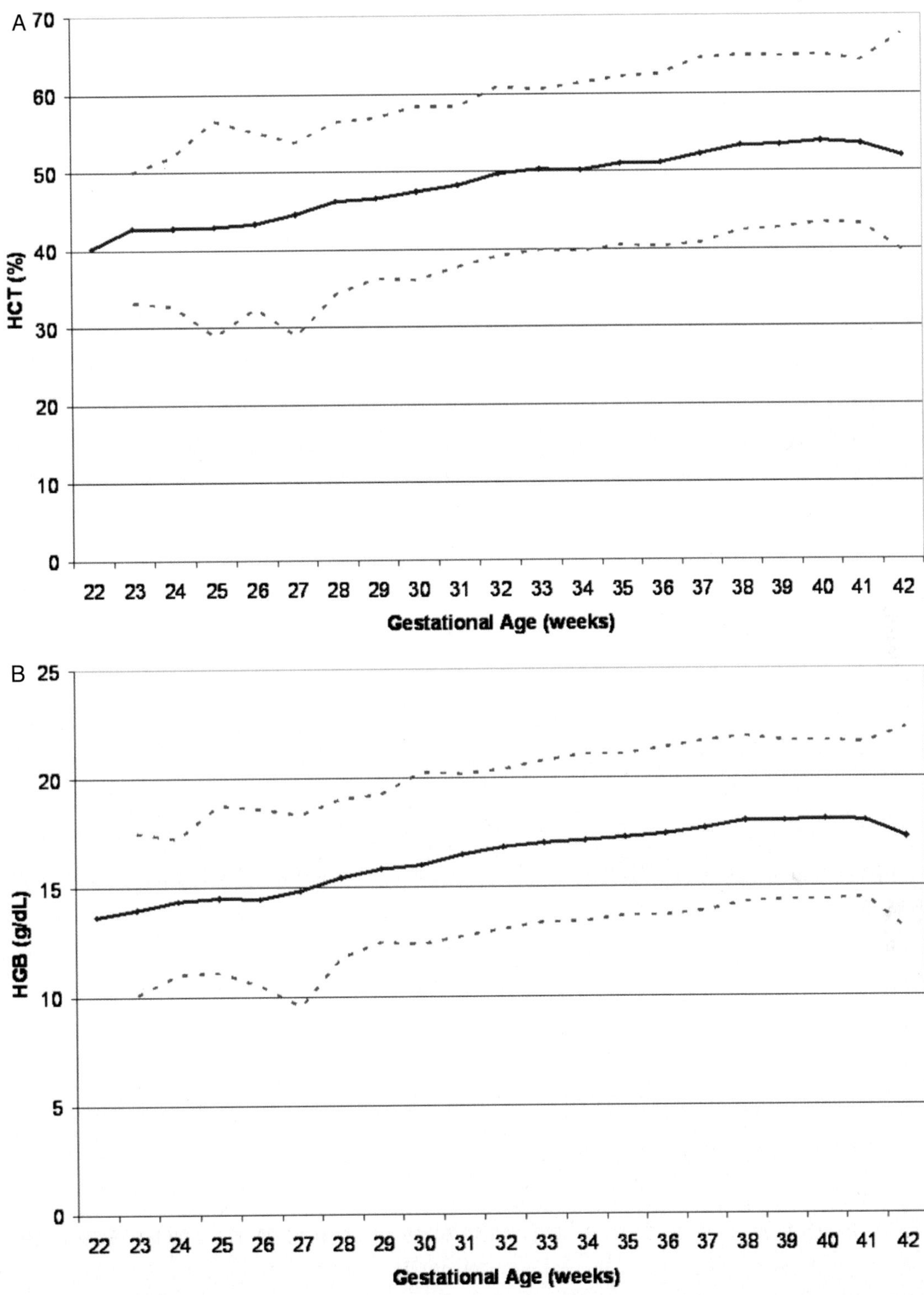

Fig. 43.1 Reference Intervals for Hematocrit and Blood Hemoglobin Concentration on the Day of Birth. (A) Hematocrit (HCT, %). (B) Hemoglobin (HGB, g/dL).Values are shown as a function of gestational age. The lower reference interval is the 5th percentile of the reference database and the upper reference interval is the 95th percentile. Values below the 5th percentile define "anemia" and those above the 95th percentile define "polycythemia," according to gestational age. (From Jopling J, Henry E, Wiedmeier SE, Christensen RD. Reference ranges for hematocrit and blood hemoglobin concentration during the neonatal period: data from a multihospital health care system. *Pediatrics*. 2009;123[2]:e333–e337, with permission.)

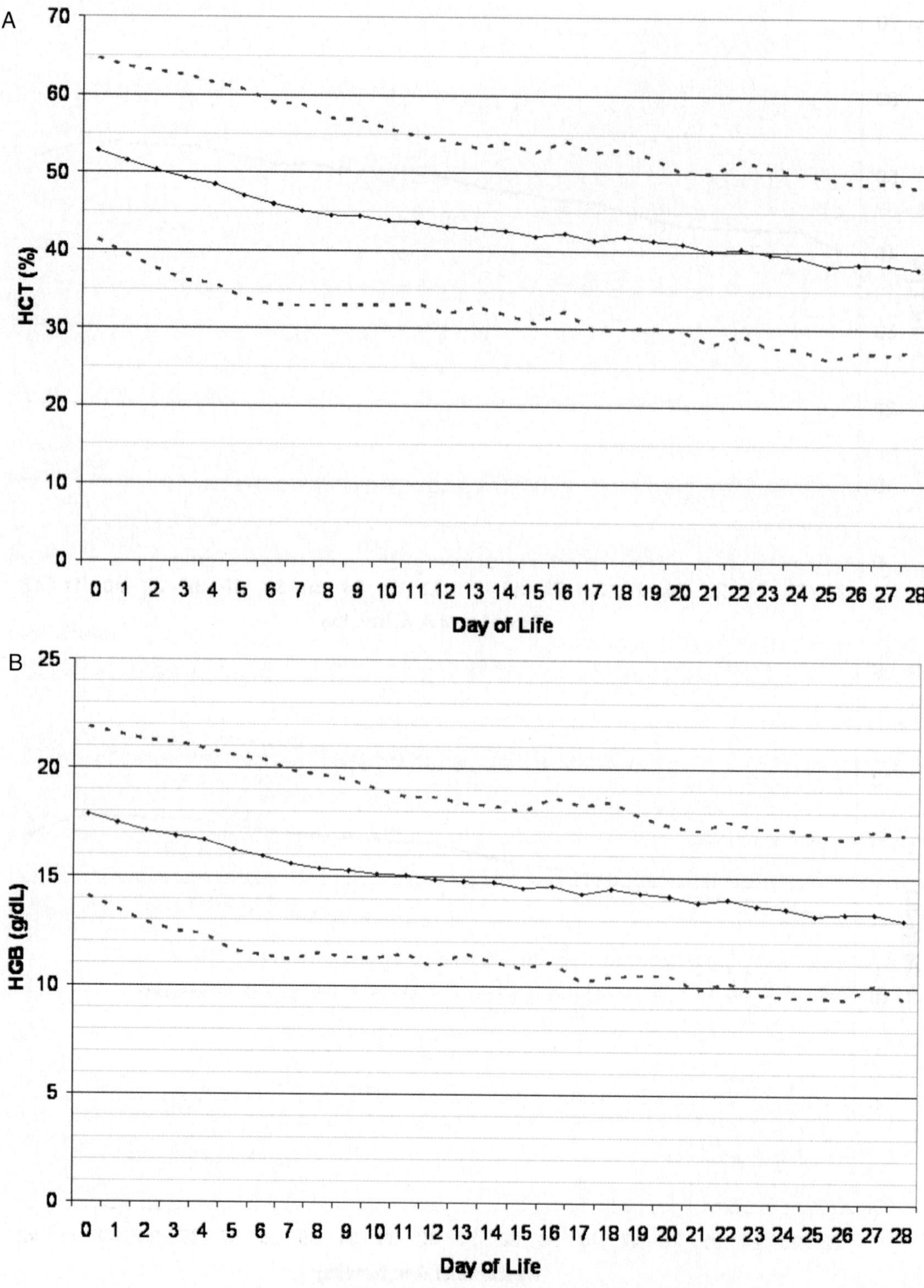

Fig. 43.2 Reference Intervals for Hematocrit and Blood Hemoglobin Concentration During the First Month After Birth. (A) Hematocrit (HCT, %) from late preterm and term neonates. (B) Hemoglobin (HGB, g/dL) from late preterm and term neonates. (C) Hematocrit (%) from preterm neonates. (D) Hemoglobin (g/dL) from preterm infants. The lower reference interval is the 5th percentile of the reference database and the upper reference interval is the 95th percentile. Values below the 5th percentile define "anemia" and those above the 95th percentile define "polycythemia," according to gestational age. (From Jopling J, Henry E, Wiedmeier SE, Christensen RD. Reference ranges for hematocrit and blood hemoglobin concentration during the neonatal period: data from a multihospital health care system. *Pediatrics*. 2009;123[2]:e333–e337, with permission.)

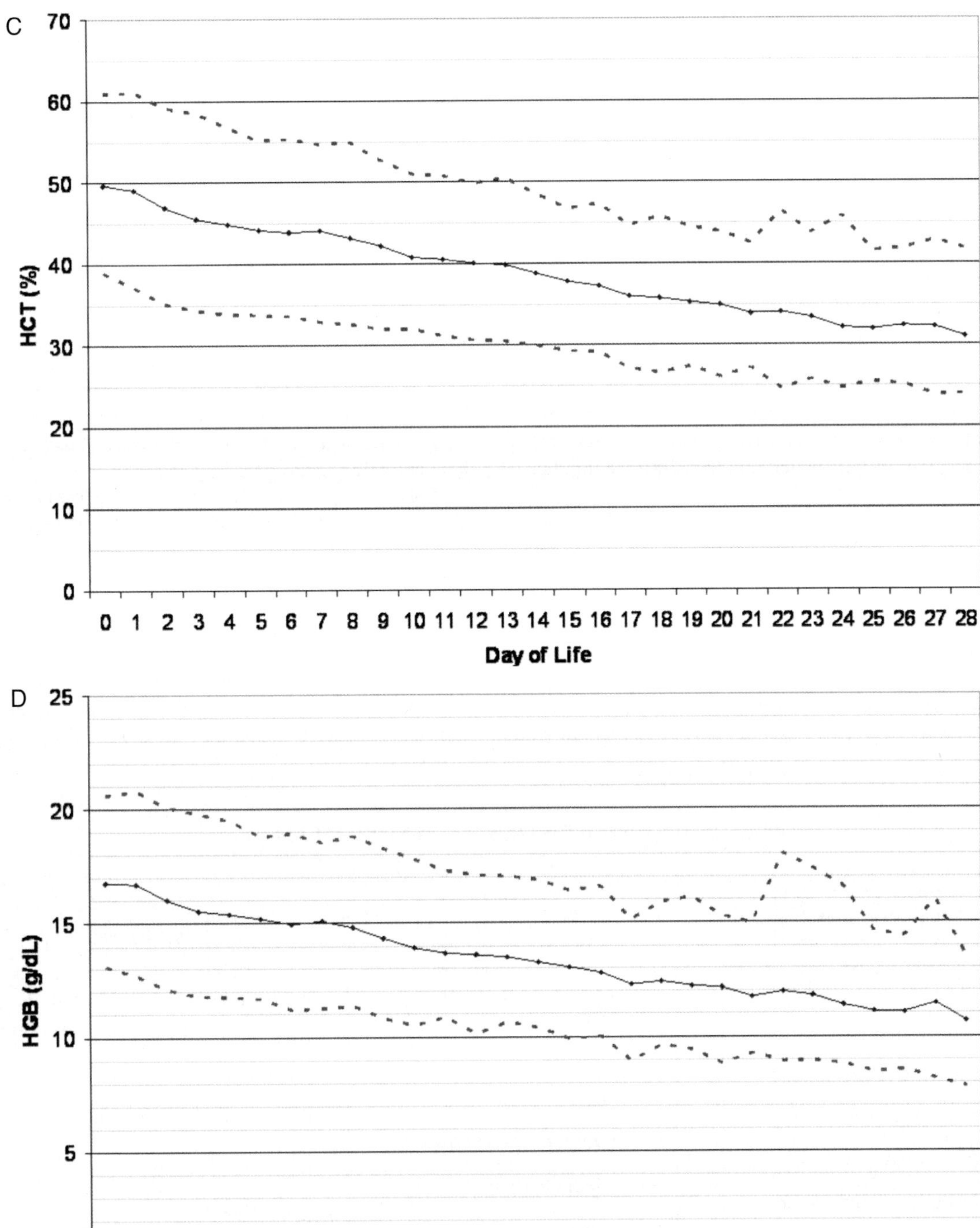

Fig. 43.2 Cont'd

body weight can be expected by delaying clamping for 30 to 60 seconds and has been claimed to reduce intraventricular hemorrhage and late-onset sepsis.[43–47]

When the Cause of Neonatal Anemia Is Not Obvious

Once anemia has been recognized in a neonate, using appropriate reference intervals, it is important to determine the cause of the anemia. In many instances, the explanation for anemia in a neonate is obvious. However, occasionally the cause is unclear. Diagnosing the cause of the anemia, not just the fact that anemia exists, is important. This is because diagnosing the cause may reveal something about the propensity for future anemia, such as with genetic hemolytic anemia. Moreover, the cause can be important to families or the obstetric management team or to quality-improvement initiatives that aim to reduce the incidence of neonatal anemia.

Thus every time anemia is diagnosed in a neonate, the cause of the anemia should be sought, and when appropriate, the cause should be documented in the medical record. An effective approach to finding the cause of the anemia in a neonate when the cause is not obvious involves careful consideration of each of the "three H's": namely, (1) hyporegenerative, (2) hemorrhagic, and (3) hemolytic (Fig. 43.3).

It can be helpful to classify whether the anemic neonate's RBCs are normal in size or are larger or smaller than normal. Similarly, it can be helpful to know whether the anemic neonate's RBC content of hemoglobin is normal or is greater or less than normal. Toward this end, reference intervals for erythrocyte indices are shown in Fig. 43.4.[48] Reference intervals for the mean corpuscular volume (MCV, measured in fL) are shown in Fig. 43.4A and for the mean corpuscular hemoglobin (MCH, measured in pg) in Fig. 43.4B. Microcytic anemia is diagnosed when the MCV is below the 5th percentile for gestational age. Thus an anemic extremely low gestational age neonate with an MCV less than about 104 fL has microcytic anemia. Likewise, an anemic term neonate with an MCV less than about 98 fL has microcytic anemia. In the way the MCV informs on red cell size, the MCH informs on erythrocyte "paleness" or hypochromia, due to an amount of hemoglobin in erythrocytes that is below normal (below the 5th percentile reference interval for gestational age). Thus an anemic extremely low gestational age neonate with an MCH less than about 35 pg would have hypochromic anemia, whereas an anemic term neonate with an MCH less than about 33 pg would have hypochromic anemia.

These reference intervals are valid for the first day of life, and probably for the first week, assuming no erythrocyte transfusion is given. However, rigorous reference intervals based on postnatal age are not yet available, and thus it is not clear precisely how the erythrocyte indices change over the weeks and months after birth. In adults, the reference interval for MCV is 88 ± 8 fL (thus an MCV less than 80fL defines microcytosis), and the reference interval for MCH is 30 ± 3 pg (thus an MCH less than 30 pg defines red cell hypochromia).

Microcytic and hypochromic erythrocytes in anemic neonates can be recognized by examining the blood smear unless they are so

WHICH OF THE THREE H'S IS CAUSING THE NEONATAL ANEMIA?

HYPOPRODUCTION	HEMORRHAGE	HEMOLYSIS
Reticulocyte count very low	Reticulocyte count elevated (if hemorrhage occurred >24 h previously)	Reticulocyte count elevated (if hemolysis began >24 h previously)
End-tidal CO normal	End-tidal CO normal	End-tidal CO elevated
Carboxyhemoglobin normal	Carboxyhemoglobin normal	Carboxyhemoglobin elevated
Haptoglobin normal	Haptoglobin normal	Haptoglobin absent
No Hgb in urine	No Hgb in urine	Hgb in urine
Careful dysmorphology exam	"External Occult" Kleihauer-Betkie may be positive	G6PD or PK enzyme levels if those deficiencies are in question
Genetic panel	"External Occult" Monozygotic Twin-Twin hgb may differ	Band 3 reduction if HS is in question
Iron studies (RET-He, soluble transferrin receptor, %Micro-R, %Hypo-He, low MCV and MCH for age, serum ferritin)	"Internal Occult" IVH, subgaleal, adrenal, hepatic	Formal schistocyte count, if microangiopathic hemolysis is in question
Blood film examination	Blood film examination	Genetic panel
		DAT
		Blood film examination

Fig. 43.3 Finding the Cause of the Neonatal Anemia, If It Is Not Obvious.

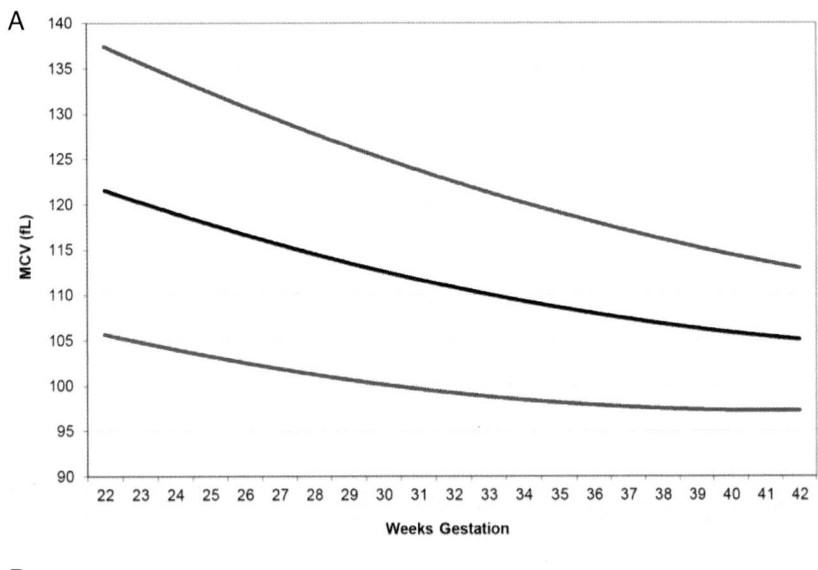

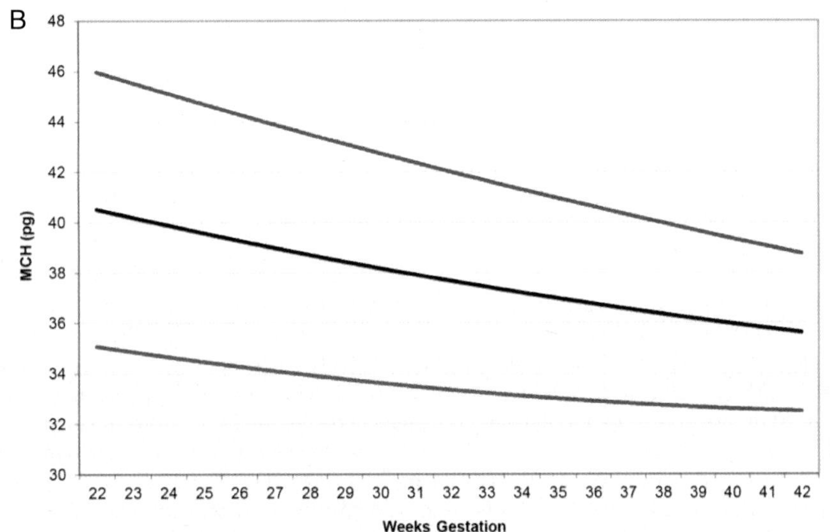

Fig. 43.4 Reference Intervals for Red Blood Cell Size and Red Blood Cell Hemoglobin Content at Birth as a Function of Gestational Age. (A) Red blood cell size (mean corpuscular volume [MCV], fL). (B) Red blood cell hemoglobin content (mean corpuscular hemoglobin [MCH], pg). For both panels, the lower reference interval is the 5th percentile of the reference database and the upper reference interval is the 95th percentile. In (A), MCV values below the 5th percentile define "microcytosis" and those above the 95th percentile define "macrocytosis." In (B), MCH values below the 5th percentile define erythrocyte "hypochromasia" and those above the 95th percentile define erythrocyte "hyperchromasia," according to gestational age. (From Christensen RD, Jopling J, Henry E, Wiedmeier SE. The erythrocyte indices of neonates, defined using data from over 12,000 patients in a multihospital health care system. *J Perinatol.* 2008;28[1]:24–28, with permission.)

mild as to be unrecognizable from normal. New complete blood cell count (CBC) parameters, besides the erythrocyte indices, give additional credence to the diagnosis of microcytosis and hypochromasia. These are the % Micro R (the percentage of RBCs with an MCV less than 60 fL) and the % HYPO-HE (the percentage of RBCs with an MCH less than 17 pg).[49] In healthy adults these parameters are both typically less than 1%, meaning that fewer than 1% of the erythrocytes are extremely microcytic or hypochromic. Precise reference intervals, based on gestational age and postnatal age, have not yet been published for neonates.

The other RBC index that can sometimes help identify the cause of an unknown variety of neonatal anemia is the mean corpuscular hemoglobin concentration (MCHC). This is a measure of the concentration of hemoglobin in red cells. Spherical erythrocytes typically have a high MCHC. Unlike the reference intervals for MCV and MCH, the reference interval for MCHC does not change with gestational or postnatal age. It should remain in the range 34 ± 1 g/dL throughout life. Fig. 43.5 illustrates MCHC histograms of three groups of neonates: (1) Coombs (direct antiglobulin test [DAT]) negative, (2) Coombs positive, and (3) neonates with a confirmed diagnosis of hereditary spherocytosis (HS). An elevated MCHC in an anemic neonate is a means, although an imperfect means, of suggesting the diagnosis of HS. As seen in the Fig. 43.5 histogram, MCHC measurements of normal neonates overlap with those with proven HS. However, anemic neonates with an MCHC greater than about 36.5 or 37 g/dL are quite likely to have HS and should be further evaluated with that diagnosis in mind.

Fig. 43.6 is a composite timeline showing typical changes in erythrocytes during the first 90 days following birth.[50] As with the other reference interval diagrams in this chapter, the lower line indicates the 5th percentile lower limit of the reference group and the upper line indicates the 95th percentile upper limit. Blood hemoglobin and reticulocyte concentrations typically decrease during the first days after birth, as does the immature reticulocyte percentage. When these values remain elevated in an anemic neonate, they suggest hemorrhage or hemolysis, reflecting an

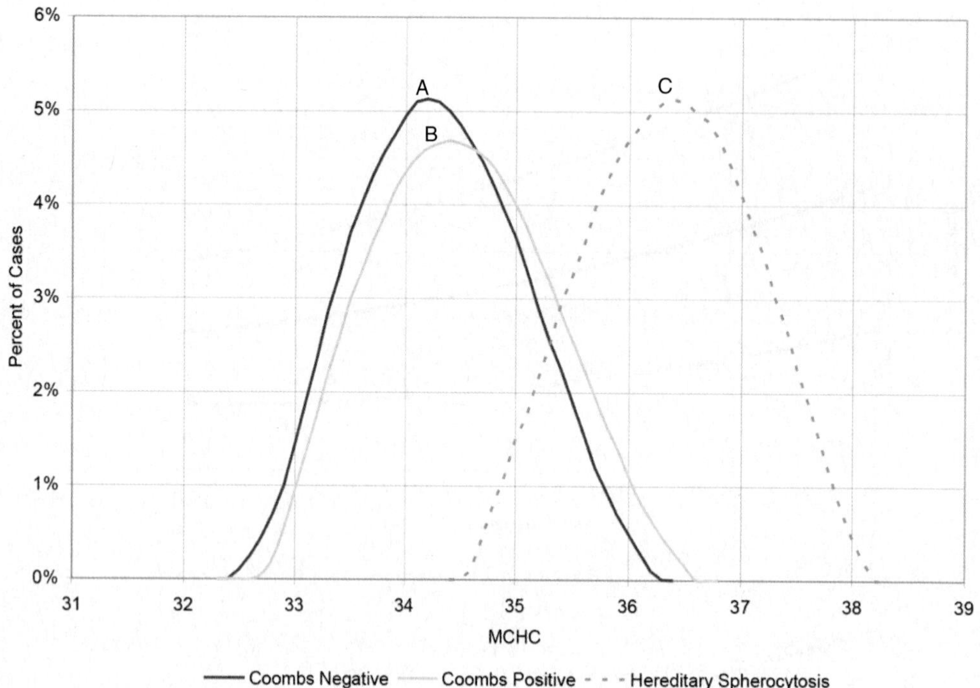

Fig. 43.5 Distribution of MCHC Measurements for Neonates With Hemolytic Jaundice. The distribution of MCHC measurements are shown for three groups of neonates with hemolytic jaundice: (A) Coombs-negative jaundice, (B) Coombs-positive jaundice, and (C) hereditary spherocytosis. *MCMH,* Mean corpuscular hemoglobin concentration. (From Christensen RD and Henry E. Hereditary spherocytosis in neonates with hyperbilirubinemia. *Pediatrics.* 2010;124[1]:120–125, with permission.)

increase in erythropoietic activity of the marrow in an attempt to compensate for the RBC loss. The reticulocyte hemoglobin content shown in the lower-most panel of Fig. 43.6 reflects the iron content of reticulocytes. Anemic neonates with reticulocyte hemoglobin below the 5th-percentile lower limit are likely to have iron deficiency.[50]

The red cell distribution width (RDW) is another way to characterize the erythrocytes of an anemic neonate.[51] The RDW describes the variation in RBC size within a blood sample. Thus it is a standard way to numerically express erythrocyte anisocytosis, meaning variance in MCV or RBC size. Fig. 43.7A shows the reference interval for RDW at birth according to gestational age. The 95th percentile upper reference interval is about 22% to 23% in extremely low gestational age neonates and 20% in those of older gestation at birth. Fig. 43.7B shows the reference interval during the first 2 weeks after birth, according to gestational age grouping. Anemic neonates with an elevated RDW (above the 95th percentile) typically have reticulocytosis because reticulocytes are larger than mature erythrocytes; thus there is more variation in RBC size. Reticulocytes are not typically measured in neonates as part of the CBC but are ordered as a separate laboratory test. However, the RDW is part of each CBC; therefore if an elevated RDW is noted in an anemic neonate, one can expect reticulocytosis, suggesting hemorrhage or hemolysis and arguing against hyporegenerative anemia.

Another parameter of interest in considering the cause of neonatal anemia is the nucleated RBC count. Fig. 43.8 shows reference intervals for nucleated red blood cells (NRBCs) shown two ways: as an absolute number of NRBCs per microliter blood and with reference to the number of NRBCs per 100 white blood cells.[30] Elevated NRBCs at birth suggest hypoxia in utero occurring 36 hours or so prior to birth.[52] Low to normal values in anemic neonates are typically seen in anemia due to erythrocyte hypoproduction.

Fragmented RBCs occur in microangiopathic conditions. In neonates these conditions are typically disseminated intravascular coagulation (DIC), necrotizing enterocolitis, and sepsis.[53–55] When erythrocytes circulate past intraluminal fibrin strands, they can be caught, tethered, and torn. After incurring this damage, the erythrocyte membrane can reseal and the damaged cell can circulate as a red cell fragment. When seen on a blood film the damaged red cells are identified as "schistocytes." Although it is not yet approved by the Food and Drug Administration in the United States, the fragmented red cells (FRCs) parameter is quantified by electronic cell counters as a routine part of the CBC. Fig. 43.9 shows reference intervals for FRCs per microliter of blood over the first 90 days after birth. Values greater than about 900,000 FRCs/μL are abnormal (above the 95th-percentile upper reference interval). Anemic neonates with an elevated FRC have hemolytic anemia from a microangiopathic condition and likely have DIC, necrotizing enterocolitis, or sepsis.[53–55]

Fig. 43.3 lists clinical and laboratory elements that indicate whether a neonate who has anemia with unknown cause is likely to have anemia due to hypoproduction, hemorrhage, or hemolysis. In the next sections, exact diagnoses under these three categories are listed and detailed.

Hyporegenerative Anemia

Impaired erythrocyte production can occur in a fetus or neonate for a variety of reasons. Lack of an appropriate marrow environment (as seen in osteopetrosis), lack of specific substrates or their carriers (e.g., iron, folate, vitamin B_{12}, or transcobalamin II deficiency), and lack of specific growth factors (e.g., decreased Epo production or abnormalities in Epo receptors) can be causative. The most common hyporegenerative anemia in neonatal intensive care unit patients is

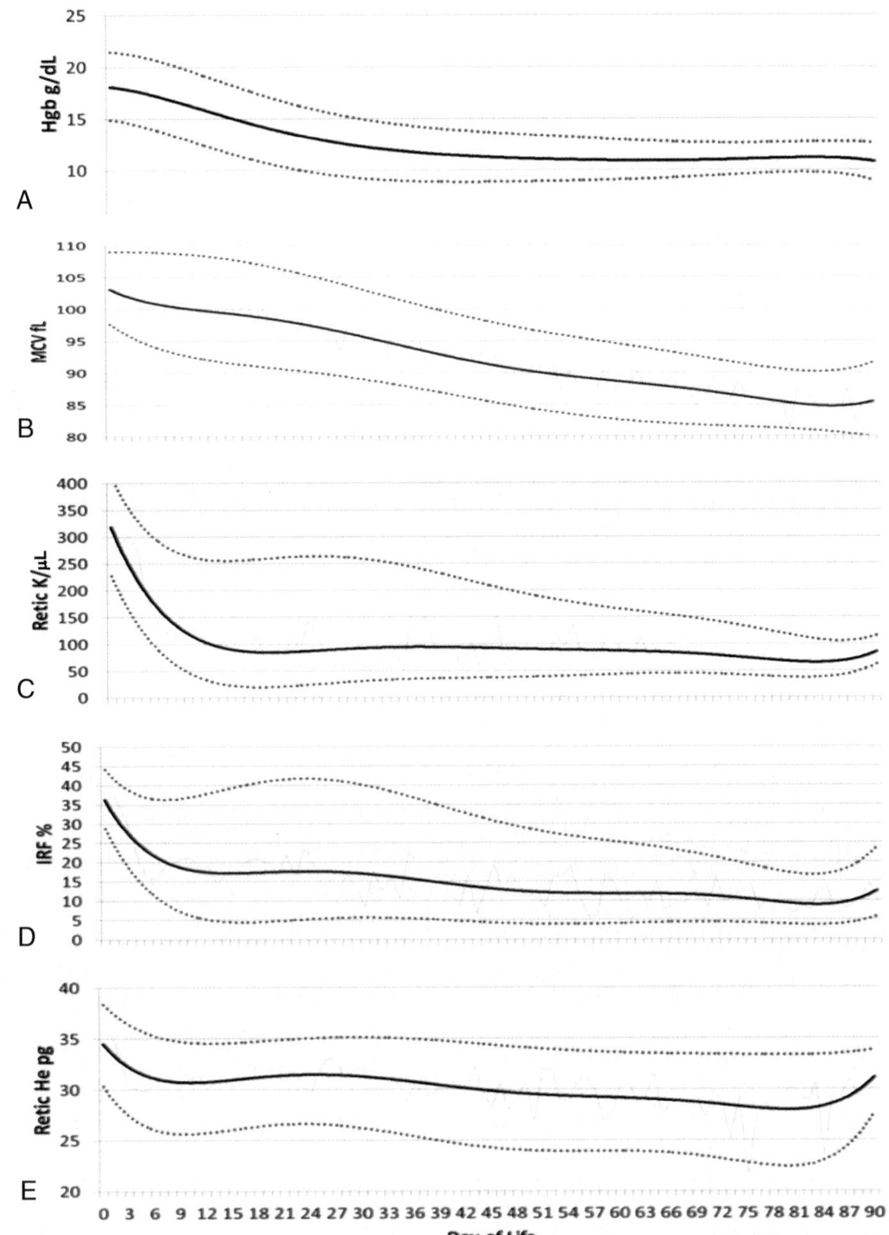

Fig. 43.6 Reticulocyte Reference Intervals From Birth to 90 Days. Reticulocyte reference intervals are displayed from the day of birth to 90 days for the following parameters: (A) blood hemoglobin concentration (g/dL), (B) erythrocyte mean corpuscular volume (MCV, fL), (C) reticulocytes (reticulocytes × 10^3/μL blood), (D) immature reticulocyte fraction (IRF, %), and (E) reticulocyte hemoglobin content (pg). The dashed lines show the 10th percentile and 90th percentile values, the solid black line shows the "smoothed" median values, and the light gray solid line shows the actual median values each day. (From Christensen RD, Henry E, Bennett ST, Yaish HM. Reference intervals for reticulocyte parameters of infants during their first 90 days after birth. *J Perinatol*. 2016;36[1]:61–66, with permission.)

"anemia of prematurity," discussed below. A rare collection of hyporegenerative neonatal anemias on a genetic basis are discussed in the section following.

Anemia of Prematurity

Infants delivered before 32 completed weeks of gestation typically develop a transient and unique anemia known as anemia of prematurity.[56] During the first week or two after birth, while in an intensive care unit, anemia secondary to phlebotomy loss is common. However, after this period has passed, a second anemia is sometimes seen, characterized as a normocytic, normochromic, hyporegenerative anemia, with serum Epo concentrations significantly below those found in adults with similar degrees of anemia.[57] This anemia is not responsive to the administration of iron, folate, or vitamin E. Some infants with anemia of prematurity are asymptomatic, whereas others have clear signs of anemia that are alleviated by erythrocyte transfusion.[56] These signs include tachycardia, rapid tiring with nipple feedings, poor weight gain, increased requirements for supplemental oxygen, episodes of apnea and bradycardia, and elevated serum lactate concentrations.

The reasons underlying the absence of an increase in serum Epo concentrations in preterm infants during this anemia are unclear. The serum concentrations of Epo do not change, but we do not know

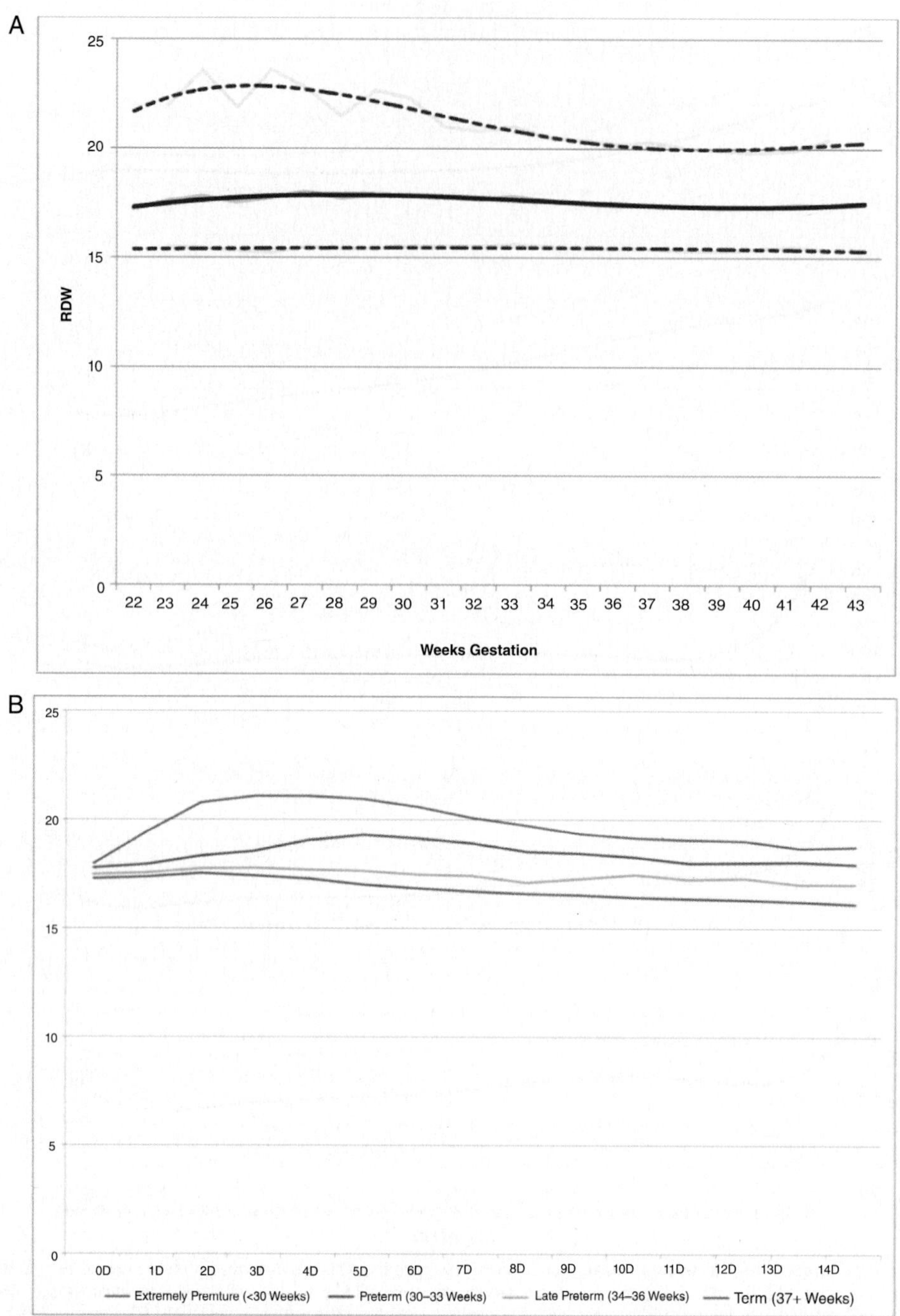

Fig. 43.7 Red Blood Cell Distribution Width (RDW) Reference Intervals. (A) RDW on the day of birth as a function of gestational age. (B) RDW over the first 2 weeks as related to gestational age at birth. The lower dashed line shows the 5th percentile reference interval limit, the solid middle line shows the mean, and the upper dashed line shows the 95th percentile reference interval limit. (From Christensen RD, Yaish HM, Henry E, Bennett ST. Red blood cell distribution width: reference intervals for neonates. *J Matern Fetal Neonatal Med*. 2015;28[8]:883–888, with permission.)

if the Epo production does not change at all or if there is a balancing change in degradation. Certainly, the erythroid progenitors remain sensitive to Epo,[58,59] and concentrations of other erythropoietic growth factors appear to be normal.[60]

The molecular and cellular mechanisms responsible for anemia of prematurity remain undefined. Some explanations include the transition from fetal to adult Hb, shortened erythrocyte survival, and hemodilution associated with a rapidly increasing body mass.[56] It is unknown whether preterm infants rely on Epo produced by the liver (the source of Epo in utero), that produced by the kidneys, or a combination of the two. Regardless of the mechanism responsible for anemia of prematurity, exogenous recombinant Epo administered to preterm infants accelerates effective erythropoiesis.[61–64] In addition, beneficial neurodevelopmental effects of recombinant Epo and darbepoetin administration have been reported in preterm infants.[65–70]

Other Hypoproliferative Anemias

Table 43.1 lists the most frequently reported of this group of rare neonatal anemic conditions. During the neonatal period, hypoproliferative anemias are rare. Diamond-Blackfan syndrome can be

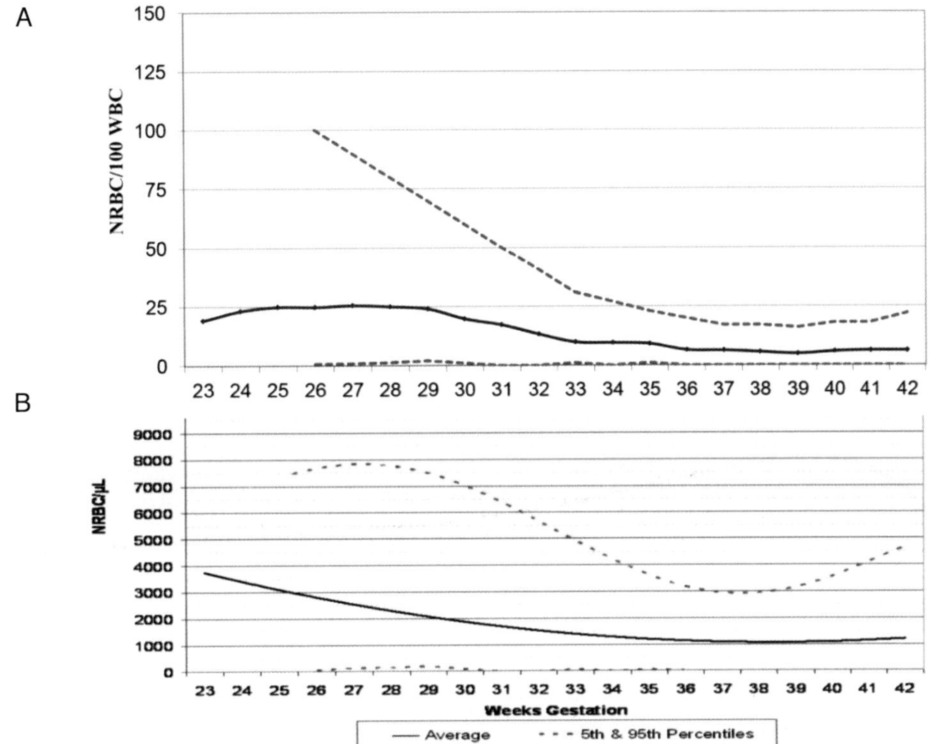

Fig. 43.8 Nucleated Red Blood Cell (NRBC) Reference Intervals on the Day of Birth According to Gestational Age. (A) The data are expressed as NRBC/µL. (B) The data are expressed as NRBC/100 white blood cells (WBC). The lower and upper lines represent the 5% and 95% limits and the middle line represents the mean value. (From Christensen RD, Lambert DK, Richards DS. Estimating the nucleated red blood cell "emergence time" in neonates. *J Perinatol.* 2014;34[2]:116–119, with permission.)

diagnosed at birth but usually is not recognized until after 2 to 3 months of age. At least 10% to 25% of infants with Diamond-Blackfan syndrome have anemia at birth,[71–73] and severe anemia with hydrops has been reported. Aase syndrome, another congenital hypoplastic anemia syndrome involving skeletal anomalies,[73,74] is sometimes classified as a variant of Diamond-Blackfan syndrome. Congenital dyserythropoietic anemia is a rare group of disorders marked by ineffective erythropoiesis, megaloblastic anemia, and characteristic abnormalities of the nuclear membrane and cytoplasm seen on electron microscopy.[75,76] Fanconi anemia is almost never manifest during the neonatal period. This autosomal-recessive disorder is characterized by marrow failure and congenital anomalies, including abnormalities in skin pigmentation, gastrointestinal anomalies, renal anomalies, and upper limb anomalies.[77,78]

Osteopetrosis involves osteoclast dysfunction, resulting in a decreased marrow space.[79,80] Developmental delay, ocular involvement, and neurodegenerative findings occur in these patients in association with hypoplastic anemia. Patients are generally treated with stem cell transplantation, but they are particularly susceptible to posttransplantation complications after myeloablation, and reduced-intensity conditioning programs may be helpful.

Pearson syndrome is a congenital hyporegenerative anemia that can progress to pancytopenia and additionally affects the exocrine pancreas, liver, and kidneys.[81] These patients can present during the neonatal period but typically do so later in infancy. Features include failure to thrive and cytopenia. The marrow examination shows characteristic vacuoles within erythroid and myeloid precursors, hemosiderosis, and ringed sideroblasts. The syndrome is caused by a loss of large segments of mitochondrial DNA.[82]

Hemorrhagic Anemia

Causes of neonatal hemorrhagic anemia are noted in Table 43.2 and are divided into (1) prenatal, (2) perinatal, and (3) postnatal varieties.

Prenatal Hemorrhage

Approximately 1 pregnancy in 400 is associated with fetal to maternal hemorrhage (FMH) of 30 mL or more, and 1 pregnancy in 2000 is associated with FMH of 100 mL or more.[83] FMH consisting of small volumes of blood is very common. Perhaps as many as 75% of pregnancies can be shown to have 0.01 to 0.1 mL of fetal blood transferred into the maternal circulation. Transfer of fetal blood cells into the mother occurs during abortions as well. This has been reported in approximately 2% of spontaneous abortions and in 4% to 5% of induced abortions.[84]

The Kleihauer-Betke stain of maternal blood evaluates the acid elution of Hb from red cells.[83,84] HbF resists acid elution to a greater degree than adult Hb. Therefore maternal cells appear clear (termed *ghost cells*), whereas any erythrocytes of fetal origin will appear pink. False positive results occur when mothers have an increase in HbF (i.e., sickle cell disease, thalassemia, and hereditary persistence of HbF). FMH can also be difficult to detect when the mother is blood group O and the infant is A, B, or AB, because fetal cells are rapidly cleared from the

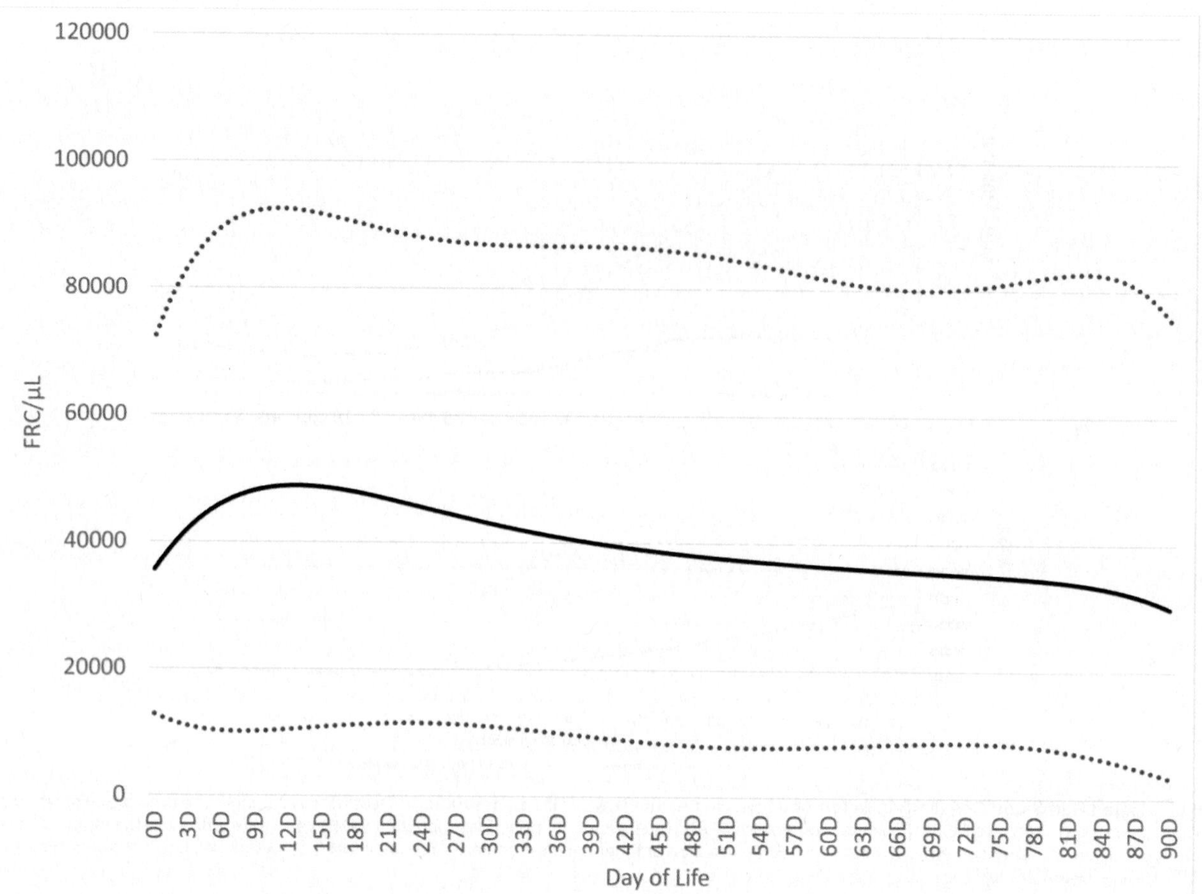

Fig. 43.9 Reference Intervals for Fragmented Red Cells (FRC/μL) Over the First 90 Days After Birth. The lower and upper dashed lines represent the 5th and 95th percentile values and the solid line represents the mean values over this interval. (From Judkins AJ, MacQueen BC, Christensen RD, Henry E, Snow GL, Bennett ST. Automated quantification of fragmented red blood cells: neonatal reference intervals and clinical disorders of neonatal intensive care unit patients with high values. *Neonatology*. 2019;115[1]:5–12m, with permission.)

maternal circulation by maternal anti-A or anti-B antibodies and therefore they do not appear on the Kleihauer-Betke stain.

Severe FMH can be suspected before delivery by decreased fetal movements and a fetal sinusoidal heart rate pattern.[84–86] Giacoia reviewed these variables to determine whether they correlated with the severity of FMH.[87] Fetal movements for a period ranging between 24 hours and 7 days were absent in 17 of 134 cases evaluated. In this group, six infants survived, five were stillborn, and five died in the neonatal period. A sinusoidal heart rate pattern was reported in 21 cases and was associated with decreased fetal movement in 40% of the cases. No significant difference was found between the cases with a hemorrhage of less than 200 mL and greater than 200 mL. Significant FMH has been described after maternal trauma.[88,89]

Neonates delivered after a significant FMH can be very pale, tachycardic, and tachypneic, but they generally do not have marked respiratory distress or a requirement for supplemental oxygen. Their Hb concentration can be as low as 4 to 6 g/dL, and a significant metabolic acidosis is often present in association with poor perfusion.[85,86] Other causes of pallor can be ruled out once the infant is stable. Infants with asphyxia or chronic anemia due to hemolysis can also present with pallor. These diagnoses can be distinguished from acute hemorrhage based on differences in clinical signs and symptoms. With chronic blood loss, the signs of shock are usually absent. Asphyxiated infants are pale, floppy, and may have poor peripheral circulation. The Hb will be stable but may decrease if DIC and internal bleeding occur.[55]

Twin-twin transfusion is a complication of monochorionic twin gestations, occurring in 5% to 30% of these pregnancies.[90–92] It involves placental anastomoses that permit transfer of blood from one twin to the other.[93] The perinatal mortality rate can be 70% or more. About 70% of monozygous twin pregnancies have monochorionic placentas. Although vascular anastomoses are present in almost all of them, not all develop twin-twin transfusion.

Acute twin-twin transfusion generally results in twins of similar size but with Hb concentrations that vary by more than 5 g/dL.[90–93] In chronic twin-twin transfusion, the donor twin becomes progressively anemic and growth retarded, whereas the recipient twin becomes polycythemic, macrosomic, and sometimes hypertensive. Both can develop hydrops fetalis; the donor twin becomes hydropic from profound anemia and the recipient twin from congestive heart failure and hypervolemia. The donor twin often has low amniotic fluid volumes whereas the recipient twin has increased amniotic fluid due to significant differences in blood volume, renal blood flow, and urine output.

Chronic twin-twin transfusion can be diagnosed by serial prenatal ultrasound measuring cardiomegaly, discordant amniotic fluid production, and fetal growth discrepancy of >20%. Percutaneous umbilical blood sampling can determine whether Hb concentration

Table 43.1 Syndromes Associated With Congenital Hyporegenerative Anemia

Syndrome	Phenotypic Features	Genotypic Features
Adenosine deaminase deficiency	Autoimmune hemolytic anemia, reduced erythrocyte adenosine deaminase activity.	AR, 20q13.11
Congenital dyserythropoietic anemias	Type I (rare): megaloblastoid erythroid hyperplasia and nuclear chromatin bridges between nuclei; type II (most common): "hereditary erythroblastic multinuclearity, positive acidified serum (HEMPAS) test, increased lysis to anti-I; type III: erythroblastic multinuclearity ("gigantoblasts"), macrocytosis."	Type I: 15q15.1-q15.3; type II: 20q11.2; type III: 15q21
Diamond-Blackfan syndrome	Steroid-responsive hypoplastic anemia, often macrocytic after 5 mo of age.	AR; sporadic mutations and AD inheritance described; 19q13.2, 8p23.3-p22
Dyskeratosis congenita	Hypoproliferative anemia usually presenting between 5–15 y of age.	X-linked recessive, locus on Xq28; some cases with AD inheritance.
Fanconi pancytopenia	Steroid-responsive hypoplastic anemia, reticulocytopenia, some macrocytic RBCs, shortened RBC lifespan. Cells are hypersensitive to DNA cross-linking agents.	AR, multiple genes: complementation; group A: 16q24.3; B: Xp22.2; C: 9q22.3; D2: 3p25.3; E: 6p22-p21; F: 11p15; G: 9p13
Osler hemorrhagic telangiectasia syndrome	Hemorrhagic anemia.	AD, 9q34.1
Osteopetrosis	Hypoplastic anemia from marrow compression; extramedullary erythropoiesis.	AR: 16p13, 11q13.4-q13.5; AD: 1p21; lethal: reduced osteoclasts
Pearson syndrome	Hypoplastic sideroblastic anemia, marrow cell vacuolization.	Pleioplasmatic rearrangement of mitochondrial DNA; X-linked or AR
Peutz-Jeghers syndrome	Iron deficiency anemia from chronic blood loss.	AD, 19p13.3
X-linked alpha-thalassemia/mental retardation (ATR-X and ATR-16) syndromes	ATR-X: hypochromic, microcytic anemia; mild form of hemoglobin H disease ATR-16: more significant hemoglobin H disease and anemia are present.	ATR-X: X-linked recessive, Xq13.3; ATR-16: 16p13.3, deletions of α-globin locus

AD, Autosomal dominant; *AR*, autosomal recessive; *RBC*, red blood cell.

Table 43.2 Causes of Neonatal Hemorrhagic Anemia

A. Prenatal
1. Twin-twin transfusion
2. Fetal-maternal hemorrhage
3. Trauma with bleeding into cord, placenta, amniotic fluid
B. Perinatal
1. Placenta previa
2. Placental abruption
3. Vasa previa
4. Velementous insertion of the umbilical cord
5. Nuchal cord
6. Trauma or incision of the cord or placenta during cesarean section
7. Rupture of the umbilical cord at delivery
C. Postnatal
1. Subgaleal hemorrhage
2. Cephalohematoma
3. Organ trauma after birth
4. Pulmonary hemorrhage
5. Intracranial hemorrhage
6. Iatrogenic blood loss

differences of greater than 5 gm/dL exist. After birth, the donor twin may require transfusions and can have neutropenia, hydrops from severe anemia, growth retardation, congestive heart failure, and hypoglycemia. The recipient twin is often the sicker of the two, with problems including hypertrophic cardiomyopathy, congestive heart failure, polycythemia, hyperviscosity, respiratory difficulties, hypocalcemia, and hypoglycemia. Neurologic evaluation and imaging are imperative because the risk of antenatally acquired neurologic cerebral lesions is 20% to 30% in both twins. The incidence of neurologic morbidity after the intrauterine death of one of the fetuses averages 20% to 25%. Morbidities include multiple cerebral infarctions, hypoperfusion syndromes from hypotension, and periventricular leukomalacia. Long-term neurologic follow-up is indicated for all survivors of twin-twin transfusion.[90–92]

Prenatal treatment for twin-twin transfusion consists of close monitoring and reduction amniocenteses to decrease uterine stretch and prolong the pregnancy. Selective feticide of the hydropic twin has been advocated by some and has resulted in the survival of the healthier twin in some studies.[74] Treatment in utero has occurred using laser ablation of bridging vessels, resulting in improved survival rates up to around 50%, with approximately 70% of the pregnancies having at least one survivor.[92,93] However, the survival rate without morbidity in the surviving twin is approximately 50%.

Perinatal Hemorrhage

Loss of blood from the fetus can occur with various complications, such as placenta previa, placental abruption, incision or tearing of the placenta during cesarean section, and cord evulsion. When a fetus undergoes significant blood loss into the placenta, the term *fetoplacental hemorrhage* is used. Placental anomalies such as a multilobed placenta and placental chorioangiomas can be a source of perinatal bleeding.[94]

Placental abruption occurs in 3 to 6 per 1000 live births. Risk factors of placental abruption include prolonged rupture of the membranes, severe fetal growth restriction, chorioamnionitis, hypertension, maternal diabetes, cigarette smoking, obesity before pregnancy, excessive weight gain during pregnancy, and advanced maternal age.[95–97] The incidence of abruption increases with lower gestational age. Neonatal mortality rates from abruption range from 0.8 to 2.0 per 1000 births, or 15% to 20% of the deliveries in which significant abruption occurs.

Women with a history of a previous cesarean birth and increased parity are at increased risk of placenta previa,[96,97] a condition where part or all of the placenta overlies the cervical os. Cigarette smoking is associated with a 2.6- to 4.4-fold increased risk of placenta previa.[98] Prenatal diagnosis of vasa previa (anomalous vessels overlying the internal os of the cervix) can be made with transvaginal color Doppler and should be suspected in cases of antepartum or intrapartum hemorrhage. Although uncommon (1 in 3000 deliveries), the perinatal death rate is high, ranging from 33% to 100% when this condition is undetected before delivery.[95–97]

Neonates delivered after placental abruption or after placenta previa can be anemic but can also have signs of hypoxia and ischemia. The majority of blood lost in an abruption or previa is maternal blood, but the neonate can have some degree of anemia as well. Therefore, when perinatal blood loss is recognized or suspected, the neonate's Hb should be measured at birth and again 12 hours or so later. A Kleihauer-Betke stain can be performed on maternal blood to determine whether fetal hemorrhage can be documented.[99] Monitoring bleeding mothers with ultrasound might detect placental abnormalities.

Cord rupture due to traction on a shortened or abnormal umbilical cord usually occurs on the fetal side. Cord aneurysms, varices, and cysts can all lead to a weakened cord. Cord infections (funisitis) can also weaken the cord and increase the risk of rupture. Infants born precipitously may be at increased risk for hemorrhage due to a ruptured cord. Cord hematomas occur infrequently (1 in 5000–6000 deliveries) and can be a cause of fetal blood loss and perinatal mortality. Intrauterine death can occur due to compression of the umbilical vessels by a cord hematoma.[100]

Subamniotic hematomas can occur when chorionic vessels get ruptured near the site of cord insertion. Most subamniotic hematomas are the result of traction on a normal or shortened umbilical cord and are not noted until after delivery. Velamentous insertion of the umbilical cord occurs when the umbilical cord enters the membranes distant from the placenta. This is present in 0.5% to 2.0% of pregnancies.[101] Blood vessels left unprotected by Wharton jelly are more likely to tear. Rupture of anomalous vessels in the absence of traction or trauma can occur even if the cord itself attaches centrally or paracentrally. The fetal mortality remains very high in this condition, often because detection by routine ultrasound is rare.[102]

Postnatal Hemorrhage

Loss of fetal blood into the placenta can occur during delivery. In fact, a net shift of blood from the fetus into the placenta is a rather common cause of low-grade neonatal anemia. At term, the fetal-placental-umbilical cord unit contains about 120 mL of blood per kg body weight. After delivery, but before the umbilical cord is severed, blood in this unit can flow predominantly toward or away from the neonate. Neonates can lose up to 20% of their blood volume when born with a tight nuchal cord, which allows blood to be pumped through umbilical arteries toward the placenta while constricting flow back from the placenta to the baby through the umbilical vein, which is more easily constricted due to its thin wall.

As shown in Fig. 43.10, blood loss can occur into the subgaleal space before or after birth. This is seen most commonly with difficult deliveries requiring vacuum or forceps assistance.[103] Subgaleal hemorrhages are potentially life-threatening and must be recognized as early as possible to prevent significant morbidity or mortality. The hemorrhage occurs when bridging veins are torn, allowing blood to accumulate in the large potential space between the galea aponeurotica and the periosteum of the skull. The subgaleal space extends from the orbital ridge to the base of the skull and can accommodate a volume equivalent to an infant's entire blood volume.

Subgaleal hematomas can form because of risk factors such as coagulopathy or asphyxia, but vacuum extraction itself is a risk factor for their development. The diagnosis should be considered in the presence of a ballotable fluid collection in dependent regions of the infant's head, coupled with signs of hypovolemia.[103–105] Treatment requires restoration of blood volume and control of bleeding. Exsanguination due to subgaleal hemorrhage has been reported. A suggested way to estimate the volume of blood lost is by following head circumference; 40 mL of blood has been lost for every 1 cm increase in head circumference that occurs. The duration of vacuum application is thought to be the best predictor of scalp injury, followed by duration of the second stage of labor and paramedian cup placement. Of those with reported subgaleal hemorrhages, 80% to 90% had some history of vacuum or instrument-assisted delivery. Those who develop

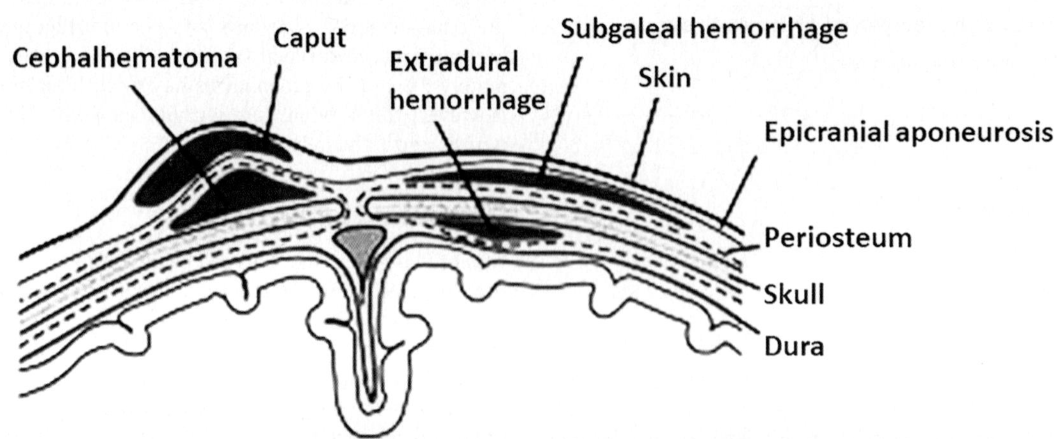

Fig. 43.10 Sites of Extracranial Hemorrhages in Neonates in Various Layers of the Scalp/Skull. (Reproduced with permission and minor modifications from Brozansky BS, Riley MM, Bogen DL. Neonatology. In: Zitelli BJ, McIntire SC, Nowalk AJ, editors. *Atlas of Pediatric Diagnosis*, 6th edition. Philadelphia: Elsevier Saunders, 2012.)

subgaleal hematomas without a vacuum or instrument delivery typically have less severe anemia and better outcomes.[106]

Anemia appearing after the first 24 hours of life in a nonjaundiced infant can be a sign of hemorrhage. Hemorrhages can be visible, such as a cephalohematoma, or occult. Breech deliveries can be associated with renal, adrenal, or splenic hemorrhage into the retroperitoneal space. Delivery of macrosomic infants, such as infants born to diabetic mothers, can result in hemorrhage. Infants with overwhelming sepsis can bleed into soft tissue and organs.

In addition to causing anemia, adrenal hemorrhage can result in circulatory collapse due to the loss of organ function. The incidence of adrenal hemorrhage is 1.7 per 1000 births.[107] Adrenal hemorrhage can also affect surrounding organs. Intestinal obstruction and kidney dysfunction have been reported in infants with adrenal hemorrhage.[108] The diagnosis can be made using ultrasonography, during which calcifications or cystic masses are noted. Adrenal hemorrhage can be distinguished from renal vein thrombosis by ultrasound, in that renal vein thrombosis generally results in a solid mass. Occasionally, both entities coexist in the same patient.

The liver of a neonate is prone to iatrogenic rupture, resulting in high morbidity and mortality.[109] Neonates with this problem can appear asymptomatic until the liver ruptures and hemoperitoneum occurs. This problem can occur in both term and preterm infants[110] and has been associated with chest compressions during cardiopulmonary resuscitation. Splenic rupture can result from birth trauma or as a result of distention caused by extramedullary hematopoiesis, such as that seen in erythroblastosis fetalis. Abdominal distension and discoloration, scrotal swelling, and pallor are clinical signs of splenic rupture; these can also be seen with adrenal or hepatic hemorrhage.[111,112]

More rare causes of hemorrhage in the newborn period include hemangiomas of the gastrointestinal tract,[113] vascular malformations of the skin, and hemorrhage into soft tumors, such as giant sacrococcygeal teratomas. Occult intraabdominal hemorrhage can occur with fetal ovarian cysts, which are usually benign and resolve spontaneously. One case of fetal anemia was diagnosed by a spontaneous hemorrhage into a fetal ovarian cyst and was managed by intrauterine blood transfusions.[114]

Hemolytic Anemia

Immune-mediated hemolytic disease of the fetus/neonate and hemolytic disease of the fetus/neonate associated with infectious diseases are reviewed separately in the final paragraphs of this chapter (Table 43.3).

Hemolysis is a pathologic shortening of the RBC life span. Hemolysis is a different process than the natural physiologic removal of red cells at the end of their normal life span by a process termed senescence.[115] Hemolysis in neonates can be the result of either inherited mutations in genes involved in erythrocyte structure or function (Fig. 43.11) or the result of acquired disorders that disrupt erythrocytes by immune-mediated mechanisms or mechanical disruption.[116] Once hemolytic disease has been identified as the cause of the neonatal anemia, the specific reason for the hemolysis can be sought, and the problems of hyperbilirubinemia and worsening anemia can be anticipated and managed expectantly.

Hemolysis should be a prime consideration whenever hyperbilirubinemia occurs "early," namely when the total serum bilirubin (TSB) exceeds the 95th-percentile hour-specific nomogram value on the first day after birth.[116] Laboratory tests to consider when hemolysis is considered the likely cause of neonatal anemia include the noninvasive measurement of end tidal carbon monoxide (CO),[117–119] or if a blood gas is needed, measuring the carboxyhemoglobin percentage.[120] Elevation in either measurement of CO can confirm hemolysis and can at the same time give a general impression of its severity, based on the degree of CO elevation.

If these tests of CO are not available, other markers of hemolysis can be used, including absent serum haptoglobin, marked hemoglobinuria, and rapidly rising indirect bilirubin. The other important second-line testing needed if hemolysis is considered as the cause of anemia is blood typing of the mother and neonate and DAT (Coombs) testing. Examination of a stained blood film specifically focusing on erythrocyte morphology can also give relevant information about hemolysis, as illustrated in Figs. 43.12–43.15 and 43.16. Some of the molecular defects are listed in Table 43.4.

If the neonatologist or hematologist looks specifically for five abnormal RBC shapes, this will often reveal the cause of the neonatal anemia. At the very least, the morphologic examination of the erythrocytes will put the clinicians on a course to identify the underlying anemia using enzymatic or genetic testing. The five abnormal shapes, discussed below, are (1) microspherocytes, (2) elliptocytes (and pyropoikilocytes), (3) bite and blister cells, (4) echinocytes, an (5) schistocytes.

Table 43.3 Causes of Neonatal Hemolytic Anemia

A. Immune mediated
1. Rh (anti-D) incompatibility
2. ABO incompatibility
3. Other blood group incompatibility—Duffy, Kell, Jka, MNS, Vw
4. Maternal autoimmune hemolytic anemia
B. Erythrocyte enzyme mutations
1. G6PD deficiency
2. Pyruvate kinase deficiency
3. Hexose kinase deficiency
4. Glucose phosphate isomerase deficiency
5. Pyrimidine 5′ nucleotidase deficiency
C. Erythrocyte membrane mutations
1. Hereditary spherocytosis
2. Hereditary elliptocytosis/ovalocytosis (Southeast Asian ovalocytosis)
3. Other membrane disorders
D. Infections
E. Hemoglobin defects
1. α thalassemia
2. γ thalassemia
F. Angiopathic hemolysis
1. Arteriovenous malformations
2. Cavernous hemangiomas
3. Disseminated intravascular coagulation
4. Large vessel thrombosis
5. Severe valvar stenosis
G. Miscellaneous causes
1. Galactosemia
2. Hypothyroidism
3. Lysosomal storage diseases

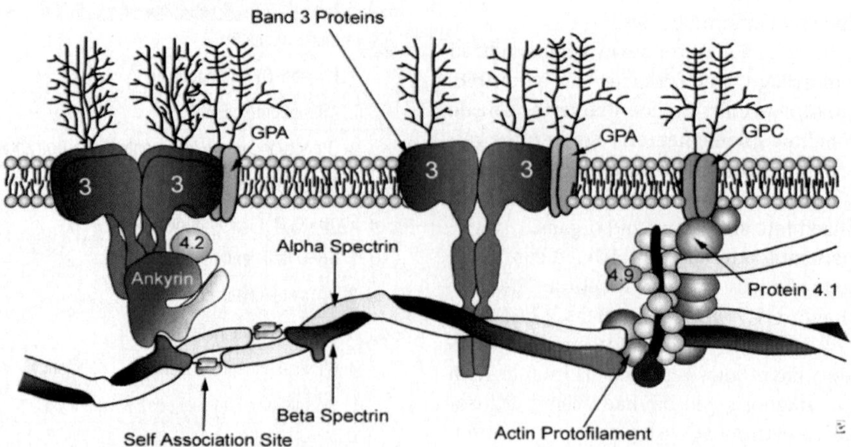

Fig. 43.11 Schematic Drawing of the Red Cell Membrane. The drawing notes the subunits described to have genetic defects as the basis for congenital abnormalities in erythrocyte shape and predisposing to neonatal hemolytic jaundice. (From Gallagher, PG. Disorders of erythrocyte metabolism and shape. In: Christensen RD, ed. *Hematologic Problems of the Neonate*. WB Saunders Co; 2000, with permission.)

Microspherocytes (Fig. 43.12)

Microspherocytes are abnormally shaped erythrocytes identified by lack of the central zone of pallor that is characteristic of normal erythrocytes and by the smaller than normal size. Microspherocytes have lost part of the cell membrane (Table 43.5) and are characterized by a low MCV with a normal hemoglobin content leading to an elevated MCHC.[121] When abundant spherocytes are observed on the smear of a neonate who has severe jaundice, two main entities should be considered: ABO hemolytic disease and HS. Although the direct Coombs test (DAT) is generally positive in the former and negative in the latter, there may

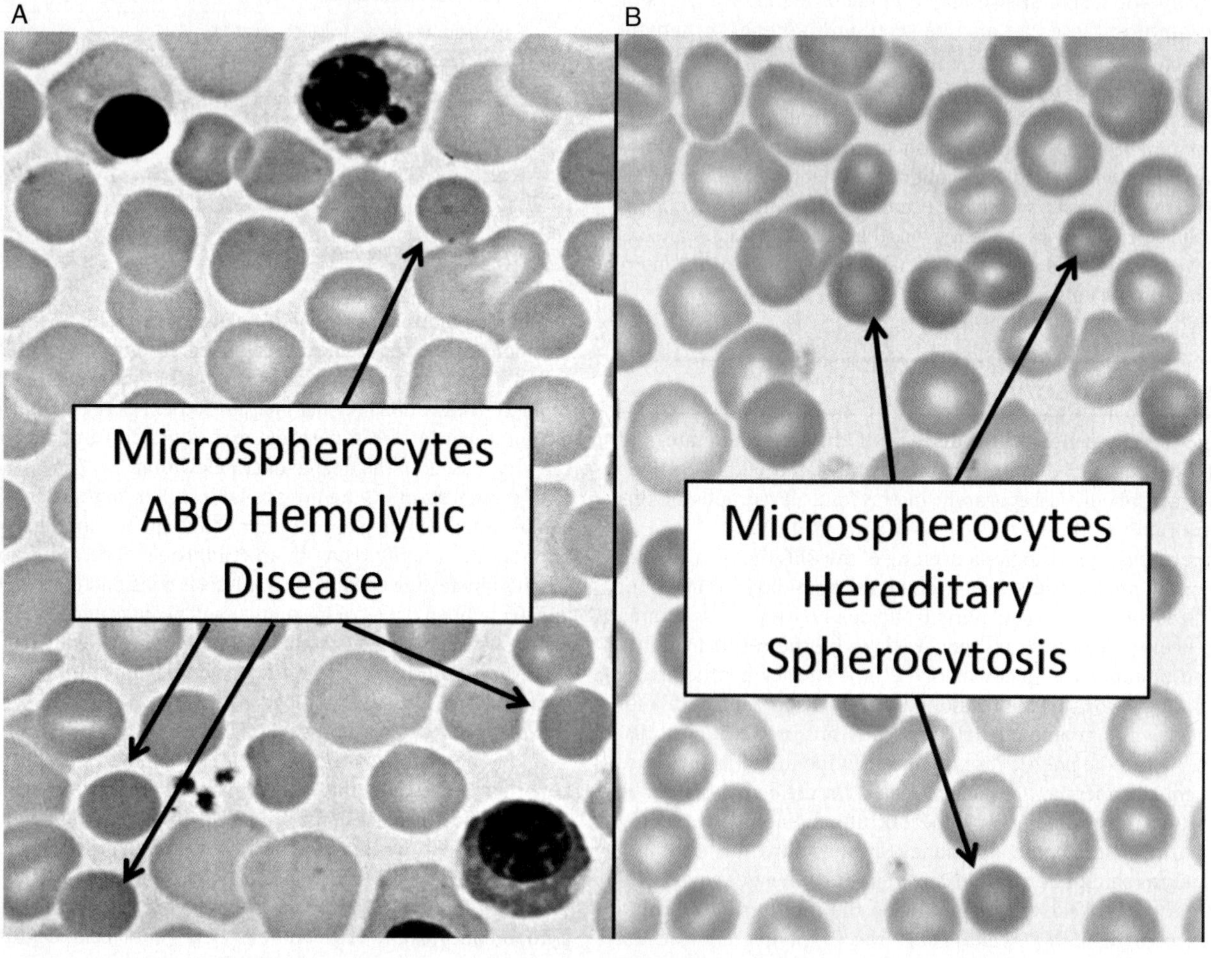

Fig. 43.12 Microspherocytes. (A) Neonate with ABO hemolytic disease. (B) Neonate with hereditary spherocytosis.

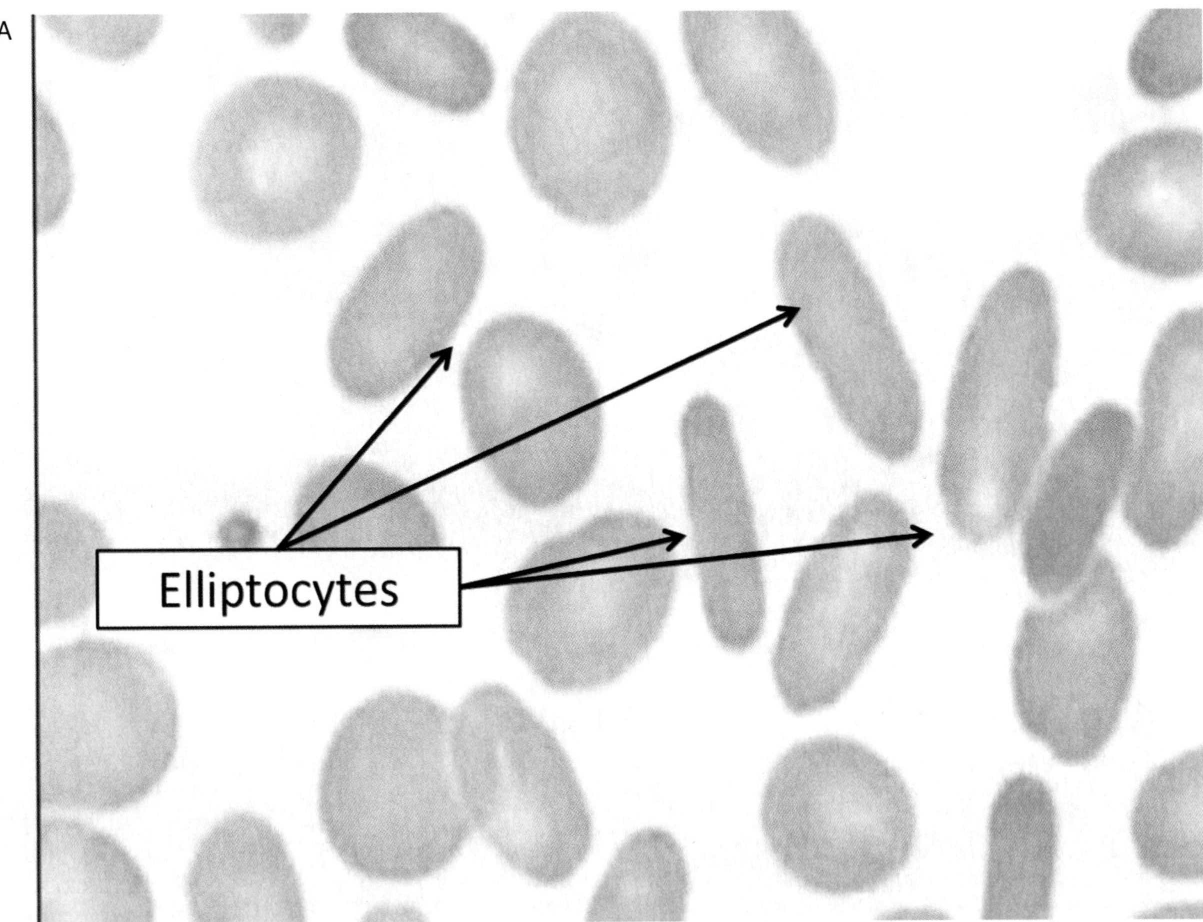

Fig. 43.13 Elliptocytes. (A) Neonate with hereditary elliptocytosis. (B) Neonate with pyropoikilocytosis.

rarely be a jaundiced neonate with ABO hemolytic disease with a negative Coombs test because of insufficient maternal antibody to render the Coombs test positive but still sufficient to result in some degree of hemolysis. Also, the DAT is sometimes negative but the indirect Coombs is positive.

The spherocytosis of ABO hemolytic disease will diminish during the first weeks and should be completely resolved 1 or 2 months after birth. In contrast, spherocytes in neonates with HS typically persist. When the mother is group O, the baby is A or B, the DAT is positive, and the baby has early hyperbilirubinemia, a blood smear may not be needed to make the diagnosis. However, we recently had a case of O/B hemolytic jaundice where the hyperbilirubinemia was so severe (TSB 41.7 mg/dL) that we deemed additional investigation needed, and indeed, HS due to a mutation in *SLC41A1* was also found.[122] The search was triggered because very large numbers of spherocytes were seen, which is not usually the case in isolated ABO hemolytic jaundice.

About 65% to 70% of neonates with HS inherit the condition in autosomal dominant fashion; thus a parent carries this diagnosis. However, sometimes a parent with HS is unaware of their own HS diagnosis.[121] This is more common with a mild phenotype or a parent who had severe jaundice only during the neonatal period. Of the remaining 30% to 35% of HS cases, some are *de novo* mutations and some are autosomal recessive varieties.[123,124]

We do not advocate obtaining an erythrocyte osmotic fragility test to confirm HS in a neonate. This test is frequently negative (normal) in a neonate with HS, only to become positive (increased fragility) after several months of age. The explanation for the frequently false-negative test in neonates involves physiologically reduced erythrocyte osmotic fragility, typical in the neonatal period because the erythrocytes are more elastic and capable of expanding in a hypotonic environment without lysing. Therefore a "normal" osmotic fragility test in a neonate with HS is common. If a confirmatory test for HS is needed, we prefer performing an eosin-5-maleimide (EMA) flow, which involves stoichiometric binding of eosin dye to Band 3 on the surface of erythrocytes. Using EMA-flow cytometry, neonates with HS can be identified by a binding pattern outside the normal "footprint."[125–127]

It is possible to determine the exact mutation in neonates to HS. However, doing so is expensive and usually adds little to the clinical care. We test for the exact mutation only in atypical or particularly severe neonatal HS cases or when neither parent has HS.[128,129]

Elliptocytes

Erythrocytes with an oval or elliptical shape (Fig. 43.13) generally occur as an autosomal dominantly inherited condition with a variety of genotypes and with phenotypes ranging from completely asymptomatic to moderately severe hemolytic anemia.[130] Mutations causing this condition result in a particular type of erythrocyte cytoskeletal instability. Erythrocytes are constantly under the influence of deforming forces as they traverse capillary spaces with a diameter narrower than themselves. They deform to pass through these spaces but reform into biconcave discs once they traverse the capillary. However, in hereditary elliptocytosis (HE), the deformation renders

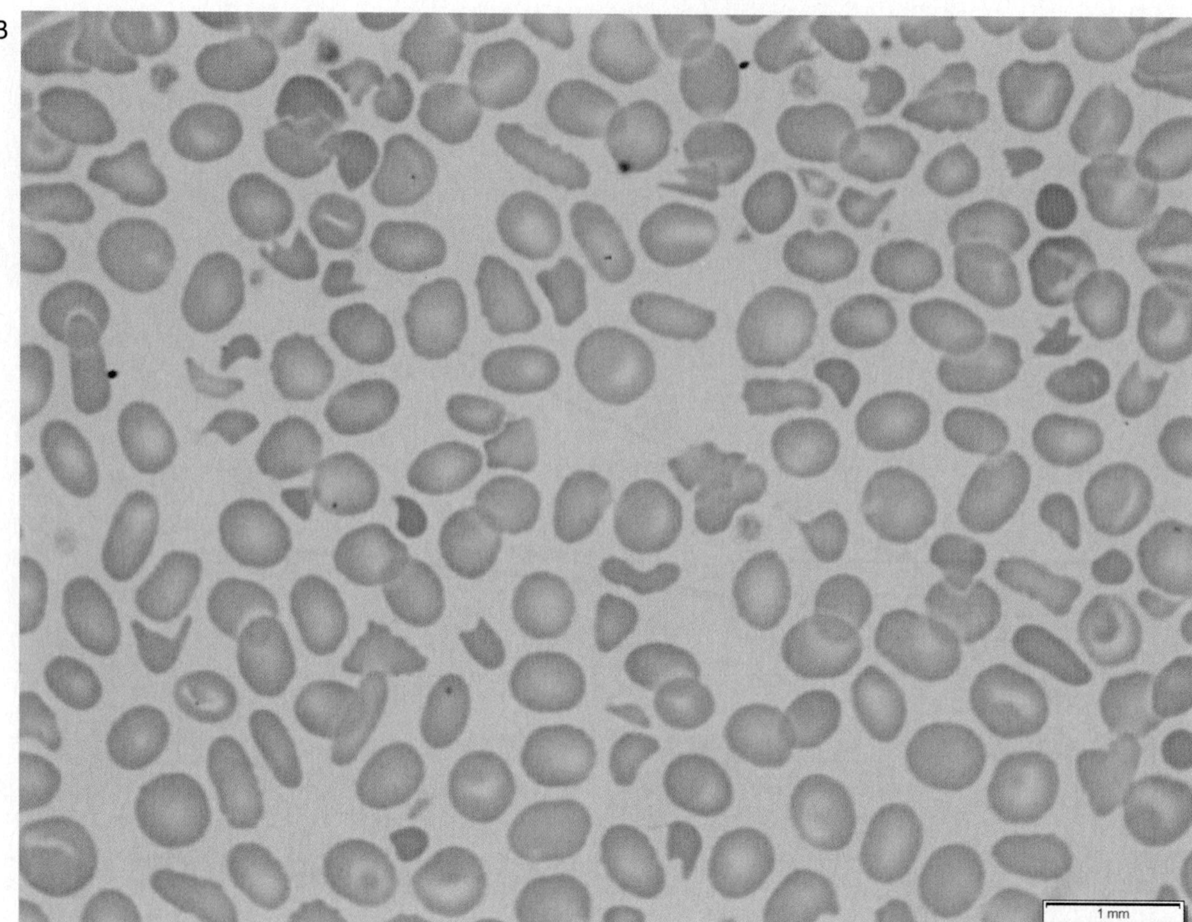

Fig. 43.13 Cont'd

the cell permanently elliptical, and these abnormally shaped cells can be culled by the spleen, shortening their survival.[131]

Unlike neonates with HS, neonates with HE lack distinctive RBC indices and are identified only by examining a blood smear. Most neonates with HE do not have significant jaundice or anemia, and the condition commonly goes undetected in the neonatal period. However, an important exception, often resulting in severe neonatal jaundice and anemia, occurs when a neonate inherits an HE mutation from one parent and also inherits a different RBC membrane defect from the other parent, similar to an autosomal recessive condition. We recently reported such a neonate in detail[130]; the condition is termed pyropoikilocytosis (see Fig. 43.13B).

Bite and Blister Cells

These abnormal erythrocytes, as their names suggest, either have a mouth-shaped bite taken from them (bite cell) or look like they have a blister on their surface (Fig. 43.14). These are erythrocytes that have lost a small portion of the hemoglobin content, leaving an empty space covered by a thin outer membrane, resembling a blister on the surface of the erythrocytes. When bite and blister cells are observed in the smear of a neonate who has hemolytic anemia/jaundice, the conclusion can be drawn that hemoglobin has precipitated at or near the membrane and that the precipitate (Heinz body) has been removed by reticuloendothelial cells. Conditions resulting in neonatal bite and blister cells include acute hemolysis triggered by unstable hemoglobins (such as hemoglobin F Poole [a gamma globin mutation] or hemoglobin Hasharon [an alpha globin mutation]).[120] Bite and blister cells can also be generated when glucose 6 phosphate dehydrogenase (G6PD) or (much less commonly) other enzymes in the same pathway are deficient, resulting in hemolytic crisis.[116] This does not occur with deficient enzymes in the glycolytic pathway (such as pyruvate kinase (deficiency), which have their own characteristic morphologic findings.

When bite and blister cells are observed, G6PD deficiency is a prime consideration, particularly if the neonate is a male and of equatorial ancestry. However, most cases of G6PD deficiency in a neonate do not have bite or blister cells. We advocate measuring G6PD enzymatic activity in all cases of unexplained severe neonatal hyperbilirubinemia. One must keep in mind that based on the severity of the defect, significantly elevated reticulocyte counts can render the G6PD enzymatic assay falsely negative, because reticulocytes are richly endowed with G6PD activity. Therefore borderline low G6PD enzymatic activity in a neonate with marked reticulocytosis and bite and/or blister cells should be interpreted as possible G6PD deficiency, and this can be confirmed later when the reticulocyte count is normal or with specific G6PD genetic testing. Females should not be excluded from consideration because of "Lyonization."

Echinocytes

These abnormal red cells are contracted and dehydrated cells with numerous, rather uniform spicules (Fig. 43.15). Sometimes echinocytes on a blood film are an artifact, but when the blood of a neonate with hemolytic jaundice has several echinocytes per high-power field

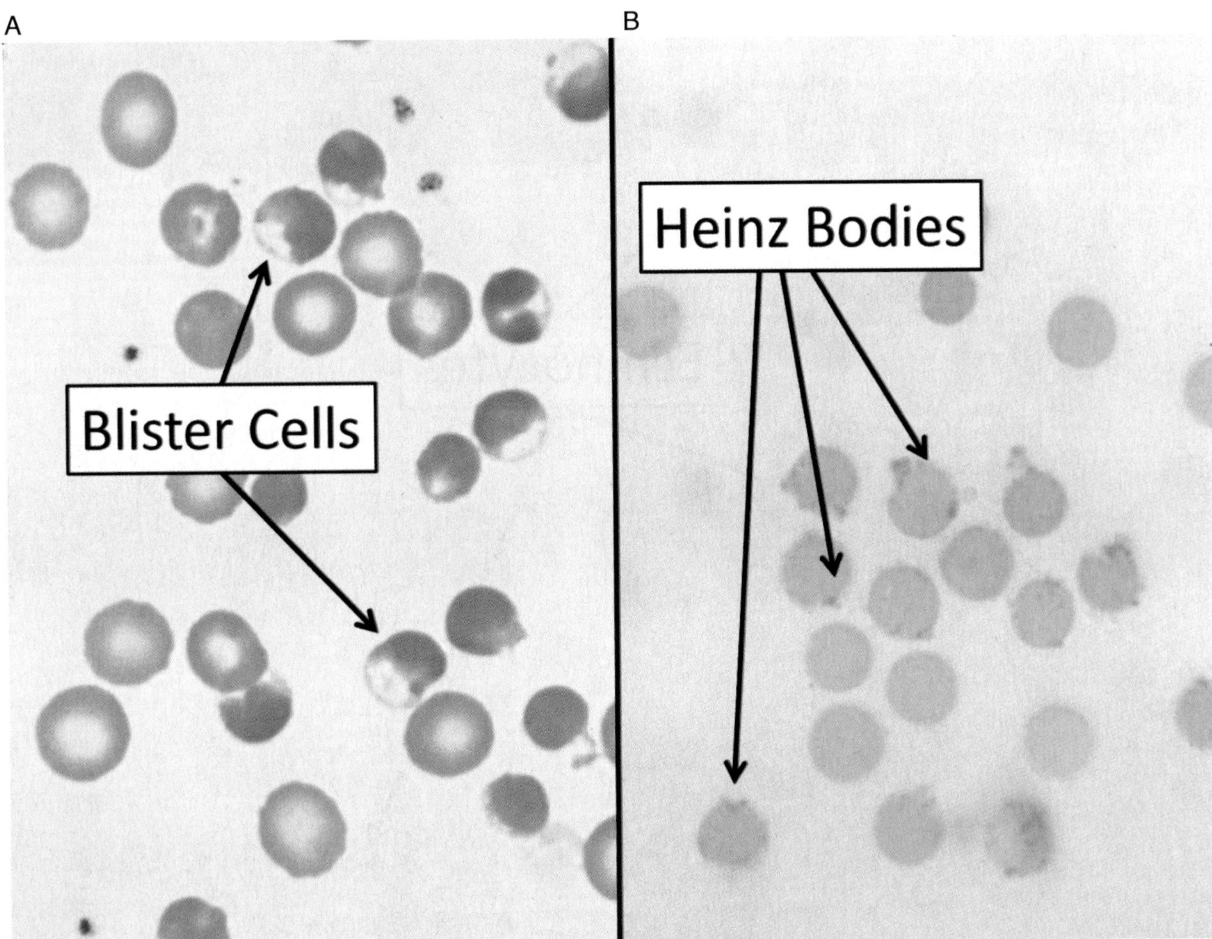

Fig. 43.14 Bite or Blister Cells. (A) Blister cells from a neonate with G6PD deficiency. (B) Heinz bodies from a neonate with G6PD deficiency. *G6PD,* Glucose 6 phosphate dehydrogenase.

throughout the blood film, associated with polychromasia, the finding is usually significant. When erythrocytes lack sufficient adenosine triphosphate to operate cell-surface ion-exchange pumps, the cells can become crenated, giving rise to some shriveled-appearing cells with spicules.[132,133] In our experience, PK deficiency is the most common condition in jaundiced neonates giving rise to these cells. Less common causes of energy failure, such as glucose-phosphate isomerase and phosphofructokinase deficiency, can also cause prominent echinocytosis.[134]

Erythrocyte PK enzymatic activity can be quantified inexpensively using small quantities of blood. PK deficiency is an autosomal recessive condition; generally the neonate is a compound heterozygote, inheriting one PK gene mutation from one parent and a different mutation in the same gene from the other parent.[132,133] Exceptions occur in consanguineous kindreds where the same mutation is inherited from an asymptomatic mother and an asymptomatic father; thus the neonate is a homozygote for the mutation.[135,136] In general, we do not seek to identify the exact mutation(s) responsible for neonates with PK deficiency. Exceptions occur as part of epidemiologic studies or other experimental studies and when the phenotype is particularly severe.[128,129]

Schistocytes

Fragments of erythrocytes, as shown in Fig. 43.16, are termed schistocytes. These suggest mechanical destruction of red cells within the vasculature. Schistocytes are not uniform in size or shape, often have a small and jagged appearance, and lack central pallor. Among neonates with severe jaundice, schistocytes on the blood film can be an artifact. However, if several schistocytes are seen per high-power field throughout the blood film accompanying normal erythrocytes, a microangiopathic condition is likely. Intravascular fibrin strands, as can occur in DIC, or large hemangiomas can cause schistocytosis when circulating erythrocytes undergo traumatic mechanical disruption.

Automated counting of schistocytes has been recommended but is not yet commonly practiced, although reference intervals are now available for neonates.[53–55] General guidelines recommend that if $>1\%$ of erythrocytes on a blood film of a full-term neonate are schistocytes, or if $>5\%$ schistocytes are found from a premature baby, the term "schistocytosis" is appropriate. Specific cell shapes qualifying for inclusion under the term "schistocyte" include the following:

- Small fragments with sharp angles or spines (triangular) and straight or distorted cytoplasmic borders; usually staining darkly, occasionally pale
- Microcrescents, which are similar to triangular forms but with a round contour on one side
- Helmet cells, which show an amputated zone of cytoplasm with a straight border and sharp angles
- Keratocytes, which show prominent spicules surrounding a concave border
- Microspherocytes (small, darkly staining spheres without central pallor); these should only be counted as schistocytes in the presence of the other schistocyte shapes

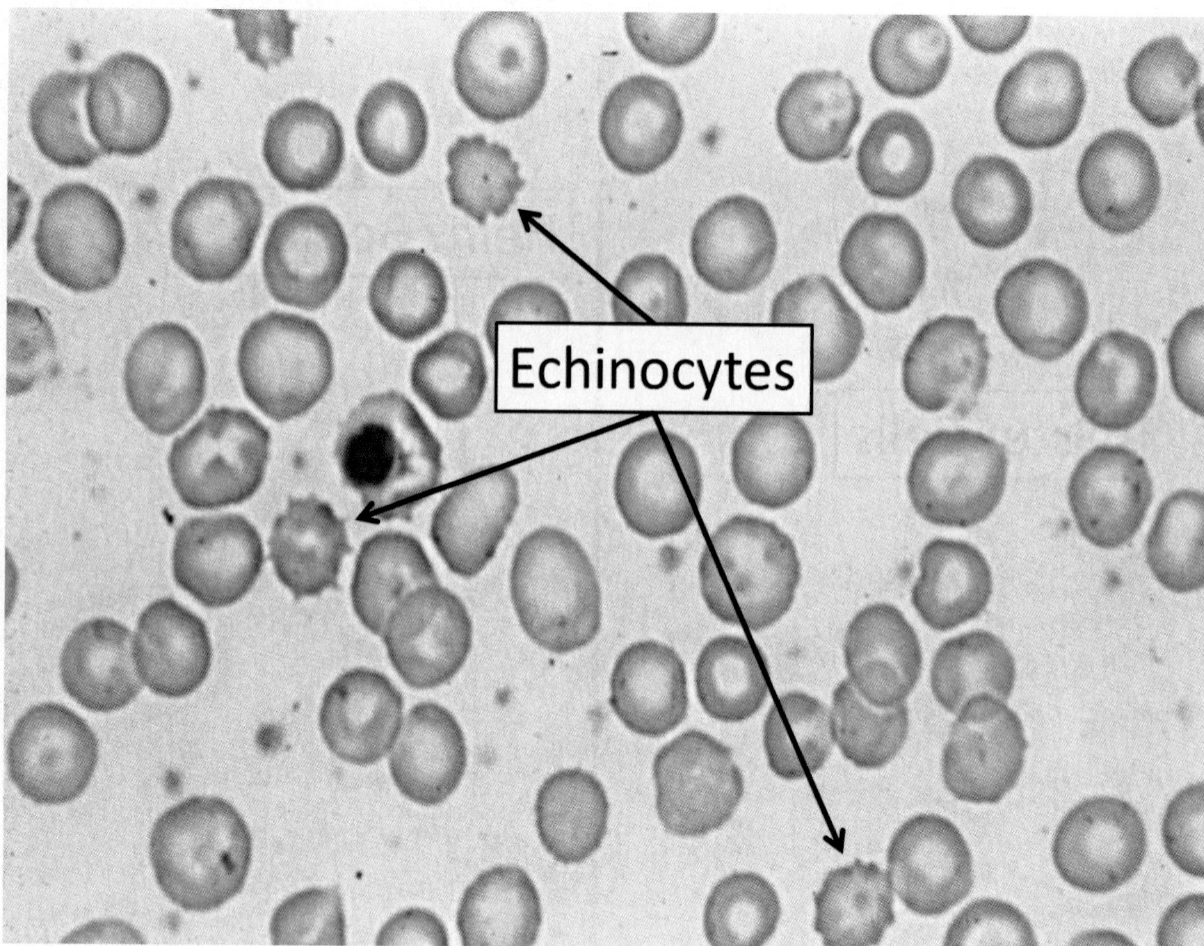

Fig. 43.15 Echinocytes From a Neonate With Pyruvate Kinase Deficiency.

The primary value of quantifying schistocytes in a jaundiced neonate is to confirm the presence of a microangiopathic condition. When thrombocytopenia is found in a jaundiced neonate with schistocytosis, several clinical conditions should be considered: (1) DIC, which can accompany perinatal asphyxia, sepsis, or other infections; (2) a congenital form of thrombotic thrombocytopenic purpura due to deficiency of the von Willebrand factor cleaving protease ADAMTS13[137]; (3) homozygous protein C deficiency[138]; (4) neonatal hemolytic uremic syndrome[139]; and (5) giant hemangioma or vascular tumors.[140]

Immune-Mediated Hemolytic Disease of the Fetus/Neonate

Rh Hemolytic Disease

Hemolytic disease of the fetus and neonate due to rhesus alloimmunization was once a major cause of perinatal and neonatal morbidity and mortality.[141] Preventing women from alloimmunization to the D antigen became possible after investigations showed that Rh-negative men who were exposed to the D antigen by transfusion with Rh-positive red cells could be protected from developing anti-D antibody if, before the transfusion, anti-D immune globulin was administered.[142] Clinical trials involving Rh-negative pregnant women demonstrated that administering Rh-D immune globulin within a 72 hour window after birth reduced the incidence of D alloimmunization from 10% to 1%–2%.[143] Later trials focused on the fact that fetomaternal hemorrhage in the third trimester contributed to the residual risk of alloimmunization during pregnancy. These new trials led to the observation that antenatal RhIG prophylaxis, combined with administration after birth, could further reduce the risk of D alloimmunization to <1%.[143]

In the 1970s the World Health Organization recommended administering Rho(D) immune globulin (RhIG) to D-negative women after delivery of a D-positive infant and after abortion. This recommendation was introduced in Canada and the United States in 1979 to 1980 and in the United Kingdom in 1998. In the United States between 1970 and 1986, the incidence of hemolytic disease of the fetus and newborn due to anti-D decreased from 40.5 to 10.6 cases per 10,000 births.[144]

Even when these highly successful recommendations are used, cases of Rh hemolytic disease of the fetus and newborn continue to occur, but in relatively low incidence compared with prerecommendation implementation. Specifically, the current incidence in the United States is about 6 cases per 1000 live births.[145] The failure of proper maternal RhIG administration to completely eliminate Rh hemolytic disease of the fetus/neonate may be due to maternal production of anti-D antibodies early in pregnancy. Countries where RhIG prophylaxis programs are not standard practice continue to have affected fetuses, stillborns, neonatal deaths, or severe brain injury that might have been prevented.[145,146]

The clinical phenotype of a neonate affected by Rh hemolytic disease ranges in severity from intrauterine hydrops fetalis to

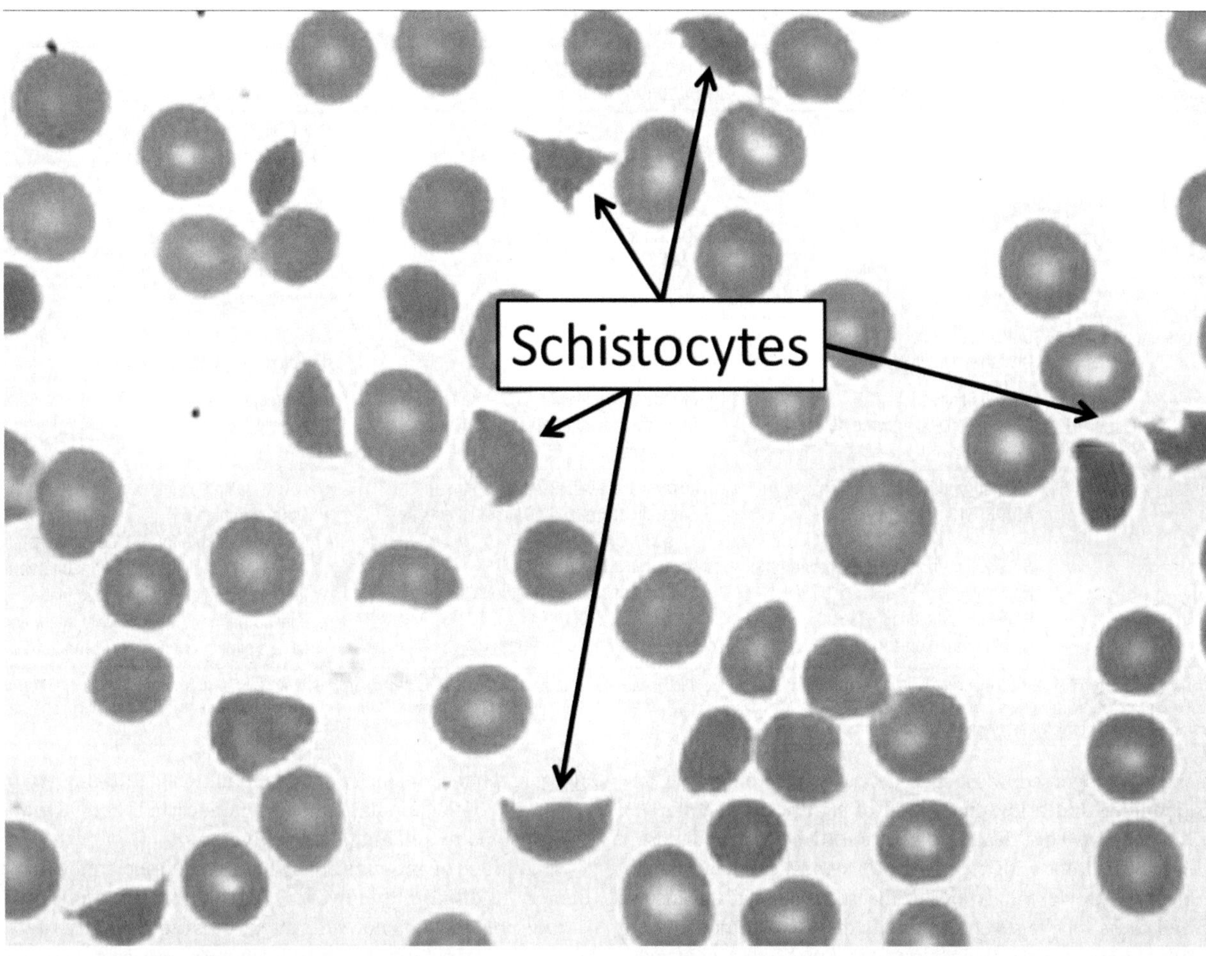

Fig. 43.16 Schistocytes From a Neonate With Disseminated Intravascular Coagulation Associated With Birth Asphyxia.

relatively mild neonatal hyperbilirubinemia and anemia. About half of neonates with detectable maternal anti-D are unaffected or only mildly affected, 30% have moderately severe hemolytic disease, and 20% are severely affected in utero.[147]

Severely affected neonates have cord blood hemoglobin concentrations <12 g/dL and cord bilirubin concentrations >5 mg/dL. If intrauterine transfusions are given, the hemolytic disease may be relatively mild and the blood type at birth may reflect the ABO and D-negative type of the transfused RBCs. Moderately severe hemolytic disease is predicted by a cord blood hemoglobin of 12 to 14 g/dL and a cord bilirubin of 4 to 5 g/dL. After birth, jaundice may occur within the first 24 hours, and bilirubin concentrations typically peak between 3 and 5 days. Mild hemolytic disease is predicted by a cord blood hemoglobin ≥14 g/dL and a cord bilirubin <4 mg/dL.

ABO Hemolytic Disease

Hemolytic disease of the newborn can occur when the maternal and fetal blood groups are discordant. Specifically, ABO incompatibility occurs when the mother is blood group O and a neonate is group A or B.[148] Most such incompatible pregnancies do not result in significant neonatal hemolysis. If the group A or B neonate born to a group O mother has a positive DAT (Coombs) and becomes sufficiently hyperbilirubinemic to qualify for phototherapy, and if no other explanation for the neonatal jaundice is identified, ABO hemolytic disease

Table 43.4 Varieties of Neonatal Hemolytic Anemia With Abnormal Erythrocyte Morphology

Defect	Disorder	Proportion With This Variety	Inheritance	Severity
Ankyrin	Spherocytosis	40%–65%	Dominant	Mild to moderate
Band 3	Spherocytosis Southeast Asian ovalocytosis	20%–35%	Dominant	Mild to moderate
β-Spectrin	Spherocytosis	15%–30%	Dominant	Mild to moderate
α-Spectrin	Spherocytosis	<5%	Recessive	Severe
Protein 4.2	Spherocytosis	<5% (Japan)	Recessive	Mild to moderate
Protein 4.1	Elliptocytosis		Dominant	Mild to moderate

Table 43.5 Morphologic Abnormalities of Erythrocytes, From Neonates With Unexplained Severe Jaundice/Anemia, as a Guide to Discovering the Underlying Cause

Abnormal Erythrocyte Morphology	Most Likely Cause(s)	Suggested Laboratory Testing/Findings	Other Features
Microspherocytes	Hereditary spherocytosis	• DAT (–) • EMA-flow (+) • Persistent spherocytosis	MCHC/MCV is elevated (>36; if >40, dx of HS is very likely)
	ABO hemolytic disease	• DAT (+) • Transient spherocytosis	MCHC/MCV is normal (<36)
Elliptocytes	Hereditary Elliptocytosis	DAT (–)	MCHC normal MCV normal
Bite and blister cells	G6PD deficiency Unstable hemoglobin	G6PD enzyme activity Heinz body prep	• Typically male • Ethnicity of equatorial origin
Echinocytes	PK deficiency Other glycolytic enzyme deficiency	PK enzyme activity Quantify activity of other glycolytic enzymes	Autosomal recessive, likely to have no family history
Schistocytes	DIC and/or perinatal asphyxia ADAMTS13 deficiency Neonatal hemolytic uremic syndrome Homozygous Protein C deficiency Giant hemangioma	Low FV and FVIII, elevated d-dimers Severely decreased ADAMTS13 activity (<0.1 U/mL) Acute renal failure Severely decreased functional protein C activity (<1%) May be internal or external	• Low or falling platelet count • Normal to high IPF • Normal to high MPV DIC, perinatal asphyxia • ADAMTS13 deficiency, early neonatal HUS, and giant hemangiomas all involve platelet consumption from endothelial injury and all have a similar neonatal presentation

ADAM, A disintegrin and metalloproteinase with thrombospondin type 1 motif 13; *DAT*, direct antiglobulin test; *DIC*, disseminated intravascular coagulation; *EMA*, eosin-5-maleimide; *FV*, factor 5; *FVIII*, factor 8; *G6PD*, glucose 6 phosphate dehydrogenase; *HS*, hereditary spherocytosis; *HUS*, hemolytic uremic syndrome; *IPF*, immature platelet fraction; *MCHC*, mean corpuscular hemoglobin concentration; *MCV*, mean corpuscular volume; *MPV*, mean platelet volume; *PK*, pyruvate kinase.

of the neonate is diagnosed. Most such neonates have only mild to moderate jaundice and a low likelihood of significant anemia.[149] However, case reports have described severe ABO hemolytic disease resulting in fetal hydrops with erythroblastosis and significant fetal/neonatal anemia.[150] However, it is possible that such cases had a second, unrecognized cause for the severe hemolytic disease and that it was not the result of ABO incompatibility alone. Similarly, severe neonatal jaundice resulting in kernicterus has been reported to result from ABO hemolytic jaundice, but this remains unproven in large case series.[151]

In the Intermountain Healthcare system, we found that ABO hemolytic disease of the newborn was not responsible for "severe" cases of neonatal jaundice.[149,152] We defined "severe" as a neonate in whom either (1) the total serum bilirubin level exceeded 25 mg/dL, (2) the patient was readmitted to the hospital for jaundice treatment, or (3) acute bilirubin encephalopathy was diagnosed. Our conclusion that ABO hemolytic disease did not result in "severe" hemolytic disease was based on identical outcomes of neonates of blood types A or B, born to group O mothers (thus at some risk of ABO hemolytic disease), versus neonates of blood type O, born to group O mothers (thus at no risk of ABO hemolytic disease).[148,152]

As illustrated in Fig. 43.12, neonates with ABO hemolytic disease typically have spherocytes on peripheral blood films, whereas neonates with other varieties of immune-mediated hemolytic disease generally do not.

Hemolytic Disease Due to Non-Rh, Non-ABO Antigens

Fetuses or neonates with hemolytic anemia due to anti-Kell antibody have lower reticulocyte counts and total serum bilirubin levels than do comparable anti-D anemic fetuses.[153,154] The level of hemolysis caused by anti-Kell antibodies is less than that caused by anti-D antibodies, but fetal erythropoiesis is blunted because Kell sensitization results in both suppression of fetal erythropoiesis and hemolysis. Anti-Kell antibodies cause fetal anemia by suppressing erythropoiesis at the level of erythroid progenitors. Unlike the RhD antigen, where a majority of the population is RhD antigen positive, a majority of the population (91% of Caucasians and 98% of African Americans) are Kell antigen negative.

High titers of anti-C antibody have been associated with neonatal hemolytic disease.[155] However, routine screening of anti-C titers during pregnancy is not warranted, because antibody titers do not accurately reflect the severity of hemolytic disease. C(w) is a low-frequency antigen in the Rh blood group system with a prevalence of about 2% among Caucasian populations (the letter C indicates its prevalence in the Caucasian population). Anti-C(w) is not too uncommon in pregnancy (0.1% incidence), but clinically significant hemolytic disease of the newborn is very unusual.[156]

Late Anemia After Hemolytic Disease of the Fetus and Neonate

Anemia can recur 2 to 10 weeks after treatment of alloimmune-hemolytic disease.[157] This variety can take one of two forms, or it can have elements of both. One form is a continued hemolytic condition on the basis of persistent maternally derived immunoglobulin G (IgG) binding to neonatal RBCs, leading to continued destruction. Hemolysis is evident by reticulocytosis, absent serum haptoglobin, presence of free hemoglobin in urine, and elevated end-tidal CO measurements. Maternal IgG can persist in the neonate for 6 weeks or longer, and even after exchange transfusion, such antibodies can remain because they may have been extravascular at the time of the exchange.

The second variety of late anemia is a hyporegenerative condition, where the reticulocyte count is low (sometimes 0%) and no evidence of hemolysis is present; serum haptoglobin is measurable, no free hemoglobin is detected in the urine, and end-tidal CO is normal, not elevated. This second variety is likely the result of fetal/early neonatal exposure to large amounts of adult hemoglobin from donor RBCs, which markedly increase oxygen delivery to tissues and suppress Epo production.[158–160]

In either variety of late-onset anemia, the hemoglobin concentration can decrease sufficiently that signs of anemia are apparent and problematic, and erythrocyte transfusion can be needed. Late transfusion can, in some instances, be avoided by the administration of recombinant Epo or darbepoetin, thereby increasing erythrocyte production, preventing severe anemia, and obviating the need for a late transfusion.[158,159]

Hemolytic Disease of the Fetus/Neonate Associated With Infectious Diseases

Sepsis in a neonate can cause anemia on the basis of DIC and hemorrhage, but some microorganisms appear to have independent hemolytic properties. Most cases of neonatal hemolytic anemia associated with infections are due to microangiopathic changes in erythrocytes; namely, mechanical disruption of red cells traversing the microvascular that has intraluminal fibrin strands associated with endothelial damage.[160] This is the principal mechanism causing hemolysis in neonates with hemolytic uremic syndrome.[161,162] However, *Clostridium perfringens* and mycoplasma are reported to cause hemolysis independent of microangiopathy.[163,164] This is because some microorganisms responsible for neonatal sepsis produce hemolytic endotoxins that result in accelerated erythrocyte destruction independent of a microangiopathic mechanism. Congenital syphilis can present with hemolytic anemia.[165] In cases of nonimmune hydrops, nontreponemal testing, if initially negative, should be repeated using serum dilutions to prevent a missed diagnosis of syphilis in women with negative syphilis serologic results.

Fetal and neonatal infection with parvovirus B19 can cause severe anemia, hydrops, and fetal demise.[166–169] This is generally a hypoplastic anemia, but hemolysis can occur as well. The virus replicates in erythroid progenitor cells and results in red cell aplasia. In utero transfusions for hydropic fetuses can be successful. Intrauterine fetal infusion of B19 IgG-rich high-titer gamma globulin has been reported to be successful.

Other fetal infections associated with neonatal anemia include malaria and HIV. Congenital malaria is seen rarely in the United States, generally in large cities where imported cases of malaria are increasing. In certain African countries, congenital malaria has been reported in up to 20% of neonates.[170,171] Congenital HIV infection in a neonate is generally asymptomatic. However, infants born to mothers on zidovudine can have hypoplastic anemia due to suppressive effects of the drug on fetal erythropoiesis.[172]

CHAPTER

44 Evidence-Based Neonatal Transfusion Guidelines

Robin K. Ohls

KEY POINTS

1. Anemia occurs when the red blood cell (RBC) mass is not adequate to meet tissue oxygen needs.
2. Target hemoglobin and hematocrit have been used as clinical indicators for RBC transfusion in preterm infants with acute and chronic anemia.
3. The minimal target hematocrit or hemoglobin that optimally balances the risks and benefits of transfusion remains unknown because a marker for transfusion need has not been identified.
4. The two largest multicenter trials evaluating liberal versus restrictive transfusion guidelines in extremely low birth weight infants were conclusive in confirming a restrictive approach to red cell transfusions.
5. In extremely low birth weight infants, a restrictive approach to transfusions should be instituted, because it results in fewer transfusions and does not increase the risk of morbidity, death, or neurodevelopmental impairment.

Introduction and Pathophysiology

Fetal and Neonatal Oxygen Delivery

Fetal hematocrit and hemoglobin concentrations gradually increase as gestation increases. Fetal erythropoiesis is stimulated by fetal erythropoietin (Epo), produced in response to the fetal hypoxic environment (Fig. 44.1), where Po_2 values range from 20 to 35 torr (Fig. 44.2). Oxygen extraction from the placental circulation is augmented by the high percentage of fetal hemoglobin, which has a greater oxygen affinity than adult hemoglobin (Fig. 44.2). Po_2 values increase once an infant is born, resulting in a rapid decline in Epo production and cessation of erythropoiesis.

Acute and Chronic Anemia

Anemia occurs when the volume of circulating red cells fails to meet the metabolic needs of tissues. Preterm infants born <1500 g (very low birth weight [VLBW]) are frequently transfused due to common clinical characteristics and features of prematurity that, compounded, result in a significant fall in hemoglobin and hematocrit in the first weeks of life. These characteristics include (1) lower hemoglobin concentrations at lower gestational ages (Fig. 44.3); (2) ongoing loss of red cells due to phlebotomy, sometimes equaling an entire blood volume (80–85 mL/kg) in the first weeks of life; (3) a shortened red cell life span of 60 to 70 days; and (4) lack adequate endogenous Epo production after birth to maintain the red cell mass. All of these characteristics lead to a fall in hemoglobin and hematocrit that is greater than that seem normally in term infants during their physiologic nadir (Fig. 44.4), resulting in frequent transfusions.

Indications for neonatal transfusions differ based on the rate of fall in hemoglobin. In an infant with acute blood loss, the need for a transfusion is generally dependent on persistent clinical signs of inadequate oxygen delivery following the restoration of intravascular volume. Infants with chronic anemia may also exhibit clinical signs of inadequate oxygen delivery such as increased resting heart rate, acidosis, poor growth, and apnea, and a need for increased respiratory support, that are often ameliorated by a transfusion.

Red cell transfusions are currently the accepted treatment for acute anemia, especially anemia due to hemorrhage, because they rapidly increase available oxygen. The oxygen content is based on the following equation:

$$\text{Oxygen content } (Cao_2) = (1.34 \times \text{Hgb}\,[\text{g/dL}] \times \%\text{ saturation}) + (0.003 \times Pao_2)$$

In this equation, 1.34 equals the mL of oxygen binding to each gram of hemoglobin, and 0.003 equals the mL of oxygen dissolved in blood per mm Hg. Oxygen availability and delivery to tissues is proportional to oxygen content and cardiac output. When cardiac output is adequate and optimized, red cell transfusions rapidly increase oxygen availability to tissues. There are, however, a growing list of risks associated with transfusions, including transmission of infection,[1] graft-versus-host disease, transfusion-related acute lung injury,[2] transfusion associated circulatory overload,[3] and toxic contamination of blood products with heavy metals.[4] In the preterm infant population, red cell transfusions may be associated with an increased risk of necrotizing enterocolitis (NEC),[5–7] extension of intraventricular hemorrhage (IVH),[8] increased mortality,[9] or impaired developmental outcome.[10,11] A causal relationship with any of these adverse events is still being determined. Neonatal transfusions can result in increases in proinflammatory cytokines such as ICAM-1, IL-1β, IL-8, IL-10, IFN-γ, IL-17, and MCP-1,[12] potentially increasing or worsening morbidities associated with prematurity. These potential complications underscore the need to carefully evaluate the need for a rapid increase in oxygen availability to tissues *prior* to ordering a nonemergent transfusion in a preterm infant. Similar to the growing emphasis on antibiotic stewardship, where antibiotics are being reassessed and more stringently prescribed, "transfusion stewardship" will hopefully provide greater focus for providers to practice evidence-based ordering of blood products for neonates.

It can be a challenge determining which neonate with a low hematocrit will benefit from a red cell transfusion. Many preterm infants can adapt to a slowly decreasing hematocrit and can be treated conservatively with supplemental iron and red cell growth factors such as Epo or darbepoetin (Darbe) to avoid the associated risks of transfusion.[13,14] Target hemoglobin and hematocrit have been used as clinical indicators for red blood cell (RBC) transfusion; however, it remains uncertain what target hematocrit or hemoglobin

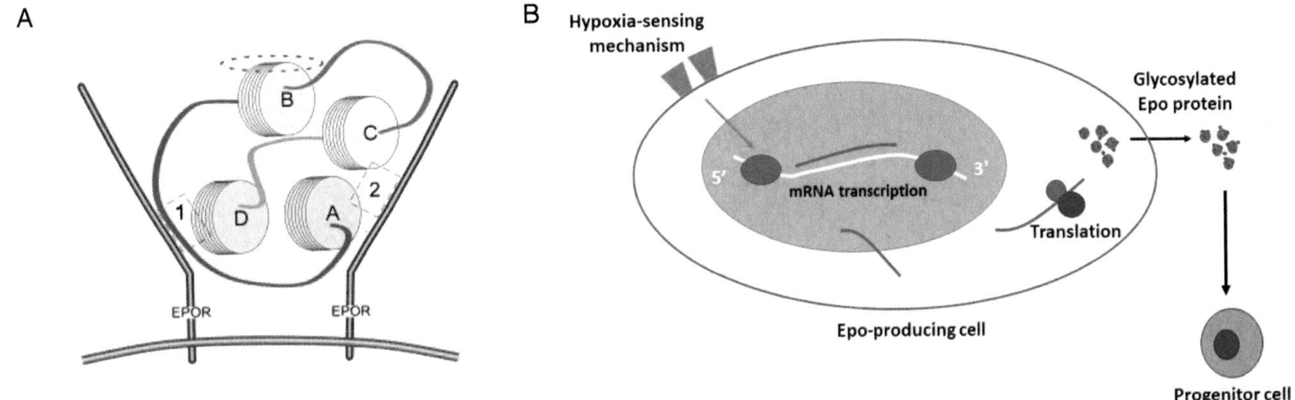

Fig. 44.1 Erythropoietin (Epo) and Downstream Signaling. (A) Epo is a globular molecule composed of four helices, where the helix B (encircled in *red*) has stayed highly conserved during evolution. Epo binds a homodimeric cognate receptor and bridges two sites *(dashed boxes)*, and the consequential conformational change results in phosphorylation of JAK2 and triggers multiple downstream molecular cascades (not shown). (Modified after permission to reproduce from Brines M. Extrahematopoietic actions of erythropoietin. In: *Textbook of Nephro-Endocrinology*, ch. 23, 411–428.) (B) Hypoxemia and anemia induce Epo expression, a process that involves the hepatic nuclear factor 4 (HNF-4) and the hypoxic inducible factor-1 (HIF-1; not shown). HNF-4 binds the Epo promoter and enhancer regions and is highly expressed in the kidneys and liver. HIF-1 is a basic helix-loop-helix transcription factor that binds the *cis*-acting hypoxia-response elements to induce Epo transcription. Although there is some evidence to suggest that HIF-1 is expressed during fetal development, the regional expression of these transcriptional activators needs further investigation.

will optimally balance the risks and benefits of this intervention. This chapter focuses on exploring the development of evidence-based transfusion guidelines in the newborn intensive care unit (NICU).

Clinical Studies

Transfusion Studies in Critical Care

Over the past 4 decades, approaches to RBC transfusions in neonates have changed significantly. In the 1980s, phlebotomy losses in NICU patients were carefully recorded in order to replace blood lost when losses reached 10 mL/kg. Transfusions were generally administered when a preterm infant's hematocrit dropped below 40%, and "top-off" transfusions (5–10 mL/kg volumes) were common in the later weeks of NICU hospitalization. Signs typical of preterm infants, such as apnea, poor feeding, tachycardia, and poor weight gain, were ascribed to anemia, and infants would be transfused frequently over a wide range of hematocrits without clear evidence of benefit.[15]

Development of transfusion guidelines in critical care became a priority for Canadian institutions after thousands of transfusion recipients were exposed to hepatitis C and HIV from contaminated blood.[16] A number of Canadian multicenter trials in populations receiving frequent transfusions ensued. The Transfusion Requirements in Critical Care (TRICC) trial randomized stable critical care patients to a restrictive hemoglobin transfusion threshold of 7 g/dL or a liberal transfusion threshold of 9 g/dL. Those in the restrictive group received fewer transfusions with better outcomes and lower in-hospital mortality (22.2% versus 28.1%).[17] In a similarly designed trial performed in stable pediatric critical care patients, a hemoglobin threshold of 7 g/dL for red-cell transfusion decreased transfusion requirements without increasing adverse outcomes.[18]

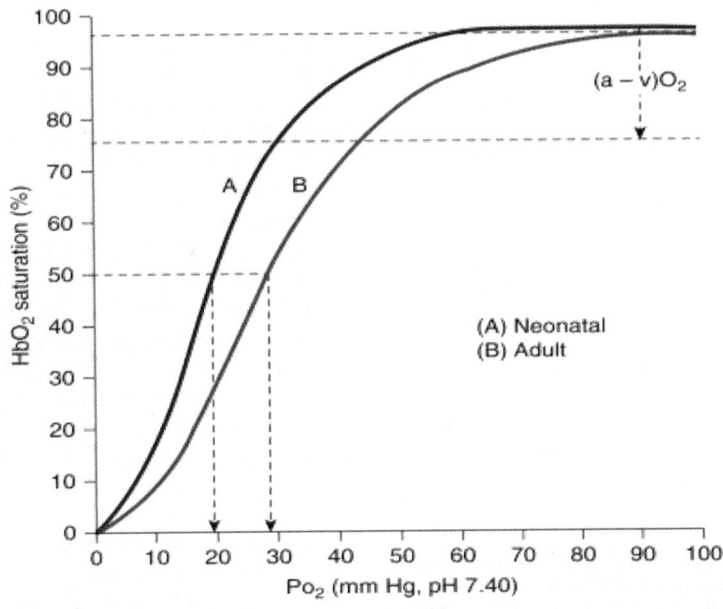

Fig. 44.2 Oxyhemoglobin (Hbo_2) Equilibrium Curves. (A) Blood from term infants at birth. (B) Blood from adults. *a*, arterial; *v*, venous.

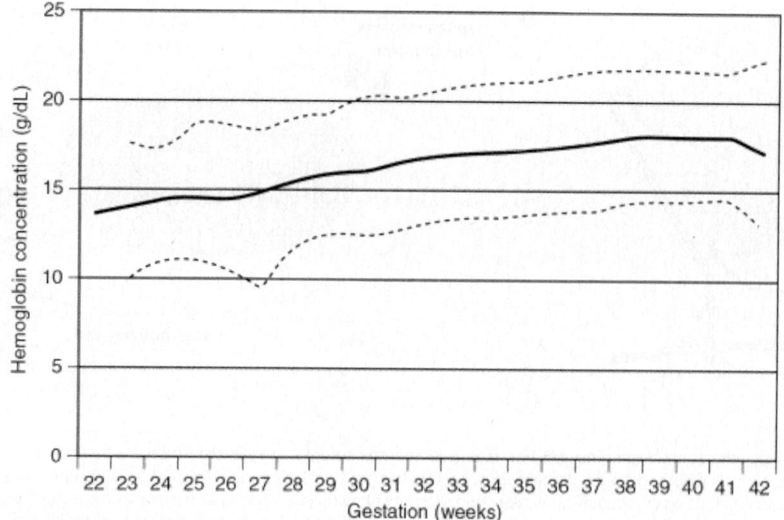

Fig. 44.3 Changes in Hemoglobin Concentration (g/dL) From 22 to 42 Weeks' Gestation. The *dotted lines* represent the 5th and 95th percentiles; the *solid line* represents the mean.

Neonatal Transfusion Studies

Neonatal transfusion practices did not begin to change until the mid-1990s, following publication of the first multicenter trial of Epo administration to VLBW infants.[19] The study implemented a transfusion protocol that was subsequently implemented in many NICUs throughout the country. As a result, the average number of transfusions administered to VLBW infants decreased significantly.[20] In order to identify strategies that would decrease the need for red blood cell transfusions and to limit donor exposure in VLBW infants, the Canadian Paediatric Society adopted guidelines that were even more restrictive than those used in the US Epo study (Table 44.1).[21] In fact, these guidelines, published in 2002, remain the most restrictive guidelines for neonates published to date.

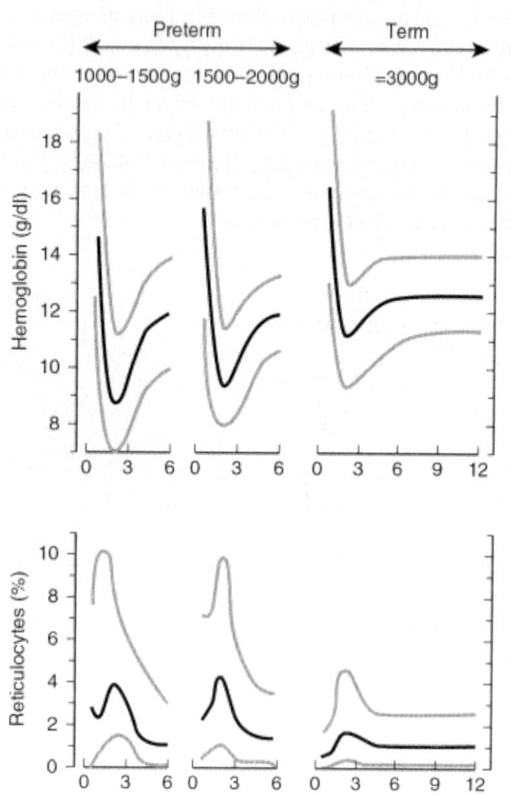

Fig. 44.4 Mean Hemoglobin and Reticulocyte Values in Term and Preterm Infants. Infants born preterm become anemic earlier in the postnatal period with hemoglobin concentrations returning to normal later. *Black*, Lower range of normal; *gray*, upper range.

Since the early 2000s, a number of studies have been performed evaluating hematocrit thresholds for transfusion in preterm infants. Bifano and colleagues were the first to compare higher and lower transfusion thresholds. They randomized 50 extremely low birth weight (ELBW) infants to maintain hematocrits above 32% or below 30%. Despite a difference in hemoglobin between groups of over 4 g/dL, they found no differences in hospital outcomes, growth, or neurodevelopment at 1 year.[15,22,23]

Bell and colleagues randomized 100 preterm infants with a birth weight of 500 to 1300 g to a liberal (higher hematocrit) or restrictive (lower hematocrit) transfusion threshold strategy, based on level of respiratory support, age, and clinical status.[24] Clinical outcomes were compared.[24] Infants in the liberal-transfusion group received more RBC transfusions (5.2 ± 4.5) compared with the restrictive-transfusion group (3.3 ± 2.9). There were no differences in pretransfusion cardiac output, hospital days, or survival to discharge. Investigators found an increase in grade 3 or 4 IVH or periventricular leukomalacia in the restrictive group (6/28 versus 0/24 in the liberal group). They concluded that more frequent major adverse neurologic imaging findings in the restrictive group suggested restrictive transfusions might be harmful.

Long-term follow-up of infants enrolled in the Iowa trial was performed on a subset of children available for evaluation at 12 years. Both cognitive function (based on developmental assessment) and magnetic resonance imaging outcomes were better in the restrictive group.[25,26]

Canadian investigators designed a large multicenter trial to evaluate transfusion thresholds on hospital outcomes. Investigators for the Premature Infants in Need of Transfusion (PINT) Study[27] randomized 451 ELBW infants to a high or low threshold transfusion strategy within 48 hours of birth. Infants in the low threshold group received fewer transfusions and were transfused at a later age. There were no differences in morbidities or mortality between the low and high hemoglobin threshold groups, resulting in no difference in the composite outcome of death or serious morbidity at the time of discharge (bronchopulmonary dysplasia, severe retinopathy of

Table 44.1 2002 Canadian Paediatric Society Neonatal Transfusion Guidelines

Red Cell Transfusions Should Be Considered for the Following Clinical Situations:
Hypovolemic shock due to acute blood loss
Hematocrit 30%–35% (hemoglobin 10–12 g/dL) associated with critical illness, where a red cell transfusion might increase oxygen delivery to vital organs
Hematocrit 20%–30% (hemoglobin 6–10 g/dL) associated with severe illness and/or mechanical ventilation with compromised oxygen delivery
Hematocrit <20% (hemoglobin <6 g/dL) associated with absolute reticulocyte count <100 × 10^3/uL, poor weight gain, respiratory distress and increased oxygen requirements, lethargy, and tachycardia (>180 bpm)

From: Red blood cell transfusions in newborn infants: revised guidelines. *Paediatr Child Health.* 2002;7:553.

prematurity, or, importantly, brain injury identified on ultrasound). At 18 to 21 months' corrected age there were no differences between the low and high target hematocrit groups in the composite outcome of death or neurodevelopmental impairment, defined as cerebral palsy, significant visual or hearing impairment, or a Bayley Scales of Infant Development II (BSID II) Mental Development Index (MDI) score <70.[28] In *post hoc* analyses using an MDI score <85 instead of <70, the primary outcome of death or neurodevelopmental impairment (NDI) was more likely in the low hematocrit group (45%) compared with the high hematocrit group (34%), leading investigators to hypothesize that maintaining a higher hematocrit would decrease the incidence of NDI in preterm infants.

A 2012 meta-analysis included both the Iowa and PINT studies and reported no difference in morbidities or mortality rates between high and low threshold transfusion groups.[29] Similar to adult and pediatric critical care populations, a restrictive (low) hematocrit threshold compared with a liberal (high) threshold (hematocrit 35%–40%) resulted in fewer transfusions with no increase in mortality or serious morbidity.[29,30] Because of concerns that long-term developmental impairment might still be associated with restrictive transfusion strategies, two similarly designed, large randomized trials were performed—one in Europe[31] and the other in the NICHD Neonatal Research Network,[32] published in 2020—that overwhelmingly confirmed the results of the previous meta-analyses. These studies are reviewed below.

TOP/ETTNO Studies

Two multicenter randomized trials were designed to definitively determine whether lower or higher thresholds for transfusing preterm infants resulted in better neurodevelopmental outcomes. The Transfusion of Prematures (TOP) trial was designed by the principal investigators of the PINT and Iowa studies to test the hypothesis that maintaining a higher hematocrit would result in decreased NDI by comparing neurodevelopmental outcomes of ELBW infants randomized to a high or low hematocrit threshold for transfusion.[31] This hypothesis was based on increased IVH in the Iowa study and the *post hoc* finding of an increased percentage of infants in the low hematocrit group scoring <85 in the PINT trial. Similarly, investigators in the Effects of Liberal versus Restrictive Transfusion Thresholds on Survival and Neurocognitive Outcomes (ETTNO) study evaluated higher and lower hematocrit strategies for red cell transfusions, testing the hypothesis that the lower hematocrit strategy would lead to an increase in the primary outcome of death or neurodevelopmental disability.[32]

Hematocrit Triggers for Transfusion

Hematocrit triggers were determined for each trial (Table 44.2). For the TOP trial, a survey of neonatologists was performed to determine an acceptable range of hematocrits that could be used to trigger transfusions.[33] Hematocrit triggers were chosen to achieve a statistical difference in hemoglobin between the low and high groups of 2 to 2.5 g/dL (hematocrit 5%–6%). In the ETTNO study, transfusion triggers were guided by current clinical practice in Germany.[34] The high and low thresholds chosen also aimed to produce a clinically relevant difference in mean hemoglobin concentrations between treatment groups of about 2 g/dL, in order to improve recognition of any effect of hemoglobin thresholds on neurocognitive outcome compared with the PINT trial, where differences between high and low thresholds were narrower.

Eligibility Criteria and Study Design

Infants in the ETTNO study had a birth weight of 400 to 999 g and were randomized at less than 72 hours of life to the high or low

Table 44.2 Transfusion Triggers for the TOP[a] and ETTNO[b] Studies

	TOP High Respiratory Support	TOP High No Respiratory Support	TOP Low Respiratory Support	TOP Low No Respiratory Support	ETTNO High Critical	ETTNO High Noncritical	ETTNO Low Critical	ETTNO Low Noncritical
0–7 days	38	35	32	29	<41	<35	<34	<28
8–14 days (TOP) 8–21 days (ETTNO)	37	32	29	25	<37	<31	<30	<24
≥15 days (TOP) >21 days (ETTNO)	32	29	25	21	<34	<28	<27	<21

Hemoglobin values were converted to hematocrit by multiplying by 2.941.

[a]For TOP: respiratory support was defined as mechanical ventilation, continuous positive airway pressure, fraction of inspired oxygen >0.35, or nasal cannula ≥1 L/min (room air nasal cannula ≥1 L/min was considered respiratory support).

[b]For ETTNO: critical was defined as the infant having at least one of the following criteria: invasive mechanical ventilation; continuous positive airway pressure with fraction of inspired oxygen >0.25 for >12 out of 24 hours; treatment for patent ductus arteriosus, acute sepsis, or necrotizing enterocolitis with circulatory failure requiring inotropic/vasopressor support; >6 nurse-documented apneas requiring intervention per 24 hours; or >4 intermittent hypoxemic episodes with pulse oximetry oxygen saturation <60%. Triggers stayed in place through 36 completed weeks of gestation (TOP) or until discharge (ETTNO).

Data from Kirpalani H, Bell EF, Hintz SR, et al. Higher or lower hemoglobin transfusion thresholds for preterm infants. *N Engl J Med.* 2020;383:2639–2651; and Franz AR, Engel C, Bassler D, et al. Effects of liberal vs restrictive transfusion thresholds on survival and neurocognitive outcomes in extremely low-birth-weight infants: the ETTNO randomized clinical trial. *JAMA.* 2020;324:560–570.

Table 44.3 Enrollment and Study Methods for the TOP and ETTNO Studies

	TOP	ETTNO
Gestation	23 0/7–28 6/7 weeks	—
Birth weight	—	400–999 g
Enrollment period	Within 48 hours of birth	Within 72 hours of birth
Length of study protocol	Transfused per protocol through 36 completed weeks	Transfused per protocol until discharge
Stratification	23–25 weeks; 26–28 weeks	400–749 g; 750–999 g
Transfusion volume	15 mL/kg	20 mL/kg
Transfusions mandated	Yes, within 12 hours of identifying transfusion trigger	Yes, within 72 hours of transfusion trigger
Erythropoietin administration allowed	No	No
Delayed cord clamping/milking	Per site guidelines; occurred in 439/1684 (25%)	Recommended for sites; occurred in 627/1011 (62%)
Follow-up blinded	Yes	Yes
Primary outcome	Death or neurodevelopmental impairment	Death or neurodevelopmental impairment

Data from Kirpalani H, Bell EF, Hintz SR, et al. Higher or lower hemoglobin transfusion thresholds for preterm infants. *N Engl J Med.* 2020;383:2639–2651; and Franz AR, Engel C, Bassler D, et al. Effects of liberal vs restrictive transfusion thresholds on survival and neurocognitive outcomes in extremely low-birth-weight infants: the ETTNO randomized clinical trial. *JAMA.* 2020;324:560–570.

group, stratified by weight (Table 44.3). Transfusions prior to enrollment did not preclude participation in the study, and approximately 25% of infants received least one transfusion prior to randomization (24% versus 25%, low versus high). The transfusion protocol remained in place through discharge or transfer from the hospital. Delayed cord clamping was recommended. Transfusions of 20 mL/kg were mandated within 72 hours of identifying a threshold hematocrit. None of the enrolled infants could receive red cell growth factors during the study.

In the TOP study, infants 22 0/7 to 28 6/7 weeks' gestation were enrolled within 48 hours of birth and randomized to the high or low group, stratified by gestation (see Table 44.3). The transfusion protocol remained in place through 36 weeks' corrected age. Transfusions could be given emergently prior to 6 hours of age (this occurred in 5% of the high group and 4% of the low group), but infants were ineligible if they received a transfusion after 6 hours of age. Transfusions of 15 mL/kg were mandated within 12 hours of identifying a threshold hematocrit. Infants could not receive red cell growth factors during the study.

Outcomes, Morbidities, and Transfusions

The primary outcome for both trials was the combined outcome of NDI or death. NDI was defined in similar fashion in both trials: cognitive score less than 85 on the Bayley Scales of Infant Development (Bayley III composite cognitive score for TOP; BSID II MDI for ETTNO); moderate or severe cerebral palsy (gross motor function classification system 2 or greater in TOP; Surveillance of Cerebral Palsy in Europe network definition for ETTNO); severe vision impairment; or severe hearing impairment.

Both trials found no differences between high and low groups in the primary outcome (Table 44.4). In fact, outcomes were basically identical between groups for both studies. Of the 1824 ELBW infants enrolled in TOP, primary outcome data were available for 92.8% (1692 infants). The primary outcome was present in 49.8% in the low group and 50.1% in the high group. There were also no differences between groups in the individual components (death or NDI) of the primary outcome. Importantly, the percentage of infants with Bayley III composite cognitive scores <85 was similar between groups: 269/695 (38.7%) in the high groups compared with 270/712 (37.9%) in the low groups, with an adjusted relative risk of 1.04 (95% confidence interval [CI], 0.91–1.18). Concerns identified in the *post hoc* analyses performed in the PINT trial[28] were alleviated by this result. Cognitive delay was the primary factor determining NDI and was identified in 97% of the infants in the high group and 91% of the infants in the low groups who were designated as neurodevelopmentally impaired. No differences between groups were identified in common neonatal hospital morbidities (bronchopulmonary dysplasia, retinopathy of prematurity, grade 3 to 4 interventricular hemorrhage or periventricular leukomalacia, or NEC; see Table 44.4). Metrics associated with severity of illness, such as length of stay, time to full feeds, length of time on a ventilator, and duration of caffeine treatment, were similar between low and high groups.

There were 1013 ELBW infants enrolled in ETTNO, and primary outcome data were available for 91.6% (928 infants) who completed the trial. The primary outcome was present in 42.9% in the low group and 44.4% in the high group. Similar to TOP, there were no differences between groups in the individual components (death or NDI) of the primary outcome. Importantly, the percentage of infants with BSID II MDI scores <85 was similar between groups (37.8% high versus 35.9% low), with an adjusted relative risk of 1.09 (95% CI, 0.81–1.46). Cognitive delay (BSID II <85) was the primary factor determining NDI and was identified in 88% of the infants in the high group and 86% of the infants in the low group who were designated as neurodevelopmentally impaired.

For both studies, the number of transfusions was significantly lower in the low group compared with the high group: 4.4 ± 4.0 versus 6.2 ± 4.3 transfusions in TOP; 1.7 versus 2.6 transfusions in ETTNO (Table 44.5). Additionally, a greater number of infants in the low threshold groups remained untransfused. For both studies, infants randomized to the low threshold groups received more transfusions outside of study protocols (see Table 44.5). These transfusions did not change the primary outcome of either trial, because analyses evaluating infants transfused per protocol yielded similar results as the main trials.

Limitations were clearly outlined by investigators for both studies.[31,32] Neither study was blinded to parents or care providers during the hospital phase, but both studies were blinded to follow-up evaluators. There was variation in blood banking procedures among participating sites, and information on donor gender was not collected. Protocol violations were greater in the low threshold groups. In the ETTNO study, the separation in hematocrit between low and high groups was less than expected.

Table 44.4 Outcomes for the TOP and ETTNO Studies

	TOP High	TOP Low	ETTNO High	ETTNO Low
Number randomized	911	913	492	521
Number evaluated for primary outcome	845	847	450	478
Death/NDI	50.1% (423/845)	49.8% (422/847)	44.4% (200/450)	42.9% (205/478)
Death by 24 months	16.2% (146/903)	15.0% (135/901)	8.3% (38/460)	9.0% (44/491)
NDI	39.6% (277/699)	40.3% (287/712)	36% (162/450)	33.7% (161/478)
Cognitive score,[a] mean	85.5±15	85.3±14.8	92.6±16.5	92.4±17.5
Cognitive score[a] <85	38.7% (269/695)	37.9% (270/712)	37.6% (154/410)	34.4% (148/430)
Cognitive score[a] <70	12.7% (88/695)	13.5% (96/712)	—	—
Cerebral palsy[b]	6.8% (48/711)	7.6% (55/720)	4.3% (18/419)	5.6% (25/443)
Hospital days[c]	96 (72–129)	97 (75–127)	93±41	92±38
NEC	10.0%	10.5%	5.3%	6.2%
ROP >grade 2	19.7%	17.2%	15.9%	13.0%
Intraventricular hemorrhage grade 3–4[d]	17.1% (146/855)	17.9% (154/859)	8.1% (40/492)	6.7% (35/521)
Periventricular leukomalacia	—	—	23/492	30/521
Bronchopulmonary dysplasia	59.0	56.3	28.4	26.0

No differences between high and low groups in each study were identified in any of the measures listed (no analyses have been performed *between* ETTNO and TOP studies).

[a]Bayley Scales of Infant Development III composite cognitive score for TOP; Bayley Scales of Infant Development II mental developmental index for ETTNO.

[b]Gross motor function classification system 2 or greater for TOP; Surveillance of Cerebral Palsy in Europe network definition for ETTNO.

[c]Values are mean and interquartile range for TOP; mean and standard deviation for ETTNO.

[d]Numbers are combined for intraventricular hemorrhage and periventricular leukomalacia for TOP.

NDI, Neurodevelopmental impairment; *NEC,* necrotizing enterocolitis; *ROP,* retinopathy of prematurity.

Data from Kirpalani H, Bell EF, Hintz SR, et al. Higher or lower hemoglobin transfusion thresholds for preterm infants. *N Engl J Med.* 2020;383:2639–2651; and Franz AR, Engel C, Bassler D, et al. Effects of liberal vs restrictive transfusion thresholds on survival and neurocognitive outcomes in extremely low-birth-weight infants: the ETTNO randomized clinical trial. *JAMA.* 2020;324:560–570.

ETTNO investigators speculated that differences in death and complications of prematurity might have reflected a healthier, more stable population than the birth weight and gestation would suggest. ETTNO recruitment extended over a period of 40 months and might have been impacted by changes in neonatal practice over time. The mean age at randomization was greater in the ETTNO study (2.5 days) than in the TOP study, and a greater number of infants received transfusions prior to study entry.

Secondary outcomes were similar in the TOP and ETTNO studies (aside from a greater incidence of bronchopulmonary dysplasia in TOP infants), and there were no differences within each study between high and low groups in the incidence of evaluated complications of prematurity. Importantly, there were no differences in NEC despite a difference in transfusions received between high and low groups. Mortality was higher in TOP (15.6%, versus 9.6% in ETTNO), which might have reflected a sicker population of ELBW infants. Fewer transfusions were administered overall in ETTNO; however, phlebotomy losses were not calculated and might have been greater in TOP infants. The overall incidence of cognitive delay, based on BSID II in ETTNO and Bayley III in TOP, was similar: 36% to 38% in ETTNO and 38% to 39% in TOP.

Summary of TOP and ETTNO

What can be concluded from these combined transfusion studies encompassing more than 2800 extremely low birth weight infants located on two continents? First, the results prove conclusively that transfusing critically ill ELBW infants at lower hematocrits did not result in adverse outcomes. Second, infants transfused at higher hematocrits did not do worse. Was there evidence that infants in either arm actually required a transfusion and improved after the transfusion? Aside from change in hematocrit, data were not collected on the efficacy of the treatment studied. Because both studies relied on consensus in determining hematocrit thresholds, both likely ended up measuring what infants *received*, rather than what they actually *needed.* In promoting transfusion stewardship, documenting evidence of benefit should be a part of future studies. In addition, cost-benefit analyses should be performed and are forthcoming on the TOP patients. Previous economic analyses performed after the

Table 44.5 Transfusions Administered for the TOP and ETTNO Studies

	TOP High	TOP Low	ETTNO High	ETTNO Low
Untransfused, %	3	12[a]	21	41[a]
Transfusions, mean	6.2±4.3	4.4±4.0[a]	2.6	1.7
Volume	—	—	40 (16–73)	19 (0–46)
Tx outside of protocol	0.8% (44/5624)	7.4% (299/4055)	5% (60/1258)	15% (137/904)

[a]$P < .05$, low versus high groups for each study.

Data from Kirpalani H, Bell EF, Hintz SR, et al. Higher or lower hemoglobin transfusion thresholds for preterm infants. *N Engl J Med.* 2020;383:2639–2651; and Franz AR, Engel C, Bassler D, et al. Effects of liberal vs restrictive transfusion thresholds on survival and neurocognitive outcomes in extremely low-birth-weight infants: the ETTNO randomized clinical trial. *JAMA.* 2020;324:560–570.

PINT trial reported less expense when infants were transfused at higher hematocrits.[35] Given the identical outcomes between the two groups and an increase in the number of transfusions administered in the higher hematocrit group, it is likely these findings will be reversed.

Evaluation and Management

Transfusions and Outcomes

Neonatal transfusion studies have focused on comparing two treatment arms, one maintaining higher hematocrits and one maintaining lower hematocrits. However, given past evidence that transfusions themselves may lead to increased morbidities in adult and pediatric studies, a number of investigators have looked at the association between the number and volume of transfusions and outcomes in preterm infants.[10,11]

We evaluated the impact of transfusions in preterm infants enrolled in a previous study.[36,37] In that trial, preterm infants were randomized to subcutaneous Epo (400 units/kg three times weekly), Darbe (10 mcg/kg once weekly), or placebo (sham injections) during their initial hospitalization, and the number and volume of red cell transfusions was recorded. Children were evaluated using standard developmental tests of cognition at 18 to 22 months (56 infants in the Epo and Darbe combined group and 24 infants in the placebo group). In a *post hoc* analysis,[10] cognitive scores on the Bayley III at 18 to 22 months were inversely correlated with transfusion volume ($P = .02$). Among placebo recipients, those receiving ≥1 transfusion had significantly lower cognitive scores than those who remained untransfused. In the erythropoiesis stimulating agent (ESA) group, cognitive scores were similar between nontransfused and transfused patients, suggesting ESAs provided neuroprotection from the effects of transfusions.

Transfusions and outcomes were analyzed in a similar fashion in preterm infants enrolled in the Preterm Epo for Neuroprotection (PENUT) trial.[11] In that study, Epo 1000 units/kg or placebo was given every 48 hours for a total of 6 doses, followed by 400 units/kg or sham injections three times a week through 32 weeks' postmenstrual age. Six hundred and twenty-eight (315 placebo, 313 Epo) patients survived and were assessed at 2 years of age. Associations between BSID-III scores and the number and volume of pRBC transfusions were evaluated in a *post hoc* analysis. Each transfusion was associated with a decrease in composite cognitive score of 0.96 (95% CI, −1.34 to −0.57), a decrease in composite motor score of 1.51 (95% CI, −1.91 to −1.12), and a decrease in composite language score of 1.10 (95% CI, −1.54 to −0.66). Significant negative associations between BSID-III score and transfusion volume and donor exposure were observed in the placebo group but not in the Epo group. Similar to the previous study,[10] transfusions in ELBW infants were associated with worse neurodevelopmental outcomes. Data from ETTNO have not been evaluated in this fashion. Analyses evaluating the association between the number and volume of transfusions and developmental outcomes in the TOP trial are forthcoming.

The search continues to determine when an infant might benefit from a transfusion. Studies focused on determining a more accurate indicator for transfusions have yet to identify a reliable and sensitive marker, preferably one that does not require a significant blood volume. Previous studies included measurement of biomarkers such as lactate or vascular endothelial growth factor,[38,39] echocardiographic evaluation of cardiovascular circulation,[40] or direct or indirect oxygen delivery (e.g., cerebral oxygen saturation, peripheral fractional oxygen extraction, and oxygen consumption).[41–44] Near infrared spectroscopy (NIRS) technology has advanced during the past 15 years and is used clinically in the NICU, especially in clinical scenarios where oxygen saturation might be impaired (not generally the case in preterm infants with gradually decreasing hematocrits). A secondary study to the TOP trial is evaluating NIRS technology to identify differences in cerebral oxygenation and fractional tissue oxygen extraction between the high and low groups during RBC transfusions, to determine whether abnormal cerebral NIRS measures are a better predictor of neurodevelopmental impairment than hemoglobin alone. As the technology improves and becomes even better suited for ELBW infants (e.g., smaller leads), this may serve to provide the nonlaboratory evidence needed to manage transfusions.[44] In the meantime, instituting red cell sparing/enhancing strategies (shown in Table 44.6)[45] and implementing restrictive transfusion guidelines similar to those in ETTNO and TOP are reasonable approaches that will decrease transfusions and support more appropriate use of blood products in the NICU. The goal of limiting red cell donor exposure to zero or one donor for each ELBW infant is definitely achievable and a good start toward improving neonatal transfusion stewardship.

Table 44.6 Measures to Decrease Red Cell Loss and Enhance Red Cell Mass in Extremely Low Birth Weight Infants
• Perform delayed cord clamping
• Obtain initial labs from the umbilical cord
• Initiate treatment with erythropoietin (Epo) or darbepoetin (Darbe) during the first day of life; administer a subcutaneous injection of 400 units/kg Epo, 10 mcg/kg Darbe, or add 200 units/kg Epo into a protein containing intravenous (IV) solution (such as a 10% dextrose solution with 2%–4% amino acids, or TPN), to run over 4–24 hours
• Administer parenteral iron (iron dextran or iron sucrose), 3–5 mg/kg once a week or 0.5–1 mg/kg/day (added to TPN or administered separately) until the infant is tolerating adequate volume feedings, then administer oral iron at 6 mg/kg/day; monitor reticulocyte hemoglobin to adjust iron supplementation
• Remove central lines
• Order labs judiciously (for example, avoid "blood gas q 6 hours" orders), and reconsider the need for screening or routine labs
• Use restrictive transfusion guidelines

TPN, Total parenteral nutrition.

Data from Ohls RK. Transfusion thresholds in the neonatal intensive care unit: what have recent randomized controlled trials taught us? In: Ohls RK, Yoder MC, eds. *Neonatology Questions and Controversies: Hematology, Immunology and Genetics.* 3rd ed. Elsevier; 2019:31–42.

CHAPTER 45

Neonatal Thrombocytopenia

Akhil Maheshwari

KEY POINTS

1. Platelets are anuclear cellular fragments that are released from megakaryocytes and are involved in primary hemostasis.
2. The normal platelet counts in newborn infants have been traditionally defined as 150 to 450 × 10^9/L. These counts decline during the early neonatal period but then begin to rise toward the end of the first week.
3. Platelet production involves the production of thrombopoietic factors such as thrombopoietin (TPO); expansion and differentiation of megakaryocyte progenitors; and production and release of platelets.
4. The safe levels of blood platelet counts in neonates are still unclear. In neonates, spontaneous bleeding from thrombocytopenia does not occur when platelet counts are >100 × 10^9/L. The risk may not be much higher even at 50 × 10^9/L and may increase only <20 × 10^9/L.
5. Thrombocytopenia is seen frequently in neonates and can occur due to a large variety of causes. Some causes are potentially more dangerous than others. These patients need to be carefully evaluated.
6. The best protocols for clinical management and platelet transfusions are a subject of ongoing debate.

Platelets are anuclear cellular fragments that are released from megakaryocytes and are involved in primary hemostasis.[1] The megakaryocyte progenitor cells differentiate under the stimulus of thrombopoietin (TPO), and once mature, generate and release platelets into the bloodstream.[2] Circulating platelets have a half-life of 7 to 10 days.[3] During primary hemostasis, the activated platelets change shape and aggregate with damaged red cells and leukocytes to seal the damaged capillary walls or completely plug the leaking vessels.[4] In secondary hemostasis, these clots get strengthened with fibrin and other products released from the coagulation cascade.[4]

Platelet Counts in Newborn Infants

The normal platelet counts in newborns and infants have been traditionally defined as 150 to 450 × 10^9/L.[5] Platelet counts decline over the first few days after birth but then begin to rise toward the end of the first week (Fig. 45.1). However, these definitions may need to be redefined with increasing survival of premature infants. Wiedmeier et al.[6] studied the platelet counts in 47,000 infants delivered between 22 and 42 weeks' gestation and showed that the mean platelet count at birth was >200 × 10^6/μL even in the most preterm infants. However, platelet counts in the 100 to 149 × 10^9/L range were not uncommon. The 5th percentile was 104 × 10^6/μL for those born at <32 weeks' gestation and 123 × 10^6/μL for late-preterm and term neonates. The platelet counts at birth increased with advancing gestational age, by approximately 2 × 10^6/μL for each week of gestation.

The true prevalence of thrombocytopenia in asymptomatic newborns is unknown. Thrombocytopenia in neonates (as in adults) has been traditionally defined as a platelet count <150 × 10^9/L, and classified as mild (100–150 × 10^9/L), moderate (50–99 × 10^9/L), and severe (<50 × 10^9/L).[7] Based on these definitions, large studies in unselected populations estimated an overall incidence of neonatal thrombocytopenia of 0.7% to 0.9%.[8] Another study of 5632 unselected newborns found platelets below 150 × 10^3/μL in approximately 1% of all neonates[9]; about one-third were term infants born after uncomplicated pregnancies and deliveries with no known maternal factors or unusual physical findings. However, the incidence was much higher in infants admitted to the neonatal intensive care unit (NICU), ranging from 18% to 35%. The incidence of thrombocytopenia is inversely correlated to the gestational age so that the most immature neonates are the most frequently affected: platelet counts less than 150 × 10^9/L were found at least once during the hospital stay in 70% of extremely low birth weight infants.[10]

Thrombocytosis is classified as mild (platelet counts 500–700 × 10^6/μL), moderate (700–900 × 10^6/μL), severe (900–1000 × 10^6/μL), and extreme (>1000 × 10^6/μL).[11] Primary thrombocytosis, a myeloproliferative disorder, is caused by monoclonal or polyclonal abnormalities of hematopoietic cells or by abnormalities in TPO biology. It is extremely rare in children and the frequency may be about 1 in 10 million. Secondary or reactive thrombocytosis is not uncommon in young infants. In a recent study, the 95th percentile upper reference range was 750 × 10^6/μL over the first 90 days of life.[6] The most common causes of reactive thrombocytosis in neonates and children are infections, tissue damage (surgeries, trauma, burns), and anemia (frequently iron deficiency). Reactive thrombocytosis has also been described in association with medications such as corticosteroids, maternal exposure to methadone or psychopharmaceutical drugs, and metabolic diseases, myopathies, or neurofibromatosis.[12]

Fetal and Neonatal Platelet Production

Platelet production involves four steps: (1) production of thrombopoietic factors such as TPO, (2) expansion of megakaryocyte progenitors, (3) differentiation of megakaryocytes through a unique endomitotic process, and (4) production and release of platelets.[1] TPO stimulates expansion of hematopoietic stem cells and downstream progenitor cells and promotes megakaryocyte differentiation and platelet production.[13] It is produced mainly in the liver but also

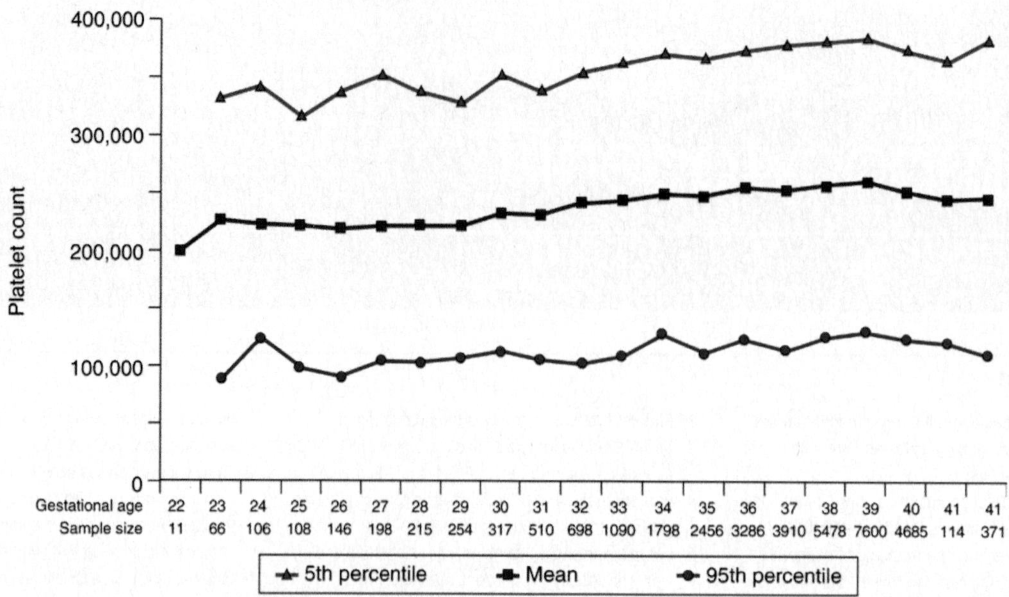

Fig. 45.1 Platelet Counts in Neonates According to Gestational Age. Reference ranges for platelet counts during the first 90 days after birth. *Middle lines* represent the mean value whereas the *lower* and *upper lines* represent the 5th and 95th percentiles. (Republished with permission from Christensen RD, Henry E, Jopling J, et al. The CBC: reference ranges for neonates. *Semin Perinatol*. 2009;33:3–11. Reproduced with permission and minor modifications from Sola-Visner and Davenport. Developmental megakaryopoiesis. *Fetal and Neonatal Physiology*, 110, 1125–1144.e6.)

in the kidney, smooth muscle, and marrow cells. Neonates have higher plasma TPO concentrations than adults. Stem cell factor, interleukin (IL)-3, IL-11, IL-6, and erythropoietin also stimulate megakaryopoiesis and thrombopoiesis.[14]

Megakaryocyte progenitors include the *burst-forming unit–megakaryocytes* (BFU-MKs) and the more mature *colony-forming unit–megakaryocytes* (CFU-MKs).[15] BFU-MKs produce large multifocal colonies containing ≥50 megakaryocytes. The CFU-MKs generate smaller (3–50 cells/colony) unifocal colonies. Megakaryocytes show typical morphologic features during endoreduplication, with large cells containing polyploid nuclei.[16] Unlike megakaryocyte progenitors, mature megakaryocytes do not generate colonies but differentiate from small mononuclear cells to large polyploid cells. Fetal/neonatal and adult megakaryocytes show important differences in morphology and biology and in the modal ploidy (the number of sets of complete chromosomes; Table 45.1).[17] Fetal/neonatal megakaryocytes are smaller in size, have lower ploidy levels, produce fewer platelets, but proliferate at higher rates. These low-ploidy but mature megakaryocytes can rapidly populate the rapidly expanding bone marrow space and blood volume in the fetus/neonate to maintain normal platelet counts. However, the reserve capacity for platelet production is lower, and neonates rapidly become thrombocytopenic during stress.

The sequence of events in platelet release from megakaryocytes is not well known. Mature megakaryocytes may migrate to a perivascular site and extend a process through the endothelium, giving rise to proplatelets, which then release platelets (Fig. 45.2).[17] An alternate mechanism may be the release of platelets in the lungs due to shear forces.

On a stained blood smear, platelets appear as dark purple spots, about 20% the diameter of red blood cells. The smear is used to examine platelets for size, shape, qualitative number, and clumping. Normal, resting platelets are disc-shaped but develop numerous long pseudopodia upon activation. These processes are important for the formation of hemostatic plugs (Fig. 45.3). Platelets contain four major types of granules, namely α-granules, dense bodies, lysosomes, and the more recently described T-granules. The constituents of each are summarized in Fig. 45.4.

Platelet Function and Primary Hemostasis

In neonates, spontaneous bleeding from thrombocytopenia does not occur when platelet counts are $>100 \times 10^9$/L. The risk may not be much higher even at 50×10^9/L and may increase only $<20 \times 10^9$/L.[18] The risk of bleeding in newborn infants may be related more to trauma sustained during the birthing process than to the platelet counts. The most feared bleeding complication is intracranial hemorrhage (ICH), due to the associated risk of adverse neurologic outcomes and mortality.

Neonatal platelets seem to be less responsive than those from adults to most agonists in terms of adhesion, aggregation, and activation.[19] This hyporeactivity is more pronounced in preterm infants. These studies have been performed with a variety of stimulants including adenosine diphosphate (ADP), epinephrine, collagen, thrombin, and thromboxane analogs (Fig. 45.5). The postulated mechanisms of this hyporeactivity include (1) fewer α_2-adrenergic

Table 45.1 Characteristics of Fetal and Adult Megakaryocytes

Parameter	Fetal/Neonatal Megakaryocytes	Adult Megakaryocytes
Size	Smaller	Larger
Polyploidy	Less polyploid (2–4N)	More polyploid (up to 16N)
Proliferation	Hyperproliferative in ex vivo culture	Less proliferative in ex vivo culture
Maturation	Express maturation markers	Express maturation markers
Proplatelet formation	Form fewer proplatelets	Form more proplatelets

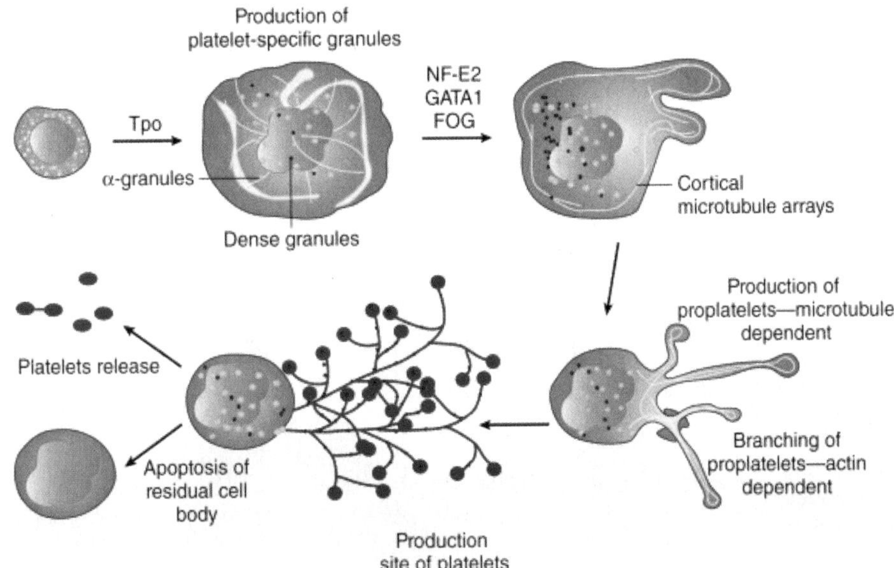

Fig. 45.2 Platelet Formation. Thrombopoietin promotes the maturation of hematopoietic stem cells into megakaryocytes by promoting the maturation of specific DNA and synthesis of platelet-specific proteins. Platelet production begins when microtubules aggregate in the cell cortex and one pole of the megakaryocyte spontaneously elaborates pseudopodia. Early pseudopodia are larger and then gradually thin out and branch into proplatelets. Platelets are assembled primarily at the ends of these proplatelets. Intracellular organelles are delivered to the platelet buds along microtubule tracks. Platelets are released from the ends of proplatelets. *FOG,* Friend of *GATA1*; *GATA1,* GATA binding protein 1; *TPO,* thrombopoietin. (Reproduced with permission and minor modifications from Italiano and Hartwig. Megakaryocyte and platelet structure. *Hematology: Basic Principles and Practice*, chap 124, 1857–1869.)

receptors, (2) impaired calcium mobilization after exposure to collagen, (3) decreased thromboxane-induced signaling, and (4) lower expression of protease-activated receptor 1.[20]

Despite these differences in responsiveness to canonical agonists, healthy full-term neonates have similar/enhanced primary hemostasis compared with adults. Bleeding times in healthy term neonates are shorter than those in adults.[21] Similarly, in in-vitro platelet function studies using Platelet Function Assay (PFA)–100, which measures the closure time taken to occlude a small aperture, the time is shorter in term neonates than samples from older children or adults.[22] This enhanced platelet/vessel wall interaction in neonates may be related to their higher hematocrits, higher mean corpuscular volumes, and higher concentrations of von Willebrand factor, all of which compensate for the hyporeactivity of neonatal platelets. Platelets from preterm infants seem less reactive than those from full-term infants, leading to longer bleeding times.[21] However, even these bleeding times were near or within the normal range for adults.

Evaluation of Neonatal Thrombocytopenia

When evaluating a thrombocytopenic neonate, the most frequent causes are listed by premature and full-term neonates by the postnatal age (Table 45.2). Infection/sepsis should always be considered

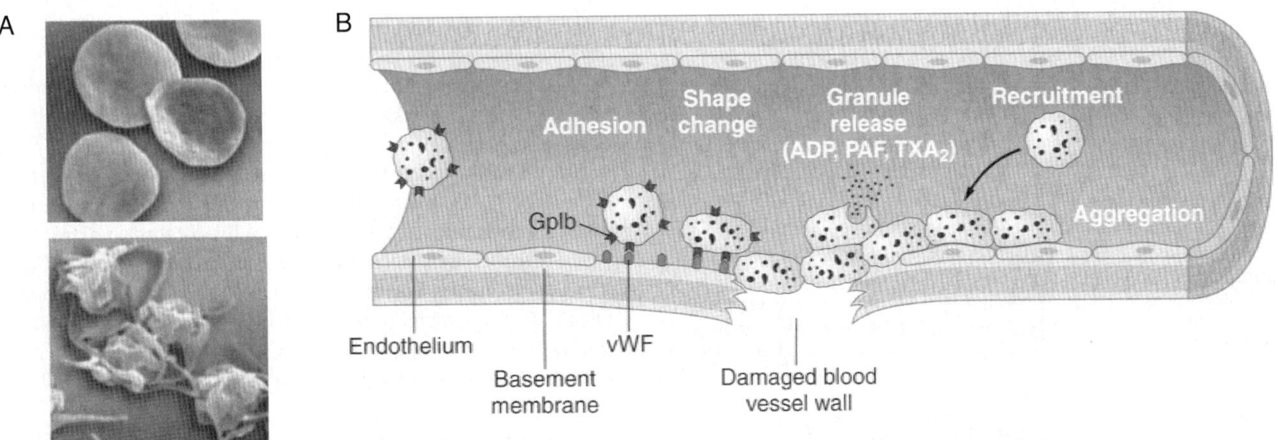

Fig. 45.3 (A) Scanning electron micrographs show platelets *(top)* with normal disc shape at rest and *(bottom)* activated morphology with numerous long pseudopodia. This morphologic change is critical for adhesion and the formation of plugs needed for hemostasis. (B) Formation of a platelet plug in a severed blood vessel. Endothelial injury and exposure of the vascular extracellular matrix facilitate platelet adhesions and activation, which change their shape and cause release of adenosine diphosphate (ADP), thromboxane A_2 (T_xA_2), and platelet-activating factor (PAF). These platelet-secreted factors recruit additional platelets (aggregation) to form a hemostatic plug. Von Willebrand factor (vWF) serves as an adhesion bridge between subendothelial collagen and the glycoprotein Ib (GpIb) platelet receptor. (A. Reproduced with permission and minor modifications from Kannan et al. Platelet activation markers in evaluation of thrombotic risk factors in various clinical settings. *Blood Reviews*. 2019;37:100583. B, Hall and Hall. Hemostasis and blood coagulation. *Guyton and Hall Textbook of Medical Physiology*, chap 37, 477–488.)

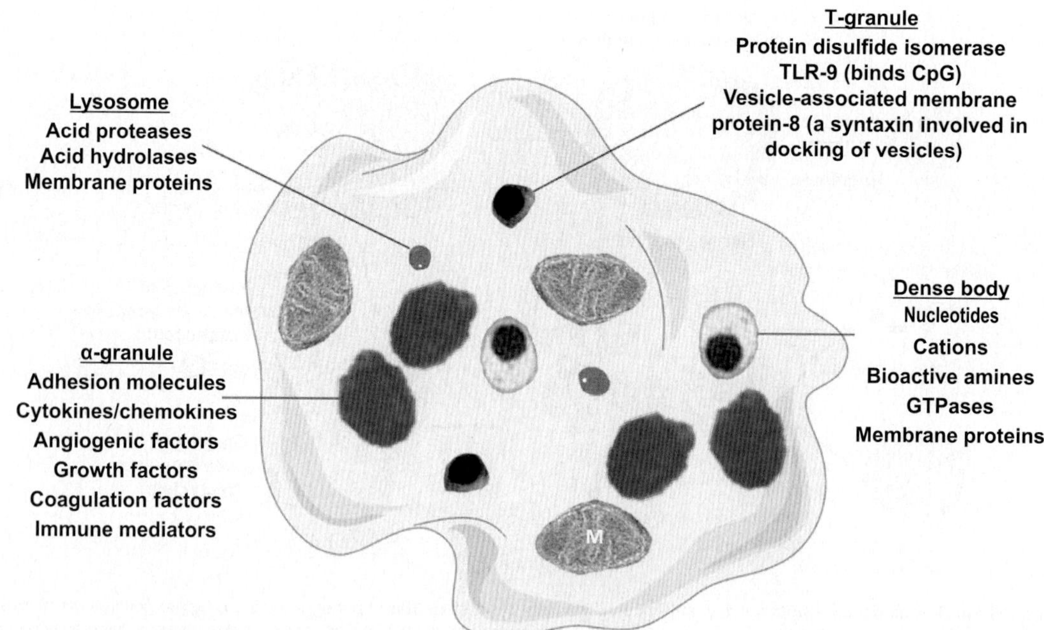

Fig. 45.4 Platelets Contain Four Major Types of Granules. The figure shows the constituents of each type. Mitochondria are labeled *M*.

(regardless of the time of presentation and the infant's appearance), because any delay in diagnosis and treatment can have life-threatening consequences.

The differential diagnosis for thrombocytopenia has been classically divided into disorders of decreased platelet production versus increased platelet consumption. However, emerging information shows that most disorders might actually be a mixture of the two mechanisms; causes that were traditionally identified to involve peripheral destruction of the platelets may actually involve the bone marrow progenitors in many cases and may also show an element of decreased megakaryopoiesis and thrombopoiesis in the bone marrow.

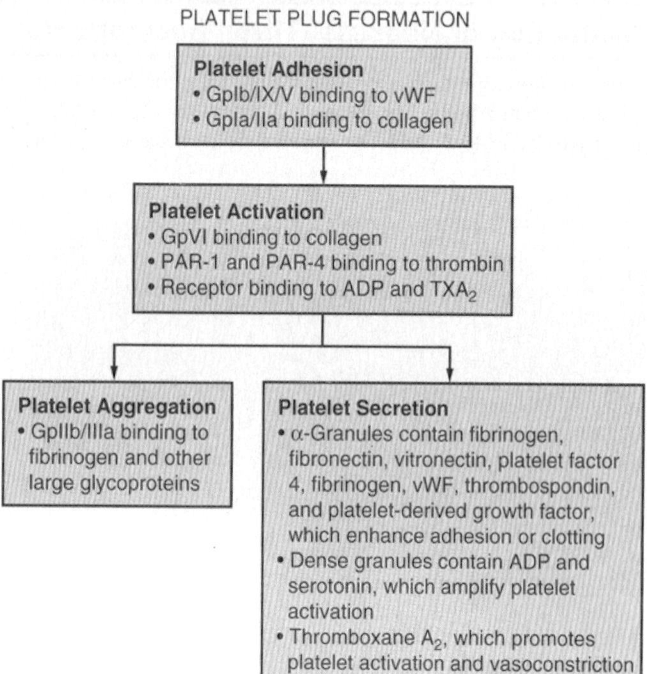

Fig. 45.5 Schematic Review of Platelet Function. *ADP,* Adenosine diphosphate; *Gp,* glycoprotein; *PAR,* protease-activated receptor; *TXA*$_2$, thromboxane A$_2$; *vWF,* von Willebrand factor. (Reproduced with permission and minor modifications from Rodger and Silver. Coagulation disorders in pregnancy. *Creasy and Resnik's Maternal-Fetal Medicine: Principles and Practice*, 53, 949–976.e8.)

Any report of platelet counts below $150 \times 10^3/\mu L$ should be confirmed with a repeat test, preferably with a blood sample obtained by venipuncture and then evaluated (Fig. 45.6). A thorough physical examination should be done to identify any cutaneous or oral petechiae or purpura. In ill infants, sepsis and disseminated intravascular coagulation are important causes of thrombocytopenia. Premature very low birth weight infants and those with gram-negative infections are also very likely to have low platelet counts. TORCH (toxoplasmosis, other agents, rubella, cytomegalovirus (CMV), or herpes simplex) infections may present with a whole range, mild to severe, of multisystem illness. In these infants, thrombocytopenia may be caused by bone marrow suppression and/or peripheral destruction. Signs of TORCH infections such as microcephaly, hepatosplenomegaly, or cutaneous "blueberry muffin" rash should be noted (Fig. 45.7). Necrotizing enterocolitis (NEC) can also cause thrombocytopenia very early in the clinical course of the disease. Critically ill infants with multisystem organ failure from any cause can develop thrombocytopenia due to destruction of platelets in various end organs such as the lung, even if they do not show laboratory evidence of diffuse intravascular coagulation. Finally, infants on extracorporeal support for oxygenation or renal replacement therapy can develop thrombocytopenia because of platelet consumption upon contact with the foreign membranes. Thrombocytopenia could appear as the initial presenting sign of sepsis, TORCH infection, or other serious condition while the baby still appears to be otherwise well.

Early Onset of Thrombocytopenia in Well-Appearing Infants

In an otherwise healthy-appearing infant, placental insufficiency may be the most likely cause of thrombocytopenia. These infants usually develop only mild to moderate thrombocytopenia ($50–150 \times 10^3/\mu L$) that resolves spontaneously within 7 to 10 days

Table 45.2 Causes of Neonatal Thrombocytopenia

Premature			**Full Term**	
Early Onset (<72 Hours)	**7–14 Days**	**>14 Days**	**Early Onset (<72 Hours)**	**Late Onset (>7 Days)**

• Placental insufficiency, pregnancy-induced hypertension, maternal diabetes
• Birth asphyxia
• Sepsis, DIC
• TORCH infections
• Chromosomal disorders
• Polycythemia
• Inherited thrombocytopenias
	• Sepsis, DIC
	• Thrombosis
	• Spontaneous intestinal perforation
	• TORCH infections
	• Fanconi anemia
	• Viral infections
	• Blood clots (such as with catheters)
		• Sepsis, DIC
		• Thrombosis
		• NEC
		• Drug-induced
		• Inborn errors of metabolism
		• Viral infections
		• Blood clots (such as with catheters)
			• Placental insufficiency
			• Birth asphyxia
			• Sepsis, DIC, NEC
			• Neonatal alloimmune thrombocytopenia
			• Autoimmune thrombocytopenia
			• TORCH infections
			• Inherited syndromes
			  • Bernard-Soulier
			  • Wiskott-Aldrich
			  • Thrombocytopenia absent radii
			  • Others
			  • Vascular tumors
			  • Kasabach-Merritt
			• Chromosomal disorders
			• Polycythemia
			• Congenital anomalies
				• Occult infection
				• Blood clots (such as with catheters)
				• TORCH infections
				• Inborn errors of metabolism
				• Fanconi anemia
				• NEC in infants with congenital cardiac defects (postoperative)
				• Viral infections

DIC, Diffuse intravascular coagulation; *NAIT,* neonatal alloimmune thrombocytopenia; *NEC,* necrotizing enterocolitis; *TORCH,* toxoplasmosis, other agents, rubella, cytomegalovirus, or herpes simplex.

after birth. This diagnosis should be considered in small-for-gestational-age infants with a history of intrauterine growth restriction or maternal hypertension, diabetes, or preeclampsia.

Well-appearing infants can show extremely low platelet counts due to immune-mediated neonatal alloimmune thrombocytopenia (NAIT)[23–28] or autoimmune platelet destruction,[23] in which maternal antibodies passed to the newborn in-utero lead to destruction of the baby's platelets. Of these, NAIT produces the most pronounced thrombocytopenia, with platelets typically $<50 \times 10^9$/L. It occurs when the fetus inherits a paternal platelet antigen not carried by the mother; this antigen then becomes a target for maternal antibodies (Fig. 45.8). Maternal platelets are not targeted and remain within normal range. NAIT affects an estimated 1 in 800 to 1000 live births. The true incidence may be higher, because milder cases might go undetected and the severe cases lead to intrauterine death.

Unlike Rh-incompatibility, NAIT frequently causes disease in a woman's first pregnancy. The severe thrombocytopenia caused by NAIT carries a significant risk of potential morbidity and mortality.

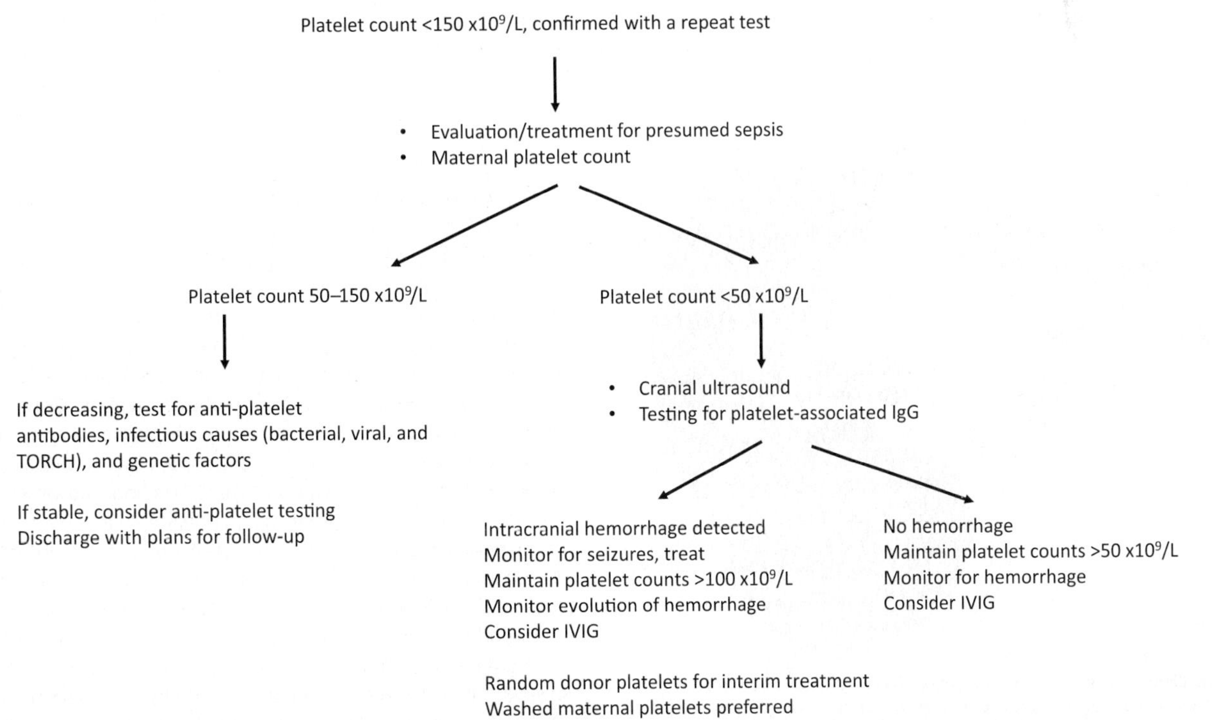

Fig. 45.6 Evaluation of Thrombocytopenia in Newborn Infants. *IVIG,* Intravenous immune globulin.

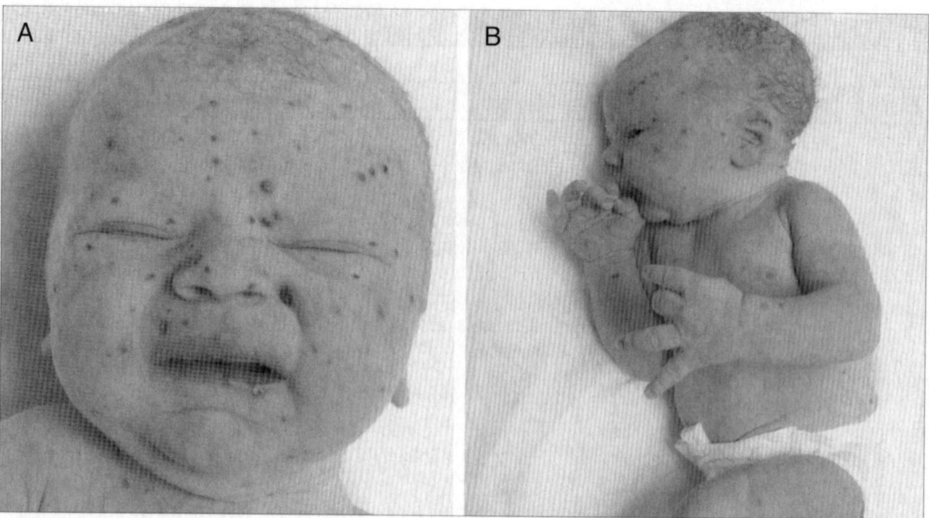

Fig. 45.7 Blueberry Muffin Rash in a Neonate. Multiple firm, nonblanching, purple papules affecting (A) the head and neck and (B) the body. (Reproduced with permission and minor modifications from Schmitt et al. Langerhans cell histiocytosis presenting as a blueberry muffin rash. *Lancet*. 2017;390:155.)

Intrauterine death or ICH may occur as early as at 14 to 16 weeks' gestation, resulting in a relatively high incidence of intrauterine ICH (>10%). Approximately 10% to 30% of newborns with NAIT will develop ICH, with about half already having developed it in utero; neurologic sequelae and death will occur in 20% and 10% of affected neonates, respectively.[6]

Immune thrombocytopenia occurs because of the passive transfer of antibodies from the maternal to the fetal circulation. There are two distinct types of immune-mediated thrombocytopenia: (1) NAIT and (2) autoimmune thrombocytopenia. In NAIT, the antibody is produced in the mother against a specific human platelet antigen (HPA) present in the fetus but absent in the mother. The antigen is inherited from the father of the fetus. The anti-HPA antibody produced in the maternal serum crosses the placenta and reaches the fetal circulation, leading to platelet destruction and apoptosis of megakaryocyte progenitors with decreased platelet production. The antigens responsible for NAIT are results of single-nucleotide polymorphisms in genes encoding any the major glycoproteins located on the platelet surface, particularly glycoprotein (GP)IIb/IIIa. The platelet antigens are named using an HPA nomenclature; antigens are numbered chronologically, according to the date of their initial report. The biallelic antigens were given an alphabetic designation of "a" or "b" in the order of their frequency (higher frequency for "a").[29–33] Sixteen HPA antigens have been identified so far. The frequency of each varies within ethnic groups: in the White population, antibodies to HPA-1a are the major cause of NAIT, followed by HPA-5a and, less frequently, HPA-9b, HPA-3a and HPA-3b, and HPA-15. Antibodies to HPA-4b are the predominant cause of NAIT in the Japanese population.

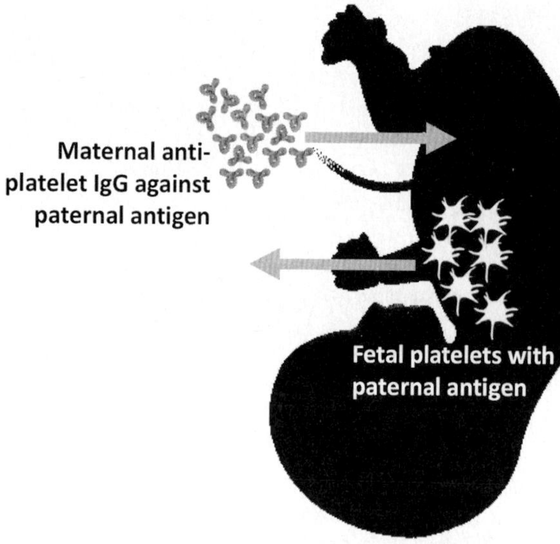

Fig. 45.8 Neonatal Alloimmune Thrombocytopenia. When fetal platelets with a paternally derived antigen cross over into the maternal circulation, the generation and transplacental passage of reactive IgG antibodies may cause thrombocytopenia in the fetus.

The diagnosis of NAIT should be considered in infants with platelet counts below 50 × 10³/μL. An infant suspected to have NAIT should be examined with a head ultrasound for ICH and followed up for any progression. In addition, the combination of severe neonatal thrombocytopenia with a parenchymal (rather than intraventricular) ICH is highly suggestive of NAIT.

If blood cannot be collected from the parents in a timely fashion, neonatal serum may be screened for the antiplatelet antibodies.[28] However, low antibody concentrations in the neonate, coupled with binding of the antibodies to the infant's platelets, can result in false-negative results. It is still unclear if there is any correlation between the affinity of the antibodies and the severity of disease.

If there is clinical suspicion for NAIT, testing for antiplatelet antibodies should be performed on the infant and/or the mother. The definitive diagnosis of NAIT involves two steps: (1) genotyping studies to identify the HPA carried by the neonate but not by the mother and (2) identification of corresponding maternal anti-HPA antibodies in the newborn by enzyme-linked immunosorbent assay.[34] If positive, both parents as well as the neonate can be genotyped for the five most frequently identified HPA types involved with NAIT. These tests can help in reproductive planning for these families, because if the fetus carries the incompatible antigen, there is a 90% likelihood of recurrence in subsequent pregnancies. Unfortunately, >80% of neonatal thrombocytopenia believed clinically to be caused by NAIT lacks demonstrable HPA incompatibility, and the information on the patterns of HPA incompatibility in non-White populations is limited.[2]

Thrombocytopenia secondary to NAIT resolves gradually because the causative maternal antibodies may take 8 to 12 weeks to be cleared.[34,35] These infants require close monitoring for hemorrhages during this period and also for developmental milestones for at least 18 months. Families of children affected by NAIT should be encouraged to receive reproductive counseling and future obstetric care at specialty centers.[27,36]

Autoimmune thrombocytopenia typically causes mild to moderate thrombocytopenia, due to maternal autoantibodies that target both maternal and fetal platelets.[23] Maternal platelet counts are expected to be low, but because the mother may carry several different types of antiplatelet immunoglobulins that may not all cross the placental barrier, the severity of her own and the neonate's thrombocytopenia may not correlate with each other. Hence, infants born to mothers with idiopathic thrombocytopenic purpura, systemic lupus erythematosus, or other autoimmune disorders should be screened for platelet counts at birth, regardless of maternal platelet count at delivery. Platelet levels eventually normalize at 2 to 8 weeks after birth as maternal autoantibodies get cleared from the baby's circulation.

In $<1\%$ of all instances, thrombocytopenia may occur as part of a genetic syndrome. These diagnoses are suspected more often in well-appearing term infants, although preterm or sicker infants are not at lower risk of these conditions. A localized skin lesion, discoloration, or palpated mass may represent a hemangioma of Kasabach-Merritt syndrome, which can consume platelets, and may also be informative.[37] Fanconi anemia and thrombocytopenia-absent-radii syndrome show upper extremity abnormalities.[38] Chromosomal abnormalities such as trisomies and Turner syndrome can be also be associated with thrombocytopenia.[39] Other genetic disorders, such as congenital amegakaryocytic thrombocytopenia (CAMT) with proximal radio-ulnar synostosis (ATRUS), can also present with thrombocytopenia.[40] If there is marked thrombocytopenia, a blood smear should be examined for abnormalities in platelet morphology, which may not be detected by automated platelet counting. Some genetic causes show abnormal platelet size, such as the small platelets in Wiskott-Aldrich syndrome (WAS) and X-linked thrombocytopenias.[41] Patients with conditions such as Bernard-Soulier syndrome or Jacobsen syndrome have large platelets (Fig. 45.9).[42]

Infants with WAS show microthrombocytopenia (platelet volume <7 μL) and later develop eczema and immunodeficiency. This is an X-linked disorder that affects 1 to 4 cases per million live male births. If clinically suspected, the diagnosis is typically made by flow cytometric assessment of WAS protein expression, followed by sequencing of the *WAS* gene. In later infancy, patients with WAS begin to show abnormalities in the humoral immune responses and may require intravenous immune globulin (IVIG) infusions.[5,41,43,44] IVIG reduces infections but does not affect platelet counts. Children with identified WAS should not receive live or attenuated vaccines but should receive all other routine immunizations at the usual schedule. All patients should also receive *Pneumocystis jirovecii* prophylaxis with trimethoprim-sulfamethoxazole or an equivalent agent.[45] Hematopoietic stem cell transplantation is currently the accepted curative treatment for WAS and preferably should be performed prior to the onset of significant infectious complications.[46]

Many inherited thrombocytopenias have characteristic abnormalities.[47,48] Most cases of Fanconi anemia develop thrombocytopenia later during childhood but may be recognized with thumb abnormalities and chromosomal fragility testing. If the infant has radial abnormalities with normal-appearing thumbs, thrombocytopenia-absent-radii syndrome should be considered. The platelet count is usually less than 50×10^9/L, and the white cell count is elevated in most patients, mimicking congenital leukemia. Infants who survive the first year of life generally do well with improvement in platelet counts to low–normal levels. The hematologic outcome of MYH-9-related disorders is good, although patients frequently develop nephritis, hearing loss, and cataracts later in life.

ATRUS should be considered if there is difficulty in rotating the forearm on physical examination. Radiologic examination shows proximal synostosis of the radius and ulna. Most cases with ATRUS show mutations in the *Hox-A11* gene and require bone marrow transplantation. Other genetic disorders associated with early-onset thrombocytopenia include trisomy 21, trisomy 18, trisomy 13, Turner syndrome, Noonan syndrome, and Jacobsen syndrome. Cases of Noonan syndrome presenting with mild dysmorphic features and very severe neonatal thrombocytopenia mimicking CAMT have been described, so genetic testing should be performed in children who present with a CAMT-like picture and no mutations in the *C-Mpl* gene.

Nonsyndromic cases of congenital thrombocytopenia often have a positive family history. These conditions belong to a heterogeneous group of diseases. Often the size of the platelets helps in the differential diagnosis. May-Hegglin anomaly, Fechtner syndrome, and Sebastian syndrome present with macrothrombocytopenia. Other congenital thrombocytopenias presenting with large platelets include Bernard-Soulier syndrome and X-linked macrothrombocytopenia. CAMT presents with normal-sized platelets and may be confused with NAIT in the newborn period. These infants often develop bone marrow failure and pancytopenia and require bone marrow transplant. The outcome of patients with congenital thrombocytopenia is variable and depends on the specific disorders.

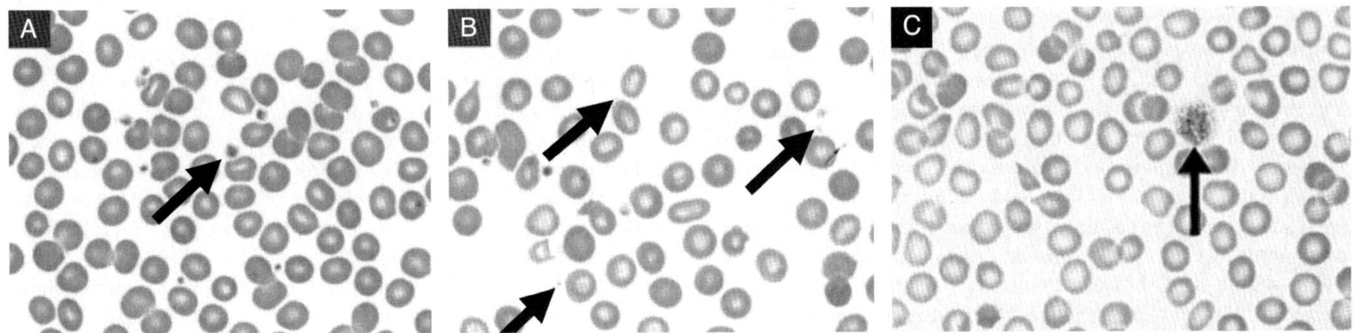

Fig. 45.9 Peripheral blood smears show *arrows* marking (A) normal, (B) microplatelets (such as in Wiskott-Aldrich syndrome), and (C) giant platelets (seen in Bernard-Soulier syndrome). (Panels A and B reproduced with permission and minor modifications from Sillers et al. Neonatal thrombocytopenia: etiology and diagnosis. *Pediatr Ann.* 2015;44[7]:e175–e180. Panel C reproduced with permission and minor modifications from Bain BJ. The peripheral blood smear. In: *Goldman-Cecil Medicine*, 148, 1020–1027.e2.)

Delayed Onset of Thrombocytopenia

Infants who develop thrombocytopenia after 72 hours of life need to be evaluated and observed for sepsis (bacterial or fungal). Full-term infants and those with congenital cardiac defects can also develop NEC. Thrombocytopenia can be the first presenting sign of these conditions.[49] Appropriate management with antibiotics, supportive respiratory and cardiovascular care, and medical/surgical treatment of NEC may be needed. In some infants the thrombocytopenia persists for several weeks. The reasons underlying this prolonged thrombocytopenia are unclear.

In some infants, viral infections such as herpes simplex virus, cytomegalovirus (CMV), or enterovirus should be considered.[50] These viral infections are frequently accompanied by abnormal liver enzymes. If the infant has or has recently had a central venous or arterial catheter, thromboses should be part of the differential diagnosis, although they only cause thrombocytopenia if the thrombus is enlarging or is infected.[51] Drug-induced thrombocytopenia is considered in some centers,[52] although we have not found this to be a major cause in our practice.

Management

Most clinicians evaluate infants with thrombocytopenia and treat them with antibiotics for 48 hours until sepsis can be excluded with negative cultures. In the absence of compelling physical findings, management of thrombocytopenia depends on the severity of the platelet count and clinical signs of bleeding (see Fig. 45.2). In newly born premature or critically ill infants, the traditional threshold for platelet transfusions has been for counts $<100 \times 10^3/\mu L$ for the first 72 hours and then is carefully lowered to $50 \times 10^9/L$. These thresholds have been chosen to counter the risk of serious ICHs. Most clinicians typically administer 10 to 15 mL/kg of a standard platelet suspension, either a platelet concentrate ("random-donor platelets") or apheresis platelets. Each random-donor platelet unit has approximately 50 mL of volume and contains approximately 10×10^9 platelets per 10 mL.

Neonatologists, particularly in the United States, have been relatively liberal in platelet transfusions, with many clinicians using prophylactic transfusions at levels above $50 \times 10^9/L$.[53] There is no clear association between thrombocytopenia and bleeding in neonates, but clinicians continue to use higher thresholds in nonbleeding preterm infants to reduce the risk of bleeding in an at-risk population, presumably to reduce clinical and medicolegal liability in the event of a bleed.[54,55]

A randomized controlled trial (1993) and a few retrospective cohort analyses showed that higher thresholds for prophylactic platelet transfusions in preterm infants did not reduce the risk of intraventricular hemorrhage (IVH) ($>150 \times 10^9/L$ versus $>50 \times 10^9/L$).[55] Kenton et al. showed that platelet transfusions did not lower the mortality or morbidity (short bowel syndrome or cholestasis) in neonates with NEC.[56] In 2007, Baer et al.[57] reviewed 1600 thrombocytopenic NICU patients and found that infants who had received platelet transfusions at any threshold had higher mortality. Sensitivity analyses suggested that transfusions were likely responsible for some of this harm.[57] Further analysis of infants with platelet counts $<50 \times 10^9/L$ showed that mortality and IVHs were predicted not by the lowest platelet counts but by the number of platelet transfusions.[10]

A 2014 structured review did not show clear evidence; the authors concluded that for critically ill preterm neonates with severe thrombocytopenia but no evidence of bleeding, the evidence for transfusions was insufficient. In 2019 Fustolo-Gunnink et al.[55] reviewed 30 studies assessing platelet count and bleeding. There were major methodological limitations in the assessment of data. Four studies showed clear temporal relationships between thrombocytopenia and bleeding; two suggested that thrombocytopenia was associated with pulmonary hemorrhage and two others suggested that low platelet counts were associated with pulmonary hemorrhage but not with bleeding at other sites. None of the studies showed platelet transfusion to reduce the risk of bleeding.

The PlaNeT-2/MATISSE study was the first randomized trial of platelet transfusion thresholds in current use to prevent bleeding in neonates.[55,58,59] There were 660 infants recruited with a median gestational age of 26.6 weeks in the United Kingdom, Ireland, and the Netherlands. The primary outcome was a composite of death or major bleeding, quantified with the use of a validated neonatal bleeding assessment tool. The study demonstrated that infants who received prophylactic platelet transfusions at a threshold of $<50 \times 10^9/L$ had a worse composite outcome of death and/or major bleeding within 28 days of randomization than those who were transfused at a threshold of $<25 \times 10^9/L$ (26% versus 19%; odds ratio [OR], 1.57; 95% confidence interval [CI], 1.06–2.32). The risk of chronic lung disease was also higher in infants transfused at the higher threshold (63% versus 54%; OR, 1.57; 95% CI, 1.06–2.32). As preterm babies often have significant acute and chronic inflammatory lung disease related to immature lung structure, platelet-derived inflammatory mediators could have contributed to lung injury. There was no difference in NEC or sepsis. A total of 146 neonates died or developed major bleeding. The internally validated C-statistic of the model was 0.63 (95% CI, 0.58–0.68). The $25 \times 10^9/L$ threshold was associated with absolute-risk reduction in all risk groups, varying from 4.9% in the lowest risk group to 12.3% in the highest risk group. These results suggest that a $25 \times 10^9/L$ prophylactic platelet count threshold can be adopted in all preterm neonates, irrespective of predicted baseline outcome risk.

In 2019, Kumar et al.[60] published their study in which they randomized preterm thrombocytopenic neonates to be transfused at platelet counts $<20 \times 10^9/L$ versus $<100 \times 10^9/L$. The primary outcome of interest was closure of patent ductus arteriosus. One limitation of the study was that the trial used platelet volumes more than routine practice; infants with platelet counts $<50 \times 10^9/L$ were given ≥ 40 mL/kg of platelets. Interestingly, the rate of intraventricular hemorrhage (IVH) was higher in the liberally transfused group: 41% of infants had any grade of IVH in the liberal transfusion group compared with 4.5% in the restrictive group. They noted a 4.3% increase in IVH for every extra 1 mL/kg volume of platelets transfused. The incidental finding of increased IVH may indicate that a hemodynamic cause for increased IVH is more likely in the setting of high or rapid volumes of transfusion. The trial included babies with early thrombocytopenia (37%), which was defined as <5 days for the purpose of the study, and late thrombocytopenia (63%). Early thrombocytopenia is often associated with placental insufficiency and in utero growth restriction.[58] It tends to be self-resolving, and values normalize by 7 to 10 days after birth on average. Despite its more "benign" nature, neonatologists often transfuse babies with early thrombocytopenia in an attempt to "prevent" IVH, because 95% of IVH occurs in the first 72 hours of life.[58,61,62] Late thrombocytopenia is typically related to NEC or sepsis, and platelets show increased rates of consumption. Although neonatologists would probably argue against exclusion of either cohort, it did lead to a heterogeneous group of infants, and with only 37% of babies showing early thrombocytopenia, this study may not be sufficient to deter early platelet transfusion in this group.[58]

Are Prophylactic Platelet Transfusions Justified?

The need for platelet transfusions in nonbleeding preterm infants needs evaluation. The PlaNeT-2/MATISSE study showed the lower threshold was less harmful but did not establish a safe threshold for platelet transfusion.[61] Adult trials have evaluated lower thresholds than those applied in the PlaNeT-2/MATISSE study, but the results cannot be easily extended to infants because of the developmental differences.[61] Future neonatal trials might consider transfusion thresholds similar to those studied in older children and adults. There are potentially significant barriers; the neonatal community may not be ready for a threshold trial at those levels and it would be difficult to recruit an adequate sample size given the infrequency of platelets $<10 \times 10^9$/L. Likelihood of protocol violation would also be a significant barrier to completion of a study of this nature.

Can Transfused Platelets Cause Inflammation?

Platelets contain inflammatory mediators and can release those following transfusions; there is clear biologic plausibility for harm.[63] Increased inflammation may explain the increase in mortality, bleeding, and lung disease demonstrated in PlaNeT-2/MATISSE, and lowering the dose in transfusions should be considered. Such inflammation and adverse complications may be more likely in premature infants. At the same time, platelets are important not only for hemostasis but also for innate immunity, inflammation, and angiogenesis. There is a need for focused studies, specifically in this population.

When making platelet transfusion decisions, it is important for neonatologists to be aware of the risks. The risk of bacterial contamination is high because platelet suspensions are stored in the blood bank at room temperature for up to 5 days, which increases the risk of bacterial growth. There is no need to pool more than one random-donor unit for a neonatal transfusion, a practice that may only increase donor exposures and activate platelets without any benefit. Other important considerations in neonatology are the prevention of transfusion-transmitted CMV infections and graft-versus-host disease. Most blood banks provide either CMV-negative or leuko-reduced products for neonates, both of which significantly reduce the risk of transfusion-transmitted CMV. Platelet transfusions can also induce transfusion-associated lung injury. Several studies also show an association between the number of platelet transfusions and the mortality rate. This association may simply reflect higher acuity of illness in these patients or may be an adverse effect of these transfusions.

Management of NAIT

The treatment of choice in NAIT is transfusion of processed maternal platelets based on the thresholds and clinical symptoms above.[24–26,36,64,65] In infants with known ICH, the targeted platelet counts should be 100×10^9/L, although this may be challenging in those with NAIT. Washing maternal platelets helps avoid adding more maternal alloantibodies to the newborn's circulation. Some patients respond to random donor platelet transfusions, and this could be used as a first line of therapy. If the patient is clinically stable and does not have an ICH, platelets are usually given when the platelet count is $<30 \times 10^9$/L. In preterm or critically ill infants, platelet transfusions can be given at platelet counts $<50 \times 10^9$/L during the first week after birth. In addition, IVIG (1 g/kg per day for 2 consecutive days) may be administered to increase the patient's own platelets and potentially to protect the transfused platelets. Because the platelet count usually decreases after birth in NAIT, IVIG may be given when the platelet count is between 30 and 50×10^9/L in a stable neonate to try to prevent a further drop.

Some infants with NAIT do not respond to random donor platelets and IVIG, and the blood bank should try to get antigen-negative platelets (either from HPA-1b1b and HPA-5a5a donors, which should be compatible in >90% of cases, or from the mother). If maternal platelets are used, these may need to be concentrated or washed to minimize the antiplatelet antibodies present in the mother's plasma.

When a neonate is born to a mother who had a previous pregnancy affected by confirmed NAIT, genotypically matched platelets (e.g., HPA-1b1b platelets) should be available in the blood bank at the time of delivery and should be the first-line treatment if the infant is thrombocytopenic.

Maternal Treatment

Mothers who have previously delivered an infant with NAIT should be followed in high-risk obstetric clinics during all future pregnancies because the reoccurrence rate is high. Fetal genetic testing should be performed. If available, noninvasive testing of cell-free DNA in maternal plasma can be reassuring. The intensity of prenatal treatment can be adjusted based on the severity of the thrombocytopenia and if there was a history of ICH in previous pregnancies. Current recommendations include maternal treatment with IVIG (0.5–2 g/kg per week) ± steroids (0.5–1 mg/kg per day prednisone), starting at 12 or at 20 to 26 weeks' gestation, depending on whether the previously affected fetus suffered an ICH during pregnancy. Most recent studies show the combination of IVIG and steroids to be effective. An elective cesarean section is recommended to avoid ICH.

Management of Autoimmune Thrombocytopenia

The diagnosis of neonatal autoimmune thrombocytopenia should be considered in any neonate who has early-onset thrombocytopenia and is born to a mother with a history of either immune thrombocytopenic purpura (ITP) or an autoimmune disease.[23] Studies show neonatal thrombocytopenia in 8% to 25%, with ICH occurring in 0% to 1.5%.[66] All neonates born to mothers who have autoimmune diseases should be tested with a platelet count at birth. If the platelet count is normal, no further evaluation is necessary. If the neonate has mild thrombocytopenia, another test should be repeated in 2 to 3 days. If the platelet count is less than 30×10^9/L, the baby should be treated with IVIG (1 g/kg, repeated if necessary). Random donor platelets, in addition to IVIG, should be provided if the neonate has evidence of active bleeding. Cranial imaging (cranial ultrasound) should be obtained in all infants with platelet counts less than 50×10^9/L to evaluate for ICH. Neonatal thrombocytopenia secondary to maternal ITP may last for weeks to months and requires long-term monitoring and sometimes a second dose of IVIG at 4 to 6 weeks of life. Antiplatelet antibodies (immunoglobulin A type) can be transferred through breastfeeding and can cause neonatal thrombocytopenia.[66]

Maternal Management

Fetal hemorrhage is rare even if the mother has severe ITP. Maternal steroid or IVIG therapy may not prevent thrombocytopenia in newborns. There is in no correlation between fetal platelet counts and maternal platelet counts, platelet antibody levels, or history of maternal splenectomy. The only reliable predictive measure of neonatal

Table 45.3 Defects in Platelet Structure and Function

Platelet Defect	Gene Defect/Chromosomal Location	Pathophysiology	Clinical and Laboratory Characteristics in Neonates	Bleeding Treatment
Platelet Structure				
Defects in Platelet Cytoskeleton				
Wiskott-Aldrich syndrome	X-linked WAS (Xp11.23–p11.22)	Loss/defective WAS protein with defective actin remodeling by actin-related protein 2/3 complex	Thrombocytopenia, small platelets Eczema Decreased intracellular WAS protein; WAS gene sequencing	Supportive care Platelet transfusion Antifibrinolytics
Actin-related protein 2/3 Complex subunit 1B (ARPC1B) deficiency	Autosomal recessive ARPC1B (7q22.1)	Loss of ARPC1B in hematopoietic cell Arp2/3 complex	Small platelets, inflammatory disease, recurrent infections, abnormal platelet function Gene sequencing	Supportive care Antifibrinolytics Platelet transfusion
Myosin heavy chain 9 (MYH9)–related disease	Autosomal dominant MYH9 (22q12–13) encoding nonmuscle myosin heavy chain IIA	Defective nonmuscle myosin IIA motor protein	Thrombocytopenia Large platelets Döhle-like inclusions and myosin IIA aggregates in neutrophils	Supportive care Platelet transfusion Antifibrinolytics THPO receptor agonists
Defects in Platelet α-Granules				
Gray platelet syndrome	Autosomal recessive Neurobeachin Like 2 (NBEAL2)	Altered α-granules	Progressive myelofibrosis Thrombocytopenia Large pale platelets with no α-granules NBEAL2 gene sequencing	Supportive care Antifibrinolytics Desmopressin Platelet transfusion Splenectomy
Arthrogryposis, renal dysfunction, and cholestasis syndrome	Autosomal dominant Vacuolar protein sorting-associated protein 33B (VPS33B), VPS33B Interacting Protein, Apical-Basolateral Polarity Regulator, Spe-39 Homolog (VIPAS39)	Abnormal intracellular vesicle trafficking and membrane fusion	Thrombocytopenia Large, pale platelets Absent α-granules VPS33B & VIPAS39 sequencing	Supportive care Platelet transfusion Antifibrinolytics
Quebec platelet disorder	Autosomal recessive Duplication of Plasminogen Activator, Urokinase (PLAU)	Increased expression urokinase plasminogen activator, gain of function defect	Delayed-onset bleeding not responding to platelet transfusion Variable thrombocytopenia Abnormal urokinase in platelets detected with immunoblot or ELISA PLAU duplication testing	Supportive care Antifibrinolytics
Paris-Trousseau/Jacobsen syndrome	Autosomal dominant Chromosome 11q23–24 deletion Hemizygous deletion of Fli-1 proto-oncogene, ETS transcription factor (FLI1)	Unknown	Thrombocytopenia Large platelets, giant α-granules Immature megakaryocytes Cognitive, cardiac, and facial abnormalities	Supportive care Antifibrinolytics Platelet transfusion
Defects in Platelet δ-Granules				
Chediak-Higashi syndrome	Autosomal recessive Lysosomal trafficking regulator (LYST)	Defective vesicular protein and membrane trafficking resulting in giant granules	Giant eosinophilic inclusions in neutrophils, Decreased δ-granules, decreased ATP release Hypopigmentation and immunodeficiency	Supportive care
Hermansky-Pudlak syndrome	Autosomal recessive Hermansky-Pudlak syndrome (HPS) 1–10, Adaptor-related protein complex 3 subunit beta 1 (AP3B1), dystrobrevin binding protein 1 (DTNBP1), biogenesis of lysosomal organelles complex 1 subunit 3 (BLOC1S3), BLOC1S6, and adaptor-related Protein complex 3 subunit delta 1 (AP3D1)	Defective intracellular biogenesis/trafficking of lysosome-related δ-granules and melanosomes	Decreased δ-granules Decreased ATP release Sequencing of 10 candidate genes Oculocutaneous albinism	Supportive care Antifibrinolytics Platelet transfusion DDAVP

Platelet Defect	Gene Defect/Chromosomal Location	Pathophysiology	Clinical and Laboratory Characteristics in Neonates	Bleeding Treatment
Platelet Function				
Defects in Platelet Activation				
Thromboxane-prostanoid receptor defects	Autosomal recessive Thromboxane A2 receptor (TBXA2R)	Abnormal response to thromboxane A2	Altered platelet aggregation TBXA2R gene sequencing	Supportive care
ADP receptor defects purinergic receptor P2Y12 (P2Y12)	Autosomal recessive P2RY12	Abnormal response to ADP, de-aggregation with high dose ADP	Altered platelet aggregation P2RY12 gene sequencing	Supportive care
Collagen receptor defects	Autosomal recessive Glycoprotein VI platelet (GP6)	Impaired response to collagen	Altered platelet aggregation: abnormal response to collagen GP6 gene sequencing	Supportive care
Defects in Platelet Adhesion				
DiGeorge syndrome	22q11.2 deletion including glycoprotein 1b-beta (GP1BB)	Defective GPIb-coagulation factor IX-factor V receptor	Thrombocytopenia, Large platelets with large α-granules; cardiac, thymus, parathyroid, facial abnormalities	Supportive care
Bernard-Soulier syndrome	Autosomal recessive mutations in GP1BA, GP1BB, Glycoprotein IX Platelet (GP9) Autosomal dominant mutations in GP1BA	Defective GPIb-IX-V receptor, impaired adhesion to VWF	Thrombocytopenia Large platelets Defective platelet aggregation	Supportive care Platelet transfusion Antifibrinolytics rFVIIa
von Willebrand disease (platelet-type)	Autosomal dominant gain of function mutations in GP1BA	Defective GPIb-IX-V, gain of function VWF-GP1bα interaction	Thrombocytopenia, large platelets, platelet clumping Altered platelet aggregation	Supportive care Platelet transfusion rFVIIa
Defects in Platelet Aggregation				
Glanzmann thrombasthenia	Autosomal recessive mutations in integrin subunit alpha 2b (ITGA2B), integrin subunit beta 3 (ITGB3)	Impaired fibrinogen-mediated aggregation, defective integrin αIIbβ3 (GPIIb/IIIa, CD41/CD61).	Normal platelet count and morphology Altered platelet aggregation. Decreased CD41 and CD61	Supportive care rFVIIa Platelet transfusion Antifibrinolytics

ADP, Adenosine diphosphate; *vWF,* von Willebrand factor.

thrombocytopenia in a mother with ITP is a history of neonatal thrombocytopenia in a previous pregnancy. There is no evidence that cesarean section is safer than uncomplicated vaginal delivery for thrombocytopenic fetuses.

Syndromic Causes of Neonatal Thrombocytopenia

Infants who continue to have thrombocytopenia beyond 2 months after birth should be evaluated for syndromic causes with examination of the bone marrow and genetic panels.[5,41,43,44,47,48,67]

Nontransfusional Therapies

Most, nearly 80%, cases of severe thrombocytopenia resolve within 14 days. About 10% continue to have low platelet counts for greater than 30 days and need multiple (>20) platelet transfusions. Two TPO mimetics, romiplostim and eltrombopag, show promise.[68] Both drugs begin to raise platelet counts in 4 to 6 days and show maximum benefit at 10 to 14 days. However, these drugs can be used only in a small subset of infants because of pharmacodynamic characteristics.

Altered Platelet Function

Etiology/Pathophysiology

Most platelet function defects seen in the NICU are acquired and can be due to medications, medical conditions, or medical interventions. Drugs that can cause platelet dysfunction include nonsteroidal anti-inflammatory drugs (indomethacin and ibuprofen), prostacyclin, certain anticonvulsants (valproic acid), and antibiotics such as beta-lactams.[69] Uremia also alters the platelet phospholipids and function.[70] Extracorporeal circuits and therapeutic hypothermia can also alter platelet function.[71]

Congenital platelet function disorders may result from defects/deficiencies in functional, structural, and regulatory proteins required for platelet function. The most severe platelet function defects involve glycoproteins located on the platelet surface. Bernard-Soulier syndrome is associated with deficiency of GPIb (the vWF receptor) and Glanzmann thrombasthenia with that of GPIIb/IIIa, the fibrinogen receptor. These can present with bleeding in neonates (Table 45.3).

Most of the other inherited platelet function defects are mild and present later in infancy or childhood. Secretory platelet disorders have defective platelet granules and cause mild to moderate bleeding. These include δ-storage pool defects (including the common ADP secretion defect and the less common absence of dense bodies associated with Hermansky-Pudlak syndrome) and α-granule defects (gray platelet syndrome). Genetic tools can help identify many defects in platelet function, such as those in *NBEAL2* with gray platelet syndrome.

Clinical Presentation and Diagnosis

Infants with platelet function disorders present with mucocutaneous or postcircumcision bleeding similar to that in thrombocytopenia. The evaluation should start with a complete blood count and a review of the peripheral blood smear. The combination of mild thrombocytopenia and large platelets (macrothrombocytopenia) is suggestive of Bernard-Soulier syndrome, which can be confirmed using flow cytometry to evaluate for the presence of GPIb on the platelet surface. Similarly, GPIIb/IIIa surface expression can be assessed to evaluate for Glanzmann thrombasthenia. Some platelet function defects show ultrastructural changes on electron microscopy. In particular, a deficiency or absence of dense bodies (δ-storage pool deficiency) or α-granules (gray platelet syndrome) can be demonstrated.

The diagnosis of platelet function disorders in neonates is problematic because the traditional platelet aggregation studies require a large volume of blood or lack reference values for neonates. These assays use a set concentration of platelet-rich plasma and assess platelet aggregation via light transmission after addition of platelet agonists such as ADP, epinephrine, ristocetin, arachidonic acid, collagen, and thrombin-related activation peptide. Neonates have reduced platelet aggregation compared with adults, and therefore the interpretation of this test in neonates is difficult. Recently, whole blood aggregometry assays have been developed and require less blood, but the neonatal reference ranges are still needed.

Evaluation

The tools for evaluation of platelet function are relatively limited. Bleeding time is still seen as the most reliable test.[72] The availability of the PFA-100 for in-vitro evaluation has shown some promise.[73] More recently, a high-throughput sequencing platform targeting 63 genes relevant for bleeding and platelet disorders was generated, which may enable the molecular diagnosis of platelet disorders in some infants.

Treatment

Drug treatment of congenital platelet dysfunction is a complicated issue. In acquired conditions, reversal of the condition that caused platelet dysfunction should be helpful, but this is not always possible. In such situations, the approach to management of bleeding is mostly based on platelet transfusions.

Medications such as desmopressin, antifibrinolytic agents, and recombinant activated factor VIIa (rFVIIa) have been used to enhance hemostasis. Desmopressin can improve platelet function in many congenital disorders, in uremia, and during cardiopulmonary bypass. However, it has not been used in young infants because it can lead to hypotension, hyponatremia, and seizures.

rFVIIa can be helpful in severe platelet function defects, such as Glanzmann thrombasthenia, that are refractory to platelet transfusions.[74] However, there is a risk of thrombosis. Thus it has to be used very cautiously only in patients with severe, refractory bleeding. It has been used in neonates, but there is a considerably enhanced risk of thrombosis. The efficacy is still uncertain.

Platelet transfusions are still the mainstay for platelet function defects, including in Bernard-Soulier syndrome and Glanzmann thrombasthenia. There is some concern about the risk of alloimmunization to GPIb and GPIIb/IIIa in patients with Bernard-Soulier syndrome and Glanzmann thrombasthenia, respectively. Once these antibodies develop, future platelet transfusions are likely to be ineffective. Thus it is imperative to withhold platelet transfusions except in life-threatening hemorrhage.

SECTION 9

Neurological Disorders

OUTLINE

Section 9

CHAPTER 46 Management of Hypoxic-Ischemic Encephalopathy Using Therapeutic Hypothermia

Joanne O. Davidson, Alistair J. Gunn

KEY POINTS

1. A healthy fetus has considerable aerobic and anaerobic reserves to successfully adapt to transient or mild hypoxia. Prolonged or repeated severe asphyxia results in failure of adaptation and progressive hypotension and hypoperfusion. The severity of brain injury is consistently related to the severity and duration of hypotension.
2. There is no intrinsic, physiologic relationship between the amount of systemic anaerobic metabolism (as reflected by metabolic acidosis) and the development of neuronal injury. The crude clinical correlation between acidosis and encephalopathy simply reflects that hypoxic-ischemic damage occurs under anaerobic conditions.
3. Hypoxia-ischemia can trigger multiple intracellular, apoptotic, and necrotic pathways and secondary inflammation in a latent phase after reperfusion that ultimately lead to delayed cell death. Many of these pathways are effectively suppressed by mild hypothermia.
4. Optimally, therapeutic hypothermia needs to be induced as soon as possible in first 6 hours after hypoxia-ischemia; brain temperature should be reduced by approximately 3.5°C, and cooling should be continued for approximately 72 hours. It is important to avoid pyrexia during or after resuscitation, before initiation of treatment.
5. It is likely but unproven that further improvements in outcome will arise from combining therapeutic hypothermia with other neuroprotective strategies. For now, clinical care should focus on timely identification and early treatment of infants who may benefit from therapeutic hypothermia.

Introduction

Impaired placental oxygen and glucose delivery can occur before or during birth at any gestational age and lead to moderate to severe acute, evolving hypoxia-ischemia and disturbed brain function (i.e., hypoxic-ischemic encephalopathy [HIE]). In the developed world it occurs in approximately 1 to 3 per 1000 live births.[1,2] HIE is associated with high rates of adverse outcomes. For example, the Western Australian Cerebral Palsy register reported that approximately 15% of infants with cerebral palsy born at term had had acute encephalopathy at birth.[3] Rates are even higher in low- and middle-income countries, so that HIE at birth and during the first 28 days of life is estimated to contribute one-tenth of all disability-adjusted life-years.[4] HIE is of course only one cause of neonatal encephalopathy. Nevertheless, HIE is the single most common cause of neonatal seizures.[5] The key link between exposure to hypoxia-ischemia as shown by metabolic acidosis and subsequent neurodevelopmental impairment is early onset of evolving encephalopathy.

Therapeutic hypothermia is now well established in clinical practice,[6] based on compelling evidence from large randomized controlled trials that it improves survival without disability in infancy and into middle childhood.[2,7] This improvement is partial; standard protocols were shown to reduce the combined risk of death and severe disabilities at 18 months of age by approximately 12%, from 58% to 46%.[8] The key challenge is now to further improve outcomes after treatment. We will dissect the known mechanisms of action of hypothermia and the evidence that current protocols for therapeutic hypothermia are essentially optimal.[9]

The Pathogenesis of Brain Cell Death

In a fetus, hypoxia-ischemia is commonly secondary to profound hypoxemia, which leads to cardiac compromise with secondary hypotension and hypoperfusion.[10] Compared with hypoxia alone, hypoperfusion reduces delivery of substrate as well as oxygen and thus accelerates depletion of cerebral high-energy metabolites, dramatically increasing the risk of subsequent injury. These concepts help explain the consistent observation that most cerebral injury after acute perinatal insults occurs in association with hypotension and consequent tissue hypoperfusion. By contrast, although asphyxial brain injury involves anaerobic metabolism, there is only a crude correlation between the severity of systemic acidosis and subsequent injury across experimental models.[10] Notably, this very weak relationship between severity of acidosis and injury is also seen clinically. For example, in a large, single-center cohort study,[11] 412 of 27,028 infants had an arterial cord blood pH $\leq$7.10. Of these, just 35 of 85 infants who developed HIE had an arterial cord blood pH $<$7.00, compared with 34 of 327 infants with pH between 7.00 and 7.10.

This reflects, at least in part, that the effects of asphyxia depend on the nature and pattern of the insult and the condition of the fetus.[10] The fetus is highly adapted to hypoxia, and injury occurs only in a very narrow window between intact survival and death. Immediate, catastrophic asphyxia due to events such as cord prolapse and placental abruption contribute to approximately 25% of cases of HIE.[12] The impact of the profound hypoxia on the fetus can be greatly potentiated by fetal blood loss leading to hypotension, as occurs during abruption. Approximately two-thirds of cases of HIE at term are associated with repeated, short periods of deep hypoxia,[12] reflecting the inherent intermittent reduction in utero-placental blood flow during contractions and reduced placental and intervillous perfusion.[13] Finally, approximately 10% of cases of moderate to severe HIE have been reported to be associated with abnormal fetal heart rate recordings before the start of labor, suggesting that the fetus had already been exposed to hypoxia-ischemia.[12,14]

As well as the pattern of hypoxia-ischemia, not surprisingly, maternal condition can affect outcomes. For example, maternal hyperthermia was independently associated with neonatal morbidity, including risk of death, HIE, and stroke, in multiple studies.[15–18]

What Initiates Neuronal Injury?

At the most fundamental level, injury requires a period of insufficient delivery of oxygen and substrates such as glucose (and other substrates in the fetus) such that neurons and glia cannot maintain supplies of high-energy metabolites and thus cannot sustain homeostasis. When this happens, the energy-dependent mechanisms of intracellular homeostasis, such as the sodium/potassium adenosine triphosphate–dependent pump, fail, leading to neuronal depolarization. This creates an osmotic and electrochemical gradient that in turn favors cation and water entry, leading to cell swelling (cytotoxic edema). If sufficiently severe, this may lead to immediate lysis.[19] Importantly, these edematous neurons may still recover, at least temporarily, if the hypoxic insult is reversed or the environment is manipulated. Multiple factors can cause cell injury during and after depolarization. These include the extracellular accumulation of excitatory amino acid neurotransmitters due to impairment of energy-dependent reuptake, which promotes further receptor-mediated cell swelling, excessive intracellular calcium entry, and the generation of oxygen free radicals and inflammatory cytokines.[20] These excitatory factors are balanced by a disproportionate release of inhibitory neurotransmitters such as gamma-aminobutyric acid and adenosine.[21,22] These inhibitory factors suppress the metabolic rate (termed adaptive hypometabolism) and protect the brain by delaying the onset of cell depolarization. The duration of neuronal depolarization in turn critically determines the severity of neural injury.[23]

Cerebral Injury Evolves Over Time

The central concept that enabled modern studies of neuroprotection is that although brain cell death can occur during sufficiently severe hypoxia-ischemia (termed the "primary" phase of injury), even after surprisingly severe events, many cells can initially reestablish oxidative metabolism in a so-called latent phase, followed by progressive secondary failure of oxidative metabolism and cell death over hours to days.[24,25] Studies using magnetic resonance spectroscopy demonstrated that many infants with evidence of moderate to severe asphyxia show initial, transient recovery of cerebral oxidative metabolism after birth, followed by secondary deterioration as shown by delayed cerebral energy failure from 6 to 15 hours after birth.[26] The severity of the secondary deterioration is closely correlated with neurodevelopmental outcome at 1 and 4 years of age.[27] Conversely, infants with HIE who did not show initial recovery of cerebral oxidative metabolism had extremely poor outcomes.[26]

An identical pattern of initial recovery of cerebral oxidative metabolism followed by delayed (secondary) energy failure was confirmed after hypoxia-ischemia in piglets, rats, and fetal sheep and is closely correlated to the severity of neuronal injury.[24,28,29] The timing of energy failure after hypoxia-ischemia is closely linked to the appearance of cell death on brain histology.[30] Continuous measurements of cytochrome oxidase, the terminal electron acceptor in the mitochondrial transport chain, using near-infrared spectroscopy demonstrated that after severe asphyxia in fetal sheep, there was initial recovery of cytochrome oxidase to sham control values, followed by a progressive fall that started after approximately 3 to 4 hours and continued until approximately 48 to 72 hours after asphyxia.[29] Delayed loss of mitochondrial activity was associated with a marked *increase* in relative intracerebral oxygenation, strongly indicating impaired ability to use oxygen.[29] This evidence of a "latent" phase of transient recovery during oxidative recovery offered the tantalizing possibility that therapeutic intervention *after* hypoxia-ischemia might be possible.

The timing and physiologic events during these phases of injury are now well described in preclinical studies. After restoration of circulation and oxygenation the initial hypoxic depolarization-induced suppression of cerebral oxidative metabolism, cytotoxic edema and accumulation of excitatory amino acids resolve over approximately 30 to 60 minutes.[21,31] Despite recovery of oxidative cerebral energy metabolism and mitochondrial activity,[29] electroencephalographic (EEG) activity remains depressed.[32] Cerebral blood flow initially recovers but typically shows a delayed, transient reduction below control values within hours after reoxygenation.[29,31] During the secondary deterioration from approximately 6 to 15 hours after moderate to severe hypoxia-ischemia, delayed seizures develop and then continue for several days,[29,31] accompanied by secondary cytotoxic edema,[31] accumulation of excitotoxins,[21] failure of cerebral mitochondrial activity,[24,29] and ultimately, cell death.[31] Secondary edema and seizures are not seen after milder insults that do not cause cortical injury.[33] By contrast, more severe hypoxia-ischemia typically accelerates the evolution of neuronal loss.[34]

As well as evolving over time, cell death spreads outward from the most severely affected regions toward less severely affected regions.[35] In piglets exposed to transient hypoxia-ischemia, the cerebral apparent diffusion coefficients normalized almost completely by 2 hours after resuscitation, followed by a fall in apparent diffusion coefficients beginning in the parasagittal cortex and then spreading through the brain. This pattern likely reflects both severity of injury and active mechanisms such as the opening of astrocytic connexin hemichannels on the cell surface, which can facilitate waves of spreading depression that can trigger cell death in less-injured tissues.[36] The secondary phase resolves over approximately 3 days after severe hypoxia-ischemia into a tertiary phase of ongoing injury, involving chronic inflammation and epigenetic changes affecting repair and reorganization that may last weeks to months and even years.[37]

These concepts—that an acute, global period of hypoxia-ischemia can trigger evolving cell death and that characteristic events are seen at different times after the insult—are central to understanding the causes and treatment of HIE. The initial triggers of the delayed death cascade during exposure to hypoxia-ischemia, including exposure to oxygen free radical toxicity, excessive levels of excitatory amino acids, and intracellular calcium accumulation down the concentration gradient due to failure of energy-dependent pumps during hypoxia and opening of channels linked to the excitatory neurotransmitters.[19] However, these events rapidly resolve during reperfusion from the insult and thus cannot readily be related to the effects of postinsult interventions such as cooling. It is striking that *in vitro* neuronal degeneration can be prevented by cooling initiated well after exposure to an insult.[38] Thus the key therapeutic targets must involve secondary consequences of hypoxia-ischemia, such as the intracellular progression of programmed cell death (apoptosis), the inflammatory reaction, and abnormal receptor activity.[20]

Intracellular Mediators of Delayed Cell Death

Multiple factors are involved in delayed development of cell death despite initial recovery of oxidative metabolism after

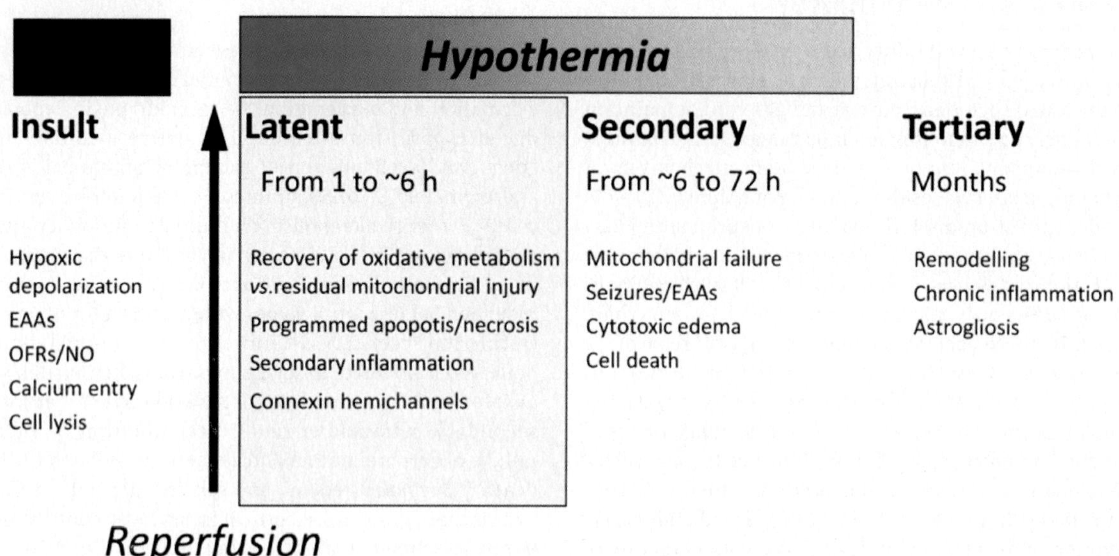

Fig. 46.1 Flow Chart Illustrating the Relationship Between the Mechanisms Active in the Pathophysiologically Defined Phases of Cerebral Injury After Moderate to Severe Hypoxia-Ischemia. During the immediate *reperfusion* period, lasting approximately 30 to 60 minutes, cellular energy metabolism is restored, with resolution of hypoxic depolarization and cell swelling. This is followed by a *latent* phase, with near-normal oxidative cerebral energy metabolism as measured by magnetic resonance spectroscopy but with depressed electroencephalographic activity and often a delayed fall in cerebral blood flow. The latent phase is associated with the intracellular components of the apoptotic cascade. This may be followed by *secondary* deterioration with delayed seizures and cytotoxic edema, extracellular accumulation of potential cytotoxins (such as the excitatory neurotransmitters), and 4 to 15 hours after the asphyxia, failure of oxidative metabolism and damage. The changes in the secondary phase may take 3 days or more to resolve. Effective neuroprotection requires that therapeutic hypothermia is started as soon as possible in the latent phase, before the onset of the secondary deterioration. *EAAs*, excitatory amino acids; *NO*, nitric oxide; *OFRs*, oxygen free radicals.

hypoxia-ischemia, including activation of cell death pathways, withdrawal of trophic factors, and secondary inflammation (Fig. 46.1). The cell death pathways are stimulated by entry of calcium during anoxic depolarization, exposure to reactive oxidative species during reperfusion, and likely other factors.[39]

There is good histologic evidence that activation of preexisting programmed cell death pathways contributes to posthypoxic cell death in the developing human brain.[39] The pattern of cell death is not purely apoptotic but rather includes elements of apoptotic and necrotic processes, with one or the other being most prominent depending on factors such as maturity and the severity of insult.[40] Consistent with the hypothesis that apoptotic processes are a key therapeutic target, postinsult hypothermia started after severe hypoxia-ischemia was reported to reduce apoptotic cell death but not necrotic cell death in the piglet.[41] Similarly, protection with posthypoxic-ischemic hypothermia in fetal sheep has been closely linked with suppression of activated caspase-3.[42]

Inflammatory Second Messengers

Brain injury also induces the inflammatory cascade with increased release of cytokines.[43] These compounds are believed to exacerbate delayed injury, whether by direct neurotoxicity, triggering apoptosis, or promoting stimulation of leukocyte adhesion and infiltration into the ischemic brain. Experimentally, cooling can potently suppress this inflammatory reaction.[44] For example, *in vitro*, hypothermia inhibits proliferation and superoxide and nitric oxide production by cultured microglia, and in adult rats, hypothermia suppresses the posttraumatic release of interleukin-1β and accumulation of polymorphonuclear leukocytes. Similarly, neuroprotection with postinsult hypothermia was associated with suppression of microglial activation in fetal sheep.[42,45,46]

Other receptor- and nonreceptor-mediated toxic factors are likely to contribute to neural injury in the latent phase. For example, there is some evidence from preterm fetal sheep of delayed production of oxygen free radicals after hypoxia-ischemia,[47] which may be particularly associated with death of oligodendroglia.

Excitotoxicity After Hypoxia-Ischemia

In contrast with their role during the primary phase, the importance of excitotoxins *after* reperfusion is questionable given that extracellular levels rapidly return to baseline values.[21,48] Pathologically elevated levels of extracellular excitatory amino acids such as glutamate are seen in a biphasic pattern. The initial increase occurs *during* hypoxia-ischemia and resolves rapidly after reperfusion, to control values.[21] Levels remain low throughout the latent phase and then secondarily rise many hours later, in association with delayed seizures and cytotoxic edema.[21,49] In near-term fetal sheep, for example, intense seizures are seen from approximately 9 ± 2 hours to 30 ± 3 hours after cerebral ischemia. It is important to appreciate that completely suppressing these large-amplitude seizures with a selective glutamate antagonist was associated with very limited reduction in neuronal damage in more mildly affected regions but with no effect on infarction of the parasagittal cortex and no improvement in recovery of EEG activity.[50] Moreover, combined antiglutamate treatment and mild whole-body hypothermia after severe asphyxia did not show additive neuroprotection in preterm fetal sheep.[51]

The preclinical studies of therapeutic hypothermia that involved subsequent clinical protocols were structured around these observations.

The Determinants of Neuroprotection With Therapeutic Hypothermia

Timing of Starting Hypothermia: The Earlier the Better

There is extensive preclinical evidence that hypothermia must be started as early as possible within the latent phase for optimal benefit.[9] In turn, this pattern is highly consistent with progressive mitochondrial failure during the latent phase, demonstrated by magnetic resonance spectroscopy after moderate to severe hypoxia-ischemia in human infants,[26,27] piglets,[52] and near-infrared spectroscopy in preterm fetal sheep.[29] Immediate initiation of hypothermia is protective across species and many paradigms of hypoxia-ischemia.[9] For example, in anesthetized piglets exposed to either hypoxia with bilateral carotid ligation or to hypoxia with hypotension, either 12 hours of mild whole-body hypothermia (35°C) or 24 hours of head cooling with mild systemic hypothermia started immediately after hypoxia prevented delayed energy failure, reduced neuronal loss, and suppressed posthypoxic seizures.[52,53]

Increasing the duration of hypothermia until resolution of the secondary phase of injury after approximately 72 hours can enable neuroprotection despite delayed initiation. In near-term fetal sheep, cerebral hypothermia induced 90 minutes after reperfusion from a severe episode of cerebral ischemia, that is, in the early latent phase, and continued until 72 hours after ischemia prevented secondary cytotoxic edema and improved electroencephalographic recovery.[31] There was a concomitant dramatic reduction in cortical infarction and improvement in neuronal loss scores in all regions. Comparable neuroprotection was seen when treatment was delayed until 3 hours after the end of ischemia.[54] By contrast, when the start of hypothermia was delayed until just before the onset of secondary seizures (5.5 hours after reperfusion), only partial neuroprotection was seen.[55] With further delay until after seizures were established (8.5 hours after reperfusion), there was no electrophysiological or overall histologic protection with cooling.[56]

Similar results have been reported in other paradigms. In nonanesthetized 21-day-old rat pups, mild hypothermia (a 2°C to 3°C decrease in brain temperature) for 72 hours after hypoxia-ischemia prevented cortical infarction, whereas cooling delayed until 6 hours after the insult had an intermediate, nonsignificant effect.[57] More recently, in 7-day-old rat pups, hypothermia induced either immediately or at 3 hours was neuroprotective after a "moderate" duration of hypoxia-ischemia (90 minutes).[58] By contrast, even immediate hypothermia did not improve outcomes after very prolonged hypoxia-ischemia (150 minutes). This illustrates that the window of opportunity for therapeutic hypothermia is critically dependent on the severity of the primary period of hypoxia-ischemia.

How Cold Is Too Cold?

The critical depth of hypothermia required for protection may be affected by multiple factors such as the delay before initiation and the severity and nature of the insult. There is some evidence from studies of moderate to severe ischemia that when cooling is delayed until 6 hours in both adult rodents and fetal sheep, greater functional and histologic neuroprotection may be seen with a 5°C reduction in brain temperature than with a 3°C reduction.[31,59] By contrast, in 7-day-old rat pups, there was no additional protection with cooling after hypoxia-ischemia to rectal temperatures below 33.5°C.[60] Similarly, in neonatal piglets exposed to global cerebral ischemia, whole-body hypothermia with a reduction in body temperature of either 3.5°C or 5°C was associated with significant (and highly similar) overall neuroprotection, whereas a reduction of 8°C was detrimental.[61]

If Some Is Good, Is More Better?

There is now compelling preclinical evidence that continuing cooling for approximately 72 hours provides optimal neuroprotection.[46,54] Broadly, and critically for clinical practice, the greater the delay before starting cooling or the more severe the insult, the greater the duration of cooling required for protection. For example, in adult gerbils, when the delay before initiating a 24-hour period of cooling was increased from 1 to 4 hours, neoronal survival in the CA1 region of the hippocampus after 6 months of recovery fell from 70% to 12%.[62] Subsequent studies demonstrated that protection could be restored by extending the duration of moderate (32°C to 34°C) hypothermia to 48 hours or more, even when the start of cooling was delayed until 6 hours after reperfusion.[63] Similarly, in near-term fetal sheep, cooling that started after 5.5 hours and continued until 72 hours was still partially protective.[55] Finally, in the same paradigm, although delayed cooling from 3 hours after ischemia until 48 hours was partially protective, it was substantially less effective for both recovery of EEG power and neuronal survival than cooling for 72 hours.[54]

Given this compelling evidence that hypothermia must be continued for at least 72 hours in large animals and humans, there has been interest in whether further prolonging the duration of hypothermia may be associated with greater benefit. However, in near-term fetal sheep, when delayed hypothermia starting 3 hours after ischemia was continued for 5 days compared with 3 days, there was no further improvement in electrophysiological recovery or neuronal survival or further reduction in cortical microglial induction.[46] Indeed, post-hoc analysis suggested that extended cooling was associated with a small reduction in neuronal survival in the parasagittal cortex and the dentate gyrus.

Clinical Evidence for Therapeutic Hypothermia

The large body of experimental evidence discussed above[44] supported the development of large randomized controlled trials of mild, induced hypothermia for moderate to severe neonatal HIE.

Evidence From Randomized Controlled Trials

A systematic meta-analysis of 11 randomized controlled trials of either selective head cooling or whole-body cooling initiated within 6 hours of birth and involving 1505 term and late preterm infants with moderate/severe HIE found consistent beneficial effects after hypothermia.[2] Mild hypothermia was associated with reduced mortality or severe neurodevelopmental disability by 18 months of age (relative risk [RR], 0.75; 95% confidence interval [CI], 0.68–0.83). Cooling reduced mortality (RR, 0.75; 95% CI, 0.64–0.88; 11 studies, 1468 infants), with reduced neurodevelopmental disability in survivors (typical RR, 0.77; 95% CI, 0.63–0.94; 8 studies, 917 infants).

Long-term follow-up of these studies is ongoing; the available evidence suggests a similar improvement in outcomes in middle childhood after mild induced hypothermia for HIE.[64–66] For example, the Total Body Hypothermia for Neonatal Encephalopathy Trial (TOBY) showed that significantly more children in the mild hypothermia group survived with an IQ score of 85 or more compared with the control group (52% versus 39%; RR, 1.31; P = .04) and that more children in the hypothermia group survived without neurologic abnormalities than in the control group (45% versus 28%; RR, 1.60; 95% CI, 1.15–2.22).[65] Further, there was a significant reduction in the risk of cerebral palsy (21% versus 36%, P = .03) and of moderate or severe disability (22% versus 37%; P = .03). Moreover, recent cohort studies of infants cooled for HIE showed a lower incidence of epilepsy at 2 years of age compared with the cooling trials,[67] as well as reduced severity of cerebral palsy.[68] The reader should note that it is not possible to exclude the possibility that infants with less severe HIE were recruited once therapeutic hypothermia became standard care. Nevertheless, these studies used the same criteria for hypothermia as the original cooling trials, including amplitude integrated EEG (aEEG) monitoring.

Is It Possible to Further Optimize Therapeutic Hypothermia?

Although therapeutic hypothermia significantly reduces the risk of death or disability, current protocols for therapeutic hypothermia were partially neuroprotective in meta-analysis, with a number needed to treat of about 7 (95% CI, 5–10; 8 studies, 1344 infants).[2] As already discussed, the experimental efficacy of hypothermia is highly dependent on *the timing of initiation*, *depth*, and *duration* of cooling.[9] Thus potentially, it may be possible to further optimize regimens for therapeutic hypothermia.

Although there have been no randomized trials of early initiation of hypothermia, in a cohort study, infants who were treated within 3 hours after birth had significantly better motor outcomes than those treated after 3 hours.[69] Few infants were started within that time frame in the large randomized controlled trials and thus there was limited power to assess the effect of earlier treatment. For example, in the CoolCap trial, hypothermia was started in only 12% of infants within 4 hours of birth, and many infants were already showing electrographic seizures.[70] This is an earlier onset of seizures than is typically seen in preclinical studies.[71] The likely reason is that many hypoxic-ischemic insults evolve over time before birth and thus the timing of the insult is often not clearly known.[12] This strongly suggests that there is considerable potential to further improve outcomes by starting hypothermia earlier than in the original trials.

There is encouraging emerging evidence that outcomes may have improved further now that therapeutic hypothermia is routine care for moderate to severe HIE. For example, in a large randomized controlled trial of 347 infants with follow-up data who were randomized to different cooling protocols, the rate of death or disability at 18 months of age in infants treated with cooling to 33.5°C for 72 hours was 29.3%[72] compared with 44% in infants receiving the same cooling protocol and recruited using the same criteria in a previous trial from the National Institute of Child Health and Human Development (the NICHD trial).[73] The factors behind this apparent improvement are unclear. In part, it might be related to recruiting infants with slightly less severe HIE,[69] but it might also be related to earlier initiation of cooling, with increasing use of passive cooling while infants are assessed for active cooling.[74]

These studies suggest that current protocols of whole-body cooling to 33.5°C for 72 hours are reasonably close to optimal; thus the most effective way to further improve outcomes from therapeutic hypothermia in infants with HIE is to initiate cooling earlier, as soon as possible in the first 6 hours after birth. Alternatively, cooling plus other pharmacologic neuroprotective agents may enable further improvements in outcome. There is currently considerable interest in such options, based on the endogenous induction of potentially neuroprotective compounds in the body as well as exogenous agents.[75]

Is More Better?

A large, randomized clinical trial of 364 infants with moderate to severe HIE who were randomized either to prolonged duration (120 hours versus 72 hours), increased depth of therapeutic hypothermia (32°C versus 33.5°C), or both was abandoned due to lack of effect and safety concerns.[72,76] The adjusted risk ratio for death in the neonatal intensive care unit after cooling for 120 hours compared with 72 hours was 1.37 (95% CI, 0.92–2.04), and for cooling to 32°C compared with 33.5°C, it was 1.24 (95% CI, 0.69–2.25). Furthermore, there was no significant overall effect of longer or deeper cooling on death or disability at a mean age of 18 months.[72] These consistent clinical and preclinical findings suggest that there is a relatively broad range of temperatures that are beneficial for the brain after hypoxia-ischemia and that, reassuringly, it should not be necessary to reduce core temperatures by more than approximately 3.5°C.

Is There Benefit From Cooling Started More Than 6 Hours After Birth?

The preclinical and clinical studies reviewed above consistently suggest that hypothermia should be started as early as possible in the first 6 hours of life to achieve optimal outcomes. However, some infants are unable to be started within this time window because of late diagnosis or being born in areas that cannot provide support for cooling. Even though it is not optimal, should these infants be offered therapeutic hypothermia after 6 hours of life? A recent randomized controlled trial conducted by the Neonatal Research Network centered in the United States compared 83 term infants who were cooled starting at 6 to 24 hours after birth (at a mean of 16 ± 5 hours) with 85 noncooled infants (range, 36.5°C to 37.3°C). Death or moderate to severe disability were seen in 24.4% of cooled infants, compared with 27.9% of noncooled infants (P = .23). Thus, although very delayed treatment was not harmful, this trial strongly suggest that it is critical to focus on initiating treatment as early as possible within the first 6 hours after birth.

Should We Cool Infants With "Mild" HIE?

The large, randomized controlled trials of therapeutic hypothermia excluded infants who had "mild" HIE in the first 6 hours of life in order to increase the rates of unfavorable outcome, so the potential benefit of treating these infants with therapeutic hypothermia is unknown. In cohort studies, some infants with mild HIE as defined using the trial criteria in the first 6 hours of life have material risk of disability. The exact results have been rather variable, likely because of variable criteria for "mild," retrospective identification, less formal neurologic examinations than used in the prospective trials, or not using aEEG criteria. The definition of "mild" HIE varies markedly between studies. The CoolCap and TOBY studies simply specified the clinical Sarnat criteria on a gestalt basis but also required that infants had moderate to severe changes on an aEEG recording before randomization.[70,77] The NICHD trial used only clinical criteria and excluded infants who did not have three or more criteria for moderate/severe HIE[73]; thus infants with one or two moderate or severe criteria were defined as having "mild" HIE. This suggests that some of these infants actually had "moderate" HIE even though they were excluded from the trial and raises the important possibility that it may be possible to refine the clinical criteria to more reliably identify infants who are at risk of disability.

A meta-analysis of studies with well-defined HIE grading at birth and standardized neurodevelopmental assessment at 18 months or older suggested that 86 of 341 infants (25%) with "mild" HIE in the first 6 hours of life had an adverse outcome,[78] defined as death, cerebral palsy, or neurodevelopmental test scores that were more than 1 standard deviation below the mean. Although most of these studies recruited infants solely on clinical criteria, a prospective cohort study of infants who were not treated with therapeutic hypothermia found that infants with mild HIE, determined by both early EEG and clinical examination, had adverse cognitive and neuromotor outcomes at 5 years of age compared with healthy controls.[79] Although survival was much greater after mild than moderate or severe HIE, survivors with mild HIE showed no significant difference in cognitive outcomes compared with those who had had moderate HIE.

Given that this population of infants with "mild" HIE in the first 6 hours is heterogeneous, the balance of clinical risk and benefit is unclear. Treating all cases of "mild" HIE would lead to a considerable increase in the number of infants being separated from their parents for at least 3 days and receiving invasive treatments such as central lines, invasive respiratory support, sedation, and delayed oral feeding. It is reasonable to reflect that there is evidence from young rodents that therapeutic hypothermia seems to be more protective after milder hypoxia-ischemia.[58] Taken as a whole, it is likely that established protocols for therapeutic hypothermia will also reduce cell loss in infants with milder clinical HIE in the first 6 hours of life. Given that there are roughly as many infants with mild HIE as there are with moderate to severe HIE, it is critical that the benefits of treatment for this group are now formally tested.

Conclusion

Therapeutic hypothermia is now established as standard care to partially improve neurologic recovery in infants with moderate to severe HIE. Further improvements in neurodevelopmental outcomes are likely to come from combining hypothermia with endogenous or exogenous neuroprotective agents. Tantalizingly, autologous or external stem cells may have potential to promote long-term neurorepair through reducing neural inflammation and promoting release of trophic factors.[80,81] While awaiting the results of further research, it is important not to forget that the most effective ways to optimize treatment with hypothermia are to avoid hyperthermia during resuscitation and to identify infants with HIE and start treatment as soon as possible after birth.[82] EEG recordings and other early biomarkers can help identify patients who would benefit from treatment in such a limited time frame.[83]

Acknowledgments

The authors' work reported in this review was supported by grants from the Health Research Council of New Zealand (17/601, 18/225, 22/559), the Lottery Health Board of New Zealand, and the Auckland Medical Research Foundation.

Section 9

CHAPTER 47

Management of Hypoxic-Ischemic Encephalopathy Using Measures Other Than Therapeutic Hypothermia

Jennifer Burnsed, Raul Chavez-Valdez

KEY POINTS

1. Neonatal encephalopathy is an alteration in consciousness or neurologic exam in newborn infants. Hypoxic-ischemic encephalopathy accounts for nearly 50% of all cases.
2. Clinical presentation depends on the duration, timing, and severity of the insult and may evolve over the subsequent hours to days. Clinical staging of encephalopathy is usually based on the Sarnat criteria.
3. Disruption of blood flow causes ischemic injury; abrupt disruption typically damages the basal ganglia and thalamus, whereas subacute, less severe loss of perfusion may damage the watershed areas.
4. Patients may be stratified for risk using factors such as gestational age, encephalopathy scores, electroencephalography signatures, near infrared spectroscopy, imaging, and biomarkers.
5. Current clinical management is largely supportive. Seizure control is important. Several potential therapeutic strategies are under investigation, which brings hope for the future.

Definition, Diagnosis, and Differential

Definition

Neonatal encephalopathy (NE) is an alteration in consciousness or neurologic exam in the neonate. The possible etiologies of NE are broad (Table 47.1) but it is most commonly (approximately 50%) caused by hypoxic-ischemic encephalopathy (HIE).[1,2] The following sections are focused on HIE, although many details are applicable to other NE etiologies.

Diagnosis

The initial diagnosis of HIE relies on evidence of an acute or subacute (prolonged) perinatal event leading to brain injury and exam findings consistent with encephalopathy. Initial evaluation of an infant with suspected HIE should include perinatal history, neurologic exam, and in some cases, electroencephalogram (EEG) and imaging, when available.

Perinatal History

Evidence of intrauterine distress such as an abnormal biophysical profile, decreased fetal movements, fetal bradycardia, or acidosis on umbilical cord/initial infant blood gas (within 1 hour of birth), along with need for extensive resuscitation and/or low Apgar scores (<5) at 5 and 10 minutes, are needed for the diagnosis.[3,4]

Neurologic Examination

The clinical presentation depends on the duration, timing, and severity of the insult and may evolve over the subsequent hours to days. Although it is not the only scoring system,[5–8] clinical staging of encephalopathy is often based on the Sarnat criteria (Table 47.2).[9] Using the modified Sarnat criteria, which do not include EEG, the current recommendations are to offer therapeutic hypothermia (TH) to infants with moderate to severe encephalopathy, although the efficacy of TH in severe encephalopathy is the subject of ongoing studies (see Chapter 32). The Sarnat score was used as an inclusion criterion in the first randomized controlled trials of TH[8,10,11] and is still used by most neonatal intensive care units for evaluation of the neonate needing TH. Longitudinal follow-up of Sarnat scoring suggests that worsening staging regardless of the initial staging is more predictive than the initial score alone.[12]

EEG

EEG was part of the originally described Sarnat score, but it is not included in the modified version, now the most often used. Regardless, in cases where there is clinical suspicion for HIE but the neurologic examination is equivocal, early EEG is useful for encephalopathy staging. Early EEG (<6 hours after birth) was used as an inclusion criterion for many of the early randomized controlled trials on TH.[10,11] A normal or mildly abnormal EEG background is highly predictive of normal neurodevelopmental outcomes at age 2 years.[13]

Pathophysiology

Acute Phase

The fetal brain requires blood flow to deliver oxygen and glucose for cellular energy and metabolic homeostasis. Interruption of blood flow leads to hypoxemia and eventually decreases cardiac output. Depending on the severity and timing of the disruption of blood flow, cerebral injury may occur and lead to HIE. Abrupt disruption of cerebral blood flow is classically associated with deep grey matter (basal ganglia and thalamus) injury. Chronic and less severe (partial) disruption of cerebral blood flow is associated with cortical injury, particularly in the watershed regions.[14–17]

The initial disruption of cerebral blood flow leads to mitochondria failure. The resulting adenosine triphosphate (ATP) depletion and lactic acid build-up impairs the function of excitatory amino acid transporters within the astrocytic membrane forming the synaptic cleft. As a result, excitatory amino acids such as glutamate accumulate and activate N-methyl-D-aspartate and α-amino-3-hydroxy-5-methyl-4-isoxazolepropionic acid receptors, leading to an intracellular influx of sodium, calcium,

Table 47.1 Major Causes of Neonatal Encephalopathy

Hypoxic-ischemic encephalopathy
Metabolic derangements (inborn errors of metabolism, hypoglycemia)
Intracranial hemorrhage
Perinatal stroke
Kernicterus
Infection
Sinovenous thrombosis
Maternal toxins

and water. Cell death results from the progression of cytotoxic edema, protease activation, and free radical production (Fig. 47.1).[18]

Latent/Chronic Phase

Restoration of cerebral blood flow, or reperfusion, after disruption and injury begins the latent phase of injury.[19] The latent phase is the therapeutic target of TH. Secondary energy failure, which signals the end of the latent phase, is marked by irreversible mitochondrial failure[20] and involves oxidative stress, intracellular calcium accumulation, inflammation, and cell death. This neuronal death includes cell death along the entire cell death continuum, including apoptosis, autophagy, continuum cell death, necroptosis, and necrosis.[21] Many of the therapeutic agents tested in the past decade have targeted many of these downstream mechanisms (Figs. 47.2 and 47.3).

Stratification of Patients by Risk

Gestational Age/Prematurity

HIE is classically reported in full-term and late preterm infants and rarely in preterm infants. Although HIE occurs at all gestational ages, the assessment of encephalopathy in preterm infants is difficult and the clinical presentation of seizures may be subtle. There have been several small studies on preterm HIE,[19,22] which have found that due to differences in neurodevelopmental stage, injury mechanisms and patterns differ from those of the full-term neonate. Oligodendrocyte maturity, vascular and blood-brain barrier permeability, and selective vulnerability of certain cell lines such as developing oligodendroglia, astrocytes, and microglia likely determine the severity and type of injury.[22] Preterm infants appear to exhibit greater susceptibility to white matter injury, most often associated with concurrent basal ganglia and thalamic injury, than do full-term infants (see Fig. 47.8 ahead).[23]

Encephalopathy Score

Multiple scoring systems have been developed to assess severity of encephalopathy and predict long-term risk of neurodevelopmental disability (see Table 47.2). The first of these was the Sarnat scoring system.[9] Clinically, in settings where other prognostic tools (magnetic resonance imaging [MRI], EEG) can be used, these scores are most commonly used to assess eligibility for TH. Regardless of the scoring or staging system used, trending the score/exam over time while in the acute period is important, because the examination will evolve over time and persistently high encephalopathy scores are generally predictive of worse outcomes.[5] Of note, administration of sedation and/or antiepileptic drugs may alter the exam, which should considered.

Findings of moderate or severe encephalopathy on exam are inclusion criteria for treatment with TH; traditionally, children with mild encephalopathy were not thought to be at significant risk for neurodevelopmental disability, but there is growing evidence that neonates with mild encephalopathy may be at risk for long-term neurodevelopmental abnormalities. Neonates with mild HIE have been described to have abnormal short-term outcomes such as longer time to reach full feeds, seizures, need for a surgical feeding device, or abnormal MRI or neurologic exam findings at discharge.[24] In a retrospective analysis of

Table 47.2 Encephalopathy Scores

	Sarnat Score From 1976[9]	Thompson Score From 1997[5]	Encephalopathy Score From 2004[7]
Scoring	Three stages of encephalopathy: mild, moderate, severe	Score 0 (best) to 2 or 3 (worst) on each component (max 22, >7 moderate-severe encephalopathy)	6 categories, scored 0–1 (total possible score 6)
Components			
Consciousness	X	X	X
Reflexes	X	X	X
Tone	X	X	X
Autonomic function	X		
Seizures/EEG	X[a]	X	X
Respiratory drive		X	X
Fontanelle		X	
Feeding			X
Prognostic use	Higher stage associated with "major disability" during early adolescence[173] Associated with 18-month ND outcomes[174]	Day 3 score >15 with high specificity (96%) for abnormal outcome at 1 year (sensitivity 71%, PPV 92%, NPV 82%)[5] Day 1 score linked with mortality and morbidity[175] Peak score associated with IQ, motor outcome, survival without ND impairment in 4- to 5-year-olds[176]	Higher score associated with worse 30-month ND outcomes[7] Max score in first 3 days of age highly associated with outcome[7]

[a]Modified Sarnat staging does not include seizures/EEG findings.
EEG, Electroencephalogram; *ND*, Neurodevelopmental; *NPV*, Negative predictive value; *PPV*, Positive predictive value.

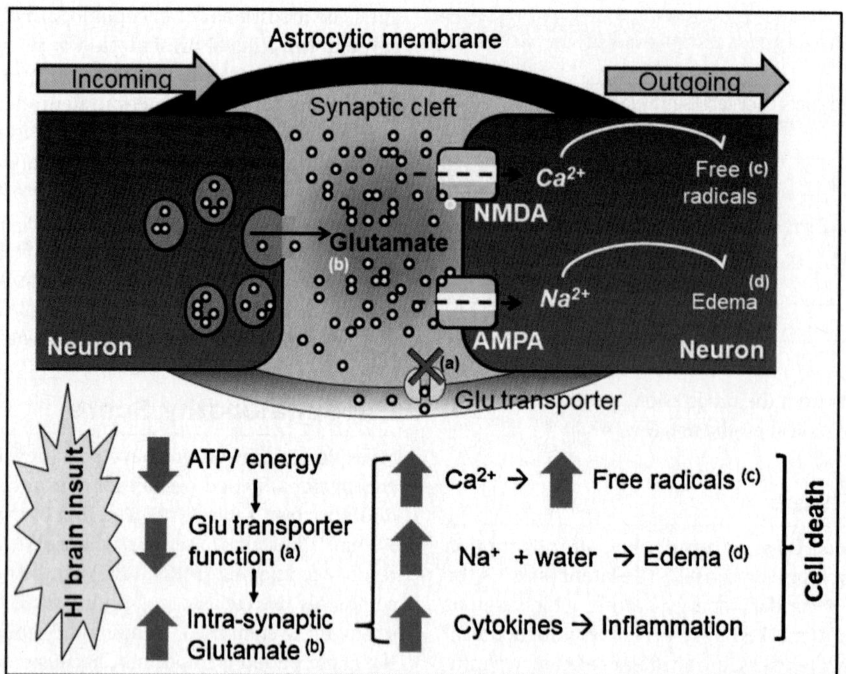

Fig. 47.1 After Neonatal Hypoxic-Ischemic Brain Insult, ATP Production Is Impaired Due to Decreased Oxygen and Glucose Delivery and Mitochondrial Failure. The function of glutamate (glu) transporters with the astrocytic membrane is adenosine triphosphate (ATP)-dependent, and thus energy failure results in (A) impaired function of these transporters and (B) glutamate accumulation within the synaptic cleft. The resulting glutamate excitotoxicity activates NMDA and AMPA receptors. (C) NMDA receptor activation facilitates Ca^{2+} influx followed by activation of synthases and production of free radicals from oxygen (i.e., superoxide) or nitrogen (i.e., nitric oxide). (D) Activation of AMPA receptors produces influx of Na^{2+} and water, with it inducing cytotoxic edema. These events and the resulting cell death will initiate and perpetuate neuroinflammation. *AMPA*, α-Amino-3-hydroxy-5-methyl-4-isoxazolepropionic acid; *NMDA*, N-methyl-D-aspartate.

infants who had received TH, MRI abnormalities after TH were equally common among infants with mild HIE compared with those with moderate or severe HIE.[25] Mild encephalopathy on early EEG is associated with lower IQ at age 5 years.[26] The PRIME (Prospective Research in Infants with Mild Encephalopathy) study revealed that over half of infants with mild HIE had an abnormal short-term outcome.[27] A recent meta-analysis showed that 20% of infants with mild encephalopathy have adverse neurologic outcomes at 18 months.[28] Study of long-term outcomes in infants with mild HIE as well as the efficacy of TH for this group is ongoing.

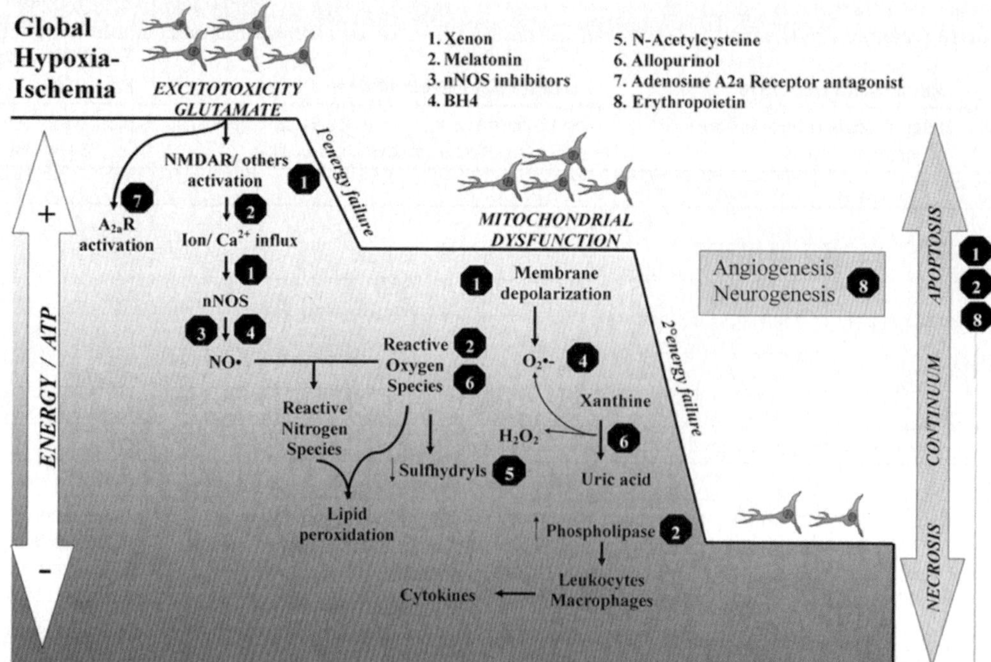

Fig. 47.2 Downstream Mechanisms of Several Therapeutic Agents Being Tested Over the Last Decade for Hypoxic-Ischemic Encephalopathy. (Robertson et al. Which neuroprotective agents are ready for bench to bedside translation in the newborn infant? *J Pediatr*. 2012;160:544–552.e4.)

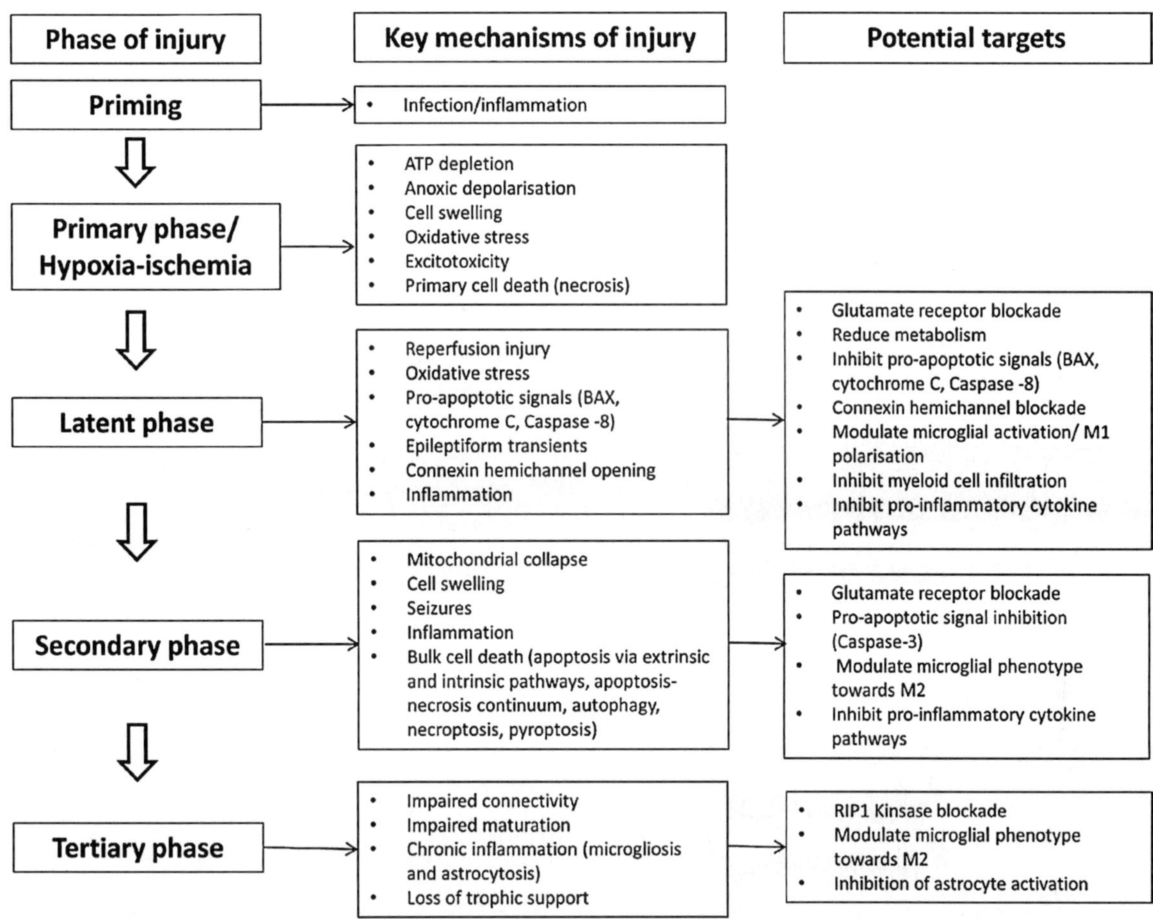

Fig. 47.3 Flow Chart Showing the Mechanisms Contributing to Each Phase of the Evolution of Neonatal Encephalopathy Over Time. (Davidson et al. *Seminars in Fetal and Neonatal Medicine*, article 101267.)

Amplitude Integrated EEG/Continuous Video EEG

Encephalopathy on neonatal EEG has been standardized by the American Clinical Neurophysiology Society.[29] Depending on available resources and setting, amplitude integrated EEG (aEEG; Fig. 47.4) or full montage EEG can be used (Table 47.3). A normal or mildly abnormal early EEG background is highly predictive of normal neurodevelopmental outcomes at age 2 years.[13] Recovery of EEG background within the first 24 hours is associated with better outcomes.[30] Persistently abnormal EEG background activity 36 to 48 hours after injury has been associated with worse neurodevelopmental outcomes.[31] aEEG is used by units particularly when continuous full montage neonatal EEG services are not available for monitoring throughout TH. A systematic review of aEEG use in HIE including 17 studies (both with and without TH) concluded that the aEEG background during the first 72 hours after HI injury has strong predictive value for long-term neurologic outcome.[32]

Near-Infrared Spectroscopy

Near-infrared spectroscopy (NIRS) is a bedside monitoring technique that continuously provides information on mixed arterial and venous saturations in the brain. In some cases cerebral saturations may be compared with control tissue such as the kidney (Fig. 47.5). Mixed saturation (rSO_2) is a measure of the differential between oxygen delivery to the brain tissue and oxygen extraction by the brain tissue. Small studies have examined the use of NIRS in infants with HIE undergoing TH, with varying results. Higher rSO_2 values in the first 10 hours of TH were associated with injury on MRI[33]; however, other studies have not found a relationship between rSO_2 values during TH and 18-month outcomes.[34] Ongoing studies are examining the use of NIRS both in guiding management of blood pressure and cerebral autoregulation as an neuroprotective strategy and as a prognostic tool[35] and in trending a number of NIRS parameters as a prognostic tool.[36,37]

Imaging

Head Ultrasound

Although much of the literature regarding imaging in HIE has focused on MRI, head ultrasound has been shown to be a useful tool for prognosis and evaluation of severity. Signs of HI injury that may be detectable on head ultrasound include small, effaced ventricles, which may be indicative of cerebral edema (although they can be a normal variant); echogenicity of the basal ganglia and thalamus can also be a sign of ischemia. Doppler measurements of the anterior cerebral artery resistive index have been associated with 2-year neurodevelopmental outcomes.[38,39] The ratio of white matter to gray matter echogenicity has also been described as a prognostic tool (Figs. 47.6 and 47.8).[39]

Magnetic Resonance Imaging

When available, MRI is the gold standard imaging technique in neonates with HIE. A specific MRI protocol for neonates is

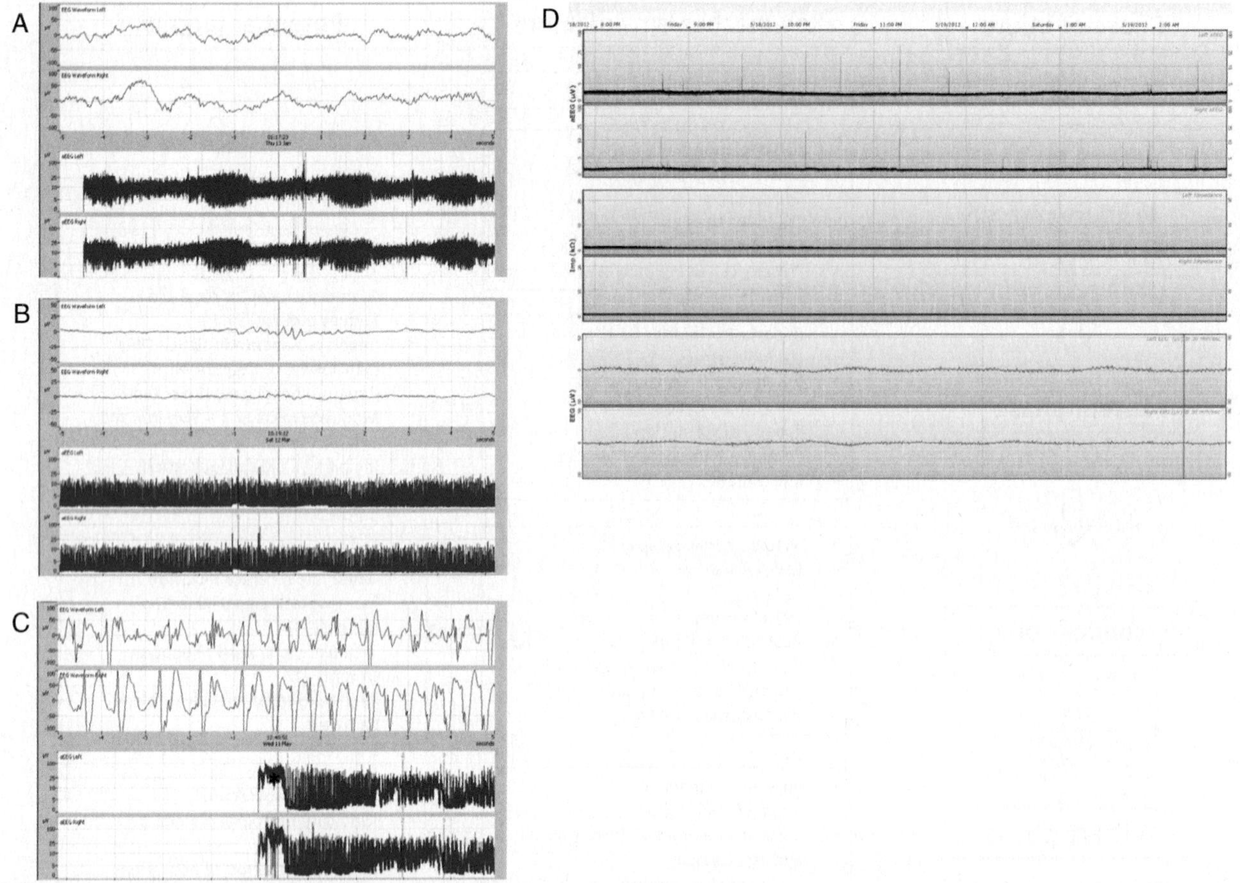

Fig. 47.4 Common Amplitude-Integrated Electroencephalography Patterns in Infants With Neonatal Encephalopathy. (A) Normal sleep-wake cycling in a full-term infant with a Sarnat score of 0 at admission to the neonatal intensive care unit. Periods with voltage from 5–25 μV alternate with periods exceeding those limits. (B) Burst-suppression pattern in an infant with severe hypoxic-ischemic encephalopathy (Sarnat score of 3) cycling between periods of profound suppression of electrical activity and usually short bursts of increased activity. (C) Pattern of rhythmicity compatible with neonatal seizures in an infant with moderate encephalopathy (Sarnat score of 2), with typical elevation of baseline exceeding 10 μV. (D) Low voltage background pattern in an infant with a Sarnat score of 2. (Courtesy Charlamaine Henson, RN coordinator for the Johns Hopkins University—Neuroscience Intensive Care Program.)

important and should be discussed with pediatric neuroradiology. Depending on the timing of imaging after injury, findings will be present on different sequences. Restricted diffusion on diffusion weighted imaging (DWI) will be present for the first 3 to 5 days after injury, with the exact timing dependent on the severity of injury. Evolution of the MRI findings occurs over the first several weeks; nearing the end of the first week, pseudonormalization may occur. Pseudonormalization of the MRI is when the diffusion weighted changes are no longer visible and injury on T1/T2 sequences are not yet apparent.[40,41] There are two major patterns of HI injury, depending on the length and severity of the insult. Acute, more complete compromise results in basal ganglia-thalamic involvement, and more prolonged, less severe compromise is associated with a watershed/cortical injury pattern. In severe, prolonged hypoxic-ischemic events, extensive HI injury, which affects both the deep gray matter and the cortex, may be present. EEG and MRI may be useful in preterm infants to assess long-term risk for neurodevelopmental deficits.[23]

Certain findings and scoring systems on MRI in HIE have been predictive of outcome. One highly predictive finding on MRI is abnormalities of the apparent diffusion coefficient in the posterior limb of the internal capsule, which is highly associated with survival and

Table 47.3 Amplitude-Integrated EEG Versus Full Montage EEG

	Amplitude Integrated EEG	Full Montage EEG
Measurement	Superficial, biparietal electrodes Derived from reduced EEG	Multielectrode array Greater depth of detection
Advantages	Greater accessibility—unit staff can place electrodes and interpret information	Greater information (more channels, depth of detection)
Disadvantages	Limited information provided (few electrodes, reduced depth)	Requires specialized staff to place electrodes and interpretation by a neurologist
Ideal clinical scenario	During transport Limited-resource settings	Larger centers with support staff and neurologists available

EEG, Electroencephalogram.

↓ O_2 extraction
C > 85%
R < 75%

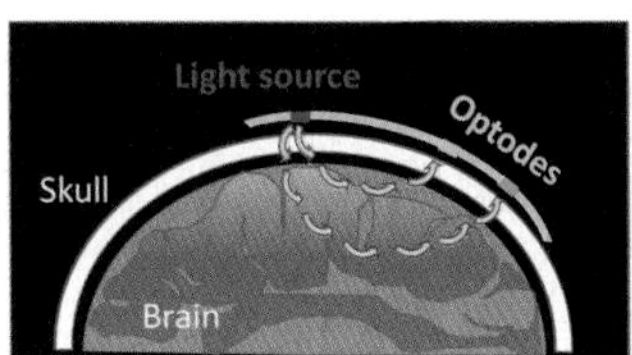

↓ Brain perfusion
C < 50%
R < 75%

Fig. 47.5 Near-Infrared Spectroscopy Is a Noninvasive Technology for Assessing Cerebral Hemodynamics. The probe emits light at a particular wavelength that passes through the scalp, skull, and brain tissue up to 1 to 2 cm. This light is absorbed by receiving optodes at two different wavelengths reflecting oxygenated and deoxygenated hemoglobin. Regional cerebral tissue oxygen saturation is calculated by the ratio between oxygenated and total hemoglobin. In some cases, cerebral saturations (labeled by the letter *C*) may be compared with a control tissue (in this case renal, labeled by the letter *R*). This is only appropriate when injury of the kidney or the control organ is minimal. Normal cerebral saturation ranges are between 65% and 75%. High cerebral oxygen saturation suggests decreased brain oxygen extraction but also occurs during therapeutic hypothermia because the brain metabolism is decreased. In contrast, low cerebral saturation suggests low brain perfusion.

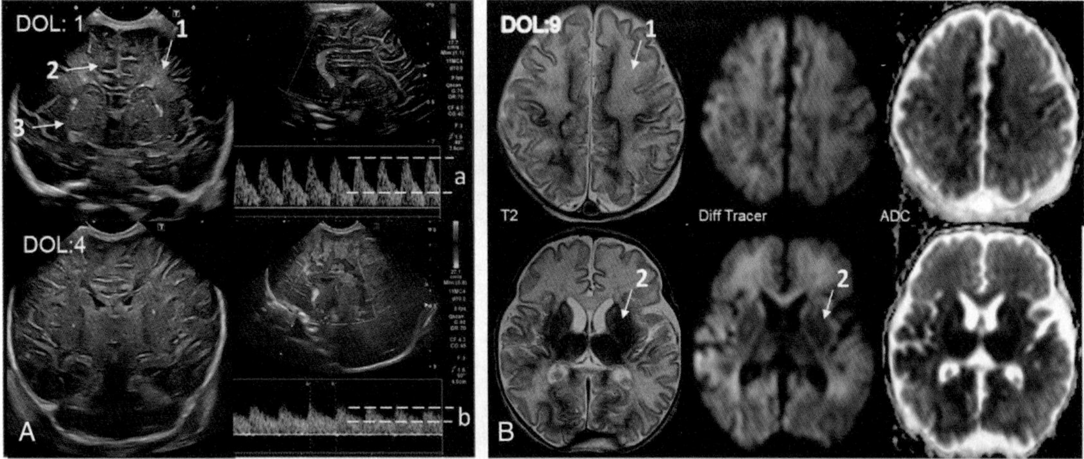

Fig. 47.6 Full-Term Infant With Severe Hypoxic-Ischemic Encephalopathy (HIE) Due to Placental Abruption. (A) Head ultrasound obtained at day-of-life (DOL) 1 demonstrates bilateral symmetric increased echogenicity of the white matter (*1*) with pronounced gray/white matter differentiation (*2*) and increased echogenicity of the basal ganglia and thalamus (*3*). At DOL 4, the above-described findings are more conspicuous and there is reduced resistive index (*b* versus *a*). (B) Brain magnetic resonance imaging at DOL 9 demonstrates diffuse increased T2 signal of the white matter (*1*), restricted diffusion and decreased T2 signal in the bilateral basal ganglia and thalami (*2*), and Rolandic gyri, mesial occipital cortices, insular and temporal polar cortices, and subcortical white matter. Prolonged pseudonormalization can be seen in neonates treated with therapeutic hypothermia with severe HIE (NICHD score of 3). (Courtesy Dr. Aylin Tekes, Director, Pediatric Radiology and Pediatric Neuroradiology, Johns Hopkins Hospital.)

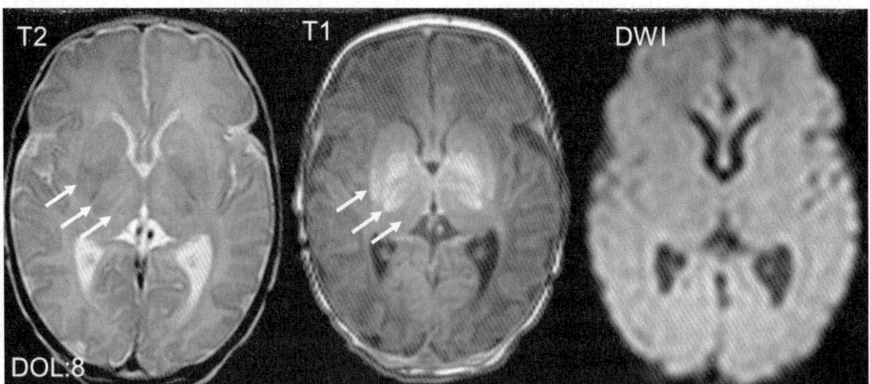

Fig. 47.7 Hypoxic-Ischemic Brain Injury in Term Infant. Infant with history of profound and brief anoxia A. An 8-day-old full-term infant with a classic central pattern of injury; note the bilateral symmetric high T2 and T1 signal in the posterior aspect of the putamen, posterior limb of the internal capsule, and ventrolateral thalami *(arrows)*. At day-of-life (DOL) 8, the diffusion tracer image (diffusion weighted imaging [DWI]) no longer demonstrates high signal due to pseudonormalization (no restricted diffusion). (Courtesy Dr. Aylin Tekes, Director, Pediatric Radiology and Pediatric Neuroradiology, Johns Hopkins Hospital.)

neuromotor outcome in infants with HIE.[15] One MRI scoring system, specifically the grey matter injury score, is highly predictive of adverse motor and cognitive outcomes at age 2 and at school age.[31] Conversely, absence of injury on MRI is not necessarily predictive of a favorable outcome, because infants with minimal or no injury on MRI may still have moderate to severe delays (see Figs. 47.6, 47.7, and 47.8).[42]

Biomarkers

The search for a reliable, testable biomarker for outcome in HIE is the topic of ongoing research.[43] A number of serum biomarkers have undergone investigation, with mixed prognostic utility. Those with the greatest evidence are summarized in Table 47.4. Ongoing trials are examining various biomarkers for feasibility of testing,

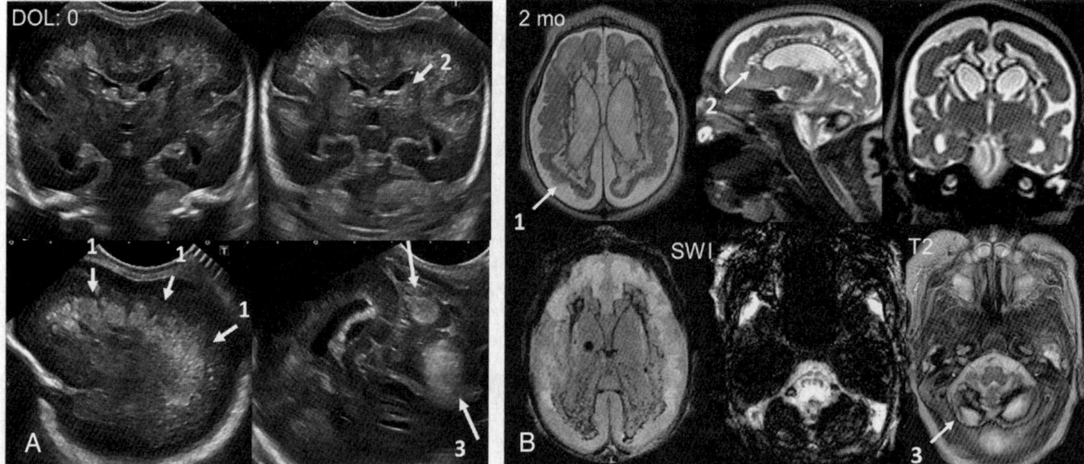

Fig. 47.8 Patterns of Hypoxic-Ischemic Brain Injury in Preterm Infants. A male infant of 26 4/7 weeks' gestational age with OEIS complex (omphalocele-exstrophy-imperforate anus-spinal defects) and severe congenital anemia. (A) Head ultrasound at day-of-life (DOL) 0 demonstrates bilateral symmetric increased echogenicity of the white matter (*1*) and the basal ganglia and thalami (*2*). Transmastoid views demonstrate bilateral focal hyperechogenicities consistent with cerebellar hemorrhages (*3*). (B) Infant at 2 months of age: brain magnetic resonance imaging showed marked periventricular white matter volume loss (*1*), severe cystic encephalomalacia in the residual periventricular white matter, and cystic necrosis in basal ganglia. Note microhemorrhages in the periventricular white matter as demonstrated in the susceptibility weighted image (SWI) (*2*). Bilateral cerebellar hemorrhages are replaced by volume loss and cystic encephalomalacia and hemosiderin straining (*3*). (Courtesy Dr. Aylin Tekes, Director, Pediatric Radiology, Johns Hopkins Hospital.)

specificity, and sensitivity for long-term neurodevelopmental outcomes (BiHiVE2 NCT 02019147; BANON study NCT03357250).

Transport

Neonates with HIE should be cared for at a tertiary care center in order for appropriate monitoring, treatment, and follow-up to occur. Because subclinical seizures are common in this population, especially after the administration of antiepileptic drugs, continuous EEG monitoring is crucial throughout TH and rewarming. EEG monitoring with either full montage neonatal EEG or aEEG is important, as is interpretation by a pediatric neurologist. In addition, the ability to obtain MRI with a neonatal-specific sequence protocol is important, and interpretation with pediatric neuroradiology maximizes yield from the study. Besides pediatric neurology and neonatology, involvement of other pediatric specialists in the care and follow-up of infants with HIE is important and should include developmental pediatrics, pediatric neuropsychology, pediatric therapies (physical therapy, occupational therapy, and speech-language pathology), and pediatric neurology.

Transport of infants with HIE undergoing TH has a special set of challenges. Prompt initiation of TH is key and has been linked to better outcomes.[44–46] For infants requiring TH who are born at referral hospitals, this means cooling should be initiated prior to and during transport to a tertiary care center.[47,48] Caution should be exercised in providing passive cooling, because infants, particularly those with severe encephalopathy, may become severely hypothermic.[48,49] If possible, active cooling during transport is optimal, because this is associated with reaching target temperatures quicker and maintaining the temperature in the goal range.[48,50]

Supportive Management

Multiorgan dysfunction is present in up to 50% to 88% of infants with HIE.[51] A summary of supportive management by system is presented in Table 47.5.

Neuroprotective Strategies

Seizure Control

Status epilepticus, seizures lasting >5 minutes, or more than two 30-second seizures per hour are accepted guidelines to start antiseizure drugs, particularly when encephalopathy is secondary to stroke.[52] Phenobarbital is the most common agent used to control seizures in this setting, but evidence guiding the duration and the combination with other antiseizure drugs is limited. One of the few points of agreement among experts is that the duration of phenobarbital (and phenytoin) treatments should be as brief as possible after controlling the initial seizures, due to the suspected harmful effects on the developing brain.[53] Between 45% and 70% of clinical seizures respond to phenobarbital (loading of 20 mg/kg), and its metabolism is grossly unchanged by TH.[54] In rodent models of neonatal HI injury, the addition of phenobarbital to TH may provide additional protection concerning the early extent of the injury, although it does not prevent motor impairments.[55] This lack of motor protection may be because phenobarbital, along with valproate and phenytoin, produces increased neuronal loss, even without a superimposed brain insult.[56–59] Thus, other alternatives such as levetiracetam and topiramate, which do not have those effects, are being explored in the developing brain.

Levetiracetam (Roweepra, Spritam, and Keppra)

Although levetiracetam appears to be as effective as phenobarbital in controlling pediatric seizures,[60–67] the preliminary results of the NEOLEV2 trial (www.clinicaltrials.gov; NCT01720667), in which 280 infants diagnosed with neonatal seizures were randomized to phenobarbital or levetiracetam, suggested superior effectiveness of phenobarbital in achieving 24-hour seizure control (80% versus 28%).[68] Regardless of those findings, levetiracetam may provide neuroprotective effects not fully linked to the control of seizures.[69] Although still controversial,[70] levetiracetam does not appear to increase neuronal death as valproate, phenobarbital, and phenytoin do,[56] and in fact it decreases cell death and injury after neonatal hypoxic-ischemic (HI) brain insult in rodents.[71] Furthermore, levetiracetam used after termination of status epilepticus with

Table 47.4 Biomarkers

Biomarker	Outcome Association
Brain derived neurotrophic factor (BDNF)	12 months ND outcomes[105]
Glial fibrillary acidic protein (GFAP)	MRI injury[177,178] Moderate to severe HIE[178,179] Abnormal Bayley III scores at 5–10 months[178] and 15–18 months[179]
S100B	MRI injury score[105] Clinical grade of encephalopathy[180–182]
Myelin basic protein (MBP)	
Ubiquitin carboxy-terminal hydrolase-L1 (UCH-L1)	MRI injury score[105,178] Clinical grade of encephalopathy[178,179,183] Abnormal Bayley III scores at 5–10 months[178]
Tau protein	MRI injury score[105] 12 months ND outcomes[105,184]
Phosphorylated axonal neurofilament heavy chain (pNF-H)	MRI injury[183]
Interleukin (IL)-1β	MRI injury score[105,185] Abnormal Bayley III scores at 15–18 months [179]
IL-6	MRI injury score[105,185] Abnormal Bayley III scores at 15–18 months[179] Death or severe MRI injury[185]
IL-8	Abnormal Bayley III scores at 15–18 months[179]
IL-10	MRI injury score[105,185] Death or severe MRI injury[185]
IL-13	MRI injury score[105,185]
IL-16	All perinatal asphyxia, including those who develop HI; did not correlate to grade of HIE or 2-year ND outcomes[186]
Interferon (IFN)-γ	Abnormal Bayley III scores at 15–18 months[179,185]
Tumor necrosis factor (TNF)-α	Abnormal Bayley III scores at 15–18 months[179,185]
Vascular endothelial growth factor (VEGF)	Abnormal Bayley III scores at 15–18 months[179]

HIE, Hypoxic-ischemic encephalopathy; *MRI*, magnetic resonance imaging; *ND*, Neurodevelopmental.

benzodiazepines provides neuroprotection against functional failure of the blood-brain barrier and neuroinflammation in rodents.[72] Accordingly, the antiseizure effect of benzodiazepines, specifically diazepam, is enhanced by levetiracetam in rodent models of status epilepticus.[73] Of note, the metabolism of levetiracetam during the first 7 days of life changes significantly.[74] The mean half-life of levetiracetam, after a 20- to 40-mg/kg bolus followed by 5 to 10 mg/kg/day as maintenance, decreases between day 1 and 7 of life from 18.5 to 9.1 hours, suggesting that more frequent dosing is required in older infants to maintain stable levels in blood.[74] The effects of TH on the pharmacokinetics of levetiracetam in neonates with NE, specifically HI insult, are unknown. Currently there are no randomized controlled trials (RCTs) studying the neuroprotective effects of levetiracetam in patients suffering from HIE.

Topiramate (Trokendi XR, Qudexy XR, and Topamax)

Case reports suggest that topiramate controls neonatal seizures refractory to phenobarbital and other first-line antiseizure agents.[53,75] Similar to levetiracetam, topiramate has demonstrated neuroprotective effects[76,77] if used immediately after injury at doses of 20 mg/kg, followed by maintenance at 10 mg/kg, in small and large animal models of neonatal HI brain injury.[78,79] Of note, high doses of topiramate (50 mg/kg) increase neuronal death in the white matter after neonatal HI in some of these studies.[79,80] From the few human studies, it is known that the metabolism of topiramate at a dose of 5 mg/kg/day is not altered by moderate hypothermia[81] and does not have significant short-term adverse effects.[82] Except for incidence of epilepsy, which is lower in patients treated with topiramate during TH (NeoNATI trial, NCT01241019), there are no differences in the degree of injury on MRI or in blindness, hearing loss, or neurodevelopmental disability at 18 to 24 months of age.[83] However, the most significant limitation of this RCT is the small sample size (n = 44); thus the result of the other ongoing phase 1 and phase 2 RCTs (NCT01765218) may provide additional information about the safety and neuroprotective effects of this drug.

Shivering Control

Shivering exacerbates brain injury in large animal models of neonatal HI brain injury,[84] likely due to increased glucose metabolism.[85] Morphine is often used to control shivering in the setting of NE in many neonatal intensive care units, following the protocols used in large RCTs. However, opiates do not specifically target the mechanism of shivering and have significant adverse effects including respiratory depression, hypotension, and later withdrawal, effects that are potentiated due to impaired clearance during TH after an HI insult.[86] α-2-Agonist agents such as clonidine or dexmedetomidine control shivering and thus may be potential adjuvant therapies to TH.[87,88] Although studies are limited, treatment with clonidine has been shown to decrease brain injury after neonatal HI in rodents.[89] Similarly, neonatal clonidine treatment delays the development of epilepsy kindling in rodent models.[90] One phase 1/2 RCT studying clonidine in NE has been completed supporting the safety of intravenous (IV) clonidine up to 1 μg/kg/dose every 8 hours in neonates receiving TH, with

Table 47.5 Management of Multiorgan Failure by Systems

	Associated Diagnosis/ Comorbidity	Pathophysiology/Clinical Signs	Management
Respiratory	Meconium aspiration syndrome/ respiratory failure	Meconium-stained amniotic fluid → aspiration Respiratory distress/hypoxemia	Support oxygenation and ventilation to achieve normoxemia and normocarbia Adjust blood gas values based on temperature during TH[187–190]
	Central apnea	Injury to respiratory control centers (brainstem injury—severe HI injury)[191] Respiratory depression secondary to medications (antiepileptic, sedation) Seizures	Mechanical ventilation Close monitoring of blood gases
Cardiovascular	Myocardial ischemia and dysfunction[192–194]	Ischemia to myocardium → ventricular dysfunction → shock/hypotension[192] Elevated cardiac enzymes (troponin I or CKMB)[192]	Echocardiogram Pressor support for hypotension/shock
	Persistent pulmonary hypertension	Initial hypoxia prevents normal relaxation of pulmonary vascular bed → pulmonary hypertension Hypoxemia associated with longer length of stay and higher mortality[195]	Pulmonary vasodilators Extracorporal membrane oxygenation[196–200]
Fluid, electrolytes, nutrition, gastrointestinal	Fluid overload	Fluid resuscitation Acute kidney injury	Gentle fluid restriction (60–80mL/kg/day) Monitor urine output, electrolytes, and weight
	Nutrition/feeding	Ischemic gut injury	NPO Total parenteral nutrition[201] Some evidence that small-volume enteral feeds may be safe in stable infants during TH[202,203]
	Hepatic injury	Ischemic liver injury → elevated liver enzymes (peak 24–72 hours after injury, normalize in 6–12 days)[204,205] Synthetic dysfunction → coagulopathy	Monitoring liver enzymes and coagulation studies Correct coagulopathy with products
	Electrolyte disarray[8,11]	Hypo- or hyperglycemia (adrenal insufficiency, or stress response) Hypocalcemia (intracellular influx during excitotoxicity) Hypercalcemia (secondary to decrease influx in patients receiving TH) Hypomagnesemia (consumption or renal loss)	Aim for euglycemia Both hypo- and hyperglycemia have been associated with worse ND outcomes[127,206] Electrolyte management with supplementation and TPN
Hematology	Coagulopathy	Liver injury → synthetic dysfunction → coagulopathy	Closely monitor clotting studies in the first 48–72 hours (PT, PTT, INR, fibrinogen) Transfuse products (FFP, cryoprecipitate) as needed Goal INR <2 or if symptomatic[203]
	Thrombocytopenia	Bone marrow suppression secondary to ischemia Effects of therapeutic hypothermia[207]	Monitor platelet counts Transfuse for platelets <50,000 or bleeding (transfusion thresholds unit dependent and controversial)[208]
	Leukopenia	Bone marrow suppression secondary to ischemia	Monitor CBC with differential
Renal	Acute kidney injury	HI injury to kidney → ATN → oliguria → fluid overload and electrolyte disarray[192,209,210]	Close monitoring of urine output, electrolytes, weight, and creatinine (peaks in first 24–48 hours, declines over next week)[211] Gentle fluid restriction Nephrology consultation and follow-up[211,212] AKI associated with worse ND outcomes[209,213]
	Syndrome of inappropriate antidiuretic hormone	CNS HI injury → disordered release of ADH → oliguria/hyponatremia	Fluid restriction and sodium correction Close monitoring of urine output, electrolytes, weight
Neurologic	Shivering/sedation	Shivering during TH—may increase metabolic rate → counteract neuroprotective effects of TH[84,214] Agitation (especially in acute phase of mild HIE)	Use of routine sedation is controversial and practices vary Morphine is most commonly used and some data show improved ND outcomes[215] Other medications (clonidine, dexmedetomidine) are being studied[91,99]
Immunologic, infectious disease	Sepsis	Maternal and neonatal infection is a risk factor for/is associated with HIE[216] NE has been linked to worse injury[217,218] and ND outcomes[219] TH may not be as neuroprotective in the context of infection[195]	Infectious work-up as clinically indicated

ADH, antidiuretic hormone; *AKI*, acute kidney injury; *CBC*, complete blood count; *CKMB*, creatine kinase-MB; *CNS*, central nervous system; *FFP*, fresh frozen plasma; *HI*, hypoxic-ischemic; *INR*, international normalized ratio; *NE*, neonatal encephalopathy; *NPO*, nil per os; *PT*, prothrombin time; *PTT*, partial thromboplastin time; *TH*, therapeutic hypothermia; *TPN*, total parenteral nutrition.

decreased need for morphine PRN (NCT01862250),[91] and a second RCT is still enrolling (SANNI project, NCT03177980).

A second α-2-agonist agent under evaluation is dexmedetomidine. The results in different rodent models of perinatal brain injury and analysis of neurodegeneration suggest dexmedetomidine has neuroprotective properties,[92–96] with an unknown link to the control of shivering. However, in a piglet model of neonatal HI, dexmedetomidine at clinically relevant doses (loading of 2 μg/kg at 10 minutes followed by 0.028 μg/kg/h for 48 hours) and plasma levels (within 1 μg/L) in combination with 48 hours of TH produced significant cardiovascular instability, increased mortality, and worsened neuronal death.[97] Additionally, in a case report, dexmedetomidine (without TH) was temporally associated with development of seizures in an infant diagnosed with NE.[98] An early phase 1 clinical study assessing the pharmacokinetics of dexmedetomidine (the Cool DEX study; NCT02529202) demonstrated slower rise in dexmedetomidine in patients receiving TH, with a good safety profile up to a dose of 0.4 μg/k/h.[99] Until more safety data are available, caution must be exercised in the routine use of dexmedetomidine and clonidine.

Future Adjuvant Therapies

A search in the World Health Organization's International Clinical Trials Registry Platform (http://apps.who.int/trialsearch/default.aspx, which includes studies in the US-based www.clinicaltrials.gov) using the search term "neonatal encephalopathy" provided information about 36 unique active clinical trials worldwide (Table 47.6). Therapies with greater progress toward translation to the clinical arena are summarized in more detail in the following sections and in Figs. 47.2 and 47.3.

Epoetin-α/Darbepoetin-α

In the phase 1 multicenter open-label dose-escalation (NEAT) study (NCT00719407), Wu et al. reported that epoetin-α (EPO) at 1000 U/kg/dose IV along with TH was well tolerated and produced plasma levels similar to those needed for neuroprotection in animal models, without serious side effects in infants with NE.[100,101] EPO clearance is slower than in infants not treated with TH.[100] In a phase 2 RCT (NCT01913340), a similar dose of EPO on days 1, 2, 3, 5, and 7 decreased injury size shown on brain MRI and improved 1-year outcomes.[102,103] Neuroprotection by EPO appears to be more robust in asphyxiated infants whose placentas do not show chronic changes.[104] However, EPO treatment in this population does not change the upregulation of S100B, Tau, ubiquitin carboxy-terminal hydrolase-L1, and proinflammatory cytokines 24 hours after the insult, which was associated with injury on MRI, and did not prevent the downregulation of brain derived neurotrophic factor levels 5 days after the insult, which was associated with worse neurodevelopmental outcomes at age 1.[105] A recent systemic review including nine RCTs concluded that EPO is neuroprotective, improving long-term neurobehavioral outcomes in neonates receiving TH for HIE.[106] Two large, multicenter RCTs, one in the United States and a second in Australia, are ongoing. The HEAL trial (USA, NCT02811263) found that administration of erythropoietin during therapeutic hypothermia did not lower the risk of death or neurodevelopmental deficits at 22–36 months of age.[106a] The PAEAN trial (Australia, NCT03079167) included 300 infants and closed enrollment in December 2021.

Longer-acting darbepoetin-α (DARBE) is biologically similar to EPO.[107] DARBE clearance is inversely correlated to gestational age in infants treated with TH for NE.[108] In a phase 1 and 2 RCT (DANCE trial; NCT0147015), DARBE treatment at either 2 or 10 μg/kg IV started within 12 hours of life, with a second dose at 7 days of life, had a similar safety profile to placebo.[109] Other results have not been reported thus far. Because 39% of infants with mild encephalopathy have an abnormal EEG, brain MRI, or neurologic exam at discharge and 25% had disabilities at age 5 years in the PRIME study (NCT01747863),[27,110] the MEND study (NCT03071861) is studying the effect of DARBE alone in a cohort of 40 newborns with mild encephalopathy. Enrollment for this study closed in October 2019.

Caffeine

Caffeine is a nonspecific adenosine receptor antagonist and a phosphodiesterase inhibitor that produces immunomodulatory effects[111–115] and provides protection against cerebral palsy and bronchopulmonary dysplasia in premature infants.[116–119] The effects of caffeine in full-term infants are not well characterized. Although near-term and full-term rodent models of neonatal HI suggest that caffeine is a potential neuroprotectant,[120–122] the side effects of blocking the effects of adenosine in preventing injury by hypoxia need consideration.[123–125] No large-animal data are available. A phase 1 clinical trial (NCT03913221) closed in June 2021 after enrolling 18 neonates cooled for NE and treated with a load of caffeine citrate at 20 mg/kg followed by 2 doses of 5 or 10 mg/kg/day IV. Further studies are needed.

Magnesium Sulfate

Perinatal magnesium sulfate supplementation is neuroprotective in preterm infants by attenuating excitotoxicity,[126] but its use in full-term infants suffering from NE remains controversial. Although magnesium blood levels are lower in neonates suffering HIE than in controls,[127] the results from animal studies using magnesium supplementation are inconsistent and confounded by magnesium-induced hypothermia.[128] Magnesium-induced hypothermia and control of shivering need further study as an alternative in low-resource regions of the world, where TH is not feasible.[129,130] Combinatorial studies are including magnesium sulfate. A feasibility study in Japan reported no adverse effects in the use of EPO at 300 U/kg, magnesium sulfate at 250 mg/kg, and TH for 72 hours in 9 patients with NE.[131] Magnesium sulfate-enhanced TH (NCT02499393) was a phase 2 and 3 RCT with a prospected enrollment of 75 neonates with pending results. A major consideration when using postnatal magnesium sulfate in patients suffering from NE is a published trend toward greater mortality and morbidity.[132,133]

Sildenafil

In rodent models of HI brain injury, sildenafil promotes recovery by enhancing neurogenesis and inducing collateral vessel patency.[134–136] Sildenafil also decreases the size of injury in a rodent stroke model via antiinflammatory mechanisms.[137] In humans, sildenafil at a 2 mg/kg/dose twice daily from day of life 2 to 9 is being tested in 80 participants with HIE treated with TH in the SANE trial, a phase 1 clinical trial (NCT02812433; Canada) with a prospected end date of June 2022. However, extreme caution should be exercised in the use of sildenafil; overdoses of >3 mg/kg/day increased mortality in RCTs for persistent pulmonary hypertension (PPHN).[138]

Autologous Cord Blood

Autologous transfusion of stem cells from cord blood has significant therapeutic potential in developmental brain injury from NE,

Table 47.6 List of Registered Clinical Trials to Study Adjuvant Therapies to Therapeutic Hypothermia

NCT Number (Date of Completion)	Phase Sample Size Randomized (Masking)	Primary Outcomes	Secondary Outcomes	References
Epoietin				
NCT02811263 (09/22/2019)	3 500 Y (Q)	Death or neurodevelopmental impairment at 22–26 months of age	• Cerebral palsy • Level of gross motor function (GMFCS) • Bayley III cognitive and language scores • Epilepsy • Behavioral abnormalities (Child Behavior Checklist)	Wu et al.[100] Wu et al.[102] Juul et al.[220]
NCT01913340 (09/01/2016)	1 & 2 50 Y (Q)	Markers of organ function	• Alberta Infant Motor Score (AIMS) at 12 months of age	Wu et al.[100] Wu et al.[102] Mulkey et al.[103]
NCT00719407 (11/01/2012)	1 24 N	Serious adverse event within 14 days of life	• Pharmacokinetic parameters	Wu et al.[100] Rogers et al.[221] Shankaran et al.[222]
NCT02499393 (12/01/2014)	2 & 3 75 Y (N)	Death to discharge	• Neurologic status within 7 days and 2 years	Merchant et al.[223]
NCT03163589 (06/01/2020)	3 40 Y (N)	Death or long-term major neurodevelopmental disability according to Griffith score at age 1	• Cerebral palsy • Epilepsy • Brain injury in MRI at 2–3 weeks of age • Brain injury in EEG at 1 week of life • Adverse effect of EPO at age 1 • Seizure until 2 weeks of life	Murray et al.[13] Frymoyer et al.[101] Kurinczuk et al.[224] Jacobs et al.[225] Zacharias et al.[226] Zhu et al.[227] Elmahdy et al.[228] Cirelli et al.[229] Bednarek et al.[230]
NCT03079167 (12/01/2021)	3 300 Y (Q)	Composite measure of death or moderate/severe disability at age 2	• Death by age 2 • Cerebral palsy • Moderate/severe motor deficit • Moderate/severe cognitive deficit • Supplemental respiratory support • Supplemental nutritional support • Major cortical visual impairment • Requirement for hearing aids • Autism spectrum disorder • Epilepsy • Cost of healthcare and service use • Frequency of selected adverse events by 30 days of age	No results posted
NCT01732146 (12/01/2017)	3 120 Y (T)	Survival without neurologic sequelae at age 2	• Mortality rates • Rate of moderate and severe sequelae • Aspect of brain lesions on MRI • Tolerance of treatment	Zhu et al.[227] Goodarzi et al.[231]
NCT01471015 (01/01/2014)	1&2 30 Y (T)	Pharmacokinetic profile of darbe after the first and second dose	• Adverse events until hospital discharge	Roberts et al.[108] Baserga et al.[109] Rogers et al.[221] Rangarajan et al.[232] Davidson et al.[233] Juul et al,[234] Nair et al.[235] Larpthaveesarp et al.[236] Messier et al.[237] Schober et al.[238]

NCT Number (Date of Completion)	Phase Sample Size Randomized (Masking)	Primary Outcomes	Secondary Outcomes	References
NCT03071861 (No reported)	2 40 Y (Q)	Neurodevelopmental outcome at age 1	• Adverse events • Seizure • Gavage or gastrostomy at discharge home • Ages and Stages Questionnaire • Height measurement • Weight measurement • Head circumference measurement	No results posted
Caffeine				
NCT03913221 (06/01/2021)	1 18 N	Area under plasma concentration-time for caffeine	• Incidence of seizures and necrotizing enterocolitis • Abnormal MRI brain findings based on NICHD Neonatal Research Network score • Bayley Scales of Infant Development (BSID-III) cognitive, language, or motor composite score <85 at age 2	Shankaran et al.[239]
Magnesium sulfate				
NCT02499393 (12/01/2014)	2 & 3 75 Y (N)	Death	• Neurologic status during first 7 days of life and at 24 months of age	Davidson et al.[223]
Sildenafil				
NCT02812433 (06/01/2022)	1 80 Y (Q)	Serious adverse events between day 1–14	• Plasmatic concentrations of sildenafil and N-desmethyl sildenafil from day 2–10	No results posted
Autologous cord blood				
NCT00593242 (01/01/2017)	1 52 N	Adverse event rates	• Preliminary efficacy as measured by neurodevelopmental function at 4–6 months and 9–12 months of age • Neuroimaging at age 6 months	Cotten et al.[142]
NCT02256618 (02/01/2018)	1 6 N	Adverse event rates during the first 3 days of life	• Efficacy at 18 months of age	Tsuji et al.[240] Ohshima et al.[241] Taguchi et al.[242]
NCT02551003 (12/01/2019)	1 & 2 60 Y (S)	Mortality and disability rate	• Bayley subscales and structural injury on MRI • Levels of IL-1β and TNF-α in serum	No results posted
NCT02881970 (09/01/2020)	1 & 2 20 N	Adverse clinical or paraclinical event rates	• Preliminary efficacy as measured by neurodevelopmental function	No results posted
NCT02434965 (1/01/2022)	2 20 N	Infusion reaction as a measure of safety and tolerability	• Improvement in neurologic condition at age 2	No results posted
NCT03352310 (12/01/2020)	1 40 N	Mortality rate Change from baseline hematocrit	• Hammersmith Infant Neurologic Examination • Griffiths Mental Development Scale • Child Behavior Checklist for Attention Deficit	No results posted

Continued

Table 47.6 List of Registered Clinical Trials to Study Adjuvant Therapies to Therapeutic Hypothermia—Cont'd

NCT Number (Date of Completion)	Phase Sample Size Randomized (Masking)	Primary Outcomes	Secondary Outcomes	References
Melatonin				
NCT02621944 (01/01/2022)	1 40 N	Tolerance to maximum dose of melatonin Bayley-III Index Scores Peak plasma concentration (Cmax) of melatonin	• Bayley-III Index Scores subscales at 18–20 months • MRI results between 7–12 days	No results posted
NCT03806816 (12/01/2022)	1 & 2 100 Y (S)	Bayley III scale	• Brain MRI • Continuous aEEG • Plasma concentration of melatonin • ATG5 plasma concentration	No results posted
Allopurinol				
NCT03162653 (12/01/2020)	3 846 Y (Q)	Death or severe neurodevelopmental impairment versus survival without severe neurodevelopmental impairment at age 2	• Death or neurodevelopmental impairment and/or death • Cerebral palsy • GMFCS score • Subscale scores (Bayley III)	Maiwald et al.[149]

aEEG, Amplitude integrated electroencephalogram; *EPO*, epoetin; *D*, double masking; *Darbe*, darbepoetin; *MRI*, magnetic resonance imaging; *N*, nonrandomized; *Q*, quadruple masking; *R*, randomized; *S*, single masking; *T*, triple masking; *Y*, randomized.

traumatic brain injury, and hydrocephalus.[139–141] Feasibility and safety of fresh autologous cord blood cells have been confirmed in 23 infants treated with TH for NE.[142,143] In this trial (NCT0593242), 74% of cell-recipient infants survived with neurodevelopmental (Bayley III) scores >85 at 1 year versus only 41% of concurrent infants treated with TH alone.[142] The final report of phase 1 for this trial including 52 participants is not available as of yet, but the follow-up multisite phase 2 study (NCT02612155), which planned to enroll 160 participants, was suspended in June 2019 for low enrollment (funding was withdrawn). Several other RCTs are ongoing, including NCT02551003 (phase 1 and 2; 60 participants by December 2019; China), NCT02256618 or JPRN-UMIN000014903 (phase 1; 6 participants by February 2018; Japan), NCT02881970 (phase 1 and 2; 20 participants by September 2020; France), NCT02434965 (phase 2; 20 participants by January 2022; United States), and NCT03352310 (phase 1; 40 participants by December 2020; China).

Melatonin

In piglets, melatonin at 5 mg/kg/h for 6 hours started 10 minutes after resuscitation followed by a second dose 24 hours later augmented the neuroprotection provided by TH alone, as assessed by MR spectroscopy and histology.[144] In a prospective RCT including 15 healthy controls, 15 patients with NE treated with TH, and 15 patients treated with TH and melatonin (5 daily doses of 10 mg/kg), melatonin decreased the incidence of seizures on EEG and white matter injury on MRI at 5 days of life and improved neurodevelopmental outcomes at 6 months of age.[145] Several clinical trials are ongoing. An early phase 1 dose escalation study (NCT02621944) will enroll 40 infants cooled for NE and receiving melatonin at doses between 0.5 and 5 mg/kg, monitoring for adverse events and neurodevelopment at 18 to 24 months, recruitment is ongoing. The MELPRO study (NCT03806816) plans to enroll 100 participants by December 2022.

Allopurinol

Allopurinol is an inhibitor of xanthine oxidase and dehydrogenase. Because allopurinol crosses the placenta, prenatal strategies may be effective. In a clinical trial (NCT00189007), 58 pregnant women developing evidence of fetal hypoxia during labor received 500 mg of allopurinol IV immediately prior to delivery, which resulted in plasma concentrations ≥2 mg/L (therapeutic for antioxidant effect) in more than 95% of the newborns by 5 minutes after maternal infusion was finished.[146] The phase 3 clinical trial showed no benefit of the prenatal intervention; however, the neurodevelopmental follow-up was greatly limited and likely underpowered (138 out of 222 participants).[147] Postnatal allopurinol at 40 mg/kg within 4 hours after birth followed by a second dose 12 hours later similarly did not provide overall protection against NE except in the subset of patients with moderate encephalopathy.[148] The ALBINO study (NCT03162653) is a quadruple-blinded phase 3 RCT evaluating allopurinol in two IV doses (20 mg/kg within 30 minutes of life followed 12 hours later by 10 mg/kg) in 846 infants treated with TH for NE.[149] A caveat is that mannitol is the placebo in the control group, and mannitol is not the standard of care in most neonatal intensive care units in the setting of hypoxia-ischemia. Although mannitol adds no benefit to treatment of cerebral edema in infants with NE,[150] mannitol may open the blood-brain barrier with undefined effects in this vulnerable population.[151]

Others

Cannabinoids

Cannabidiol (CBD) may be neuroprotective based on data derived from small-animal models.[152–154] Although in studies in lambs, using WIN55212-2 (a cannabinoid agonist) decreased apoptotic cell death after partial umbilical cord occlusion, studies in anesthetized piglets undergoing HI showed conflicting results. Pazos et al. reported decreased excitotoxicity, oxidative stress, and inflammation using low CBD doses (1 mg/kg IV) without TH.[154] To the contrary, Garberg et al. reported no neuroprotection by CBD at 1 mg/kg or with higher doses (10, 25, or 50 mg/kg) IV, although TH was neuroprotective.[155,156] There are no ongoing clinical trials.

Nanoparticles

The blood-brain barrier limits the delivery of drugs to the central nervous system and thus their effectiveness in the treatment of many neurologic disorders. Nanoparticles created by ligating pharmacologic agents to dendrimers may overcome this limitation.[157,158] Thus it is not surprising that these constructs are being used to deliver antiinflammatory agents (e.g., N-acetylcysteine [NAC], polyamidoamine [PAMAM]) directly to the activated microglia after neonatal HI brain injury in animal models.[159] Additionally, dendrimer nanoparticles also have transplacental effects, decreasing markers of inflammation in mouse models of intrauterine infection, preterm birth, and perinatal brain injury.[160] These constructs are an effective and efficient way to deliver drugs and may also be a platform to deliver gene therapy.[161] Nanoparticles are a new frontier for the treatment of perinatal brain injury and the resulting sequelae.[162] No clinical trials are registered to this date.

Postacute Care Follow-Up

To determine the most appropriate postacute care plan after NE, the provider needs to answer three main questions: (1) Was the etiology established? (2) Did the patient respond reasonably well to the therapy? and (3) Are there any persistent symptoms to manage? All of these questions must be answered in a rigorous manner by the neonatologist along with a multidisciplinary team that includes a pediatric neuroradiologist, pediatric neurologist, and epileptologist along with neurodevelopment and neurophysiology specialists and occupational and physical therapy.[163] The role of an experienced pharmacologist in assisting the neonatologist in monitoring of medications in neonates whose metabolism may be impaired needs special attention.[164]

Etiology

Hypoxic-ischemic brain injury represents 50% of all cases of NE. If evidence of a perinatal event, findings from brain MRI, and results in the full montage continuous video EEG all suggest HIE, then no further diagnostic evaluation may be needed. If any of these pieces of evidence suggest another potential etiology for NE, then specific follow-up and further work-up are needed. As a general rule, after the first full neonatal MRI with DWI, diffusion tensor imaging, and susceptibility weighted imaging has been performed, follow-up MRI after discharge is not needed unless clinically indicated (e.g., significant neurodevelopmental impairments not explained by previous brain MRI and concerns for secondary stroke or brain injury, among others). If a stroke, arterial or venous, is identified in the DWI with apparent diffusion coefficient sequence,[165] then additional imaging with MRA and MRV may be necessary to clearly identify the distribution. A pediatric hematology consult is necessary only when a strong suspension for a hypercoagulable state exists; however, as a general rule for neonatal arterial ischemic stroke, studies for thrombophilia and other disorders of the coagulation system are not recommended acutely.[165] Infectious causes need to be ruled out prior to discharge from the hospital, with an appropriate diagnostic battery (e.g., lumbar tap, blood titers, and brain imaging) for timely treatment. Genetic and metabolic disorders, which typically present with a picture of NE out of proportion to the perinatal history, may have specific MRI and EEG patterns. When these etiologies are suspected, a genetics consultant should be involved to recommend further work-up and management.

Clinical Progress

Rapid normalization of abnormal EEG patterns and cerebral edema assessed by a head ultrasound are markers of good prognosis. Although all patients diagnosed with NE and treated with TH need neurodevelopmental and early intervention follow-up, those with persistent, late, or ongoing neonatal seizures also need follow-up by a pediatric neurologist. Monitoring of the neurologic exam has significant prognostic value. No improvement in muscle tone, activity, and feeding after weaning off sedation is a marker of poor prognosis.[166]

Persistent Deficits

Persistent hypotonia and impaired per os feeding are well-known markers of serious neurodevelopmental impairment.[167] Similarly, autonomic manifestations such as apnea, temperature dysregulation, and arrhythmia are manifestations of severe injury and may increase mortality.[168] Hearing and vision impairment occur in 8% to 10% of survivors, and TH does not prevent these deficits.[169,170] Similarly, cognitive and memory impairments are not attenuated by TH.[171,172]

CHAPTER 48

Management of Encephalopathy of Prematurity

Sandra E. Juul, Niranjana Natarajan, Ulrike Mietzsch

KEY POINTS

1. Encephalopathy of prematurity reflects white and gray matter injury combined with neuronal-axonal abnormalities impacting preterm infants.
2. Key risk factors include hypotension and the need for inotropes, hypoxia, and inflammation.
3. Evaluation of high-risk infants in the neonatal intensive care unit (NICU) includes use of neuroimaging and neurobehavioral assessments such as the General Movements Assessment.
4. Management starts prior to birth and continues throughout the NICU stay and is geared toward prevention and treatment of risk factors.
5. After NICU discharge, management is geared toward use of developmental surveillance, parental support, and physical and occupational therapy.

Introduction

Encephalopathy of prematurity is the result of altered brain development and brain injury after preterm birth. The term "encephalopathy of prematurity" describes a phenomenon that results from a variety of different pathophysiologic factors that occur either alone or in combination. These affect the development and maturation of white and gray matter, both of which undergo crucial development during the third trimester.[1–4] Infants at highest risk are very low birth weight infants (<1500 g) and to a greater extent extremely low birth weight infants (<1000 g). Periventricular leukomalacia (PVL) combined with neuronal-axonal injury is the hallmark of encephalopathy of prematurity.[4,5] These findings can be seen either in isolation or in conjunction with other forms of preterm brain injury, such as periventricular-intraventricular hemorrhage, intraparenchymal hemorrhage, or cerebellar injury.[6]

White matter involvement can be focal or diffuse, both involving damage to the preoligodendrocytes and disruption of developmental myelination. Consequences of this white matter injury include motor deficits such as cerebral palsy, affecting about 5% to 10% of very low birth weight infants and much more commonly visual, cognitive, and neurobehavioral abnormalities including autism, which can be seen in up to 25% to 50% of patients.[7] Although white matter injury most commonly affects infants born prior to 32 weeks' gestation, similar injury patterns have been associated with intrauterine chronic hypoxic states including placental insufficiency and cyanotic heart disease.

As implied by the name, encephalopathy of prematurity affects mainly preterm infants. The overall rate of prematurity, defined as birth before 37 weeks of gestation, is 10.6% worldwide; of those, 15.4% are born before 32 weeks' gestation.[8] In the United States, the rate of preterm birth decreased from 12.5% in 2004 to a low of 9.57% in 2014 but has since increased to 10.0% in 2018, with a stable rate of birth before 32 weeks of 2.75%.[9–11]

The incidence of cystic PVL has decreased overtime, but diffuse white matter injury remains prevalent and is now the most common manifestation of encephalopathy of prematurity. The incidence of any degree of white matter injury has been reported in some studies to be as high as 72%.[12] Abnormal neurodevelopmental outcome is strongly correlated to the degree of white matter injury, in particular moderate to severe white matter injury.[12–14]

Pathophysiology

White Matter Injury

Periventricular leukomalacia is the hallmark of encephalopathy of prematurity, defined by the pathologic characteristics of focal necrosis in the periventricular area combined with diffuse reactive gliosis and activation of microglia cells in the surrounding white matter. Large areas of necrosis (>1 mm) may evolve over weeks into macroscopic cysts, termed cystic PVL.[4] This occurs in less than 5% of preterm infants in the current era. Diffuse PVL is characterized by small focal necrotic areas measuring ≤1mm, surrounded by reactive astrocytosis and microgliosis. These smaller or microscopic areas of necrosis, caused by injury to immature oligodendrocytes, evolve into glial scars. Punctate white matter lesions and diffuse white matter injury represent the most common imaging manifestations of white matter injury.[2] Both patterns result in damage to the preoligodendrocytes and thus result in impaired maturation of preoligodendrocytes and dysfunctional oligodendrocytes. Oligodendrocytes derive from neuroglial stem cells, which differentiate sequentially into oligodendrocyte precursors and premyelinating oligodendrocytes before becoming mature myelinating oligodendrocytes.[15] As a result, hypomyelination can be observed. Myelin surrounds the axons and facilitates signal transmission and developmental migration. Abnormal myelination can result in axonal damage and modification of the white matter tracts.[16–18] Oligodendrocytes also play an important role in axonal development, and impaired function of the mature oligodendrocyte has been associated with abnormal axonal development.[19,20]

Neuronal-Axonal Injury

White matter injury has historically been described as an appearance of cysts alongside the ventricles, termed cystic PVL, occurring

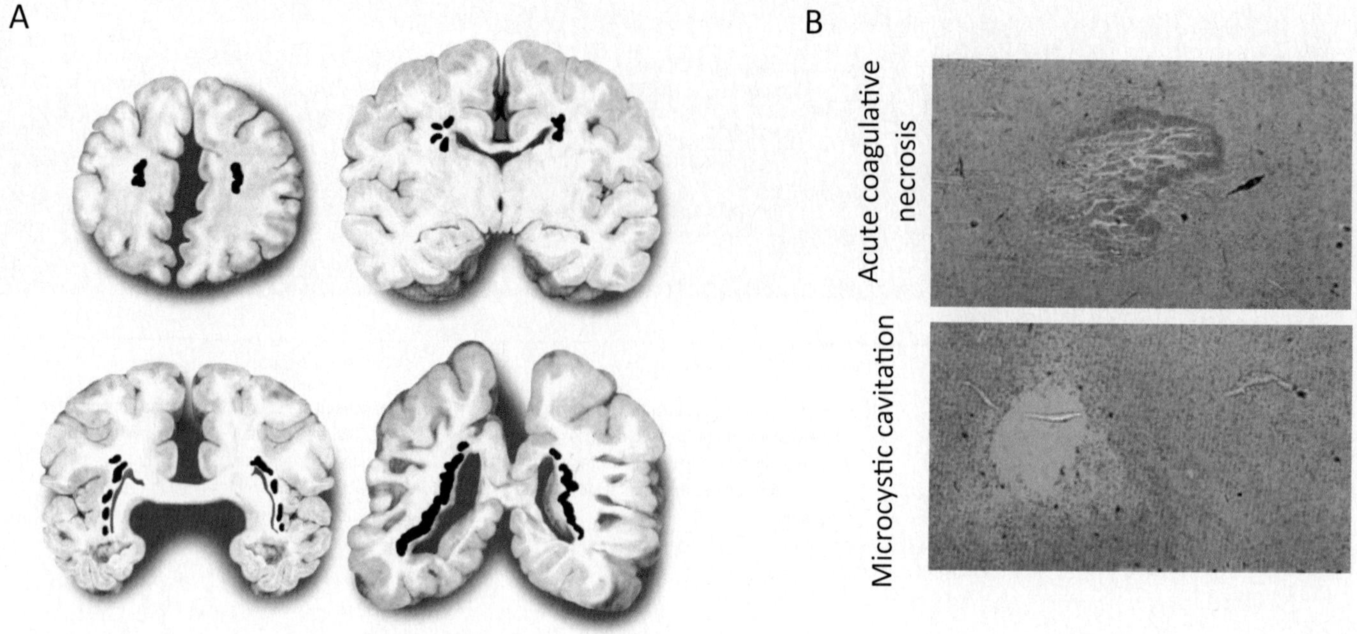

Fig. 48.1 Periventricular Leukomalacia. (A) Topographic location *(solid black ovals)*. (B) Focal necrosis <2 mm in periventricular white matter. (Reproduced with permission from Kinney and Volpe. Encephalopathy of prematurity: neuropathology. In: *Volpe's Neurology of the Newborn*; ch. 14, 389–404.)

approximately 10 days to 2 weeks after an insult. These cysts may disappear over the following weeks, replaced with glial tissue, which can be detected on later brain magnetic resonance imaging (MRI) as diffuse white matter lesions, now the most common form of preterm brain injury (Fig. 48.1).[21] Several risk factors have been associated with a higher risk of PVL, including hypoxia-ischemia, prolonged hypercapnia, inflammatory states, and transient impairment of cerebrovascular autoregulation.[22]

A combination of neuronal and axonal injury is commonly found in conjunction with PVL.[23] White matter injury can generate abnormalities in the gray matter as a result of terminal axonal injury. Axonal guidance is required for developing and migrating neurons to reach their target destination. Interruption of such guides results in abnormal migration, most commonly seen as reduction of neurons and pyramidal cells in cortical layer V.

One of the underlying pathophysiologic mechanisms of preterm brain injury is related to impaired cerebrovascular autoregulation and the resulting pressure passive state. Cerebrovascular autoregulation refers to the ability to maintain a stable cerebral blood flow independent of systemic blood pressure. This mechanism, however, is not fully developed in preterm infants and may result in a pressure-passive state where systemic blood flow correlates linearly with cerebral blood flow (Fig. 48.2). This is particularly common in the most critically ill patients.[24–26] The pressure-passive state can be observed in nearly all preterm neonates for some period of time, and the duration of time spent in a pressure-passive state correlates with an increased risk for brain injury. Near infrared spectroscopy in combination with blood pressure monitoring can be used to evaluate cerebral blood flow and thereby identify the infants at highest risk.[27] Predisposing factors for a pressure passive state include extreme prematurity, hypocarbia ($PCO_2 < 30$ mm Hg), and hypercarbia ($PCO_2 > 55$ mm Hg). Three injury types have been described in the setting of impaired cerebral autoregulation: focal cystic necrosis, incidence $\leq 5\%$; focal microscopic necrosis, incidence 15% to 20%; and diffuse nonnecrotic injury, incidence $\geq 50\%$.[28]

Gray Matter Injury

The gray matter component of encephalopathy of prematurity is characterized by neuronal loss combined with reactive gliosis. Synaptic connections formed during brain development are also altered by preterm birth, resulting in altered functional connectivity that persists through adolescence and is a significant risk factor of neurodevelopmental impairment.[29–31]

The patterns of injury are heterogeneous and reflect different types of injury. The disruption of normal cortical development can result in a delay in cortical folding of >2 weeks and volume loss.[14,32] Gray matter lesions are most commonly found in the subcortical area and cerebellum.[23] Fig. 48.2 illustrates the interactions that result in encephalopathy of prematurity. A summary of the mechanisms

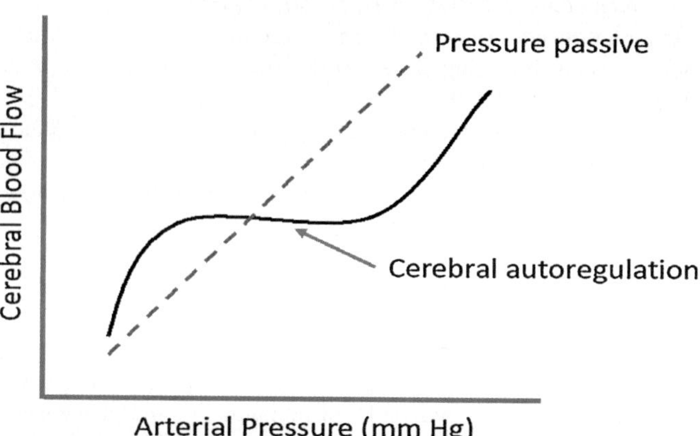

Fig. 48.2 Regulation of Cerebral Blood Flow.

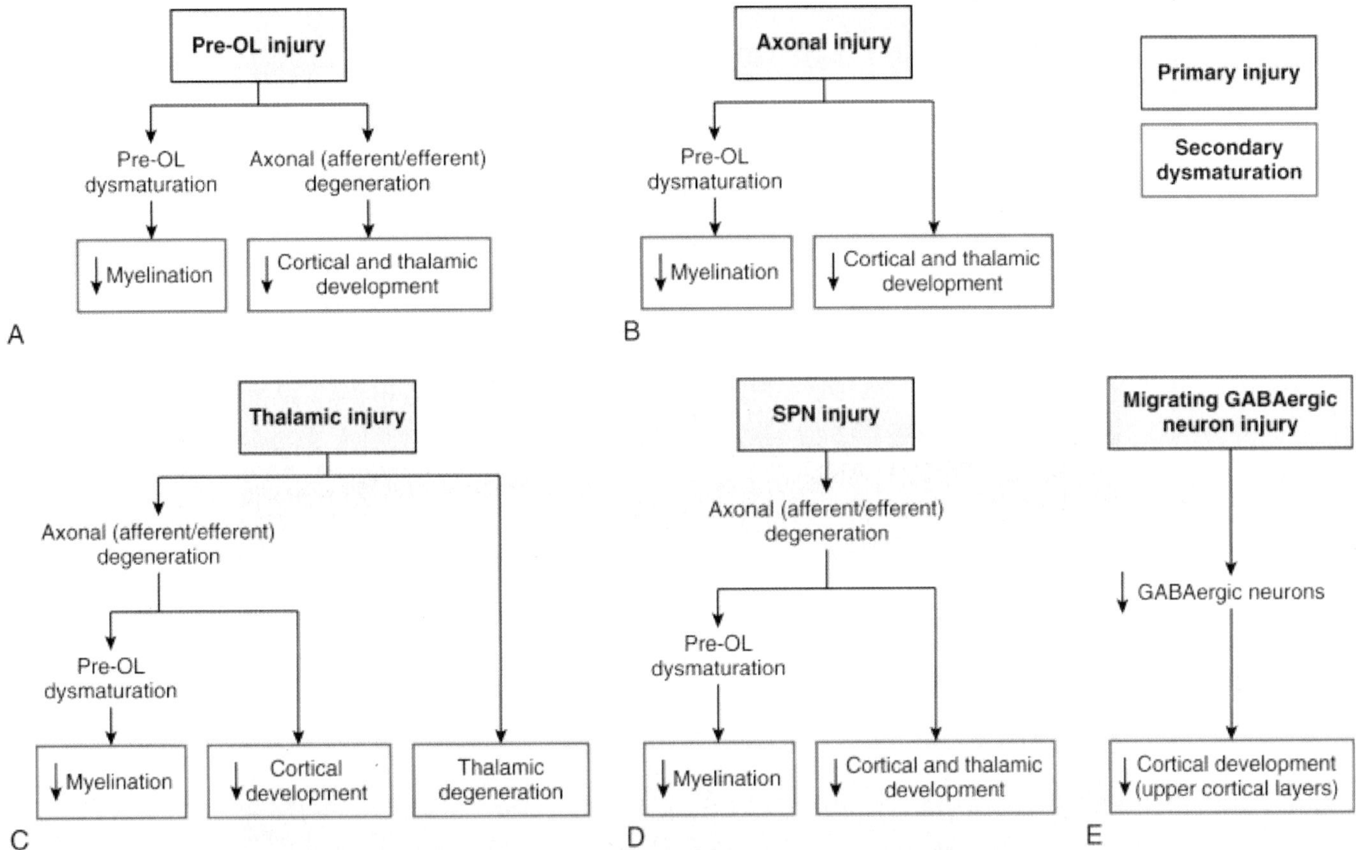

Fig. 48.3 Potential Sequences of Events in Encephalopathy of Prematurity. Each sequence illustrates the progression from primary injury (in *yellow*) to secondary dysmaturational events that lead to structure changes that can be seen on magnetic resonance imaging *(red-outlined boxes)*. *Pre-OL,* Preoligodendrocyte. (Reproduced with permission from Kinney and Volpe. Encephalopathy of prematurity: neuropathology. In: *Volpe's Neurology of the Newborn*; ch. 14, 389–404.)

implicated in the pathogenesis of encephalopathy of prematurity is shown in Fig. 48.3.

Clinical Features and Evaluation

The early clinical features of preterm infants with encephalopathy of prematurity and related white and gray matter abnormalities are often challenging to detect clinically. Thus knowledge of the risk factors associated with encephalopathy of prematurity and routine surveillance methods should be employed to aid in early identification and subsequent management.

Neonates at greatest risk for encephalopathy of prematurity are those exposed to a combination of prenatal and postnatal inflammatory insults, difficult resuscitation, and ongoing hypoxic events as shown in Table 48.1. The risk is inversely related to gestational age. The presence of prolonged premature rupture of membranes or chorioamnionitis and associated inflammatory states is associated with higher risk for PVL.[33,34] Infections, intraventricular hemorrhage (IVH), and seizures during the neonatal intensive care unit (NICU) stay have been associated with impaired motor outcome and higher incidence of PVL.[22,35] Furthermore, infants with periventricular white matter injury are more commonly found to have IVH and seizures.[36] Clinically, routine examination may not clearly detect those neonates who will develop symptomatic encephalopathy of prematurity, and thus heightened awareness of the diagnosis and involvement of ancillary services such as physical, occupational, and feeding therapists is necessary to detect those with subtle features requiring longer-term evaluation.

Clinical and Imaging Evaluation

Examination with the General Movements Assessment (GMA) by a trained professional within the NICU can aid in identifying infants at risk for sequelae of encephalopathy of prematurity. GMA utilizes observation of the spontaneous movements of the newborn at key time points, with the theory that these spontaneous movements provide insight into the integrity of the neurologic system at key

Table 48.1 Neuroprotection Considerations

Prenatal	Perinatal	Postnatal
Magnesium sulfate	Delayed cord clamping	Euglycemia
Antenatal steroids		Caffeine
		Minimize prolonged hypocarbia
		Avoid prolonged hypercarbia

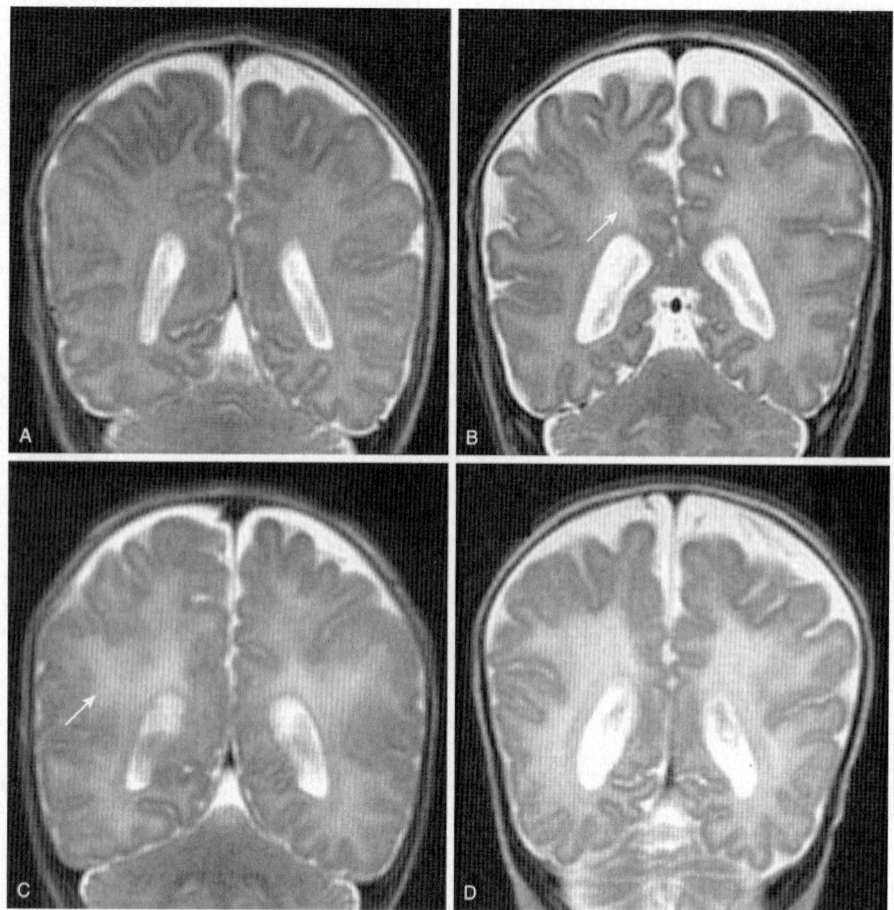

Fig. 48.4 Magnetic Resonance Imaging (MRI) Scans (T2-Weighted) of "Nonnecrotic/Noncystic" Cerebral White Matter Injury in Preterm Infants. (A) A normal scan for comparison. (B) Abnormally increased signal in periventricular regions. (C, D) Extensively increased signal in cerebral white matter or beyond (diffuse excessive high signal intensity). (Reproduced with permission from Kinney and Volpe. Encephalopathy of prematurity: neuropathology. In: *Volpe's Neurology of the Newborn*; ch. 14, 389–404.)

points of early development.[37,38] Work by the Prechtl group suggests that the spontaneous movements of preterm infants are reflective of the cortical subplate and its projections to central pattern generators.[39] Thus, injury to these areas by encephalopathy of prematurity affect the spontaneous movements observed. As the brain matures, the spontaneous movements noted evolve from "writhing movements" that occur until 45 weeks' postmenstrual age to "fidgety movements"; these are typically noted up to 60 weeks' postmenstrual age, theorized to reflect the maturation of projections from the subplate neurons.[39] Absence of fidgety movements on the GMA has been strongly correlated with later development of cerebral palsy,[40] minor neurologic dysfunction,[41,42] attentional disorders, and cognitive disabilities.[43]

Utilization of the GMA in the NICU is increasing because abnormal cramped synchronous movements in the writhing period are associated with abnormal neurodevelopmental outcomes but are less specific compared with abnormalities later with absent fidgety movements in the postneonatal period (48–60 weeks' postmenstrual age), which can be highly predictive for later neurodevelopmental seque lae.[38,40,44–51] Use of this early diagnostic tool can allow for earlier identification and therapeutic intervention for symptomatic infants.

Neuroimaging plays a role in the evaluation of the preterm infant at risk for neurodisability. Although ultrasonography is excellent for detecting IVH and historically was used for detection of cystic periventricular leukomalacia, it is not optimal for detecting noncystic white matter disease or cerebellar injury.[52–54] There is therefore an increasing role for the use of term-equivalent MRI (TE-MRI) in the evaluation of preterm infants to help stratify risk of neurodevelopmental impairment beyond cerebral palsy and cognitive sequelae (Fig. 48.4). White matter injury noted on TE-MRI is predictive of neurodevelopmental impairment in the first years of life.[12,55,56] TE-MRI obtained at or after 36 weeks' postmenstrual age can detect white matter injury including white matter lesions, reduced white matter volumes, reduced gray matter volume, and ventriculomegaly.[4,57] In addition, MRI can detect cerebellar hypoplasia or microhemorrhages typically not well appreciated by ultrasound.

Advanced MRI techniques of diffusion tractography have been studied to look specifically at white matter tracts and the effects of signal changes in long-term development. The corticospinal tracts, corpus callosum, thalamic connections, and optic radiations among other pathways have been evaluated. Changes in diffusivity with lower fractional anisotropy values in the corticospinal tracts and corpus callosum have been associated with lower psychomotor scores on developmental testing.[58]

Diffuse excessive high signal intensity (DEHSI) can be detected on TE-MRI and is reported in up to 75% of preterm infants imaged at term.[59] Because increased white matter signal can be subjective, studies have demonstrated poor inter- and intraobserver reliability[60]; thus researchers have attempted to better grade the extent of high signal abnormality.[61] The significance of DEHSI remains debated, with uncertainty as to whether it represents a developmental state[62] versus a biomarker of later neurocognitive sequelae.[63]

Given the frequency with which DEHSI is identified, there has been interest in determining its relevance for developmental outcome. Several studies have looked at presence or absence of DEHSI, whereas others have looked at DEHSI grading and outcome. Although initial studies demonstrated a correlation between the presence of DEHSI and later neurodevelopmental outcome at 18 to 36 months,[63] multiple studies subsequently did not find that neurodevelopmental outcomes correlated with DEHSI.[59–62,64–66] Newer studies have raised the suggestion that abnormal signal in the posterior crossroads (the posterior periventricular white matter representing commissural white matter pathways and projection associations) may correlate with outcome; however, this remains uncertain.[64,67]

Utilization of TE-MRIs for all preterm neonates remains controversial,[68,69] with some families of former preterm infants noting the adverse psychological impact of this knowledge on the family[70,71] and others questioning the added value of such a study over ultrasound. Although white matter injury on TE-MRI correlates with adverse neurodevelopmental outcome, a significant cohort of patients with white matter injury do not manifest significant developmental impacts.[12,55,72] Concomitant use of a neurologic exam marginally increases both the positive and negative predictive values for neurodevelopmental outcome.[73] A TE-MRI with normal or minor abnormalities in conjunction with a normal neurologic exam can marginally increase the negative predictive value for a later reassuring standardized neurologic exam (from 99% to 100%), suggesting that a reassuring MRI and exam together would portend a favorable outcome. In contrast, a TE-MRI with moderate or severe abnormalities alone has a positive predictive value for neurologic impairment at 2 years of age of 27%. With an abnormal neurologic exam at discharge, the positive predictive value for neurologic impairment at 2 years of age increases to 35%.[73] Ultimately, TE-MRI can provide insight into those patients at risk for developing cerebral palsy and neurocognitive sequelae and, if obtained, should be used to advocate for early introduction of physical and occupational therapy through early intervention services and close neurodevelopmental surveillance while acknowledging the uncertainty that remains regarding outcome. Discussion with both clinicians and caregivers regarding MRI should acknowledge the limitations of imaging in prognostication. A combination of MRI findings and GMA may further refine prediction, and if abnormal, heighten concern for sequelae from prematurity such as cerebral palsy,[46,74,75] promoting early referral to therapy services.

Management

Management of the neonate at risk for encephalopathy of prematurity is multipronged and includes neuroprotective measures prenatally and in the NICU and long-term follow-up with developmental therapies.

Prenatal Treatments: Antenatal Corticosteroids and Magnesium Sulfate

Two doses of antenatal corticosteroids within a week of preterm birth can reduce the incidence of PVL and IVH by up to 50%, even in neonates as young as 23 weeks' gestation.[76–78] A single dose is not as effective.[79] The mechanism of action is direct, by stabilizing the vasculature of the germinal matrix, and indirect, mediated by a reduction in severity of respiratory distress syndrome and improved cardiovascular stability, particularly in the first 24 hours of life.[80–83] Multiple studies have shown that repeating a two-dose course of prenatal steroids after 14 days if preterm delivery is still a concern confers additional benefit.[84] The American College of Obstetricians and Gynecologists (ACOG) currently recommends repeat administration of prenatal steroids every 7 to 14 days as a rescue treatment if delivery prior to 34 weeks is impending.[85] Caution must be used, however, because a large randomized controlled trial examining the effect of repeat courses of antenatal steroids found four or more courses to be associated with a higher rate of cerebral palsy or death at the 2- to 3-year follow-up (5.6% versus 1.4%). No difference in Bayley scores or head circumference was detected.[86]

Magnesium sulfate has been given to pregnant women for a variety of indications, most commonly to prevent preeclampsia, and early observational data suggested exposure to magnesium sulfate might have a neuroprotective effect on the preterm brain.[87,88] Several randomized controlled trials and meta-analyses have now been conducted, including over 4000 neonates.[89–95] Although none of the studies showed a difference in PVL, a reduction in the combined outcome of death and severe gross motor dysfunction was reproduced in the trials. When combining the trials in meta-analyses, magnesium sulfate also appears to decrease risk of cerebral palsy. In 2009, antenatal magnesium sulfate was recommended with a number to treat (NNT) of 63 to prevent 1 preterm baby from developing cerebral palsy.[96] In 2017, a meta-analysis including over 4000 neonates showed a decrease in the NNT of 46 to prevent cerebral palsy and an NNT of 42 to prevent impaired neurodevelopmental outcome.[97] The ACOG affirmed the findings of these studies and supports the short-term use of magnesium sulfate for neuroprotective measures in fetuses at risk for delivery prior to 32 weeks' gestation.[98] In 2013, the Food and Drug Administration recommended against the use of magnesium sulfate for more than 5 days due to concerns for osteopenic changes in bone mineralization.[99] The mechanisms of action are not completely understood, but amelioration of free radicals or reduction of hypoxic-ischemic events through the stabilization of cerebral blood flow have been proposed.[100] Modulation of N-methyl-D-aspartate (NMDA) glutamate channels has also been proposed as a mechanism of reducing NMDA receptor-mediated injury.[101]

Intrapartum Management—Delayed Cord Clamping

Delayed cord clamping has been investigated as a potential protective mechanism for several decades. In a small randomized controlled trial in the 1980s, a reduction in IVH was demonstrated that inspired further investigations.[102] Since then, delayed cord clamping has been shown in multiple studies to improve and stabilize blood pressure, blood glucose, and temperature and decrease the rate of late onset sepsis, all factors associated with an increased risk for encephalopathy of prematurity.[103–107] A reduction in red blood cell transfusion has also been shown in some trials, further reducing exposure to an inflammatory state and various cytokines, which could possibly contribute to the decreased rate of brain injury seen in this population.[21,105,108,109]

Improved hemodynamic status and thus fewer fluctuations in blood pressure and cerebral blood flow in the first 24 hours after delivery is of particular interest, because this is the highest risk period for the occurrence of an IVH. Delayed cord clamping is also associated with improved cerebral oxygenation during the first 24 hours of life.[104] In a randomized controlled trial of 200 neonates between 27 and 34 weeks of gestation, no difference was demonstrated in the rate of IVH or PVL. This study was originally designed to include less mature neonates; however, the mean gestational age of participants was >30.5 weeks, so the study was likely underpowered to identify decreased incidence of IVH and PVL.[110] In a larger Australian study, delayed cord clamping was associated with a trend toward decreased death, but major morbidities including significant brain injury were comparable between groups.[111] The overall analysis and assessment of the studies resulted in a 2012 ACOG recommendation to delay cord clamping by a minimum of 30 seconds in infants born at <32 weeks, with the prospect of potentially reducing IVH by as much as 50%, endorsed in 2017 by the American Academy of Pediatrics and the Neonatal Resuscitation Program and reindorsed by ACOG in 2020.[112–115] A meta-analysis published in 2018 confirmed the findings of the Cochrane Review from 2012 that delayed cord-clamping was associated with decreased mortality but not with a significant decrease in IVH or PVL, and a more recent randomized controlled trial showed a significant risk reduction of severe IVH by more than 50% with delayed cord clamping versus cord milking.[109,116,117]

Postnatal Management

Glucose Control

Targeted euglycemia is recommended because both absolute levels of blood glucose and glucose variability contribute to preterm brain injury. Hypoglycemia stresses energy metabolism, and in the resultant state of deprivation, oligodendrocytes and neurons become injured, sometimes severely enough to result in necrosis.[118] Hyperglycemia during the first 24 hours of life has also been associated with an increased risk of death and white matter injury on MRI.[119] These findings likely reflect an underlying event that results in a significant stress response, displayed as hyperglycemia. Stress-associated hyperglycemia results in an overall improvement of the infants' energy state but has detrimental effects on astrocytes, leading to intracellular acidosis and targeted damage.[118] In a small study conducting continuous glucose monitoring during the first week of life, no difference in outcome in regard to IVH and PVL could be demonstrated.

Hypercarbia and Hypocarbia

Both hypo- and hypercarbia are detrimental to the developing brain and can potentiate white matter injury. Hypocarbia decreases cerebral blood flow and therefore increases the risk of ischemic white matter injury. Although no definite cutoff values have been identified, persistent $PaCO_2$ <25 mm Hg has been shown in several studies to decrease cerebral blood flow with concomitant decreased oxygen delivery.[120] In a large sample of preterm infants, Shankaran et al. described a dose response relationship between time spent in a hypocarbic state ($PaCO_2$ <35 mm Hg) during the first 7 days of life and periventricular leukomalacia, with those experiencing the most exposure to hypercarbia having a more than fivefold increase in incidence of PVL.[121]

Hypercarbia has vasodilatory effects that in turn cause alterations in cerebral blood flow, placing the infant at risk for hemorrhagic injury. Ventilated preterm infants who have a $PaCO_2$ >45 mm Hg demonstrate a dose dependent increase in cerebral blood flow and subsequently have progressive loss of autoregulation.[122]

Caffeine

The neuroprotective effects of methylxanthines are mediated through inhibition of adenosine receptors, resulting in protection from energy failure and subsequent cell death.[123,124] Caffeine has neuroprotective effects and improves long-term neurodevelopmental outcomes of preterm infants, in particular motor outcome.[125] Furthermore, chronic caffeine exposure appears to preserve the maturation and development of the microstructural white matter.[126] In a large randomized controlled trial, caffeine exposure was associated with improved motor outcome and decreased cognitive impairment. The NNT to prevent 1 preterm baby from having an adverse outcome was 16 based on this study.[125] However, these benefits did not consistently persist with age. At the 5-year follow-up visit, the incidence of cerebral palsy was not different between groups, but there was a significant improvement in developmental coordination disorders in the caffeine group.[127] Brain structural differences were no longer evident at 11 years,[128] yet the caffeine group continued to show improved motor development compared with placebo-treated infants.[129,130]

Caffeine has a wide toxicity margin; however, safety of dosing must still be considered: in a randomized pilot study of 74 preterm infants comparing the standard loading dose of caffeine to a dose four times higher, increased cerebellar injury and motor abnormalities including hypertonicity were observed.[131] A higher loading dose has also raised concern for an increased incidence of seizures and a threefold increase in seizure burden.[132]

Seizures and Role of Electroencephalography

Recognition of seizures in preterm infants requires a high degree of suspicion because they may be clinically silent ("subclinical" or "electrographic-only"), and the use of electroencephalography (EEG) to appropriately recognize seizure is needed.[133] Risk factors for seizures in preterm neonates include sepsis, meningitis, IVH, and encephalopathy. This forms the basis of the recommendation to monitor patients with high-grade IVH, meningitis, or encephalopathy for development of seizures.[133] Reports of seizure rates in preterm populations vary from 4% to 48%.[134–139] Neonatal seizures are a risk factor for subsequent epilepsy, cognitive impairment, and mortality.[140–142] A recent publication from the extremely low gestational age newborns (ELGANs) study demonstrated a 12% risk of at least one seizure and a 7% risk of epilepsy; infants more likely to develop epilepsy included those with more cerebral white matter injury, initial instability, severe bronchopulmonary dysplasia, and postnatal hydrocortisone.[143] EEG background is also associated with cognitive outcomes,[144–148] particularly when combined with findings from term-equivalent MRI.[149]

Early Developmental Therapy

After addressing neuroprotective measures, the introduction of developmental assessments while neonates are in the NICU is imperative. This not only aids in detection of patients at risk for neurodisability but also provides the opportunity to begin early introduction of therapies geared toward improving outcome. The beneficial effects of early intervention therapies and programs on motor outcomes persist through infancy, and systematic reviews suggest that the cognitive benefits remain through preschool.[150–152]

The home environment and parental interaction play an important role in neurodevelopment and are impacted by stressors related to the NICU. Teaching of parenting skills and involvement of parents in developmental care, starting in the NICU and continuing through early intervention, can help through 36 months' age.[153]

Outcome

Preterm infants require long-term developmental follow-up for assessment of motor, cognitive, and behavioral development, thus allowing appropriate interventions to be instituted in a timely manner to improve outcome.

CHAPTER 49

Neonatal Seizures

Melisa Carrasco, Carl E. Stafstrom

KEY POINTS

1. Seizures are very common in the neonatal period and constitute a neurologic emergency.
2. Specific aspects of the physiology of the developing brain make it highly susceptible to hyperexcitability and seizure occurrence.
3. Brain injury often causes or contributes to seizures. Among premature infants, seizures are most often triggered by intraventricular hemorrhage; in term babies, hypoxic-ischemic encephalopathy and stroke are the leading causes of seizures.
4. Electrolyte derangements are a frequent and readily treatable cause of neonatal seizures; work-up of the newborn with seizures should assess serum glucose, calcium, magnesium, and sodium.
5. Genetic mutations and inborn errors of metabolism may cause seizures in newborns and should be considered, especially in patients not responsive to antiseizure drug treatment.
6. "Everything that shakes is not a seizure"—A wide differential diagnosis should be considered, including jitteriness, benign neonatal sleep myoclonus, and drug exposures, especially when the electroencephalogram (EEG) does not confirm the presence of seizures.
7. Continuous video (v)-EEG is the current gold standard for seizure monitoring of newborns. Amplitude-integrated EEG (aEEG) is a useful bedside screening technique.
8. Phenobarbital remains the first-line antiseizure drug for newborns. When unsuccessful, additional drugs should be considered promptly, including fosphenytoin and levetiracetam. Infants in status epilepticus should be treated aggressively with those established antiseizure drugs. Status epilepticus refractory to those medications should be treated with a midazolam infusion and a pyridoxine trial.
9. Given the potential for adverse effects, antiseizure drugs should be discontinued as soon as clinically appropriate, ideally prior to hospital discharge.
10. Patients with neonatal seizures have an increased risk of epilepsy, intellectual disability, and neuropsychiatric disorders later in life.

Introduction

Seizures are more common during the neonatal period than at any other age, occurring at a rate of 1.5 to 3 per 1000 live births.[1] They should be considered a neurologic emergency and require prompt recognition and treatment.

Seizures can be recognized on an electroencephalogram (EEG) as rhythmic activity lasting at least 10 seconds and consisting of an obvious onset, evolving frequency and amplitude over time, and a definitive offset.[2] In term newborns, seizure activity is characterized by the presence of rhythmic sharp waves and spikes. In preterm infants, seizures are often characterized by low frequency (often approximately 1 Hz) focal discharges, often constrained to a limited area of cortex.[3,4] Due to immature myelination, seizures in neonates propagate slowly to other cortical areas. Status epilepticus is diagnosed if electrographic seizure activity exceeds 50% of a 1-hour (or longer) recording epoch.[5]

In full-term infants, seizures can be either "electroclinical" (characterized as having an associated clinical manifestation, such as apnea or rhythmic limb movements, along with EEG evidence for seizure) or "electrographic-only" (also referred to as "subclinical," i.e., without an observable clinical change). In extremely premature infants, seizures are almost always electrographic only. EEG monitoring is an essential part of neonatal intensive care unit (NICU) care, as many seizures in this age range are clinically silent.

Pathophysiology

The increased susceptibility of the neonatal brain to seizures is due to a combination of extrinsic and intrinsic factors.[6] Extrinsic factors include all of the pathologies to which a newborn may be subjected, such as hypoxia-ischemia, intracranial hemorrhage, infection, inborn and acquired metabolic errors, and congenital brain malformations. Intrinsic factors are those related to aspects of brain maturation, including ion channels, synapses, and circuits (Fig. 49.1; Table 49.1).

At any age, seizure occurrence can be conceptualized as an imbalance between excitation (E) and inhibition (I) in neurons, synapses, and brain circuits. When E increases and/or I decreases, either temporarily or on a chronic basis, the balance of E/I tips toward excessive excitability.[7] However, this E/I imbalance concept is oversimplified and seizure generation is likely mediated by additional signaling mechanisms.[8] For a seizure to happen, hyperexcitability must be coupled with hypersynchronous neuronal firing to cause the abnormal excitation (i.e., seizure) to propagate and lead to a clinical event. In neonates, a seizure may involve clinical changes such as rhythmic motor activity or altered vital signs, but often, a seizure on EEG may not have any associated clinical correlate.

During brain development, the regulation or expression of physiologic factors governing neuronal excitation evolve, and a seizure can be generated by different mechanisms and manifestations at different postconceptual ages.[9] A couple of the major concepts are summarized here; for details, the reader is referred to comprehensive reviews.[4,6,10,11]

Ion Channels

Neuronal action potentials are generated by influx of sodium ions (Na^+) and terminated by efflux of potassium ions (K^+). Mutation of genes controlling either Na^+ or K^+ channels can predispose to hyperexcitability and seizure generation. For example, mutations in the gene that codes for one type of voltage-dependent potassium channel, *KCNQ2* (responsible for action potential frequency adaptation), underlies both a relatively benign epilepsy (benign familial

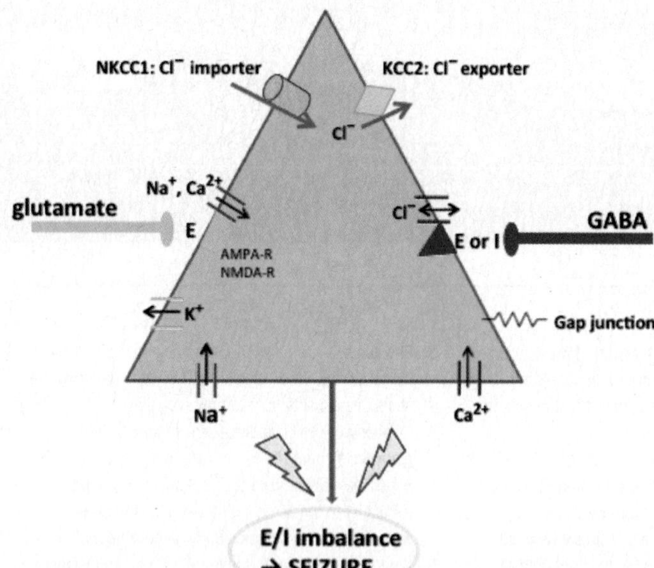

Fig. 49.1 Hypothetical Cortical Neuron *(Triangle)* With Ion Channels, Synaptic Inputs, and Chloride Transporters, Illustrating Sites That Might Predispose the Neonatal Brain to Increased Excitability and Seizures. *AMPA-R,* Alpha-amino-3-hydroxy-5-methyl-4-isoxazolepropionic receptor; *Ca^{2+},* calcium; *Cl^-,* chloride; *E,* excitation; *GABA,* gamma-aminobutyric acid; *I,* inhibition; *K^+,* potassium; *KCC2,* potassium-chloride cotransporter type 2; *Na^+,* sodium; *NKCC1,* sodium-potassium-chloride cotransporter type 1; *NMDA-R,* N-methyl-D-aspartate receptor.

Table 49.1 Some Factors Favoring Hyperexcitability and Seizures in the Neonatal Brain

Ion channels	Earlier development of Na^+, Ca^{2+} channels
	Delayed development of K^+ channels
Neurotransmitters and synapses	Electrical synapses (gap junctions) common in early development
	Excitatory synapses appear before inhibitory synapses
	Overexpression of excitatory synapses during critical period
	NMDA and AMPA receptor subunit configurations favor greater excitability early in life
	GABA is excitatory in the prenatal and early postnatal period
Circuits and networks	Underdeveloped myelination favors focal seizure onset and limited seizure spread

AMPA, Alpha-amino-3-hydroxy-5-methyl-4-isoxazolepropionic acid; *Ca^{2+},* calcium; *GABA,* gamma-aminobutyric acid; *K^+,* potassium; *Na^+,* sodium; *NMDA,* N-methyl-D-aspartate.

neonatal epilepsy) and a severe epileptic encephalopathy.[12] Likewise, mutation in the gene *SCN1A*, which codes for voltage-dependent sodium channels, underlies Dravet syndrome, in which seizures typically begin in the toddler age range but could occur in neonates.[13] Of note, development of ion channels mediating depolarization (Na^+, calcium [Ca^{2+}]) develop earlier than those mediating repolarization (K^+).[14]

Ion Gradients

During the premature period and possibly extending shortly beyond term, the basal intracellular chloride ion (Cl^-) concentration exceeds the extracellular Cl^- concentration. Therefore, when Cl^- channels open as a result of GABAergic (gamma-aminobutyric acid) synaptic transmission, Cl^- exits from the cell, depolarizing it and causing neuronal excitation (and potentially, seizure activity). As development proceeds, the Cl^- gradient reverses, and the extracellular Cl^- concentration becomes much higher than the intracellular Cl^- concentration; in that case, activation of GABA receptors promotes an influx of Cl^- into the neuron, which hyperpolarizes it, causing inhibition (Fig. 49.2). The reason for the different internal Cl^- concentrations at different gestational ages relates to membrane chloride-cation transporters whose differential expression over time leads to the variable Cl^- concentrations. During prenatal life, the sodium-potassium-chloride cotransporter 1 (NKCC1) predominates and intracellular Cl^- accumulates. By term or shortly thereafter, the expression of NKCC1 declines and there is increased expression of another transporter, potassium-chloride cotransporter 2 (KCC2), which leads to a net efflux of Cl^-, leaving the neuron with a lower basal concentration of Cl^-. In summary, in the fetal or preterm brain, GABA binding to its receptor results in Cl^- efflux, depolarizing the neuron. Postterm, GABA binding results in Cl^- entry into the cell, hyperpolarizing it. Hence the physiologic "paradox" of early GABA-induced depolarization (and excitation) is a consequence of the age-related expression of Cl^- cotransporters and variable internal Cl^- concentrations (see Fig. 49.2). Depolarizing GABA plays key trophic roles in the developing brain and is essential for normal synaptogenesis and circuit formation, but this situation comes at the price of increased excitability and seizure predisposition during early brain development.

Synaptic Receptors

GABAergic transmission is excitatory rather than inhibitory in the preterm and early postterm infant, leading to the "paradoxical" GABA excitation just described. This physiologic situation has clinical implications, possibly accounting for the failure of GABAergic drugs (phenobarbital, benzodiazepines) to fully stop neonatal seizures. Studies are ongoing to establish whether specific blockers of NKCC1 (e.g., bumetanide) can ameliorate neonatal seizures by preventing excessive intracellular Cl^- accumulation (see Fig. 49.2). Hopefully, other rational therapies can be developed based on the specific physiologic idiosyncrasies of early brain development.

There is also a developmental sequence for excitatory neurotransmitters and receptors; excitatory transmission develops earlier than inhibitory transmission. Brain excitation is largely mediated by glutamate, which binds to two classes of glutamate receptor: alpha-amino-3-hydroxy-5-methyl-4-isoxazolepropionic (AMPA) and N-methyl-D-aspartic acid (NMDA) (see Fig. 49.1). AMPA receptors mediate fast excitatory transmission and NMDA mediates relatively prolonged excitatory responses. Subunit expression of both AMPA and NMDA receptors favors excessive excitation in neonates.[9,11]

Other Factors Favoring Hyperexcitability in the Developing Brain

Additional physiologic factors in the developing brain promote susceptibility to seizures. Intercellular communication via gap junctions (electrical synapses) plays a pivotal role in neuronal development; fast-acting electrical transmission via gap junctions can facilitate rapid synchrony of neuronal networks and facilitate seizures.[15] Gap junctions are most active prior to chemical synapse formation. Other factors that play a role in early brain excitability include homeostatic regulation of glial K^+ and the sodium-potassium pump.[9]

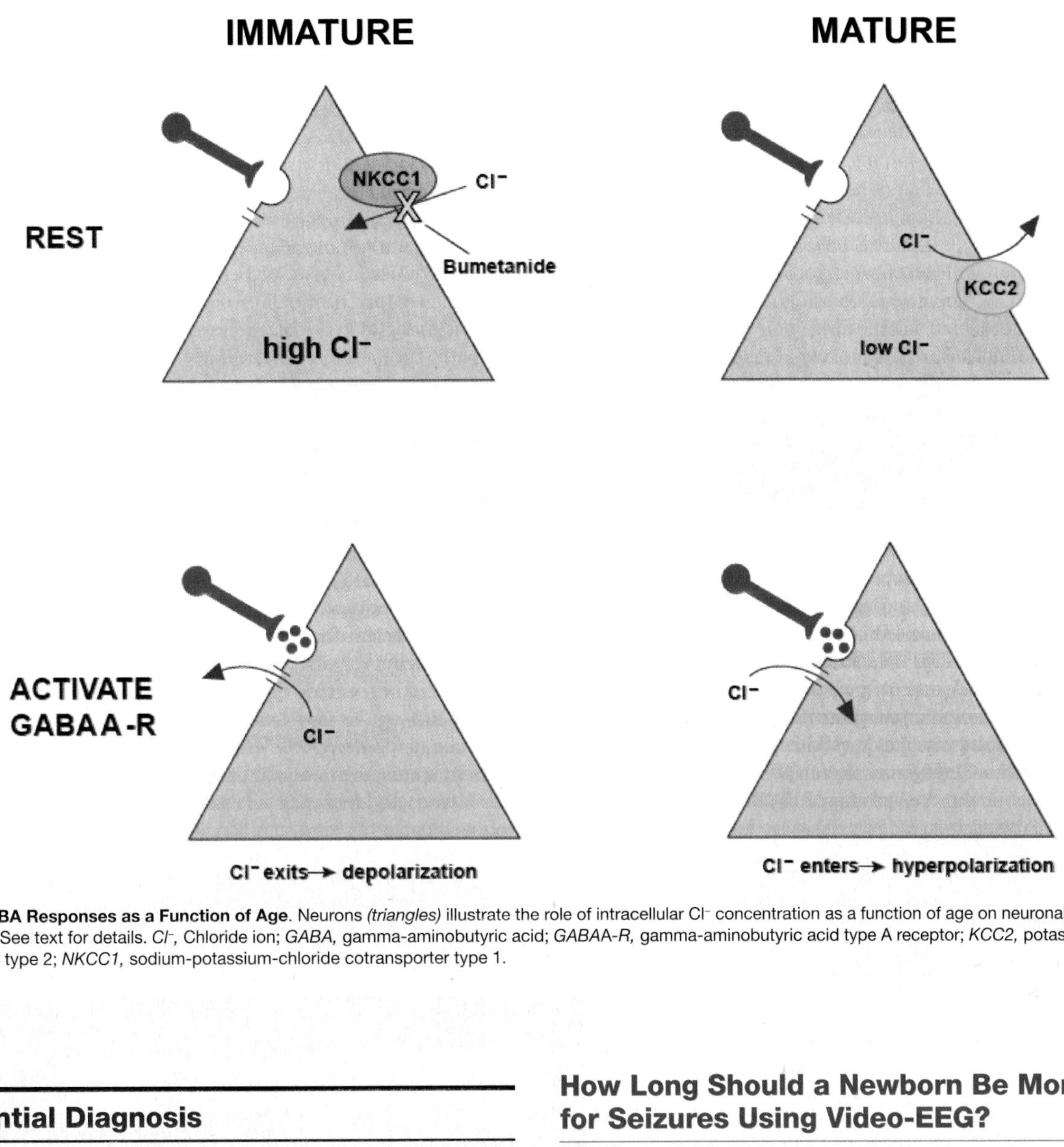

Fig. 49.2 GABA Responses as a Function of Age. Neurons *(triangles)* illustrate the role of intracellular Cl^- concentration as a function of age on neuronal responses to GABA *(dots)*. See text for details. *Cl^-*, Chloride ion; *GABA,* gamma-aminobutyric acid; *GABAA-R,* gamma-aminobutyric acid type A receptor; *KCC2,* potassium-chloride cotransporter type 2; *NKCC1,* sodium-potassium-chloride cotransporter type 1.

Differential Diagnosis

Seizures during the neonatal period are often provoked by acute brain injury, usually in the setting of stroke, intracranial hemorrhage, or hypoxic-ischemic encephalopathy (Fig. 49.3). In addition, a myriad of genetic mutations, inborn errors of metabolism, and other metabolic derangements can lead to neonatal seizures (see Fig. 49.3 and Tables 49.2–49.6). Not all rhythmic movements in newborns are due to seizures. Nonepileptic causes of paroxysmal events should be considered, especially when episodes of concern are not verified as seizures on EEG (Table 49.7).

Evaluation

Seizure occurrence should be followed closely with EEG monitoring (Table 49.8). Continuous video (v)-EEG is the gold standard for seizure identification and monitoring,[40] yet the interpretation of neonatal recordings is challenging, even for experienced readers. There is also considerable interobserver variability[41] and a continuing tendency to treat patients lacking electrographic evidence of seizures.[42] Prompt laboratory and imaging work-up to search for possible etiologies should be pursued (Table 49.9).

How Long Should a Newborn Be Monitored for Seizures Using Video-EEG?

There are no published data addressing this question.[46] We recommend monitoring infants with continuous v-EEG for 24 to 48 hours after their last electrographic seizure to ensure seizure responsiveness to the treatment chosen.

When to Consider an Inborn Error of Metabolism as a Potential Seizure Cause?

Seizures caused by primary inborn errors of metabolism or genetic causes are often difficult to diagnose based on initial clinical presentation alone. Inborn errors of metabolism should be considered if (1) seizures fail to respond to typical antiseizure drugs, (2) seizures persist in a baby with ongoing clinical deterioration in spite of appropriate sepsis coverage and cardiorespiratory support, (3) the EEG shows burst suppression, and (4) magnetic resonance imaging (MRI) findings are atypical, such as evidence of atrophy or features that do not conform to common causes of seizures in this age range.[24] Babies exhibiting tonic seizures alone should raise concern for a genetic epilepsy. Strokes occurring outside of arterial or venous territories should raise suspicion for a metabolic etiology.

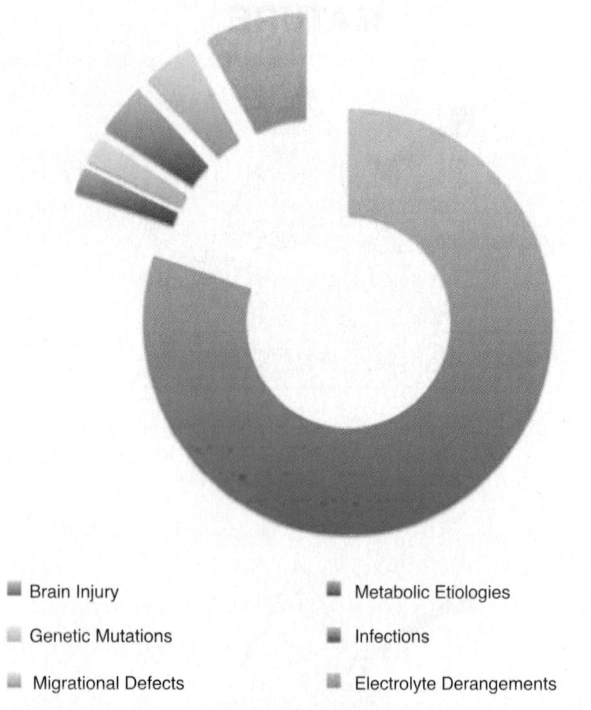

Fig. 49.3 Common Neonatal Seizure Etiologies. Multiple causes of neonatal seizures have been identified. The majority of causes are secondary to brain injury (e.g., hypoxic-ischemic encephalopathy, hemorrhage), infection, or electrolyte derangement.

Early testing is crucial, because some inborn errors of metabolism are treatable and treatment delays may contribute to a worse outcome (e.g., pyridoxine in the case of pyridoxine-responsive seizures; ketogenic diet in the case of glucose transporter type 1 deficiency). Support groups are available for families with a baby affected by metabolic and genetic epilepsies: the Rare Epilepsy Network (https://www.epilepsy.com/make-difference/research-and-new-therapies/engagement/rare-epilepsy-network-ren) and the Epilepsy Leadership Council (https://www.epilepsyleadershipcouncil.org/).

Genetic Work-Up

Expedited genetic work-up should be considered in newborns in whom initial laboratory and imaging-work-up fails to reveal a cause for seizures. A number of genetic variants (including single gene mutations and chromosomal abnormalities) can lead to early seizures. In a recent study, more than 80% of infants with epileptic encephalopathy who underwent genetic testing were found to have a genetic etiology, with *KCNQ2* variants being a frequent etiology.[16] Genetic testing may be especially helpful in cases involving severely ill newborns (e.g., those with burst suppression EEGs and those with dysmorphic features) to aid in diagnosis and prognosis.[47,48]

A rational approach to genetic testing in neonates with seizures entails targeted versus single-gene testing when the history and examination point toward a specific syndrome.[49] Gene panels and chromosomal microarrays can be pursued when considering two or more candidate genes as part of the differential. When initial genetic

Table 49.2 Specific Brain Injuries Contributing to Neonatal Seizure Development[16–20]

PRETERM INFANTS		
Injury	**Description**	**Sample MR Image**
Intraventricular hemorrhage (IVH)	• Intraventricular and periventricular hemorrhages are common due to fragile germinal matrix. • Intraparenchymal hemorrhages secondary to venous infarction are highly associated with seizure occurrence.	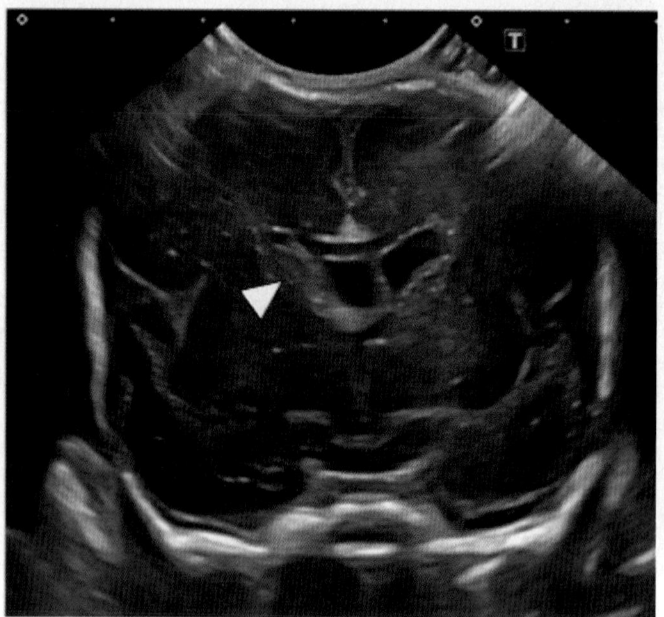 Head ultrasound obtained from patient with a right-sided germinal matrix hemorrhage (*arrowhead*).

Table 49.2 Specific Brain Injuries Contributing to Neonatal Seizure Development—cont'd		
TERM INFANTS		
Injury	**Description**	**Sample MR Image**
Hypoxic-ischemic encephalopathy	• Most common cause of seizures in term newborns (accounts for 40%–60%).	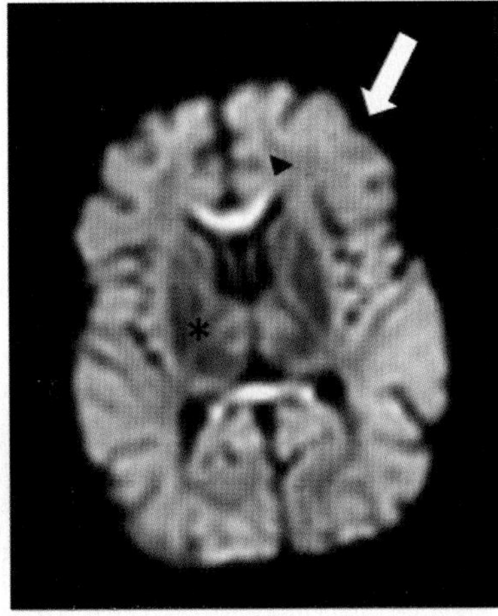 Diffusion-weighted image obtained from a patient with severe hypoxic-ischemic encephalopathy. Note the diffuse supratentorial (*arrow*), callosal (*black arrowhead*), and basal ganglia (*asterisk*) involvement.

Stroke	• Second most frequent cause of neonatal seizures in term newborns.
	• Subcategories include:
	  • arterial ischemic strokes.
	  • ischemic strokes secondary to cerebral sinovenous thrombosis.
	• One-third of children with perinatal arterial ischemic stroke will develop epilepsy.
		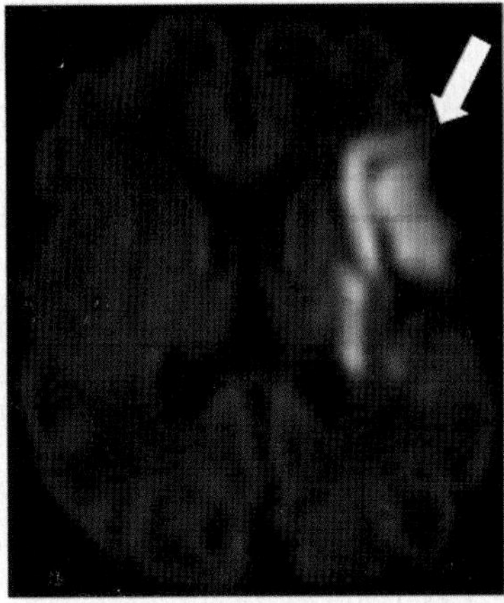 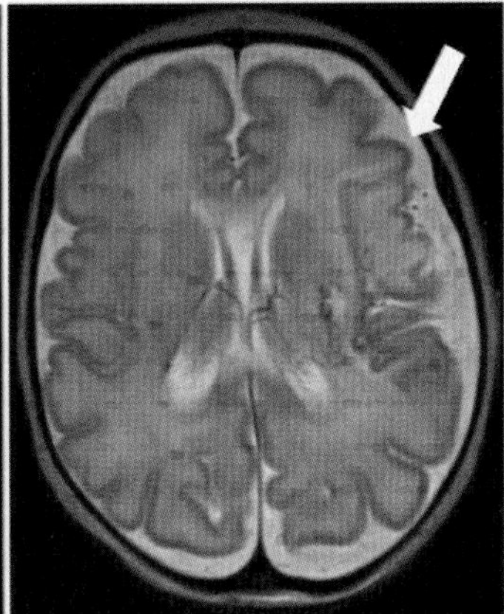 MR images (diffusion-weighted and T2-weighted) were obtained from a term patient with a left-sided middle cerebral artery stroke (*arrows*).

Intracranial hemorrhage	• Parenchymal hemorrhages, including those secondary to:
	  • hemorrhagic conversion of ischemic infarction of arterial or venous origin.
	  • less common causes include vascular malformations and genetic causes (e.g., *COL4A1* mutation) and trauma. Coagulopathies may in theory lead to parenchymal hemorrhage, but these are rare in the neonatal period.
		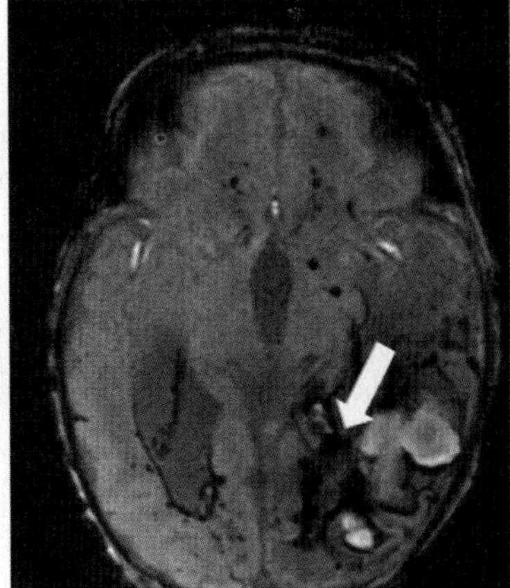 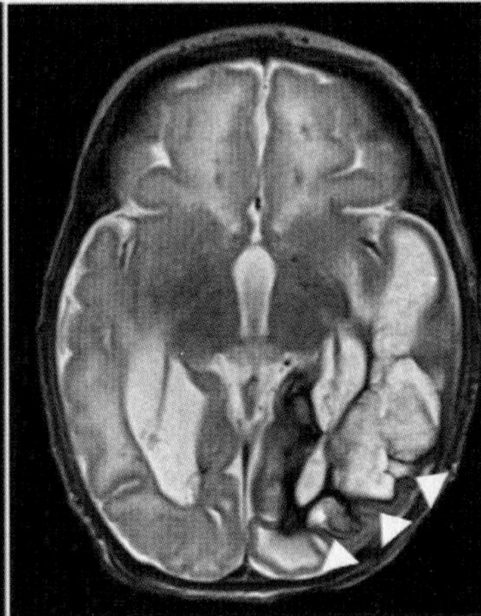 MR images (susceptibility-weighted and T2-weighted images) were obtained from a patient with extensive hemorrhagic injury (*arrow*). Also visible: cystic encephalomalacia and associated volume loss in the left temporal lobe (*arrowheads*).

Continued

Table 49.2 Specific Brain Injuries Contributing to Neonatal Seizure Development—cont'd

TERM INFANTS		
Injury	**Description**	**Sample MR Image**
	• Subdural hemorrhages.	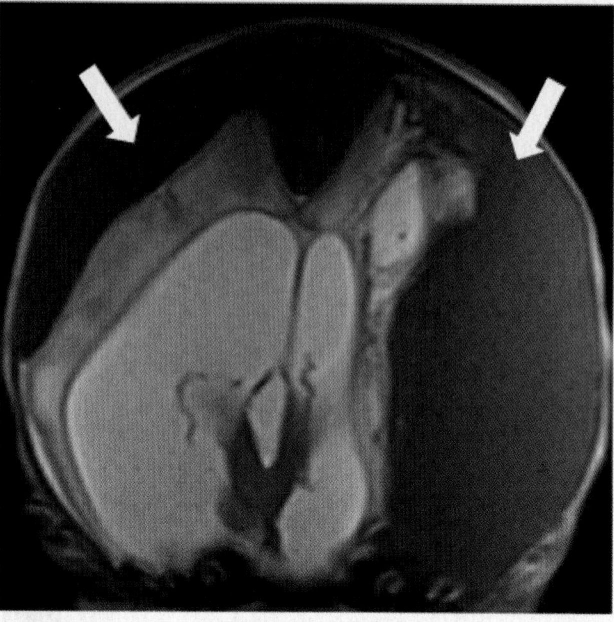 MR image showing bilateral large subdural hematomas (*arrows*) compressing both cerebral hemispheres; hematomas were secondary to coagulopathy at birth.

MR, Magnetic resonance.

Table 49.3 Electrolyte Abnormalities Causing Neonatal Seizures[21,22]

Hypoglycemia	• Especially at risk are newborns who are critically ill, preterm, small for gestational age, and/or born to diabetic mothers. • Hypoglycemia is often associated with adverse neurodevelopmental outcomes. Severe hypoglycemia may result in injury to the posterior limb of the internal capsule and occipital cortex, which is appreciable on MRI. Patients may go on to develop epilepsy. • Mechanism: Hypoglycemia promotes seizures by contributing to brain edema. • Treatment: Correct with 10% dextrose solution.
Hypocalcemia/hypomagnesemia	• Especially at risk are newborns who are born to diabetic mothers and/or low birth weight. • Suspect diabetes insipidus, DiGeorge syndrome (22q11 deletion) in infants with late-onset derangements. • Mechanism: Decreased surface charge screening secondary to hypocalcemia decreases the threshold for depolarization and contributes to increased excitation. • Treatment: Correct electrolyte imbalance with calcium gluconate. Also address concurrent hypomagnesemia.
Hypernatremia/hyponatremia	• Especially high risk in extremely premature or very low birth weight newborns. • In term infants, severe hypernatremia is associated with early discharge from hospital before breastfeeding is fully established. • Mechanism: Fluid changes contributing to edema (in the case of hyponatremia). The mechanism contributing to encephalopathy and seizures secondary to hypernatremia is unknown. • Treatment: Correct electrolyte imbalance with fluid resuscitation.

MRI, Magnetic resonance imaging.

Table 49.4 Inborn Errors of Metabolism Commonly Associated With Neonatal Seizures[23,24]
Nonketotic hyperglycinemia
Pyridoxine-responsive seizures
Folinic acid–responsive seizures
Biotinidase deficiency
Urea cycle disorders
Pyruvate dehydrogenase deficiency
Glucose transporter deficiency type 1 (GLUT1)
Peroxisomal disorders
Congenital disorders of glycosylation

Table 49.5 Selected Gene Mutations Associated With Neonatal Seizures[9,25–29]

Gene	Description
HCN1	• Observed with severe epileptic encephalopathy.
KCNT1	• Observed with epilepsy of infancy with neonatal-onset migrating focal seizures. • Quinidine is the current treatment of choice.
KCNQ2, KCNQ3	• Observed in a wide spectrum of phenotypes, including benign familial neonatal seizures, as well as severe epileptic encephalopathy.
SCN1A	• Observed in severe myoclonic epilepsy of infancy.
SCN2A	• Observed in benign familial neonatal seizures.
STXBP1	• Presents with both epileptic spasms and focal seizures.
STXBP1, KCNQ2, ARX, CDKL5	• All associated with burst-suppression, in the setting of early infantile epileptic encephalopathy (EIEE).

Table 49.6 Selected Structural Etiologies Contributing to Neonatal Seizures[30–36]

Malformation	Description	Sample MRI Image
Neuronal migration disorders	Schizencephaly • Neonates may present with hypotonia and early seizures. Associated with developmental delay. • Associated gene mutations include *EMX2, SIX3,* and *COL4A1.*	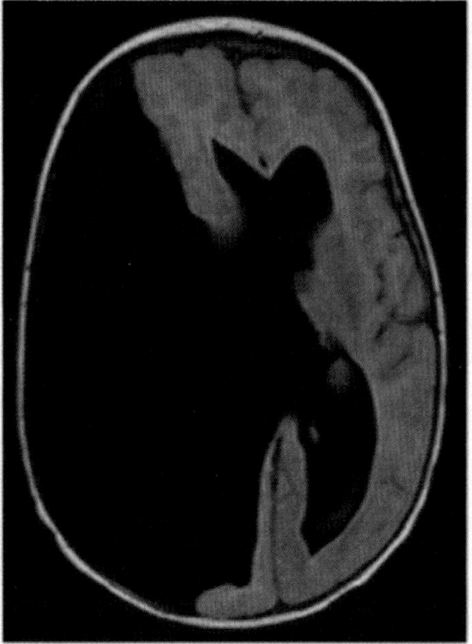 T1-weighted MR image from a patient with right-sided schizencephaly.
	Polymicrogyria • Results in increased formation of gyri. • Associated mutations include *ADGRG1, TUBA8, TUBB2B,* and *TUBB3.* Subcortical band heterotopias and periventricular nodular heterotopias	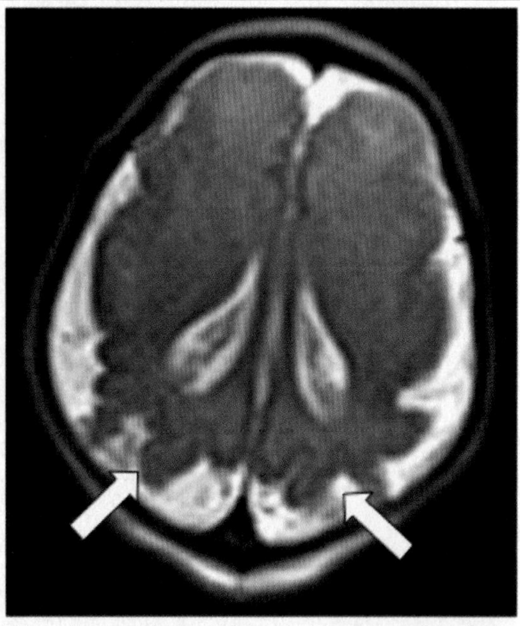 T2-weighted MR image from a patient with bilateral parietal and occipital polymicrogyria (*arrows*).

Continued

Table 49.6 Selected Structural Etiologies Contributing to Neonatal Seizures—cont'd

Malformation	Description	Sample MRI Image
	Focal cortical dysplasia (FCD) • Frontal lobe localization or early seizures due to FCDs are associated with a higher risk for epileptic spasms. • Can be amenable to early surgery.	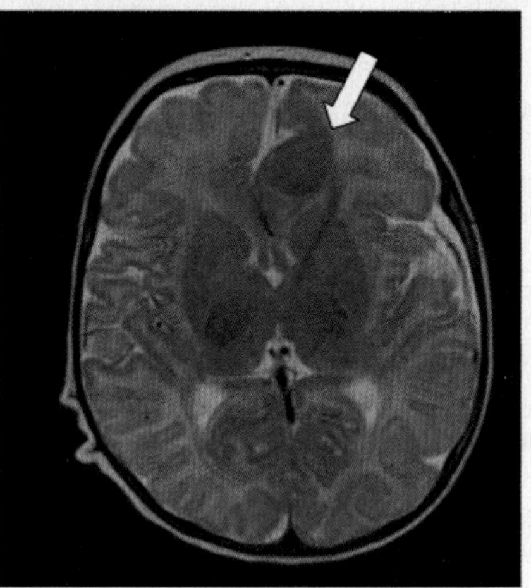 T2-weighted MR image from a patient with a left frontal cortical dysplasia (*arrow*).
Neurocutaneous syndromes	Tuberous sclerosis complex • Screen for signature skin findings (hypopigmented macules) in newborns; among older children: epilepsy, infantile spasms, and developmental delays. • Associated gene mutations: *TSC1, TSC2.* • Diffusion tensor imaging may help identify epileptogenic tubers when considering epilepsy surgery.	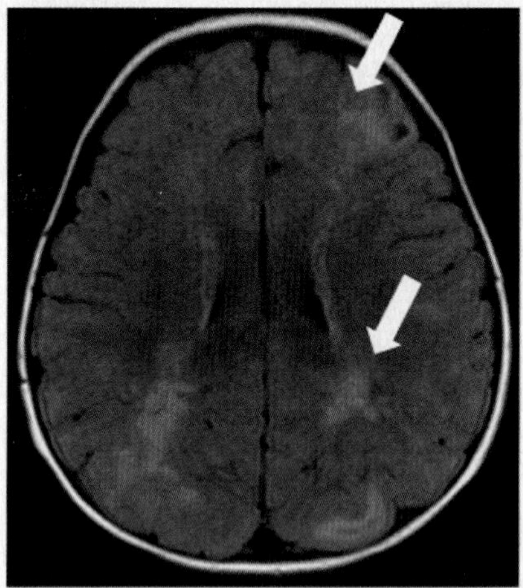 T1-weighted MR image from a patient with tuberous sclerosis (*arrows* indicate individual tubers).

Table 49.7 Mimics of Neonatal Seizures[37–39]
Jitteriness
Benign neonatal sleep myoclonus
Neonatal tremor
Hyperekplexia
Drug exposure • Selective serotonin reuptake inhibitors (SSRIs) • Caffeine • Drugs of abuse (e.g., heroin/opiates, cocaine) • Neonatal alcohol withdrawal syndrome
Motor automatisms
Dystonic posturing secondary to reflux/Sandifer syndrome
Apnea, cardiovascular dysfunction

Table 49.8 Electrophysiological Monitoring[42–44]

Technique	Advantages	Disadvantages
Amplitude-integrated EEG (aEEG)	• Economical • Readily available • Easy lead placement • Ongoing bedside evaluation	• Limited number of electrodes • Lower sensitivity, especially when seizures are brief and distant from recording leads • Very vulnerable to artifacts, which are especially prevalent in preterm infants
Continuous video (v)-EEG	• Current gold standard for seizure detection	• Time intensive • Not available at all institutions • Interpretation requires specially trained personnel

EEG, Electroencephalogram.

Table 49.9 Neonatal Seizure Work-Up (With Prioritization of Studies)[24,45]

Initial labs	Prioritize: Arterial blood gas, basic metabolic panel, complete blood count, transaminases, calcium, magnesium, glucose
Infectious work-up	Prioritize: • Blood, urine, and CSF cultures • Consider TORCH screen (the acronym TORCH complex or TORCHes infections refers to the congenital infections of toxoplasmosis, others [syphilis, hepatitis B, varicella-zoster, and Zika virus], rubella, cytomegalovirus [CMV], and herpes simplex) • Septicemia without meningitis may also cause seizures
EEG	Prioritize: Continuous EEG if available (otherwise consider aEEG)
Imaging	Prioritize: Head ultrasound If available and when patient is stable: Magnetic resonance imaging Consider: Magnetic resonance angiography and venography if clinically indicated
Metabolic work-up	Prioritize: Ammonia, lactate, pyruvate, acylcarnitine profile, plasma amino acids, urine organic acids, urine sulfites If indicated: • CSF amino acids (pair with plasma) • CSF glucose (pair with plasma), pyruvate, lactate • CSF neurotransmitters Consider: • Genetic testing for *ALDH7A1* mutations, often as part of a panel Alternatively: Consider urine alpha-aminoadipic semialdehyde (deficiency contributes to pyridoxine-dependent epilepsy)
Additional considerations	Important: Placental pathology (in cases of suspected hypoxic-ischemic encephalopathy or arterial stroke) If possible: Expedite newborn screen results Consider: • Expedited genetic work-up

aEEG, Amplitude-integrated electroencephalogram; *CSF*, cerebrospinal fluid; *EEG*, electroencephalogram; *HSV-2*, herpes simplex virus type 2.

testing is inconclusive, it is worthwhile to consider expedited whole-exome sequencing, which may reveal a diagnosis, guide subsequent prognostic discussions, improve treatment efficacy, and decrease costs long-term.[50] Genetic counseling should be offered if available.[49]

Management

Evidence-based guidelines for the management of neonates with seizures are limited and have changed little over the past decade.[51] All antiseizure medications commonly used in neonates have potential side effects, including possible adverse effects on long-term neurodevelopment.[52] No antiseizure drug has received approval from the US Food and Drug Administration for use in neonates.[53] Phenobarbital remains the first-line antiseizure drug for newborns and is superior to all other treatments, including levetiracetam.[54] Unfortunately, phenobarbital stops seizures in only about half of patients.[55]

If phenobarbital is unsuccessful, additional drugs should be considered promptly (Fig. 49.4). The order of second-line agents (fosphenytoin, levetiracetam) varies between institutions as well as between individual clinicians. Small trials have shown that both levetiracetam and fosphenytoin can be efficacious, including in term infants and older children with hypoxic-ischemic encephalopathy (HIE).[56,57]

In spite of best efforts, current standard therapy for neonatal seizures is imperfect. A recent prospective cohort of more than 500 neonates showed that only one-third of patients with acute symptomatic seizures had a complete response when treated with an initial antiseizure medication.[58] Recent data also suggest that the effectiveness of phenobarbital, fosphenytoin, and levetiracetam can be limited in neonates suffering from refractory seizures.[59] Among neonates with status epilepticus refractory to phenobarbital, fosphenytoin, and levetiracetam, treatment with oxcarbazepine, pyridoxine, or a midazolam infusion can be tried (see Fig. 49.4). In Europe, lidocaine is often used for refractory status.[60] Options for patients requiring maintenance antiseizure medications are listed in Table 49.10.

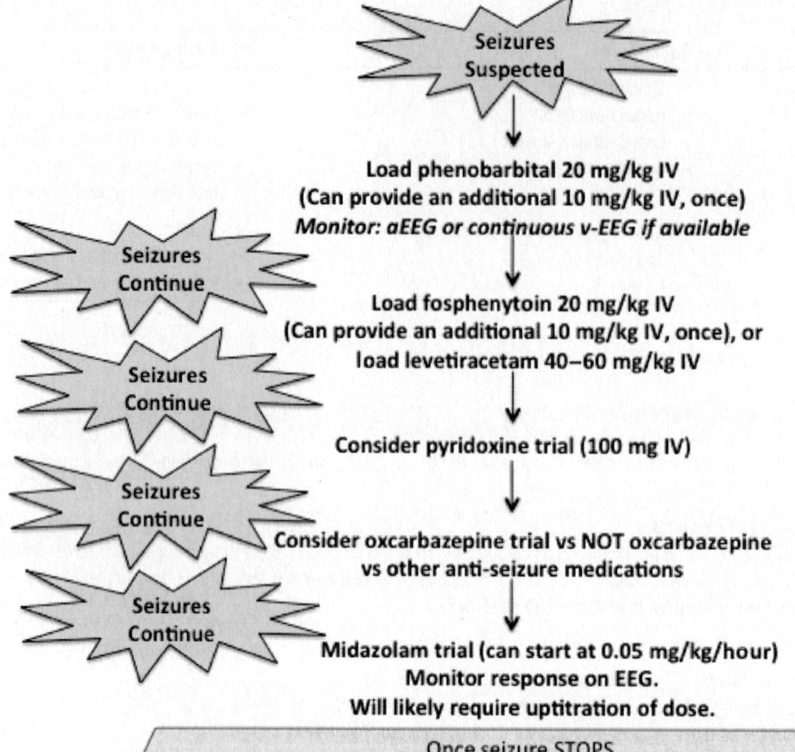

Fig. 49.4 Neonatal Seizure Protocol. Phenobarbital is the first-line drug for newborns. When unsuccessful, additional drugs should be considered promptly, as indicated. *a-EEG,* Amplitude-integrated electroencephalogram; *HIE,* hypoxic-ischemic encephalopathy; *IV,* intravenous; *v-EEG,* video electroencephalogram.

Table 49.10 Maintenance Therapy: Treatment Options[51,61–68]

Drug	Maintenance Dosing	Advantages	Disadvantages
Phenobarbital	5–7 mg/kg/day divided every 12 hours	• First-line therapy • Best efficacy • Inexpensive	• May produce sedation • May induce changes in cardiac and respiratory function • Animal data suggest increased risk of apoptosis and effect on synapse maturation, which may affect learning and memory • May worsen previously existing neuronal injury when utilized to treat status epilepticus
Levetiracetam	30–60 mg/kg/day divided every 8 hours	• Increased use in recent years • Safe • Considered second-line • Neuroprotective effects possible • Neuronal apoptosis has not been reported in animal models	• Possible side effects: irritability, drowsiness, feeding dysfunction
Fosphenytoin	5–8 mg/kg/day divided every 8 hours	Fairly good effectiveness	• Drug-drug interactions common • Less likely to contribute to vital sign instability and cardiac side effects (compared with phenytoin) • Requires switch to oral formulation (which is poorly absorbed) prior to discharge • Does not follow linear kinetics
Additional antiseizure medicine (ASM) options: • Topiramate • Lacosamide • Oxcarbazepine		• Topiramate may be neuroprotective • Lacosamide can be utilized for treatment of *SCN2A*-associated neonatal seizures • Oxcarbazepine is useful in infants with seizures due to mutations in *KCNQ2*, including infants with benign familial neonatal epilepsy	—

When to Discontinue Antiseizure Medications?

In neonates with seizures resulting from acute injury (e.g., HIE, hemorrhage, stroke, infection), the World Health Organization suggests that antiseizure medications be discontinued once a neonate has been seizure-free for 72 hours, if the neurologic exam is normal and the infant is no longer exhibiting seizures.[46]

A small retrospective study showed that a normal EEG can be a helpful prognosticator for discontinuing antiseizure drugs in most infants.[69] Discontinuing antiseizure medications in the NICU prior to hospital discharge has not been linked to an increased risk for seizures once the infant goes home.[70] Longer phenobarbital use does not decrease the occurrence of epilepsy.[71] Given the available data, it is prudent to wean antiseizure medications prior to discharge from the NICU if possible. Of note, antiseizure therapies should not be stopped in babies diagnosed with a neonatal epilepsy syndrome or with seizures secondary to genetic or metabolic etiologies, as these tend to require antiseizure therapy long-term.

Long-Term Outcomes

Neonatal seizures are associated with significant morbidity and mortality; worse behavioral, cognitive, and language outcomes; and an increased incidence of epilepsy later in life.[4,72–75] Furthermore, babies with elevated seizure burden are at greater risk for persistent abnormal neurologic function.[59] Although therapeutic hypothermia conveys neuroprotection in newborns with HIE, no targeted neuroprotective agent confers brain protection in neonates with active seizures.[61] Current research is focusing on potential neuroprotective therapies such as melatonin, ganaxolone, and some interleukins.[61]

Animal models have shown that early recurrent seizures can have detrimental effects on neurogenesis.[76] Neonatal seizures may also have secondary effects on synaptic organization (including sprouting of the hippocampal CA3 and supragranular regions) as well as distribution of glutamate receptors.[77] How these specific mechanisms contribute to long-term outcomes after neonatal seizures is an active area of research.

CHAPTER

50 Stroke in Neonates

Ryan J. Felling, Lisa R. Sun

KEY POINTS

1. Perinatal arterial ischemic stroke most often results from the convergence of multiple stroke risk factors specific to the perinatal period and has a low risk of recurrence.
2. Neonatal arterial ischemic stroke refers to the most common presentation of perinatal stroke when focal seizures or diffuse neurologic signs lead to diagnosis soon after birth. A subset of patients remain undiagnosed in the neonatal period and present as having presumed perinatal arterial ischemic stroke, with emerging neurologic deficits later in infancy.
3. Cardiac disease, although present in a minority of cases, is a risk factor for stroke recurrence and should be investigated with echocardiography after perinatal stroke diagnosis.
4. In the absence of multiple thromboembolic events and/or a family history of thrombosis, extensive thrombophilia evaluations are generally not recommended because they do not predict recurrence or alter management.
5. Management of perinatal stroke should focus on supportive care with the primary goal of promoting adequate perfusion to the brain and minimizing extension of the injury. Although the presentations of perinatal stroke and hypoxic-ischemic encephalopathy may overlap, treatment with hypothermia should not be delayed if hypoxic-ischemic encephalopathy is suspected.

Introduction

The perinatal period represents one of the highest-risk times of life for stroke, and the consequences are significant in terms of neurologic morbidity across the lifespan. In 2007 an international workshop convened by the National Institutes of Neurological Disorders and Stroke defined ischemic perinatal stroke as a "group of heterogeneous conditions in which there is focal disruption of cerebral blood flow secondary to arterial or cerebral venous thrombosis or embolization, between 20 weeks of fetal life through the 28th postnatal day, confirmed by neuroimaging or neuropathologic studies."[1] Perinatal stroke can be divided into distinct syndromes based on the pathophysiology, presentation, and developmental stage at which it occurs. Neonatal arterial ischemic stroke (NAIS), cerebral sinovenous thrombosis (CSVT), and neonatal hemorrhagic stroke typically present acutely in the neonatal period, whereas presumed perinatal arterial ischemic stroke (PPAIS), periventricular venous infarction, and presumed perinatal hemorrhagic stroke occur pre- or perinatally but frequently do not manifest until later in infancy (Fig. 50.1).[2]

Epidemiology

Ischemic perinatal stroke occurs in 1 in 2300 to 5000 live births, with most presenting within the first week of life, significantly higher than the weekly risk of stroke in an adult with known risk factors.[3–6] Arterial strokes represent the majority of these, with most presenting acutely in the neonatal period (NAIS).[7] The incidence of CSVT is less common, occurring in 2.6 per 100,000 births.[8,9] A male predominance has been demonstrated in multiple studies of perinatal stroke.[6,10] Hemorrhagic stroke is significantly less common in the perinatal population and is often excluded from studies of perinatal stroke, but one study identified a population prevalence (excluding isolated germinal matrix hemorrhage) of 6.2 in 100,000 live births over a 10-year period, also with a male predominance.[11]

Pathogenesis

The cause of perinatal stroke is thought to be multifactorial, with convergence of multiple risk factors specific to the peripartum period creating conditions ripe for thrombosis and clot embolization to the cerebral arteries. First, pregnancy is a hypercoagulable state. Hemostatic changes occur throughout pregnancy, with increases in procoagulant factors, decreases in anticoagulant factors, and decreases in intrinsic fibrinolytic activity.[12] These changes are essential for maintaining placental function during pregnancy and defending against hemorrhage during delivery, while predisposing to thrombosis. Thrombosis of the placental vessels that normally occurs as the placenta separates at the time of birth may lead to direct embolization into the fetal circulation.[13] Second, the fetal circulation allows for direct embolization of a venous clot across right-to-left cardiac shunts (such as patent foramen ovale) to the aorta and directly to the cerebral circulation. The rapid and complex transition from fetal to postnatal circulation results in significant alterations in blood flow that may contribute to the pathogenesis of perinatal stroke. Third, in addition to thrombosis at the level of the placenta, the placenta may play a larger role in neonatal stroke through cytokine release, thereby creating an inflammatory, procoagulant environment that promotes systemic thrombus formation.[14]

Multiple additional risk factors specific to the pregnancy and the peripartum period have been associated with perinatal stroke, without a clear causative role being established.[7,10,14–21] The most consistently demonstrated risk factors include chorioamnionitis, maternal fever, and neonatal sepsis or meningitis, highlighting an important role of inflammation in perinatal stroke. Male sex has also been a consistently demonstrated risk factor for perinatal stroke, although the reason for this association is unknown.[10,17,20–22] Numerous other risk factors have been proposed but without being consistently demonstrated. Proposed prepartum risk factors include primiparity, prior fetal loss, intrauterine growth restriction/small for gestational age, oligohydramnios, gestational hypertension or preeclampsia, and maternal diabetes, among others.[7,10,17,18–21] Proposed intrapartum risk factors include prolonged rupture of

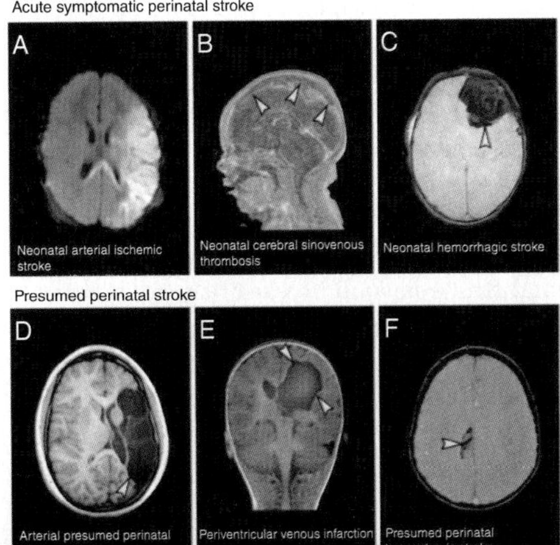

Fig. 50.1 Acute Perinatal Stroke Diseases as Seen on Magnetic Resonance of Imaging (MRI). (A) Neonatal arterial ischemic stroke features acute restriction on axial diffusion-weighted MRI in an arterial territory; diaschisis of the splenium of the corpus callosum is also evident. (B) Neonatal cerebral sinovenous thrombosis is evident as a filling defect on sagittal MR venogram (shown), in this case, in the superior sagittal sinus *(arrows)*. (C) Neonatal hemorrhagic stroke detectable on gradient echo or susceptibility-weighted MRI *(arrow)*. (D) Arterial presumed perinatal ischemic stroke in a child with hemiparesis is diagnosed by focal encephalomalacia on CT or MRI (axial T1-weighted MRI shown) in an arterial territory *(arrow)*. (E) Periventricular venous infarction presents with congenital hemiparesis with a focal lesion affecting the periventricular white matter with sparing of the cortex and basal ganglia, shown on coronal T1-weighted MRI (porencephaly indicated with *arrows*). (F) Presumed perinatal hemorrhagic stroke with a focal area of remote parenchymal injury showing hemorrhage (gradient echo, *arrow*). *CT*, Computed tomography. (Reprinted from Dunbar M, Kirton A. Perinatal stroke: mechanisms, management, and outcomes of early cerebrovascular brain injury. *Lancet*. 2018;2:666–676, Fig. 2, 668.)

membranes, prolonged second stage of labor, complicated delivery, abnormal fetal heart tracing, birth asphyxia, fetal hypoglycemia, and a low 5-minute Apgar score (less than 7), though whether these are the cause or the result of the perinatal brain injury is unclear.[7,16–18,20,21] The risk of perinatal stroke has been shown to increase significantly when multiple risk factors are present.[21]

The idea that multiple risk factors confined to the perinatal period converge to create a high-risk time for perinatal stroke is consistent with the low recurrence rate of perinatal stroke. However, there are some risk factors that confer ongoing stroke risk to the child, and their identification is essential to proper management. Hypercoagulable disorders have been thoroughly investigated in studies of perinatal stroke, and the results are inconsistent. Early studies examining the role of prothrombotic risk factors in perinatal stroke demonstrated high rates of prothrombotic abnormalities in infants with perinatal stroke. A large case-control study of infants with perinatal stroke showed that 68% of neonates with stroke had at least one abnormality on thrombophilia testing compared with 24% of age- and sex-matched healthy controls.[23] In two studies of mother-child pairs, more than 50% of both the infants with perinatal stroke and their mothers had prothrombotic abnormalities on testing in the neonatal period.[24,25] These abnormalities included low protein C or S, elevated lipoprotein(a), elevated homocysteine, methylene tetrahydrofolate reductase mutations, factor V Leiden, prothrombin G20210A mutations, or antiphospholipid antibodies. A prospective study of children with perinatal stroke showed that although the risk of a recurrent symptomatic thromboembolic event was low, about 3%, the risk of a second event was higher if prothrombotic risk factors were identified.[26] A meta-analysis including six studies that exclusively evaluated perinatal stroke likewise concluded that thrombophilia was a risk factor for neonatal arterial ischemic stroke, but the authors noted the paucity of eligible studies with control subjects, which limited the conclusions that could be drawn.[27] Despite these findings, more recent, larger studies have suggested that there is only a minimal association between perinatal stroke and thrombophilia.[28,29] Importantly, abnormal testing in these studies did not predict stroke recurrence, leading the authors to conclude that hypercoagulability evaluations should not be routinely completed in infants with perinatal stroke. Even if disordered coagulation is identified in the perinatal period, it is often transient, confined to the perinatal period or related to the thrombus itself. Regardless, multiple thromboembolic events and/or a family history of thrombosis should prompt consideration of a thorough thrombophilia evaluation.

In contrast, cardiac disease, although present in a minority of cases, is a risk factor with a clearer causal link to stroke and is associated with a substantially increased recurrence risk.[30] Imaging studies of children with congenital heart disease have found that 10% to 30% of infants can have stroke, with at least half occurring preoperatively.[31,32] In another study of children with congenital heart disease, the stroke recurrence rate was 14% after a neonatal sentinel stroke.[33] In addition, compared with older children, neonates are at higher risk for stroke associated with extracorporeal membrane oxygenation.[34]

Although arteriopathy is the most common risk factor for childhood arterial ischemic stroke,[35] its role in perinatal stroke is minimal. Rare cases of arteriopathic stroke in the perinatal period have been published, with etiologies felt to be congenital or traumatic.[36–39] Incidence of arteriopathy in association with perinatal stroke may be underestimated due to inconsistency in the use of vascular imaging.[37]

Table 50.1 Presenting Signs and Symptoms of 248 NAIS Patients in the International Pediatric Stroke Study Registry

Presenting Signs	Percentage
Seizure	72
Level of consciousness	39
Tone	38
Focal neurologic signs	30
Respiratory difficulty	26
Feeding difficulty	24

NAIS, Neonatal ischemic stroke.

Data from Kirton et al. Symptomatic neonatal arterial ischemic stroke: the International Pediatric Stroke Study. *Pediatrics*. 2011;128;e1402.

Presentation

Perinatal stroke can present at different times from fetal to postnatal life, with distinct clinical presentations depending on when the stroke is discovered. Therefore perinatal stroke can be subclassified into different types, including fetal, neonatal, and presumed perinatal arterial ischemic stroke.

Fetal strokes are typically hemorrhagic, although arterial ischemic stroke is increasingly being diagnosed with advancement of imaging including high-quality fetal ultrasound and fetal magnetic resonance imaging. In these cases, pregnancy often proceeds normally and the child's parents may present before the child is born for counseling on prognosis.[40]

Neonatal stroke is the subclassification of perinatal stroke that applies to children who present in the in the first 28 days of life.

Neonatal stroke typically presents with acute symptomatic seizures or diffuse neurologic signs on the first days of life (Table 50.1).[30] Seizures are focal and often refractory to treatment in the first few days of life, but they typically spontaneously remit outside of the acute period. Diffuse neurologic signs most commonly include abnormal tone or decreased level of arousal. Respiratory distress and feeding difficulties can also be part of the presentation of perinatal stroke. Focal findings are uncommon in the neonatal period. Typically, these children will be discharged home appearing well, although seizures may recur and neurologic deficits may emerge over time.

The diagnosis of PPAIS is given to children who present after the first 28 days of life with clinical or radiologic evidence of stroke that is presumed to have occurred in the perinatal period (between the 20th week of fetal life and the 28th day of postnatal life). Typically, pregnancy, delivery, and postnatal periods are medically unremarkable, and these children are often discharged from the nursery without suspected neurologic concerns. Often, PPAIS presents around 3 to 12 months of age with emerging focal deficits which may include early handedness, unilateral fisting, increased tone on one side, or visual field cut. Alternatively, children may present later in childhood with focal seizures, and they may or may not have subtle focal findings on a careful neurologic examination. These clinical findings often prompt neuroimaging that reveals evidence of a chronic infarction, which in the absence of a history of acute-onset neurologic deficits after the first month of age allows for a retrospective diagnosis of PPAIS. PPAIS is thought to occur by the same mechanisms as neonatal stroke, and why different children present in different ways is a question that deserves further investigation.

Evaluation and Management

Stroke should be on the differential diagnosis for any term infant presenting with focal seizures or encephalopathy soon after birth. An algorithm for the diagnosis and management of perinatal stroke is presented in Fig. 50.2. There can be some overlap in the presentation of infants with hypoxic-ischemic encephalopathy (HIE) and stroke. One study comparing infants with these diagnoses found a lower frequency of sentinel events and acidosis in the perinatal stroke group compared with the HIE group.[41] Nevertheless, HIE has a specific time-dependent treatment in hypothermia, and therefore, if HIE is suspected this should take precedence. It remains unclear whether hypothermia is beneficial or harmful for infants with stroke. Treatment with hypothermia should not be delayed when there is suspected HIE.

The diagnosis of perinatal stroke is made by neuroimaging. Magnetic resonance imaging (MRI) is the gold standard for evaluating infants with suspected stroke. Serial MRI can also provide important information about the evolution of the lesions (Fig. 50.3). Although computed tomography is fast and widely available, if provides far less information than MRI and has the additional concern of radiation exposure.[42] Diffusion weighted imaging will demonstrate infarcted brain tissue very early in the course. We recommend including sequences that are sensitive for blood products such as gradient echo or susceptibility weighted imaging. Vessel imaging with magnetic resonance (MR) angiography and venography can be included to identify arteriopathies or CSVT, which can be difficult to distinguish based on clinical presentation alone. All of these studies can be performed without the use of gadolinium, although MR venography will benefit from contrast administration.

Evaluation of risk factors has become more controversial in recent years. In a study by the International Pediatric Stroke Study registry, 18% of neonatal stroke patients had a concomitant cardiac diagnosis; thus evaluation of cardiac structure and function with echocardiography is recommended. The other group of infants that have a high risk of recurrence are those with severe thrombophilia, but testing for these risk factors is cumbersome and rarely yields findings that change management. One case-control study that evaluated infants with perinatal stroke beyond 1 year of age found that they had no increased incidence of prothrombotic laboratory findings than the general population.[28] Perinatal stroke presents a unique challenge in terms of stroke management because of the common absence of focal deficits that typically define time of onset. Recanalization strategies that have transformed the treatment of stroke in older children and adults are time-dependent and thus generally not applicable in perinatal stroke because the time of onset is often unknown. Management strategies thus focus on supportive care with the primary goal of promoting adequate perfusion to the brain and minimizing extension of the injury. This includes avoiding dehydration, targeting normal to moderately high blood pressures between the 50th and 99th percentile for gestational age (permissive hypertension), and maintaining normoglycemia.[43]

Antithrombotic therapies such as antiplatelet agents and anticoagulation are generally not indicated in neonatal arterial ischemic stroke because the risk of recurrence is exceedingly low. Exceptions would be infants with congenital heart disease or severe systemic thrombophilia in whom antithrombotic treatment should be tailored individually by a multidisciplinary team including neonatology, neurology, cardiology, and hematology. In older children and adults, anticoagulation is recommended for CSVT to prevent thrombus propagation and worsening symptoms, which may occur in approximately 30% of patients.[43,44] This is more controversial in neonates with CSVT due to uncertain benefits and risks. In a single-center study of neonatal CSVT, 51% of neonates received anticoagulation, including 30% of those with intracranial hemorrhage.[45] In this cohort there was no difference in increased hemorrhage between those who were anticoagulated and those who were not anticoagulated (5.3% versus 3% incidence, respectively). Our approach is to consider anticoagulation in these patients at diagnosis, but if perceived hemorrhage risk is felt to be too high, then to follow closely with repeat neuroimaging to monitor for thrombosis propagation.

Management of seizures in perinatal stroke is an important topic that has garnered increasing attention. Seizures are frequently the first or only presenting sign of stroke in neonates, and acute symptomatic seizures, defined as those occurring within 7 days of stroke, are much more common in neonates than in older children. A recent prospective study identified acute symptomatic seizures as a risk factor for the development of later epilepsy.[46] It remains unproven whether treatment of acute seizures can prevent epileptogenesis after perinatal stroke, but this nonetheless is an important part of the acute management of stroke in the newborn. Acute symptomatic seizures are often self-limited; thus we favor dosing with single boluses of antiseizure medicine for prolonged or recurrent seizures. Treatment options in the neonate include phenobarbital 20 mg/kg intravenous (IV), levetiracetam 60 mg/kg IV, and fosphenytoin 20 mg/kg IV. For refractory seizures, maintenance doses of either phenobarbital or levetiracetam are commonly used, but we typically try to wean to monotherapy by discharge and off completely soon after.

Because our options for acute treatment of perinatal stroke are limited, attention has turned to rehabilitation and early intervention service as the optimal strategy for improving neurologic outcomes.[47]

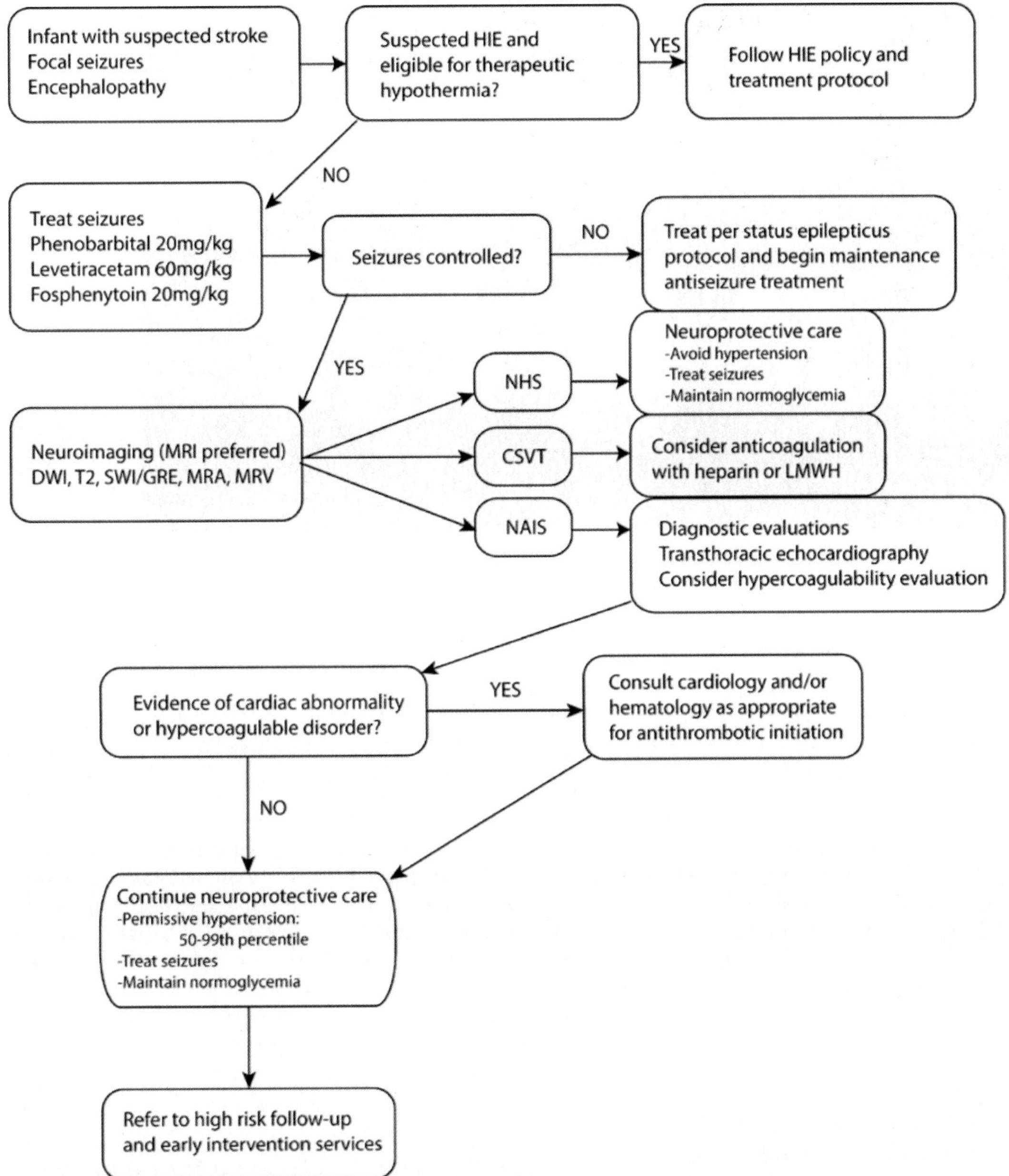

Fig. 50.2 Algorithm for the Evaluation and Management of Newborns With Suspected Perinatal Stroke Syndromes. *CSVT*, Cerebral Sinovenous Thrombosis; *DWI*, Diffusion Weighted Imaging; *GRE*, Gradient Echo; *HIE*, Hypoxic Ischemic Encephalopathy; *LMWH*, Low Molecular Weight Heparin; *MRA*, Magnetic Resonance Angiography; *MRV*, Magnetic Resonance Venography; *NAIS*, Neonatal Arterial Ischemic Stroke; *NHS*, Neonatal Hemorrhagic Stroke; *SWI*, Susceptibility Weighted Imaging.

In this regard perinatal stroke also presents unique challenges. Clinical and basic/translational science has demonstrated that the early period after stroke represents an important time for regeneration and remodeling that forms the basis of clinical recovery. In adults most motor recovery is complete by 1 month after stroke. Presumably this would be the time when therapies aimed at improving recovery would be most effective. Unfortunately, most therapies available today are targeted to rehabilitating a clinical deficit, and in infants with perinatal stroke those deficits are frequently not evident until several months after the stroke has occurred. Despite this apparent paradox, many experts in the field are advocating for early referral to rehabilitation and early intervention. The benefits of this include early therapy and environmental enrichment to promote neurodevelopment. The potential downside is that prediction of deficits and disability remains a challenge, and perhaps such early intervention may place an undue burden on families whose infants may do very well without it. Trials are currently underway to investigate the effectiveness of early and intensive rehabilitation. We also advocate for continued longitudinal follow-up of children in a multidisciplinary setting to identify emerging deficits early and implement strategies to improve development in these areas.

Outcomes

Understanding outcomes after perinatal stroke is challenging because many studies involve small series of children evaluated at varying time points. Overall, global outcomes can be quite good, although specific impairments in a variety of neurologic domains are common (Table 50.2).[2,48]

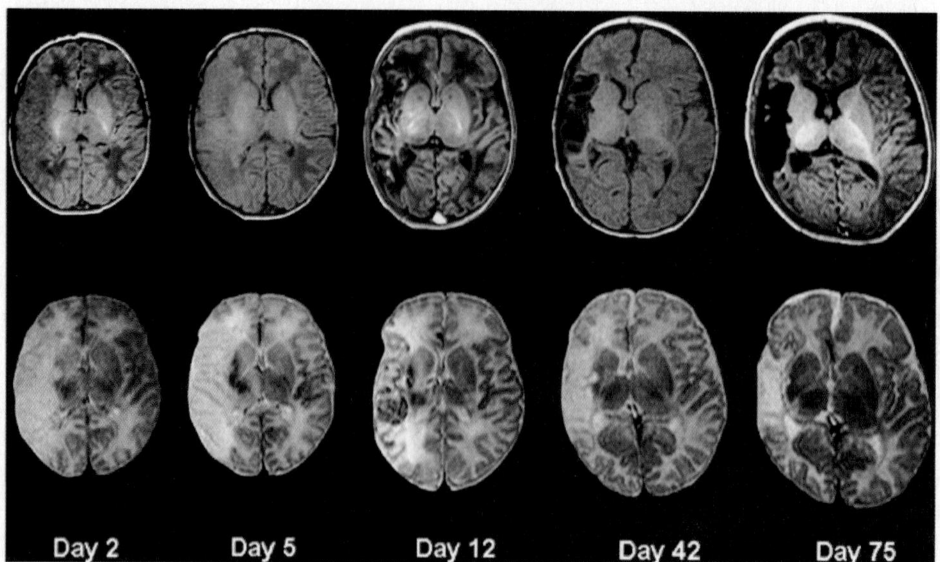

Fig. 50.3 Serial Imaging After Neonatal Stroke. Serial T1-weighted *(upper row)* and T2-weighted *(lower row)* sequences within the first 3 months after perinatal stroke at term, involving the right middle cerebral artery (MCA) in its cortical area and sparing deep grey matter (complete pial MCA stroke). Serial T1-weighted imaging (T1WI) and T2-weighted imaging (T2WI) showed increased signal intensity (SI) in the affected cortex and white matter. Vasogenic edema in combination with cytotoxic edema increased the overall water content in the infarcted tissue, resulting in prolonged T2 relaxation times. On T1WI the affected cortex exhibited low SI in the first week, from about day 2 after the onset of stroke. Next, from 1 week to 1 month, high SI was seen in the cortex on T1WI and low cortical SI on T2WI. The low cortical SI seen on T2WI is believed to be due to petechial hemorrhages, release of myelin lipids, and/or calcifications. An intermediate variegated or "checkerboard" pattern of mixed high and low SI in the areas of infarction can appear after 2 to 3 weeks in the neonate and subsequently progress into areas of cystic tissue loss after 1 to 2 months. (Reprinted from Dudink J, Mercuri E, Al-Nakib L, et al. Evolution of unilateral perinatal arterial ischemic stroke on conventional and diffusion weighted MR imaging. *AJNR Am J Neuroradiol*, doi:10.3714/ajnr.A1480.)

Recurrence

One of the guiding principles in stroke management is secondary prevention of recurrence. As described above, the perinatal period has many intrinsic risk factors that are unique and isolated to that time period. Recurrence of stroke in children with perinatal stroke is extremely rare, reported in about 3% of patients.[49] The most significant exception is those with congenital heart disease, who have a known significant risk of recurrent stroke.[33]

Neurologic Outcomes

Perinatal stroke, in particular arterial ischemic stroke, is the leading cause of hemiplegic cerebral palsy, and sensorimotor deficits are the most commonly reported sequelae in these infants, reported in more than 50%.[50] The vast majority of children learn to walk with some mild delay, with bilateral infarcts being the only predictor of lack of independent walking.[51] Language delay has been identified in 20% to 34% of patients.[2,52] Interestingly, the laterality of infarct does not significantly impact this, but the pattern and trajectory of language development is significantly altered, highlighting the plasticity underlying language acquisition after perinatal brain injury.[53] Although high incidences of specific neurologic deficits are frequently reported after perinatal stroke, the severity of neurologic outcomes is quite variable. Studies report moderate to severe neurologic deficits in 9% to 30% of patients after perinatal stroke, depending on age of assessment.[48,54] This is a significant fraction of patients who will, in all likelihood, have some degree of lifelong disability. Recent advances in the identification of neuroimaging predictors of clinical motor function are exciting (Fig. 50.4). As shown in these images, the investigators were able to measure structural connectivity via white matter tractography of the bilateral cortical spinal tract.

Cognitive and Behavioral Impairment

Cognitive and behavioral effects of perinatal stroke are important to recognize. While many studies show that perinatal stroke patients have IQ scores within the normal range, they are often lower compared with control groups.[55] Furthermore, perinatal stroke patients may be more at risk of deficits in full-scale IQ, verbal IQ, and working memory than children with strokes later in childhood.[56] Cognitive impairment may

Table 50.2 Neurologic Morbidity Following Perinatal Arterial Ischemic Stroke

Sequela	Incidence Range (%)	References
Cerebral palsy	37–54	Felling et al.,[48] Kirton and deVeber[50]
Language delay	25–34	Wagenaar et al.,[52] Trauner et al.[53]
Neuropsychological impairment	23–60	Kirton and deVeber,[2] Wagenaar et al.,[52] Kolk et al.,[55] Westmacott et al.,[56] Westmacott et al.[57]
ADHD	15	Williams et al.[58]
Epilepsy	19–54	Fox et al.,[60] Billinghurst et al.,[61] Wusthoff et al.[62]

ADHD, Attention deficit and hyperactivity disorder.

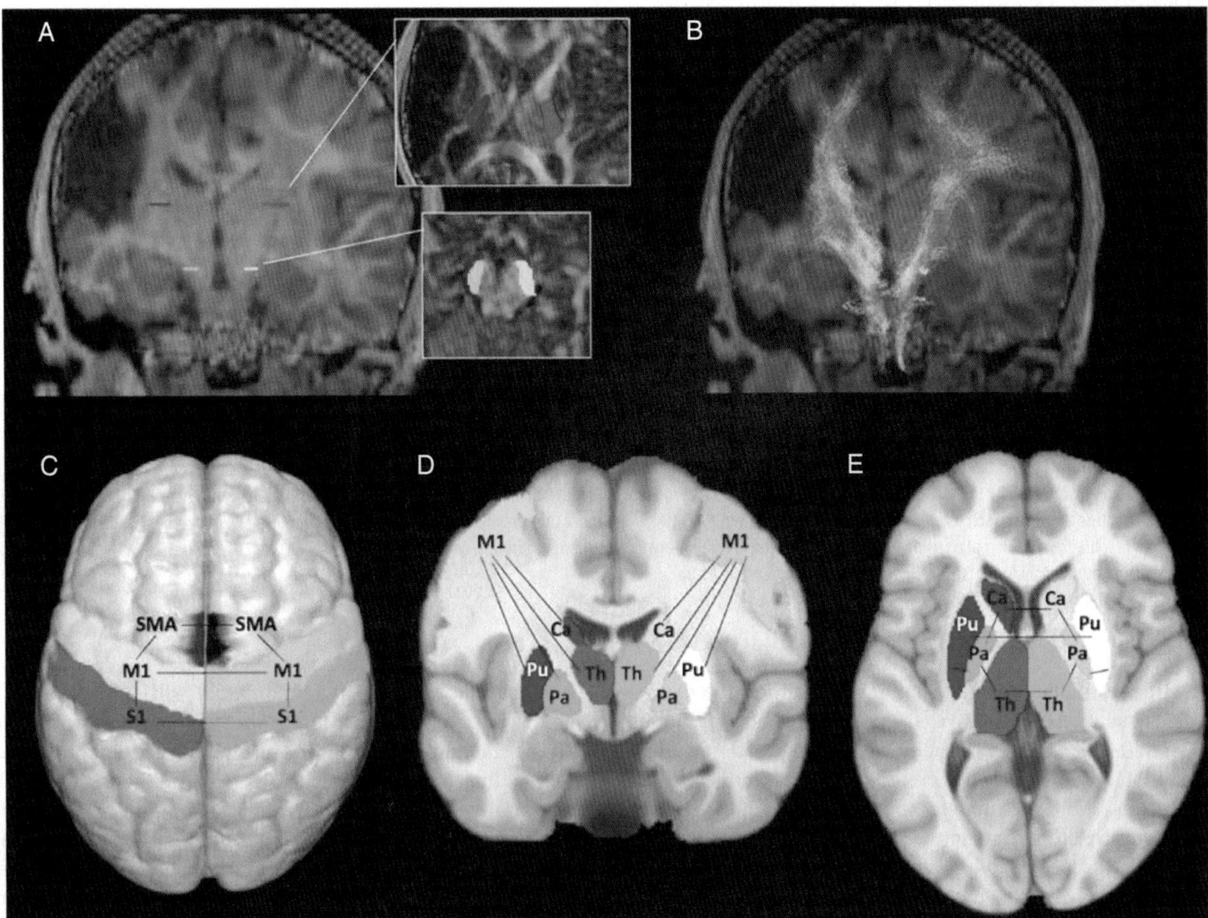

Fig. 50.4 Neuroimaging Predictors of Clinical Motor Function. Structural connectivity was measured via white matter tractography of the bilateral cortical spinal tract (CST). (A) Regions of interest (ROIs) included the posterior limb of the internal capsule (*red/pink* ROIs) and the cerebral peduncles (*yellow/cyan* ROIs). Underlying diffusion characteristics (mean FA, MD, RD, and AD) were extracted from CST masks overlaid on the diffusion maps (B). Functional connectivity was measured between cortical motor areas (C), cortico-subcortical areas (D), and within subcortical areas (E). *AD,* Axial diffusivity; *Ca,* caudate; *FA,* fractional anisotropy; *M1,* primary motor cortex; *MD,* mean diffusivity; *Pa,* pallidum; *Pu,* putamen; *RD,* radial diffusivity; *S1,* primary sensory cortex; *SMA,* supplementary motor area; *Th,* thalamus. (Reprinted from Carlson et al. Structural and functional connectivity of motor circuits after perinatal stroke: a machine learning study. *NeuroImage Clin.* 2020;28:102508. https://doi.org/10.1016/j.nicl.2020.102508.)

become more manifest over time as children age and are expected to master increasingly challenging material.[57]

Attention deficit and hyperactivity disorder (ADHD) is increasingly being recognized in children after stroke. In one cohort, 15% of perinatal stroke patients were diagnosed with ADHD, and this significantly impacted overall IQ compared with both perinatal stroke patients without ADHD and ADHD patients without stroke.[58] Further research is needed to determine whether there is a differential response to conventional treatments including pharmacologic and behavioral approaches in this specific population.

The occurrence of cognitive and behavioral impairments after perinatal stroke is often overlooked because the sensorimotor and epilepsy outcomes are more obvious. These are important, however, to be aware of because they can significantly impact quality of life. In one study, 15% of perinatal stroke survivors were rated as having a poor overall quality of life at least 3 years after their stroke, and one of the significant predictors of this was cognitive/behavioral impairment.[59] Longitudinal follow-up in multidisciplinary clinics is important to screen and diagnose patients with these impairments and provide the necessary resources and treatment.

Epilepsy

Epilepsy is an important adverse outcome after perinatal stroke that can significantly impact quality of life and other domains of neurologic function.[60–62] Infants with neonatal stroke are at higher risk for development of remote epilepsy than older children, with 10-year cumulative rates of unprovoked remote seizures of 54% after neonatal stroke compared with 33% after childhood stroke.[63,64] Substantially fewer are classified as “active epilepsy” after 10 years, suggesting that long-term outcomes of epilepsy itself may be more optimistic than the incidence of remote seizures.[65] Epilepsy can manifest as focal seizures or as infantile spasms.[61] The occurrence of acute symptomatic seizures, which occur in the majority of infants with NAIS, are predictive of the development of later epilepsy.[46,64] It remains unknown whether these both reflect the innate hyperexcitability of the immature brain or whether acute symptomatic seizures actually contribute to epileptogenesis. In the latter case, they may represent an important therapeutic target for preventing the development of epilepsy.

CHAPTER

51 Using Biomarkers for Management of Perinatal Brain Injury

Allen D. Everett, Ernest Graham, Melania M. Bembea

KEY POINTS

1. Hypoxic-ischemic encephalopathy (HIE) is a major cause of neonatal morbidity and mortality. More than 50% of all infants with HIE will die or have severe neurologic disabilities by the age of 2 years.
2. The need to institute therapies such as whole-body hypothermia in a timely fashion make rapid identification of neurologic injury critically important.
3. The focus of biomarker development in neonatal brain injury has been on the identification of moderate to severe injury, which is most likely to be treatable.
4. Glial biomarkers such as glial fibrillary acidic protein (GFAP) holds the most promise. GFAP is a cytoskeletal intermediate filament protein seen mainly in astroglial cells.
5. A single biomarker may not be sufficient to estimate the severity of a multifaceted complex disease such as HIE or traumatic brain injury. A combination with other potential brain injury biomarkers or with clinical tools may help.

Worldwide it is estimated that 1.15 million babies develop hypoxic-ischemic encephalopathy (HIE) every year.[1] Up to 60% of infants with HIE will die or have severe disabilities by the age of 2, including mental retardation, epilepsy, and cerebral palsy.[2] The costs related to HIE exceed $11 billion annually in the United States.[3] HIE is defined by a constellation of symptoms in the neonate, but no definitive diagnostic test is available.[4] One of the greatest challenges in perinatal medicine is assessing the fetus during labor and the neonate shortly after birth for evidence of brain injury. The presence of meconium, nonreassuring fetal heart rate tracing, Apgar scores, umbilical artery blood gases, and physical exam are tools currently used to identify brain injury in the fetus and neonate, but all of these lack precision.

The availability of therapies such as whole-body hypothermia, which must be instituted within 6 hours of birth, make the rapid identification of a baby with neurologic injury critically important. How to rapidly and objectively identify the fetus and neonate with brain injury may be solved by borrowing an approach from traumatic brain injury research. Extensive effort has been applied in the field of traumatic brain injury to identify acute blood biomarkers as diagnostics to identify these patients, discriminate severity, and monitor treatment efficacy and as prognostics for recovery and long-term disabilities.[5] Although urine can be obtained noninvasively, and due to its rich source of proteins may contain many potential biomarkers, severely asphyxic newborns shunt blood away from their kidneys, which can lead to acute renal injury and oliguria, making interpretation of urinary biomarkers difficult. Biomarkers of brain injury can also be obtained from cerebrospinal fluid (CSF); however, obtaining CSF is more invasive and potentially complicated than obtaining blood and is not amenable to serial sampling.

The focus of biomarker development in traumatic brain injury has been on the identification of moderate to severe injury[6]; however, the greatest potential impact of blood biomarkers to change clinical practice in perinatology is for mild injury because diagnostic and prognostic challenges presented for mild injuries are more difficult to identify and monitor.[5] There is no current standard therapy for mild injury, and increasingly late follow-up suggests that mild injury results in identifiable pathology in children.

It is unlikely that a single biomarker will reflect the full picture of the injured brain for a multifaceted, complex disease such as HIE or traumatic brain injury.[5] Combining biomarkers from multiple cellular pathways has shown superior sensitivity and specificity in the identification of traumatic brain injury.[5] Simultaneous measurements of neuronal and glial biomarkers may complement each other to identify distinct injury mechanisms and determine the timing of injury. A study of severe traumatic brain injury found that glial biomarker elevations are primarily a reflection of focal mass lesions and that diffuse injuries primarily result in neuronal biomarker elevations.[6] Because patients with diffuse injuries may require different therapies than patients with focal lesions, such a combination of biomarkers may enable us to select patients for targeted therapies.[5,7] In perinatal medicine this might allow differentiation of large major vessel stroke from more diffuse hypoxic-ischemic injuries. The ideal biomarker panel may include multiple biomarkers produced by different brain cell types, and currently available multiplex immunoassay platforms make it possible to measure up to 10 biomarkers with a high degree of sensitivity from small volumes of plasma.[5] Investigators have proposed developing a point-of-care handheld device that can quickly and accurately measure brain injury biomarkers, similar to the handheld dextrometer for diabetic patients that can measure a glucose level within seconds.[8]

Optimally, the level of the brain injury biomarkers should correlate with the size, location, and severity of the lesion, clinical outcome, and response to treatment.[9] Ideally, serum biomarkers should provide information on the pathophysiology of injury, improve stratification of patients by injury severity, assist in the monitoring of secondary insults and injury progression, monitor response to treatment, and predict functional outcome.[10] Circulating brain injury biomarker levels in neonatal HIE could indicate brain injury and reflect the extent of damage, solving a clinical dilemma in the discrimination of mild versus moderate-severe injury.[11] Neonatal brain injury is also complex, with the initial hypoxic-ischemic injury followed by secondary injury, which maybe inflammatory in nature. Biomarkers that can discriminate acute injury and interrogate secondary injury are likely to be the most helpful for outcome prognostication and discriminating treatment effects (Box 51.1).

■ Box 51.1 Desired Characteristics of an Ideal Biomarker of Central Nervous System Injury

- Early change in blood levels that show mild-moderate injury in its early phase, which might be potentially treatable
- Combinations of neuronal and glial biomarkers might improve sensitivity and specificity
- Combinations of biomarkers from multiple cellular signaling pathways might improve sensitivity and specificity
- Ease of measurement, possibly with a portable, handheld device
- Blood change linearly with increasing severity of injury
- Identify secondary insults and injury progression
- Identify response to treatment and predict eventual outcome
- Clear understanding of the significance of levels in blood versus the cerebrospinal fluid

Because currently there is no gold standard for diagnosing mild traumatic brain injury, not even by conventional assessment through neuroimaging techniques,[12] these approaches have been applied to identify brain-specific markers of injury (Fig. 51.1). During brain injury, neural proteins or their breakdown products are released into the extracellular environment, reaching the CSF in relatively high concentration and the bloodstream via the compromised blood-brain barrier.[13] In premature infants in particular, the blood-brain barrier is particularly fragile, potentially increasing the likelihood that brain proteins may reach the circulation after injury.[14] The clearance and half-life of the biomarkers contribute to the final concentration that can be measured in blood.[13]

Of the numerous candidate biomarkers for traumatic brain injury, glial fibrillary acidic protein (GFAP) holds the most promise.[13] One of the main strengths of GFAP as a brain injury biomarker is that it is only found within the central nervous system.[15] GFAP is a cytoskeletal intermediate filament protein that forms networks that support astroglial cells and is found only in the astroglial cytoskeleton.[13] Astrocytes are important to brain injury because their foot processes compose part of the blood-brain barrier, and with disruption after injury, astrocyte damage results in early release of GFAP.[13,16] GFAP levels peak at 1 to 2 days following severe brain trauma and are normal in patients with other trauma that does not include traumatic brain injury, an indication of GFAP's brain specificity.[17] In neonates, serum GFAP levels have been shown to be significantly elevated at the time of birth and during the first week of life in term and near-term infants with HIE who have abnormal brain magnetic resonance imaging (MRI) scans at 1 week of life[18–20] and in premature neonates who develop periventricular white matter injury.[21] In addition, GFAP may provide insights into the pathobiology of therapeutic hypothermia because significant elevations in GFAP occur after rewarming from therapeutic cooling for HIE in the neonates that later have an abnormal MRI, suggesting that the neonates with severe injury manifest reperfusion injury after therapeutic cooling.[17] This may offer an opportunity to discriminate mild from moderate to severe HIE and triage high-risk neonates to evolving adjunctive therapies.

Blood biomarkers discovered in traumatic brain injury could significantly improve the management of neonates with HIE, particularly those with mild and moderate injury, by providing more accurate early diagnosis and prognosis and by monitoring therapies in the acute care setting.[10] Biomarkers could help determine the severity and mechanism of injury and quantitatively measure injury progression, which would provide major opportunities for clinical research.[10]

Several potential epilepsy biomarkers have been proposed in recent years, including blood biomarkers of inflammation, blood-brain barrier damage, and brain injury. Given the complexity of epilepsy, it is unlikely that a single biomarker is sufficient for predicting epileptogenesis, but a combinatorial approach may be able to identify appropriate biomarkers at different stages of the evolution of the disease.[22]

The pathology of perinatal HIE is very heterogeneous, and one "magic" biomarker may not be the solution, but a panel of biomarkers may prove to be most useful in distinguishing the different pathologic-anatomic processes that compose the injury.[10] The brain consists of many elements, and depending on the mechanism and severity

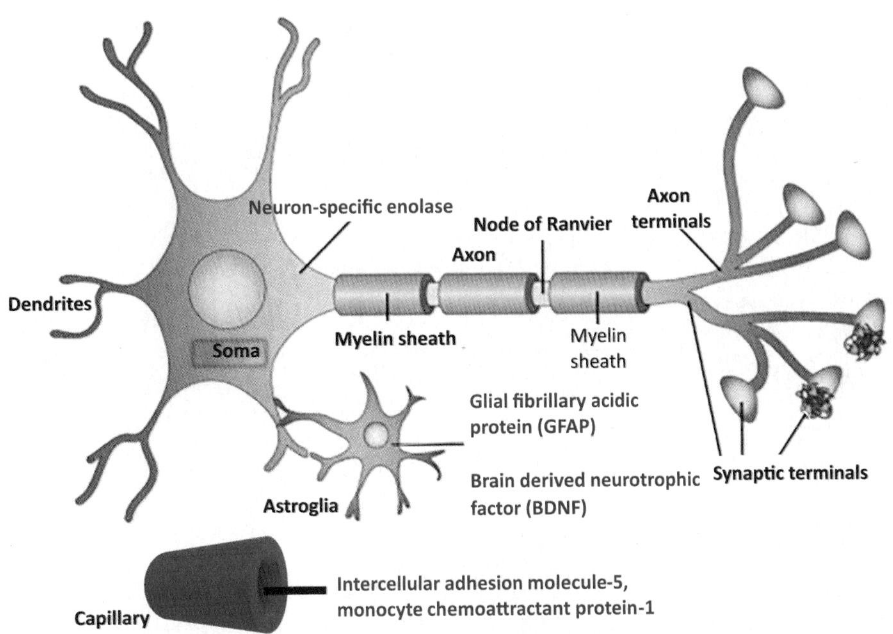

Fig. 51.1 Sources of Potential Biomarkers (in *Red Font*) of Central Nervous System Injury in Neonates.

of injury, various damage patterns may be reflected by different combinations of biomarkers.[23] Biomarkers will probably supplement existing tools such as the Glasgow Coma Scale and neuroimaging for the initial classification of brain injury in the near future.[10] Because the hypoxic injury pattern on MRI is not diagnostic for 7 to 14 days, a blood biomarker that could fill the clinical gap for predicting current and worsening neurologic status or long-term disability would have great clinical utility. With the combinations of different pathophysiology related to each biomarker, a multibiomarker analysis would seem to be the most effective way to assess brain injury and would likely increase diagnostic accuracy.[24]

Blood biomarkers offer an objective and quantitative way to identify and follow a neonate with brain injury. They could be used to triage neonates to the current standard of 72 hours of hypothermia as well as investigational therapies such as erythropoietin, xenon gas, melatonin, and stem cell treatment. Blood biomarkers could possibly provide information about the extent of injury in the acute phase before ultrasound or MRI can identify abnormalities and determine the timing of injury as well. Rather than imprecise measures of fetal and neonatal brain injury, such as fetal heart rate abnormalities, meconium, cord gas at delivery, and Apgar scores, a multiplex combining glial and neuronal biomarkers could provide objective evidence of the extent and pattern of injury that would lead to improved identification of the brain-injured fetus or neonate and triage to appropriate therapy after birth and would serve as an objective measure of the effectiveness of treatment.

Applications for circulating brain injury biomarkers may also become clinically relevant in the future for infants who suffer severe cardiopulmonary failure or cardiac arrest in the neonatal period. Interventions employed in the neonatal intensive care unit may contribute to additional risk of neurologic injury in these scenarios. One such intervention is extracorporeal life support in the form of extracorporeal membrane oxygenation (ECMO) used in the neonatal period for infants with severe refractory persistent pulmonary hypertension of the newborn, meconium aspiration syndrome, congenital diaphragmatic hernia, congenital heart disease, and other more rare indications.[25] Over 30,000 neonatal ECMO cases have been reported to the Extracorporeal Life Support Organization (ELSO) registry from inception in 1989 to July 2019.[26] Although the number of neonatal ECMO cases has stabilized, there has been a continued and steady increase in the number of cardiac and extracorporeal cardiopulmonary resuscitation neonatal ECMO cases reported to the ELSO registry in the past decade.[26] Despite this increase in the total number of ECMO cases, survival in the past 5 years has remained stable at 68% for neonatal respiratory ECMO cases, 50% for neonatal cardiac ECMO cases, and 43% for neonatal extracorporeal cardiopulmonary resuscitation cases.[26] ECMO is associated with high risk for neurologic injury, including intracranial hemorrhage and stroke.[25] Both complications have been shown to be associated with reduced survival.[25] Therefore, neurologic monitoring is paramount for prompt diagnosis of brain injury with implementation of neuroprotective interventions, and after ECMO decannulation, of rehabilitation interventions. Several neurologic monitoring methods have been deployed in neonatal ECMO patients with varying success, including daily head ultrasounds, amplitude integrated electroencephalography, standard or continuous electroencephalography, transcranial Doppler ultrasound, cerebral oximetry monitoring, and circulating brain injury biomarkers.[27] Serial monitoring of brain-specific proteins circulating in blood has been shown to be associated with abnormal neuroimaging findings during or immediately after ECMO support, with survival after critical illness requiring ECMO support, and with neurofunctional status at hospital discharge in former ECMO patients.[28,29] Given the heterogeneity of injury encountered during ECMO support, efforts were made to develop panels of brain injury biomarkers in this population that have the ability to reflect neuronal injury (e.g., neuron specific enolase [NSE], brain derived neurotrophic factor), astrocytic injury (e.g., GFAP, S100b), and neuroinflammation (e.g., monocyte chemoattractant protein 1 [MCP1], intercellular adhesion molecule-5). In a study of 80 neonatal and pediatric patients, the performance characteristics for a combination of biomarkers of brain injury included an area under the receiver operating characteristic curve that reached significance for GFAP, MCP1, NSE, and S100b (0.71, 0.64, 0.68, and 0.66, respectively).[28] A model for unfavorable outcome prediction that removed collinear biomarker predictors yielded an improved area under the curve of 0.73 for the combination of GFAP and NSE.[28] It is foreseeable that neonates requiring intensive care interventions will, in the future, be monitored with serial measurements of circulation brain injury biomarkers during periods of high risk for injury, including ECMO, cardiopulmonary bypass for congenital heart disease repair,[30–32] or after cardiac arrest.[33–35]

CHAPTER 52

Intraventricular Hemorrhage and Posthemorrhage Hydrocephalus

Venkat Reddy Kallem, Akhil Maheshwari

KEY POINTS

1. Very-low-birthweight infants are at risk of spontaneous germinal matrix–intraventricular hemorrhages (GM-IVHs).
2. GM-IVHs usually originate within the subependymal germinal matrix lining the ventricles and progress outwards into the ventricles. IVH occurs most frequently during the first 72 hours after birth.
3. A subset of infants with IVH develop periventricular hemorrhagic infarction, posthemorrhagic ventricular dilatation, and posthemorrhagic hydrocephalus (PHH).
4. Posthemorrhagic ventricular dilatation is noted in 30% to 50% of infants with IVH of grade III or IV and can damage the surrounding white matter due to increased pressure. One-third of these infants recover, but others require intervention.
5. The definitive treatment of PHH is usually the placement of a ventriculoperitoneal shunt, where the catheter has a proximal end in the ventricular system of the brain that is connected to a valve underneath the skin to control cerebrospinal fluid flow. Several other treatment modalities are being investigated.

Introduction

Premature infants with a birth weight < 1500 g (very low birth weight infants) are at risk of spontaneous germinal matrix–intraventricular hemorrhages (GM-IVHs).[1–3] These hemorrhages usually originate within the subependymal germinal matrix lining the ventricles,[1,4] a highly vascularized region rich in neuronal-glial precursor cells in the periventricular regions in the developing brain,[5] and can progress outward.[6] The etiology of IVH is multifactorial, but as currently understood, it can be ascribed primarily to frequent, accentuated fluctuations in the cerebral blood flow[7] and the fragile vasculature of the germinal matrix.[8] A subset of infants with IVH develop periventricular hemorrhagic infarction and posthemorrhagic ventricular dilatation (PHVD).[9,10] The ventricular dilatation may reflect hydrocephalus *ex vacuo* from encephalomalacia in some and symptomatic progressive posthemorrhagic hydrocephalus (PHH) with increased intracranial pressure in others.[11,12] Despite all the improvement in the frequency of neonatal morbidities and mortality in the past 2 decades, the incidence if IVH has not changed. GM-IVH is associated with increased mortality and abnormal neurodevelopmental outcomes in the form of posthemorrhagic hydrocephalus, cerebral palsy, epilepsy, severe cognitive impairment, and visual and hearing impairment.[13]

In this chapter, we review the pathophysiology of IVH and PHVD, outline the medical and surgical management, and discuss interventions for prevention of IVH. In addition to data from our own unpublished quality-improvement/outcome-monitoring studies, this chapter includes information from an extensive literature review of the PubMed, EMBASE, and Scopus databases. To avoid bias in identifying studies, keywords were short-listed *a priori* from anecdotal experience and PubMed's Medical Subject Heading (MeSH) thesaurus.

Incidence and Timing of GM-IVH

GM-IVH is seen most frequently in premature infants, and both the incidence and severity of hemorrhage are inversely related to birth weight and gestational age. The incidence of IVH is highest is extremely low birth weight infants, although this varies by center and ranges between 5% to 52% of grades 3 to 4 and 5% to 19% of grade 2, respectively.[14] Overall, the incidence of some of form of IVH in very low birth weight infants ranges from 20% to 25%.[15] IVH occurs most frequently during the first 72 days after birth; nearly 50% of all IVHs occur within the first 24 hours, 25% on the 2nd day, and 15% on the 3rd day.[16]

Neuropathology

Normal Cerebrospinal Fluid Pathways

Cerebrospinal fluid (CSF) is normally produced in the ependyma and choroid plexus. It flows from the lateral ventricles and passes through the foramina of Monro and then into the third ventricle. From there, it travels down the aqueduct of Sylvius and into the fourth ventricle. It then leaves the ventricular system through the foramina of Luschka and Magendie, entering the subarachnoid space of the basal cisterns. The flow continues up over the cerebral convexities to the arachnoid granulations, where it is resorbed into the venous system by a pressure-dependent mechanism.[17] These details are shown in Fig. 52.1.

Germinal Matrix-Intraventricular Hemorrhage

In GM-IVH, the bleeding originates in the germinal matrix, the region of the brain located just outside ependymal lining of the ventricles.[2] The groove between the head of the caudate nucleus and the thalamus is the most frequently involved site[18,19]; this region is a rich source of neuroblasts that migrate outwards from developing fetal brain (Fig. 52.2).[20,21] The germinal matrix is largest during midgestation at 23 to 24 weeks' gestation and then gradually involutes by 36 weeks.[22] The capillary bed in the germinal matrix is highly vascular[23] and is composed of relatively large, irregular endothelial-lined vessels.[24] The high propensity for hemorrhage in the germinal matrix is due to characteristic features including exuberant angiogenesis,[23] which could possibly be related to the high vascular endothelial

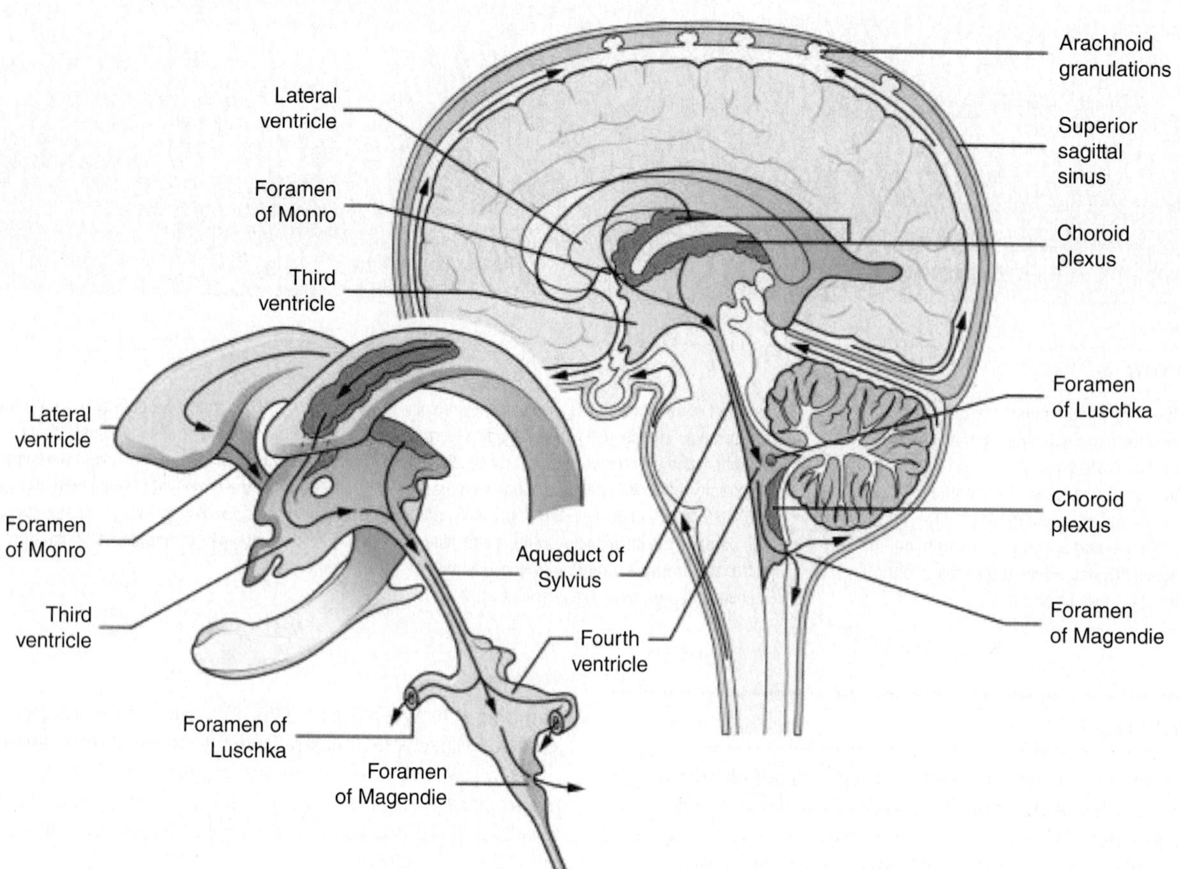

Fig. 52.1 Normal Cerebrospinal Fluid Pathways. (Reproduced with permission and after modifications from Bonow et al. Hydrocephalus in children. In: *Principles of Neurological Surgery*, 8, 133–147.e3.)

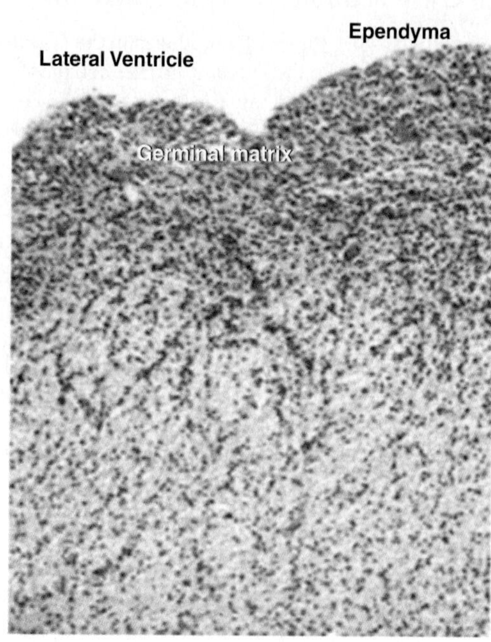

Fig. 52.2 Germinal Matrix in the Brain of a 20-Week-Gestation Fetus. This area is located directly adjacent to the ependyma of the lateral ventricles and is densely populated with neuronal precursors. The germinal matrix diminishes and eventually disappears in the first year of postnatal life. (Reproduced with permission and minor modifications from Brat DJ. Normal brain histopathology. In: *Practical Surgical Neuropathology: A Diagnostic Approach*. 2017:19–37.)

growth factor and angiopoietin levels,[25] discontinuous glial end-feet of the blood-brain barrier,[26] paucity of pericytes,[27] immaturity of the basal lamina,[1] and developmentally regulated vascular wall characteristics such as a high morphometric ratio of diameter to wall thickness.[28] In most cases of germinal matrix hemorrhage, the blood enters the lateral ventricles and spreads throughout the ventricular system (see Fig. 52.1). This blood may trigger obliterative arachnoiditis over the next few days and may hamper CSF dynamics, leading to obstruction of CSF flow.[29,30] Neuropathological consequences of IVH include germinal matrix destruction, cerebral white matter injury/dysmaturation, cerebral gray matter dysmaturation, cerebellar dysmaturation, periventricular hemorrhagic infarction, and posthemorrhagic hydrocephalus.[31–35]

The pathogenesis of GM-IVH is multifactorial and it is primarily related to intravascular factors (related to regulation of blood flow), vascular factors (related to fragility of germinal matrix vasculature), and extravascular factors (related to platelet and coagulation disturbances; Table 52.1). The risk of hemorrhage can be partially explained on the basis of vascular anatomic features (Fig. 52.4). However, because all premature neonates do not develop IVH, additional factors are likely involved.

The increased risk of IVH in premature infants can be ascribed to multiple pathophysiological factors (see Fig. 52.3).

1. Anatomic and developmentally regulated structural risk factors in the local vascular supply[24,36] (Fig. 52.4):
   a. The arterial supply to the subependymal germinal matrix is derived particularly from the anterior cerebral artery (through the Heubner artery), the middle cerebral artery (through the

Table 52.1 Risk Factors for GM-IVH

Major Pathogenetic Mechanism	Probable Mechanism	Risk Factors
Intravascular factors (dysregulation of cerebral blood flow)	Fluctuation in cerebral blood flow/altered autoregulation	Hypercarbia Hypoxia Asynchrony on mechanical ventilation Suctioning PDA Agitation Hypovolemia
	Pressure-passive circulation	Hypertension Hypotension Rapid volume expansion Hypercarbia Decreased hematocrit Decreased blood glucose
	Increase in cerebral venous pressure/altered autoregulation	Labor and vaginal delivery Asphyxia Respiratory disturbances Pneumothorax
Vascular factors (fragility of germinal matrix)	Maturational changes/structural weakness of capillaries (involuting and remodeling capillary bed, deficient vascular lining, large surface area of the vascular lumen)	Prematurity
	Vulnerability of GM to hypoxic, ischemic injury (vascular border zones, high metabolism)	Prematurity Hypoxic ischemic insult Sepsis
Extravascular factors (platelet dysfunction, immature coagulation)	Immature vascular structure Abnormal fibrinolytic activity	Prematurity Thrombocytopenia Disseminated intravascular coagulation

GM, Germinal matrix; *GM-IVH*, germinal matrix–intraventricular hemorrhage; *PDA*, patent ductus arteriosus.

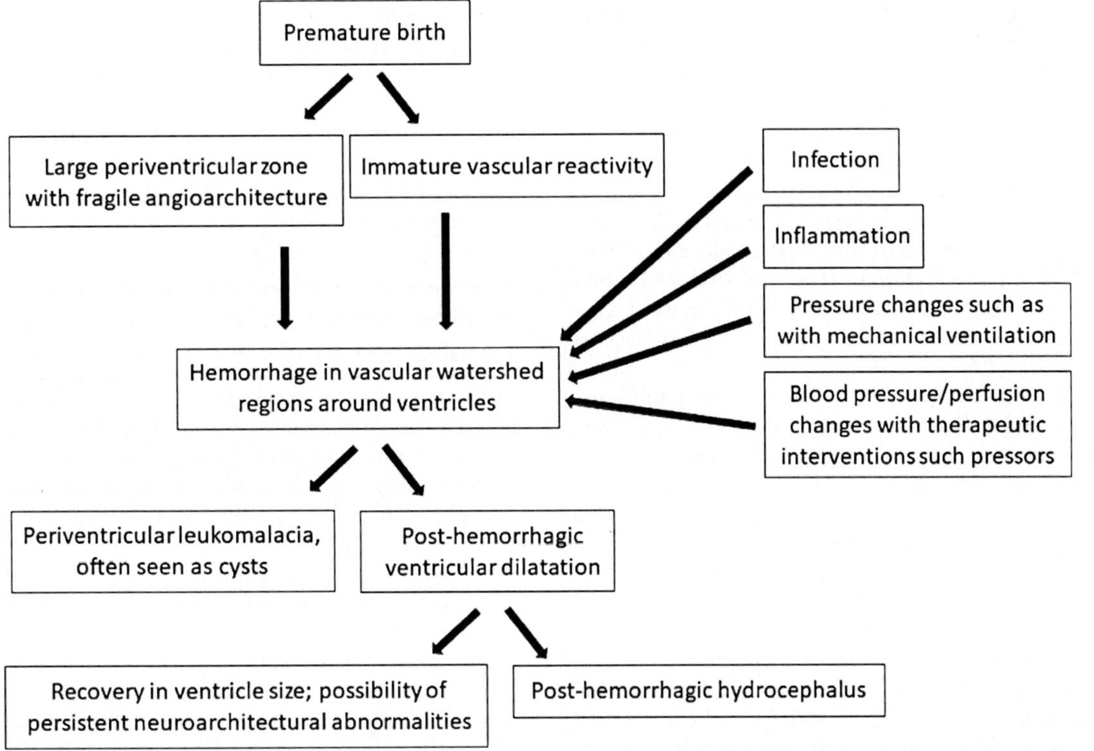

Fig. 52.3 Pathogenesis of IVH-PVHI in Premature Infants. *IVH*, Intraventricular hemorrhage; *PVHI*, periventricular hemorrhagic infarction.

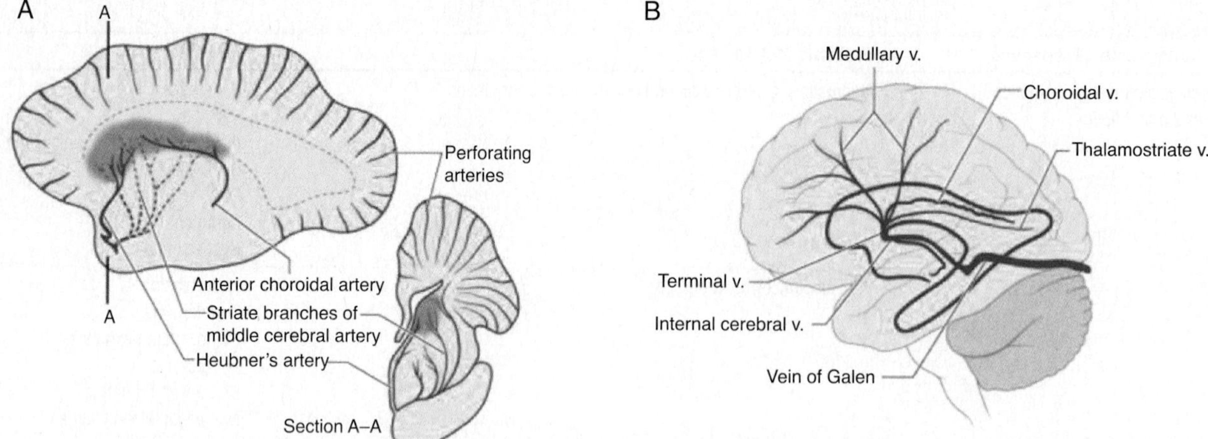

Fig. 52.4 Anatomic and Structural Vascular Risk Factors for Germinal Matrix Hemorrhage in Preterm Infants. (A) Arterial supply to the subependymal germinal matrix at 29 weeks of gestation. (B) Veins of the galenic system, midsagittal view. Note that the medullary, choroidal, and thalamostriate veins come to a point of confluence to form the terminal vein. The terminal vein, which courses through the germinal matrix, empties into the internal cerebral vein, and the major flow of blood changes direction sharply at that junction. (A, From Hambleton G, Wigglesworth JS. Origin of intraventricular hemorrhage in the preterm infant. *Arch Dis Child.* 1976;51:651–659; B, the composite figure was produced with permission and after modifications from the figures in Inder et al. Preterm intraventricular hemorrhage/posthemorrhagic hydrocephalus. In: *Volpe's Neurology of the Newborn*, ch. 24, 637–698.e21.)

deep lateral striate branches and the penetrating branches from the surface meningeal branches), and the internal carotid artery.[37–39] The terminal branches of the Heubner artery and the lateral striate arteries constitute a vascular end zone and cause vulnerability to ischemic injury.[38]

b. The arterial supply feeds an elaborate capillary bed in the germinal matrix. These capillaries are fragile; they are relatively large, irregular, endothelial-lined vessels that show discontinuous glial end-feet of the blood-brain barrier, relative lack of pericytes, immature basal lamina characteristics, and developmentally regulated characteristics including a high morphometric ratio of the vascular diameter to wall thickness.[26,31]
c. The rich microvascular network drains into a deep venous system, which eventually terminates in the great cerebral vein of Galen. At the usual site of germinal matrix hemorrhage, the direction of blood flow in the venous system changes in a peculiar U-turn.[24,36] This feature may increase the risk of GM-IVH and even periventricular hemorrhagic infarction.

2. Perinatal clinical factors: birth asphyxia, subtle cranial trauma due to vaginal/forceps delivery, severity of prematurity-related respiratory distress, and the use of hypertonic solutions such as bicarbonate.
3. Physiologic immaturity: fluctuating cerebral perfusion volumes due to the mismatch between the systemic and cerebral blood flow and regional variations in blood flow velocities in different parts of the brain. In addition to cranial trauma during birth, fluctuations in regional and overall cerebral perfusion during resuscitation at birth and subsequent intubation, ventilation, and periods of hypo-/hyperoxia have been implicated. Periods of systemic hypotension, patent *ductus arteriosus*, and hypercarbia may also contribute to the risk.[6,16,40–42] In term infants, intracranial and IVH can occur if the infant has coagulation abnormalities, arteriovenous malformations, and sinovenous thromboses. Genetic abnormalities in the formation of extracellular matrix components can also increase the risk.[43,44]

Pathogenesis of Periventricular Hemorrhagic Infarction

Nearly 15% of all cases of GM-IVH develop periventricular hemorrhagic infarction (PVHI), lesions composed of hemorrhagic necrosis in the periventricular white matter dorsal and lateral to the external angle of the lateral ventricles (see Fig. 52.5).[11] The incidence of PVHI is inversely related to gestational age; extremely low birth weight infants are at the highest risk.[35,45] The main pathologic event in the development of PVHI is GM-IVH; the sequence of events is obstruction of terminal veins, impaired blood flow in the medullary veins, and venous infarction.[3] Microscopically, the lesions show perivascular hemorrhages in a fan-shaped distribution, arising from the medullary veins in periventricular white matter.[46,47] The most frequent sequelae of PVHI are one or more porencephalic cysts that may or may not communicate with the lateral ventricle (Fig. 52.6).[47] The severity of periventricular leukomalacia can be graded by several systems,[48–50] one of which is shown in Table 52.2.[51]

Posthemorrhagic Ventricular Dilatation and Posthemorrhagic Hydrocephalus

PHVD and PHH may occur after GM-IVH.[11] When ventricular dilatation occurs secondary to periventricular leukomalacia or PVHI or both, this entity is called PHVD. It progresses gradually over several weeks and is typically not associated with raised intracranial pressure or rapid changes in head circumference. When IVH obstructs the CSF flow at any point along the ventricular system with impaired CSF dynamics, the term PHH is used.

Many infants with PHH have had inflammatory ependymitis, obstruction of the aqueduct of Sylvius or the fourth ventricle by blood clot(s), and/or basilar arachnoiditis.[52] As expected, the incidence of PHH is higher in premature infants surviving severe IVH, and it increases with the severity of IVH (grades II–IV).[11] However, the predictors of PHH are still not well known.[53] Once IVH has been noted, serial sonograms should be performed to monitor ventricular

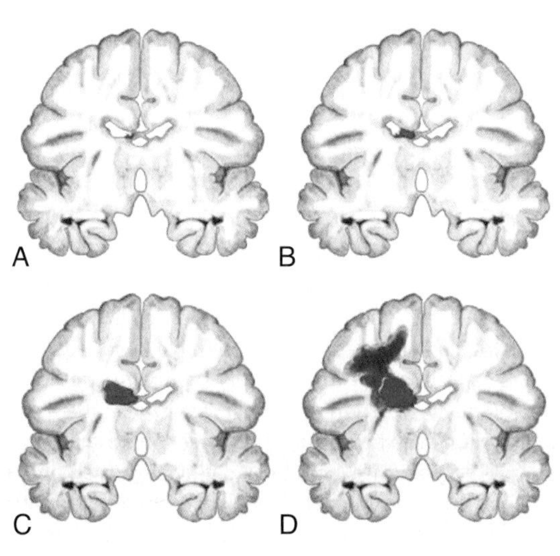

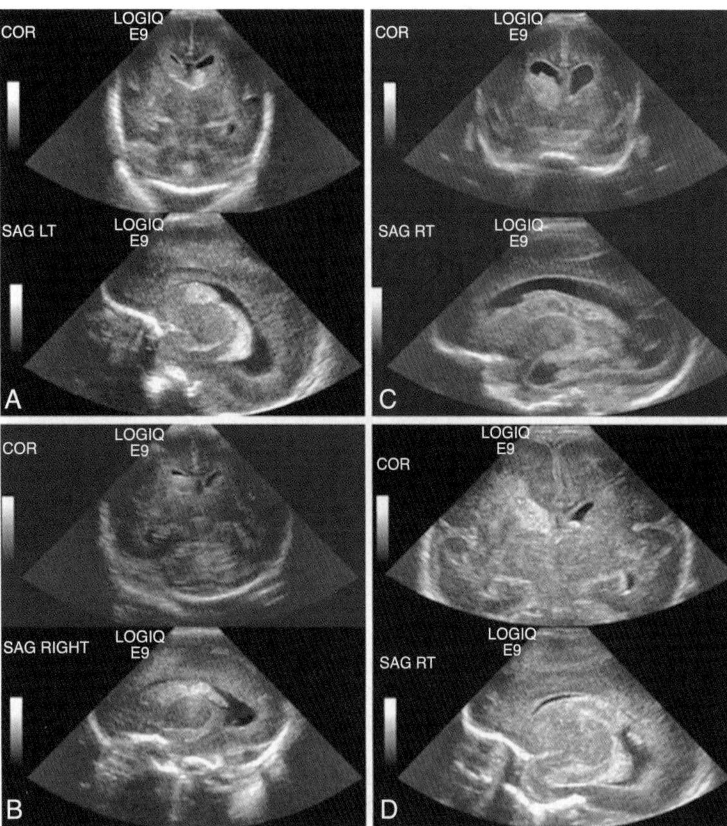

Fig. 52.5 Severity Grades of Intraventricular Hemorrhage Shown in Schematic *(Left)* and Cranial Ultrasound Images *(Right)*. (A) Grade I hemorrhage involves less than 10% of the ventricular volume of the lateral ventricles. (B) Grade II involves 10% to 50% of the ventricular volume and no ventricular dilatation. (C) Grade III involves more than 50% of the ventricular volume and is frequently associated with ventricular dilatation. (D) Hemorrhage is associated with periventricular hemorrhagic infarction. (Schematic imaged *[top]* reproduced with permission and after modifications from Garfinkle and Miller. In: *Bradley and Daroff's Neurology in Clinical Practice*, 110, 2022–2039.e5; Cranial sonographic images *[bottom]* reproduced with permission and after modifications from Merhar and Thomas. Nervous system disorders. In: *Nelson Textbook of Pediatrics*, ch. 120, 913–925.e1.)

size until it has either stabilized or hydrocephalus has progressed to a point that treatment is necessary.[54] A time lag between ventricular dilatation and rapid head growth is noted because of a paucity of cerebral myelin, relative excess water content in white matter, and a relatively large subarachnoid space. This can be detected by serial ultrasound scans.[54]

Clinical Features

The usual clinical scenario in a case of GM-IVH is a preterm infant with respiratory distress syndrome requiring mechanical ventilation.[55] The three basic modes of presentation are:

1. Clinically silent presentation
   a. Most common presentation
   b. Very subtle
   c. Not apparent clinically
   d. Picked up by a routine ultrasound scan or an unexplained fall in hematocrit
2. Saltatory presentation
   a. Second most common presentation
   b. Progresses over a period of many hours
   c. Stuttering course
   d. Usual presenting signs noted are alteration in level of consciousness, decreased spontaneous movements, abnormal eye position and movement, and abnormal popliteal angle (tightness due to meningeal irritation)
3. Catastrophic presentation
   a. Least common presentation
   b. Progresses very fast over a period of minutes to hours
   c. Neurologic features noted are encephalopathy (ranging from stupor to coma), apneas, seizures, decerebrate posturing, fixed

Table 52.2 Ultrasonographic (US) Diagnosis of Periventricular Leukomalacia

Sonographic Appearance	Temporal Evolution	Neuropathological Correlation
Echogenic foci, bilateral, posterior > anterior	1 week	Necrosis with congestion and/or hemorrhage (size >1 cm)
Echolucent foci ("cysts")	1–3 weeks	Cyst formation secondary to tissue dissolution (size >3 mm)
Ventricular enlargement, often with disappearance of "cysts"	≥2–3 months	Deficient myelin formation; gliosis, often associated with collapse of the cyst

From Neil JJ, Volpe JJ. Encephalopathy of prematurity: clinical-neurological features, diagnosis, imaging, prognosis, therapy. In: *Volpe's Neurology of the Newborn.* 6th ed. Philadelphia,: Elsevier; 2018.

gaze and fixed pupils, flaccid quadriparesis, and bulging anterior fontanelle

d. Systemic features noted are hypotension, bradycardia, temperature instability, and metabolic acidosis

Diagnosis

Cranial ultrasound is the most reliable screening tool to detect and assess the severity of IVH. Advantages of ultrasound are its high resolution, portability, lack of radiation, and cost-effectiveness. The grading scale developed by Papile in 1978 and later modified by Volpe, with the addition of a grade IV, is used most frequently (see Fig. 52.5).[3]

Clinical Management

Prevention of GM-IVH

The following interventions may protect against IVH[1,15,56–61]:

1. Antenatal interventions:
   a. Antenatal glucocorticoids, particularly when given ≤48 hours prior to delivery.
   b. Antenatal magnesium sulfate may protect through antiinflammatory effects, not against IVH; may be considered in deliveries at <34 weeks' gestation within 24 hours.
2. Interventions during delivery:
   a. Delivery in a tertiary care perinatal center.
   b. Delayed cord clamping by 30 to 60 seconds in vigorous preterm infants.
   c. Postnatal interventions.
   d. Prophylactic indomethacin may protect against patent ductus arteriosus and IVH; a Cochrane review suggests that prophylactic indomethacin may protect against or lower the incidence of IVH, including severe IVH, although there is some inconsistency in long-term benefits.
3. Postnatal interventions—may lower fluctuations in cerebral perfusion and improve autonomic stability in the first 72 hours, the period of highest risk for IVH:
   a. Neutral head positioning using gel pillows during the first 72 hours of life, which may reduce cerebral blood flow fluctuations. Head positioning toward one side can alter cerebral perfusion by altering jugular blood flow. The effect of these interventions is not conclusive yet. Elevated head positioning, defined as the head raised 30 degrees above the bed, aims to reduce cerebral venous pressure and improve oxygenation. Two studies examining the combination of these strategies continued for 4 days showed decreased progression to PVHI in premature infants weighing <1000 g but not an overall reduction in the incidence of IVH.
   b. Minimal handling during care and procedures, which can promote autonomic stability. Although not proven,[62] this intervention is logical and does not seem to have negative effects. Minimizing stimulation can definitely reduce fluctuations in cerebral blood flow. Minimizing painful procedures is also logical and may even have a positive effect on brain development; multiple painful experiences could negatively impact the development of white matter and subcortical gray matter. Reducing heel sticks, venous blood draws, routine tracheal suctioning, lumbar punctures, and other procedures is easy and humane. Umbilical arterial catheters for blood draws can also help monitor hemodynamic stability and reduce unnecessary noxious stimuli. There may be benefits of reducing unnecessary stimulation even with procedures as innocuous as diaper changes.
   c. Promoting cerebral autoregulation. Prevention of hypotension and hypoperfusion can reduce fluctuations in cerebral perfusion. Maintaining mean BP >30 mm Hg can lower the risk of severe IVH. Examination of cutaneous perfusion and monitoring of urine output can help assess blood flow to internal organs, although the best perfusion, be it the use of fluid boluses or vasopressors, needs careful consideration. The impact of these measures on systemic blood flow is better known than on cerebral perfusion.
   d. Gentle ventilation, with a safe degree of hypercapnia in the first 3 days. If possible, the use of percutaneous measurements

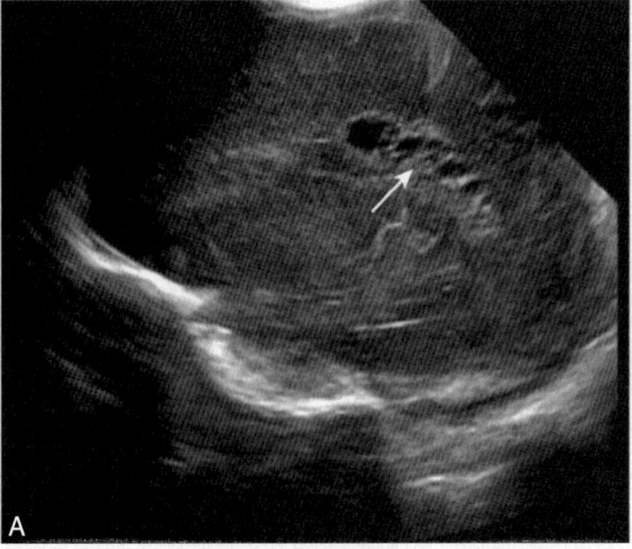

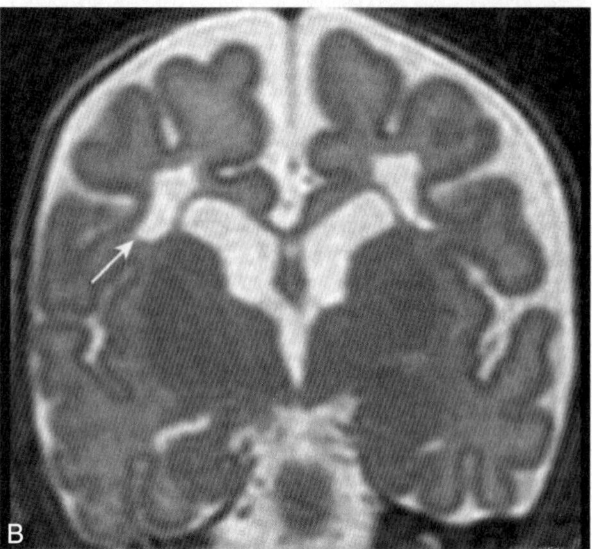

Fig. 52.6 Severe Cystic Periventricular Leukomalacia. (A) Parasagittal ultrasound image showing numerous large cysts superolateral to the lateral ventricle *(arrow)*. (B) Coronal T2-weighted MR image in which cysts are present superolateral to the lateral ventricles *(arrow)*. (Reproduced with permission and after modifications from Merhar and Thomas. Nervous system disorders. In: *Nelson Textbook of Pediatrics*, ch. 120, 913–925.e1.)

such as pulse oximetry and transcutaneous CO_2 measurements can be helpful.

Posthemorrhagic Hydrocephalus (PHH)

Posthemorrhagic ventricular dilatation is noted in 30% to 50% of infants with grade III or IV IVH and can damage the surrounding white matter due to increased pressure.[10] One-third of these infants recover, but others require intervention. Infants with obstructive changes, such as those with aqueductal clots, develop ventricular dilatation more frequently.[63] Others with nonobstructive changes develop ventriculomegaly over longer periods. There is no consensus on the best therapeutic measures[64]; some centers are relatively conservative and carefully monitor these infants, whereas others use a more aggressive approach with an initial lumbar puncture followed by surgical insertion of a ventricular access device such as an Ommaya reservoir to stop ongoing damage to the white matter.[65–67] Ventriculoperitoneal shunts are utilized in infants with progressive PHVD after early intervention.[68]

PHVD can be identified with increasing ventriculomegaly on serial cranial ultrasounds.[69] Infants <32 weeks' gestation are at higher risk. The ventricular index (VI), or width, or the *Levene index* is used to monitor ventricular size (Fig. 52.7).[70,71] It is a measurement of the distance from the falx to the lateral border of the lateral ventricle in a coronal view taken at the level of the foramen of Monro. Although originally described as an "index," it is actually a measurement of width, not an actual ratio. The VI is the distance between the falx and the lateral wall of the anterior horn in the coronal plane at the level of the third ventricle. The anterior horn width (AHW) is the width of the distance from the medial walls of the lateral ventricles at the widest points.[72] Intervention should be considered when patients show severe dilatation with measurements the VIs measuring higher than the 97th percentile +4 mm, and the AHWs more than 10 mm.

Doppler ultrasound can help measure the resistive index (RI) in the assessment of the need for ventricular drainage.[73–75] The RI is a calculation of the systolic and diastolic velocities in the cerebral arteries. Normal RI values are 0.65 to 0.85. A high RI (>0.85) may indicate low blood-flow velocity and high resistance in patients with PHVD, suggesting a need for ventricular drainage.

There are several possible approaches to protect from white matter injury. Nonsurgical management may involve serial lumber punctures to relieve CSF pressure and remove debris from the ventricles.[76] A typical therapeutic lumbar puncture is performed to remove 10 mL/kg of CSF on 2 to 3 consecutive days, and ultrasound surveillance is used to monitor the VI and AHW. If the VI and AHW decrease appropriately, weekly ultrasound surveillance is continued until the infant is ≥32 weeks' GA and the ventricles are stable. If ventricular dilation persists, surgical intervention is considered. There are several options for neurosurgical management of progressive PHVD.

If the infant is too small or clinically unstable, a temporizing procedure is often performed first.

There are 3 options for temporary surgical management of PHVD (Fig. 52.8):

1. Ventriculosubgaleal shunt.[77] A catheter is placed with the proximal tip in the lateral ventricle of the brain and the distal end in a pocket in the subgaleal space to divert the CSF flow. This closed system can decompress the ventricular system without the need for frequent spinal taps. The risk of electrolyte abnormalities is low. However, some infants may have overdrainage, hemorrhages, CSF leaks, or infections (see Fig. 52.4).

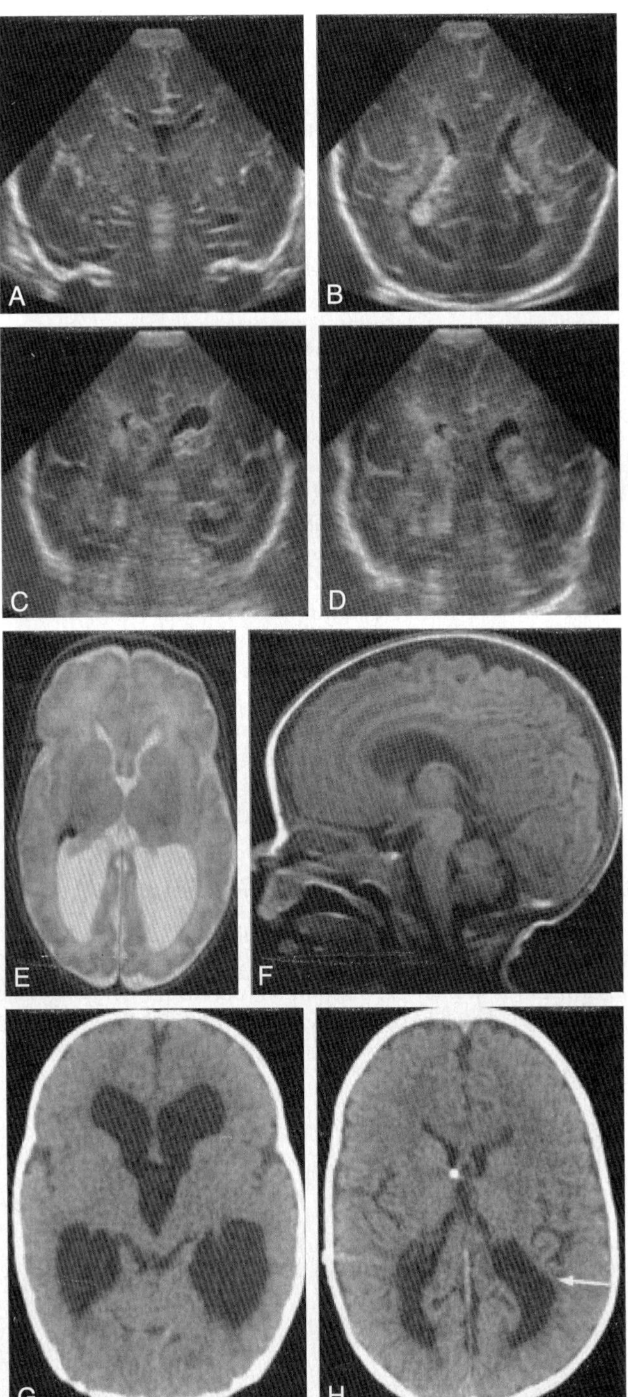

Fig. 52.7 Evolution of Posthemorrhagic Hydrocephalus Resulting From Germinal Matrix Hemorrhage in a Preterm Infant Born at 27 Weeks' Gestation. (A, B) Cranial ultrasonography (US) in the (A) coronal and (B) axial planes at 12 hours of life shows minimal abnormalities. (C, D) Repeat US 2 days later reveals bilateral grade IV intraventricular hemorrhage, also termed *periventricular hemorrhagic infarction.* The infant did not develop signs of symptomatic hydrocephalus as a neonate. (E, F) At term equivalent, magnetic resonance imaging showed (E) a paucity of white matter, suggesting the diffuse form of periventricular leukomalacia; (F) also note the small cerebellum, a typical finding among former preterm infants. (G) At 8 months of age the infant developed symptomatic hydrocephalus with an enlarging head circumference and dilated ventricles on a computed tomography (CT) scan. (H) Several months later a baseline CT scan shows well-decompressed ventricles, but the paucity of white matter remains *(arrow)*. (Reproduced with permission and after modifications from *Youmans and Winn Neurological Surgery*. Winer and Robinson. 2017:1595–1601.e2.)

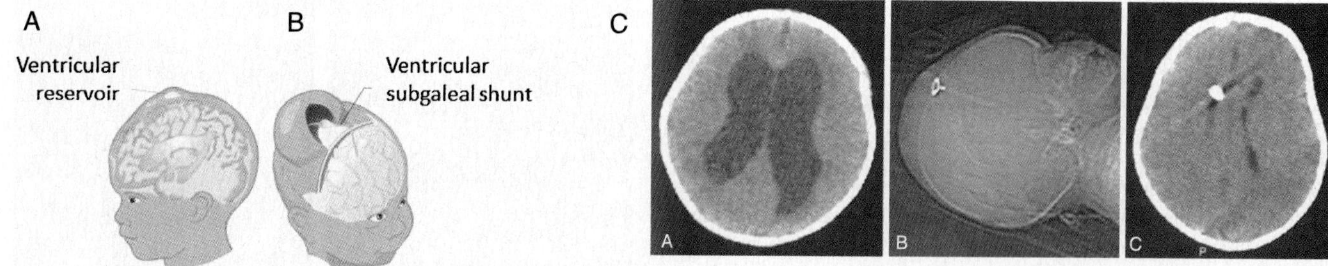

Fig. 52.8 Temporizing Measures for PHVD. (A) Ventricular reservoir: a computed tomography (CT) scan demonstrates ventriculomegaly in a child with posthemorrhagic hydrocephalus. (B) A lateral skull radiograph demonstrates placement of a ventricular subgaleal shunt. (C) Subgaleal reservoir: an axial CT scan 1 month postoperatively demonstrates interval decrease in the size of the ventricles. *PHVD*, Posthemorrhagic ventricular dilatation. (B, Reproduced with permission and after minor modifications from El-Dib et al. *J Pediatr.* 2020;226:16–27.e3; C, reproduced with permission and after minor modifications from Bonow et al. Hydrocephalus in children. In: *Principles of Neurological Surgery*, 8, 133–147.e3.)

2. External ventricular drain (EVD).[78] A drain is placed into the ventricular system and tunneled under the skin to exit the scalp into an external collection chamber. The EVD eliminates the need for percutaneous tapping and allows controlled CSF removal. There are risks of infection and electrolyte abnormalities related to CSF removal. EVD insertion is generally used for specific clinical situations such as meningitis (see Fig. 52.5)
3. Ventricular access device.[65] A catheter is placed with the proximal end in the ventricular system and the distal end attached to a silicone dome implanted in a subgaleal pocket. It allows for serial, percutaneous CSF aspirations through the dome. There is a small but measurable risk of infection with these serial taps (Fig. 52.6).

Long-Term Neurosurgical Management

Some infants require a more definitive hydrocephalus treatment (Fig. 52.7). Early removal of debris due to IVH may prevent permanent impairment of normal CSF absorption, but nearly 60% of infants treated with a temporizing procedure will need long-term CSF diversion (Fig. 52.8).[65,77,79] The timing of treatment may be based on the infant's weight (≥2 kg), gestation, and comorbidities. The definitive treatment is usually the placement of a ventriculoperitoneal shunt (Fig. 52.9), where the catheter has a proximal end in the ventricular system of the brain that is connected to a valve underneath the skin to control CSF flow.[68] The valve is then connected to another catheter that has its distal end in the peritoneal cavity. Enough tubing is placed during the initial insertion to accommodate growth to full adult height. The tubing is tunneled entirely under the skin through incisions on the head and abdomen. Shunting can generally be considered after the infant has reached a weight ≥2 kg, because the risk of infection and hardware complications is higher in smaller infants.

In patients who are not able to accept a peritoneal shunt because of abdominal comorbidities such as severe necrotizing enterocolitis, a ventriculoatrial shunt ending in the atrium of the heart can be considered.[80] There may be more complications such as migration, cardiac arrhythmias, thrombus formation, and nephritis.

CSF shunts have a 5% to 10% risk of infection, which is seen most often within the first 6 months after placement.[81] Shunt malfunction

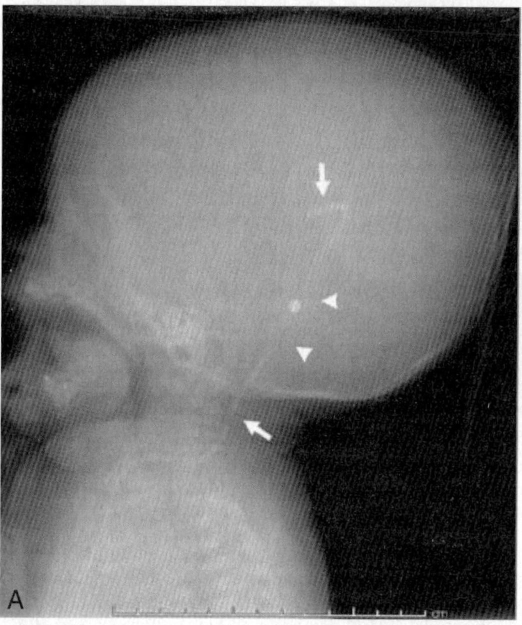

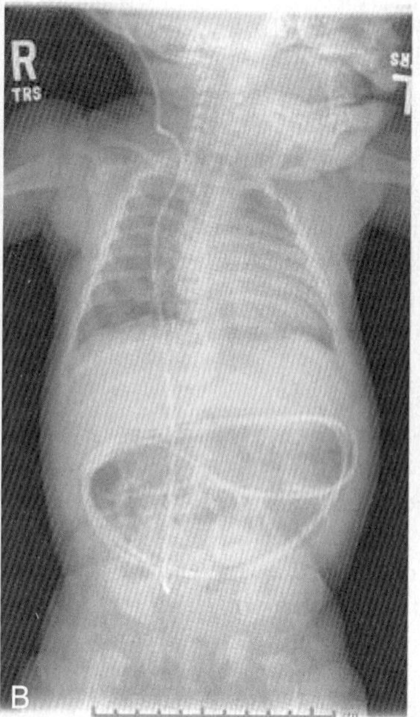

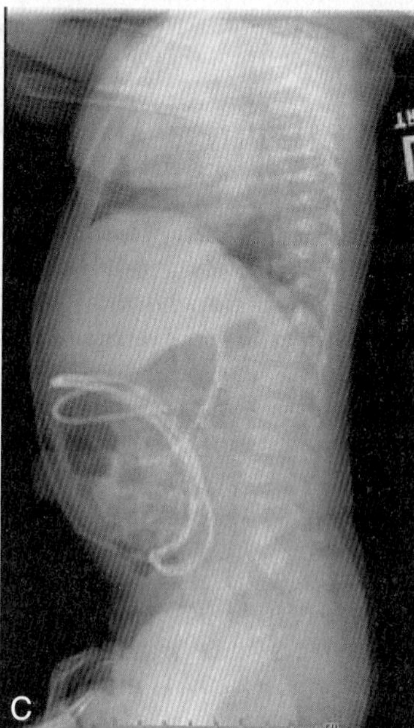

Fig. 52.9 Ventriculoperitoneal Shunt. (A) Lateral view of the intact shunt tubing *(arrows)*; a normal area of radiolucency is seen in areas of connections around the shunt valve *(arrowheads)*. (B) Anteroposterior view of the intact shunt tubing. (C) Lateral view of the intact shunt tubing. (Reproduced with permission and after minor modifications from Vezzedtti R. Don't lose your head: ventriculoperitoneal [VP] shunt issues. In: *Pediatric Imaging for the Emergency Provider*, 27, 125–129.)

may also occur because of obstruction, migration, and fractured tubing.[82] Infants with shunts are more likely to have multiple hospitalizations and neurosurgical procedures.[83] Twenty to forty percent require at least one shunt revision by 2 years of age.[84]

An alternative for surgical management of hydrocephalus is an endoscopic third ventriculostomy (ETV) with or without choroid plexus cauterization.[85] The procedure creates a stoma in the third ventricle to divert fluid out of the ventricular system into the basal cisterns. Choroid plexus cauterization is sometimes added to ETV surgery to improve the efficacy by cauterizing as much as possible of the choroid plexus, where CSF is produced, to reduce the overall circulating volume of CSF. This treatment is useful in some forms of hydrocephalus but is not used very often in young infants with PHH because of high failure rates. Nearly 80% infants treated with ETV go on to require a shunt.

Conclusions

The neurodevelopmental outcome for infants with IVH and PHVD depends on the gestational age and the size and location of the hemorrhage and of the parenchymal injury. Cerebral palsy occurs more often with white matter injury. IVHs of grade III or higher have a 50% risk of neurodevelopmental sequelae, and PVHI has a ≥75% risk. The best management approach is still not clear.

Section 9

CHAPTER

53 Management of Neurotrauma

Joaquin Hidalgo, Eric M. Jackson

KEY POINTS

1. Childbirth is a traumatic event; the head of the neonate is subject to multiple forces that, in turn, may result in clinically relevant neurologic injuries.
2. Extracranial scalp traumatic injuries are the most common type of neonatal head trauma.
3. Scalp lesions may hinder the diagnosis of more serious intracranial lesions, such as depressed skull fractures.
4. Intracranial hematomas can be found in asymptomatic neonates, with a strong association with forceps-assisted deliveries. The management of neonates with intracranial hemorrhage depends on both clinical manifestations and radiologic findings.
5. Head ultrasound can be a useful screening method for head injuries. MRI, the imaging modality of choice, avoids ionizing radiation and provides high-definition imaging of soft tissues, neurologic structures, and associated injuries such as hematomas.
6. Timely medical stabilization and appropriate work-up of the injuries and possible associated conditions (coagulopathy, congenital malformations) is the main goal of the neonatologist. Surgical interventions are seldom needed; however, neurosurgical consultation should be considered in certain cases.

Introduction

Neonatal neurotrauma can be defined as disturbances of nervous (cerebrum, spinal cord, nerves) and adnexal tissues (meninges, spine, cranium, or scalp) due to mechanical forces exerted during birth (labor, delivery, cesarean section) or within the first 4 weeks of life.

Delivery (vaginally or cesarean section) can be a traumatic event with common injuries arising from it with varying degrees of clinical significance. The treatment of such injuries should be dictated by the clinical presentation and impact to the patient. Traumatic injuries from mechanical force can result in injury to any part of the neonatal nervous system. Even during uncomplicated deliveries, the neonate is exposed to several forces that can cause neurotrauma, which will be discussed further.

Epidemiology

Traumatic birth injuries of the central nervous system have become less common in the current era with the increased use of cesarean delivery in anticipated difficult vaginal delivery. The rate of birth trauma in the United States has been estimated at about 29 per 1000 births, with the most common birth related lesions being scalp injuries.[1] Intracranial hemorrhage in full-term neonates has been found to be as prevalent as 26% of patients born via vaginal delivery.[2] Skull fractures can also occur related to birth and delivery. Uncommonly, fractures can cause brain compression and significant neurologic and aesthetic damage if not treated effectively and promptly.[3]

Neonatal Neurotrauma Anatomical Classification

1. Head injuries
   a. Scalp injuries and hematomas
      - Cephalohematoma
      - Caput succedaneum
      - Subgaleal hematoma (SGH)
   b. Skull fractures
2. Intracranial hematomas
   a. Extraaxial hematomas
      - Subdural hematoma
      - Epidural hematoma
   b. Intraaxial hematomas
3. Spine and spinal cord injuries

Head Injuries

Scalp Injuries

The most common birth-related neonatal traumatic injuries are scalp lesions. In order to discuss scalp lesions it is important to understand the basic scalp layered structure, which is often remembered by the mnemonic "SCALP": Skin, dense Connective tissue (where most of the vasculature lies), Aponeurosis *(Galea aponeurotica)*, Loose areolar tissue, and Periosteum (Fig. 53.1). Hematomas are termed according to the layer of the scalp in which they reside. Scalp lacerations, in turn, are graded based on the extent of layers they violate and the presence or absence of a skull fracture.

Scalp Hematomas

Caput Succedaneum

Caput succedaneum is the hemorrhagic edema of the scalp layers above the periosteum caused by head pressure against the birth canal or vacuum extractor. This pressure leads to obstruction of the venous return of the scalp and the consequent extravasation of fluid into the interstitial tissue.[4] This edema of the scalp is usually soft and can cross suture lines of the cranium and the midline.

The management of caput succedaneum is expectant, requiring imaging only in cases of progression of the edema after 24 hours or failure of resolution after 48 to 72 hours. In cases of progression, the diagnosis of caput succedaneum should be questioned. Typical imaging can include a head ultrasound or a rapid sequence magnetic resonance image (MRI) of the head. In most cases, the correct diagnosis can be made by physical examination with determination that the edema (usually pitting) crosses suture lines and/or the midline.

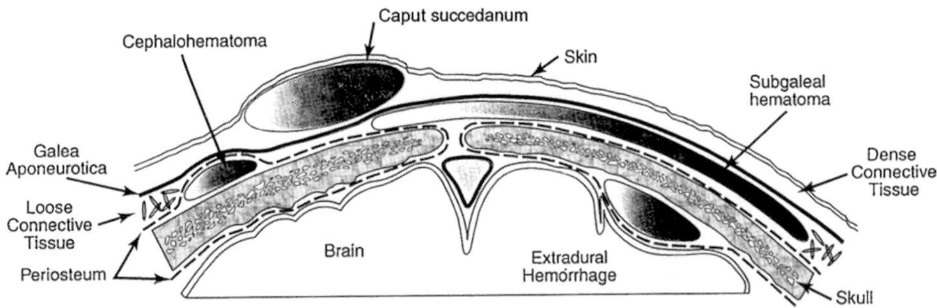

Fig. 53.1 Schematic Representation of the Layers of the Scalp, Skull, Meninges, and Brain and the Relation of Different Types of Hematomas in the Neonate.

Pharmacologic treatment is usually not necessary and the condition usually resolves within a week of birth.[5] Placement of scalp IVs are not contraindicated in cases of isolated caput succedaneum.

Cephalohematoma

A cephalohematoma is a collection of blood between the periosteum and the skull (Fig. 53.2). The hematoma is contained to a focal area of the cranium by the periosteal attachments to the sutures of the skull. Cephalohematoma occurs in about 1% to 2 % of all deliveries. The rate is higher with forceps-assisted (5%) and vacuum-assisted (4%) deliveries. Other significant risk factors for cephalohematoma include cephalo-pelvic disproportion, occipital-posterior and occipital-transverse presentations, large size, a primigravida mother, and placement of fetal scalp electrodes.[6] Regardless of the cause, the hematoma is thought to develop from the disruption of emissary or diploic veins as the periosteum is lifted away from the skull when the head of the neonate moves with significant pressure against another surface (e.g., birth canal, forceps).[7]

Management

1. Diagnosis
   a. Physical examination: The diagnosis should be suspected on physical examination of the head of the neonate. A finding of disproportionate head shape with a nonpedunculated subcutaneous mass that does not cross suture lines or leave pitting edema and is isolated to a region of the calvaria strongly suggests a diagnosis of cephalohematoma. Head circumference measurement and size of the hematoma must be documented and serially measured to establish stability or progression of the hemorrhage. A thorough neurologic examination should always be obtained, looking for associated deficits that can indicate a more serious lesion.
   b. Imaging and laboratory workup: Head ultrasonography can be a practical bedside method to obtain objective measurements of the hematoma; it can also identify associated intracranial hemorrhage such as epidural hematoma. The use of higher-resolution techniques can further delineate the morphologic characteristics and the extent and location of the hematoma(s). The use of limited (rapid sequence T2-HASTE technique) MRI is of particular value in the sense that it provides more detailed images of the brain and scalp without exposing the neonate to ionizing radiation via computerized tomography (CT). In the setting of a cephalohematoma that is rapidly enlarging or larger than 5 cm, laboratory evaluation for coagulopathy, platelet dysfunctions, progressive anemia, or hyperbilirubinemia should be considered with abnormalities corrected accordingly.
2. Treatment: By the end of the first week of life, the majority of neonates will show signs of dissolution (decreasing size or softening) of the hematoma, and complete resolution can be seen in

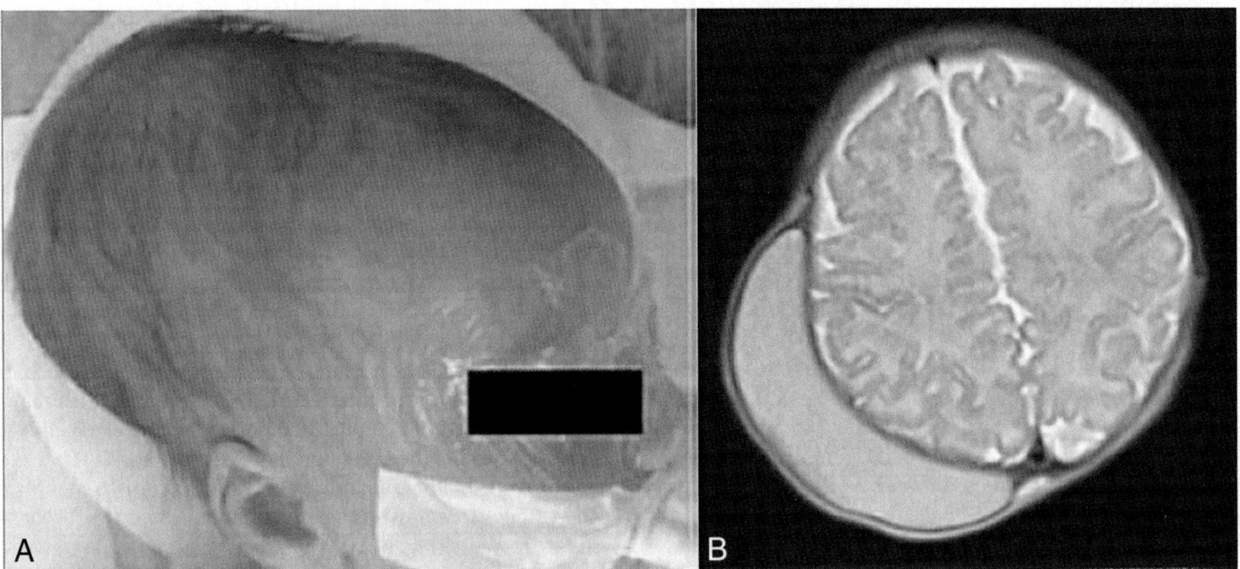

Fig. 53.2 (A) In situ cephalohematoma on a 2-week-old neonate. (B) T2-HASTE magnetic resonance image demonstrating large acute cephalohematoma.

most cases by the end of the second week without any intervention.[8] Delayed increasing size or appearance of neurologic deficits should trigger neurologic consultation for evaluation.[7]

3. Complications: The main reported complications of cephalohematoma arise from nonabsorption of the hematoma.
   a. Infection: Several cases of infection of the hematoma have been reported in the literature. In the setting of infection, treatment consists of washout and antibiotic therapy. Of note, in a neonate who meets criteria for sepsis without a known source and a history of cephalohematoma, drainage of the hematoma should be considered to obtain microbiological analysis.
   b. Calcification: Calcification of the residual cephalohematoma (after 4–6 weeks from birth) is part of the expected natural history of these lesions. Significant head deformities can arise in large collections if left untreated, although they often remodel over time (Fig. 53.3). In this situation, patients can be referred to a craniofacial surgeon or neurosurgeon for drainage or evaluation for cranioplasty at a later age.[9]

Subgaleal Hematoma/Hemorrhage

SGH is an accumulation of blood between the galea aponeurotica (aponeurosis) of the scalp and the periosteum of the skull. SGHs are usually caused by the rupture of emissary veins or arterioles of the scalp during delivery or another traumatic event in a newborn.[10] The peculiarity of this "virtual" space of the scalp is that there is no strong adhesion between the aponeurosis and the pericranium; therefore a significant amount of blood can accumulate (over 250 mL).[10,11] SGH can represent a significant threat for an actively bleeding neonate, given the small intravascular volume. The incidence of neonatal SGH increases significantly with the use of vacuum devices during delivery, from 0.4 in 1000 vaginal deliveries without the use of vacuum or forceps to 5.9 in 1000 in vacuum-assisted deliveries.[12]

Management

1. Diagnosis
   a. Neonates diagnosed with SGH the day of admission appear to have better prognosis than those diagnosed the following day.[10] SGH should be suspected on the grounds of examination and characteristics of delivery. Prolonged labor and vacuum extraction should trigger the neonatologist to look for signs of scalp lesions to establish the appropriate diagnosis. Differentiating SGH from cephalohematoma and caput succedaneum can usually be achieved by physical examination. Cephalohematoma, as discussed above, does not cross the midline or suture lines, whereas SGH usually does. In fact, SGH can involve the entire head circumference and it may displace the ear and the skin over the orbital rims. Cephalohematomas are usually tense to palpation and do not change with variations in head position, whereas SGHs palpate as a fluctuant (boggy) mass that can migrate to dependent areas when the position of the neonate is changed. SGH, in comparison to caput succedaneum, usually does not produce scalp pitting edema on palpation and takes longer to resolve than caput succedaneum, which tends to resolve as the swelling starts to dissipate within hours to days.
   b. Head imaging such as head ultrasound and MRI of the brain can be obtained to rule out associated intracranial hemorrhage and pathology. Still, this imaging should not delay other diagnostic tests and measures in the setting of a potentially life-threatening hemorrhage or an unstable neonate. The use of head CT is discouraged given the exposure of the neonate to ionizing radiation and should be avoided if possible, depending on the urgency and medical center capabilities. Close monitoring for signs of hypovolemia, anemia, acidosis, and hyperbilirubinemia should be established, and related laboratory studies including coagulation studies should be obtained at baseline.
2. Treatment
   a. The mainstay of treatment for patients with SGH is avoidance of complications related to acute blood loss. Patients with suspected SGH or strong risk factors for SGH, such as prolonged vacuum-assisted deliveries, should be closely monitored. In the setting of proven SGH, hourly vital sings, neurologic checks, and recurring examination of the hematoma should be established. Blood transfusions, correction of acidosis, and other supportive measures should be promptly instituted. Surgical intervention is not typically indicated in the setting of isolated SGH. Some practitioners have advocated head wrapping to tamponade the hemorrhage and reduce the subgaleal space, but one must be careful because this can result in elevated intracranial pressure if the head wrap is too tight.[11] Furthermore, the head wrap may make proper examination of the hematoma more difficult. Neurosurgical evaluation can be considered in the setting of an associated intracranial hemorrhage or skull fracture.

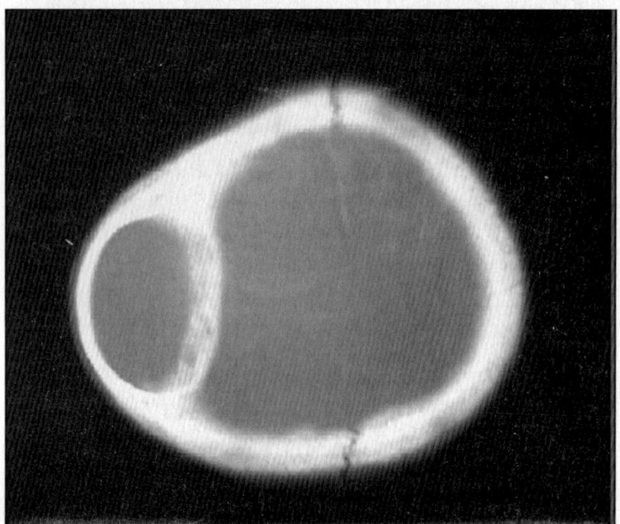

Fig. 53.3 Computed Tomography of the Head Without Contrast Demonstrating Right Parietal Calcified Cephalohematoma on a 3-Year-Old Female Patient.

Skull Fractures

Skull fractures are usually classified as either linear or displaced. In linear fractures there is a separation of the skull bone without variation of the circumferential shape of the skull (Fig. 53.4). They can be simple (single line of fracture) or complex (comminution of the bone or multiple ramifications of the line of fracture). In displaced fractures, the shape of the skull bone becomes irregular by depression or elevation of the fracture edges. Depressed fractures may cause pressure on the intracranial contents, whereas elevated fractures move away from the intracranial contents.

In the neonatal population and early infancy (6 months of age and younger), depressed fractures are usually "ping-pong" or "greenstick" fractures (Fig. 53.5). The name comes from the inversion of the cranial convexity to a concavity at the site of the fracture, reminiscent of an indentation on a ping-pong ball. This type of fracture

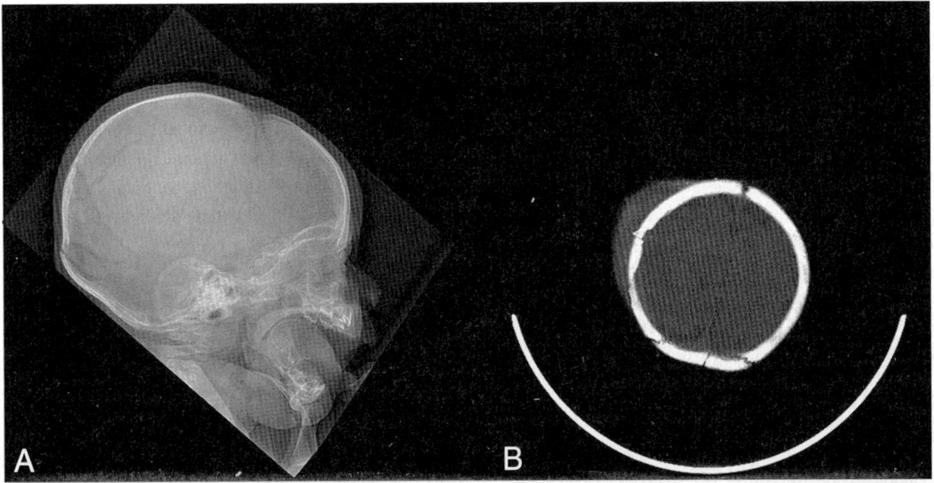

Fig. 53.4 (A) Plain lateral skull x-ray on a 3-day-old newborn who presented to the emergency room with delayed right parietal scalp swelling; a parietal linear skull fracture is appreciated. (B) Computed tomography of the head with and without contrast was performed confirming the findings; there was no associated underlying hematoma.

occurs in the neonatal population due to the immaturity of the skull bones, because they have more elastic capabilities and resilience to physical separation. This type of fracture is the most common depressed skull fracture in the neonatal population,[13] whereas linear skull fractures are the most common skull fracture in the neonatal age overall.[6]

The incidence of congenital skull fracture has been estimated to be between 2% and 3% of every 100,000 deliveries.[6,14] It is unclear, however, the true incidence of skull fractures in this population; some fractures may have minimal symptoms and the diagnosis can be missed because patients are, appropriately, not routinely radiologically screened for such lesions.

Management

Diagnosis

Clinical Manifestations. It is important to differentiate between skull remodeling from labor and delivery and a skull fracture. Skull fractures are associated with a focal hematoma in more than 25% of cases,[6] whereas skull remodeling occurs by overriding of the sutures of the skull and is a normal self-limited consequence of labor and delivery. Skull remodeling is often symmetric versus asymmetric with an isolated unilateral defect for skull fractures. An indentation defect can be palpated in most cases of depressed skull fractures. Associated clinical manifestations of skull fractures in the neonate can include seizures, focal motor deficits, and pupillary abnormalities.[6]

Diagnostic Testing. The gold standard test for identification of a skull fracture is CT without contrast. CT is also helpful to identify associated hemorrhage intra- or extracranially. The drawback of CTs is the exposure of the neonate to radiation; thus CT should be reserved for patients with a high suspicion of skull fracture. Other imaging techniques, such as HASTE sequence MRI (also known as rapid sequence or ultrafast MRI), can be used as an initial test for a suspected traumatic injury,[15] although the bone anatomy may not be as clear as with CT. Skull x-rays can be used if more advanced diagnostic studies are not available. Information about associated hemorrhage and intracranial tissue involvement is limited, and x-rays are not as sensitive as head CT for identification of linear skull fractures.[14] Therefore, the use of skull x-rays is of limited utility in neonatal trauma.

Treatment. The identification of a skull fracture should prompt the neonatologist to consider a consultation with a neurosurgeon, although most identified skull fractures do not require a neurosurgical intervention. Criteria for surgical intervention of a neonatal skull fracture vary from case to case. Linear skull fractures without associated hematomas are managed nonoperatively. A depressed skull fracture may require surgical elevation if the depression is greater than 5 mm or significant brain compression is present.

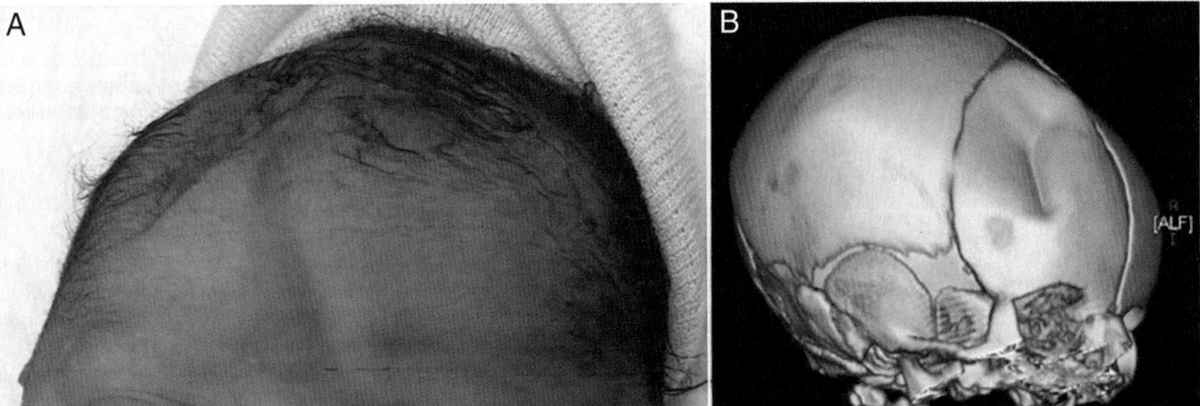

Fig. 53.5 (A) Image of a newborn scalp after an instrumented forceps delivery complicated with a right frontal depressed skull fracture. (B) Three-dimensional reconstruction computed tomography of the same newborn demonstrating a "greenstick" type of fracture.

"Ping-pong" fractures can be successfully treated with suction devices by the neurosurgical team[13]; however, in more complex depressed skull fractures, surgical exploration and elevation should be considered.

Complications

Growing Skull Fracture: Skull fractures can disrupt the meninges covering the brain at the time of injury. In nonhealed meningeal defects, the growing brain and cerebrospinal fluid can herniate through the defect, creating a meningocele or meningoencephalocele. Patients with a neonatal skull fracture (formally diagnosed or not) can present with delayed neurologic deficits or skull deformity due to this phenomenon, often months after the injury. Therefore, any patient with an identified skull fracture should be followed to rule out development of a growing skull fracture.

Seizures: Seizures are of concern, particularly with depressed skull fractures and/or intracranial hematomas, due to potential cerebral cortical irritation.

Intracranial Hematomas

Hematomas related to trauma can occur in any of the different compartments of the intracranial space (both supra- or infratentorial): epidural, subdural, subarachnoid, intracerebral, or intraventricular.[16] Intracranial hematoma in the setting of neonatal trauma has a different pathogenesis than intraventricular hemorrhage seen in premature neonates (germinal matrix hemorrhage) as well as other intracranial hematoma from nontraumatic medical conditions.

Risk factors for traumatic intracranial hematomas in neonates include assisted vaginal delivery, breech presentation, large fetal weight, and prolonged duration of labor.[17] However, it has also been shown that intracranial hemorrhages can be commonly found in asymptomatic neonates after vaginal deliveries.[2] There has likely been an increase in the identification of neonatal intracranial hemorrhages due to the availability of more advanced imaging techniques; however, the true incidence and repercussion of these hemorrhages is not fully known or understood.[2,18] Ultimately, given its close association with hypoxic-ischemic injury and other medical conditions, significant morbidity has been historically associated with hemorrhagic brain injuries.

As mentioned above, hematomas can occur in any compartment of the intracranial space. Table 53.1 depicts a summary of the anatomic location, radiologic characteristics, and pathogenesis of intracranial hemorrhage. In the neonate, hemorrhages can commonly be seen in multiple compartments.

Epidural Hematoma

The more commonly seen supratentorial epidural hematoma associated with head trauma from middle meningeal artery injury is rarely seen in the neonatal population.[18] More commonly, in the neonatal population, epidural hematoma is related to venous sinus injury, epidural bleeding from an adjacent skull fracture, or scalp hematoma that has percolated to the epidural space through a suture.

Subdural Hematoma

Subdural hematoma has been reported as the most commonly found intracranial infratentorial hematoma related to trauma in the neonate.[2] The tearing of dural sinuses secondary to molding skull forces on the tentorium during labor and delivery is the presumed etiology of these bleeds.[19]

Subarachnoid Hemorrhage

The most commonly diagnosed traumatic supratentorial hematoma of the newborn.[20]

Intraventricular and Intracerebral Hemorrhage

Although seen in the setting of trauma, these locations are more closely related to intracranial hemorrhages of prematurity,

Table 53.1 Summary of Neuroanatomic-Based Intracranial Hemorrhage in Term Newborns

Intracranial Hemorrhage Type[a]	Definition	Cranial Computed Tomographic Scan Characteristics	Comments or Pathogenesis
Epidural	Blood between the skull and outside the dura	Lentiform hyperattenuation along inner side of calvarium	Rare, because the middle meningeal artery moves freely away from displacements of the skull
Subdural	Blood between the dura and arachnoid membrane	Crescent-shaped hyperattenuation conforming to the adjacent brain	Most common; vertical molding of skull causes tearing of blood vessels of tentorium
Subarachnoid	Blood between the arachnoid and the pia membrane	Hyperattenuating fluid in basal subarachnoid spaces or along cerebral sulci	Most common type; tearing of bridging blood vessels or dural sinuses during labor
Intraventricular[b]	Blood in lateral, third, or fourth ventricles	Hyperattenuating fluid typically seen as layering within the ventricles	Uncommon hemorrhage of choroid plexuses; extension of thalamic or subependymal matrix
Intraparenchymal	Blood within brain (intraaxial) parenchyma	Hyperattenuating focus within the cerebral or cerebellar hemispheres, with varying amount of surrounding vasogenic edema	Less frequent; primary hemorrhage must be distinguished from secondary intraparenchymal hemorrhage

[a]Location of intracranial hemorrhage may be supratentorial or infratentorial.

[b]Unlike term newborns, 80% of preterm newborns with intraventricular hemorrhage have associated germinal matrix hemorrhagic infarction. Occurrence of intraventricular hemorrhage in term newborns is a poor predictor of neurologic outcome.

From Gupta SN, Kechli AM, Kanamalla US. *Intracranial Hemorrhage in Term Newborns: Management and Outcomes.* Elsevier; 2009.

hypoxic-ischemic disease, sinus thrombosis, and other nontraumatic diseases or conditions.[16]

Grading

Although there is no specific grading system for intracranial hematomas in the neonatal population, clinically relevant data typically include the size/volume of the hemorrhage, the amount of neural tissue compressed, and the presence of hydrocephalus or increased intracranial pressure.[16]

Management

Diagnosis

Clinical Manifestations

Seizures have been reported as the most common symptomatic presentation of intracranial hemorrhage in neonates. Apnea, bradycardia, and irritability are other common presenting symptoms.[20] Often, with less significant traumatic events, no symptoms are identified.[2,5]

In patients with concern for intracranial hemorrhage, the physical examination must include special attention to tension of the anterior fontanelle, head circumference, and pupillary and motor examination. Other sites of profuse bleeding such as the mucosa, skin, or other bodily compartments should raise the concern of a hematologic disorder.

Diagnostic Testing

1. Radiologic assessment
   a. Head ultrasound can usually be obtained without transferring the patient outside the neonatal unit; however, the sensitivity has been reported as inadequate to be used as a screening tool for neonatal intracranial hemorrhage, particularly for small hematomas.[21] From the authors' experience and practice, the head ultrasound remains a valid tool in patients who are too unstable to be transferred to a CT or MRI scanner, as well as for serial hematoma volume follow-up in patients in whom the diagnosis has already been established but concern for enlargement triggers frequent imaging.
   b. CT of the brain allows for rapid evaluation to confirm or rule out an intracranial hemorrhage, as well as overall assessment of associated skull fractures, ventricular size, and cerebral edema. As mentioned above, CT exposes the neonate to ionizing radiation, and therefore, it should be used judiciously. Conventional MRI of the brain can provide further anatomic information between the hemorrhage and intracranial contents (i.e., intradural versus extradural) and associated neural injuries.
2. Other pertinent tests
   a. Hematologic work-up should be performed to timely identify platelet or coagulation disorders. Electroencephalography should be considered in patients with poor mental status or clinical evidence of seizure activity.

Treatment

The mainstay of treatment in intracerebral hematomas is supportive medical management assuring adequate ventilation and metabolic and vital sign stabilization. Basic hematologic laboratory parameters should be maximized with a minimum platelet count of >50,000/mm^3 and replacement of deficient coagulation factors or vitamin K. Hematology consultation should be considered.

Neurosurgical consultation can be obtained once the diagnosis of intracranial hemorrhage has been established, even though surgical intervention is rarely necessary.[2]

Spine and Spinal Cord Injuries

Spine or spinal cord injuries are exceedingly rare in neonates because the viscoelastic properties of the immature neonatal bones and ligaments can accommodate for significant external traumatic forces. The most common causes of spine and spinal cord injury are related to musculoskeletal congenital malformations/disorders (e.g., osteogenesis imperfecta or atelosteogenesis) or extremely forceful delivery.[22] Similar to intracranial injuries, intraspinal hematomas can also occur in the neonate. These hemorrhages are usually related to congenital clotting or platelet disorders and forceful deliveries. The severity of these hematomas is directly proportional to the size and amount of spinal cord compression along with neurologic manifestations.

Distraction injuries such as cranio-cervical or cervico-thoracic dislocation can occur during hyperextension of the joints as the fetus is delivered from the birth canal. This distraction can result in isolated osteo-ligamentous injuries or in association with spinal cord or peripheral nerve (brachial plexus) stretch or transection injuries.[22]

Management

Diagnosis

Clinical Manifestations

Neurologic examination can herald spinal cord and peripheral nerve injuries with flaccid paresis of the corresponding extremities, depending on the level of the neurologic injury. In cervico-medullary or high cervical spine injuries, stridor, respiratory distress, or dysphagia can occur along with flaccid quadriparesis or quadriplegia. In injuries of the lower cervical spine or below, paraparesis or paraplegia can be seen. Monoparesis (upper or lower extremity) is often associated with peripheral nerve stretch injuries. Other physical examination clues to spinal injury include torticollis, cervical or thoracolumbar deformities, and perispinal subcutaneous masses.

Diagnostic Testing

Radiologic Assessment. In contrast to neonatal head ultrasound, spinal ultrasound is a poor screening tool for the examination of spine or spinal cord injuries.[22] Spinal CT or x-rays can be more helpful for osteo-ligamentous injuries (e.g., dislocation, fracture). For evaluation of neurologic structures and intraspinal hematomas, MRI of the spine without contrast is the test of choice and should be the initial radiologic test of choice in the setting of motor paralysis.[22]

Treatment

In the rare event of a suspected spinal injury, spinal precautions should be instituted with immediate bed rest and avoidance of manipulation of the neonate's head or torso until further information is available to ascertain spinal stability. Neurosurgical consultation should be obtained if a traumatic spinal injury is suspected.

With the advent of fetal MRI and advanced ultrasonography, congenital musculoskeletal defects can be identified before delivery, which allows multidisciplinary prenatal evaluation and planning to prevent or decrease the severity of peripartum spine traumatic injuries in predisposed patients.

CHAPTER

54 Management of Myelomeningocele and Related Disorders of the Newborn

Mari L. Groves, Jena L. Miller

KEY POINTS

1. Spina bifida is the most common nonlethal birth defect of the central nervous system and occurs when the vertebral column fails to close, resulting in neurologic impacts from both the abnormal formation and ongoing damage to the exposed nervous tissue.
2. The underlying cause of spina bifida is multifactorial, involving genetic, metabolic, and environmental influences.
3. The Chiari II malformation is classically associated with open neural tube defects (NTDs) due to ongoing loss of cerebral spinal fluid from the lesion and herniation of the brainstem through the foramen magnum, resulting in obstructive hydrocephalus.
4. Prenatal ultrasound is the primary diagnostic tool, and amniocentesis is offered to all patients to assess for genetic abnormalities.
5. Fetal surgery has emerged as a treatment strategy that decreases the need for postnatal ventriculoperitoneal shunt placement for selected cases, but the majority of newborns will undergo postnatal surgery.
6. Delivery is recommended at a site where both neonatal and neurosurgical services are available.
7. Patients should be followed by a multidisciplinary team to help maximize recovery of function and to prevent further decline of motor, sphincter, and orthopedic function.

Introduction

Open spina bifida aperta, or open myelomeningocele (MMC), is a midline vertebral defect that may occur anywhere along the spinal column, resulting in exposure of the contents of the spinal column to the outside environment.[1] It is the most common nonlethal congenital birth defect of the central nervous system, occurring in approximately 3 to 4 per 10,000 live births in the United States annually.[2] Improved treatments have helped decrease mortality, but long-term morbidity exists secondary to medical concerns including hydrocephalus, Chiari II malformations, spinal cord tethering, neurogenic bowel and bladder, and orthopedic abnormalities. Consequently, children with spina bifida require complex multispecialty care to help maximize their quality of life and prevent serious long-term sequelae.

Pathophysiology

Open neural tube defects (NTDs) are caused by a spontaneous failure of neurulation occurring within the first 3 to 4 weeks of gestation. There is likely a multifactorial etiology based in both genetic predispositions and environmental influences. Up to 16% of NTDs may be associated with a chromosomal anomaly (Table 54.1). Genes that seem to be associated with NTD include the retention and metabolism of folate and vitamin B_{12}, the methylation cycle and transulfuration, glucose transport and metabolism, oxidative stress, retinoid metabolism, transcription factors, and DNA repair. Folate (vitamin B_6) has been shown to play a particularly important role. In the 1980s, folate use was shown to play a critical role in a methylation cycle. Because the effects on the methylation cycle occur before a pregnancy is detected, public health efforts were initiated to introduce folate fortification for the general public. Although this reduced some degree of the incidence of NTDs between the years 1984 and 1994, the incidence has remained 0.7 to 0.8 per 1000 live births, with some regional variation, since 2004.[2,3] In the United States, this ranges between 0.3 and 1.43 per 1000 live births.

Spina bifida occulta encompasses a variety of etiologies that result from a malformation of the midline dorsal neural, mesenchymal, and cutaneous ectodermal structures during embryogenesis.[4] Unlike spina bifida aperta, the dorsal dysraphism is skin covered and does not require immediate intervention at the time of delivery. Although there is a wide array of etiologies (Table 54.2), if they cause clinical symptoms it is typically due to impairment through tethering of the spinal cord, neuronal compression, or myelodysplasia. Symptoms may develop over time due to tethering, which can cause progressive symptoms through tension on the spinal cord, leading to vascular abnormalities. However, this clinical course can vary drastically. Progressive symptoms are sometimes responsive to intervention, although some patients have baseline neuronal deficits due to the aberrant formation of the neural placode during development. Even after the initial surgical repair, progressive symptoms of tethering may recur in a delayed fashion. For the purposes of this chapter, we will primarily describe spina bifida aperta, as it is most often dealt with during the acute perinatal period.

Spinal development occurs during three basic embryologic stages: gastrulation, primary neurulation, and secondary neurulation. Gastrulation occurs during the second or third week of development and involves the differentiation of the embryonic disc into the ectoderm, mesoderm, and endoderm. During primary neurulation, which occurs during the third and fourth week of development, the notochord and overlying ectoderm then form the neural plate. This then folds to form the neural tube and closes in a bidirectional, zipper-like manner. Secondary neurulation, which occurs during weeks 5 to 6 of development, thus further differentiates the neuronal tissue and undergoes cavitation to form the conus medullaris and filum through retrogressive differentiation. Typically, spina bifida aperta occurs when the caudal end of the notochord incompletely fuses and leads to a persistent and exposed neural placode.

Table 54.1 Associated Etiologies With Neural Tube Defects

Genetic	Genetic disorders • Meckel-Gruber syndrome • Roberts syndrome • Jarcho-Levin syndrome • HARD (hydrocephalus, agyria, and retinal dysplasia) • Trisomy 13 • Trisomy 18 • PHAVER syndrome • VATER syndrome • X-linked neural tube defects
Environmental	Maternal associations • Alcohol use • Caffeine use • Elevated glycemic index • Gestational diabetes mellitus • Low maternal folate and methionine intake • Low levels of zinc, vitamin C, vitamin B_{12}, and choline • Maternal smoking • Maternal fever or hypothermia or sauna or hot tub use during the first trimester Environmental factors • Air pollution • Disinfectant byproducts in drinking water • Exposure to organic solvents • Pesticides • Nitrate-related compounds • Polycyclic aromatic hydrocarbons

PHAVER, Pterygia, heart defects, autosomal recessive inheritance, vertebral defects, ear anomalies, and radial defects; *VATERL* vertebrae, anus, heart, trachea, esophagus, kidney, and limbs.

Clinical Features

Clinical manifestations of open spina bifida occur due to the initial primary failure of neuronal closure and aberrant nervous tissue formation as well as secondary insults to the exposed nervous tissue.[5] The original neural placode can have relatively normal neuronal tissue. However, throughout gestation and exposure to the amniotic fluid, the exposed nervous tissue may become hemorrhagic and die.[6] Spina bifida aperta likely has associated brain malformations and hydrocephalus due to the effects of ongoing exposure of the placode and loss of cerebrospinal fluid (CSF).

Chiari II malformations compose the majority of brain anomalies associated with MMCs. Ongoing development with a surrounding small posterior fossa as well as ongoing CSF loss caudally leads to herniation of the cerebellum through the foramen magnum. This is often associated with distortion of the midbrain, or tectal beaking, in 65% of infants. The medulla can additionally be elongated and kinked at the spino-medullary junction for 70% of infants.[7] Other brain anomalies include underdevelopment of the corpus callosum in up to 50% of infants.[8] This suggests that some disruption of neuronal migration typically occurs in the second trimester. Hydrocephalus can develop throughout the course of gestation from obstruction of the CSF flow. Several hypotheses have been proposed, but most likely this occurs due to obstruction of the fourth ventricle through herniation and crowding of the cerebellum due to ongoing rostral CSF loss through the defect.

Neurologic deficits can affect the innervation of the bladder, leading to neurogenic bladder. Abnormalities in storage and emptying of urine can lead to high pressure and cause secondary deterioration in renal function. Renal deterioration can be seen in patients with noncompliant bladders with high intravesical pressures. Neurogenic bowel can also be seen and can complicate urologic function as well. The majority of infants will require some degree of support to optimize bowel and bladder function. Congenital and acquired orthopedic anomalies result largely from muscular imbalance, paralysis, and decreased sensation. Both hip dislocation and foot deformities should be primarily assessed early in life.

Diagnosis

Prenatal Diagnosis and Counseling

Ultrasound detection of fetal open NTDs is possible beginning in the first trimester by evaluation of the posterior brain in the same midsagittal plane of the fetal profile used for screening for trisomy 21.[9] Features of the Chiari II malformation, including compression of the fourth ventricle and obliteration of the cisterna magna as well as an increase in the brainstem to brainstem occipital bone distance, can be observed. If the posterior brain appears abnormal, further investigation of the fetal central nervous system can be performed.[10]

Second-trimester ultrasound is the primary diagnostic test for fetal NTDs, with a detection rate of up to 96% for open lesions. The characteristic findings reflect the impact of physiology of the Chiari II malformation and include indentation or narrowing of the frontal bones (lemon sign) and semicircular shape of the cerebellum (banana sign), with or without obliteration of the normal fluid-filled spaces of the posterior fossa and ventriculomegaly.[11–13] Rigorous assessment of the fetal spine follows identification of the level of the lesion,[14] visualization of the placode, and any additional bony abnormalities[15] (Fig. 54.1). Detection is easiest when the lesion is raised, but identification of small or flat lesions can be challenging. Most cases of spina bifida occulta do not have the associated brain abnormalities, so a lack of the secondary brain findings can help differentiate between open and closed lesions.[16] Evaluation for any additional fetal anomalies is important to determine whether the NTD is isolated or associated with an underlying genetic or more complex condition.

Amniocentesis is offered as the standard of care and allows diagnostic analysis for genetic abnormalities, amniotic fluid alpha-fetoprotein (AFP), and acetylcholinesterase (AchE).[17] Both amniotic fluid AFP and AchE are elevated in >99% of cases with open NTDs, but false positives can occur in the setting of fetal abdominal wall defects, other major structural anomalies, congenital nephrosis, blood

Table 54.2 Etiologies of Spina Bifida Occulta

Thickened filum terminale	Thickening of the filum terminale
Fatty filum	Some degree of fat causing thickening or infiltrating the filum terminale
Diastematomyelia	Split cord malformation where there is either a bony or fibrous attachment causing formation of two spinal cords
Lipomyelomeningocele	Fat attached to the surface of the spinal cord or nerve roots that may cause incomplete closure of the spinal cord and may be connected to the subcutaneous fat
Dermal sinus tract	A band of tissue extending from the cutaneous surface through the dura and attaching to the spinal cord
Meningocele	Skin-covered out-pouching of the dura with fluid without neuronal components

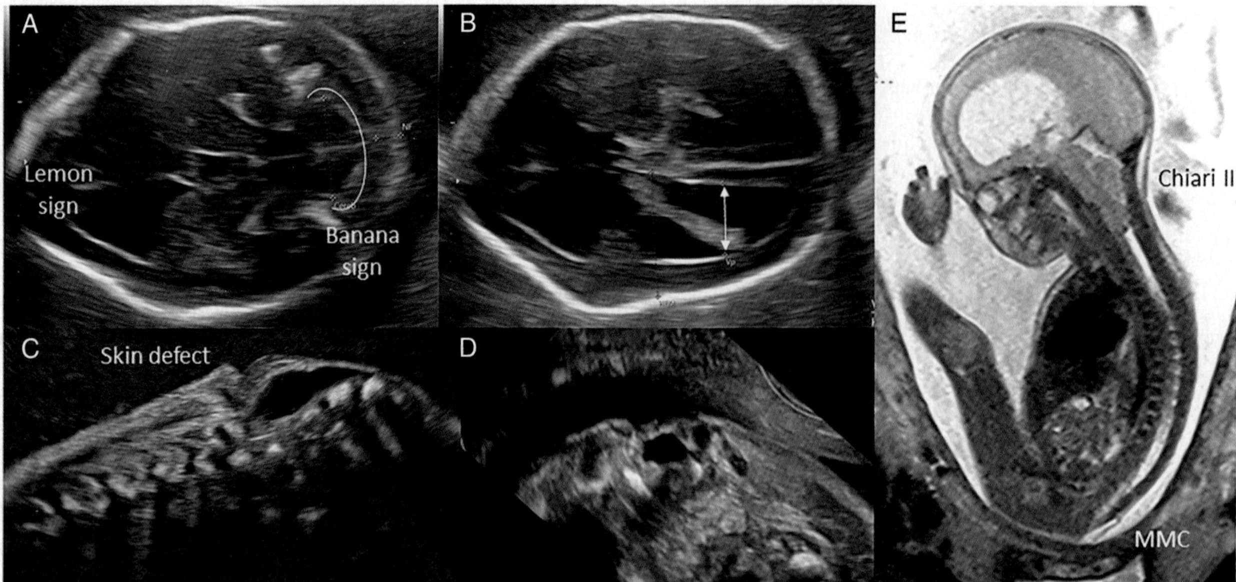

Fig. 54.1 Prenatal Ultrasound and Magnetic Resonance Imaging (MRI) of a Lumbosacral Fetal Myelomeningocele. High-resolution ultrasound demonstrates the characteristic brain findings including (A) bitemporal indentation of the frontal bones (lemon sign) and the concave shape of the cerebellum (lemon sign), (B) ventriculomegaly, (C) sagittal views of the lumbosacral spine with the myelomeningocele sac, and (D) coronal view showing stretched neural elements extending to the surface of the lesion. (E) Corresponding MRI demonstrating evidence of the Chiari II malformation and myelomeningocele (MMC).

contamination, and impending miscarriage.[18] Maternal serum screening for AFP performed at 16 to 18 weeks of gestation is the least sensitive as a primary screening tool. This test is only 75% sensitive for detecting an open NTD.[19] False-positive results may occur in cases of underestimated gestational age, multiple pregnancies, or fetal abdominal wall defects. False-negative results may result from spina bifida occulta lesions such as myelocystoceles.

Prenatal counseling aims to help parents understand the spectrum of outcomes possible for individuals with NTDs. Perinatal mortality is uncommon with proper treatment. Most mortalities within the first year of life are secondary to respiratory complications (poor effort or apnea) associated with symptomatic Chiari II malformation.[20] In addition, morbidity may contribute significantly to a patient's quality of life. Ambulation, urinary and bowel continence, hydrocephalus, limitations of cognitive function, and spinal cord tethering remain significant challenges for these patients throughout the course of their lives.

Up to 70% to 80% of patients with an open MMC have historically required a ventricular shunt, with up to 50% to 75% of shunts timed within the initial perinatal stay. Shunt malfunction rates have been reported as high as 30% to 40% within the first year, 60% within the first 5 years, and up to 85% at 10 years. Patients with hydrocephalus requiring shunt placement have been described as having a lower IQ. However, this may be related to underlying cortical dysplasias or serial shunt malfunctions, which are well documented to be associated with cognitive loss. In their series, Hunt and colleagues described that 89% of patients without a shunt had a high level of achievement, whereas only 69% of patients with a shunt but no revisions achieved the same level. This population dropped to 50% of those requiring shunt revisions before 2 years of age and 18% in those patients who required shunt revisions beyond 2 years of age.[21] Despite the overwhelming majority of patients obtaining a normal intelligence quotient (IQ, 70%–75%), hydrocephalus may negatively impact both IQ and cognitive function[22] and the ability to live independently.[23]

Ambulation and functional mobility of the lower extremities does correlate with the sensorimotor level, which can correlate with the bony dehiscence. Patients with lesions higher than spinal level L3 are typically nonambulatory.[24] The majority of preadolescent children are ambulatory, although the majority of patients in the series[21] had a lumbosacral lesion. Ambulation does decline as patients age, however, partially due to the efficiency of wheelchair use but also to the children's inability to carry additional weight as they grow.[25,26]

Management

Once the diagnosis is confirmed prenatally, referral to a tertiary care center is advised for multispecialty counseling and care coordination. The initial evaluation is aimed to determine the level of the lesion, which correlates with the degree of impairment as well as any associated anomalies, presence of a Chiari II malformation, and degree of ventriculomegaly. Assessment of fetal motor function can be performed to evaluate the potential for ambulation.[27] Fetal magnetic resonance imaging is complementary to the ultrasound examination to assess for callosal or migrational disorders. Genetic counseling and amniocentesis should be offered to exclude chromosomal anomalies. Multidisciplinary, objective counseling and discussion of management options should be done by a team experienced with spina bifida and include specialists in maternal fetal medicine, neurosurgery, neonatology, developmental pediatrics, and social work. Management options include pregnancy continuation with postnatal repair, fetal surgical closure for selected cases, or termination of pregnancy.[28]

For continuing pregnancies planned for neonatal repair, ongoing prenatal care aims to provide parent education and support about the fetal condition with the goal to achieve a term delivery. Serial ultrasound surveillance is done to assess interval fetal growth and head size that may affect the mode of delivery.[29] There has been substantial controversy about the optimal mode of delivery for fetal spina bifida. A recent meta-analysis demonstrated that cesarean delivery was not protective for neurologic function for unrepaired fetal spina bifida[30]; however, a substantial proportion of patients are delivered by cesarean section for obstetric indications such as breech presentation and macrocephaly.[31] The American College of Obstetricians and Gynecologists recommends that decisions about delivery mode and timing be individualized based on the specific case characteristics.[32]

Maternal fetal surgery is reserved for cases of fetal spina bifida without any additional anomalies and a normal karyotype. The landmark Management of Myelomeningocele Study demonstrated that prenatal closure of the fetal lesion via maternal laparotomy and hysterotomy before 26 weeks' gestation decreased the risk of death or need for shunt within the first year of life to 40% and improved the rate of independent ambulation at 30 months from 21% to 42%.[33] However, prenatal surgery increases the risk for obstetric complications and the rate of preterm birth and maternal complications, primarily related to the uterine incision, in both the current and all future pregnancies.[34] Accordingly, all women who undergo a hysterotomy for fetal surgery should be delivered by cesarean section expeditiously if there is concern for preterm labor or electively at 37 weeks due to the risk for uterine rupture.[35] An alternative is the fetoscopic approach, which is minimally invasive to the uterus. It is performed using two to four small ports either completely percutaneously or with assistance of a maternal laparotomy. This aims to preserve the fetal benefits while avoiding the risks of a hysterotomy (Fig. 54.2). Although the optimal technique remains a matter of debate, an international registry cohort demonstrated similar outcomes for shunting within the first 12 months of life, allowing the option for vaginal delivery and avoiding the risk for uterine dehiscence at the surgical site.[36] Regardless of whether the surgical closure is performed prenatally or planned after birth, delivery is recommended at a site where neonatal and neurosurgical services are available.[37]

Acute Perinatal Management for Open NTD

After delivery, initial assessment should proceed to ensure that the infant is hemodynamically stable, breathing appropriately, and meeting baseline neonatal criteria for stabilization. When positioning a neonate with an open NTD, care should be taken to keep direct pressure off the open lesion. The patient should be placed in an infant warmer with the head of the bed level to keep the MMC defect level. This avoids additional gravitational pull of the CSF toward the lesion, which ultimately can leak out of the open defect. A sterile, saline-soaked gauze should be used to cover the defect. Larger lesions may be susceptible to significant loss of body heat and fluid and so electrolyte and fluid status should be monitored closely. Temperature regulation may require not only an infant warmer but even covering the patient in a plastic drape to help trap body heat.

With active exposure of CSF to the unsterile environment, broad-spectrum intravenous antibiotics with CSF penetration should be instituted early. This has been shown to significantly reduce the likelihood of ventriculitis until the lesion is closed. The most common contaminants are *Escherichia coli*, group B *Streptococcus*, or *Staphylococcus*.[38] Some series have reported a high rate of shunt malfunction due to infection in infants who are concurrently shunted at the same time of their MMC closure.[39]

Initial newborn evaluation should examine whether there are other signs for a genetic or developmental syndrome because 15% will have clinically significant anomalies outside of the central nervous system.[40,41] A thorough examination of other organ systems should be conducted, including the cardiovascular, gastrointestinal, pulmonary, and genitourinary systems. While most coexisting anomalies are not immediately life-threatening, severe anomalies may portend a poor prognosis. Parents of infants with a known underlying chromosomal anomaly may choose not to proceed with closure or have limited interventions. Adequate prenatal workup and diagnosis in conjunction with the neonatal team may help establish a birth and treatment plan to help ease the burden on families after delivery.

Echocardiogram and renal ultrasound should be obtained to evaluate any physiologic dysfunction. If infants have had an adequate prenatal echocardiogram or do not manifest any clinical symptoms such as cyanosis or cardiac murmur, the echocardiogram may be delayed until after surgery. Most children with an MMC will have a neurogenic bladder, although this is rarely emergent in the immediate perinatal period and should not delay spinal closure. Additional preoperative considerations include hormonal and metabolic response to stress, adequate complete blood count, and nutrition. Preoperatively, enteral nutrition may be held, and if so, parenteral nutrition should be considered. Adequate enteral nutrition should be started as soon as possible but is dependent on several factors including hemodynamic and respiratory stability, extubation, gastrointestinal tract recovery from anesthesia, and in infants with a Chiari II malformation, aspiration risk or difficulty swallowing.

Sensorimotor function should be assessed to help determine the physiologic lesion level. Lower-extremity contractures may signal muscle imbalance that can lead to fixed hip flexion, knee extension, or ankle dorsiflexion. Hydrocephalus may manifest as a full fontanelle with split cranial sutures. Over time, rapid increase in head circumference or limitation of upward movement of the eyes, or "sunsetting eyes," may represent increased intracranial pressure. Brainstem dysfunction may manifest as bradycardia, apnea, swallowing deficits, weak cry, vocal cord palsies, and global hypotonia. Persistent brainstem dysfunction during the early perinatal period may represent symptomatic hydrocephalus as well as abnormal neuronal development within the brainstem itself.

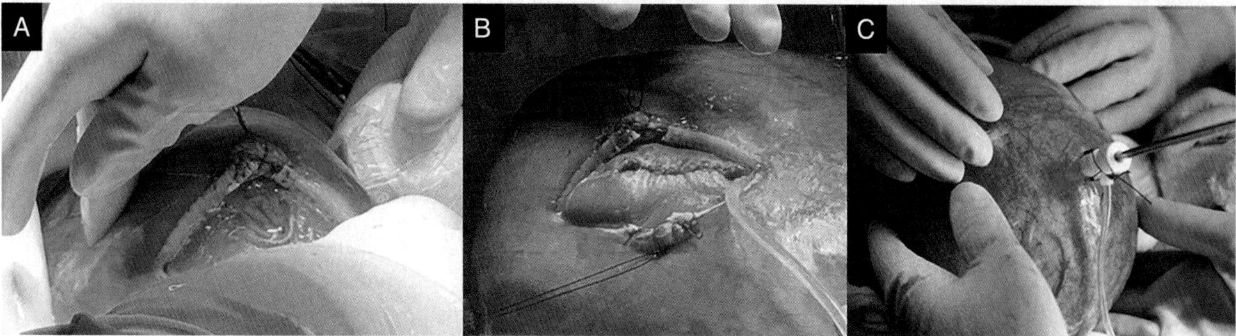

Fig. 54.2 Maternal Fetal Surgery for Spina Bifida Closure Via Hysterotomy and Fetoscopy. After maternal laparotomy and hysterotomy, (A) the fetal lesion is initially exposed and then (B) a multilayer closure is performed. (C) For the laparotomy-assisted fetoscopic approach, two to four small ports are inserted into the uterus using ultrasound guidance to perform the fetal closure.

Other routine preoperative preparation should include routine workup for neonates. Most neonatal infants have a high hematocrit and adequate intravascular volume. Routine monitoring of weight, blood pressure, and electrolyte status can help manage appropriate fluid and electrolyte management.[42] Other perioperative considerations include hypothermia and hypoglycemia. Neonates may experience a quick drop in their normal core body temperature due to evaporative heat loss and exposed body surfaces. This can be combated by wrapping all exposed surfaces intraoperatively that are not included in the operative field and using warmed intravenous solutions and agents for inhalation.

Historical series have looked at early versus late closure of MMCs. Unrepaired infants who are fed but denied antibiotics have a survival rate of 40% to 60%, albeit with significant impairment. With the addition of antibiotics, morbidity and mortality will fall for those infants repaired within the first 24 hours. Delaying the initial closure may have some benefit in families where there are significant underlying comorbidities in socially complex situations to allow for better surgical counseling. The current standard of care is for closure within 72 hours of birth to reduce the risk of complication.

Infants with MMCs are at greater risk than the general population of developing latex allergies, most likely due to latex immunoglobulin E antibiotics that develop throughout multiple operations and exposures.[43] Martinez and colleagues reported a prevalence of latex allergy in spina bifida patients ranging between 10% and 73%.[44] Clinical allergic reactions may be as high as 20% to 30% and may manifest with urticaria, bronchospasm, laryngeal edema, and systemic anaphylaxis.[1] Allergy may be related to age, the number of operations, and perhaps and underlying genetic predisposition. In our institution, all patients with MMC are listed as having a latex sensitivity, and procedures should be conducted in a latex-free environment.[45]

Operative Technique for Open NTD

Infants with MMCs undergo administration of general endotracheal anesthesia. When placed in a supine position, the midline spinal defect is generally protected by placing padding surrounding the lesion to alleviate any direct pressure or contact. Peripheral access is generally achieved without the need for central access. The infant is then placed in the prone position with bolsters or gel rolls under the chest and along the anterior iliac crest. Patients with a high lesion and contractures within the hips or knees may require additional padding or higher bolsters to allow for adequate tension-free positioning. Intravenous antibiotics should be initiated at birth with broad central nervous system coverage and are continued during the immediate perioperative period. The operative table should be placed in slight Trendelenburg position to avoid excessive drainage of CSF. The ambient room temperature should be elevated to minimize the difference with core temperature. In addition, a warming device should be placed underneath the infant to maximize surface area contact. Intravenous and irrigating fluids should be warmed as well to help maintain core body temperature.

When preparing and sterilizing the skin, the neural placode should be avoided. Alcohol or iodine can be caustic to the neural tissue but may be applied up to the junctional zone to help cleanse the skin. Draping should be generous because rotational flaps or relaxing incisions may sometimes be necessary for skin closure. The placode is first sharply dissected along the junctional zone to separate the skin from the perimeter of the open neural placode to avoid any subsequent inclusion dermoids (Fig. 54.3). Vascular input to the neural placode is important, and any traversing small feeding arteries or draining veins should be preserved if possible. Once free, the anterior projecting nerve roots can be seen exiting the neural placode and will appear to be completely released and tension free (Fig. 54.4). The rostral extent of the spinal cord may be seen entering the spinal canal. The lateral edges of the placode should be approximated with the use of a fine suture to reconstitute the neural tube.

Once the placode is closed, the dura can be reflected from the underlying fascia (see Fig. 54.3). In premature infants, or in cases where the dura is exceedingly thin, this may be reflected down to the paraspinal musculature and fatty plane. Dural grafts are rarely necessary, because the fascial incision can be done laterally enough to avoid strangulating the placode with a standard running suture.

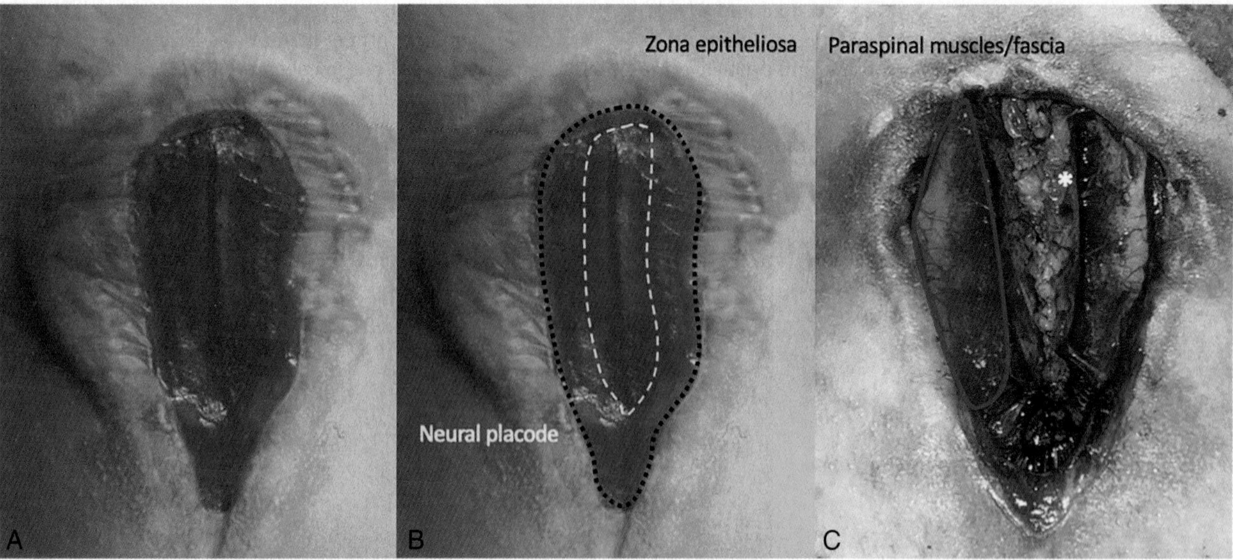

Fig. 54.3 Dorsal Nonannotated (A) and Annotated (B) View of the Neuroplacode at the Time of Operative Closure. The neuroplacode is seen as part of a fluid-filled sac containing cerebrospinal fluid. The sac is formed dorsally by the pia and disorganized neural tissue, which are fused to the epidermis at the zona epitheliosa. Following transection of this (C), the deeper layers of the dura are encountered, and these can be reflected to recreate the dural sac (*). Disorganized paraspinal muscles with investing fascia may be seen laterally, which can be incised to reflect additional closure.

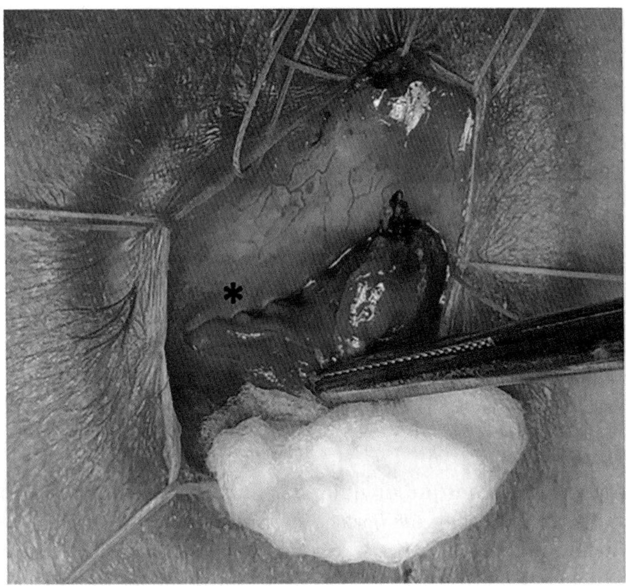

Fig. 54.4 Ventral Exiting Nerve Roots Through the Neuroforamina (*).

The lumbodorsal fascia may then be reflected over to create a myofascial flap closure over the dural closure to further reduce the incidence of CSF leak. Varying types of skin closures have been described, including vertical, horizontal, and a Z-plasty closure.[46] A vertical closure most closely mimics traditional midline spinal incisions and minimizes wound complications if future surgery is necessary. Care should be taken to avoid undermining the skin too laterally to avoid compromising the perforating vascular supply to the skin from the underlying fascia. If aggressively undermined, the skin may become necrotic due to loss of these perforators and could cause further wound complications.

Initial treatment of hydrocephalus is typically considered in a delayed fashion for several days to ensure there is no underlying infection. However, patients with considerable hydrocephalus evident at birth may require daily fontanelle taps to minimize wound leakage from the lumbar wound. CSF diversion at the time of repair has some advantages including avoiding a future procedure with intubating and decreasing the potential for CSF leakage. Miller and colleagues showed that placement of a ventriculoperitoneal shunt at the time of MMC closure compared with shunting in a delayed fashion reduced wound complications and spinal fluid leakage from 17% to 0%.[47] However, with simultaneous placement there was a higher percentage of patients who developed a shunt malfunction (19%, compared with 8% in the delayed shunt treatment group).

Postoperative Management for Open NTD

Postoperatively, infants are observed in the neonatal intensive care unit and should continue to follow routine best practices for critically ill newborns. Consideration for prior concerns including thermoregulation, cardiorespiratory monitoring, stress response, and fluid and electrolyte management should be maintained for all critically ill newborns. Specific postoperative concerns including pain management and nutritional status will be addressed in more detail. Infants will need to be monitored daily for the development of worsening hydrocephalus, infection, or concern for wound healing.

Nutritional status can be challenging in some infants with MMC due to prolonged intubation or multiple procedures that may delay or interrupt enteral feeding. Gastrointestinal function should be monitored to assess for paresis or delayed emptying due to anesthesia or pain medication by monitoring for abdominal distension or the passage of stool. In addition, brainstem dysfunction may manifest with swallowing difficulty or poor latch and/or suck reflexes, signaling a risk for aspiration. Babies might be noted to choke on liquids or have significant nasal regurgitation or vomiting. If there is a concern, a nasogastric tube can be inserted for gavage feeding, and this can be done in conjunction with a nutritionist and gastroenterologist. In infants who have ongoing surgical procedures for which gavage feeding may not be possible, parenteral nutrition should be considered.

Postoperative positioning should avoid pressure points over any tenuous areas of closure over the spine. Some closures may necessitate a prolonged period of time in the prone position, and this would include nursing in a manner that reduces pressure overlying the skin closure. Wound infections may manifest with erythema, swelling, tenderness at the site, or purulent drainage. In such cases, wound debridement may be necessary with initiation of systemic broad-spectrum antibiotics.[48] In their series, Charney and colleagues describe only 1% of infants receiving preoperative prophylactic antibiotics developing ventriculitis, compared with 19% of infants who did not receive antibiotics.[38] Ventriculitis may relate to wound breakdown or CSF fistulation at the site of closure.[48] Care should be taken to keep the operative site clean after repair, because infants with a neurogenic bladder and bowel may have a high rate of contamination of an incision that lies within the diaper itself.

Long-Term Outcomes

Long term care for infants with MMC are best managed with a multidisciplinary clinic that can address the myriad of medical concerns that will surround this patient population. Neurosurgery, orthopedic, urologic, physical therapy, occupational therapy, and neurocognitive specialists may be helpful. The long-term prognosis of children with spina bifida varies widely based on the level of lesion and presence of associated anomalies. In general, more than 90% of infants will survive beyond infancy.[25] Mortality within the first year is most commonly related to the Chiari malformation and underlying brainstem dysfunction as well as shunt malfunction or infections. Overall mortality has a significant range between 24% and 60%, typically highest within the first 5 years at 15% to 34% and decreasing to 9% to 26% after the 5-year mark.[49,50]

Neurosurgical

Hydrocephalus

Hydrocephalus and rates of ventricular shunting are somewhat variable throughout the literature, with rates ranging from 80% to 90% in some series to only 60% to 70%.[51] There may be geographic variability as well as an increased tolerance for ventriculomegaly in more contemporary series. In addition, the advent of endoscopic third ventriculostomy as an alternative to shunting has been introduced during the past few decades and has shifted treatment paradigms for hydrocephalus. Success rates for patients with MMC may reach as high as 70% among eligible patients who meet the following criteria: evidence of noncommunicating hydrocephalus, minimal or no discernible subarachnoid space, and a third ventricle at least 4 mm in width.[52] Shunted patients experience a shunt failure rate at 40%, 60%, and 85% at 1, 5, and 10 years after shunting, respectively. Shunt infection rates have fallen during the past three decades, but patients shunted before 6 months of age have a higher likelihood of malfunction and complication. Any neurologic clinical deterioration that is seen in children with MMC with shunted hydrocephalus may be attributed to the shunt. Therefore, evaluation of the neuraxis should always begin with a full assessment of the shunt.

Characteristic cognitive strengths and weaknesses in children with open spina bifida are highly variable. Neurocognitive difficulties may stem from anomalies within the corpus callosum that typically are associated with reduced interhemispheric communication and difficulties integrating information in language, reading, and social domains. In general, procedural learning and attention functions involving sustained attention and persistence are generally preserved.[53] General deficits in timing, attention, and movement can be seen as early as 6 months of age and can continue to affect infants over the course of their lifetime. Assembled processes, such as learning to construct and assimilate information, can be challenging. In contrast, children often have greater strengths with associative processing, such as associative and procedural learning.[54] The severity of the malformation and hydrocephalus can lead to significant variability within these findings.

Chiari II Malformation

Up to 70% to 80% of infants with MMC will have a radiographic Chiari II malformation, with herniation of the cerebellar vermis, brainstem, and fourth ventricle. Typically infants will present with lower cranial neuropathies, disordered eye movements, swallowing dysfunction, or disordered breathing compared with the more commonly seen Chiari I malformation that may manifest with occipital, exertional headaches.[55] Although Chiari malformation is commonly seen radiographically, most children are asymptomatic and only one-third of patients will require surgical intervention due to progressive symptoms.[55–59] In patients who present with progressive failure to thrive, clinicians should have a low threshold to evaluate for swallowing dysfunction. Other concerning signs may include disordered breathing, central or obstructive apnea as seen on a sleep study, inspiratory stridor, vocal cord paralysis, and a hoarse, weak, or high-pitched cry. Patients who have stridor and apnea at the time of delivery have a poorer outcome and higher overall mortality rate than patients who develop these symptoms in a more delayed fashion.[60] Older children may present with such signs as spasticity or weakness of the extremities, headaches and neck pain, cerebellar dysfunction, oculomotor dysfunction, and scoliosis.[57]

In patients in whom there is concern for a symptomatic Chiari malformation, care should first assess whether there is any underlying hydrocephalus or shunt malfunction. If there is any concern, shunt insertion or revision should be considered prior to decompression of the Chiari malformation. Additional workup should include a formal swallowing study, direct laryngoscopy to evaluate vocal cord paresis, and pulmonary studies such as a sleep study to evaluate the degree of dysfunction of apnea. Treatment hinges on the severity and on the age of presentation. Some series argue against treatment of a Chiari malformation in infants due to a historically high mortality rate that is no better than the natural history of the underlying disease process.[57,61] However, other studies have shown improvement in outcomes for infants treated early and aggressively. In general, newborns with underlying brainstem dysfunction often may require tracheostomy and gastrostomy with Nissen fundoplication. Neonates with less brainstem involvement and older children have a lower rate of surgical morbidity and mortality as well as improved overall outcomes.[62,63]

Tethered Cord Syndrome

Clinical neurologic deterioration has been described in children with MMC, with up to one-third of patients requiring surgical untethering in childhood.[64] Tethering is thought to cause symptoms due to ongoing stretching of the spinal cord that leads to an overall decreased blood flow. This then shifts to anaerobic metabolism with reduced glucose metabolism and mitochondrial failure that can lead to progressive neuronal loss with time. Increased pull occurs during periods of rapid growth, and this can lead to additional stretch of an already compromised spinal cord.[65,66] Releasing this tension can result in stability and some improvement in neurologic function, urologic function, and orthopedic deformities.

All patients with an MMC have some degree of radiographic tethering. Therefore, tethered cord syndrome is based on the development or progression of clinical symptoms. Patients may manifest with axial back pain, radicular pain, motor deterioration or worsening spasticity, sensory changes, worsening bowel or bladder function, and progressive orthopedic deformities such as pes cavus, equinovarus, hip dislocations, or scoliosis.

Urologic

Urologic anomalies are ubiquitous with spina bifida and do not always correlate with the level of spinal involvement. Typical urodynamic findings include decreased bladder capacity, decreased compliance, detrusor overactivity, detrusor-sphincter dyssynergia, bladder outlet obstruction, and complete denervation. Goals of management include ensuring safe bladder storage pressures and adequate bladder emptying at low pressures. Early recognition and management are critical to preventing progressive deterioration; however, the timing and interpretation of urodynamic studies or initiation of clean intermittent catheterization are controversial.[67] A thorough urologic evaluation includes a renal and bladder ultrasound, voiding cystourethrography, functional imaging such as a radionuclide scan, and urodynamics, once feasible. These help establish a baseline appearance and function of the upper and lower urinary tracts for future comparison. Infants should undergo evaluation with renal and bladder ultrasonography early to determine the postvoid residual urine. This additionally will help detect early signs of upper tract deterioration to help prevent additional renal damage. Renal and bladder ultrasound can help identify any worrisome findings such as hydronephrosis, ureteral dilation, renal size discrepancy, or bladder wall thickening and can help determine the need for antibiotic prophylaxis.

Early management is controversial. Some centers perform expectant management, where patients are monitored clinically and interventions such as catheterization are only performed if there is evidence of clinical deterioration. Other centers follow a more proactive approach and initiate catheterization early. Outcomes have been largely mixed in the literature, and there is no clear consensus. Lifetime goals include preserving renal function and achieving continence. This may require a combination of catheterization, anticholinergics, intradetrusor botulinum toxin A injections, bladder neck bulking agents, or reconstruction with bladder augmentation and/or a bladder neck procedure. As children grow, preventing bladder perforation, chronic renal disease, and kidney stone disease are important clinical factors.[68]

Neurogenic bowel dysfunction is also a common comorbidity and has been associated with a significant decrease in quality-of-life measures. Psychosocial metrics such as depression, discrimination of peers, decreased school attendance, and lower rates of employment have all been linked to poor management of neurogenic bowel incontinence.[69–71] Up to 80% of patients with MMC will require a bowel management program for constipation or fecal continence.[72] Interventions to help achieve some degree of control include oral medications, digital rectal stimulation through suppositories or enemas, large-volume enemas, Peristeen, antegrade enemas, or pouched fecal diversion. Overall fecal continence remains low at 30% to 65% despite interventions[73] but remains an important goal given the hope to maintain healthy self-esteem and improved quality of life.

Orthopedic

Scoliosis, or a curvature of the spine, may be seen in up to 90% of children with MMC and is more prevalent in patients with thoracic or upper lumbar lesions.[74–76] In neuromuscular cases of scoliosis, paravertebral muscle weakness as well as sensorimotor imbalance and muscle contractures may all contribute to spinal deformity progression. In patients with midlumbar-level lesions, with a curvature less than 45 degrees, curve stabilization may be obtained through untethering the spinal cord. Curvatures that present at 45 or 55 degrees are less likely to respond to untethering, and spinal deformity correction should be considered to obtain the best possible stabilization. Patients with spinal deformities beyond 80 or 90 degrees may develop pulmonary or cardiac compromise, and surgical morbidity is less in more modest spinal curvatures.

Other orthopedic concerns include hip or pelvic and severe foot deformities. Hip deformities or instability may be the result of muscle imbalance and paralysis around the hip joint. Approximately up to 50% of infants may develop instability or dislocation by 1 year of age. This results from unopposed action of the flexor and adductor muscles given paralysis of hip extensor and abductor muscles. Ultrasound can be used to evaluate the infant hip because the acetabulum and femoral head are cartilaginous. After 1 year of age, this can be followed with x-rays. Hip anomalies can be further exacerbated by hip contractures and subluxation and dislocation. If left untreated, pelvic obliquity can result and can drive sitting imbalance and scoliosis formation. Knee, tibia, and fibula deformities can lead to rotational issues that may make fitting of orthotics more challenging. These should be assessed with x-rays or magnetic resonance imaging when indicated. Congenital and acquired foot deformities are common, occurring in 80% to 95% of infants. Intrauterine paralysis is the major cause of congenital deformities, with malposition and intrauterine pressure leading to additional abnormalities. Talipes equinovarus, or club foot, is also commonly seen due to muscle paralysis or structural anomalies. Initial treatment consists of serial casting as early as possible, and surgical correction can be performed after a year of life if indicated.

In conclusion, NTDs remain the most common congenital birth defect of the central nervous system that results in lifelong morbidity from local nerve damage and the secondary effects of hydrocephalus from the Chiari II malformation. Due to the multisystem impacts of the condition, multidisciplinary care beginning during pregnancy allows for prenatal characterization of the lesion, assessment of ventriculomegaly, consideration of maternal fetal surgery for selected cases, and initial pediatric consultations. Postnatal management involves early surgical closure for children unrepaired at birth and management of associated hydrocephalus and urologic and orthopedic sequelae. Goals of treatment are targeted to optimize baseline function and enhance quality of life.

CHAPTER

55 Treating Neonatal Abstinence Syndrome in the Newborn

Jessie R. Maxwell, Sandra Brooks, Tamorah R. Lewis, Jessie Newville, Gabrielle McLemore, Estelle B. Gauda

KEY POINTS

1. In the United States an infant is born every 15 minutes who will develop symptoms of neonatal abstinence syndrome (NAS); each year, about 32,000 infants are estimated to develop NAS.
2. The exposure of the developing fetus to stimulants, alcohol, cannabinoids, and antidepressant medication can all have a negative impact. To refer specifically to the impact of opioids, the term neonatal opioid withdrawal syndrome (NOWS) is preferred.
3. We have summarized the information on the impact of transplacentally transferred opiates on the developing fetus. Various therapeutic options that are currently available for the management of NOWS or are under evaluation have been discussed.
4. The effects of transplacentally transferred pharmacologic stimulants such as cocaine, methamphetamine, and prescription drugs; herbal stimulants such as kratom tea; alcohol; cannabinoids; and antidepressant medications have been described in separate sections.

Introduction

In the United States an infant is born with neonatal abstinence syndrome (NAS) every 15 minutes, with an estimated 32,000 babies with NAS born every year.[1] This estimates only the infants with symptomatic withdrawal after prenatal opioid exposure. Additional use of substances during pregnancy, such as stimulants, alcohol, cannabinoids, and antidepressant medication, can all result in negatively impacting the developing fetus. Thus it is paramount to understand the mechanism of how each substance can result in exposure to the fetus and if any known therapies are effective to mitigate these changes.

Opioids

Opioids are a class of drugs that are usually used to reduce pain. This can include prescription medication, such as oxycodone, hydrocodone, fentanyl, morphine, and methadone, as well as illicit substances such as heroin. Use of these drugs by pregnant women can result in adverse outcomes such as stillbirth or preterm birth, NAS, and birth defects. From 1999 to 2014, across the United States, the rates of opioid use disorder at the time of delivery more than quadrupled.[2] Infants exposed to opioids throughout pregnancy develop a dependence on the drug, with a resultant withdrawal once the drug is no longer present.[3] The withdrawal was previously referred to as NAS, which is now more specifically termed neonatal opioid withdrawal syndrome (NOWS).[4] Opioids can cross the placenta, thus resulting in exposure to the fetus. The following describes placental transport of opioids, the resultant symptoms in infants after birth, current therapeutic options, and the resultant impact on development.

Mechanism of In Utero Exposure

One puzzling aspect of neonatal opiate withdrawal is the lack of association between the maternal opiate dose during pregnancy and the incidence or severity of NOWS. A recent systematic review confirms the results of many smaller studies, namely that there is no currently known relationship between the maternal dose of methadone and the incidence or severity of NOWS.[5] This lack of association is likely because the current thinking on the maternal–fetal–neonatal transfer and effect of opiate medications is oversimplified and does not account for the potential impact of drug metabolism and drug target variability. This drug metabolism and drug target variability is influenced by maternal and fetal genetics as well as the stage of gestation and fetal development. There have been some important efforts to understand the pathogenesis of NOWS (Fig. 55.1), but we still do not have all the answers.

Many factors can affect the amount of free drug in the maternal circulation available for transplacental fetal transfer at any given time. It is known that maternal drug metabolism changes through different trimesters and that environmental factors such as maternal comedication and cigarette use can alter rates of drug metabolism and placental transport.[6,7] In addition, there is known genetic variation in opiate metabolism.[8–10] The efficiency of placental metabolizing enzymes and placental opiate transport proteins such as multidrug resistant protein 1 (MDR1) and breast cancer resistance protein can dictate how much drug reaches the fetus for any specific mother-infant pair.[11–13]

MDR1 is a known placental transporter for methadone. Using a single layer of placental cells in a dual perfusion model, Nanovskaya et al. showed that methadone transfer to the fetal circuit was increased by 30% by different MDR1 inhibitors.[12] The authors concluded based on this experiment that the concentration of methadone in the fetal circulation is likely affected by the expression and activity of placental MDR1. Data from experiments in an *ex vivo* placental model provides evidence that buprenorphine transport across the placenta is not mediated by MDR1[14] but rather via passive diffusion. Buprenorphine crosses placental cells into the fetal circuit to a lesser degree than methadone, with less than 10% of initial maternal concentrations detected on the fetal side of the circuit after a 4-hour equilibration.[13] This decreased transfer of buprenorphine is thought to be secondary to its highly lipophilic nature and significant tissue accumulation within the placenta compared with both the maternal and fetal compartments.

The fetal and neonatal blood-brain barrier also contribute to the risk of developing NOWS. On postmortem samples from gestational age 20 weeks to postmenstrual age 3 months, it was found that p-glycoprotein expression is very limited in the fetal and neonatal period compared with older infants and adults.[15] This is important

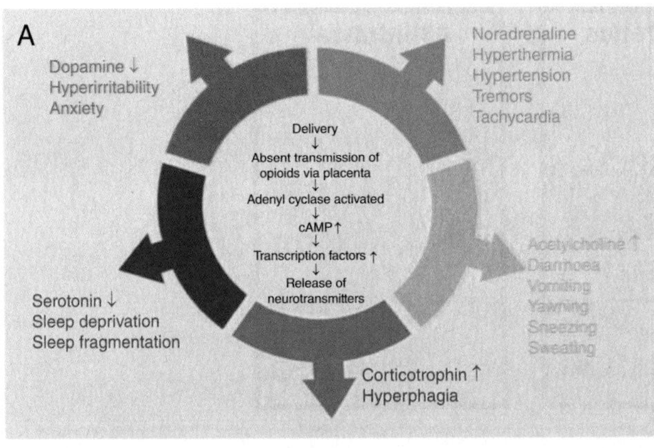

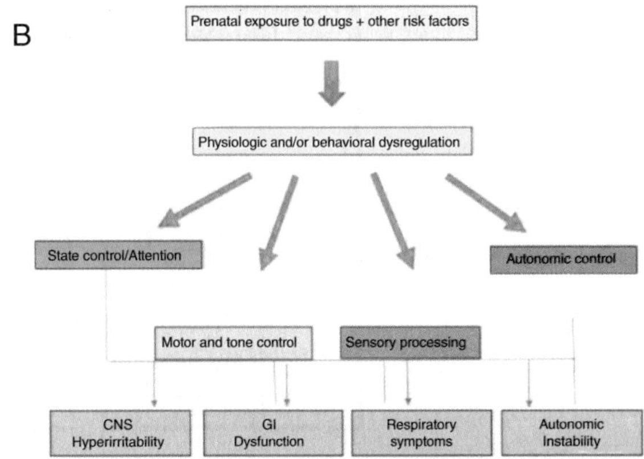

Fig. 55.1 Pathophysiology of Neonatal Abstinence Syndrome (NAS), Which May Be More Appropriately Termed Neonatal Opiate Withdrawal Syndrome (NOWS). (A) At a mechanistic level, the clinical manifestations can be understood in terms of altered levels of different neurotransmitters; (B) in clinical assessment, NOWS is marked by dysregulation in four domains of functioning. (B, Reproduced with modifications from Jansson and Patrick. *Pediatric Clinics of North America*. 2019;66:353–367.)

because p-glycoprotein plays a critical role in efflux of opiates from the central nervous system (CNS) back into the systemic circulation. There are currently no studies in humans to elucidate the extent of methadone or buprenorphine accumulation in the CNS.

Neonatal Opioid Withdrawal Syndrome Symptoms

Chronic in utero opiate exposure leads to activation of the fetal brain μ-opioid receptor. This leads to intracellular adaptations, including decreased adenylyl cyclase activity and decreased cyclic adenosine 3′,5′-cyclic monophosphate (cAMP) and release of excitatory neurotransmitters. After umbilical cord ligation at birth, there is an abrupt cessation to opiate exposure, which, as the newborn metabolizes and clears the maternal opiate, leads to an abrupt increase in adenylyl cyclase activity and downstream effects (Fig. 55.2).[3] This leads to a large increase in central sympathetic outflow, resulting in the symptoms of newborn opiate withdrawal. These symptoms include autonomic signs such as diarrhea, emesis, yawning, sneezing, and sweating. They also include CNS excitatory signs such as hyperirritability, tremors, hyperthermia, tachycardia, and poor sleep (Fig. 55.3). In extreme and untreated cases of newborn opiate withdrawal, the neuroexcitatory neurotransmitter milieu of epinephrine and norepinephrine can lead to clinical seizures.

The duration of opiate withdrawal symptoms is highly variable and depends in part on which drugs were part of in utero exposure (Table 55.1).[3] NOWS as a result of methadone or buprenorphine tends to last longer than heroin or short-acting prescription drugs, but polypharmacy and multiple in utero exposures are common, and the way these modify NOWS severity and duration are poorly understood. The treatment of NOWS symptoms includes opiate replacement and slow weaning of postnatal treatment, providing the deranged CNS pathways time to reset and return to normal. Current research about optimal NOWS therapy seeks to find a balance between control of symptoms and avoiding prolonged and excessive opiate exposure.

Treatment of Neonatal Opioid Withdrawal Syndrome

Nonpharmacologic Treatments

The most optimum treatment of NOWS is still a matter of debate. However, most clinicians agree on the need for adopting one standardized protocol and following this with close follow-up to optimize it for the particular clinical unit and the local patient population (Fig. 55.4). There is universal agreement that nonpharmacologic treatments should be implemented prior to use of medications to alleviate NOWS. A simple yet critically important first step is to maintain the mother-infant dyad if possible. Many infants are moved to a newborn intensive care unit, which will then separate the pair. A meta-analysis of 6 studies and 549 patients showed a decrease in hospitalization by 10 days when rooming-in, or maintaining the mother-infant dyad, occurred.[16] These infants had a reduction in the use of pharmacotherapy by 63%.[16] Additional environmental measures such as minimizing stimulation through dim lighting and optimizing comfort through swaddling should be considered standard treatment for this patient population. Observing the infant's response to environmental stimuli is critical to determine the best interventions to minimize overstimulation. Various signs of stress in the infant can be used to identify a stimulus as stressful, such as hiccups, color change (mottling, perioral cyanosis), excess gas, and even changes in breathing patterns.[17]

If a woman is prescribed methadone or buprenorphine, the levels measured in breast milk have been observed to be low.[18] This does not seem to be impacted by the maternal dose, and thus breastfeeding is considered safe.[18] It has also been observed that breastfeeding can result in a shorter hospital stay and decreased need for pharmacologic treatment. Breastfeeding should be encouraged, although a recent review found that many women on opioid maintenance therapy did not breastfeed.[19] There is discussion that it may be related to schedule demands on the woman; however, societal stigma may result in a lack of patient support, even in hospitals with the Baby-Friendly designation.[19]

Mechanism of Action for Pharmacologic Treatments

Opiates are the mainstay of pharmacologic therapy for NOWS, although other nonopiate drugs such as clonidine show great promise as either monotherapy or adjunct therapy. Pharmacologic therapy is indicated for infants who fail nonpharmacologic interventions and display significant and persistent signs of opiate withdrawal, as quantified by a validated NOWS scoring tool.

Morphine and Methadone

Morphine and methadone are the most commonly used opiate to treat NOWS, but there are increasing data about buprenorphine as a primary modality.[20] Morphine is a short-acting μ-opiate receptor

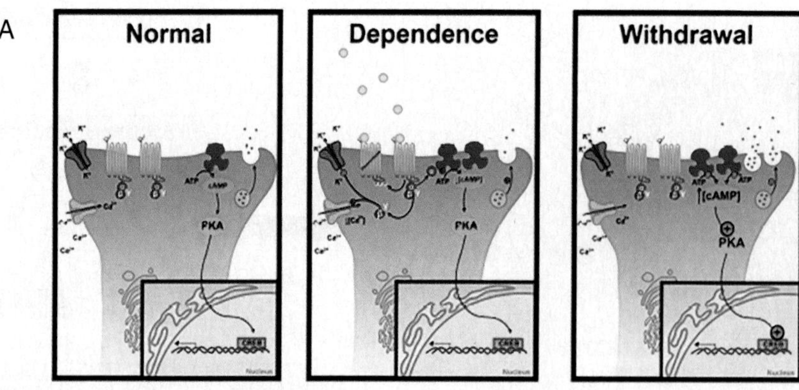

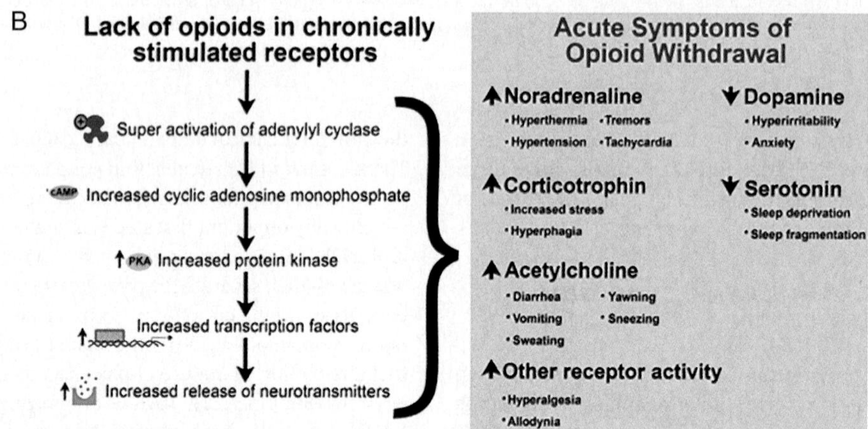

Fig. 55.2 (A) A schematic illustration of cellular signaling in an opioid-sensitive neuron under normal conditions that are altered under conditions of opioid dependence and withdrawal. Chronically stimulated μ-opioid receptors lead to reduced responsiveness to opioid agonists and a g-protein–regulated decrease in calcium ion concentration. Importantly, chronic stimulation results in overactivation of g-protein–coupled receptors, suppression of adenylyl cyclase activity, and ultimately, reduced cyclic adenosine monophosphate (cAMP) concentrations. These opioid-induced effects produce an adaptive up-regulation of adenylyl cyclase machinery and superactivation of adenylyl cyclase under conditions of withdrawal, leading to elevated cAMP and phospho-cAMP-response element binding protein (CREB). (B) Step-by-step summary of molecular events that lead to altered production and release of various neurotransmitters responsible for the acute symptoms of opioid withdrawal. (Adapted from Kocherlakota P. Neonatal abstinence syndrome. *Pediatrics*. 2014;134:e547–e561.)

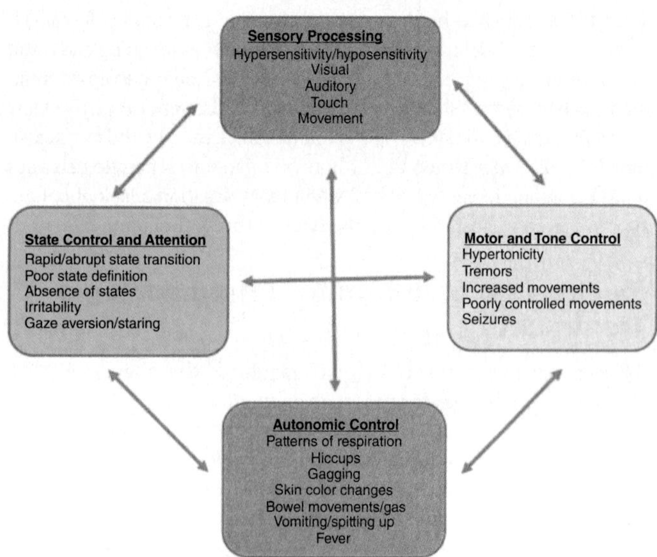

Fig. 55.3 Signs of Neonatal Opiate Withdrawal Syndrome Expression in the Four Major Domains of Functioning. Each domain can influence expression in other domains. (Reproduced with modifications from Jansson and Patrick. *Pediatric Clinics of North America*. 2019;66:353–367.)

agonist. Because of the short half-life of morphine, the best outcomes have been demonstrated when morphine doses are given no longer than 4 hours apart (generally with feedings). Methadone is a long-acting μ-opiate receptor agonist. The longer half-life of methadone provides less of a flux between peak and trough levels while also providing ease of administration at less frequent intervals. However, the long half-life necessitates waiting 48 to 72 hours to see the full effect of dosing changes; thus there is concern that it is less "easily titratable" than short-acting morphine.

Multiple studies have evaluated the differences in treating with morphine or methadone in an attempt to determine superiority. One such meta-analysis reviewed five studies and found no significant difference in opioid treatment days, length of hospital stay, and duration of treatment between morphine or methadone.[21]

Buprenorphine

Buprenorphine is emerging as a safer and more efficient drug for adult detoxification and maintenance programs and has been studied during pregnancy as an alternative to methadone. Overall, it is showing great promise as a therapeutic agent for the treatment of NAS. Buprenorphine is a long-acting partial μ-opioid receptor agonist. At the molecular level, there are three well-described opioid receptors (μ-opioid receptor, δ-opioid receptor, and κ-opioid receptor). Morphine and methadone are among the opioids that act as agonists

Table 55.1 The Onset of Withdrawal Symptoms, Frequency of Withdrawal Occurrence After Exposure, and Duration of Withdrawal Caused by Various Substances

Onset, Duration, and Frequency of NAS

		Onset (h)	Frequency (%)	Duration (d)
Opioids	Heroin	24–48	40–80	8–10
	Methadone	48–72	13–94	Up to 30+
	Buprenorphine	36–60	22–67	Up to 28+
	Prescription medication	36–72	5–20	10–30
	Kratom tea (high dose)	6–33	Unknown	5–12+
Stimulants	Methamphetamine	24	2–49	7–10
	Cocaine	48–72	6	Up to 7
Depressants	THC	24–72	Unknown	7–30
	Alcohol	3–12	2–5	Up to 3
SSRIs	Prescription medication	24–48	20–30	2–6

NAS, Neonatal abstinence syndrome; *SSRI,* selective serotonin reuptake inhibitor; *THC,* Δ^9-tetrahydrocannabinol.

Adapted from Kocherlakota P. Neonatal abstinence syndrome. *Pediatrics.* 2014;134:e547–e561.

at each of these receptors, but buprenorphine differs because it has an antagonistic effect at the κ-opioid receptor.[22] This molecular characteristic is thought to allow for less sedation and less respiratory depression among buprenorphine users.

The effect on neonates of the maternal use of buprenorphine during pregnancy has been well studied. A double-blind, double-dummy, flexible dosing, randomized controlled trial found that infants exposed to prenatal buprenorphine versus methadone had required significantly less morphine therapy (mean dose, 1.1 mg versus 10.4 mg; $P < .0091$), had a significantly shorter hospital stay (10.0 days versus 17.5 days; $P < .0091$), and had a significantly shorter duration of treatment for NAS (4.1 days versus 9.9 days; $P < .003125$) with no difference in neonatal or maternal adverse outcomes.[23] A recent retrospective study showed similar results with less use of phenobarbital as adjunct therapy in infants exposed to buprenorphine prenatally.[24] The first published use of buprenorphine for the treatment of NAS dates back to 2008 when Kraft and colleagues randomized 13 infants to receive sublingual buprenorphine (initial dose of 13.2 mcg/kg/day divided in three doses) and compared them to the same number of infants who were managed with their standard-of-care oral opium solution. There were no adverse effects noted in the buprenorphine-treated group. The mean length of treatment and the overall mean length of hospital stay were shorter in this group as well (mean length of treatment of 22 days compared with 32 days and overall mean length of hospital stay of 38 days compared with 27 days).[25]

Additional studies have compared buprenorphine with other commonly used drugs in the treatment of NAS. A single-site, randomized, open-label trial was published in 2011 and compared buprenorphine at a dose of 15.9 mcg/kg/day given in three divided doses to morphine at a dose of 0.4 mg/kg/day in six divided doses. There were 12 infants in each arm, and again the results were in favor of treatment with buprenorphine. Infants had a 40% reduction in length of treatment (23 days versus 38 days) and a 24%

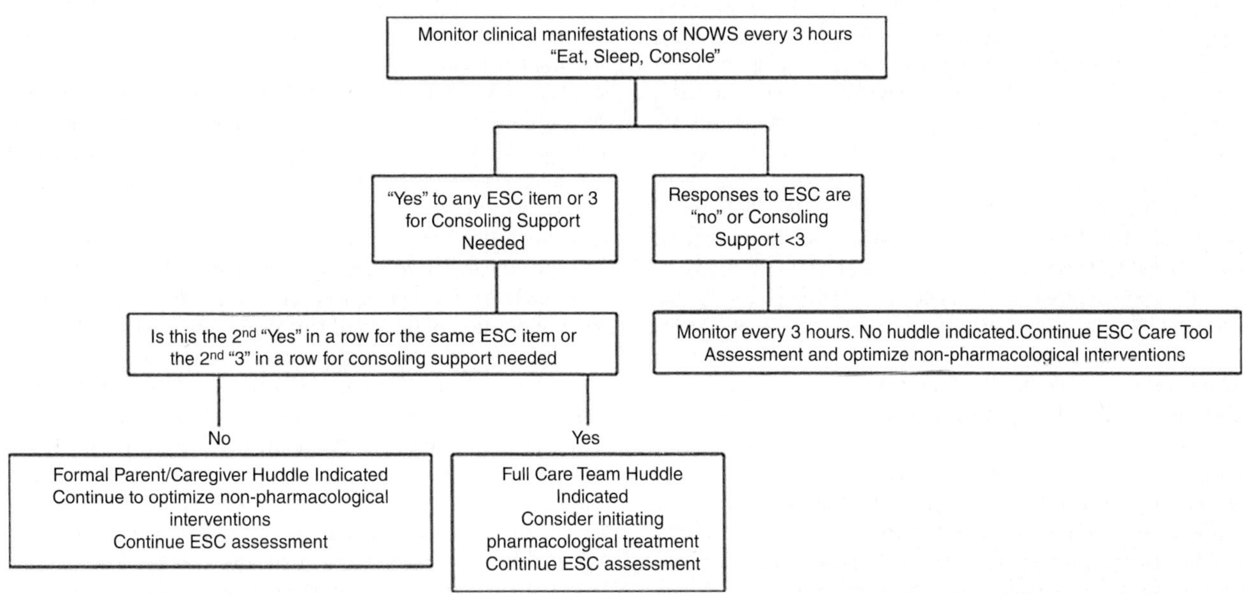

Fig. 55.4 One Possible Strategy for Standardized Management of Neonatal Opiate Withdrawal Syndrome.

reduction in length of hospital stay (32 days versus 42 days).[26] Similar findings were seen among 126 infants in a single-site, double-blind, double-dummy clinical trial (BBORN), with infants randomly assigned in a 1:1 ratio to either receive sublingual buprenorphine or oral morphine and the corresponding placebo. Buprenorphine doses ranged from 15.9 mcg/kg/day to a maximum of 60 mcg/kg/day in three divided doses, and morphine sulfate ranged from 0.4 mg/kg/day to 1.0 mg/kg/day in six divided doses. The median duration of treatment was significantly shorter with buprenorphine than with morphine (15 days versus 28 days), as was the median length of hospital stay (21 days versus 33 days; $P < .001$ for both comparisons). Adjunctive phenobarbital was administered in 5 of 33 infants (15%) in the buprenorphine group and in 7 of 30 infants (23%) in the morphine group ($P = .36$). Rates of adverse events were similar in the two groups.[20] Extensive analyses of blood samples obtained from these infants have allowed extrapolation of a pharmacokinetic model for both buprenorphine and norbuprenorphine and identification of a novel relationship in the pharmacokinetics and pharmacodynamics of buprenorphine administration in NAS, thus paving the way to work toward optimization of buprenorphine dosing in future clinical trials.[27]

Of note, buprenorphine use has also been compared with methadone therapy in a multicenter, retrospective cohort analysis in southwest Ohio where 38 infants treated with buprenorphine were compared with 163 treated with methadone after intrauterine exposure to short-acting opioids or buprenorphine. Buprenorphine therapy was associated with a significantly shorter course of opioid treatment (9.4 days versus 14.0 days) and a significantly decreased hospital stay (16.3 days versus 20.7 days) compared with methadone therapy. No difference was detected in the use of adjunct therapy (23.7% versus 25.8%) between treatment groups. The initiation dose of buprenorphine was 13.2 mcg/kg in three divided doses.[28] At the time of this publication, an industry-sponsored phase 2, multicenter, double-blind, double dummy, randomized, two-arm parallel study is underway to evaluate the efficacy, safety, and pharmacokinetics of buprenorphine in babies with NAS.

Adjunctive Therapies

Phenobarbital and clonidine are also used in the treatment of withdrawal. Phenobarbital is no longer considered a first-line option for treatment for withdrawal due to higher incidence of seizures and need for longer treatment duration.[29] As a gamma-aminobutyric acid (GABA) receptor agonist, phenobarbital has sedative effects, making some feel it is of benefit if infants have also been exposed to benzodiazepines.[30] Clonidine is an α_2-adrenergic receptor agonist and thus can impact the heart rate. A retrospective review found a decrease in heart rate in infants receiving clonidine and a mild increase in blood pressure once clonidine was discontinued that did not seem clinically significant.[31] A review of three clinical trials and five observational studies concluded that clonidine did have effectiveness in both monotherapy and combinational therapy with minimal side effects.[32] A study of 190 infants treated from 2005 to 2015 compared outcomes when using phenobarbital versus clonidine as adjunctive therapy to morphine.[33] The length of morphine therapy and the length of stay was significantly decreased using clonidine compared with phenobarbital.[33] Thus there may be a continued role for the use of phenobarbital and particularly for clonidine as adjunctive treatment in infants undergoing withdrawal.

A recent abstract in the Cochrane review library[34] summarized the findings of all randomized controlled trials comparing different modes of pharmacologic therapy (Table 55.2). Most practicing neonatologists would agree that more than *which* opiate agonist is chosen as primary therapy, having an evidence-based and agreed upon protocol for diagnosis and management of infants with NOWS is the most important tool for optimizing therapy.

Long-Term Impact of Neonatal Opioid Withdrawal Syndrome

There remains a paucity of data in the neurodevelopmental outcomes of children following in utero opioid exposure with resultant withdrawal syndrome. However, studies are following these patients as they age with resultant outcomes. In Finland, buprenorphine is the most commonly used opiate, with 60% of infants exposed late in the pregnancy developing NOWS.[35] One study followed this cohort until age 3 years and found that 11% had eye disorders, 5% had major congenital anomalies, and there was an increased incidence of dental caries and poor cognitive abilities. Lind and colleagues noted an increased incidence of congenital malformations such as oral clefts, ventricular septal defects and arterial septal defects, spina bifida, and congenital talipes equinovarus.[36] Isolated cleft palate and isolated cleft lip were noted to have a higher prevalence in infants with NOWS compared with the general live population.[37] Continued research is needed on neurodevelopmental outcomes of this high-risk population following in utero exposure to opiates.

Stimulants

According to reports from the U.S. Department of Health and Human Services report from 2015, stimulants, including cocaine, methamphetamines, and prescription stimulants, are the second most widely used and abused substances in the United States.[38] The use of stimulants among pregnant women, particularly methamphetamine, has increased over time,[39] an alarming trend as evidence mounts that these agents may negatively impact both maternal and fetal health.[38] Results from the Infant Development, Environment, and Lifestyle (IDEAL) study across four clinical centers in the United States indicate that 6% of pregnant women used methamphetamine,[40] a pattern similar to other regions of the world.[41] Interestingly, one study found that 63% of methamphetamine-using pregnant women reported using throughout pregnancy.[42]

Although cocaine has a short half-life (0.7–1.5 hours), its effects throughout the body are potent because it binds and blocks presynaptic monoamine reuptake transporters, resulting in the accumulation in the synaptic cleft of dopamine, serotonin, and norepinephrine, leading to enhanced and prolonged sympathetic effects.[43] Cocaine rapidly crosses from maternal to fetal circulation and across the fetal blood-brain barrier by simple diffusion.[44] Under normal circumstances, cocaine is rapidly metabolized by cholinesterase in the plasma and liver; however, cholinesterase is diminished in pregnant women and is even lower in the fetus,[43] potentially resulting in increased exposure. After transfer from maternal to fetal circulation, preclinical evidence suggests that cocaine and its metabolites accumulate in the liver and brain.[45] Mechanistically, cocaine results in acute and delayed vasoconstriction of maternal and fetal vessels, which can also result in an increased incidence of placental abruption.

Withdrawal after prenatal exposure to stimulants has not been thoroughly characterized, although a few studies have described withdrawal symptoms of stimulant-exposed neonates. In an early small retrospective study of 166 infants, with 74 infants exposed to amphetamine prenatally, exposed infants experienced increased levels of drowsiness during the first months of life, which resolved at the 1-year follow-up.[46] Consistent with the previous study, the larger IDEAL study, which enrolled 412 patients across four centers in the United States, found that assessment within the first 5 days of life

Table 55.2 Summary of Clinical Studies Investigating Pharmacologic Treatments of Neonatal Abstinence Syndrome

Studies on Diagnosis & Treatment of NAS

First Author, Year	Study Design	No.	Intervention	Comparator	Outcomes	Conclusions
Brown, 2015[46a]	Prospective, randomized	n = 78	Methadone	Morphine	Duration of treatment of NAS	Methadone resulted in shorter treatment compared with morphine
Bada, 2015[46b]	Prospective, randomized	n = 31	Morphine	Clonidine	Neurobehavioral performance	Clonidine may be a more favorable alternative to morphine for NAS treatment
Nayeri, 2015[46c]	Randomized, open-label	n = 60	Oral morphine sulfate	Phenobarbital	Duration of treatment Duration of hospital stay Requirement of adjunctive treatment	No significant difference between treatments
Raith, 2015[46d]	Prospective, randomized	n = 28	Acupuncture with pharmacologic treatment	Pharmacologic treatment alone	Duration of treatment	Acupuncture with pharmacologic treatment reduced duration of morphine treatment
Surran, 2013[46e]	Prospective, nonblinded, block randomized	n = 68	Clonidine	Phenobarbital	Duration of treatment	Clonidine resulted in shorter therapy time compared with phenobarbital
Kaft, 2010[46f]	Randomized, open-label, active-control	n = 24	Sublingual buprenorphine	Morphine	Safety Duration of treatment Duration of hospital stay	Sublingual buprenorphine was safer and more effective compared with morphine
Agthe, 2009[46g]	Randomized, controlled, double blind	n = 80	Clonidine	Placebo	Safety Duration of treatment Effectiveness	Clonidine reduced the duration of pharmacotherapy without causing short-term adverse cardiovascular outcomes
Kaft, 2008[25]	Randomized, open-label, active-control	n = 13	Sublingual buprenorphine	Neonatal opium solution	Safety Duration of treatment	Sublingual buprenorphine was determined safe to treat NAS

NAS, Neonatal abstinence syndrome.

Adapted from CADTH Rapid Response Report: Summary of Abstracts. 2017. The diagnosis and treatment of neonatal abstinence syndrome: clinical effectiveness and guidelines. *CADTH.* Ottawa.

with the NICU Network Neurobehavior Scale revealed decreased arousal, increased stress, and poor quality of movement at birth.[47] Importantly, this same study reported a dose-response of prenatal methamphetamine exposure, with increased CNS stress. Similarly, cocaine exposure has been associated with increased CNS stress, poor movement, poor visual and auditory following, hypertonicity, and drowsiness at birth.[48,49]

Interestingly, in multiple other studies investigators employed scoring systems that were designed to evaluate NAS following opioid exposure. For example, one study found symptoms consistent with opioid withdrawal, including irritability, hyperactivity, and tremors,[50] occurring between day of life 2 and 3.[51] These results are consistent with a study of 104 methamphetamine-exposed or cocaine-exposed infants demonstrating altered neonatal behavioral patterns, as assessed by the Finnegan scoring system, similar to those of infants with neonatal opioid withdrawal.[52] In a retrospective study of neonates whose mothers used methamphetamines during pregnancy, matched to unexposed controls, the incidence of methamphetamine-exposed infants with evidence of withdrawal symptoms was 49%, with 4% exhibiting severe withdrawal symptoms requiring pharmacologic intervention.[42] Methamphetamine-exposed infants may develop jitteriness, drowsiness, and respiratory distress suggesting withdrawal; pharmacologic intervention is rarely indicated.[42,52]

The paucity of new research aimed at characterizing neonatal abstinence after preterm stimulant exposure or avenues of pharmacologic treatment to better support these infants warrants attention from preclinical and clinical investigators.

Kratom Tea

Mitragyna speciosa, commonly called kratom, is a plant that grows in parts of Southeast Asia including Thailand, Malaysia, Indonesia, and Papua New Guinea. The plant leaves are used to make a tea, smoked, or made into a powder, and it is a widely available herbal supplement that is often advertised as a treatment for opioid withdrawal.[53] While not classified as an opioid, it is an herbal alkaloid that has agonistic effects on μ-opioid receptors, similar in action to morphine. At the time of this publication, there are no U.S. Food and Drug Administration–approved uses for kratom and the safety profile continues to be evaluated.[54] A recent survey of 3024 current and former users of kratom reported using the substance primarily for pain relief (48% of the respondents) and to help cut down on opioid use and/or relieve withdrawal (10% of the cases).[53] Thus pregnant women are starting to use the herb, and reports of withdrawal symptoms in infants are beginning to be reported.

One such case was an infant born to a mother with history of opioid abuse but who had successful rehabilitation and a negative urine drug screen at hospital admission.[54] The infant developed symptoms consistent with opioid withdrawal, including sneezing, jitteriness, irritability, a high-pitched cry, and hypertonia and required pharmacologic treatment.[54] Another case of neonatal withdrawal following kratom exposure in utero resulted in oral morphine treatment for 2 months.[55] There remain no diagnostic tests to screen for kratom use, and the impact on neonates and development continue to be researched.

Depressants

Alcohol

The current leading preventable cause of birth defects and intellectual and neurodevelopmental disabilities is prenatal alcohol exposure (PAE), which has led the American Academy of Pediatrics to state that no amount of alcohol is safe during pregnancy.[56] Exposure to alcohol in utero may result in fetal alcohol spectrum disorder (FASD), which is a comprehensive term that includes PAE diagnoses, including fetal alcohol syndrome, alcohol-related birth defects, alcohol-related neurodevelopmental disorder, and neurobehavioral disorder associated with PAE.[56] The impact of PAE was first described by Jones et al. in 1973; they reported patterns of craniofacial, limb, and cardiovascular defects in 8 children born to mothers who were chronic alcoholics.[57] Diagnosis of fetal alcohol syndrome is now made by observing three characteristic facial features (smooth philtrum, thin vermillion border, and small palpebral fissures), growth deficits, and CNS abnormalities in the setting of maternal alcohol use. A recent study estimated the prevalence of FASD to range from 1.1% to 5.0% in the United States.[58]

Alcohol readily crosses the placenta, which allows direct impact on the fetus during development. A review of 13 articles showed that multiple organ systems are impacted after PAE, including the brain, heart, kidneys, liver, gastrointestinal tract, and endocrine system.[59] Aside from the facial abnormalities described above, additional abnormalities may occur including maxillary hypoplasia, cleft palate, and micrognathia.[56] Unfortunately, PAE can also result in fetal death and is associated with sudden infant death syndrome.[56] Cases of withdrawal in infants with alcohol exposure have been reported, with symptoms typically including irritability, tremors, seizures, abdominal distention, and opisthotonos.[60] Additional signs of withdrawal may include a high-pitched cry, jitteriness, and a poor sleeping pattern.[61] These symptoms may persist for up to 18 months.[61]

Long-term impacts following PAE are better studied than other drugs used during pregnancy. A secondary analysis conducted from the Canadian component of the World Health Organization International Study on the Prevalence of FASD found individuals with FASD had impairments in perceptual reasoning, verbal comprehension, visual-motor speed and motor coordination processing speed, attention and executive function, visuospatial processing, and language, in combination with rule-breaking behavior and attention problems.[62] Similar to preclinical models,[63] a virtual water maze test in 10-year-old children found deficits in spatial navigation in those children heavily exposed to alcohol during pregnancy.[64]

Cannabinoids

Cannabinoids (CBs) are a class of chemical compounds that act on CB receptors, including CB1R and CB2R. The ligands for the receptors include the endogenous CBs (endocannabinoids: anandamide; 2-arachidonoylglycerol) and the exogenous phytoCBs that are constituents of the hemp plant *Cannabis sativa* (lipophilic and psychoactive Δ^9-tetrahydrocannabinol [THC]).[65] Finally, synthetic CB analogs include WIN 55, 212-2, HU-210, and JWH-133. We have previously discussed the "double-hit hypothesis" as it relates to prenatal cannabis exposure (PCE). We contended that PCE, like a neurodevelopmental teratogen, delivers the "first hit" to the endocannabinoid signaling system (ECSS), which is composed in such a way that a second hit (i.e., postnatal stressors) will precipitate the emergence of a specific phenotype. We concluded that perturbations of the intrauterine milieu via exogenous CBs alter the fetal ECSS, predisposing the offspring to abnormalities in cognition and altered emotionality. We argued that young women who become pregnant should immediately take a "pregnant pause" from using cannabis.[66] Here we will discuss the state of PCE during fetal and adolescent development and subsequent epigenetics alterations. We will highlight epigenetic alterations and fetal malprogramming in adults exposed to cannabis in utero and in adolescence and in subsequent generations conceived by individuals with germ cell cannabis exposure.

According to a 2018 Pew Research Center survey, 62% of Americans were in favor of legalizing cannabis compared with 31% in 2000,[67] which reflects an increase in societal permissiveness toward cannabis and coincides with the growing perception that cannabis is safe[68] and, therefore, believed to have no adverse effects on fetal or adolescent development. There are several reasons why cannabis use during pregnancy and cannabis use disorder are on the rise, including legalization of medical and recreational cannabis use in approximately 50% of U.S. states,[69] selective breeding for more potent cannabis strains containing higher levels of THC and lower levels of cannabidiol (CBD),[70,71] increased amount of THC delivered in cigar-sized blunts versus joints,[70] and attenuation of pregnancy-induced nausea and vomiting.[72,73] Additionally, substantiated childhood maltreatment[74]; increased cannabis use in disabled adults, the never-married, low income groups, and urbanites[69]; and maternal stressors such as psychopathology, healthcare access, and nutritional, social, and underrepresented group member statuses[66] all contribute to increased use of cannabis. Cannabis is the illicit drug most commonly used by Americans aged 18 to 25 years,[75] and from 2002 to 2017, the incidence of cannabis use during pregnancy grew at an alarming rate.[76–78] Societal permissiveness toward cannabis use highlights the importance of elucidating the long-term consequences (inter/transgenerational epigenetic alterations) of PCE on fetal and adolescent neurodevelopment and neuroplasticity, which may lead to cognitive, behavioral, emotional, and psychological consequences and a predisposition to drug abuse in adulthood and in subsequent offspring. To date, evidence regarding the effects of PCE remains inconsistent or inconclusive due to comparisons between less potent cannabis strains of yesteryear versus today, confounding genetic, environmental, and polysubstance use variables, and limited sample sizes or methodological issues.[79] Conversely, although data connecting cannabis exposure in utero and in adolescence is far from unequivocal, enough evidence has been amassed to make tight associations between fetal and adolescent cannabis exposure and adulthood mental health abnormalities.[80] Much consternation and no unequivocal preponderance of evidence exists demonstrating an association between PCE and transgenerational epigenetic inheritance (i.e., parent-child-grandchild transmittance of information, who were never exposed to cannabis, which affects phenotypic traits without altering the DNA sequence).[81]

Epigenetic perturbations, induced by PCE, during critical fetal and adolescent developmental periods can lead to persistent alterations in gene expression via DNA methylation (DNA Me), remolding, and posttranslational histone modifications of the nucleosome core particle, consisting of approximately 146 base pairs of DNA wrapped around a histone octamer (2 × each core histone: H2A, H2B, H3, and H4).[80,82] Additional small RNAs (<200-nucleotide-long, noncoding,

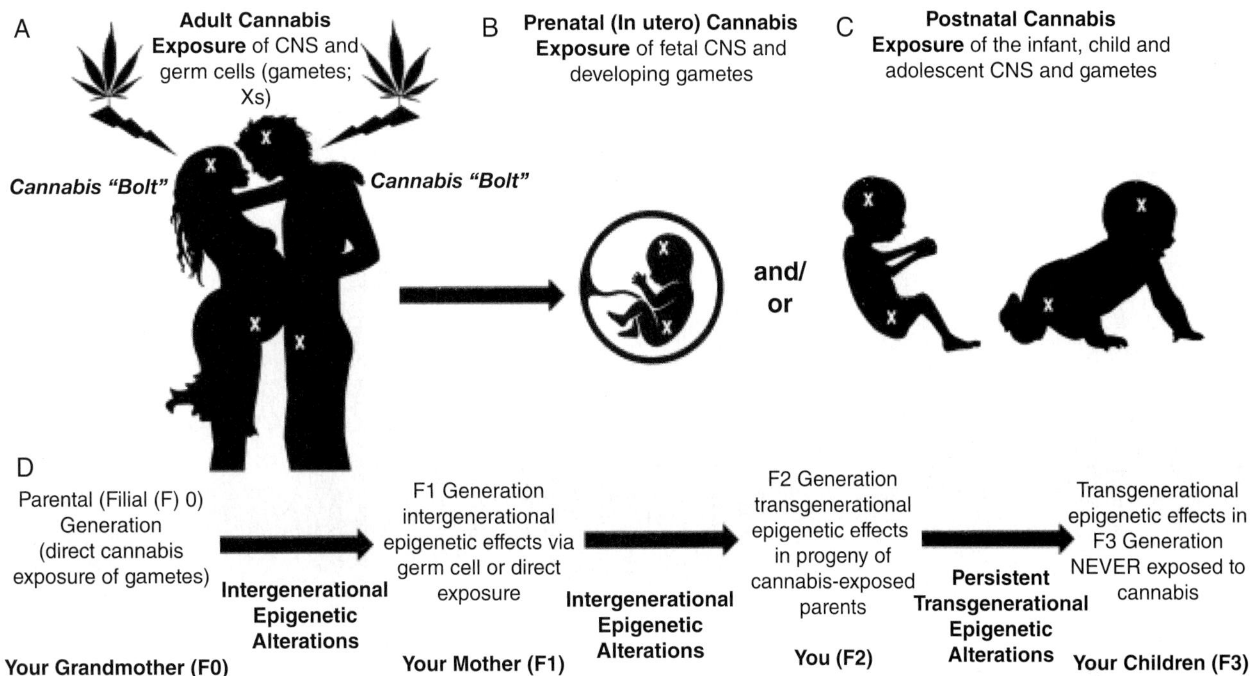

Fig. 55.5 Theoretically, Epigenetic Effects From Adult Cannabis Exposure Could Influence Subsequent Generations Via Intergenerational and Transgenerational Inheritance. (A) Adult cannabis exposure *(Cannabis "Bolt")* could directly affect the central nervous system (CNS) and the germline cells (gametes; egg and sperm) of the parental (F0) generation. The gametes (germ cells) would produce the F1 generation (i.e., intergenerational epigenetic transmission [IT]), because progeny would be directly exposed to cannabis. IT could occur with the direct exposure to cannabis of the F0 and the F1 generations via the developing germ cells or fetus in utero. (B) Prenatal (in utero) cannabis exposure of a F1 generation fetus. The exposure of germline cells of the F1 and F2 generations to cannabis would represent IT. Adult cannabis use could not only expose the developing F1 fetus to cannabis but could expose the F1 fetal germline is exposed as well, ultimately resulting in IT to the F2 generation. (C) Cannabis exposure of a F1 generation during postnatal development. (D) Transgenerational epigenetic transmission (TT) could occur when the effects of parental exposure to cannabis during pregnancy are still present in the F3 generation, the first generation that is not directly exposed to cannabis. Similar to in utero exposure, these F1 and F2 generations would be directly exposed to cannabis, representing IT, with the following F3 generation representing transgenerational transmission (TT). (Modified from Klengel T, Dias BG, Ressler KJ. Models of intergenerational and transgenerational transmission of risk for psychopathology in mice. *Neuropsychopharmacology*. 2016;41:219–231.)

RNA-silencing molecules; microRNA, miRNA) regulate gene expression by changing chromatin structure into transcriptionally permissive euchromatin or inactive heterochromatin.[83] DNA Me at specific gene loci is known to persist during germ cell maturation,[84,85] making these methylation loci potential candidates for inter/transgenerational and, perhaps, multigenerational inheritance of cannabis effects.[80] Nucleosomal modification has been associated with the persistent effects of cannabinoids in the nucleus accumbens and hippocampal neurons and glioma and lymph node cells.[80,86–90] Histone lysine (K) Me has been shown to produce persistent alterations in gene expression.[91] MiRNAs have been deemed important regulators of multigenerational inheritance in *Caenorhabditis elegans*,[80,92] and the epigenome, comprising chemical compounds that covalently bond to DNA without altering the sequence and modulate gene expression, has been shown to persist through cell division and may be inherited multigenerationally, providing the cellular bull's eye for perinatal cannabis exposure, thereby rendering the epigenome a significant candidate for the perpetuation of abnormal neurodevelopment and neuroplasticity. Szutorisz and colleagues state that evidence suggests that the ECSS modulated via CB1R and CB2R mediates cellular functions in different tissues via epigenetic modifications via DNA Me,[80,93] histone methylation,[86] and miRNAs,[94] highlighting the role of the ECSS system in regulating cellular functions via epigenetic alterations, and they suggest that modulation of these mechanisms with cannabis use may have life-long neurobiological and functional impact. D'Addario et al. reviewed epigenetic regulation of the ECSS in detail.[95] Figs. 55.5 and 55.6 show how epigenetic effects from adult cannabis exposure can influence subsequent generations of offspring via intergenerational and transgenerational inheritance.[96] Table 55.3 is a detailed compilation of evidence of epigenetic modifications and fetal malprogramming induced by cannabinoid exposure in utero and in adolescence.

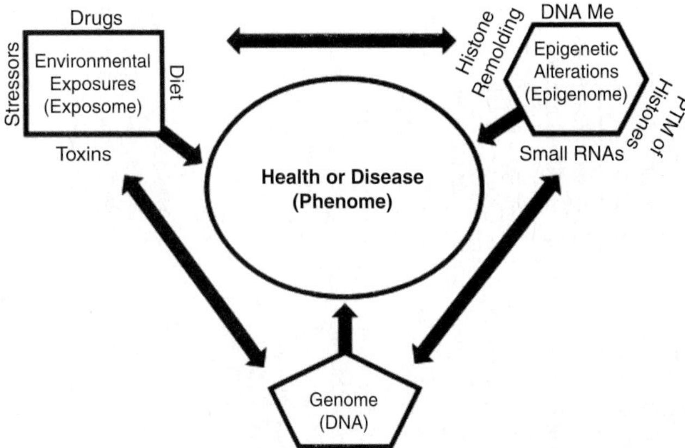

Fig. 55.6 Interactions Between The Big 3: The Genome, Epigenome, and Exposome in Determining Wellness and Health or Illness and Disease (the Phenome). Epigenetic alterations induced by cumulative environmental and lifestyle exposures (e.g., drugs, diet, toxins, and stressors) and leading to alterations in the germline of the exposed individual can be transmitted to the subsequent generations. The multifaceted interaction between environmental exposures and the genome is represented by the exposome, which alters the epigenome (comprising the chemical compounds that covalently bond to DNA), altering the genome without altering the DNA sequence, and modulate gene expression, which alters the phenome, the representation of the sum total of all phenotypic traits. *PTM*, Posttranslational modifications. (Redrawn from PAOLONI-GIACOBINO, A. 2011. Post genomic decade–the epigenome and exposome challenges. *Swiss Med Wkly.* 141, w13321.)[108]

Table 55.3 Compilation of Detailed Evidence of Epigenetic Modifications and Fetal Malprogramming Induced by Cannabinoid Exposure In Utero and in Adolescence[96a,b]

To Briefly Recollect, the Basal Ganglia Include the Striatum (Comprising a Dorsal Part with the Caudate Nucleus and Putamen and a Ventral Part That Includes the Nucleus Accumbens and Olfactory Tubercle), Globus Pallidus, Ventral Pallidum, Substantia Nigra, and Subthalamic Nucleus

Cannabinoid	Mode of Exposure	Epigenetic Modification/ Fetal Malprogramming	Biologic Target	Results Summary	References
Cannabis (abuse or dependence but not used during month before study)	Adulthood exposure	Increased C-phosphate-G (CpG) DNA methylation (DNA Me) at the promotor's transcription start site (TSS)	Human whole peripheral blood (WPB)	DNA methylation of some proinflammatory genes in WPB altered in schizophrenics; hyper- or hypomethylation pattern protects against reality distortion systems	J Lui et al., 2014
Cannabis (use in past 4 weeks); no cannabis (nonusers); cannabis use ≤ 4 × (low-frequency users); cannabis use >4 × (high-frequency users)	Adolescent exposure (adolescents with Met Met Cate-chol-O-methyltrans-ferase [COMT] genotype)	Membrane bound (MB)-COMT promoter CpG DNA Me	Human adolescent WPB	Adolescents with the Met/Met genotype and increased MB-COMT promoter CpG DNA methylation rates had decreased likelihood of being high-frequency cannabis users than adolescents with the Val/Val or Val/Met genotype	LJ van der Knapp et al., 2014
Δ^9-tetrahydrocannabinol (THC) (1.5 mg/kg IP every 3rd day from postnatal day [PND] 28–49)	Adolescent exposure	HSA behavior (fixed ration-1; 3-h sessions) from young (PND 57) to full adulthood (PND 102)	Long-Evans adult male rats (PN-102) nucleus accumbens shell (NAcsh) in the basal ganglia; HSA and opioid neural systems	THC exposure (30 mg/kg/infusion) increased HSA, opiate sensitivity, and striatal expression of proenkephalin in NAc shell; heroin intake increased μ-opioid receptor (mOR) GTP-coupling in the brainstem in the mesolimbic and nigrostriatal regions	M Ellgren et al., 2007
THC (0.15 mg/kg IV) daily from GD5-PND 2	Human fetal brain specimens (18–22 weeks' gestation) and prenatal rat exposure	Demethylated lysine 9 (2MeH3K9) and trimethylated lysine (3meH3K4) on histone H3; promoter, gene body, which increased gene transcription	Adult rat (PN 62) NAc (brain)	THC reduced methylation patterns in the dopamine receptor genes (both D1 and D2); in the Drd2 gene, THC increased 2meH3K9 and decreased 3meH3K4; in the Drd1 gene, there was no change in 2meH3K9 and a reduction in 3meH3K4. THC suppressed the expression of DNA polymerase Pol II; there was no change in the expression of Drd1, but THC reduced the expression of Drd2 and Drd2 D2R binding sites, which increased adulthood sensitivity to opiate reward	JA DiNieri et al., 2011
THC (1.5 mg/kg ip) every 3rd day from PND 28–49	Adolescent exposure	me3H3K4, me2H3K9; promoter, gene body	Adult rat brain NAc brain shell (NAcsh); the targets are the striatopallidal neurons (to recapitulate, the striatopallidal neurons projecting from the striatum to the globus pallidus are mainly confined to the putamen [unlike the striatonigral neurons projecting to substantia nigra that are located in the caudate nucleus])	THC expression suppresses the expression of the proenkephalin gene in striatopallidal neurons, which leads to decreased heroin self-administration (SA); THC-naïve adolescent rats treated with THC exposure showed increased PENK expression via decreased histone H3 lysine 9 methylation (meH3K9) in the NAcsh	HC Tomasiewicz et al., 2012

THC (1.5 mg/kg ip) every 3rd day from PND 28–49	Adolescent exposure	CpG DNA Me downstream of promoter's TSS and in intergenic regions (genomic "dark matter") and gene bodies	Adult rat brain NAc	Differentially methylated regions (DMRs) are associated with neurotransmission and synaptic plasticity; DMR-associated genes in the Dlg4 network (Dlgap2, Kcna5, Begain, Grin2a, and Dlg4) exhibit differential mRNA expression in the NAc of adolescent THC-exposed adult F1 offspring	CT Watson et al., 2015
THC (1.5 mg/kg ip) every 3rd day from PND 28–49	Adolescent parental germline exposure	DNA Me	Adult rat brain NAc	THC exposure increased heroin SA, altered stereotyped and approach-avoidance behaviors, decreased long-term depression (LTD) in adult male F1 offspring, and consequently altered synaptic plasticity	H Szutorisz et al., 2014
THC (20 mg/kg)	Juvenile exposure	H3K4me3, H3K9me3, H3K27me3, H3K36me3; promoter, intergenic regions, gene bodies	Differentiating mouse popliteal lymph node (LN) cells	Increased genome-wide histone modifications in dysregulated genes and noncoding RNAs(SEB): THC reduced the effects of Staphylococcal enterotoxin B on cell proliferation and immune responses in vivo and genome-wide (promoter TSS, intergenic region, and gene bodies) alterations in histone H3 methylation profiles • me3H3K4—most enriched in the promoter regions and increased near the TSS of genes; this reduces the signal density • me3H3K27, which is mostly located in the gene body and intergenic regions • me3K36—mainly found in the gene body • me3H3K9—mainly found in intergenic regions • H3K9ac—increased near the TSS of genes	X Yang et al., 2014
THC (0.3–30 μM in 0.1% ethanol; 48 h)		Histone deacetylase 3 (HDAC3) expression	Human choriocarcinoma cell line (BeWo)	BeWo cell cultures THC (48 h): THC reduced the BeWo cell confluency and number; there was an increase in histone deacetylase 3 (HDAC3) expression THC (15 mM) modulated genes encoding for growth, apoptosis, cell morphology, and ion-exchange pathways	M Khare et., 2006
Chronic THC (0.32 mg/kg IM 2 × daily), 28 days before inoculation with simian immunodeficiency virus (SIV) strain: mac521; 100 × TCID50 (50% Tissue Culture Infective Dose; 0.18 mg/kg, IV)	Adult exposure	DNA Me at CpG islands in tissues considered to be critical checkpoints for HIV/SIV replication and pathogenesis miRNAs (miR-142-3p, -142-5p, and -150) in CD4+ cells	SIV-infected Rhesus macaque cerebellum and peripheral T-cells (brain)	Altered DNA methylation changed mRNA and miRNA expression profiles	PE Molina et al., 2011
THC (25 ng/kg ip) to induce CD11b+ Gr-1+ myeloid-derived suppressor cells (MDSCs) from mouse peritoneal exudates	Adult exposure (8–10 weeks)	mRNA exposure profile of CD11b+ Gr-1+ functional MDSCs	Female C57/BL6 (WT) mouse MDSCs	THC altered mRNA, miRNA, and differentiation profiles in CD11b+ Gr-1+ functional MDSCs; it altered cell growth and proliferation and myeloid differentiation miRNAs with potential functional role in MDSC development and function	VL Hegde et al., 2013
THC (0.05 mL/kg) 4 weeks before SIV infection; 0.18 mg/kg	Chronic exposure	Global miRNA expression profile of duodenal tissue	Age- and weight-matched male SIV-infected Indian rhesus macaque intestines	THC increased the antiinflammatory miRNA expression profile in the gut epithelium, increased miR-99b expression, and decreased NADPH oxidase 4+; selective upregulation of antiinflammatory miRNA expression contributes to THC-mediated suppression of gastrointestinal homeostasis and inflammation	LC Chandra et al., 2015

Continued

Table 55.3 Compilation of Detailed Evidence of Epigenetic Modifications and Fetal Malprogramming Induced by Cannabinoid Exposure In Utero and in Adolescence—Cont'd[96a,b]

To Briefly Recollect, the Basal Ganglia Include the Striatum (Comprising a Dorsal Part with the Caudate Nucleus and Putamen and a Ventral Part That Includes the Nucleus Accumbens and Olfactory Tubercle), Globus Pallidus, Ventral Pallidum, Substantia Nigra, and Subthalamic Nucleus

Cannabinoid	Mode of Exposure	Epigenetic Modification/ Fetal Malprogramming	Biologic Target	Results Summary	References
Exogenous anandamide (AEA; 1 μM)	Adult human skin cell culture (HaCat-spontaneously immortalized keratinocytes)	Genomic DNA Me in differentiating keratinocytes	Human keratinocytes	AEA suppressed keratinocyte differentiation by increasing DNA Me via a CB1R-mediated, p38, and p42/44 MAPK-dependent pathway; this signaling pathway activated NDA methyltransferase activity and increased genomic DNA Me	Paradisi et al., 2008
Exogenous AEA; 40 mg/kg	Female adult C57/BL6 mice	miRNA from draining lymph nodes (LN)	Murine LN cells	Decreased T-helper 17 (Th17)-mediated delayed type hypersensitivity response by increasing IL-10, which in turn increased miRNAs that target proinflammatory pathways	AR Jackson et al., 2014
Synthetic cannabinoid agonists: HU-210 (30 nM) and JWH-133 (1.5 mg/kg) daily to subcutaneous gliomas	Glioma-derived stem-like cells (GSC) derived from glioblastoma multiforme (GBM) biopsies and the human glioma cell lines U87MG and U373MG normal neural stem cell-like neurospheres	H3K4 me3; global levels	GSC-GBM biopsies and glioma cell lines U87MG and U373MG that express cannabinoid type 1 receptors (CB1Rs) and CB2Rs; the transient receptor potential cation channel subfamily V member 1 (TRPV1), also known as the capsaicin receptor, fatty acid amide hydrolase (FAAH), and monoacylglycerol lipase (MAGL)	Cannabinoid agonists targeted the stem cell-like compartment of brain tumors, promoted CBR-induced GSC differentiation, and reduced gliomagenesis in vivo; ex vivo, there was a decrease in neurosphere formation and secondary xenograft cell formation, gliomas derived from CB-treated cancer stem-like cells, and nestin expression	T Aguado et al., 2019
HU-210 (100 μg/kg) daily	Adolescent exposure: combination treatment of prenatal polyribocytidylic acid (poly I:C maternal immune activation [MIA]: GD 15) with adolescent HU-201 (PND 35–49)	Whole-genome miRNA expression of entorhinal cortex (EC)	Adolescent male Wistar rat brain EC	Combined treatment: altered left hemisphere EC-associated differences in miRNA expression that are highly overrepresented in a single imprinted locus on chromosome 6q32, which is syntenic to the 14q32 locus in humans; these loci encode miRNA that are differentially expressed in schizophrenic peripheral blood lymphocytes	SL Hollins et al., 2014
WIN55212.2 (WIN) CB1R/ CB2R agonist (0.5, 1, or 3 mg/kg), 3 weeks	Adolescent exposure: C57/BL6/J male mice (5 weeks) and adult mice (13 weeks of age) underwent behavioral testing	DNA methylation	Adult mouse hippocampus	Cognitive impairment (as seen in Morris Water Maze and Fear Conditioning Tests) and persistently increased hippocampal CA region AEA levels; increased DNA methylation at the Rgs7 locus and decreased Rgs7 mRNA level regulation (epigenetic and transcriptional alteration)	J Tomas-Roig et al., 2016
THC Acute in vivo exposure: Dams given 20 or 50 mg/kg on GD16 Subchronic in vivo exposure: Dams given 25 mg/kg on GD 16 and 10 mg/kg daily until delivery (total of 55 mg/kg)	Acute perinatal exposure	—	Pooled fetal or pup thymi (GD17, GD18, and PD1); examined cell lines and organ cultures; evaluated immunity to HIV-1; also examined for T-cell infiltration	Acute perinatal THC exposure caused cannabinoid receptor apoptosis and alterations in fetal thymus T-cell subsets, which persisted for several days after exposure Acute perinatal THC exposure reduced immunity to HIV-1 p17/p24/gp120 Subchronic perinatal THC exposure led to thymic and splenic atrophy in 1-week-old pups; there was a reduction in the total number of T-cells but no change in T-cell subsets	CL Lombardi et al, 2011

Marijuana ± nicotine, alcohol, opiates, and/or selective serotonin reuptake inhibitors	Human prenatal marijuana exposure: human infants 2–6 weeks	Whole-brain functional connectivity maps	Human hippocampus, insula, amygdala, caudate, putamen, and thalamus seed regions (center voxel + face-connected neighboring voxels) due to increased CBIR expression levels in adult and neonatal brain	MJ+ infants showed decreased functional connectivity between bilateral caudate-cerebellar/vermis, left anterior insula-cerebellum, and right caudate-occipital fusiform; these changes may contribute to deficits in motor and visual visual-spatial activity, integration and coordination, attention, and social-emotional stability in children and adolescents in PME The inhibitory control network was attenuated in the striatum, the cerebellum, and the frontal regions; these changes may disrupt networks in which the insula may serve as a central hub for processing and integrating external information with visceral, cognitive, and affective states to determine salience and guide drug-seeking behavior	K Grewen et al., 2015
WIN (0.5 mg/kg SC) daily or THC mg/kg	Prenatal exposure	—	—	Adult male PCE rats: decreased sniffing and playing social interaction behaviors with unchanged locomotion, anxiety, and cognition; systemic administration of CDPPB (3-cyano-N-[1,3-diphenyl-1H-pyrazol-5-yl] benzamide), a positive allosteric modulator of the metabotropic glutamate receptor subtype 5 (mGluR5), may restore LTD and normalize social interaction via cannabinoid 1 receptor (CB1R) and TRPV1 activation; in vivo, the administration of URB597 (FAAH inhibitor) normalized social deficits; blocking AEA degradation may also normalize social deficits via CB1R eCB-mediated LTD in the medial prefrontal cortex (mPFC) was absent; URB597-treated mPFC slices showed restored eCB-LTD; SR141716, which is a CB1R antagonist, blocked the URB597 rescue; there was increased excitability of deep layers in the mPFC pyramidal cells; there was a mild increase in mGlu1 and mGlu5 mRNA levels; CDPPB restored the ability of excitatory mPFC synapses to express LTD, and preincubation with either SR141716AQ or capsazepine prevented the rescue of synaptic plasticity Adult female PCE rats showed decreased TRPV1, mGlu5, and DAGLa mRNA levels; TRPV1R antagonist suppressed the induction of eCB-LTD	A Barra et al., 2018
THC (5 mg/kg ip) or WIN (0.75 mg/kg ip) from embryonic day E10.5–18.5	Prenatal exposure	Cell morphology and behavioral analysis	Mouse hippocampal neurons	Adult prenatally THC- or WIN-exposed mice showed fewer cholecystokinin-containing interneurons in the CA1 hippocampus; the cellular changes in the hippocampus may begin early during fetal life with decreased dendritic complexity and loss of perisomatic synaptic boutons; depolarization-induced feedback inhibition loops also seemed to have been affected	GA Vergish et al, 2017

AEA, anandamine (N-arachidonoylethanolamine; *GD*, gestational day; *GTP*, guanosine-5'-triphosphate; *HSA*, heroin self-administration; *IL-10*, interleukin 10; *IM*, intramuscular; *IP*, intraperitoneal; *IV*, intravenous; *PCE*, prenatal cannabis exposure; *PME*, prenatal marijuana exposure; *SC*, subcutaneous; *SEB*, staphylococcal enterotoxin B

During the developmentally sensitive perinatal period, complex, symphonic, ontogenetic regulatory movements between genomic DNA sequences, transcription factors, and epigenetic modifiers, all of which determine gene expression, are orchestrated with far-reaching consequences that can be negatively impacted by cannabis exposure. This magnificent symphony of movements is harmonized throughout an individual's development and lifespan and within cellular compartments during differentiation of various cells, tissues, and organs.[80] Brown contends that although attention has focused on pregnancy (in utero exposure) as a vulnerable period during which to sustain neurodevelopment insults, it is likely that cannabis use in adolescence alters critical developmental events, causing waves of dysregulation from the molecular level up through neural networks, which lead to widespread disruption of neurophysiology and increased susceptibility to psychotic episodes.[97]

It is apparent that epigenetic alterations are tantamount to a causal link between genomic DNA (nature) and environment factors (nurture). Epigenetic mechanisms have been shown to underlie drug-induced neuroplasticity by orchestrating gene expression throughout the brain. The epigenome provides a direct mechanism for PCE to influence the genetic symphony involved in the development and heritability of addiction in subsequent generations.[98] Szutorisz et al. demonstrated that exposure of male and female adolescent rats before mating (i.e., germline exposure) leads to molecular malprogramming and behavioral aberrations in subsequent unexposed offspring.[99] These studies revealed that THC-naïve adult offspring exerted increased determination to self-administer heroin, demonstrating that adolescent cannabis exposure induced preconception epigenetic alterations in the parental germline, and these molecular marks (i.e., the epigenome) were transferred to the gametes, thereby influencing future offspring (i.e., inter/transgenerational gateway hypothesis).

Finally, to amass an unequivocal preponderance of evidence demonstrating a causal relationship between PCE and transgenerational epigenetic inheritance, legions of researchers from the fields of biochemistry, bioinformatics, biology, biomedical technology, environmental epidemiology, exposure science, genetics, psychology, public heath, etc. must focus on the broader definition of the exposome (i.e., *"the cumulative measure of environmental influences and associated biologic responses throughout the lifespan, including exposures from the environment, diet, behavior, and endogenous processes"*) and work collaboratively to expand the Human Exposome Project. Longitudinal multigenerational cohort studies need to be conducted that link scans of the exposome and phenome (the sum total of an organism's phenotypic traits) of ancestral and parental generations to grandchildren, delineate global loss of DNA methylation in the aged, and use extensive epigenome analysis and metastable epialleles (i.e., variably expressed alleles in monozygotic twins).[100] Although a causal relationship between PCE and transgenerational epigenetic inheritance remains to be firmly established, the fact that any evidence exists that cannabis use during pregnancy may be detrimental to fetal and adolescent development and that these maladaptations may be passed on to subsequent generations should be reason enough for why pregnant women should err on the side of caution and take a pregnant pause from pot.

Selective Serotonin Reuptake Inhibitors

Selective serotonin reuptake inhibitors (SSRIs) are a class of antidepressant medications including sertraline, citalopram, escitalopram, fluoxetine, and fluvoxamine. To assess for congenital malformation, 23 studies were reviewed and included 9,085,854 births.[101] There was an increased risk of overall major congenital anomalies and congenital heart defects, with similar associations between women using citalopram, fluoxetine, and paroxetine.[101] Sertraline was associated with cardiac septal defects and respiratory system defects.[101] Interestingly, a review of 11 studies found exposure to SSRIs during pregnancy was associated with an increased risk for persistent pulmonary hypertension of the newborn.[102] Of the drugs reviewed, sertraline had the lowest risk for persistent pulmonary hypertension of the newborn, which suggested to the authors a better safety profile for use in pregnancy.[102]

Infants with SSRI exposure in utero may experience withdrawal symptoms within a few hours or days after birth. The symptoms include irritability, jitteriness, shivering, fever, hypertonia, tachypnea, feeding difficulty, hypoglycemia, and seizures.[103] Treatment guidelines are lacking at many institutions, with only 4 of 112 units in the United Kingdom having a specific protocol to guide management of SSRI-exposed infants.[104]

Long-term outcomes following SSRI exposure in utero continues to be investigated. A population-based case-cohort study of 117,475 infants found that SSRI-exposed children had significantly delayed school entry compared with unexposed children; however, there was no difference in the need for special education support.[105] Other reviews have found no differences in neurodevelopmental outcomes at follow-up.[106] Therefore, use of SSRIs during pregnancy should be considered because treatment discontinuation may have risks to the mother that outweigh the risks of exposure.

Conclusions

Multiple substances continue to be used by adults, with pregnant women being no exception. Among women of reproductive age in the United States, polysubstance use is highly prevalent, with 89% of all women using nonmedical opioids reporting polysubstance use.[107] Each substance has a unique withdrawal profile as discussed here, although many will result in infants requiring admission to the newborn intensive care unit. Although pharmacologic therapies exist for certain withdrawals, others require supportive care treatment both short- and long-term. Additionally, multiple areas continue to require ongoing research to determine the impact on infants so that the highest-quality care can be provided to ensure the best possible outcome for this highly vulnerable population.

SECTION 10

Immunology

OUTLINE

CHAPTER 56 Neonatal Immunity

Akhil Maheshwari, Sundos Khuder, Shelley M. Lawrence, Robert D. Christensen

KEY POINTS

1. The fetal-neonatal immune system becomes activated at birth to play a role in host defense and eliminate environmental pathogens but also to tolerate self-antigens, nutrients, and commensals.
2. The innate immune system is comprised of neutrophils, the monocyte-macrophage lineage, natural killer cells, and the noncytotoxic innate lymphoid cells.
3. Neutrophils are the most numerus subgroup of leukocytes, but unlike in the adult, these cells are developmentally deficient in many host defense functions such as migration, phagocytosis, and microbial killing.
4. Increasing heterogeneity is being recognized in the macrophage system.
5. Cord blood contains a higher number and proportion of plasmacytoid dendritic cells than adult peripheral blood, but there are important functional differences.
6. The adaptive immune system also displays innate-like properties to compensate for limitations in antigen-specific acquired immune responses. T cells show important limitations in the repertoire of the antigenic specificity but show rapid maturation after birth. The immunoglobulin repertoire is relatively restricted in the fetus and neonate.
7. The B-1 lymphocytes show broad poly-specificities and may have a role in innate, not adaptive, immunity.
8. Fetal and neonatal natural killer (NK) cells have a significantly lower cytolytic activity than in adults. These cells should not be confused with the natural killer T cells, a heterogeneous group of T cells that express an alpha beta T-cell receptor besides some of the NK cell markers.
9. Noncytotoxic innate lymphoid cells are morphologically similar to other lymphocytes, but unlike adaptive T and B cells, they do not show antigen specificity. These cells function more as innate immune cells.

In the developing immune system, birth is an important functional watershed. The fetus is continuously exposed to maternal antigens in utero and its immune responses must remain suppressed for survival. In the neonatal period, the immune system is exposed to a diverse set of environmental antigens and needs a dichotomous set of responses to "contain" certain microorganisms on various cutaneous and mucosal surfaces, and at the same time, develop tolerance to other commensals and dietary macromolecules. Some components of the immune system are reasonably mature at birth, but other arms are yet to gain full functional reactivity. The deficient responses could be viewed as a developmentally regulated state of immunodeficiency. This chapter highlights the quantitative and qualitative differences in major leukocyte subsets (Fig. 56.1) during the neonatal period.

Leukocyte Populations in the Fetus and the Neonate

During development, most leukocyte lineages can be traced back diverging from hematopoietic stem cells during the embryonic and fetal period (Fig. 56.2). Downstream, during the neonatal period and beyond, the leukocyte subsets show increasing heterogeneity with multiple, specialized subsets (Fig. 56.3). We have recognized many of these subsets of T cells for some time, including the T-helper cells, regulatory T cells, cytotoxic T cells, and γδ T cells.[1–6] The two B-cell lineages, B-1 and B-2, which may be involved in innate and adaptive immune responses, respectively, have also been known.[7] We, and others, have investigated the role(s) of various macrophage subclasses.[8–10] The antigen-specific heterogeneity of lymphocytes has also been studied.[11] Emerging information on the functional proficiency of innate lymphoid cells (ILCs) during the neonatal period, when adaptive immunity is still immature, is exciting. There is evidence that some of these subsets, such as the group 3 ILCs (ILC3), can be modulated by the microbiome and inflammation.[12] Most recently, some heterogeneity has been noted in neutrophils in patients with malignancies; there may be two distinct neutrophil lineages, N-1 and N-2, that play different roles in immune regulation.[13] This polarization could very well extend to the normal immune system. These details are discussed later in the chapter.

Innate Immune System

This section outlines the development and functional maturation of various cellular lineages in the innate immune system (as mentioned above; see Fig. 56.3) (Box 56.1).

Neutrophils

During development, hematopoiesis begins in the extraembryonic yolk sac in about the third week of embryogenesis. The two major hematopoietic progenitors committed to the neutrophil lineage are the colony-forming units-mix, which give rise to a mixture of various leukocyte populations, and the CFU-GEMM, which produce granulocytes, erythrocytes, megakaryocytes, and macrophages.[14–16] Early hematopoiesis gets activated at about 7 to 8 weeks' gestation with hematopoietic stem cells derived from the intraembryonic endothelial cells in the descending aorta. These hematopoietic stem cells subsequently seed the liver and the bone marrow later in gestation.

The neutrophil lineage can be viewed in a proliferating pool of early precursors, the neutrophil proliferating pool (NPP) that may have a capacity for 4 to 5 cell divisions, and a postmitotic neutrophil storage pool (NSP) that continues to differentiate (Fig. 56.4A). In adults, the NPP contains about 2×10^9 cells/kg body weight and the NSP contains about 6×10^9 cells/kg body weight.[17] The NPP and NSP comprise nearly 90% of all neutrophils in the body; the other

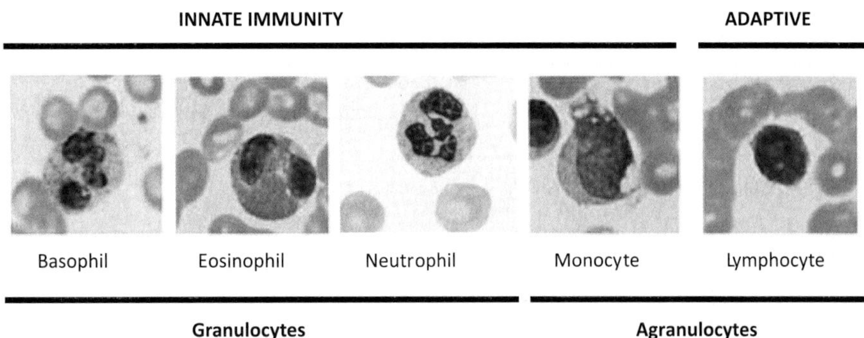

Fig. 56.1 Leukocytes in Innate and Adaptive Immune Systems. (Figure uses images reproduced after permission and minor modifications from Ananthi and Balasubramaniam. A new thresholding technique based on fuzzy set as an application to leukocyte nucleus segmentation. In: *Computer Methods and Programs in Biomedicine*. 2016;134:165–177. The image of the neutrophil is from Maheshwari's laboratory.)

10% of neutrophils (Fig. 56.4B) are either flowing in the circulation or are marginated (loosely attached to the microvascular endothelium). During late gestation and at birth, the blood contains 10- to 50-fold higher concentrations of CFU-GM than in adults,[18] but the overall size of the pool of neutrophil progenitors is much smaller than in adults and gets easily exhausted during stress, such as during sepsis.[19,20] The NPP is only about one-tenth the size (per kilogram of body weight) seen in adults.[21,22]

During acute inflammation, neutrophils are released first from the NSP, and once these limited stores are exhausted, progressively immature cells are mobilized (the "left" shift of sepsis). After circulating for 6 to 8 hours, neutrophils move into the tissues and can then stay there for up to a few days. In the fetus, as in the adult, the NSP is contained in the marrow, with some portion within the liver and spleen.

Function

Transendothelial Migration

Circulating neutrophils leave the intravascular compartment to enter the tissues in three major steps: *margination and rolling* on vascular endothelium, *attachment* to the endothelial cells, and *transendothelial* migration (Fig. 56.5).[23–25] In the inflamed tissues, neutrophils are recruited through regional differences in vascular flow and along

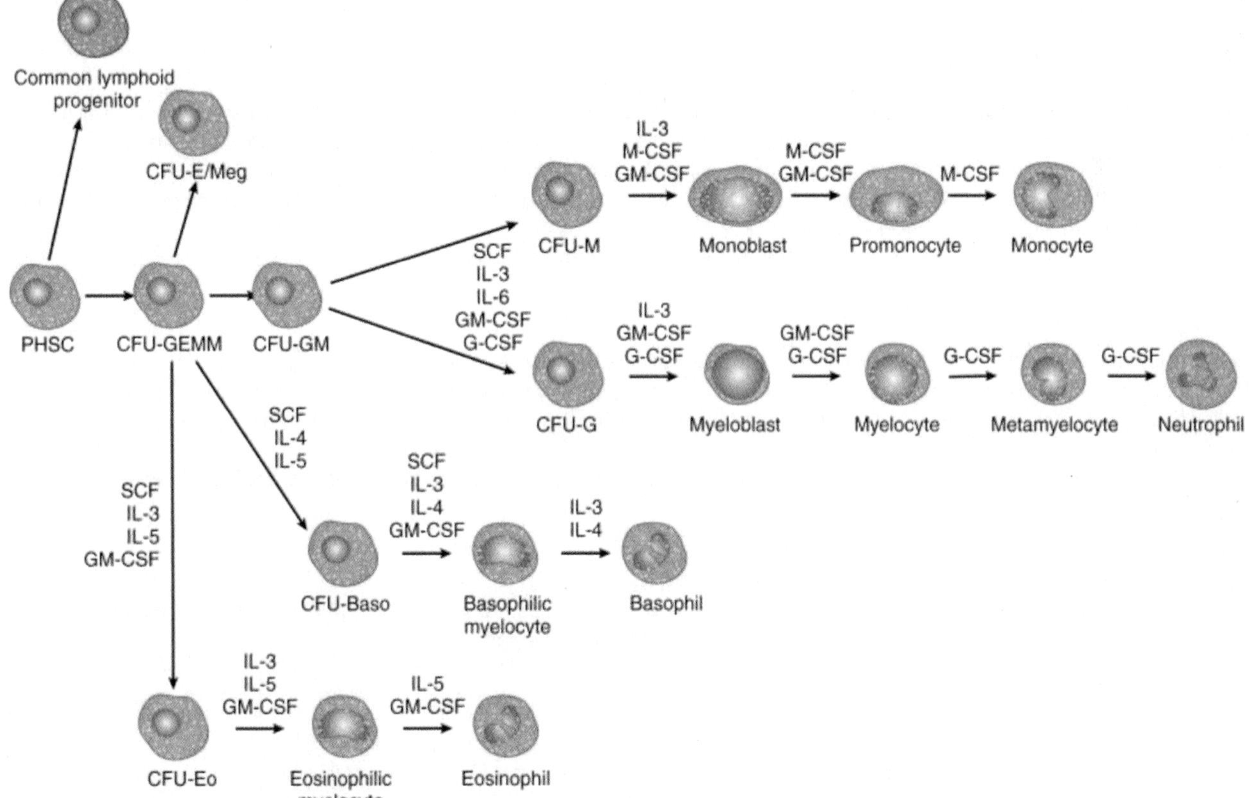

Fig. 56.2 Differentiation of Granulocytic Subsets. *CFU-Baso,* Colony-forming unit-basophil; *CFU-E/Meg,* colony-forming unit-erythrocyte/megakaryocyte; *CFU-Eo,* colony-forming unit-eosinophil; *CFU-G,* colony-forming unit-granulocyte; *CFU-GEMM,* colony-forming unit-granulocyte/erythrocyte/macrophage/megakaryocyte; *CFU-GM,* colony-forming unit-granulocyte/macrophage; *CFU-M,* colony-forming unit-macrophage; *G-CSF,* granulocyte colony-stimulating factor; *GM-CSF,* granulocyte–macrophage colony-stimulating factor; *IL,* interleukin; *M-CSF,* monocyte colony-stimulating factor; *PHSC,* pluripotent hematopoietic stem cell; *SCF,* stem cell factor. (From Khanna-Gupta and Berliner. Granulocytopoiesis and monocytopoiesis. In: *Hematology: Basic Principles and Practice*. Ch. 27, 321–333.e1.)

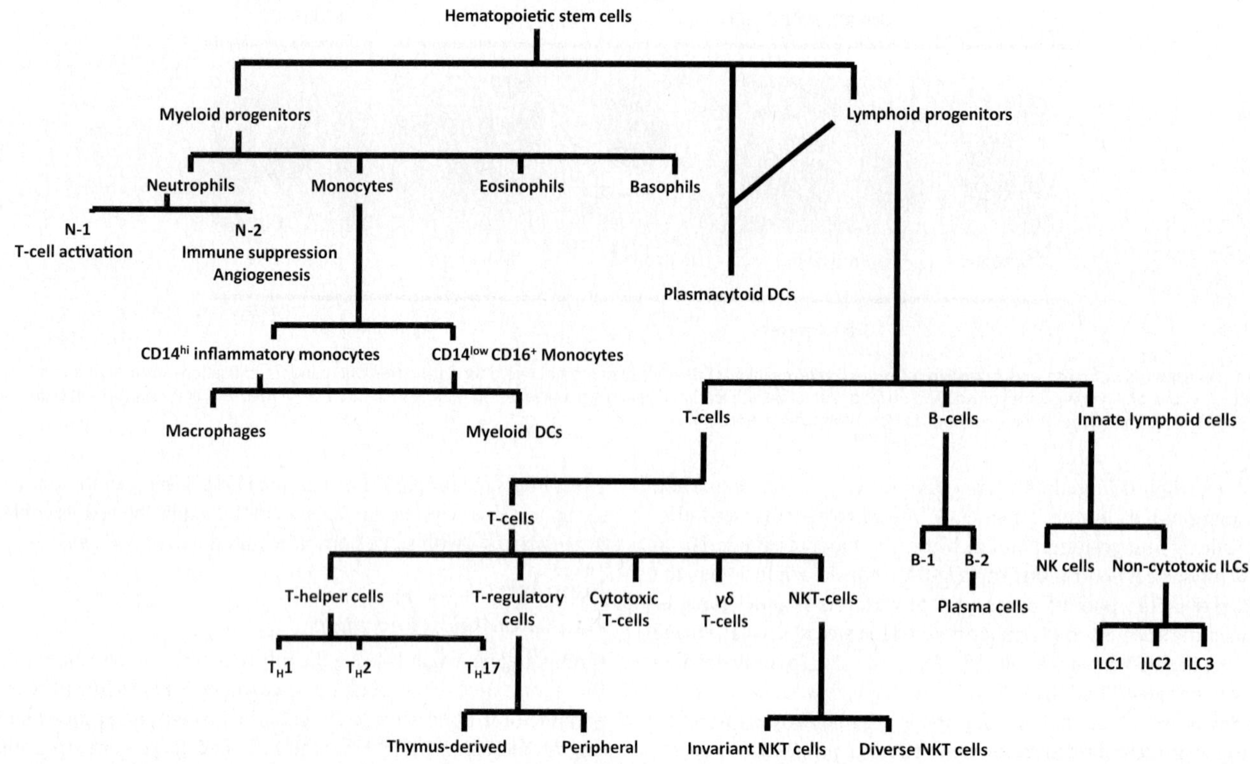

Fig. 56.3 Heterogeneity in Various Leukocyte Subsets. *DCs*, Dendritic cells; *ILCs*, innate lymphoid cells; *NK*, natural killer; *NKT*, natural killer T cell.

■ Box 56.1 Major Subsets of Leukocytes

Neutrophils

- Neutrophil function includes emigration from the bloodstream, phagocytosis, and microbial killing
- Neutrophils from both term and preterm neonates adhere poorly to endothelium; neonatal neutrophils have less selectin and β_2-integrin (Mac-1/CD11b) expression; transendothelial migration, which is dependent on cell deformability, is comparable to adults
- Neonatal neutrophils show impaired chemotaxis; term neutrophils show normal chemotaxis at 2 weeks; late preterm infants achieve normal function at term PCA; neutrophils from very low birth weight (VLBW) neonates begin to mature at 2–3 weeks after birth and progress very slowly
- Neutrophils from preterm neonates phagocytose slowly and ingest fewer bacteria; corrects by term PCA
- Preterm neutrophils display poor respiratory burst and impaired killing of *Staphylococcus aureus* or *Escherichia coli*; improves by 2 months postnatal; term neonates are normal in this regard

Monocytes

- Preterm monocytes show slightly impaired chemotaxis; however, activated monocytes show normal trafficking and adhesion molecule expression
- Preterm monocytes can kill pathogens (*Staphylococcus aureus*, *S. epidermidis*, *E. coli*, and *Candida albicans*) comparable to adult monocytes
- During sepsis, neonatal monocytes express TLRs and cytokines at levels similar to adults; monocytes from VLBW neonates may be slightly more impaired than in term infants
- Skewed pattern of cytokine expression with low levels of Th1-polarizing cytokines such as interleukin (IL)12p70 and interferon-α, and more of the antiinflammatory cytokine IL-10

Dendritic Cells (DCs)

- Cord blood contains fewer DCs (0.5%) than adult blood (1%)
- Neonatal myeloid DCs are immature (lower CD83, CD86 expression) and produce less IL-12 and IFN-γ but more IL-10 than adult DCs
- Neonatal DCs also perform poorly as accessory cells for T-cell mitogenic responses

T Cells

- Most T cells carry a T-cell receptor (TCR) composed of α and β chains, but in about 5% of all T cells, the TCR is composed of γ and δ chains
- Each TCR protein chain contains an immunoglobulin-like extracellular region with a variable (V) domain at its N-terminal and a constant (C) domain at the C-terminal end; TCR diversity results from recombination of variable (V), diversity (D), and joining (J) gene segments in individual T cells
- Term infants have more T cells in peripheral blood than adults; neonates have CD4/CD8 ratios of 5:1, which decline to adult values (2:1) by 4 years of age
- Preterm infants have lower $CD4^+$ and $CD8^+$ counts than term infants
- 80% T cells in cord blood have a naïve CD45RA phenotype, compared with <50% of circulating T cells in adults; memory CD45RO T cells reach adult levels in adolescence

■ Box 56.1 Major Subsets of Leukocytes—Cont'd

T-Helper Cells

- Naïve CD4+ cells differentiate into three effector T-helper (Th) subsets: Th1, Th2, and Th17
- Th1 cells defend against intracellular pathogens and virus-infected cells and produce IL-2, IFN-γ, TNF, IL-13, and GM-CSF
- Neonates have low Th1 function, produce less IL-12 and IFN-γ, and express less CD154 (CD40 ligand) than adults
- Th2 cells participate in allergic reactions; they produce IL-4, IL-5, IL-9, IL-10, IL-12, and IL-13
- Th17 cells protect against infections and activate neutrophils and macrophages; they produce IL-17A, IL17-F, IL-21, IL-22, and IL-26; cord blood T cells show limited capacity to produce IL-17

Regulatory T Cells

- Derived from naïve $CD4^+$ cells; suppress immune responses by expressing IL-10, TGF-β, cytotoxic molecules, and modulators of cAMP
- Two populations: thymus-derived (tT-regs) and peripherally derived T-regs (pT-regs)
- In the fetus/preterm infant, T-regs are tolerogenic and promote self-tolerance
- During midgestation, $CD4^+CD25^+$ Fox $P3^+$ T-regs constitute 20% of all $CD4^+$ cells in lymphoid tissues; represent <5% of $CD4^+$ cells in cord blood from term infants and in the adult blood
- Preterm and term T-regs are less functional than adults; they limit contact between DCs and effector T cells, causing decreased DC immunogenicity and impaired T-cell activation

Cytotoxic T Cells (CTLs)

- $CD8^+$ T cells can differentiate into cytotoxic T lymphocytes; they protect against intracellular pathogens—cause cytotoxicity by releasing pore-forming mediators (perforin/granzyme) or by activating fas-mediated apoptosis
- Neonatal CTLs are less efficient than in adults; circulating αFP and prostaglandins may inhibit CTL activity in neonates
- γδ T Cells
- γδ T cells respond to nonpeptide microbial metabolites, show cytotoxicity, and produce interferon-γ and TNF. γδ IELs protect epithelial tissues from injury
- Constitute 10% of circulating T cells during midgestation, but the number declines to about 3% at term in skin and mucosa
- In the intestine, 30% of IELs, 10% of mucosal lymphoid tissue lymphocytes, and 5% of LPLs have the γδ TCR

Natural Killer T Cells (NKTs)

- NKT cells express TCR-αβ chains and NK cell markers; classified into two main subsets, that is, type I or invariant NKT cells and type II or diverse NKT cells
- Invariant NKT cells have limited TCR diversity and recognize lipid antigens such as α-galactosylceramides in the context of the major histocompatibility complex (MHC)-like molecule CD1d; this works similar to PRRs, but for microbial lipids; I-NKT cells secrete anti- and proinflammatory cytokines and activate adaptive immune responses
- Diverse NKT cells express a variety of TCRs and may recognize lipid antigens with cross-reactivity between mammalian and microbial phospholipids, possibly representing the adaptive immune arm for lipid antigens

B Cells

- Preterm and term neonates have more circulating B cells than adults; B-cell counts peak at 3 months and then decline to adult levels by 6 years of age
- More than 90% of B cells in the fetus/neonate express CD5 and are called B-1 cells; the proportion drops to 75%–80% during infancy and to the 25% adult levels by late adolescence; they express activation markers (CD25) and a $CD11b^+$ $sIgM^{high}$ $sIgD^{low}$ phenotype
- Localize in the spleen and peritoneum; broad polyspecific specificities; the restricted immunoglobulin repertoire suggests a role in innate, rather than in adaptive, immunity
- Respond to T-cell-independent, carbohydrate antigens (unlike follicular B-2 cells that respond to protein antigens)
- Preterm infants produce antibodies but may not respond to all antigens in a vaccine; may remain limited to immunoglobulin M (IgM) with delayed isotype switch and may produce antibodies of low affinity
- Postnatal age is a better predictor of antibody response than gestation; both preterm and term infants respond weakly to diphtheria toxoid in the first week and better at 1–2 months of age; premature infants respond poorly to the hepatitis B vaccine in early infancy but are comparable to term infants in later infancy

Immunoglobulin Production

- Most immunoglobulins in cord blood are derived from maternal IgG (particularly IgG1 and IgG3)
- Preterm infants have lower IgG levels; term infants have serum IgG levels (1000 mg%) similar to or higher than those in maternal serum
- Immunoglobulin levels drop to 300–500 mg% at 3–5 months, when the infant starts producing more; this nadir is reached earlier and is lower in preterm infants

Innate Lymphoid Cells (ILCs)

- Noncytotoxic ILCs are derived from the common lymphoid progenitor but do not exhibit antigen specificity
- ILC1s express Th1-associated cytokines such as IFN-γ and TNF to protect against intracellular bacteria and parasites
- ILC2s express Th2 cytokines (including IL-4, IL-5, IL-9, and IL-13); detectable in cord blood and are implicated in intestinal inflammation in gastroschisis

Continued

■ Box 56.1 Major Subsets of Leukocytes—Cont'd

- ILC3s express Th17 cytokines IL-17A, IL-17F, IL-22, GM-CSF, and TNF, to promote antibacterial immunity and inflammation; abundant in gut mucosa and may be involved in enhancing IgA production and in shaping the local microbiome

Diagnosis of Primary Immunodeficiency in Neonates

- Neutrophil defects, T-cell defects, severe combined immunodeficiency, and bone marrow failure syndromes can present in the neonatal period
- T-cell defects may include DiGeorge syndrome, hyper-IgM syndrome, and ZAP-70 tyrosine kinase defects
- SCID includes purine nucleoside phosphorylase deficiency (viral infections, severe varicella, GVHD), cartilage hair hypoplasia, IL2Rα defects, X-SCID (Jak3), and AR SCID (ADA, RAG1/2, IL7Ra)
- B-cell defects present only after maternally derived antibody levels drop during infancy
- Transient hypogammaglobulinemia of infancy may be considered after 6 months; low basal but normal stimulated Ig responses

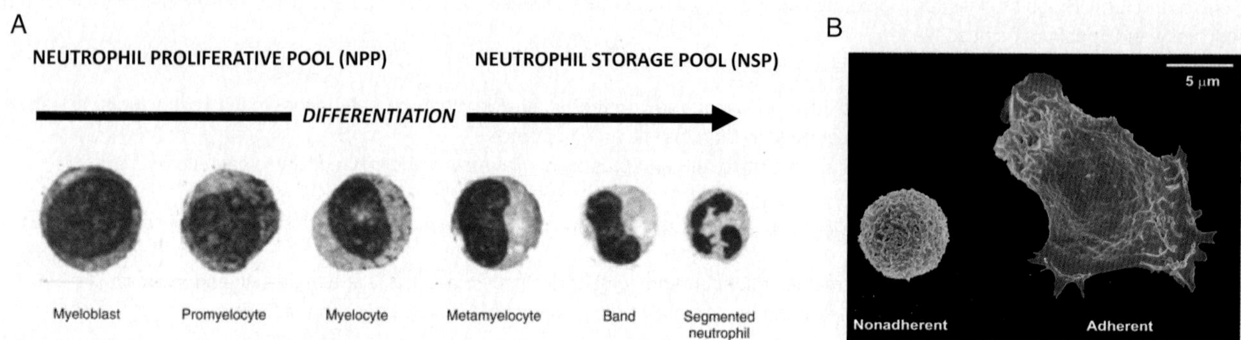

Fig. 56.4 (A) Neutrophil maturation stages. (B) Scanning electron micrographs of nonadherent and adherent neutrophils. (A, Reproduced after permission and minor modifications from Khanna-Gupta and Berliner. Granulocytopoiesis and monocytopoiesis. In: *Hematology: Basic Principles and Practice*. Ch. 27, 321–333.e1. B, Reproduced after permission and minor modifications from DeLeo and Nauseef. Scanning electron micrographs of nonadherent and adherent neutrophils. Granulocytic phagocytes. In: *Mandell, Douglas, and Bennett's Principles and Practice of Infectious Diseases*. 2020.)

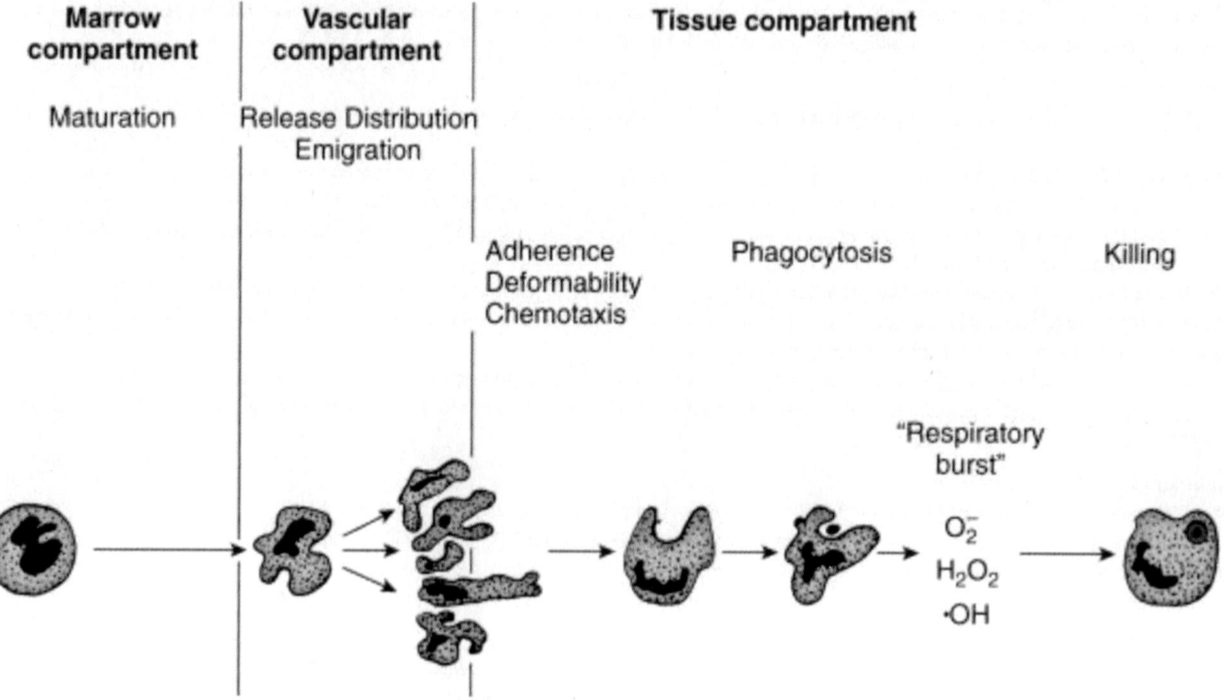

Fig. 56.5 Overview of Neutrophil Functions. Neutrophils are produced and mature in the bone marrow over a 2-week period. On release from the marrow, neutrophils circulate for 6 to 8 hours before emigrating into tissues. At sites of infection, chemotactic factors enhance neutrophil adhesion to and emigration through the vascular endothelium, and neutrophils migrate in a directed fashion (chemotaxis) toward the pathogens. Phagocytosis of the offending organisms stimulates an increase in production of oxygen metabolites (respiratory burst), which facilitates neutrophil killing of the ingested microbes. (Reproduced after permission and minor modifications from Benjamin and Maheshwari. Developmental immunology. In: *Fanaroff and Martin's Neonatal-Perinatal Medicine*. 47, 752–788.)

concentration gradients of chemokines (Fig. 56.6, some members in Table 56.1), chemotactic tripeptides such as *N*-formylmethionyl-leucyl-phenylalanine (*N*-fMLP), complement fragments (C5a), and leukotrienes (LTB_4). Among chemokines, the CXC subfamily with a glutamate-leucine-arginine tripeptide sequence (such as interleukin-8 [IL-8/CXCL8]) are most important.[25,26] *N*-fMLP is an endogenous, chemotactic peptide derived from mitochondria in dying cells that attracts and activates neutrophils and macrophages. It mimics *N*-formyl oligopeptides released by bacteria and attracts and activates circulating blood leukocytes by binding to specific G-protein–coupled receptors on these cells.

In inflamed tissues, alterations in the endothelial surface, with increased leukocyte-binding receptors, and increased gradients of the CXC motif-bearing chemokines (see Fig. 56.5 and Table 56.1) promote neutrophil emargination. This process is mediated through a process of repetitive binding and release of selectins (L-selectin on neutrophils, E- and P-selectin on endothelium; Fig. 56.7).[27] Rolling neutrophils slow down and attach to endothelium through the binding of β_2-integrins to cognate receptors on endothelial cells.[28] The β_2-integrins expressed on neutrophils include the leukocyte function-associated antigen 1 (LFA-1) ($\alpha_L\beta_2$, CD11a/CD18), CR3

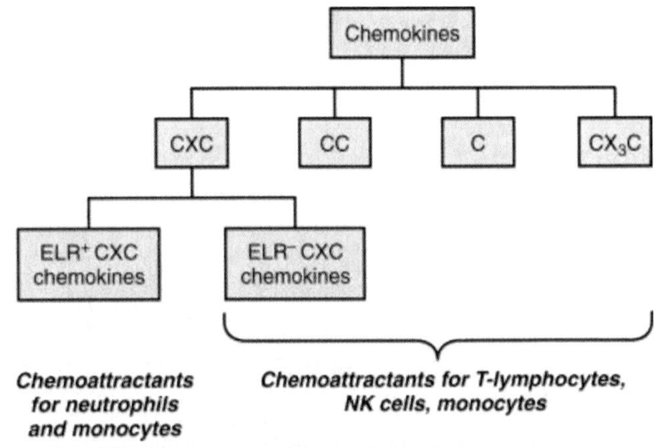

Fig. 56.6 Chemokines Are Classified According to the Position of Conserved Cysteine Residues Near the *N*-Terminus. In CXC chemokines, two conserved cysteine (C) residues are separated by a variable amino acid (X). CC and C-chemokines have conserved cysteines, whereas the CX3C chemokine, fractalkine, has two cysteines separated by three variable amino acids. (Reproduced after permission and minor modifications from Benjamin and Maheshwari. Developmental immunology. In: *Fanaroff and Martin's Neonatal-Perinatal Medicine*. 47, 752–788.)

Table 56.1 Human CXC and CC Chemokines and Relative Receptors

Chemokines	Leukocytes Recruited	Systematic Name	Chemokine Receptors
Growth-related oncoprotein (GRO)-α	Neutrophils and monocytes	CXC-motif ligand (CXCL) 1	CXC receptor (CXCR) 2
GRO-β	Neutrophils and monocytes	CXCL2	CXCR2
GRO-γ	Neutrophils and monocytes	CXCL3	CXCR2
Epithelial neutrophil chemoattractant (ENA-78)	Neutrophils and monocytes	CXCL5	CXCR2
Granulocyte chemoattractant protein (GCP)-2	Neutrophils and monocytes	CXCL6	CXCR2, CXCR1
Neutrophil-activating peptide (NAP)-2	Neutrophils and monocytes	CXCL7	CXCR2
IL-8	Neutrophils and monocytes	CXCL8	CXCR2, CXCR1
Monokine induced by gamma interferon (MIG)	Monocytes and lymphocytes	CXCL9	CXCR3
Interferon-gamma-inducible protein 10 (IP-10)	Lymphocytes	CXCL10	CXCR3
Interferon-inducible T-cell alpha chemoattractant (I-TAC)	Lymphocytes	CXCL11	CXCR3
Stromal cell-derived factor 1 (SDF-1)	Lymphocytes	CXCL12	CXCR4
B-cell chemoattractant (BCA-1)	Lymphocytes	CXCL13	CXCR5
Monocyte chemoattractant protein (MCP)-1	Monocytes and lymphocytes	CCL2	CCR2
MCP-2	Monocytes and lymphocytes	CCL8	CCR3
MCP-3	Monocytes and lymphocytes	CCL7	CCR1, CCR2, CCR3
		CCL13	CCR2, CCR3
Macrophage inflammatory protein (MIP)-1α	Monocytes and lymphocytes	CCL3	CCR1, CCR5
MIP-1β	Monocytes and lymphocytes	CCL4	CCR5
RANTES (regulated upon activation, normally T-expressed, and presumably secreted)	Monocytes and lymphocytes	CCL5	CCR1, CCR3, CCR5
Eotaxin-1	Eosinophils	CCL11	CCR3
Eotaxin-2	Eosinophils	CCL24	CCR3
Eotaxin-3	Eosinophils	CCL26	CCR3
Liver and activation-regulated chemokine (LARC)	Monocytes and lymphocytes	CCL20	CCR6
Thymus expressed chemokine (TECK)	Monocytes and lymphocytes	CCL25	CCR9
Cutaneous T-cell-attracting chemokine (CTACK)	Monocytes and lymphocytes	CCL27	CCR10
T-cell-directed CC chemokine (TARC)	Monocytes and lymphocytes	CCL17	CCR4
Macrophage-derived chemokine (MDC)	Monocytes and lymphocytes	CCL22	CCR4
Dendritic cell-specific chemokine (DC-CK1)	Monocytes and lymphocytes, dendritic cells	CCL18	Not known
Epstein-Barr virus–induced molecule 1 ligand chemokine (ELC)	Monocytes and lymphocytes, dendritic cells	CCL19	CCR7
Secondary lymphoid tissue chemokine (SLC)	Monocytes and lymphocytes, dendritic cells	CCL21	CCR7
Fractalkine	Monocytes and lymphocytes, dendritic cells	CX3CL1	CX3CR1

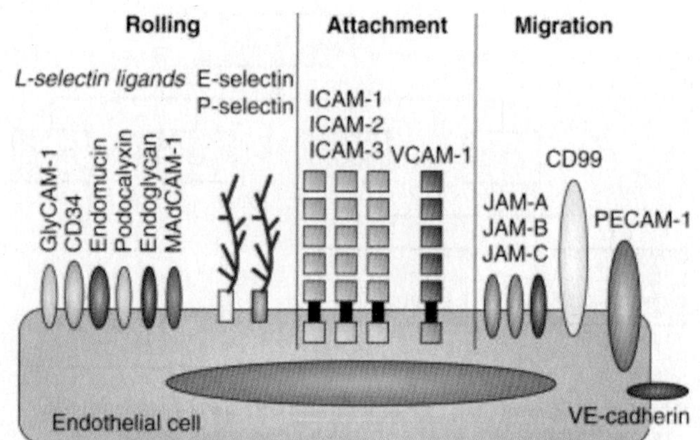

Fig. 56.7 Adhesion of White Blood Cells to Endothelial Cells Is Mediated by Several Receptor–Ligand Pair Interactions. A distinct set of endothelial molecules is involved in each stage of leukocyte recruitment (rolling, attachment, and transendothelial migration). In the rolling phase, L-selectin receptors on neutrophils bind to one of several ligands on the endothelial cells. Similarly, in the attachment phase, neutrophil β-integrins bind to the ICAM 1 to 3 or VCAM-1 receptors. *ICAM*, Intercellular adhesion molecule; *VCAM*, vascular cell adhesion molecule. (Reproduced after permission and minor modifications from Benjamin and Maheshwari. Developmental immunology. In: *Fanaroff and Martin's Neonatal-Perinatal Medicine*. 47, 752–788.)

(Mac-1, $\alpha_M\beta_2$, CD11b/CD18), and p150, 95 ($\alpha_X\beta_2$, CD11c/CD18), which bind endothelial receptors such as the intercellular adhesion molecule 1 and 2 (ICAM-1 and ICAM-2) and vascular cell adhesion molecule 1 (VCAM-1). LFA-1 binds to both ICAM-1 and ICAM-2, whereas Mac-1 and p150, 95 bind exclusively to ICAM-1. These neutrophils undergo activation on the endothelial surface and migrate through the capillary/venular wall, a process that involves the platelet-endothelial cell adhesion molecule (PECAM1, CD31), the integrin-associated protein (CD47), and other junctional molecules (Fig. 56.8).[29]

Compared with neutrophils from adults, neonatal neutrophils adhere less avidly to the endothelium. Neonatal neutrophils have lower selectin expression than adults,[30] which might be further reduced by perinatal stress such as in birth asphyxia.[31] In addition, neonatal neutrophils display defective shedding of L-selectin.[30] These properties impair neutrophil rolling on the endothelial surface and thereby the tissue recruitment of these cells. Neutrophil-endothelial adherence and neutrophil transmigration is also limited in neonates due to a developmental deficiency of mac-1 (CD18/CD11b), one of the β_2 integrins.[32] The transendothelial migration of neutrophils is also limited due to less deformability of neonatal neutrophils.[33]

Chemotaxis

Once outside the blood vessel, neutrophils migrate (see Fig. 56.5) along concentration gradients of chemoattractants such as IL-8 and other chemokines, f-MLP, and C5a.[26] These chemotaxins bind high-affinity G-protein–coupled receptors on the leukocyte surface. Bacterial products may be more potent chemoattractants than host chemokines.[34] Neonatal neutrophils migrate slower than do adult neutrophils until 2 to 3 weeks after birth[35–38] and achieve normal chemotaxis only by 40 to 42 weeks of postconceptional age or later.[35,39] Although minor infections may enhance chemotaxis in neonates, the migratory responses of neonatal neutrophils may become further depressed during systemic gram-negative sepsis.[40,41]

Neonatal neutrophils bind various chemoattractants normally, but chemoattractant-induced membrane depolarization, calcium transport, and sugar uptake are less efficient. These chemotactic defects occur because neonatal neutrophils may have a larger, poorly motile neutrophil subpopulation, impaired calcium mobilization, and aberrations in intracellular signaling pathways such as NF-κB activation.[42,43] Lower Mac-1 expression can also impede chemotaxis due to impaired neutrophil interaction with the extracellular matrix.[42,44] Inability to effectively direct neutrophils to the bacterial source contributes to the neonatal vulnerability to septicemia.

Phagocytosis

Phagocytosis is a specialized form of endocytosis directed at engulfing solid particles into an internal phagosome, which then "matures" through interactions with the endosomal compartment and eventually fuses with a lysosome for killing of internalized microorganisms and terminal degradation of the cargo (see Fig. 56.5).[45] Phagocytosis is more efficient when the target is opsonized by specific immunoglobulin (IG) G. Neutrophils express receptors for IgG ($F_{c\gamma}$ receptors I-III, or CD16,

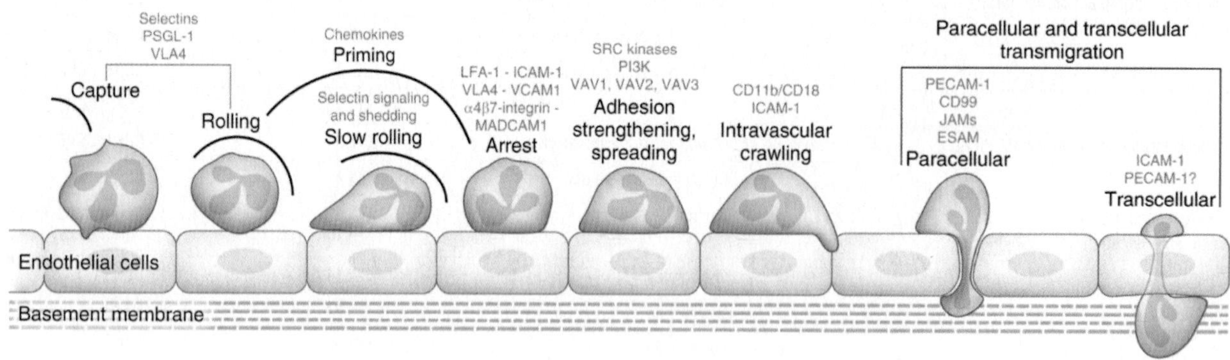

Fig. 56.8 Emigration of Neutrophils From the Vascular Space. Effector molecules are indicated in gray text. Initial capture is mediated by interactions between neutrophil/leukocyte (L)-selectin and endothelial cell (E, P)-selectins and their respective carbohydrate ligands on the opposing cell surface (e.g., P-selectin glycoprotein ligand-1 [PSGL-1]), whereas integrins (e.g., very late antigen 4 [VLA4]) are responsible for firm adherence. Selectin-mediated signaling slows the rolling or tumbling neutrophils, partially countering the shear forces resulting from blood flow. Chemokines diffusing into the bloodstream from sites of microbial invasion in the tissues bind to specific receptors and activate the neutrophil, which is then arrested by integrin-dependent interactions. The activated neutrophil flattens against the endothelium and crawls along the luminal surface of the vessel wall. Platelet-endothelial cell adhesion molecule-1 (PECAM-1), junctional adhesion molecules (JAMs), and endothelial cell-selective adhesion molecule (ESAM) localized to interendothelial cell junctions interact with PECAM-1 and CD99 on the neutrophil surface to permit neutrophil migration between and through endothelial cells. Once in the tissues, the polarized neutrophils move up the mediator concentration gradient to reach the site of microbial invasion. See text for further details. *ICAM-1*, Intercellular adhesion molecule; *LFA-1*, leukocyte function–associated antigen; *MADCAM1*, mucosal addressin cell adhesion molecule 1; *PI(3)K*, phosphatidylinositol-3-phosphate kinase; *SRC*, sarcoma; *VAV1*, vav1 guanine nucleotide exchange factor; *VCAM1*, vascular cell adhesion molecule 1. (Reproduced after permission and minor modifications from DeLeo and Nauseef. Scanning electron micrographs of nonadherent and adherent neutrophils. Granulocytic phagocytes. In: *Mandell, Douglas, and Bennett's Principles and Practice of Infectious Diseases*. 2020.)

CD32, CD64), C3b (CR1), and iC3b (CR3). In some instances, microorganisms may be ingested without opsonization through lectin-carbohydrate (lectins on bacterial fimbriae interact with neutrophil glycoproteins), protein-protein (proteins such as filamentous hemagglutinin that express the arg-gly-asp or RGD amino acid sequence bind to integrins), and hydrophobic-protein (bacterial glycolipids and neutrophil integrins) interactions.[45,46] The interaction of IgG or complement (Fig. 56.9) receptors on the neutrophil surface with the opsonized particle trigger cytoskeletal rearrangements to enclose the opsonized particle within a phagosome. Phagocytosis is most efficient when organisms are coated with opsonins such as IgG and C_3, which interact with cognate receptors (see Fig. 56.5). Neutrophils also express integrin receptors for matrix proteins such as fibronectin, laminin, and collagen.[45,47,48]

Preterm neutrophils have impaired phagocytosis, which corrects only in the late third trimester.[36] Preterm neutrophils ingest particles more slowly and ingest fewer bacteria (such as *Escherichia coli*). The lack of opsonic activity with a lower concentration of specific antibodies may be a contributing factor.[49] Preterm neutrophils also have lower expression of CD16 ($F_{c\gamma}$RIII) and CD32 ($F_{c\gamma}$RII), which bind IgG.[50] The expression of CD16, but not that of CD32, may improve during the neonatal period.[51]

Intracellular Killing

The phagolysosome exposes the ingested microorganism to toxic substances such as reactive oxygen species (ROS) in an enclosed space (see Fig. 56.5).[45] The production of ROS utilizes a "respiratory burst," where an NADPH-dependent oxidase localized on the phagosome membrane reduces molecular oxygen (O_2) to superoxide anion ($O{\bullet}_2^-$)[52] and leads to subsequent generation of peroxide (H_2O_2). The hydroxyl radical (OH•, formed in the presence of iron) also contributes to the microbicidal capacity of neutrophils.[53] The oxygen-dependent bactericidal mechanisms can be broadly divided into myeloperoxidase (MPO)-independent (such as H_2O_2) and MPO-dependent (MPO catalyzes reactions between H_2O_2 and halides to form highly reactive products).[54] H_2O_2 is a relatively weaker bactericidal agent than the MPO-H_2O_2-halide system.[53]

Neutrophils also have many nonoxidative killing mechanisms such as low pH (as low as 6.0), broad-spectrum antimicrobial peptides such as defensins, bactericidal/permeability-increasing protein (BPI), lactoferrin, lysozyme, and a variety of cationic proteins.[55] BPI binds lipopolysaccharide and can damage the outer membrane of gram-negative bacteria.[56] Lactoferrin, as an iron chelator, is bacteriostatic and is also involved in neutrophil degranulation and in granulocytopoiesis. Lysozyme hydrolyses bacterial cell wall peptidoglycan. The neutrophil primary granules also contain other cationic antibacterial proteins such as azurocidin, indolicidin, and cathelicidin.[45,57]

Preterm neutrophils have a less active respiratory burst, which reduces the efficiency of intracellular bacterial killing (in addition to low opsonic activity).[36,58–61] The neutrophil respiratory burst in preterm infants improves postnatally as a function of chronologic age in about 2 months but continues to have an overall weaker oxidative burst than adults.[62] The antiviral activity of neonatal neutrophils is also diminished.

Neutrophil extracellular traps (NETs) (Fig. 56.10), which are composed of extracellular strands of decondensed DNA bound to histones, elastase, myeloperoxidase, lactoferrin, and defensins, add to the extracellular antimicrobial defense ability of neutrophils.[63,64] The formation of NETs, usually referred to as NETosis,[65] usually involves two major pathways: (1) an NADPH oxidase-dependent production of ROS[66,67] and (2) the complement system.[68,69] The NET-forming ability of term and preterm neonates is less than that in adults,[70,71] possibly because of inhibitory mediators such as the NET-inhibitory factor and its related peptides.[72,73]

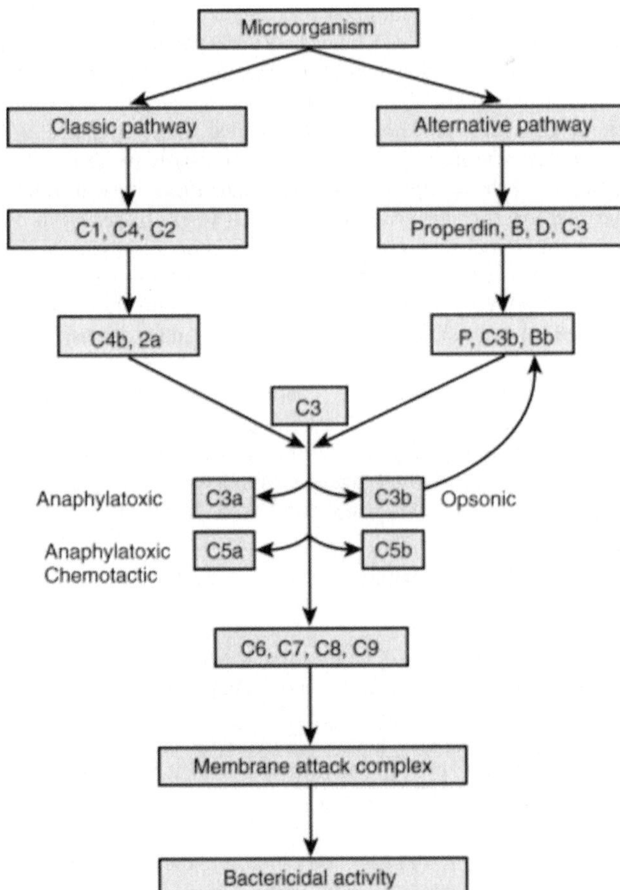

Fig. 56.9 Complement System Activation Cascade. Activation of the classic pathway *(left)* and the alternative pathway *(right)* causes generation of soluble factors that amplify phagocyte functions and produce a membrane-bound attack complex that damages cell membranes. (Reproduced after permission and minor modifications from Benjamin and Maheshwari. Developmental immunology. In: *Fanaroff and Martin's Neonatal-Perinatal Medicine*. 47, 752–788.)

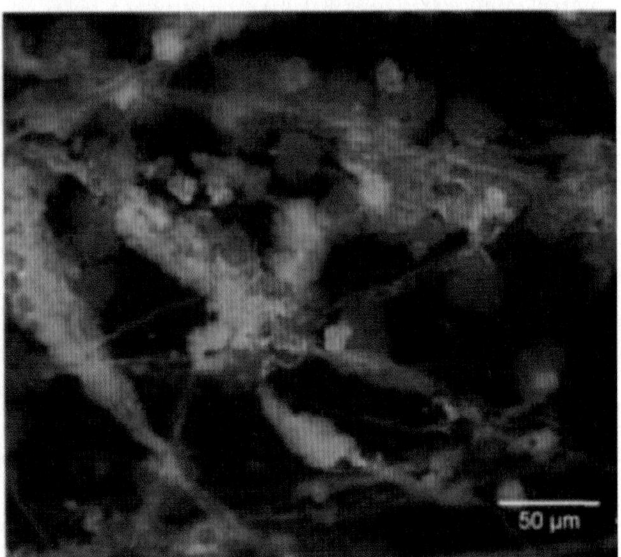

Fig. 56.10 Neutrophil extracellular traps (NETs) are blue weblike structures. In this merged image, the circular blue structures are nuclei. (Reproduced after permission and minor modifications from Baines et al. Biology of neutrophils. In: *Middleton's Allergy: Principles and Practice*. 17, 267–277.e1.)

Degranulation

Neutrophil granules (Fig. 56.11) are of at least four types: (1) the "azurophilic" or primary granules (stain with the azure A dye), (2) "specific" or secondary granules, (3) tertiary or gelatinase granules, and (4) secretory vesicles. Azurophilic granules contain MPO (peroxidase-positive granules); proteases such as cathepsins, proteinase-3, and elastase; and antimicrobial proteins such as defensins and the BPI. These granules release their contents into the phagolysosomes for intracellular killing. Specific granules contain antibacterial agents such as lactoferrin, lysozyme, and receptors for complement components. These granules play an important role in extracellular killing and fuse with the cell membrane to release their contents, such as integrins, cytochrome-*b*558, receptors for chemotactic agents, and opsonins, to the cell surface by exocytosis.[74]

Neutrophils from term neonates contain granules and show degranulation responses similar to adults.[75] However, those from preterm infants release less BPI, elastase, and lactoferrin.[36,76] Collectively, developmental deficiencies in neutrophil function explain, in part, the susceptibility of neonates to invasive bacterial infections.

Monocytes and Macrophages

Development

Embryonic macrophages appear in the yolk sac during the third week of gestation.[77] These large histiocytic cells develop prior to the first appearance of monocytes.[78–80] During the fourth week, some progenitors also start appearing as erythro-myeloid progenitors in the yolk sac and some in the aorta-gonad-mesonephros zone. At 5 weeks of gestation, two distinct cell lineages with a dendritic/macrophage structure can be identified in the yolk sac, mesenchyme, fetal liver, and bone marrow. Most are major histocompatibility complex II (MHC II)-negative. MHC II-negative cells also appear in the thymic cortex, in the marginal zones of lymph nodes, in the splenic red pulp, and in the bone marrow.[81] Some MHC II-positive cells appear in the liver at 7 to 8 weeks, the lymph nodes at 11 to 13 weeks of gestation, and the T-cell area's thymic medulla by 16 weeks of gestation. Subsequently, MHC class II-positive cells are also seen in the skin and gastrointestinal tract.[81,82]

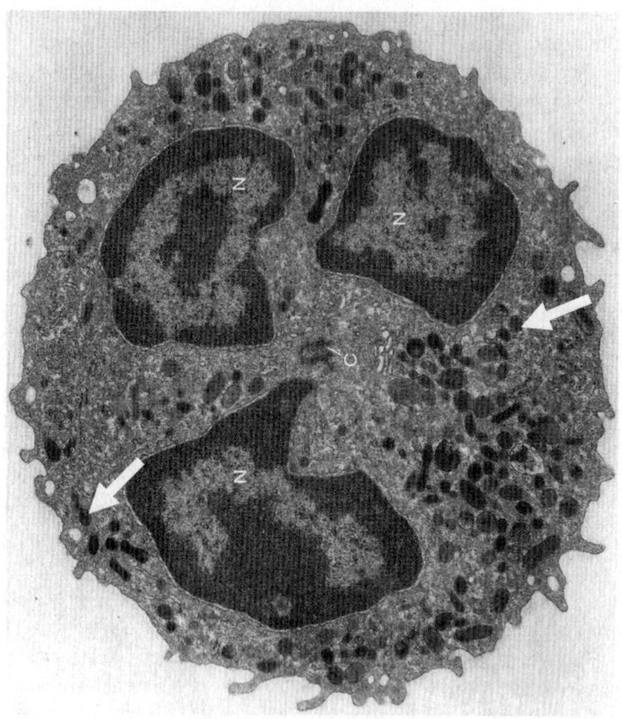

Fig. 56.11 Neutrophils Contain Many Granules. The cell here looks trinucleated because the connections between the three lobes are outside the fields of view. The granules are marked by *arrows*. There is a centrally located centriole (C). The azurophilic granules *(white arrows)* are electron-dense and contain myeloperoxidase, proteolytic enzymes, antibacterials such as defensins, and bactericidal permeability-increasing protein. Specific granules are relatively electron-lucent and contain lactoferrin, lysozyme, receptors for complement fragments, and f-MLP. The tertiary granules contain gelatinase. The secretory vesicles contain surface membrane-bound receptors. (Image reproduced after permission and minor modifications from Gartner. Blood and hemopoiesis. *Textbook of Histology*. 10, 217–248.e2.)

During the 4- to 8-week period, hematopoiesis starts in the fetal liver and the bone marrow and monocytes appear in proportions as high as 70% of all hematopoietic cells.[83] These monocytes differentiate into macrophages (Fig. 56.12). During the next 6 weeks, this proportion falls to 1% to 2%.[83] The first monocytes appear in circulation in the fifth month of gestation[83–85] and increase toward term when there is a relative monocytosis. The absolute monocyte counts rise during the early neonatal period and then decrease slightly in the third week of postnatal life. The absolute monocyte counts average about 1400/μL at 40 weeks of gestation.[86]

Peripheral blood monocytes are composed of at least two subpopulations: (1) "classic" $CD14^+$ $CD16^-$ monocytes, which express CCR2, CD64, and CD62L, represent nearly 80% of all blood monocytes, have phagocytic activity, and produce cytokines when exposed to bacteria; and (2) "nonclassic" $CD14^{low}$ $CD16^+$ monocytes that lack CCR2.[87] These are poorly phagocytic and mainly patrol the circulation to remove senescent endothelial cells and extravasate during tissue healing.[88] Monocytes in term infants are fairly functional. These show strong adherence, random migration, chemotaxis, bactericidal activity, and phagocytosis.[89–91] Fetal and neonatal monocytes kill a variety of pathogens including *Staphylococcus aureus, S. epidermidis, E. coli,* and *Candida albicans* at levels similar to monocytes in adults.[89,92]

The size of the macrophage pool varies in different organ systems. Intestinal macrophages can be seen at 10 weeks of gestation and form a sizable pool by midgestation.[80,93–97] However, the fetal lung shows only a few alveolar macrophages, and these expand after birth.[93,94,96–104] Macrophages are also polarized into the classically activated M1 macrophages that express various inflammatory signals and the more-recently described M2 macrophages that function with an antiinflammatory profile.[105] These macrophages are active in immunoregulation, maintain tissue integrity after injuries and in chronic infections, and promote angiogenesis.[106] The M2 macrophages are a relatively heterogeneous group composed of five subcategories (M2a, M2b, M2c, M2d, and M2f)[9] (Table 56.2).

Natural Killer Cells

Development

Natural killer (NK) cells are large granular lymphocytes (Fig. 56.13) and have characteristic surface markers including the CD56/neural cell adhesion molecule and CD16/Fcγ receptor IIIa (FcγRIIIa), a low-affinity IgG receptor. They also express CD2, LFA-1, and cytokine receptors such as $IL\text{-}2R_{\beta\gamma c}$, IL-12R, interferon (IFN)-γR, and $IL\text{-}15R_{\alpha}$.[107] NK cells share some T-cell markers[108–110] and may share a common progenitor.[111,112]

NK cells appear at 6 weeks of gestation, and the number increases progressively until birth. Fifty to eighty percent of fetal NK cells express CD3γ, ε, λ, and σ proteins, which is much higher than at term or in adults, and express much less CD16 than adults.[111] However, these cells mature rapidly and constitute 10% to 15% of all circulating lymphocytes at term, which is similar to that in adults.[111] Similarly, CD56 and CD57 are expressed poorly on fetal or

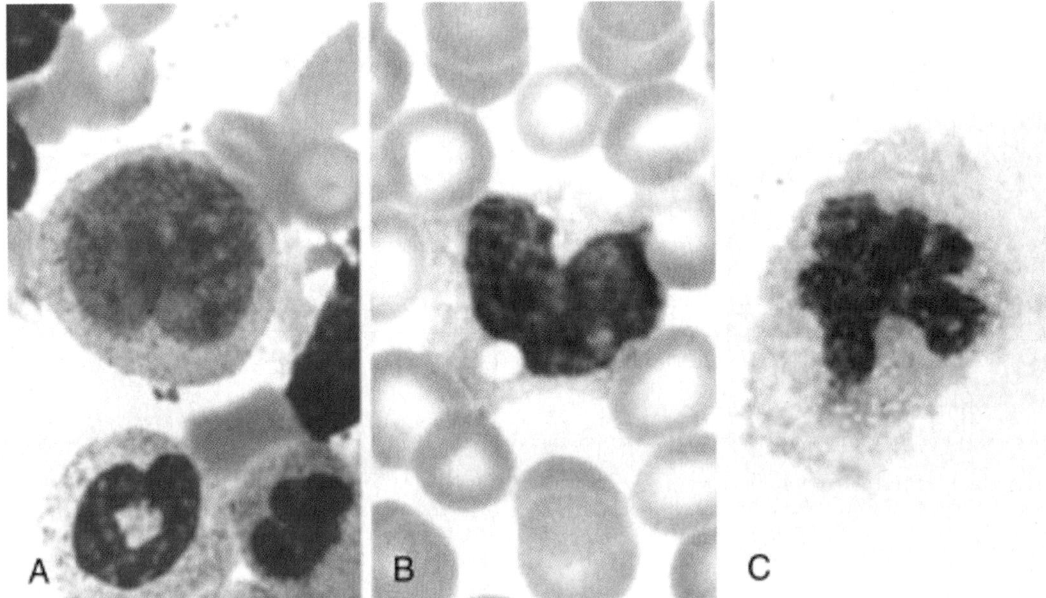

Fig. 56.12 Differentiating Monocytes. (A) Promonocytes have a slightly folded nucleus and have nucleoli. Cytoplasm is moderately abundant and blue/gray with very faint granules. (B) Monocytes in blood typically have more folded or horseshoe-shaped nuclei and more abundant gray cytoplasm, frequently with vacuoles and rare granules. (C) Macrophages are larger with irregular nuclei. (Reproduced after permission and minor modifications from Khanna-Gupta and Berliner. Granulocytopoiesis and monocytopoiesis. In: *Hematology: Basic Principles and Practice*. ch. 27, 321–333.e1.)

neonatal NK cells, compared with nearly 50% positivity in adult NK cells.[111,113]

Function

NK cells recognize viral-infected and tumor cells by the absence or decreased expression of MHC class I molecules on the cell surface.[114–116] Their MHC-unrestricted killing is mediated by perforin/granzyme apoptotic pathways.[117] The other mechanism of cytolysis is antibody-dependent cell-mediated cytotoxicity (ADCC), where target cell-bound IgG1 or IgG3 triggers the FcγRIIIa receptor on the NK cell.[116,118] NK cells are also believed to play a key role in maintaining immunologic tolerance at the maternal-fetal interface.[119]

Fetal NK cells have significantly lower cytolytic activity (including ADCC) against tumor-cell target cell lines than do those of adults, but cytolytic activity increases with gestational age parallel to increasing expression of CD56 and CD16.[111,120] However, even at term, the cytolytic activity is only 50% to 80% of adult levels.[112]

NK cells should not be confused with the natural killer T cells, a heterogeneous group of T cells that express an alpha beta T-cell receptor besides some of the NK cell markers. Many of these cells

Table 56.2 Subtypes of Macrophages

M1 macrophages—classically activated, proinflammatory: Surface expression of TLR2, TLR4, CD80, CD86, MHC-II Signaling mediators: NF-κB; STAT-1, -5; IRF-1, -2, -5	Express TNF, IL-1α, IL-1β, IL-6, IL-12, CXCL9, CXCL10	• Inflammation • Phagocytosis • Killing of intracellular pathogens
M2 macrophages—alternatively activated, immunoregulatory Surface expression of mannitol receptor, CD206, CD163, CD209, FIZZ1, Ym1/2, TLR1, and TLR8; signaling mediators: JAK-1, -3; STAT-1, -3, -5, -6; Ras; SP-1		
M2a	Express both inflammatory and noninflammatory cytokines (Type 2 pattern): IL-1β, IL-10, TGF-β, CCL17, CCL18, CCL22	• Inflammation • Killing of intracellular pathogens • Allergy • Recruitment of pericytes
M2b	Express IL-10, CCL1, CCL20, and CXCL1	• Immunoregulation • Phagocytosis of apoptotic cells
M2c	Secrete matrix metalloproteinases (MMPs) Express IL-10, TGF-β, CCL16, and CCL18	• Immunoregulation • Matrix deposition • Tissue remodeling • Phagocytosis of apoptotic cells • Suppress angiogenesis
M2d	Express IL-10 and vascular endothelial growth factors	• Angiogenesis
M2f	—	• Immunoregulation • Phagocytosis of apoptotic cells • Smooth muscle cell differentiation • Pericyte differentiation • Suppress vascular permeability

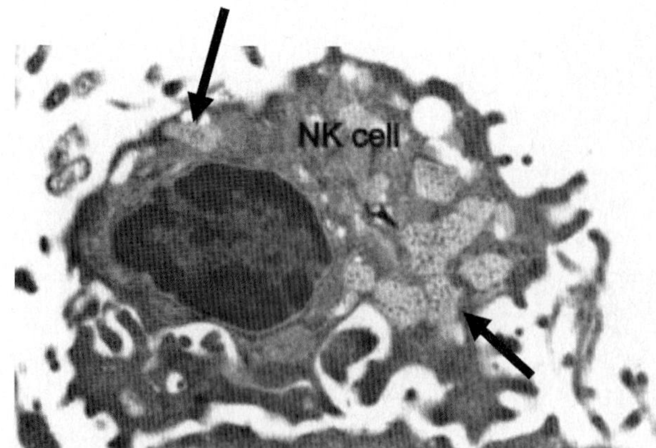

Fig. 56.13 Natural Killer (NK) Cells. Electron micrograph. The *black arrows* within the NK cell cytoplasm point to destructive granules containing pore-forming proteins that have been labeled with colloidal gold particles. (Reproduced by permission from the Encyclopedia of Immunology (Second Edition), 1998, Electron Microscopy: Immunological Applications by Matthew A. Gonda. Micrograph was contributed by J. Ortaldo, K. Nagashima, and M. A. Gonda.)

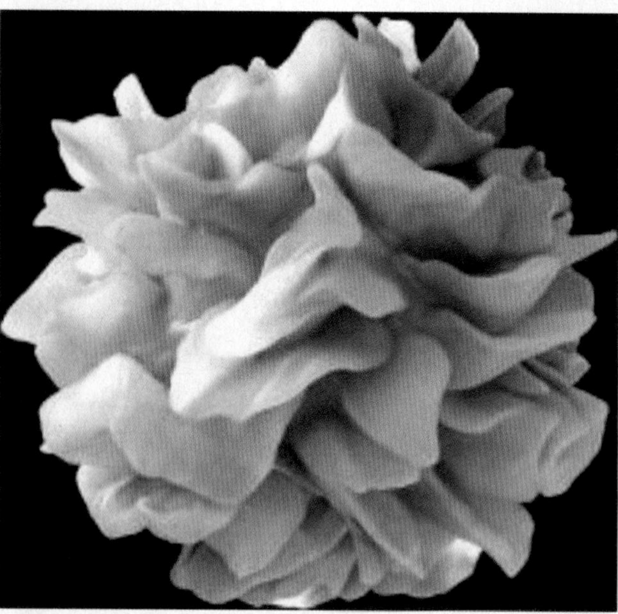

Fig. 56.14 High-Resolution 3D Rendition of a Dendritic Cell (Immature). (Reproduced after permission and minor modifications from Russo et al. A new hypothesis for the pathophysiology of complex regional pain syndrome. *Med Hypotheses.* 2018;119:41–53.)

recognize the nonpolymorphic CD1d molecule, an antigen-presenting molecule that binds self- and foreign lipids and glycolipids. NK T cells constitute only 0.2% of all peripheral blood T cells. These cells play an important role in mucosal immunity and in the pathogenesis of inflammatory/allergic conditions; the role during fetal life remains unclear.[121] Imbalances in this system produced by chronic inflammation may be involved in the presentation of the acquired forms of hemophagocytic lymphohistiocytosis in the neonatal period.

Noncytotoxic Innate Immune Cells

Development

Noncytotoxic ILCs are morphologically similar to other lymphocytes, but unlike adaptive T cells and B cells, they do not show antigen specificity and function more as innate immune cells.[122] The common lymphoid progenitor[123] differentiates into three subgroups: ILC1, ILC2, and ILC3. There are some similarities with T-helper cells in cytokine expression and function, but these cells have differential requirements for transcription factors during development, cytokine expression, and other functions.[28,122] ILC1s may protect against intracellular bacteria and parasites; ILC2s may be active during tissue repair, allergic disorders, and antihelminth immunity; and ILC3s may promote antibacterial immunity, chronic inflammation, or tissue repair.

Function

There is limited information on ILCs in the fetus and neonate. ILC2 cells can be seen in cord blood.[124] In another study, ILC3s were implicated as a source of increased IL-17 levels seen in patients with preeclampsia and gestational/chronic diabetes.[125]

Adaptive Immune System

Dendritic Cells

Dendritic cells (DCs) are a leukocyte subset specialized for antigen-presenting function. DC populations have been differentiated from a common granulocyte-monocyte-dendritic cell progenitor.[126] Cells with a dendritic/macrophage structure are present in the yolk sac, mesenchyme, and liver at 4 to 6 weeks of age. DCs are detectable in skin by 6 to 7 weeks of gestation.[127] These cells were named based on their distinctive morphology, with numerous fine dendritic cytoplasmic processes penetrating epithelial-bound organ surfaces (Fig. 56.14). These cells stimulate T cells, are home to T cell–dependent lymph node areas, show active pinocytosis, and display characteristic cell-surface antigens.[128]

During hematopoiesis, DC precursors differentiate into two subgroups[129,130]: (1) myeloid DCs (or mDCs), derived from pre-DC1, are $CD11c^+$ cells that express myeloid markers such as CD13, CD33, CD1a-d, and CD11b; and (2) plasmacytoid DCs (or pDCs), derived from pre-DC2, are $CD11c^-$ and have a plasmacytoid morphology with well-developed rough endoplasmic reticulum and Golgi apparatus.[131]

Function

Neonatal DCs compose about 0.3% of all mononuclear cells. Cord blood contains a higher number and proportion of pDCs than does adult peripheral blood, with pDC:mDC ratios of 1 to 3:1 (usually 1:2 in adults).[132] Compared with pDCs from adults, cord blood DCs exhibit low expression of costimulatory molecules CD40, CD80, or CD86, show an impaired maturational response after stimulation with agonists for various toll-like receptors (measured as increase in the expression of costimulatory molecules and production of IFN-alpha, TNF-alpha, IL-1, IL-6, and IL-12), and perform poorly at accessory function.[133,134] Neonatal DCs have lower expression of ICAM-1 and MHC antigens and are poorer activators of lymphocytes than those from adults.[133]

T Lymphocytes

Development

The thymus develops at about 6 weeks of gestation, with the ectodermal layer developing into a cortex and the endodermal layer into the medulla.[135,136] Lymphoid cells migrate into the thymus first from the yolk sac and fetal liver and then from the bone marrow over the next 2 to 3 weeks.[137–143] These prothymocytes proliferate actively and differentiate with expression of the first T cell–specific surface molecules (e.g., CD2, and later CD4 and CD8).[140,144,145] The most immature thymocytes are found in the subcapsular cortical region, and cells move into the deeper layers as they mature.[135] Early prothymocytes do not express CD3, the T cell receptor (TCR), CD4, or CD8 and are often referred to as "triple-negative thymocytes."[146] The progeny continues to divide and rearrange their TCR genes, and because these cells express both CD4 and CD8, they are now called "double-positive."[135,146] These cells undergo *positive selection* by self-MHC restriction, and more than 95% of the cells die each day during this stage.[146] *Negative selection* occurs next and is mediated by the bone marrow–derived antigen-presenting cells (such as dendritic cells and macrophages), which eliminate autoreactive cells either by *clonal deletion* or *clonal anergy*.[147,148] As these thymocytes mature and reach the medulla, they express only one of the CD4 or CD8 antigens. These single-positive T cells migrate from the thymus to the peripheral lymphoid organs at about 14 weeks of gestation.[135] By 15 weeks, human thymocytes express a complete set of TCRs.[135,149] During fetal life, the thymus is the largest lymphoid tissue in terms of body proportions. At birth, it is about two-thirds of its mature weight. It reaches full size at 10 years, then gradually involutes and is replaced by adipose tissue.[150]

T Cell Receptor (TCR) Repertoire

The TCR is composed of two distinct functional subunits, each specialized for a different function.[151] The first, highly polymorphic, is structured unique for each T cell for antigen recognition; it is composed of two polypeptide chains, α and β (except in a specific T-cell subset where it consists of γ and δ chains).[151,152] The second, also known as CD3, is a trimolecular complex, involved in signal transduction and cellular activation. The extracellular region of the TCR resembles an Ig Fab fragment and derives its structural diversity from recombinatorial permutations involving a set each of variable (V), diversity (D), and joining (J) gene segments (Fig. 56.15).[153,154] The variable domain is situated in the N-terminal end of the α/β (or γ/δ) chains, whereas the C terminal is the constant region.[151] The variable domains consist of V, D, and J elements in the β chain, and V and J in the α chain.[155] The antigen-binding sites are formed by three "complementarity-determining regions" (CDRs). CDR3, the most extensive of these segments, serves as a key site for antigen recognition.[156]

By midgestation, all the TCR Vβ families (V here refers to the variable domain of the β chain, not the V gene segments mentioned above) are expressed, but they have shorter CDR3 regions, and consequently, premature neonates have less CDR3 heterogeneity.[157] In term infants, the T-cell Vβ repertoire begins to resemble that in adults.[156,158] T cells are important in the maturation of the immune system.

Circulating T Cells

T cell subpopulations expand beyond 19 weeks' gestation and peak at about 6 to 9 months after birth. The numbers decline subsequently to adult levels at 6 to 7 years of age.[159,160] In term neonates, CD4+ cells constitute a higher proportion of T cells than in adults. There are fewer CD8+ cells, and this number does not change much with age. Therefore, with decreasing CD4+ cells, the CD4/CD8 ratio of 4.9:1 during the perinatal period declines to adult values of approximately 2:1 by 4 years of age.[159–162]

In neonates, 80% to 90% of the circulating T cells are naïve (CD45RA phenotype), compared with only 40% to 60% in adults.[163,164] The percentage of memory T cells (CD45RO) increases in healthy infants during the first few years of life.[163] The ratios and relationships of T-cell subtypes during development need further clarification.

During development, naïve T cells differentiate into effector T-helper (Th) subsets. These differentiated T cells were originally categorically designated Th1 and Th2 cells based on distinct functional properties and the cytokines that drive their development.[165] Th1–type cytokines such as IFN-γ and IL-2 play a key role in initiating early resistance to pathogens, and induction of cell-mediated immunity. Th2 cytokines drive the system toward immune tolerance rather than toward defense from microbial infections. A differentiated T-cell population, Th17 cells, plays a protective role in immunity to infection but may also have a pathogenic role in allergic and other chronic inflammatory diseases.[166–168] Neonatal Th17 cells have a relatively limited capacity to produce IL-17.[169]

The fetus occupies a unique immunologic position where the Th2 phenotype predominates in utero and transitions to a more Th1 functionality after birth. This may be a core process of evolutionary significance where both the mother and fetus maintain a high level of immunologic suppression to enable continuation of pregnancy.

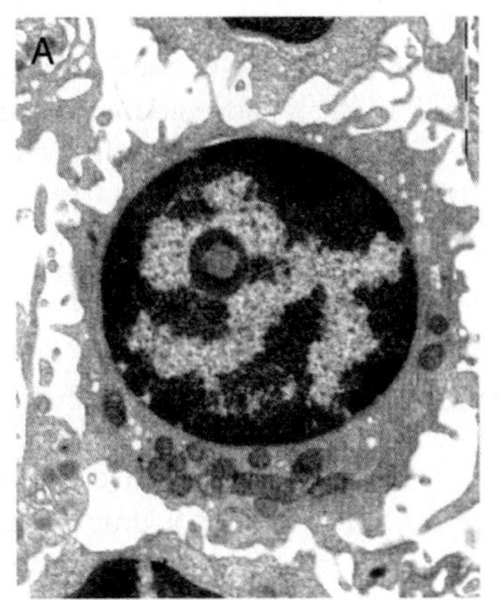

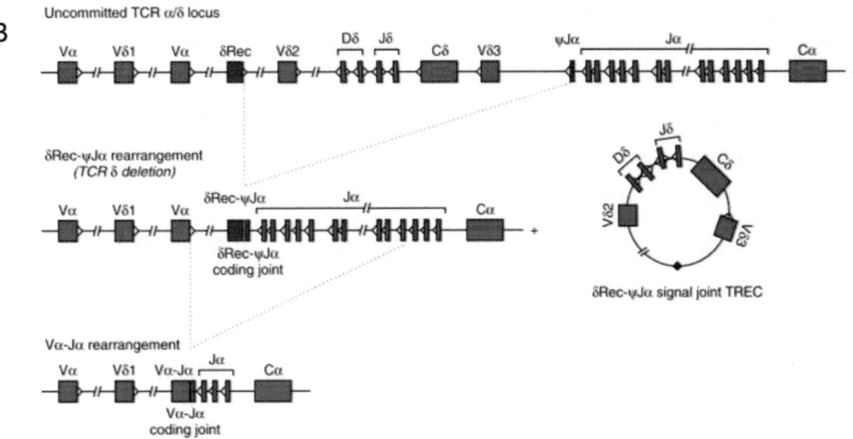

Fig. 56.15 Lymphocytes. (A) Ultrastructure. (B) Sequential rearrangements in the T-cell receptor (TCR)-α/δ locus generate signal joint T-cell receptor excision circles (sjTRECs) and Vα-Jα rearrangements. Rearrangement of the δRec to the Jα segment results in a commitment to the αβ-TCR lineage because this deletes the C and J segments that are necessary to encode a productive TCR-δ chain. The δRec-ψJα rearrangement also generates an sjTREC, which is commonly used for monitoring peripheral T-cell populations for their recent thymic origin. The δRec-ψJα rearrangement is followed by TCR-α (Vα-Jα) rearrangements, which if productive result in expression of an αβ-TCR on the thymocyte cell surface. Most thymocytes that express αβ-TCRs have molecular evidence of nonproductive rearrangements of portions of the TCR-δ gene locus (not shown). (Reproduced after permission and minor modifications from Hong and Lewis. Developmental immunology and role of host defenses in fetal and neonatal susceptibility to infection. In: *Remington and Klein's Infectious Diseases of the Fetus and Newborn Infant*. 4, 81–188.)

Function

Proliferation

T cells from premature infants have a limited capacity for proliferation, but these defects are corrected by full term.[163,170–173] These responses improve as the numbers of peripheral blood memory T cells increase. When tested with allogeneic cells (mixed lymphocyte reaction), however, cord blood lymphocytes respond better, although still somewhat less than cells from adult subjects.[163,171,174–176]

Cytokine Production

Neonatal concentrations of proinflammatory cytokines such as IL-1, IL-6, TNF, IFN-α, and IFN-β are comparable to those in adults.[177–181] Premature infants, however, are known to produce less TNF and IFN-α than those born at term.[182–184] Among the cytokines involved in adaptive immunity, IL-2 levels are comparable, but those of IL-4, IL-5, IL-10, IL-15, and IFN-γ are lower than adults.[183–188] Transforming growth factor β_1 and macrophage inflammatory protein 1α, which normally suppress hematopoiesis, are also present in lower concentrations.[189]

The concentrations of hematopoietic colony stimulating factors (CSFs) including IL-3, GM-CSF, and monocyte-CSF are lower than adults.[190,191] Chemokine levels are comparable, including those of IL-8/CXCL8, epithelial neutrophil attractant-78/CXCL5, growth-related oncoprotein-α/CXCL1, eotaxin/CCL11, and RANTES (regulated upon activation, normal T cell expressed and secreted)/CCL5.[192] Most of these deficiencies are caused by altered regulation of posttranscriptional mRNA processing[189] and a relative paucity of memory T cells, and possibly by genetic factors.[193–195]

Antigen-Specific Responses

The response of T cells to specific antigens can also be assessed in terms of proliferation or cytokine production. These responses usually require previous exposure to the corresponding antigen and are generally not detected at birth or from cord blood unless there was an intrauterine exposure. Neonatal T cells do, however, respond well to certain antigens such as tetanus/diphtheria toxoids, influenza, and mycobacterial antigens.[171] In response to superantigens, cord blood T cells produce lesser amounts of IL-2.[196] However, after stimulation, the percentage of $V\beta_2$+ T cells (which determine potential reactivity to superantigens) and the number of memory T cells increase significantly just like in adults.[196,197] However, unlike adult T cells, cord blood T cells are unable to respond if restimulated with the superantigen. This tolerance induction in cord blood T cells may be due to the underlying immunologic naïvete.[196,198]

Other Subgroups (See Fig. 56.3)

Cytotoxic T Lymphocytes

Cytotoxic T lymphocytes (CTLs) are important in host defense against intracellular infections, in allograft rejection, and in tumor cell surveillance.[199,200] CTLs induce cell lysis by either releasing extracellular mediators (such as the pore-forming perforin/granzyme system) or via a second fas/fas ligand-dependent pathway that leads to target cell apoptosis.[201,202] CTL cytotoxicity becomes recognizable by 18 weeks' gestation but is less efficient than in adults even in neonates born at term (< 20% of adult CTL activity).[176,203]

γδT Cells

The γδ T cells represent a distinct functional subset, with a majority lacking surface expression of both CD4 and CD8.[204–206] These cells are present mainly on skin and mucosal surfaces.[206] The exact function of these T cells is not well understood, but they can lyse target cells with the perforin/granzyme system like the cytotoxic T cells and can secrete cytokines such as IFN-γ and TNF upon activation. The cytotoxicity of neonatal γδ T cells is significantly less than in adults.[207]

These cells are detectable in the fetal liver as early as 5 to 6 weeks of gestation[208] and in the fetal thymus after 8 weeks of gestation[209] and compose nearly 10% of the peripheral blood T cells at 16 weeks.[208,210] Subsequently, the numbers decline gradually to reach about 3% at term.[211] By 20 to 30 weeks of gestation, Vγ9Vδ2+ T cells dominate the γδ repertoire.[209] V1 + T-cell generation increases later in gestation, and the majority of the γδ repertoire in cord blood and the pediatric thymus is composed of Vδ1 + T cells.[212] Fetal γδ T cells have a more diverse repertoire than adults. This diversity is retained throughout the first year of life and then decreases gradually during the first decade of life.[207] Overall, however, γδ T cells have a relatively restricted repertoire in comparison with the αβ T cells or B cells.[213]

T-Regulatory Cells

T-regulatory cells (T-regs) downregulate T-cell responses to both foreign and self-antigens, thereby playing an important role in regulating Th1/Th2 effector lineages.[214,215] T-regs, including both natural $CD4^+$ $CD25^+$ T-regs and the IL-10–producing T-regs, express the forkhead/winged-helix family transcriptional repressor-p3 (Foxp3),[216] a commonly used but not entirely specific marker for T-regs.[217] T-regs have been detected in neonatal blood, but information about T-reg function in early life is limited.

B Lymphocytes

Development

B-cell progenitors, pro-B cells, are derived from pluripotent hematopoietic cells in the bone marrow.[218] The first recognizable B-cell progenitor, the large pre-B cell, is characterized by the presence of cytoplasmic μ heavy chains.[218] Immature B cells undergo a selection process analogous to that of T cells to eliminate self-identifying clones *(clonal selection, clonal deletion)*, although other mechanisms to maintain self-tolerance may also be active.[219,220] Once B cells begin to express surface IgM (sIgM), they are ready to leave the bone marrow to enter the peripheral circulation.[221]

Pre-B cells can be identified in the fetal liver as early as 7 weeks' gestation and in the marrow by 12 weeks. sIgM+ B cells are found in the fetal liver by 9 weeks and in the bone marrow, peripheral blood, and spleen by 12 weeks. B cells with sIgA, sIgG, and sIgD isotypes appear between 10 and 12 weeks.[222] There is also increased traffic to the lymphoid tissues, and by 22 weeks, the proportion of B cells in the spleen, peripheral blood, and bone marrow resembles that in adults.[222,223] By 30 weeks, the bone marrow becomes the exclusive site for B-cell maturation. Plasma cells are first seen at about 20 weeks' gestation. IgM/IgD+ B cells are seen in lymph nodes at 16 to 17 weeks' gestation and in the spleen at 16 to 21 weeks.[223,224]

Immunoglobulin Repertoire

Receptor diversity in the antigen binding site originates from DNA recombination involving various V, D, or J gene segments, giving rise to a large number of V(D)J permutations.[154] Additional receptor diversity is generated by imprecise gene segment joins, additional nucleotides added to the splice junction of the VDJ joins by the enzyme terminal deoxynucleotidyl transferase, and somatic mutations (for B cells only, not T cells). Thereafter, these VDJ or VJ (light chains) units join to their respective constant region gene segments.[225,226]

The Ig repertoire is relatively restricted in the fetus and neonate. During early and midgestation, some selected heavy-chain V gene segments are preferentially expressed.[94] Early in fetal life, the most J_H proximal V_H gene segments are used preferentially, and consequently, the CDR3 region of the rearranged VDJ gene segment is shorter than that in adults. This leads to relatively limited junctional diversity, but this altered architecture of the antigen-binding site may also allow greater polyspecificity of antigen binding.[227,228] The utilization of V_H gene families becomes even more with increasing gestation. However, even at term, cord blood B cells have higher use of the V_H1 and V_H5 families than do adult B cells.[229] In general, the antibody response in neonates consists primarily of low-affinity IgMs. The somatic mutation of the heavy and light Ig variable region genes and the selection of higher affinity antibody-producing B cells is limited at birth but increases very slowly after 10 days.[230]

Circulating B Cells

At birth, the proportion of B cells resembles that in adults. The absolute number of B cells is higher at birth,[231] peaks at about 3 to 4 months, and then declines to adult levels by 6 to 7 years of age.[232] The number of B cells in preterm infants resembles that in term infants.[233] Unlike adults, most B cells in neonates express activation markers (CD25, CD23, transferrin receptor).[234]

Function

Immunoglobulin Production

The fetus and the neonate can produce antigen-specific antibody responses, although at lower levels than in adults.[235–239] However, this response remains immature,[224] and they may not be able to respond to all the antigens in a vaccine or may have a delayed isotype switch.[240] The postnatal age may be more important as a determinant of antibody response than the gestational age. Both preterm and term infants responded better to diphtheria toxoid immunization if the vaccination was deferred until 1 to 2 months of age.[240] However, with other antigens such as hepatitis B, premature infants may show a poorer early response than their term counterparts. These deficiencies correct during later infancy.[241]

Serum Immunoglobulin Levels

Serum Ig levels remain low until 18 to 20 weeks' gestation. Most of the newborn's serum immunoglobulins are derived from active transplacental transfer of maternal IgG (particularly IgG1 and IgG3) during later pregnancy.[242–244] In the full-term neonate, serum IgG levels are equal to or even higher than maternal serum IgG levels, but in the preterm neonate, who failed to receive these maternal antibodies, the levels are lower.[243,245] The levels fall after birth (through normal catabolism) to a nadir of 300 to 500 mg/dL between 3 and 5 months of age, when the infant starts producing increasing amounts of her/his own. This nadir may be much lower, and earlier, in preterm infants.[246] Cord blood Ig levels also tend to be lower in growth-retarded neonates.[247] In comparison, serum levels of IgA, IgM, and IgE are very low in newborn infants because these antibodies do not cross the placenta. However, when faced with an intrauterine infection, the fetus can produce appreciable amounts of IgM.[248]

Other Subgroups

CD5 Expressing B Cells

Many neonatal B cells express CD5, which is a T-cell antigen. These CD5+ B cells have been labeled as the "B-1" subset of cells, distinct from the conventional adult "B2" population. These cells appear earlier in ontogeny, have greater capacity for bone marrow-independent self-renewal, and express the signal transducer and activator of transcription-3 gene (STAT3).[249,250] B-1 cells express B-cell markers CD19 and CD45R but have lower levels of CD45R than do B-2 cells.[251–253] B-1 cells in the peritoneal and pleural cavities can be identified by their unusual CD11b+ $sIgM^{hi}$ $sIgD^{low}$ phenotype and can be further subdivided on the basis of differential expression of the cell-surface antigen CD5, into CD5+ CD11b+ $sIgM^{hi}$ $sIgD^{low}$ B-1a cells and CD5− CD11b+ $sIgM^{hi}$ $sIgD^{low}$ B-1b cells.[254]

In the fetus, B-1 cells are the predominant type of B cells and are localized in the spleen, lymph nodes, and peritoneal cavity.[255,256] Adults show CD5 expression on 25% to 35% of all B cells, unlike >90% of neonatal B cells. This number falls to 75% to 80% during infancy and then gradually drops over 15 years.[255,256]

Function

The exact function of B-1 cells is not clear. These cells show unique localization, and with broad polyspecific specificities, they may have a role in innate, not adaptive, immunity.[257] Unlike follicular B-2 cells that coordinate with T cells to respond to protein antigens, B-1 cells respond mainly to carbohydrate antigens independent of T cells.[251–253] B-1 cells may be composed of two subsets; B-1a cells spontaneously secrete IgM to defend against certain encapsulated bacteria such as *Streptococcus pneumoniae*, whereas B-1b cells may have a role in pathogen clearance and long-term protection.[254,258,259]

T- and B-Cell Interaction

T-cell signals are crucial for the proliferation, differentiation, and survival of B cells and include both antigen presentation and humoral signals.[260] Several receptor-ligand molecular pairs may be involved, including the CD40-CD40 ligand (CD40L) in B-cell immunoglobulin isotype switching and others like B7/CD28, CD11a (LFA-1)/CD54 (ICAM-1), and CD58 (LFA-3)/CD2 in T- and B-cell activation.[260] These functions are served by T cells after these have had antigen exposure and have developed memory subsets.[120,261] In general, neonatal T cells are less efficient at providing humoral and CD40-dependent activation signals.[262–265]

Recruitment of Various Leukocyte Subpopulations

In the above sections, we have attempted to describe an ever-increasing diversity in the leukocyte population seen during normal, healthy development and during disease. The coordinated recruitment of these cells into various tissues is a closely controlled process and follows patterns, both temporal and in cellular subtypes. The most widely accepted models of inflammation recognize four distinct, sequential phases: (1) initial tissue damage and local activation of inflammatory factors; (2) recruitment of inflammatory leukocytes, which is determined by the specific insult, and the temporal course; (3) a phase of consolidation, when the infectious organisms/inciting factors are largely eliminated; and (4) engagement of tissue-repair responses that promote tissue repair and restoration. In some cases, the transition between steps 3 and 4 may get altered with the onset of secondary immunopathology that may not resolve along expected timelines and may continue to cause tissue damage and scarring. Further work is needed, and is indeed ongoing, to answer some of these questions.

Section 10

CHAPTER

57 Immunodeficiency Syndromes Seen During the Neonatal Period

Keyur Donda, Benjamin A. Torres, Jolan Walter, Akhil Maheshwari

KEY POINTS

1. At birth, the fetal-neonatal immune system gets activated. It is critical for survival to recognize and eliminate all the potentially dangerous pathogens in the infant's external and its own enteric environment.
2. The innate arm is particularly necessary because the adaptive immunity is still developing.
3. In immunodeficiency states, the aberrant development of the immune system puts the infant at risk of infections, and all the chaotic attempts at host defense often cause dysregulated and excessive inflammation.
4. The neutrophils are the first line of defense against invading pathogens. There are known defects in adhesion and transepithelial migration, cellular life span, chemotaxis, and bacterial killing.
5. Most defects in the monocyte-macrophage system are parts of multisystem disorders and are recognized in the neonatal period more often due to manifestations in other organs.
6. Most defects in adaptive immunity in term infants manifest later in infancy once the maternally derived immunoglobulins fade away.
7. Severe combined immunodeficiency (SCID) presents early in life with severe infections such as respiratory infections, diarrhea, and sepsis; it is a genetically heterogeneous disorder that is comprised of many genetic defects. The most frequently seen subtype is inherited as an X-linked trait and is T– B+ NK–. Fifty to seventy percent of infants have lymphopenia, particularly in T cells. Early recognition of SCID syndromes can help in survival. Testing for these conditions is part of the neonatal screening.

Introduction

At birth, the fetus suddenly moves out of a relatively sterile intrauterine sanctuary into an open environment that is full of microflora. In utero, the fetal immune system is hypoactive and tolerant, which may actually be beneficial in evading recognition as an allograft by the maternal immune system. However, after birth, the same fetal-neonatal immune responses become critical for survival, to recognize and eliminate all the potentially dangerous pathogens in the external and the enteric environment. The innate arm is particularly necessary because the adaptive immunity is still developing. There is also a need for a functional dichotomy in the innate immunity that will help harmonize with the friendlier commensals but at the same time "contain/eliminate" the confrontational pathogens. In immunodeficiency states, the aberrant development of the immune system puts the infant at risk of infections, and with all the chaotic attempts at host defense, it often causes dysregulated and excessive inflammation.

In this review, we present an overview of various immunodeficiency syndromes that present during early infancy. We have included evidence from our own studies and from an extensive literature search in the databases PubMed, Embase, and Scopus. To avoid bias in the identification of studies, keywords were short-listed *a priori* from anecdotal experience and PubMed's Medical Subject Heading thesaurus.

Innate Immune System

Neutrophils are the first line of defense against invading pathogens. Once activated by infection and/or associated inflammation, this amphibious "naval" force of leukocytes patrolling in the bloodstream gets rapidly deployed into the affected tissues. The activated neutrophils emarginate out of the circulation, attach to the vascular endothelium, migrate across the capillary walls, move rapidly with focused chemotaxis, and then eliminate the pathogens through phagocytic ingestion or extracellular killing. The major limitations in the role of neutrophils in host defense can be due to decreased neutrophil number and/or function.

Neutropenia

In neonates, neutropenia is a frequent occurrence. It is defined as an absolute neutrophil count (ANC) $< 1000/\mu L$ or an ANC less than the 5th percentile for age.[1,2] There are existing norms for gestational and postnatal age-dependent neutrophil counts.[3–5] Neutropenia is frequently seen in extremely premature infants, with some studies having noted it in as many as half of all very low birth weight infants in the first week after birth.

In terms of kinetics, neutropenia can be secondary to decreased neutrophil production, increased destruction, or a combination of these mechanisms. Based on etiology, duration, and severity, neonatal neutropenia can be broadly classified into several groups:

1. Transient neonatal neutropenia of the neonate: Small-for-gestational-age infants, particularly those born to mothers with preeclampsia or pregnancy-induced hypertension, are frequently neutropenic in the first 3 to 5 days after birth.[2] These infants may have some inhibitors of normal granulocyte colony stimulating factor (G-CSF) production and consequent suppression of neutrophil production. Neutropenia may also be seen for 2 to 3 days after birth in donor twins in twin-twin transfusion syndromes.

Table 57.1 Congenital Neutropenia Syndromes[a]

Neutropenia Syndrome	Gene	Inheritance	Hematologic Features	Nonhematologic Features	Treatment
Severe congenital neutropenia	ELANE	AR	Neutropenia	—	rG-CSF[56]
Kostmann disease	HAX1	AR	Neutropenia	—	rG-CSF[57]
Severe congenital neutropenia—AD forms	GFI1 PRDM5 PFAAP5	AD	Neutropenia	—	rG-CSF
Cyclic neutropenia	ELANE	AD	Neutropenia	—	rG-CSF[6]
Barth syndrome	TAZ1	X-linked	Neutropenia	Cardiomyopathy, growth retardation, muscle weakness	rG-CSF[58]
Shwachman-Bodian-Diamond syndrome	SDBS	AR	Neutropenia, anemia, thrombocytopenia	Pancreatic insufficiency, skeletal anomalies, short stature, failure to thrive, delay in development	rG-CSF, HSCT[59]
Warts, hypogammaglobulinemia, infections, and myelokathexis (WHIM) syndrome	CXCR4	AD	Neutropenia, lymphopenia, thrombocytopenia, myelokathexis	Cardiac anomalies	rG-CSF[60], CXCR4 antagonist[61]
Hermansky-Pudlak syndrome type 2	AP3B1	AR	Neutropenia, platelet dysfunction	Albinism	
Glycogen storage type IB	G6PT1	AR	Neutropenia, neutrophil dysfunction	Hypoglycemia, lactic acidemia, hyperlipidemia	rG-CSF
Cartilage hair hypoplasia	RMPR	AR	Neutropenia, lymphopenia, macrocytic anemia	Short stature, aganglionic megacolon, fine sparse hair	rG-CSF[62]
Chediak-Higashi syndrome	LYST	AR	Neutropenia, giant neutrophil granules, bleeding diathesis	Albinism, peripheral neuropathy, hemophagocytic syndrome	HSCT[63]
Cohen syndrome	VPS13B	AR	Neutropenia	Facial dysmorphism, retinochoroidal dystrophy, delay in development	
Schimke immuno-osseous dysplasia	SMARCAL1	AR	Neutropenia, lymphopenia	Spondyloepiphyseal dysplasia, postnatal growth failure, proteinuria	G-CSF[64], HSCT[65]

[a]Genetic causes, clinical features, and current treatment modalities for disorders with congenital neutropenia are highlighted.

AD, Autosomal dominant; *AR,* autosomal recessive; *HSCT,* hematopoietic stem cell transplant; *rG-CSF,* recombinant granulocyte colony stimulating factor.

2. Congenital neutropenia syndromes: Neutropenia may be severe and protracted with ANCs as low as <200 µL/mL.[6] These conditions are rare and are noted only when these infants have recurrent infections and are noted to be severely neutropenic. Table 57.1 summarizes important congenital neutropenia syndromes. Kostmann disease is an important example that is caused by mutations in *HAX1*,[7] with consequent arrest of neutrophil maturation at the promyelocytic stage. Cyclic neutropenia is a rare autosomal dominant condition with mutations in the *ELANE* gene. These patients have regular drops in ANCs to levels <250 µL/mL at 3-weekly intervals. Bone marrow studies in these patients demonstrate an arrest in neutrophil maturation that precedes or coincides with severe neutropenia.[6]

3. Immune-mediated neonatal neutropenias: These conditions should be considered in infants with persistent neutropenia. Neonatal alloimmune neutropenia (NAIN) occurs when the mother develops antibodies against fetal red blood cells carrying a paternally derived human neutrophil antigen,[2] and these antibodies are then transmitted across the placenta back into the fetus to cause neutropenia. NAIN can be severe and protracted. Neonatal autoimmune neutropenia results when mothers have antineutrophil autoantibodies that cross the placental and bind fetal neutrophils. This form of neutropenia is usually milder than NAIN.[2] In addition to allo- and autoimmune neutropenia, some patients have been reported with the so-called autoimmune neutropenia of infancy. This relatively transient form of immune neutropenia is caused by antineutrophil autoantibodies produced by the neonate's own immune system.[8]

4. Sepsis: Neonates, particularly those born preterm, can become neutropenic during sepsis[2] due to exhaustion of neutrophil reserves. Neonates have a limited neutrophil storage pool in the bone marrow.[9] In the proliferative pool, the progenitors have a higher steady-stage rate of proliferation at baseline, which reduces the ability of these cells to substantially increase production when needed, resulting in neutropenia.
5. Idiopathic neutropenia of prematurity: This is seen in some growing premature infants, possibly because a large fraction of the marrow progenitors is committed to erythroid differentiation to compensate for anemia of prematurity. This is a benign form of neutropenia that typically presents after the early neonatal period (week 4–10). Neutropenia is usually transient and recovers spontaneously in these patients.[10]

Diagnosis and Laboratory Evaluation

A complete blood count with differential leukocyte counts is important in the initial evaluation of patients with neutropenia. Concomitant presence of anemia and thrombocytopenia would indicate marrow failure syndromes. On the other hand, an increased number of immature neutrophils and a high immature/total ratio indicates increased neutrophil destruction and marrow that is actively proliferating to restore neutrophil numbers. In comparison, a normal immature/total ratio may indicate decreased neutrophil production. If autoimmune or alloimmune neutropenia is being considered, maternal anti-NAIN antibody titers and typing for NAIN antigens in the mother, father, and infant is indicated. In infants with prolonged neutropenia (2 weeks to months), a bone marrow biopsy should also be considered.[1]

Management

Therapy with recombinant granulocyte colony stimulating factor (rG-CSF) and recombinant granulocyte-macrophage colony stimulating factor (rGM-CSF), which are myeloid growth factors, can be used in neutropenic infants. Unlike G-CSF, which primarily affects neutrophil populations, GM-CSF stimulates proliferation of both neutrophil and macrophage precursors. Both G-CSF and GM-CSF can increase neutrophil counts, but G-CSF is more effective. G-CSF (rG-CSF) can also raise neutrophil counts in many patients with congenital neutropenia, such as those with Kostmann syndrome and cyclic neutropenia, and it can reduce the frequency of infections.[10] G-CSF is also an effective therapy in immune-mediated neutropenia.[2]

Recombinant G-CSF treatment has been evaluated in neonatal sepsis. Smaller studies have shown some success, but no convincing effects were seen in a Cochrane review by Carr et al.[10–12] Intravenous immunoglobin can mobilize neutrophils from the storage pool into circulation and has been tried.[13] Similarly, the efficacy of granulocyte transfusions in sepsis is uncertain.[14]

Defects in Adhesion and Transepithelial Migration

Leucocyte Adhesion Deficiency

Leucocyte adhesion deficiency (LAD) is a rare autosomal recessive (AR) disorder impairing adhesion, migration, and phagocytic ability of neutrophils (Fig. 57.1). Many infants present with delayed separation of the umbilical cord and sometimes omphalitis. Some infants go on to have recurrent bacterial infections, recurrent skin and periodontal infections, and deep tissue abscesses. In a patient with typical clinical features, neutrophilia raises the clinical suspicion, which can be confirmed by flow cytometry of peripheral blood leukocytes to measure CD18 expression on neutrophils.

There are three types of LAD. LAD-1 results from mutation in the integrin β_2 *(ITBG2)* gene, which is located on chromosome 21q22.3 and encodes the CD18 subunit of β_2 integrins. More than 100 mutations have been reported in the *ITGB2* gene, including many that are missense, involving the splice site, small deletions, large deletions, and nonsense mutations. The degree of clinical severity and prognosis depends on CD18 expression, and hence, LAD1 can be classified into mild (CD18 expression >30%), moderate (2%–30%), and severe (<2%).[15] The clinical suspicion can be confirmed by flow cytometry for lack of expression of CD18 on neutrophils or by genetic testing.

Hematopoietic stem cell transplantation (HSCT) is the treatment of choice, although it is used mostly in patients with severe LAD1. Recently, adipose tissue-derived mesenchymal stem cells have shown some promise in improving wound healing in murine LAD1 via adaptive release of transforming growth factor beta (TGF-β1).[16] Similarly, gene therapy studies using different vectors have shown promising short- as well as long-term results in canine LAD1. These findings have increased the enthusiasm for future research in humans.[17,18]

LAD-2 is an extremely rare AR disorder caused by mutations in the Solute Carrier Family 35 Member C1 *(SLC35C1)* gene, which encodes the guanosine diphosphate–fucose transporter 1. The clinical hallmark of LAD2 is recurrent bacterial infections (less severe than LAD1) and developmental abnormalities including psychomotor and mental impairment, dysmorphic facies (coarse facial features, broad nasal tip, hypertelorism, and microtia), and short stature (not seen

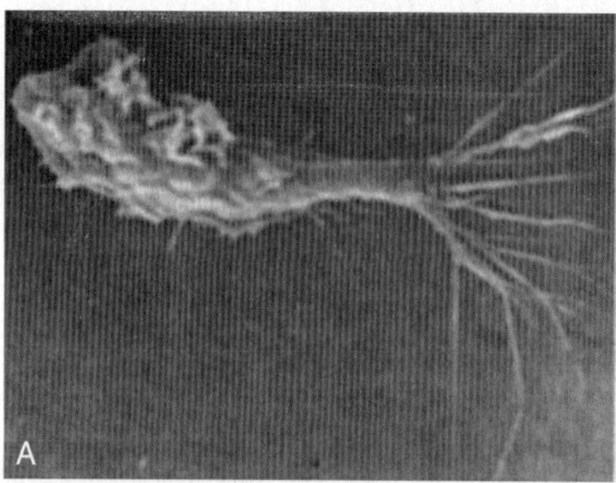

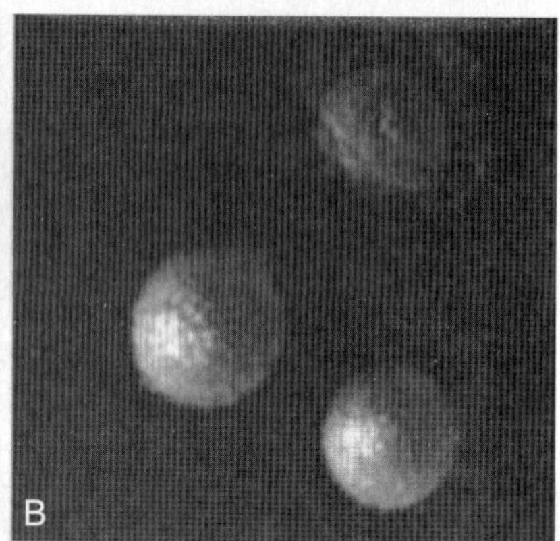

Fig. 57.1 Scanning Electron Micrographs. The scanning electron micrographs show attachment and spread of (A) control and (B) leukocyte adhesion deficiency neutrophils through cell surface integrins. (Reproduced with permission and minor modifications from Letterio et al. Hematologic and oncologic problems in the fetus and neonate. In: *Fanaroff and Martin's Neonatal-Perinatal Medicine*, 79, 1416–1475.)

in LAD1).[19,20] The *SLC35C1* gene is located on chromosome 11p11.2, and mutations result in decreased expression of fucosylated glycans on the cell surface, including the sialyl Lewis X ligand that binds selectins. Therefore LAD2 is also known as congenital disorder of glycosylation type IIc. Flow cytometry can confirm the diagnosis by showing a lack of sialyl Lewis X (CD15s) expression on the leukocyte cell surface and the absence of H antigen on the red blood cell surface (Bombay blood type). Oral supplementation with high-dose fucose has benefitted some patients, but the effect is not consistent.[20]

LAD3 is also a very rare AR disorder resulting from mutations in the *FERMT3* (FERM Domain Containing Kindlin 3; F for 4.1 protein, E for ezrin, R for radixin, and M for moesin) gene located on chromosome 11q13.1. *FERMT3* mutations lower the expression of kindlin-3, causing impaired integrin activation and impaired leukocyte and platelet adhesion. LAD3 shares the clinical features with LAD1 with an additional platelet aggregation defect; the diagnosis is suspected when a patient presents with typical clinical manifestations but flow cytometry shows normal expression of β_2-integrins. Therefore confirmation of diagnosis requires next-generation sequencing looking at mutation in the *FERMT3* gene. The high tendency for bleeding (even in the intracranial area) and risk of infections qualifies these patients for early HSCT.

Defects in Chemotaxis and Cellular Life Span

Hyper-Immunoglobulin E Syndromes (HIES)

Hyper-immunoglobulin E (IgE) syndromes are a group of rare primary immunodeficiency disorders characterized by neonatal-onset, chronic, atopic-like dermatitis and recurrent cutaneous, mucocutaneous, and lung infections due to *Staphylococcus aureus* and *Aspergillus*; musculoskeletal anomalies including hyperextensible joints, scoliosis, and recurrent fractures; and dental anomalies such as retained primary teeth. Reduced neutrophil chemotaxis, most likely due to defects in protein signaling related to signal transducer and activator of transcription 3 (STAT3), is recognized. There are also variable T-cell defects. Serum IgE levels are high. In infancy, many of these characteristic features could still be absent, and dermatitis develops with exposure to pathogens at about the first 2 weeks of life. Unlike neonatal acne, the dermatitis progresses to other areas of the body and resembles eczema. IgE levels and worsening dermatitis can be prevented by meticulous skin hygiene.

These diseases are known to follow autosomal dominant (AD), AR, and X-linked patterns in some families, but most reported cases have been sporadic. Loss-of-function missense and in-frame insertion/deletion mutations with a dominant negative effect in the *STAT3* gene is the prototype of these disorders and is also known as Job syndrome. The *STAT3* gene, located on chromosome 17q21.2, plays a crucial role in modulating inflammatory response as well as regulation of matrix metalloproteinases. Recently, loss-of-function mutations with a dominant negative effect in the Erbb2-interacting protein *(ERBB2IP)* gene, located on chromosome 5q12.3, and in the caspase recruitment domain containing protein-11 *(CARD11)* gene, located on 7p22.2, have been described in patients with hyper Ig-E syndromes.[21,22] HIES resulting from AR mutations are rare, including deficiencies in the interleukin 6 (IL6) receptor and IL6 signal transducer, ZNF341, phosphoglucomutase-3 (located on chromosome 6q14.1, causing severe dysmorphic features), and SPINK5 (Comel-Netherton syndrome). Lastly, unique variants of HIES are related to abnormal TGFBR1 or TGFBR2 signaling and result in Loeys-Dietz syndrome with characteristic aortic aneurysms. Although in the past, genes affected by AR mutations in dedicator of cytokinesis 8 (DOCK8, located on chromosome 9p24.3) and tyrosine kinase 2 (located on chromosome 19p13.2) were categorized in the HIES group, currently they are grouped with syndromic combined immunodeficiencies.[23] As the name suggests, elevated serum IgE levels ($\geq$2000 IU/mL) are a universal laboratory finding and begin to rise after birth and normalize with advancing age. Eosinophilia is also common. The serum IgE level of degree of eosinophilia does not correlate with disease activity. The diagnosis is confirmed by DNA testing. Treatment is mainly supportive, aiming at meticulous skin care and prophylactic antistaphylococcal antibiotic and antifungal treatment to prevent infections. Success of HSCT depends on underlying mutation and gene involvement; the best results have been reported in infants with AR mutations of DOCK8.[24–26]

Defects in Chemotaxis and Bacterial Killing

Chédiak-Higashi Syndrome

Chédiak-Higashi syndrome (CHS) is a rare AR disease characterized by an accumulation of enlarged lysosome and granules in various cell types including neutrophils, lymphocytes, melanocytes, and platelets (Fig. 57.2). Clinically, the characteristic features of CHS include recurrent skin, lung, and gingival *S. aureus* infections, oculocutaneous albinism, bleeding tendencies, and progressive neurodegeneration. Almost all patients with CHS who survive childhood eventually develop hemophagocytic lymphohistiocytosis (HLH), commonly known as accelerated phase. Patients with HLH present with high fever, pancytopenia, lymphohistiocytic infiltration causing lymphadenopathy, and hepatosplenomegaly. The HLH is the primary cause of mortality in CHS.

CHS neutrophils show giant granules and impaired chemotaxis, phagocytosis, and intracellular killing. The disease involves mutations in the lysosomal trafficking regulator *(LYST)* gene, located on chromosome 1q42.3. Due to the large size of the *LYST* gene, numerous mutations including nonsense, missense, frameshift, and splice-site mutations have been reported throughout the gene. The diagnosis is confirmed by identification of mutation(s) in the *LYST* gene by genetic testing. The treatment is limited to supportive care. Timely

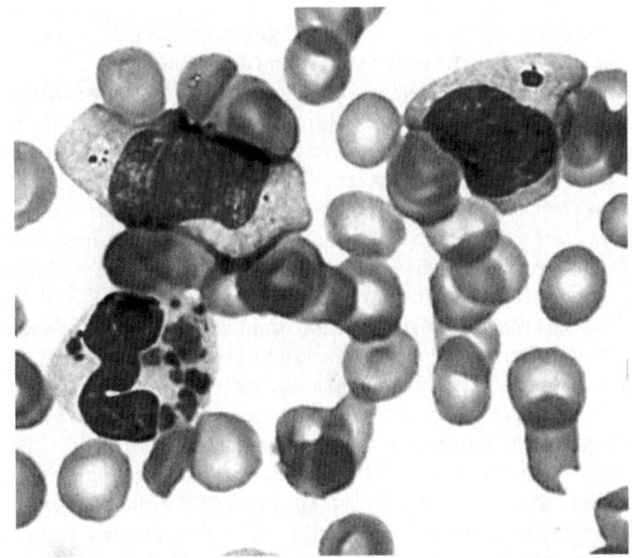

Fig. 57.2 Chédiak-Higashi Neutrophils and Lymphocytes With Large Granules. (Reproduced with permission and minor modifications from Nasr et al. Hematologic and oncologic problems in the fetus and neonate. In: Nasr MR, Hutchison RE. *Henry's Clinical Diagnosis and Management by Laboratory Methods*. January 1, 2022.)

diagnosis and early initiation of HSCT are the key in patients with HLH. Despite HSCT, neurodegeneration in HLH remains inevitable. Due to the size of the *LYST* gene and the wide distribution of mutations on the already large *LYST* gene, gene therapy remains elusive in patients with CHS.

Warts, Hypogammaglobulinemia, Infections, and Myelokathexis Syndrome

The neonatal presentation of a syndrome characterized with warts, hypogammaglobulinemia, infections, and myelokathexis is known as WHIM syndrome. A subset of these patients has cardiac abnormalities in infancy. Predisposition for warts secondary to susceptibility for human papilloma virus may occur later in life. However, early presentation is dominated by neutropenia and lymphopenia, and patients may be identified by newborn screening for severe combined immunodeficiency with low T-cell receptor excision circle (TREC) levels. The genetic defect is mostly in the C-X-C Motif Chemokine Receptor 4 *(CXCR4)* gene and results in gain-of-function increased signaling that retains the neutrophils and lymphocytes in the bone marrow. A pathognomonic finding of myelokathexis is reflective of this process; however, because it is an invasive and operator-dependent diagnostic tool, patients often are recognized late. Depending on the level of neutropenia and antibody deficiency syndrome, treatment approach may include granulocyte stimulating hormone and immunoglobulin replacement therapy. In select cases, patient may also quality for HSCT.

Chronic Granulomatous Disease

Chronic granulomatous disease (CGD) is a rare genetic syndrome that presents clinically with recurrent bacterial and fungal infections, particularly during early infancy, and involving various body organs including the skin, soft tissue, lungs, lymph nodes, liver, bones, and gastrointestinal tract. The most frequently encountered species include *S. aureus, Burkholderia cepacia, Nocardia, Serratia marcescens, Salmonella,* and *Aspergillus,* most of which are catalase-positive microorganisms that are often hard to identify with common microbiological testing and are difficult to eradicate effectively because they require a prolonged treatment course (3–6 months). A novel approach with sequencing for pathogenic DNA can be of high importance in CGD patients with active disease, and this method is gaining importance among patients with complex fungal diseases.

Most patients with CGD have defect(s) in the nicotinamide adenine dinucleotide phosphate (NADPH) oxidase complex that impair the intracellular bactericidal properties of neutrophils. The NADPH oxidase has five essential structural components: NOX2 (also known as $gp91^{phox}$), $p22^{phox}$, $p47^{phox}$, $p67^{phox}$, and $p40^{phox}$. $Gp91^{phox}$ is the main enzymatic component that needs $p22^{phox}$ for stability. Together, these proteins form the NADPH-binding flavocytochrome b_{558} in the plasma membrane. During the resting state, the binding site is not available for NADPH. At the time of infection or inflammation, a complex of cytosolic proteins $p47^{phox}$, $p67^{phox}$, and $p40^{phox}$ bind with NOX2/$p22^{phox}$ dimer, make the NADPH binding site accessible, and activate NADPH oxidase. Once active, NOX2/$p22^{phox}$ accepts an electron from NADPH and makes it available for reactive oxygen species (ROS) generation.[27] Mutations involving any of these five components can impair the function of the NADPH complex, impairing ROS availability in the phagocytic vacuoles and causing CGD. The most common form of CGD results from mutations of the cytochrome b (558) subunit beta *(CYBB)* gene located on X-chromosome Xp21.1-911.4 and encoding $gp91^{phox}$. The second most common cause of CGD is mutations in the neutrophil cytosolic factor 1 *(NCF1)* gene on chromosome 7q11.23, encoding $p47^{phox}$. Most other forms are inherited AR and involve mutations in *NCF2* on chromosome 1q25.3, *CYBA* on chromosome 16q24.2, and NCF4 on chromosome 22q13.3, encoding $p67^{phox}$, gp22phox, and p40phox, respectively.[27]

CGD is diagnosed by flow cytometry assay by measuring neutrophil oxidant production. Normal activated neutrophils oxidize dihydrorhodamine 123 and increase fluorescence. Historically, the diagnosis of CGS was based on the nitroblue tetrazolium test (NBT); normal neutrophils produce superoxide and reduce NBT, but this does not occur consistently in CGD. Molecular genetic testing to test all the five genes is available. If prior family testing is available, other testing options can be explored.

Management of CGD patients requires antibiotic and antifungal prophylaxis. Prophylactic trimethoprim-sulfamethoxazole given daily reduces the burden of bacterial infection, and similarly, itraconazole daily reduces the fungal infection rate. Interferon-γ three times a week has been shown to reduce serious bacterial and fungal infections and can be considered.[28] Once infection develops, clinicians must cautiously evaluate for deep-seated infections. HSCT is the mainstay of CGD treatment. Recently, gene therapy for X-linked CGD has been evaluated for safety and efficacy. The study demonstrated restored NADPH-oxidase activity with infection-free time.[29] However, further studies are needed.

Myeloperoxidase Deficiency

Myeloperoxidase (MPO) deficiency is an inherited, autosomal recessive disorder of phagocytes with mutations in the MPO gene on chromosome 17q22, impairing MPO-dependent generation of bactericidal ROS such as the H_2O_2-halide system. However, MPO-independent mechanisms to generate ROS also exist, which often makes MPO deficiency clinically silent. MPO deficiency is diagnosed by measuring neutrophil peroxidase activity. Most patients are asymptomatic, and hence, prophylactic antibiotics are not warranted.

Macrophages Derived From Tissue Progenitors and From Monocytes

In neonates, tissue macrophages are derived from progenitors first in the yolk sac from myeloblasts and erythro-myeloid progenitors and then from the vascular endothelium in the aorta-gonad-mesonephros zone. These cells subsequently develop in the liver and bone marrow, and some subgroups are seen in specific organs such as the gastrointestinal system. These macrophages are important for host immunity, inflammation, cellular homeostasis and turnover, tissue remodeling during development, and tissue repair.

Defects in monocyte maturation have been noted in lysosomal diseases such as Gaucher disease, mucopolysaccharidoses, osteopetrosis, and metachromatic leukodystrophy; defects in pathways for the synthesis of complement components; and defects in microbicidal activity such as chronic granulomatous disease (conditions with defects seen in other leukocytes such as neutrophils). Most of these conditions present first with multisystem organ dysfunction, not isolated immune deficiencies.

Adaptive Immune System

The adaptive immune system, including T and B cells, starts its diversification and selection against self-reactivity at a very early age in utero. The preimmune B-cell repertoire further evolves with exposure to foreign antigens such as infections and food antigens to eventually shape the full immune repertoire needed to fight infection. Defects in early B-cell development result in full or near absence of

B cells and circulating antibodies, except maternally acquired IgG. Unlike B cells, T-cell receptor diversification is solely located in the thymus; however, in the periphery, unique T-cell subsets develop to help antibody response (CD4+ Th), antiviral cytotoxicity (CD8+ T), and regulation of immune responses. Full absence of functional T cells may be a consequence of either defects in primary T-cell development or thymic environment. Regulatory T cells are essential during early infancy to prevent autoimmune complications and tendency for atopic diseases. Newborn screening with T-cell receptor excision circle (TRECs) is available in the United States and allows for the early detection of an abnormal adaptive immune system, specifically T-cell deficiency, severe combined immunodeficiency, DiGeorge syndrome, and other forms of primary immunodeficiencies.

Antibody Production Defects

Selective IgA Deficiency

Selective IgA deficiency is the most common primary immunodeficiency, but it usually presents after infancy.[30] The prevalence varies worldwide from 0.006% to 0.6% depending on the race and ethnicity of study population.[31–33] The underlying genetic defects vary and may include maturation defect of B and/or T cells. Clinically, most patients are asymptomatic, possibly because of compensatory overproduction of other immunoglobulins. Patients who develop severe symptoms usually present with recurrent sinopulmonary, gastrointestinal, or urogenital tract infections because IgA plays a vital role in mucosal immunity. Allergies and autoimmune diseases are also prevalent in this patient population.[30]

X-Linked Agammaglobulinemia

X-linked agammaglobulinemia (XLA), also known as Bruton agammaglobulinemia, is one of the more common primary immunodeficiency disorders. It is caused by mutations in the Bruton tyrosine kinase (BTK) gene located on chromosome Xq22.1. BTK is a Tec family tyrosine kinase involved in B-cell maturation and generation of plasma cells and immunoglobulins. Although rare, autosomal recessive and autosomal dominant inheritance patterns have been reported causing agammaglobulinemia.[34]

Clinical manifestations of XLA are recurrent bacterial infections from pyogenic organisms including *Streptococcus pneumoniae*, *Hemophilus influenzae*, and *Pseudomonas* spp. Viral infections from echoviruses, coxsackieviruses, hepatitis viruses, and enterovirus have been reported. Usually, the infant is protected from infections by maternal IgG antibodies during first 6 to 9 months of life. Diagnostic criteria include (1) flow cytometry showing <2% CD19+ and CD20+ B cells and hypogammaglobulinemia; (2) BTK gene mutation and/or defective BTK protein expression; and (3) family history of a maternally related male with XLA.[35] The mainstay of XLA treatment consists of lifelong immunoglobulin replacement therapy.[36] Prophylactic antibiotics may be considered in patients with recurrent life-threatening infections despite immunoglobulin replacement therapy. The role of HSCT in XLA management is not well studied. Gene therapy remains in the early phase of exploration with promising results.[37] Recently, Gray et al.[38] showed nearly physiological levels of BTK expression after clustered, regularly interspaced short palindromic repeats-associated protein 9 (CRISPR-Cas9)–mediated gene editing of XLA. This provides a foundation for future research.

Transient Hypogammaglobulinemia of Infancy

Transient hypogammaglobulinemia of infancy (THI) is characterized by transient drops in IgG levels 2 standard deviations below expected levels during infancy. Physiologically, transplacentally acquired IgG from the mother starts plunging down in the first 6 months of infancy, during which most infants begin to produce IgG. Due to unknown reasons, some infants have a protracted nadir of IgG levels. As the name suggests, this protracted nadir of IgG is transient and resolves without any intervention. Most patients remain asymptomatic. THI is suspected in an infant with recurrent respiratory, gastrointestinal, and urinary trach infections. In such symptomatic patients, common variable immunodeficiency and XLA must be excluded. One important clue for a THI diagnosis can be preserved responses to vaccines.

Hyper-Immunoglobulin M Syndrome

Hyper-immunoglobulin M syndrome (HIGM) is a rare primary immunodeficiency characterized by normal or elevated serum IgM levels and low or absent levels of IgA, IgG, and IgE, suggesting an underlying defect in the class switch recombination process. The most common clinical manifestation seen in patients with HIGM is severe infection. The most common site of involvement is the respiratory tract, followed by the gastrointestinal tract; pneumonia is the most common infection. The patients are susceptible to opportunistic pathogens including *Pneumocystis (carinii) jiroveci*, *Cryptococcus*, *Candida*, *Mycobacterium*, and *Histoplasma*.

Genetically, HIGM is heterogenous with X-linked, AR, and AD inheritance involving numerous genes. The X-linked hyper-IgM accounts for 70% of all HIGM cases and is caused by mutation in the *CD40L* gene located on chromosome Xq26.3. *CD40L* is expressed on Th cells, and such mutations impair the class switch in B cells, resulting in these cells producing only IgM. Autosomal recessive HIGM is caused most often by mutations in activation-induced cytidine deaminase on chromosome 12p13.31, uracil DNA glycosylase on chromosome 12q24.11, and CD40 on chromosome 20q13.12. Autosomal recessive HIGM is characterized by B-cell intrinsic defects. Autosomal dominant mutations in various genes have also been described.[39,40] Evaluation includes quantitative assessment of immunoglobulins to confirm a normal or elevated IgM level with associated low IgG, IgA, and IgE levels. The laboratory assessment should be complemented with targeted gene panels.

The management of HGIM is based on the underlying genetic defect. Infectious complications are managed by antimicrobial agents, and some may require monthly antibiotic prophylaxis and intravenous immunoglobulins. Neutropenia can be treated with granulocyte colony stimulating factor. Despite all these measures, mortality is high in patients with X-linked HIGM, and therefore, stem cell transplant is used frequently. Gene therapy focused on CD40L expression is being tried.[41–46]

T-Cell Defects

Chromosome 22q11.2 Deletion Syndrome

Chromosome 22q11.2 deletion syndrome (22q11 DS) is the most common T-cell disorder with multiorgan involvement. Most patients with 22q11 DS have a 3-Mb deletion on chromosome 21 affecting >100 genes. The resulting haploinsufficiency of many genes is well described, including key roles of T-box transcription factor 1 (TBX1) and DiGeorge Critical Region 8 (DGCR8) in most of the clinical phenotypes.[47] The phenotype is variable with facial dysmorphisms; congenital cardiac defects (mainly conotruncal and aortic arch defects); velopharyngeal insufficiency with or without cleft palate, causing speech delay; thymic hypoplasia; parathyroid hypoplasia presenting as hypocalcemia; developmental delay; and renal, ocular, and skeletal malformations. Thymic

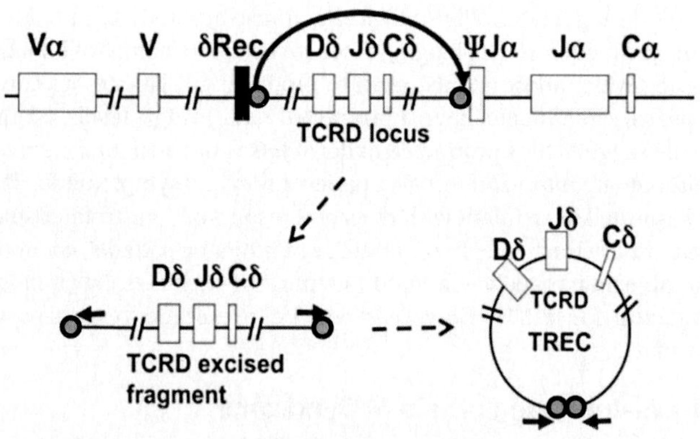

Fig. 57.3 T-Cell Receptor Excision Circle (TREC) Assay. TRECs are small circles of DNA created in T cells during their passage through the thymus as they rearrange their T-cell receptor (TCR) genes. Their presence indicates maturation of T cells; TRECs are reduced in severe combined immunodeficiency disease. T cells can recognize an enormous range of antigens because the TCRs are formed thorough recombination of multiple gene segments known as variable (V), diversity (D), and joining (J) regions that lie close to the constant regions. During TCR rearrangement, a series of enzymes introduce double-stranded DNA breaks at specific sites, rejoin different segments, and then process and repair the segments. The excised DNA fragments, which are not incorporated into the TCR, can form a variety of circular DNA structures known as TRECs. The figure shows generation of the δRec-ψJα TRECs (*REC*, receptor excision circle). The germline configuration of the T-cell receptor α (TCRA) locus, with T-cell receptor delta (TCRD) embedded, is shown at the top of the illustration, which also shows the points *(gray dots)* at which the DNA is cut to excise the TCRD locus in T-lymphocyte progenitors destined to express the α and β TCRs. After excision *(lower left)* and ligation *(lower right)* of the δRec-ψJα fragment to form a TREC, PCR primers *(horizontal arrows)* can amplify a DNA junction fragment containing the joint. (Reproduced with permission from Taki et al. Newborn screening for severe combined immunodeficiency. From: *Pediatric Clinics of North America*. 2019;66:913–923. The legend has been modified.)

hypoplasia/aplasia with consequent T-cell developmental impairment is the cause for immunodeficiency in 22q11 DS. It is crucial to identify such newborns early because they are born with profound immunodeficiency and are at risk for various infections due to opportunistic pathogens. Besides the characteristic but variable clinical presentation of dysmorphism, newborn screening for SCID with TREC may contribute to early recognition of these patients.

A newborn metabolic screen may identify many infants with TREC (Fig. 57.3). Newborns with hypocalcemic seizures, severe conotruncal cardiac anomalies, and severe immunodeficiency should raise clinical suspicion. The diagnostic method of choice is fluorescence in situ hybridization for 22q11.2 microdeletions. Immunodeficiency in 22q11 DS requires reconstitution of the immune system. In patients with complete thymic aplasia, thymic tissue transplant is warranted. Infection prevention is important and can be achieved by hand hygiene, prophylactic antimicrobials, and immunoglobulin replacement therapy. Patients with complete 22q11 DS are at risk for graft-versus-host disease after blood transfusion; therefore such patients must receive leukoreduced, cytomegalovirus (CMV)–negative, irradiated blood products.

Immune Deficiency Affecting Multiple Cell Lineages

Severe Combined Immunodeficiency

Severe combined immunodeficiency (SCID) is a heterogenous group of disorders primarily impairing T cells in combination with primary or secondary defects in development of B and/or natural killer (NK) cells (Table 57.2, Fig. 57.4). The International Union of Immunological Societies' primary immunodeficiency diseases committee categorized SCID into T-B+ and T-B− phenotypes. In the general population with no consanguinity the most frequently seen are X-linked mutations involving interleukin 2 receptor subunit gamma (IL2RG) located on chromosome Xq13.1. Other common mutations are AR recombination activating gene 1 (RAG1, located on 11p12), RAG2 (located on 11p12), and adenosine deaminase (ADA, located on chromosome 20q13.12). There is a shift of the frequency of the most common phenotype in hypomorphic (partial) SCID variants and in populations is high rate of consanguinity.

The pathogenesis of SCID due to ADA deficiency is unique because there is a clearly known enzymatic defect, and therefore, the treatment for ADA-deficient SCID differs from traditional SCID management (Fig. 57.5). ADA deficiency leads to accumulation of its toxic substrates, adenosine (Ado) and 2′-deoxyadenosine (d-Ado), in lymphocytes causing apoptosis.[48] These substrates can also disrupt cellular functions in the lungs, brain, bones, liver, and kidneys.[49] The current standard of care is characterized by enzyme replacement therapy to all ADA-SCID patients as an immediate stabilizing measure and as a bridge for definitive HSCT or HSC gene therapy.[49] Enzyme replacement therapy restores ADA activity and reestablishes B-cells, T-cells, and antibodies within 2 to 4 months of therapy. However, long term lymphocyte reconstitution is not sustained and therefore, ADA-SCID patient will ultimately need HSCT or HSC gene therapy. Lentiviral HSC gene therapy is promising with markedly improved survival at 36 months of follow-up.[50]

The impact of early diagnosis of SCID and timely treatment is significant because infectious complications, survival outcomes, and healthcare burden differ substantially if proper treatment including transplant can be instituted within 3.5 months of life.[51,52] In the United States, SCID screening is included in newborn

Table 57.2 Clinical Manifestations Frequently Associated With Severe Combined Immunodeficiency (SCID)
SCID presents early in life with severe infections such as respiratory infections, diarrhea, and sepsis.
Fifty to seventy percent of infants have lymphopenia compared with age-specific normal ranges.
T-cell lymphopenia is notable. In some cases, absolute B and NK lymphocytopenia may also be noted. Some infants may show maternally derived T lymphocytes, which can thrive in infants with SCID, and hence, a normal ALC does not rule out SCID.
Most states in the US now enumerate TRECs to screen for SCID (see Fig. 57.3). TRECs are numerous in newly generated T cells and scarce when T cells are absent or when maternally engrafted T cells are present.
SCID is a genetically heterogeneous disorder that is composed of many genetic defects. The most frequently seen subtype, inherited as an X-linked trait, is T− B+ NK−.
Adenosine deaminase deficiency frequently presents with few/no lymphocytes (T− B− NK− SCID). Testing for the ADA enzyme level is critical, because if confirmed to be absent, treatment with PEG-ADA can have therapeutic value.

ADA, Adenosine deaminase; *ALC*, absolute lymphocyte count; *NK*, natural killer cell; *PEG-ADA*, polyethylene glycol-modified adenosine deaminase; *TREC*, T-cell receptor excision circle.

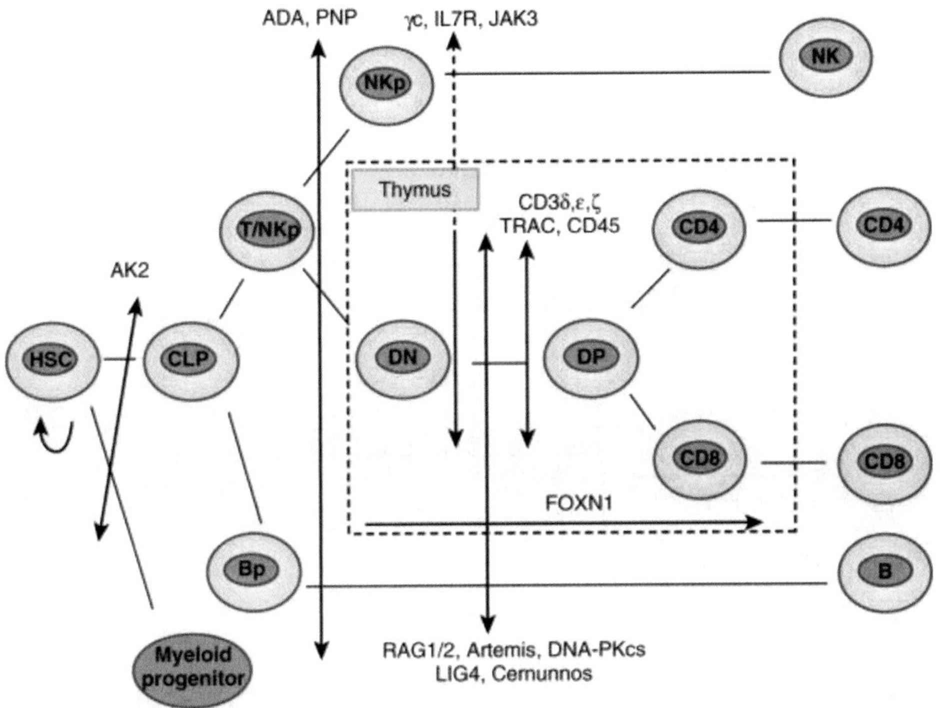

Fig. 57.4 Genetic Defects Associated With Severe Combined Immune Deficiency. Schematic representation of blocks *(arrows)* in lymphoid development associated with genetic defects responsible for severe combined immunodeficiency. *Dashed line* indicates that the generation of NK lymphocytes is compromised in γc and JAK3 deficiency but not in IL7R deficiency. *ADA,* Adenosine deaminase; *AK2,* adenylate kinase 2; *B,* B cell; *Bp,* B-cell progenitor; *CLP,* common lymphoid progenitor; *DN,* double-negative thymocyte; *DNA-PKcs,* DNA protein kinase catalytic subunit; *DP,* double-positive thymocyte; *γc,* common gamma chain; *HSC,* hematopoietic stem cell; *IL7R,* interleukin-7 receptor; *JAK3,* Janus-associated kinase 3; *LIG4,* DNA ligase IV; *NK,* natural killer cell; *NKp,* natural killer cell progenitor cell; *PNP,* purine nucleoside phosphorylase; *RAG,* recombinase activating gene; *T/NKp,* common progenitor of T and natural killer lymphocytes; *TRAC,* T-cell receptor alpha constant chain.

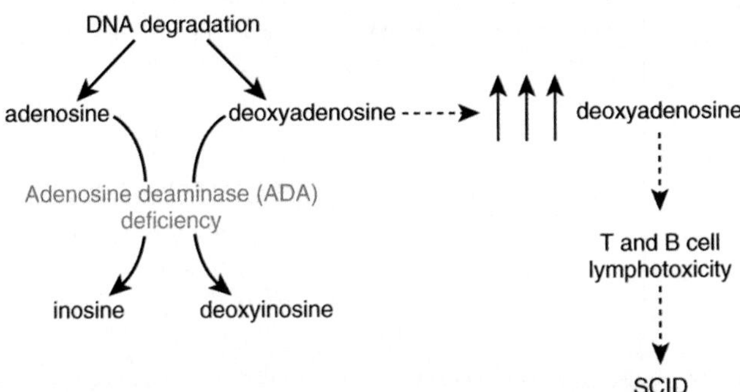

Fig. 57.5 Adenosine Deaminase (ADA) Converts Adenosine to Inosine and Deoxyadenosine to Deoxyinosine. In ADA deficiency, deoxyadenosine accumulation in lymphocytes is lymphotoxic, killing the cells by impairing DNA replication and cell division to cause severe combined immunodeficiency. (From Nussbaum et al. The treatment of genetic disease. In: *Thompson and Thompson Genetics in Medicine*, ch. 13, 257–282.)

screening programs, focused on TREC, a marker for naïve T cells, from dried spot blood (see Fig. 57.3). The test may yield false positive results suggesting low levels of TREC in prematurity and in infants with trisomy 21, DiGeorge syndrome, ataxia telangiectasia, trisomy 18, and CHARGE (coloboma, heart defects, atresia choanae, growth retardation, genital abnormalities, and ear abnormalities) syndrome. There may also be some false negative results, and such infants may present later with failure to thrive, chronic diarrhea, and recurrent mucocutaneous/systemic infections with atypical pathogens including *Pneumocystis jirovecii*, *Cryptosporidium*, *Mycobacteria*, and/or *Candida* (Fig. 57.6). The biggest challenge for detection of patients with SCID is among patients with prematurity and/or intrauterine growth retardation (IUGR). Normally, SCID patients are born full-term in an asymptomatic stage. Because preterm infants often are detected with low TREC levels, the possibility of SCID in this group could be overlooked. In particular, in patients with a combination of prematurity and IUGR, it could be the result of intrauterine infection and maternal stressors (drugs) without SCID. However, a unique group of SCID disorders linked to DNA repair defects may present with a combination of prematurity, IUGR, and extralymphatic complications. Radiosensitivity and genetic testing are key diagnostic modalities to identify these patients in time. The specific diagnosis could also alter preparations for conditioning.

After a positive newborn screen or typical clinical presentation, diagnosis is confirmed by one of two criteria: (1) a low absolute number of T cells (< 300 CD3 T cells/mm^3) and (2) impairment as measured by proliferation of T cells on mitogen stimulation. Although not required for diagnosis, evaluating lymphocyte subpopulations such as B cells and NK cells and quantitative assessment of immunoglobulins are important because they help in the classification of these patients. Similarly, genetic testing by next-generation sequencing can provide information for counseling and antenatal testing.

The goal of clinical management of SCID is early diagnosis, prevention of infection, and early initiation of HSCT to improve survival. *Pneumocystis jirovecii* prophylaxis with trimethoprim-sulfamethoxazole can be started within the first week of life. Antifungal prophylaxis is indicated with additional risk factors. Monoclonal antibody palivizumab may be needed to prevent respiratory syncytial virus infections during high-risk seasons. Care must be taken to limit blood

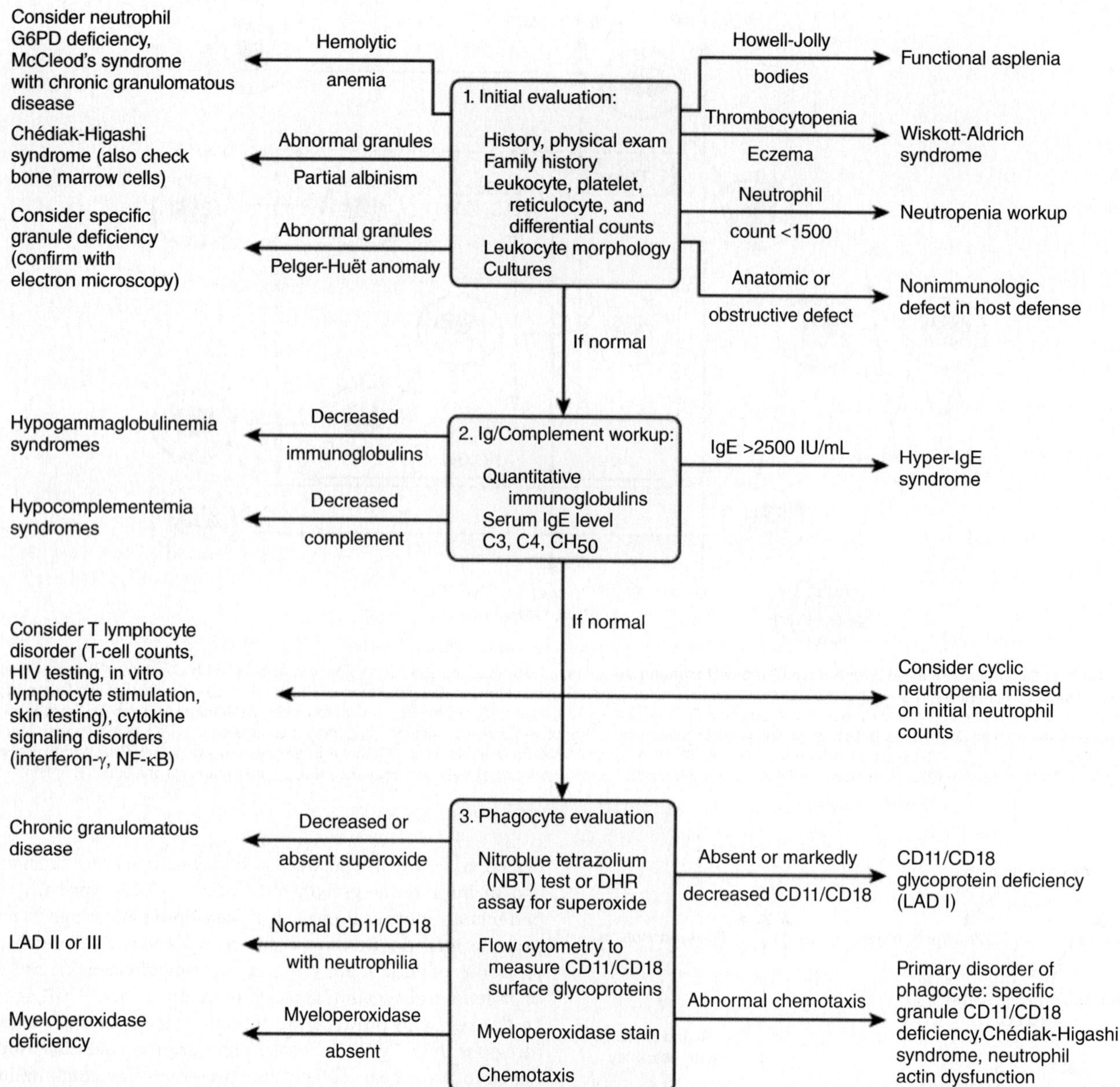

Fig. 57.6 Algorithm for the Workup of a Young Infant With Recurrent Infections. Units for the neutrophil count *(box 1)* are neutrophils/mm³. *DHR,* Dihydrorhodamine; *G6PD,* glucose-6-phosphate dehydrogenase; *HIV,* human immunodeficiency virus; *Ig,* immunoglobulin; *LAD,* leukocyte adhesion deficiency; *NBT,* nitroblue tetrazolium; *NF-κB,* nuclear factor κB. (Reproduced with permission and minor modifications from Dinauer et al. Phagocyte system and disorders of granulopoiesis and granulocyte function. From: *Nathan and Oski's Hematology and Oncology of Infancy and Childhood*, ch. 22, 773–847.e29.)

product transfusions, and if needed, the blood products must be leukoreduced, CMV negative, and irradiated to prevent CMV infection and later graft-versus-host reaction. Monthly intravenous infusions can help maintain optimum levels of IgG. The definitive treatment of SCID is hematopoietic stem cell transplant prior to the onset of severe infections.[51–53] Gene therapy for X-linked SCID is still in the experimental phase. Gene therapy using retroviral or lentiviral vectors can help normalize T-cell counts and reduce the risk of opportunistic infection,[54] but some patients may have increased risk of leukemia.[54] Further work is needed.[55]

SECTION 11

Kidney

OUTLINE

CHAPTER

58 Neonatal Acute Kidney Injury

Heidi J. Steflik, David T. Selewski, Alison Kent, Cherry Mammen

KEY POINTS

1. Acute kidney injury (AKI), previously referred to as "acute renal failure", is defined by an abrupt change in the glomerular filtration rate with rising serum creatinine levels or decrease in urine output. AKI is associated with adverse outcomes.
2. The newborn kidney undergoes a number of physiologic and functional changes after birth that impact its function and increase the susceptibility to AKI.
3. The risk of AKI is higher in premature and critically ill infants; those with systemic illness due to birth asphyxia, sepsis, or necrotizing enterocolitis; and infants with congenital heart disease under/after treatment with extracorporeal membrane oxygenation or after cardiac surgery/cardiopulmonary bypass.
4. AKI has been associated with nephrotoxic medications, including antibiotics such as aminoglycosides and vancomycin, nonsteroidal antiinflammatory drugs, and diuretics.
5. The KDIGO (Kidney Disease: Improving Global Outcomes) classification is a useful tool for early identification of AKI severity.
6. Several ongoing research studies seek to measure/monitor kidney function, determine the risk of AKI and the impacts of its early identification, and identify potential treatment options.

Introduction

During the past decade, there have been extraordinary advances in our understanding of neonatal acute kidney injury (AKI). During this time, it has become clear that AKI occurs commonly in critically ill neonates and is associated with adverse outcomes irrespective of the specific neonatal population studied. AKI is no longer considered a symptom of illness severity but instead an independent risk factor for adverse outcomes, impacting short-term outcomes (length of mechanical ventilation, length of stay, and mortality) as well as long-term kidney health (subsequent chronic kidney disease [CKD] and hypertension).

Neonates with AKI represent some of the most challenging patients encountered in the intensive care unit. A firm understanding of AKI risk factors and pathophysiology is necessary for neonatal providers as well as an appreciation of the unique characteristics of neonatal AKI. This chapter provides a comprehensive overview of neonatal AKI including developmental considerations, definitions, epidemiology and risk factors, evaluation, novel approaches, management, and long-term outcomes.

Developmental Considerations

In order to appreciate the intricacies of neonatal AKI, an understanding of nephrogenesis and the dynamic kidney function changes that occur after birth is critical. A detailed understanding of these processes is outside the scope of this chapter, but this section will serve as a primer to better understand the pathophysiology and potential impact of neonatal AKI on outcomes.

Nephrogenesis

Nephrons are the functional units of the kidney, and their development occurs until 36 weeks' gestation.[1] At 15 weeks' gestation there are on average 15,000 nephrons and by 40 weeks of gestation, 745,000 nephrons, with 60% of nephrogenesis occurring in the third trimester.[2]

Animal models and neonatal autopsy studies have shed light on the impact of premature birth on nephron endowment and structure. Altered glomerular structure in 0.2% to 18% of glomeruli in the outer renal cortex has been found in a preterm baboon model.[3] Premature mice models have shown reduced nephron number with subsequent development of reduced glomerular filtration rate (GFR), proteinuria, and hypertension in adulthood.[4] In a postmortem study of human preterm neonatal kidneys, infants who were born preterm and survived for a period of time were noted to have accelerated maturation and abnormal glomerular morphology in comparison with stillbirth controls.[5] Abnormal glomerular morphology may result in later glomerular loss, resulting in hypertension and CKD. This altered glomerular morphology and function in the preterm neonatal kidney is associated with a reduced capacity to respond to insults and an increased susceptibility to injury. As a result, premature birth results in lower nephron endowment, placing the kidney at risk for adverse short- and long-term outcomes.

Dynamic Changes in Renal Blood Flow and Physiology After Birth

After birth, the newborn kidney undergoes a number of physiologic and functional changes that impact function and susceptibility to AKI. At birth, the kidneys receive only 2.5% to 4% of total cardiac output compared to 20% to 25% in adults. This increases to 6% at 24 hours of life, 10% at the end of the first week, and 15% to 18% at 6 weeks of age.[6–9] These changes are driven by increased peripheral vascular resistance and decreased renal vascular resistance. Perfusion in the newborn kidney is dependent on a delicate balance of vasodilatory and vasoconstrictive factors. The greater reliance on factors such as prostaglandins and angiotensin to maintain renal blood flow in the neonatal kidney explains the most potent, adverse impact of medications such as nonsteroidal antiinflammatory drugs and angiotensin converting enzyme inhibitors on kidney function.

Changes in kidney function parallel increases in renal blood flow. GFR is also considerably lower at birth than later in life. In term infants, GFR is 10 to 20 mL/min/1.73 m^2, increasing to 30 to 40 mL/min/1.73 m^2 by the second week of life and increasing steadily during the ensuing months to reach an adult level by 2 years of age.[10–12] Preterm neonates have an even lower GFR at birth that increases at a slower rate compared with term infants. Due to tubular immaturity, preterm neonates excrete higher amounts of sodium and have less ability to concentrate urine than do healthy, term infants and adults.[13–15] This has implications for susceptibility to AKI because increased sodium excretion can be accompanied by significant diuresis, leading to hypovolemia. This risk for AKI is potentially compounded by exposures to nephrotoxic medications in the face of volume depletion.

Definitions of Neonatal AKI

AKI, previously referred to as "acute renal failure," is defined by an abrupt change in GFR (Fig. 58.1) identified by a rise in serum creatinine (SCr) or decrease in urine output. SCr is known to be an imperfect clinical biomarker for AKI but remains the gold standard for diagnosis at this time. In general, SCr is a delayed marker of AKI (elevated 48–72 hours after insult) and reflects changes in function rather than ongoing tubular damage. Defining AKI in neonates is further complicated by dynamic changes in renal physiology after birth, as noted above, and the presence of maternal SCr. With the increase in GFR that occurs in the first weeks of life, SCr slowly decreases.[16–18] However, the trajectory of declining SCr is also highly dependent on gestational age (GA) with a slower decline seen in lower GA infants.[13,15]

During the past two decades there has been a transition from threshold-based definitions of AKI to staged definitions that represent the entire spectrum of injury that typifies AKI. These definitions include the Risk, Injury, Failure, Loss, and End stage renal disease (RIFLE), the Acute Kidney Injury Network classification (AKIN), and most recently, the Kidney Disease: Improving Global Outcomes (KDIGO) definition.[19–22] A multitude of studies have been performed using these staged definitions of AKI in a variety of neonatal populations.[23–25] This important work led to the development of a consensus neonatal definition of AKI.

In 2013, an expert working group consisting of neonatologists and nephrologists at a National Institutes of Health–sponsored neonatal AKI workshop agreed that the neonatal modified KDIGO

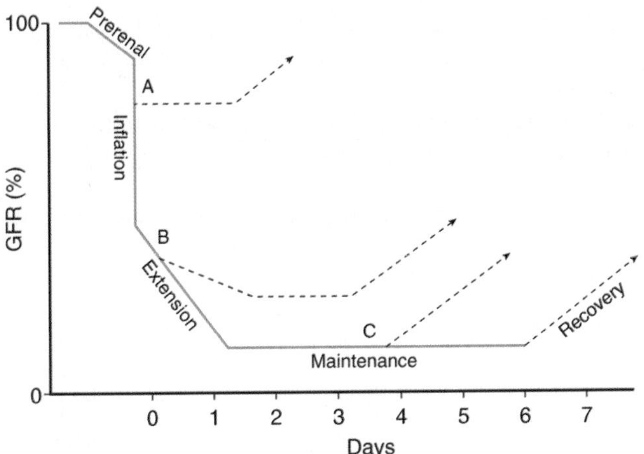

Fig. 58.1 Phases of Acute Kidney Injury. *GFR*, Glomerular filtration rate. (Reproduced with permission and after minor modifications from Kliegman et al. Renal failure. *Nelson Textbook of Pediatrics*, chap. 550, 2769–2779.e1.)

Table 58.1 Neonatal Acute Kidney Injury KDIGO Classification

Stage	SCr Criteria	Urine Output Criteria[a]
0	No change in SCr or rise < 0.3 mg/dL	>0.5 mL/kg/hour
1	SCr rise ≥ 0.3 mg/dL within 48 hours or SCr rise ≥ 1.5–1.9 × reference SCr[b] within 7 days	<0.5 mL/kg/hour for 6–12 hours
2	SCr rise ≥ 2–2.9 × reference SCr[b]	<0.5 mL/kg/hour for >12 hours
3	SCr rise ≥ 3 × reference SCr[b] or SCr ≥ 2.5 mg/dL or Receipt of dialysis	<0.3 mL/kg/hour for >24 hours or anuria for >12 hours

[a]Urine output for the AWAKEN study was collected over a 24-hour period and differed slightly from these criteria.

[b]Reference SCr, defined as the lowest previous SCr value.

KDIGO, Kidney Disease: Improving Global Outcomes; *SCr*, serum creatinine.

definition should be used as a consensus definition for neonatal AKI (Table 58.1).[26] The modifications of the neonatal KDIGO definition include a reference SCr value, defined as the lowest previous SCr value and an absolute SCr cutoff of ≥2.5 mg/dL (221 μmol/L) to define severe AKI (stage 3). Using this definition, single-center studies and the multicenter AWAKEN (Assessment of Worldwide Acute Kidney Injury Epidemiology in Neonates) study have clearly shown AKI occurs commonly in the neonatal intensive care unit (NICU) and is associated with adverse outcomes.[27]

In discussions about AKI definitions, it is critical to consider urine output. Although urine output criteria have been included in every AKI staging iteration, they have rarely been systematically studied. This largely stems from the challenges of quantifying urine output and retrieving this data from medical records. As a result, the contribution of urine output to AKI has largely been ignored in the AKI literature until recently. Recent multicenter work in critically ill children and neonates has clearly shown that AKI as defined by urine output identifies distinct episodes of AKI associated with adverse outcomes that would have been missed by SCr-based criteria alone.[27,28] Although there remain important questions about the optimal threshold and duration of oliguria, it is clear that urine output is a critical component to the definition of neonatal AKI.[29]

It is important to appreciate that the authors of the consensus statement acknowledge the fact that the neonatal modified KDIGO definition represents a starting point for an iterative process in defining neonatal AKI. In an effort to begin to interrogate the current definition of neonatal AKI, a secondary analysis of the AWAKEN study data was undertaken to evaluate optimal definitions based on GA.[27] The study identified a number of opportunities for optimization of the neonatal AKI definition, including unique SCr rise cutoffs for different GAs.[30] The optimal absolute SCr rise thresholds to predict mortality were ≥0.3 mg/dL (≥26.5 μmol/L) for <29 weeks' GA and ≥0.1 mg/dL (≥8.85 μmol/L) for ≥29 weeks GA. Further prospective studies are needed to determine the optimal SCr-based neonatal AKI definition for both clinicians and researchers. Until further work is done and subsequent consensus modifications of the neonatal AKI definition are published, it is recommended that clinicians and researchers use the neonatal modified KIDGO criteria to define neonatal AKI.

Epidemiology and Risk Factors for Neonatal AKI

Despite the many recent advances in our understanding of neonatal AKI, there are no evidence-based treatments for AKI. As a result, it is critical to understand which neonatal populations are at highest risk to develop AKI. Single-center work has clearly shown that there are identifiable patient factors and disease characteristics that predispose neonates to AKI. The AWAKEN study has provided a large, multicenter, retrospective review of risk factors for AKI in both the early (first 7 days) and later neonatal period.[31,32]

Several specific populations of neonates are known to be at high risk for AKI, including premature neonates (particularly very low birth weight [VLBW, i.e., birth weight <1,500 g] and extremely low birth weight [ELBW, i.e., birth weight <1,000 g] infants) and infants with specific diseases processes including sepsis, necrotizing enterocolitis (NEC), and hypoxic-ischemic encephalopathy (HIE), as well as those infants who reuire extracorporeal membrane oxygenation, and those with congenital heart disease requiring cardiac surgery. Preterm infants, especially VLBW and ELBW infants, are known to be at particularly high risk for AKI given the dynamic changes in renal blood flow and physiology after birth compounded by lower nephron endowment as described above. These vulnerable patients are also known to have prolonged hospitalizations with potential for multiple episodes of AKI and are particularly sensitive to other perinatal factors and nephrotoxins. Table 58.2 includes epidemiologic study findings for premature, VLBW, and ELBW infants, specifically. The epidemiology, as well as the pathophysiology believed to be underlying the increased risk for AKI in each of these conditions, is shown in Table 58.3.

Table 58.2 Epidemiology of Neonatal Acute Kidney Injury in Premature, Very Low Birth Weight, and Extremely Low Birth Weight Infants

Classification	Study	Incidence of AKI	Findings
Premature infants	Ladeiras 2018[101] (n = 106)	22.6%	• Lower GA was an independent risk factor for AKI (aOR, 0.39; 95% CI, 0.2–0.76; *P* = .006)
	Shalaby 2018[100] (n = 214)	56%	• Those with AKI had lower GA (AKI: 35±3 weeks vs. no AKI: 32±4 weeks; *P* < .001) • Lower GA was independently associated with increased risk of AKI (RR, 4.8; 95% CI, 3–9) • AKI was independently associated with mortality (RR, 5.49; 95% CI, 2–14)
	Elmas 2018[102] (n = 105)	20%	• Lower GA was an independent risk factor for AKI (aOR, 3.21; 95% CI, 1.12–9.30; *P* = .032)
	Stojanovic 2017[103] (n = 195)	44%	• Infants with AKI had a lower GA compared with infants without AKI (27.6±3.8 weeks vs. 30.3±3.9 weeks; *P* < .001) • AKI was an independent risk factor for mortality (OR, 7.49; 95% CI, 3.19–17.58)
	Nagaraj 2016[104] (n = 450)	12%	• Functional kidney failure rate[a]: 48.14% • Intrinsic kidney failure rate[b]: 51.85%
	Weintraub 2016[105] (n = 357)	30.3%	• GA was associated with early AKI (OR, 0.51; 95% CI, 0.40–0.65; *P* < .001)
	Stoops 2016[106] (n = 125)	30.5%	• AKI was associated with an increased risk of grade II or higher IVH (HR, 3.55; 95% CI, 1.39–9.07) and grade III or higher IVH (HR, 4.34; 95% CI, 1.43–13.21)
	Stojanovic 2014[107] (n = 150)	26%	• Lower GA was associated with AKI (AKI: 27.3±3.1 weeks vs. no AKI: 31.3±3.3 weeks; *P* < .001)
VLBW and ELBW infants	Askenazi 2015[107a] (n = 122)	30%	• AKI was independently associated with increased risk of oxygen requirement or of dying at 28 days of life (RR, 1.45; 95% CI, 1.07–1.97; *P* < .02).
	Chowdhary 2018[108] (n = 483)	60%	• Mortality was higher in infants with advanced AKI regardless of the AKI definition used[c]
	Srinivasan 2018[109] (n = 457)	19.5%	• Infants with AKI had significantly higher mortality (25/89 [28%] vs. 15/368 [4%]; *P* < .001)
	Daga 2017[110] (n = 115)	22.6%	• Lower GA was associated with AKI (AKI: 25 weeks [IQR, 24–27 weeks] vs. 29 weeks [IQR, 27–30 weeks]); *P* < .001)
	Lee 2017[111] (n = 276)	56%	• Lower GA was an independent risk factor for AKI (aOR, 0.7; 95% CI, 0.58–0.83; *P* < .001) • Severe AKI (KDIGO stage 3) was associated with increased mortality (HR, 10.6; 95% CI, 2.1–53.7)
	Carmody 2014[112] (n = 455)	39.8%	• Rate of multiple episodes of AKI: 16.5% • AKI was independently associated with mortality (aOR, 4.0; 95% CI, 1.4–11.5; *P* = .01)
	Rhone 2014[34] (n = 107)	26.2%	• Inverse relationship between BW and nephrotoxic medications received per day (R^2, 0.169; *P* < .001) • Infants with AKI received more nephrotoxic medications per day than infants who did not have AKI (0.24 vs. 0.15; *P* = .003)
	Koralkar 2011[23] (n = 229)	18%	• AKI was associated with mortality (crude HR, 9.3; 95% CI, 4.1–21.0; *P* < .001)

[a]Functional kidney failure was defined as all cases without oliguria but with persistently deranged kidney function (i.e., a minimum of two abnormal values taken 24 hours apart) and cases of oliguria that responded to a challenge test, with kidney sonography not revealing any abnormality and with no persistent biochemical derangement.

[b]Intrinsic kidney failure was defined as cases with oliguria responding to a challenge test but having either persistent biochemical derangement of kidney function or kidney sonography demonstrating altered echo texture.

[c]See study for specific data points.

AKI, Acute kidney injury; *aOR*, adjusted odds ratio; *BW*, birth weight; *CI*, confidence interval; *ELBW*, extremely low birth weight; *GA*, gestational age; *HR*, hazard ratio; *IQR*, interquartile range; *IVH*, intraventricular hemorrhage; *KDIGO*, kidney disease: improving global outcomes criteria; *RR*, relative risk; *VLBW*, very low birth weight.

Table 58.3 Epidemiology and Pathophysiology of Neonatal Conditions Associated With Increased Risk of Acute Kidney Injury

High AKI Risk Conditions	Pathophysiology	Epidemiology: Study	Epidemiology: Findings
Sepsis	• Kidney hypoperfusion, ischemia, direct injury of kidney tubule cells, inflammation, and apoptosis all play a significant role[113] • Effects on the microcirculation are associated with organ dysfunction[114,115] • AKI can occur despite maintenance of systemic BP and RBF in septic episodes[114,115]	Vachvanichsanong 2012[116] (n = 139)	• AKI rates: 0.9%–6.3% • Sepsis was the most common cause of AKI (30.9%) • Sepsis-associated AKI independently increased risk of mortality (aOR, 13.7; 95% CI, 3–63.5; $P < .001$)
		Mathur 2006[117] (n = 200)	• AKI rate: 26% • AKI was associated with increased mortality (70% vs. 25%; $P < .001$)
NEC	• May be associated with bacteremia, systemic inflammation; animal models show widespread kidney inflammation, disruption of tight junction proteins, and AKI[118]	Bakhoum 2019[119] (n = 77)	• AKI rates: 42.9% • AKI was associated with increased mortality (HR, 20.3; 95% CI, 2.5–162.8; $P = .005$)
		Criss 2018[120] (n = 181)	• AKI rates: 54% • AKI was independently associated with mortality (HR, 2.4; 95% CI, 1.2–4.8; $P = .009$)
HIE	• During the hypoxic event, blood is diverted to critical organs, resulting in decreased perfusion and oxygen supply to the kidneys • Renal parenchymal cells have limited ability to perform anaerobic metabolism and increase susceptibility to reperfusion injury[121]	Chock 2018[122] (n = 38)	• AKI rate: 39% • Patients with AKI had higher Rsats compared with those without AKI after 24 hours of life ($P < .01$)[a]
		Medani 2014,[123] Karlo 2014,[124] Matyanga 2013[125]	• AKI rate: 33.3%–56%
		Alaro 2014[126] (n = 60)	• AKI rate: 11.8%–51.6%, depending on severity of HIE • 24-fold increases risk of death in neonates with AKI ($P = .001$)
		Sarkar 2014[127] (n = 88)	• AKI rate: 39% • AKI during therapeutic hypothermia was predictive of abnormal brain MRI findings at postnatal day 7–10 (OR, 2.9; 95% CI, 1.1–7.6)
		Selewski 2013[25] (n = 96)	• AKI rate: 38% • AKI was associated with prolonged duration of mechanical ventilation (aR2, 0.292; $P < .001$) and NICU stay (aR2, 0.279; $P < .001$)
ECMO	• Risk factors for AKI that are inherent to their critical illness (underlying disease, hypotension, nephrotoxic medication, etc.) • Unique aspects of ECMO that increase the risks of AKI include systemic inflammation after cannulation, a hypercoagulable state, and hemolysis[128]	Mallory 2019[71] (n = 424)	• AKI rate: 47.4% • AKI was associated with in-hospital mortality ($P = .02$)
		Fleming 2016[129] (n = 832)	• AKI rates: 66%–74% depending on definition used • AKI was independently associated with ECMO duration (AKI: 149 hours vs. No AKI: 121 hours; $P = .01$) and mortality (aOR, 1.52; 95% CI, 1.04–2.21; $P = .03$)
		Zwiers 2013[130] (n = 242)	• AKI rate: 64% • High-stage AKI was independently associated with mortality ($P < .001$)[a]
		Askenazi 2011[131] (n = 7941)	• AKI was independently associated with mortality in neonates (aOR, 3.2; 95% CI, 2.6–4.0; $P < .0001$) and pediatrics patients (aOR, 1.7; 95% CI, 1.3–2.3; $P < .001$)

Continued

Table 58.3 Epidemiology and Pathophysiology of Neonatal Conditions Associated With Increased Risk of Acute Kidney Injury—Cont'd

High AKI Risk Conditions	Pathophysiology	Epidemiology: Study	Epidemiology: Findings
Congenital heart disease and cardiac surgery	• Multifactorial in nature: ∘ Nephrotoxic exposures, ∘ Ischemic-reperfusion injury ∘ Systemic inflammation[132,133] • Defined risk factors for AKI in those undergoing cardiac surgery: ∘ Age <1 year ∘ Risk Adjustment in Congenital Heart Surgery (RACHS) category score ≥4 ∘ Bypass time ≥90 minutes ∘ Single ventricle physiology ∘ Preoperative inotrope support ∘ Preoperative AKI[134,135]	SooHoo 2018[136] (n = 95)	• AKI rate: 40% (44% with correction for FO) • Use of modified Blalock-Taussig shunt (aOR, 9.38; 95% CI, 1.68–52.56; *P* = .01) and higher VIS score on postoperative day 1 (aOR, 1.20; 95% CI, 1.06–1.35; *P* = .003) were associated with increased risk of AKI
		Mah 2018[137] (n = 117)	• AKI rate (≥stage 2 AKI): 21% • Patients with greater FO were more likely to have ≥stage 2 AKI (<10% FO: 9.8 vs. 10%–20% FO: 18.2 vs. >20% FO: 52.4%; *P* = .013)
		Kumar 2016[138] (n = 102)	• AKI rate: 0%–8% depending on stage of AKI • Higher STAT category was an independent risk factor for AKI (aOR, 3.43; 95% CI, 1.59–7.42; *P* < .01)
		Piggott 2015[139] (n = 95)	• AKI rate: 45% • AKI was associated with increased LOS (AKI: 22 days [IQR, 29 days] vs. no AKI: 5 days [IQR, 9 days]); *P* = .002) and postoperative ventilator days (AKI: 22 [IQR, 29] vs. no AKI: 5 [IQR, 9]; *P* < .001)
		Alabbas 2013[140] (n = 122)	• AKI rate: 62% • Severe AKI associated with mortality (OR, 6.7; 95% CI, 1.1–41.5) and longer PICU stay (HR, 9.09; 95% CI, 1.35–60.95)
		Morgan 2013[141] (n = 264)	• AKI rate: 64% • AKI was independently associated with longer times to extubation (*P* < .0001), ICU discharge (*P* = .0001), and hospital discharge (*P* = .001)[a] • AKI was independently associated with mortality (aHR, 7.3; 95% CI, 1.6–33.4; *P* = .01)
		Blinder 2012[135] (n = 430)	• AKI rate: 52% • Severe AKI was associated with mortality, increased duration of mechanical ventilation, and inotrope support[a]

[a]See study for specific data points.

aHR, Adjusted hazard ratio; *aR2*, adjusted R-squared value; *AKI*, acute kidney injury; *aOR*, adjusted odds ratio; *BP*, blood pressure; *CI*, confidence interval; *ECMO*, extracorporeal membrane oxygenation; *FO*, fluid overload; *HIE*, hypoxic ischemic encephalopathy; *HR*, hazard ratio; *ICU*, intensive care unit; *IQR*, interquartile range; *LOS*, length of stay; *MRI*, magnetic resonance imaging; *NEC*, necrotizing enterocolitis; *NICU*, neonatal intensive care unit; *OR*, odds ratio; *PICU*, pediatric intensive care unit; *RACHS*, risk adjustment for congenital heart surgery; *RBF*, renal blood flow; *Rsats*, renal saturations; *STAT*, Society of Thoracic Surgeons Congenital Heart Surgery mortality categories; *VIS*, vasoactive-inotropic score.

Incidence and Outcomes: AWAKEN Study

Single-center NICU studies using modern, staged definitions of neonatal AKI, similar to the modified neonatal KDIGO classification, have clearly shown that AKI occurs commonly and is associated with adverse outcomes. The AWAKEN study, the only large multicenter NICU study to date including more than 2000 infants, revealed a similar AKI incidence to prior single-center studies at 29.9% using SCr and urine output KDIGO criteria.[27] AKI incidence varied by GA groups (22–29 weeks': 49.7%; 29–36 weeks': 18.3%; and >36 weeks': 36.7%). When classified according to highest AKI stage, 46.4%, 23.6%, and 29.9% of patients with AKI were classified as stages 1, 2, and 3, respectively. After adjusting for several potential confounders, infants with AKI had 4.6 times higher odds of mortality (95% CI, 6.1–11.5 times) and stayed in hospital 8.8 days longer (95% CI, 6.1–11.5 days). Data from this landmark study confirm the strong association of the neonatal KDIGO definition with poor outcomes observed in single-center studies.

Perinatal Risk Factors

There are a multitude of perinatal risk factors that predispose neonates to AKI. These can be broadly characterized as prenatal exposures, demographics, and perinatal events. Patient characteristics

Table 58.4 Commonly Used Nephrotoxic Medications in the NICU and Their Mechanism of Injury

Medication	Mechanism of Nephrotoxic Injury
Aminoglycosides (e.g., gentamicin)	Proximal tubular toxicity, resulting in accumulation of the drug in lysosomes, rise in intracellular reactive oxygen species, phospholipidosis, and cell death; toxicity also includes intrarenal vasoconstriction and glomerular/mesangial cell contraction
Nonsteroidal antiinflammatory medications (e.g., ibuprofen, indomethacin)	Inhibition of prostaglandin production causes afferent arteriole constriction and subsequent reduction in GFR
Diuretics (e.g., furosemide)	May cause intravascular volume contraction and reduced kidney blood flow with subsequently reduced GFR; increased risk of nephrocalcinosis with long-term use of loop diuretics
Vancomycin	Unclear cause of nephrotoxicity; may be due to proximal tubular injury with generation of reactive oxygen species
Angiotensin converting enzyme inhibitors (e.g., enalapril)	Decreased angiotensin II production results in dilation of the efferent arteriole, resulting in decreased GFR
Acyclovir	Urinary drug precipitation that is increased in low flow and hypovolemia states; results in renal tubular obstruction and decreased GFR
Amphotericin B	Distal tubular toxicity, vasoconstriction, and subsequent reduced GFR
Radiocontrast agents	Produce increased reactive oxygen species resulting in kidney tubular toxicity

GFR, Glomerular filtration rate.

associated with increased risk of AKI include earlier GA and lower birth weight. Perinatal events that predispose neonates to AKI include intubation, need for epinephrine during resuscitation, lower Apgar scores, and events that result in HIE (discussed below.) The AWAKEN study confirmed that these perinatal factors are associated with AKI and identified some novel factors that were protective against the development of AKI, including multiple gestation and scheduled cesarean section.[33]

Admission to the NICU invariably results in exposure to nephrotoxic medications—the most common being aminoglycosides, nonsteroidal anti–inflammatory drugs, diuretics, and vancomycin. Nephrotoxic medications are consistently shown to be a risk factor for the development of AKI and represent an important modifiable risk factor. However, there is little epidemiologic data on the burden of nephrotoxic medication exposures in critically ill neonates. Rhone et al. published the most comprehensive evaluation to date in a single-center study of 107 VLBW neonates. In this report, 87% of VLBW infants were exposed to at least one nephrotoxic medication during their hospital stay; for the entire cohort, VLBW infants experienced an average of 2 weeks of nephrotoxic medication exposure during their hospitalization.[34] The mechanisms of nephrotoxic injury for the most common nephrotoxins encountered in the NICU are provided in Table 58.4.

Efforts should be made to minimize nephrotoxin exposure, and a multidisciplinary approach using specially trained clinical pharmacists is critical in these patients. A more detailed discussion of surveillance strategies and the Nephrotoxic Injury Negated by Just-in-time Action (NINJA) project are discussed below.

Evaluation: Prevention and Mitigation of Neonatal AKI

The first crucial step in the evaluation and management of neonatal AKI is to recognize AKI early using the modified KDIGO classification. Next, a thorough evaluation to attempt to determine the underlying etiology is needed to guide efforts to reverse the process believed to be causing the AKI when possible. Clues to the underlying etiology can be gained from the maternal history, perinatal and postnatal course, laboratory results, and radiographic information. The evaluation and management of the consequences of AKI drives most of the interventions.

Although there have been significant advances in our understanding of the epidemiology, risk factors, and outcomes associated with neonatal AKI, there currently are no established treatments for AKI. As a result, the most successful strategy to improve outcomes in critically ill neonates is a multimodal strategy of prevention, early recognition, and comprehensive supportive care. These efforts aim to prevent AKI or to mitigate AKI when it occurs and thus lower the risk of associated morbidities and increased mortality.

Nephrotoxin Avoidance

In recent years, it has become clear that AKI induced by exposure to nephrotoxic medications is independently associated with increased costs and adverse outcomes in hospitalized children.[35–39] Furthermore, nephrotoxin-associated AKI may have long-standing consequences.[35,40] In a recent cohort of 100 noncritically ill children, nephrotoxic medication–induced AKI was associated with reduced estimated GFR, proteinuria, and/or hypertension at a 6-month follow-up in 70% of patients.[35]

In an effort to decrease nephrotoxin exposures in hospitalized children, electronic medical record (EMR) surveillance initiatives have been created and studied. In 2013 Goldstein et al. described the development and implementation of an EMR surveillance initiative aimed at decreasing the rates of nephrotoxic medication–induced AKI, termed the NINJA study.[41] Using the EMR, investigators were able to successfully identify patients at risk of nephrotoxic AKI (defined by exposure to aminoglycosides for $\geq$3 days or $\geq$3 nephrotoxic medications simultaneously). Once these patients were identified, clinicians were reminded of the exposure and encouraged to monitor kidney function (i.e., Scr) daily. In this seminal single-center prospective study, a multidisciplinary effort led to a sustained decrease in AKI rate and improved outcomes. In a recent study using the same systematic surveillance program in a single-center NICU, the authors demonstrated a reduction in high nephrotoxic medication exposure (i.e., $\geq$3 nephrotoxic medications within 24 hours or $\geq$4 calendar days of an intravenous aminoglycoside) from 16.4 to 9.6 per 1000 patient-days ($P = .03$).[42] They also demonstrated a reduction in the percentage of nephrotoxic medication–related AKI (30.9%–11.0%; $P < .001$) and in AKI intensity (9.1–2.9 per 100 susceptible patient-days; $P < .001$) and estimated they prevented

100 AKI episodes during an 18-month period. It is clear from both of these important studies that a multidisciplinary approach involving clinicians and pharmacists, using the best available evidence, is crucial.

Kidney Function Monitoring

An important step in improving outcomes in neonates with AKI is the early identification of those with AKI. At the heart of early recognition is regular surveillance of kidney function, which remains an area of great practice variation. One of the most enlightening findings of the AWAKEN study was the variation in center SCr surveillance practices. The SCr counts per patient at each of the 24 centers in the study varied from a median of one SCr check during the 3-month study period (IQR, 1–1 check) to 11 checks (IQR, 3–26 checks).[27] This study also showed that seven institutions checked a median of ≤2 SCr values during a patient's entire NICU stay. Not surprisingly, the rates of AKI and outcomes varied significantly by institution based on how frequently the institution measured SCr; the site with the lowest AKI rate also had the lowest number of Scr checks and the site with the highest AKI rate had more frequent Scr checks. It is possible, as the authors acknowledge, that the true incidence of AKI may have been underestimated, underlying the importance of AKI surveillance protocols.

This practice variation was further highlighted in a survey of 375 neonatologists and nephrologists that showed only one-third of institutions had protocols to monitor kidney function in neonates receiving aminoglycosides.[43] The development of standardized monitoring protocols and more frequent monitoring of kidney function in those at risk are some of the most feasible ways to improve outcomes in neonatal AKI and are critical areas for education, collaboration, and future research.

Novel Approaches to Determining AKI Risk and Kidney Function

Although it remains critical to standardize kidney-function surveillance protocols in order to diagnose AKI earlier, discoveries that allow for the earlier detection of AKI are paramount. At the heart of this issue is the imperfect nature of SCr as a biomarker of kidney function; it is a marker of lost function and not of ongoing damage. This shortcoming likely explains some of the lack of success in interventional trials in AKI that rely on SCr as a biomarker. Investigators have begun to overcome these issues by using risk stratification based on patient characteristics to identify patients most vulnerable to AKI, studying novel biomarkers of kidney injury, and evaluating other assessments of kidney function.

Risk Factor Assessment: Renal Angina Index

At the crux of identifying AKI early is patient risk stratification, using patient characteristics present on admission or that develop during the intensive care unit (ICU) course to aid in identifying patients at high risk of developing AKI. This concept is embodied in the concept of the renal angina index. The renal angina index is calculated using a scoring system based on patient characteristics combined with markers of kidney dysfunction and stratifies patient risk for the development of subsequent severe AKI. This concept has been developed and validated in critically ill children.[44] Although a similar scoring system remains to be developed and validated in neonates, the concept is critical to improving outcomes.

Novel Biomarkers

There has been a significant amount of research done during the past decade to identify "novel" urine and serum AKI biomarkers that improve our ability to diagnose impending AKI in a timely manner. These biomarkers share the common characteristic of detecting tubular damage, rather than changes in function, and include urine neutrophil gelatinase-associated lipocalin, kidney injury molecule-1, interleukin 18, liver fatty acid binding protein, and others. These biomarkers each have shown the characteristic of rising 2 to 12 hours after an insult and predict the development of SCr-based AKI at 48 hours. Although these novel biomarkers were frequently developed and most commonly studied in children undergoing cardiopulmonary bypass, where the timing of an insult is known, there has been a significant amount of study in a variety of NICU populations.[45–47] As with any biomarker, the sensitivity and specificity of the novel biomarkers is optimized when used in conjunction with a strategy of pointed use based on patient characteristics and risk stratification. Despite promising results, further study is needed to understand how to begin to use novel biomarkers in neonates.

Kidney Function Assessment

One of the more practical advances in AKI diagnosis and management is the use of functional assessments of kidney function. Furosemide is a loop diuretic that is frequently used in efforts to encourage urine output in patients who have developed fluid overload or AKI. The "furosemide stress test" represents a functional test of kidney function that uses a single dose of furosemide followed by quantifying urine output response for 6 hours to identify patients at risk for severe AKI. Although this test was initially developed and validated in critically ill adult populations, single-center work in a variety of pediatric populations has shown similar results.[48] To date there have not been any studies in neonates, but neonatologists should understand the potential prognostic significance of furosemide response.

Management of Neonatal AKI

Supportive Care

AKI is characterized by an abrupt impairment in kidney function that can lead to significant retention of multiple endogenous and exogenous toxins and dysregulation of extracellular fluid volume, electrolytes, and acid-base homeostasis. In the absence of proven treatments for AKI, the care of neonates with AKI is centered on preventing worsening kidney injury and minimizing these sequelae. To achieve this, a multidisciplinary approach that includes neonatologists, nephrologists, dieticians, nurses, and pharmacists is optimal.

Medication Dosing

In order to prevent further kidney injury, it is imperative to understand the nuances of dosing medication in neonates of varying GAs and to involve clinical pharmacists with expertise in this area. Neonates have important differences in their kidney development and maturational variances in their kidney function that significantly impact drug dosing and clearances. This can be further complicated by AKI. For example, in perinatal asphyxia (i.e., HIE), both therapeutic hypothermia and asphyxia itself can alter gentamicin pharmacokinetics, prolonging the clearance of this known nephrotoxin and increasing the risk of AKI.[49,50] As a result, the daily evaluation of patient medications by a team of clinicians and pharmacists with expertise in neonatal AKI and medication dosing is a critical component of AKI prevention and management.

Electrolyte Management

Neonates with AKI are predisposed to electrolyte and acid-base abnormalities including but not limited to metabolic acidosis, hyperphosphatemia with associated ionized hypocalcemia, dysnatremia, and hyperkalemia. In these patents, regular electrolyte monitoring is indicated until kidney function has recovered. Regular assessment and adjustment of enteral and parenteral nutrition in consultation with a nephrologist, dietician, and/or pharmacist to prevent and/or treat significant electrolyte perturbations is necessary.

As the result of impairments in excretion of acid and regeneration of bicarbonate, AKI is commonly associated with metabolic acidosis. Acidosis can sometimes be worsened by the underlying AKI etiology (i.e., poor perfusion from sepsis, diarrhea, and heart failure). If the patient experiences significant metabolic acidosis, treatment to improve the acidosis may be necessary. Cautious correction of acidosis during AKI is recommended, because aggressive treatment with sodium bicarbonate may result in sodium excess, worsening fluid overload, and symptomatic hypocalcemia.

Infants with AKI are also at risk to develop hyperphosphatemia due to impaired phosphorus (PO_4) excretion, with secondary hypocalcemia from increased binding of free calcium (Ca^{++}). Compared with older children, neonates have significantly higher serum phosphate levels at baseline, making the management of AKI-associated hyperphosphatemia particularly challenging in neonates.[51] If enterally fed or receiving total parenteral nutrition, all nutritional options must be reviewed to minimize PO_4 content until hyperphosphatemia and AKI resolve. Concentrated preterm formulas and human milk fortifier are designed to contain high amounts of PO_4 and Ca^{++} to assist in bone development; infants receiving these feeds should be switched to plain breast milk or specifically designated low PO_4 formulas if available. If the PO_4 content of a formula is too high or a low PO_4 formula is not available, pretreating the formula with calcium carbonate (PO_4 binder) or a non–calcium-based binder such as sevelamer is an option.[52–54] Due to risks of an elevated PO_4/Ca^{++} product and extraskeletal calcification, secondary hypocalcemia should not be treated unless severe and/or symptomatic.

Hypo- or hypernatremia may occur depending on the underlying cause of AKI, the infant's fluid balance status, and the presence of oliguria, sodium (Na^+) intake, and the ability of the kidneys to retain Na^+ appropriately. In the face of hyponatremia, where a net Na^+ loss is suspected, Na^+ delivery may be increased. If the problem is excess water accumulation, interventions are necessary to achieve a negative water balance. The etiology of hypernatremia most often is due to a free water deficit as opposed to Na^+ excess. Interventions to make the patient net fluid positive by increasing total fluid delivery using enteral feeds or more hypotonic intravenous fluids may be appropriate in this scenario. Use of daily patient body weights and the clinical examination and history is paramount to distinguishing the etiology and guiding the treatment of hypo- and hypernatremia.

Hyperkalemia is one of the most dangerous complications of AKI and can lead to cardiac arrhythmias, cardiac arrest, and death. Neonates, especially VLBW and ELBW infants, are more prone to hyperkalemia due to low GFR, concurrent acidosis, reduced Na^+/potassium (K^+) pump activity, and reduced tubular K^+ secretion secondary to aldosterone insensitivity.[55–58] If significant hyperkalemia (>6.0 mmol/L) is confirmed, the K^+ content of all available nutritional options should be reviewed and any exogenous K^+ administration must be immediately discontinued. Nutritional supplements such as human milk fortifier may increase K^+ content considerably. If any electrographic changes are observed, cardiac stabilization should begin under electrocardiogram surveillance with treatment options including diuretics (furosemide), insulin with or without dextrose, bicarbonate infusion, and calcium administration. If concurrent metabolic acidosis is present, correction of acidosis may also improve hyperkalemia via intracellular shifting.

Nutrition Management

AKI represents a catabolic state, and providing adequate nutrition to neonates with AKI is critical to their recovery. Although there have been no studies in neonates specifically, a recent study in critically ill children suggests that those with AKI often do not receive adequate nutrition.[59,60] Even though not well studied in neonates, important metabolic abnormalities are induced by AKI, including activation of protein catabolism with excessive release of amino acids and sustained negative nitrogen balance, peripheral glucose intolerance/increased gluconeogenesis, and inhibition of lipolysis with altered fat clearance. Caloric and protein needs of neonates tend to be quite high to support growth and development and should be maintained in catabolic states including AKI.[61,62] Meeting nutritional goals can be a serious challenge in the face of neonatal AKI. When oliguria accompanies AKI, it can be difficult to provide enough nutrition without progression of fluid overload. Inability to remove waste products will lead to increases in blood urea nitrogen and other uremic toxins. In order to optimize nutritional status and improve outcomes, the treatment of neonates with AKI should involve a dietician with expertise in the area. As will be discussed in a later chapter, the inability to provide adequate nutrition remains an indication for renal replacement therapy (RRT).

Fluid Management

Fluid management in AKI is critical. The assessment and measurement of fluid balance is an integral step. There are two methodologies reported in the literature to measure fluid balance: (1) based on cumulative fluid balance or (2) based on changes in body weight.[24,63–67] Weight-based methodologies may be of particular value in neonatal populations, where insensible losses may be more profound and outputs may be difficult to accurately quantify (diaper weight, etc.).[68] This is of particular importance when one considers that a single missing value in cumulative fluid balance calculations makes accurate calculation impossible. An evaluation of the impact of fluid balance in 645 term/near-term neonates in the AWAKEN study demonstrated that only 74% had complete input and output data to accurately calculate fluid balance.[69] As such, the following formula should be used in critically ill neonates to calculate fluid balance:

$$\%\text{Fluid Overload} = \frac{\text{Daily Weight} - \text{Birth Weight or Growth-adjusted Weight}}{\text{Birth Weight or Growth-adjusted Weight}} \times 100$$

Fluid management in neonates with AKI is one of the most challenging problems the clinician will face in managing neonatal AKI. This represents a delicate balance between ensuring adequate intravascular volume to maintain organ perfusion without suffering the deleterious impact of fluid overload. Neonates with AKI may be predisposed to abnormalities in fluid balance for a multitude of reasons including oliguria, iatrogenic fluid administration, systemic inflammation and capillary leak, and disordered fluid homeostasis. Maintaining adequate intravascular kidney perfusion is critical to maintain urine output. The clinician should look for signs of fluid excess or deficit and determine whether there is a component of AKI that is responsive to intravenous fluids. This fluid-responsive AKI, or what was previously labeled "vasomotor nephropathy," is common in neonates and potentially reversible.[70] The fractional excretion of sodium can be a useful tool to identify oliguric neonates who may benefit from intravascular volume expansion; however, normal (or non-low) fractional excretion of sodium in preterm infants does not necessarily indicate adequate intravascular volume due to the limited ability of immature tubules to reabsorb sodium. Irrespective, it may be reasonable to perform a trial of a bolus of isotonic fluids and monitor the urine output response if the patient is not significantly fluid overloaded. If there is no response to the initial fluid challenge, the patient's volume status should be re-evaluated and more conservative fluid management strategies may be considered. This may include use of functional echocardiography to assess cardiac function and filling to help guide fluid management.

The deleterious state of fluid overload has been clearly shown to adversely impact the outcomes in critically ill pediatric populations.[69,71–74] Until recently there have been limited data in neonates evaluating the relationship between AKI and abnormalities in fluid balance. In a study of 58 sick term/near-term neonates, Askenazi et al. demonstrated that neonates with AKI had a higher median percentage of fluid overload at day of life 3 (8.2% [IQR, 4.4%–21.6%] versus −4% [IQR, −6.5% to 0.0%]); $P < .001$).[24] In the AWAKEN study cohort, the impact of fluid balance and AKI was evaluated in 645 term/near-term neonates during the first postnatal week. This study showed that those with AKI had significantly higher median peak fluid balance in the first postnatal week (2.7% [0%–7.4%] versus 0.5% [−0.8% to 4.0%]); $P < .0001$).[69] Furthermore, on adjusted analysis, peak fluid balance in the first postnatal week predicted the need for mechanical ventilation on postnatal day 7.

As mentioned previously, one of the biggest challenges that remain in AKI is the absence of treatments for AKI. While trials of various diuretic regimens have failed to show that diuretics improve outcomes in AKI, it is agreed on that a time-limited trial of diuretics is reasonable in oliguric AKI. In the KDIGO Clinical Practice Guidelines for Acute Kidney Injury, the only recommended use for diuretics in the setting of AKI is in the management of volume overload.[75] A critical component to this recommendation is the time-limited nature of the trial, which may use a loop diuretic such as furosemide. If this trial is not successful, clinicians should manage sequelae as noted above and consider renal replacement therapies.

Evolving Research on Specific Therapeutics

Although there are currently no medical interventions approved for the treatment of AKI, several medications, specifically adenosine receptor antagonists, have been reported to ameliorate the effects of or in some cases prevent neonatal AKI. Adenosine is released in response to hypoxia and ischemia. Adenosine contributes to a fall in GFR by inducing renal vasoconstriction. In turn, adenosine-receptor antagonists have been shown to improve renal perfusion and subsequent kidney function and have shown promise in neonatal cohorts at high risk for AKI, including term infants with perinatal asphyxia, premature infants, and infants requiring congenital cardiac surgery. Theophylline has been studied in perinatal asphyxia. Six trials in asphyxiated infants found that a single prophylactic dose of intravenous theophylline, a methylxanthine with adenosine receptor antagonism properties, had a kidney-protective effect.[76–80] In a metanalysis of these six trials, the pooled estimates suggested a 60% reduction in the incidence of AKI compared with placebo (relative risk, 0.35; 95% CI, 0.25–0.49).[81] A significant limitation in the generalizability of these data is that theophylline has yet to be studied in a population undergoing hypothermia, which is known to alter pharmacokinetic clearance of other drugs. Consequently, the KDIGO guidelines for the management of AKI suggest that a single dose of theophylline should be considered in severely asphyxiated infants at high risk for AKI.[81,82,109] In preterm infants <32 weeks' gestation with respiratory distress syndrome who received daily theophylline for 3 days, there was improved kidney function in the first 2 days of life compared with placebo, including significantly higher urine output (theophylline: 2.4 mL/kg/hour versus placebo: 1.6 mL/kg/hour; $P = .023$) and significantly decreased SCr (theophylline: 0.76 mg/dL versus placebo: 1.0 mg/dL; $P = .025$).[83]

The effect of a more commonly used methylxanthine, caffeine, on AKI has been explored in several studies in premature infants.[34,84–86] Caffeine is commonly used prophylactically in a protocolized manner in premature neonates as a respiratory stimulant to prevent apnea of prematurity. After the previously mentioned positive studies of methylxanthines and perinatal asphyxia, there was interest in evaluating the impact of caffeine on kidney function and subsequent AKI in preterm neonates. Carmody et al. first evaluated this in a single-center retrospective study of 140 VLBW neonates exposed to caffeine in the first postnatal week. In this study, AKI was less common in neonates who received caffeine (17.8% versus 43.6%; $P = .002$). In adjusted analysis, exposure to caffeine was independently associated with less AKI (adjusted odds ratio [aOR], 0.21; 95% CI, 0.07–0.64) with a number needed to treat of 2.9 to prevent a single case of AKI.[86] Subsequently, Harer et al. explored 675 premature infants enrolled in the AWAKEN multicenter retrospective study.[84] Infants who received caffeine in the first 7 days after birth developed AKI less frequently than neonates who did not (11.2% versus 31.6%; $P < 0.01$). After multivariable adjustment, receipt of caffeine remained associated with reduced odds of developing AKI (aOR, 0.20; 95% CI, 0.11–0.34), and for every 4.3 neonates exposed to caffeine, one case of AKI was prevented. Caffeine receipt has also been studied in premature infants with NEC and spontaneous intestinal perforation. Of 146 patients with NEC and spontaneous intestinal perforation, AKI occurred less frequently among patients who received caffeine than in infants who did not receive caffeine (aOR, 0.08; 95% CI, 0.01–0.42).[85]

Although uric acid is not frequently measured in neonates, several case series have shown that rasburicase, a recombinant urate oxidase, may help infants with hyperuricemia and AKI.[87–89] In the largest series, Hobbs et al. reported on seven neonates who received a single intravenous dose of rasburicase (mean dose of 0.17 ±0.04 mg/kg of body weight).[89] Within 24 hours, serum uric acid decreased from a mean of 13.6 to 0.9 mg/dL, SCr decreased from a mean of 3.2 to 2.0 mg/dL, and urine output increased from a mean of 2.4 to 5.9 mL/kg per hour (all $P < .05$). Prior to the use of rasburicase, glucose-6-phosphate dehydrogenase (G6PD) deficiency should be ruled out. Hemolytic anemia is likely to occur in G6PD-deficient patients due to their inability to break down hydrogen peroxide during the oxidation of uric acid to allantoin.[90]

It is critical to note that all of these specific therapies require more extensive testing and evidence from clinical trials research before they are broadly adopted.

Indications for Renal Replacement Therapy

RRT remains a treatment option for neonates with advanced stages of AKI. The details surrounding RRT use in neonates are discussed in Chapter 59. The timing of RRT is one of the most controversial topics in acute-care nephrology. Like any other intervention, the right time to start is when the potential benefits outweigh the potential risks. RRT should be considered when there is impending harm to the patient if the physiologic needs of the patient are not being met under maximal medical management. There are no specific SCr or blood urea nitrogen thresholds that signal the need to initiate RRT. Rather, an evaluation of the trajectory of consequences resulting from the inability of the kidneys to perform their physiologic functions drives the decision to initiate RRT. RRT is indicated when conservative management has failed to adequately control any of the following conditions[33,91]:

1. Fluid overload
2. Hyperkalemia
3. Hyponatremia
4. Refractory metabolic acidosis
5. Hyperphosphatemia
6. Inability to provide necessary blood products, drugs, and/or nutrition without progressive fluid overload
7. Toxicity of certain medications
8. Hyperammonemia related to inborn errors of metabolism

Long-Term Outcomes After Neonatal AKI

The survival of critically ill neonates has improved drastically during the past 30 years. As the survival of the most critically ill and fragile neonates has improved, care has shifted to understanding the pathologic changes in more detail and optimizing their long-term outcomes (Fig. 58.2). Epidemiologic studies have clearly shown that prematurity and perinatal characteristics are risk factors for subsequent CKD later in life.[92,93] The Chronic Kidney Disease in Children Study is a longitudinal study of North American children with CKD. In this study, individuals in the cohort were more likely than the general population to be low birth weight, small for GA, premature, and have a history of a NICU stay.[93,94] This study confirmed previous work that has suggested that events around the time of birth contribute to the risk for CKD later in life.

The concept of fetal origins of adult diseases was first put forward by David Barker.[95] Epidemiologic data have shown that low birth weight neonates are known to be at increased risk of insulin resistance, hypertension, obesity, and coronary artery disease later in life. As mentioned previously, there is likely a similar link between fetal and perinatal events and the risk of CKD later in life for NICU survivors. The pathophysiology is multifactorial with contributions from the disruption of normal nephrogenesis and events in the postnatal period that impact kidney function. The final trimester represents a critical time for nephron development, with more than 60% of

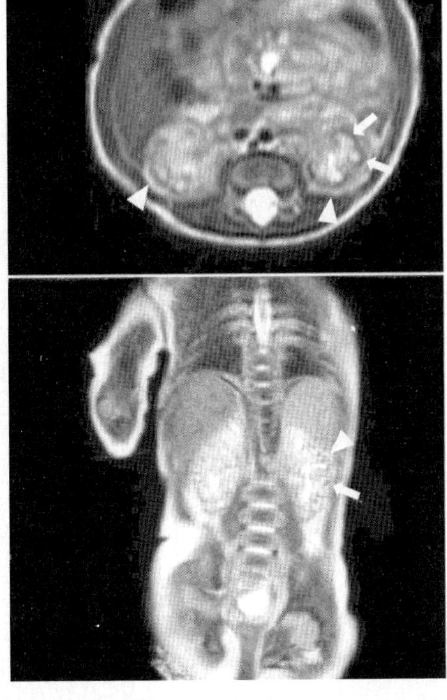

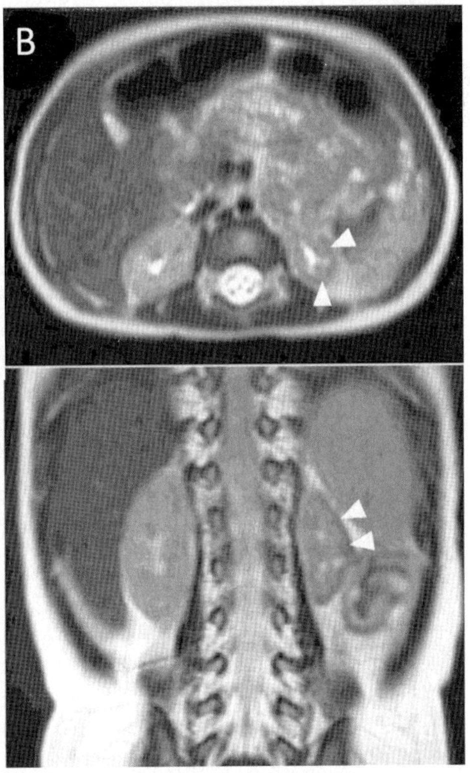

Fig. 58.2 Magnetic Resonance Imaging (MRI) of Renal Cortical Necrosis After Asphyxia. (A) T2-weighted MRI taken on day 13 after birth shows a dark signal rim at the inner cortex *(arrow)*. A relatively high signal intensity of the outer cortex is identifiable *(arrowheads)*. (B) T2-weighted MRI on the sixth month. The left kidney is shrunken and a dark signal intensity rim of the cortex was noted *(arrowheads)*. (Reproduced with permission and after minor modifications from Nishijima et al. Renal impairment following perinatal asphyxia. *Pediatr Neonatol*. 2021;62:451–452.)

nephrons formed during this time period. Furthermore, the extrauterine environment does not allow for proper development. Animal studies and autopsy data have clearly shown that premature neonates have a lower nephron endowment than term infants. While the pathophysiologic link between prematurity and the subsequent risk of CKD is becoming increasingly clear, less is known about the contribution of postnatal events, such as episodes of AKI, to the risk of CKD.

During the past decade it has become clear that discrete episodes of AKI may predispose individuals to subsequent CKD. Several adult studies have shown that AKI is a discrete risk factor for the development of subsequent CKD. This work culminated in a meta-analysis published by Coca et al. demonstrating that adults who suffer AKI have an adjusted hazard ratio of 8.8 (95% CI, 3.1–25.5) of developing subsequent CKD.[96] Recent work in children with congenital heart disease and critically ill general pediatric patients has shown a similar link between discreet episodes of AKI and evidence of chronic kidney damage.[35,97,98]

In recent years the link between neonatal AKI and subsequent CKD has been identified. Charlton et al.[99] recently performed a follow-up study of 34 VLBW neonates at a median age of 5 years. This study showed that those with AKI had higher risk of subsequent kidney dysfunction (65% versus 14%; $P = .01$). These findings are particularly interesting when one considers the recent study of 214 neonates by Shalaby et al., who showed that almost 28% of those with AKI were discharged with abnormal SCr for age.[100] Although these data point to a link between perinatal events and subsequent CKD, a longitudinal study of CKD and kidney outcomes following AKI is needed.

Currently there are no specific guidelines for follow-up to monitor the kidney health of neonates discharged from the NICU. Of note, premature neonates represent one of the high-risk populations that warrant blood pressure checks prior to age 3. Guidelines for follow-up of AKI have been proposed by the KDIGO group and they recommend kidney function testing within 3 months of discharge for individuals after an episode of AKI. The development of neonatal specific follow-up guidelines for kidney function monitoring is a priority.

Summary

AKI occurs commonly in critically ill neonates and has significant impact on short- and long-term outcomes. To begin to improve the outcomes of neonatal AKI, it is critical to understand high-risk populations, improve surveillance, and develop strategies aimed at early identification and AKI prevention. A multidisciplinary approach is critical to the management of neonates with established AKI to prevent the development of sequelae related to AKI. Finally, long-term follow-up of neonates with AKI is critical to improve long-term kidney health in neonates after NICU discharge.

CHAPTER 59

Renal Replacement Therapy

Julie E. Goodwin, Ashok Kumar, Jorge Fabres, Akhil Maheshwari

KEY POINTS

1. Renal replacement therapy (RRT) is an effective therapy for treating neonates with acute kidney injury (AKI) and inborn errors of metabolism with hyperammonemia.
2. Peritoneal dialysis is used most frequently to treat AKI in neonates, although intermittent hemodialysis and continuous renal replacement therapy (CRRT) are important alternatives.
3. Timely initiation of RRT may improve outcomes in neonates with AKI and volume overload.
4. RRT can be an important temporizing option in infants with chronic issues such as congenital anomalies of the kidney and urinary tract and inherited cystic diseases until transplantation is possible/available.
5. Treatment of hyperammonemia with dialysis may help reduce neurotoxicity.
6. CRRT can be useful in various combinations of ultrafiltration with hemodialysis.

Recent advances in the safe application and availability of renal replacement therapy (RRT) have changed the management of premature and young infants with acute kidney injury (AKI) or severe congenital anomalies of the kidney and urinary tracts. In the 1990s, only 41% of infants younger than 1 month of age were eligible to receive RRT.[1] This number has steadily increased. This article reviews the available RRT options for neonates to treat AKI, inborn errors of metabolism with hyperammonemia, and renal structural anomalies until more definitive treatment becomes available.

Renal Replacement Therapy in Infants With Acute and Chronic Renal Failure

As described in other chapters in this section, the survival of infants with AKI and chronic renal failure is increasing. AKI is being recognized in up to 18% of very low birth weight infants, 23% to 52% of neonates being treated with cardiopulmonary bypass, and 71% of infants receiving extracorporeal membrane oxygenation (ECMO).[2] The survival rates of infants with congenital anomalies of the kidney and the urinary tract (CAKUTs) and inherited cystic anomalies are also increasing.[3] Encouragingly, many of these infants can be supported using RRT.

In RRT, the primary idea is to mimic the normal, physiologic renal system, where blood in the afferent arteriole enters the glomerular system for filtration and then exits through the efferent arteriole (Fig. 59.1). Three RRT systems are currently available to support these infants with AKI and/or chronic renal failure. These systems include acute peritoneal dialysis (PD), intermittent hemodialysis (HD), and continuous renal replacement therapy (CRRT; Fig. 59.2).[4] RRT can efficiently remove endogenous and exogenous toxins and maintain fluid, electrolyte, and acid-base balance in safe ranges until renal function recovers or a kidney transplantation is feasible/available (Table 59.1).[5]

In neonates, the determinants of the efficacy of RRT in AKI or chronic kidney disease (CKD) are still being determined.[4] Factors such as gestation, birth weight, the cause of kidney injury, the severity of metabolic derangements, hemodynamic changes, and nutritional needs are important.[6] There is a need to understand the severity of renal failure and its progression to predict the need for RRT. The cause, the overall disease severity, its tempo, secondary changes in the fluid/electrolyte balance, and nutritional deficits are important. The renal injury may be underestimated because the lower muscle mass found in neonates may cause baseline levels of the traditional indicators such as blood urea nitrogen (BUN) and serum creatinine to be lower.[7] These infants may also be less responsive to diuretics to excrete fluids and electrolytes and may develop fluid overload. The need for enteral feedings/hyperalimentation to support nutritional needs may be an important consideration for the initiation of RRT.[8]

Peritoneal Dialysis

PD is an important therapy for AKI and CKD in neonates, even extremely low birth weight infants, in whom stable vascular access can be difficult to maintain.[9] PD is relatively easy to perform; it only requires surgical insertion of a PD catheter, an intact peritoneal membrane that functions as the filter for dialysis, dialysis fluids, and connecting tubing and drainage bags. There is infrequent need for heparinization, and hemodynamic stability is not an absolute need. If needed, PD can be initiated soon after placement of the catheter using low-fill volumes such as 10 to 20 mL/kg, and the volumes can be increased as needed, although a period of catheter immobilization and healing of approximately 2 weeks is most ideal. The procedure can be used for long periods of time. The efficiency can be increased by increasing the frequency of exchanges as often as every hour and using dialysate with higher glucose concentrations.

The peritoneal cavity is accessed using a Tenckhoff catheter.[10] Very low birth weight neonates can also be dialyzed using a 14-gauge vascular catheter to access the peritoneal fluid.[11] Commercially available 1.5%, 2.5%, and 4.25% glucose solutions that have been warmed to body temperature should be used in PD (Table 59.2). PD can be started in neonates with volumes of 5 to 10 mL/kg body weight, and the volumes can be gradually increased based on the need for solute and fluid removal and with safety based on the cardiovascular and respiratory status.[12] Neonates with lactate acidosis should be dialyzed using a bicarbonate-buffered dialysate solution.[13]

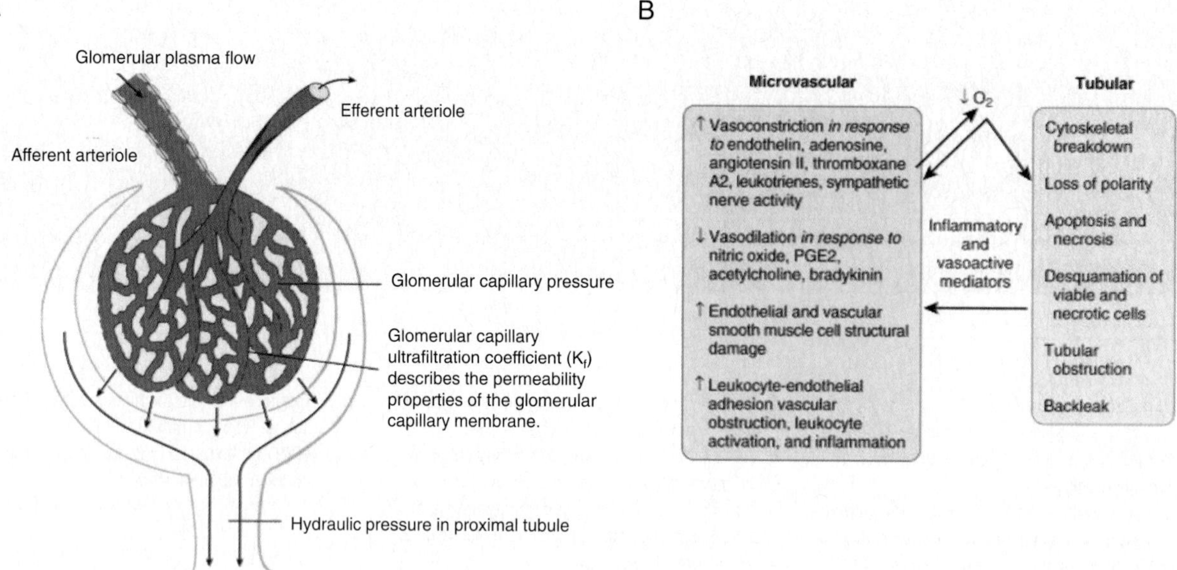

Fig. 59.1 (A) Glomerular filtration is determined by the rate of glomerular plasma flow (GPF) entering the afferent arteriole, the difference between the hydraulic pressure within the glomerular capillary and the hydraulic pressure in the proximal tubule, and the glomerular capillary ultrafiltration coefficient. (B) Pathophysiology of ischemic acute kidney injury. *PGE2,* Prostaglandin E_2. (Figure modified and reproduced from Jetton et al. Pathophysiology of neonatal acute kidney injury. In *Fetal and Neonatal Physiology*, 165, 1668–1676.e3.)

PD may be slower to correct metabolic derangements, and there is a risk of peritonitis. Patients who have had recent abdominal surgery and have massive organomegaly or intraabdominal masses as well as ostomies may be less suitable for PD. There may be some difficulties related to fluid and electrolyte imbalances, particularly when using frequent exchanges. Prolonged use of hypertonic glucose solutions can cause hyperglycemia, hypernatremia, and hypovolemia. Some patients can also develop peritonitis (dialysate white blood count >100/mm^3) and should be treated with intraperitoneal antibiotics.[14] Hypokalemia or hypophosphatemia during the course of dialysis can be treated by adding 3 to 5 mEq/L of potassium chloride[15] although this would be managed more frequently though dietary supplementation.

Osmotic Agents

The usual osmotic agent used in dialysis fluids is dextrose monohydrate (the bioavailable D-form of glucose).[16] These high concentrations of dextrose create an osmotic gradient to draw water from the peritoneal capillaries to the peritoneal cavity. Amino acids or icodextrin can be added in chronic dialysis to reduce the toxic effects of the dextrose on the peritoneal membrane.[17]

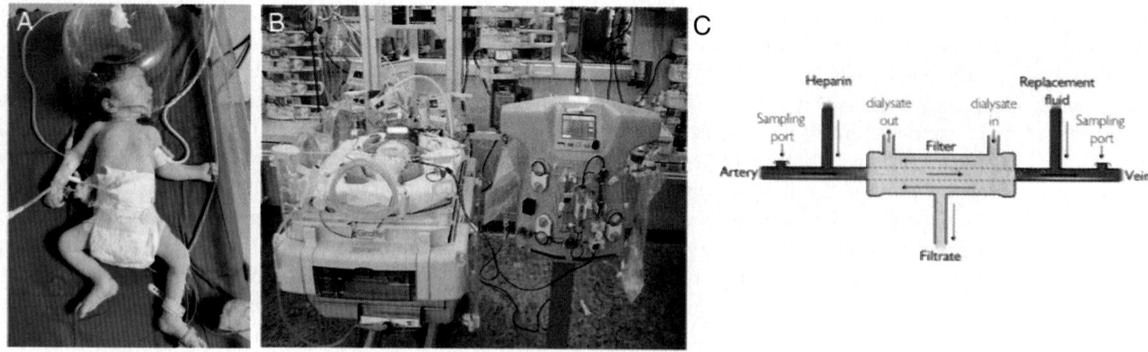

Fig. 59.2 Renal Replacement Therapies for Infants. (A) Peritoneal dialysis (PD). (B) Hemodialysis (HD). (C) Schematic showing hemofiltration and hemodiafiltration. In PD, the peritoneal lining acts as a natural filter. PD fluid is infused into the peritoneal cavity and then removed at protocol-defined intervals. HD, or hemofiltration, can be used if PD is not possible due to procedural difficulties such as with severe respiratory distress, disease-related issues (in inborn errors of metabolism), or primary conditions that led to renal failure (such as necrotizing enterocolitis). In these procedures, blood is cycled through an artificial kidney machine. HD can remove small solutes by diffusion across a membrane. An artery (umbilical or femoral) and a vein (umbilical, femoral, or jugular) are cannulated, and blood is driven across a filter by the patient's systemic blood pressure (SBP). An SBP ≥40 mm Hg can maintain flow across the filter. If necessary, a volumetric infusion pump can be inserted into the circuit, and ultrafiltration rates may be increased up to 5 mL/kg/hour. Replacement fluid and parenteral nutrition can be infused into the venous port of the circuit. Continuous arterio-venous hemofiltration (CAVH) removes solutes by convection (not diffusion) and can eliminate even larger molecules such as myoglobin or cytokines. If needed, such as in patients with increased urea generation, diffusive clearance can be added by running dialysis fluid through a filter in the opposite direction to blood flow. CAVH may not be effective in patients with hypotension or poor cardiac function. Most infants will tolerate maximum extracorporeal removal of 10% of their blood volume. Hemofiltration with or without dialysis can help process fluids rapidly; the disadvantages are the need for heparinization, blood priming of the circuit in small infants, and the risk of severe fluid and electrolyte imbalance. In infants who are clinically more stable, veno-venous dialysis may also be possible.

Table 59.1 An Overview of Available RRTs

	PD	Hemodialysis	Continuous Veno-Venous Hemofiltration/Hemodiafiltration
CLINICAL FEASIBILITY			
Ease of access	+++	–	–
Respiratory compromise	++	–	–(+)
Peritonitis	++++	–	–
Hypotension	+	+++	+++(+++)
Need for hemodynamic stability	–	+++	–(+)
PHYSIOLOGIC EFFECTIVENESS			
Solute removal	+++	++++	+(+++)
Fluid removal	++	+++	+++(+++)
Toxin removal	+	++++	–(+)
Removal of potassium	++	++++	+(++)
Removal of ammonia	+	++++	+(+++)
CONVENIENCE/RISK			
Need for anticoagulation	–	++	–/+(–/+)
Continuous	+++	–	+++(+++)
Disequilibrium	–	+++	–(–)?
Reverse osmosis water	–	++++	–(–)?

PD, Peritoneal dialysis; *RRT*, renal replacement therapy; *?*, per current information (need for more data).

Electrolytes

PD fluids contain sodium concentrations that may be slightly lower than that in plasma and enhance the diffusion of sodium to the dialysate fluids to prevent hypernatremia. Standard PD solutions can be high-calcium (1.75 mmol/L) or low-calcium (1.25 mmol/L). The high-calcium dialysis fluids may be used to create a positive calcium balance if appropriate; however, neonates are prone to hypercalcemia and most commonly are dialyzed with lower calcium solutions.

Table 59.2 Composition of a Typical Commercially Available PD Fluid[a]

OSMOTIC AGENTS	
Dextrose	1.5–4.25 g/dL
Icodextrin	7.5 g/dL
Amino acids	1.1 g/dL
ELECTROLYTES	
Sodium	135 mmol/L
Calcium	1.25 mmol/L
Magnesium	0.25–0.75 mmol/L
Chloride	96–109 mmol/L
BUFFER	
Lactate	35–40 mmol/L
Bicarbonate	25 mmol/L
Lactate/bicarbonate	30–40 mmol/L

[a]The dialysis fluid is generally composed of an osmotic agent, a buffer, and electrolytes. These components can be modified to affect blood purification and fluid removal via ultrafiltration.

PD, Peritoneal dialysis.

Buffers

Lactate is rapidly absorbed and converted to bicarbonate by the liver. This gain of bicarbonate is designed to counterbalance the simultaneous loss of blood bicarbonate into the relatively acidotic (pH 5.5–6.5) dialysis fluid. Newer PD fluid bags now contain either pure bicarbonate or a mixture of bicarbonate and lactate buffer. Bicarbonate-containing PD fluids can effectively correct metabolic acidosis and cause less inflammation than lactate-only PD fluids.[18]

Hemodialysis

HD has also been used for several years in the treatment of AKI and CKD. It also can correct metabolic abnormalities and hypervolemia by rapid ultrafiltration. There are some difficulties such as the need for heparinization and skilled personnel and for maximally purified water and a reverse osmosis system. The procedure can also be used to treat associated metabolic disorders such as hyperammonemia in urea cycle defects (Fig. 59.3).[19] It is harder to do in cases of hemodynamic instability or hemorrhage.

In neonates, the umbilical vessels can be used for vascular access. Later, a catheter may have to be placed in the internal or external jugular veins or in the femoral vein. To avoid hypotension, the total volume of the dialysate circuit, including the dialyzer and tubing, should not exceed 10% of the estimated blood volume.[20] A starting blood flow rate of 3 mL/kg/min is targeted, but depending on the patient's weight and the specifications of particular dialysis machines, blood flow of up to 10 mL/kg/min may be used. During HD, rapid ultrafiltration can cause hypotension and renal ischemia and can increase renal injury.[20] Rapid removal of BUN and other uremic products can also cause dialysis disequilibrium with seizures and altered sensorium, particularly if the starting

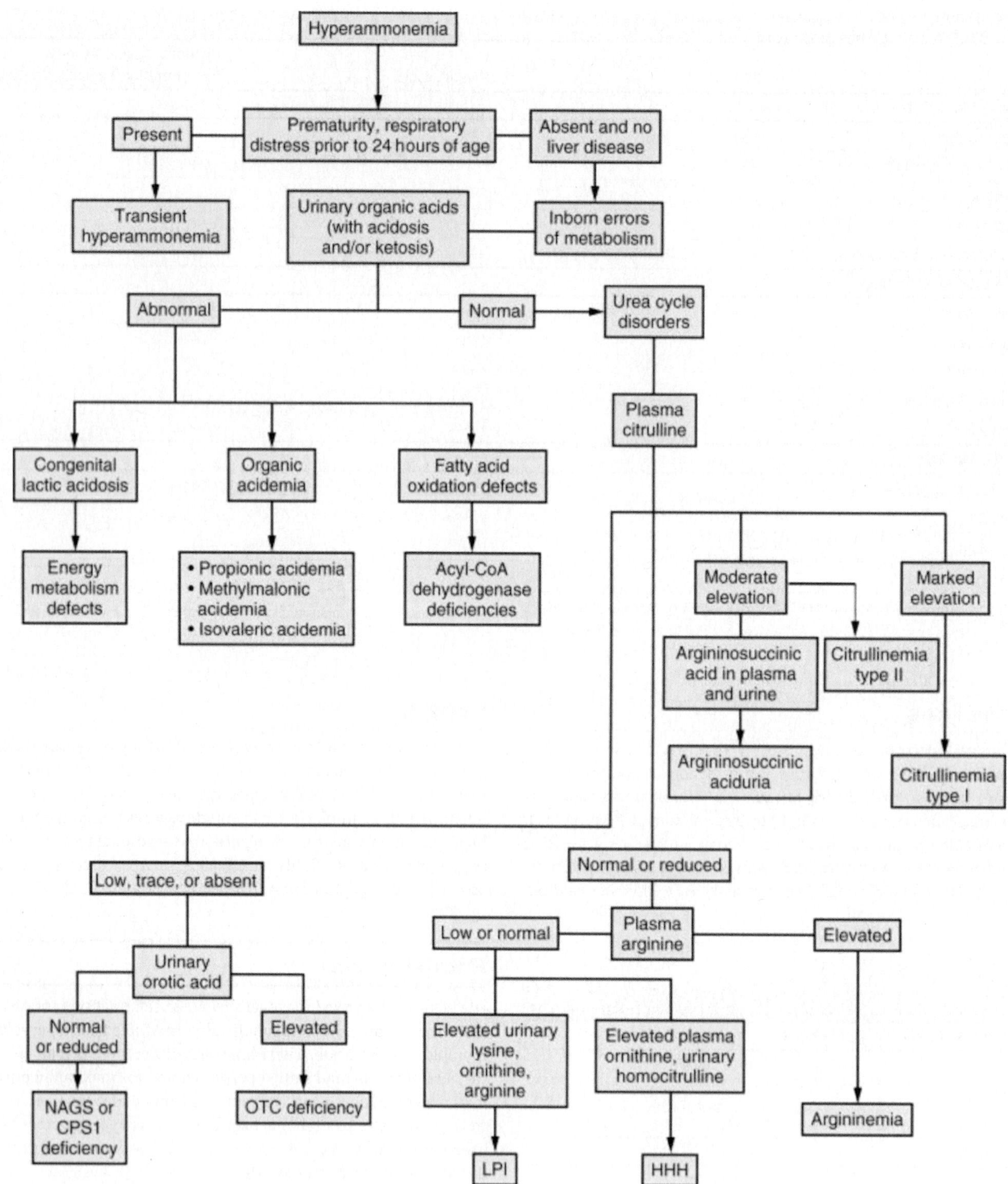

Fig. 59.3 Algorithm for Differential Diagnosis of Hyperammonemia. Plasma amino acids, serum lactate, and urinary excretion of orotic acid and organic acids are measured. *Acyl-CoA,* Acyl coenzyme A; *CPS1,* carbamoyl-phosphate synthase 1; *HHH,* hyperornithinemia-hyperammonemia-homocitrullinuria syndrome; *LPI,* lysinuric protein intolerance; *NAGS,* N-acetylglutamate synthase; *OTC,* ornithine transcarbamylase. (From Nagamani and Lichter-Konecki. Inborn errors of urea synthesis. In: *Swaiman's Pediatric Neurology*, 38, e720–e732.)

BUN is >120 mg/dL.[21] These symptoms could be related to removal of urea from the blood while brain levels decline more slowly. To maintain adequate control of azotemia and to allow for adequate veno-venous nutrition during AKI, frequent HD (as often as daily) may be needed in neonates.[22]

CRRT

Even though PD is usually efficient at blood purification and fluid removal, it cannot be used in infants with abdominal wall defects or after recent abdominal surgical procedures or skin infections.

Moreover, some of the more severely fluid-overloaded neonates may not have adequate ultrafiltration with PD. Technological advances during the past several years have enabled CRRT in neonates. There are four different modalities of CRRT[23]: (1) slow continuous ultrafiltration, which is better for removal of fluids than solutes; (2) continuous veno-venous hemofiltration (CVVH), where solute removal is accomplished by convection and a replacement fluid is required; (3) continuous veno-venous HD, where solute removal occurs by diffusion against a dialysate fluid gradient; and (4) continuous veno-venous hemodiafiltration, where both a replacement fluid and a dialysis fluid are used and solute removal occurs by both convection and diffusion. The blood flow rate in neonates is usually upwards of 6 mL/kg/min and often as high as 8 to 12 mL/kg/min. The combined dialysis and replacement rate is 2000 to 3000 mL/hour/1.73 m^2. Two forms of anti-coagulation are possible. If using the regional citrate approach, the citrate is delivered at 1.5 times the blood flow rate and a separate line to deliver CaCl must be established. The calcium infusion rate is generally started at 0.4 times the citrate infusion rate with goals of an ionized calcium level in the circuit of 1.0 to 1.4 mg/dL and an ionized calcium level in the patient of 4.4 to 5.2 mg/dL. When using citrate anti-coagulation, dialysis and replacement solutions must be calcium-free. The other form of anti-coagulation is heparin-based in which calcium-containing dialysis and replacement solutions must be selected. In this case a heparin bolus of 10 U/kg is given at initiation and then an infusion of 5 to 20 U/kg/hour is continued to maintain circuit activated clotting times (ACT) of 180 to 220 seconds. CRRT is used in nearly 75% of infants on ECMO to prevent volume overload or to correct electrolytes and is particularly useful because these infants can become hemodynamically unstable.[25]

CVVH is a continuous procedure that does not cause rapid solute and fluid shifts but can remove large quantities of ultrafiltrate from plasma with replacement of an isosmotic electrolyte solution.[23] It can also remove solutes via an added dialysis circuit. Hemodynamic stability is not a requirement. Hemofiltration and hemodiafiltration can allow good control of fluid, electrolyte, and acid-base balance and have been used to treat inborn errors of metabolism. CVVH can also be performed in neonates being treated with ECMO by adding a filter in the ECMO circuit or by inserting a CRRT machine.[23]

There are some difficulties. As in HD, catheterization of a large vessel such as the internal or external jugular veins or the femoral vein is needed. There is also a need for constant anticoagulation, and there is some risk of fluid and electrolyte abnormalities due to the large fluid shifts. In neonates at risk of bleeding, there is some new hope from the use of regional anticoagulation using citrate.

In a report from the Prospective Pediatric CRRT Registry, the mortality rate was 57% among infants weighing <10 kg and 36% in infants weighing >10 kg.[26] The mortality rates did not differ among patients weighing <5 kg versus those weighing between 5 and 10 kg. Survivors in this report were more likely to start CRRT sooner after intensive care unit (ICU) admission and were less fluid overloaded at CRRT initiation than were the nonsurvivors. Infants who were able to achieve dry weight during CRRT were more likely to survive than those who were not. These data suggest that clinical management strategies to prevent fluid overload and early initiation of CRRT for ultrafiltration may improve the outcome in these infants.

CRRT treatment requires an access line, hemofilter and tubing, anticoagulation, and replacement and dialysate fluids. The presence of a functional, optimally sized vascular access is important.[27] To maximize blood flow, the largest-gauge catheter that can be placed safely is ideal. A 7 French dialysis catheter can usually be placed successfully in 3- to 6-kg infants in the femoral/internal jugular veins.[28] Subclavian catheters should be avoided because of the risk of venous stenosis, which may limit the option of HD if needed.[29] Double- and triple-lumen catheters are acceptable. The goal is to use the smallest possible circuit volume to minimize the extracorporeal blood volume. A blood prime is necessary if the extracorporeal circuit exceeds 10% to 15% of the total blood volume.[20] The most frequently used anticoagulation protocols are systemic heparin and circuit regional anticoagulation using citrate.[30] Serial activated clotting times are used for monitoring.

For neonates, CRRT systems are still being adapted from those designed for adults. The ultrafiltration volume error range of some CRRT machines is 20 to 190 mL, which may be difficult for neonates.[31] The Cardio-Renal Pediatric Dialysis Emergency Machine was developed for the treatment of neonates between 2 and 10 kg with circuit volumes not exceeding 41.5 mL, and the errors of ultrafiltration seem acceptable.[32] Similarly, the Newcastle Infant Dialysis and Ultrafiltration System (NIDUS) has also been used in young infants.[33] Low-volume CRRT circuits are also being designed to provide the low extracorporeal volumes (50 mL) needed for neonates.[23]

RRT is Changing the Prognosis of Acute AKI in Neonates

The incidence of AKI in neonates and young infants may be up to 3.9/1000 admissions.[34] The inpatient mortality in children with AKI was higher in infants <1 month of age compared with those older than 1 month (31.3% versus 10.1%).[34] The other groups with similarly high mortality were children admitted to the ICU, with an in-hospital mortality of 32.8% versus 9.4% in patients not admitted to the ICU, and children on dialysis, with a rate of 27.1% versus 14.2% in children not requiring dialysis.

The prognosis of neonates with AKI eventually depends on the primary cause of their illness. Recent studies show that AKI, as an indicator of the severity of illness, is also a predictor of mortality. Other predictors may include multiorgan failure, hypotension, need for pressors, hemodynamic instability, and mechanical ventilation.[35] Overall, neonates with AKI may have mortality rates as high as 10% to 61%, and rates are particularly high in neonates with multiorgan failure.[36] Infants with non-oliguric renal failure are at a lower risk of death compared to those with oliguria or anuria (20% versus 64%).[37] Long-term follow-up showed that neonatal AKI predicted death and kidney sequelae such as CKD at 3 to 5 years.

AKI in neonates is associated with kidney disease later in life.[8] There is a growing body of evidence confirming the development of CKD in preterm and low birth weight infants and in those who suffer from AKI during their neonatal course.[38] Mammen et al.[39] analyzed the long-term risk of CKD in children admitted to the ICU who developed AKI and noted that 30 of their 126 patients were neonates. In their prospective cohort study, they used the Acute Kidney Injury Network (AKIN) criteria[40] to define stages of AKI and observed an overall incidence of CKD 1 to 3 years after AKI of 10.3%. The long-term effect of AKI in neonates is potentially compounded when the insult occurs before the full complement of nephrons has developed in utero.[37] Because nephrogenesis proceeds until 34 to 35 weeks' gestation, AKI before this time may result in a reduced nephron number.[41] Indeed, it has been shown that preterm neonates with AKI have a higher incidence of low glomerular filtration rate (GFR) and increasing proteinuria several years later, and morphologic studies have shown a decreased nephron number and glomerulomegaly. Several studies in animal models and some human studies have documented that hyperfiltration of the remaining nephrons may eventually lead to progressive glomerulosclerosis.[42] Typically, the late development of CKD first becomes apparent with the development of hypertension and proteinuria, and eventually, elevated BUN and creatinine.[43] A systemic review and meta-analysis of observational studies performed by White et al.[44] demonstrated that low birth weight is associated with a long-term risk of CKD. Subsequent prospective studies appear to confirm this finding. However, despite all the risks, there is also hope. In one study, most infants who had undergone long-term PD showed normal development, attended regular school, and had good growth and development.

The IRENEO study was a single-center, prospective, controlled study in France to assess the outcome of premature infants born at <33 weeks with a diagnosis of AKI.[45] These patients were evaluated at 3 to 10 years of age. There was no difference in estimated GFR (eGFR; using serum creatinine), urinary microalbumin, or blood pressure. Children with AKI did appear to have a trend toward lower renal volume. However, of all the children included, 10.8% had microalbuminuria and 23% had an eGFR <90 mL/min per 1.73 m^2. There may have been some issues related to the small sample size, and there is a need for further study.

Neonates with congenital anomalies of the kidney and urogenital tract, cortical necrosis, or cystic kidney diseases are at risk for later development of CKD.[46] Hypoxic-ischemic and nephrotoxic insults can also result in later kidney disease.[47] When premature neonates were investigated during childhood (ages 6.1–12.4 years), there was lower tubular reabsorption of phosphorus. Urinary calcium excretion was also higher in children born prematurely compared with control children. Some of these changes could be ascribed to aminoglycoside nephrotoxicity. Low birth weight is also a risk for focal segmental glomerulosclerosis. In addition, extrauterine and intrauterine growth retardation may also be associated with impaired renal function in preterm infants during follow-up. Neonates with AKI and nephrotoxic insults may need careful monitoring of their kidney function and blood pressures.[48]

RRT may also be needed in infants who have been treated with cardiopulmonary bypass.[49] AKI has been reported in 23% to 52% of these infants, and RRT may be needed in 2.1% to 17% of infants, with mortality rates up to 40%.[50] PD is the most commonly used RRT modality to treat the consequences of AKI in this population. The approach was relatively conservative with careful observation and initiation of RRT when signs of volume overload were seen. Based on data from adult patients and early neonatal studies, this practice is now becoming more proactive, with initiation of RRT early in the course of AKI. These studies suggest that starting RRT early after cardiac surgeries may reduce in-hospital mortality and hospital stay, shorten the duration of RRT, and reduce the dependence on dialysis.[51]

The Impact of RRT on CAKUTs and Inherited Cystic Kidney Diseases

Compared with RRT for AKI, the number of neonates requiring chronic dialysis as treatment for end-stage kidney disease (ESKD) is smaller.[52] The most common reasons for neonatal ESKD are CAKUTs, notably renal dysplasia or hypoplasia and obstructive uropathy.[53,54] However, RRT is changing the outlook in many structural kidney diseases that typically led to renal failure in the past. The encouraging impact of RRT has been briefly discussed in Chapter 61 that is dedicated to these disorders.

Section 11

CHAPTER

Neonatal Hypertension 60

Janis M. Dionne, Joseph T. Flynn

KEY POINTS

1. Blood pressure should be measured with the proper cuff size on the right upper arm with attention to technique when using oscillometric devices in neonates.
2. Blood pressure is rapidly changing during the first weeks of life, especially in premature neonates, and measured values need to be compared with appropriate normal values.
3. In premature infants, the most common causes of hypertension are related to complications of prematurity or iatrogenic causes, whereas in term infants hypertension is most often due to an underlying condition.
4. A cause or risk factor for neonatal hypertension can be determined in most infants after review of the perinatal and postnatal history, physical examination, and some basic investigations.
5. Antihypertensive medications should be used judiciously in hypertensive neonates, given the lack of good evidence on efficacy and safety in this population.
6. Most prematurity-related neonatal hypertension will resolve during the first years of life, but premature and intrauterine growth restricted infants are at risk of kidney and cardiovascular disease later in life.

Introduction

Neonatal hypertension is far less common than is neonatal hypotension, and because of its infrequency, clinicians are less used to identifying and managing high blood pressures in neonates. Left unrecognized, neonatal hypertension could lead to serious cardiac, vascular, and neurologic consequences. Part of the difficulty in diagnosing high blood pressure likely comes from the fact that newborn blood pressures are naturally rapidly changing during the first weeks of life, especially in premature infants. In addition, blood pressure values by routine nursing care can be variable if not done with a proper blood pressure measurement technique.

Fortunately, when neonatal hypertension is properly identified, an underlying risk factor or cause for the hypertension is often found. A review of the perinatal and postnatal history, examination of the infant, and some basic investigations can often reveal the etiology. Although antihypertensive medications are not approved for use in this population, clinicians have been treating infants with a variety of antihypertensive medications for decades. Fortunately, most neonatal hypertension will resolve during the first months and years of life if a chronic condition is not identified. In this chapter we will describe the best evidence-based recommendations for blood pressure measurement and norms and for the diagnosis, evaluation, and management of neonatal hypertension.

Proper Blood Pressure Measurement

Although intraarterial blood pressure measurement remains the gold-standard technique and most common method in critically ill neonates, oscillometric devices are used more commonly for the majority of neonates within a neonatal intensive care unit (NICU). The evidence supporting oscillometric devices for blood pressure measurement in neonates and infants is conflicting, yet the potential for measurement error with oscillometric devices needs to be balanced against the risks of invasive monitoring with intraarterial catheters.[1]

Intraarterial measurement of blood pressure should be used in critically ill and unstable neonates and strongly considered in those whose mean arterial pressure is <30 mm Hg. Lalan and Blowey evaluated almost 1500 paired intraarterial and oscillometric measurements in 101 ill neonates and found that oscillometric measurements overestimated radial arterial values by 4 to 8 mm Hg.[2] Compared with umbilical arterial values, oscillometric mean values were similar for the mean arterial pressure (MAP), higher for systolic pressures, and lower for diastolic pressures, although the standard deviations of the measurements were large and clinically significant at approximately 10 mm Hg. Troy et al. also found differences in blood pressures of extremely low birth weight neonates of 10 to 18 mm Hg between intraarterial and oscillometric methods, which represented a blood pressure percent difference of 39% to 43%.[3] Several other studies have similar findings,[4–7] and although a few found good correlation between the two measurement methods,[8,9] there was often a large standard deviation of measured values. In addition, several studies have shown that the oscillometric method does not correlate well with intraarterial values at a lower range of blood pressures, and in particular, when the MAP is <30 mm Hg.[9–11] In this setting, the oscillometric device may underestimate hypotension. A systemic review of neonatal blood pressure studies has shown that oscillometric MAP correlated best with intraarterial values, compared with systolic or diastolic blood pressure.[1] The MAP is the only blood pressure value measured by the oscillometric device, whereas a computational algorithm determines systolic and diastolic values. Therefore, MAP should be the primary blood pressure value compared with normative data, because it is the most accurate parameter.

Blood pressures should be measured in the right upper arm using a proper cuff size with a cuff width approximately 50% of the infant arm circumference. Several early studies assessed the effect of cuff size on accuracy of blood pressure values with recommendations for using a cuff-width-to-arm-circumference ratio of 0.44 to 0.55,[12] 0.45 to 0.70,[13] and 0.36 to 0.64.[14] Lum and Jones stated a rule of cuff width of 50% of the arm circumference was a reasonable estimate for proper cuff size, and this recommendation has also been endorsed by the International Neonatal Consortium after systematic evaluation of the literature.[1,14] Studies that have compared calf blood pressure measurements to upper arm measurements have found the calf values are more variable and the blood pressure differences between

Table 60.1 Protocol for Oscillometric Device Blood Pressure Measurement in Neonates and Infants
Position infant prone or supine
Choose cuff with cuff width approximately 50% the arm circumference
Apply cuff to right upper arm
Leave infant undisturbed for 15 minutes
Measure blood pressure when infant is asleep or quiet awake
Take three blood pressure readings at 2-min intervals
1.5 hours after a feed or medical intervention when possible

Adapted from Nwankwo MU, Lorenz JM, Gardiner JC. A standard protocol for blood pressure measurement in the newborn. *Pediatrics.* 1997;99:E10.

locations increases with increasing postnatal age.[5,15–18] Crapanzano et al. found that calf blood pressure was slightly less than arm values in young infants but that by 6 to 9 months of age the calf pressures exceeded arm values.[15] In addition, the right upper arm is the preferred location for measurement in case of coarctation of the aorta.[19]

Blood pressures should be measured in neonates and infants using a standardized blood pressure measurement technique.[1] Several studies have shown that blood pressure values are more variable with "routine nursing care."[3,7,20] Infant pressures may vary significantly based on state of arousal, position, sucking, and feeding.[20,21] Nwankwo et al. compared blood pressure values in low birth weight infants using routine nursing care with a measurement protocol and found blood pressures were significantly higher and more variable by routine care.[20] In addition, first readings were higher than third readings in their protocol, which included three readings at 2-minute intervals for each measurement period (Table 60.1). Because many factors may affect blood pressure readings, using a standard blood pressure measurement protocol should improve the accuracy of the measurements.

Physiology of Blood Pressure in Neonates

Blood pressure values at birth can be affected by maternal, perinatal, and infant factors. Maternal factors may include maternal blood pressure, diabetes, and obesity, whereas perinatal factors may include antenatal steroids, complications of pregnancy, and mode of delivery.[22] In premature infants, the blood pressure on day 1 of life is primarily determined by the gestational age at birth and birth weight. Both Pejovic et al.[23] and Zubrow et al.[24] have shown a linear correlation of blood pressure on day 1 of life with birth weight and gestational age, with the most premature and lowest weight neonates having the lowest blood pressures at birth (Fig. 60.1). Although other factors may play a minor role, gestational age and birth weight are consistently the strongest determinants of neonatal blood pressure on day 1 of life.

In premature infants, blood pressure rapidly changes during the first weeks of life. In fact, Pejovic et al. found that in infants born at less than 28 weeks' gestational age, the MAP increases by 26% in the first week and >50% during the first month of life.[23] They found the most rapid rate of increase in the most premature infants. Kent et al. determined that the phase of most rapid increase in blood pressure occurred during the first 2 to 3 weeks of life in infants born at less than 32 weeks' gestation and only during the first week of life in infants born at 32 to 36 weeks' gestation (Fig. 60.2).[25] They noted that the blood pressure after the rapidly increasing phase is similar to that of term infants at birth. For most term infants, blood pressure increases significantly from the first to second day of life but only modestly each day afterward.[26] Lurbe et al. found that term infants born small for gestational age also had a lower blood pressure at birth compared with those born appropriate for gestational age but then had a rapid increase in their blood pressure during the first month of life to reach values similar to those of other neonates.[27] These various patterns of blood pressure changes during the first months of life are illustrated in Fig. 60.3.[22]

After the initial rapid rise in blood pressure, premature infants settle into a phase of slower, steadily increasing blood pressure. Zubrow et al. found that after 5 days of life, neonates increase their systolic blood pressure by about 1 mm Hg every 4 days whether born premature or term.[24] Zubrow and the Philadelphia Neonatal Blood Pressure Study Group developed user-friendly graphs of blood pressure by postconceptional age, although unfortunately, MAP was not included.[24] More recently, Dionne et al. synthesized blood pressure data from the literature into a reference table of infant blood pressure values after 2 weeks' postnatal age by current postmenstrual age.[28] The table provides the 50th, 95th, and 99th percentile values for systolic, mean, and diastolic blood pressure for infants 26 to 44 weeks postmenstrual age (Table 60.2). Unfortunately, most blood pressure studies in neonates have modest patient numbers and use heterogeneous populations and measurement methods, so a large multicenter prospective study of neonatal blood pressure is greatly needed.

Incidence of Hypertension

The incidence of neonatal and infant hypertension is about 1% to 2% in the NICU and has been stable over time. In 1978 Adelman published a report on neonatal hypertension, citing an incidence of 2.5% in a single NICU and describing risk factors including umbilical artery catheters, patent ductus arteriosus, and congenital heart disease.[29] In 1992, Singh et al. found an incidence of hypertension of 0.8% in their NICU population with risk factors that included umbilical artery catheters, chronic lung disease, patent ductus arteriosus, and intraventricular hemorrhage.[30] A recent study of a national database by Blowey et al. found an overall NICU incidence of hypertension of 1% after exclusion of congenital heart disease.[31] Risk factors for hypertension in this study included higher severity of illness, expiry prior to discharge, extracorporeal membrane oxygenation (ECMO), kidney failure or kidney disorder, and lower birth weight. Sahu et al. also noted a similar incidence of 1.3% hypertension in their NICU population, noting that 74% of affected infants were preterm.[32] They also found that the term infants presented earlier, at an average of 38 days compared with 121 days in infants born at less than 28 weeks' gestation. The actual definition of hypertension did vary in some of the early studies, but currently the most accepted definition of hypertension is a blood pressure that is consistently greater than the 95th percentile based on postmenstrual age.[28]

One exception to the above studies is data from the Assessment of Worldwide Acute Kidney Injury Epidemiology in Neonates (AWAKEN) study, which confirmed an incidence of diagnosed hypertension of 1.8% but also found that another 3.7% of neonates had undiagnosed hypertension based on recorded blood pressure values.[33] Of note, the AWAKEN authors used an internally generated table of normative blood pressure values, not the previously published data in Table 60.2. Further study is needed to determine whether the higher incidence of hypertension in AWAKEN was seen because of the normative data used or whether neonatal hypertension is truly underdiagnosed.

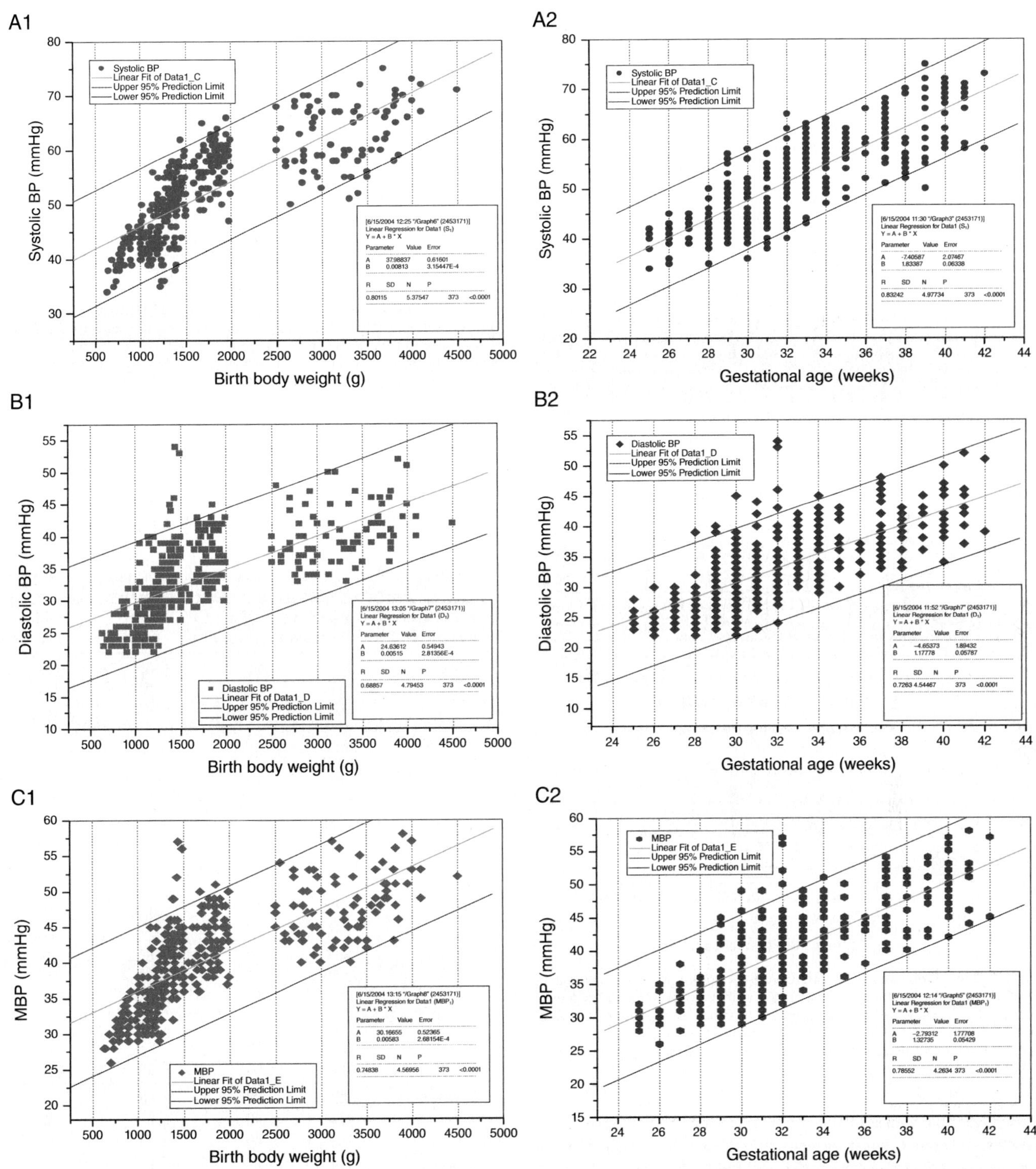

Fig. 60.1 Neonatal Blood Pressure on Day 1 of Life by (1) Birth Weight and (2) Gestational Age. (A) Systolic, (B) diastolic, and (C) mean blood pressure (MBP). (Reproduced with permission from Pejovic B, Peco-Antic A, Marinkovic-Eric J. Blood pressure in noncritically ill preterm and full-term neonates. *Pediatr Nephrol.* 2007;22:249–257.)

Etiology of Hypertension

The causes of hypertension in neonates and infants are most commonly related to kidney or cardiac abnormalities, renovascular anomalies, iatrogenic causes, and/or prematurity. A summary of the common and uncommon causes of hypertension are provided in Table 60.3. Depending on the study population, kidney causes account for 25% to 50% of infant hypertension, renovascular causes for 15% to 25%, cardiovascular causes for 4% to 8%, neurologic causes for 9% to 15%, and medications for 8% to 9%.[30,34–36] Because the hypertension associated with chronic lung disease usually develops after several months of life and even after hospital discharge, the incidence is more difficult to determine because many studies are of short duration.[37] In analyses that included longer follow-up and/or multiple predisposing factors for the hypertension, chronic lung disease accounted for as much as 60% of infant hypertension in these studies.[32,36]

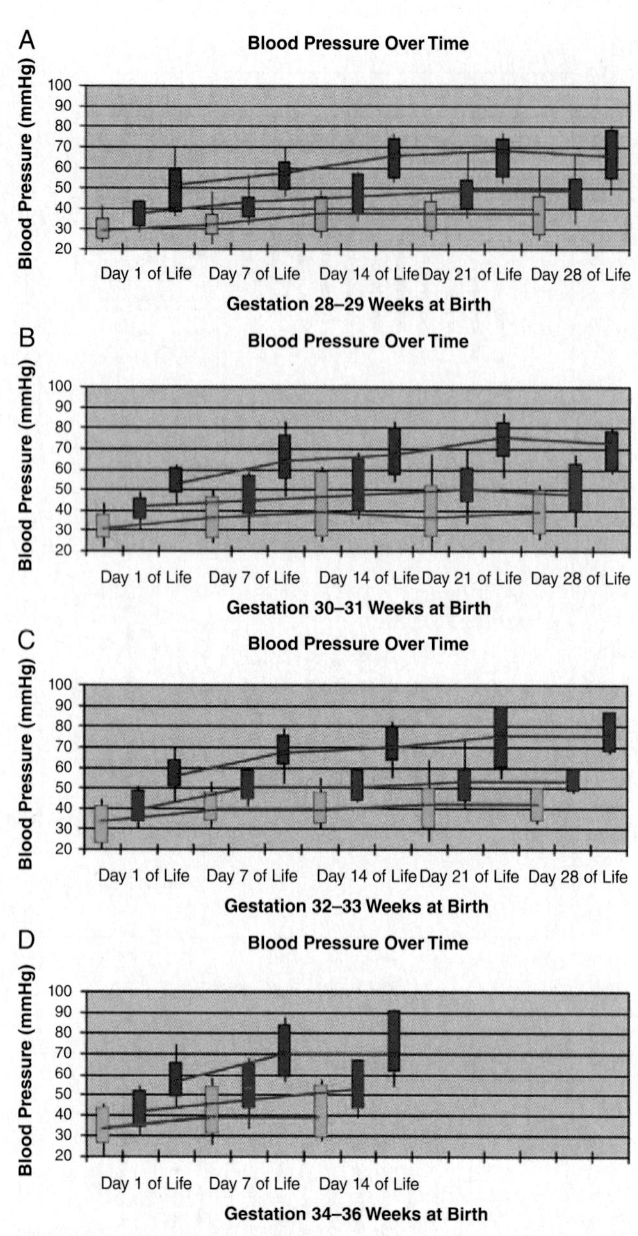

Fig. 60.2 Blood Pressure by Gestational Age Group During the First Weeks of Life. Bars represent the 10th to 90th percentile blood pressures for diastolic *(green)*, mean *(red)*, and systolic *(blue)* blood pressure. (Reproduced with permission from Kent AL, Meskell S, Falk MC, Shadbolt B. Normative blood pressure data in non-ventilated premature neonates from 28 to 36 weeks gestation. *Pediatr Nephrol.* 2009;24:141–146.)

Renovascular causes include renal artery thrombosis, renal artery stenosis, and renal vein thrombosis. Renovascular problems have been associated with use of umbilical catheters in neonates because they were found to cause aortic and renal thrombosis, stenosis, or emboli in about 30% of infants in early studies that routinely scanned all catheters.[38,39] Renal vein thrombosis may be associated with risk factors including perinatal asphyxia, dehydration, and maternal diabetes mellitus, and unfortunately, most affected kidneys become atrophic over time, with further risk of hypertension.[40] Renal parenchymal causes may be congenital, such as dysplasia or autosomal recessive polycystic kidney disease, associated with a urologic abnormality such as posterior urethra valve, or acquired, such as acute tubular necrosis or cortical necrosis (see Table 60.3). Cardiovascular causes most commonly include coarctation of the aorta and patent

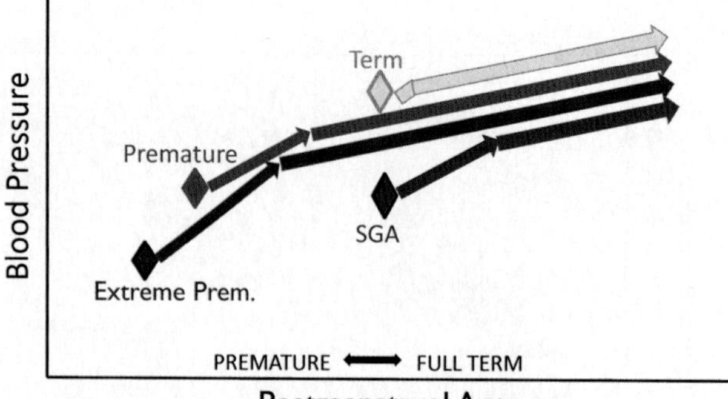

Fig. 60.3 Blood Pressure Patterns During the First Months of Life for Infants Born Term, Premature, Extremely Premature, and Small for Gestational Age (SGA). (Reproduced with permission from Dionne JM. Neonatal and infant hypertension. In: Flynn JT, Ingelfinger JR, Redwine K, eds. *Pediatric Hypertension.* 4th ed. New York, NY: Springer International Publishing; 2018:1–26.)

ductus arteriosus. In addition, ECMO is associated with hypertension in 10% to 38% of infants when used in a NICU population.[31,41] Pain, seizures, and intraventricular hemorrhage are the most common neurologic causes of neonatal hypertension. Medications that

Table 60.2 Infant Blood Pressures by Postmenstrual Age

Postmenstrual Age	Blood Pressure	50th Percentile	95th Percentile	99th Percentile
44 weeks	SBP	88	105	110
	MAP	63	80	85
	DBP	50	68	73
42 weeks	SBP	85	98	102
	MAP	62	76	81
	DBP	50	65	70
40 weeks	SBP	80	95	100
	MAP	60	75	80
	DBP	50	65	70
38 weeks	SBP	77	92	97
	MAP	59	74	79
	DBP	50	65	70
36 weeks	SBP	72	87	92
	MAP	57	72	77
	DBP	50	65	70
34 weeks	SBP	70	85	90
	MAP	50	65	70
	DBP	40	55	60
32 weeks	SBP	68	83	88
	MAP	49	64	69
	DBP	40	55	60
30 weeks	SBP	65	80	85
	MAP	48	63	68
	DBP	40	55	60
28 weeks	SBP	60	75	80
	MAP	45	58	63
	DBP	38	50	54
26 weeks	SBP	55	72	77
	MAP	38	57	63
	DBP	30	50	56

DBP, Diastolic blood pressure; *MAP,* mean arterial pressure; *SBP,* systolic blood pressure.

Reproduced with permission from Dionne JM, Abitbol CL, Flynn JT. Hypertension in infancy: diagnosis, management and outcome. *Pediatr Nephrol.* 2012;27:159–160.

Table 60.3 Common and Uncommon Causes of Neonatal and Infant Hypertension

Common	Uncommon
Renovascular Renal artery thrombosis Renal artery stenosis Renal vein thrombosis	Renovascular Midaortic syndrome Congenital rubella syndrome Idiopathic arterial calcification of infancy Renal myofibromatosis
Renal parenchymal Congenital Dysplasia Unilateral hypoplasia Polycystic kidney disease	Renal parenchymal Congenital Multicystic dysplastic kidney Congenital and infantile nephrotic syndrome Renal tubular dysgenesis Atypical hemolytic uremic syndrome
Associated with urologic abnormality Obstructive uropathy Ureteropelvic junction obstruction	Associated with urologic abnormality Neurogenic bladder Megaureter
Acquired Acute tubular necrosis Cortical necrosis	Acquired Pyelonephritis Interstitial nephritis Nephrocalcinosis
Cardiovascular Coarctation of the aorta Patent ductus arteriosus ECMO	Cardiovascular Congenital ductus arteriosus aneurysm Congenital aortic aneurysm
Respiratory Chronic lung disease	Respiratory Pneumothorax
Neurologic Pain Seizures Intracranial hypertension	Neurologic Familial dysautonomia Subdural hematoma
Medications/drugs Corticosteroids Adrenergic agents Caffeine Theophylline Excess salt/saline	Medications/drugs Phthalates Phenylephrine Erythropoietin Pancuronium Vitamin D intoxication Maternal cocaine or heroin
	Endocrine Congenital adrenal hyperplasia Cushing syndrome Neonatal hyperthyroidism Hyperaldosteronism Pheochromocytoma Aldosterone synthase deficiency Argininosuccinate lyase deficiency
	Neoplastic Neuroblastoma Wilms tumor Mesoblastic nephroma Adrenocortical carcinoma
	Heritable hypertension Liddle syndrome Apparent mineralocorticoid excess Glucocorticoid-remediable aldosteronism
	Other causes Hypercalcemia Total parenteral nutrition Closure of abdominal wall defect Adrenal hemorrhage Traction

ECMO, Extracorporeal membrane oxygenation.

clinicians prescribe may also be the cause of neonatal hypertension, with the most common offenders including corticosteroids, adrenergic agents, caffeine or theophylline, and excess salt or saline. Exposure to phthalates, which are ubiquitously present in intravenous tubing and respiratory equipment used in the NICU, has recently been associated with the development of hypertension in premature neonates.[42] In addition, there is a long list of uncommon causes of hypertension that includes endocrine causes, neoplastic causes, and genetic forms of hypertension that are likely best investigated by pediatric subspecialists most familiar with the rare etiologies (see Table 60.3).

Clinical Presentation

Most neonatal and infant hypertension presents with nonspecific features or is asymptomatic, with identification of the issue primarily by repeated blood pressure measurement. Infants may present with irritability, poor feeding, vomiting, or restlessness.[29,43] They can also present with neurologic signs and symptoms such as lethargy, tremors, seizures, apnea, and hemiparesis that may be difficult to distinguish from an intracranial pathology.[29] Kidney findings may include hematuria, proteinuria, oliguria or polyuria, and acute kidney injury.[43,44] The cardiovascular system can be affected by hypertension, with typical symptoms such as tachycardia, tachypnea, abnormal pulses or perfusion, and pulmonary congestion.[29,44] Occasionally, infants present with hypotension in decompensated heart failure, and only after cardiac function improves is the hypertension identified.[45,46]

Evaluation of Hypertension

In many cases of neonatal hypertension, one or more potential risk factors or causes may be identified by review of the infant's perinatal and postnatal medical history, medication list, and physical examination. If an obvious cause is not identified to direct further evaluation, basic investigations for kidney, renovascular, and cardiovascular causes should identify an etiology in the majority of cases (Table 60.4). Recommended investigations include electrolytes, kidney function, urinalysis, complete blood count, kidney ultrasound with Doppler, and echocardiography. Buchi and Siegler found an abnormality in kidney function, urinalysis, plasma renin activity, or echocardiogram in 62% of infants who had neonatal hypertension in their early study.[34] More recently, studies have documented abnormalities on kidney ultrasound in about 25% of infants with hypertension, and a cause or risk factor for the hypertension was identified in most infants.[32,47] Sahu et al. found that the factors varied based on if the infants were term or preterm. Hypertension in the preterm infants was associated with chronic lung disease and iatrogenic factors such as medication and ECMO, whereas term infants were more likely to have a cardiac or systemic disease.[32] Occasionally, more specific investigations such as endocrine studies or detailed kidney scans may be needed but should be directed in consultation with specialists most familiar with the investigations.

Management of Hypertension

Once a diagnosis has been established, potential treatments can be considered. When a cause of hypertension with a known specific treatment has been identified, initiation of treatment is straightforward and should be commenced without delay. Common examples of conditions causing neonatal hypertension with known specific treatments are summarized in Table 60.5. Most of these do not involve the administration of antihypertensive medications; many result in complete correction of the hypertension.

However, many other causes of neonatal hypertension do not have known specific treatments, so the use of antihypertensive medications must be considered. With the exception of infants with symptomatic severe hypertension (see below), criteria for drug treatment of hypertension in neonates are uncertain because there are no data on whether drug treatment improves outcomes compared with no treatment. Additionally, there is no specific guidance available on what level of blood pressure elevation necessitates drug treatment—this is especially vexing because many hypertensive neonates have relatively mild hypertension that is detected on routine monitoring of vital signs.

It is reasonable to consider initiation of pharmacologic therapy in neonates with moderate, sustained, asymptomatic hypertension (blood pressure ≥99th percentile; see Table 60.2) or in those with

Table 60.4 Diagnostic Investigations for Neonatal and Infant Hypertension

Common Investigations	Abnormality May Suggest Etiology Due to
Serum electrolytes (Na, K, Cl, HCO_3)	Renovascular, kidney, endocrine, heritable hypertension
Blood urea nitrogen, creatinine	Renovascular, kidney
Urinalysis	Renovascular, kidney
Complete blood count	Renovascular, kidney, neoplastic
Kidney ultrasound with Doppler	Renovascular, kidney, neoplastic
Echocardiography	Cardiovascular, end organ damage
Specific Investigations	
Plasma renin activity, aldosterone	Renovascular, kidney, endocrine, heritable hypertension
Head ultrasound	Neurologic
Serum calcium	Medications, endocrine, other
Cortisol, thyroid studies	Endocrine
Renal scintigraphy (MAG3, DTPA)	Kidney
Angiography	Renovascular

Cl, Chloride; *DTPA*, Tc 99m diethylenetriamine pentaacetic acid; *HCO_3*, bicarbonate; *K*, potassium; *MAG3*, Tc 99m mercaptoacetyl-triglycine; *Na*, sodium.

Table 60.5 Causes of Neonatal Hypertension With Specific Treatments

Cause	Treatment
Coarctation of the aorta	Surgical repair
Congenital adrenal hyperplasia	Glucocorticoids
Drug (corticosteroids, vasopressors)	Discontinue or reduce dose
Neonatal hyperthyroidism	Methimazole, propranolol
Pain	Improve analgesia
Pneumothorax	Chest tube
Renal arterial or venous thrombosis	Anticoagulation, nephrectomy
Tumor (Wilms, neuroblastoma)	Surgical removal
Urinary obstruction	Drainage catheter, surgery
Volume overload	Fluid restriction, diuretics

lesser degrees of blood pressure elevation who are symptomatic or known to have end organ involvement such as left ventricular hypertrophy. Observation may be appropriate if the blood pressure does not reach this level or if there is no evidence of target-organ involvement. As discussed earlier, careful blood pressure measurement is crucial in deciding to initiate pharmacologic therapy—such decisions should ideally be based on blood pressure measurements in the upper arm using correct technique.[1]

No clinical trials of antihypertensive medications have been conducted in neonates; therefore none are labeled by the US Food and Drug Administration or any other governmental agency for use in this age group. Choice of antihypertensive medication is therefore empiric and dependent on practitioner expertise. During the past several decades, many case series have appeared describing the use of a wide variety of agents to treat persistent neonatal hypertension.[31,32,47] Agents that have been reported effective include vasodilators, calcium channel blockers, diuretics, beta-blockers, and angiotensin converting enzyme (ACE) inhibitors. Some agents may be contraindicated depending on the neonate's postmenstrual age and concurrent medical conditions; examples would include avoidance of ACE inhibitors in neonates less than 44 weeks' postmenstrual age and avoidance of noncardioselective β-adrenergic blockers in infants with significant chronic lung disease.

The other important aspect of medication treatment is choosing the most appropriate route of administration. Some neonates have severe, symptomatic hypertension with target-organ manifestations such as congestive heart failure or encephalopathy; this is termed "acute severe hypertension" and has been discussed in detail elsewhere.[48] Neonates with acute severe hypertension require controlled blood pressure reduction using a continuous intravenous infusion and require continuous blood pressure monitoring to avoid excessively rapid blood pressure reduction. Neonates with less severe blood pressure elevation may be treated with oral medications unless they are nil per os for other reasons such as necrotizing enterocolitis. Pharmacologic therapy is typically initiated with a single drug, increasing the dose gradually until the blood pressure is controlled or the maximum dose is reached. If hypertension persists or adverse effects of the first drug develop, a second drug should be added. Dosing recommendations for selected antihypertensive medications in neonates can be found in Table 60.6.

Given the lack of outcome data mentioned earlier, there is no guidance on the optimal goal blood pressure for hypertensive neonates once treatment has been initiated. It is reasonable to target the 95th percentile in most hypertensive neonates unless the underlying condition would benefit from a lower blood pressure—for example, blood pressures below the 50th percentile may be beneficial in patients with known chronic kidney disease.[49] Neonates treated with antihypertensive therapy will need to have ongoing monitoring of their blood pressure to ensure that treatment goals are being met. Laboratory monitoring may also be needed as appropriate, depending on the choice of agent (e.g., diuretics or ACE inhibitors). Duration of antihypertensive therapy will be influenced by the underlying cause of hypertension. Although hypertension may resolve over time in many neonates, allowing discontinuation of antihypertensive medications, some infants will require long-term treatment.

Long-Term Outcomes

Fortunately, most neonatal hypertension related to prematurity resolves during the first couple years of life. Sahu et al. found that 85% of infants with neonatal hypertension required antihypertensive medication at discharge.[32] Buchi and Siegler followed up their NICU hypertensive population and found that two-thirds were normotensive by 6 months of age and more than 80% by 1 year.[34] Others have shown that almost all neonatal hypertension resolves by 2 years of life,[50,51] although some infant hypertension may present during NICU follow-up related to chronic lung disease or previously undiagnosed kidney, cardiac, or neoplastic conditions.[50,51] Hypertension associated with chronic lung disease presented in a follow-up clinic in 45% of patients in a study by Anderson et al., with a mean age of onset of 5.9 months and duration ranging from 0.5 to 25.7 months.[52] NICU hypertension related to chronic kidney conditions such as autosomal recessive polycystic kidney disease or hypodysplasia may not resolve over time.[53,54] In repaired coarctation of the aorta, some hypertension is slow to resolve and other times it reappears when restenosis occurs.[55] If an underlying condition is responsible for the neonatal hypertension, blood pressures should be monitored at every healthcare encounter through infancy and childhood, as recommended by the American Academy of Pediatrics Clinical Practice Guideline for Screening and Management of High Blood Pressure in Children and Adolescents.[49]

The American Academy of Pediatrics Clinical Practice Guideline also recommends regular blood pressure assessment in all infants and children who have graduated from the NICU, particularly those who were premature, small for gestational age, or very low birth weight.[49] There is increasing evidence for the development of hypertension, cardiovascular disease, and kidney disease in adolescents and adults who were born premature and intrauterine growth restricted. Neonates born preterm or very low birth weight have

Table 60.6 Dosing of Selected Antihypertensive Medications for Treatment of Hypertensive Neonates

Class	Drug	Route	Dosing	Interval
ACE inhibitors	Captopril	Oral	<3 months: 0.01–0.5 mg/kg/dose Max 2 mg/kg/day >3 months: 0.15–0.3 mg/kg/dose Max 6 mg/kg/day	TID
	Enalapril[a]	Oral	0.08–0.6 mg/kg/day	QD-BID
	Lisinopril[a]	Oral	0.07–0.6 mg/kg/day	QD
α and β antagonists	Labetalol	Oral	0.5–1.0 mg/kg/dose Max 10 mg/kg/day	BID-TID
		IV	0.20–1.0 mg/kg/dose 0.25–3.0 mg/kg/hour	Q 4–6 h Infusion
	Carvedilol	Oral	0.1 mg/kg/dose up to 0.5 mg/kg/dose	BID
β Antagonists	Esmolol	IV	100–500 mcg/kg/min	Infusion
	Propranolol[a]	Oral	0.5–1.0 mg/kg/dose Max 8–10 mg/kg/day	TID
Calcium channel blockers	Amlodipine[a]	Oral	0.05–0.3 mg/kg/dose Max 0.6 mg/kg/day	QD–BID
	Isradipine	Oral	0.05–0.15 mg/kg/dose Max 0.8 mg/kg/day	QID
	Nicardipine	IV	1–4 mcg/kg/min	Infusion
Central α agonist	Clonidine	Oral	5–10 mcg/kg/day Max 25 mcg/kg/day	TID
Diuretics	Chlorothiazide[a]	Oral	5–15 mg/kg/dose	BID
	Hydrochlorothiazide	Oral	1–3 mg/kg/dose	QD
	Spironolactone	Oral	0.5–1.5 mg/kg/dose	BID
Direct vasodilators	Hydralazine	Oral	0.25–1.0 mg/kg/dose Max 7.5 mg/kg/day	TID–QID
		IV	0.15–0.6 mg/kg/dose	Q 4h
	Minoxidil	Oral	0.1–0.2 mg/kg/dose	BID-TID
	Sodium nitroprusside	IV	0.5–10 mcg/kg/min	Infusion

[a]Commercial suspension available.

ACE, Angiotensin converting enzyme; *BID*, twice daily; *BPD*, bronchopulmonary dysplasia; *IV*, intravenous; *Q*, every; *QD*, once daily; *QID*, four times daily; *TID*, three times daily.

higher systolic blood pressure than term neonates during childhood, adolescence, and adulthood.[56,57] Infants born with intrauterine growth restriction or small for gestational age already have stiffer blood vessels and more hypertension during childhood.[58–60] The mechanism seems to be related to being born with a lower nephron endowment, leading to glomerular hyperfiltration and injury.[61,62] Given the increasing population of premature neonates surviving to older ages, routine blood pressure monitoring is a simple way to detect early risk of future cardiovascular and kidney disease. All NICU graduates, whether hypertensive or not, should be encouraged to have lifelong regular blood pressure measurements during routine health exams.

CHAPTER 61

Altered Development of the Kidneys and the Urinary Tract

Julie E. Goodwin, Akhil Maheshwari

KEY POINTS

1. Congenital renal anomalies account for one-fourth of all congenital anomalies.
2. Early pre- or postnatal detection can facilitate appropriate, timely management.
3. Many infants will require coordinated, multispecialty treatment.
4. Renal abnormalities are being increasingly recognized in four broad groups: (1) congenital anomalies of the kidney and the urinary tract (CAKUTs), such as renal agenesis, kidney hypodysplasia, and abnormalities of the draining systems; (2) functional disorders such as congenital nephrotic syndrome and renal tubular acidosis; (3) low nephron counts and glomerular volume, which may be an isolated condition or may be seen in association with CAKUT; and (D) inherited cystic disorders, which can be autosomal recessive or autosomal dominant.
5. Infants with inherited renal abnormalities require long-term specialty care to assess both urologic and renal function.

Altered Development of the Kidneys and the Urinary Tract

The two kidneys begin developing at approximately the 3rd week, and despite some ethnic variation, they can each contain more than 1 million nephrons by the 36th week.[1] The normal renal system filters waste and excess liquid from the blood, produces hormones that help strengthen bones, controls blood pressure, and directs the production of red blood cells.[2] The filtered waste, in the form of urine, drains from the kidneys to the bladder through the ureters and is excreted from the bladder through the urethra. Prenatally, the fetal bladder may be first visible at 10 to 12 weeks' gestation, and by midgestation, it fills and empties every 30 to 60 minutes.[3] Fetal urine production begins by 9 to 10 weeks of gestation and increases by 14 to 16 weeks, such that after this point the bulk of amniotic fluid is made of fetal urine.[4,5]

The kidneys and urinary tract often show birth defects that can affect the form and function of these organs. There are four major types of congenital renal abnormalities: (1) anatomic disruptions that are grouped together as the congenital anomalies of the kidney and the urinary tract (CAKUTs), such as renal agenesis, kidney hypodysplasia, and abnormalities of the draining systems[6,7] (the etiology of all CAKUTs is not yet clearly known, but genetic and environmental risk factors are being identified[6]; anomalies at the most severe end of the spectrum, such as renal agenesis, may be inconsistent with survival, but many less severe defects may remain asymptomatic until later childhood or even adulthood); (2) functional disorders such as congenital nephrotic syndrome and renal tubular acidosis; (3) low nephron counts and glomerular volume,[8,9] which may be an isolated condition or may be seen in association with CAKUT; (4) inherited cystic disorders, which can be autosomal recessive or autosomal dominant.[10] Most patients with autosomal dominant polycystic kidney disease do not develop symptoms until adulthood, although some infants are now increasingly being identified earlier.

In this chapter, we seek to illustrate lesions involving the renal system, including pathologic alterations associated with various syndromes, and to analyze the more recent therapeutic interventions that may modify the natural history of some of these severe conditions. We have included evidence from our own clinical experience and from an extensive literature search in the databases PubMed, Embase, and Scopus. To avoid bias in identification of existing studies, key words were short-listed prior to the actual search, both from anecdotal experience and from PubMed's Medical Subject Heading (MeSH) thesaurus.

Congenital Abnormalities of the Kidney and the Urinary Tract

The congenital anomalies of the kidney and the urinary tract, frequently grouped together and described using the acronym CAKUT,[6,7] comprise 20% to 30% of all major birth defects.[1,4,11] More than 200 clinical syndromes currently include CAKUTs as a component of the phenotype.[4] There are three major types:

- Renal abnormalities include uni- or bilateral renal agenesis, malpositioned kidney(s), renal hypoplasia, structural abnormalities with renal dysplasia, and anatomic abnormalities such as in horseshoe kidney.[12]
- Ureters may show blockage at the ureteropelvic junction or the ureterovesicular junction with the formation of a ureterocele; vesicoureteral junction reflux; or ureteral duplication, where one of the two ureters may show reflux or obstruction.[13]
- Downstream abnormalities may occur in the bladder and urethral valves. The bladder may not be visualized prenatally in the case of a bilateral severe kidney anomaly with no kidney function. A large bladder may result from either bladder outlet obstruction or may indicate neurogenic dysfunction with poor emptying capacity.[14]

Any blockages in urinary flow can result in renal enlargement, as in hydronephrosis. These changes can start in utero and can be seen in prenatal sonography. The severity may vary; mild abnormalities can result in hydronephrosis or recurrent urinary tract infections, whereas the more severe ones can result in life-threatening kidney failure and end-stage renal disease.

The inheritance of CAKUTs is complex and not completely understood. These anomalies are seen at a frequency of 1 in 100 to 500

Table 61.1 Genes Associated With CAKUT in Humans

Type of Malformation	Renal Phenotype	Gene	Cause
Renal agenesis	Absence of the ureter and kidney	*RET, GDNF, FGF20, FRAS1, FREM2*	Lack of interaction between the ureteric bud and MM
Renal hypoplasia	Reduced number of ureteric bud branches and nephrons; small kidney size, often associated with dysplasia	*Pax2, Sall1, Six2, BMP4, HNF1B, UMOD*	Aberrant interaction between ureteric bud and MM
Renal dysplasia	Reduced number of ureteric bud branches and nephrons; undifferentiated stromal and mesenchymal cells, cysts, or cartilage	*PAX2, HNF1B, UMOD, Nphp1 BMP4, Six2, XPNPEP3*	Aberrant interaction between ureteric bud and MM
MCDK	Absent glomeruli and tubules	*HNF1B, UPIIIA, PEX26, ELN, HNF1B, ALG12, FRG1, FRG2, CYP4A11*	Aberrant interaction between ureteric bud and MM
Duplex ureters	Duplex ureters and kidneys or duplex ureters and collecting systems	*Robo2, FoxC1, FoxC2, BMP4*	Supernumerary ureteric bud budding from the MD
Horseshoe kidney	Kidneys are fused at inferior lobes and located lower than usual	*HNF1B*	Defects in renal capsule
VUR	Urine refluxes to various degrees from bladder up into the collecting system	*PAX2, ROBO2, SIX1, SIX5, SOX17, TNXB, CHD1L, TRAP1*	Aberrant insertion of ureter into bladder wall
Renal tubular dysgenesis	Absence of or incomplete differentiation of proximal tubule	*ACE, AGT, AGTR1, REN*	Impaired tubular growth and differentiation

CAKUT, Congenital anomalies of the kidney and urinary tract; *MCDK,* multicystic dysplastic kidney; *MD,* mesonephric duct; *MM,* metanephric mesenchyme; *VUR,* vesicoureteral reflux.
Reproduced with minor modifications from Song R, Yosypiv IV. Genetics of congenital anomalies of the kidney and urinary tract. *Pediatr Nephrol. 2011*; 26:353–364.

neonates, are familial in 10% to 20% of cases, can be uni- or bilateral, and constitute approximately 20% to 30% of all anomalies identified in the prenatal period.[15] These conditions lead to 30% to 50% of all pediatric chronic kidney disease and are the most common cause of end-stage renal disease requiring renal replacement therapy in children.[16]

When inherited, most CAKUTs follow an autosomal dominant pattern with reduced penetrance. Some anomalies show an autosomal recessive pattern.[17] In many cases, the inheritance pattern is unknown or the condition may not be inherited. Some patients may have non-motile ciliopathies and other syndromes associated with renal malformations, such as Meckel–Gruber, short rib, Bardet–Biedl, asplenia/polysplenia, hereditary renal adysplasia, Zellweger, trisomies, the VACTER-L association (vertebral defects, anal atresia, cardiac defects, tracheo-esophageal fistula, renal anomalies, and limb abnormalities), Potter, caudal dysplasia, and sirenomelia.[16] A list of the best-known genes involved in CAKUTs is provided in Table 61.1.

Renal Agenesis

Unilateral kidney agenesis is a relatively frequent, multifactorial anomaly.[18] Most cases result from the involution of a multicystic dysplastic kidney or as a primary developmental anomaly. Sometimes, it may reflect an earlier renal infarction due to inadequate vascular supply or an involuted unilateral dysplastic kidney. The clinical outcomes of infants with a solitary functioning kidney are generally favorable if there are no other forms of CAKUT. Some infants are at risk for hyperfiltration injury[19] and may require follow-up. However, the surviving kidney in most patients will undergo compensatory hypertrophy, which is due to an increase in nephron hypertrophy, not a change in nephron number.

Bilateral renal agenesis is considered a form of CAKUT. Historically this was considered to be a fatal condition, incompatible with extrauterine life. There are reports of amnioinfusion to support lung development, and studies are currently underway to assess this intervention and its outcomes. It is critical to note that even if lung development is adequate, the neonate will have end-stage kidney disease, and amnioinfusions increase the risk for preterm delivery, both of which will contribute to morbidity and mortality.[20,21]

Renal Ectopia

Ectopic kidneys can be located anywhere in the body other than the typical renal fossa and may be noted prenatally, postnatally, or later if imaging is obtained for another purpose. The most frequently noted site is the pelvis, and very rarely, the thorax.[4]

Similar to horseshoe kidneys, crossed-fused renal ectopia is also a fusion anomaly and results in both kidneys being located on one side. The ureter of the ectopically located kidney inserts orthotopically into the bladder, on the original side.[4]

Multicystic Kidney Dysplasia

Kidneys with multicystic kidney dysplasia show areas with abnormal tissue organization and multiple noncommunicating cysts, which may be of variable size and location. These affected regions do not have function; some cysts may involute over time, but many persist.[14] Some cases also show a dilated renal outflow tract, although it may be unclear whether this dilatation is yet another primary developmental abnormality or is a secondary manifestation related to compression from the cysts. In these cases, functional scanning using dimercaptosuccinic acid (DMSA) or mercaptoacetyltriglycine (MAG3) can help determine the likely effectiveness of intervention.

Horseshoe Kidney or Renal Fusion

In most cases, the kidneys are fused at the lower pole (Fig. 61.1). These anomalies have been associated with trisomy 18 and male gender. Anatomically, fused kidneys may be positioned lower than normal and may have associated ureteropelvic junction (UPJ) obstruction; the clinical manifestations may include urinary tract infections, abdominal mass, and/or hematuria.[22]

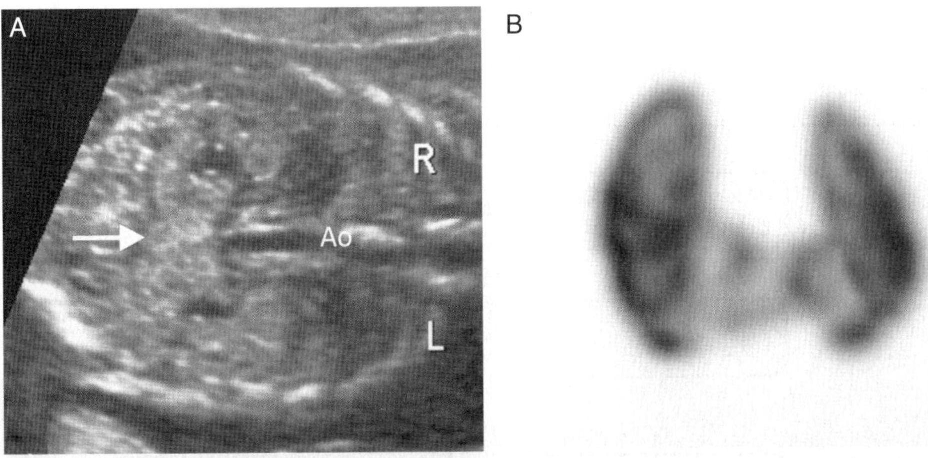

Fig. 61.1 Horseshoe Kidney. (A) A coronal ultrasound image in a 19-week fetus shows the bridge of renal parenchyma *(arrow)* connecting the lower poles of the kidneys, anterior to the aorta (Ao). (B) A technetium-99m-dimercaptosuccinic acid scan from a different patient demonstrates fusion of the kidneys inferiorly by an isthmus, forming a horseshoe kidney. (A, Reproduced with permission and minor modifications from Fong et al. The fetal urogenital tract. In: *Diagnostic Ultrasound*, ch. 39, 1336–1375; B, Reproduced with permission and after minor modifications from Ayyala et al. Genitourinary imaging. In: *Pediatric Radiology: The Requisites*, ch. 6, 141–190.)

The treatment is surgical. Some infants may be treatable with transperitoneal laparoscopy, which may permit exploration of the pyelocalyceal system and detection of anatomic anomalies such as crossing vessels, and if needed, procedures such as pyeloplasty.

Duplex Kidneys

The term duplex kidney indicates the presence of duplicated ureters or a duplicated collecting system (Fig. 61.2A). Such duplications comprise a spectrum of disorders that range from incomplete changes in a small segment of the ureter to complete doubling of the ureter(s), where two ureteral tubes join at the bladder. Incomplete duplication may involve a bifid collecting system. Complete ureteral duplication is when there are two separate ureters that continue and enter the urinary bladder.[23,24]

A ureterocele is a cystic dilation of the ureter at the bladder entrance (see Fig. 61.2B).[25] These anomalies may follow an autosomal dominant inheritance with incomplete penetrance. The risk of infections, including pyelonephritis, may be increased.[26,27] Conjoint ureters may be more frequent than complete ureteral duplication and may have a female predilection.[28] In some cases, a duplex system may be associated with hydronephrosis, obstruction, reflux, and infections,[29] which may lead to chronic renal disease.

Prenatally Diagnosed Hydronephrosis

Antenatal urinary tract dilation is diagnosed in 1% to 5% of all pregnancies. As many as 36% to 80% of the less severe cases recover postnatally, but the most severely afflicted infants may not. Mutations in the hepatocyte nuclear factor 1B *(HNF1B)* gene are identified in up to 50% infants with kidney anomalies.[1,30] Other frequently detected mutations include those in the paired box gene 2 *(PAX2)* and the eyes absent homolog 1 *(EYA1)* genes. A schematic diagram

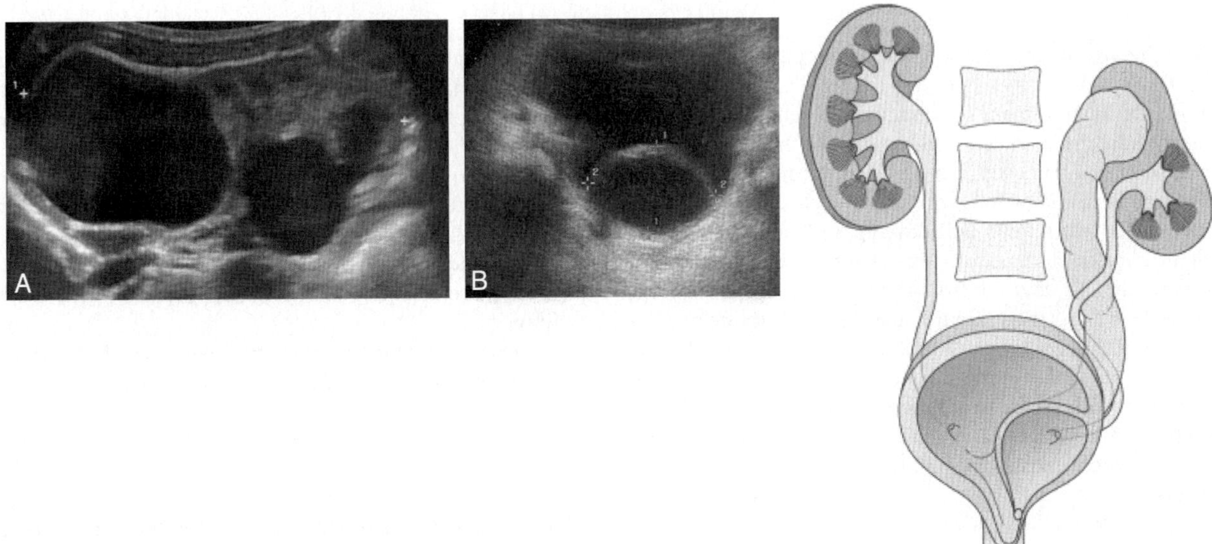

Fig. 61.2 Renal Anomalies. (A) Duplex kidney. Ultrasound shows grossly dilated upper moiety of the right kidney, with milder dilatation of the lower moiety. (B) A large ureterocele is identified on ultrasound within the bladder. Schematic figure shows the same on the right. (Reproduced with permission and minor modification from Arthurs et al. Imaging of the kidneys, urinary tract and pelvis in children. In: *Grainger & Allison's Diagnostic Radiology*, 72, 1846–1885.)

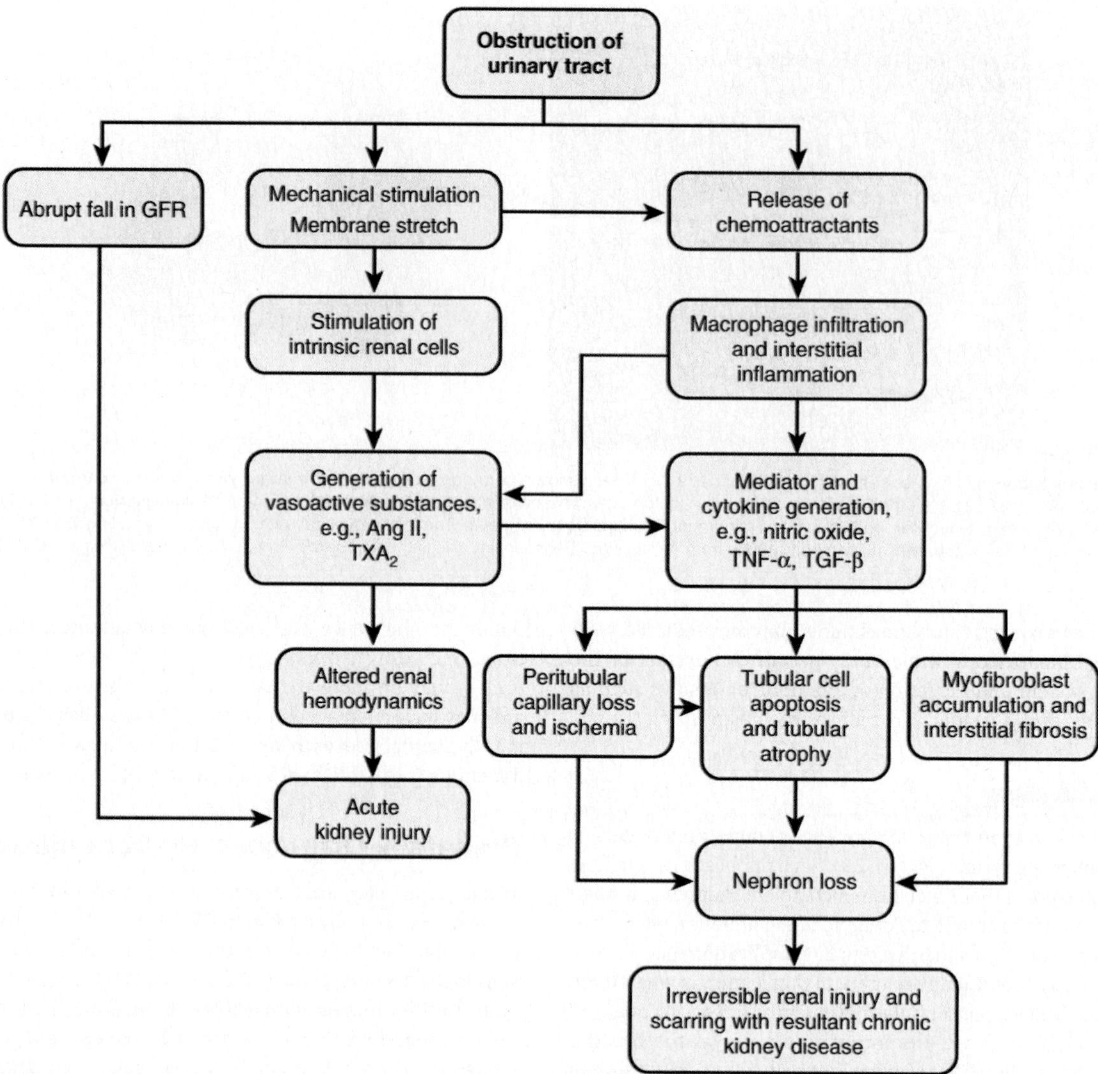

Fig. 61.3 Pathophysiology of the Loss of Renal Function and Chronic Structural Damage in Obstructive Nephropathy. *Ang II,* Angiotensin II; *GFR,* glomerular filtration rate; *TGF-β,* transforming growth factor-β; *TNF-α,* tumor necrosis factor α; *TXA_2,* thromboxane A_2. (From Gallaghar and Hughes. Urinary tract obstruction. In: *Comprehensive Clinical Nephrology*, 58, 704–716.e1.)

for the loss of renal function in obstructive nephropathy is shown in Fig. 61.3.

The postnatal management of antenatally diagnosed hydronephrosis is not fully resolved yet.[31] The severity of the urinary tract dilation in the third trimester can be classified in several ways (Figs. 61.4 and 61.5). However, mild hydronephrosis is likely to be transient; <5% of infants will develop vesicoureteral reflux (VUR) or urinary tract infections. These infants do not require antibiotic prophylaxis, and the first postnatal ultrasound may be safely delayed for 1 to 2 weeks. In the subgroup with severe hydronephrosis, about 20% will have VUR and 10% to 40% will likely develop urinary tract infections during infancy. Even in the absence of VUR, children with severe hydronephrosis are at risk of urinary tract infections. The need for a voiding cystourethrogram (VCUG) and antibiotic prophylaxis in moderate to severe hydronephrosis is controversial.

Ureteropelvic Junction Obstruction

UPJ obstruction is one of the most frequently seen CAKUTs; the incidence may vary somewhere between 1 in 1000 to 1500 newborns and is a common cause of antenatal hydronephrosis.[13] Longstanding obstruction may lead to pyelonephritis, hydronephrosis, and renal failure. The pathophysiology of UPJ obstruction is unknown, but some possibilities have been noted:

1. Obliteration-recanalization: transient obliteration of the developing ureteric duct (future ureter) followed by recanalization. This hypothesis has lost some support.
2. Developmental abnormalities with insertion anomalies of the ureters, ureteral muscular hypertrophy, and/or peripelvicalyceal fibrosis.
3. Extrinsic obstruction by abnormal blood vessels: the developing ureters may have a positional kink or compression due to abnormal large vessels.
4. Genetic anomalies: this is a possibility; homozygous and heterozygous *Id2* mutations in rodents have been associated with hydronephrosis due to congenital UPJ obstruction. It is more frequent in males and unilateral, in the right kidney that is positioned higher.
5. Some investigators have suggested a role of smooth muscle cell apoptosis and defective neural development in congenital UPJ obstruction.

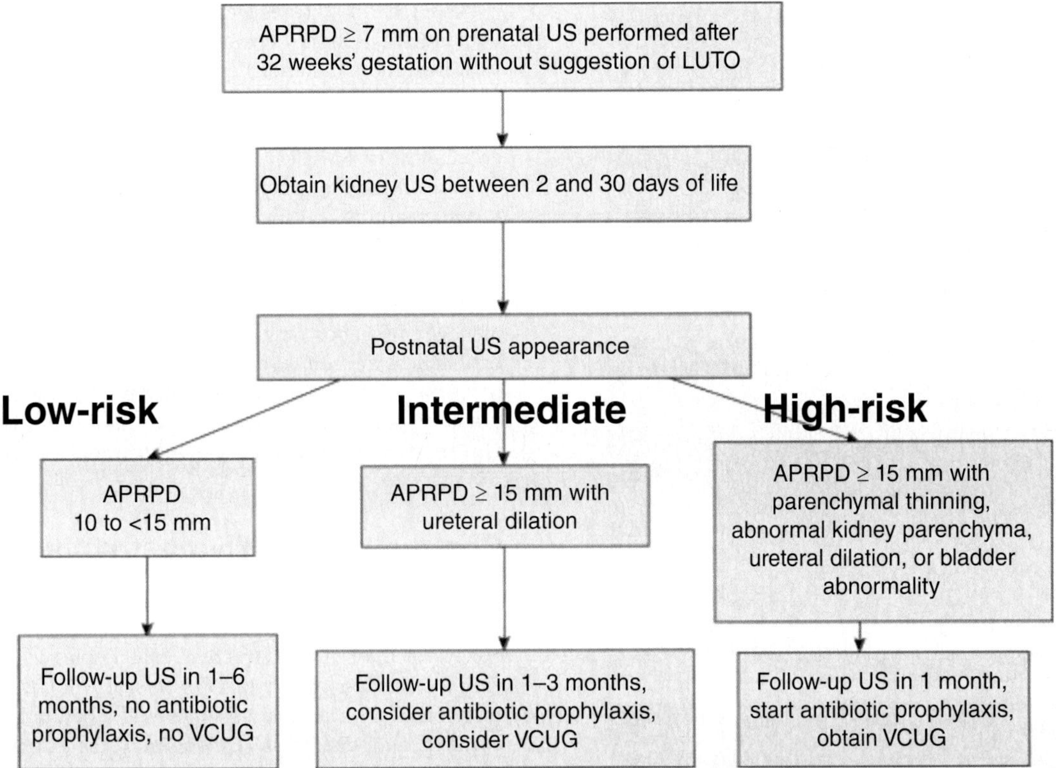

Fig. 61.4 Urinary Tract Dilatation Classification With Suggested Postnatal Management of Antenatal Hydronephrosis. The classification includes three categories with increasing risk. *APRPD,* Anterior posterior renal pelvic dilation; *LUTO,* lower urinary tract obstruction; *US,* ultrasound; *VCUG,* voiding cystourethrogram. (Reproduced with permission and minor modifications from Vogt and Springel. The kidney and urinary tract of the neonate. In: *Fanaroff and Martin's Neonatal-Perinatal Medicine*, 93, 1871–1895.)

UPJ obstruction results from intrinsic stenosis, fibrosis, or a crossing vessel leading to ureteral compression. Less severe cases are often asymptomatic and may not be identified during infancy. Most infants do not require surgery in the neonatal period, except those with severe abnormalities without a normal contralateral kidney or in cases of bilateral UPJ obstruction. Surgery may be needed if the renal function, size of the kidney, or drainage parameters are worsening over time. The best practice for unilateral cases with a normal contralateral kidney is still not defined. Some cases related to genetic abnormalities/familial CAKUT need evaluation.[30]

Primary Megaureter

Megaureter refers to an enlarged ureter, which may be due to an intrinsic abnormality, external obstruction, or VUR.[32] Many cases resolve during the first 1 to 3 years of age, but infants with megaureter are still at risk for pyelonephritis and kidney scarring. Thus infants with megaureters with VUR are often treated with prophylactic antibiotics. Secondary megaureters due to a neurogenic bladder or urethral issues such as posterior urethral valves may have to be treated for the specific etiology. Ureterovesical junction obstruction may result from a primary obstructive process or secondarily in cases of bladder hypertrophy, often associated with bladder outlet obstruction.

Vesicoureteral Reflux

VUR is the retrograde flow of urine from the bladder upward into the ureters and kidneys, resulting from anomalous anatomy of the ureterovesical junction. VUR is graded by VCUG on a scale of 1 to 5 (Fig. 61.6). The degree of vesicoureteral reflux is poorly correlated with the degree of urinary tract dilation seen on ultrasound, and therefore, voiding studies are required for assessment.[33] Severe VUR and pyelonephritis can increase the risk of kidney scarring. High-grade VUR can also lead to bladder dysfunction over time.

Posterior Urethral Valves and Prune Belly Syndrome

Posterior urethral valves (PUVs) are seen in about 4 per 100,000 male infants and are the most frequently seen cause of lower urinary tract obstruction in male infants.[34] Because fetal urine contributes to the total amniotic fluid volume, PUVs and related urinary tract obstruction are often associated with oligohydramnios. The urethral obstruction causes urethral dilatation (megalourethra); a dilated, dysfunctional bladder (megalocystis); VUR; megaureters; bilateral hydronephrosis; and obstructive renal dysplasia. The urinary bladder frequently shows a hypertrophic muscular wall. Subsequent pressure over the abdomen produces atrophy of the abdominal muscles and leads to an abdomen covered only by skin and peritoneum or by an extremely atrophic muscular layer. These changes have been described as the prune belly or the Eagle–Barrett syndrome (Fig. 61.7); Fig. 61.8 shows various types of renal cysts. The diaphragmatic elevation into the thoracic space causes pulmonary hypoplasia and respiratory insufficiency, which is an important predictor of survival. Many patients have undescended testes and intestinal malrotation due to the bladder distention that impedes normal bowel positioning or testicular descent. The full oligohydramnios sequence may include low-set ears, a flat nose, folds under the eyes, and *varus* deformities of the feet.

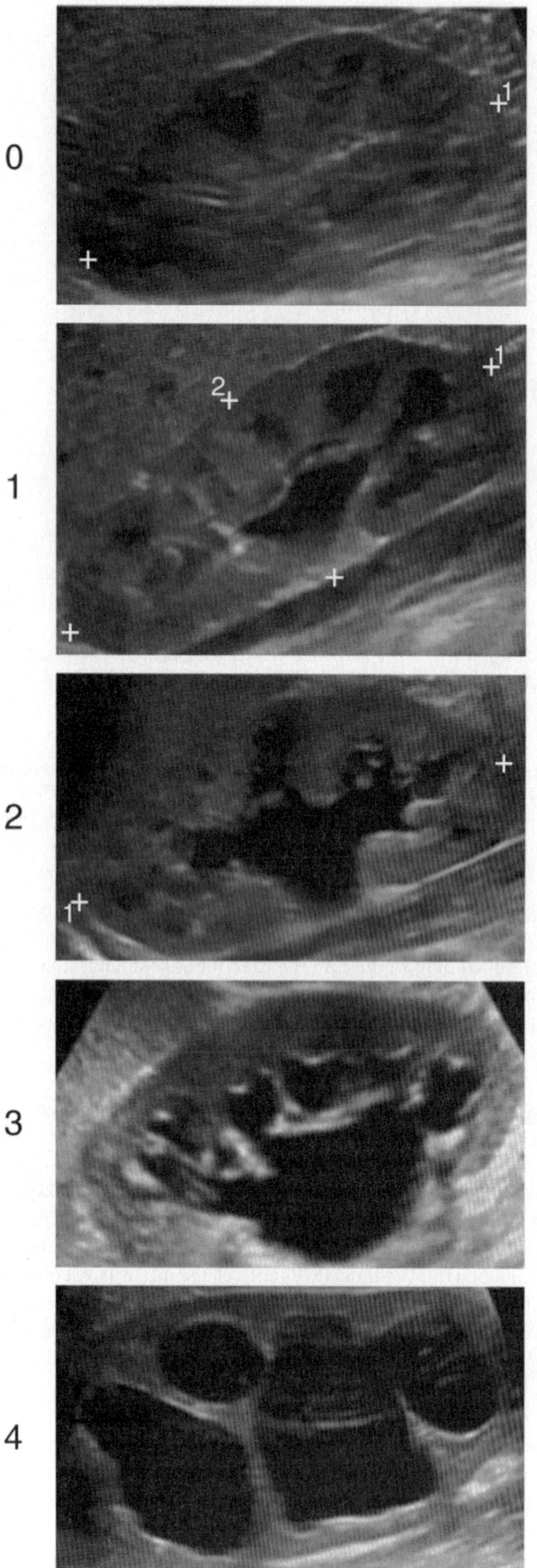

Fig. 61.5 **Congenital Hydronephrosis.** The Society for Fetal Urology (SFU) criteria as demonstrated in postnatal sonograms. Grade 0 shows no central renal dilation. In grade 1, the renal pelvis only is visible; in grade 2, major calices can be identified; in grade 3, major and minor calices can be identified; and grade 4 has features of grade 3 but with parenchymal thinning as well. (Reproduced with minor modifications from Pohl. Pediatric urogenital imaging. In: *Campbell-Walsh-Wein Urology*, 24, 403–425.e2.)

About 3% of all cases with prune belly syndrome are associated with mutations in the hepatocyte nuclear factor 1β *(HFN1β)* gene.[35] However, these mutations are not specific; similar mutations have been seen in infants who either did not have these anomalies or had the VACTER-L association. One report also noted these mutations in an infant with a Müllerian anomaly and a solitary kidney.

Assessment of outcomes for infants with PUVs reveal that a nadir serum creatinine ≥1 mg/dL is associated with progression to end-stage kidney disease in childhood.[36] The urinary bladder can be drained by placing a vesico-amniotic shunt in utero or by vesicocentesis after birth. Fetal lower urinary tract obstructions have also been managed by endoscopic placement of a vesico-amniotic shunt to drain fetal urine into the amniotic sac, which may reduce the severity of the oligohydramnios and associated pulmonary hypoplasia. Unfortunately, some infants with these shunts can develop bilateral obstructive renal dysplasia leading to chronic renal failure.

Obstructive and Nonobstructive Renal Dysplasia

Renal dysplasias can be obstructive (in nearly 60% of cases) or nonobstructive.[37] The obstructive renal dysplasias may be associated with a distended urinary bladder (megacystis), which can be identified on fetal ultrasound. In some mild cases, only the renal pelvis or the ureter is distended. Histologically, the kidneys show evidence of hydronephrosis but with medullary compression by the urine accumulated within the pelvis. Histopathologically, the renal medulla and even the cortex may show some fibrosis.

Nonobstructive renal dysplasias can be either syndromic or nonsyndromic. The molecular mechanisms involved are not well known; a minority have documented genetic mutations. Mutations in the transforming growth factor-β gene are plausible but have not been studied in large cohorts. Some cases with multicystic renal dysplasia have been noted to have overexpression of the insulin growth factor.[38] Other cases have been documented to have mutations in the hepatocyte nuclear factor-1 β *(HNF1β)*, paired box gene 2 *(Pax2)*, uromodulin *(UMOD)*, and eyes absent homolog 1 *(Eya1)* genes.[39] A large study by Saisawat et al. applied massive parallel exon resequencing of 30 candidate genes in pooled DNA from 40 patients with CAKUT and identified seven novel mutations in four genes: *RET*, *BMP4*, *FRAS1*, and *FREM2*.[40]

Nonmotile Ciliopathies and Congenital Renal Diseases

Primary ciliary dysfunction has been noted in many genetic conditions. There are several types of cilia in the human body, and their functions differ from one other. The embryonic node is a motile monocilium involved with laterality. Renal tubular cells have been noted to have nonmotile monocilia,[41] and these have been implicated in renal dysplasia associated with Meckel–Gruber syndrome, Joubert syndrome, short rib syndrome, asplenia/polysplenia syndrome, and VACTER-L.

Meckel–Gruber Syndrome

Meckel–Gruber syndrome is an autosomal recessive condition that includes large cystic kidneys in combination with microcephaly with occipital encephalocele, cleft palate, and polydactyly, undescended testes, or ambiguous genitalia.[42] The chromosomal anomalies have been noted on 17q22, 17q12.2, 8q22.1, 12q21.32, 16q12.2, 4p15.32, 3q22.1, and 12q24.31.[42–45]

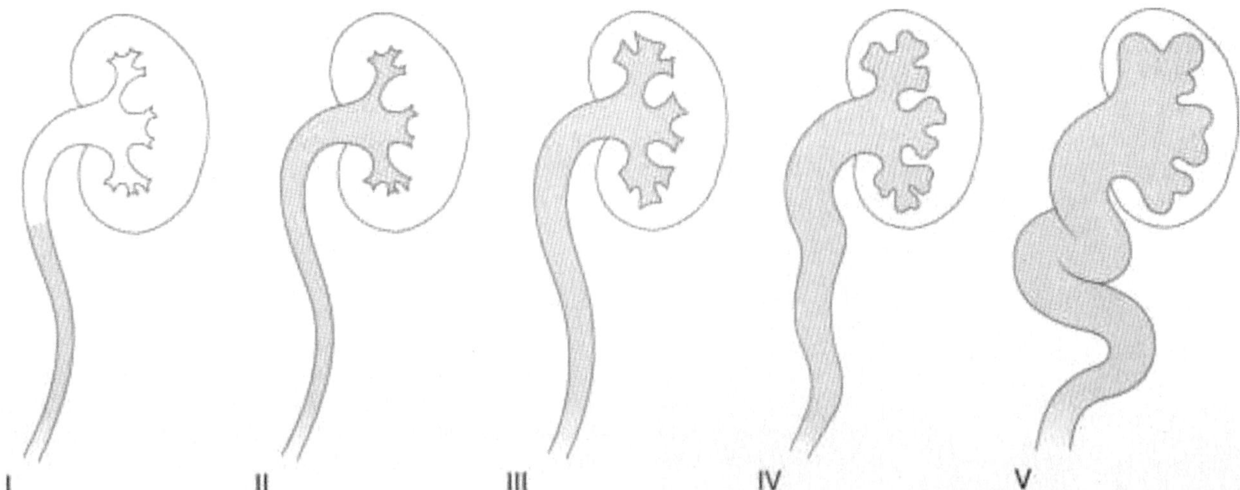

Fig. 61.6 Vesicoureteral Reflux Grading. A schematic drawing demonstrating the vesicoureteral reflux grading system on a voiding cystourethrogram. (I) Ureter and upper collecting system without dilatation; (II) mild or (III) moderate dilatation of the ureter and mild or moderate dilatation of the renal pelvis but minimal blunting of the fornices; (IV) moderate dilatation and/or tortuosity of the ureter with moderate dilatation of the renal pelvis and calyces and obliteration of the sharp angle of the fornices but maintenance of papillary impression in the majority of calyces; (V) gross dilatation and tortuosity of ureters, renal pelvis, and calyces; papillary impressions are not visible in the majority of calyces. (Reproduced with permission and minor modifications from Karmazyn, Boaz; Brown, Brandon P. Vesicoureteral Reflux. In: Caffey's Pediatric Diagnostic Imaging. Published January 1, 2019. Pages 1148–1156.e3.)

Joubert Syndrome and Related Disorders

These conditions are autosomal recessive conditions where cystic renal dysplasia and nephronophthisis (tubulointerstitial nephritis and cysts at the cortico-medullary junction) may be associated with hypoplasia of the cerebellar vermis, retinal dystrophy, ocular coloboma, rotatory nystagmus, polydactyly, and congenital hepatic fibrosis. The presenting renal abnormalities in these infants may include elevated creatinine and polyuria, which may eventually lead to renal failure. The prevalence of kidney problems in Joubert syndrome and related disorders may be as high as 30%. When children are followed long term, the percentage is even higher.[46]

Joubert syndrome may be rooted in ciliary disorders with some overlap in clinical presentations with Meckel and Bardet–Biedl syndromes. Mutations have been noted in the ciliary/basal body genes: *INPPFE, AH11, NPHP1, CEP290, TMEM67/MKS3, RPGR1P1L, ARL13B*, and *CC2D2A*.

Short Rib Syndrome

Short rib syndrome is a lethal, autosomal recessive osteochondrodysplasia and has been traditionally divided into four types (I–IV). Many patients have bilateral cystic renal dysplasia, associated with thoracic, gastrointestinal, facial, eye, and brain abnormalities. The syndrome has been associated with mutations in *TTC21B*, which encodes the retrograde intraflagellar transport protein IFT139. This can explain the nephronophthisis and asphyxiating thoracic dystrophy.[47]

Bardet–Biedl Syndrome

Bardet–Biedl syndrome is an autosomal recessive condition that shows renal dysplasia in association with retinitis pigmentosa, polydactyly, and hypogenitalism. The possibility of renal insufficiency increases with age. Fetal ultrasound can assist with prenatal diagnosis with detection of polydactyly and renal cysts. Eighteen genes have been associated with Bardet–Biedl syndrome: *BBS1, BBS2, ARL6 (BBS3), BBS4, BBS5, MKKS (BBS6), BBS7, TTC8 (BBS8), BBS9, BBS10, TRIM32 (BBS11), BBS12, MKS1 (BBS13), CEP290 (BBS14), WDPCP (BBS15), SDCCAG8 (BBS16), LTZFL1 (BBS17)*, and *BBIP1 (BBS18)*. Histologically, the kidneys show extensive replacement of parenchyma by round cysts lined by flat to cuboidal epithelium. The glomeruli are preserved. Persistent fetal lobulations have been noted, suggesting a maturational defect.[48]

Renal-Hepatic-Pancreatic Dysplasia (RHPD) and Asplenia/Polysplenia

RHPD is an autosomal recessive condition that is sometimes associated with situs inversus and polysplenia or asplenia. The kidneys show cystic dysplasia.[49] At the molecular level, two types of RHPDs have been described: (1) a homozygous or compound heterozygous mutation in the *NPNP3* gene on chromosome 3q22 and (2) a homozygous mutation in the *NEK8* gene on chromosome 17q11. The kidneys in RHPD and polysplenia tend to be grossly more solid than kidneys with multicystic dysplasia.

Hereditary Renal Adysplasia or Renal Hypodysplasia/Aplasia (RHDA)

RHDA is an autosomal dominant condition with variable penetrance and is characterized by unilateral renal agenesis and contralateral dysplasia. This combination is often lethal due to oligohydramnios and pulmonary hypoplasia. RHDA1 syndrome has been associated with mutations in the *ITGA8* gene (chromosome 10p13) and *RHDA2* with *FGF20* (chromosome 8q22). The disease spectrum may include unilateral renal agenesis, double ureters, renal cyst, hydronephrosis, and unilateral multicystic kidneys.[50]

Zellweger Syndrome and Peroxisomal Disorders

Peroxisomes are ultrastructural organelles involved in biosynthesis of membrane phospholipids, cholesterol, and bile acids; amino acid degradation; reduction of hydrogen peroxide; and regulation of oxalate synthesis (abnormalities may increase the risk of calcium oxalate synthesis and nephrolithiasis). The best known peroxisomal disorder is Zellweger syndrome, also known as cerebrohepatorenal syndrome. This is an uncommon autosomal recessive, lethal condition, seen in about 1 in 25,000 to 50,000 infants. In addition to cystic renal dysplasia with persistent fetal lobulations, horseshoe kidney, and urethral duplication, these infants may have hypotonia, a long and narrow forehead, small whitish or grayish-brown spots in the

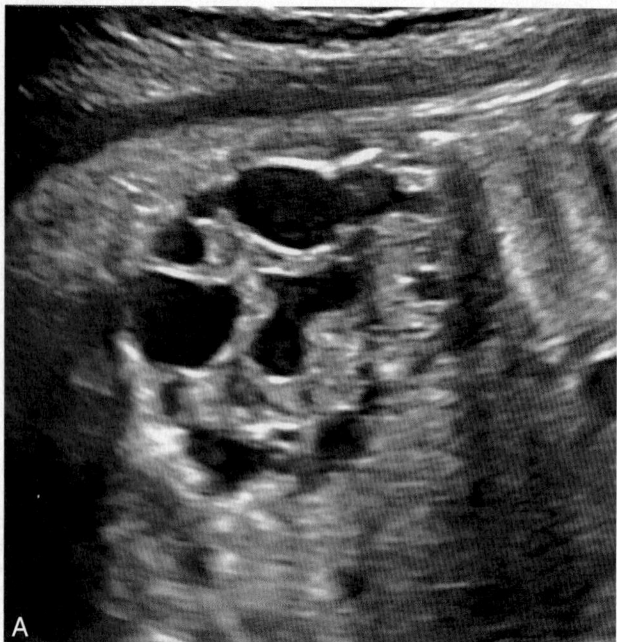

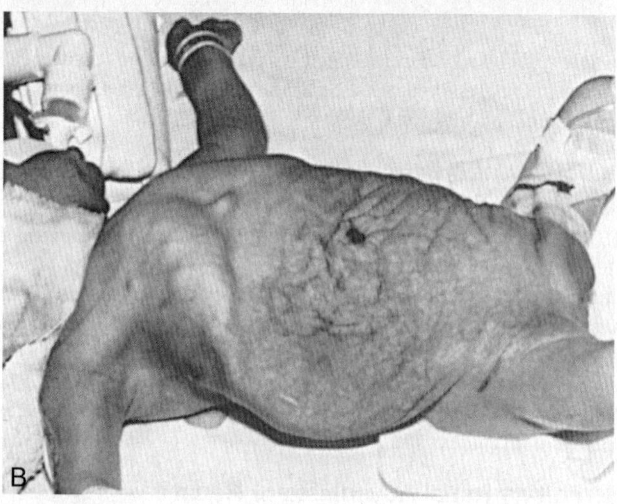

Fig. 61.7 Obstructive Renal Dysplasia and Prune Belly Syndrome. (A) An ultrasound image from an infant with bilateral ureteropelvic junction shows cortical and parenchymal cysts. (B) Photograph of a 1600-g newborn with the prune-belly syndrome. The lack of tonicity of the abdominal wall and the wrinkled appearance of the skin are notable. (A, Reproduced with permission and after minor modifications from Kamaya et al. Genitourinary imaging. In: *Pediatric Radiology: The Requisites*, ch. 6, 141–190. B, Reproduced with minor modifications from Elder JS. Obstruction of the urinary tract. In: *Nelson Textbook of Pediatrics*, ch. 555, 2800–2810.e1.)

iris (Brushfield spots), hypoplastic supraorbital ridges, epicanthal folds, abnormal brain gyri, and seizures. Histopathologically, the kidneys contain small cortical cysts and occasionally dilated tubules.[51]

Trisomies and Congenital Anomalies of the Kidneys

Infants with trisomies 13, 18, and 21 may show hydronephrosis, horseshoe kidney, a duplex kidney/collecting system, cortical cysts and/or cystic dysplasia, glomerular microcysts, or renal hypoplasia. However, no specific histopathological abnormalities have been identified with these syndromes. About 25% of trisomy 18 patients have duplicated collecting systems and horseshoe kidney. Some may have cortical cysts (17%) and hydronephrosis (15%). In trisomy 21, infants may have renal involvement ranging from cortical microcysts, simple cysts, renal hypoplasia, and immature glomeruli deep in the cortex. These children may also develop obstructive uropathy.[52]

VACTER-L Association

Infants with a VACTER-L association may have a range of renal abnormalities, including hypoplasia, histopathological glomerular and medullary abnormalities, and renal agenesis. This is most likely to be a group of disorders, not a single entity, so there is considerable variation in the clinical features and histopathology of the urinary tract.[53]

Bilateral Renal Agenesis (Potter Syndrome)

Complete absence of both kidneys is one of the most severe congenital renal anomalies. The "Potter facies," with folds under the eyes, a flat nose, a receding chin, and low-set ears, as well as pulmonary hypoplasia, wide hands, and rocker-bottom feet are mechanical deformities produced by the oligohydramnios sequence. The syndrome is likely a group of several genetic abnormalities; one involves recessive mutations in the integrin α8 *(ITGA8)* encoding gene. This gene has a crucial role in renal development and it is expressed in the metanephric mesenchyme surrounding the ureteric bud.[28]

Caudal Dysplasia Syndrome

Renal anomalies include bilateral renal agenesis, renal dysplasia, and horseshoe kidney. These infants may have hypoplastic lower extremities, caudal vertebrae, sacrum, neural tube, and urogenital system. Many also have an imperforate anus.

Infants of diabetic mothers have a 3 to 4 times increased incidence of congenital malformations, including the caudal dysplasia syndrome. Many infants can also have abnormal development of the genitourinary tract.[28]

Sirenomelia

Infants with sirenomelia are born with a single lower extremity. They may have bilateral or unilateral renal agenesis with absent ureters and urinary bladder, renal dysplasia, and renal hypoplasia, with a range of abnormalities including imperforate anus, either ambiguous or absent external genitalia, and a single umbilical artery. The face may show the oligohydramnios sequence with a flat nose, receding chin, and low-set ears, and these infants may have a hypoplastic thorax and broad hands.[54]

Evaluation

Infants with CAKUT warrant close examination to evaluate renal anomalies and various associated anomalies in the cardiac, genital, skeletal, colorectal, and other systems. Birthmarks, branchial cleft cysts, or skeletal anomalies may offer insight into an underlying genetic condition. Severe congenital renal anomalies may be associated with loss of urine output and consequent oligohydramnios and pulmonary hypoplasia. In some cases, serial amnioinfusion and postnatal dialysis have been successful, although these findings need further investigation.

In most cases, postnatal imaging should be delayed until the first void or for 24 hours to avoid underestimating the severity of findings due to physiologic low urine output in the first few days after birth. In 2014 a consensus statement was released including recommendations for classification of prenatal and postnatal urinary tract dilation and general guidelines for postnatal assessment based on the findings.[55] Figs. 61.1 and 61.2 classify patients into risk categories, depending on whether the urinary tract dilation was noted prenatally or postnatally, which then informs further decision-making. Infants with suspicion for high-grade VUR or obstruction should receive prophylactic antibiotics to prevent urinary tract infections.

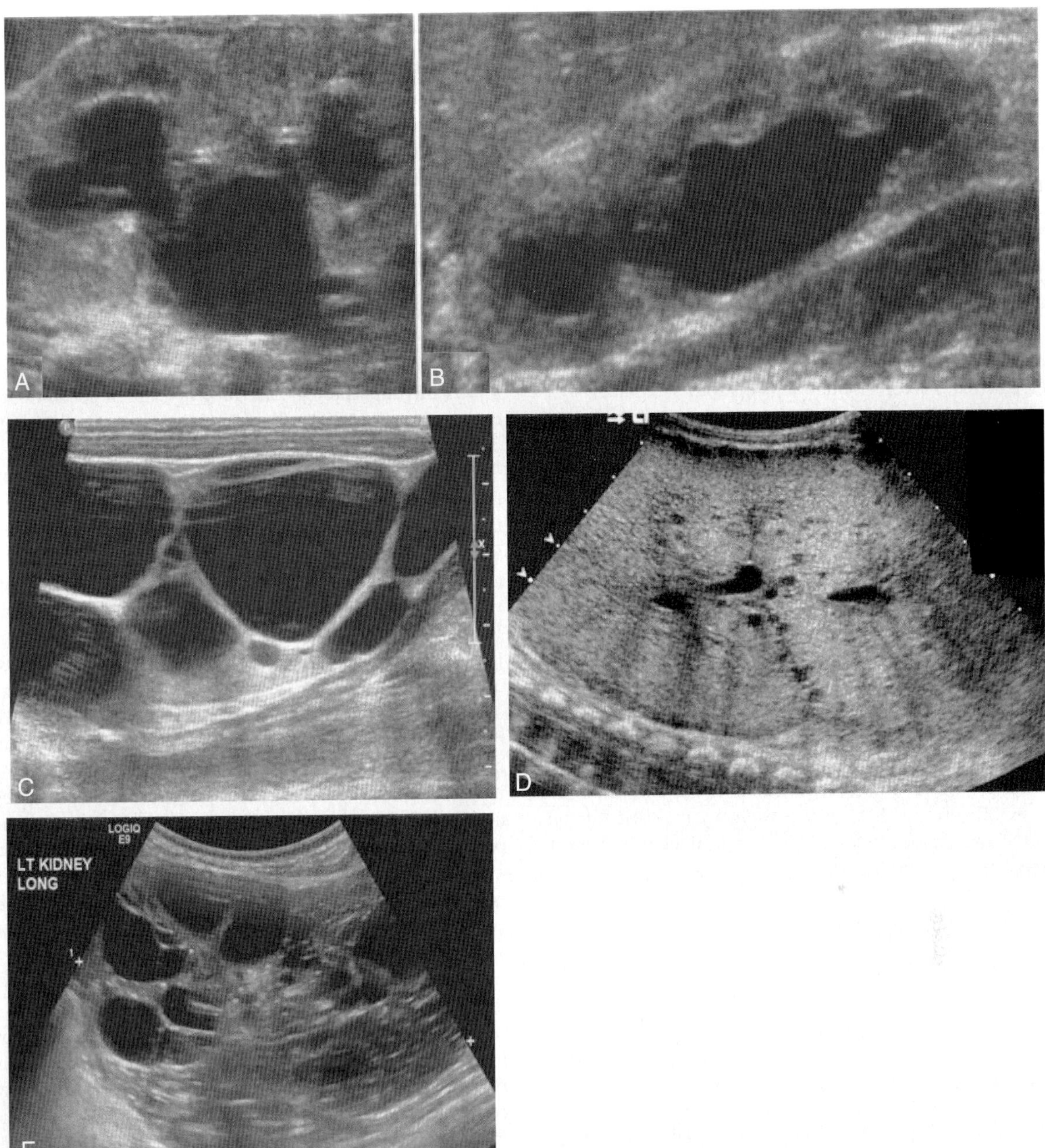

Fig. 61.8 Cystic Diseases of the Neonatal Kidney. (A, B) Obstructive renal dysplasia in an infant with posterior urethral valves. Ultrasound images show bilateral hydronephrosis and thinning of renal cortices. (C) Multicystic dysplasia in the right kidney (MCDK) is marked by cysts of varying size that have replaced the renal parenchyma. (D) Autosomal recessive polycystic kidney disease. Longitudinal view through the kidney demonstrates renal enlargement and lack of normal renal architecture. Note numerous small cysts diffusely. (E) Autosomal dominant polycystic kidney disease. The disorder can be occasionally seen in young infants. Longitudinal view through the kidney demonstrates renal enlargement with cysts in the cortex. (C, Reproduced with permission and after minor modifications from Ayyala, et al. Genitourinary imaging. In: *Pediatric Radiology: The Requisites*, ch. 6, 141–190. D, Reproduced with permission and after minor modifications from Berlin S. Diagnostic imaging of the neonate. In: *Fanaroff and Martin's Neonatal-Perinatal Medicine*, 38, 608–633. E, Reproduced with permission and minor modification from Arthurs et al. Imaging of the kidneys, urinary tract and pelvis in children. In: *Grainger & Allison's Diagnostic Radiology*, 72, 1846–1885.)

Ultrasound is the most convenient study because it can be performed at the bedside. In complicated cases, more invasive studies such as a VCUG, radionuclide cystogram, magnetic resonance urography (MRU), MAG3 scan, and DMSA scan can be done. For longitudinal follow-up, ultrasound is commonly used because it is safe and also can be performed serially at the bedside. Voiding contrast-enhanced ultrasound can also be as useful as VCUG. VCUG has been traditionally used to assess for VUR and possibly ureteroceles and bladder diverticulae. A radionuclide cystogram is used to follow vesicoureteral reflux but will not give anatomic detail of the urethra, ureterovesical junction, or bladder. Thus, when suspecting posterior urethral valves, ureterocele, or another anatomic anomaly, VCUG is preferred as the initial study. MRI/MRU can be used to evaluate for obstructive lesions, anomalies external to the urinary tract, and detail regarding cysts and other anomalies.[56]

A MAG3 scan is a nuclear medicine test used to evaluate for obstruction and differential kidney function by assessing the diuretic function of each kidney. A DMSA scan consists of administering a short-lived radioisotope that is taken up by kidneys. This test provides information regarding the size, function, shape, and position of the kidneys. It is typically used to detect renal scarring, pyelonephritis, and infarction. Both MAG3 and DMSA depend on uptake of the kidneys and hence are performed after 3 months of age.[57]

Functional Disorders

Congenital Nephrotic Syndrome

Congenital nephrotic syndrome (CNS) presents with heavy proteinuria, hypoalbuminemia, hyperlipidemia, and edema. The condition occurs in about 1 in 8200 live births, usually with autosomal recessive inheritance in infants with Finnish ancestry. Some cases occur sporadically or with other conditions such as the Denys–Drash or Pierson syndromes. Sometimes, infants with intrauterine infections or those born to mothers with lupus erythematosus can also develop nephrotic syndrome.[58]

Mothers carrying infants with CNS often have elevated serum or amniotic fluid α-fetoprotein levels due to fetal urinary protein losses. Many fetuses may also show placental edema, ascites, or hydrops. The placenta is typically large, weighing >25% of the infant's birth weight.

CNS type I is caused most often by mutations in the nephrin *(NPHS1)* gene, a component of the glomerular slit diaphragm that plays an important role in urinary filtration. These patients have mesangial hypercellularity, tubular microcysts, and immature glomeruli demonstrating prominent cuboidal epithelial cells. Other genes such as podocin, Wilms tumor suppressor gene *(WT-1)*, and laminin β2 *(LAMB2)* have also been associated with CNS.

The treatment of CNS is complex. Primary CNS is resistant to corticosteroids and immunosuppressive agents, and current treatment is limited to supportive measures such as albumin infusions, nutritional support, and treatment of infectious and thromboembolic complications. Bilateral nephrectomy is typically required for the management of protein loss, followed by peritoneal dialysis support and early renal transplantation.

Neonatal Bartter Syndrome

Neonatal Bartter syndrome is an autosomal recessive inherited hypokalemic tubulopathy that may include classic Bartter syndrome and Gitelman syndrome. The incidence of neonatal Bartter syndrome is 1 in 50,000 to 100,000 live births. These infants typically present with profound salt wasting, polyuria, hypokalemia, and hypercalciuria.[59]

Inborn errors of metabolism such as cystinosis and Fanconi syndrome may present with tubulopathies. These should be excluded in infants with unexplained glucosuria, phosphaturia, and metabolic acidosis.

Renal Tubular Acidosis

Renal tubular acidosis (RTA) is caused by a defect in the reabsorption of bicarbonate or in the secretion of hydrogen ions that is not related to a decrease in the glomerular filtration rate. RTA should be suspected in infants with persistent hyperchloremic metabolic acidosis. There are three forms of RTA: proximal (type II), distal (type I), and hyperkalemic (type IV). RTA may be sporadic or inherited as a classic mendelian trait.[60]

Low Nephron Counts and Glomerular Volume

Nephron development occurs during 5 to 26 weeks' gestation. Intrauterine factors can cause subtle renal structural abnormalities or limit the nephron count, which reduces the filtration surface area in the kidneys with decreased ability to excrete sodium, relative hypervolemia, and increased risk of hypertension and renal disease later in life. Nephron counts show a complex interplay between genetics, genomic imprinting, and the environment.[1]

Numerous studies suggest that the renal nephron count can be lower due to prematurity; intrauterine growth restriction; female gender; maternal diets deficient in protein, iron, or vitamin A; uterine artery ligation; maternal hyperglycemia; and prenatal exposure to glucocorticoids and drugs such as gentamicin, cyclosporin, β-lactams, ethanol, and cox2 inhibitors. One large study calculated that each 1-kg increase in birth weight may add 257,426 glomeruli.[61] The Brenner hypothesis proposes that patients with congenital reduction in the number of nephrons have greater likelihood of developing cardiovascular disease and renal failure in adulthood.

Several important genetic pathways are important in nephrogenesis, such as the glial cell-derived neurotrophic factor (GDNF)/ret proto-oncogene (RET), fibroblast growth factors, paired box gene 2 *(PAX2)*, and hereditary hemochromatosis. The AAA haplotype of the *PAX2* gene can cause a 10% reduction in kidney volume.[62] RET is required for branching nephrogenesis, and a polymorphic variant, RET^{1476A}, can also impair renal development. Mutations in major histocompatibility complex (MHC) class I polypeptide-related sequence B (Imx-1), EYA transcriptional coactivator and phosphatase 1 (Eya-1), SIX homeobox 1 (Six1), spalt-like transcription factor 1 (Sall1), and HNF1 homeobox B (Hnf1b) can also reduce nephron number and disorganize kidney tissue.[63]

In animal models such as rats, interventions during critical phases of development can improve nephron counts.[63] Adequate postnatal nutrition, achieved by cross-fostering growth-restricted pups onto normal lactating females at birth, can restore nephron number and abrogate development of subsequent hypertension. Similarly, supplementation of a maternal low-protein diet with glycine, urea, or alanine during gestation normalized the nephron number in all rat offspring, although blood pressure was only normalized in those supplemented with glycine. Postnatal hypernutrition in normal rats was found to increase the nephron number by 20%, but these rats went on to develop hypertension and glomerulosclerosis with age, likely as a result of obesity. Vitamin A deficiency has been shown to reduce the nephron number in a dose-dependent manner, but encouragingly, a single dose of retinoic acid, administered during early nephrogenesis, was enough to restore nephron numbers to levels of control rats in pups exposed to a low-protein diet in utero. Interestingly, administration of ouabain was also found to abrogate the effect of serum starvation and a low-protein diet on nephron development. Thus there is a possibility that carefully designed, timely interventions may improve nephron counts.

Inherited Renal Cystic Disorders

In addition to the obstructive renal dysplasia and multicystic dysplastic kidneys described above, the autosomal recessive polycystic kidney disease (ARPKD) is also seen in neonates. Fig. 61.8 shows all these types together for comparison.

ARPKD

ARPKD occurs in 1 in 20,000 to 40,000 live births and has a heterozygous carrier rate of 1 in 70. Hence it is a less frequent ciliopathy than autosomal dominant polycystic kidney disease (ADPKD).[64] This disease is associated with mutation(s) in the polycystic kidney and hepatic disease genes, *PKHD1* (chromosome 6p21) and *PKHD2*. The former produces the severe form of the disease and its gene product, polycystin-1, is a receptor-like integral membrane protein involved in cell–cell matrix interactions and calcium homeostasis through physical interaction with the protein product of *PKD2*.[65] Genetic testing through direct sequencing can detect 80% of all cases. Parents of infants born with ARPKD are gene carriers and may be offered preimplantation genetic diagnosis.

Prenatal or early neonatal ultrasonography shows enlarged, echogenic kidneys (see Fig. 61.8D). The renal cysts are in the collecting tubule, appear elongated, and are oriented with the long axis perpendicular to the capsule. Many pregnancies are marked by oligohydramnios in the late second trimester. Infants with ARPKD typically present with Potter facies, enlarged kidneys, hypertension, and renal insufficiency. Pulmonary hypoplasia and consequent respiratory failure are common. Congenital hepatic fibrosis becomes progressively more prominent during later infancy and beyond. Of the neonatal survivors, approximately 40% have severe liver fibrosis and renal disease. Thirty percent present with severe renal and mild hepatobiliary disease and the other 30% with severe hepatobiliary and mild renal disease.

Clinical management is supportive. Neonates with pulmonary hypoplasia need ventilatory support. Hypertension and electrolyte imbalances such as hyponatremia also need treatment. Unilateral nephrectomies may provide some relief and improve feeding issues. Nearly 70% of neonates respond to supportive care, and about 80% of neonatal survivors are alive at 10 years of age. Many patients develop complications of chronic kidney disease such as growth failure, chronic liver disease such as portal hypertension and ascending cholangitis, and chronic lung disease later in the first decade of life. In infants with severe renal and hepatobiliary disease, the combined renal-liver transplant looks promising.

ADPKD

ADPKD is seen in 1 of every 400 to 1000 live births and accounts for approximately 10% of patients with chronic renal failure requiring dialysis or transplant.[66] Typically, ADPKD occurs as a systemic disorder in adult patients. This disease typically also involves the liver, gastrointestinal tract, aorta, and cerebral vessels.

ADPKD is one of the primary ciliopathies with mutations in the polycystin-1 (*PKD1* gene) protein that is involved in maintaining tubular phenotype and in injury repair.[67] The allele from the normal parent produces enough polycystin-1 to maintain the tubules relatively healthy for many years, but the levels fall below the required amounts by adulthood. The disease is managed by dialysis or transplantation, although recently there is new hope with the availability of an arginine-vasopressin–V_2 receptor inhibitor to treat individuals with subclinical disease. The collecting ducts and distal nephrons affected in ADPKD are sensitive to vasopressin, and an arginine-vasopressin receptor inhibitor can delay cyst formation and may be helpful.

Medical Management of Renal Anomalies

Infants with congenital renal issues are at risk for decreased kidney function and metabolic derangements. Some patients may progress to chronic kidney disease and show metabolic acidosis, anemia, and mineral and bone derangements leading to secondary hyperparathyroidism, hypertension, and growth impairment. Laboratory measurements should include electrolytes, blood urea nitrogen, creatinine, complete blood counts, levels of parathyroid hormone and 25-hydroxy vitamin D, and iron stores. Cystatin C measurements may be useful; cystatin C is produced by all nucleated cells and is freely filtered and less affected by muscle mass, age, and gender than serum creatinine.[14] The frequency of laboratory assessment needs to be decided based on the severity of renal dysfunction. Infants with renal anomalies show frequent changes in urine output, and if so, they may need laboratory assessment and supportive treatment.

In many disorders, the care providers may have to consider certain specific issues. Infants with one normal kidney and one abnormal kidney (agenesis or multicystic dysplasia) rarely require urgent evaluation or intervention. Those with bilateral anomalies have increased risk of decreased kidney function and complications, therefore requiring a higher level of monitoring and assessment.[55] Figs. 61.3 and 61.4 outline management for infants with urinary tract dilation, depending on when the urinary tract dilation was first detected.

UPJ obstruction frequently improves over time in those in whom it is detected prenatally. Infants with unilateral UPJ obstruction frequently do not require intervention, unless there is a resultant urinoma causing compression of the ureter. In such cases, a nephrostomy tube or other intervention to drain the renal pelvis may be required. Those with bilateral UPJ obstruction require monitoring for oliguria, decreased kidney function, and electrolyte derangements. If such complications develop, drainage or diversion may be required.

As discussed above, ureterovesical junction obstruction is seen frequently in the setting of bladder outlet obstruction. Management of VUR includes antibiotic prophylaxis in many cases to prevent urinary tract infections. Many cases of VUR will improve over time, and not all children require surgical repair. Indications for repair typically include infections despite receiving antibiotic prophylaxis and no improvement in or worsening of VUR by age 4 to 6 years.

Duplex kidneys usually require no intervention and may be monitored by renal ultrasound. In cases which involve a ureterocele and in infants with a ureterocele without a duplex kidney, incision of the ureterocele is often required to avoid obstruction within the bladder.

Infants with prune belly syndrome should not be catheterized unless absolutely necessary. They may have issues with bladder emptying given the lack of musculature; however, the degree of hydronephrosis will determine the need for intervention. These patients may require additional procedures to correct reflux and/or megaureters as well as orchidopexy for undescended testes.

Infants with suspected PUV should have a urinary catheter placed soon after birth. If a catheter cannot be placed, the bladder can be accessed either by a suprapubic tube or vesicostomy.

In the long term, infants with CAKUT and other renal disorders need guidance for dietary modifications and careful, continued clinical monitoring for growth and development, renal function, cardiovascular health, and proteinuria. They also need psychological support and partnership during the long-term care needed by these infants.

SECTION

12 Eye Disorders

OUTLINE

CHAPTER 62

Retinopathy of Prematurity

Prolima G. Thacker, Michael X. Repka

KEY POINTS

1. Retinopathy of prematurity (ROP) is a disease characterized by altered vascularization of the immature retina of premature infants and is common cause of reduced vision in the developed world.
2. The first, obliterative phase of ROP occurs from birth to a postmenstrual age of about 30 to 32 weeks and is characterized by suppressed growth/obliteration of retinal vessels due to relative hyperoxia.
3. The second, vasoproliferative phase of ROP begins at approximately 32 to 34 weeks' postmenstrual age with altered blood vessel growth at the junction of the vascularized and the avascular zones of the retina.
4. The International Classification of Retinopathy of Prematurity (ICROP) is a standard way to describe ROP based on extent and severity.
5. The management of ROP is focused on three components: prevention, interdiction, and correction. Each component is a subject of intense preclinical, translational, and clinical study.
6. Current management of ROP is based on the ablation of the avascular zones by cryotherapy or laser photocoagulation. Ongoing studies are evaluating the use of antibodies to suppress the effects of biologic mediators such as vascular endothelial growth factors (VEGF). Once ROP has progressed to stage 4 or beyond, vitreoretinal surgery is the only option.

Introduction

Retinopathy of prematurity (ROP) is a disease affecting the retina of premature infants. It is a very common cause of reduced vision in the developed world. ROP is characterized by neovascularization of the immature infant retina. The spectrum of ROP outcomes varies from the most minimal sequelae without affecting vision to bilateral, irreversible, total blindness. Improving neonatal care has resulted in improved survival rates of the smallest premature infants, who are at the greatest risk for ROP. ROP was first identified by Terry in 1942.[1] He termed the condition retrolental fibroplasia. Serial examination of premature infants led to the revelation that the condition develops after birth. The term ROP was coined by Heath in 1951.[2] ROP soon became the largest cause of childhood blindness in the developed world and exceeded all other causes of childhood blindness in the United States.[3]

The incidence varies with birth weight but is reported in approximately 50% to 70% of infants whose weight is less than 1250 g at birth.[4] Fielder studied infants weighing less than 1700 g and noted development of ROP in 51%.[5] In general, more than 50% of premature infants weighing less than 1250 g at birth show evidence of ROP, and about 10% of the infants develop stage 3 ROP. Significant ROP rarely develops after 30 weeks' postmenstrual age.

The median age of onset of ROP is at 35 weeks' (range, 31–40 weeks') postmenstrual age. Risk factors for development of threshold ROP include preeclampsia, birth weight, pulmonary hemorrhage, duration of ventilation, and duration of continuous positive airway pressure.[6]

An observational study compared the characteristics of infants with severe ROP in countries with low, moderate, and high levels of development and found that the mean birth weight of infants from highly developed countries was 737 to 763 g compared with 903 to 1527 g in less-developed countries. The mean gestational ages of infants from highly developed countries were 25.3 to 25.6 weeks compared with 26.3 to 33.5 weeks in less-developed countries.[7] Thus larger and more mature infants develop severe ROP in less-developed nations. This suggests that individual countries need to develop their own screening programs with criteria suited to their local population.

As early as the 1950s, high oxygen saturation was identified as the cause for development of ROP.[8] However, as the natural history of the disease was better understood, other factors including low birth weight, gestational age, sepsis, necrotizing enterocolitis, intraventricular hemorrhage, sepsis, bronchopulmonary dysplasia, respiratory distress, and hypotension were recognized to have a role too.

Pathophysiology

Retinal blood vessels develop through vasculogenesis at the optic nerve opening in the sclera.[9] Beginning at approximately 15 weeks' gestation[10] and continuing through 22 weeks' gestation, these precursor cells become angioblasts and form a vascular network in the inner retina extending from the optic nerve. After 22 weeks' gestation, additional development of the retinal vasculature occurs through budding angiogenesis. Astrocytes sense physiologic hypoxia[11] and up-regulate vascular endothelial growth factor (VEGF). Endothelial cells proliferate and migrate along the gradient of VEGF and thereby extend the inner vascular plexus toward the peripheral retina. Besides astrocytes, glial cells, Müller cells, and neurons such as ganglion cells are also important.[12–14] Of the many factors involved in retinal vascular development, VEGF is essential.

Normal retinal blood vessel development in humans commences at the optic nerve at approximately 15 to 16 weeks' gestation, proceeding in a centripetal manner at about 0.1 mm/day.[15] The nasal retina is completely vascularized by about 36 weeks' postmenstrual age, whereas the temporal retina is completed near term.[4]

The development of ROP has two phases, obliterative and vasoproliferative (Fig. 62.1). The first phase of ROP (obliterative) occurs from birth to a postmenstrual age of approximately 30 to 32 weeks. During this phase retinal vascular growth slows, along with some regression of retinal vessels.[15] The relative hyperoxia of the

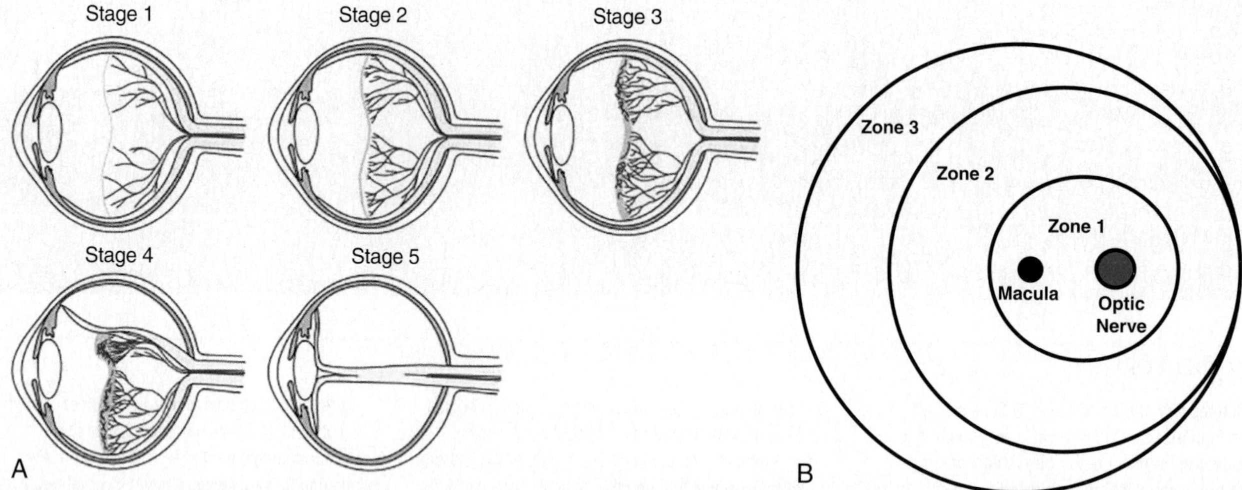

Fig. 62.1 Zones and Stages of Retinopathy of Prematurity (ROP). (A) The zones in the right eye. (B) The severity of ROP is classified in stages. The disease progresses in two phases, obliterative (stages 1 and 2) and vasoproliferative (≥stage 3). Stage 1 is characterized by a thin line of demarcation between the vascularized and nonvascularized retina, stage 2 by a ridge, stage 3 by extraretinal fibrovascular proliferation, stage 4 by partial retinal detachment, and stage 5 by total retinal detachment. In stage 3, extraretinal neovascularization can become severe enough to cause retinal detachment (stages 4–5), which can cause blindness. (B) The retina is divided into three concentric zones: zone 1 (the innermost zone) consists of the most posterior retina limited by a circle, zone 2 extends from the edge of zone 1 nasally to the ora serrata, and zone 3 is the crescent of the temporal retina anterior to zone 2. (Hellström et al. *Lancet*. 2013;382:1445–1157.)

extrauterine environment and supplemental oxygen are thought to be responsible for this process. Normally in utero, the blood is only approximately 70% saturated compared with 100% in full-term infants on room air. PaO_2 in utero is 30 mm Hg, whereas a normal infant breathing room air will have a PaO_2 of 60 to 100 mm Hg.[16] The relative hyperoxia results in down-regulation of VEGF and other factors, leading to cessation or regression of vasculogenesis. The inner retinal blood vessels are vulnerable to injury and may be obliterated by stressors including excessive oxygen supply, decreased VEGF, and the scarcity in cytoprotective factors, notably insulinlike growth factor (IGF).[17]

As the child ages the relatively avascular retina becomes increasingly hypoxic due to an increased metabolic demand of the developing retina. This sets the stage for the second phase (vasoproliferative) of ROP. This phase begins ophthalmoscopically at approximately 32 to 34 weeks' postmenstrual age. The relative hypoxia increases expression of VEGF and blood vessel growth.[18] New but abnormal vessels form at the junction between the vascularized retina and the avascular zone of the retina. These vessels may, weeks later, produce a fibrous scar on the surface of the retina. Contraction of the scar tissue can in some cases produce a retinal detachment and blindness, while in others it can involute.

Role of Growth Hormone and IGF-1 in ROP

Biochemical mediators in addition to VEGF are likely involved in ROP. Inhibition of VEGF does not completely halt development of hypoxia-induced retinal neovascularization. Even with much improved management of supplemental oxygen, the disease persists.

IGF-1 is important to normal development of retinal vessels.[19] Reduced IGF-1 is associated with lack of vascular growth and subsequent proliferative ROP. IGF-1 controls maximum VEGF activation of an endothelial cell survival pathway.[20] Low postnatal serum levels of IGF-1 are directly correlated with the severity of clinical ROP.[20–23]

A hypothesis for retinal vessel development and ROP has emerged. Retinal vessel growth requires both IGF-1 and VEGF. In premature infants, IGF-1, which is normally supplied by the placenta and the amniotic fluid, is at very low levels after birth because the infant cannot replace the loss. Retinal vessel growth slows or stops because IGF-1 is required for VEGF to promote vascular endothelial growth. When supplemental oxygen is provided after birth, VEGF is also suppressed. Thus prematurity and oxygen administration contribute to the suppression of vessel growth and vessel loss. As the infant grows and the retina begins to mature without an adequate supply of oxygen, hypoxia develops, which induces increased expression of VEGF. In addition, the infant's liver begins to produce IGF-1, allowing the elevated levels of VEGF to stimulate blood vessel growth.

Other Factors With Possible Roles in Pathogenesis of ROP

Hypoxia-Induced Factor 1

During fetal development, low oxygen concentrations increase local hypoxia-induced factor (HIF)–1α and VEGF levels, which promote normal vascularization.[24] Exposure to relative hyperoxia after premature birth suppresses HIF-1α levels, thus reducing VEGF expression and reducing the number of retinal capillaries. As HIF-1 increases, vasoproliferation ensues.[25]

Erythropoeitin

The administration of erythropoeitin prevents the loss of retinal vasculature in the obliterative stage.[26] In contrast, treatment during the vasoproliferative stage might exacerbate the disease by promoting endothelial cell proliferation.

Genetics

Although ROP has the same incidence rates in White and African American populations, the progression to severe stages is more common in White than in African American infants and in males than in females.[27–29] There is an increased frequency of polymorphisms of β-adrenoreceptors (β-ARs) in Black compared with Caucasian infants. Several gene variants such as those of the Wnt pathway (frizzled 4, lipoprotein-related receptor-related protein 5, and Norrie disease protein) have been implicated.[30]

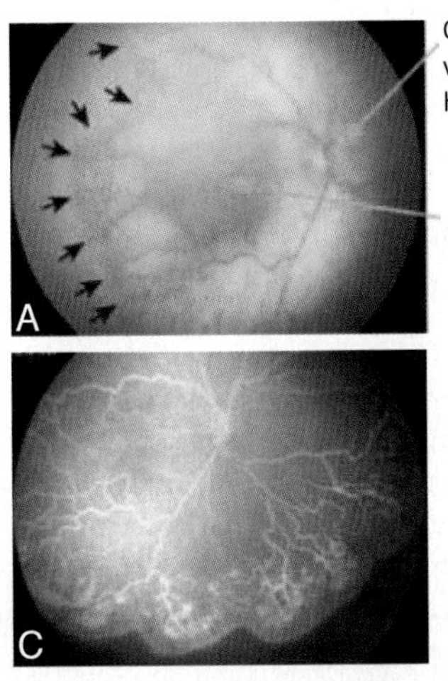

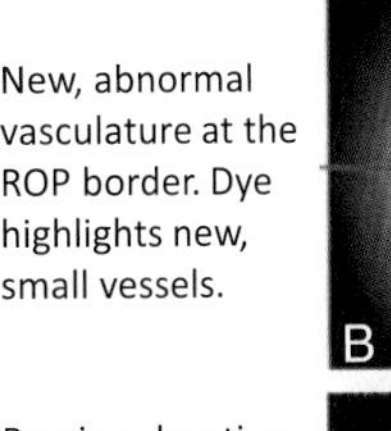

New, abnormal vasculature at the ROP border. Dye highlights new, small vessels.

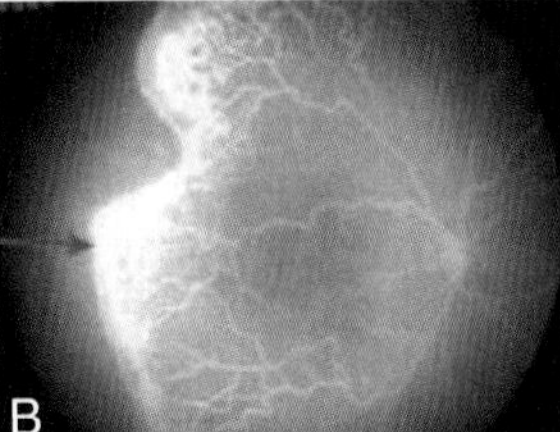

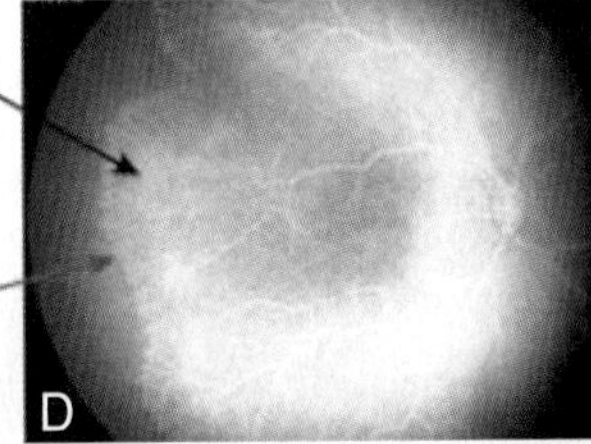

Fig. 62.2 Retinopathy of Prematurity (ROP) in Stage 3, Zone 1, With Signs of Plus Disease. (A) *Small arrows* show the border between vascular and avascular parts of the retina. The thick *red line* at the border highlights neovascularization. (B) Fluorescein angiography shows the retinal vasculature. The bright border highlights the border between the vascular and avascular parts of the retina. (C) Fluorescein angiography shows the lower part of the retina. The neovascularization is seen as small clumps. (D) Anti-VEGF therapy was given; 1 month later, fluorescein angiography showed growth of the normal retinal vasculature and resolution of neovascularization and plus disease (dilation and tortuosity of vessels). *VEGF,* Vascular endothelial growth factor. (Sun et al. Retinopathy of prematurity. In: *Fanaroff and Martin's Neonatal-Perinatal Medicine*; Jan 2020.)

Oxidative Stress

The premature retina is relatively deficient in antioxidants. Consequently, oxidative stress may induce peroxidation, damaging the retinal microvasculature and leading to vaso-obliteration.[31]

Adrenergic Receptors

Angiogenesis is controlled by the adrenergic system through its regulation of proangiogenic factors. β-ARs are widely expressed in vascular endothelial cells,[32] and β-adrenoreceptors (β-ARs) can regulate angiogenesis in response to ischemia. β-AR up-regulates VEGF, thereby promoting the vasoproliferative phase of ROP. β-blockers might represent useful drugs in the treatment of ROP.[33]

Adenosine and Apelin

These agents have been found to regulate vasculogenesis of the developing retina. In animal models, these chemicals are found in low concentrations in the vaso-obliterative phase and are increased in the proliferative phase of ROP.

Omega 3 Lipids

Notably, docosahexaenoic acid (DHA) and eicosapentaenoic acid (EPA) have been found to exert a number of beneficial biologic properties such as cytoprotection of neural tissue, decreased oxidant stress, and decreased inflammation.[34,35] Premature newborns are relatively deficient in omega-3 lipids, and supplementation with DHA and EPA has been found to improve visual acuity.[36]

Clinical Features of ROP

The International Classification of Retinopathy of Prematurity (ICROP) is a standardized way to describe ROP.[37,38] The key aspects of the classification include (1) the location of retinal involvement by zone, (2) the extent of retinal involvement by clock hour, (3) the stage of retinopathy at the junction of the vascularized and avascular retina, and (4) the presence or absence of dilated and tortuous posterior pole vessels, termed plus disease (Fig. 62.2).

Stages

There are five stages of acute ROP. The stage of disease represents the changes seen at the vascular-avascular junction in the retina. In an eye, the stage often differs in different portions of the retina. The retina is subdivided into zones and clock hours (discussed below). The patient is described by the most advanced stage that occurs in at least one clock hour of the retina.

Stage 0

No active disease is seen; the vascularized retina blends seamlessly into the avascular retina. Some vascular changes can be apparent prior to the development of ROP, such as dilatation of the vessels or vessels positioned in a circumferential pattern.

Stage 1: Demarcation Line

A whitish line is observed separating the vascular from the avascular retina. Abnormal branching of vessels can be seen leading up to the demarcation line, which is flat.

Stage 2: Ridge

The ridge has volume (height and width). It may be white or pink. Associated vascular abnormalities include isolated, vascular tufts at the retinal plane lying posterior to the ridge, called popcorn vessels.

Stage 3: Extraretinal Neovascularization

Neovascularization extends from the ridge on the surface of the retina into the vitreous. Typically, it has a pink color.

Stage 4: Partial Retinal Detachment

After the development of neovascularization, the vascular change can involute or develop fibrosis. The scarring causes traction on the retina toward the center of the base at the area of fibrosis. Stage 4 is subdivided into the following:

- Stage 4A: partial retinal detachment not involving the macula.
- Stage 4B: partial retinal detachment involving the macula.

Stage 5: Total Retinal Detachment

The detachment is most commonly tractional but can be exudative in nature too. It is usually funnel shaped. The most common is the open funnel, which is open both anteriorly as well as posteriorly.

When more than one ROP stage is present in an eye, staging for the eye as a whole is determined by the most severe stage identified. For purposes of recording the examination, ROP is drawn with the extent of each stage in clock hours on a drawing.

Zone

The retina is divided into three concentric zones centered on the optic disc. Zone 1 (the innermost zone) consists of the most posterior retina limited by a circle. The radius of the circle extends from the center of the optic disc to twice the estimated distance from the optic disc to the macula. This is closely approximated by the field of view using a 28 D indirect ophthalmoscopy lens. Zone 2 extends from the edge of zone 1 nasally to the ora serrata. Zone 3 is the crescent of the temporal retina anterior to zone 2. Zones 2 and 3 are mutually exclusive. By convention, ROP should be considered to be in zone 2 until it is determined that the nasal-most two clock hours are vascularized to the ora serrata.[39,40]

Extent of Disease: Clock Hours

The extent of each stage of disease is recorded for a total of 12 clock hours (or as 30° sectors). These can be contiguous or not contiguous. For instance, when the disease is not contiguous, the hours of stage 3 may be added together, with the total termed "cumulative" (e.g., four cumulative clock hours of stage 3). In general, for the same number of clock hours, contiguous disease is considered more severe than noncontiguous disease.

Plus Disease

Plus disease describes venous dilation and arteriolar tortuosity of the posterior retinal vessels in at least two quadrants.[41] A + symbol is added to the ROP stage to designate plus disease. For example, stage 2 ROP with plus would be written as stage 2+ ROP.

Preplus Disease

A recent version of the ICROP defined preplus disease as vascular abnormalities of the posterior pole insufficient for the diagnosis of plus disease but having more arterial tortuosity and venous dilatation than normal. Preplus disease may progress to plus disease or regress.

Aggressive-Posterior ROP

Aggressive-posterior ROP (AP-ROP) is an uncommon, rapidly progressing form of ROP that is posterior with prominent plus and poorly defined disease. This rapidly progressing retinopathy has been referred to previously as "Rush disease."[42] AP-ROP is observed most commonly in zone 1 but may occur in posterior zone 2. AP-ROP does not progress through the classic stages 1 to 3, instead reaching stage 3 very rapidly.

Regression of ROP

Most ROP regresses or involutes spontaneously. However, this is determined retrospectively. One of the first signs of involution of acute-phase ROP is failure to progress to the next stage during serial visits or a change to a more peripheral zone.[43] In some cases the regression is accompanied by fibrosis of the areas of preretinal neovascularization. This scar may produce traction on the retina, varying from minor distortions of foveal architecture to dragging the retina peripherally, usually temporally, producing macular ectopia and pulling the superior and inferior retinal vascular arcades toward the horizontal meridian. This often causes some visual loss. Finally, axial traction on the retina can produce a traction or rhegmatogenous retinal detachment.

Management

Management of ROP includes three components: (1) prevention, (2) interdiction, and (3) correction.[44] Prevention of ROP is the most effective, and the best preventive measure is to reduce preterm births through comprehensive prenatal and obstetric care. Additional methods aimed at the prevention of ROP include vitamin E supplementation, ambient light reduction, oxygen supplementation, and inositol supplementation. It was hoped that vitamin E supplementation would mitigate the effects of free-radical damage caused by hyperoxia. However, studies had contradictory results, and supplementation is standard.[45,46] Excessive visible light is also associated with free-radical generation and possibly increases the chances of ROP.[47] However, the LIGHT-ROP study, a randomized, multicenter trial of light reduction with goggles worn by very low birth weight premature infants, did not demonstrate any effect of light reduction on the incidence of ROP.[48]

STOP-ROP was a multicenter trial conducted to determine whether supplemental oxygen would decrease the progression to threshold ROP when administered to infants with prethreshold ROP, reducing the hypoxic drive for neovascularization.[49] Infants with prethreshold ROP were randomized to a conventional oxygen arm with pulse oximetry targeted at 89% to 94% saturation or an oxygen supplemental arm with pulse oximetry targeted at 96% to 99% saturation. The study found no benefit to increasing the oxygen. In fact, supplemental oxygen increased the risk of adverse pulmonary events including pneumonia and/or exacerbations of chronic lung disease and the need for oxygen, diuretics, and hospitalization at 3 months' corrected age.

A randomized controlled trial was conducted to determine the efficacy and safety of myo-inositol to reduce type 1 ROP among infants younger than 28 weeks' gestational age.[50] Treatment with myo-inositol for up to 10 weeks did not reduce the risk of type 1 ROP or death compared with placebo.

For the past 10 years there has been interest in reducing the oxygen levels of babies to reduce the rate of ROP while not increasing the mortality rate.[51] The SUPPORT Study Group conducted a trial for children requiring supplemental oxygen to determine if a more hypoxic target range of 85% to 89% was better than the commonly used 91% to 95%. The primary outcome, a composite of death and ROP, was not different; however, the lower range was associated with greater mortality and less severe ROP, whereas the higher range showed the opposite.

Screening for ROP

ROP screening programs are established to identify infants who need treatment and to ensure follow-up upon neonatal intensive care unit discharge/transfer. Because undiagnosed or treatment-delayed ROP may lead to blindness, it is important that all infants at risk be screened. Current consensus guidelines recommend that timing be scheduled based on the gestational age of the infant and that the follow-up be determined by the severity of the ROP. The American Academy of Pediatrics guidelines recommend ROP screening for[52]

- all infants with a birth weight of ≤1500 g or a gestational age of 30 weeks or less (as defined by the attending neonatologist) and
- infants with a birth weight between 1500 and 2000 g or a gestational age >30 weeks who are believed to be at risk for ROP (such as infants with hypotension requiring inotropic support, infants who received oxygen supplementation for more than a few days, or infants who received oxygen without saturation monitoring).

The screening should be performed by a trained ophthalmologist with pupillary dilation of the infant using binocular indirect ophthalmoscopy and scleral depression. Pupillary dilatation can be achieved with 1.0% phenylephrine hydrochloride and 0.5% cyclopentolate or tropicamide 1.0%, instilled twice after a gap of 5 to 15 minutes, taking care to wipe off the excess drops from the medial canthi to decrease the systemic absorption of these drugs.[53] Multiple doses can adversely affect the cardiorespiratory and gastrointestinal status of the infant. Sterile instruments should be used to examine each infant.

The use of wide-angle retinal photography in the nursery, which captures images that can be transmitted electronically and read remotely, may improve the availability of screening in the community and may be used for improved documentation.[54,55] Digital retinal photography, when quality images can be obtained, has high accuracy for detection of clinically significant ROP.[56] Remote grading has excellent inter- and intragrader agreement and would be one objective way to standardize ROP protocols, guidelines, and care delivery.[57,58]

The results of the examinations and imaging should be available for the nursery team and, as appropriate, communicated with the parents of the infant.

Timing of Screening

The initial screening should be performed based on postmenstrual age, rather than postnatal age. This reduces the examinations for the youngest babies during a period when there is no risk of serious ROP. Table 62.1 follows current consensus screening guidelines.[52]

Current screening guidelines by design have very high sensitivity and poor specificity. For children weighing less than 1250 g, older data found that approximately 10% of those screened will require treatment.[59] For the whole group weighing less than 1500 g, approximately 6% will develop type 1 ROP and require treatment.[60] Approximately 6% will have type 2 ROP and require careful monitoring.

Due to the high exam burden on the neonatal intensive care unit and the examining ophthalmologists, newer algorithms are being developed to select the most at-risk infants for screening and reduce the overall number of exams. These include WIN-ROP[61], CO-ROP,[62,63] CHOP-ROP,[64] and G-ROP and take additional factors such as the rate of weight gain into account. Substitution of these algorithms for the professional society consensus guidelines is not yet justified by current literature.

Subsequent examinations of infants are determined by the treating ophthalmologist depending on the severity of ROP. The actual follow-up timing in practice will vary based on factors such as postmenstrual age and prior exam results.

Table 62.1 Timing of Initial ROP Exam

Postmenstrual Age at Birth, week	Postmenstrual Age at Initial ROP Exam, week	Chronologic Age at First-Suggested ROP Exam, week
22	31	9
23	31	8
24	31	7
25	31	6
26	31	5
27	31	4
28	32	4
29	33	4
30	34	4

ROP, Retinopathy of prematurity.

One Week or Shorter Follow-Up

1. Zone 1, no disease (stage 0).
2. Zone 1, stage 1 or stage 2 ROP.
3. Suspected AP-ROP.

One- to Two-Week Follow-Up

1. Posterior zone 2: immature vascularization.
2. Zone 2, stage 2 ROP.
3. Zone 1, unequivocally regressing ROP.

Two-Week Follow-Up

1. Zone 2, stage 1 ROP.
2. Zone 2, stage 0 ROP.
3. Zone 2, unequivocally regressing stage 2 or 3 ROP.

Two- to Three-Week Follow-Up

1. Zone 3, stage 0, 1, or 2 ROP.
2. Zone 3, regressing ROP.

Discontinuation of ROP Examinations

There is no absolute postmenstrual age or levels of disease at which to stop examinations; some are suggestive.

1. Full retinal vascularization (close proximity to the ora serrata for 360°—usually approximately two disc diameters). This criterion should also be used for all cases treated for ROP solely with anti-VEGF medications.
2. Zone 3 retinal vascularization without previous zone 1 disease (any stage) or zone 2, stage 3 ROP. If anti-VEGF medications were used, ROP evaluations should be performed until a postmenstrual age of at least 65 weeks. Very late recurrences of proliferative ROP have been reported after VEGF treatment.[65–67]
3. Regression of ROP.

Treatment of ROP

Two randomized clinical trials form the evidence basis for ablative treatment of acute ROP. These included Cryotherapy for Retinopathy of Prematurity (CRYO-ROP)[68–70] and Early Treatment for Retinopathy of Prematurity (ETROP). CRYO-ROP used the ICROP classification, a standard photograph of plus disease, and a (consensus) threshold severity of disease, defined as five contiguous clock hours or eight noncontiguous (cumulative) clock hours of stage 3 ROP with plus disease in zone 1 or zone 2. Children's eyes were randomized to cryotherapy to the avascular retina or observation at threshold ROP. The basis of treatment was that retinal ablation would decrease VEGF production by the hypoxic nonvascularized anterior retina. Reduced VEGF would translate to regression of ROP.

CRYO-ROP demonstrated a significant reduction in unfavorable anatomic outcomes. At the 1-year follow-up, unfavorable outcomes were reported for 47.4% of control eyes and 25.7% of treated eyes.[71] At 15 years of age, 30% of treated eyes and 52% of control eyes had unfavorable anatomic outcomes.[72] Unfavorable visual acuity outcomes (20/200 or worse) were found in 45% of treated eyes versus 64% of control eyes.

Although effective, cryotherapy was not uniformly associated with good outcomes, which many clinicians felt could be improved with earlier treatment. The tradeoff for treating earlier would mean the treatment of some children who would not need to be treated. To study this question, ETROP was launched.[73] For purposes of the study, high-risk disease was determined using a risk model based on CRYO-ROP data. In addition, technology allowed a shift from cryotherapy to laser ablation with the indirect ophthalmoscope. Laser has fewer associated local and systemic adverse effects, including pain and swelling, and does not require conjunctival incision.[74] Early treatment was associated with a reduction in unfavorable visual acuity outcomes, from 19.8% to 14.3% ($P < .005$). Unfavorable structural outcomes were also reduced from 15.6% to 9.0% ($P < .001$) at 9 months. To translate to clinical practice, where a mathematical model was not available, the ETROP investigators recommended treatment for newly defined "type 1 ROP," defined as zone 1, any stage of ROP with plus disease; zone 1, stage 3 ROP without plus disease; or zone 2, stage 2 or 3 with plus disease. However, the analysis supported close monitoring for "type 2 ROP," defined as zone 1, stage 1, and 2 without plus disease or zone 2, stage 3 without plus disease. These eyes should be considered for treatment only if they progress to type I ROP or worse.[73]

After the publication of ETROP, treatment with a portable indirect laser became the standard of care. ROP treatment is performed with sedation or general anesthesia. The entire avascular retina from the disease or end of the vascularized retina to the ora serrata is treated with laser burns spaced about half a burn width. After treatment, infants are followed closely for resolution of disease. If plus disease persists after approximately 10 days, additional laser treatment is performed for any areas that were not adequately treated.

Despite the improving outcomes after ETROP and early treatment becoming the norm, unfavorable outcomes were still seen with posterior zone 1 disease, APROP, a gestational age <29.5 weeks, and presence of preretinal hemorrhage before treatment.[75] Laser photocoagulation may be challenging or the outcomes after laser poor despite confluent laser treatment. Such situations include poor pupillary dilatation due to severe tunica vasculosa lentis or rubeosis iridis, vitreous haze, or vitreous hemorrhage.

As discussed earlier, VEGF has been recognized as a key factor in retinal vascular development. The use of the anti-VEGF inhibitor bevacizumab (Avastin; Genentech, San Francisco, California), a recombinant humanized monoclonal antibody, was first reported for treatment of ROP in 2007.[76] Shortly thereafter, Bevacizumab Eliminates the Angiogenic Threat of Retinopathy of Prematurity (BEAT-ROP),[77] a randomized multicenter study, was conducted in infants with stage 3+ ROP who were randomized to intravitreal bevacizumab (IVB) (0.625 mg in 0.025 mL) or indirect laser. The dosage was a convenience dose typically administered to adults. The primary outcome was recurrence of the retinopathy in one or both eyes requiring retreatment before 54 weeks' postmenstrual age. Recurrence was seen in four infants in the bevacizumab group (4%) and 19 infants in the laser-treated group (22%) ($P = .002$). A beneficial treatment effect was found for zone 1 disease ($P = .003$) but not for zone 2 disease ($P = .27$). In addition, the study described that development of peripheral retinal vessels continued after treatment with IVB, whereas conventional laser therapy led to permanent destruction of the peripheral retina. There appeared to be less high myopia (≥8.00 diopters) with IVB compared with conventional lasers.[78] Although no systemic or local toxic effects attributable to bevacizumab were observed, the study concluded that the population size was too small to assess the safety of the drug.

VEGF is needed for normal pulmonary, brain, and kidney development.[79] Lien et al. have shown that VEGF levels in ROP infants were depressed for up to 8 weeks after IVB.[80] In addition to potential systemic effects, there is concern regarding persistence of peripheral avascular retina after IVB acting as a source of VEGF, leading to persistence of abnormal angiogenesis and thereby resulting in late recurrences of ROP with anti-VEGF monotherapy. Studies have reported reactivation of ROP 4 to 5 weeks after IVB. Therefore long-term monitoring needs to be assured upon discharge or back-transport in infants treated with IVB. (See the follow-up guidelines earlier in this chapter.)

Surgery

Once ROP has progressed to stage 4 and beyond, vitreoretinal surgery is the only option. The technique depends on the stage of ROP and the extent and location of the traction. Those surgeries include scleral buckling or lens-sparing vitrectomy for stage 4 and lensectomy with vitrectomy for stage 5. Lack of prior treatment such as laser, a late presentation, and a higher incidence of narrow-narrow funnel configuration are predictors for poor surgical outcome. The anatomic success rates of lens sparing vitrectomy for stage 4A ROP have been reported to vary from 84% to 100% whereas those for stage 5 ROP range from 14.3% to 45.5% in various series.[81–83] Visual results are quite poor.[84,85]

Sequelae of Treated ROP

A number of structural sequelae occur in eyes treated for ROP. These include moderate and high myopia, vascular tortuosity, narrowing of the vascular arcades, a temporal myopic crescent, macular heterotropia, disc drag, vitreous membranes, visual field constriction, and peripheral tractional retinal detachment. Long-term follow-up of these children is required for the assessment of refractive errors, strabismus, anisometropia, and amblyopia.

Future Direction

Although timely ablation treatments can reduce the incidence of blindness by 25% in infants with late-stage disease, the patients often still have poor visual acuity after treatment. The development of preventive and less destructive therapies for ROP, including nutritional supplements such as omega-3 fatty acids[86] and the potential administration of cytoprotective growth factors such as erythropoietin and/or IGF-1[87,88] and granulocyte colony stimulating factor,[89] could be more desirable than treatment of an established disorder. However, although promising, other than limiting postnatal hemoglobin-oxygen saturation, the other modalities remain speculative. Other than pharmacologic and nutritional strategies, cell-based strategies for vascular repair are likely to emerge from advances in regenerative medicine using stem cells and gene therapy.[90]

CHAPTER

63 Developmental Anomalies of the Globe and Ocular Adnexa in Neonates

Jefferson J. Doyle, Mireille Jabroun

KEY POINTS

1. Major structural abnormalities of the eye in neonates include anophthalmos (no ocular tissues), microphthalmos (small, disorganized eye), nanophthalmos (small but relatively normally structured eye), and buphthalmos (whole eye is enlarged).
2. Major eyelid defects in neonates include complete fusion of the upper and lower eyelids and a "hidden" eye (cryptophthalmos), focal fusion of the upper and lower eyelids (ankyloblepharon), focal defects in either or both eyelids (eyelid coloboma), or abnormal shape of the lower eyelid (euryblepharon).
3. Causes of a narrowed palpebral fissure (space between the eyelids) with or without upper eyelid drooping (ptosis) in neonates include blepharophimosis, congenital ptosis, or congenital Horner syndrome.
4. There are a number of known genetic causes for many of the above disorders, which are discussed throughout the chapter. In some cases these anomalies may occur sporadically and/or in isolation, whereas in other instances they may point to and help guide workup of a number of underlying systemic conditions.
5. Management is challenging and case dependent. Consultation with an ophthalmologist is advisable prenatally if the condition is identified on prenatal imaging or soon after birth. Overarching principles include creating a clear visual axis to optimize visual development and restoring functional eyelids to help cover the eye and avoid corneal scarring and/or exposure.

Introduction to the Eye and Adnexal Structures

The upper eyelids form by fusion of the medial and lateral frontonasal processes, whereas the lower eyelids form by fusion of the medial nasal and maxillary processes. The eyelids play a critical role in protecting the eye from mechanical injury, generating some components of the tear film, and opening and closing to facilitate tear distribution and adequate hydration of the cornea and conjunctiva. Each eyelid contains a fibrous plate called a tarsal plate that gives it structure and shape. The tarsal plates contain Meibomian glands, which open onto the surface at the eyelid margin; these produce an oily secretion that covers the aqueous layer of the tear film generated by the lacrimal glands and reduces evaporative tear loss. The inner side of the tarsus and the anterior white of the eye (sclera) are lined by conjunctiva, a mucous membrane that provides protection and lubrication to allow the eyes to move smoothly under the eyelids. The outer aspect of the tarsus is covered by the orbicularis oculi muscle, which permits blinking. The superior aspect of the tarsus attaches to the levator and Muller's muscles, both of which contribute to eyelid opening. The orbicularis muscle and lacrimal gland are innervated by the seventh cranial nerve. The levator muscle is innervated by the third cranial nerve and the Muller's muscle by the sympathetic nervous system.

The anterior segment of the eye includes the cornea, iris, ciliary body, and lens. The lens develops from surface ectoderm, whereas the cornea has both surface ectoderm and neural crest components. The iris and ciliary develop from both neuroectoderm and neural crest, whereas the drainage angle is neural crest in origin. Light enters the eye through the cornea and is refracted by both the cornea and the lens to help focus it on the retina at the back of the eye. The pupil alters in size to allow more or less light into the eye, depending on ambient illumination. The iris contains radial (dilating) and circular (constricting) muscles that adjust the size of the pupillary aperture. The ciliary body produces aqueous humor that flows from behind the iris through the pupil and to the anterior chamber and drains into the anterior chamber angle (i.e., trabecular meshwork). A delicate balance between production and drainage of aqueous humor maintains the intraocular pressure within normal limits. Light that has passed through the cornea, aqueous humor, and lens makes its way through the vitreous humor in the vitreous cavity to the retina at the back of the eye. Photoreceptors in the retina receive the light, convert it to an electrical signal, and transmit it to the brain via the optic nerve.

Developmental anomalies can occur in each of these structures. This chapter will focus on those that are identifiable on fetal imaging, apparent during standard clinical examination by a nonophthalmologist in the neonatal period, and/or are important enough to cause functional consequences if not recognized early and referred for further evaluation.

Abnormal Eye Structure

Absent or Small Disorganized Eye: Anophthalmos and Microphthalmos (Fig. 63.1)

Clinical Features

Anophthalmos and microphthalmos encompass a spectrum of disease ranging from a complete absence of ocular tissues (anophthalmos) to a variable reduction in the size of the eye and degree of disorganization of the ocular structures (microphthalmos). In both conditions, the adnexal elements (brow, eyelids, palpebral fissure, and eyelashes) remain normal. Primary anophthalmos is extremely rare and patients clinically suspected of having this usually have some rudimentary structures present. Microphthalmos can be associated with uveal (iris, ciliary body, and choroid) and/or optic nerve colobomas. In some instances, a cyst may form through the area of defective closure (microphthalmia with cyst) (see Fig. 63.1). In these patients, the eye may be displaced superiorly with bulging of cysts in the inferior lid.[1]

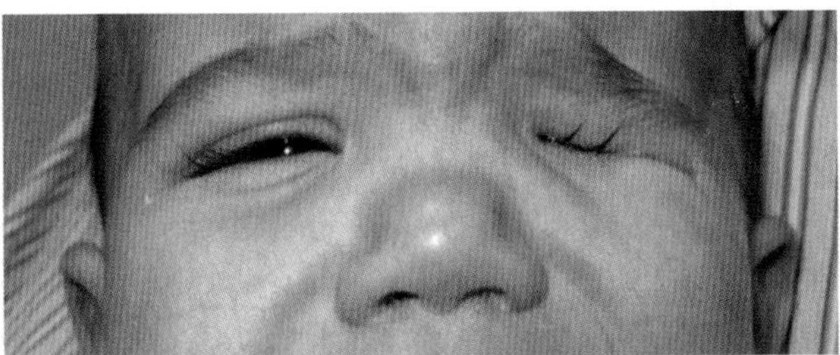

Fig. 63.1 Left Anophthalmia With Asymmetry and Phimosis of Eyelids. (Reproduced with permission and minor modifications from Cruz et al. Orbital developmental disorders. In: Fay and Dolman, eds. *Diseases and Disorders of the Orbits and Ocular Adnexa*. 2017;117.)

Systemic abnormalities co-occur with both conditions.[2] Up to 90% have associated conditions such as amniotic band sequence, **C**oloboma of the eye, **H**eart defects, **A**tresia of the choanae, **R**estriction of Growth and development, and **E**ar abnormalities and deafness (CHARGE) syndrome, Meckel-Gruber syndrome, **V**ertebral defects, **A**nal atresia, **C**ardiac defects, **T**racheo-**E**sophageal fistula, **R**enal anomalies, and **L**imb abnormalities (VACTERL) association, and less-defined musculoskeletal, cardiovascular, and central nervous system anomalies. Genetic counseling should be considered, because there is approximately a 10% chance of either anophthalmos or microphthalmos presenting in a sibling.[3] This is more likely in those with bilateral disease and those who have optic fissure closure defects or colobomas.[4]

Pathophysiology

The incidence of microphthalmos is 10 to 11 in 100,000, and of anophthalmos, 1 to 2 in 100,000.[2–7] There is no sex predilection; however, risk increases with greater maternal age.[5,6] Both can be seen in the setting of trisomy 13 or 18.[7] Only a minority (10%–20%) of cases have an identifiable genetic cause.[5,6] Mutations in *SOX2* are the most common cause of bilateral and severe anophthalmos. Relatively consistent systemic associations with *SOX2* mutations include learning disability, seizures, brain malformations, specific motor abnormalities, male genital tract malformations, mild facial dysmorphism, and postnatal growth failure.[8] Sensorineural hearing loss has been described more recently.[9] Mutations in *STRA6, ALDH1A3, VSX2, RAX,* and *FOXE3* have been implicated in consanguineous families with bilateral eye disease, with *VSX2* mutations being specific to individuals of Middle-Eastern descent.[10]

Evaluation

Ophthalmologic assessment should ideally be done in the first 2 weeks of life, especially if there are severe ocular anomalies. Functional determination of visual potential using electrophysiology can be performed when visual assessment is limited by age. Visual function does not always correlate with phenotypic findings, but vision is important in guiding treatment.[11]

Magnetic resonance imaging (MRI), computed tomography (CT) scan, and/or ultrasound can confirm the absence of ocular tissues or determine abnormalities in those that are present. MRI and CT offer the advantage of simultaneously imaging cranial structures. Although CT imaging avoids the use of general anesthesia, MRI offers higher-resolution images with the ability to detect possible communication between a cyst and the brain. Ultrasound has the advantage of being quick and noninvasive and has been shown to detect microphthalmia as early as 18 weeks in utero.[12]

Management

Management focuses on increasing the socket volume in the first 2 to 4 years of life. A microphthalmic eye with an axial length of less than 16 mm is not likely to promote orbital growth resulting in facial asymmetry.[11] Multiple orbit expanders are used, including hard spherical implants, inflatable soft-tissue expanders, hydrogel osmotic expanders, and dermis-fat graft implants. Each have advantages and disadvantages. Hard spherical implants require multiple returns to the operating room to be replaced as the patient grows. Inflatable and self-inflating expanders are at risk of extrusion. Dermis-fat grafts grow with the child but require a second surgical site for harvest and have the risk of atrophy before achieving adequate orbit size.[11]

Eye-socket conformer or prosthesis use can maintain socket shape. Caregivers must be counseled as to the importance of continuous use, because unnecessary removal may lead to contracture of the fornix. Prosthesis use is not as critical if there is a large orbital cyst (>16 mm) because this will also maintain orbital volume. At approximately age 4 years, when the orbit has fully matured, the cyst may be excised and a permanent orbital implant may be placed.[11] Close follow-up is necessary throughout life for these patients. Microphthalmic eyes are prone to developing angle-closure glaucoma, resulting in vision loss and pain.[11]

Small but "Normally Structured" Eye: Nanophthalmos (Fig. 63.2)

Clinical Features

In contrast to microphthalmos, in which the eye is small and its contents are disorganized, nanophthalmos refers to a small eye with (relatively) normally structure. Eye growth is compromised after the embryonic fissure has closed. Because the eye does not grow to a normal size, it typically exhibits a high degree of far-sightedness (hyperopia)[13,14] and is at a greater risk of angle closure glaucoma (because the anterior segment drainage angle is narrower than normal) and ocular surgical complications (e.g., intraoperative expulsive hemorrhage, choroidal effusion).

Due to its small size, the eye usually appears deeply set in the orbit (enophthalmos), with mild ptosis due to the upper eyelids hanging down over the eyes. The cornea can often be smaller than normal (microcornea) but not always. Various retinal abnormalities have been documented, including underdevelopment of the fovea (the part of the retina which permits good vision),[15] schisis-like changes,[16] midperipheral yellow spots, and pigmentary retinal degenerative changes.[17] Patients can develop unilateral or bilateral amblyopia, nystagmus, and/or turning in of the eyes (esotropia),[18] the latter of which can often be improved with glasses.

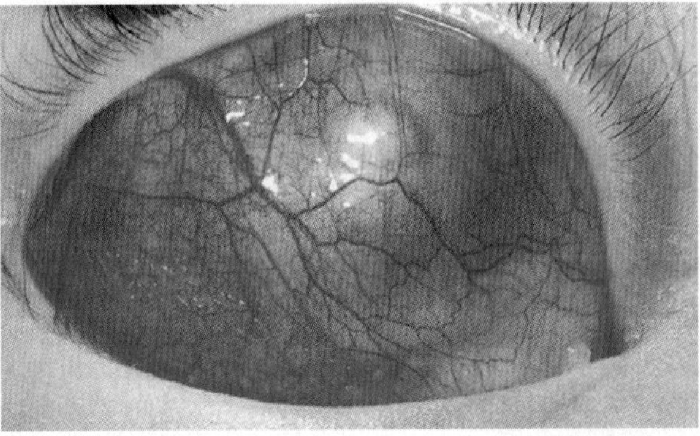

Fig. 63.2 Microphthalmia With Cyst. The eye is small and malformed, and a cyst is contiguous with the globe. The cyst is formed from proliferating retina. (Reproduced with permission and minor modifications from Krachmer and Palay. Normal anatomy and developmental abnormalities of the cornea. In: *Cornea Atlas 2014*; 88.)

Pathophysiology

Nanophthalmos is usually bilateral and symmetric in most cases and can be inherited in a sporadic, autosomal dominant, or autosomal recessive manner. Two loci have been identified for autosomal dominant nanophthalmos (NNO1 and NNO3),[19,20] whereas the autosomal recessive form can be caused by mutations in the *MFRP* gene at the NNO2 locus.[17] *MFRP* is expressed predominantly in the retinal pigment epithelium in humans and only after approximately 20 weeks of gestation, which is relatively late during ocular development, consistent with the relatively normal structure of these eyes.[21] Nanophthalmos can be associated with a number of syndromes including autosomal dominant vitreoretinochoroidopathy, oculo-dento-digital dysplasia syndrome, and Kenny-Caffey syndrome (see below).

Evaluation

Patients should undergo a complete ophthalmologic exam in the first few months of life. This should include axial length, corneal diameter, refraction, slit-lamp examination of the anterior segment, dilated fundus exam of the retina, and ideally gonioscopy of the anterior segment drainage angle (only possible in older children and adults, unless under anesthesia). Optical coherence tomography of the retina can help delineate subtle retinal changes in the macula. Electroretinography can identify varying degrees of scotopic (rod-mediated) or photopic (cone-mediated) retinal dysfunction. Patients require long-term follow-up because some of the complications, such as angle-closure glaucoma, may not appear for several decades.[22]

In the absence of syndromic involvement, nanophthalmos is not typically associated with systemic findings, although there is a report of its coincidence with cryptorchidism.[23] Autosomal dominant vitreoretinochoroidopathy with nanophthalmos is caused by mutations in the *BEST1* gene and usually manifests ocular findings.[24] Patients with oculo-dento-digital dysplasia syndrome present with syndactyly and/or camptodactyly of the fingers, aplasia or hypoplasia of the middle phalynx of the fifth fingers and toes,[25] tooth enamel hypoplasia, and a narrow nose.[26] It usually shows autosomal dominant inheritance and is caused by mutations in *GJA1*, which encodes connexin-43, a protein involved in channel assembly or conductivity.[27] Patients with Kenny-Caffey syndrome can show proportionate growth retardation, macrocephaly, and episodic hypocalcemia with hyperphosphatemia.[28,29] Patients with the recessive form may also have mental retardation, microcephaly, micrognathia, cryptorchidism, and small hands/feet.[30,31]

Management

The high to extreme degree of hyperopia usually seen in patients may be correctable with high-power glasses. This can result in moderate to good visual acuity but should be corrected beginning early in life because it can be very amblyogenic. Refractive correction with glasses may also help with the strabismus that these patients develop because their eyes often turn in as a result of them having to accommodate so hard to see even at distance. Residual esotropia not correctable with glasses may require surgery. Depending on the vision in each eye, patients may require amblyopia treatment, including patching and optical and/or pharmacologic penalization.[32] These patients are at risk of lifelong eye issues, including angle closure glaucoma and spontaneous, intraoperative, or postoperative choroidal congestion, choroidal detachment, and/or exudative retinal detachment, so they should be counseled accordingly and followed chronically.

Enlarged Eye: Buphthalmos

A diffusely enlarged eye with an enlarged cornea most commonly is due to congenital glaucoma (please see the glaucoma chapter for further information).

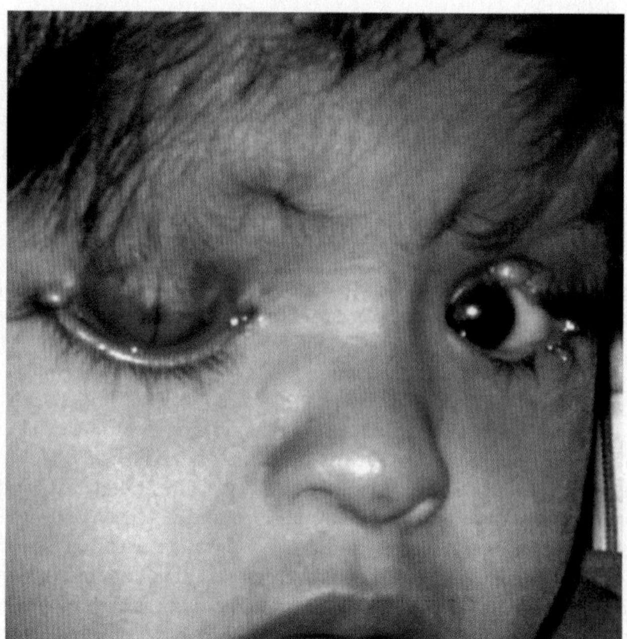

Fig. 63.3 Cryptophthalmos. A 2-year-old girl with cryptophthalmos, right eye. The upper eyelid is maldeveloped, containing no lid margin structures, and completely fused with the ocular surface. The coloboma also involves the ipsilateral eyebrow. A cleft is present in the contralateral upper eyelid. (Reproduced with permission and minor modifications from Revere et al. Eyelid developmental disorders. In: Fay and Dolman, eds. *Diseases and Disorders of the Orbits and Ocular Adnexa*. 2017; 139.)

Abnormal Eyelid Structure/Function

Absence of Eyelids, Adnexal Structures, and "Hidden Eye": Cryptophthalmos (Fig. 63.3)

Clinical Features

In the "complete" form of cryptophthalmos, skin extends from the forehead to the cheek with no recognizable adnexal structures, including brow, eyelids, eyelid margin, eyelashes, meibomian glands, tear glands, or tear ducts.[33] The eye is usually hidden underneath the skin and is often malformed, ranging from defects in the anterior chamber to the whole eye. There are also "incomplete" forms that show varying degrees of residual adnexal structures, but these too are usually associated with significant ocular malformations.[33] Cryptophthalmos can also occur rarely in isolation, in which the eyelids and all adnexal structures form but are abnormal.

Pathophysiology

The isolated form can be inherited in an autosomal dominant fashion.[34] More commonly, cryptophthalmos is inherited in an autosomal recessive manner and occurs in conjunction with systemic abnormalities as part of cryptophthalmos syndrome, cryptophthalmos-syndactyly syndrome, or Fraser syndrome. Systemic features include mental retardation, dyscephaly with skull malformations, and/or anomalies of the ears, nose, larynx, digits, kidneys, or genitals.[35,36] Fraser syndrome can be caused by mutations in *FRAS1* or *FREM2*, which are thought to encode putative extracellular matrix proteins that interact with and stabilize epithelial basement membranes.[37]

Evaluation

Ophthalmologic assessment should be performed in the first few weeks of life to determine the visual potential. The skin directly overlying the eye can show a small depression, and sometimes a

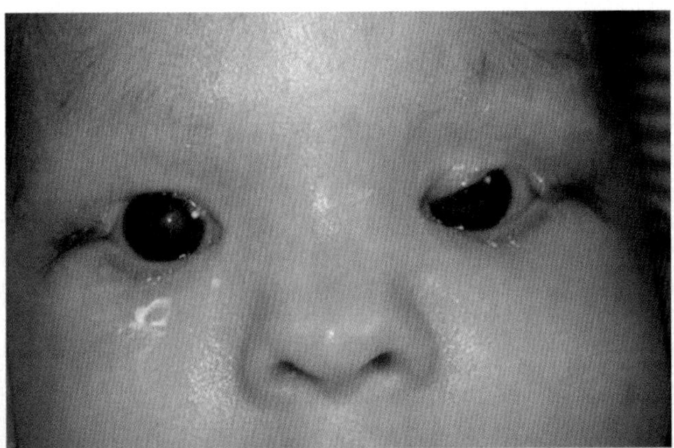

Fig. 63.4 Eyelid Colobomas. Neonate with bilateral upper eyelid colobomas, which extend into the eyebrows. (Reproduced with permission and minor modifications from Revere et al. Eyelid developmental disorders. In: Fay and Dolman, eds. *Diseases and Disorders of the Orbits and Ocular Adnexa*. 2017; 140.)

response to bright light can be observed (in the form of periocular muscle contraction). In its more complete forms, visual prognosis is usually very guarded, even if a response to light is observed. MRI, CT, ultrasound, and electrophysiology (visual evoked potential [VEP] and electroretinography) can be used to determine the visual potential.

Management

If visual potential can be demonstrated, surgical intervention can be considered. The goals of surgery are to create a clear visual axis to optimize vision and some sort of functioning eyelids to help cover the eye and avoid corneal exposure. Success depends on the extent of preexisting ocular malformation and adnexal structures. Full-thickness corneal transplants tend to do poorly due to the absence of conjunctiva and a normal ocular surface. An artificial cornea (keratoprosthesis) can be a choice, although these carry their own substantial risks.[38]

Focal Eyelid Defect: Coloboma (Fig. 63.4)

Clinical Features

Coloboma is a full-thickness defect in the eyelid due to failure of the mesodermal folds to fuse correctly during development. Severity ranges from a small notch at the eyelid margin to near absence of an eyelid. It can be unilateral or bilateral and can involve the upper, lower, or both eyelids. The defect can be triangular or rectangular, with the eyelashes and tarsal plate typically being absent in the affected area. The majority of defects involve the upper eyelids, are usually more nasal, and are at greater risk of corneal exposure. Lower-eyelid defects are less common, more temporal, and have a lower risk of corneal exposure. Nasal lower-eyelid defects are often associated with tear-drainage-system (nasolacrimal) defects.[39]

Pathophysiology

Eyelid colobomas can occur in isolation or as part of a craniofacial syndrome such as Goldenhar or Treacher Collins (Fig. 63.5). Goldenhar syndrome is caused by defects in structures derived from the first and second branchial arches and first branchial cleft. Features include upper-eyelid coloboma in up to 20% of patients, limbal epibulbar dermoids, preauricular skin tags, deafness, small ears, and vertebral anomalies.[40,41] Congenital cranial nerve dysinnervation issues (e.g., Duane syndrome) are also more common in Goldenhar syndrome than in the general population. Treacher Collins syndrome is inherited in an autosomal dominant manner, is caused by mutations in *TCOF1* that lead to impaired neural crest precursor development,[42] and represents the most extensive developmental abnormality of the first branchial arch.[43] Features include lower-eyelid colobomas in 75% of patients, downward-sloping palpebral fissures, mandibular and malar hypoplasia, malformed external ears, deafness in 50% of patients, unusual hair growth patterns, and normal intelligence.[44]

Evaluation

Ophthalmologic assessment should ideally be performed in the first few days of life to determine the risk of corneal exposure, decompensation, and/or permanent scarring from the eyelid defect(s). Fluorescein testing can rule out corneal epithelial defects. Other ocular anomalies that could infer a systemic condition should be carefully evaluated. Limbal dermoids confer a significant risk of astigmatism, so patients should undergo careful refraction.

Management

Artificial tears or artificial tear ointment can be used to provide additional ocular lubrication. Definitive surgical intervention depends on the shape, size, and location of the eyelid coloboma.[45] Defects smaller than 50% of the eyelid can often be repaired by mobilizing the lateral canthus, moving the tissue nasally, and directly

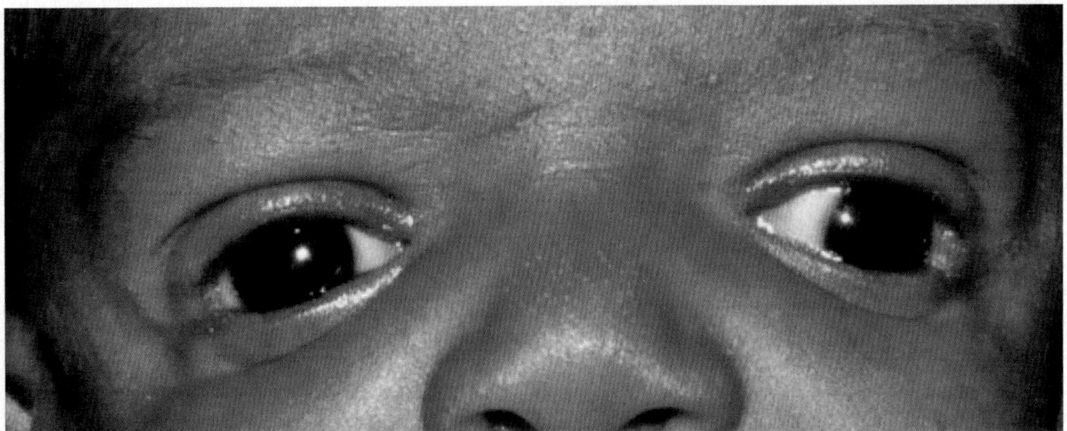

Fig. 63.5 Treacher Collins Syndrome. Bilateral zygomatic defect with underdeveloped maxillae and downward slanting eyes. (Reproduced with permission and minor modifications from Cruz et al. Orbital developmental disorders. In: Fay and Dolman, eds. *Diseases and Disorders of the Orbits and Ocular Adnexa*. 2017; 123.)

closing the defect. For defects larger than 50% of the eyelid, sliding or rotational flaps are generally preferred in place of eyelid-sharing techniques, because the latter run the risk of causing deprivational amblyopia in infants.

Abnormal Eyelid Fusion (Ankyloblepharon) or Shape (Euryblepharon) (Figs. 63.6 and 63.7)

Clinical Features/Pathophysiology

Ankyloblepharon refers to adhesions between the upper and lower eyelids. Ankyloblepharon filiforme (which presents with fine fibrovascular strands) can be isolated or be part of popliteal pterygium syndrome along with abnormal digits and genitals[46] or Van der Woude syndrome along with cleft lip/palate, hypodontia, lower lip paramedian pits, or mucous cysts.[47] Both are autosomal dominant syndromes caused by mutations in *IRF6*. They can also occur in conjunction with trisomy 18,[48] isolated cleft lip/palate,[49] in the setting of CHANDS syndrome (curly hair, ankyloblepharon, nail dysplasia),[50] or AEC syndrome (ankyloblepharon, ectodermal dysplasia, and cleft lip/palate),[51] the latter of which is inherited in an autosomal dominant fashion and caused by mutations in the *TP73L/P63* gene.[52]

Euryblepharon refers to an abnormal horizontal widening of the palpebral fissure, resulting in sagging of the lower eyelid and poor apposition to the globe. This can result in corneal exposure and chronic tearing. It can occur in isolation or may be part of systemic conditions such as Kabuki syndrome or blepharocheilodontic syndrome.[53,54] The former includes distinct facial features, mental retardation, and skin, skeletal, renal, and urinary tract anomalies.[55,56] Other ocular features include blue sclera, ptosis, strabismus, microphthalmia, coloboma, and/or corneal abnormalities.[57] Blepharocheilodontic syndrome includes euryblepharon, out-turned eyelids (ectropion), cleft lip/palate, and dental issues.[58] Other ocular features include incomplete eyelid closure (lagophthalmos), a second row of eyelashes (distichiasis), and widely spaced eyes (hypertelorism).[58]

Evaluation

Ophthalmologic assessment should ideally be performed in the first few weeks of life. Any eyelid fusion that appears to impede the visual axis should be surgically divided to avoid deprivation amblyopia. Other ocular anomalies that could infer a systemic condition should be carefully evaluated. There are rare cases of ankyloblepharon in association with anterior segment dysgenesis and early-onset glaucoma[59]; hence testing for eye pressure, corneal diameter, refractive error, and optic nerve appearance should be performed at the same time. Fluorescein testing can rule out corneal exposure in euryblepharon.

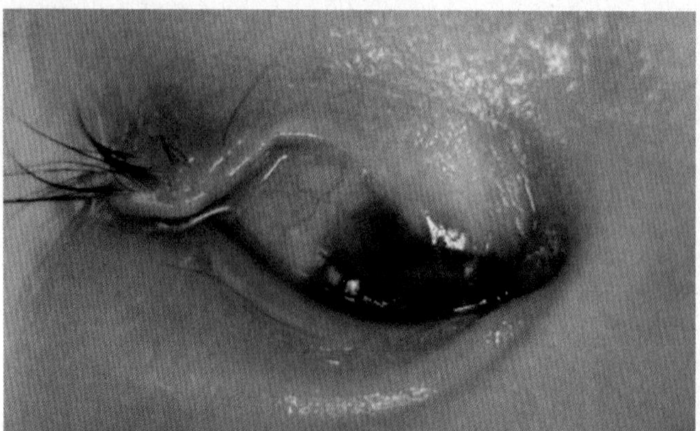

Fig. 63.6 Ankyloblepharon. Persistent adhesions are seen between the upper and lower lid temporally, representing failure of normal separation of the eyelids at 6 to 7 months' gestation. (Reproduced with permission and minor modifications from Revere et al. Eyelid developmental disorders. In: Fay and Dolman, eds. *Diseases and Disorders of the Orbits and Ocular Adnexa*. 2017; 141.)

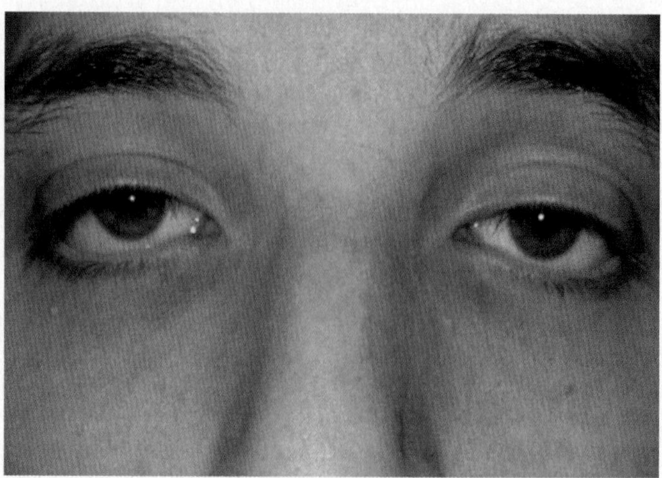

Fig. 63.7 Euryblepharon. The lateral one-third of the lower eyelid is displaced downward, producing an enlarged fissure that is wider laterally than medially. (Reproduced with permission and minor modifications from Revere et al. Eyelid developmental disorders. In: Fay and Dolman, eds. *Diseases and Disorders of the Orbits and Ocular Adnexa*. 2017; 148.)

Management

Fine ankyloblepharon strands may be breakable by traction, although surgical division may be necessary and more controlled. Conservative management of corneal exposure includes use of artificial tears or artificial tear ointment. Definitive intervention for euryblepharon includes surgical repair in the form of horizontal eyelid tightening, with superior displacement of the lateral canthal tendon.

Abnormally Narrow Eyelid Opening (Palpebral Fissure): Blepharophimosis (Fig. 63.8)

Clinical Features/Pathophysiology

Blepharophimosis is an abnormally small palpebral fissure in both the vertical and horizontal planes and forms part of a tetrad along with ptosis (eyelid drooping with poor eyelid opening), epicanthus inversus (upward fold of lower-eyelid skin near the inner cornea of the eye), and telecanthus (increased distance between the inner corners of the eyes), known as BPES (blepharophimosis-ptosis-epicanthus syndrome). It is caused by mutations in *FOXL2*[60] and is inherited in an autosomal dominant fashion with incomplete penetrance.[61] BPES is divided into two forms based on the presence or absence of premature ovarian failure in females. Affected patients are at greater risk of other ocular anomalies involving the eye (e.g., microphthalmos, optic disc colobomas), eyelids (e.g., euryblepharon), tear drainage system (nasolacrimal ducts), strabismus, and amblyopia.[62]

Evaluation

Ophthalmologic assessment should ideally be performed in the first few weeks of life. The most concerning feature from a functional perspective is the eyelid drooping (ptosis) and the risk of impaired

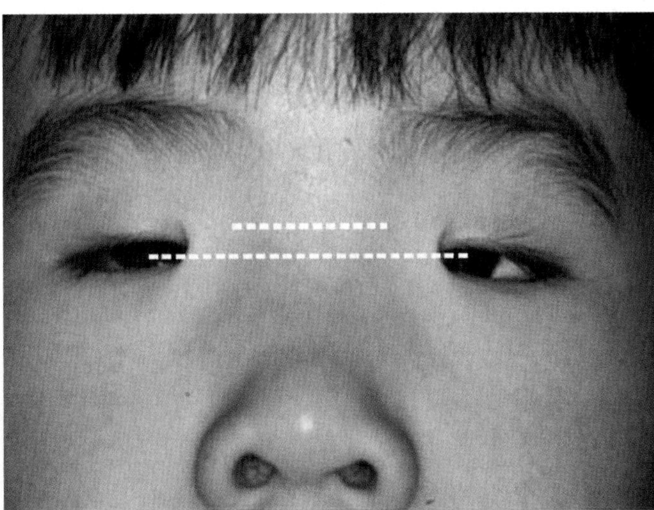

Fig. 63.8 Blepharophimosis, Ptosis, and Epicanthus-Inversus Syndrome (BPES). *Telecanthus* refers to a wider intercanthal distance but with normal position of the eye and orbital structures. In this child, the interpupillary distance, depicted by the *lower, longer white dotted line*, is normal, whereas the intercanthal distance is wider than the expected distance, depicted by the *upper, shorter white dotted line.* (Reproduced with permission and minor modifications from Dolman and Goold. Clinical evaluation and disease patterns. In: Fay and Dolman, eds. *Diseases and Disorders of the Orbits and Ocular Adnexa*. 2017; 42.)

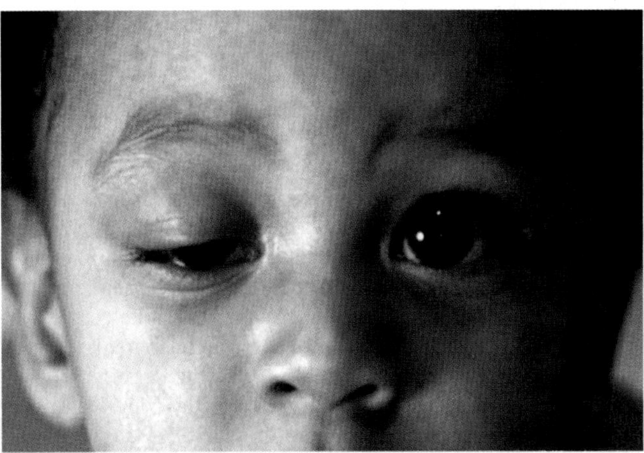

Fig. 63.9 Congenital Ptosis. Unilateral right-sided. The lid crease is typically diminished, and the frontalis is often used in an attempt to elevate the eyelid. A chin-up head position may also be observed. (Reproduced with permission and minor modifications from Revere et al. Eyelid developmental disorders. In: Fay and Dolman, eds. *Diseases and Disorders of the Orbits and Ocular Adnexa*. 2017; 150.)

vision from deprivation amblyopia if the eyelids block the visual axis. Patients often develop a chin-up head position to allow them to see through their small palpebral fissures, which may help preserve vision, although it can cause long-term neck muscle contracture with pain and movement restriction. Visual function should be monitored over time to ensure amblyopia does not develop in one or both eyes, which guides the need and timeline for surgical intervention. Female patients with BPES should also undergo endocrinology evaluation and genetic counseling.

Management

Surgical correction of the eyelid drooping may be necessary if visual function is being compromised or the chin-up head posture is causing functional, social, or neck issues. The timing of ptosis repair remains controversial. Early intervention may reduce the risk of amblyopia but is less predictable, with overcorrection risking corneal exposure from incomplete eyelid closure. Later repair can be more predictable and may be preferable if visual function is preserved. There are several approaches to epicanthus and telecanthus repair.[63] Both may improve with age, so delayed repair may be advisable, although some surgeons advise repairing all three at the same time.[63] Ovarian failure is best managed by an endocrinologist and includes consideration of estrogen-deficiency symptoms, emotional health, fertility, sexual function, and bone and cardiovascular health.

Eyelid Drooping: Congenital Ptosis (Fig. 63.9)

Clinical Features/Pathophysiology

The upper eyelid is raised by both the levator palpebrae (major effector) and Muller's muscle (minor effector). Congenital ptosis is most commonly caused by a developmental defect of striated muscle fibers in the levator. It is unilateral in 75% of cases and usually sporadic, although there may be a family history. Eyelid closure may also be incomplete (lagophthalmos), increasing the risk of inferior corneal exposure. Patients are also at greater risk of refractive amblyopia from astigmatism in the affected eye, because children's eyes and eyelids are more pliable and the drooping eyelid distorts the cornea more than the unaffected side.

An elevation deficit in the same eye as the ptosis is known as double elevator palsy (DEP) or monocular elevation deficiency. This results from defective innervation of both the levator palpebrae and superior rectus muscle on the same side. A chin-up head position in these cases may be driven by the limitation of elevation of the eye rather than the eyelid droop and hence should be carefully evaluated to ensure that ptosis surgery for a chin-up head position is justified and likely to be effective; it can also limit the ability of the eye to elevate when the eyelid closes (Bell's phenomenon) and hence increases the risk of corneal exposure if ptosis surgery is performed but this is not identified. Ptosis can also occur as part of congenital Horner syndrome, so this should be excluded as part of the workup (see later section).

Evaluation

Ophthalmologic assessment should ideally be performed in the first few weeks of life and at defined intervals thereafter, depending on laterality and severity. Impaired vision can result from deprivation amblyopia if an eyelid blocks the visual axis or refractive amblyopia due to astigmatism in the ptotic eye(s), even if the ptosis is only mild. Corneal exposure from lagophthalmos should also be monitored. A chin-up head position, or horizontal corrugations in the forehead on the side of the ptosis due to frontalis muscle overaction raising the brow and hence the eyelid, are reassuring features in unilateral ptosis that the patient is trying to use the eye. If the ptosis is bilateral, the child will likely develop these features to allow them to see out of one or both eyes. However, fatigue can limit the effectiveness of frontalis overaction, and a chin-up head posture runs the risk of long-term neck issues. Visual function should be reevaluated over time because testing accuracy improves with age and helps guide the need for surgical intervention.

Management

Astigmatism is typically in the vertical axis and can be corrected by glasses. If there is concern for amblyopia, patching of the unaffected eye can be instigated to force the brain to use the affected eye. The intensity of the patching depends on the severity of the amblyopia. Glasses in combination with patching may be necessary for the child to see out of the affected eye when the unaffected eye is patched. If the infant refuses to wear a patch, atropine can be instilled in the unaffected eye 2 days per week to blur the vision (as long as the child is far-sighted, which most are; this will not work if they are near-sighted or have no refractive error).

Surgical correction of the ptosis may be necessary if visual function is being compromised or the chin-up head posture is causing functional, social, or neck issues.[64] Early intervention (e.g., 6–12 months of age) may reduce the risk of amblyopia but is less predictable, with overcorrection risking corneal exposure from lagophthalmos and/or DEP-related impaired Bell's phenomenon. Later repair (e.g., 5–6 years of age) can be more predictable and may be preferable if visual function has been preserved. The type of repair depends on the severity of the ptosis and the amount of residual levator muscle function.[65] If the ptosis is more severe and/or there is very limited levator muscle function, a sling procedure that tethers the upper eyelid to the frontalis muscle in the forehead may be preferable (this helps the patient use their frontalis muscle to raise the eyelid). If the ptosis is less severe and/or levator muscle function is relatively preserved, shortening (resecting) the levator muscle can give a more natural appearance to the eyelid contour and avoids the use of implanted material. After any surgery, the patient must be carefully monitored to ensure corneal exposure does not develop, and aggressive corneal lubrication is typically started and then slowly tapered. If the patient also requires strabismus surgery for DEP, operating on the vertical muscles can alter eyelid position, and thus strabismus surgery may be performed prior to ptosis surgery if possible.

Eyelid Drooping: Congenital Horner Syndrome (Fig. 63.10)

Clinical Features/Pathophysiology

Horner syndrome is due to defective sympathetic innervation to the eye and adnexal structures. About 1 in 6250 babies are born with Horner syndrome, with less than 5% of cases being truly congenital.[66] The most common cause of congenital Horner syndrome is birth trauma.[65] Potentially fatal causes include thoracic and cervical neuroblastoma, internal carotid artery agenesis, and perinatal surgical complications. Carotid artery aneurysm and traumatic carotid dissection are rare but have been reported in congenital cases,[67] as have postviral damage and fibromuscular dysplasia.[68,69] Signs include eyelid droop (ptosis), small pupil (miosis), and absent flushing during crying. Congenital cases associated with sympathetic dysgenesis (not birth trauma) can also cause the affected eye to have a lighter colored iris, because both sympathetic ganglion cells and iris melanocytes are of neural crest origin.

Evaluation

Ptosis due to Horner syndrome can usually be distinguished from congenital ptosis because of the associated ocular and adnexal findings, especially the pupil. Diagnosis can be challenging in infants. The heterochromia may only become apparent as the iris of the unaffected eye acquires more pigment, and pharmacologic testing of pupils in infants can be difficult to evaluate and/or may yield equivocal results.[70] Different reports have recommended varying degrees of investigation.

A clear history of birth trauma helps guide diagnosis. Factors include forceps use, vacuum extraction use, shoulder dystocia, fetal rotation, and/or limb manipulation. Klumpke paralysis is infrequently present.[69] Asymmetric facial flushing is usually absent in these cases, indicating a postganglionic lesion. Hydroxyamphetamine testing can be used to confirm the lesion location, although it may only generate partial dilation.[71] Apraclonidine testing may be performed in older infants to see if it reverses the miosis; however, it can cause extreme drowsiness in young infants (<6 months),[72] so is not advisable in this age group. A full clinical examination should be performed to identify any abdominal or other masses or additional cranial neuropathies. Asymmetric facial flushing can help localize the lesion to the preganglionic neuron. Iris heterochromia, which can be present in nearly 80% of cases, is typical of congenital Horner syndrome, although it can also develop if a lesion is acquired before age 2 years.[73]

Cervical or mediastinal neuroblastoma is the most significant treatable cause of Horner syndrome, and prognosis is better if it is identified prior to 1 year of age.[74] It can be associated with congenital Horner syndrome.[75] Thus in an infant with no clear history of birth trauma or surgery, urinary vanillylmandelic acid (VMA) (which is raised in up to 95% of cases) and MRI of the brain, neck, and chest should be considered.[76] Despite extensive testing, a significant number of pediatric Horner syndrome patients show no identifiable cause, even in the presence of longer-term follow-up.[68,73]

Management

From a systemic perspective, treatment depends on the location and cause of any lesion or tumor and is beyond the scope of this chapter. As with congenital ptosis, indications for surgical

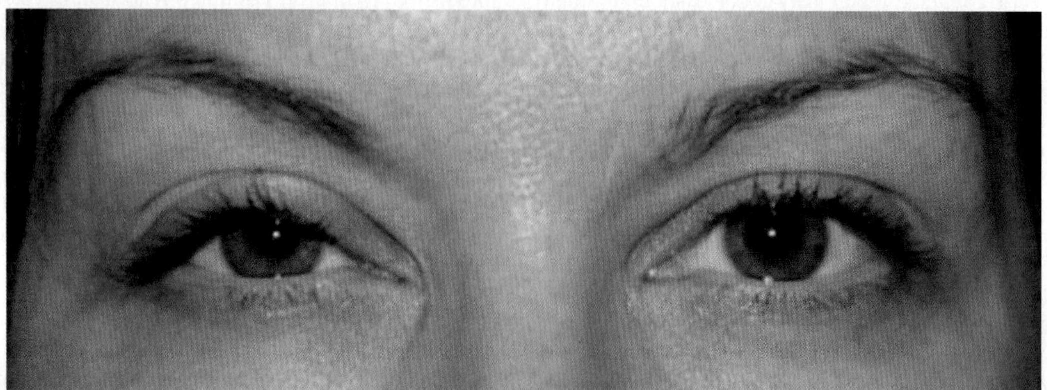

Fig. 63.10 Congenital Horner Syndrome. Right miotic pupil and ptosis in a 16-year-old female with Horner syndrome dating from birth-related trauma. The slightly paler iris color confirms that onset was before 2 years of age. (Reproduced with permission and minor modifications from Dolman and Goold. Clinical evaluation and disease patterns. In: Fay and Dolman, eds. *Diseases and Disorders of the Orbits and Ocular Adnexa*. 2017; 39.)

intervention of ptosis in Horner syndrome are amblyopia and issues resulting from a chin-up head position. However, ptosis in Horner syndrome is much milder than that in congenital ptosis, because it results from Muller's muscle inactivation rather than levator dysfunction. Because Muller's muscle is a minor effector of eyelid elevation, the ptosis may be less severe. If intervention in needed, response of the ptosis to instillation of phenylephrine drops (a sympathetic agonist) can help simulate the effect of surgical intervention on Muller's muscle. If deemed sufficient, there are several approaches to Muller's muscle tightening.[77,78] If not sufficient to correct the ptosis, other approaches similar to those used in congenital ptosis can be performed.

CHAPTER

64 Developmental Anomalies of the Cornea and Iris in Neonates

Rachel R. Milante, Jefferson J. Doyle

KEY POINTS

1. Causes of primary neonatal corneal opacification include congenital hereditary endothelial dystrophy (CHED), posterior polymorphous corneal dystrophy, congenital hereditary stromal dystrophy (CHED), and corneal dermoid. Secondary causes include trauma (e.g., forceps), infection, metabolic disorders, and congenital glaucoma. Corneal opacification requires further workup to diagnose the underlying cause and to help plan any surgical intervention.
2. Primary megalocornea is defined as a horizontal corneal diameter of >12 mm at birth or >13 mm by 2 years of age in the absence of elevated eye pressure. Congenital glaucoma must be ruled out; isolated cases do not usually require intervention. Microcornea is defined as a clear cornea of normal thickness with a horizontal corneal diameter of <9 mm in newborns and <10 mm after 2 years of age. It is commonly associated with other ocular and/or systemic findings.
3. Developmental anomalies of the iris include diffuse underdevelopment (congenital aniridia, including its association with Wilms tumor), focal developmental defects (coloboma), failed involution of the central iris (prepupillary membrane), iris cysts (and their association with thoracic aortic aneurysm), bilateral hypopigmentation (e.g., albinism), asymmetric pigmentation (heterochromia, e.g., Waardenburg syndrome, congenital Horner syndrome), iris atrophy (e.g., Axenfeld-Rieger anomaly), and displaced pupil (corectopia) with or without lens displacement (ectopia lentis), both of which can occur in isolation or in association with systemic causes such as neonatal Marfan syndrome.

Cornea: Abnormal Appearance or Size

Congenital Corneal Opacification (CCO)

Clinical Features

Primary congenital corneal opacifications include congenital hereditary endothelial dystrophy (CHED), posterior polymorphous corneal dystrophy, congenital hereditary stromal dystrophy (CHSD), and corneal dermoids.[1]

CHED manifests as bilateral, often symmetric, diffuse corneal cloudiness from edema (Fig. 64.1).[2] CHED1 (which is now known as CHED) usually presents with clear corneas at birth that tend to become progressively cloudier during the neonatal period, along with new-onset light sensitivity but no nystagmus. By contrast, CHED2 (which is now considered a neonatal variant of posterior polymorphous corneal dystrophy) usually presents with corneal cloudiness from birth that is nonprogressive and with nystagmus (due to lack of visual input from birth) but no light sensitivity.[3] CHED may also be seen as part of Harboyan syndrome, which presents with CCO and sensorineural deafness.

CHSD presents with limbus-to-limbus corneal clouding and flake-like opacities in the corneal stroma but no corneal vascularization.[4] Corneal dermoids are choristomas (normal cells in an abnormal location) and present as creamy nodular opacities that are classically located at the periphery of the cornea, where they can cause significant visual impairment from astigmatism. Sometimes they can obstruct the visual axis directly or cause ocular surface dryness and thinning (dellen) from tear film disruption.

Peters' anomaly (Fig. 64.2) and "sclerocornea" (Fig. 64.3) have historically been used to describe certain types of CCO, although these terms are now discouraged due to their nonspecific nature.[1] Because many prior reports utilize such terms, it is still important to note that Peters' anomaly traditionally refers to abnormal adhesions between the cornea and iris (and is one form of anterior segment dysgenesis [ASD]). This impairs the ability of the inner layer of the cornea (endothelium) to successfully pump fluid out of the cornea in areas of adhesion, the process it uses to maintain clarity. As a result, Peters' anomaly typically presents with cloudiness in part of the cornea from birth, which often slowly improves over a matter of months to years. Some cases also involve the lens and have congenital cataract. Peters' plus syndrome includes additional systemic features such as short disproportionate stature, developmental delay, dysmorphic facial features, and cardiac, genitourinary, and central nervous system malformations.[5]

Sclerocornea describes a nonprogressive, noninflammatory ingrowth of opaque sclera extending into the peripheral cornea, causing an indistinct border between the two tissues. It can occur in isolation or along with other ASD syndromes such as Peters' anomaly.[6] It can be complete, where the whole cornea is opaque and flattened, or it can spare the central cornea and only affect the peripheral part.

Mucolipidosis IV is the only true metabolic cause of neonatal CCO.[1] This rare metabolic storage disease is inherited in an autosomal recessive pattern and is associated with progressive psychomotor retardation.

Acquired corneal opacification that presents early in life includes trauma from accidental or nonaccidental causes. Forceps injury should be kept in mind because this is a well-recognized etiology of postnatal corneal opacification. It is almost always unilateral and is associated with fine streaks (breaks) in the inner cornea,[1] which are only visible with magnification. Viral or bacterial infection may both present with corneal clouding in the neonatal period[7,8] but are often accompanied by other findings such as eyelid swelling, corneal ulcer, and/or muco-purulent discharge. Corneal clouding also occurs as part of primary congenital glaucoma (discussed in the glaucoma chapter).

Pathophysiology

CCO has a prevalence of 3 in 100,000 newborns, or 6 in 100,000 when congenital glaucoma is included.[9] Many of the primary forms are inherited. CHED can be passed on in an autosomal dominant (CHED1) or autosomal recessive (CHED2) manner.[2,3] Primary dysfunction of the corneal endothelium increases permeability, causing hydration by aqueous humor and hence clouding. Harboyan syndrome is due to mutations in *SLC4A11*.[10] CHSD is caused by disruption of collagen

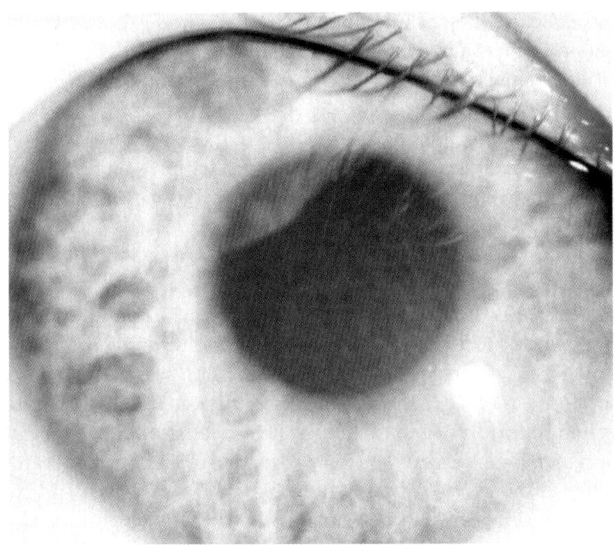

Fig. 64.1 Congenital Hereditary Endothelial Dystrophy (CHED). Diffuse stromal edema is present at birth or develops in the first decade of life. This creates a diffuse corneal haze that typically involves the entire cornea. (Reproduced with permission and minor modifications from Krachmer and Palay. Corneal dystrophies, ectatic disorders, and degenerations. In: *Cornea Atlas*. 2014:170.)

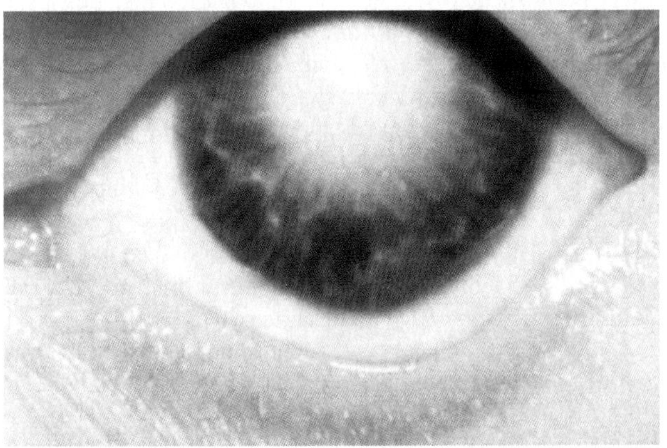

Fig. 64.2 Peters Anomaly. There is central opacification of the corneal stroma with relative clearing in the corneal periphery. In mild cases, adherent strands of iris tissue extend from the pupillary margin to the posterior cornea. In severe cases the iris is markedly abnormal and the lens may adhere to the posterior cornea. Glaucoma is often present. (Reproduced with permission and minor modifications from Krachmer and Palay. Normal anatomy and developmental abnormalities of the cornea. In: *Cornea Atlas*. 2014:96.)

organization due to mutations in *DCN* (which encodes decorin).[11,12] Peters' anomaly can occur sporadically, but dominant and recessive forms have been reported.[13] It can be caused by mutations in *PAX6*, *PITX2*, *FOXC1*, *CYP1B1*, *MAF*, or *MYOC* and is associated with trisomy 13. Peters' plus syndrome is recessively inherited and can be caused by mutations in *B3GALTL*.[14,15] Causes of sclerocornea show significant overlap with other forms of ASD and include mutations in *FOXE3*, *RAX*, *SOX2*, *PITX3*, *PAX6*, and *PXDN*.[15] Mucolipidosis type IV is caused by mutations in *MCOLN1*; mucolipin-1 dysfunction impairs lipid and protein transport, causing their accumulation in lysosomes. Viral infection early in the neonatal period is often caused by herpes simplex. When accompanied by purulent discharge, *Neisseria gonorrhea* should be considered due to the high rate of progression and risk of perforation.

Evaluation

Diagnosing the cause of neonatal CCO based on clinical appearance alone is hard, because different entities present similarly. High eye pressure helps distinguish primary congenital glaucoma from other causes. Corneal thickness measurement by pachymetry helps distinguish CHED (increased due to edema) from CHSD (normal thickness). Imaging using ultrasound biomicroscopy (UBM) and anterior segment optical coherence tomography (AS-OCT) helps identify cornea-iris or cornea-lens adhesions suggestive of Peters' anomaly and also aids in preoperative planning.[16] Genetic testing can help identify underlying genetic etiologies. Corneal lesions suspicious for infectious causes must be scraped and sent for microbiologic testing.

Management

Primary corneal diseases without significant ASD can undergo full thickness corneal transplant (penetrating keratoplasty [PKP]) and have fair outcomes, albeit not as good as adults.[1] For disorders that only affect specific layers of the cornea (e.g., CHSD), selectively transplanting that layer (i.e., deep anterior lamellar keratoplasty [DALK]) may be an option.[17] Corneal dermoids can be managed by PKP or DALK, depending on their size.[18,19] Corneal transplants are avoided in patients with active infection, but once the infection and associated inflammation have resolved, the residual scar can be replaced with a PKP or DALK.[1,17] Conjunctival transplantation may help corneal clouding due to mucolipidosis IV.[20]

Corneal Crystals

Clinical Features

Examples of disorders with corneal crystal deposits include cystinosis and tyrosinemia type 2. Crystals appear as bifringent stromal opacities that may be visually significant.[21] Patients can have light sensitivity due to light scattering by the crystals or redness and irritation

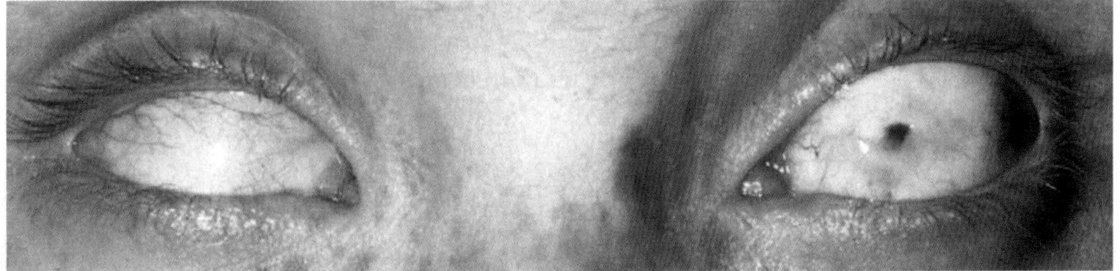

Fig. 64.3 Sclerocornea. There is diffuse whitening (scleralization) of the cornea. The cornea may be totally opaque, as in the right eye of this patient, or there may be a central relatively clearer area, as seen in the left eye. The central cornea is flat because it reflects the curvature of the sclera. There are usually associated ocular abnormalities, and the prognosis for vision with corneal transplant is poor. (Reproduced with permission and minor modifications from Krachmer and Palay. Normal anatomy and developmental abnormalities of the cornea. In: *Cornea Atlas*. 2014:89.)

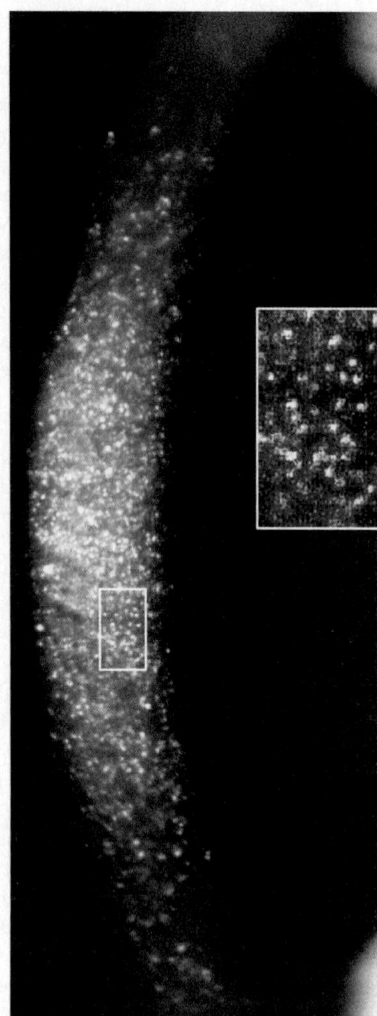

Fig. 64.4 Cystinosis. Crystals containing cysteine are deposited in the corneal epithelium and stroma. The crystals are polygonal, refractile, and polychromatic *(inset)*. (Reproduced with permission and minor modifications from Krachmer and Palay. Corneal manifestations of systemic disease and therapy. In: *Cornea Atlas*. 2014:105.)

from an uneven corneal surface. Fifty percent of infants with cystinosis present with light sensitivity.[22] Tyrosinemia type 2 can also present with corneal epithelial defects that resemble herpes simplex dendrites (pseudodendrites).

Cystinosis occurs in 1 in 100,000 newborns.[23] There is no gender or racial predilection. It is the most common cause of pediatric renal Fanconi syndrome and accounts for 5% of pediatric renal failure cases.[23] It is divided into three types, including nephropathic, intermediate, and nonnephropathic (ocular) forms (Fig. 64.4). The nephropathic form is the most common and severe form and develops in infancy; it presents with light sensitivity and renal failure. The nonnephropathic form only affects the cornea.

Tyrosinemia type 2 results from elevated blood tyrosine levels, and affects the eyes, skin, and intellectual development. Symptoms include eye pain, redness, excess tearing, and light sensitivity as well as painful skin lesions on the palms and soles (palmoplantar hyperkeratosis). Fifty percent of patients have intellectual disability.[24]

Pathophysiology

Cystinosis is inherited in an autosomal recessive manner. All forms are caused by mutations in *CTNS*, which encodes lysosomal membrane protein cystinosin.[21] Impaired cystinosin function results in lysosomal cysteine accumulation due to impaired export; the accumulated crystals damage affected tissues.

Tyrosinemia type 2 is inherited in an autosomal recessive manner. It is caused by mutations in the gene tyrosine aminotransferase *(TAT)*; this results in impaired function of the enzyme tyrosine aminotransferase, one of the enzymes required for tyrosine breakdown. Impaired tyrosine aminotransferase function causes accumulation of tyrosine crystals in affected tissues.[24]

Evaluation

White blood cell cysteine levels of 3 to 20 nmol half-cysteine/mg protein is diagnostic of cystinosis.[25] Molecular testing for mutations in the gene Cystinosin, Lysosomal Cystine Transporter *(CTNS)* can be performed. AS-OCT shows hyperreflective and iridescent deposits involving the corneal epithelium and corneal stroma but typically sparing the inner corneal layers.[26,27] Tyrosinosis is confirmed by high urinary elimination of tyrosine and tyrosine derivatives and high serum tyrosine levels up to 52 mg/100 mL.[24]

Management

In cases where corneal deposition is nonprogressive, complaints of light sensitivity may decrease over time, so observation is reasonable.[26] Oral cysteamine treatment depletes systemic cysteine levels and is used to improve renal function; of note, it does not help with corneal crystal deposits or eye symptoms due to the cornea being avascular.[28] Cysteamine eye drops do help decrease corneal crystal density and associated symptoms,[29] although to date, existing eye drop preparations require up to hourly instillation and are hence challenging for patient treatment adherence. Crystals found only in the corneal epithelium can sometimes be managed by removal of the outer corneal layers (superficial keratectomy).[27]

Large Cornea: Megalocornea

Clinical Features

Megalocornea is defined as a corneal diameter >12 mm at birth or >13 mm after 2 years of age in the absence of elevated eye pressure (Fig. 64.5).[30] It is usually bilateral and may be isolated or associated with other ocular or systemic disorders.[31]

Pathophysiology

Isolated megalocornea is most commonly inherited in an X-linked recessive pattern (90%) and thus occurs mostly in males.[32] It can

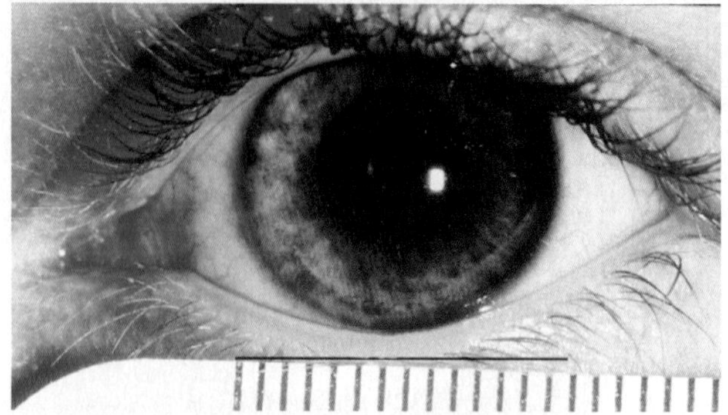

Fig. 64.5 Megalocornea. The corneal diameter is greater than or equal to 12 mm at birth or 13 mm after the age of 2 years in the absence of elevated eye pressure. It is most commonly transmitted as an X-linked recessive disorder, with 90% of affected patients therefore being male. It is associated with numerous ocular and systemic disorders. (Reproduced with permission and minor modifications from Krachmer and Palay. Corneal manifestations of systemic disease and therapy. In: *Cornea Atlas*. 2014:89.)

be inherited in an autosomal recessive manner or very rarely in an autosomal dominant fashion. It is associated with several gene mutations including *CHRDL1* (X-linked megalocornea), *LTBP2*, *SH2PXD2B*, *NOTCH2*, *PIK3R1*, *ZNF469*, and chromosome 16 duplication.[32]

Evaluation

Clinical measurement of horizontal corneal diameter is diagnostic. It is important to rule out congenital glaucoma by measuring eye pressure, axial globe length, and refraction and assessing the ocular structures, especially corneal clarity and optic nerve cupping (all of which are affected in glaucoma but not megalocornea).

Management

Intervention is not needed for isolated megalocornea, because it is nonprogressive. Dryness due to exposure can be treated with artificial tears. Treatment of associated ocular or systemic issues are determined by a multidisciplinary team.

Small Cornea: Microcornea

Clinical Features

Microcornea is defined as a clear cornea of normal thickness with a diameter <9 mm at birth or <10 mm after 2 years of age (Fig. 64.6).[33] It is most commonly associated with other ocular findings such as cataract, coloboma, iris maldevelopment, retinal underdevelopment or outpouching, nystagmus, and/or ptosis.[33] Various systemic findings such as skeletal, cardiac, genitourinary, and neurologic defects have been reported in association with microcornea.

Pathophysiology

Isolated microcornea is very rare. It is thought to represent an arrest of corneal growth after differentiation is complete in the fifth month age of gestation. Genetic association is poorly defined,[34,35] but mutations in *PAX6*,[36] *CRYBB1*,[37] *ZNF408*,[38] and *WDR37*[39] have been reported. It has been associated with an *FBN1* mutation in one case of severe neonatal Marfan syndrome and bilateral ectopia lentis.[40] In utero exposure to cytomegalovirus has also been implicated.[41]

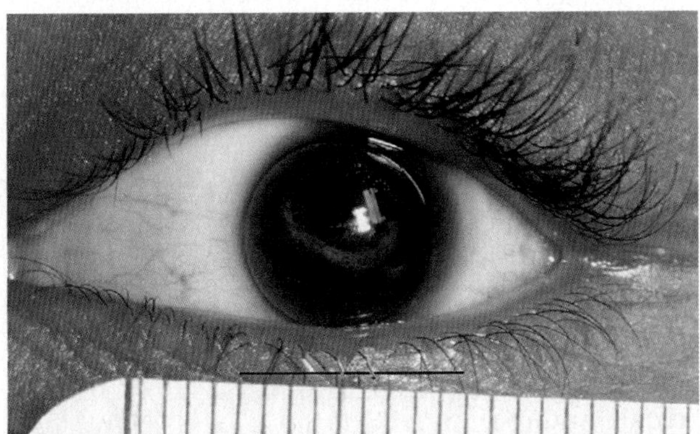

Fig. 64.6 Microcornea. Microcornea is defined as a clear cornea of normal thickness with a diameter less than 9 mm at birth or 10 mm after 2 years of age in an eye of normal size. If the entire eye is small, the condition is termed nanophthalmos. This patient with microcornea had congenital cataracts removed and is wearing an aphakic contact lens. (Reproduced with permission and minor modifications from Krachmer and Palay. Corneal manifestations of systemic disease and therapy. In: *Cornea Atlas*. 2014:88.)

Evaluation

Clinical measurement of horizontal corneal diameter is diagnostic. Because it rarely occurs in isolation, further investigation to uncover associated ocular or systemic features is warranted. Eye pressure, portable slit-lamp biomicroscopy, and dilated fundus exam should be performed in the first few weeks of life. Further imaging, such as AS-OCT or UBM, may be advisable depending on clinical findings.

Management

Isolated microcornea does not warrant intervention if the cornea remains clear. However, given the small anterior chamber, patients are at risk of glaucoma, so long-term eye pressure monitoring is advisable. Medical and surgical interventions will depend on associated findings.

Iris and Pupil: Congenital Abnormalities

Diffuse Iris Underdevelopment: Aniridia

Clinical Features

Iris hypoplasia may be total (aniridia) or partial (coloboma). Although aniridia directly translates to absence of iris tissues, congenital aniridia is considered a panocular abnormality involving the iris, cornea, anterior chamber angle, lens, retina, and optic nerve (Fig. 64.7).[42] Of note, there is usually a small peripheral stump of iris tissue that is visible both on clinical exam and histologically. The most common accompanying ocular finding is cataract.[42] Other lens changes (subluxation, coloboma, posterior lenticonus, and microspherophakia), corneal opacification, micro- or megalocornea, glaucoma, and foveal hypoplasia can co-occur with aniridia. Especially in cases with no family history, Wilms tumor must be ruled out.[43,44]

Pathophysiology

Congenital aniridia prevalence is estimated to be 1 in 40,000 to 1 in 96,000 newborns.[45,46] It may be sporadic or inherited either in isolation due to *PAX6* mutations or as part of Wilms

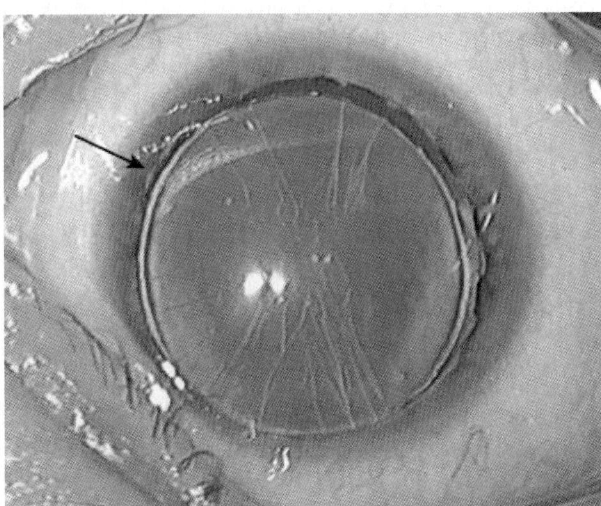

Fig. 64.7 Aniridia. This patient has remnants of iris tissue and consequently the appearance of a significantly dilated pupil. The lens edge is visualized circumferentially at the pupil border, which is not usually possible in normal eyes. (Reproduced with permission and minor modifications from Orge. Examination and common problems in the neonatal eye. In: *Fanaroff and Martin's Neonatal-Perinatal Medicine*, 95, 1934–1969.)

tumor–aniridia–genital anomalies–retardation (WAGR) syndrome; the latter is due to 11p13 deletions that affect both *PAX6* and adjacent *WT1* genes.[47,48] Aniridia has also been associated with mutations in *FOXC1* and *CYP1B1*.[49]

Evaluation

A complete ophthalmologic examination should be performed in the first few weeks of life. Cataract and glaucoma are seen at an early age,[42] so regular monitoring of lens opacities and eye pressure is necessary. Genetic testing can be used for diagnosis confirmation, familial counseling, and early detection of children at risk for Wilms tumor.[50] The nature of the *PAX6* mutation and the degree to which PAX6 protein function is impaired influence disease severity. Some patients only have partial iris defects, no foveal hypoplasia, and relatively normal vision; others are more severely affected. Renal ultrasound can be obtained while awaiting genetic testing results.

Management

Treatment will depend on the ocular findings. Refractive correction with protection for light sensitivity is advised. If eye pressure is raised it should be treated, initially with eye drops and often then with surgery. Cataracts can undergo removal as needed. Because both the anterior and posterior segments of the eye are often affected,[42] visual impairment tends to be significant. Low-vision aids, educational accommodations, and multidisciplinary supervision are needed for long-term care.

Focal Iris Underdevelopment: Iris Coloboma

Clinical Features

Iris coloboma classically presents as a keyhole-shaped iris defect (Fig. 64.8). These defects most commonly involve the inferonasal iris and can be unilateral or bilateral, symmetric or asymmetric. They can occur in isolation or in conjunction with colobomas involving other ocular structures such as the ciliary body, choroid, retina, and/or optic nerve. If only the iris is involved, visual prognosis is usually good; patients can have glare/light sensitivity due to light scatter through the peripheral lens in the area of the iris defect, or occasionally double vision. If there is retinal or nerve involvement, vision may be more severely impaired and will depend on the size and location of the coloboma(s).

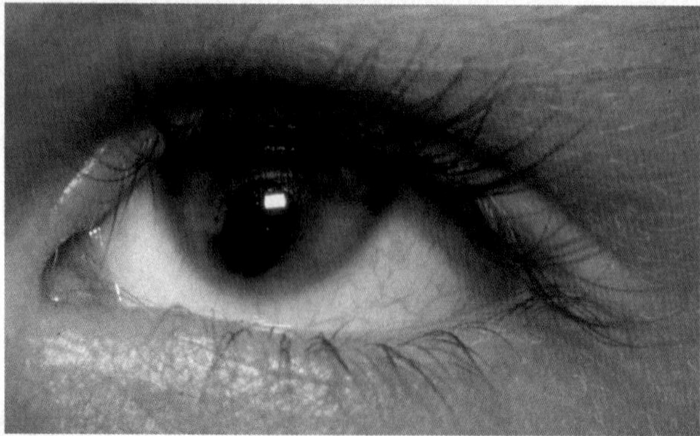

Fig. 64.8 Iris Coloboma ("Keyhole Pupil"). The photo depicts an inferonasal coloboma—the most common location for it to occur. (Reproduced with permission and minor modifications from Olitsky and Marsh. Abnormalities of pupil and iris. In: *Nelson Textbook of Pediatrics*, ch. 640, 3349–3353.e1.)

There are a number of syndromes associated with ocular colobomas. CHARGE syndrome is an acronym for coloboma of the eye, heart defects, nasal choanae atresia, growth/development retardation, genitourinary anomalies, and ear issues/deafness. Cat eye syndrome describes the vertical colobomas reminiscent of a cat pupil seen in these patients. Patau syndrome can include iris and/or retina/nerve colobomas as well as microphthalmia, Peters' anomaly, cataract, retinal dysplasia, optic nerve hypoplasia, and nystagmus. Treacher Collins syndrome has classic facial features including iris colobomas, downslanting eyelid margins, ear anomalies, and/or micrognathia.

Pathophysiology

Ocular colobomas affect <1 in 10,000 births. They are usually caused by failure of the embryonic fissure to close in the fifth week of gestation and can be associated with mutations in *PAX2*.[51] CHARGE syndrome is an autosomal dominant condition caused by mutations in *CHD7*. Cat eye syndrome is caused by trisomy/tetrasomy of part of chromosome 22. Patau syndrome results from trisomy of chromosome 13. Treacher Collins syndrome is caused by mutations in *TCOF1*.

Evaluation

Complete ophthalmologic examination in the first few weeks of life can help define the size and symmetry of iris colobomas and also identify any other associated ocular anomalies that may impact vision. If the eyes are asymmetrically involved, amblyopia can develop in the more affected eye, in which case early prophylactic therapy (e.g., patching) can be instigated. Eyes with additional colobomas may need further workup and/or treatment (e.g., chorioretinal colobomas can cause retinal detachment[52] and may benefit from prophylactic laser to prevent a future occurrence or surgery to treat an existing one). Genetic testing can be used for diagnosis confirmation, familial counseling, and early detection in future pregnancies. Involvement of other services for systemic workup and management is important.

Management

Treatment depends on the degree of involvement. Asymptomatic isolated iris coloboma(s) may only require observation. Light sensitivity can be treated with tinted glasses. Surgical repair of an iris defect may be possible by bringing together the two edges of the coloboma to create a more rounded pupil; this can help with both cosmesis and glare/light sensitivity and can be performed in young patients who still have their native lens. However, it may not be possible in patients with larger defects. If the ocular lens is involved (e.g., ciliary body colobomas can cause a focal lens zonular defect and resultant astigmatism), refractive correction should be used. Cataracts can undergo removal as needed. If vision is significantly impaired, low vision aids, educational accommodations, and multidisciplinary supervision may be necessary.

Diffuse Bilateral Iris Hypopigmentation: Albinism

Clinical Features

Albinism encompasses a heterogenous group of inherited disorders that share a defect in melanin biosynthesis. Whereas cutaneous and/or iris hypopigmentation are obvious external signs, other less evident ocular features include underdevelopment of the central retina (foveal hypoplasia), resulting in delayed visual development, reduced vision, nystagmus, and eye misalignment (Fig. 64.9).[53]

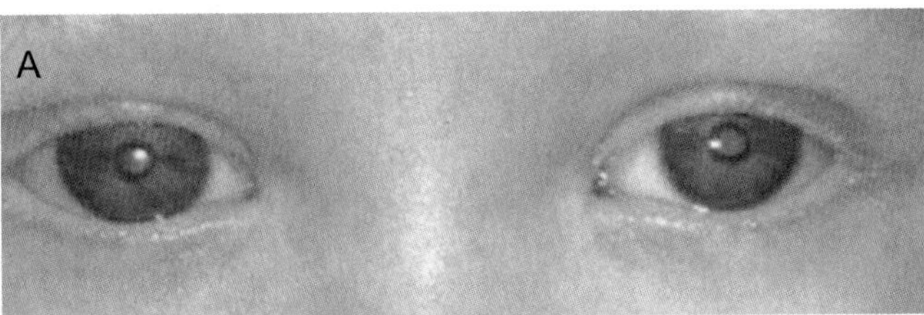

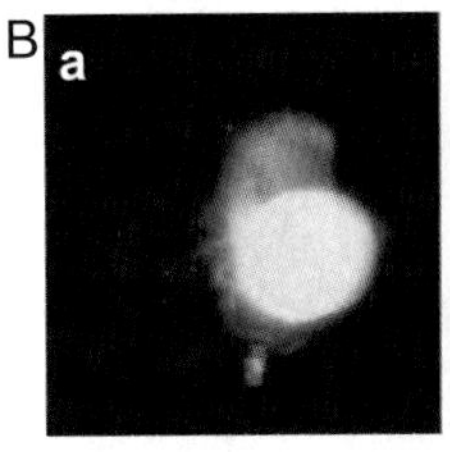

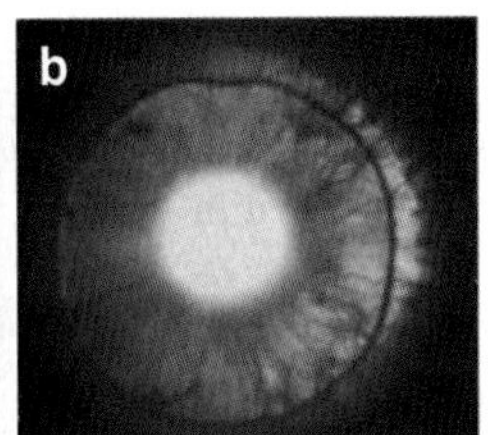

Fig. 64.9 Albinism. (A) Very light irides in both eyes showing transillumination defects (*red-orange* hue from light shone through the pupil and reflected back off the retina is visible through the iris, which is not seen in normal eyes). (B) On greater magnification, *(a)* the edge of the lens cannot be visualized through the undilated pupil in a normal eye but *(b)* can be seen in albinism.

Pathophysiology

Current classification is based on pathologic genes. X-linked ocular albinism is due to *GPR143* mutations on Xp22.3,[54] whereas autosomal recessive oculocutaneous albinism (OCA) is caused by mutations in genes encoding several different proteins (OCA1: tyrosinase; OCA2: P protein; OCA3: TYRP1A; and OCA4: SLC45A2).[53] *TYR* mutations in OCA1 have a more severe effect on pigmentation (and hence phenotype) than mutations in the genes encoding GPR143 or P protein.[55]

Evaluation

Iris transillumination defects can be evaluated by transscleral illumination with a pen-light placed directly on the bulbar conjunctiva or by directing a strong slit beam through an undilated pupil. In albinism, the thin iris will allow incident light to be reflected not only through the pupil but also through the iris itself.[54] In preverbal children, visual acuity can be tested using Teller Acuity Cards. Cycloplegic refraction should be performed to determine refractive errors that require glasses correction. Retinal OCT can be used to show a lack of foveal umbo (the normal dip in the central retina required for good acuity). AS-OCT can demonstrate a thin iris, specifically the posterior epithelium.[56] A special visual-evoked potential technique can be performed to show excess optic nerve fiber crossing at the chiasm that is highly sensitive for albinism.[57] Absence of nystagmus, detectable depth perception, melanin pigment in the macula, and some degree of foveal reflex are predictors of better future vision.[53]

Management

Annual follow-up for patients under 16 years old is recommended to update their glasses prescription and ensure adequate filter for light sensitivity.[54] Prosthetic iris implants are now approved by the US Food and Drug Administration[54a] and have shown better safety and effectiveness profiles in patients with albinism compared with other iris pathologies (e.g., trauma, aniridia, and uveitis), so they may be considered to reduce glare.[58] Many children with nystagmus develop an abnormal head position where the nystagmus is least prominent and hence vision is best (null point). If the abnormal head position causes neck muscle issues or interferes with daily activities or socialization, surgery to bring the null point into the primary visual axis (i.e., straight ahead) can be performed (Kestenbaum-Anderson procedure).[59,60] This is often delayed until the infant is older to allow more accurate preoperative measurements. Oral levodopa (L-DOPA) therapy has proved beneficial in albino mice,[61,62] but a prospective randomized controlled trial failed to find benefit in humans.[63]

Asymmetric Iris Pigmentation: Heterochromia (Fig. 64.10)

Clinical Features

A difference in color between the two eyes at birth may be due to Waardenburg syndrome or congenital Horner syndrome. Waardenburg syndrome is defined by iris heterochromia, eyelid and tear drainage system abnormalities, narrow eyelid fissures (blepharophimosis), prominent broad nasal root, nasal eyebrow overgrowth, a white forelock, and deaf-mutism.[64] Partial or complete iris heterochromia occurs in approximately 30% of patients.[65] Waardenburg syndrome has four types (I, II, III, IV), of which type II is most commonly associated with iris heterochromia.[65,66] Congenital Horner syndrome presents with heterochromia, ptosis, miosis, and facial anhidrosis (reduced flushing on the affected side of the face during crying in neonates).[67,68]

Pathophysiology

Waardenburg syndrome is inherited in an autosomal dominant (type I, II, III, and some type IV) or autosomal recessive (remaining type IV) manner.[67] Causal genes affect melanocyte development from the primitive neural crest. Types I to III are mostly caused by *PAX3* mutations, with 15% of type II due to *MITF* defects.[66] Type IV can be caused by endothelin-3 *(EDN3)*, endothelin-receptor B *(EDNRB)*, or *SOX3* mutations.[66,69] Iris heterochromia in congenital Horner syndrome results from disruption of sympathetic postganglionic neurons, leading to iris melanocyte dysgenesis.[70]

Evaluation

Audiologic testing should be performed early in cases of suspected Waardenburg syndrome,[69] even while awaiting genetic testing results. Further imaging and diagnostic tests are dictated by individual phenotypic expression of the disease. Gastroenterology referral, abdominal x-ray, barium enema, and rectal biopsy may be needed in patients who are suspected of having associated Hirschsprung disease.[71]

Management

Intervention for Waardenburg syndrome depends on disease manifestations. Hearing aids must be introduced early to mitigate effects on speech and socialization. Hypopigmentation is addressed with sun protection. Musculoskeletal deformities are life-long and managed with physical and occupational therapy. Treatment for

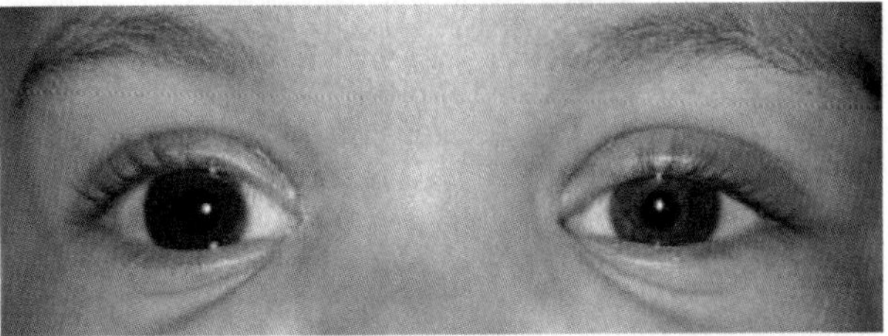

Fig. 64.10 Iris Heterochromia in an Infant With Congenital Horner Syndrome. The left eye shows a lighter iris and smaller pupil and left upper eyelid ptosis. (Reproduced with permission and minor modifications from O'Keefe et al. Pediatric iris disorders. In: *Taylor and Hoyt's Pediatric Ophthalmology and Strabismus*, ch. 39, 378–384.)

Hirschsprung disease will depend on severity and may entail surgical resection of the aganglionic colon.[71] See the "Congenital anomalies of the globe and ocular adnexa" (Chapter 63) for evaluation and management of congenital Horner syndrome.

Atrophic or Distorted Iris: Anterior Segment Dysgenesis

Clinical Features

The term anterior segment dysgenesis (ASD) spans an array of ocular disorders caused by aberrant development of neural crest, mesoderm, surface ectoderm, and/or neuroectodermal derivatives of the eye.[72] Nomenclature has been challenging due to overlapping causal genes and complicated phenotypes.[1,72] The prototypical ASD is Axenfeld-Rieger anomaly (ARA).

Axenfeld anomaly is defined by posterior embryotoxon (a fine white ring around the cornea just inside the limbus [Fig. 64.11]), with attached iris strands that cause drainage angle distortion and glaucoma.[73] Rieger anomaly refers to iris abnormalities including corectopia (displaced pupil), polycoria (multiple pupils), and iris atrophy.[73] Rieger anomaly plus systemic findings such as redundant umbilicus, hypoplastic teeth, maxillary hypoplasia, or pituitary issues is referred to as Rieger syndrome (Fig. 64.12).[72] Approximately 50% of patients with ARA develop glaucoma.[74] Alagille syndrome is a multisystem disorder characterized by pulmonary artery hypoplasia, pale skin and hair, triangular facies, butterfly vertebral arches, intellectual disability, and growth retardation.[75] It prominently includes posterior embryotoxon, although patients can also have microcornea, iris hypoplasia, optic disc drusen, and/or retinal pigment changes.[76,77]

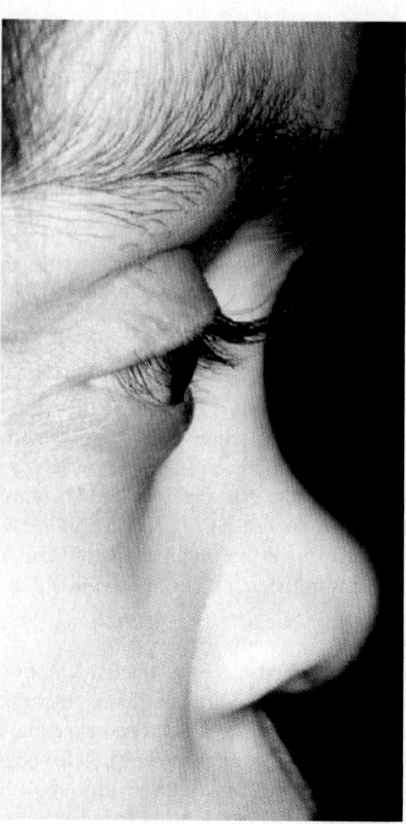

Fig. 64.12 Axenfeld-Rieger Syndrome: Flat Nasal Bridge With Maxillary Hypoplasia. The figure shows a combination of Rieger's anomaly and systemic abnormalities, which include microdontia, a flat nasal bridge with maxillary hypoplasia, and hypospadias. (Reproduced with permission and minor modifications from Normal anatomy and developmental abnormalities of the cornea. In: *Cornea Atlas*. 2014:95.)

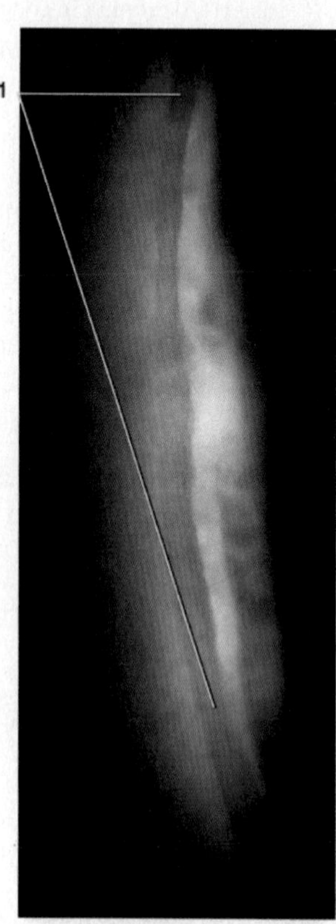

Fig. 64.11 Posterior Embryotoxon. Enlargement and anterior displacement of Schwalbe's line (1), which represents the termination point of the inner layers of the cornea. It is seen in up to 30% of normal eyes but is commonly seen in Axenfeld anomaly and other genetic conditions (e.g., Alagille syndrome). (Reproduced with permission and minor modifications from Normal anatomy and developmental abnormalities of the cornea. In: *Cornea Atlas*. 2014:93.)

Pathophysiology

ARA is usually inherited in an autosomal dominant manner, although it can occur sporadically. There is significant genetic overlap between ARA and other ASDs such as Peters' anomaly (see earlier section).[72] *FOXC1* and *PITX2* mutations most commonly cause ARA,[78,79] although *PAX6*,[80] *FOXO1A*, and *CYP1B1* have also been implicated. Notably, the underlying genetic abnormality remains undefined in up to 60% of cases.[81] Alagille syndrome is an autosomal dominant disorder caused by heterozygous mutations in *JAG1* or *NOTCH2*.[76,77]

Evaluation

Complete ophthalmologic examination should be performed in the first few weeks of life, including corneal diameter, refraction, axial length, eye pressure, pachymetry, gonioscopy, and dilated fundus exam. Characterization of the dysgenesis with AS-OCT or AS-UBM is paramount. Patients should be followed regularly to identify and treat glaucoma. Given genetic heterogeneity in ASDs, broad genetic testing with microarray and next-generation sequencing is suggested.[72] In suspected Axenfeld-Rieger and Alagille syndromes, patients should be examined carefully to elicit systemic involvement (e.g., dental, facial, skeletal, hepatobiliary, cardiac, or pulmonary issues).

Management

Current treatment for ARA is directed at managing glaucoma with medical, laser, and/or surgical control of eye pressure. The prognosis depends on how early optic nerve damage is detected and how successful efforts are to control eye pressure. Patients with Alagille syndrome are managed mainly for hepatobiliary issues.

Excess Iris Tissue: Primary Iris Cysts, Iris Flocculi, and Persistent Pupillary Membrane

Clinical Features

Primary iris cysts (Fig. 64.13) are classified as pigmented (derived from the iris pigment epithelium) or nonpigmented (derived from the iris stroma).[82] Pigmented iris cysts (flocculi) are multiple smooth, hyperpigmented, grape-like nodules around the pupil margin. Iris stromal cysts are unilateral, solitary lesions with a transparent capsule.[83] Small or collapsed cysts are often asymptomatic, but larger ones may cause visual axis obstruction, corneal opacity, ocular inflammation, or elevated eye pressure.

Persistent pupillary membrane (PPM) is a common congenital eye anomaly that appears as fine residual iris strands that traverse the pupil and attach either to the iris at both ends (type 1) or connect the iris to the lens capsule (type 2). The vast majority are fine diaphanous strands that do not cause symptoms, but occasionally dense PPMs can impair vision.[84] In asymmetric presentations, deprivation amblyopia is a concern.

Pathophysiology

Iris flocculi are rare in the adult population but can occur in up to 3.5% of newborns; 85% will resolve or become less apparent by 2 months of age.[85] Lesions that fail to resolve must be differentiated from congenital ectropion uveae,[86] iris stromal cysts, nevi, melanocytoma, pigmented adenoma, or melanoma.[85] Patients with bilateral iris flocculi should undergo workup for thoracic aortic aneurysm with autosomal dominant inheritance[87,88] and associated *ACTA2* mutation.[89,90] These patients may also present with congenital pupil dilation but no flocculi.[89] Both the aortic and iris issues are speculated to result from connective tissue weakness.[91] Iris stromal cysts are congenital in 50% of cases.[83] They represent 16% of iris cystic tumors in infants and can enlarge after initial identification.[92]

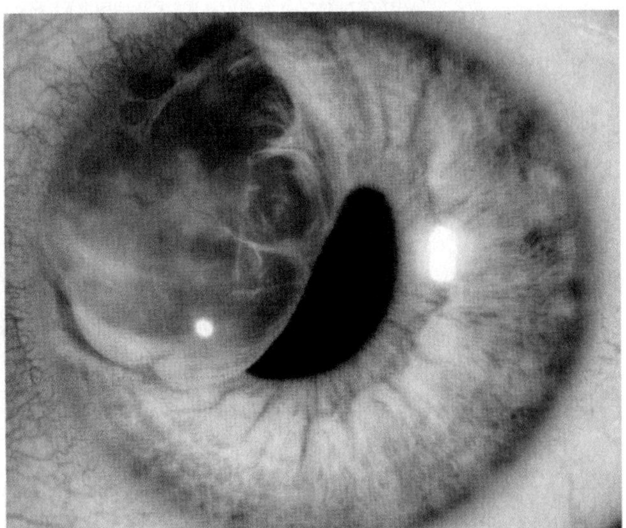

Fig. 64.13 Congenital Iris Stromal Cyst. These are congenital lesions that can remain stable for many years and then suddenly enlarge. The iris is thinned and lacks its normal architecture. (Reproduced with permission and minor modifications from Krachmer and Palay. Corneal manifestations of systemic disease and therapy. In: *Cornea Atlas*. 2014:286.)

PPMs are a remnant of the tunica vasculosa lentis, a structure that provides nourishment to the avascular lens during development. Normally, this structure fully regresses by birth or in the first few weeks of life, although residua can be seen in 30% to 95% of newborns.[93,94] Failure to fully regress leads to PPMs, which can occur in isolation or in association with other eye findings (e.g., small flat cornea, foveal hypoplasia).[95] A case of bilateral PPMs with congenital heart disease has been reported.[96]

Evaluation

Clinical examination entails careful evaluation of the cornea, anterior chamber, and iris lesion(s) in the first few weeks of life. Corneal diameter and eye pressure must be measured. Gonioscopy must be performed to reveal accompanying angle dysgenesis. AS-OCT and UBM help characterize the iris lesion(s) and are often diagnostic. Iris flocculi consist of fluid-filled, single-cell membrane cysts originating from the posterior iris surface at the pupil margin.[89,97] Iris stromal cysts have a thin wall with medium reflectivity, contain fluid with suspended particles, and show underlying iris deformity.[83] PPM can vary in laterality, size, density, and configuration; they must also be evaluated for lens adhesions that can affect vision even after PPM removal.[98]

Management

The majority of primary iris cysts are nonprogressive and can be managed conservatively. Regular monitoring for elevated eye pressure and/or signs of ocular inflammation is sufficient in asymptomatic cases. For cysts that are enlarging or causing symptoms, fine-needle aspiration with careful injection of autologous blood, alcohol, or antimitotic agent or surgical excision with or without lensectomy may be needed.[83] Recurrence can occur if excision is incomplete.[99]

PPM management depends on membrane size and density and pupil aperture. Because most patients have good vision,[100] conservative treatment with dilating drops, refraction, and/or amblyopia therapy (patching) often suffices.[101] Yag laser PPM lysis has been reported, but risks include bleeding, iris pigment dispersion, increased eye pressure and cataract formation.[102] Surgical excision, with or without lens removal,[103,104] can be performed, although it carries the same risks, as well as those of anesthesia and intraocular infection.[84] For PPMs that interfere with vision, it is important to intervene early to prevent deprivation amblyopia, especially if they are bilateral but asymmetric.

Abnormal Iris Lesions: Juvenile Xanthogranuloma and Brushfield Spots

Clinical Features

Nodular iris lesions in neonates may be due to juvenile xanthogranuloma (JXG), a rare non-Langerhans cell histiocytosis with cutaneous and extracutaneous (CNS, liver, spleen, lung, and/or eye) nodules.[105] The eye is the most common extracutaneous location, with involved sites including the iris, drainage angle, limbus, and/or conjunctiva (Fig. 64.14).[106] Spontaneous unilateral hyphema (blood in the anterior chamber) is the most common presenting sign in infants and young children.[107] Patients may have an enlarging yellowish mass on the iris surface,[106] along with uveitis (redness, light sensitivity).[106,108] Even if an iris nodule is not readily apparent, the iris may appear bumpy, with pigmented material in the peripheral iris and drainage angle on gonioscopy.[108] Secondary glaucoma may develop later in the course.[109]

Iris nodules seen in infants with Down syndrome are known as Brushfield spots (Fig. 64.15).[110] These are 0.1- to 1-mm discrete or coalescing hypopigmented white or grayish-brown nodules that form a ring at the junction of the middle to outer third of the iris.[111]

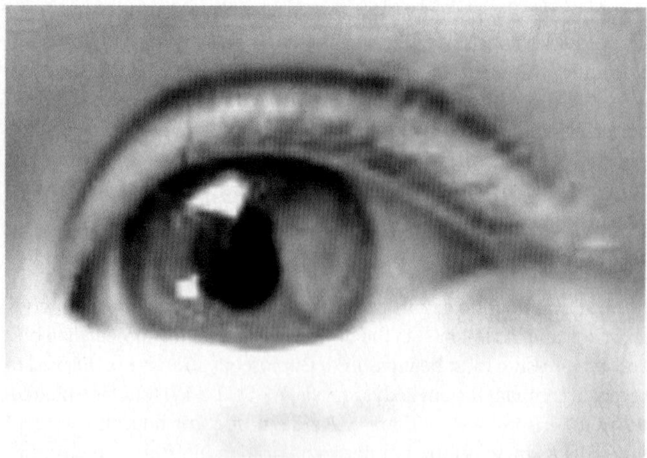

Fig. 64.14 Juvenile Xanthogranuloma (JXG). The ocular lesion of JXG is usually visualized as a fleshy, yellowish-brown tumor on the surface of the iris. The lesions are vascular, bleed easily, and can cause spontaneous hyphema. (Reproduced with permission and minor modifications from Winter and Lyons. Complete resolution of iris juvenile xanthogranuloma in an infant with topical corticosteroid treatment only. *CJO*. 2021. https://doi.org/10.1016/j.jcjo.2021.04.022. https://www.canadianjournalofophthalmology.ca/article/S0008-4182(21)00166-6/fulltext#articleInformation.)

Pathophysiology

JXG is a non-Langerhans cell histiocytic inflammatory disorder characterized by multinucleated giant (Touton) cells. It is most common in children aged 2 years and younger, with a median age at diagnosis of 1.3 years.[112] Eye involvement occurs in approximately 10% of patients with cutaneous JXG.[113]

The prevalence of Brushfield spots in Down syndrome varies depending on the population (and eye color). Studies in patients with dark irides from South Asia and the Middle East report a prevalence of 3% to 9%,[114,115] but in patients with light irides from Europe, the prevalence can be as high as 17% to 31%.[116,117] Iris imaging using near-infrared light has better sensitivity to detect Brushfield spots in dark irides, increasing the prevalence to 67% in such populations.[118] The spots are thought to represent an accumulation of excess collagen fibrils,[119] which are made more conspicuous by the adjacent iris being hypolastic.

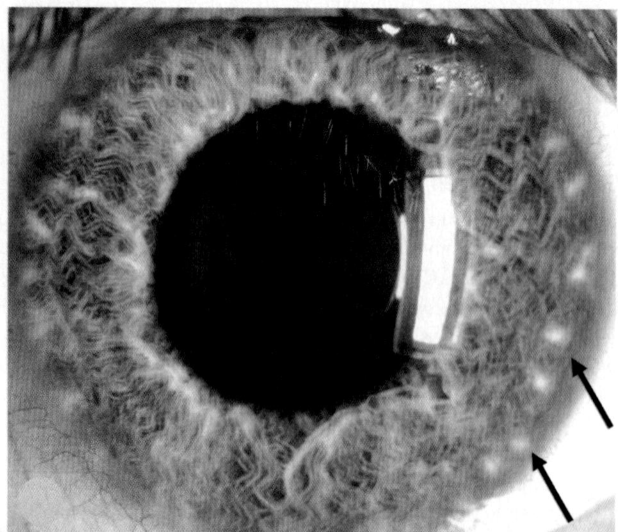

Fig. 64.15 Brushfield Spots. Small, whitish, peripheral iris speckles arranged in a concentric ring, occurring particularly in Down syndrome although also representing a normal finding in blue eyes. They consist of focal areas of mildly hyperplastic iris tissue surrounded by a ring of hypoplasia. (Reproduced with permission and minor modifications from Salmon. Ocular tumors. In: *Kanski's Clinical Ophthalmology*. 2020;20:827–880.)

Evaluation

XG is diagnosed by histopathology and immunohistochemistry. Cutaneous lesions should be biopsied; the presence of Touton giant cells in hematoxylin and eosin stains, positive CD68 staining, and negative S-100 and CD1a staining confirms JXG.[106,107] AS-UBM may show a single iris nodule, a localized area of minimal thickening, diffuse homogenous thickening, or a generalized bumpy iris contour.[106,108] AS-UBM is also valuable in determining the relationship of nodules to surrounding tissues and in serial monitoring of size and location before and/or after treatment.[106] No workup is necessary for Brushfield spots.

Management

Bleeding from JXG that involves the iris should be treated to prevent corneal blood staining, glaucoma, and amblyopia.[108] Topical corticosteroids are the mainstay of treatment. They are instilled every 2 hours, then slowly tapered over a period of 3 to 4 months.[107] Eye pressure must be regularly monitored and treated, because it can result from either the disease process or the treatment (steroid-response). Systemic steroids are used only for refractory cases. Focal lesions on the ocular surface can be surgically excised.[106] Brushfield spots are benign and hence do not need intervention.

Displaced Pupil and/or Lens: Corectopia and/or Ectopia Lentis

Clinical Features

The pupil is normally situated 0.5 mm inferonasally from the center of the iris, and minor deviations up to 1.0 mm are usually cosmetically and functionally insignificant. Corectopia refers to a displaced pupil. Idiopathic tractional corectopia is an isolated, progressive corectopia in infants (Fig. 64.16).[120] It is characterized by a fibrous strand that tethers the pupil to the peripheral iris[121] and can progress during the first 6 months of life.[120] Corectopia also occurs with other

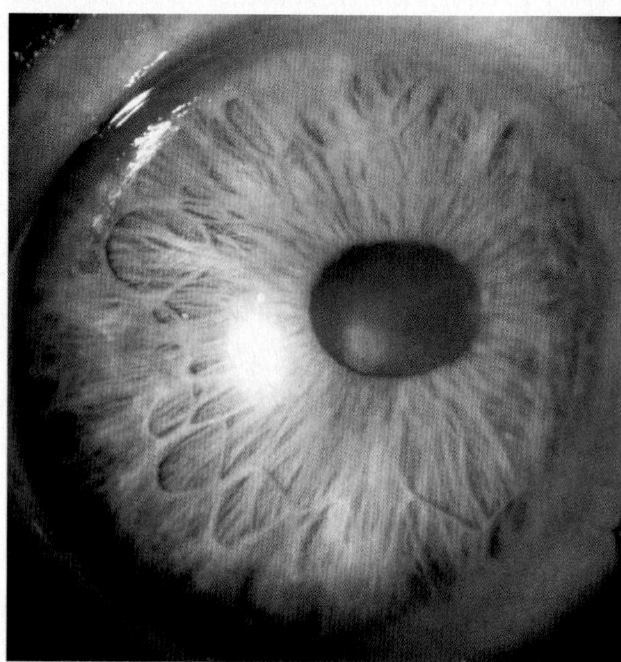

Fig. 64.16 Corectopia. Displacement of the pupil away from the center of the cornea. It can be associated with congenital or acquired conditions. (Reproduced with permission and minor modifications from Krachmer and Palay. Corneal dystrophies, ectatic disorders, and degenerations. In: *Cornea Atlas*. 2014:166.)

systemic findings (galactosemia, facial dysmorphism, and cyanotic heart disease)[122] or ocular conditions (cataract, lens subluxation, and myopia).[123] When accompanied by lens dislocation (ectopia lentis et pupillae), the pupil is usually displaced in the opposite direction to the lens.[124,125] This can be accompanied by PPM, cataract, iris dilator muscle hypoplasia, optic nerve hypoplasia, myelinated nerve fibers, or corneal issues.[126]

Pathophysiology

The exact etiology of idiopathic tractional corectopia is unknown, although it is thought to represent a membrane derived from ectopic iris tissue that is formed by aberrant neural crest cell migration.[127] Ectopia lentis may result from persistent remnants of the tunica vasculosa lentis that mechanically interfere with development of the lens zonules, leading to lens dislocation.[128] Alternatively, ectopia lentis et pupillae may result from localized persistence of the secondary vitreous, which forms a marginal bundle that tethers the iris to the anterior vitreous face, while also causing zonular disruption.[124]

Evaluation

A complete ophthalmologic exam will help differentiate isolated corectopia from ectopia lentis et pupillae. This should be done in the first few weeks of life, because blockage of the visual axis by a severely displaced pupil or the astigmatism created by a displaced lens can both be very amblyogenic. Cycloplegic refraction must be performed to evaluate the need for glasses correction. Gonioscopy, eye pressure measurement, and a dilated fundus exam, along with AS-OCT or UBM, can help aid in the diagnosis. Systemic examination, including the cardiovascular, central nervous, and musculoskeletal systems, should be performed.

Management

Treatment depends on the severity of the pupil displacement and whether the lens is also involved. Therapeutic options include topical dilating drops, Yag laser lysis of tethering strands, and/or surgery to enlarge the pupil (sphincterotomy or sectoral pupilloplasty).[120,121] Amblyopia therapy (patching, or atropine penalization if patching fails) should be initiated early. Lens displacement can result in visual impairment from severe myopia, astigmatism, cataract, and/or retinal detachment.[125] Close monitoring by an ophthalmologist for regular refraction, slit-lamp examination to evaluate for lens displacement and/or opacification, eye pressure monitoring, and a dilated retinal exam are essential. Significant lens opacification, refractive error that is uncorrectable with glasses, or ectopia lentis-induced glaucoma warrant lens removal. Many patients can be treated successfully with either aphakic contact lenses or aphakic glasses once their native lens has been removed. Delayed placement of an artificial intraocular lens that is attached to either the iris or sclera can be considered down the line but is generally not recommended for patients in the neonatal or infantile period.

Section 12

CHAPTER 65 Cataract and Glaucoma

Rachel R. Milante, Courtney L. Kraus

KEY POINTS

1. Cataracts are inherited or sporadic; congenital or acquired; isolated or in a syndrome.
2. Size, density, and location of lens opacity influence its visual significance.
3. Timing of cataract surgery is important; earlier detection and surgery have better outcomes.
4. Primary congenital glaucoma is the most common form of glaucoma in infants. It usually requires surgical treatment.
5. Some forms of infantile glaucoma may be managed with topical antihypertensives but may also require surgery.

Congenital Cataract

Cataracts develop due to disturbances in the normal highly ordered cellular arrangement of the crystalline lens. Pediatric cataracts remain a significant cause of preventable blindness.[1] However, the related vision loss can be greatly mitigated with prompt identification and treatment of significant lens opacities. In the United States, prevalence is estimated at 13.6 per 10,000 infants,[2] with 3.0 to 4.5 per 10,000 being visually significant.[3] The role of the neonatologist and pediatrician in early detection and prompt treatment cannot be overstated.

Presentation

History

Because congenital cataracts are often associated with genetic diseases or syndromes, a comprehensive history assists in diagnosis and management. Concerns about a white spot in the pupil, nystagmus, strabismus, asymmetric size of one eye relative to the other, photophobia, or visual inattentiveness should prompt referral. A detailed medical history includes documenting the onset of symptoms, such as whether prior exams documented a normal red reflex, birth weight, prematurity, evidence of maternal infection (especially TORCH infections [toxoplasmosis, other agents, rubella, cytomegalovirus, or herpes simplex], rash, or febrile illness during pregnancy), pertinent prenatal and perinatal history (i.e., radiation, alcohol, or drug exposure), maternal travel, history of ocular trauma, and corticosteroid therapy.[4]

Family history is important. A complete ocular examination is needed within the first few weeks after birth in infants with a family history of childhood cataract, particularly if it is bilateral. Hereditary bilateral cataracts are often inherited in an autosomal dominant (AD) pattern with a high degree of penetrance. A history of consanguinity can help in identifying the risk of genetic disorders associated with congenital cataracts.

Examination

For infants with bilateral cataracts, parents and caregivers can provide information on visual interest. In neonates, the significance of a cataract is determined primarily by examination. Later, visual fixation, following faces,[4] and reaching for objects are important milestones. For monocular cataracts, squinting, crossing, or wandering of an eye, a face turn, or opposition to blocking vision in one eye can allude to poor vision in the setting of lens opacity.

The Bruckner Red Reflex Test can be used to detect and determine the density of a lens opacity. Both eyes are viewed using a direct ophthalmoscope at a distance of approximately 3 feet to compare the red reflexes. The light reflex is normally symmetric in both eyes.

Infants with uni- or bilateral cataracts can develop nystagmus due to poor vision. Those with bilateral, dense cataracts often develop nystagmus by 3 months of age, which is when the fixation reflex normally develops.[4]

Congenital cataracts can be classified based on morphology, location, laterality, and/or etiology (Fig. 65.1). Although a detailed description of each type of cataract is beyond the scope of this text, the neonatologist must remember several characteristics that make cataracts more visually significant and thus amblyogenic: large and dense opacities, central and posterior location, unilaterality, or association with a persistent fetal vasculature (PFV). Cataract type is a critical determinate of outcome and can assist in narrowing a genetic diagnosis.

AD-inherited bilateral nuclear cataracts are usually an isolated finding (see Fig. 65.1); these can be variable in density and visual significance and are often visible with a simple bedside penlight exam as a centrally located, white opacification obscuring the visual axis. In a recent large, US-based cataract registry, family history was present in 18% of 994 children.[5]

In contrast, PFV cataracts are typically unilateral and the eye is often microphthalmic. A fibrovascular stalk may connect the posterior lens capsule to the optic nerve and can cause a tractional retinal detachment if it extends to the retina. Angle closure glaucoma may also occur if the retrolenticular membrane contracts.[6] Aphakic glaucoma commonly occurs after removal of a PFV cataract. Visual outcomes are generally quite poor.

Many hereditary cataracts present at birth, although many worsen with age and may be detected only in later years. Cataracts may be the first, or a later, presenting sign of a systemic disorder. Lamellar or zonular cataracts are usually inherited in an AD fashion and are among the most common type of inherited childhood cataracts (see Fig. 65.1). Usually bilateral, the opacities are not visually significant unless they progress to involve the lens cortex or nucleus.[6] Table 65.1 summarizes inherited cataracts related to systemic disorders. Physical examination can help tailor investigations to identify syndromic associations.

In-utero maternal infections, trauma, and exposure to therapeutic agents (i.e., corticosteroids or radiation) are noninherited causes of

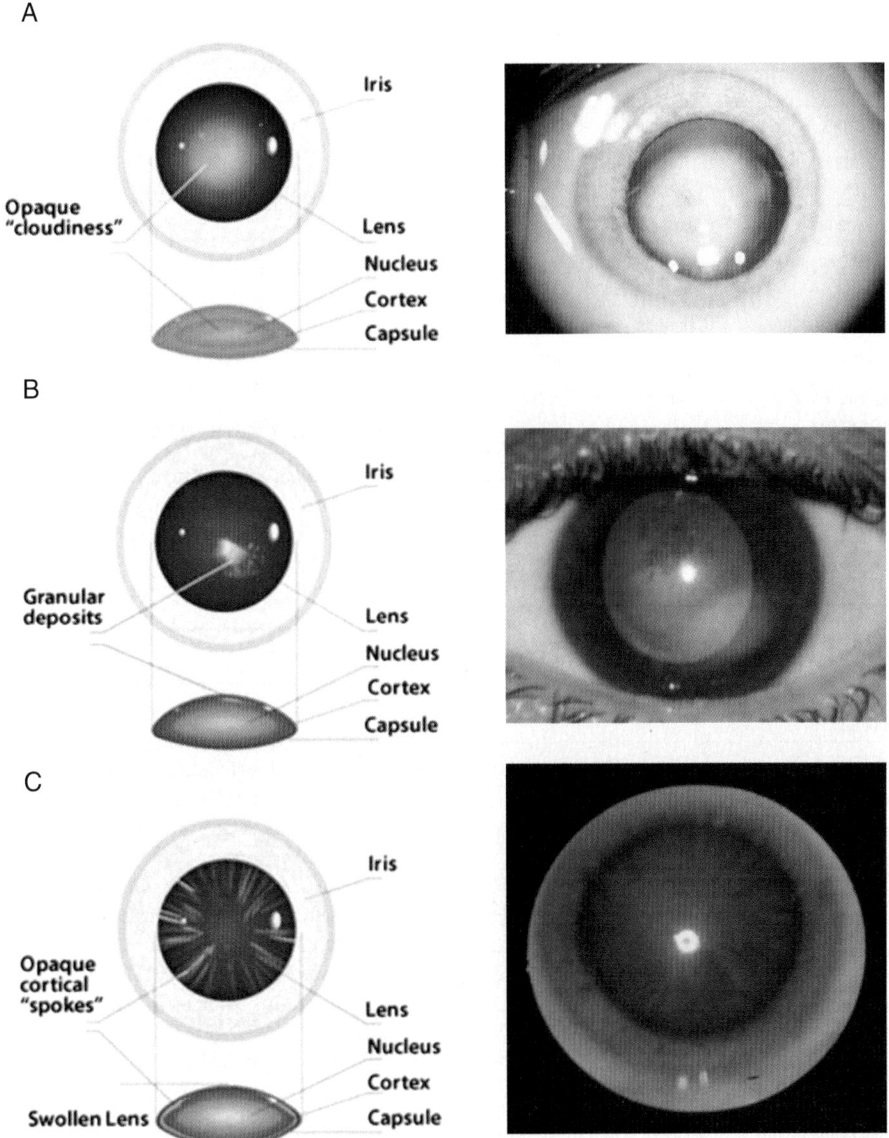

Fig. 65.1 (A) Nuclear cataract in a 3-month-old infant. (B) Posterior subcapsular cataract in a 5-year old. (C) Cortical cataract viewed with retroillumination. ([B] From Thompson J et al: Cataracts. Prim Care. 42(3):409–23, 2015.)

congenital cataracts. Lens opacities tend to develop later in neonates exposed to steroids or radiation. Traumatic injury to the lens has been reported to occur in infants treated for retinopathy of prematurity.[7]

Workup and Management

Laboratory Investigations and Tests

Please see the online version for details. Most congenital cataracts are idiopathic, especially when unilateral.[8] Up to 86% of unilateral and 68% of bilateral cataracts have no discernable cause.[9] There may be associated eye anomalies in up to one-fourth of eyes with cataracts.[5]

TORCH screening should be done in infants with maternal TORCH infections or if microcephaly, thrombocytopenia, and hepatomegaly are present. Bilateral cataracts, hypotonia, failure to thrive, and developmental delay may indicate a possibility of a metabolic disorder. Next-generation sequencing may be useful.[10] A genetics consultation is important for these infants.

Examination Under Anesthesia

An exam under anesthesia (EUA) is recommended with preparation for possible cataract removal, with measurement of intraocular pressure, corneal diameter, a complete eye examination with refraction, and retinoscopy. Determination of corneal curvature and globe axial length helps in surgical planning, intraocular lens power calculation, and prognostication. If there is poor view to the posterior pole, B-scan ultrasonography is done to make sure that there is no associated retinal pathology or PFV prior to proceeding with surgery.

Preoperative Planning

Please see the online version for details. Lens opacities obscuring >3 mm of the red reflex are visually important. Cataract extraction earlier than 4 to 8 weeks may have more ocular complications, especially glaucoma.[11–14] The surgeon can wait until 4 to 6 weeks in unilateral and up to 10 weeks in bilateral cases with less risk of amblyopia and glaucoma development. In infants with bilateral cataracts, the second eye surgery should be performed within 1 to 2 weeks.[15]

Table 65.1 Systemic Diseases Associated With Cataracts and/or Glaucoma

Condition		Ocular Findings
METABOLIC		
	Galactosemia	Cataracts (lamellar)
	Fabry disease	Cataracts (posterior subcapsular)
	Hyperglycemia	Cataracts
	Mannosidosis	Cataracts (posterior subcapsular)
	Refsum disease	Cataracts
	Wilson disease	Cataracts (sunflower)
	Multiple sulfatase deficiency	Cataracts
RENAL		
	Lowe syndrome	Cataracts (multiple forms), glaucoma
	Alport syndrome	Cataracts (anterior lentiglobus)
MUSCULOSKELETAL		
	Myotonic dystrophy	Cataracts (Christmas tree)
	Chondrodysplasia punctate	Cataracts
	Stickler syndrome	Cataracts, glaucoma
	Albright hereditary osteodystrophy	Cataracts
	Robert syndrome	Cataracts
	Majewski syndrome	Cataracts
DERMATOLOGIC		
	Cockayne syndrome	Cataracts
	Rothmund-Thomson syndrome	Cataracts
	Sturge-Weber syndrome	Glaucoma
	Juvenile xanthogranu-loma	Glaucoma
	Neurofibromatosis	Cataracts (PSC), glaucoma
	Oculodermal melanocytosis	Glaucoma
OTHER		
	Rubinstein-Taybi syndrome	Cataracts, glaucoma
	Smith-Lemli-Opitz syndrome	Cataracts
	Cerebro-oculo-facial-skeletal syndrome	Cataracts
	Kabuki syndrome	Glaucoma
CHROMOSOMAL ABNORMALITIES		
	Trisomy 13	Cataracts, glaucoma
	Trisomy 18	Cataracts
	Trisomy 21	Cataracts
	Turner syndrome	Glaucoma

PSC, Posterior subcapsular cataract.

Operative Approach and Issues

The objective of surgery is to clear the visual axis by removing the opacified lens. The details of the surgical procedures are outlined in the online version.[16–19]

Postoperative Management

After surgery, an eye patch and/or shield is placed over the operated eye for 24 hours, and close monitoring is needed. The infant needs to wear corrective lenses and adhere to amblyopia therapy to lower the risk of later strabismus.[20,21] Please see the online version for details.

Complications and Long-Term Prognosis

Posterior capsular opacification, glaucoma, intraocular hemorrhage, inflammation, infectious endophthalmitis, and retinal detachment can occur after cataract surgery. Please see the online version for details.[5,11,12,22–27]

Glaucoma

Infantile glaucoma includes a heterogeneous group of eye disorders characterized by optic neuropathy, increased intraocular eye pressure (IOP), vision/visual field loss, and anatomic changes related to this pathophysiology. Although rare in children without cataract, it can have irreversible vision-threatening consequences if not addressed promptly.

Glaucoma may occur in infants due to an abnormality in aqueous outflow, often with a genetic etiology. Secondary glaucoma results from an underlying ocular or systemic disease, trauma, or medication. Some glaucoma in childhood can have both primary and secondary origins, such as in Sturge-Weber syndrome or neurofibromatosis.[28]

Primary congenital glaucoma (PCG) is a frequently seen cause of primary glaucoma in infants (1 in 10,000–20,000 live births; Fig. 65.2).[29] Most cases (>75%) present with bilateral disease, although the severity may be asymmetric.[30] About 15% of cases present with a classical triad of photophobia, epiphora (tearing), and blepharospasm (frequent blinking). More frequently, the condition is seen as a hazy or cloudy cornea and buphthalmos (see Fig. 65.2). "Buphthalmos," or eye enlargement, is derived from the Greek word *bous* (ox or cow) due to the resemblance of eyes in infants with high IOP to large bovine eyes. *CYP1B1* mutation in the GLC3A locus and *LTBP2* mutation in the GLC3C locus have been linked to PCG.[31]

Secondary glaucoma with anterior segment dysgenesis can occur in up to 50% of those with aniridia, Axenfeld-Rieger syndrome, and Peters' anomaly and 15% of those with posterior polymorphous dystrophy.[28] Glaucoma has been linked with abnormalities in many genes, including *PITX2, PITX3, FOXC1, FOXE3, PAX6, LMX1B*, and MAF.[31]

Aniridia refers to bilateral congenital hypoplasia of the iris and can present with high IOP in infants (Fig. 65.3). Many infants may also have microcornea, cataracts, angle abnormalities,[32] and foveal and optic nerve hypoplasia.[33] Careful systemic and genetic evaluation is necessary even in sporadic cases; there are known associations with *PAX6* mutations and Wilms tumor, genitourinary abnormalities, and mental retardation (WAGR syndrome).[34]

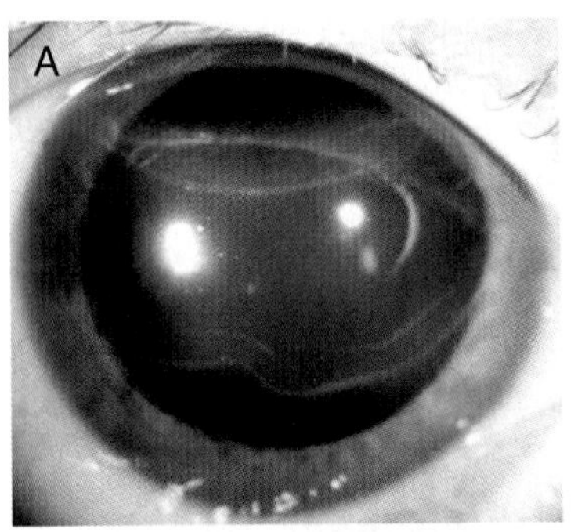

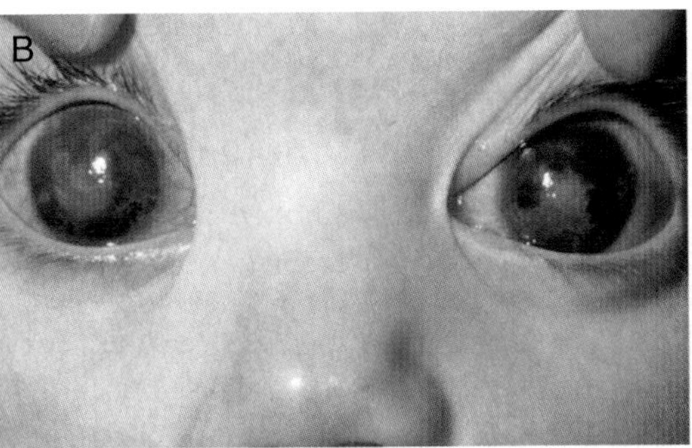

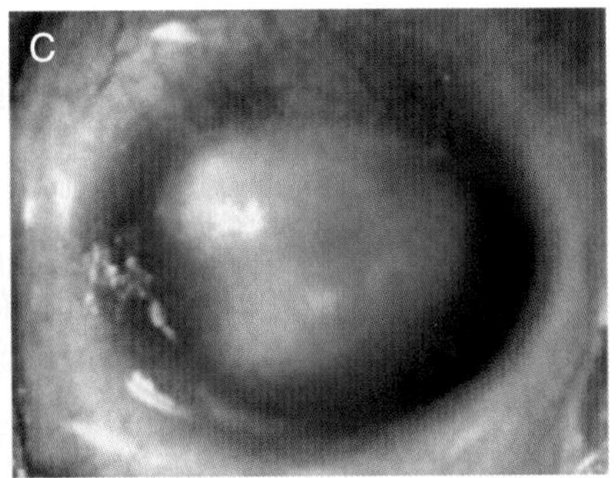

Fig. 65.2 (A and B) Bilateral congenital glaucoma in an infant with enlarged corneal diameters (>12 mm), corneal haze (bluish coloration of iris), and haab striae. (C) Peter's anomaly featuring congenital glaucoma and cloudy cornea.

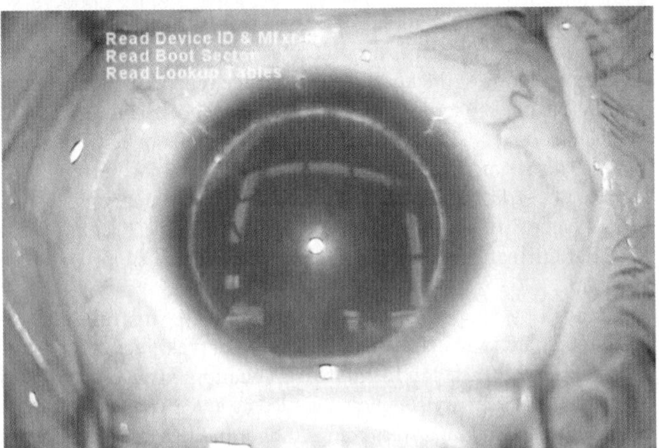

Fig. 65.3 Aniridia. Eye has undergone cataract extraction and is aphakic.

Axenfeld-Rieger syndrome is a spectrum of developmental anomalies[35] in the anterior segment of the eye involving the cornea (posterior embryotoxon), angle (iridotrabecular and iridocorneal processes), iris (corectopia), and lens. Systemic associations include dental anomalies (oligodontia, anodontia), skeletal and skull dysplasia, and umbilical abnormalities.

Peters' anomaly is a congenital defect in the Descemet membrane in the cornea, which causes opacities with variable lens involvement and iris adhesions. It can occur as an isolated ocular disorder or with associated congenital abnormalities such as colobomatous microphthalmia, persistent fetal vasculature, and retinal detachment.[36,37] Peters' plus syndrome can be associated with developmental delay, short stature, facial dysmorphism, cleft lip/palate, external ear abnormalities, congenital heart disease, and genitourinary and neurologic structural defects.[37] Glaucoma management is complicated by a limited view through the opacity. Successful long-term outcome is also limited by inherent challenges of corneal transplantation in children.

Posterior polymorphous dystrophy is an AD condition involving the Descemet membrane and endothelium causing vesicular changes in the cornea. Infrequently, iridocorneal adhesions are present.[38]

The IOP may rise during early infancy due to anterior chamber malformations or later in childhood due to elevated episcleral venous pressure.[39] Regular IOP measurements and fundus examinations can help monitor for choroidal hemangiomas that may be seen in up to 40% of cases and can cause macular edema and exudative retinal detachment (Fig. 65.4).[28]

Table 65.1 summarizes various systemic diseases associated with glaucoma. Glaucoma is the most common ocular morbidity (30%–70%) in Sturge-Weber syndrome. Childhood glaucoma can also

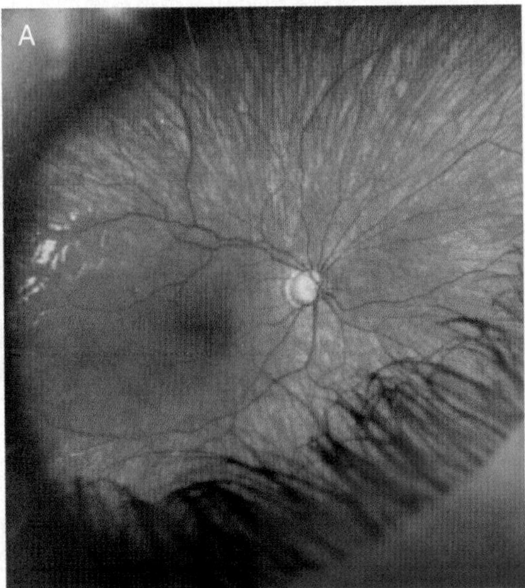

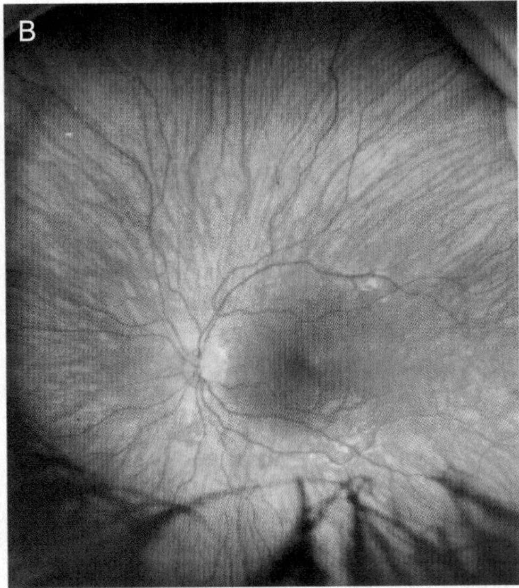

Fig. 65.4 (A) Affected right eye demonstrating reddish hue consistent with diffuse choroidal hemangioma in a patient with right-sided port-wine stain. Cupping of the optic nerve consistent with glaucoma can be seen. (B) Left eye uninvolved.

Table 65.2 Differential Diagnoses in Addition to Congenital Glaucoma Based on Specified Clinical Findings[44]

Clinical Finding	Possible Condition
High IOP	Poor cooperation (squeezing/straining) Lid speculum Elevated intrathoracic pressure from endotracheal tube Thick corneas (i.e., aphakia, pseudophakia, aniridia)
Globe enlargement	Megalocornea without glaucoma Corneal ectasia High myopia Proptosis Lid retraction or contralateral ptosis
Descemet tears/ bands	Birth injury secondary to forceps Corneal ectasia Hypotony Endothelial infection (i.e., rubella, syphilis)
Corneal haze/ scarring	Congenital hereditary endothelial dystrophy Corneal dystrophy Mucopolysaccharides and other storage disease
Optic nerve cupping	Physiologic cupping in large optic nerve heads Papillorenal syndrome Optic nerve hypoplasia in periventricular leukomalacia

IOP, Intraocular pressure.

develop in association with other eye diseases such as retinoblastoma, inflammatory conditions such as antinuclear antibody-associated uveitis, steroid use, lens pathology (angle closure induced by lens subluxation in Weill-Marchesani syndrome or Marfan syndrome), neovascularization (sickle retinopathy), or retinopathy of prematurity.[28,40] Glaucoma can occur after cataract surgery in about 30% of infants by 5 years of age; the risk is higher if there is associated microphthalmia and/or after congenital cataract surgery at <7 months of age.[12,41]

Presentation

History

In primary congenital glaucoma, symptoms result from stretching of ocular tissues due to the elastic collagen fibers in the young eyeball. Enlargement of the eye with resulting corneal edema causes irritation, so infants will demonstrate tearing, light sensitivity, and blepharospasm.[42] For secondary glaucoma, diagnosis with any of the associated conditions will lead a child to have routine monitoring for glaucoma.

Examination

Early-onset glaucoma and rapid corneal enlargement may break the Descemet membrane (Haab's striae) with consequent corneal clouding or edema in many cases. Refractive errors can be suggestive of glaucoma, because increased IOP can cause corneal scarring and increase axial length with consequent myopia and astigmatism.[28] If the optic nerve can be visualized, an increased cup-to-disc ratio is suggestive. Cup-to-disc ratios >0.3 and/or marked asymmetry between the two eyes are indicative of glaucoma.[43] However, these signs are not specific and can be seen in other conditions that may be mistaken as childhood glaucoma (Table 65.2).[44]

IOP measurements can help in the diagnosis and management of glaucoma. The average IOP in infants ranges from 8 to 15 mm Hg and is lower than in adults.[45] The use of anesthesia may be helpful in uncooperative infants who need measurements of IOPs, corneal thickness (pachymetry), and axial length (ultrasound) and for characterizing angle anatomy (gonioscopy).

Workup and Management

Laboratory Investigations and Tests

Laboratory testing should be considered for bilateral disease to rule out systemic conditions such as TORCH infections and metabolic diseases. Genetic testing can be useful for family counseling, although it does not change management.

Examination Under Anesthesia

An EUA provides an opportunity to perform diagnostic tests in uncooperative infants. Sedatives, narcotics, and inhalational anesthetic agents typically lower the IOP,[46] whereas laryngoscope insertion and endotracheal intubation can increase the pressures.[47] Pressure measurements must be obtained as soon as possible after induction but before intubation. Central corneal thickness also affects the reliability of tonometry such that IOP is higher in thicker corneas. In children 6 to 23 months of age, the normal central corneal thickness is approximately 540 μm.[48]

Anterior-segment inspection with a microscope or portable slit-lamp can help distinguish between primary and secondary glaucoma. Measurements of the horizontal corneal diameter (Fig. 65.5) and axial length can help monitor eye enlargement in progressive glaucoma.[30]

Gonioscopy can help in visualizing internal eye structures including the iris, angle structures, and the optic nerve. Placing the gonioprism on the cornea can facilitate examination through a slit-lamp or microscope. Primary congenital glaucoma and juvenile open-angle glaucoma have distinct morphologic abnormalities in the angle and iris insertion. A closed or narrow angle suggest a secondary etiology and the need for urgent intervention.

Imaging Techniques and Functional Testing

EUA can allow imaging of the optic nerve in infants with limited attention spans or nystagmus.[41] Hand-held optical coherence

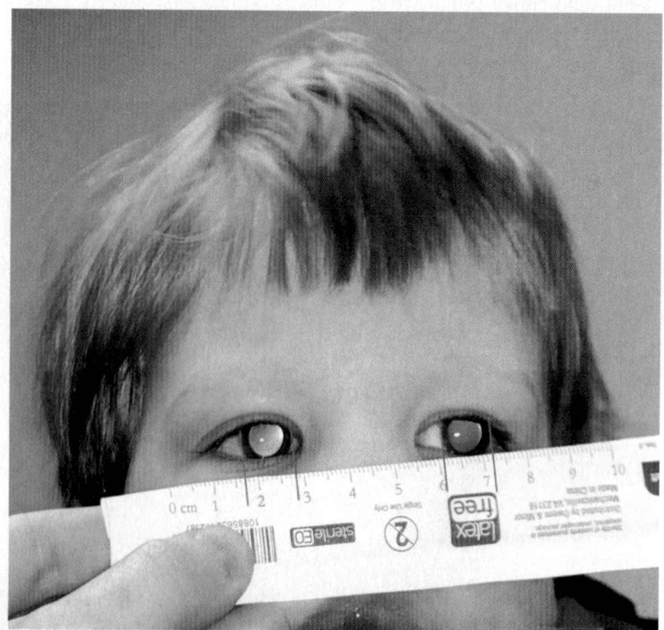

Fig. 65.5 Ocular Findings. Measuring the horizontal corneal diameter in an uncooperative child can be performed by taking a photo with a ruler as shown. This toddler's horizontal corneal diameters are 11 mm on both eyes.

Table 65.3 Ocular and Systemic Adverse Effects of Pediatric Glaucoma Drugs[59]

Class	Drugs	Ocular Adverse Effects	Systemic Adverse Effects
Beta blockers	Timolol, betaxolol, carteolol	Burning, pain, itching, erythema, dry eyes, allergic reaction, occasional corneal disorders	Hypotension, bradycardia, bronchospasm, apnea, light-headedness, depression, masked hypoglycemia in diabetics
Carbonic anhydrase inhibitors (topical)	Dorzolamide, brinzolamide	Burning, stinging, itching, blurred vision, lacrimation, conjunctivitis, superficial punctate keratitis, eyelid inflammation, anterior uveitis, corneal edema	Metabolic acidosis
Carbonic anhydrase inhibitors (oral)	Acetazolamide	Transient myopia	Headache, dizziness, paresthesia, asthenia, sinusitis, rhinitis, nausea, hypersensitivity reaction, bitter taste, epistaxis, urolithiasis, growth suppression
Alpha-2 agonists	Brimonidine (apraclonidine)	Frequent hyperemia, burning, stinging, blurring, pruritus	Central nervous system toxicity, somnolence, respiratory depression, apnea, and coma
Prostaglandin analogs	Latanoprost, travoprost, bimatoprost	Transient conjunctival redness, blepharitis, brown pigmentation of the iris, ocular irritation, transient punctate epithelial erosion, skin rash and darkening, thickening and lengthening of eyelashes	Uncommon dyspnea and asthma exacerbation, sleep disturbance, and sweating

tomography can be used for sequential measurement of the optic nerve head retinal fiber layer thickness.[49,50] Unlike in adults, perimetry testing cannot be used in infants with glaucoma for quantifying visual fields.[51]

Treatment Options

Medications and Special Considerations

Medical management of infantile glaucoma is often a temporizing measure until surgical intervention. Many IOP-lowering drugs are not approved by the US Food and Drug Administration for use in children, and the dosing needs to be customized based on the child's age and general health, the type of glaucoma, and the known efficacy and safety profiles of each medication.[52]

Beta-blockers, carbonic anhydrase inhibitors, alpha-adrenergic agonists, parasympathomimetics, and prostaglandin analogs can be useful in infants (Table 65.3). Monotherapy with beta-blockers such as timolol and prostaglandin analogs such as latanoprost can be useful but may need to be avoided in heart failure, high-degree atrioventricular block, sinus bradycardia, and bronchospasm.[53,54] Alpha-adrenergic agonists such as brimonidine are avoided in infants due to frequent side effects. Combination preparations, most commonly timolol-dorzolamide, are preferred to simplify the treatment regimen.

Oral acetazolamide (10–20 mg/kg/day in divided doses) lowers IOP more than topical forms. Systemic side effects including loss of appetite, sleepiness/listlessness, nausea, and a need for metabolic monitoring reduce its use for refractory cases.[28]

Surgical Approaches

Angle surgery may help some patients with PCG.[55–57] The details are provided online.[58]

Long-Term Management

After treatment for the acute increase in IOP, repeated EUAs are needed to monitor for disease progression. Amblyopia therapy with patching or penalization is required. Subsequently, refractive correction of significant myopia and astigmatism may be needed. In addition to optic neuropathy, corneal opacity, refractive error, and strabismus, amblyopia is one of the most common reasons for permanent visual loss in glaucoma.[42]

SECTION

13 ENT and Auditory Conditions

OUTLINE

Section 13

CHAPTER 66

Neonatal Tracheostomy

Jonathan Walsh

KEY POINTS

1. Chronic cardiopulmonary and neurologic disorders are the most common indications for neonatal tracheostomy, overtaking upper airway obstruction.
2. Noninvasive ventilation of neonates is likely reducing indications and the need for tracheostomy.
3. Neonatal tracheostomy is associated with high overall mortality and morbidity and lower quality of life.
4. Postoperative and long-term care is necessary to help mitigate and manage the increased risks associated with neonatal tracheostomy.
5. Tracheostomies have impact in all domains of neurodevelopment.

Introduction

Tracheostomy has played a critical role in the care of infants since the early 1900s. Prior to the 1800s, tracheostomies were viewed with skepticism and criticism because these procedures were performed for acute airway obstruction and associated with high mortality rates. The relative success of tracheostomy in the treatment of children with diphtheria helped increase acceptance of the procedure.[1–5] Holinger published a 30-year review of infant tracheostomy in 1965, demonstrating more acceptance of the procedure, improved technology of tracheostomy tubes, and an increasing list of indications, primarily for airway obstruction.[6] Unfortunately, the mortality changed very little during that time period, with mortality rates approximately 30% for these infants.[6–10]

The mid 1900s heralded great advances in neonatal resuscitation and ventilation. In 1953 Donald and Lord published a description of an infant mechanical ventilation device.[2,7] In 1965, McDonald and Stocks demonstrated success in longer-term intubation and ventilation in neonates.[3,8] Continuous positive pressure ventilation for respiratory distress of newborns was published in 1971.[4] The 1960s also saw the establishment of the first neonatal intensive care units, and more infants were surviving conditions that in decades past were considered fatal.

The history of neonatal tracheostomy has been an evolving story of changing indications, technological advancements, and improvements in survival.

An understanding of the history of neonatal tracheostomy and neonatal care provides insight into the current evidence-based management of neonatal tracheostomy and the challenges now faced. The landscape of neonatal tracheostomy is changing. Very low birth weight preterm infants are now surviving, and noninvasive methods of respiratory support for these infants are reducing morbidity. Young children with severe chronic cardiopulmonary or neurologic disorders are managed with ventilators both in the neonatal intensive care unit (NICU) and out of the hospital. Some of the questions we now face for neonatal tracheostomy center on appropriate timing for tracheostomy, improving postoperative care pathways, decreasing morbidity of the procedure and subsequent care, facilitating adaptive neurodevelopment and communication, and improving quality of life after tracheostomy.

Pathophysiology

Multiple factors impact the pathophysiology and indications of neonatal tracheostomy. Unique neonatal anatomy, physiology, and medical conditions associated with prematurity influence tracheostomy decisions in the neonatal period.

The infant and neonatal airway diameter and length will vary by gestational age. The narrowest portion of the infant airway is at the glottis and subglottis, and these locations are the most common sites of postintubation stenosis. For a newborn, the subglottis has a 3.5- to 4-mm inner diameter. The tracheal length from glottis to carina is about 40 mm. Premature infants may have a subglottic airway of less than 3 mm.[5] Airflow and effective ventilation in these small airways are influenced by Bernoulli's and Poiseuille's equations. Small changes in airway size will have significant effects on airway pressure, dynamic collapse, and resistance to flow. The clinical implication for many preterm infants is that airway edema or stenosis changes at the 1-mm level or less can destabilize effective ventilation, requiring increased support or tracheostomy. Subglottic stenosis occurred in 12% to 20% of infants with prolonged intubation in the 1960s. With contemporary neonatal respiratory care, rates of stenosis are typically around 1%.[11,12] Tracheostomy can be used to bypass levels of stenosis or decrease the need for respiratory support by removing upper airway resistance.

Typical indications for neonatal tracheostomy are prolonged ventilation, facilitation of ventilator weaning, upper airway obstruction, subglottic stenosis, or infectious etiologies.[13–24] Although Holinger demonstrated infectious etiologies and airway obstruction as the most common indication for neonates in the 1960s, chronic cardiopulmonary and neurologic disorders are now the primary indications for tracheostomy. Multiple studies have described this shift from infectious indications for tracheostomy to cardiopulmonary and neurologic indications in neonates who have comorbid conditions.[6,15,16,22,24,25]

Clinical Features and Indications

When tracheostomy is required, the decisions of timing and patient selection are critical to reduce morbidity. However, a limiting factor is the size of the neonatal airway in relation to the smallest available tracheostomy tube outer diameter (OD). The inner diameter of a full-term neonatal trachea is approximately 3.5 to 4 mm. Extremely premature infants may have an inner diameter of 2 mm or smaller. Currently the smallest OD tracheostomy tube is the 2.5 Tracoe with an OD of 3.6 mm or a 2.5 NEO Bivona TTS cuffed trach with an OD of 4.0 mm. Tracheal length also may be a factor in being able to accommodate the 30 mm of length of the tracheostomy tubes. These anatomic constraints are critical when considering airway interventions prenatally. Since the 1990s, ex utero intrapartum treatment procedures created the possibility of prenatal airway management for cases of congenital high airway obstruction (CHAOS), airway tumors, laryngeal and tracheal stenosis, and lymphatic malformations.[26]

In addition to tracheal size and gestational age, patient weight is a consideration. Studies of other procedures have shown increased morbidity and mortality in procedures performed in neonates weighing less than 2.5 kg.[27–29]

There is no established weight requirement for a tracheostomy procedure.[16–18] Tracheostomy performed in infants with weights between 2.0 and 2.5 kg is common. Rawal et al. did not find increased morbidity when comparing infants <2.5 kg and >2.5 kg in an American College of Surgeons National Surgical Quality Improvement Program–Pediatric (ACS NSQIP-P) Database study.[30] The data regarding appropriate timing of tracheostomy in infants is based on retrospective studies.[31] It appears that the timing of tracheostomy does not decrease the duration of mechanical ventilation in the majority of infants.[31–33]

Advances in noninvasive ventilation of newborns have improved morbidity and mortality through decreasing intubations and related iatrogenic lung and laryngotracheal injury. Systematic reviews have demonstrated the efficacy and safety of these methods compared with traditional orotracheal intubation.[34–38] The implications of these advances for neonates requiring tracheostomy are varied. The total number of infants requiring tracheostomy may be decreasing, along with the aforementioned decrease in subglottic stenosis rates.[11,12] However, tracheostomy rates may be increasing in certain subpopulations of very low birth weight premature infants with more severe cardiopulmonary disease.[18,39] In some of these critical ill neonates, the risk of tracheostomy may be unacceptable. Highly unstable pulmonary hypertension or cardiopulmonary disease can be relative contraindications.[23] If the neonate is unable to be transported safely to the operating room, be manipulated and positioned for surgery, and tolerate exchange of the endotracheal tube to a tracheostomy tube, then surgery should be delayed or deferred. Table 66.1 lists common indications and relative contraindications for neonatal tracheostomy.

Management

Discussion of management can be organized into preoperative planning, intraoperative procedure, postoperative care, and long-term care.

Preoperative

Preoperative planning is crucial for neonates with complex and critical medical status who require a tracheostomy. The workup for tracheostomy should be tailored to the indications and status of the infant. Neurologic evaluation, magnetic resonance and computed tomography imaging, echocardiography, chest x-ray, laryngoscopy, bronchoscopy, and laboratory studies may all be used for preoperative workup. Coordination with a multidisciplinary team of neonatologists, pulmonologists, cardiologists, surgeons, social workers, and family can expedite care and improve quality of care.[33] For infants with critical congenital cardiac disease that requires repair, tracheostomy may be deferred to reduce wound infections and morbidity.[40,41]

Early family integration in the decision, planning, and timing of the tracheostomy helps counseling of both short- and long-term implications of a neonatal tracheostomy on family care. Estimated 2-year healthcare costs associated with infants receiving tracheostomy range from $1643 to $112,608, with costs for the care of some children much higher.[42] In addition to cost, there is a social and personal burden and decreased quality of life for families and caregivers.[43–45] Family counseling and tracheostomy care education are important in the success and safety of neonatal tracheostomies. Families should be prepared for routine and emergency care of infants with tracheostomy, with early guidance to assist with expectations and to avoid misconceptions before the surgery is performed.[46,47] Families and caregivers may experience a significant burden in quality-of-life, financial, social, and relational domains. Quality of life is lower in families of neonates with tracheostomy compared with neonates without tracheostomy. Neonates with tracheostomy are more likely to have readmissions, outpatient visits, and fewer parents with full-time employment.[43–45,48]

Procedure[49]

In a standard neonatal tracheostomy, the patient is positioned with a small shoulder roll and extended neck position. The critical landmarks of the sternal notch, trachea, cricoid, and thyroid cartilage are palpated and marked. Careful palpation deep to the sternal notch is performed to identify any abnormally high location of large vessels. The proposed incision is injected with lidocaine and epinephrine with a dose as appropriate for weight. The patient is then prepped and draped in a sterile fashion but should be draped in a manner to allow access to the endotracheal tube for removal at the time of tracheostomy tube placement. Typically, a 1.5-cm horizontal incision is made just below the cricoid in the midline. Subcutaneous fat is removed to expose the cervical fascia and strap muscles. The midline raphe is identified to separate the strap muscles vertically, being careful to remain in midline. The cricoid cartilage and thyroid gland isthmus are identified and the isthmus is divided. Tracheal rings 2 through 4 are isolated and identified using the cricoid cartilage as a landmark (Fig. 66.1). The endotracheal tube cuff is deflated to

Table 66.1 List of Common Indications and Relative Contraindications for Neonatal Tracheostomy

Indications	Contraindications (Relative)
Chronic cardiopulmonary disease (bronchopulmonary dysplasia, pulmonary hypertension, etc.)	Critically ill and unable to tolerate general anesthesia or transportation to the operating room
Neurologic disorders, congenital and acquired	Critical mid to low tracheal stenosis or agenesis
Acquired or congenital glottic, subglottic, or tracheal stenosis	Craniofacial and cervical dysmorphia that prevents surgical access
Craniofacial syndromes and disorders (Robin sequence, Treacher Collins, Goldenhar, etc.)	Congenital cardiac disease requiring sternotomy, which may be contaminated by presence of tracheostomy
CHAOS (congenital high airway obstruction syndrome)[a]	
Vascular malformations or tumors	

[a]Via ex utero intrapartum treatment (EXIT) procedure.

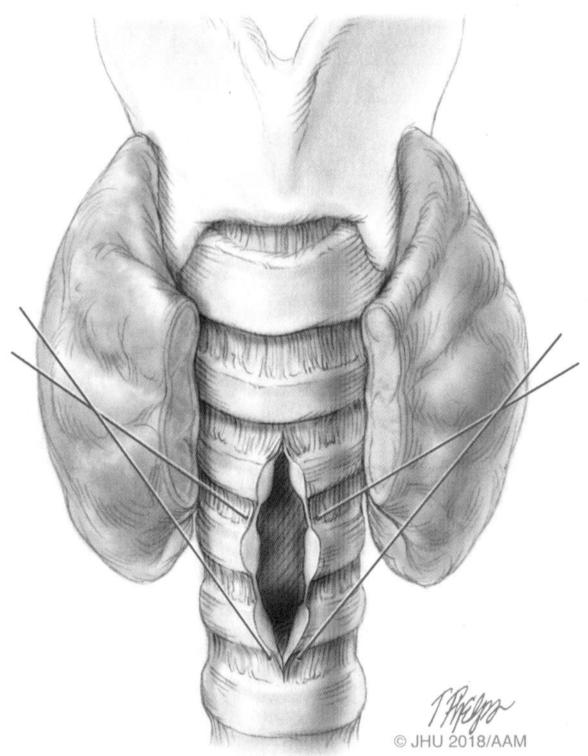

Fig. 66.1 In the Tracheostomy Surgical Procedure, a Vertical Incision Is Made Through Tracheal Rings 2 Through 4. (From: Chapter 1, authored through Elsevier. *Clinics in Perinatology: Diagnosis and Management of Pediatric ENT Conditions*. Dec 2018.)

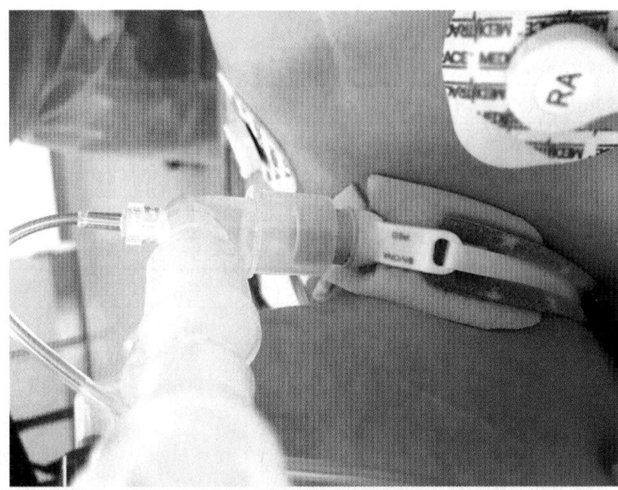

Fig. 66.2 The Tracheostomy Tube Is Secured With Ties, and Skin-Protecting Dressing Can Be Applied to the Neck, Chin, and Chest to Limit Skin Breakdown During the Healing Process.

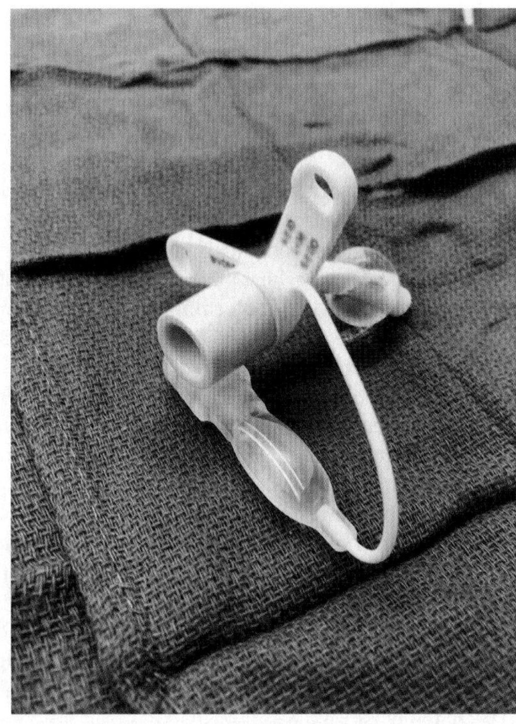

Fig. 66.3 Neonatal Tracheostomy Tubes Are Available From Several Manufacturers, With Both Cuffed and Uncuffed Options.

avoid inadvertent cuff puncture, and tracheal retraction sutures are placed through 2 tracheal rings oriented vertically with 3-0 Prolene "stay" sutures. They are labeled with "left" and "right" identifiers. These stay sutures are placed to facilitate tube reinsertion should accidental decannulation occur postoperatively.

Using 5-0 chromic sutures, the skin edges can be tacked to the superior and inferior edges of the trachea to help mature[50] the tracheostomy stoma. Next, a vertical incision is made through tracheal rings 2 through 4 in the midline between the two retraction sutures. Simultaneously, the endotracheal tube is pulled back just above the tracheostomy site. A tracheostomy tube is then placed into the incision, and confirmation of correct placement is made with auscultation of lung fields, end tidal CO_2 measurement, and visualization through the tracheostomy tube lumen using a small fiberoptic scope. The tracheostomy tube is then secured with ties, and skin-protecting dressing (DuoDERM, Mepilex) to limit skin breakdown during the healing process can be applied to the neck, chin, and chest (Fig. 66.2).

Tracheostomy Tube Sizes

Neonatal tracheostomy tube choices vary by diameter size and length. The principal manufacturers in the United States are Smiths Medical Bivona, Shiley, and TRACOE. These manufacturers offer both cuffed and uncuffed options (Fig. 66.3). The decision for type and style of tracheostomy may depend on ventilation pressure requirements and the size of the trachea for a given infant. The numeric sizes of the tracheostomy tubes are in reference to their inner diameter. Additionally, designations of NEO (neonatal) versus PEDs (pediatric) tracheostomy reflect differences in overall length of the tracheostomy tube. Even small changes in diameter from 2.5 mm to 3.0 mm will have a dramatic effect on airflow resistance according to Poiseuille's law. Length also affects resistance but to a lesser degree. Table 66.2 lists neonatal tracheostomy tube options.

Postoperative Complications

Neonatal tracheostomies have high intermediate- and long-term morbidity and overall mortality. Mortality of infants and children with tracheostomies is reported between 1.5% and 8.9%.[42,51–53] However, tracheostomy-specific mortality is lower, reported to be 0.7%.[51] Intraoperative complications such as decannulation,

Table 66.2 List of Neonatal Tracheostomy Tube Options

Tracheostomy Tube	ID (mm)	OD (mm)	Distal Length (mm)	Cuff Option	Material	Suction Size
BIVONA (NEONATAL)						
2.5	2.5	4	30	Y	Silicone	6 Fr
3	3	4.7	32	Y	Silicone	6–8 Fr
3.5	3.5	5.3	34	Y	Silicone	8 Fr
4	4	6	36	Y	Silicone	8 Fr
SHILEY (NEONATAL)						
2.5	2.5	4.2	28	Y	PVC	6 Fr
3	3	4.8	30	Y	PVC	6–8 Fr
3.5	3.5	5.4	32	Y	PVC	8 Fr
4	4	6.0	34	Y	PVC	8 Fr
4.5	4.5	6.7	36	Y	PVC	8 Fr
TRACOE						
2.5	2.5	3.6	30	Y	Silicone/PVC[a]	6 Fr
3	3	4.3	32	Y	Silicone/PVC	6–8 Fr
3.5	3.5	5.0	34	Y	Silicone/PVC	8 Fr
4	4	5.6	36	Y	Silicone/PVC	8 Fr

[a]Both soft silicone and PVC options are available.
ID, Inner diameter; *OD*, outer diameter.

pneumothorax, bleeding, laryngeal injury, and skin burns have been reported to be approximately 3%.[42,51–54]

Short-term postoperative complications include skin pressure ulceration, accidental false tracking and accidental decannulation, mucous plugging, neck infection, bleeding, or tracheal or carinal ulceration. Analysis of the ACS NSQIP database in 2016 and 2019 described major and minor complications.[30,53] The highest major complications were a 7.55% rate of sepsis and a 6.45% rate of reoperation. Death occurred in 4.24% of infants.[30] Minor complications included a 1.66% rate of skin infection.[30] Skin infection and ulceration can occur due to unintended pressure by the ventilator tubing, tracheostomy tube and flanges, or trach ties.[55] To prevent accidental decannulation and false tracking, the tracheostomy tube must be well secured during the early healing period. This vigilance may also create conditions where skin breakdown can occur. Meticulous perioperative care from the surgical, nursing, and respiratory therapy team is needed to prevent such morbidity. Protective dressings and standardized postoperative care can reduce morbidities of accidental decannulation and pressure ulcers.[55–57]

When considering long-term complications and associated comorbidities, the overall morbidity associated with an infant through the first years after placement is high, reported to be between 19.9% and 63%.[42,51–53] Reported long-term complications can be stoma bleeding or granulomas, accidental decannulation, tracheostomy mucous plugging, tracheomalacia, pneumonia, tracheitis, trachea-esophageal fistula, trachea-innominate fistula, or respiratory failure leading to death.[42,51–53] Infants with significant congenital cardiac disease in addition to tracheostomy had increased morbidity and complications compared with infants without cardiac disease.[40,41,53] These infants likely have lower cardiopulmonary reserve to tolerate morbidities when they occur, and long-term care should be delivered with vigilance due to their higher risk.

An improperly sized tracheostomy tube or overly aggressive tracheal suctioning can lead to granulation of tracheal tissue, ulceration, and erosion. Chronic infections, tracheitis, and suprastomal granulomas can occur. Tracheostomy tubes, as indwelling foreign bodies, are prone to biofilm and bacterial colonization and tracheitis.[58,59] Chronic infection of the tracheal cartilage can be a risk factor for secondary tracheal stenosis. With growth of an infant, the initial tracheostomy tube size and length may be inadequate for the neck anatomy, leading to accidental decannulations or pressure with the tracheal wall. Severe erosion through the tracheal wall can lead to a tracheo-innominate artery fistula or a tracheoesophageal fistula, especially with long-term tracheostomy or concomitant tracheal and/or thoracic pathology. Long-term routine tracheostomy care and follow-up are needed to help prevent these complications.[46,47,60]

Postoperative Care

Important considerations in postoperative tracheostomy care are the frequency/method of suctioning, maintenance of secure tracheostomy ties, and timing of the first trach change. There are no comprehensive, universally accepted guidelines for tracheostomy care, but many institutions have created protocols and care pathways to reduced morbidity. The American Academy of Otolaryngology published a clinical consensus statement on tracheostomy care for both pediatric and adult patients. Statements addressed the timing of the first tracheostomy tube change within the first 5 to 7 days postoperatively as well as decannulation pathways.[61] Specific protocols for routine care and tracheostomy maintenance should be modified for each patient's needs to limit mucous plugging, pressure ulceration, accidental decannulation, false tracking, and long-term complications.[51,52,61]

Saline installation and suctioning is performed to a predetermined appropriate depth based on the length and position of the tracheostomy tube, and this is done for pulmonary toilet and to prevent mucous plugging. Daily wound and peristomal/neck skin examinations should be performed and protective dressings should be used to minimize risk for and severity of skin ulcerations (see Fig. 66.2).[55–57] Timing of the first tracheostomy tube change may depend on patient anatomy, medical and ventilator status, and surgical site healing. The first tracheostomy tube change can occur between postoperative day 2 and day 7.[62,63] Timing of the first change seeks to balance the goals of adequate surgical site healing for safe tube exchange with reducing patient immobilization and decreasing skin ulceration risk. Even before the first tracheostomy tube change, families and caregivers can begin structured training for tracheostomy care.[46,47]

Long-Term Outcomes

With the complex medical comorbidities of neonates with tracheostomy, longer-term mortality has been shown to be 8.9% in a study following such children in a Medicaid population during a 2-year period.[42] When looking at tracheostomy-specific long-term outcomes in children, there are adverse effects on speech, language, feeding, neurodevelopment, Eustachian tube function, quality of life, financial burden, and caregiver burden.[64–71]

Speech and language development can be significantly affected by tracheostomy in children.[65–67] Between 40% and 80% of children with tracheostomy, even without neurologic disorders, may have such delays.[65–67] Adaptive communication technologies, integrative speech and language therapy, and early use of speaking valves may help mitigate some risk.[72,73] In some infants, a speaking valve may be able to be used in the first months of life.[72] Speaking valve tolerance can be increased by drilling side holes in the valve.[74] This technique has been described to decrease subglottic pressure for infants who do not have an adequate airway for a standard speaking valve. It requires an "off-label" modification of a device, which may compromise vocalization with the device. Education and care should be taken if device modification is to be performed.

Although the presence of a tracheostomy in and of itself does not preclude oral feeding in neonates, dysphagia is a significant comorbidity in infants with tracheostomy tube placement. One study showed that only 43% of infants with a tracheostomy tube had an oral diet at discharge, and 57% required nasogastric or gastrostomy tube feeding.[64] In another study, 70% of infants had demonstrated problems with the oral or pharyngeal phase of swallowing and 43% showed aspiration.[75]

A large multicenter study evaluating neurodevelopment impairment outcomes in 8683 preterm infants found increased impairment associated with patients who received a tracheostomy (odds ratio, 4.0).[65] Neurodevelopmental impairment was present in 81% of preterm infants receiving a tracheostomy compared with 36% without a tracheostomy. Additionally, in the same cohort of preterm infants, those with tracheostomy had higher rates of cognitive delay (77%), motor delay (68%), visual impairment (4%), and hearing impairment (8%).[65] However, in a cohort of preterm infants with severe bronchopulmonary dysplasia, infants who received tracheostomy had improved growth and increased participation in physical therapy activities.[76]

The family and financial burdens associated with the care of infants with tracheostomy cannot be overlooked. Families of infants with tracheostomies had lower quality of life, increased social isolation, and financial burden.[43,44,48,70] Nursing support, educational programs, and caregiver intervention can help provide the needed support and resources for these families.[77–82]

Summary

The indications for tracheostomy in young infants have changed, and the rates of tracheostomy in newborns are decreasing.[15,16,19,22] Neonatal care has had significant advances in noninvasive methods of respiratory support, and more extremely preterm and very low birth weight infants are surviving NICU care. Management of severe chronic cardiopulmonary or neurologic disorders both in the NICU and at home has become more common, and neonates with tracheostomy have highly complex needs. As a result, neonatal tracheostomy has high mortality rates and substantial morbidities. Due to these high morbidities, the ACS NSQIP data analysis has demonstrated neonatal tracheostomy as a surgical procedure that would benefit from increased outcomes research and quality improvement.[53,54] To mitigate these risks and improve outcomes, multidisciplinary care pathways, teaching and training protocols, and improved long-term outpatient resources and support for families and caregivers will likely have the greatest impact.

Section 13

CHAPTER

67 Stridor and Laryngotracheal Airway Obstruction in Newborns

Elaine O. Bigelow, David E. Tunkel

KEY POINTS

1. Stridor is a sound caused by obstruction of the upper airway, usually from abnormalities within one or more of the subsites of the larynx (supraglottis, glottis, and subglottis) or in the trachea.
2. Stridor is a physical sign and not a diagnosis. It can be characterized by its presence during inspiration or expiration (or both), by its pitch and loudness, and by its change with activity or position.
3. Laryngomalacia is the most common cause of neonatal stridor, and most cases will improve over the first 12 to 18 months of life.
4. The second most common cause of neonatal stridor is vocal cord paralysis, but it is the likely diagnosis when stridor is observed immediately after delivery.
5. Subglottic stenosis presents with stridor and airway obstruction and can be either congenital or acquired from prior endotracheal intubation.
6. Subglottic hemangiomas should be suspected when stridor develops in infants 1 to 2 months of age, especially when cutaneous hemangiomas are also seen.

Introduction

Stridor describes the sound caused by turbulent airflow within the large airways during respiration. Stridor is typically high-pitched, although the sound can vary with changes in shape and caliber of the airway and with respiratory effort. Stridor can be inspiratory, expiratory, or biphasic, and this quality can indicate the likely site of obstruction. Inspiratory stridor is associated with extrathoracic airway obstruction, typically at the level of the vocal cords or above. Expiratory stridor may be seen with intrathoracic obstruction within the middle or distal trachea. Biphasic stridor indicates obstruction at the level of the vocal cords, subglottis, or upper trachea and is characterized by noise during both inspiration and expiration, although the inspiratory component often predominates. Stridor must be differentiated from stertor: a low-pitched, gurgly, inspiratory or expiratory sound caused by reverberation of redundant soft-tissue or secretions within the oropharynx, nose, or nasopharynx. Stridor and stertor may coexist or be present in isolation.

Stridor in neonates is most commonly caused by laryngomalacia. The other likely causes of stridor in newborns are vocal cord paralysis and subglottic stenosis. Stridor may present immediately at birth or within days to months. Stridor is a sign, not a diagnosis, and persistent stridor in a neonate necessitates formal diagnostic evaluation. Although laryngomalacia, the most common cause of neonatal stridor, typically has a favorable course and requires little intervention, stridor may signal a potentially progressive airway lesion that mandates urgent action. However, with proper evaluation and management, most infants with neonatal stridor have a good prognosis.

Pathophysiology and Clinical Features

Stridor can emanate from obstruction at any level of the larger airways. It can be explained using the Bernoulli principle: when airway diameter decreases at the level of an obstruction, air flow velocity increases exponentially, resulting in negative pressure and airway collapse behind it. Therefore typical laminar flow is disrupted and the turbulent flow results, vibrating the surrounding upper airway soft tissues with resultant stridor.[1]

The larynx has three subsites: the supraglottis, glottis, and subglottis (Fig. 67.1). The supraglottis includes the cartilaginous structures above the true vocal cords, including the epiglottis and arytenoid cartilages and the false vocal folds. The glottis includes the true vocal cords. The subglottis is the area just below the true vocal cords and includes the cricoid cartilage. Stridor may also be a result of narrowing of the trachea, which is composed of C-shaped cartilaginous rings with a muscular membrane posteriorly.

Clinical features of a newborn with stridor often suggest the site of obstruction and likely pathology (Table 67.1). A careful clinical assessment will allow appropriate timing and selection of diagnostic studies.

Supraglottic Larynx

The presence of inspiratory stridor most often portends supraglottic obstruction. The supraglottis is involved with respiration and with airway protection during swallowing and as such has several moving parts.

Laryngomalacia is the inspiratory collapse of supraglottic soft tissues and accounts for most cases of neonatal stridor (Fig. 67.2). Multiple etiologic theories have been proposed, with roles for supraglottic anatomic abnormalities, immature supraglottic cartilages, neuromotor abnormalities, or gastroesophageal reflux disease (GERD).[2] One prospective study of 201 infants with laryngomalacia supports abnormal sensorimotor integrative function as an etiologic theory, with laryngeal tone and sensorimotor integrative function found to be altered and correlated with disease severity.[3]

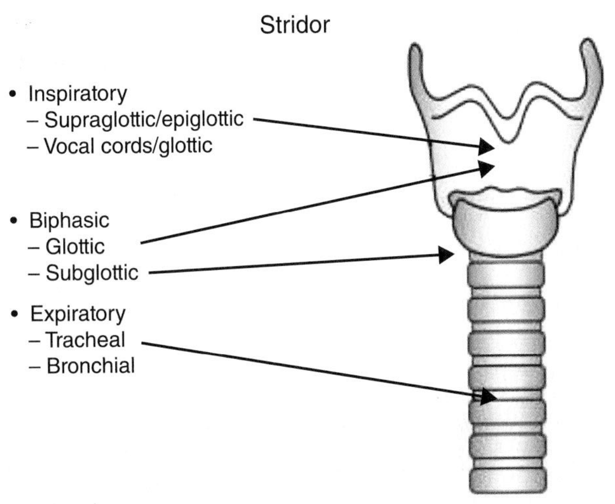

Fig. 67.1 Depiction of Laryngotracheal Anatomic Sites Related to Stridor.

Laryngomalacia is characterized by high-pitched, inspiratory stridor that manifests within the first 2 weeks of birth. Stridor is exacerbated with agitation or exertion and typically worsens while supine and improves when prone or upright. Stridor may be associated with feeding difficulties (including coughing, choking, and regurgitation). Laryngomalacia often coexists with gastroesophageal reflux. One systematic review examining the relationship between laryngomalacia and gastroesophageal reflux found an overall reflux prevalence of 59% among infants with laryngomalacia, with three studies finding increased prevalence of reflux among infants with more severe laryngomalacia.[4] However, a causal relationship with GERD and laryngomalacia cannot be inferred, at least with existing studies. Laryngomalacia may also coexist with other comorbidities including neurologic disease (such as seizure disorders, cerebral palsy, microcephaly, and Chiari malformation), synchronous secondary airway lesions (such as tracheomalacia or subglottic stenosis), congenital heart disease, or genetic disorders (commonly Down syndrome).[5]

Laryngomalacia is characterized as mild, moderate, or severe based on the degree of airway obstruction and of feeding impairment. Most infants with laryngomalacia have mild disease, consisting of stridor without signs of respiratory difficulties (such as retractions, nasal flaring, tachypnea, etc.) and no major feeding symptoms. In the majority of infants with mild laryngomalacia, it resolves by age 12 to 18 months. Infants with moderate laryngomalacia have stridor that is associated with frequent feeding-related symptoms, including coughing, choking, and transient periods of respiratory distress. Infants with moderate laryngomalacia typically improve with acid suppression therapy and feeding modification strategies, including upright positioning or thickened feeds. Infants with severe

Table 67.1 Clinical Features

Condition	Clinical Presentation	Symptom Onset, Severity, and Progression	Key Diagnostic Procedure and Additional Tests to Consider
SUPRAGLOTTIS			
Laryngomalacia	• High-pitched, inspiratory stridor, worse with agitation or when supine, better at rest or when prone • Feeding problems/GERD • May be associated with OSA, FTT, ALTEs, or neuromotor disease	**Onset:** first 2 weeks of life **Severity:** most commonly mild, but can be severe **Progression:** may initially worsen; typically resolved in 6–18 months	Fiberoptic laryngoscopy • Swallowing evaluation (VFSS/FEES) • Polysomnography • Imaging or direct laryngoscopy/ bronchoscopy to rule out second airway lesions
Cysts (saccular, ductal, vallecular)	• Inspiratory stridor (may mimic laryngomalacia by causing supraglottic obstruction or epiglottis prolapse into airway) • May have associated abnormal cry/ feeding difficulties	**Onset:** at birth **Severity:** variable with size/location of mass **Progression:** stable	Fiberoptic laryngoscopy • Imaging or direct laryngoscopy/ bronchoscopy to rule out second airway lesions
GLOTTIS			
Vocal cord paralysis	• Unilateral: mild high-pitched inspiratory stridor, hoarse or weak cry • Bilateral: inspiratory stridor from birth (may be severe), respiratory distress; typically a normal cry • May be associated with neck or chest/cardiac surgery or CNS abnormalities (e.g., Chiari malformation, hydrocephalus)	**Onset:** congenital paralysis manifests at birth; acquired paralysis may present after extubation or after neck/chest procedure **Severity and progression:** variable; many cases resolve over time	Fiberoptic laryngoscopy • Unilateral paralysis may warrant echocardiogram or other tests of cardiac anatomy • Congenital bilateral paralysis warrants CNS imaging
Glottic web	• Abnormal cry (high-pitched or weak) • Biphasic stridor and airway obstruction, worse with larger webs • May be associated with 22q11 deletions (VCFS, DiGeorge)	**Onset:** at birth **Severity:** variable **Progression:** stable	Fiberoptic laryngoscopy • Genetic testing • Tests of cardiac anatomy if VCFS is suspected • Laryngoscopy/bronchoscopy to look for SGS
Iatrogenic vocal cord injury	• Inspiratory or biphasic stridor, abnormal/hoarse cry • Associated with airway manipulation	**Onset:** within hours to days of extubation **Severity and progression:** variable	Fiberoptic laryngoscopy

Table 67.1 Clinical Features—Cont'd

Condition	Clinical Presentation	Symptom Onset, Severity, and Progression	Key Diagnostic Procedure and Additional Tests to Consider
SUBGLOTTIS			
Subglottic stenosis and subglottic cyst	• Inspiratory or biphasic stridor • Barky cough or repeated croup-like illnesses • Acquired SGS or cysts associated with history of intubation or extubation failure	**Onset:** congenital SGS may manifest at birth or later; acquired SGS or cysts may present within hours to days of laryngeal manipulation or extubation **Severity and progression:** variable	Laryngoscopy and bronchoscopy in operating room
Subglottic hemangioma	• Inspiratory or biphasic stridor • Barky cough or recurrent croup-like illnesses • May be associated with cutaneous hemangioma or PHACES	**Onset:** 4–6 weeks after birth **Severity and progression:** rapidly progressive within several months of diagnosis if not treated	Laryngoscopy and bronchoscopy in operating room
TRACHEA			
Tracheomalacia	• Expiratory stridor, wheezing, apneic events if severe • Feeding difficulties, possible recurrent respiratory infections • Extubation failure • May be associated with cardiovascular anomalies	**Onset:** at birth if severe; may be within weeks to months **Severity and progression:** variable	Flexible tracheobronchoscopy during spontaneous respiration • PFTs • Consider airway fluoroscopy • Chest imaging if suspicious of cardiothoracic abnormalities
Vascular rings	• Expiratory stridor, respiratory distress, apneic spells • Feeding difficulties • May be associated with genetic disease or cardiovascular anomalies	**Onset:** at birth **Severity:** may be severe **Progression:** typically stable	CT or MR angiography • Laryngoscopy and bronchoscopy in operating room • Echocardiogram
Tracheal stenosis	• Expiratory or biphasic stridor • Respiratory distress, apneas dependent on degree of obstruction • Often associated with cardiovascular abnormalities, bronchial anatomic abnormalities, genetic conditions	**Onset:** at birth **Severity and progression:** variable	Laryngoscopy and bronchoscopy in operating room • Chest CT

ALTE, Apparent life-threatening event; *CNS,* central nervous system; *CT,* computed tomography; *GERD,* gastroesophageal reflux disease; *FEES,* fiberoptic endoscopic evaluation of swallow; *FTT,* failure to thrive; *MR,* magnetic resonance; *OSA,* obstructive sleep apnea; *PFT,* pulmonary function test; *PHACES,* posterior fossa malformations–hemangiomas–arterial anomalies–cardiac defects–eye abnormalities–sternal cleft and supraumbilical raphe; *SGS,* subglottic stenosis; *VCFS,* velocardiofacial syndrome; *VFSS,* video fluoroscopic swallow study.

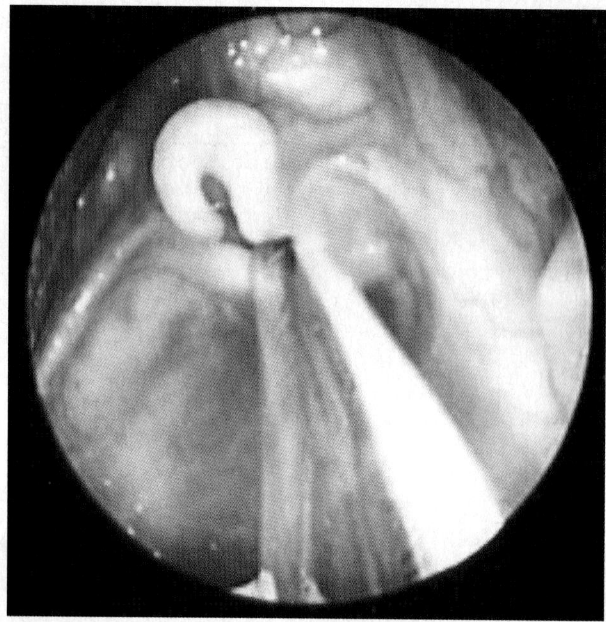

Fig. 67.2 Laryngomalacia. Note the curled, omega-shaped epiglottis seen in a patient intubated for surgery.

laryngomalacia are those who have stridor associated with severe respiratory and feeding symptoms, including apneic spells, aspiration, recurrent cyanosis, and failure to thrive. Infants within this category often require surgical intervention.[2]

Congenital laryngeal cysts are a rarer cause of supraglottic obstruction, with an estimated incidence of 1.8 to 3.5 per 100,000 live births. They may be saccular or ductal.[6] Saccular cysts arise within the laryngeal saccule just above the vocal cords and may result from atresia or obstruction of the laryngeal ventricular opening. They may be contained to the larynx or may extend to extralaryngeal tissues.[7] Ductal cysts result from obstruction of submucosal salivary ducts, leading to mucous-retention cysts. Vallecular cysts are a type of ductal cyst that arise within the space at the base of the tongue that marks the boundary between the pharynx and larynx. Vallecular cysts originate outside the supraglottis, but they can cause supraglottic obstruction by posterior displacement of the epiglottis (Fig. 67.3). Histologic analysis of laryngeal cysts may reveal either squamous or respiratory epithelium.

Infants with congenital laryngeal cysts may present with inspiratory stridor and respiratory distress soon after birth. Infants with smaller cysts may not have significant stridor and may instead present later with feeding difficulties or incidentally.[6,7]

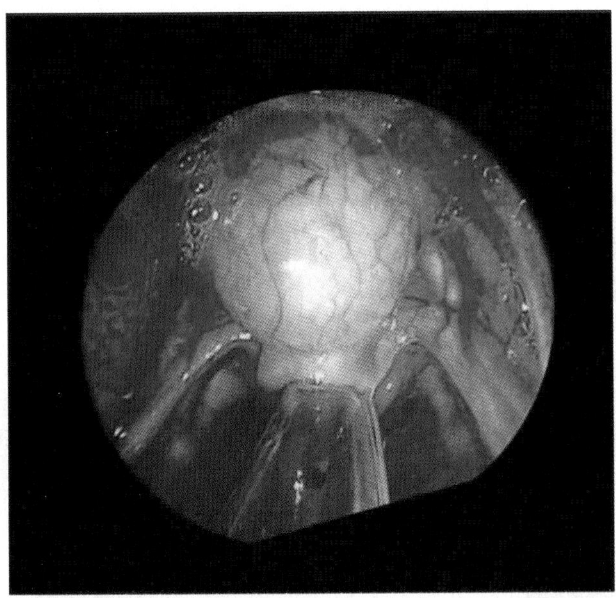

Fig. 67.3 Vallecular Cyst Causing Posterior Displacement of the Epiglottis.

Glottic Larynx

Vocal cord paralysis is the second most common cause of neonatal stridor. Vocal cord paralysis can be unilateral or bilateral, and it can be congenital or acquired. Congenital vocal cord paralysis may be related to anomalies of the central nervous system that cause dysfunction of the vagus nerve (such as Chiari malformation, hydrocephalus, or cerebral palsy)[8] or idiopathic. Unilateral vocal cord paralysis is more likely to be acquired and may be associated with birth difficulties such as difficult forceps delivery or nuchal umbilical cord.[9] Unilateral vocal cord paralysis can be seen after cardiothoracic surgery or treatment with extracorporeal membrane oxygenation therapy (ECMO), because these procedures can cause recurrent laryngeal nerve injury in the neck or the chest.[10,11] Bilateral and unilateral vocal cord paralysis have also been seen after periods of endotracheal intubation.

Infants with bilateral vocal cord paralysis may present with severe inspiratory or biphasic stridor and even respiratory distress. The cry is typically normal because the vocal cords usually can oppose, but they do not abduct for adequate respiration. Infants with unilateral paralysis rarely are distressed and they present with a hoarse cry.

Anterior glottic webs are a less common cause of neonatal stridor at the glottic level, accounting for approximately 5% of congenital laryngeal abnormalities (Fig. 67.4).[12] Glottic webs occur when the laryngeal lumen fails to recanalize during embryologic development, a process that occurs between weeks 8 and 10.[13] Glottic webs range from mild (<35% of the glottis) to severe (up to 90% of the glottis); the degree of dysphonia and airway distress correlates with the extent of vocal cord involvement of the web. Additionally, large glottic webs can be associated subglottic stenosis. An estimated 65% of anterior glottic webs are associated with velocardiofacial syndrome, which occurs in 1 in 4000 live births, commonly associated with a deletion at chromosome 22q11.2.[14] Laryngeal atresia may also occur, essentially a complete glottic web with life-threatening airway obstruction, requiring prompt heroic interventions.

Patients with glottic webs typically present with a hoarse voice and a degree of inspiratory or biphasic stridor shortly after birth.

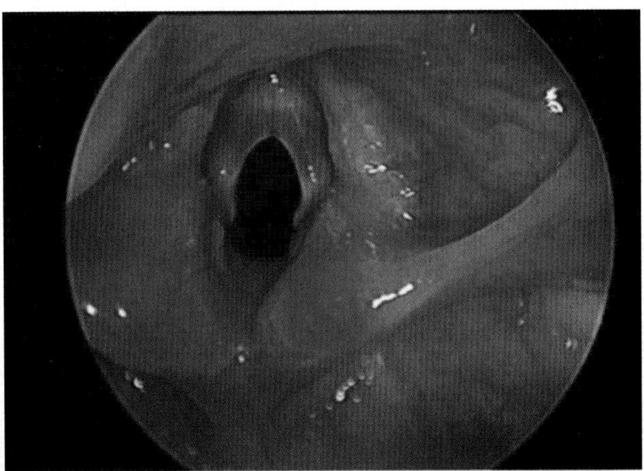

Fig. 67.4 Congenital Anterior Glottic Web.

Severity of symptoms is dependent on the extent of vocal cord involvement. The Cohen classification categorizes glottic webs into type 1 (thin anterior web involving ≤35% of the glottis, which causes minimal airway obstruction); type 2 (thin or moderately thick anterior web involving 35%–50% of the glottis, which causes some airway obstruction); type 3 (thick anterior web involving 50%–75% of the glottis, often associated with subglottic narrowing and with moderately severe airway obstruction); and type 4 (thick glottic web involving up to 75%–90% of the glottis, with subglottic extension and severe airway obstruction).[12]

Glottic obstruction may also result from injury from traumatic or prolonged intubation. Secondary glottic lesions related to intubation injury include vocal cord avulsion, glottic scar, granulomas, or paralysis.

Subglottic Larynx

Subglottic stenosis is the third most common cause of neonatal stridor. The subglottis contains the cricoid, which is the narrowest part of the neonatal airway and is the only complete cartilaginous ring in the airway. The cricoid is resistant to expansion, is not well vascularized, and is prone to scar formation after trauma. Congenital subglottic stenosis results from failure of airway recanalization through the cricoid cartilage, leading to malformation of the lumen or an abnormal relationship of the cricoid cartilage and the first tracheal ring. Congenital subglottic stenosis is commonly associated with genetic or syndromic diagnoses such as trisomy 21, CHARGE (coloboma, atresia choanae, retardation of growth, genitourinary abnormalities, and ear abnormalities) syndrome, and 22q11 deletion.

Acquired subglottic stenosis is nearly always related to endotracheal intubation (Fig. 67.5). In older children, subglottic stenosis may also be associated with a history of a high tracheotomy, laryngeal burn, and neck trauma or tumors.[15] Endotracheal tubes can cause pressure necrosis in the adjacent subglottis, and the resulting ulceration predisposes the area to infection or perichondritis. As the injured site heals by secondary intention, granulation tissue accumulates and a thick, fibrotic scar may result.[16] The current risk of developing subglottic stenosis with appropriate endotracheal tube selection is estimated to be as low as 1% among neonates intubated longer than 48 hours.[17] However, that risk increases with a larger endotracheal tube diameter; unexpected extubations, reintubations, or tube exchanges; excessive movement of the endotracheal tube (i.e., undersedation); duration of intubation; infection; and the presence of gastroesophageal reflux.[17,18]

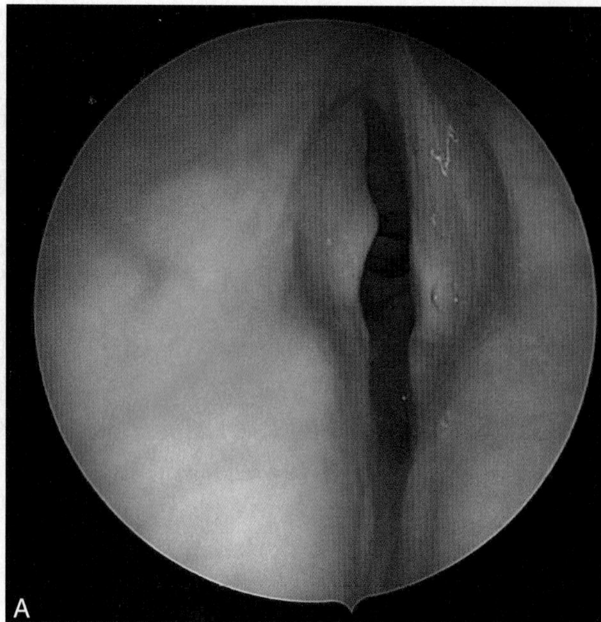

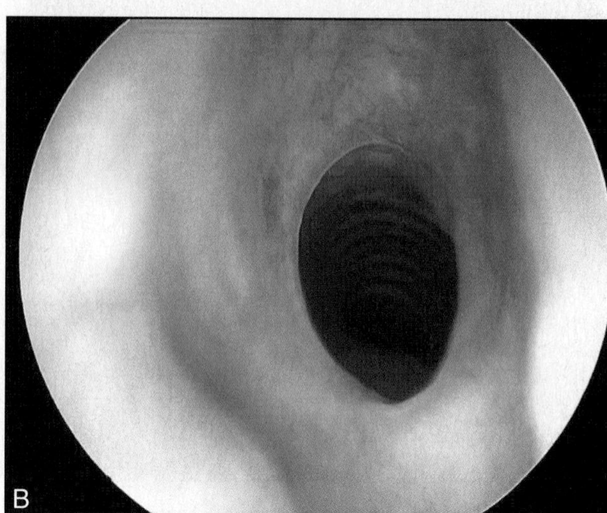

Fig. 67.5 (A) Acquired glottic scarring with subglottic stenosis. (B) Circumferential subglottic stenosis.

Infants with congenital subglottic stenosis typically present with biphasic stridor and respiratory distress, with the severity and timing of onset variable based on the severity of the obstruction. Subglottic stenosis is categorized using the Cotton-Myer grading system: grade I (≤50% stenosis), grade II (51%–70% stenosis), grade III (71%–99% stenosis), and grade IV (complete obstruction).[19]

Subglottic hemangioma is another cause of neonatal stridor. Although infantile hemangiomas are a relatively common tumor of infancy, congenital airway hemangiomas are relatively uncommon, composing 1.5% of congenital laryngeal anomalies in one 1967 series.[20] The pathogenesis of subglottic hemangioma involves endothelial cell hyperplasia, although the cause remains unknown. A popular theory suggests that embryonic endothelial precursor cells deposit in the subglottis and proliferate due to angiogenic stimuli.[21] Subglottic hemangiomas are commonly associated with beard-distribution facial hemangiomas and PHACES (posterior fossa malformations, hemangiomas, arterial anomalies, cardiac defects, eye abnormalities, sternal cleft, and supraumbilical raphe) syndrome.[22]

Subglottic hemangiomas typically present with inspiratory or biphasic stridor during weeks 4 to 6 of life, then enter a rapid proliferation phase for several months. Untreated, growth can be extensive and may require surgical intervention or tracheotomy. They typically begin a spontaneous, slow involution at 18 months, and most resolve by 5 to 7 years.[23,24]

Trachea

Tracheomalacia occurs when there is abnormal increased collapsibility of the trachea, which can result from intrinsic cartilage defects or from extrinsic compression. Tracheomalacia can be congenital or acquired and is a distinct entity that is far less common than laryngomalacia. Congenital causes include prematurity, cartilaginous abnormalities (e.g., chondromalacia or Ehlers Danlos syndrome), several genetic syndromes, congenital anomalies (e.g., tracheoesophageal fistula), or idiopathic causes. Secondary tracheomalacia may result from prolonged intubation or tracheostomy or compression from anatomic anomalies (such as cardiomegaly or vascular rings), skeletal malformations (such as pectus excavatum or scoliosis), or tumors or other masses.[25]

Tracheomalacia, if severe or extensive, may present soon after birth with expiratory stridor that may be low-pitched or honking in quality. Otherwise, symptoms may manifest weeks or months after birth, with stridor, wheezing, recurrent respiratory distress especially with exertion, and in some cases, recurrent respiratory infections due to ineffective cough.

Vascular rings are another cause of stridor. Vascular rings occur when a vessel from an abnormally developed aortic arch completely encircles the trachea and/or esophagus and causes airway compression.[26] The most common vascular rings are double aortic arch, right aortic arch with aberrant left subclavian artery, and ligamentum arteriosum. Vascular rings present with stridor, respiratory distress, and often, feeding difficulties. Vascular rings may also cause or be associated with tracheomalacia.

Tracheal stenosis may result from membranous webs or from complete tracheal rings. A complete tracheal ring results from abnormal growth of one or more cartilaginous rings in relation to the posterior membranous trachea. Whereas normal tracheal rings are C-shaped and allow for expansion and growth, complete tracheal rings cause narrowed tracheal segments and stenosis.[27] Infants with tracheal stenosis present with symptoms depending on the degree of obstruction and the length of the involved stenotic trachea. They may present within hours or days of birth with stridor, cyanosis, and respiratory failure. Symptoms may occur later in infancy as activity increases (typically around 12 months of age), and some rings are diagnosed incidentally later in childhood or adolescence. Common symptoms of tracheal stenosis include expiratory or biphasic stridor, respiratory distress wheezing, apneas, difficulty with intubation, or extubation failure. Tracheal stenosis and complete tracheal rings are often associated with cardiovascular abnormalities (71% in one series),[28] genetic conditions, and abnormal bronchial branching patterns.

Evaluation (Clinical, Laboratory, and/or Imaging)

History

A detailed clinical history is key to the evaluation of a neonate with stridor, helping to focus on likely diagnoses. Birth history should include gestational age at birth, birth weight, mode of delivery, and difficulty of delivery (e.g., forceps, vacuum). Infants with a history of prematurity or low birth weight may have been cared for in the neonatal intensive care unit and may have received aggressive or prolonged respiratory support. A detailed history of respiratory interventions and instrumentation should include history of suctioning, mode of instrumentation, endotracheal tube size, duration of intubation, and history of tube exchanges or unexpected extubations. Even infants who are intubated only for a few moments, such as for meconium suctioning after birth, may have laryngeal trauma and develop stridor as a result.[29]

The timing of symptom onset also sheds light on the etiology of stridor. All congenital airway lesions may cause stridor soon after birth, but each lesion varies in its time of presentation. Generally, any fixed congenital narrowing of the larynx, such as laryngeal webs, congenital subglottic stenosis, or bilateral vocal cord paralysis, will present with stridor at birth, potentially severe. In contrast, stridor due to dynamic lesions such as laryngomalacia may not occur for days or weeks after birth, and subglottic hemangiomas typically do not cause stridor until 4 to 6 weeks of life.

Feeding history should also be obtained. The presence of feeding difficulties (e.g., slow feeding, frequent pauses for breathing, frequent cough, or emesis) or poor weight gain in an infant with stridor may signal the presence of a more extensive airway lesion. Feeding difficulties in a stridorous infant may stem from direct impairment of swallowing (e.g., from a mass, such as a laryngeal cyst) or from poor swallow coordination because of increased respiratory effort. Gastroesophageal reflux or aspiration may also contribute to feeding difficulties, because acidic reflux contents may irritate and inflame the larynx.

An abnormal cry or voice suggests a glottic (vocal cord) lesion. This includes hoarseness, a high-pitched cry, or aphonia. The degree of voice change is based on the size and extent of true vocal cord involvement and the ability of the vocal cords to oppose each other.

History of a barky cough or repeated croup-like illnesses elicits concern for subglottic pathology. Congenital subglottic stenosis or subglottic hemangioma may present in this way. Acquired subglottic stenosis may also present with these symptoms, especially in infants with a history of endotracheal intubation or laryngeal instrumentation.

Other aspects of the neonatal history are also informative. Family history should be obtained with special attention paid to any syndromic or genetic diagnoses, many of which may have associated airway abnormalities. Additionally, comorbid conditions may shed light on the etiology of stridor, such as the presence of central nervous system abnormalities and congenital heart anomalies. Finally, past surgical history can be informative; for example, patent ductus arteriosus closure or ECMO are both associated with unilateral vocal cord paralysis due to injury of the left recurrent laryngeal or cervical vagus nerves.[11,30]

A useful mnemonic for evaluating a patient with stridor is SPECS, as outlined by Holinger and colleagues.[31] The components are: S—severity (presence of retractions, respiratory effort); P—progression (changes in quality over time); E—eating (feeding difficulties, failure to thrive, aspiration, reflux); C—cyanotic spells (apparent life-threatening events); and S—sleep (change in quality of stridor with sleep; retractions during sleep).

Physical Examination

Physical examination of a stridorous infant provides insight into the severity of the airway lesion. Routine vital signs should be obtained, including pulse oximetry. Special attention should be paid to the infant's respiratory effort. If stridor is accompanied by tachypnea, severe retractions, cyanosis, or lethargy, the neonate will likely require urgent airway evaluation and support and possibly operative intervention.

A complete head and neck examination is necessary. Note should be made of any craniofacial abnormalities, including obvious deformities of the ears, nose, midface, or jaw. Facial hemangiomas, particularly in the "beard" distribution (lower cheeks, mouth, chin, and neck) should be documented. Nasal cavities may be assessed for patency by passing a catheter through each side. The oral cavity and oropharynx should be assessed for palate anomalies, masses, and abnormalities in tongue shape or position. The neck should be examined for masses.

The infant should also be examined for abnormalities of the chest wall or respiratory dynamics. Lung fields and the neck should be auscultated. Additionally, one should consider evaluation of the infant in upright, prone, and supine positions, because stridor may vary by position. For example, with laryngomalacia, infants tend to have improvement in their symptoms when prone or upright compared with when supine.

Special Diagnostic Procedures

Flexible fiberoptic laryngoscopy (FOL) is the gold standard to provide a dynamic assessment of the upper airway from nose to glottic larynx. FOL is typically performed by an otolaryngologist using a flexible fiberoptic scope passed through the nose. It is performed without sedation as an outpatient or inpatient bedside procedure while the infant is awake, usually held upright in an assistant's lap. It allows for inspection of the nasal cavities, palate, pharynx, hypopharynx, supraglottis, and glottis and can detect the presence of laryngomalacia, vocal cord paralysis, or any fixed lesions or masses of the supraglottis or glottis. The subglottis may be partially visualized during full abduction of the vocal cords. Of note, FOL may be performed in conjunction with speech and language pathology evaluation of swallowing in a fiberoptic endoscopic evaluation of swallowing examination.

Direct laryngoscopy with bronchoscopy is a diagnostic procedure performed in the operating room using general anesthesia. Operative laryngoscopy and bronchoscopy are required for full evaluation of the subglottis, trachea, and bronchi and allow for palpation of structures, measurement of airway caliber, and operative treatments of endoscopically treatable obstructive lesions. Typically, this procedure should be undertaken with the most likely diagnoses in mind and possible interventions planned; however, emergency operative action is occasionally necessary. Coordination and expertise of pediatric otolaryngologists and anesthesiologists are paramount to success of this procedure.

Imaging and Laboratory Tests

Radiologic examination may be considered in the evaluation of neonatal stridor if the results are expected to impact either treatment or prognosis. Care should be taken to limit ionizing radiation exposure for young infants. With that said, plain radiographs of the neck ("high kV" or "soft-tissue" images) or chest may give insight into tracheal caliber, pulmonary or cardiac abnormalities, and soft tissues of the neck and pharynx. Contrast esophagrams or modified barium swallow studies may be considered in infants with feeding problems or suspected esophageal disease. Ultrasound has a limited role in evaluation of stridor but may have some utility in evaluating vocal cord movement in infants.[32] Computed tomography or magnetic resonance imaging studies generally should not be first-line diagnostic tools; rather, they may be pursued if high-resolution images are needed to inform treatment after history, physical, and airway endoscopy have been completed. If vascular ring is suspected, computed tomography or magnetic resonance angiography should be performed.

Laboratory testing is not typically utilized in the evaluation in otherwise healthy infants with stridor, with the exception of genetic testing when there is clinical suspicion of genetic/syndromic disease.

Management and Long-Term Outcomes

The severity of airway obstruction and the clinical impression of an infant's respiratory distress guide the pace of planned interventions and management (Table 67.2). Often, a well-appearing infant with mild stridor but no major respiratory distress or feeding problems can be managed observantly in an outpatient setting, whereas an infant with severe respiratory distress requires urgent evaluation and intervention. With the occasional exception of some newborns with classic mild laryngomalacia, an infant with stridor requires evaluation by an otolaryngologist. Additionally, management of neonatal airway lesions may require multidisciplinary coordinated efforts of pediatric otolaryngology, pediatric surgery, gastroenterology, and pulmonology.

Table 67.2 Management

Condition	Management
SUPRAGLOTTIS	
Laryngomalacia	
Mild	• Observation • Positioning • Antireflux treatment if feeding problems or confirmed GERD
Moderate	• Antireflux treatment and GERD management • Consider supraglottoplasty if feeding problems severe • Look for second airway lesions
Severe	• Supraglottoplasty • Look for second airway lesions • Tracheostomy rarely necessary
Vallecular or saccular cysts	• Surgical excision (endoscopic approaches most common)
GLOTTIS	
Vocal cord paralysis	• Swallowing evaluation
Unilateral	• May observe if mild • If persistent, consider medialization or reinnervation procedure with aspiration or dysphonia
Bilateral	• May observe if symptoms are mild and expected to improve • Address neurologic condition if present • May require tracheostomy if symptoms are severe; if persistent, additional surgical interventions may include cordotomy, posterior cricoid split/graft, arytenoidectomy, or lateralization
Glottic web	• Mild webs with good voice: observe • Extensive webs with dysphonia: endoscopic division • Severe webs with associated subglottic stenosis: open airway reconstruction
Iatrogenic vocal cord injury	• Observation versus surgical management
SUBGLOTTIS	
Subglottic stenosis	• May observe if stridor is not severe and stenosis is mild • Tracheostomy is indicated with severe stenosis if prolonged mechanical ventilation is anticipated, other surgical interventions fail, or the presence of multiple comorbidities limits options • Surgical management ranges from endoscopic dilations with or without cricoid split to laryngotracheal reconstruction or cricotracheal resection
Subglottic cyst	• Surgical endoscopic excision
Subglottic hemangioma	• Propranolol therapy (inpatient for infants <8 weeks or with comorbidity) • Consider steroids (intralesional or systemic) or surgical excision if refractory (endoscopic preferred)
TRACHEA	
Tracheomalacia	• Observe • Noninvasive positive airway pressure as needed • Consider hypertonic saline nebulizers, inhaled corticosteroids, and other supportive therapy • Surgical intervention if severe (aortopexy, tracheostomy with positive pressure ventilation)
Vascular rings	• Surgical correction of vascular anomaly • Supportive care of residual tracheomalacia
Tracheal stenosis	• May observe if mild • Surgical intervention if severe (tracheal resection, slide tracheoplasty)

GERD, Gastroesophageal reflux disease.

Supraglottic Larynx

Laryngomalacia

For mild and moderate laryngomalacia, treatment generally involves observation and perhaps GERD treatment, with consideration of surgical intervention if feeding difficulties or growth problems persist. In one prospective series of 201 infants with congenital stridor and laryngomalacia, the authors found that half of the infants with mild laryngomalacia had a feeding symptom and GERD that improved with antireflux medications, and most patients had resolution of symptoms by 12 months.[3] Infants with mild laryngomalacia who also had two or more comorbidities all progressed to moderate or severe laryngomalacia. Infants with moderate laryngomalacia had severe feeding symptoms, and although antireflux treatment led to improved coughing and choking symptoms, infants within this category required a longer course of treatment than those in the mild group; additionally, some infants required multimodality antireflux therapy. Antireflux treatment included omeprazole, ranitidine, and Nissen fundoplication. Of the infants with moderate laryngomalacia in this series, 28% required supraglottoplasty, most commonly for feeding problems. Supraglottoplasty is a surgical procedure performed through the mouth that removes redundant supraglottic tissue and relieves airway obstruction. Of the infants with severe laryngomalacia in this series, 97% required surgical intervention with supraglottoplasty or, in rare instances, tracheostomy.

One case series examined whether gestational age affects outcomes of supraglottoplasty in premature infants with laryngoplasty. The series included 325 consecutive infants <12 months of age who underwent supraglottoplasty between 2004 and 2012 (excluding patients with syndromes or neurologic or cardiac comorbidities).[33] They found that supraglottoplasty was equally successful at resolving airway symptoms in term and preterm infants (≥90%); the remaining infants required revision supraglottoplasty or tracheostomy.

Of note, any infant with severe laryngomalacia should be evaluated for synchronous airway lesions. In one series of 52 infants with severe laryngomalacia who underwent supraglottoplasty, 58% had synchronous airway lesions (most frequently subglottic stenosis, tracheomalacia, or bronchomalacia).[34] Nearly two-thirds of patients in this series, especially those with neurologic conditions or subglottic stenosis, required postoperative nonsurgical airway support. The presence of second airway lesions in infants with mild laryngomalacia is debated but likely far less common, so operative bronchoscopy and imaging should be used judiciously.

Laryngomalacia typically resolves by 1 to 2 years of age with observation and antireflux treatment. Patients have no major long-term sequelae after supraglottoplasty. In patients with severe laryngomalacia who required tracheostomy, comorbidities predict a longer duration of tracheostomy placement.

Laryngeal Cysts

Large congenital laryngeal cysts may cause significant airway obstruction and therefore present acutely after birth, requiring urgent intubation, whereas smaller ductal cysts or vallecular cysts may have a more subtle presentation or be found incidentally. Regardless of presentation, once identified, laryngeal cysts require surgical treatment. Several surgical methods have been used, including needle aspiration, endoscopic marsupialization, endoscopic excision, laser treatment, and resection via external open approach. Several series advocate for full cyst excision rather than needle aspiration or marsupialization, citing increased risk of recurrence with the latter modalitites.[35,36] Occasionally, patients who have significant extralaryngeal extension of their cyst require an open-approach resection.[7] For patients who have laryngeal cysts with complete resection, no long-term sequelae are expected.

Glottic Larynx

Vocal Cord Paralysis

Treatment of vocal cord paralysis depends on the severity of symptoms. An infant in acute distress related to vocal cord paralysis requires urgent respiratory support and intubation, whereas an infant with mild symptoms may, at least initially, be managed conservatively, undergo a formal feeding assessment, and be observed with aspiration precautions.

One retrospective series of neonates with vocal cord paralysis identified 61 infants with unilateral vocal cord paralysis and 52 infants with bilateral vocal cord paralysis, 10 of whom required tracheostomy.[37] The other patients were managed expectantly, with nearly three-quarters of infants with unilateral paralysis and half of those with bilateral paralysis achieving symptom resolution. In another series of 22 patients with congenital bilateral vocal cord paralysis, 68% required tracheostomy.[38] A third series looked at factors associated with tracheostomy among 102 infants with complete or partial bilateral vocal fold paralysis and found that approximately two-thirds required tracheostomy, which was more common among patients with concomitant airway disease and vocal cords paralyzed in the paramedian position.[39] Infants with persistent unilateral vocal cord paralysis may eventually undergo a vocal cord medialization or reinnervation procedure to improve voice. Patients with persistent bilateral vocal cord paralysis may eventually undergo additional procedures including cordotomy, arytenoidectomy, or lateralization to improve airway patency; however, such procedures are not usually done in infants and toddlers.

Long-term outcomes among patients with vocal cord paralysis are varied. Patients with bilateral congenital vocal cord paralysis may have spontaneous recovery of function (64% in one series of 22 patients[39] and 52% in a series of 19 patients[37]). Some patients with bilateral vocal cord paralysis related to Chiari malformation may have resolution after neurosurgical decompression.[8] Patients with acquired vocal cord paralysis related to birth trauma have an improved prognosis, with one pooled analysis suggesting a 91% recovery and 68% recovery in unilateral and bilateral paralysis, respectively.[9] In a meta-analysis of patients with vocal cord paralysis after cardiothoracic surgery, the spontaneous recovery rate was approximately 64%, although only a small number of patients were included.[10] Patients with neurogenic causes of vocal fold paralysis (such as Chiari malformation) have a poor chance of recovery (14% in one series of 113 patients).[39]

Anterior Glottic Web

Management of glottic webs is dependent on severity of symptoms and the extent of the web. Many infants with mild glottic webs may be observed through infancy and treated later in childhood. The treatment for glottic webs is surgical and ranges from simple incision and dilation for mild webs to extensive open surgical approaches including complete laryngotracheal reconstruction for severe webs. Generally, after ensuring initial airway stabilization (which may require tracheostomy), open surgical approaches can be pursued later in childhood once growth and other comorbidities are optimized. In one series of 51 infants with glottic webs, infants with type 1 webs were observed; infants with type 2 webs were often observed throughout infancy and later treated via endoscopic surgical approach; infants with type 3 webs required either tracheostomy or serial surgical incision and dilations; and neonates with type 4 webs required tracheostomy soon after birth.[12] Another series reviewed 14 patients with type 3 and 4 webs, 12 of whom required tracheostomy at a median of 32 days.[40]

With appropriate surgical intervention, good airway and voice outcomes may be achieved. Most patients who undergo airway reconstruction achieve tracheostomy decannulation. Patients with severe type 3/4 webs may have moderate to severe residual dysphonia despite reconstruction.[40]

Subglottic Larynx

Subglottic Stenosis

Treatment of subglottic stenosis depends on the grade of obstruction and the severity of symptoms. Definitive treatment for subglottic stenosis is surgical, with techniques ranging from endoscopic procedures (including balloon dilation with or without cricoid split) to extensive open airway procedures (including cricotracheal resection or laryngotracheal reconstruction). Prevention of acquired subglottic stenosis is possible with selection of appropriate endotracheal tube sizes, management of sedation to prevent excessive tube movement or unintended extubations, and use of noninvasive ventilation techniques in neonates.[41]

Generally, subglottic stenosis of Cotton-Myer grade I and II may be managed conservatively in neonates. Symptoms and airway diameter may improve as the child grows, and definitive surgery may be delayed or deferred. Conversely, grade III or IV disease is likely to require operative management. A tracheostomy secures the airway, allowing for prolonged mechanical ventilation (if needed) and management of medical comorbidities and optimization prior to definitive surgical airway reconstruction. However, cricoid split, laryngeal reconstruction, and endoscopic dilation have been performed in infants with subglottic stenosis to avoid tracheostomy in many cases.

Several series have examined the outcomes of various treatments of congenital and acquired subglottic stenosis.[42–51] The median age of definitive surgical intervention in these studies ranged from approximately 3 to 42 months for endoscopic interventions and 7 to 50 months for open approaches. For neonates, the primary objective is to ensure a safe airway for the infant, whether by close observation or tracheostomy, with definitive surgical management deferred until the child has grown. However, among infants with acquired subglottic stenosis related to intubation injury, surgical intervention performed earlier rather than later (i.e., prior to scar maturation) may improve outcomes.[44,46] In a systematic review of infants with subglottic stenosis, patients who underwent one or more endoscopic balloon dilation procedures for grade II or III subglottic stenosis had a 65% likelihood of long-term success, with improved likelihood for lower severity of stenosis.[52] In more severe stenosis that requires endoscopic expansion surgery or open airway surgery, rates of tracheostomy decannulation have been reported between 54% and 96%.[49,51,53,54]

Subglottic Hemangioma

The core treatment principle for subglottic hemangiomas is to maintain an adequate airway and attempt to reduce the size of the hemangioma while awaiting growth of the child and expected natural regression of the lesion. The preferred treatment for subglottic hemangioma is medical therapy with propranolol, with corticosteroids (systemic or intralesional) and surgery as secondary options. In 2015 a double-blinded, placebo-controlled randomized controlled trial of propranolol efficacy in 460 infants with subglottic hemangioma found propranolol treatment was effective at 3 mg/kg per day for 6 months, with a small percentage of patients requiring additional treatment.[55] There are consensus guidelines for initiating propranolol safely in infants, which recommend the following: (1) pretreatment electrocardiogram and cardiology consultation in infants with baseline bradycardia, suspected arrhythmia, family history of arrhythmia, or maternal history of connective tissue disease; (2) vital sign assessment before, 1 hour after, and 2 hours after treatment initiation (because beta-blockade on heart rate and blood pressure peaks within 1–3 hours); (3) discontinuance of propranolol during times of illness to avoid hypoglycemia with decreased oral intake; (4) initiation of propranolol as an inpatient for neonates <8 weeks (gestationally corrected age) or who have comorbid conditions; and (5) for infants with PHACES, obtaining a neurology consultation prior to propranolol initiation to assess stroke risk.[56]

If propranolol is ineffective in reducing the size of the lesion, corticosteroids may be used, although data suggest steroids are less effective than beta blockers. In one 2013 systematic review and meta-analysis of 56 studies comparing propranolol with corticosteroids, corticosteroids were found to have a pooled efficacy rate of 69% compared with 97% for propranolol.[57] Oral corticosteroids were typically dosed between 2 and 3 mg/kg/day for 4 to 8 weeks. Side effects were reported in 18% of patients, including altered growth, moon facies, osteoporosis, fungal infection, and hypertension.

Surgical treatment is a third option. In one 2005 review, the authors analyzed 28 case series between 1986 and 2002 that included 372 infants.[24] In this review, tracheostomy was often performed either as the sole treatment followed by observation or as the first step prior to definitive interventions with CO_2 laser, steroids, and/or surgical excision. They concluded that use of the CO_2 laser had an 89% success rate and shortened tracheostomy duration and that surgical excision in patients as young as 2.5 months was successful in 98% of cases, although adverse effects were noted with each of these treatments. With contemporary use of propranolol for airway hemangioma, surgery is rarely needed aside from initial laryngoscopy and bronchoscopy for diagnosis.

For subglottic hemangioma, with proper securement of the airway, whether through treatment with propranolol, corticosteroids, surgical resection, or tracheostomy (or a combination thereof), patients have good outcomes, and hemangiomas are expected to regress early in childhood.

Trachea

Tracheomalacia

Many infants with tracheomalacia may be observed expectantly. Infants with severe symptoms of tracheomalacia may require urgent intubation and airway support, including possible surgical intervention. Historically, treatment for severe tracheomalacia included tracheostomy and sustained mechanical ventilation; however, noninvasive positive airway pressure techniques such as continued positive airway pressure or biphasic positive airway pressure are effective in maintaining tracheal patency during expiration and may avoid the need for surgery. Other surgical interventions vary by the cause of obstruction, and as such, they may require correction of compressive cardiovascular abnormalities or, in some cases, resection of the malacic tracheal segment.

Medical interventions for tracheomalacia may include use of hypertonic saline nebulizers to thin mucus and improve clearance of secretions, inhaled corticosteroids to reduce airway inflammation, use of ipratropium bromide inhalers, and a low threshold for initiation of antibiotics during respiratory infections.[25] A 2012 Cochrane review assessed current treatment practices including surgical approaches and noninvasive positive pressure airway support modalities and noted an absence of evidence to support any specific therapy over another based on available data.[58]

In the majority of infants with mild or moderate tracheomalacia, it improves by 1 to 2 years of age as the trachea grows and stiffens with age.

Vascular Rings

Management of vascular rings requires cardiovascular surgical intervention, with the approach dependent on the anatomy of the specific abnormality and the presence of coexisting cardiac defects. However, secondary tracheomalacia related to the vascular compression may take months to improve. In fact, in some series, up to approximately one-fourth of patients have persistent symptomatic tracheomalacia 10 years after surgery, with symptoms including stridor or recurrent respiratory infections.[59,60]

Tracheal Stenosis

Tracheal webs may be managed with endoscopic surgical intervention. Patients with mild tracheal stenosis may be observed, and some patients may outgrow their condition, with tracheal diameters approaching normal measurements later in childhood.[61,62] One study retrospectively used computed tomography to assess tracheal diameter among infants with congenital tracheal stenosis and found that if the narrowest segment was >40% of the normal-for-age tracheal diameter, then conservative management may be appropriate.[63]

Patients with severe tracheal stenosis who present soon after birth require urgent airway support. Endotracheal intubation may be difficult in cases of severe obstruction, because even the smallest endotracheal tube may not pass the stenotic segment; in these cases, noninvasive airway support may be attempted and ECMO may be required. Patients who present acutely within the neonatal period are a high-risk group, with mortality after surgical management in one series cited at 73% among infants less than 1 month old.[64] Mortality in this series remained significant but lower among infants repaired after 1 month of age, cited at 19%. For severe tracheal stenosis, the only definitive treatment is surgical, with the slide tracheoplasty technique usually the preferred procedure.[28] Symptoms improve for many patients after reconstruction, but some patients require further airway surgery (such as dilations or stenting) later in life.

Section 13

CHAPTER

68 Pierre-Robin Sequence/Cleft Palate-Related Airway Obstruction Seen in Neonates

Anita Deshpande, Mai Nguyen, Steven L. Goudy

KEY POINTS

1. Pierre Robin sequence (PRS) is an association of congenital micrognathia, glossoptosis, and cleft palate that presents with tongue-based airway obstruction.
2. Infants with PRS can present with a host of findings ranging from severe respiratory distress to mild feeding difficulties.
3. Evaluation of an infant found to have PRS should include direct visualization of the airway with flexible laryngoscopy, assessment of adjunctive measures to relieve airway obstruction (e.g., prone positioning, nasal trumpet), and evaluation of feeding and weight gain.
4. Nonsurgical treatment options include prone positioning, oropharyngeal or nasopharyngeal airway, continuous positive airway pressure, and endotracheal intubation.
5. Surgical options considered if nonsurgical management fails include tongue-lip adhesion, subperiosteal release of floor of mouth, mandibular distraction osteogenesis, and tracheostomy.
6. The majority of infants with PRS can be managed nonsurgically, although many will initially require nasogastric tube feeding and possibly gastrostomy tube placement; however, most will be successfully consuming an oral diet by 3 years of age.

Introduction

Pierre Robin sequence (PRS) was named after Dr. Pierre Robin, a French stomatologist who first described its features in 1923. PRS is an association of congenital micrognathia, glossoptosis, and airway obstruction.[1] The association of a wide, U-shaped cleft palate was added to the sequence in 1934. PRS is not considered a syndrome in itself but rather a sequence, where multiple anomalies result from a sequential chain of malformations.[2] Patients typically present with respiratory distress, feeding difficulties, and failure to thrive. Mortality rates of 2% to 26% have been described historically, but recent studies report a mortality rate of 10% significantly associated with syndromic PRS and the presence of neurologic anomalies.[3]

Overall, the estimated incidence of PRS is approximately 1 in 8000 to 14,000 individuals.[2] The highest rate of incidence is found in the United States, where it is estimated to occur in 1 in 3120 individuals.[4] PRS affects males and females equally. There appears to be a genetic basis for this sequence due to the high incidence of twins with PRS, and studies have shown that family members of infants with PRS have a higher incidence of cleft lip and palate.[1] Additionally, 50% to 62% of PRS cases are syndromic. The three most common syndromes include velocardiofacial, Treacher Collins, and Stickler syndromes, which account for 65% of cases.

Pathophysiology

Genetic Contributions to PRS

PRS is a heterogenic entity and can be found as isolated disease (nonsyndromic PRS) or in association with other syndromes (syndromic PRS). Nonsyndromic PRS is linked to the *SOX9* gene.[5] The *SOX9* gene is located on the long (q) arm of chromosome 17 at position 23 (17q23). *SOX9* is an HMG-box transcription factor that regulates chondrogenesis and testis development.[6] In humans, haploinsufficiency in the coding sequence of *SOX9* causes campomelic dysplasia, a semilethal, rare, autosomal-dominant disorder involving shortening and bowing of long bones, skeletal malformations, and male-to-female sex-reversal.[7] Disruptions upstream or downstream of an intact *SOX9* coding region result in milder phenotypes including the nonsyndromic form of PRS.

To date, the Online Mendelian Inheritance in Man (OMIM) database identifies 34 conditions related to syndromic PRS.[8] Stickler syndrome is a frequent cause of syndromic PRS and is due to an autosomal-dominant connective-tissue disorder caused by mutations in COL genes (*COL2A1*, *COL9A1*, *COL11A1*, or *COL11A2*), which affect type 2 and type 11 collagen.[9] It is characterized by ocular, orofacial, auditory, and skeletal manifestations. The characteristic facial appearance includes midface hypoplasia, micrognathia, elongated philtrum, and palatal abnormalities such as cleft palate, bifid uvula, or high arched palate.

Velocardiofacial syndrome is an autosomal-dominant disorder caused by a microdeletion from chromosome 22 at the q11.2 band.[10] It has an extremely expansive phenotypic spectrum, and no single clinical feature occurs in 100% of cases. Common features include congenital heart defects, facial anomalies, palatal anomalies, neonatal hypocalcemia, speech and learning disabilities, and hypoplastic thymus.

Treacher Collins syndrome derives from mutations in the *TCOF1*, *POLR1C*, and *POLR1D* genes.[11] These genes play a critical role in the early development of structures that become bones and tissues of the face. Treacher Collins syndrome can be inherited in an autosomal dominant or autosomal recessive manner. Typical features include bilateral and symmetric downslanting palpebral fissures, malar hypoplasia, micrognathia, retrognathia, and external ear abnormalities.

There are three major embryologic hypotheses to explain the sequence of events resulting in PRS:

1. Mandibular hypoplasia: During normal palatal development, the tongue lies between the two palatal shelves. The mandible starts growing ventrally and inferiorly during week 7 of development, pulling the tongue in the same direction. Due to a defect in Meckel's cartilage, which is involved in the formation and growth of the mandible, the hypoplastic mandible results in the developing tongue being forced upward and backward (glossoptosis).[6,12] Glossoptosis subsequently prevents fusion of the vertical palatal shelves, leading to the development of a wide, U-shaped cleft palate. This was demonstrated in animal (zebrafish and murine) models. There is thought

to be mandibular catch-up growth by 1 year of age, suggesting that ex utero, the mandible growth can normalize.[13]

2. Neurologic maturation theory: The inability of the developing fetus to engage in mandibular exercise prevents the tongue from descending, leading to mandibular hypoplasia.[14] In PRS patients, delays in neurologic maturation have been noted on electromyography of the tongue, the pharyngeal pillars, the palate, and hypoglossal nerve conduction. Fetal oral muscular activity (including swallowing) is thought to be required for normal mandibular growth.[15] The spontaneous correction with age supports this theory. Additionally, PRS is associated with several other conditions that are characterized by hypotonia.
3. Compression of mandible in utero: This may be the etiology for a small percentage of infants born with PRS. The fetal head is flexed with the growing mandible against the chest during the first 6 weeks of development. The gradual extension of the head results in a normal outgrowth of the mandible. Factors that could result in intrauterine restriction, such as oligohydramnios, twin pregnancies, or an abnormal embryonic implantation site, may lead to micrognathia.[13] In addition, studies show a higher incidence of PRS in twins than in the general population.

Clinical Features

Pierre Robin sequence is a triad of congenital micrognathia, glossoptosis, and airway obstruction. Micrognathia is often accompanied by overjet measurement >4 mm. Overjet is defined as the extent of anterior-posterior overlap of the maxillary central incisors over the mandibular central incisors. Glossoptosis causes airway obstruction at the level of the tongue base, and the severity of obstruction varies greatly between patients.[16] Obstruction can happen spontaneously, with feeding, and while awake or asleep. Airway obstruction may also be progressive, so serial airway evaluations (flexible versus rigid endoscopy) are important.[17–19] Polysomnography may demonstrate the presence of obstructive sleep apnea, and serial capillary gases can be used to evaluate for CO_2 retention.[12] Patients can present with stridor, retractions, and cyanosis. Severe obstruction can lead to feeding difficulties and failure to thrive, so it is important to follow daily weight gain. Feeding difficulties are prevalent in 25% to 45% of patients with PRS, and these difficulties are secondary to airway obstruction and cleft palate. Infants cannot form the negative intraoral pressure required for adequate suck. Infants with PRS may need nasogastric tube feeding for several months, and some may even require gastrostomy tube placement.[20] The prevalence and severity of feeding difficulties are higher in syndromic compared with nonsyndromic cases.[21] It is important to note that infants may have feeding difficulties without airway obstruction, or these difficulties may persist even after airway obstruction has been corrected.

The overall goals of PRS treatment are airway maintenance, adequate feeding, and weight gain. If untreated or inadequately treated, infants with PRS can suffer from chronic hypoxia with CO_2 retention, increased pulmonary vascular resistance, cor pulmonale, and malnutrition/failure to thrive.

Evaluation

The approach to evaluation of an infant suspected to have Pierre Robin sequence should include not only direct assessment of the airway with flexible endoscopy but also the degree of airway obstruction, feeding difficulties, and presence of reflux disease, along with potential investigation for comorbid abnormalities with genetics consult, ophthalmology consultation, and audiogram, given the high likelihood of hearing loss and otitis media with effusion.

Direct airway evaluation should initially take place with flexible nasolaryngoscopy, which can allow for examination of the upper airway structures, identification of abnormalities, and localization of the site of obstruction. Evaluation of the infant should include assessment of the nasal cavities, the choana, the pharynx including the tongue base, and the larynx. Obstruction at the level of the tongue base is a characteristic feature of PRS, but other associated abnormalities include laryngomalacia, vocal cord paralysis, and less frequently, tracheomalacia, choanal atresia/stenosis, and hypoplastic epiglottis.[22–25]

Because approximately 8% of infants with PRS have been shown to have lower airway abnormalities, rigid or flexible bronchoscopy should be considered to evaluate the subglottis, trachea, and bronchi.[17,22] Bronchoscopy should occur prior to other (nonairway) surgical procedures or surgical correction of tongue base obstruction and in cases with persistent obstruction after surgical correction.[17]

Drug-induced sleep endoscopy (DISE) can also be performed in the operating room to determine the site of dynamic airway obstruction during inspiration while asleep. Obstruction of the level of the tongue base is seen in PRS, but other sites of obstruction that can lead to pediatric sleep-disordered breathing or obstructive sleep apnea include inferior turbinate hypertrophy and laryngomalacia.[26] Findings elicited during DISE not only can be utilized for initial surgical planning but can also help elucidate the etiology of persistent obstruction after surgical correction of a tongue base obstruction.[17]

Objective data should be measured to quantify hypoxemia and hypercapnia. Initially, pulse oximetry can help determine oxygen saturation in arterial blood. Repeated airway obstruction has also been shown to lead to elevated partial pressure of carbon dioxide (P_{CO_2}), and capillary P_{CO_2} testing can be followed longitudinally.[17,26] Polysomnography has long been considered the gold standard for the diagnosis of obstructive sleep apnea/hypopnea syndrome and can help quantify the severity of airway obstruction.

Given the prevalence of feeding difficulties seen in infants with PRS, a feeding assessment and objective swallowing evaluation should be performed. Often these are performed by or in conjunction with a speech-language pathologist. An infant who demonstrates low oral intake with inadequate weight gain, prolonged feeding time, fatigue, and coughing or gagging with feeds may benefit from nasogastric tube placement.[17] Infants may appear to have clinically satisfactory feeding outcomes but be silently aspirating, so a feeding assessment should be performed in all infants with PRS. Objective evaluation can be performed with videofluoroscopic swallowing studies or fiberoptic endoscopic evaluation of swallowing.

Additionally, there is a high prevalence of gastroesophageal reflux disease (GERD) in the PRS population and objective evaluation should be strongly considered, especially in the case of persistent airway obstruction after intervention.[27,28] Standard tests for evaluation of GERD in infants include barium swallow, esophagoscopy, and pH monitoring.[29]

Genetics consultation should be considered early once an infant with PRS has been identified, given its association with multiple syndromes. Depending on the presence of any syndromes and associated abnormalities, routine ophthalmology and audiology assessments may be crucial and lead to early interventions.

Management

There are a variety of nonsurgical and surgical options that can be used to treat airway obstruction, with management decisions individualized

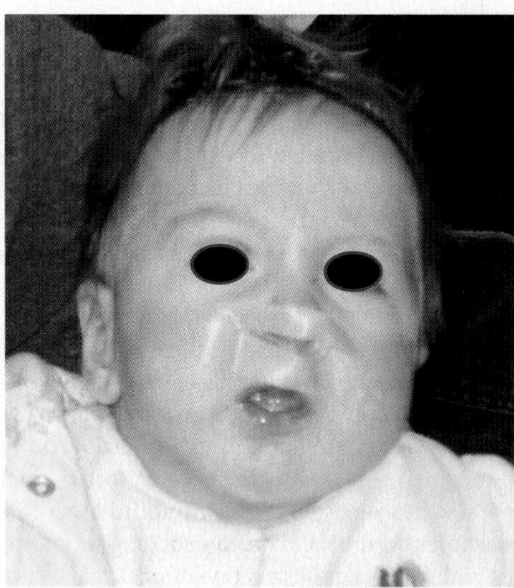

Fig. 68.1 Pierre Robin Sequence Patient With Nasal Airway Taped in Left Nares.

and based on the severity of respiratory feeding difficulties and comorbidities.[30] Nonsurgical options include prone positioning, oropharyngeal or nasopharyngeal airway, orthodontic appliance, continuous positive airway pressure (CPAP), and endotracheal intubation.[31] Surgical options include tongue-lip adhesion (TLA), subperiosteal release of the floor of the mouth, mandibular distraction osteogenesis (MDO), and tracheostomy.[31] Several studies have been performed to risk-stratify patients with PRS, and certain patient factors are predictive of need for surgical intervention, including prematurity, need for intubation or tracheotomy in the first 24 hours of life, CPAP/bilevel positive airway pressure (BiPAP) use, and the presence of comorbid neurologic disease.[32,33]

The first-line intervention, which is simple to perform and can lead to rapid benefit, is prone positioning. This maneuver allows for forward movement of the mandible and tongue, which can relieve tongue-base obstruction. Prone positioning has been shown to be successful in 40% to 70% of children with PRS.[17,21] Drawbacks to prone positioning include the difficulty of monitoring an infant for signs or symptoms of airway obstruction and its association with sudden infant death syndrome.[34]

Placement of a nasopharyngeal airway, either a nasal trumpet or a modified endotracheal tube placed intranasally and positioned in the oropharynx, has also been shown to relieve high upper airway obstruction.[35–37] This technique can be taught to the infant's parents or caregivers, and if successful, it can act as an effective temporizing measure for months as the mandible grows (Fig. 68.1). One drawback to this method, however, is that it often precludes oral feeding, necessitating nasogastric or gastric tube placement for enteral feeding. Polysomnography can be performed to assist in determining the timing of removal, with the average duration of nasopharyngeal airway use being approximately 8 months.[37]

CPAP is not often used in the long-term management of PRS due to the difficulty in utilizing this technique in infants, the infeasibility of using this method long-term, and the paucity of data regarding the success of the method in relieving airway obstruction.[17] Furthermore, prolonged CPAP use has been shown to lead to acquired maxillary hypoplasia.[38]

For infants who have moderate to severe obstruction that does not resolve with noninvasive interventions, surgical procedures must be considered. The majority of these target airway obstruction at the level of the tongue base. Flexible nasolaryngoscopy must be performed in all infants who are being considered for surgical intervention to help determine the level of obstruction and thus the surgical procedure most likely to have benefit.

TLA can be utilized for obstruction isolated to the tongue base. This procedure anchors the anterior tongue to the lip and the posterior tongue to the mandible. The genioglossus can also be released from the floor of mouth.[39] There does exist controversy regarding the success of TLA in relieving airway obstruction, and there is a lack of long-term objective data in the literature.[17] A small study demonstrated a drop in the mean apnea-hypopnea index from 37.6 to 21.6, indicating that despite an improvement, infants who underwent TLA still had persistent severe airway obstruction.[40] Furthermore, this study also demonstrated that 4 out of 15 patients who underwent TLA ultimately required tracheostomy. Those who underwent mandibular distraction osteogenesis did not require postprocedure tracheostomy.[40] The GILLS score has been proposed to predict the likelihood of TLA success by assigning 1 point to each of the following: gastroesophageal reflux, intubation preoperatively, late operation (older than 2 weeks), low birth weight (< 2500 g), and syndromic diagnosis.[41] TLA demonstrates a success rate of 100% in infants with a GILLS score of 2 or less and a failure rate of 43% in infants with a GILLS score of 3 or more.

MDO is the only surgical procedure addressing mandibular hypoplasia. It involves creating a bilateral mandibular osteotomy and then gradually advancing the mandible forward to relieve tongue-base obstruction. It is being performed more frequently in place of tracheostomy, although it does have contraindications and should not be performed in a child with absent mandibular condyles, absent coronoid processes, and a poorly defined glenoid fossa.[17,42] Preoperatively, lateral and anteroposterior cephalograms, an orthopantomogram, and, when necessary, three-dimensional computed tomography imaging should be performed to determine the vector of distraction.[42] Using the three-dimensional models, virtual surgical planning is used to plan the mandibular correction procedure (Figs. 68.2 and 68.3).

Tracheostomy is the definitive management option when other interventions have failed to relieve severe airway obstruction and may also be used as a bridging procedure.[17] Although relief from airway obstruction can be immediate, the procedure is associated with significant morbidity and mortality when performed in the pediatric population due to its associated complications including tracheostomy tube obstruction and decannulation. Furthermore, compared with MDO, tracheostomy may lead to higher treatment costs, mainly due to prolonged hospital stay.[43,44]

The approach to PRS patient management is detailed in Table 68.1. Table 68.2 lists the relative advantages and disadvantages of each intervention.

Feeding Management

Apart from airway management and alleviation of respiratory difficulties, infants with Pierre Robin syndrome often require feeding support due to swallowing challenges posed by the cleft palate, the increased prevalence of esophageal motility disorders, and the presence of GERD, which is a known comorbidity.[45,46] It is estimated that the prevalence of feeding problems in the PRS population ranges from 25% to 45% in typically developing children and 33% to 80% in those with developmental delays.[47–49] Correcting airway obstruction does not always improve feeding and swallowing difficulties, because 42% of infants with PRS who have successful treatment of airway obstruction with positional maneuvers still demonstrate feeding difficulty.[21]

The etiology of feeding difficulties is multifactorial. Infants with PRS have altered suction abilities due to the presence of cleft palate, because the cleft decreases the infant's ability to satisfactorily establish the

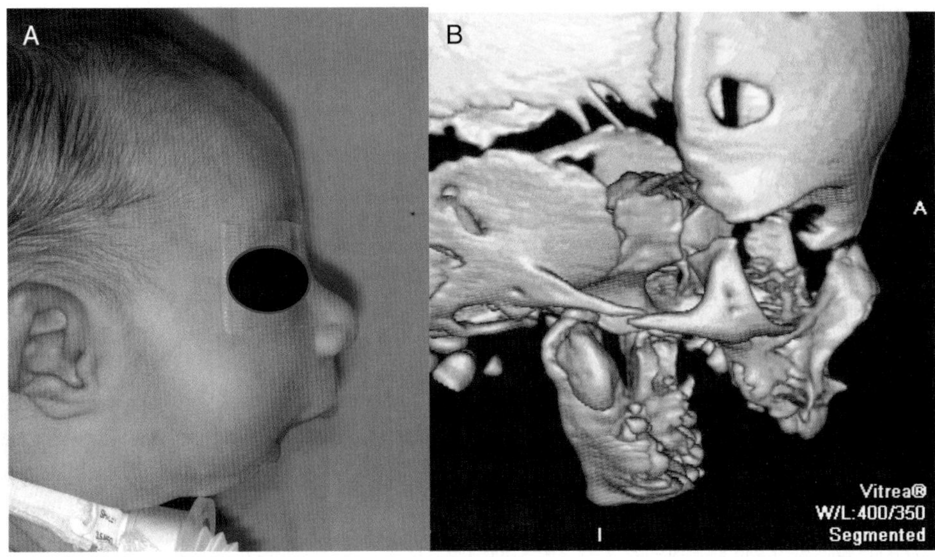

Fig. 68.2 Child With Pierre Robin Sequence. (A) Lateral view. (B) Corresponding 3-D computed tomography scan of the mandible.

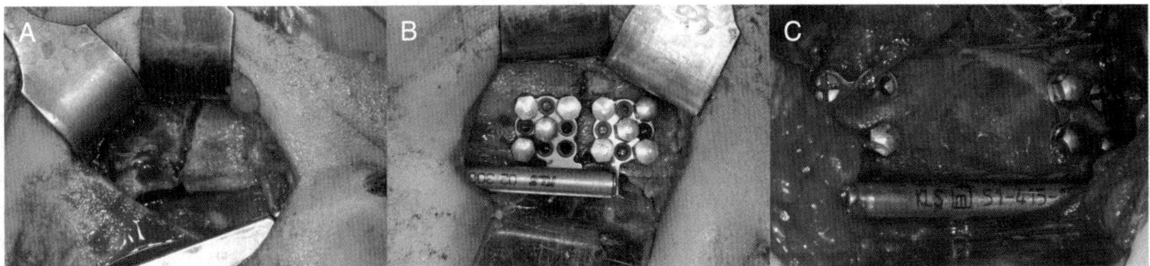

Fig. 68.3 (A) Cervical incision with osteotomy. (B) Distractor device in place. (C) Regenerated bone.

negative intraoral pressure required to suck milk from a breast or standard bottle, leading to disorganized bolus formation and transit.[46] These infants may derive significant benefit from specialized bottles and nipples, such as the Mead Johnson Cleft Nurser, the Pigeon Cleft Bottle, Dr. Brown's Specialty Feeding System, or the Haberman Special Needs Feeder.[46] Other techniques to facilitate feeding include using pacifiers, massage to relax and anteriorize the tongue, rhythmic movement of the nipple in the oral cavity, and feeding of the infant in the global symmetric position, with upper extremities positioned along the midline and lower extremities and the head semiflexed, or in a side-lying position.[50] Additionally, administration of a hypercaloric diet can lead to an improvement in nutritional status, which can contribute to improved respiratory conditions.[51]

Ultimately, however, infants with PRS may require nasogastric or gastrostomy tube placement for enteral feeding, with one study demonstrating that tube feeding was required in 53% of children with isolated PRS, 67% of children with syndromic PRS, and 83% of children with unique PRS, which was defined as children with PRS who also had a variety of abnormalities not meeting criteria for existing syndromes.[21] Infants with isolated or syndromic PRS more often required a short (0–3 months) or intermediate (4–18 months) duration of tube feeding, with infants with unique PRS more commonly requiring long-term (more than 18 months) gastrostomy tube feeding.[21] The need for enteral feeding, however, tends to resolve, with 91% of patients with isolated PRS, 92% of those with syndromic PRS, and 78% of those with unique PRS consuming an oral diet by 3 years of age.[21] Performance of mandibular distraction osteogenesis has been shown to lead to the avoidance of gastrostomy tube placement.[52]

Table 68.1 Interventions to Manage High Upper Airway Obstruction in Infants With Pierre-Robin Sequence

PRS Intervention	1st Line	2nd Line	3rd Line	4th Line	5th Line
Positioning	xxx				
Trumpet		xxx			
Tongue-lip adhesion			xxx		
Mandible distraction				xxx	
Tracheostomy					xxx

PRS, Pierre Robin sequence.

In infants with PRS, sucking-swallowing electromyography and esophageal manometry have revealed dysfunction in the motor organization of the tongue, pharynx, and esophagus, even in the absence of clinically apparent feeding difficulties.[53] Additionally, there is a high prevalence of GERD in the PRS population, which can exacerbate tongue-based airway obstruction.[27,28] Prophylactic medical treatment of GERD is recommended, because sequelae include laryngeal edema, which can increase airway obstruction.[46]

Long-Term Outcomes

The immediacy of airway obstruction can vary based on which method of intervention is utilized. Nonsurgical intervention may take months to show improvement in airway obstruction, whereas

Table 68.2 Relative Advantages and Disadvantages of Various Interventions Available to Manage High Upper Airway Obstruction in Infants With Pierre-Robin Sequence

Intervention	Advantages	Disadvantages
Prone positioning	Easy to do No instrumentation or surgery	May not help Concern about "back to sleep" issues
Nasal airway	Easy to do Readily available	Usually precludes oral feeding Tubes may occlude Nasal trauma Difficult to send home with
Tongue-lip adhesion	Less invasive surgery	Requires take down later Effectiveness questionable
Mandibular distraction	Increasing track record of success May avoid trach and G tube	Scars, tooth damage Airway maintenance during distraction may be tenuous
Tracheostomy	Secure airway for severe upper airway obstruction Useful for patients with multilevel airway obstruction or pulmonary disease	Long-term care issues and complications of tracheostomy (1% mortality per year with trach)

tracheostomy may yield almost immediate relief. Côté et al summarize the reported success of various interventions as follows[17]:

- Prone position—47% to 73%
- Side position—26%
- Nasopharyngeal airway—57% to 100%
- CPAP—69%
- Orthodontic appliance—91% to 100%
- TLA—27% to 100%
- Subperiosteal release of floor of mouth (FOM)—50% to 84%
- Mandibular distraction osteogenesis—88% to 100%

Often, infants with PRS do show resolution or improvement in respiratory difficulties, due to the increase in airway dimensions occurring in the first 2 years of life.[17] A cephalometric study has shown that infants with PRS have a shorter tongue and mandibular length, narrower airway, smaller tongue area, and more posteriorly and inferiorly positioned hyoid compared with normal control infants. This distinction narrows with increasing age and results from an increased mandibular growth rate in infants with PRS that results in improved airway dimensions.[54]

As discussed above, most feeding issues improve with time. A majority of children with PRS do require nasogastric or gastrostomy tube feeding, with the incidence of enteral feeding being higher and the duration being longer in children with syndromic PRS or those with other associated anomalies. However, most are able to successfully achieve an oral diet by 3 years of age.[21]

There is controversy regarding the presence and potential etiology of long-term neurocognitive deficits in children with PRS, which have been thought to be due to underlying congenital disorders or repetitive hypoxia resulting from severe airway obstruction.[17] A longitudinal prospective study analyzed long-term developmental outcomes in children with isolated PRS or PRS associated with Stickler syndrome, finding that at 15 months of age, 56% of children had language delay, with the incidence of language delay decreasing to 46% at 3 years of age.[54,55] Hypernasality was present in 69% of children at 6 years of age. This study also found that 85% of children could be fed orally by 12 months of age, with 74% displaying normal eating behavior by 15 months and 94% by 6 years of age. Cognitive scores were within normal ranges, and although global developmental quotient scores were lower in children with associated Stickler syndrome, this difference was not statistically significant.

Summary

Pierre Robin sequence (PRS) is an association of congenital micrognathia, glossoptosis, and cleft palate. Infants with PRS can present with a host of findings ranging from severe respiratory distress to mild feeding difficulties. An infant found to have PRS should undergo thorough airway and feeding evaluations. Initially, conservative management should be sought, with nonsurgical options including prone positioning, oropharyngeal or nasopharyngeal airway placement, continuous positive airway pressure (CPAP), and endotracheal intubation. If nonsurgical management fails, surgical treatment options include TLA, MDO, and tracheostomy. The majority of infants with PRS can be managed nonsurgically, and although many may initially require enteral feeding, most will be successfully consuming an oral diet by 3 years of age.

CHAPTER 69

Congenital Hearing Loss Seen in Neonates

Kavita Dedhia, Albert Park

KEY POINTS

1. All newborns must have a hearing screen by the age of 1 month, a diagnostic audiologic test at 3 months if they do not pass their hearing screen, and a referral for early intervention by 6 months if they are diagnosed with hearing loss.
2. Genetic factors are the most common causes of hearing loss, accounting for approximately 65% of congenital sensorineural hearing loss (SNHL).
3. The most common environmental cause of hearing loss is congenital cytomegalovirus (cCMV).
4. The optimal time to perform cCMV testing is prior to 3 weeks of age.
5. Ototoxicity is an important cause of hearing loss, especially in children exposed to aminoglycosides.
6. Clinicians should follow-up after a failed newborn hearing screen in children with middle ear fluid, because approximately 10% may also have SNHL.
7. Auditory neuropathy will be missed in children who have a hearing screened using otoacoustic emissions only. Because this condition is prevalent in neonatal intensive care infants, hearing screening in these infants should include automated auditory brainstem response testing.
8. Because progressive SNHL may develop in children despite a normal newborn hearing screen, clinicians should refer children with SNHL risk factors for additional audiologic testing at 24 to 36 months of age.

Introduction

The most common congenital condition is hearing loss, with a reported prevalence of 3 out of 1000 infants. Prior to the year 2000, only children who were considered high risk underwent hearing screening prior to discharge from the newborn nursery. However, with this "high-risk" screening process, approximately 50% of children with hearing loss were not identified. In 1994 the Joint Committee on Infant Hearing recommended universal newborn hearing screening (UNHS) prior to hospital discharge for all infants. This did not take effect until after the year 1999 in most states, until sufficient evidence was found and it was approved by the US Preventive Services Task Force. Since that time, several states followed suit, and now all states have UNHS programs.[1–4]

UNHS follows the 1 to 3-6 rule. The infant must undergo hearing screening prior to 1 month of age. Children who do not pass the hearing screen must get diagnostic testing to confirm if they do or do not have hearing loss by the age of 3 months. If the child is diagnosed with hearing loss, they should be referred for early intervention (EI) by 6 months of age. Using the 1 to 3-6 rule, children with congenital hearing loss have been identified and treated earlier.

Since the initiation and acceptance of UNHS, there has been dramatic improvement of early identification of children with hearing loss, because approximately 50% of newborns with hearing loss have no readily identifiable risk factors.[5] Prior to UNHS, the average age of suspicion of hearing loss was 18.8 months, with confirmation at 26 months and hearing aids at 30 months. With the early implementation of UNHS the age of intervention has decreased to 6 months, and in a study performed in Colorado, the average age for fitting hearing aids was 5 weeks.[3,6,7]

In addition to UNHS, other advances in diagnosis and management of pediatric sensorineural hearing loss (SNHL) should be noted. The advent of genetic testing panels allows evaluation of more than 100 genes to increase the likelihood of identifying a causative genetic disorder. High-resolution imaging of the temporal bones with computed tomography (CT) and magnetic resonance imaging (MRI) has allowed detailed analysis of inner ear anatomy for children with hearing loss. Furthermore, more birthing hospitals and states are adopting congenital cytomegalovirus (cCMV) testing prior to 3 weeks of age, increasing the possibility of identifying children with cCMV.

Early recognition of hearing loss in young children has led to EI and management with preferential school seating, hearing aids, bone-anchored hearing aids, and cochlear implants. Such EIs recognize the critical period for optimal language skills to develop, and with EI, patients have better outcomes. The literature suggests that diagnosis and intervention prior to 6 months can improve speech and language outcomes.[4,6,8–12] In this chapter we will discuss etiology, diagnosis, and management of children who fail their newborn hearing screen.

Etiology and Pathophysiology of Sensorineural Hearing Loss

There are four types of hearing loss: conductive, mixed, sensorineural, and auditory neuropathy. Conductive hearing loss is caused by middle ear fluid or an abnormality of the ossicles and/or the external auditory canal. SNHL is due to malformations or malfunction of the cochlea or cochlear nerve. Mixed hearing loss has components of both conductive hearing loss and SNHL. Auditory neuropathy is due to lack of proper synchronized auditory input from the cochlear nerve to the brain, with or without a normal cochlea. In this chapter we will focus mainly on SNHL.

There are several causes of congenital hearing loss (Fig. 69.1).[13] Genetic mutations account for approximately 50% to 68% of congenital hearing loss, and of these, nonsyndromic causes represent approximately 70%.[13,14] The most common genetic cause of SNHL is a mutation in the gene coding for connexin 26, a protein responsible for maintaining endolymphatic potential through potassium ion transport. The gene locus coding for this protein is the gap junction beta-2 *(GJB2)* gene. There are approximately 400 syndromes that are associated with SNHL; some of the common syndromic causes are listed in Table 69.1.

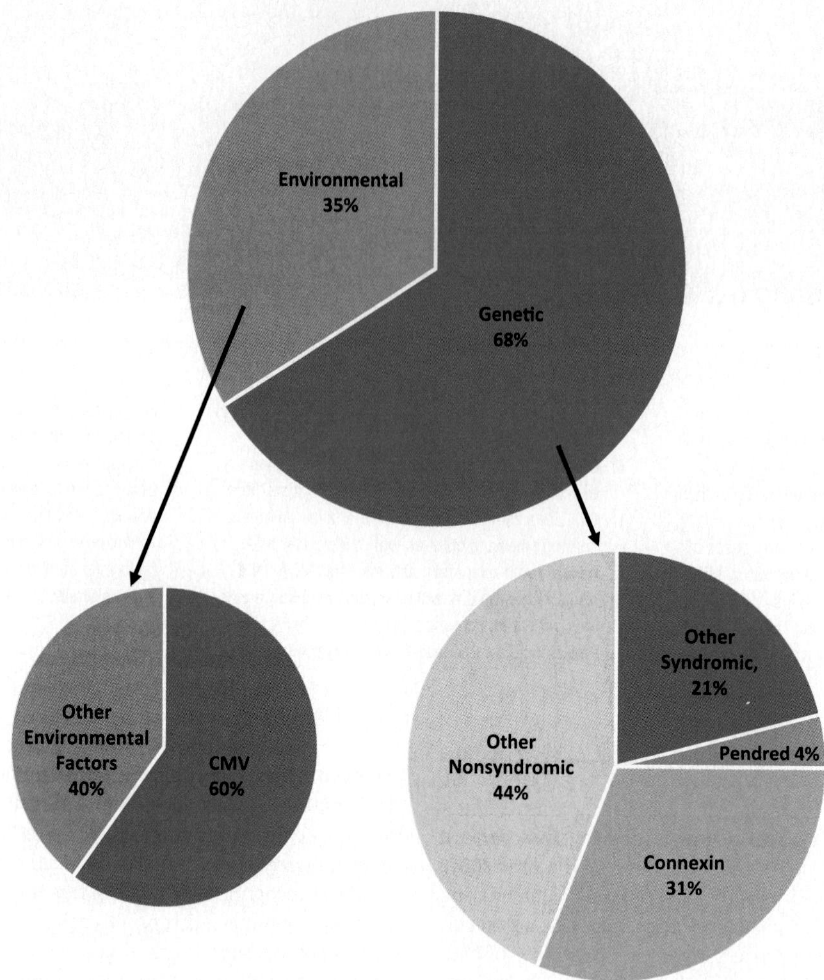

Fig. 69.1 Estimated Etiology of Sensorineural Hearing Loss at Birth in the United States. *CMV,* Cytomegalovirus.

Environmental etiologic factors cause 35% to 50% of SNHL, of which cCMV infection is the most common. We will discuss cCMV in further detail later in this chapter. Other prenatal infections such as toxoplasmosis, rubella, herpes, and syphilis can cause SNHL. Furthermore, prematurity, hypoxia, hyperbilirubinemia, meningitis, and ototoxic medications have been identified as environmental factors associated with congenital SNHL.

Ototoxicity is a special consideration in newborns, given that antibiotic regimens used to treat neonatal sepsis often contain aminoglycosides. The proposed mechanism of ototoxicity is from free-radical formation that damages the hair cells in the cochlea. Initially, high-frequency hearing is impacted, and then it may progress to include lower frequencies.[16] Factors associated with aminoglycoside ototoxicity are coadministration of vancomycin, loop diuretics, or neuromuscular blockers; underlying disease; prior aminoglycoside exposure; and drug peak and trough concentration. Furthermore, individuals who have mitochondrial mutations, especially mtDNA A155G, are highly susceptible to ototoxicity from these medications even without high drug concentration levels in the blood.[16,17] This mutation has been observed in 17% of Caucasians and 10% to 30% of Asians with aminoglycoside ototoxicity.[17]

There is currently no standard for monitoring infants for ototoxicity. Although the American Speech and Language Association recommends obtaining a baseline hearing test, the frequency and urgency of empiric aminoglycoside treatment may make such baseline testing impractical prior to starting treatment. Furthermore, the UNHS protocols do not test higher than 4K Hz, which is an early characteristic of ototoxic hearing loss. However, distortion product otoacoustic emissions can be measured at high frequencies and may have better potential in ototoxic monitoring in this population. Another challenge is the difficulty in interpreting results in very premature neonates due to an immature auditory system, stenotic ear canals with debris, and noise in the neonatal intensive care unit that can interfere with results. Further research is needed to identify the best protocol for evaluating these children and identifying how to decrease potential ototoxicity in this population.[18]

Newborn Hearing Screen (NHS)

There are two types of hearing screen tests for young infants: otoacoustic emissions (OAEs) and automated auditory brainstem response (AABR). All newborns must undergo this evaluation prior to 1 month of age, and it is usually performed in the birth hospital prior to discharge. One type of screening is the evoked OAE (EOAE), which tests the outer hair cells and is a measure of only cochlear function. EOAE testing does not evaluate the entire auditory pathway. There are two main types of EOAEs performed: transient (TEOAE) and distortion product (DPOAE). Small microphones are placed into the external auditory canal, and a series of clicks at a sound pressure level of

Table 69.1 Common Etiology of Syndromic Hearing Loss[13–15]

Name	Inheritance Pattern	Gene	Phenotype	Expected Hearing Loss
Pendred	AR	*SLC26A4*	Bilateral enlarged vestibular aqueduct, enlarged thyroid	Severe to profound Mild to moderate progressive
Alport	X-linked or AR	*COL4A3, COL4A4, COL4A5*	Kidney disease and eye abnormalities	Late-onset high frequency
Usher type 1	AR	*USH1A, MYO7A, USH1C, CDH23, USH1E, PCDH15, USH1G*	Vestibular symptoms, retinitis pigmantosa	Profound
Usher type 2	AR	*USH2A, USH2B, USH2C, ADGRV1, WHRN*	Retinitis pigmentosa	Mild to severe
Usher type 3	AR	*USH3, CLRN1*	Variable vestibular symptoms, late-onset retinitis pigmentosa	Progressive
Waardenburg type 1	AD	*PAX3*	White forelock, heterochromic irises, dystopia canthorum	Normal or moderate to profound
Waardenburg type 2	AD or AR	*MITF, SNAI2*	White forelock, heterochromic irises	Normal or moderate to profound
Waardenburg type 3	AD	*PAX3*	Same as type 1 with limb defects	Normal or moderate to profound
Waardenburg Type 4	AR	*SOX10, EDN3, EDNRB*	Increased risk of Hirschsprung disease in carriers and homozygotes	Normal or moderate to profound
Jervell and Lange-Nielsen syndrome	AR	*KCNE1, KCNQ1*	Prolonged QT	Profound
Branchio-otorenal	AD	*EYA1*	Renal abnormalities, preauricular pits or other external/middle ear abnormalities, branchial fistula/cyst	SNHL/CHL/MHL, mild to profound

AD, Autosomal dominant; *AR*, autosomal recessive; *CHL*, conductive hearing loss; *MHL*, mixed hearing loss; *SNHL*, sensorineural hearing loss.

approximately 80 dB are used to elicit a response when performing TEOAEs. If emissions are present, this indicates hearing of at least 20 to 40 dB hearing loss in the 500 to 4K Hz range, essentially excluding hearing losses greater than mild.[19] When two pure-tone stimuli, one low frequency and the other high frequency, are presented at moderate levels (55–65 dB sound pressure level) to the ear, the cochlea generates DPOAE, which occurs somewhere between the low- and high-frequency stimuli.[20] EOAEs are only accurate when both the external ear and the middle ear are clear of debris and/or fluid.

Another type of screening test is the AABR. This screening test evaluates the entire auditory pathway, from the cochlea to the brainstem. When performing the AABR, transient acoustic stimuli are generated and detected with probes that are placed in the ear canal and surface electrodes that are placed in the head and neck region (e.g., vertex, mastoid region). A rapidly repeated click stimulus is presented at 30 to 45 dB hearing loss to evaluate the auditory pathway. The automated test will give a pass or fail result. Because the AABR is actually a measurement of a summated evoked potential over time, background noise and movement of the infant can adversely affect testing.[1,21]

Currently there is no consensus on which screening test should initially be performed in the newborn nursery. The type of test used varies across states, cities, and even at the hospital level. The Joint Committee on Infant Hearing recommendations note that the type of screening program will depend on what is practical and suitable for the program, based on both cost and availability of resources.[22] The only instance where AABR must be performed in all children is in the neonatal intensive care unit (NICU), because auditory neuropathy occurs more frequently in this population. The first hearing screen should be performed at least 12 hours after birth, preferably as close to discharge as possible in order to decrease the referral rate from amniotic fluid or debris in the ear canal. For infants who "refer" after the first screen, a repeat screen is recommended prior to diagnostic testing. Several studies have shown that testing infants at least 24 to 48 hours after birth will lead to decreased false-positive results.[23–25]

In general, EOAEs are easier and faster to perform; however they only evaluate the cochlea and are adversely impacted by middle and outer ear pathology such as vernix, cerumen, and middle ear fluid.[26] AABR is more time consuming, but it is generally reported to have a lower false-positive rate.[27] In a study by Lin and colleagues, the referral rate was 5.8% for TEOAE, 1.6% for two-step TEOAE and AABR, and 0.8% for AABR only.[27] Clarke et al. compared the results of AABR and TEOAE in 81 newborns undergoing NHS. They found the probability of a newborn passing the AABR was much higher than for TEOAE on both the first and second screens.[25] Despite the lower referral rates with AABR only, the increased technical difficulty and cost are barriers to implementation in many settings.

A two-stage protocol using EOAEs and subsequent AABR in cases where the newborn refers the EOAEs is also used at many birthing centers. A number of investigators have reported that this approach reduces the false-positive rate and will minimize unnecessary referrals,[28–33] although other studies have shown that infants who have undergone the two-stage NHS protocol may be at increased risk of a missed hearing-loss diagnosis.[34] Optimizing the screens and decreasing false positives will decrease the need for subsequent follow-ups, superfluous testing, cost, and the potential of parental anxiety.

A pass on the NHS does not mean that the child will continue to have normal hearing. Currently, if children pass their NHS, they will not undergo a repeat hearing screen until the age of 4. The literature reports that up to 22% to 30% of children diagnosed with hearing loss had previously passed their NHS. For this reason, it is important to reevaluate children at risk for future SNHL by the age of 24 to 30 months (Table 69.2).[22] With this second screen, children would be identified prior to preschool, and intervention could be started earlier to improve speech and language outcomes.[22] Additionally, per the

Table 69.2 Risk Indicators Associated With Permanent Congenital, Delayed-Onset, or Progressive Hearing Loss in Childhood[22]
Caregiver concern regarding speech, language, or developmental delay
Family history of permanent childhood hearing loss
Neonatal intensive care (NICU) of >5 days
NICU for any period of time with the following: Extracorporeal membrane oxygenation (ECMO), assisted ventilation, exposure to ototoxic medications or loop diuretics, and hyperbilirubinemia requiring exchange transfusion
In utero infections: Toxoplasmosis, rubella, cytomegalovirus, herpes, syphilis
Craniofacial anomalies including those that involve the pinna or ear canal, ear tags, ear pits, and temporal bone anomalies
Physical findings associated with syndromes known to include sensorineural or permanent conductive hearing loss
Syndrome associated with hearing loss
Neurodegenerative disorders
Culture-positive postnatal infections associated with sensorineural hearing loss (meningitis)
Head trauma, especially basal skull/temporal bone fracture requiring hospitalization
Chemotherapy

From Flint, Haughey, Lund, Robbins, Thomas, Lesperance, and Francis. Early detection and diagnosis of infant hearing. In: *Cummings Otolaryngology Head and Neck Surgery*. Ch. 193, p. 42. 9780323611794. Permission obtained.

American Academy of Pediatrics, all children should be monitored during their well-check visits at 9, 18, 24, and 30 months for middle-ear disease, auditory and speech skills, and developmental milestones, using the validated global screening tool. If there is parent or physician concern for hearing, speech, or language delay, the assessment should be performed earlier.[22]

Each state has a local Early Hearing Detection and Intervention chapter responsible for ensuring that the NHS guidelines are followed. NHS data are reported to the national chapter, which is part of the Centers for Disease Control and Prevention (CDC), and these data are aggregated and reported, most recently in 2017. The average percentage of newborns who were screened by the recommended 1 month was 97.1% (ranging from 94.3% to 100%), which is reassuring. The most common reasons for no documented hearing screen were infant death, home birth, or the family declining testing. After the screening, an average of 24.6% of infants nationally (range, 0%–86.7%) did not undergo diagnostic testing due to loss to follow-up/documentation. The average rate of infants with diagnosed hearing loss being enrolled into EI by 6 months was reported to be quite low at 43.4% (range, 8.1%–83.3%). Reasons identified by Early Hearing Detection and Intervention were mainly due to families declining EI, families being contacted for follow-up but not responding, inability to contact families, families being nonresidents or moving out of state, or families being ineligible for Part C Medicaid. Overall, even though screening is most likely performed in almost all newborns in the United States, improvements still need to be made in achieving diagnostic testing by 3 months and starting EI for hearing loss by 6 months of age.[35]

Special NHS Considerations

Prematurity

Due to the improvement in modern technology, we are fortunate to sustain life in extremely premature infants. However, there are no guidelines detailing when to evaluate hearing and interpretation of diagnostic tests in this group. Myelination of the cochlear nerve and auditory pathway does not begin until the third trimester of pregnancy (27 weeks). At this time, the fetus may start moving to sounds, although this response may be more consistent at 28 to 29 weeks, when evoked responses may be present. Full cochlear maturity is achieved a few weeks prior to term birth.[36] Given the time course for development of the auditory system, it is important to consider gestational age when interpreting the auditory brainstem response (ABR) results.[37] Delayed maturation of the auditory pathway in premature infants may lead to abnormal ABR results, which may improve with time in this population.[38–42] It is important to consider obtaining repeat evaluations in this population. Hof and colleagues described a series of nine infants with improved hearing prior to 80 weeks' gestation.[38] Another case series described 23 infants diagnosed with severe to profound hearing loss at 3 months who significantly improved within the first year of life.[43] Although there are no strong data at this time, both studies identified that severely preterm infants should have frequent hearing evaluations until at least 80 weeks of gestational age, especially when evaluating cochlear implantation candidacy.[38,43]

Interpretation of the Effects of Middle Ear Fluid

Otitis media with effusion (OME) is a common finding in infants who fail their newborn hearing screening. Several large studies have reported that between 15% and 65% of infants who failed their NHS have OME.[44–47] Eavey reported mesenchyme, amniotic fluid, purulent otitis media, and blood in a significant number of neonatal temporal bones.[48] He also found that autologous keratin in a gerbil model provided histologic findings similar to those seen in the human neonatal temporal bones. OME may seem reassuring to the primary care provider and family because this finding may explain why the newborn failed the hearing screening test. In fact, Boudewyns et al. noted that none of 64 infants with OME and a failed NHS were found to have underlying SNHL.[45] In contrast, Boone et al. detected underlying SNHL in 11% of infants who presented with a failed NHS and middle-ear fluid.[44]

Boone et al.'s finding is higher than that reported by Boudewyns et al. but does appropriately illustrate the importance of considering SNHL in such patients. One must not assume that the infant who fails his or her NHS and has OME will not also have SNHL. This motivation to avoid a delay in SNHL detection is the rationale for a recommendation in a clinical practice guideline from the American Academy of Otolaryngology–Head and Neck Surgery Foundation that states that "clinicians should document in the medical record counseling of parents of infants with OME who fail a newborn hearing screen the importance of follow-up to ensure that hearing is normal when OME resolves and to exclude an underlying SNHL."[49]

The best approach for the infant with OME and a failed NHS is not known. A prolonged period of surveillance may not be ideal. Boudewyns et al. noted that only 15 of 64 infants with middle-ear effusion presenting at an average age of 49 days had resolution of their fluid by 4.8 months of age.[45] Doyle et al. have noted that neonatal OME is a risk factor for subsequent chronic otitis media through the first year of age.[50] In addition, we have reported a high level of parental dissatisfaction with the NHS process, predominantly because of the number of repeated clinic visits and delays in treatment.[51] This level of frustration probably accounts for some of the high rates of loss to follow-up seen in many hearing programs.[3,52] Korres et al. reported that two-thirds of families of newborns with failed hearing screening did *not* return for follow-up testing.[53]

Weber et al. recommend prompt operative intervention with diagnostic myringotomy with intraoperative ABR in this situation.[54] They noted that children who underwent this procedure in the operating room were diagnosed approximately 3 months earlier than children in the nonoperative observation group. A clinical practice guideline on OME states that referral to an otolaryngologist is appropriate for all infants with documented persistent hearing loss after a failed NHS, even if the cause is presumed to be secondary to OME.[49] The approach at our institution is to permit a 3-month period for OME to resolve but then to proceed with tympanostomy tube placement if the fluid does not resolve. Other at-risk groups such as those with Down syndrome or NICU graduates also undergo tympanostomy tube insertion at this time. We may also consider tympanostomy tube placement and an intraoperative ABR but will try to avoid this approach because we have detected discrepancies between these threshold measures and subsequent behavioral threshold responses.[55] This discrepancy may be related to a temporary threshold shift from suctioning, bleeding, inadequate removal of fluid, and/or residual inflammation from the middle-ear disease. The infant is typically evaluated 3 to 4 weeks after tube placement and undergoes otoacoustic emission testing. If the result is normal, the child will be followed in 6 months for future behavioral hearing testing. If the test is abnormal, the child may need to undergo a diagnostic ABR. Further evaluation and treatment are determined by the results of the ABR.

Auditory Neuropathy Spectrum Disorder

Auditory neuropathy spectrum disorder (ANSD) is a heterogeneous disease characterized by behavioral thresholds that do not match with other auditory measures such as ABR or speech discrimination scores. Prevalence of this condition may be up to 10% of patients previously considered to have profound SNHL.[56] There are multiple etiologies including genetics (e.g., mutation of the otoferlin or pejvakin genes), ototoxicity, anatomy (e.g., cochlear nerve hypoplasia), and hyperbilirubinemia. The auditory system is particularly sensitive to hyperbilirubinemia, with moderately elevated bilirubin levels leading to auditory neuropathy.[57] The site of pathology may involve the auditory nerve fibers, the inner hair cells, or their synapses with the auditory nerve terminals.[58] The earliest cases of ANSD were attributed to "high risk" infants—specifically premature infants admitted to the NICU or those who sustained a prolonged or difficult delivery.[59]

Diagnosis requires testing of both outer hair cell activity (OAEs and cochlear microphonics) and auditory nerve function (ABR). Typically the OAEs and cochlear microphonics are present with an absent or abnormal ABR waveform.[60] Pure tone threshold responses are variable, from normal to profound loss and with variable word recognition in quiet and generally poor responses in noise.[61] An important challenge with this condition is that a commonly used screening tool for hearing diagnosis, transient OAE, can miss this diagnosis because patients with ANSD may have emissions present. Because this condition can be found frequently in premature infants or those admitted to the NICU, automated or diagnostic ABRs must be used to screen these patients (Table 69.3).

Another important nuance of ANSD is treatment. Unlike in the typical child with SNHL, hearing aids may not be consistently helpful. Berlin et al. reported the management outcomes of 260 patients with ANSD.[60] Hearing aids were tried in 85 of these patients. Approximately 15% reported some benefit from hearing aids. Some will demonstrate hearing threshold improvement over time.[58,62] Harrison et al. reported that of 75 ANSD patients evaluated at the Hospital for Sick Children in Toronto, 1 in 5 showed some threshold recovery that allowed adequate speech and language development without the need for amplification.[63] EI and regular audiological assessments are crucial. If the child has normal behavioral and speech reception thresholds, hearing aids are not indicated. If behavioral responses are poor, then we will often consider hearing aids but with a conservative stimulus to avoid high-intensity amplification. Some of these children will become candidates for cochlear implantation, although results can be unpredictable. There is a great need to develop preoperative tools that can predict cochlear candidacy and outcome. Shearer and Hansen have proposed using a nuanced molecular classification of ANSD based on the molecular site of lesion.[63a] Sharma and Cardon have proposed using cortical auditory evoked potentials as prognostic indicators of success of clinical intervention in ANSD patients.[63b]

Table 69.3 Audiologic Test Results in Auditory Neuropathy Spectrum Disorder in Children

Test	Outcome
OAEs	Typically present
Cochlear microphonics	Present
ABRs	Absent (75%) or severely abnormal
Pure tone thresholds	Normal to severe/profound hearing loss
Word recognition in quiet	Variable
Word recognition in noise	Generally poor
Middle ear muscle reflexes	Typically absent (90%)

ABR, Auditory brainstem response; *OAE,* otoacoustic emission.

From Farinetti A, Raji A, Wanna B, et al. International consensus (ICON) on audiological assessment of hearing loss in children. *European Annals of Otorhinolaryngology.* 2018;135:S46. With permission.

Definitive Diagnosis

Diagnostic Auditory Brainstem Response

If newborn screening suggests a possible hearing loss, diagnostic testing is required to confirm and characterize the severity of the loss. This is most commonly done through a threshold ABR that measures responses to clicks and frequency-specific tone-bursts. ABR testing can be a very useful noninvasive tool because estimation of pure-tone thresholds can be compared with the waveform outputs from normative data and from the child's contralateral ear.[64] Most infants under age 4 months can be tested during natural sleep and do not require sedation. Scheduling of tests near nap times, preventing sleep prior to the appointment, absence of siblings at the appointment, and feeding on arrival may all increase likelihood of a successful nonsedated ABR.[65,66] ABRs are performed by placement of electrodes on the forehead and mastoid processes and either headphones or inserts for the child's ears. The protocol for ABR varies by institution and audiologist, with the goal to obtain thresholds at as many useful frequencies as possible while the child remains asleep.[67] If hearing loss is determined, bone conduction studies should be performed to distinguish between conductive and sensorineural losses.

Behavioral Testing

Visual reinforced audiometry is the behavioral diagnostic method of choice in children who are developmentally 6 months to 2 years of age.[68] Visual reinforced audiometry involves presenting a sound to the child and rewarding appropriately timed head turns with a picture or other visual stimulus.[69] Inserts or headphones can be used to obtain ear-specific information, with inserts being preferred to avoid collapsing canals. Inserts are more reliably tolerated in children older than 18 months of age, although a number of pediatric centers have reported excellent success in obtaining individual thresholds in even younger children.[70] Ideally 500-, 1000-, 2000-, and 4000-Hz thresholds should be obtained if possible. A positive response generally requires a 90-degree head turn, and normative data by age are available for interpretation.[71]

Conditioned play audiometry is used for children developmentally 2 to 5 years of age. For this test, the child is first conditioned to ensure understanding of the task and participation. The chosen task may vary based on child interest and cooperation—for example, putting a peg in a board, tossing a block in a box, or a digital task in response to hearing a sound.[72] Again, frequencies are chosen to maximize the useful information obtained prior to patient fatigue.

Management of Newborns With SNHL

To provide adequate management of these patients, it is important to identify the etiology of their hearing loss and work as a multidisciplinary team. Each patient should undergo a thorough history and physical exam and audiogram/hearing evaluation. Studies have shown that routine laboratory evaluation of all patients has low diagnostic yield and should only be performed when there is clinical suspicion.[73,74] The only critical test that should be ordered early is cCMV testing, because this infection is the most common environmental cause of hearing loss. If cCMV testing is negative, genetic testing can be pursued in children with bilateral symmetric SNHL or imaging in children with asymmetric or unilateral hearing loss. A consensus statement published in 2016 provides an algorithm for testing of newborn SNHL (Fig. 69.2).[75]

Components of the History in an Infant With SNHL

The history of a child who fails the NHS is crucial and can help identify the etiology of hearing loss and direct hearing loss

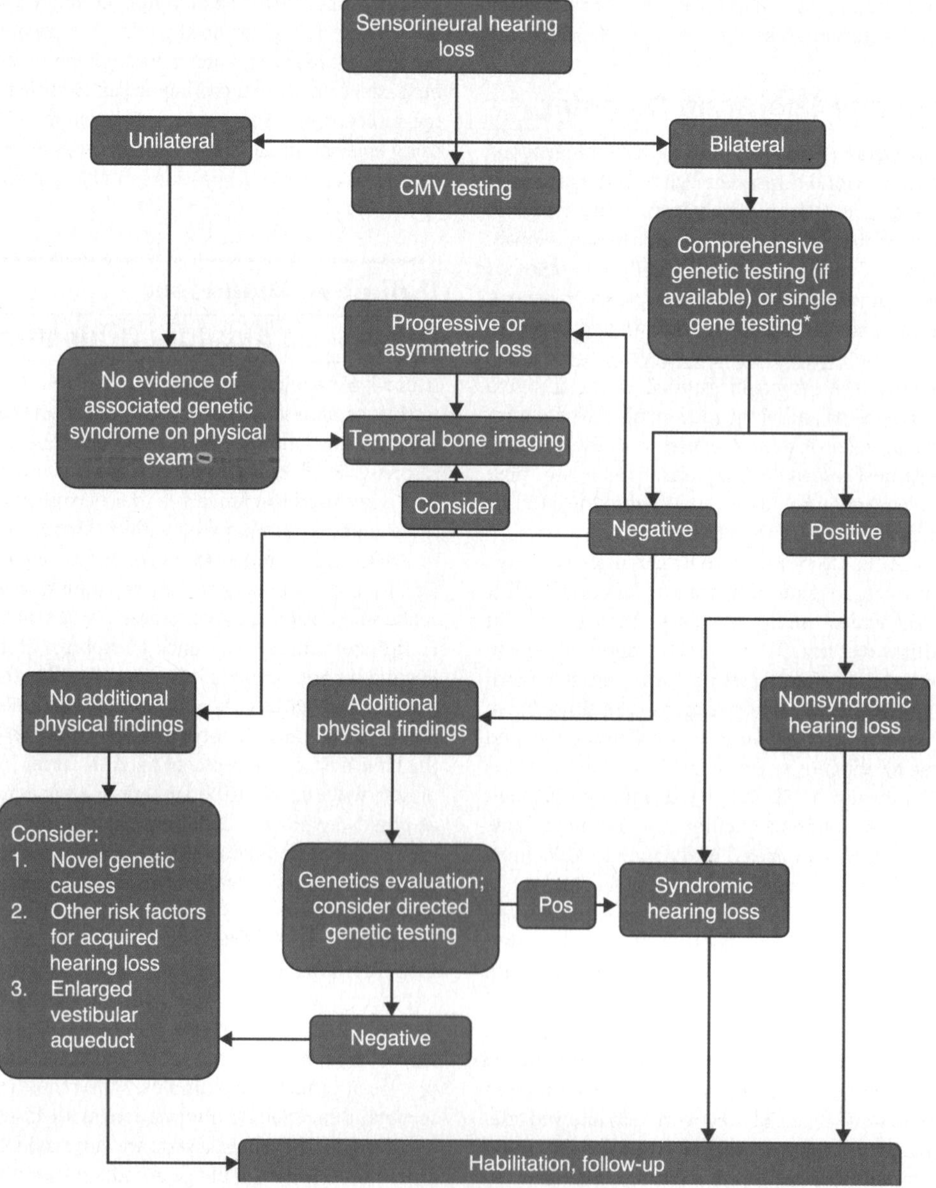

Fig. 69.2 Evaluation of Hearing Loss in Infants. *If clinical features suggest a single-gene related syndromatic diagnosis. *CMV,* Cytomegalovirus; *Pos*, positive. (From Liming BJ, Carter J, Cheng A, et al. International Pediatric Otolaryngology Group [IPOG] consensus recommendations. *Int J Pediatr Otorhinolaryngol*. 2016.)

management. It is important to ask the mother about prenatal risk factors, especially in regard to exposure to TORCH syndrome (toxoplasmosis, other agents, rubella, cytomegalovirus, or herpes simplex), smoking, alcohol use, and illicit drug and/or prescription medication use. There are also multiple factors in the birth history that in themselves are risk factors for hearing loss. Children with a history of preterm birth, severe hypoxia, intubation, low birth weight, neonatal intensive care for longer than 5 days, severe jaundice requiring blood transfusion, intravenous antibiotics (namely aminoglycosides), cCMV, renal abnormalities, craniofacial abnormalities, and/or the need for extracorporeal membrane oxygenation are at higher risk of hearing loss. It is important to obtain the presence of the above factors in the initial evaluation. Furthermore, a family history of hearing loss or sudden death is also important. If the child has a family history of hearing loss, the etiology may be genetic, and it is important to test siblings of the child. If there is a history of sudden death in the family, one should consider the possibility of Jervell and Lange-Nielsen syndrome and immediately obtain an electrocardiogram with possible cardiology referral based on the results.

Hearing Aids and Early Intervention

Once a diagnosis of hearing loss has been established, it is essential to immediately refer the child for both hearing aids and EI. EI will give children with hearing loss tools to improve speech and language and should start as soon as hearing loss is diagnosed. EI programs are available through the state for children with hearing loss who are aged 0 to 3. After the age of 3, speech services are provided to the family through the public school system.

A referral must be made to the audiologist to start the hearing aid process. Contrary to popular belief, it is never too early for a child to wear hearing aids. In fact, the earlier a child starts with hearing aids, the better their speech outcomes and acceptance of the hearing aids. The audiologist will fit the child with the proper size of hearing aids and will also frequently see the child to reevaluate hearing (with and without amplification) and ensure the hearing aids are programmed appropriately for the level of hearing loss.

Children who have severe to profound SNHL may not always benefit from hearing aids. In cases where the hearing aids are not helpful, the child may be a candidate for a cochlear implant. A cochlear implant is a surgical procedure where an electrode is inserted into the cochlea to provide a signal directly to the cochlea. Auditory rehabilitation to optimize the cochlear implant settings and learn to communicate with this device is essential to success of the surgery. Young children have the best results after cochlear implantation, even those with severe to profound hearing loss.[76]

Diagnostic Testing

Congenital Cytomegalovirus Screening, Diagnosis, and Management in Pediatric SNHL

cCMV is the most common congenital infection worldwide, the number one cause of nongenetic SNHL, and a leading cause of central nervous system defects in newborns.[77–79] While patients and their families directly experience the devastating speech and language delays associated with this disease, cCMV infection also carries a massive economic burden of approximately 4 billion dollars annually in the United States.[80]

The prevalence of cCMV varies by population but is believed to be 0.58% overall (95% CI, 0.41%–0.79%).[81] Thus, in 2018, it was estimated that approximately 20,000 infants were born with cCMV in the United States. Although approximately 10% of newborns with cCMV present with symptomatic infection at birth (jaundice, hepatosplenomegaly, hydrocephalus, petechiae, etc.), the majority (90%) are asymptomatic. Within this asymptomatic cohort, between 9.4% and 16.3% either present with or develop SNHL over time.[81] Because this group lacks overt signs of an infection, patients with CMV-induced SNHL who are otherwise asymptomatic are at risk for delayed diagnosis. Delay in diagnosis and initiation of intervention puts children at increased risk for speech, language, and learning delays.[82–84] Addressing hearing loss at the earliest age possible allows for auditory, education, speech, and potentially medical intervention while the child is still in early stages of development.[83,84]

Critically, to diagnose most forms of cCMV, infants need to be identified through CMV screening. Screening requires testing of saliva or urine via DNA detection of the virus through polymerase chain reaction (PCR) or via a culture before 3 weeks of age. Later testing *cannot* distinguish congenital from postnatal infection, which does not cause SNHL. Saliva is easier to collect; however, there is a risk for a false-positive result, presumably from breast milk.[85,86] For that reason, it is recommended that saliva testing be delayed at least 90 minutes after breastfeeding.[87] Even with this approach, false positives have been observed by our team. Although urine is more difficult to obtain, it may be a better test because results are not confounded in breastfed infants. Currently, a confirmatory urine sample should be done whenever a child is found to have a positive saliva PCR CMV result.[87,88]

A child older than 3 weeks of age can potentially be diagnosed via CMV-DNA detection of archived neonatal dry blood spots (DBSs) (samples are obtained for all newborns in the United States). This approach has several drawbacks because the blood spots are often not well maintained, are only stored for a short period of time, or are inaccessible. The other limitation is the sensitivity of the assay, which has been reported to be as low as 28%.[89] There is an ongoing CDC-funded study comparing saliva CMV PCR to DBS PCR.[90] Of 12,554 individuals enrolled, 56 newborns were confirmed to have cCMV. Combined DBS results from either of the 2 institutions demonstrated a sensitivity of 85.7%.[90] This study indicates a higher analytical sensitivity compared with prior studies and suggests that as more-sensitive PCR methods emerge, DBS-based screening may become a viable, low-cost screening option in the future.

The efficacy of different approaches to screen for the presence of congenital CMV is debated. Examples of these approaches include universal CMV screening of all newborns, targeted screening based on clinically evident symptoms present at birth, and hearing-targeted screening for infants who fail their NHS. A hearing-targeted cCMV screening approach (HT-cCMV) was initiated at Parkland Memorial Hospital 19 years ago.[79] The outcomes of this approach over a 5-year period (1999–2004) showed that 5% of infants (24 of 483) who failed their NHS and were screened for cCMV tested positive for the presence of the virus. In this study, the majority of infants with cCMV-induced hearing loss (75%) were identified to have this infection based only on their abnormal NHS.[79]

A similar approach was implemented statewide in Utah. A retrospective review of 509 infants who failed their NHS in Utah in 2017, 24 months after the enactment of HT-cCMV legislation, showed that 62% of the infants were tested for cCMV within 21 days of birth. Of this group, 6% (14 of 234) tested positive for cCMV. Of the 14 infants with CMV-positive PCR results, 6 (43%) were shown to have SNHL.[91] Despite an incomplete assessment of all infants who failed their NHS (62%), 14 infants were diagnosed with cCMV and likely would not have been identified without the implementation of HT-cCMV screening in Utah. Of note, the odds of achieving a timely diagnostic hearing evaluation (≤90 days) increased from 56% to 77% after the implementation of this hearing-targeted approach. This result suggests improvement in the timing of the diagnostic workup for all infants who fail their NHS. Delays in the diagnosis and treatment of hearing loss are a major challenge for all UNHS programs and can have adverse repercussions for speech and language development.[11,92–96]

In addition to clinical demand and potential childhood health benefits, the cost-effectiveness of these screening methods must be considered. Gantt et al.[96a] described the expected costs and outcomes of universal and HT-cCMV screening. To identify one case of cCMV-associated hearing loss, this study estimated costs at $27,460 by universal screening or $975 by targeted screening. This study describes a model that provides evidence for a net cost benefit in the use of an HT-cCMV approach in screening for cCMV.

Although a comparison of the cost-effectiveness between universal and HT-cCMV screening methods is necessary, it is important to consider the practicality of each method. A universal approach would require the screening of approximately 4 million newborns, which could be a labor-intensive undertaking. The HT-cCMV testing approach would involve between 52 to 80,000 newborns (1.4%–2% failure rate of newborn hearing screening [NBHS]),[53,97,98] a more manageable population to screen for symptoms of cCMV-related hearing loss. Either approach, however, requires an adequate infrastructure for successful screening.

A supplemental approach that may be used to improve detection of cCMV-infected infants involves a protocol that would initiate CMV testing in infants who present with known signs or symptoms of this infection. Prior studies have reported poor detection in centers that lack a screening protocol for symptomatic CMV-infected newborns.[82] The impact is problematic, because ganciclovir and valganciclovir have been shown to improve hearing and neurocognitive outcomes in symptomatic newborns and are currently recommended for newborns with confirmed cCMV and involvement of at least one end organ.[99,100] Since 2016, this targeted approach has been implemented at two large birth hospitals and three NICUs in Utah.[101] In addition to failed NHS, infants with microcephaly, intrauterine growth restriction, unexplained hepatosplenomegaly, transaminase elevation, petechial rash, persistent thrombocytopenia, or intracranial abnormalities (e.g., calcifications, polymicrogyria) undergo screening for cCMV. Out of 349 patients who underwent screening, 19 tested positive for CMV (5.4%). Currently, the results indicate that 19 symptomatic infants were diagnosed with cCMV, and without this program, they may not have been diagnosed appropriately.

Implementation of this expanded targeted cCMV screening approach for symptomatic infants is currently being implemented at all university and intermountain hospitals in Utah and Idaho. Parkland Hospital in Dallas, Texas, follows a similar approach, completing CMV testing in clinically symptomatic infants, those who do not pass newborn hearing screening (HT-CMV screening), and infants born to HIV-positive mothers.[79,102] In a 5-year review of this protocol (conducted in 2010), 50 infants were identified with cCMV. Of these, 22 were identified due to clinical signs (symptomatic), 19 due to failed newborn hearing screening, and 9 due to maternal HIV infection.[102] Future studies on this approach will need to be performed to determine its impact.

Once a child is diagnosed with cCMV, a multidisciplinary approach is recommended to determine the severity and extent of disease.[103] A head ultrasound is performed in children without obvious central nervous system involvement; MRI is performed if the ultrasound is abnormal or for children with central nervous system signs. The battery includes a complete blood count with differential, comprehensive metabolic profile, ophthalmology evaluation, EI, and a diagnostic ABR study. We categorize the groups into asymptomatic, isolated SNHL, or symptomatic (Fig. 69.3).

Genetics

Genetic mutations are the most common cause of SNHL. There are more than 130 genes and nearly 8000 genetic variations associated with nonsyndromic deafness.[104] For many years, single-gene testing was favored; however, single-gene sequencing is costly and time consuming and has a relatively low diagnostic yield compared with massively parallel sequencing, which is becoming the standard of care for the genetic evaluation of children with SNHL. The expected yield from genetic testing has continued to improve. The Genetics of Hearing Loss Clinic at the Children's Hospital of Philadelphia reported on their outcomes of 660 individuals with hearing loss between July 2008 and July 2015.[105] Testing included a single-nucleotide polymorphism chromosomal microarray and a hearing loss next-generation sequencing panel. Six hundred twelve patients (93%) presented with a nonsyndromic form of hearing loss. Of those with syndromic presentations, Usher and Waardenburg syndromes were the most commonly noted. A definitive diagnosis was established in 23.8% of tested patients using molecular analyses, clinical examination, and laboratory testing. We suggest that patients with idiopathic bilateral congenital hearing loss who are cCMV negative and with no obvious syndromic features be worked up with genetic testing. Children with unilateral hearing loss should undergo genetic testing only if they are cCMV negative and have normal imaging.

Imaging

Radiologic imaging is an integral component for evaluation of pediatric SNHL, because approximately 27.4% to 49% of infants will have radiologic abnormalities.[106–109] There are two main types of radiographic testing of the temporal bones: high-resolution CT (HRCT) and MRI. Both of these modalities have advantages and disadvantages. CT has been the more commonly used modality because of low cost, rapid image capture, decreased sedation needs, and provision of superior bone detail. MRI, on the other hand, has better soft-tissue detail and no radiation exposure.[110] There is no clear consensus regarding which test should be used, and it is usually patient and provider dependent, in most cases.

Historically, HRCT has been considered the investigation of choice for patients with hearing loss due to its ability to provide superior detail of the bony labyrinth.[111–113] However, approximately 57% of soft-tissue abnormalities of the inner ear may not be identified with a CT scan.[114] This result is especially important when determining the presence or absence of the cochlear nerve.[113] Clemmens et al. have reported that 26% of children with unilateral SNHL will have a hypoplastic cochlear nerve.[115] Although cochlear nerve canal stenosis has previously been used to predict the integrity of the cochlear nerve, it is not always sensitive enough.[112,116]

Recently, MRI of the internal auditory canal has become the more popular imaging modality. Despite the length and expense of the test compared with HRCT, avoiding ionizing radiation and visualizing the cochlear nerve are compelling reasons for ordering this study. The diameter of the cochlear nerve is especially important when a cochlear implant is being considered. An absent cochlear nerve is a relative contraindication for cochlear implantation, because a functioning cochlear nerve is critical for a successful outcome. Children with hypoplastic cochlear nerves will have poorer hearing outcomes compared with those with normal-sized nerves.[117]

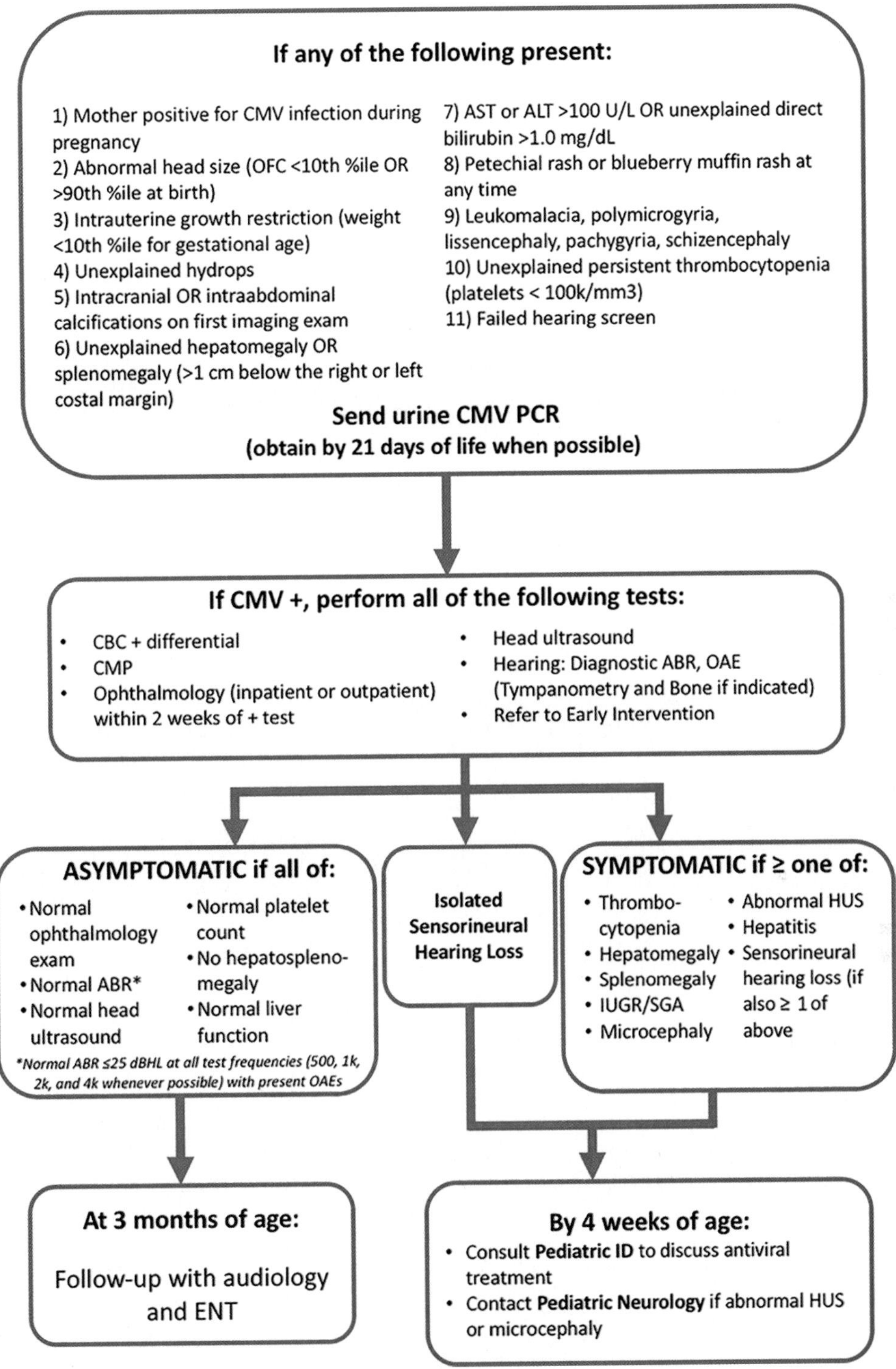

Fig. 69.3 Cytomegalovirus Workup. *%ile*, Percentile; *ALT*, alanine transaminase; *AST*, aspartate transaminase; *CBC*, complete blood count; *CMP*, comprehensive metabolic panel; *ENT*, ear, nose and throat; *HUS*, head ultrasound; *ID*, infectious disease; *IUGR*, intrauterine growth retardation; *OFC*, fronto-occipital circumference; *PCR*, polymerase chain reaction; *SGA*, small for gestational age. (From Early detection and diagnosis of infant hearing loss. *Cummings Otolaryngology Head and Neck Surgery*. 2020. With permission.)

Imaging is recommended as the first diagnostic test in the following circumstances: asymmetric, unilateral, or progressive SNHL or auditory neuropathy. The most common radiographic abnormality is an enlarged vestibular aqueduct, which is associated with progressive SNHL and Pendred syndrome. The most common radiographic abnormality for unilateral SNHL is a hypoplastic cochlear nerve. Therefore, in our opinion, MRI should be the initial imaging modality of choice in this patient population. There is no clear consensus on when imaging should be obtained; it is provider dependent and usually depends on patient factors and sedation needs.

Conclusion

During the past decade there have been significant changes in management of pediatric hearing loss. Newborns should be screened for hearing loss prior to 1 month of age, and this is happening in over 95% of cases in most states. However, there continue to be significant issues with loss to follow-up for confirmatory audiologic testing and for EI. Recent cCMV initiatives have shown promise in improving the rates of loss to follow-up. The implementation of targeted cCMV testing has identified cases of previously missed cCMV and improved time to diagnosis and treatment in all children who fail their NHS. Also, the improvement in both imaging technology and genetic testing has helped identify the etiology of hearing loss in more children. Most importantly, earlier hearing aid use and cochlear implantation have significantly improved speech and language outcomes for young children, even those with profound hearing loss.

CHAPTER 70

Nasal Obstruction in Newborn Infants

Marisa A. Ryan, David E. Tunkel

KEY POINTS

1. Nasal obstruction in neonates can cause respiratory distress and feeding difficulty, as newborns rely heavily on nasal breathing.
2. Mild cases of nasal obstruction can be observed, but severe obstructive lesions can be life-threatening and usually require early surgical intervention.
3. Further workup may be needed to identify any associated conditions and syndromes.
4. Neonatal rhinitis may respond to short-term intranasal corticosteroid treatment.
5. Early reduction of severe neonatal nasal septal deformity can relieve nasal airway obstruction.
6. Ophthalmology and otolaryngology evaluations are helpful for the management of dacryocystoceles.
7. Infants with congenital pyriform nasal aperture stenosis and midnasal stenosis can often be observed, but severe cases of obstruction may require intranasal surgery with stenting.
8. Choanal atresia is usually repaired through a transnasal endoscopic approach, and bilateral choanal atresia is repaired in the neonatal period.
9. A neonate with an intranasal mass requires imaging with computed tomography and/or magnetic resonance imaging before biopsy or excision to define anatomy and look for intracranial extension.

Introduction

Neonates are generally considered obligate, or at least preferential, nasal breathers.[1] The neonatal upper airway anatomy predisposes to such obligate nasal breathing (Fig. 70.1). The tongue sits in contact with the soft and hard palate, which obstructs oral breathing. The larynx is higher, putting the epiglottis superior to the soft palate and separating the nasal breathing passage from the passage of liquid from the mouth. This neonatal anatomy maximizes the ability to breathe during oral feeding. Neonatal nasal obstruction may not be apparent until respiratory difficulties are noted during oral feeding. Nasal obstruction in a newborn usually requires prompt evaluation, typically with otolaryngology consultation. Although the potential underlying causes of nasal obstruction are numerous, congenital and traumatic causes are most common (Table 70.1).

The following causes of neonatal nasal obstruction will be reviewed more in depth: neonatal rhinitis, nasal septal deviation, nasolacrimal duct cyst/dacryocystocele, congenital nasal pyriform aperture stenosis (CNPAS), midnasal stenosis, choanal atresia, and midline congenital nasal masses.

General Clinical Features and Recommended Evaluations for Neonatal Nasal Obstruction

Neonatal nasal obstruction can present with various signs of abnormal breathing and feeding (Table 70.2).

Initial Examination

When nasal obstruction is suspected, examination should begin with evaluation of the external nasal and facial appearance. The exam should focus on the nasal contour and identifying any other facial anomalies. Anterior rhinoscopy can be performed with an otoscope or nasal speculum. Attempts should be made to pass a 5 or 6 French suction catheter through each side of the nose into the nasopharynx. Because these catheters may coil in the nose against an obstruction, visualizing the catheter in the posterior pharynx is reassuring. Attempts to pass a catheter should not be made if there is any concern for a skull base defect. An alternative is the mirror test, where a mirror is placed in front of each nostril; fog should appear if the nasal airway is patent. If a catheter cannot be passed or other concerning findings are present, then an otolaryngology consultation should be obtained.

Nasal Endoscopy

The consulting otolaryngologist will likely examine the nasal cavities and nasopharynx with nasal endoscopy with a flexible fiberoptic scope. This is a simple bedside procedural examination that can be performed without sedation and with minimal risks. Endoscopy may be done before and after decongesting with topical oxymetazoline or phenylephrine to determine the impact of mucosal edema compared with a fixed, anatomic obstruction.

Imaging

Imaging is usually performed before surgical intervention on any nasal mass or congenital obstruction, with the exception of septal deviation. Computed tomography (CT) scan is best to delineate bony anatomy and is usually the best initial study when CNPAS, midnasal stenosis, or choanal atresia are suspected. Magnetic resonance imaging (MRI) is preferred for lesions that may extend intracranially, such as dermoid cysts, gliomas, or encephaloceles (Table 70.3).

Fetal imaging, including ultrasound and/or MRI, may suggest craniofacial anomalies or airway obstruction prior to delivery. When severe anomalies are present and airway obstruction at delivery is predicted, ex-utero intrapartum treatment at delivery can be planned to secure the airway while maintaining maternal-fetal circulation before completing delivery.[2] Ex-utero intrapartum treatment is not usually needed for anomalies that are limited to the nose.

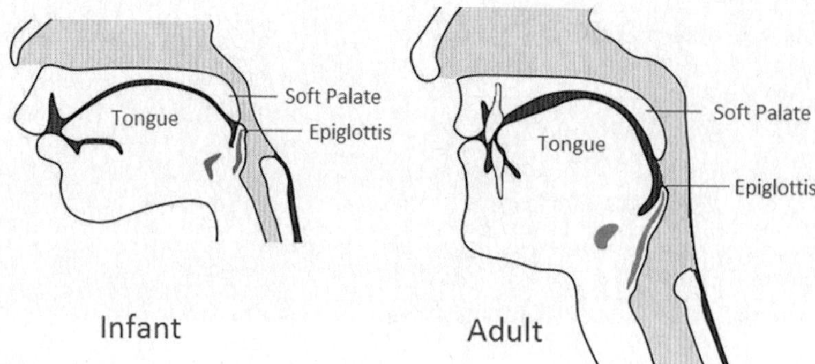

Fig. 70.1 Anatomic Comparison Between the Infant and Adult Airway. (From Kwong KM. Current updates on choanal atresia. *Front Pediatr.* 2015;3:52. Copyright © 2015 Kwong. This is an open-access article distributed under the terms of the Creative Commons Attribution License [CC BY]. The use, distribution, or reproduction in other forums is permitted, provided the original authors(s) or licensor are credited and that the original publication in this journal is cited, in accordance with accepted academic practice. No use, distribution, or reproduction is permitted which does not comply with these terms.)

Table 70.1 Differential Diagnosis of Nasal Obstruction

Congenital
- Nasolacrimal duct cyst/dacryocystocele
- Midnasal stenosis
- Congenital pyriform aperture stenosis (CNPAS)
- Choanal atresia
- Midfacial hypoplasia
- Nasal hypoplasia
- Nasal dermoid
- Glioma
- Encephalocele
- Thornwaldt cyst
- Cleft lip nasal deformity

Traumatic
- Nasal septal deviation from intrauterine pressure or difficult delivery

Iatrogenic
- Nasal septal deviation from assisted delivery
- Irritation and scarring from:
  - traumatic nasal suctioning
  - nasal cannula or noninvasive positive pressure ventilation prongs
  - nasogastric tubes
- Rhinitis medicamentosa from long-term topical decongestant use

Infectious
- Viral or bacterial upper respiratory infection
- Vertical transmission of sexually transmitted infection (chlamydia, gonorrhea, syphilis)
- Neoplasms
- Teratoma
- Hamartoma
- Sarcoma
- Neurofibroma
- Lipoma
- Chordoma
- Lymphoma
- Hemangioma
- Lymphovascular malformations

Endocrine
- Rhinitis from circulating maternal estrogen
- Hypothyroidism

Other
- Rhinitis
- Idiopathic

Evaluation for Other Airway and Pulmonary Lesions

Additional airway or pulmonary abnormalities should be identified. Stridor, wheezing, and persistent hypoxia are unusual for isolated nasal obstruction and should raise suspicion for another condition.

Table 70.2 Clinical Signs of Neonatal Nasal Obstruction
Noisy breathing—stertor or snoring
Grunting or snorting
Nasal flaring
Retractions
Cyclic respiratory distress that is temporarily relieved with crying
Perioral cyanosis, may be cyclic
Apnea
Difficulty feeding
Nasal drainage
Inability to pass a suction or scope through the nose and into the pharynx
External nasal deformity
Epiphora

Table 70.3 Indications for MRI in Evaluation of Neonatal Nasal Obstruction

- Evaluate for holoprosencephaly and pituitary deficiency in CNPAS
- Evaluate for an intracranial connection and better characterize any midline nasal mass
- Better evaluate intracranial anatomy after suspicious intracranial findings on initial CT

CNPAS, Congenital nasal pyriform aperture stenosis; *CT,* computed tomography; *MRI,* magnetic resonance imaging.

Pulmonary/Sleep Medicine Consultations

In cases of mild or unilateral nasal obstruction, the need for and timing of intervention may be unclear. Polysomnography can be performed to determine the severity of obstruction during sleep and the presence of apnea/hypopnea, oxygen desaturation, or hypercarbia. A normal polysomnogram can support initial observation rather than early surgery for newborns with low-grade nasal obstruction.

Swallowing/Feeding Evaluation

Many neonates with nasal obstruction may not be able to coordinate breathing and effective swallowing. Swallowing dysfunction can persist even after treatment of the nasal obstruction.[3] A clinical swallowing assessment by a speech-language pathologist or occupational therapist should be considered, supplemented by a videofluoroscopic swallow study or fiberoptic endoscopic evaluation of swallowing when swallow dysfunction is apparent. Severe feeding difficulties may indicate earlier surgery for correctable nasal lesions.

Gastroenterology

Gastroesophageal reflux (GERD) is seen in many newborns with airway obstruction. Airway obstruction for nasal pathology can increase intrathoracic pressure and worsen GERD. Untreated GERD may contribute to restenosis of a nasal obstruction after surgical management if refluxate comes in contact with the healing surgical site. Pharmacologic and nonpharmacologic management of GERD should be considered, as well as gastroenterology consultation in recalcitrant cases.

Genetics

Genetics evaluation with appropriate testing is indicated for many neonates with nasal obstruction as we recognize the association of some nasal pathology with syndromic diagnoses. Specific indications will be reviewed in this chapter as related to specific clinical findings.

Considerations for Initial Management of Neonatal Nasal Obstruction

Initial management of any critical nasal airway obstruction involves maintaining an adequate airway with either appropriate positioning, an oral airway, a McGovern nipple (an oropharyngeal airway made by cutting off the end of a large feeding nipple and securing it in the mouth with tape around the head), or intubation. When using an oral airway or McGovern nipple, feeding can be done with intermittent removal of the airway or with gavage feeds. Nasal trumpets (for newborns with narrow but not totally occluded nasal airways), and noninvasive positive pressure ventilation can be used to temporize until definitive treatment or resolution of the obstruction.

Epidemiology, Pathophysiology, Clinical Features, Evaluation, and Management of More Common Causes of Neonatal Nasal Obstruction

Neonatal Rhinitis

Epidemiology

Neonatal rhinitis is considered the most common cause of neonatal nasal obstruction.[4] More neonates present with this in the fall and winter months.[5] There is no apparent race or gender propensity.[5]

Pathophysiology

Inflammation of the nasal mucosa in neonatal rhinitis can range from mild to severe and be due to both maternal and neonatal factors (Table 70.4).[2,6,7]

Clinical Features

Anterior rhinoscopy and nasal endoscopy show edematous nasal mucosa and rhinorrhea. However, a 5 or 6 French suction catheter can still be passed through the edematous soft tissue.

Table 70.4 Etiologic Factors in Neonatal Rhinitis
Viral upper respiratory infection
Vertical transmission of sexually transmitted infection (chlamydia, gonorrhea, syphilis)
Maternal estrogen
Maternal medications (methimazole, methyldopa, opiates, tricyclic antidepressants, propranolol)
Maternal cocaine
Cow's milk allergy
Gastroesophageal reflux
Cystic fibrosis
Kartagener's syndrome
Hypothyroidism
Idiopathic

Evaluation/Management

Close observation is recommended because resolution is common. A short trial of topical decongestant (oxymetazoline or phenylephrine) may be helpful. Phenylephrine has been given safely to infants 3 weeks to 12 months of age for viral bronchitis in a randomized controlled trial.[8] Hemodynamic effects on blood pressure and heart rate have been seen intraoperatively and postoperatively with oxymetazoline use in surgery.[9] Oxymetazoline has been given safely to children in an observational study of nasolacrimal surgery and a randomized controlled trial of nasal surgeries on the sinuses, turbinate, and adenoids, but clinical studies have not evaluated it in neonates.[10,11] These medications should be dosed judiciously in neonates who are also being clinically monitored. Regular use of topical decongestants for more than a few days should be avoided because of the risk of causing rhinitis medicamentosa with worsened nasal obstruction.[12]

Nasal saline drops and suction can help, especially in the setting of thick or dried nasal drainage. If breathing and feeding do not improve, then dexamethasone ophthalmic drops in the nose usually result in a rapid improvement over days.[5] The majority of 20 neonatal intensive care unit patients in one case series showed improvement with this stepwise medical management of nasal saline and topical decongestants and then a topical steroid for persistent symptoms.[5] Imaging is not usually needed but is reserved for cases where symptoms persist and other obstructive lesions need to be ruled out.

Long-Term Outcomes

Resolution is expected over time with appropriate medical management.

Nasal and Septal Deviation

Epidemiology

The incidence of neonatal nasal septal deviation ranges from 0.6% to 31%, but some of these cases may be asymptomatic and go unnoticed.[13] It is more common after "difficult" vaginal deliveries.[14] Significant dislocation of the nasal septum off the maxillary groove occurs less frequently, in 0.6% to 0.93% of neonates.[15]

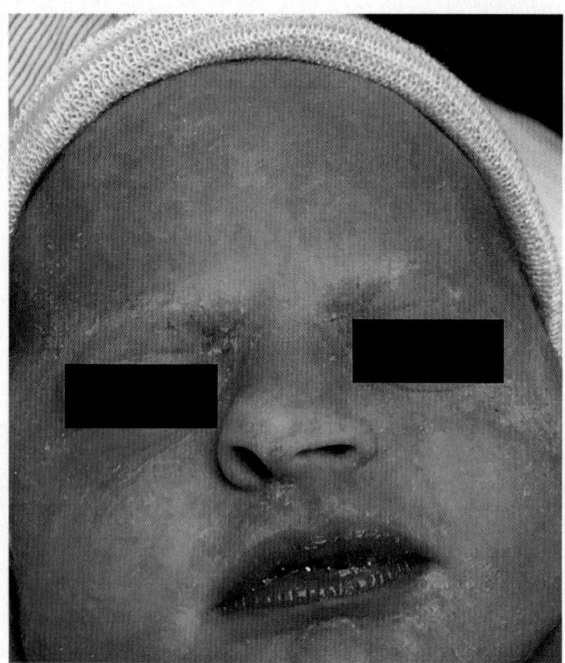

Fig. 70.2 Nasal and Septal Deviation in a Neonate Attributed to Intrauterine Forces After an Atraumatic Cesarean Section Delivery.

Pathophysiology

Septal deviation can develop from in-utero pressure, pressure during delivery, or iatrogenic force during assisted deliveries.[16]

Clinical Features

In nasal and septal deviation there is lateral deviation of the nasal tip, asymmetry of the nostrils, an oblique position of the columella, and easy flattening of the nasal tip with pressure (Fig. 70.2).

Evaluation/Management

External inspection and palpation are followed by anterior rhinoscopy. Nasal endoscopy maybe indicated to evaluate posterior deviations. A CT scan is usually not necessary. Minor degrees of septal deviation often improve within weeks without any treatment.

Severe symptomatic septal deviations can be corrected with early closed reduction at the bedside. This can be done with a curved hemostat shielded with rubber catheters without general anesthesia.[17] This has also been successfully performed in neonates in the operating room under general anesthesia with short-term nasal packing.[18] The benefits of resolving the nasal obstruction under anesthesia need to be weighed with the risk of anesthesia in the neonatal period. In rare cases of severe deviation that cannot be reduced with closed reduction, operative septoplasty in neonates has been described with favorable results maintained through infancy.[14]

Long-Term Outcomes

Nasal septal deviation may lead to compromised nasal breathing, snoring, sinusitis, epistaxis, eustachian tube dysfunction, and cosmetic concerns. A study of closed nasal septal reduction during the first 2 days of life found 46 of 49 children had satisfactory anatomic and functional results, with a follow-up period of 13 years.[17] Interestingly, one study described no significant functional or cosmetic differences over 8 years of follow-up between patients who were corrected early, those who were not corrected, and control individuals who did not have any nasal septal deformity at birth.[19]

Nasolacrimal Duct Cyst/Dacryocystocele

Epidemiology

Nasolacrimal duct obstruction is a common condition affecting up to 30% of neonates.[20] In contrast, a dacryocystocele in the nasal cavity, associated with nasolacrimal duct blockage, is much less common. Congenital dacryocystocele was diagnosed in 1 in 3884 births in one US population.[21] They are usually unilateral, but bilateral cases have been reported.[22–24]

Pathophysiology

With most nasolacrimal duct obstruction there is a single site of obstruction in the nasolacrimal system. Most cases resolve spontaneously without intervention or with conservative measures. In contrast, persistent nasolacrimal duct cysts likely occur from additional, more distal obstruction at the valve of Hasner, likely due to a persistent membrane after in-utero lacrimal system canalization. This results in a cyst in the anterior-inferior nasal cavity (Fig. 70.3).

Clinical Features

Anterior rhinoscopy or nasal endoscopy shows a cystic mass in the inferior meatus (Fig. 70.4). There can be a visible and palpable bluish mass or swelling near the medial canthus and epiphora. Dacryocystitis or preseptal cellulitis may develop if the fluid contained in the cyst becomes infected. Unilateral cases rarely require urgent intervention, but bilateral large cysts can cause respiratory compromise in newborns and are addressed promptly.

Evaluation/Management

Dacryocystoceles are evaluated with otolaryngology and ophthalmology consultations. Conservative treatment with a combination of massage and warm compresses can be used for nasolacrimal duct obstruction without nasal extension. A CT of the midface and orbits is the preferred imaging modality. A CT scan will detail the dilated nasolacrimal duct, an intranasal cyst, and a medially displaced

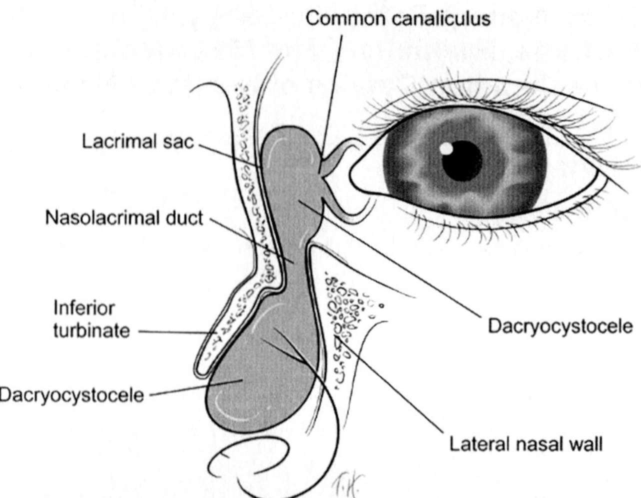

Fig. 70.3 Schematic Drawing of a Left Congenital Dacryocystocele Extending Into the Nasal Cavity and Displacing the Inferior Turbinate Medially. (From Fig. 2 in Becker BB. The treatment of congenital dacryocystocele. *Am J Ophthalmol*. 2006;142:835–838. Epub September 20, 2006.)

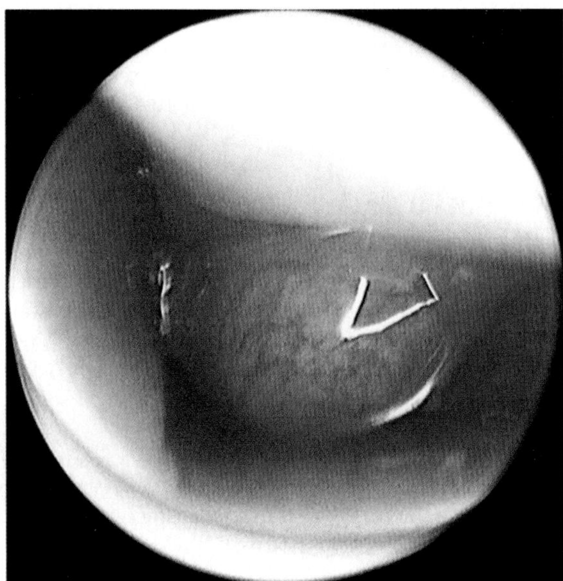

Fig. 70.4 Endoscopic View of a Left Dacryocystocele Lateral and Inferior to the Inferior Turbinate Resulting in Superomedial Displacement of the Turbinate. (From Fig. 7 in Gnagi SH, Schraff SA. Nasal obstruction in newborns. *Pediatr Clin North Am.* 2013;60:903–922. doi: 10.1016/j.pcl.2013.04.007. PubMed PMID: 23905827. Epub July 3, 2013. Review.)

inferior turbinate (Fig. 70.5). In some cases, probing of the duct and puncture of the intranasal cyst through the lacrimal puncta may resolve the obstruction. Systemic antibiotics should be started if dacryocystitis or preseptal cellulitis develops.

If the cyst does not resolve or there is substantial nasal obstruction, the cyst should be marsupialized or excised using transnasal endoscopic instrumentation. Intraoperatively an ophthalmologist will often probe the lacrimal system. In a recent case series, half of the neonates tolerated an endoscopic intranasal cyst marsupialization and nasolacrimal duct probing at the bedside without general anesthesia, with excellent results at 6 months.[25]

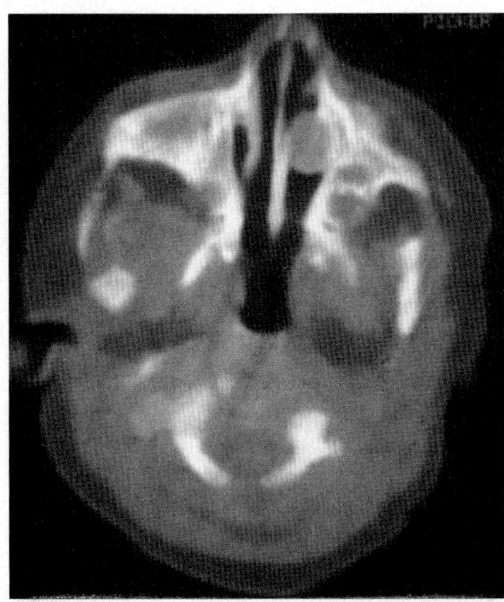

Fig. 70.5 Axial Computed Tomography Scan of Nasolacrimal Duct Cyst. (From Fig. 7 in Rajan R, Tunkel DE. Choanal atresia and other neonatal nasal anomalies. *Clin Perinatol.* 2018;45:751–767. doi: 10.1016/j.clp.2018.07.011. Epub September 18, 2018. Review.)

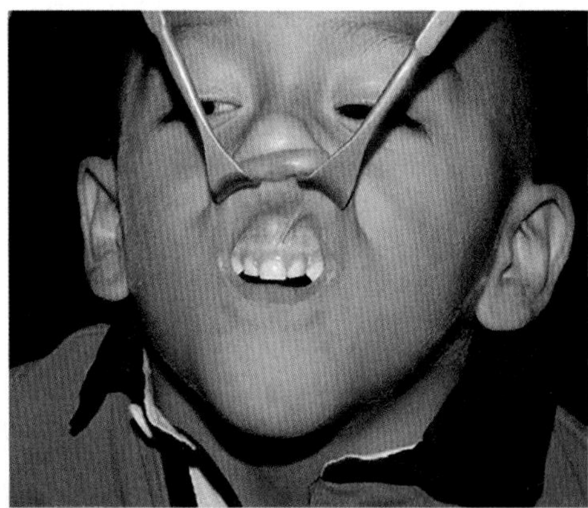

Fig. 70.6 Single Central Megaincisor in a Child With Congenital Nasal Pyriform Aperture Stenosis. (From Fig. 3 in Tate JR, Sykes J. Congenital nasal pyriform aperture stenosis. *Otolaryngol Clin North Am.* 2009;42:521–525. doi:10.1016/j.otc.2009.03.006.)

Long-Term Outcomes

Long-term outcomes have not been reported, but recurrence seems rare.

Congenital Nasal Pyriform Aperture Stenosis

Epidemiology

CNPAS is rare overall and occurs in about 1 in 25,000 births.[26] There are no reported race or sex predilections.

Pathophysiology

The pyriform aperture is the bony opening of the anterior nasal cavity. It is the narrowest portion of the nasal cavity and formed by the nasal bones, the horizontal maxillary processes, and the nasal processes of the maxilla. In CNPAS there is obstruction of the aperture from either prominent or medialized nasal processes of the maxilla. This has been postulated to occur at 4 months of gestation, when maxillary ossification occurs.

Clinical Features

CNPAS is associated with a central single megaincisor in up to 60% of cases (Fig. 70.6).[27] It is associated with several other anomalies, particularly other midline anomalies of the central nervous system (Table 70.5).[28,29]

Evaluation/Management

On anterior rhinoscopy the inferior turbinates are often seen in contact with the anterior nasal septum. Nasal endoscopy can be

Table 70.5 Anomalies Associated With Congenital Nasal Pyriform Aperture Stenosis
Central single megaincisor
Absent upper lip frenulum
Submucous cleft palate
Hypoplastic maxillary sinuses
Absence of anterior pituitary
Holoprosencephaly
Absent corpus callosum

performed to evaluate the posterior nasal airway, but even the small 2.7-mm scopes may not fit through the pyriform aperture. A CT scan will define the bony anatomy (Fig. 70.7).

Concomitant central nervous system issues may cause disorders of respiration that do not improve even with correction of the nasal aperture size. This should be considered to avoid unnecessary interventions and to help predict surgical outcomes. Pituitary dysfunction is present in up to 40% of CNPAS, and its identification is important to minimize perioperative risk, particularly hypoglycemia, and ensure appropriate follow-up.[30,31] Endocrine testing and follow-up should be considered in patients with CNPAS.[31] Genetic evaluation should also be considered, especially when midface anomalies and a central megaincisor are found.

Initial medical treatment includes humidified air, atraumatic suctioning, a topical decongestant and/or steroid drops, and close observation.[29] This is advocated for at least 2 weeks if possible.[32] If respiratory support is needed, feeding difficulties are present, or failure to thrive occurs, then surgical intervention is indicated, but many cases do not require surgery.[33] A pyriform aperture of <11 mm is considered diagnostic for CNPAS, but this does not solely determine the need for surgical correction. Different case series suggest that widths less than 5.5 to 6.3 mm will likely need surgery.[29,34–36] However a systematic review of CNPAS concluded that the size of the aperture alone did not predict the need for surgery.[33] One case series suggested that additional measurements of the angle between the anterior maxilla and the anterior-posterior nasal axis may predict need for surgical management.[37] In some cases of CNPAS there is also nasal cavity narrowing posterior to the pyriform aperture that requires management.[38]

Surgery involves drilling away the prominent maxillary nasal processes through a sublabial approach. Indwelling nasal stents or packs are usually left up to weeks after surgery to allow swelling to resolve. The stents can occlude and even cause anterior nasal necrosis if not carefully cleaned and monitored. Postoperative saline instillation and steroid drops are used to prevent granulation and restenosis.[39] A case report showed no complications and good long-term outcomes with off-label placement of a steroid-eluting stent (designed to keep the sinus ostia patent after sinus surgery in adults) rather than traditional nasal trumpet or endotracheal tube stents.[40] This off-label medical device use may show promise but needs further study.

A sublabial approach can be avoided in some cases. In one series, endonasal dilation with Hegar cervical dilators was successful.[41] Endonasal balloon dilation with postoperative stenting with nasal trumpets has also been described.[42] Rapid expansion of the maxilla/nasal base with an expansion device fixed to the palate has been successful in one reported case.[43]

Long-Term Outcomes

CNPAS tends to improve with time because nasal cavity growth follows craniofacial growth. Therefore good long-term outcomes can be expected, and recurrence has not been reported after early success with surgery.

Midnasal Stenosis

Epidemiology

A diagnosis of midnasal stenosis may be overlooked because there is less awareness of it compared with other forms of congenital bony nasal obstruction, that is, CNPAS and choanal atresia. The exact incidence is not known, but it is likely less common than CNPAS and choanal atresia.

Pathophysiology

Midnasal stenosis occurs from overgrowth of the lateral nasal sidewalls or excessive thickening of the nasal septum midway through the intranasal cavity.

Clinical Features

Midnasal stenosis is identified by bony nasal obstruction with a patent pyriform nasal aperture and choanae. It can be an isolated condition, but it is often seen in newborns with fetal alcohol syndrome, midface hypoplasia, CNPAS, and syndromic craniosynostoses.[44]

Evaluation/Management

A scope can be passed beyond the anterior end of the inferior turbinate, but the middle turbinate cannot be visualized despite the absence of septal deviation. Surgical management is reserved for failures after medical treatment and observation. Dilation with rigid dilators and subsequent stenting for weeks has been successful in a case report.[45] Endoscopic surgery can be performed and is aimed at lateralizing the inferior turbinates with postoperative nasal stenting.[46]

Long-Term Outcomes

Long-term results of interventions for midnasal stenosis are not known given the infrequency of this condition.

Choanal Atresia/Stenosis

Epidemiology

Choanal atresia occurs in approximately 1 of 5000 to 8000 live births.[47–49] It is twice as common in girls than boys.[49–51] Unilateral choanal atresia is more common than bilateral, accounting for 48%

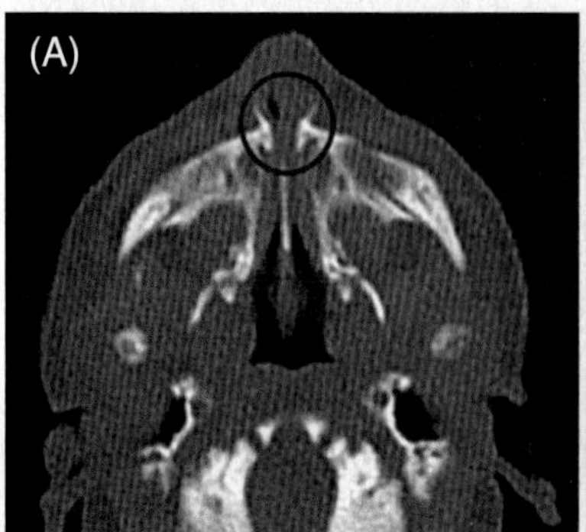

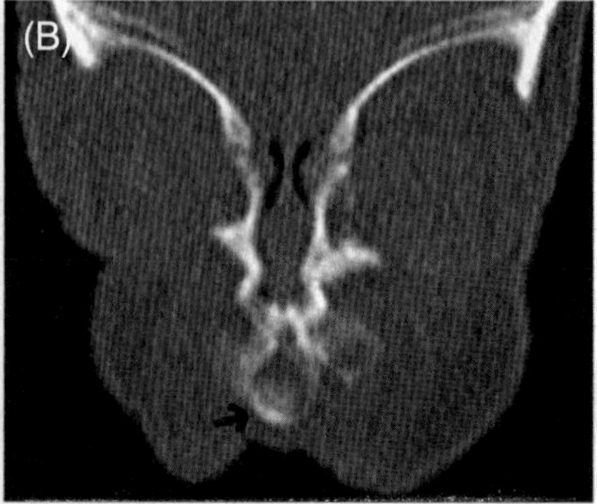

Fig. 70.7 Axial (A) and coronal (B) computed tomography of a neonate with congenital nasal pyriform aperture stenosis measuring 3 mm in diameter at its narrowest and a solitary central incisor *(black arrow)*.

to 75% of cases.[51–53] Bilateral cases are often associated with other anomalies.[54]

Pathophysiology

Choanal atresia is a complete blockage between the posterior nasal cavity and the nasopharynx. This is believed to occur when either the buccopharyngeal or nasobuccal membranes do not involute during embryologic development.[53,55] Lack of retinoic acid during development,[56,57] activation of fibroblast growth factor,[57,58] and maternal use of thionamides have been implicated in the development of choanal atresia.[59,60]

Clinical Features

One or both choanae can be narrowed or have a complete membranous, bony, or mixed bony/membranous barrier. Purely membranous choanal atresia is rare. Imaging studies have shown that 30% are complete bony obstruction and 70% have an atresia plate that is part bony and part membranous.[61] In mixed or bony choanal atresia the typical CT findings are a thickened posterior vomer, medial bowing of the lateral nasal walls, and medial expansion of thickened pterygoid plates (Fig. 70.8). Pooled nasal drainage is commonly seen collected above the atresia plate. On endoscopic view there is a blind ended pouch at the atresia plate (Fig. 70.9).

Evaluation/Management

Bilateral choanal atresia presents early with respiratory distress either immediately after birth or at the time of the first oral feed. Unilateral choanal atresia usually has more subtle symptoms of nasal congestion and/or persistent unilateral nasal secretions and therefore may not be identified until later in childhood.

The diagnosis is suspected clinically and then confirmed with nasal endoscopy and imaging. The CT images will assess the bony/membranous nature of the type of atresia plate and may show associated nasal, skull base, or nasopharyngeal anomalies that can affect the ability to perform choanal atresia repair. Additionally, images of the temporal bone may show a semicircular canal absence that is a common feature in CHARGE (colobomas, heart abnormalities, choanal atresia, growth/mental retardation, genitourinary anomalies, ear abnormalities) syndrome. CHARGE is present in up to 25% of patients with choanal atresia.[51,52] A genetics evaluation and evaluation for possible associated conditions should be performed. Choanal atresia is associated with another anomaly in up to 75% of cases, particularly other airway, brain, developmental, or heart defects, skeletal abnormalities, and hearing impairment (Table 70.6).[51–53]

An echocardiogram and a cardiology evaluation are indicated in the setting of choanal atresia because of the association with CHARGE. Even in the absence of CHARGE or other syndromes there is an increased incidence of congenital heart defects in the setting of choanal atresia.[52]

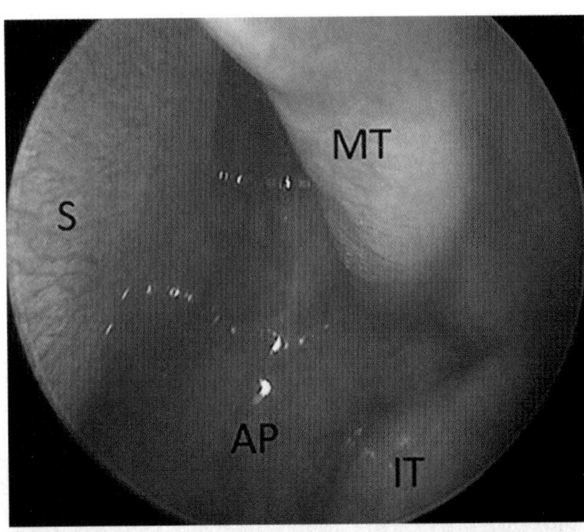

Fig. 70.9 Endoscopic View of the Left Atresia Plate in Choanal Atresia. *AP,* Atresia plate; *IT,* inferior turbinate; *MT,* middle turbinate; *S,* septum.

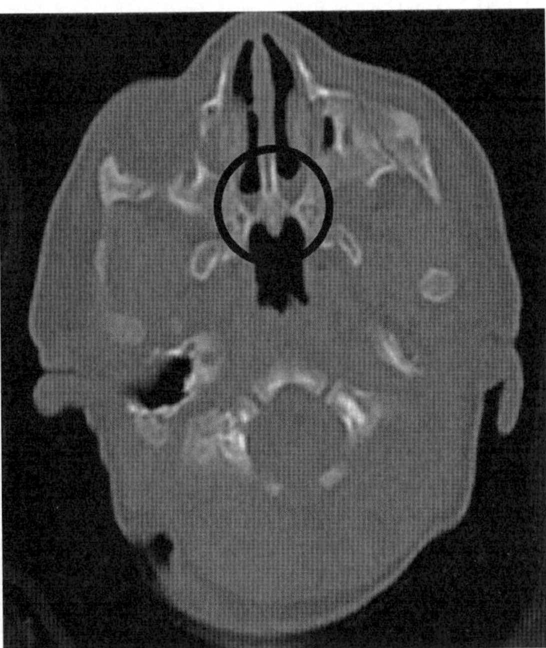

Fig. 70.8 Axial Computed Tomography Scan of a Neonate With Bilateral Bony Choanal Atresia. (Adapted from Fig. 1 in Rajan R, Tunkel DE. Choanal atresia and other neonatal nasal anomalies. *Clin Perinatol*. 2018;45:751–767. doi: 10.1016/j.clp.2018.07.011. Epub September 18, 2018. Review.)

Table 70.6 Syndromes and Anomalies Associated With Choanal Atresia

SYNDROMES
CHARGE
Crouzon
Trisomy 21
22q11.2 deletion
Treacher Collins
Fetal alcohol
ANOMALIES
Craniosynostosis
Microcephaly
Meningocele
Facial asymmetry
Cleft palate
Hypertelorism
Other nasal anomalies
Auricular anomalies
Polydactyly
Genital and renal anomalies
Heart defects

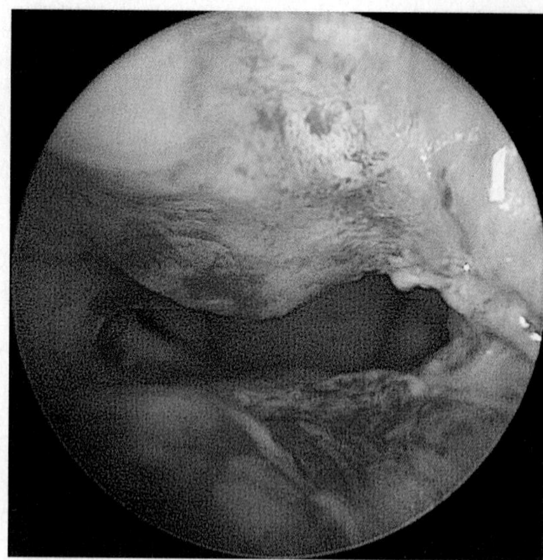

Fig. 70.10 View of Nasopharynx Through Posterior Septectomy and Neo-Choana After Repair of Bilateral Choanal Atresia in a Neonate.

The timing of the repair, surgical approach, postoperative stenting, postoperative adjuvants, and plan for managing restenosis need to be considered. Surgery may be urgent but is never emergent and should always occur after a thorough evaluation and management of comorbid conditions. Surgery is performed early for neonates with bilateral atresia and airway compromise. It should not be performed in neonates with asymptomatic unilateral atresia.[51] Children with unilateral atresia can undergo elective repair when older to alleviate nasal obstruction and the thick rhinorrhea before entering school.

Transpalatal and transseptal approaches have been described and used to repair the stenosis, but the majority of repairs are now performed through the nose with endoscopes. Such endoscopic repair affords excellent visualization with wide opening of the atresia plate and fewer complications. High-arched palate, cross-bite deformities, and excessive surgical blood loss are potential complications of the transpalatal approach.[62] With the transnasal endoscopic technique the atresia plate is taken down with the goal to create as large of an opening as possible by removing the atresia plate and surrounding bone (Fig. 70.10). Another goal is to avoid raw mucosal surfaces that may promote scarring. There is a significant risk of restenosis and scarring after surgery.

There are several techniques employed to minimize restenosis. Mucosal flaps can be laid down to reline the opening with a low incidence of restenosis in a case series.[63] Postoperative stents made of silastic tubing or endotracheal tubes are used by some surgeons to minimize restenosis. In a recent systematic review and meta-analysis the success of the repair was similar with and without stent use, and stents may be associated with more complications.[64] Two recent case series showed no complications and good long-term outcomes with off-label placement of a steroid-eluting stent in the choana after repair.[65,66] The use of topical mitomycin C intraoperatively to reduce postoperative scarring has been reported, but a systematic review found a lack of evidence to support its use.[64]

A 2012 Cochrane Review of choanal atresia repair identified no high-level evidence to support any particular surgical approach or postoperative adjuvants; therefore management plans are based on case series and clinical experience.[67] Subsequent to that, the only randomized controlled trial for choanal atresia found no difference in long-term outcomes in endoscopic repair with a mucosal flap and no stenting versus no mucosal flap and stenting.[68] Regardless of the technique and adjuvants used, parents should be counseled that multiple procedures are often necessary to achieve an adequate nasal airway. Use of topical saline, an antibiotic, and topical steroid drops may minimize the need for reoperation by minimizing granulation tissue and scarring.

When severe airway obstruction from bilateral choanal atresia repair is not anatomically feasible or is unlikely to be successful because of medical comorbid conditions, tracheostomy should be performed. This should also be considered in some patients with CHARGE, who may have worse outcomes from initial repair of the atresia due to a narrower nasopharynx and poor tongue/pharyngeal muscle control.[51,69,70] Delayed repair of the atresia can then be performed when appropriate.

Long-Term Outcomes

The risk of restenosis is high in the short and intermediate term. In one series with a mean follow-up of 5.2 years, 26 out of 50 cases needed some revision surgery.[71] Recurrence was especially common in bony atresia and CHARGE syndrome.[71]

Midline Congenital Nasal Masses

Epidemiology

Midline congenital nasal masses or frontonasal masses are rare, affecting 1 in every 20,000 to 40,000 births. Dermoid cysts are the most common of the midline congenital masses. They have a male predominance and can cluster in families.[72] The incidence of encephaloceles is declining with increased intake of prenatal folic acid consumption before and during pregnancy.[73] The incidence is estimated to be 1 in 30,000 to 40,000 live births in North America and Europe and 1 in 5000 to 6000 in Asian populations.[74] Gliomas occur more in males and do not have familial inheritance.

Pathophysiology

Midline congenital nasal masses include dermoids, encephaloceles, and gliomas, which have a shared embryologic origin. Fig. 70.11 highlights the locations and potential intracranial connections of these nasal masses.

In utero the dura projects through an opening in the anterior skull base called the foramen cecum. As the nasal and frontal bones form during the seventh week of gestation, the dura and neurocranial tissue usually regress.[74] When they do not, a dermoid, encephalocele, or glioma may develop. Failure of closure of the anterior neuropore is implicated in this aberration.[75]

A nasal dermoid contains ectodermal and mesodermal derivatives from persistent embryonic neuroectoderm. It is a cyst of skin appendages that develops in the prenasal space because of skin pulled internally through the anterior neuropore. A sinus tract usually connects to the cyst, which contains epithelium, sebaceous material, and/or hair. Encephaloceles and gliomas are related in that they are derived from defects in the skull base allowing tissue that would normally be intracranial into the nasal cavity (see Fig. 70.11). Encephaloceles are usually connected with the cerebrospinal fluid (CSF) space. Meningoceles contain dura and CSF, but unlike encephaloceles they do not contain brain tissue. Gliomas consist of glial tissue that has been disconnected from the subarachnoid space and CSF. They may have a fibrous stalk that can extend intracranially. They are also more accurately referred to as nasal glial heterotopia.

Clinical Features

Dermoids are usually heralded by a midline dorsal nasal dimple, sometimes with drainage, swelling, or hair growth (Fig. 70.12). They

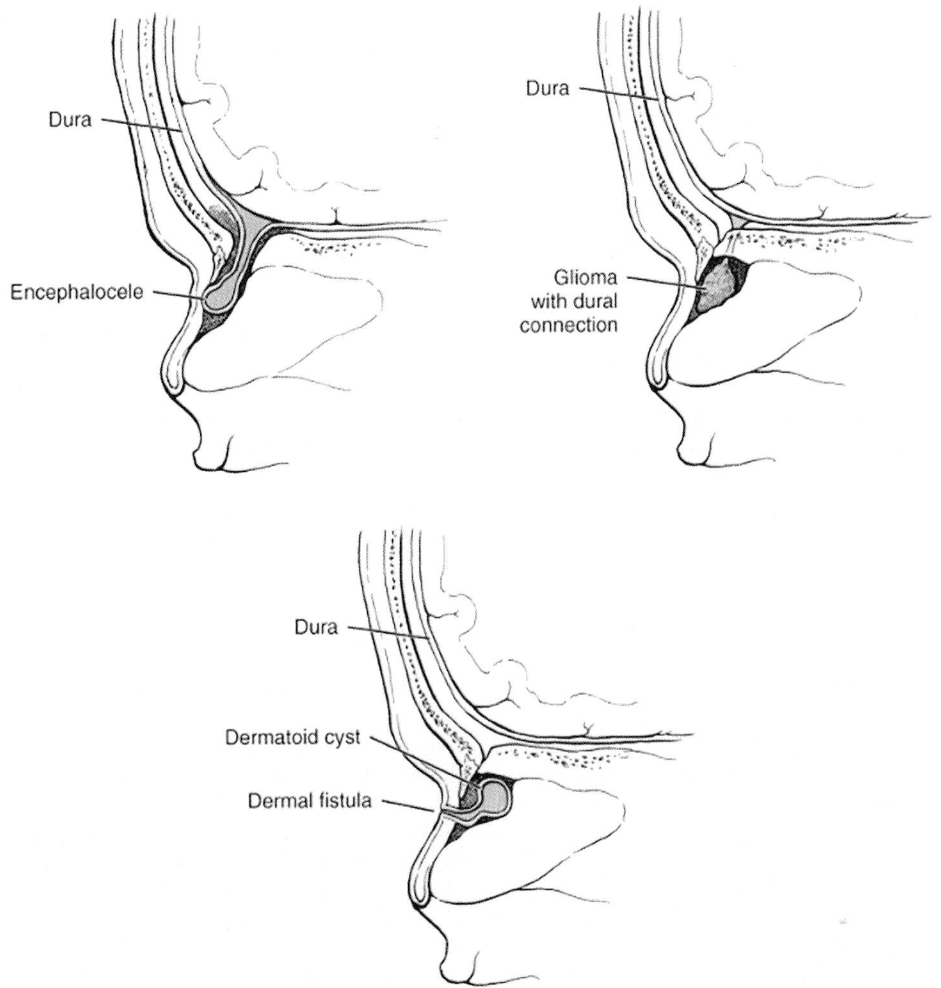

Fig. 70.11 Sagittal Depictions of Development of Midline Nasal Masses Including an Encephalocele With Dura Extending Into the Prenasal Space, a Glioma Attached to a Fibrous Stalk That Extends Intracranially, and a Dermoid in the Prenasal Space With a Tract Connecting to the Skin. (From Fig. 189.1 in Flint PW, Haughey BH, Lund V, et al., eds. *Cummings Otolaryngology–Head & Neck Surgery.* 6th ed. Philadelphia: Elsevier Saunders; 2015.)

are usually isolated anomalies. Intracranial extension with attachment to the dura varies from 5% to 45%.[76] Encephaloceles are strongly associated with other anomalies, especially intracranial anomalies.[77] Sincipital encephaloceles are usually evident at birth, but basal encephaloceles are entirely intranasal and may not be immediately evident. Gliomas can be described as extranasal (60%), intranasal (30%), or combined (10%).[78] Extranasal lesions are smooth, firm, and noncompressible masses. Intranasal gliomas are pale masses that may protrude from the nostril and can cause substantial nasal obstruction. In some cases there can be a widened nasal bridge or wide-set eyes. Physical findings vary based on the type of lesion because of the differing contents and central nervous system connections (Table 70.7).

Evaluation/Management

Imaging should always precede biopsy of midline nasal masses because there can be a risk of bleeding and CSF leak. CT provides the best definition of bony anatomy of the skull base, and MRI is ideal to evaluate potential central nervous system soft-tissue connections or abnormalities.

Otolaryngology consultants can perform nasal endoscopy to evaluate the intranasal appearance and extent and can help advise about imaging methods. Earlier intervention is advocated for masses with

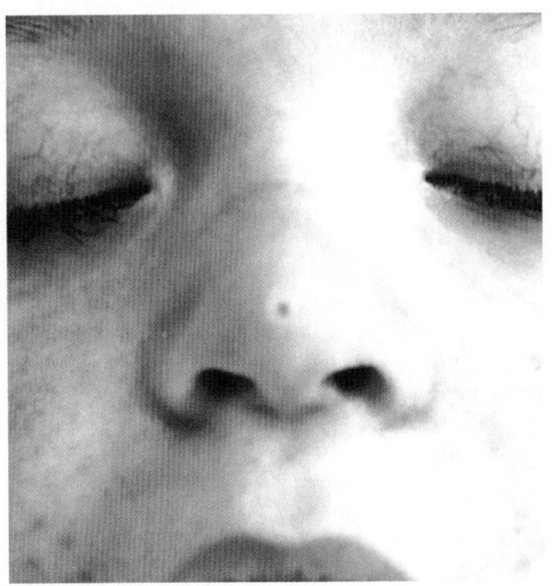

Fig. 70.12 Nasal Dermoid Cyst With Characteristic Midline Pit. (From Fig. 8 in Rajan R, Tunkel DE. Choanal atresia and other neonatal nasal anomalies. *Clin Perinatol.* 2018;45:751–767.)

Table 70.7 Clinical Characteristics of Midline Congenital Nasal Masses

Lesion	Encephalocele	Glioma	Dermoid
Contents	Meninges ± neural tissue	Glial tissue	Skin appendages
Location	Glabella, nasal dorsum, intranasal	Glabella, nasal dorsum, nasal tip, intranasal	Nasal dorsum, typically with a hair or pit
Intracranial communication	Yes	Possible	Possible
Expansion when crying, straining, or with ipsilateral jugular vein compression (Furstenberg sign)	Yes	No	No
Transilluminates	Yes	No	No

Adapted from Table 1 in Rajan R, Tunkel DE. Choanal atresia and other neonatal nasal anomalies. *Clin Perinatol.* 2018;45:751–767.

intracranial extension to avoid infection and deformity. However, surgery is rarely urgent. Most gliomas and dermoids can be monitored and removed later in childhood to minimize perioperative risks of neonatal surgery.

Neurosurgery consultation should be obtained for any lesions with suspected or documented intracranial extension. The surgical goal is to remove the entire mass and resolve all intracranial connections to avoid postoperative CSF leak and meningitis. Small intranasal lesions can be removed endoscopically or with an open approach to the nose. For larger lesions with intracranial extension, combined approaches with nasal endoscopy, open nasal surgery, and craniotomy are used to achieve complete resection. Postoperative epistaxis, CSF leak, meningitis, hydrocephalus, scarring, and poor cosmetic outcome are potential risks of removing midlines nasal masses.

Long-Term Outcomes

Recurrence of midline nasal masses is possible but not common. Additional nasal reconstruction may be needed in older children if there are persistent functional or cosmetic nasal issues.

Conclusions

The causes of nasal obstruction in the newborn are diverse, and many require close observation while resolution occurs. The initial evaluation includes a clinical assessment to ensure safe ventilation, followed by more specialized assessments including nasal endoscopy and imaging. Surgery for congenital anomalies such as choanal atresia are successful in restoring normal nasal airflow. Some conditions require evaluation for syndromes and comorbid diagnoses.

SECTION 14

Orthopedic Conditions

OUTLINE

CHAPTER 71 Upper Extremity Conditions in the Neonate

Jessica G. Shih, Lahin M. Amlani, Laura Lewallen

KEY POINTS

1. Congenital upper extremity differences are relatively rare but numerous and complex in nature.
2. Refer to a pediatric hand surgeon for management if an upper extremity congenital anomaly is suspected.
3. Some of the relatively more common conditions include syndactyly, polydactyly, and radial longitudinal deficiency or thumb hypoplasia.
4. Diagnosis is usually made based on clinical examination; however, further investigation may be warranted to rule out associated syndromes and conditions. Radiographs are helpful in certain conditions to visualize underlying bony structure.
5. Timing of surgical management varies; however, the majority of initial reconstruction procedures occurs at 12 to 18 months of age.
6. Satisfaction with overall functional and esthetic outcomes following reconstructive surgery with the described conditions is generally high.

Introduction

Several complex congenital anomalies are seen in the upper extremities. This chapter will provide an introduction and overview of several of these anomalies that are seen relatively more frequently. The Oberg, Manske, and Tonkin Classification of congenital hand and upper limb anomalies provides a framework for placing conditions in one of three groups based on limb embryogenesis: malformations, deformations, and dysplasias.[1] Malformations represent the majority of congenital upper extremity differences (74%–90% of total diagnoses), examples of which include syndactyly, polydactyly, thumb hypoplasia, radial/ulnar/central longitudinal deficiencies, and symbrachydactyly. Deformations are subdivided into constriction ring sequence, trigger digits, and not otherwise specified. Dysplasias are subdivided into hyperplasia such as macrodactyly and tumorous conditions such as vascular tumors/malformations, connective tissue tumors, and skeletal tumors.[2,3] A comprehensive list of anomalies and associated syndromes is described according to the Oberg, Manske, and Tonkin Classification[1] (Table 71.1).

Congenital abnormalities of the upper extremities can occur in isolation or with associated syndromes and can be sporadic or inherited. There are numerous congenital upper extremity anomalies that occur as a result of changes in limb embryogenesis. They are often clinically evident at birth and therefore may be recognized and diagnosed by the primary care team. However, specialist referral to pediatric hand surgeons within plastic surgery or orthopedic surgery is recommended for management of congenital upper extremity pathology.

Embryology

Limb bud formation begins at approximately 4 weeks' gestation and is complete at approximately 8 weeks (days 26–52).[4] The majority of limb abnormalities take place during this time.[5] The upper limbs develop approximately 24 hours sooner than the lower limbs, because the embryo forms cranially to caudally.[6] Both the paraxial mesoderm and parietal plate mesoderm participate in limb development. Limbs initially form as paddle-like structures (appearing at day 33), flattened mediolaterally and hugging the body. As the limb develops and takes on a more recognizable structure, a delicate balance of differential cell growth and selective cell death must be obtained.

Fibroblast growth factor 10 is a signaling molecule that migrates from the lateral plate mesoderm across formerly mesodermal tissue, now undifferentiated mesenchyme, to ectodermal tissue to initiate limb formation (limb bud appears at day 26).[7] Bones of the limb originate from somatic lateral plate mesoderm. All bony structures in the limb, except the clavicles, originate via endochondral ossification, a process by which bone invades a preformed cartilaginous model with bone precursors (osteoblasts). The paraxial mesoderm forms bundles, called somites, along the length of the body. Somitic cells may differentiate into somitic myotome, eventually resulting in limb muscle.[7] A portion of the myotome will divide into two factions: a dorsal muscle mass and a ventral muscle mass.[8] The masses will surround bone in the limb on either the dorsal or ventral sides as their names suggest. They will transition to myoblasts (muscle precursor cells) and eventually mature muscle cells. This process provides an explanation as to the different innervations of the two muscle groups. Motor axons from the neural tube diverge into anterior and posterior ventral rami and take the path of least resistance, avoiding dense connective tissue. Somatic fibers trigger myoblast differentiation. Sensory axons take a permissive path; they follow the path motor neurons took because it offers the least resistance, with minimal tissue interference. These developmental steps explain why the sensory and motor neurons are located in the same place within limbs.

The development of limbs can be thought of as occurring in three spatial axes: proximal-distal, cranial-caudal, and dorsal-ventral.[9] Along the edge of the distal limb bud is a ridge of ectodermal tissue called the apical ectodermal ridge (AER). It is believed that the AER gives a signal to differentiate proximal and distal structures; however, the exact mechanism is unclear. The progress zone model, a timing-based model, and the early allocation and progenitor expansion model, a prespecification model, are believed to be possible

Table 71.1 Oberg, Manske, and Tonkin (OMT) Classification

Malformations

1. Failure of axis formation/differentiation—entire upper limb
   a. Proximal-distal outgrowth
      - Brachymelia with brachydactyly
      - Symbrachydactyly
      - Transverse deficiency
      - Intersegmental deficiency
   b. Radial-ulnar (anteroposterior) axis
      - Radial longitudinal deficiency
      - Ulnar longitudinal deficiency
      - Ulnar dimelia
      - Radioulnar synostosis
   c. Dorsal-ventral axis
      - Nail-patella syndrome
2. Failure of axis formation/differentiation—hand plate
   a. Radial-ulnar (anteroposterior) axis
      - Radial polydactyly
      - Triphalangeal thumb
      - Ulnar polydactyly
   b. Dorsal-ventral axis
      - Dorsal dimelia (palmar nail)
      - Hypoplastic/aplastic nail
3. Failure of axis formation/differentiation—unspecified axis
   a. Soft tissue
      - Syndactyly
      - Camptodactyly
   b. Skeletal deficiency
      - Brachydactyly
      - Clinodactyly
      - Kirner deformity
      - Metacarpal and carpal synostoses
   c. Complex
      - Cleft hand
      - Synpolydactyly
      - Apert hand

Deformations

1. Constriction ring sequence
2. Arthrogryposis
3. Trigger digits
4. Not otherwise specified

Dysplasias

1. Hypertrophy
   - Macrodactyly
   - Upper limb
   - Upper limb and macrodactyly
2. Tumorous conditions

Adapted with permission from Oberg KC, Feenstra JM, Manske PR, Tonkin MA. Developmental biology and classification of congenital anomalies of the hand and upper extremity. *J Hand Surg Am.* 2010;35:2066–2076; adapted from Tonkin MA, Tolerton SK, Quick TJ, Harvey I, Lawson RD, Smith NC, Oberg KC. Classification of congenital anomalies of the hand and upper limb: development and assessment of a new system. *J Hand Surg.* 2013;38:1845–1853.)

explanations for proximal-distal differentiation.[10,11] Cranial-caudal axis formation is centered around a chemical located on the caudal side of the developing limb, sonic hedgehog (SHH). The area expressing SHH is called the zone of polarizing activity. SHH from the zone of polarizing activity radiates across the developing limb bud in every direction from the caudal side.[12] The signal is weaker further from the origin, resulting in a morphogenetic gradient. The thumb develops on the cranial side, where there is greater not-caudal character. Finally, the dorsal-ventral axis involves Wnt signaling, although this pathway is poorly understood. This axis is not the result of a gradient. Instead, through the Wnt signaling pathway, a signaling molecule, Lmx-1, is expressed on the dorsal side of the limb, causing the mesenchyme to adopt dorsal characteristics while the ventral side expresses a signaling molecule, En-1, whose product essentially stops the dorsal signaling by blocking the Wnt signaling pathway.[13]

Segmental separation occurs to achieve the definitive structure of the limb. Constriction of the presumptive wrist and elbow, flattening of the hand plate in a dorsal-ventral fashion, and division of the AER and apoptosis in the interdigital spaces are all consequences of selective cell death of the limb. Finally, limb rotation gives rise to the adult dermatome structure.

Pathophysiology

Limb development is tightly controlled and regulated. Molecular and biochemical alternations occur in a precise and transient manner as to trigger the next stage in a cascade of events through limb development. Therefore it is fitting that even small alterations affecting morphologic processes in limb development can result in abnormal structure. Teratogens, genetic components, and metabolic poisons can all adversely affect the delicate process of limb development leading to the conditions described in this chapter.

The exact cause of syndactyly remains unclear. Four areas of caudal divisions of the AER from apoptosis result in a typical five-digit hand. Deviations from the typical programmed cell death that yields five distinct digits can result in syndactyly. Digits in the hand become apparent on days 41 to 43 and are fully separated by day 53 in a typical hand.[14–16] Apoptosis is mediated by bone morphogenic protein 4.[2,17] Disturbance of these molecular mechanisms may result in atypical hand plate formation. Syndactyly has been reported in some cases to be transmitted in an autosomal-dominant manner with incomplete penetrance.[18,19]

Polydactyly can be a product of disruptions in the cranial-caudal axis, leading to additional caudal divisions and subsequently extra digits. Polydactyly has shown an autosomal dominant form of transmission, and genetic defects have been noted in chromosome 2.[20] Polydactyly has also been linked to chromosome 7, where the regulatory element of SHH is located.[2]

Thalidomide was previously given to pregnant women for relief of nausea and morning sickness; however, it has been shown to be associated with a high incidence of skeletal deformities including radial longitudinal deficiency when given to women between days 38 and 45 of fetal development.[21] For this reason, it is no longer used. Other teratogens have also been associated with radial longitudinal deficiency, including fetal alcohol syndrome.[22]

Clinical Features, Evaluation, Management, Long-Term Outcomes, and Conditions

Syndactyly

Clinical Features

Syndactyly refers to an anomalous connection between two or more digits. It is the second most common congenital malformation of the hand.[23,24] Overall prevalence of syndactyly ranges from 1 in 1000 to 1 in 2500 live births.[23,25,26] It is more common in males than females and occurs with equal frequency unilaterally and bilaterally.[27–30] Syndactyly occurs most commonly between the ring and middle fingers (40%–50%), second most commonly between the ring and small fingers (25%–28%), and least commonly between the index

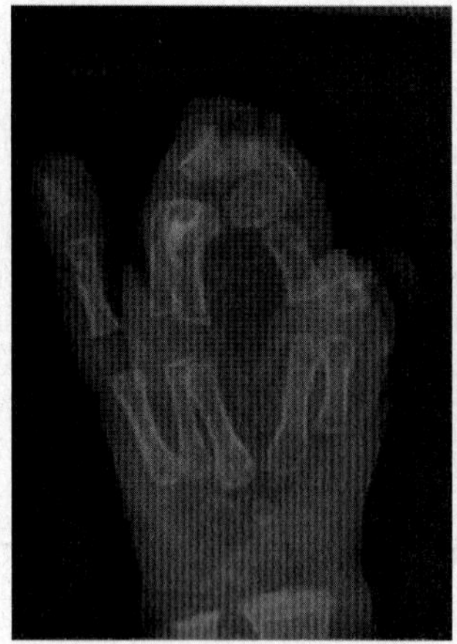
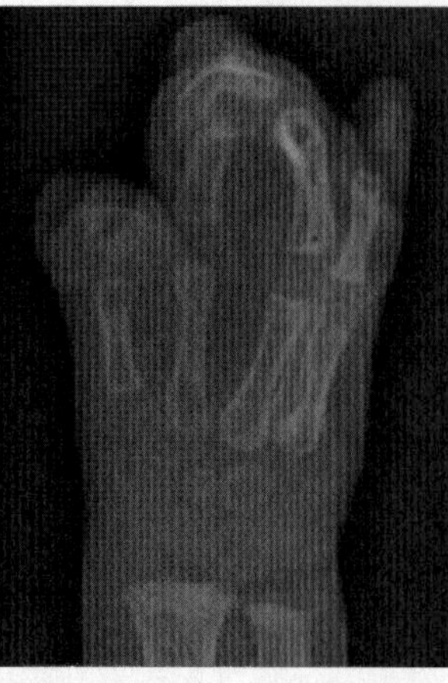

Fig. 71.1 A 2-Year-Old Male With Apert Syndrome and Complex Syndactyly Who Underwent Bilateral Staged Reconstruction During the Course of 2 Years.

and middle fingers or the thumb and index finger.[31–37] Syndactyly of the fingers is typically an isolated condition. However, it may be associated with other conditions such as syndactyly of the toes, polydactyly, and club foot and with syndromes such as Apert syndrome (Fig. 71.1), Poland syndrome, and acrosyndactyly.[38,39]

Syndactyly is classified according to whether the connection between two or more digits is partial, creating a webbed digit, or fully extending to the tip (incomplete versus complete, respectively), whether the connection involves skin only or bone also (simple versus complex, respectively), and whether there is abnormal bone structure with rudimentary bones, missing bones, extra bones, abnormal joints, or more than one synostoses (complicated).[14,40–42]

Evaluation

Clinical examination of the digits can often distinguish between the types of syndactyly. Incomplete versus complete syndactyly can be easily distinguished clinically by whether the skin connection involves only a proximal portion of the digit compared with the complete length of the digit. Differential movement of the digits is indicative of a simple syndactyly with skin connection only and lack of bony fusion. Connection of the nail between the digits is a sign of underlying bony connection between the distal phalanx of the two digits. X-rays of the hand can help determine whether a bony connection exists but is not necessary and should be avoided in the early neonatal period to prevent radiation exposure. X-rays may be performed closer to the planned surgical date at 12 to 18 months of age if required.

Management

Surgical intervention for syndactyly in the upper extremity is not medically necessary; however, syndactyly release allows functional improvement with independent, differential digit motion, prevention of growth abnormalities and contractures of affected digits, and esthetic and social normalcy.[39,40,43] The timing of surgical intervention depends on both the type of syndactyly and the digits affected.[27,38,43–49] Simple syndactyly between the middle and ring fingers does not require urgent correction. Timing of simple or incomplete syndactyly involving the middle and ring fingers is somewhat arbitrary and can occur anywhere between 18 months and several years of age.[27,40] Prognosis may be worse if correction is performed after 2 years of age, because cerebral cortical patterns may require retraining, and correction should be performed prior to school age.[47] Earlier intervention for simple cases can result in web migration distally,[26] involves potential increased anesthetic risk of operating on infants less than 6 months of age,[50,51] and is more technically difficult due to the smaller size of the digits. Complete syndactyly without involvement of the border digits can be performed between 12 and 18 months to balance risks of earlier surgical intervention and differential growth of the digits based on bony connections.[52] Border digits with involvement of the index or small fingers should be released relatively early, between 6 and 12 months of age, because the differential lengths of the connected digits are more likely to result in angular, rotational, and flexion deformities without early correction.[26,40,52] Earlier intervention between 4 and 6 months can be considered if multiple digits including border digits are involved, requiring staged reconstruction. Staged reconstruction, by operating on only one side of a digit and returning to the operating room 6 months later to release the other side of the digit, prevents the risk of vascular compromise of the digit.[26,38,45,49]

Surgical correction involves separation of the digits using opposing zig-zag incisions, creating a web space commissure that is deep and wide and covering any areas of skin deficit with skin grafts.[26,40,43] A variety of surgical techniques are described. Full-thickness skin grafting helps prevents scar contracture and web creep.[38] Several options are available including the antecubital fossa, wrist flexion crease, or groin (lateral third of inguinal crease).[24] Postoperative care involves a long arm cast from the fingertips to the shoulder, with the elbow flexed approximately 90 degrees. The cast is typically left in place for 2 weeks until the first postoperative wound check, with additional dressings or immobilization for a total of 4 to 6 weeks as needed.[26,40]

Long-Term Outcomes

Syndactyly release may successfully improve function with independent finger motion and hand appearance.[53] Long-term follow-up into adolescence is important to follow the most common reason for reoperation, which is web creep.[26] Reoperation usually involves scar release and correction with tissue rearrangement such as Z-plasty or additional full-thickness skin graft.[38] Rates of revision surgery are higher with border digits, complex syndactyly, and releases performed before 18 months of age.[26,27,53–56]

Polydactyly

Clinical Features, Evaluation, and Management

Polydactyly in the upper extremity refers to one or more extra digits that can range from a rudimentary digit to a fully formed digit on the radial, ulnar, or central hand. This condition is most often found in isolation but is also associated with certain genetic syndromes.[57] Polydactyly is twice as prevalent in males compared with females.[58] Ulnar, or postaxial, polydactyly is the most common form of polydactyly,[59] with central polydactyly the least prevalent (5%–15% of all polydactylies).[60,61] Ulnar polydactyly is 10 times as prevalent among children of African descent, ranging from 1 in 100 to 1 in 300 live births,[59,62] is more likely to be bilateral, and is usually of autosomal-dominant inherence compared with children of Caucasian descent (1 in 1500 to 1 in 3000, unilateral, and sporadic).[20,62] Radial, or preaxial polydactyly, also known as thumb duplication, is more common in children of Caucasian and Asian descent and is often unilateral.[20] The prevalence is approximately 1 in 1000 live births.[51]

Ulnar/Postaxial Polydactyly/Small Finger Duplication

Ulnar polydactyly is typically classified as either Type A (well-formed digit) or Type B (small, rudimentary, or underdeveloped digit). Type B polydactyly is more common than Type A.[20,57,62]

Type A polydactyly typically requires surgical excision of the accessory digit with reconstruction of the ulnar collateral ligament and abductor digiti minimi in the operating room. This is usually performed around 12 to 16 months of age, when the anesthetic risk is lower and the larger size of digit is technically easier to reconstruct.[20,50,51,57,63] Preoperative x-rays of the hand should be obtained in Type A polydactyly with potential osseous involvement.[57]

Type B polydactyly often presents as a pedunculated accessory digit or small nubbin of soft tissue at the base of the small finger[64,65] (Fig. 71.2). This is most often treated in the office setting with ligation at the base of the digit (using suture or hemoclip). This results in necrosis of the digit over the following days or weeks.[57,64] A residual bump or skin tag is the most common complication and is reported in up to 80% of patients.[59,65,66] The residual tissue may contain nerve tissue that can form a sensitive neuroma.[64,67,68] Other complications of suture ligation include infection and cyst formation.[65,69] Therefore some authors recommend performing surgical excision of the stalk and accessory digit with traction neurectomy of the accessory digital nerve away from the skin edge.[57,65,67,70] This can be performed either at an early age (under 2–3 months) under bottle anesthesia if the infant is cooperative or in the main operating room at approximately 12 months of age. Bottle anesthesia refers to pacifying the infant with either sugar water or feeding from a bottle of milk while a small volume of local anesthesia is injected at the base of the small finger.[57] Radiographs are not usually needed in Type B polydactyly.[57]

Radial/Preaxial Polydactyly/Thumb Duplication

Radial polydactyly, or thumb duplication, is most often classified using the Wassel classification system.[57] The additional digit is located at the level of the thumb distal phalanx for type I (bifid) and type II (duplicated), the proximal phalanx for type III (bifid) and type IV (duplicated), and the metacarpal for type V (bifid) and type VI (duplicated). Type VII is a triphalangeal thumb.[71] Type IV is the most common (40%–50%), with type II being second most common (15%–20%).[20,72]

X-rays of the hand can help classify thumb duplication based on the anatomic location and whether the digit is bifid versus duplicated but should be delayed until the preoperative stage to avoid early radiation exposure. Thumb duplication is rarely associated with syndromes; therefore screening for genetic syndromes is not routinely recommended.[57]

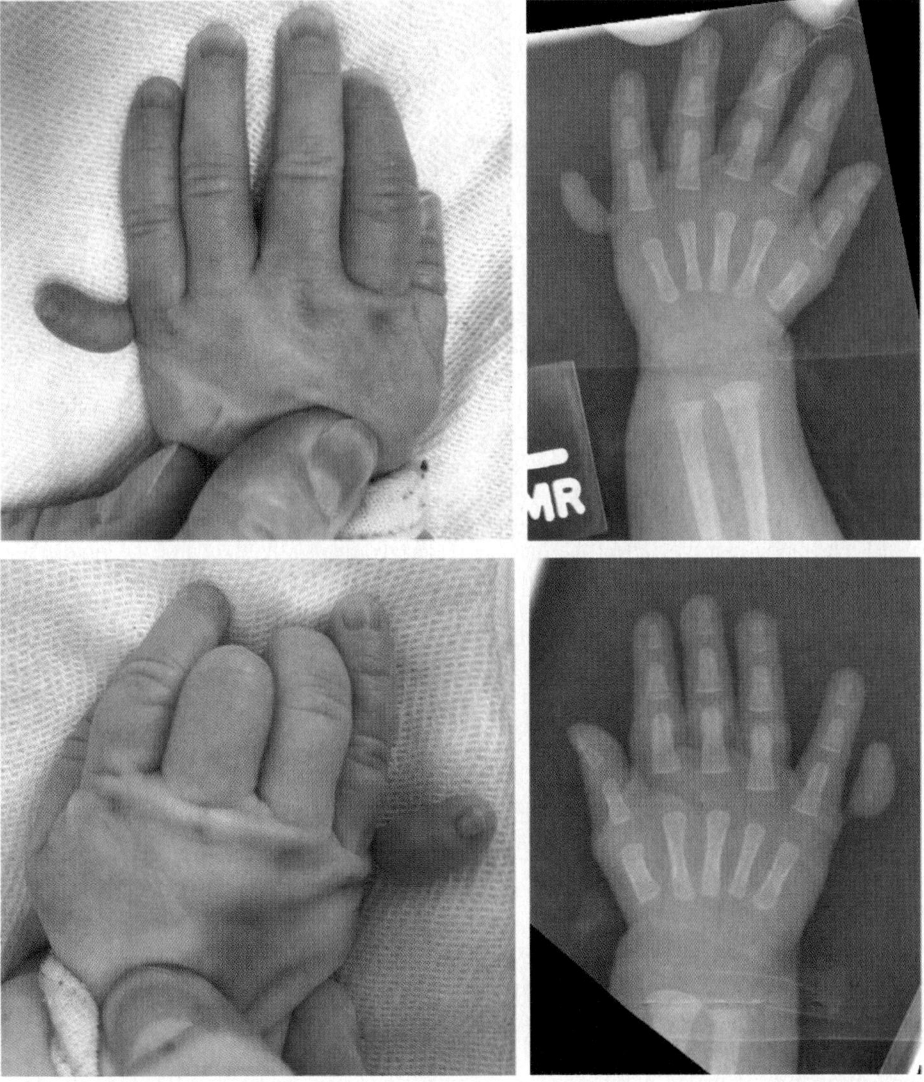

Fig. 71.2 Clinical Photos and Radiographs of a 6-Week-Old Patient With Bilateral Postaxial Polydactyly, Type B.

Surgical management of thumb duplication often requires reconstruction of the collateral ligaments and musculature as well as bony realignment to ensure a functional, stable thumb.[57,73] Timing of reconstruction around 12 months of age allows for assessment of function and stability of the remaining thumb to ensure removal of the relatively less functional thumb does not interfere with function. This also allows for greater development of fine motor skills.[50,51,57] It is important to counsel parents that the remaining thumb is often smaller, weaker, and less functional compared with the unaffected side.[41,57,74]

Central Polydactyly

Central polydactyly is relatively rare. Surgical reconstruction can be challenging and may involve multiple surgeries. Outcomes are less predictable than for radial and ulnar polydactyly reconstruction.[57,61,75]

Long-Term Outcomes

Surgical excision of ulnar polydactyly typically results in satisfactory outcomes with minimal functional or esthetic concerns.[57,76] Ligation of small-finger duplication can result in a sensitive neuroma that may require further nonsurgical or surgical management. Results of thumb duplication are more variable, with long-term complications including unsatisfactory cosmetic appearance, residual angular deformity, stiffness, weakness, and instability.[57,77,78] Satisfactory functional and esthetic outcome is difficult to achieve in central polydactyly, with nearly all reconstructions requiring multiple/revision surgeries.[57,61]

Radial, Ulnar, and Central Longitudinal Deficiencies

Clinical Features

Longitudinal deficiencies refer to hypoplasia or absence of a specific portion of the limb. In the upper extremity, they are most often classified into radial, ulnar, or central longitudinal deficiency. Radial longitudinal deficiency occurs along a spectrum ranging from thumb hypoplasia to partial or complete absence of the radial-sided hand and/or radius.[20,79,80] Hypoplastic thumbs are usually classified into 5 categories, based on the recommendations from Blauth (circa 1967) and later modifications by Manske (circa 1995).[81–84] *Type I* hypoplasia is a minor, but generalized hypoplasia that may affect the thenar muscles and may limit intricate hand functions in later life. *Type II* hypoplasia is characterized by hypoplasia of the thenar muscles that are innervated by the median nerve. Muscles innervated by the ulnar nerve are partially intact. These infants retain some metacarpophalangeal joint flexion, although the joint may show some laxity. Lister classified these patients into those who had uni- or multiaxial instability. *Type III* hypoplasia is more severe with added deficiencies of extrinsic extensors and flexors. There is some loss of active movement at both the metacarpophalangeal and interphalangeal joints. *Type IV* hypoplasia is a profound deficiency known as a *pouce flottant*, or *floating thumb*. The thumb remnant is attached to the hand solely by a narrow bridge of skin containing a single neurovascular element. The thumb is floppy and is entirely ignored during prehension. And *Type V* hypoplasia is complete absence of the thumb. A small nubbin of skin can be noticed in some infants. This classification system helps guide decision making in the management of thumb hypoplasia. The stability of the thumb carpometacarpal joint helps in deciding between the possibility of thumb stabilization and ligament reconstruction versus the need for reconstruction with index pollicization.

Table 71.2 Classification of Radial Longitudinal Deficiency

Type	Definition	Description
1	Short distal radius	Distal radial epiphysis present but delayed, little radial deviation, thumb hypoplasia almost always present
2	Hypoplastic radius	Growth defective in proximal and distal radial epiphyses, radius in miniature
3	Partial absence of the radius	Defect can be proximal, middle, or distal third, but most frequently proximal; hand is radially displaced, wrist is unsupported
4	Total absence of the radius	Most common type; hand is usually severely radially displaced

Radial longitudinal deficiency is also classified along a spectrum of severity (Tables 71.2 and 71.3).[80] This is helpful in guiding treatment. Radial longitudinal deficiency is more common (1 in 5000 to 1 in 100,000 live births)[85–87] than ulnar deficiency (1–7 in 100,000 live births)[88,89] or central deficiency (1 in 10,000 to 1 in 90,000 live births).[39,90–92] Radial longitudinal deficiency is most often sporadic, although it may also be associated with Holt-Oram syndrome, thrombocytopenia-absent radius, VACTERL (vertebral defects, anal atresia, cardiac defects, tracheo-esophageal fistula, renal anomalies, and limb abnormalities) association, and Fanconi anemia.[20,81] Approximately two-thirds of patients with radial longitudinal deficiency have abnormalities involving other organ systems (gastrointestinal, genitourinary, cardiovascular, or hematopoietic systems).[83,88,90,91,93]

Ulnar longitudinal deficiency clinically presents as partial or complete absence of the ulnar-sided hand and/or ulna or complete syndactyly, smaller digits, or absent digits on the ulnar side.[94] Syndromes associated with ulnar longitudinal deficiencies include ulnar-mammary, Cornelia de Lange, and femur-fibula-ulna syndromes.[14,95,96] Approximately one-third of patients with ulnar longitudinal deficiency have associated musculoskeletal conditions such as proximal femoral focal deficiency, hip dysplasia, fibular deficiency, absent patella, club foot, scoliosis, spina bifida, and mandibular defects.

Table 71.3 Modified Classification of Radial Longitudinal Deficiency

Type	Thumb	Carpus	Distal Radius	Proximal Radius
N	Hypoplastic or absent	Normal	Normal	Normal
0	Hypoplastic or absent	Absence, hypoplasia, or coalition	Normal	Normal, radioulnar synostosis, or congenital dislocation of the radial head
1	Hypoplastic or absent	Absence, hypoplasia, or coalition	>2 mm shorter than ulna	Normal, radioulnar synostosis, or congenital dislocation of the radial head
2	Hypoplastic or absent	Absence, hypoplasia, or coalition	Hypoplasia	Hypoplasia
3	Hypoplastic or absent	Absence, hypoplasia, or coalition	Physis absent	Variable hypoplasia
4	Hypoplastic or absent	Absence, hypoplasia, or coalition	Absent	Absent

Adapted from James M, McCarroll R, Manske PR. The spectrum of radial longitudinal deficiency: a modified classification. *J Hand Surg Am*. 1999;24:1145–1155.

Central longitudinal deficiency, also known as "cleft hand," presents with partial or complete deficiencies of the second, third, or fourth rays.[97] Patients typically have bilateral hand and foot involvement. Clinically, central longitudinal deficiency presents as a V-shaped cleft in the center of the hand rather than a U-shaped cleft more representative of symbrachydactyly.[63] Central longitudinal deficiency is most often autosomal dominant in nature.[63,83,88]

Evaluation

Due to the possible associated conditions, it is important to perform a complete history and physical examination and radiographs of the affected limb at 6 to 12 months of age. Further investigations to screen for associated conditions in radial longitudinal deficiency include complete blood cell count, echocardiogram, renal ultrasound, and spine x-rays. If a syndrome is suspected in the infant, further consideration for genetic counseling is also important.[83] Diepoxybutane testing for Fanconi anemia detection is advocated by some at the time of initial evaluation due to its association with radial longitudinal deficiencies.[5]

Management

Functional concerns of longitudinal deficiency include stability of the wrist or elbow, grip and pinch strength, and ability of the hand to reach the mouth.[97,98] When radial or ulnar longitudinal deficiency is detected at birth, occupational therapy should be initiated to begin range of motion and stretching exercises for the wrist. Once of appropriate size and age, splinting can also be helpful.[20,83] Surgical intervention for radial, ulnar, or central longitudinal deficiencies includes a variety of different procedures. Treatment decisions are based on the severity and type of deficiency.[20,84] The goals of surgery are to optimize function and esthetics of the upper extremity. Potential surgical options include tendon transfers, opponensplasty, thumb metacarpophalangeal stabilization, first web space deepening, index pollicization, cleft closure, stabilization and centralization of the wrist, rotational osteotomy, and limb lengthening.[22,20,81,99,100] Timing of surgical management is often between 12 and 18 months of age or later. This allows for the opportunity to assess the optimal functional position of the hand and wrist once the child begins to grasp objects.[83]

Long-Term Outcomes

Range of motion in patients with index pollicization is diminished compared with the normal hand[101–103]; however, hands undergoing pollicization tend to develop at a rate comparable to age-matched controls in terms of strength and dexterity.[101,104,105] The main risk in patients undergoing surgical reconstruction of radial longitudinal deficiency is recurrence of the deformity.

CHAPTER

72 Newborn Spine Deformities

Alexandra M. Dunham, Paul D. Sponseller

KEY POINTS

1. Spina bifida usually can be diagnosed prenatally with screening and in the early neonatal period by physical exam. Early diagnosis and intervention may improve outcomes.
2. Assessment of vertebral anomalies is best done in early childhood. The first available film should be analyzed and used for subsequent comparisons.
3. Associated anomalies occur with neonatal spine disorders. Additional tests other than those that serve to evaluate the spine are necessary, and collaboration between medical and surgical teams is important for optimization.
4. Progressive deformation is due to imbalance in spine growth. The pattern of deformity is correlated to risk of progression and risk of thoracic insufficiency and impacts time to intervention.
5. Bracing has almost no effect on congenital spine curves.
6. Surgery should usually be performed as early as practical to prevent secondary structural changes.

Introduction

Neonatal spine deformities encompass a wide-ranging breadth of pathologies, some of which can be diagnosed in the prenatal and neonatal periods. A working knowledge of spinal development, musculoskeletal and neurologic examination, and imaging findings help the savvy neonatal provider make an assessment regarding a patient's abnormal spine. Conditions can be described by the resultant deformity in alignment (scoliosis, kyphosis), may allude to the anatomic abnormality (myelodysplasia, hemivertebrae, sacral agenesis), or may be part of a syndrome (musculoskeletal dysplasia).[1–3]

Although much of the technical management for spine deformity is ultimately under the purview of orthopedic or neurosurgical specialists, the neonatologist or pediatrician plays an integral role in the medical care and overall health of the patient. The high association of multiple medical comorbidities with spine deformities makes surgical treatment challenging.[4,5] Multiple musculoskeletal differences are also associated with neonatal spine deformities, and orthopedic management becomes a life-long part of many patients' care. A multidisciplinary approach is essential in the management of these multifaceted deformities.

Identification and Treatment in Early Life

In few instances, prompt identification and early surgical intervention is crucial to life. This is particularly true for diagnoses such as myelomeningocele, where early coverage of the defect, ideally within the first few days of life, is important to minimize the risk of infection and further neurologic damage.[6] In some selected centers, fetal surgery can be performed in utero for myelomeningocele, which offers a rare, albeit investigational, opportunity to potentially improve the outcome for the developing patient.[6,7] However, most cases of spinal deformity are surgically addressed later in infancy or early childhood.

Early childhood intervention may be recommended due to the progressive nature of the deformity and the subsequent neurologic, respiratory, or even vascular complications that can ensue from the deformity.[8–10] The main goal of orthopedic surgical intervention is to maximize function and independence. For the vast majority cases, this is directly related to the level of neurologic involvement. The timing of surgical interventions must be carefully balanced in regard to the patient's growth potential. Despite an ever-expanding variety of growth-friendly surgeries, relative equipoise remains on when to best operate on the spine that requires early intervention—many patients begin with serial nonoperative interventions in an attempt to delay surgery as much as reasonable prior to early surgery on the fewest vertebrae possible.

Appraisal Literature and Evidence-Based Guidelines

Spina bifida, in comparison with other neonatal spine deformities, is a more common deformity, so there is good literature regarding its natural history, evaluation, assessment, and management. However, for the remaining less common neonatal deformities, there are usually several accepted options for management[11–13] (Table 72.1). Unfortunately, there are few high-level studies regarding most neonatal spinal deformities.[14] This is partially due to the relatively low incidence of each disorder and the heterogeneity present within each disorder.

There is often high-level evidence about the natural history of newborn spine deformity.[1,2,8,9] Historically, most treatment studies are of evidence level four or five, with the rare level-three evidence study. With the advent of growth-friendly surgical techniques and the relatively new opportunity to compare long-term outcomes, there is now a growing number of level-two evidence studies in the literature.[14,15] With continued advancement of our knowledge of spinal development and the emergence of new techniques, so too will evidence emerge to improve management of this complex and diverse patient population.

Pathophysiology

Neonatal spine deformities are three-dimensional (3D) abnormalities of the spine due to congenitally anomalous vertebral development. The bony malformations contributing to deformity typically occur during the fourth through sixth week of gestation. This timing is of

Table 72.1 Prevalence/Incidences of Neonatal Spine Deformities Covered in This Chapter[6,14,31,32,34]

Anomaly	Incidence
Spina bifida	3.4 per 10,000
Congenital vertebral malformations	1–3 per 10,000
Caudal regression syndrome	0.1–0.25 per 10,000
Skeletal dysplasia	
Nonlethal	
Spondyloepiphyseal dysplasia	3–4 per 1 million people
Diastrophic dysplasia	1 per 500,000 in US (1 per 33,000, Finland)
Larsen syndrome	1 per 100,000
Metatropic dysplasia	<1 per 1,000,000
Achondroplasia	1 per 25,000
Lethal	15 per 100,000

critical importance given that it represents a vulnerable period of fetal organogenesis, leading to the association of additional anatomic differences. Depending on the abnormality, spine growth and morphology will be varied. Spine development results in an imbalance of the longitudinal growth of the spine, which is typically progressive in nature. Whether the ultimate cause of the anomaly is due to environmental factors, genetic differences in embyrologic pathways, or a mutation affecting multiple organ systems, understanding how the spine develops in utero is an important first step in understanding how to take care of these patients.

Embryologic Development of the Spine[16,17]

At approximately the gestational age of 20 days, the neural plate folds to form the neural tube. As the lateral-edge closure proceeds both cranially and caudally toward each neuropore, the neural tube is effectively pinched off from the epidermis. The cranial neuropore closes at about day 24; the caudal neuropore, day 28. The neural tube will go on to develop as the spinal cord and the rest of the central nervous system. The notochord persists as the nucleus pulposus in intervertebral discs.

In somitogenesis, the paraxial mesoderm condenses in pairs on either side of the notochord. Each somite gives rise to a ventral sclerotome and a dorsolateral dermomyotome. In the fourth week of gestation, a portion of each sclerotome migrates ventrally to fully engulf the notochord. Ventrally migrated cells will go on to form the vertebral body; the dorsal cells will form the vertebral arch and costal processes. The cranial half of one sclerotome and the caudal half of the adjacent sclerotome fuse, each contributing a portion of cells to the development of a single vertebra. Thus a single vertebra results from the proper formation and migration of cells from two somite levels.

During the first year of life, the vertebral arches join together. The arches then go on to join the vertebral bodies, beginning cervically at about 3 years of age and completing distally by 6 years of age.

Environmental Etiology of Spinal Malformations[17]

Maternal exposure to medications or toxins such as carbon monoxide, alcohol, boric acid, and/or valproic acid may cause congenital scoliosis. Aberrations in the developmental milieu have also been associated with vertebral malformations, hyperglycemia, hypoxia, and hyperthermia. However, in most cases, an individual cause cannot be found.

Similarly, it is also appreciated that the developmental milieu must also have sufficient presence of certain factors. The most notable of these is folic acid for proper neurulation. The decrease in incidence of infants born with neural tube defects has been attributed to prenatal screening and now widely accepted maternal perinatal supplementation. In populations where perinatal supplementation is limited and where the cultural diet contains less enriched foods, incidence of neural tube defects is higher.

Growth and Development[18,19]

The neonatal spine will nearly triple in length from birth to adulthood. The vertebral apophysis at the superior and inferior vertebral endplates contributes to two rapid growth periods—from birth to about 5 years of age and during puberty. Each thoracic vertebrae, of two apophyses per vertebrae, contributes approximately 1 mm per year to vertebral column height. The more rapid growth velocity is from birth to 5 years of age, when the spine gains about 10 cm in vertebral column length. The growth of the spine, thoracic cavity, and lungs is intimately associated. Significant disturbance of normal spinal growth or thoracic cavity development will impair pulmonary maturation, potentially severely decreasing pulmonary function.

Clinical Features

Spina Bifida[20–22]

Spina bifida disorders, or myelodysplasias, are neural tube defects characterized by failure of formation, affecting the dorsal vertebral elements, and a defect of the overlying skin, allowing for exposure of the meninges and spinal cord. In the most common and most severely disabling form of spina bifida, myelomeningocele, examination reveals a protruding sac containing neural elements. With meningocele, the protruding sac does not contain neural elements. Lipomeningocele refers to an open distal lumbar bony canal with intact dermis and epidermis. There is fatty infiltration of the canal, often causing tether. Hydrocephalus is rare. In spina bifida occulta, despite an underlying defect in the vertebral arch, the meninges and cord are normal and the bony defect has no clinical significance.

In addition to intrinsic malformation, exposure of the spinal cord and nerve roots to the toxic amniotic fluid leads to neurogenic bladder, bowel dysmotility, and motor and sensory deficits below the level of the lesion. Asymmetry of sensory loss or weakness is common. Other lesions exist in conjunction with spina bifida that can affect neurologic function, including Chiari malformation, cerebellar hypoplasia, hydrocephalus, tethered cord, syringomyelia, or diastematomyelia. Congenital manifestations of spina bifida including kyphosis, scoliosis, hip dislocation, clubfoot, or vertical talus are often present at birth and can worsen with development. Additional musculoskeletal pathology such as contracture, bony deformity, fracture, and wounds may develop with time due to chronic muscular imbalances, disuse osteopenia, paralysis, and sensation deficit.

Congenitally Abnormal Vertebrae[1,2,8,9,11,13,23]

Congenitally abnormal vertebrae collectively describe abnormal bony development seen in congenital scoliosis, congenital kyphosis, rib and scapular fusions, clefted vertebrae, and vertebral agenesis. Three basic types of vertebral anomalies occur: failures of formation, failures of segmentation, or a mixed deformity (Fig. 72.1). Failures of

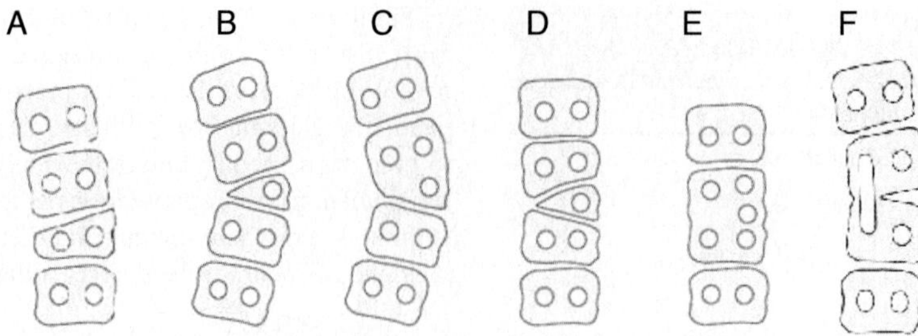

Fig. 72.1 Subclassification of Congenital Vertebrae Anomalies. Failures of formation include (A) wedge vertebrae–partial unilateral failure resulting in bilateral pedicles but asymmetric vertebral height and hemivertebrae of a complete unilateral failure with a single pedicle with variable growth potential, (B) segmented, (C) semisegmented, (D) incarcerated, and (E) nonsegmented. Failure of segmentation can manifest as (F) bar, a partial fusion between vertebrae, that prevents normal longitudinal growth on the fused side.[24]

formation and segmentation both may manifest as lateral-based structures, causing scoliosis; dorsal, causing lordosis; ventral, causing kyphosis; or a combination of these positions.

Failure of formation can be partial, which causes wedged vertebrae with intact pedicles, or complete, which causes hemivertebrae with a unilateral pedicle or occasionally complete absence of a vertebral segment. Subtypes of failure of formation abnormalities are named for their effect on the end plate, and therefore growth (see Fig. 72.1). Failure of segmentation during somatogenesis manifests as a spectrum. As with other bar malformations in the body, the bony vertebral bar resulting from a partial failure in segmentation will restrict growth in the same plane of direction as the bar. Vertebral anomalies often exist in conjunction as "mixed" deformity. Anomalies can be found on several levels. Multiple abnormal vertebrae may significantly complicate deformity or may functionally balance the curve. The natural history of congenital vertebral anomalies relates to the type of deformity, location, number and span of deformities, initial severity of curve, global growth potential, and balance of the spine.

Effects on Pulmonary Function[10,25–28]

Congenital abnormalities of vertebrae often occur with rib abnormalities. Rib fusion in the setting of an abnormal spine can lead to growth restriction of the thoracic cavity during a period of crucial pulmonary development. Alveolar development primarily occurs before 5 years of age, so ensuring that growth can occur as much as possible during this time is crucial. Should the growth abnormalities lead to enough restriction such that the tissue is unable to sufficiently develop, thoracic insufficiency syndrome (TIS) may develop. Early spine fusion before age 9, especially in patients requiring longer fusions, puts patients at risk for the development of restrictive pulmonary disease.

Associated Anomalies[4,29,30]

Because the development of the spine coincides with the development of many other organ systems, associated anomalies occur in 30% to 60% of children with congenital spine malformations. Many associated anomalies are part of the VACTERLS association. The acronym includes various deficiencies: vertebral defects (V), anal atresia (A), cardiac defects (C), tracheoesophageal fistula (TE), radial limb reduction and renal defects (R), limb defects (L), and single umbilical artery (S) (Table 72.2). Additional testing other than those that serve to evaluate the spine are necessary. Collaboration with the patient's primary care provider and other specialties will serve to prepare the surgical team and optimize the patient for surgery.

The most common anomalies involve the spinal cord, the genitourinary tract, and the cardiac system. Intraspinal anomalies include problems such as tethered cord, diastematomyelia, syringomyelia, Chiari malformations, and intradural lipomas. The most common genitourinary defects are horseshoe kidney, renal aplasia, ectopic kidney, duplication, reflux, and hypospadias. Congenital heart defects range from the more common atrial and ventricular septal defects to the more complex tetralogy of Fallot or transposition of the great vessels.

Caudal Regression Syndrome[31]

Caudal regression syndrome, or sacral agenesis, manifests as the complete or partial absence of the sacrum and lower spine with corresponding distal absence or abnormalities of the nerves at that level. The pelvis and lower extremities are underdeveloped. Additional associated conditions include VACTERLS manifestations. Similar to spina bifida, motor deficits correspond to level of abnormality. However, in contrast to spina bifida, sensation distally is intact, which protects against pressure injuries and wounds. Caudal regression syndrome has been associated with maternal diabetes.

Skeletal Dysplasias[32]

Skeletal dysplasias represent a diverse group of disorders characterized by disordered bone and/or cartilage growth. Several skeletal dysplasias are commonly accompanied by spinal problems, some of which can be appreciated in the neonatal period. Developmental and degenerative abnormalities can result in spinal cord compression and impingement on associated neural elements. Resulting neurologic complications, including pain and paralysis, significantly reduce patient quality of life and life expectancy.

Evaluation

Physical Exam[30]

The physical examination of a patient with neonatal spine deformity is guided by the knowledge of a high frequency of other structural and neural anomalies. Maternal and perinatal history and developmental milestones must be fully explored. Presence of a dimple, nevi, hemangiomas or hairy patches, and/or any other cutaneous mark on the back should be noted. The sagittal plane balance and coronal balance, shoulder malalignment, and any deviation of the head and trunk from the center of the pelvis should be checked. The cervical spine should be especially examined, including range of neck motion. In addition, it is

Table 72.2 VACTERLS–Associated Pathologies and Relative Frequencies[14,29,30,34,41]

Associated Anomaly	Incidence	Type of Manifestations	Initial Tests
Intraspinal	35%	Tethered cord Diastematomyelia Syringomyelia Chiari malformation Intradural lipoma	Physical exam (motor and reflex) Ultrasound spine MRI spine
Anal atresia	36%	Spectrum	Physical exam (inspection) History (failure to pass meconium, constipation) Ultrasound of abdomen Radiograph (dilated colon)
Congenital heart defects	25%	Atrial and ventricular septal defects Tetralogy of Fallot Transposition of the great vessels	Physical exam (auscultation) Echocardiogram Cardiac CT or MRI
Tracheoesophageal fistula	23%	—	Ultrasound (polyhydramnios) History (breathing/eating difficulty) Radiograph
Renal malformations	20%	Horseshoe kidney Renal aplasia Ectopic kidney Renal duplication Reflux Hypospadias	Labs (can be normal) Ultrasound (pre- and postnatal) Cystourethrogram
Limb deficiency	27%	Radial limb reduction	Ultrasound (prenatal) Physical exam (inspection, power, range of motion) Radiographs
Single umbilical artery	20%	Can be first clue to diagnosis	Ultrasound (prenatal) Physical exam (inspection)

CT, Computed tomography; *MRI,* magnetic resonance imaging; *VACTERLS,* vertebral defects, anal atresia, cardiac defects, tracheoesophageal fistula, radial limb reduction and renal defects, limb defects, and single umbilical artery.

critical to assess and document the neurologic status, including strength, reflexes, the presence of atrophy, and the existence of latent ataxia or myelopathy. Flexibility of the deformity, trunk shortening, and limb-length inequality should be checked. Pain, if present, should be localized when able. The examiner should search for other anomalies of the extremities (particularly limb malformation).

Ultrasound[33,34]

Ultrasound in the prenatal and postdelivery perinatal period can be a useful tool in the early diagnosis of spine deformity. In addition to the other early screening methods, ultrasound offers a noninvasive, radiation-free, cost-effective, and reliable diagnosis for pathologies such as spina bifida and some skeletal dysplasias. The spine itself can be imaged in sagittal, axial, and coronal planes starting in the late first trimester (Fig. 72.2). Additional musculoskeletal features including limb length and talipes can also been seen via ultrasound. Early diagnosis of spine pathology is advantageous to aid in family discussion and guidance, appropriately prepare the delivery team for prompt neonatal care, and potentially provide in utero therapy.

Radiographs[35–38]

Plain radiographs remain the standard for the diagnosis, classification, and longitudinal monitoring of congenital spine deformities. Ideally, radiographs are obtained prior to 4 years of age (Fig. 72.3).

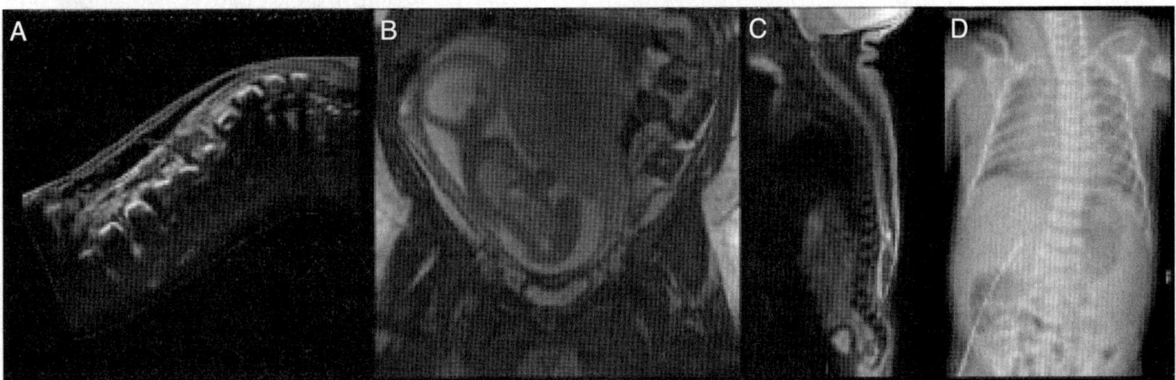

Fig. 72.2 Spina Bifida With Open Myelomeningocele as Seen in Multiple Modalities Demonstrating Large Defect in the Lumbosacral Area Beginning at L1. (A) Sagittal ultrasound view of a fetus. (B) In utero sagittal magnetic resonance image (MRI) prior to repair. (C) Saggital MRI after postbirth repair. (D) Radiograph demonstrating widened lumbar interpedicular distance.

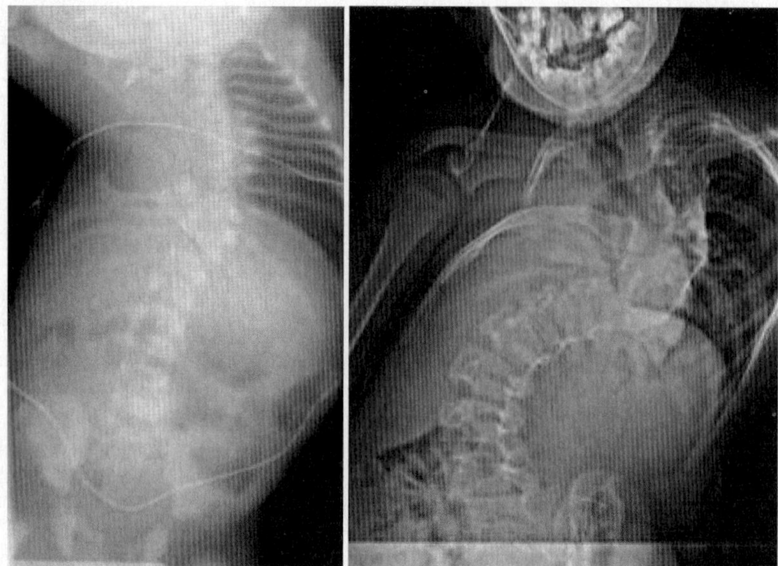

Fig. 72.3 Congenital Anomalies Are Easier to Analyze in Radiographs Obtained Earlier in Development. Radiograph A, taken early in infancy, shows abnormalities in eight ribs on the right side and thoracic vertebrae. Radiograph B was taken later in childhood; the abnormalities are obstructed by the bony deformity and progressive curvature.

After this time period, it may be difficult to fully appreciate the deformity because vertebrae are more ossified, especially in the areas of fusion or bars. Prior radiographs of the chest and abdominal or renal studies are typically available given the neonatal medical management that many patients require and are useful tools in assessing early development. Subtle findings such as the presence and spacing of pedicles and fused, atretic, or absent ribs provide clues about underlying deformity. Radiographs are more time-, cost-, and radiation exposure–efficient means of assessing bony spine differences compared with serial advanced imaging studies.

In spina bifida, spinal deformity correlates with the level of neurologic involvement. For patients with high-level lesions, it is recommended to obtain spine radiographs at least annually to evaluate any deformity. Patients with low-level involvement have a comparatively low incidence of scoliosis, so development of abnormal curvature should raise the possibility of an underlying tethered cord.

Computed Tomography[37,39,40]

Computed tomography (CT) with 3D reconstruction can be used to more completely and more consistently identify spinal abnormalities, especially posterior element abnormalities, in complex cases. Additionally, the spatial relationship of each structure can be better demonstrated with CT. Reconstruction into 3D modeling aids in the evaluation of the TIS and highlights deformities including rib synostoses, rib hypoplasia or agenesis, and intracanal protrusions through the radicular foramina (Fig. 72.4).

Magnetic Resonance Imaging[30,41–44]

Magnetic resonance imaging (MRI) serves to evaluate intraspinal anomalies that are often associated with neonatal spine disorders. Because general anesthesia is often needed to obtain MRI in young children, it should be ordered only when it may affect treatment or prior to a planned surgical procedure. Careful physical examination can suggest underlying spinal dysraphism. However, a normal physical exam dose not rule out neuraxial malformations. MRI of the spine will also typically demonstrate the presence or absence of renal anomalies.

Patients who have congenital scoliosis with cervical and thoracic hemivertebrae tend to have more intraspinal abnormalities than those with lumbar hemivertebrae. The most common anomalies reported are tethered cord, syringomyelia, and diastematomyelia. Clinically relevant MRI findings for spina bifida occulta include low conus medullaris, dermal sinus tract, lipomyelomeningocele, neuroenteric cyst, and spinal cord malformation. Some of these may require neurosurgical treatment for their own sake (e.g., a

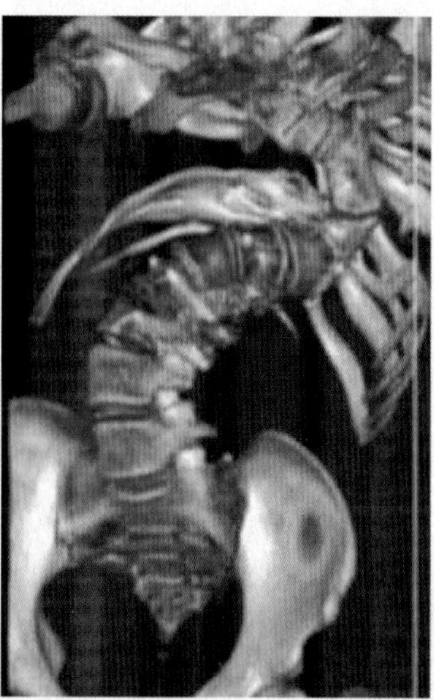

Fig. 72.4 Three-Dimensional Computed Tomography Reconstruction of Congenital Spine Disorder Helps the Surgeon More Fully Appreciate Complex Deformities.

large syrinx), whereas others need may require neurosurgical collaboration if corrective orthopedic surgery is planned (e.g., diastematomyelia).

Management

The management of musculoskeletal spine abnormalities begins with surgical specialty consultation with pediatric orthopedic or neurologic surgery. In most cases, the initial phases of management include close monitoring of deformity and caregiver counseling. More involved patients will require multiple interventions throughout infancy and childhood, ranging from bracing to serial surgical procedures. Because of the high association of additional musculoskeletal differences in patients with congenital spine abnormalities, interventions on pathologies such as clubfoot or hip dysplasia often begin prior to addressing the spine deformity itself. Orthopedic management becomes a life-long part of many patients' care. Early consultation will help develop a meaningful relationship between the family, patient, and provider teams.

Myelomeningocele Repair[20,45–48]

Early coverage of myelomeningocele defects, ideally within the first days of life, is important to minimize the risk of infection and further neurologic damage. Some centers perform fetal surgery in utero. Although the procedure cannot restore lost neurologic function, it offers a rare opportunity to potentially prevent additional loss from occurring.

Deformity Management Principles[1,29,49–52]

Congenital vertebral anomalies require close clinical monitoring at periodic intervals during growth. Malformations with low progression rates should be periodically evaluated for possible progression. In complex, progressive malformations, early treatment is often more straightforward and safer.

Contrary to idiopathic scoliosis, brace treatment has little value in congenital scoliosis.[53,54] Only a small number of cases, characterized by long and flexible curves, may be temporized by bracing to slow the progression of the curvatures. However, these curves will predictably eventually decompensate and ultimately require surgical stabilization. Congenital scoliosis progresses because the growth potential of the spine is imbalanced.

In general, careful monitoring every 4 to 6 months with regular examination and radiographic evaluation is prudent in curves measuring up to 40 degrees. Other factors including deformity type, growth profile, and pulmonary, cardiac, or neurologic function may require earlier surgical intervention. Without any treatment, 50% of patients with congenital scoliosis will have a curve greater than 45 degrees by maturity.

Age is not necessarily a limiting factor for surgery. For example, spines with successive, fully segmented hemivertebrae concomitant with additional severe deformities of the rib cage will go on to cause TIS. In this case the patient would be recommended for surgical intervention earlier, regardless of the Cobb angle, to allow for growth of the thoracic region.

In situ fusion is an option to stabilize but not correct the deformity. Therefore, in situ fusions are restricted to small curves and should be performed shortly after documented progression as a prophylactic treatment that prevents further progression. The corrective strategy seeks to straighten the spine and restore more anatomic alignment and can be applied to longer curvatures.

The goal of surgical treatment of spinal curvature in patients with congenital deformity is four-fold: (1) achieve a straight spine, with or without deformity reduction; (2) restore a physiologic sagittal profile while maintaining flexibility; (3) limit curve progression; and (4) preserve normal spinal growth as much as possible by only fusing a short segment.

Several operations have been described: posterior spine fusion,[50,51,55,56] combined anterior and posterior spine fusion,[50,57] convex hemiepiphysiodesis,[58–64] hemivertebra excision,[65–70] osteotomies,[71–73] vertebral column resection,[74–77] and guided growth procedures.[78–85] Correction of deformity should occur early to allow the correction of the fewest vertebrae possible and to protect against continued, severe structural spine decompensation. The appreciation of the need to preserve pulmonary function and to allow maximum spinal height has spurred the development of growth-preserving surgical alternatives to traditional spinal fusion, including growing rods, guided growth, epiphysiodesis, and distraction thoracoplasty (Fig. 72.5).

Growth Preservation Strategies[78–85]

Thoracic cavity growth and chest wall development are often restricted in patients with complex congenital deformities due to the extent of vertebral abnormalities tethering normal longitudinal and circumferential growth. The exact timing of surgical intervention to address these complex deformities remains a topic of debate. On one hand, early spinal fusion has the advantage of preventing further growth restriction. On the other hand, early spinal fusion restricts growth and development beyond the time of fusion.

In a young patient with progressive deformity, growing rods provide progressive correction of the curve and the expansion of the thorax. By using expandable devices and serial surgeries for

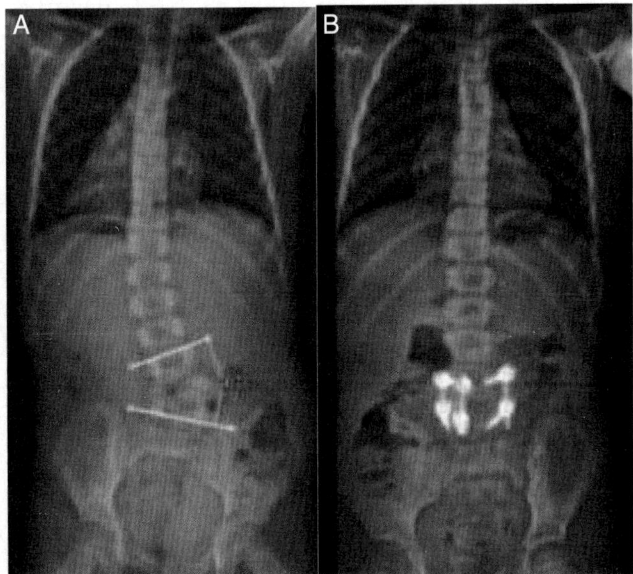

Fig. 72.5 Radiographs demonstrate localized lumbar scoliosis meeting operative indications in a 6-year-old (A) and postoperative correction after hemivertebrae excision and anterior and posterior spinal fusion with instrumentation at 1 year's follow-up (B).

lengthening, one can free the abnormal tethering restricting thoracic growth while also permitting for continued growth after the first surgery. This strategy seeks to prevent deformity progression, maximize growth, and delay definitive fusion for as long as possible (Fig. 72.6).

Both in patients with and without rib anomalies, vertical expandable prosthetic titanium rib guided growth has been shown to be effective in improving the Cobb angle and allowing for increasing thoracic height.

Magnetic controlled growing rods (MCGRs) continue to expand the possibilities for guided growth procedures. Rather than continued reoperation with exchange of implants, as is needed with conventional growing rods, MCGRs can facilitate curve control, maintain growth along the spine, and spare the patient multiple reoperations by using nonsurgical distraction methods. Preliminary data on MCGRs are promising both from a safety and an efficacy standpoint.

The medical and surgical teams must be aware of potential complications unique to expandable implants. Migration of spinal anchors, infection, postoperative pain, device fracture due to stress fatigue, brachial plexus palsy, and neurologic injury occur at high rates compared with traditional implant techniques.

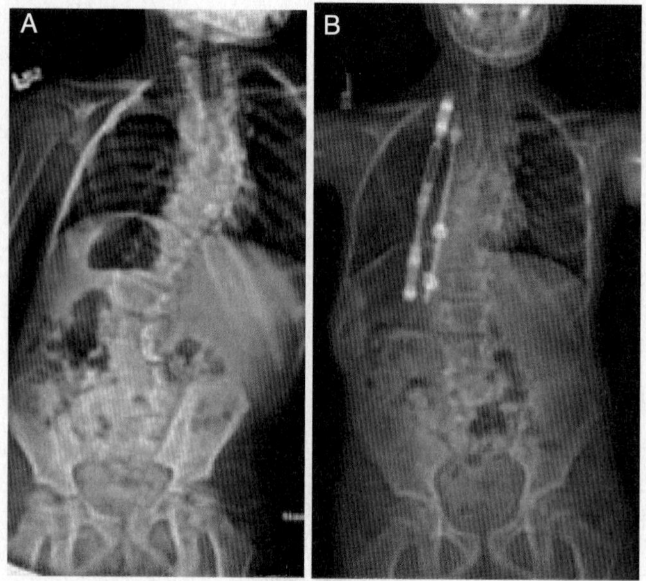

Fig. 72.6 Radiographs of a 5-year-old with congenital scoliosis who underwent growth-preserving corrective surgery with an expandable device along the left ribs (A) and the resultant correction at 12 years old (B).

CHAPTER 73

Hip and Lower Extremity Deformities

Erin Honcharuk

KEY POINTS

1. Early diagnosis of abnormalities in the lower extremities is important for normal musculoskeletal and neurologic development.
2. Developmental dysplasia of the hip starts early in the embryonic period and continues after birth. It includes a range of abnormalities including acetabular dysplasia with deficient development of the acetabulum, subluxation with displacement but some maintained contact between the femoral head and acetabulum, and complete dislocation with no contact between the two surfaces.
3. Congenital talipes equinovarus, also known as clubfoot, is a congenital dysplasia in the structures distal to the knee. The talus is shortened with greater acute angulation than normal. The navicular is also medially and plantarly deviated.
4. The calcaneovalgus foot is a soft-tissue positional contracture; it is usually a flexible deformity in which the foot is hyperdorsiflexed at the ankle and there is a mild subtalar eversion.
5. Congenital vertical talus or rocker-bottom foot is a rigid dorsal dislocation of the talonavicular joint with a fixed hindfoot equinus. A less severe manifestation is the oblique talus, where the navicular can be reduced in certain foot positions.
6. Congenital hyperextension of the knee describes a spectrum of disease, from hyperextension to subluxation to true dislocation of the knee.
7. Fibular hemimelia is a congenital deficiency of the fibula. Tibial hemimelia is a spectrum of disease with varying degrees of deficiency of the tibia and associated bones in the knee and the foot. Some patients may show tibial bowing in various planes. Some infants may show a spectrum of femoral shortening and deformity.

Developmental Dysplasia of the Hip

Developmental dysplasia of the hip (DDH) covers a spectrum of abnormal development of the hip that starts during embryology and continues after birth. It ranges from dysplasia, or deficient development of the acetabulum, through subluxation, with displacement but some maintained contact between the femoral head and acetabulum, to complete dislocation, with no contact between the two surfaces.[1,2] The incidence of DDH is about 1 per 1000.[3]

Pathophysiology

There are a few known risk factors associated with DDH.[4] These include being female, a family history of DDH, breech positioning, first-born children, and oligohydramnios. However, the etiology of DDH is certainly multifactorial. Ligamentous laxity, which can be hereditary, increases the risk of DDH. This has been confirmed in several animal models, in which changes to the hip capsule and ligamentum teres leads to DDH whereas removing the bony acetabulum does not. Additionally, newborns, especially females, respond to maternal relaxin hormone during delivery, and this may explain the higher rates of DDH in female children.

There is also a higher rate of DDH in infants born in a breech position.[4] This is particularly true for those in a frank breech position. This may be because the hamstrings pull across the flexed hips and straight knees and act as a dislocating force.[5] The increase in DDH in first-born children or pregnancies affected by oligohydramnios further supports the effect intrauterine positioning, in this case uterine crowding, has on DDH.[6] Other postural orthopedic conditions such as torticollis and metatarsus adductus add to the evidence that positioning has an effect on hip development. Postnatal positioning can also lead to DDH. Positioning that keeps the hips in full extension, such as seen in cultures that use cradleboards, increases the rate of DDH.

If DDH is not treated, the hip will continue to develop improperly. The posterosuperior rim of the acetabulum loses its sharp curve over the femoral head and flattens out. This allows the femoral head to slide in and out. Over time, further changes occur, which can in fact block reduction. Pulvinar, a fatty tissue in the acetabulum, can develop and thicken.[7] The ligamentum teres will elongate but also thicken. Both of these take up room within the acetabulum itself. The transverse acetabulum ligament, at the base of the acetabulum, can also thicken and impair spontaneous reduction. The inferior hip capsule changes shape to that of an hourglass. This reduces the opening through which the femoral head can fit. The iliopsoas, pulling across the capsule, is partially responsible for this. If treatment is started at an appropriate time, many of these changes are reversible and the contact between the femoral head and acetabulum allow for proper development of both.[7]

Clinical Presentation

The first step in evaluation is a hip exam. A normal hip will have wide abduction symmetric with the contralateral sign. Limited range of motion (ROM) is concerning for DDH. The Barlow and Ortolani tests are best done one hip at a time and in a patient who is calm and relaxed (Fig. 73.1).[8] The examiner flexes the knees and hips and during the Barlow maneuver attempts to subluxate or dislocate the hip in a posterior direction with the hip slightly adducted. If positive, the examiner will feel the hip slide out of the acetabulum. The hip may reduce spontaneously with decreased force on the hip. During an Ortolani maneuver, the hip is abducted with pressure on the greater trochanter to try to reduce the femoral head. The examiner may feel a clunk on a positive test. These are often the earliest findings on exam.

Over time, as the hip progresses along this spectrum and becomes subluxated or dislocated without the ability to reduce it, other signs start to appear. The dislocated femoral head, located proximal to the other side, causes shortening of the thigh. This can cause asymmetric skin folds, a positive Galeazzi sign, or a positive Klisic test. In the Galeazzi sign, both hips and knees are flexed to 90 degrees with the feet flat on the exam table; the affected knee will appear

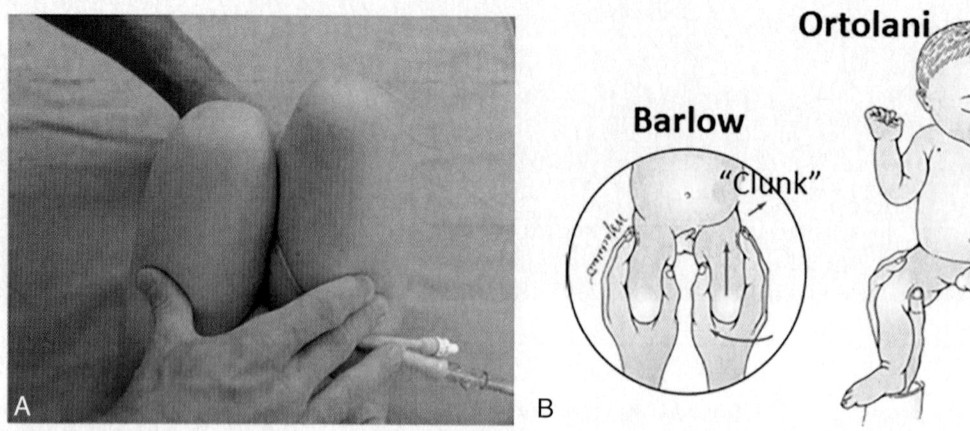

Fig. 73.1 Developmental Dysplasia of the Hip. (A) Presence of Galeazzi sign. (B) Ortolani (left) and Barlow (right) maneuvers. The Ortolani sign (reducing a dislocated hip) is the most sensitive examination finding in patients younger than 3 months. ([A] Reproduced after permission and minor modifications from Grottkau BE et al. Common neonatal orthopedic ailments. In: Taeusch HW et al., eds. *Avery's Diseases of the Newborn*. 8th ed. 2005:1423–1435, Fig. 94.1; [B] Reproduced after permission and minor modifications from Swartz MH. The pediatric patient. In: Swartz MH, ed. *Textbook of Physical Diagnosis*. 7th ed. Philadelphia, PA: Saunders; 2014:671–742, Figs. 21–22.)

shorter.[8] For the Klisic test, the examiner places one finger on the greater trochanter and another on the anterior superior iliac sign and creates an imaginary line connecting these points. A test is negative if that line, continuing on, hits at or below the umbilicus. One that continues above the umbilicus is positive. The Klisic test is especially useful with bilateral DDH, as compared with a normal comparative side in which it is not required.[8]

As a child with unilateral DDH begins to walk, their gait may include toe walking because one leg is shorter. They may also have a Trendelenburg gait, in which they lean over the unaffected side while walking. Again, it can be more difficult to evaluate a child with bilateral DDH, because both legs are shortened. However, there may be increased lumbar lordosis and a waddling gait.

Further evaluation is done with imaging.[9–11] At birth through 4 to 7 months of age, the femoral head is cartilaginous. Therefore ultrasound is used initially, although this should not be done prior to 6 weeks of age because it can increase the rate of false positives.[10] The alpha angle, the angle between a line down the ilium and a line down the bony acetabulum, should be higher than 60 degrees, although 50 to 60 degrees can be considered borderline in infants less than 3 months. The percentage of the femoral head covered by the bony acetabulum is also measured and should be greater than 50% (Fig. 73.2). A dynamic ultrasound uses the Barlow and Ortolani maneuvers to evaluate the degree of subluxation during stress.[11] Once the femoral head starts to ossify, radiographs can be used to evaluate for DDH (Fig. 73.3).[10] Fig. 73.4 shows the appearance of a hip with DDH and useful lines and angles measured on an anteroposterior (AP) pelvis. A break in Shenton lines suggests proximal migration of the femur. The acetabular index decreases over time and should be less than 20 degrees by age 2.

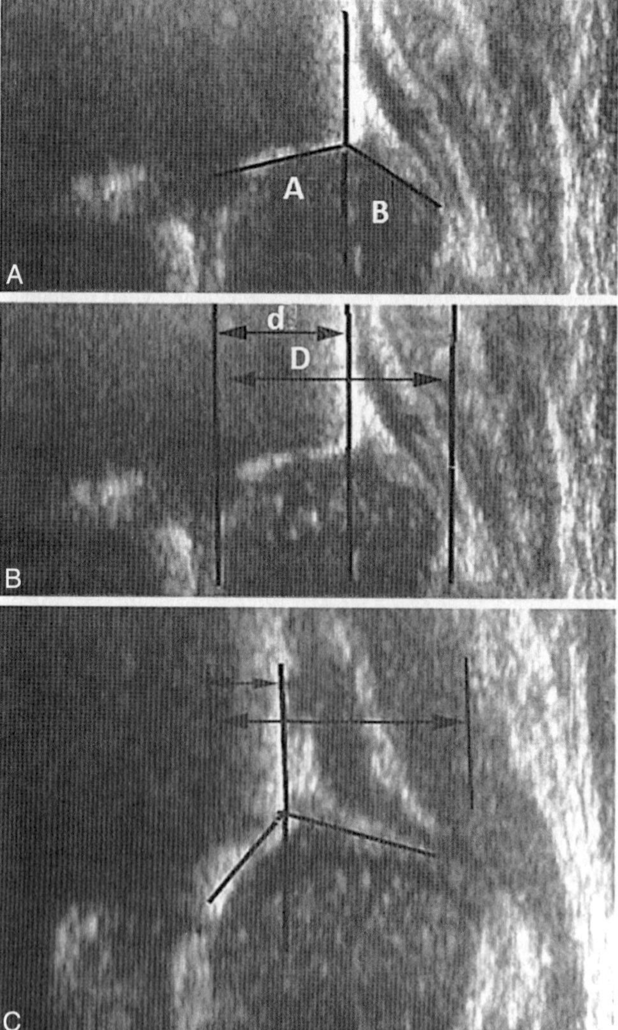

Fig. 73.2 Standard Coronal Plane Ultrasonogram of a Normal Infant's Hip. (A) The alpha angle *A* corresponds to the bony acetabular roof (normal, >60 degrees). The beta angle *B* represents the cartilaginous roof (normal, <50 degrees). (B) Method for determining percentage of coverage of the femoral head: d/D × 100 (normal, ≥50%). (C) Coronal plane ultrasonogram of a dysplastic hip. The alpha angle was 40 degrees; the femoral head was subluxated with only 25% coverage. (Reproduced after permission and minor modifications from Kayes and Didelot. Major congenital orthopedic deformities. In: *Pediatric Surgery*, ch. 129, 1699–1710.)

Treatment

In a child less than 6 months of age diagnosed with DDH, treatment with a Pavlik harness is initiated (Fig. 73.5).[12,13] In the harness, the hips are flexed beyond 90 degrees, sometimes up to 120 degrees, and with the hips abducted, although not in forced abduction. The child is maintained in the harness until reduction is ensured and usually at least 6 weeks. They are monitored in clinic for any issues pertaining to the harness and with ultrasound to ensure improvement of the hips. It is vital to make sure the child continues to kick their legs, because excessive hip flexion can cause a femoral nerve palsy and loss of that motion. If that occurs, the harness should be removed

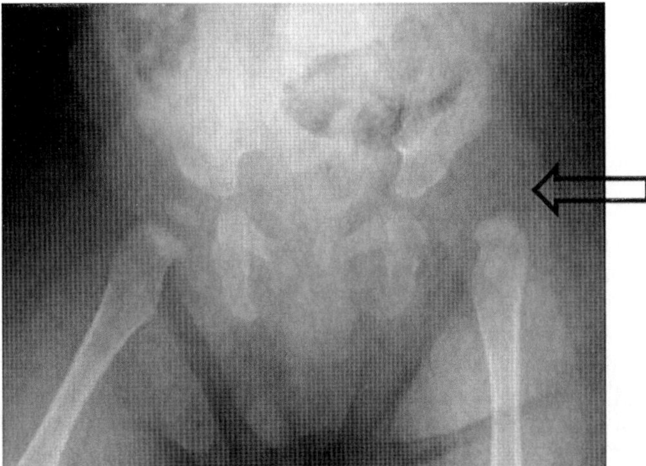

Fig. 73.3 Anteroposterior Radiograph of a 6-Month-Old Infant With Developmental Dysplasia of the Hip. The dysplasia of the left hip is notable with missing ossification in the femoral nucleus, superior and lateral dislocation, and a small, steep acetabulum (highlighted with the *arrow*). (Reproduced after permission and minor modifications from Schwend RM et al. Evaluation and treatment of developmental hip dysplasia in the newborn and infant. *Pediatr Clin North Am.* 61(6):1095–1107, 2014, Fig. 2.)

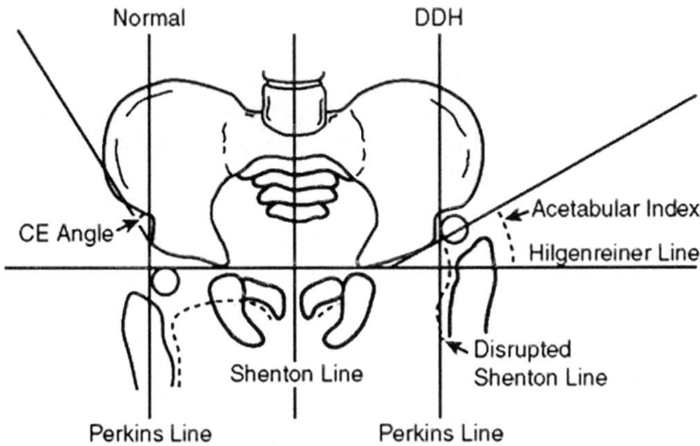

Fig. 73.4 Diagram of Radiographic Measurements. Hip development starts with the femoral head and acetabulum being formed as a block of cartilaginous cells. At 7 to 8 weeks a cleft develops between the head and acetabulum; the joint starts as "reduced" in the socket. The joint is completely developed by 11 weeks of gestation. An ossific nucleus begins to be formed in the cartilaginous femoral head at about 4 months after birth. The hip is dependent on the femoral head and acetabulum maintaining concentric reduction for normal development. If the femoral head is not concentrically reduced, the joint is less likely to develop with a normal anatomy at maturity. The acetabulum undergoes considerable remodeling and development during infancy. In DDH, the adductor muscle becomes contracted and the iliopsoas muscle can be a major block to reduction of a completely dislocated hip. It becomes contracted and can exert a powerful obstacle to reduction by forming an hourglass-shaped constriction of the anterior medial capsule. The ligamentum teres, connecting the fovea of the femoral head to the acetabulum, can hypertrophy and also pose a block to a good concentric reduction. The pulvinar is an accumulation of fat and fibrous tissue in the space next to the medial wall of the acetabulum, which can keep the femoral head lateralized during a reduction attempt. The labrum or cartilaginous rim of the acetabulum can become infolded and blunted and also block the femoral head. The anterior-medial joint capsule can become constricted. The transverse acetabular ligament spanning the inferior portion of the hip between the medial and posterior walls can also limit reduction inferiorly. All these problems may become more marked as the child gets older and may pose more difficulty in achieving an adequate reduction. *CE*, Center edge; *DDH*, developmental dysplasia of the hip. (Reproduced after permission and modifications from Kayes and Didelot. Major congenital orthopedic deformities. In: *Pediatric Surgery*, ch. 129, 1699–1710.)

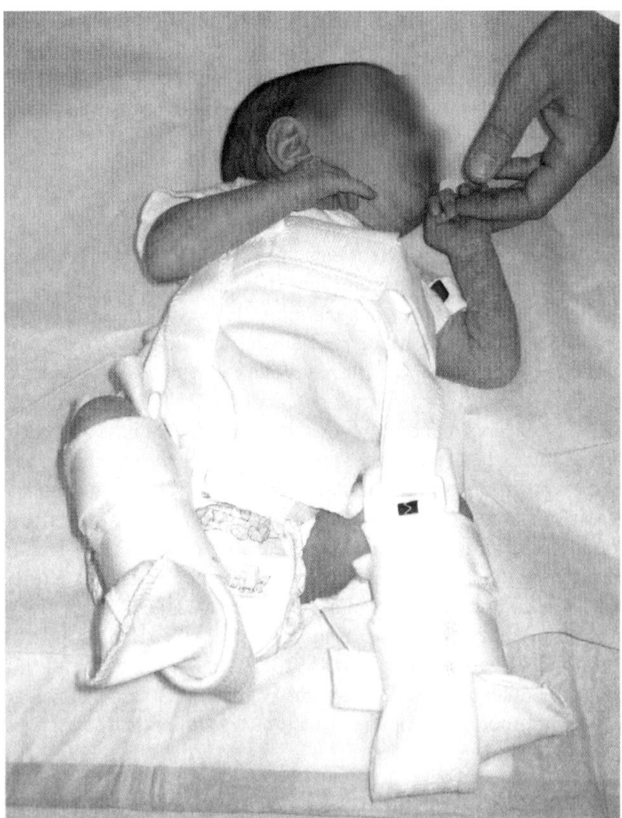

Fig. 73.5 Pavlik Harness. The transverse chest strap should be placed just below the nipple line. The hips should be flexed to 120 degrees, and the posterior straps should not produce forced abduction. (Reproduced after permission and minor modifications from *Developmental Dysplasia of the Hip*. Elsevier Point of Care. Updated December 29, 2021.)

until quad muscle function returns. Abduction ensures good contact between the developing acetabulum and femoral head, but forced abduction can cause avascular necrosis (AVN) of the femoral head. Pavlik harness treatment is highly successful, with success rates over 90%, albeit somewhat lower in hips that are irreducible. If the harness does not show reduction of the femoral head, other, more rigid abduction braces can be used and have reported variable degrees of success based on the reducibility of the hip.

In an infant who presents after 6 months of age or who fails treatment with a Pavlik harness, closed reduction in the operating room is indicated.[13] This includes an arthrogram, where dye is injected into the hip, which allows for better fluoroscopic evaluation of the femoral head and the reduction. The practitioner will also evaluate how easily the hip reduces, if at all, and the range of abduction in which the hip maintains a stable reduction. If that window is too narrow, an adductor tenotomy can be performed to widen that range. If the reduction is adequate, the patient is placed in a spica cast. They are usually taken back once or twice for repeat evaluations in the operating room and cast exchanges.

If the hip is irreducible or is not adequate, an open reduction will be performed. This can be done through two approaches, an anterolateral or a medial approach, both with their pros and cons. In patients who present after 18 to 24 months, most surgeons will primarily do an open reduction. This approach can be combined with a pelvic or femoral osteotomy. A pelvic osteotomy will increase coverage of the femoral head and can reorient or decrease the size of the acetabulum depending on the type of osteotomy performed.

A femoral osteotomy usually includes shortening of the femur, which decreases the force needed to reduce the hip. It can also derotate the femur if required. These procedures are also followed with a period of spica casting and possibly followed with abduction bracing afterward.

Long-Term Outcomes

Most studies support excellent outcomes of DDH treatment even into adulthood. This is true even for hips that show radiographic abnormalities or signs of early degeneration. However, the biggest and potentially most devastating risk during any of these treatments, including the use of a Pavlik harness, is AVN, which causes a growth disturbance of the proximal femoral physis.[13] This is most often caused by excessive abduction in either the brace or cast. Increasing abduction has been shown to decrease blood flow into the femoral head, even in a normal population. Forceful reductions can also increase tension between the femoral head and acetabulum, reducing blood flow and thus also creating AVN. Mild AVN leads to minimal changes in the femoral head and is often well tolerated without long-term sequelae in children. However, more severe forms of AVN significantly alter the shape of the hip joint, potentially leading to alterations in gait and early arthritis.[14,15] Therefore, it is vital to be vigilant about positioning of infants in harnesses and casts and to include a femoral shortening osteotomy if the reduction required significant force.

Talipes Equinovarus

Congenital talipes equinovarus, better known as clubfoot, is a congenital dysplasia of all the structures distal to the knee.[16–19] This leads to a situation of an abnormal foot in an abnormal position. The goals of treatment are to place the foot in a functional position, although the underlying differences in the musculoskeletal structures are still present. However, outcomes can still be exemplary and allow the patient to lead a normal, fully active lifestyle.

Pathophysiology

Although there have been several genes that increase the likelihood of clubfoot, there is no one specific gene that definitively causes it. Other proposed etiologies include a neuromyogenic imbalance, an arrest in embryologic development, and a fibrotic response causing contraction of the foot. Studies have both supported and refuted these hypotheses. Additionally, there does seem to be a hereditary pattern to clubfoot, albeit not following a specific hereditary pattern. This suggests that clubfoot is multifactorial but does lead to abnormal development during embryologic development.[16–19]

The pathoanatomy demonstrates significant abnormality of the talus, which becomes shortened and has more of an acute angulation than normal. Additionally, the entire bone itself is medially and plantarly deviated.[17,18] Although the calcaneus and navicular are less abnormal, there are articular changes related to their relationships with the talus. The navicular in particular, which is also medially and plantarly deviated, can create false articulations with the medial malleolus and often leaves the talar head undercovered. Furthermore, there are often contractions of joint capsules, ligaments, and tendons. Because this is a dysplasia starting at the knee, the gastrocsoleus is often smaller than a contralateral, unaffected side. Lastly, reports of absent dorsalis pedis and posterior tibialis artery have been reported in idiopathic clubfeet.

Evaluation

The typical clubfoot is often easily diagnosed at birth and can sometimes be seen on prenatal ultrasound scans.[16,17] The foot is equinus and inverted compared with the tibia with hindfoot varus (Fig. 73.6). There is also cavus and adduction of the forefoot. Even at this young age, the unilateral clubfoot is often already smaller than the contralateral side, and this is important to point out to parents. The smaller size becomes more apparent over time, but noting this early on will avoid any concerns that treatment caused a stunting of growth. Postural clubfoot can sometimes masquerade as clubfoot, but its flexibility and ability to correct to neutral, especially without any fixed equinus, helps differentiate it.

Clubfoot can be idiopathic or associated with a variety of conditions, and therefore a thorough evaluation is required. A drop-toe sign, where the toes are held in plantarflexion even with plantar stimulation, may indicate an underlying neurologic condition.[20] Certain conditions such as arthrogryposis, myelodysplasia, diastrophic dysplasia, and fetal alcohol syndrome are known to have resistant clubfoot.[21] There are multiple classification systems available for use, and they can help predict response to treatment and outcomes over the next several years.

Management

The current initial treatment of clubfoot is nonoperative and follows the Ponseti method, developed by Ignacio Ponseti in the 1940s, although it was not universally adopted until several decades later. Other treatments including physical therapy with stretching and taping have been used; however, the easier applicability of the Ponseti method has led to its being the dominant strategy for clubfoot management.[22] The treatment includes weekly casts that gradually address the underlying deformities. The cavus is addressed first; the varus and adductus are addressed next and at the same time. To prevent recurrence, the foot is brought into abduction of 60 to 70 degrees, which can often be alarming to parents and other family members. Adequate explanation of the goals and expectations of casting can help allay concerns. The equinus is addressed last and is usually not fully corrected with casting alone. Therefore, a percutaneous tendoachilles tenotomy is required and can often be done in the clinic, although some practitioners prefer to do this in the operating room. The final cast is left in place for several weeks and then the patient is transitioned to a foot abduction brace to hold the foot in its new, corrected position. Patients initially wear this full time and then transition to nighttime wear for several years.

For patients who present with an underlying syndrome associated with resistant clubfoot, are of an older age, or have a recurrence, Ponseti casting can still be attempted.[22] The foot can often achieve the same result or at least lessen the required surgical intervention. These procedures may include repeat Achilles tenotomy or lengthening, posterior capsular release or a more extensive posteromedial release, and osteotomies.

In children older than 2 or 3 years, the appearance of a dynamic supination, such that the foot inverts only during the swing phase of gait or while they are dorsiflexing the ankle, may appear. This increases weight bearing on the lateral border of the foot, and over time it can lead to hindfoot varus. This is not a true recurrence and not related to compliance during brace wear but is related to the underlying pathology of the clubfoot itself, with imbalance between the relatively stronger tibialis anterior compared with the weaker peroneal tendons and tibialis posterior. In these cases, a transfer of the tibialis anterior from the first metatarsal to the lateral cuneiform is indicated.[21]

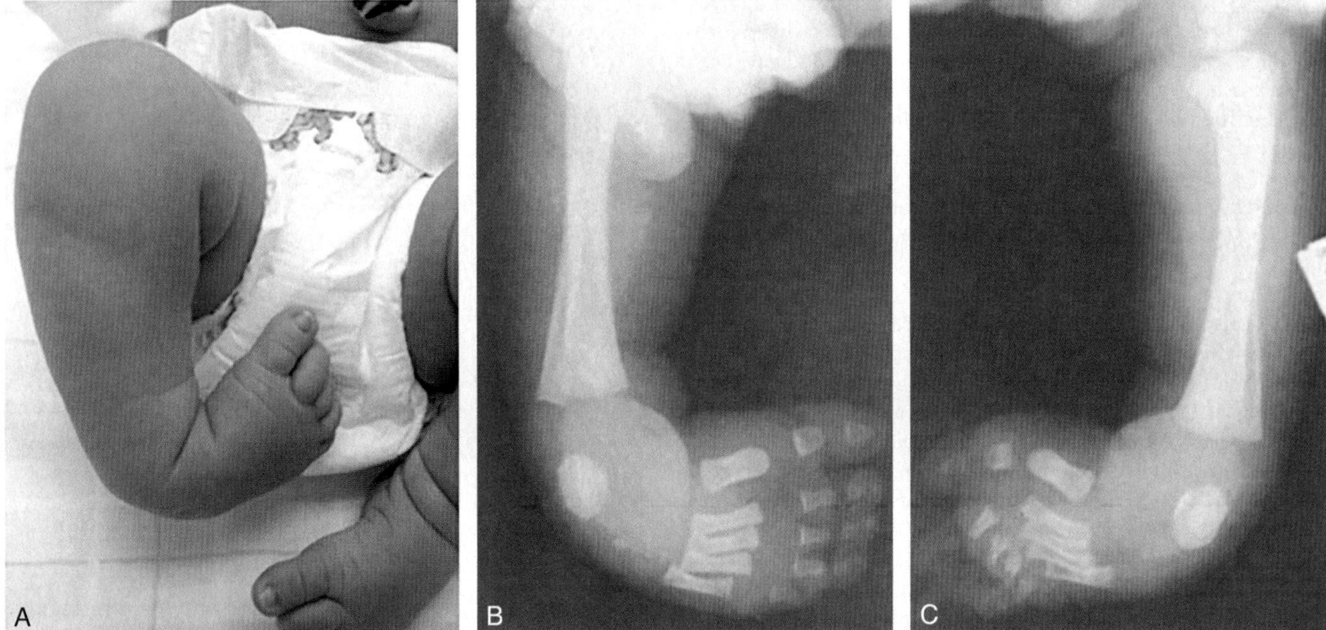

Fig. 73.6 Talipes Equinovarus in a Newborn. (A) Clinical appearance of an untreated clubfoot. (B, C) Initial radiographic appearance of bilateral untreated clubfeet. (Reproduced after permission and minor modifications from Winell and Davidson. The foot and toes. From *Nelson Textbook of Pediatrics*, ch. 694, 3597–3606.e2.)

Long-Term Outcomes

The Ponseti method has a 95% success rate of initial correction of the clubfoot.[22] However, there is at least a partial recurrence in one of every 3 such feet over the next couple of years, most frequently due to poor compliance with brace wear or delayed presentation. Still, long-term outcomes are excellent, with one long-term study showing 85% of patients with normal or good outcomes. Strength was comparable with that of the contralateral normal side, whereas motion was decreased.

Increased surgery, especially intraarticular surgery, does seem to worsen outcomes. The capsulotomies stiffen the joints with further loss of motion.[23] Additionally, overcorrection into significant hindfoot valgus is reported, especially with a full posteromedial release. Although poor brace compliance increases the need for these procedures, a more severe clubfoot at birth may also prognosticate increased need for surgery. Worse outcomes, therefore, are difficult to fully differentiate between these two groups and there is most likely overlap. There is no study comparing initial operative versus nonoperative treatment, and only further long-term studies will help delineate outcome patterns for patients with clubfeet.

Calcaneovalgus

Calcaneovalgus foot is seen in newborns and is a soft-tissue contracture problem (Fig. 73.7).[24] Positional calcaneovalgus is a flexible foot deformity in which the foot is hyperdorsiflexed at the ankle and there is mild subtalar eversion; this is caused by intrauterine positioning. It is more common in girls, first-born children, and children of young mothers.

In evaluating a patient with calcaneovalgus, it will be noted that the hindfoot externally rotates and dorsiflexes. This can cause the dorsum of the foot to come into contact with the anterior tibia. Additionally, there may be associated posteromedial bowing of the tibia, which may exacerbate the appearance of the foot dorsiflexion.

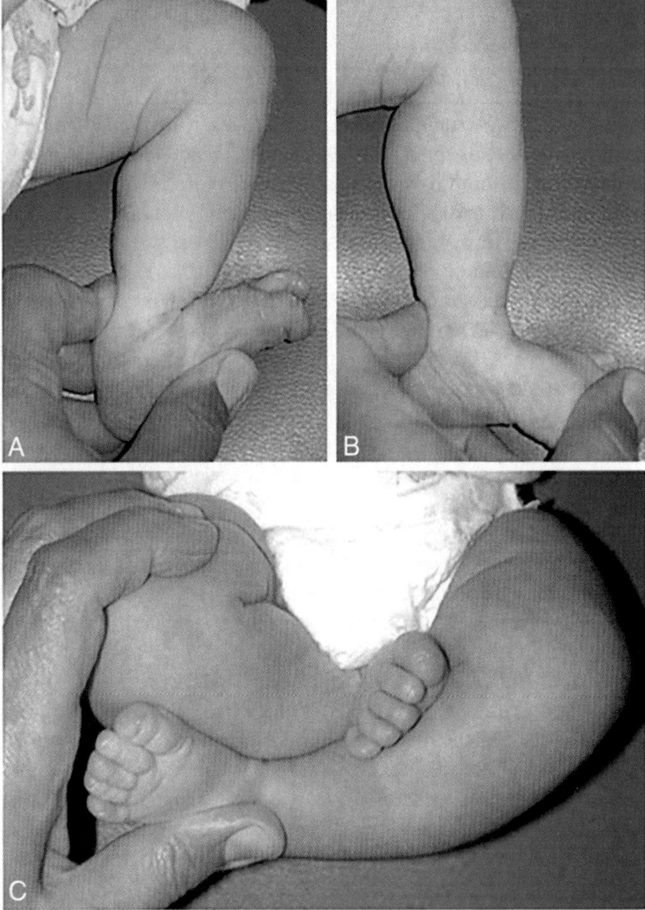

Fig. 73.7 Clinical picture of a calcaneovalgus foot (A) that is passively correctable (B) because of intrauterine positioning (C). (Reproduced after permission and minor modifications from Winell and Davidson. The foot and toes. In: *Nelson Textbook of Pediatrics*. chap 694, 3597–3606.e2).

However, posteromedial bowing of the tibia can be isolated and is sometimes misdiagnosed as calcaneolvagus foot. To distinguish between these, the apex should be determined; in calcaneovalgus, the apex is at the ankle joint, whereas in posteromedial bowing, the apex is in the tibia. The flexibility of the deformity should also be evaluated; it most often is correctable to an almost neutral position.

Radiographs are usually not indicated unless to evaluate for other diagnoses such as posteromedial bowing of the tibia or vertical talus.

The literature is mixed about the association between DDH and calcaneovalgus, but the association does appear higher in patients who have a contralateral metatarsus adductus (Fig. 73.8).

Most feet with calcaneovalgus are self-resolving, but gentle stretching of the foot into plantar flexion and inversion can be helpful. Expected improvement should occur in 3 to 6 months. Patients who also have posteromedial bowing should be counseled on the potential for a limb-length discrepancy, which may require treatment.

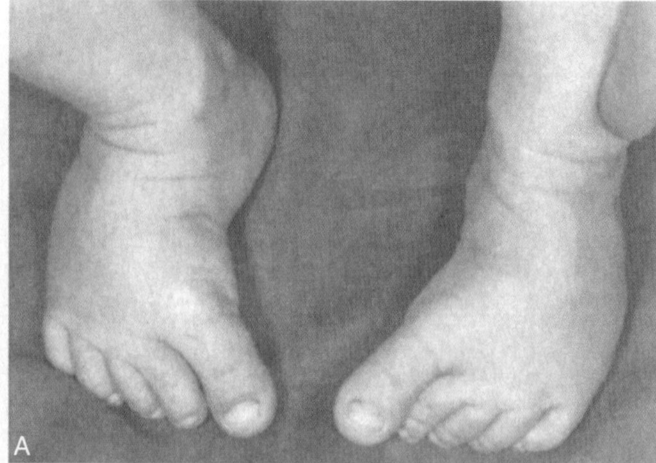

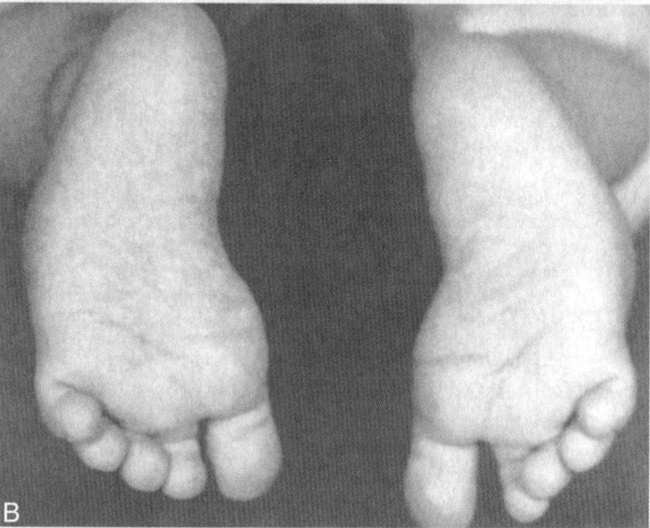

Fig. 73.8 Bilateral Mild Metatarsus Adductus. (A) Dorsal view showing medial deviation of all the metatarsals. (B) Plantar view showing the "bean-shaped" foot. This type of foot is easily corrected with serial casting. (Reproduced after permission and modifications from Ricco AI, Richards BS, Herring JA. Disorders of the foot. In Herring JA, ed. *Tachdjian's Pediatric Orthopaedics*. 5th ed. Philadelphia: Elsevier; 2014:Figs. 23–19.)

Congenital Hyperextension of the Knee and Congenital Knee Dislocation

Congenital hyperextension of the knee is often described as the knee being "backward" and describes a spectrum of disease from hyperextension to subluxation to true dislocation of the knee (Fig. 73.9).[25]

Pathophysiology

Abnormal intrauterine positioning with lack of movement from the fetus is the cause of congenital hyperextension and knee dislocation. Although congenital hyperextension is often idiopathic, syndromes associated with laxity and/or decreased fetal movement, such as Larsen, Beals, or Ehler-Danlos syndrome and arthrogryposis, are associated with congenital knee dislocation. These often have an associated hip dislocation and anterior cruciate ligament (ACL) deficiency. Idiopathic, isolated congenital knee dislocation can also occur with no associated underlying syndrome. It is thought that this abnormal positioning and decreased motion then leads to quad muscle atrophy and fibrosis.[25]

Evaluation

Diagnosis is made during prenatal ultrasounds or soon after birth, with the foot will be near the child's foot or shoulder and the femoral condyles may be palpable on the posterior knee. The correctability of the knee can also suggest where on the spectrum the diagnosis lies. If gentle stretching improves the knee flexion, it is most likely grade 1 or congenital hyperextension. Grade 2, or subluxation, shows some improvement in flexion with maintained contact between the tibial and femoral epiphysis. If there is no improvement with stretching or the tibia moves around the femur with attempted flexion, this is suggestive of a grade 3, or true congenital knee dislocation. Radiographs can also be helpful to differentiate between the three.

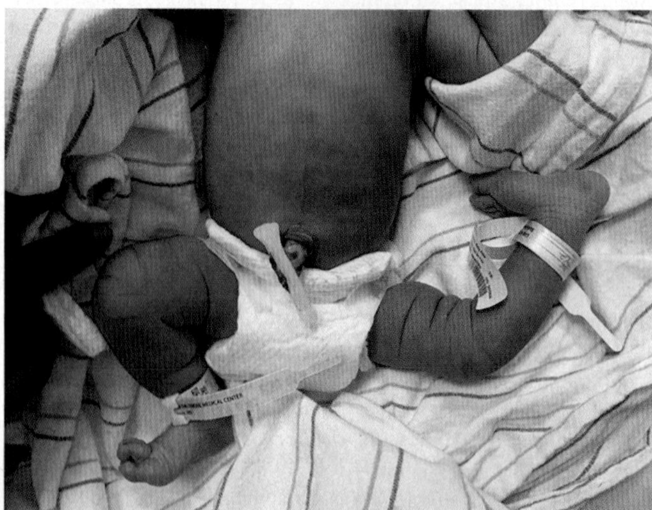

Fig. 73.9 Congenital Dislocation the Knee. Congenital dislocation the knee is a hyperextension deformity of the knee with anterior displacement of the tibia. It describes a spectrum of disease, from hyperextension to subluxation and to true dislocation of the knee.

Management

Grade 1 and 2 hyperextension can often be treated with observation, or stretching and casting to bring the knee into a flexed position.

This should be done gently and gradually to avoid fractures. If there is difficulty in obtaining reduction, botulinum toxin type A can be used as an adjunct. This is injected into the quadriceps muscle during manipulation. Splinting is used for several months and recurrence is uncommon.

For more severe knee subluxations or dislocations, surgery may be required. There are multiple different approaches for this and can include quadriceps tendon lengthening, femoral shortening, posterior capsulorrhaphy, and ACL reconstruction. Femoral shortening is particularly useful in cases of ipsilateral hip dislocation. Recently there has been less focus on quadriceps lengthening, because this can lead to a small, weakened tendon with significant scarring.

Long-Term Outcomes

In those with disorders of ligamentous laxity, there is still a concern of recurrent dislocation as the capsule and ligaments stretch out over time. This was especially true prior to the increased use of ACL reconstruction and posterior capsulorrhaphy in surgery. Recurrence is less of a concern in those without laxity syndromes such as arthrogryposis. Outcomes in idiopathic congenital knee hyperextension and dislocation are quite good, with low recurrence and ability to participate in full activities.[25]

Fibular Hemimelia

Fibular hemimelia, or congenital fibular deficiency, is the most common long-bone deficiency, although it is still quite rare at 7 to 20 per 1 million births. This disorder also encompasses several other differences in the limb, from the hip to the foot, and patients can present within a wide spectrum of the disorder. The goal of treatment is to restore function to the patient and lower extremity and can be achieved through several different means. Limb reconstruction and lengthening is usually recommended for mild to moderately severe fibular hemimelia.[26] For more severe presentations, some recommend early amputation, while others still promote limb reconstruction.

Pathophysiology

Most incidents of fibular hemimelia are sporadic. There have been some reported cases of genetic and chromosomal abnormalities associated with fibular hemimelia; vascular abnormalities have also been hypothesized and affected limb development.[26]

Evaluation

As mentioned, patients can present with different patterns and severity of fibular hemimelia.[26–28] For instance, while the fibula is always affected, it can range from mild shortening proximally and/or distally to complete absence with just a cartilaginous fibular anlage present. This often causes an anterolateral bowing of the tibia with overlying dimpling, which is caused by the tethered fibular anlage. Limb length discrepancy (LLD) is always present, especially in unilateral cases, and can range from mild to severe. Fibular hemimelia is also associated with congenital femoral deficiency, and the hip and femur should also be evaluated. Even in isolated fibular hemimelia, there is frequently lateral femoral hypoplasia, which can cause genu valgum. Other abnormalities of the knee include ACL deficiency, posterior cruciate ligament deficiency, patella alta, and hypoplastic patella. Interestingly, many of these patients, while clinically lax, are not symptomatic and may not require intervention for this. The shortened or absent lateral malleolus results in loss of the lateral buttress of the ankle, resulting in the more typical equinovalgus ankle deformity (although equinovarus is possible) and ankle instability. Other foot and ankle abnormalities include missing foot rays and tarsal coalitions. There may be a ball-and-socket ankle joint, which may be congenital or adaptive to the underlying tarsal coalitions. Many of these differences can be identified with radiographs. However, magnetic resonance imaging (MRI) is useful in infants to evaluate a cartilaginous fibular anlage and the anatomy of the nerves and vessels in that region for surgical planning. Upper extremity abnormalities can present with fibular hemimelia, especially in bilateral cases. This is important to identify because it may change the treatment algorithm.[26]

Treatment

Surgical interventions for fibular hemimelia are based on the underlying concern. For the LLD, treatment will depend on the amount of shortening. For minimal discrepancies, no intervention may be required; as the LLD increases, though, options include contralateral epiphysiodesis or ipsilateral lengthening. For significant discrepancies, sometimes multiple lengthenings with or without a contralateral epiphysiodesis may be required. For patients undergoing lengthening procedures, it is important to evaluate the stability of the knee and hip joints. Those with significant instability are at risk of subluxation and/or dislocation of the joint. To prevent this, either prophylactic reconstructive surgeries can be performed prior to lengthening or these patients must be watched closely during the lengthening process for any subtle hints of increased instability.[26–28]

Multiple reconstructive options have been described for the knee and ankle joints. Outcomes are favorable in small, shorter outcome studies. However, patients with more severe fibular hemimelia may require multiple reconstructive surgeries and lengthening procedures, all with inherent complications. Additionally, these repeated surgeries and hospitalizations come with psychological stress as well. Some families may not want to go through this extensive process, and some patients may not achieve adequate function despite all these surgeries. In such cases, early amputation may be a better alternative and should be discussed with families as a reasonable treatment option. In both reconstructive and amputation groups, genu valgum, if present, will need to be addressed. In the growing child, growth guidance with hemiepiphysiodesis plates is used, whereas in skeletally mature patients, osteotomies are necessary.

Patients with upper-extremity deformities may rely on their lower extremities to function as arms and hands. In these cases, amputation should be avoided. Reconstruction also may not be helpful, because it may stiffen the leg that is required to move in certain positions to achieve activities of daily living.[26–28]

Long-Term Outcomes

The goal for these patients is to achieve a functional lower extremity with normal limb length for functional gait. There are several ways to achieve this goal, and discussion with the families is important in decision-making. However, with both reconstruction and amputation, patients can be very functional and participate in a variety of activities and sports.[26–28]

Congenital Femoral Deficiency

Congenital femoral deficiency (CFD), also known as proximal femoral focal deficiency, refers to a spectrum of shortening and deformity of the femur. This can range from a congenital short femur to more severe instability, deformity of the bone, and shortening or absence of the bone.[29–31]

Pathophysiology

CFD is usually not associated with any genetic conditions unless there are other associated limb deformities or if it is bilateral. If there are abnormal appearances of other limbs, the facies, or the spine, genetic consultation should be considered. Femoral hypoplasia–unusual facies syndrome is an autosomal dominant malformation.[30]

Evaluation

The most telling feature is a shortened femur, although in more severe cases, there is abnormality of the shape of the proximal femur as well. This usually includes coxa vara along with flexion and external rotation of the shaft compared with the proximal femur; there is often acetabular dysplasia as well. Beyond a bony abnormality, the abductors, hip flexors, and extensors are short and may not function properly. Knee flexion can also be present, and that, along with the flexion of the femur, can overexaggerate the apparent limb-length discrepancy. Patients may have concomitant fibular hemimelia, with its associated presentation.

On imaging, patients with congenital short femur may just have a foreshortened femur. In more severe CFD, there is often an apparent disconnection between the femoral neck and shaft. This can represent a true pseudoarthrosis, but it may ossify over time. The femoral head may also be small, absent, or fused to the acetabulum. An MRI can be useful to better differentiate between these different patterns in young infants.[30]

Management

The treatment options for patients with CFD are determined by the pattern and severity of the disease with which they present. An LLD can be treated with orthotics, contralateral epiphysiodesis, or ipsilateral lengthening. Orthotics can also control motion at unstable joints while adding the necessary length to equalize the limbs. Because the other options are not often done during early childhood, orthotics are useful to allow children the ability to be active and mobile. Because there is often acetabular dysplasia and features of fibular hemimelia, including ACL deficiency, these joints and potential instability must be addressed prior to lengthening to avoid any subluxation or dislocation events. The hip is normally addressed first, during the infant or toddler years, to reconstruct the hip through soft-tissue lengthening and femoral and acetabular osteotomies. A true pseudoarthrosis can also be addressed at the same time, although some have advocated for not treating this problem. By correcting the underlying abnormalities of both bony and soft tissue, more normal joint function can be achieved with the creation of a stable hip joint for future lengthenings. The knee can be reconstructed at the same time if there is significant instability or can be closely monitored and addressed later. In hips with significant abnormality, such as an absent or fused femoral head, a rotationplasty may be a better alternative to multiple reconstructive surgeries and lengthenings that will not improve function. This does require a functional ankle, which will act like the knee joint. The remnant femur is fused to the pelvis, and the knee acts like a hip joint.[29,31]

Long-Term Outcomes

Longer-term results are starting to be published in patients with CFD, with overall positive findings. Research also suggests that patients with more severe CFD who undergo rotationplasty do better and have better function than those who undergo amputation and prosthetic management.

Tibial Hemimelia

Tibial hemimelia, or congenital tibial deficiency, is a spectrum of disease with a varying amount of absent tibia and other associated abnormalities of the knee and foot.[32,33]

Pathophysiology

There is no specific etiology for tibial hemimelia. There is no specific genetic mutation, although abnormalities along the Shh pathway have been implicated in certain cases; vascular insufficiency has also been proposed as a mechanism. In syndromic forms, there are both autosomal dominant and recessive models described. These include Werner's syndrome, tibial hemimelia diplopodia syndrome, tibial hemimelia–split hand and foot syndrome, and tibial hemimelia-micromelia-trigonobrachycephaly syndrome. Unlike the other lower-extremity congenital deficiencies, there is a high rate of associated abnormalities along the VACTERL (vertebral defects, anal atresia, cardiac defects, tracheo-esophageal fistula, renal anomalies and limb abnormalities) spectrum. Hip dislocation and femur abnormalities can also be present. Therefore tibial hemimelia does warrant a genetic and clinical workup to rule out other visceral abnormalities.[32,33]

Evaluation

Shortening of the lower leg and foot abnormalities are the most obvious clinical features of tibial hemimelia. Radiographs can further delineate the severity of the disease. There are multiple classification schemes, but most focus on type, location, and amount of deficiency. In mild forms, there is slight shortening and deformity of the tibia. The proximal or distal tibia, with the epiphysis, can also be absent, or the entire tibia can be deficient. Lastly, there can be diastasis between the fibula and tibia with the ankle positioned between the two bones. In those with deficiency of the proximal of the proximal or entire tibia, there can be associated patella deficiency and lack of an extensor mechanism. These patients may also have a knee flexion contracture, and dimpling is often seen in those with more severe tibial deficiency. Sometimes there may be delayed ossification of the proximal tibia, and an ultrasound or MRI are better imaging studies for evaluation. The fibula can be palpable proximal to the knee joint, and varus instability is clinically evident. The foot is often in varying degrees of equinovarus, and extra toes may be present.[33]

Management

The treatment approach for tibial hemimelia depends on the classification type and on discussion with the family. Both reconstruction and amputation, sometimes both, are options in treating tibial hemimelia; the family, therefore, must understand and be prepared for the treatment plan upon which they decided with the surgeon. When the proximal aspect of the tibia is present, patients do well with a fusion between the remnant tibia and the adjacent fibula. This can entail pulling the fibula distally to gain length or leaving it in its current position. Some recommend combining this with a Syme amputation and prosthetic fitting, whereas others will fuse the distal aspect of the fibula to the ankle. Proponents of amputation note the issues of instability due to the deformities about the foot and ankle. To avoid this instability, ankle fusion can be done, and those who recommend it still find excellent function because the foot is smaller and the leg is also left slightly shorter to aid in ambulation and function.[33]

When the proximal tibia is not present, a knee disarticulation is usually recommended. Some have described a procedure to reconstruct the extensor mechanism, where the patella is placed under the distal femoral condyles and fused to the proximal fibula to act as the proximal tibial epiphysis. Some short-term follow-ups show promising results, although there are limited middle- and long-term follow-ups. Complications include stiffness, pain, loss of function, and instability, with some progressing to a knee disarticulation eventually. Therefore this option is only rarely offered to patients.

In the situation of diastasis between the tibia and fibula, Syme amputation is again most commonly offered. The foot and ankle can be gradually lengthened and brought to station and the ankle reconstructed. Again, there are concerns for stiffness and instability, because the talus and calcaneus are abnormally shaped and there is a lack of a normal distal tibial articulation. Fusion between the tibia and talus can also be considered once they are properly positioned.

In all cases, the affected limb is shorter than the contralateral side, especially if it is unilateral. Therefore, lengthening may be required, either through the limb itself or through the prosthesis.

Long-Term Outcomes

Outcomes for children who undergo amputation and prosthetic fitting do very well over the long term, including those who require a cross-union between the fibula and tibia and those who undergo a knee disarticulation.

Tibial Bowing

Tibial bowing can occur in three planes: anteromedial, anterolateral, and posteromedial. Each type of bowing is associated with different syndromes, workups, and treatment plans. Each type is distinct and often easily recognizable soon after birth. Being able to distinguish between the three is beneficial in terms of guiding further management.[34]

Pathophysiology

Anteromedial bowing is most commonly associated with fibular hemimelia, which was discussed previously. Anterolateral bowing is frequently seen with congenital pseudoarthrosis of the tibia (CPT).[34,35] However, there is a rare variant that self-resolves with no progression to pseudoarthrosis. In these patients, there is often thickening of the cortical bone of the concavity of the tibia. The more common presentation of CPT does show eventual progression to pseudoarthrosis. Although patients may present with a continuous tibia, overtime, the bending worsens and there is an eventual fracture with pseudoarthrosis formation. The two ends of the bones thin to points, giving a "sucked candy" appearance. The fibula may or may not fracture. Up to 50% of patients with CPT are also diagnosed with neurofibromatosis. Interestingly, only between 5% and 25% of patients with neurofibromatosis have CPT. CPT is also associated with fibrous dysplasia in up to 15% of patients. The underlying pathology of CPT is an abnormal, thickened periosteum, known as a hamartoma, that is localized to the pseudoarthrosis. The hamartoma has been shown to have decreased osteoblastic and increased osteoclastic activity, explaining the poor healing potential in this area of bone. Additionally, others have found abnormalities of the subperiosteal blood vessels, with narrowing and absence of the vessels, further supporting poor bone healing.

Posteromedial bowing of the tibia is associated with calcaneovalgus deformity of the foot. The foot deformity was covered previously, and this section will only focus on the bowing. The underlying pathology is intrauterine positioning.[34]

Clinical Presentation

All three types of bowing are usually noticeable at birth or shortly after as the disease progresses. Not only is there bowing of the tibia, with possible dimpling over the apex, but the foot is also involved. In anterolateral bowing, the foot is often medially directed or inverted in relation to the tibia. The mobile pseudoarthrosis, when present, can also be palpable to the clinician. The foot and leg may also be smaller and shorter, and in more mild cases, these can be the only presenting symptoms. In very mild cases, the leg may appear normal, and it is only after an incidental fracture with nonunion with further workup that a diagnosis of CPT is made. Other features, particularly cutaneous, of neurofibromatosis or fibrous dysplasia should be looked for and noted. Radiographs help determine the diagnosis and follow the progression of the disease.[34,35]

As previously mentioned, the calcaneovalgus foot with posteromedial bowing can exaggerate the clinical appearance of each. The calf may also be smaller, again related to the intrauterine positioning. Radiographs are often not required but can be helpful to confirm diagnosis.

Management

Initial management of CPT can include nonoperative brace wear to try to slow progression of the bowing and ultimate fracture or more early surgical intervention. Unfortunately, once there is a fracture in CPT, it is unlikely it will heal spontaneously. This is also true with surgery, and an operation to treat a fracture that has yet to occur may propagate the progression of CPT anyway. However, there are advocates for both, and treatment algorithms have changed with more recent advances in treatment of CPT. Brace treatment usually starts at the time of ambulation and can initially include the ankle and later just involve the tibia with a clamshell orthosis. There is no research that this will prevent fracture. Before a fracture occurs, some recommend bypassing the tibia along its concavity with a structural bone graft, either the contralateral fibula or a fibular autograft. Over time this is incorporated into the tibia itself. Some early- and midterm follow-ups are positive, but angular deformities are still often present. A more recently described treatment option for prefractured anterolateral bowing is the application of growth guidance in the distal tibia in the plane of the bowing. In the short term, this has successfully improved the angulation without any resultant fractures.[34,35]

When a fracture has occurred, the goals of surgical intervention include removing the diseased periosteum, aligning the mechanical axis appropriately, and bolstering the tibia with fixation to protect against further fractures. The most recently developed procedure involves resection of the hamartoma and creates a cross-union between the tibia and fibula. This is done with a massive iliac crest bone autograft sandwiched between an autograft fascial layer and a bone morphogenetic protein 2 (BMP2) collagen sponge. At the same time, the deformity is corrected and the tibia is fixed with an intramedullary growing rod along with either a plate along the side or an external fixator; the fibula will also receive intramedullary fixation. Preoperatively, bisphosphonates are also used to improve the healing potential. Over time, the graft incorporates, connecting the tibia and fibula and protecting the tibia and fibula from future fracture. As the limb grows, the rod will lengthen and does require replacement with longer, more stout rods over time. This can be done prior to or after fracture formation.[34,35]

Similar to calcaneovalgus foot deformity, posteromedial bowing of the tibia is usually self-resolving over the first 6 to 12 months of life. However, families must be told about the potential for limb-length shortening, because this often requires treatment. Finally, not all posteromedial bowing improves, and some cases lead to proximal and distal compensatory deformities. In such cases, operative management may be preferred early on to avoid such zed (z)-deformities and to treat the LLD at the same time.

Long-Term Outcomes

Initial surgical options for CPT are often quite disappointing, with refracture rates up to 50% to 60% for all procedures. For families that have undergone multiple operations with continued failure, amputation may eventually be offered as an alternative to repeated surgeries. There is controversy as to which patients have worse outcomes, with earlier intervention and neurofibromatosis both being reported as risk factors in some studies and equivalent in others. Angular deformity, though, does portend worse functional outcomes and an increased risk of refracture.[34]

More recent procedures, including growth guidance and cross-union, have had very positive short-term outcomes, with up to 100% healing with no fracture and no angular deformity. Still, larger and longer-term studies are necessary to bear out these early results.

Posteromedial bowing has much more favorable outcomes, especially given its often resolving nature. There is no risk of fracture in this type of bowing.

Congenital Vertical Talus

Congenital vertical talus (CVT), or rocker-bottom foot, is a rigid dorsal dislocation of the talonavicular joint with a fixed hindfoot equinus. It is quite rare, occurring in less than 1 in 10,000 live births. A less severe manifestation is the oblique talus, where the navicular can be reduced in certain foot positions. CVT can be difficult to diagnose in the newborn and to differentiate from other postural foot deformities. However, early detection and treatment are helpful for the pain and disability that come with untreated CVT.[36]

Pathophysiology

The etiology of CVT is most likely multifactorial, with about half of cases associated with varying underlying neurologic or genetic syndromes and the other half occurring idiopathically. CVT can be seen in arthrogryposis, myelomeningocele, and aneuploidy of chromosomes 13, 15, and 18. Genetic counseling can be useful to further evaluate these patients. Even in idiopathic cases, a family history is found about 20% of the time, suggesting this is still a genetic, inherited condition. However, no one gene has been found to cause CVT, and other factors, such as muscle imbalance or vascular deficiency, may also play a role.[36,37]

This is supported by the pathoanatomy of CVT.[38] Multiple tendons and joint capsules around the dorsum of the foot and ankle are contracted, subsequently causing the multiple joint and bony deformities. The capsules and ligaments on the plantar aspect, conversely, are attenuated. The tendons may also be subluxed, changing their mechanism of action, for instance from plantarflexor to dorsiflexor, and further propagating joint dislocations and rigidity. The bony pathoanatomy shows the navicular dorsally dislocated and instead articulating with the dorsum of the talus. The talus is angled distally and is dysplastic in shape. The calcaneus is displaced posterolaterally, contacts the distal fibula, and is stuck in equinus. There is also dysplasia of the calcaneus with a resultant abnormal subtalar joint and articulation between the talus and calcaneus. In terms of vascular pathoanatomy, MRI studies have also reported arterial deficiencies in isolated vertical talus.

Clinical Presentation

The rigid rocker-bottom appearance of CVT includes hindfoot equinus and valgus and forefoot dorsiflexion and abduction. The rigidity, especially the hindfoot equinus, is necessary for diagnosis and helps distinguish it from other foot deformities, including oblique talus. There is a convex plantar surface, and the dorsum of the foot often has a palpable gap and deep creases. Besides examining for any flexibility or reducibility, motor function of the foot and a full clinical exam are helpful to evaluate for other underlying genetic or neurologic conditions. They can also help predict response to treatment and outcomes.[38]

Radiographs are also important in evaluating these patients and include AP and three lateral views of the foot: in neutral, maximum dorsiflexion, and maximum plantarflexion. The lateral views will demonstrate the talus in a near vertical position, whereas the plantarflexion view will show the reducibility of the talonavicular joint. If it reduces, this suggests an oblique talus; otherwise, it is a true CVT. The max dorsiflexion view will show continued rigid equinus in CVT.[38]

Management

Previously, most patients were treated with extensive surgical release of the joint capsules and lengthening of the contracted tendons.[37–41] This could be done in a single or two-stage approach. More recently, a minimally invasive approach has evolved. This includes serial casting and then a small procedure to place a pin across the talonavicular joint and an Achilles tenotomy to correct the equinus without destabilizing the talonavicular joint. The serial casting is often referred to as a "reverse Ponseti" method, because the goal just prior to surgery is to create a foot that resembles a clubfoot. Sometimes, a small capsulotomy intraoperatively to fully reduce the talonavicular joint and limited lengthening of still-contracted tendons are necessary. Patients are subsequently braced for the next several years.

Long-Term Outcomes

In untreated CVT, as patients start to weight bear, there are progressive osseous changes and callus formation on the plantar aspect of the foot. The heel never reaches the ground, and ultimately, pain and disability occur. Good to excellent outcomes have been reported for the more extensive releases. There is still concern about over- and undercorrection and wound necrosis. Over time, stiffness, arthritis, and recurrent deformity can occur. Therefore further corrective surgeries or fusions may be required. Overall, excellent outcomes, although not as long-term as with the extensive approach, have been reported for the minimally invasive approach to CVT, including minimal recurrences, better motion and function, and less pain.[37–41]

CHAPTER 74

Fractures and Musculoskeletal Infections in the Neonate

Arjun Gupta, Paul D. Sponseller

KEY POINTS

1. Fractures and musculoskeletal infections in neonates follow a distinct pathophysiology.
2. The clavicle is the most frequently injured long bone in newborns; the injury occurs most often during birth. These fractures heal and remodel well. In some infants, congenital pseudoarthrosis of the clavicle may need to be differentiated from fractures.
3. The humerus is the second most common long bone to be fractured in neonates; most fractures occur during birth or early infancy. These fractures are typically midshaft; some may be seen in proximal and distal epiphyses.
4. Neonatal femur fractures can sometimes occur during birth and have been associated with shoulder dystocia, twin pregnancies, breech presentation, prematurity, small size for gestational age, and congenital osteoporosis.
5. Musculoskeletal infections in the newborn have a unique pathophysiology and may occur in multiple locations simultaneously. The most frequently isolated organisms are *Staphylococcus aureus*, but sometimes nonstaphylococcal bacteria can also be seen.

Clavicular Fractures

Epidemiology and Risk Factors

The clavicle is the most frequently injured long bone in newborns, composing between 10% and 15% of all fractures.[1] The incidence of clavicle fractures in neonates ranges from 0.5% to 7% of all live births.[2,3] The fractured clavicle typically demonstrates excellent healing even with no intervention, and surgery is rarely indicated. The prognosis is almost always highly favorable.[3]

In the neonate, the most common mechanism of clavicular injury is during birth, whereas other traumas such as falling on an outstretched arm are predominantly responsible in older children. Previously identified risk factors for obstetric clavicle fracture include large birth weight (>4500 g), shoulder dystocia, prolonged gestational age, and difficult or complicated deliveries involving mechanical assistance.[2,4] Midshaft fractures are the most common pattern of injury in the neonate.[5] Fractures of the medial or lateral clavicle are more likely to involve the physis, although these are difficult to diagnose radiographically because the epiphyses are not yet ossified at this age. The acromioclavicular and sternoclavicular joints are relatively stable due to strong supporting ligaments, making dislocation at these joints fairly uncommon.[6]

Clinical Features and Evaluation

Neonatal clavicle fractures are most commonly detected within the first 3 days of life, although recognition and diagnosis can be challenging.[3] They are often first discovered when parents notice a lack of spontaneous movement in their infant's upper extremity, often termed "pseudoparalysis."[5] Visible callus formation within 7 to 10 days of the injury may also be one of the first clinical clues. Common signs and symptoms that aid in diagnosis include point tenderness, swelling or edema, crepitation, asymmetric bone contour, decreased active movement, crying on passive movement, and decreased Moro reflex (also known as startle reflex).[3,5] Diagnosis can also be made by palpating a spongy mass over the fracture site.[7] However, the majority of these signs may not persist beyond a few days after birth.

Initial radiographs may be negative or inconclusive, especially for minimally displaced fractures (Fig. 74.1). In such cases, repeat radiographs of the clavicle may be helpful if obtained within 7 to 10 days after callus formation and periosteal reaction have begun.[8] Ultrasonography may occasionally aid in diagnosis of occult neonatal fractures.

The most important differential diagnosis is congenital pseudarthrosis of the clavicle, which is discussed in further detail below. Unlike fractures, pseudarthroses are nontender or minimally tender. Another condition to differentiate is cleidocranial dysplasia. This

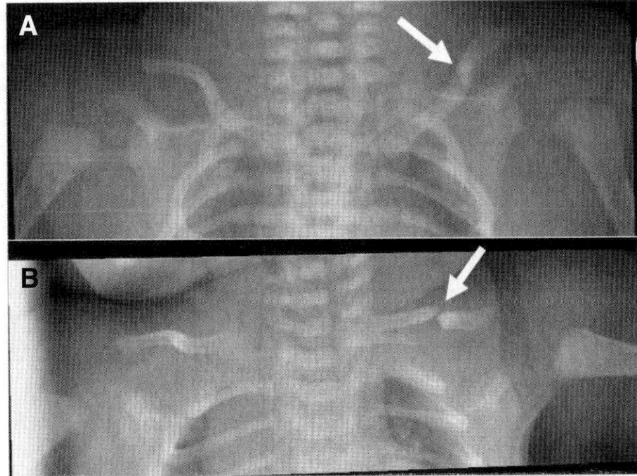

Fig. 74.1 Supine AP Radiographs of a Newborn Female With a Midshaft Fracture of the Right Clavicle Detected Shortly After Birth *(White Arrows)*. (A) The medial and lateral fragments are superimposed when arms are in neutral position. (B) When arms are abducted, the fragments are moderately displaced in the AP (anterior-posterior) view.

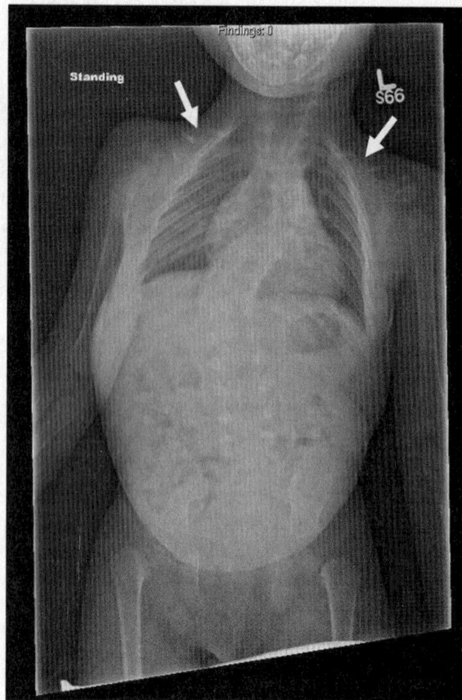

Fig. 74.2 Full Spine Standing AP (Anterior-Posterior) Radiograph of a Male Patient With Cleidocranial Dysplasia Affecting the Bilateral Clavicles *(White Arrows)*.

condition, due to a mutation in *CBFA1*, presents with large gaps in the opposing ends of both clavicles, which are also smooth (Fig. 74.2). In some cases, the clavicles are absent entirely. No treatment is needed for the clavicles themselves, although there are other skeletal deformities associated with this condition.

Long-Term Outcomes

Clavicle fractures always heal and remodel well in newborns with no residual deformity. Erb's palsy (brachial plexus injury) should also be ruled out in neonates with clavicular fracture.[9]

Management

In all cases, management can be conservative. Simple immobilization methods such as a sling, ace wrap, or shirt that holds the affected arm close to the infant's torso generally provide sufficient comfort and allow for initial stages of healing. Referral to a pediatric orthopedic surgeon can be helpful.

Congenital Pseudarthrosis of the Clavicle

Epidemiology and Risk Factors

Congenital pseudarthrosis of the clavicle (CPC) is a rare condition almost always occurs on the right side, except in patients with situs inversus. Left-sided lesions are therefore strongly associated with dextrocardia and cervical ribs.[10] A few bilateral cases have also been described, although this is exceedingly rare.[11] Some studies suggest a higher predilection for females compared with males.[10] Although the pathophysiology of CPC is poorly understood, reports of familial association suggest a potential genetic component.[11,12]

Clinical Features and Evaluation

Importantly, CPC is commonly misdiagnosed as clavicular fracture or injury due to abuse.[13] The classic physical exam finding is a painless mass or swelling over the middle third of the affected clavicle. This may be due to enlargement of the disjointed pseudoarticular ends. Notably, the mass tends to grow in size with age.[13] Absence of tenderness is a key diagnostic clue that distinguishes CPC from acute fracture, although physical activities producing compression of the lesion may produce pain in some children. Diagnosis is confirmed by the presence of smooth, tapered opposing ends of the bone, in contrast to the sharp edges of a fresh fracture (Fig. 74.3).[14]

The mass is more accentuated when patients raise the upper limb.[10,15] Upper-extremity range of motion, strength, and sensation are normal in the vast majority of cases but may be affected depending on severity of fragment misalignment and malunion. Hypermobility of the distal segment and asymmetric drooping of the scapula may be noted in some cases.

Management

The lifetime prognosis is almost always benign with no real complications beyond cosmetic deformity, with very rare occurrences of thoracic outlet obstruction in some patients after reaching adulthood.[16] No treatment is needed in the newborn period, although pseudarthroses that are symptomatic may be successfully fixed as the child ages.

Humerus Fractures

Epidemiology and Risk Factors

The humerus is the second most common long bone to be fractured in neonates, just behind the clavicle.[17] The incidence of birth-related fractures is near 0.1 out of every 1000 live births, although this figure varies widely.[17,18]

Factors associated with birth-related humerus fractures include maternal obesity, shoulder dystocia, vacuum-assisted delivery, male sex, multiple births, breech delivery, preterm birth, large size for gestational age, large birth weight (>4000 g), and brachial plexus injury.[17] Of note, humerus and other long-bone fractures can occur with both vaginal deliveries and cesarean section deliveries.[17,19] Importantly, breech presentation is the single most influential risk factor for birth-related fracture of the humerus regardless of delivery, and neonates delivered in breech position should be assessed for orthopedic injuries soon after birth.[19–21]

Additionally, 14% of humerus fractures in early infancy (age <6 months) have been associated with abuse. The high contribution of maltreatment to the incidence of population-level humerus fracture among infants is also supported by other literature.[22] As such, pediatricians and other healthcare providers must be observant for other signs indicating abuse in infants presenting with long-bone fractures, especially outside of the immediate neonatal period. In later infancy, 56% of humerus fractures could be attributed to accidental fall trauma.[18]

Clinical Features and Evaluation

The most common type of humeral fracture is transverse midshaft, followed by proximal and distal epiphyseal fractures.[23] Proximal or

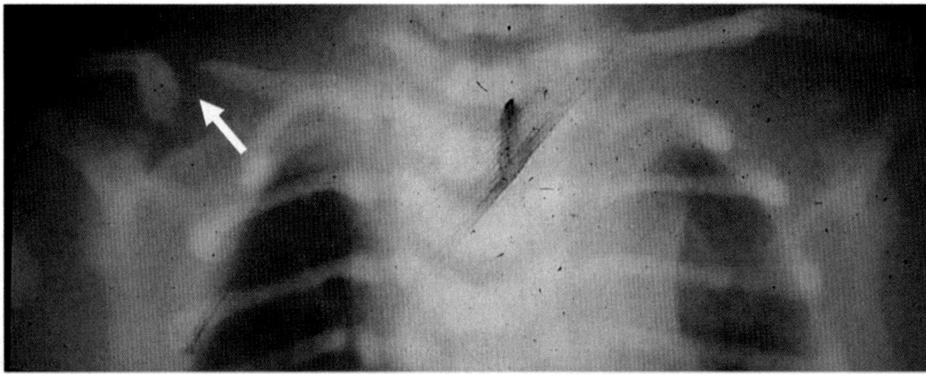

Fig. 74.3 Upper Thoracic AP (Anterior-Posterior) Radiograph of a Female Patient With Congenital Pseudarthrosis of the Right Clavicle *(White Arrow)*. Note the presence of smooth, tapered opposing ends of the bone, in contrast to the sharp edges of a fresh fracture.

distal fractures may mimic dislocations at the shoulder or elbow and are more difficult to diagnose. Radiographic confirmation of epiphyseal separations is particularly challenging in newborns. Furthermore, soft-tissue swelling may impede palpation of distal anatomic landmarks such as the olecranon and epicondyles, making such injuries difficult to ascertain through physical examination alone.[24] Thus, the chances of missed or late diagnosis are increased with physeal fracture-separations in newborns. One study reported an average time to diagnosis of 9 to 30 days after birth for distal epiphysis separations.[25] Nonetheless, some diagnostic signs that raise clinical suspicion for a distal humeral epiphysis fracture-separation include focal tenderness, swelling and edema, pseudoparalysis of the arm, and "muffled crepitus" upon movement, representing friction between preossific cartilaginous structures.[24,25]

Ultrasonography is generally the most useful imaging modality for humeral physeal fracture detection and classification in neonates. Compared with magnetic resonance imaging (MRI) and radiography, ultrasonography is readily available, inexpensive, and nonirradiating, and it can be performed easily at the bedside without the need for sedation.[24] Ultrasonography is also far more sensitive than traditional radiography for detection of physeal fractures in neonatal patients with cartilaginous epiphyses.

Management

Birth-related humerus fractures generally demonstrate good remodeling, with no observable deformity after 6 months.[17,25] The primary goals of care are comfort and immobilization, because the young bone has excellent healing potential. We recommend a conservative treatment approach involving immobilization with a splint, cast, or swaddling. No reduction is needed.[17,23,25] Although traditional slings and shoulder immobilizers are unlikely to fit an infant, a simple yet effective option for management of upper-extremity fractures in these very young patients is to pin the sleeve of the newborn to their shirt.[26]

Femoral Fractures

Epidemiology and Risk Factors

Unlike the clavicle and humerus, the femur is rarely fractured in neonates. The incidence varies from 0.02 to 0.13 per 1000 live births.[18,27,28] Infants do sustain femoral fractures more frequently after the immediate neonatal period; however, the etiologies in this age group are distinct from birth-related fractures. Like other neonatal fractures, prognosis is generally favorable. At least two studies have reported complete union by 4 weeks, with no evidence of long-term leg length discrepancy or residual deformity after appropriate treatment.[27,29]

Neonatal femur fractures have been associated with shoulder dystocia, twin pregnancies, breech presentation, prematurity, small size for gestational age, and congenital osteoporosis.[18,27] The mean gestational age reported in one study was 37.2 weeks.[29] Birth-related femur fractures have been more frequently reported in the setting of cesarean sections compared with vaginal births, especially for breech presentation babies.[27–31] This is well documented despite the widely accepted paradigm that cesarean section delivery reduces the risk of neonatal trauma. The most common pattern of injury is a diaphyseal spiral fracture of the proximal half of the femur, suggesting that excess torque applied during fetal extraction is likely responsible.[27,29] It is important for pediatricians and obstetricians to conduct a thorough assessment for signs of femoral fracture in neonates delivered by difficult cesarean section wherein traction was applied.

In utero fractures that are discovered postnatally may occur secondary to syndromic osteoporosis, such as in patients with myelomeningocele or metabolic bone disease of prematurity in neonates born after less than 28 weeks of gestation.[27,32,33] Other pathologic etiologies such as osteogenesis imperfecta and osteomyelitis have also been described.[29] In fact, underlying bone fragility is recorded in 5% of infantile femur fractures.[18] Birth-related femur fractures may therefore be a useful clinical indicator for pediatricians to screen for underlying pathologies.

Notably, 20% of femur fractures in early infancy (age <6 months) were associated with abuse.[18,22] After the immediate neonatal period, 73% of femur fractures in later infancy were associated with accidental fall trauma. As with humerus fractures, pediatricians must be observant for other signs indicating abuse in infants presenting with long-bone fractures.

Clinical Features and Evaluation

Diagnosis can be challenging due to the nonspecific presentation in newborn children. Typical signs include local swelling, point tenderness, redness, fever, lack of spontaneous movement, and crying with passive movement such as during diaper changes. Nonetheless, because the majority of femoral fractures in the neonate are midshaft injuries, plain radiograph is a reliable diagnostic tool (Fig. 74.4).

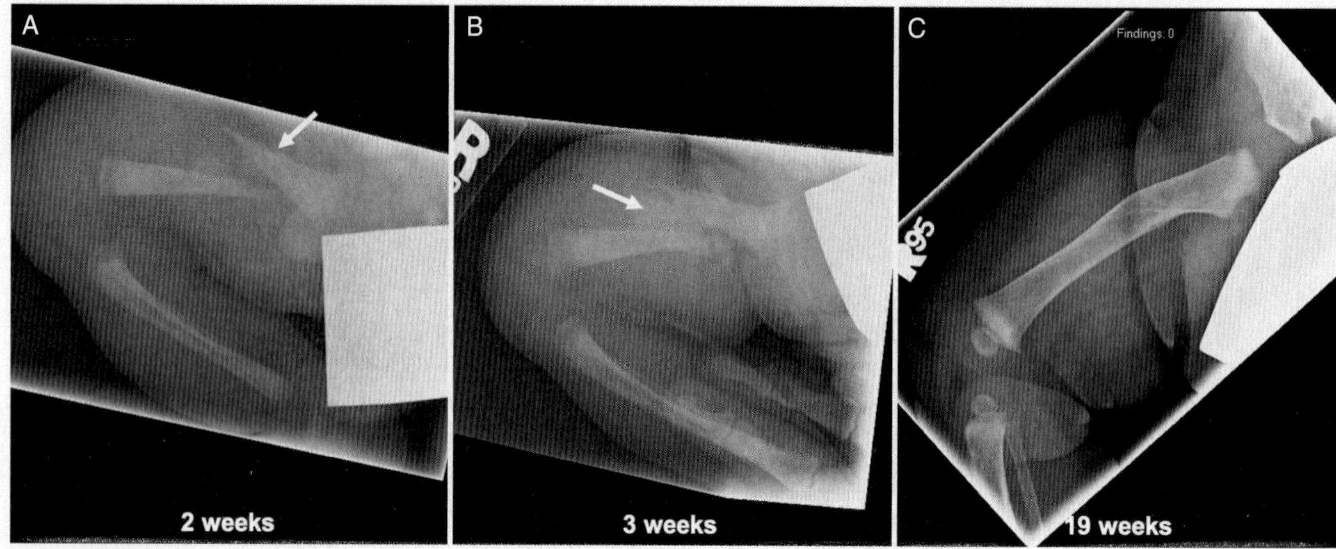

Fig. 74.4 Follow-Up Radiographs of a Male Newborn With Birth-Related Fracture of the Right Femur Who Was Placed in a Pavlik Harness at 1 Day of Life. (A) After 2 weeks, early callus formation can be seen between the distal and proximal fragments, with discernible periosteal reaction as well *(white arrow)*. (B) Rapid growth of the callus is noted by week 3 *(white arrow)*. (C) By 19 weeks after birth, the fracture has healed completely with near-anatomic reunion of the femoral shaft.

Management

The main goal of treatment is immobilization of the femoral shaft. Commonly deployed methods include spica casting and Pavlik harnesses. Adjustable harnesses enable easy at-home care and can be applied in an outpatient setting without the need for general anesthesia while still producing satisfactory fracture reduction (Fig. 74.5).[34,35] Single-leg, soft-cast spicas offer similar ease of use and may provide better comfort of the fracture site compared with Pavlik harnesses.[26]

Congenital Pseudarthrosis of the Tibia

Epidemiology and Risk Factors

Congenital pseudarthrosis of the tibia (CPT) is extremely rare, with an estimated incidence of 1 out of every 150,000 to 250,000 live births.[36,37] It is characterized by recurrent, pathologic fractures of the tibia with incomplete healing. CPT can present at birth or several months later. CPT often develops in the first 1 to 2 years of infancy and is therefore considered by some to be incorrectly classified as "congenital," although congenital cases have been reported.[36–38] Tibial fractures commonly reoccur throughout the affected child's skeletal growth phase and even into adulthood, with frequency decreasing with age. More than 50% of cases are associated with type 1 neurofibromatosis, 10% of cases are associated with fibrous dysplasia, and the rest are classified as idiopathic.[37]

Clinical Features and Evaluation

The clinical features of CPT vary greatly. The classic lower-extremity deformity seen in CPT patients is anterolateral bowing of the tibia, although frank fractures with complete nonunion may be seen in more severe cases (Fig. 74.6).[36] In less severe cases, pathologic tibial fractures may not occur until the child begins to walk, which may be the first indication of CPT. Radiographically, there may be evidence of atrophic or hypertrophic pseudarthrosis and cystic or dystrophic lesions. One important debilitating consequence of CPT is leg-length discrepancy, along with ankle stiffness, muscle contractures, and additional foot deformities. Typically, only one leg is affected, and fibular involvement is seen in more than 50% of cases.

Management

Prognosis is poor, and the treatment course typically consists of multiple orthopedic surgeries. Early referral to a pediatric orthopedic surgeon may facilitate early intervention and hinder development of recalcitrant deformity.

Bone and Joint Infections

Pathophysiology

Musculoskeletal infections in the newborn have a unique pathophysiology. Infection often occurs in multiple locations simultaneously. The most commonly isolated organism across all age groups is *Staphylococcus aureus*. Due to the immature immune system in neonates, however, causative organisms are frequently nonstaphylococcal.[39]

Because rich transphyseal vascular networks allow infections of the bone to cross the growth plate, osteomyelitis and joint infections commonly coexist in newborns. In certain bones where the epiphysis lies within the articular capsule (i.e., the proximal femur, humerus, radius, and distal tibia), joint infections may also be seen with higher frequency compared with other age groups.[40] Septic arthritis and epiphyseal involvement occur in up to 76% of neonatal/infantile osteomyelitis cases.[41]

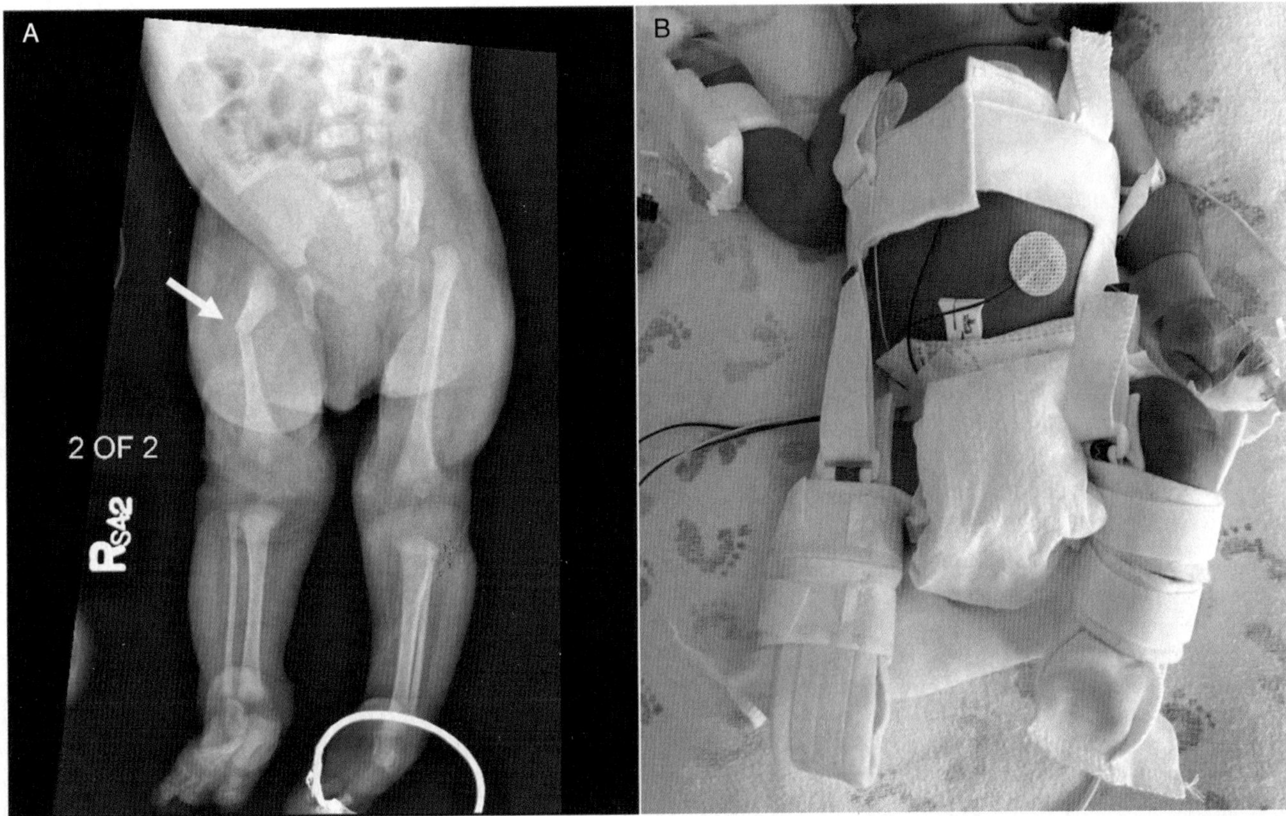

Fig. 74.5 Birth-Related Fracture of the Right Femur in a 1-Day-Old Female Neonate Treated by Immobilization of the Lower Extremity in a Pavlik Harness.

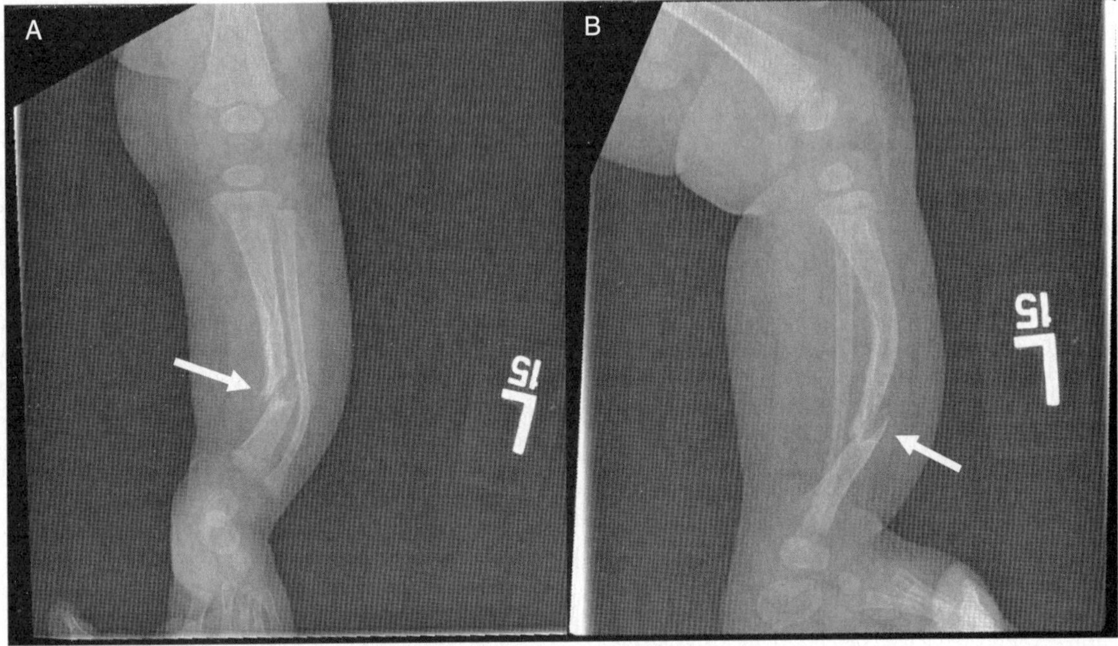

Fig. 74.6 Radiographs of the Left Lower Extremity Demonstrate the Classic Anterolateral Pattern of Tibial Bowing in a Female Infant With CPT.
(A) AP (anterior-posterior) radiograph. (B) Lateral radiograph. Pseudarthrosis formation can also be visualized, which is distinct from the sharp diaphyseal edges seen after acute fracture. *CPT,* Congenital pseudarthrosis of the tibia.

Infection of intervertebral discs, or discitis, is a relatively uncommon type of musculoskeletal infection. The cartilaginous vertebral end plates in very young children are supplied by small blood vessels that lie close to the disc space, which serve as a source for hematogenous seeding of infection in the disc.[42,43]

Epidemiology and Risk Factors

The published incidence is 28 per 100,000 infants between the ages of 0 and 2 years, which is more than three-fold higher than the incidence in older children aged 3 to 15 years.[44] Risk factors include prematurity, umbilical catheterization, preexisting bone or urinary tract disease, and dermatologic or ear infections.[42] Hematogenous seeding is the most common source of metaphyseal infection, so recent or active soft-tissue infection is fundamentally a risk factor for osteomyelitis.

Clinical Features and Evaluation

The clinical presentation of acute hematogenous osteomyelitis in newborns can be highly ambiguous. The first signs of infection are often simply crying on passive movement of the affected extremity, such as during diaper changes. Refusal by the baby to produce active movements (pseudoparalysis) may be another manifestation noticed by the parents or caretakers. Other common signs of distress such as poor feeding or irritability should be noted. The affected joint may be swollen or warm, although erythema is not often present due to the depth of the infection.

The physiologic response to infection in the neonate is not typical. Somewhat counterintuitively, fever is not part of the classic disease course, which is contrary to the presentation of osteomyelitis in children of older age.[40] Neonates with osteomyelitis or septic arthritis may present with normal leukocyte count and erythrocyte sedimentation rate.[45] However, C-reactive protein is almost always elevated in these patients. With a negative predictive value of 95%, serum C-reactive protein has robust utility in ruling out infection.[46] The normal value range for leukocyte count in the first week of life is between 9000 and 30,000 cells/mL. In the neonate, leukopenia (<5000 cells/mL) may be suggestive of infection.[8]

Imaging

Plain radiography can be an informative initial imaging modality, although there are certain limitations in neonates and young children due to the presence of cartilaginous epiphyses. Findings that increase clinical suspicion for osteomyelitis include metaphyseal radiolucency consistent with bony destruction, osteoporosis, and periosteal reaction.[42,47] However, bony destruction may not be visible on radiographs until at least one-third of the osseous matrix has been compromised, which explains why the vast majority of patients present with unremarkable x-ray findings.[48,49] Soft-tissue swelling can be detected within 48 hours of onset, although this may be less useful in the neonate due to poorly defined fascial planes.[45,50] In septic arthritis, additional findings may include widening of the joint space due to effusion and hip subluxation or dislocation, which are common sequelae of septic arthritis.[42] However, plain radiographs have a low sensitivity for detection of joint effusions.[51] This imaging modality is also useful for ruling out other differentials such as fracture.

Ultrasonography is generally the most reliable imaging modality for assessment of joint pathology in the neonate. Ultrasound can allow for visualization of joint effusion or subperiosteal abscess and is therefore extremely useful in neonates presenting with an unclear diagnosis.[47] Joint effusion seen on ultrasonography has a very high negative predictive value for hip septic arthritis, although a normal hip ultrasound does not rule out osteomyelitis.[52] In patients with a septic hip, ultrasound of the contralateral hip should be performed to rule out bilateral involvement.[47]

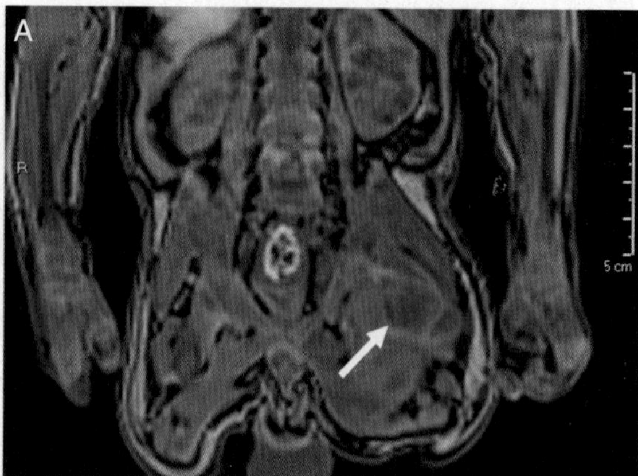

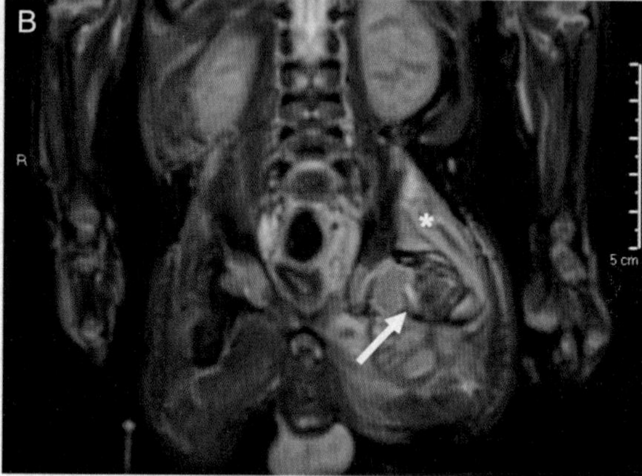

Fig. 74.7 Magnetic Resonance Images of a Left Proximal Femur Osteomyelitis With Septic Arthritis of the Hip. (A) Coronal T1-weighted image shows a focus of low signal intensity near the physis, suggestive of subperiosteal abscess *(white arrow)*. (B) The same view in the T2-STIR (Short Tau Inversion Recovery) sequence shows the abscess as a clearly defined collection returning high signal intensity *(white arrow)*. There is also high signal intensity in the adjacent soft tissue compared with the contralateral hip, indicating muscle edema and inflammation *(asterisk)*. Asymmetric positioning of the two femoral heads is a result of anterior subluxation of the affected left hip joint.

MRI is typically used to evaluate soft-tissue involvement in osteomyelitis, and it is also a particularly useful imaging modality in neonates and young children to assess cartilaginous structures such as the epiphysis and growth plate that are not well visualized on plain radiograph. Sites of infection and/or inflammation appear as foci of low signal on T1-weighted and high signal on T2-weighted and STIR (Short Tau Inversion Recovery) sequences (Fig. 74.7).[42,53] One way to distinguish isolated septic arthritis from concomitant osteomyelitis is to assess the bone marrow signal, which should be normal in the absence of osteomyelitis.[42] MRI scout images may be useful to look for other sites of infection.

Management

The single most important step in diagnosing and treating osteomyelitis is identification of the causative organism. A blood culture should be obtained promptly in any patient presenting with signs or

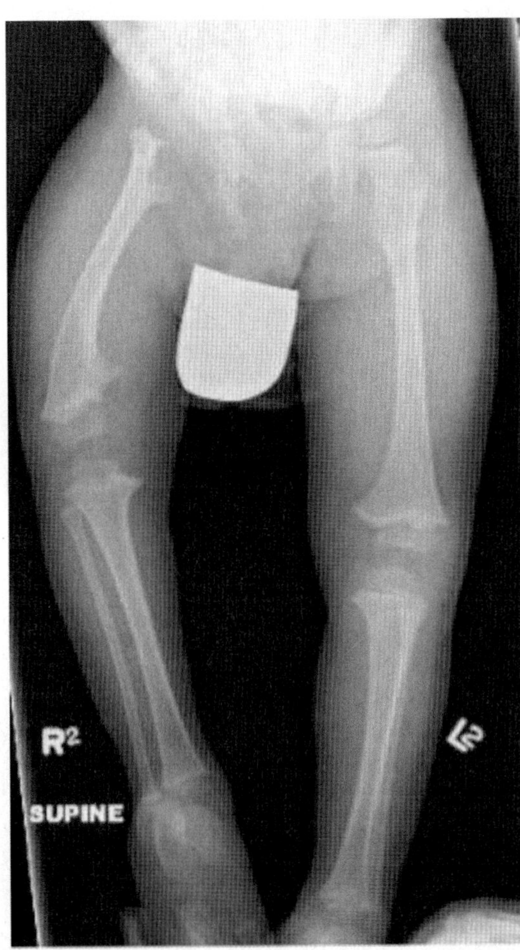

Fig. 74.8 Long-Term Deformities Resulting From Osteomyelitis. Deformities resulting from osteomyelitis of the right proximal femur are seen radiographically: epiphyseal destruction, joint dislocation, acetabular deformation, growth plate arrest, limb length discrepancy, diaphyseal bowing, and genu varum.

symptoms suggestive of infection. Empiric treatment for *S. aureus* can be initiated if there is a high index of clinical suspicion for infection before culture results are available. A specific organism should be sought if blood cultures do not yield it.[39] Aspiration of bone marrow or joint effusion fluid can then be performed to obtain a sample for culture.

Septic arthritis is a clinical emergency that demands a rapid diagnosis and prompt medical intervention to relieve pressure on the fragile cartilage. Early detection can be key to preventing long-term morbidity and preventing poor functional outcomes that would afflict the child for life. Any patient with suspected osteomyelitis or septic arthritis should prompt a consultation with orthopedic surgery. Surgery is indicated for any joint infection or osteomyelitis with abscess formation.

Long-Term Outcomes

Musculoskeletal infections can lead to degradation of fragile joint cartilage, physeal destruction, growth plate arrest, secondary limb-length discrepancy, postinfectious arthritis, and osteonecrosis or separation of the epiphysis (Fig. 74.8).[42,54] Effusion and inflammatory exudate in the joint can also cause compression of vasculature embedded in the soft cartilaginous femoral head, which may lead to avascular necrosis.[42] Additionally, because muscle tone in the neonate is not fully developed, the hip joints are particularly susceptible to subluxation or dislocation as a result of joint damage after septic arthritis.[42]

Conclusion

Given their unique orthopedic pathophysiology and anatomy, a high index of clinical suspicion, ideally supported by cultures and imaging studies, is required to promptly diagnose osteomyelitis or septic arthritis in the neonate.

SECTION

15 Inborn Errors of Metabolism and Newborn Screening

OUTLINE

CHAPTER 75

Most Frequently Encountered Inborn Errors of Metabolism

Jubara Alallah, Pankaj B. Agrawal, Alvaro Dendi, Akhil Maheshwari

KEY POINTS

1. Inborn errors of metabolism (IEMs) are inherited conditions that block metabolic pathways. As a group, these conditions could be identified in 1 out of every 1500 infants.
2. We have suspected IEMs in infants during the early neonatal period if they have progressively worsening encephalopathy with lethargy, seizures, or coma that cannot be explained as due to asphyxia or infections; unexplained severe high anion-gap metabolic acidosis; or unexplained respiratory alkalosis associated with considerable and persistently increased serum ammonia levels.
3. Infants with urea-cycle defects can present with lethargy, anorexia, hyper- or hypoventilation, hypothermia, seizures, neurologic posturing, subclinical or clinically evident seizures, or coma.
4. Congenital hypothyroidism is the most frequently detected abnormality in newborn screening programs, seen in 1 in 2000 to 4000 newborn infants.
5. Congenital adrenal hyperplasia is a group of genetic disorders affecting adrenal steroid biosynthesis and can be seen in virilizing or salt-wasting clinical presentations.
6. Infants with galactosemia have markedly elevated blood galactose and can present with subtle clinical signs such as jaundice, vomiting, and poor weight gain, lethargy and hypotonia, hepatomegaly, and sepsis, most often due to *Escherichia coli.*
7. Organic acidemias typically present within the early neonatal period with poor feeding, vomiting, hypoglycemia, irritability, lethargy, hypotonia, and seizures. Hepatomegaly may be present. Patients with infantile or late-onset forms may have failure to thrive, developmental delay, seizures, and spasticity. Laboratory tests show metabolic acidosis, ketosis, hyperlactatemia, and hyperammonemia.
8. Phenylketonuria is a rare autosomal-recessive disorder of phenylalanine (Phe) metabolism associated with Phe accumulation in the brain and other organs. The classic signs are microcephaly, hypotonia, motor deficits, eczematous rash, autism, seizures, and developmental problems.
9. Neonates with classic maple syrup urine disease present within the first few weeks of life with feeding intolerance, urine with a maple syrup odor, seizures, coma, and death.
10. Medium-chain acyl-coenzyme A (CoA) dehydrogenase deficiency is seen with altered mental status, lethargy, seizures, emesis, and even death.
11. Citrullinemia presents after the first 24 hours of life with tachypnea and respiratory alkalosis, but if untreated, these infants develop worsening lethargy, seizures, coma, hepatomegaly with increased transaminases, and eventually death.

Inborn errors of metabolism (IEMs) are inherited conditions that block metabolic pathways. Even though these disorders may be rare at an individual level, genetic screening suggests that as a group, these conditions could be identified in 1 out of every 1500 infants.[1] Disturbances in metabolic pathways usually cause a spectrum of systemic findings involving multiple organ systems. Early recognition is important because institution of definitive treatment, or at least palliation of the manageable aspects, can improve mortality and morbidity.[2,3]

We have suspected IEMs in infants during the early neonatal period, before the screening reports become available, if they have progressively worsening encephalopathy with lethargy, seizures, or coma that cannot be explained as due to asphyxia or infections; unexplained severe high anion-gap metabolic acidosis; or unexplained respiratory alkalosis associated with considerable and persistently increased serum ammonia levels.

In the United States, the newborn screening (NBS) programs include up to 52 conditions (as described in the next chapter).[2] To improve the clinical outcomes in IEMs, there may be two possible strategies. One may be focused on early diagnosis by expanding the NBS programs. There may be benefits in early institution of therapeutic measures, in supporting these families, and in finding help from social, religious, educational, and/or political leadership. The second strategy may be to strengthen the educational programs for healthcare providers for early diagnosis and management of these rare disorders. However, we still have not identified clear therapeutic measures for all these disorders. No NBS program will be sensitive enough to detect every single genetic variant of these diseases, and hence there may be a need for individualized interventions at multiple levels. We may not have the resources to do so.

In the following sections, we provide a brief summary of the most frequently seen IEMs, focusing on epidemiologic information, clinical features, available tools for diagnosis, and possible treatment(s). This chapter will have to be expanded in time as more information becomes available. We have assimilated findings from our own clinical experience with an extensive review of the literature, using key terms in multiple databases including PubMed, Embase, and ScienceDirect.

Diagnosis of Conditions With Early Neonatal Onset or Those Not Included in Screening Programs

As described above, we have suspected IEMs during the first few days after birth if there is worsening encephalopathy, unexplained severe high anion-gap metabolic acidosis, or unexplained respiratory alkalosis associated with high serum ammonia levels (Fig. 75.1).

These clinical manifestations may appear in the most severe variants and in urea-cycle defects. In the following section, we describe the clinical approach to urea-cycle defects, which are mostly not included in NBS programs.

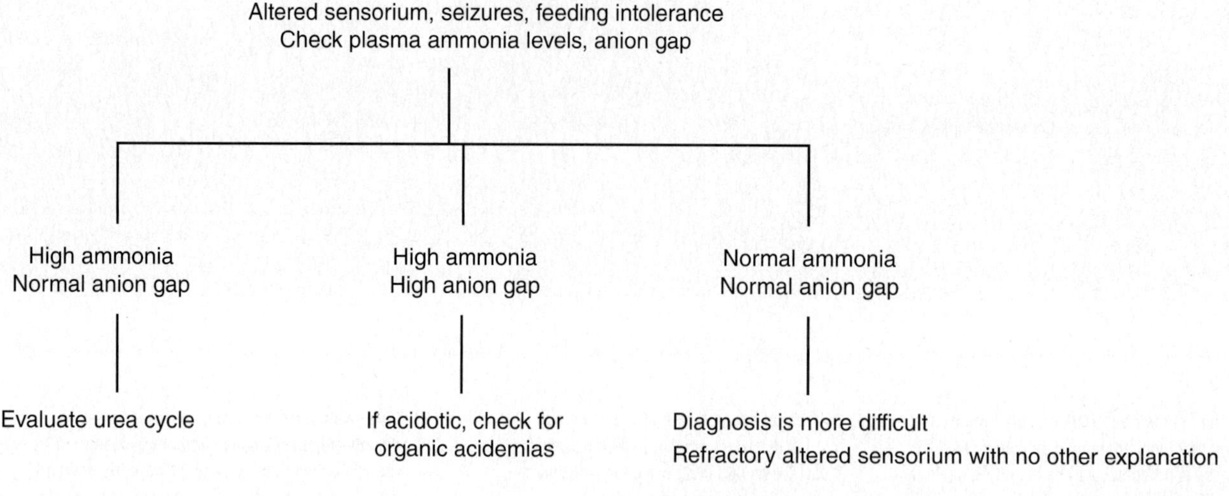

Fig. 75.1 Most Frequent Settings in Which to Suspect an Inborn Error of Metabolism Before the First Newborn Screening Reports Become Available. *MRI,* Magnetic resonance imaging.

Urea Cycle Defect

The urea cycle is composed of five core enzymes, one activating enzyme, and one mitochondrial ornithine/citrulline antiporter (Krebs-Henseleit cycle) that convert waste nitrogen generated from protein catabolism into urea, which is then excreted from the body (Fig. 75.2). Urea-cycle disorders (UCDs) result in the failure of conversion of ammonia into urea, resulting in accumulation of ammonia and other products. If not recognized and treated rapidly, this results in encephalopathy, coma, and death.

The incidence of UCDs is estimated at 1 in 35,000 births. Existing information indicates that defects in ornithine transcarbamylase (OTC) constitute nearly 60% of all UCDs. In the United States, two UCDs, argininosuccinic synthetase and lyase deficiency, are currently detected by NBS; each of these accounts for approximately 15% of the UCDs.[4] Argininosuccinate synthetase (AS) deficiency is described later in the chapter. Individuals with predicted attenuated forms of argininosuccinic aciduria seem to be overrepresented in the NBS group.[5]

Severe deficiency or total absence of activity of any of the first four enzymes in the pathway (carbamoylphosphate synthetase [CPS], OTC, ASS, and argininosuccinate lyase [ASL]) or a cofactor producer (N-acetylglutamate synthase deficiency; not shown) results in the accumulation of ammonia and other precursor metabolites and can present very early, during the first few days of life, before the results of NBS become available. Because no effective secondary clearance system for ammonia exists, complete disruption of this pathway results in the rapid accumulation of ammonia and development of related symptoms.

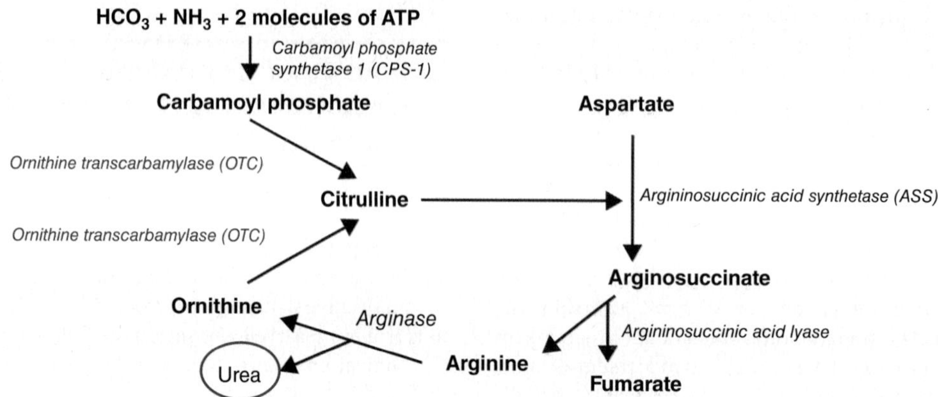

Fig. 75.2 The Urea Cycle. These five reactions convert ammonia into urea (*encircled*). The deficiency of ornithine transcarbamylase (OTC; shown in *red*) is most frequently associated with clinical manifestations. *ATP,* Adenosine triphosphate; *HCO_3,* bicarbonate; *NH_3,* ammonia.

Carbamoyl phosphate synthetase I (CPS1) deficiency is the most severe of the UCDs. Individuals with complete CPS1 deficiency rapidly develop hyperammonemia in the newborn period. Ornithine transcarbamylase deficiency in males can be as severe as CPS1 deficiency. Approximately 15% of carrier females develop hyperammonemia. ASS1 deficiency can also be associated with severe hyperammonemia.

Argininosuccinic aciduria (ASL deficiency) can also present with rapid-onset hyperammonemia in neonates. Some affected infants develop chronic hepatic enlargement and elevation of transaminases. Arginase deficiency is not typically characterized by rapid-onset hyperammonemia, but affected infants can present with spasticity and choreoathetosis. Ornithine translocase deficiency presents less frequently in neonates and has symptoms that evolve more slowly. Citrin deficiency can manifest in newborns as neonatal intrahepatic cholestasis.

Clinical Features

Infants with a UCD may appear normal at birth and may have only nonspecific symptoms in the initial few days. Most newborns are discharged from the hospital within 1 to 2 days after birth, and the symptoms of a UCD often develop when the child is at home and may not be recognized in a timely manner by the care providers.

Affected infants can rapidly develop lethargy, anorexia, hyper- or hypoventilation, hypothermia, seizures, neurologic posturing, and coma. Seizures are common in acute hyperammonemia and may result from cerebral damage, but subclinical seizures may also be common in neonates. Many infants may show hepatic dysfunction.

Diagnosis

Hyperammonemia with plasma ammonia >150 μM/L should trigger evaluation. If the anion gap is >20 or if there is hypoglycemia, then urine organic acids, plasma amino acids, and acylcarnitine profile should be checked to exclude other disorders.

Quantitative plasma amino acid analysis can be used to arrive at a tentative diagnosis. (Because the liver is not fully mature at birth, affected newborns often have plasma amino acid concentrations that are quite different from those in older children and adults.) Plasma concentration of citrulline can help distinguish between proximal and distal urea-cycle defects, because citrulline is the product of the proximal enzymes and is absent or very low in deficiency of CPS1, OTC, and N-acetylglutamate synthase (NAGS). It is a substrate for the distal enzymes (ASS1 and ASL) and is elevated in defects in these enzymes. Plasma concentration of arginine is markedly elevated in arginase 1 deficiency. It may be reduced in other UCDs.

Urinary orotic acid is normal or low in CPS1 deficiency and significantly elevated in OTC deficiency. Urinary orotic acid excretion can also be increased in argininemia (ARG1 deficiency) and citrullinemia type I (ASS1 deficiency). Urine amino acid analysis can also be helpful.

Molecular genetic testing is the primary method of diagnostic confirmation for all UCDs. If molecular testing is uninformative, CPS1, NAGS, or OTC enzyme activity can be measured in hepatocytes; ASL, ASS1, or ornithine transporter in fibroblasts; and ARG1 in erythrocytes.

Imaging changes in acute hyperammonemia can resemble those seen in hypoxic-ischemic encephalopathy. Lesions show cerebral edema and are frequently seen in deep white matter, particularly in the parietal, occipital, and frontal regions. This is best appreciated on T_2-weighted magnetic resonance imaging (MRI) sequences or on diffusion tensor imaging. MRI findings may lag behind clinical changes.

Treatment

Infants with neurologic symptoms should be treated at a tertiary center with access to specialists. The removal of ammonia is critical with whichever treatment is available; intermittent hemofiltration (arteriovenous or venovenous) and hemodialysis, extracorporeal membrane oxygenation, or continuous renal replacement therapies can all work if instituted in a timely fashion.

Nitrogen scavenger therapy (sodium phenylacetate and sodium benzoate) can be used as an intravenous infusion for acute management and an oral preparation for long-term maintenance.

Deficient urea-cycle intermediates need to be replaced depending on the diagnosis; these can include arginine (intravenous infusion) and/or citrulline (oral preparation). Reduction of the catabolic state is important.

Clinical Approach to IEMs Detected in NBS Programs

Congenital Hypothyroidism

Introduction

Congenital hypothyroidism is the most frequently detected abnormality in NBS programs, seen in 1 in 2000 to 4000 newborn infants.[6] It involves insufficient production of the thyroid hormones with dysfunction of the hypothalamic–pituitary–thyroid axis at various levels; there may be abnormal development or function of the thyroid gland, low levels of upstream regulators produced in the hypothalamus and/or the pituitary gland, or impaired thyroid hormone action in the peripheral tissue.[7]

Clinical Features

Congenital hypothyroidism may be completely asymptomatic in newborn infants. In some, symptoms may be seen or may appear in time. There may a goiter, poor feeding, constipation, hypothermia, bradycardia, edema, wide fontanelles, macroglossia, prolonged jaundice, umbilical hernia, poor growth, and developmental delay. Up to 10% of infants with congenital hypothyroidism have other congenital abnormalities if it occurs as a part of specific syndromes. If not detected timely, congenital hypothyroidism can cause neurodevelopmental delay and cognitive impairment.[6]

Diagnosis

Universal NBS is the most important tool for diagnosing congenital hypothyroidism.[8] Most screening programs measure the blood concentrations of thyroid-stimulating hormone (TSH); in some programs, T4 is also measured routinely or is requested if TSH is elevated. Screening based on TSH levels is sensitive for detecting primary hypothyroidism. However, TSH measurements may not detect newborn infants with central hypothyroidism in whom TSH is not elevated despite low T4 levels. Screening programs that include T4 measurements may have some strengths. The optimal time for TSH screening may be between 48 and 72 hours after birth because there is often a transient surge in TSH levels in the first few hours after birth and early blood samples may result in erroneous results. Genetic tests with next-generation sequencing techniques have allowed early identification of patients at risk of or with congenital hypothyroidism.[9]

Thyroid imaging (either by ultrasound or scintigraphy) may help establish a diagnosis of thyroid dysgenesis or ectopic thyroid. Measurements of serum thyroglobulin levels can provide useful information about the etiology of congenital hypothyroidism. Further evaluation may include MRI of the pituitary and hypothalamus and laboratory assessment of pituitary hormone function to investigate the possibility of central hypothyroidism. Causes of congenital hypothyroidism are summarized in Table 75.1.

Treatment

Any abnormal result on NBS should prompt immediate confirmation by measuring serum concentrations of TSH and free thyoxine (FT4). Pediatric endocrinologists should be consulted as soon as possible, and treatments should be initiated. If the screening TSH level is greater than 40 mIU/L, treatment should be started without waiting for the confirmatory test results. Levothyroxine (LT4) is the standard treatment for congenital hypothyroidism at a recommended dose of 10 to 15 mg/kg.[7,9]

Delayed initiation of treatment is associated with poor neurodevelopmental outcomes. The goal of treatment is to achieve euthyroidism rapidly. Normalization of serum TSH and FT4 levels within 2 weeks after starting therapy seems to improve cognitive outcomes. The treatment of congenital hypothyroidism is monitored by measuring serum TSH and FT4 concentrations.

Congenital Adrenal Hyperplasia

Introduction

Congenital adrenal hyperplasia (CAH) is a group of genetic disorders affecting adrenal steroid biosynthesis, resulting in decreased cortisol production from the fasciculate layer of the adrenal gland. The most frequently seen genetic defects result in decreased expression of the enzyme 21-hydroxylase (21-OH), which leads to low levels of cortisol. The consequent interruption of the normal feedback inhibition loops stimulates the pituitary to produce more adrenocorticotropic hormone (ACTH) and causes hyperplasia of the adrenal glands. The incidence has been estimated to be about 1 in 8000 newborn infants.[10]

Most cases, more than 90%, with low 21-OH expression are related to autosomal-recessive (AR) mutations in the gene encoding cytochrome P450 family 21 subfamily A member 2 protein (*CYP21A2*).[11] This causes the accumulation of its substrate, 17-hydroxyprogesterone (OHP), and increases androgen production with masculinization of the female newborn and virilization of affected males.

Depending on the severity of the enzyme deficiency, infants with 21-OH deficiency are classified into the following categories:

1. Classic (severe adrenal hyperplasia): Further subdivided into virilizing or salt-wasting forms. Many individuals with mild loss-of-function mutations present with androgen excess rather than adrenal insufficiency, which leads to an ascertainment bias that favors diagnosis in females.
2. Nonclassic (relatively milder).[11]

Patients with the classic or symptomatic nonclassic forms can be treated with glucocorticoids to suppress the excessive secretion of the corticotrophin-releasing hormone and ACTH. Recent studies suggest that there may be an advantage of detecting CAH through molecular genotyping (*CYP21A2* mutations) of fetal cells obtained by chorionic villous sampling, possibly as early as at 9 to 11 weeks' gestation. Identification of satellite DNA markers from an amniocentesis sample obtained at 15 to 18 weeks or by analyzing cell-free fetal DNA in maternal circulation can increase the diagnostic accuracy.[10]

In mothers with CAH, the sex of the fetus can be determined as early as 7 weeks' gestation, which can reduce parental anxiety and facilitate treatment planning. Gonadal hormones, particularly androgens, affect certain aspects of brain development and have permanent influences on the psychosexual identity of the patient. Hence, early detection of CAH can facilitate early initiation of treatment, even in utero. Early detection of CAH in infants born to mothers with non-classic adrenal hyperplasia due to 21-OH deficiency can reduce the severity of abnormalities in the infants (approximately 2.5%, from 14.8%, respectively).[10] Prenatal treatments for mothers with CAH, to prevent fetuses from developing ambiguous genitalia, are also available. However, some studies have discussed the long-term effects of antenatal dexamethasone treatment on verbal working

Table 75.1 Causes of Congenital Hypothyroidism
Thyroid dysgenesis (1 in 4500); isolated thyroid aplasia, hemiagenesis, hypoplasia, or ectopy mutations in transcription factors PAX-8, TTF-1, FOXE1 (TTF-2), NKX2-5, SHH, and Tbx1
Defects in thyroid hormonogenesis (1 in 35,000) • Abnormal iodide uptake (NIS, SLC5A5), concentration, organification • Abnormal TPO enzyme • Abnormal H_2O_2 generation (THOX, DUOX2) • Pendred syndrome (SLC26A4) • Defective Tg synthesis or transport • Abnormal iodotyrosine deiodinase (DEHAL1) • Abnormal thyroxine cerebral transport (MCT8)
Secondary and/or tertiary hypothyroidism (1 in 50,000–100,000) • Isolated TSH deficiency • TRH deficiency
Multiple hypothalamic hormone deficiencies • Isolated hypothalamic defect • Associated with other midline facial/brain structural defects such as septo-optic dysplasia, cleft lip/palate Pituitary abnormality • Isolated TSH deficiency (IGSF1), TRH resistance, abnormal TSHβ molecule • Multiple pituitary hormone deficiencies with eutopic posterior pituitary gland (transcription factor defect, e.g., POU1F-1, PROP1, LHX3) or ectopic posterior pituitary gland (idiopathic, transcription factor defect, e.g., HESX1, SOX3, LHX4, OTX2)
TSH resistance with mutations in the TSH receptor gene, possible postreceptor defect Thyroid hormone resistance (1 in 100,000)

TPPO, Triphenylphosphine oxide; *TRH,* thyrotropin-releasing hormone; *TSH,* thyroid stimulating hormone.

memory and certain aspects of self-perception. Some researchers recommend a flexible clinical approach.

Clinical Features

Excessive androgen production is the hallmark of this disorder. In the severe classic form, genital ambiguity is present in affected female infants. This virilization of the female fetus may begin before 11 to 12 weeks' gestation, and this disorder may be the most common cause of ambiguous genitalia in a genetically female fetus. The phenotypic virilization ranges from simple clitoromegaly, with or without partial fusion of the labioscrotal folds, to the appearance of a penile urethra. Although the genitalia of a female born with the severe form of the disease may be indistinguishable from those of a male, the important differentiating points are the absence of testes and the presence of a normal uterus and ovaries. The internal genitalia (uterus and fallopian tubes) that arise from the Müllerian duct are also normal.

Males with 21-OH deficiency do not manifest genital abnormalities at birth but may have subtle penile enlargement and some hyperpigmentation of external genitalia. These infants may continue to show accelerated virilization during childhood. The aldosterone deficiency can predispose them to salt-wasting crises.

Diagnosis

The initial laboratory evaluation should include the measurements of blood glucose, electrolytes, and a liver function panel; arterial blood gases; serum levels of cortisol ACTH, and 17-OHP; pelvic ultrasonography; karyotype; and comprehensive mutation analysis of *CYP21A2*. Genotype–phenotype correlations associated with *CYP21A2* mutations and clinical presentations are described in Table 75.2.

The measurement of 21-OH levels is an important evaluation in patients suspected of experiencing an adrenal crisis. To evaluate adrenal function and differentiate among the various potential enzymatic defects, an ACTH stimulation test should be performed. This can be done by administration of 0.25 mg of cosyntropin (a synthetic ACTH) to stimulate the adrenal glands, maximizing hormone secretion. A full adrenal profile, including measurement of 17-OHP, cortisol, deoxycorticosterone, 11-deoxycortisol, 17-hydroxypregnenolone, dehydroepiandrosterone, and androstenedione, should be obtained immediately prior to and 60 minutes after cosyntropin administration. If the total amount of blood drawn is of concern in small infants, a single sample collected at the 60-minute time point is most valuable. If the diagnosis remains unclear, it may be desirable to treat the child and retest later after partially or completely tapering the glucocorticoids.

Screening programs for CAH are also important to identify male infants with the salt-wasting type of CAH in NBS panels by measuring 17-OHP concentrations using filter paper blood-collection cards. To achieve higher sensitivity in detection, a low 17-OHP cutoff value is typically used. Preterm, sick, or stressed infants tend to have higher 17-OHP values, even when corrected for birth weight. Unfortunately, the specificity of the test is only 2%, which translates to very high false-positive rates. False negatives can also occur, and there may be reason to repeat the tests in cases with a high index of suspicion. Term infants with mildly elevated 17-OHP levels (40–100 ng/mL) should be followed up with repeat tests. If elevated potassium and decreased sodium concentrations are found, the same treatment indicated for an acute adrenal crisis should be started immediately while waiting for confirmatory laboratory studies, and a pediatric endocrinologist should be consulted for additional management. Genetic testing can allow the identification of carriers. Prenatal genetic testing is also available and can be useful in at-risk patients with known familial mutations.

Treatment

Hydrocortisone is currently the most widely used medication for replacing cortisol. To achieve a sufficient cortisol response in an infant with classic CAH who has fever, trauma, or is undergoing surgery, the maintenance dose of replacement glucocorticoids should be increased. Further work is needed to optimize the medical treatment.[12] The salt-wasting form of CAH requires mineralocorticoid replacement (fludrocortisone) and sodium chloride supplementation. Surgical correction of clitoroplasty and vaginal reconstruction is often required in affected female infants.

Organic Acidemias

Introduction

Organic acidemias occur at a rate of 3.7 to 12.6 per 100,000 births and are inherited as AR traits. The defects involve abnormal amino acid catabolism with accumulation of organic acids. Propionic acidemia (PA) occurs at a rate of 1 per 100,000 newborns and can be as high as 1 per 14,000 newborns in countries with high consanguinity.

PA and methylmalonic aciduria occur due to defects in the oxidation of the branched-chain amino acids (isoleucine, valine, threonine, and methionine), propionate produced by gut bacteria, odd-chain fatty acids, thymidine, uracil, and cholesterol (Fig. 75.3). Most mutations are in the propionyl–coenzyme A (CoA) carboxylase subunit alpha (*PCCA*) or PCC beta (*PCCB*) genes, resulting in

Table 75.2 Genotype-Phenotype Correlations in Congenital Adrenal Hyperplasia Owing to 21-Hydroxylase Deficiency

Severity	Classic Salt Wasting	Classic Simple Virilizing	Nonclassic
21-Hydroxylase enzyme activity (% normal)	0	1–2	20–50
CYP21A2 mutations (phenotype generally corresponds to the least-affected allele)	Gene deletion; mutation in Intron 2 (c.293–13C>G); Exon 3 del 8 bp; Exon 6 cluster mutations; p.Q318X p.R356W	p.I172N; mutation in Intron 2 (c.293–13C>G)	p.P30L; p.V281L; p.P453S
Aldosterone synthesis	Low	Normal	Normal
Age at diagnosis (without newborn screening)	Infancy	Infancy (46,XX individuals); childhood (46,XY individuals)	Childhood to adulthood, or asymptomatic
Virilization	Severe	Moderate to severe	None to mild

Adapted from Kliegman RM. *Nelson Textbook of Pediatrics*. 21st ed. Philadelphia: Elsevier; 2020.

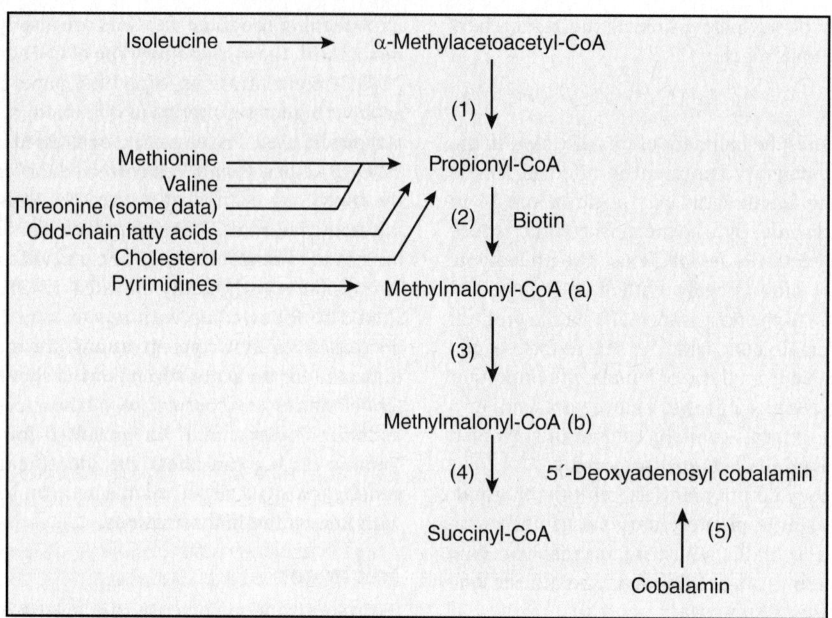

Fig. 75.3 The Propionate Pathway. (1) β-Ketothiolase. (2) Propionyl-CoA carboxylase. (3) Methylmalonyl-CoA isomerase. (4) Methylmalonyl-CoA mutase. (5) Cobalamin metabolic pathway. *CoA,* Coenzyme A. (Reproduced with permission and with minor modifications from Marcdante and Kliegman. Organic acid disorders. In: *Nelson Essentials of Pediatrics*, ch, 54, 205–207.)

decreased propionyl-CoA carboxylase activity, leading to inability to break down propionyl-CoA into methylmalonyl-CoA and decreased substrate for use in the citric acid cycle.[13]

Methylmalonic acidemia is caused by gene defects in methylmalonyl-CoA mutase (*MMUT*), metabolism of cobalamin associated A (*MMAA*), metabolism of cobalamin associated B (*MMAB*), or methylmalonic aciduria and homocystinuria type D protein, mitochondrial (*MMADHC*). The condition can be cause either by a defect in one of the above-mentioned genes or by deficient synthesis of its cofactor adenosylcobalamin.[14]

Clinical Features

Infants typically present within the early neonatal period with poor feeding, vomiting, hypoglycemia, irritability, lethargy, hypotonia, and seizures. Hepatomegaly may be present. Patients with infantile or late-onset forms may have failure to thrive, developmental delay, seizures, and spasticity.[13]

Diagnosis

Laboratory tests show metabolic acidosis, ketosis, hyperlactatemia, and hyperammonemia. When an organic acidemia is suspected, the diagnosis can be confirmed by measuring organic acids in urine.

A diagnosis of PA is made by measuring urine organic acids with the use of gas chromatography–mass spectroscopy. The results will typically show increased propionic acid and methylcitrate, but methylmalonic acid will likely be decreased. Decreased methylmalonic acid helps differentiate this disorder from methylmalonic aciduria. Standard NBS tests can identify these conditions in most infants. Prenatal diagnosis is possible by measuring enzyme activity in cultured amniotic fluid cells or chorionic villi cells. Further genetic tests can pinpoint the exact mutations for screening in the family.[15]

In methylmalonic acidemia (MMA), elevations of methylmalonic acid together with 3-hydroxypropionate and presence of 2-methylcitrate can confirm a diagnosis of MMA; a similar pattern can be seen in PA without abnormal levels of methylmalonic acid. Infants with PA often have increased tiglylglycine and propionylglycine. The diagnostic workup may be complemented with the measurement of acylcarnitines in dried blood spots or plasma.[13] In this test, a striking elevation of C3 acylcarnitine (propionylcarnitine) can be found in both MMA and PA. In addition, plasma amino acid measurements show elevated glycine levels in MMA and PA.[15]

Standard NBS tests can be used to diagnose these disorders. Prenatal diagnosis is preferentially performed by molecular analyses in fetal DNA.[16] Biochemical analyses for MMA can be used as an alternative or additional method in cases where the genetic results are inconclusive or not available. Prenatal diagnosis of MMA can be performed by measurement of MMA in dried amniotic fluid.[13] The combination of two independent methods (biochemical and genetics) increases the reliability of results.

Treatment

Early diagnosis and timely referral are essential to reduce morbidity and morbidity.[17,18] Intensive-care treatment of patients with a metabolic decompensation can be necessary if there is a severe metabolic acidosis with or without hyperammonemia and hyperlactatemia. Treatment modalities include extracorporeal detoxification. It seems appropriate to advise against the primary use of sodium phenylbutyrate as an ammonia scavenger in MMA and PA, because it can lead to decreased glutamine levels, potentially hampering tricarboxylic acid–cycle anaplerosis via 2-ketoglutarate.

Treatment includes a low-protein diet (typically 8–12 g/day). The diet may be supplemented with specialized amino-acid formula preparations that do not contain amino acids that cannot be metabolized in infants deficient in propionyl CoA carboxylase. AMMONUL is a metabolically active compound that serves as an alternative to urea for excretion of nitrogenous wastes, essential in the setting of hyperammonemia. Because there can be a relative carnitine deficiency in organic acidemias, supplemental carnitine provides a buffer to trap toxic acyl-CoA metabolites.[13] Methylmalonic acidemia is occasionally due to reduced concentrations of its cofactor, cobalamin. In this setting, hydroxocobalamin supplementation can augment the function of MMUT.

Severely affected infants often die during the newborn period or later due to metabolic derangements, hypoglycemia, or infections. Survivors are at risk of cognitive abnormalities and seizures. MRI may show changes in the basal ganglia region. Pancreatitis and osteoporosis are noted at greater frequency in patients who have PA.

For acute metabolic decompensation, the protein intake may have to be stopped for 24 to 48 hours, and the infant may have to be managed with intravenous glucose infusion with the carnitine dose increased to 200 mg/kg/day. Extensive intravenous glucose administration can be associated with lactic acidosis, potentially due to the inhibited pyruvate dehydrogenase enzyme in MMA and PA. The acid–base balance and levels of ammonia and electrolytes need to monitored closely. Hyperammonemia can be treated with sodium benzoate, and in some infants with hyperammonemia and encephalopathy, the administration of carglumic acid or extracorporeal detoxification can be considered. Some severely afflicted infants may need liver or liver and kidney transplantation.

Galactosemia

Introduction

Galactosemia is a rare, AR disorder of galactose metabolism that leads to markedly elevated blood galactose levels (Fig. 75.4). The disorder can occur due to defects in the galactose-1-phosphate uridylyltransferase (*GALT*), galactokinase (*GALK1*), and uridine diphosphate galactose 4-epimerase (*GALE*) genes, which can cause accumulation of galactose. Type I disease is caused by complete absence of GALT. Partial GALT activity is present in several variants, the most common being the Duarte variant. The severity of symptoms depends on the degree to which GALT activity is lost. If an individual has as little as 10% of normal GALT activity, symptoms may be minimal.[19] More than 230 *GALT* mutations have been identified worldwide. Further details are included in the chapter on newborn screening.

The incidence of galactosemia varies by geographic region. In the United States, some areas have shown an incidence of 1 in 60,000 births. The incidence is higher in western Europe and in Saudi Arabia. It is lower in eastern Asia (1 in 1,000,000 births in Japan).

Clinical Features

Subtle clinical signs, including jaundice, vomiting, and poor weight gain, may be present early and should trigger the consideration of an inborn error of metabolism if symptoms are not progressing as anticipated. Symptoms are the most severe with a total deficiency of GALT; affected infants often manifest symptoms in the first week after birth, especially with human milk or cow milk–based formula feedings. The most common initial findings are lethargy and hypotonia, jaundice, vomiting, and hepatomegaly. In some infants, feeding problems and poor weight gain are prominent. Hepatic damage occurs from toxic galactose metabolites, especially galactitol, and this may cause only mild elevations of liver enzymes or lead to more severe hepatic insufficiency with coagulopathy and occasionally ascites. Approximately 10% of infants with galactosemia will develop sepsis, most often due to *Escherichia coli.* Ongoing ingestion of lactose-containing feedings will cause progressive brain injury, including seizures. Jaundice associated with galactosemia is typically related to indirect hyperbilirubinemia in the first week but typically progresses to cholestasis within another week. Brain imaging in infants with galactosemia has demonstrated various abnormalities, including abnormal white matter, cerebral atrophy, and ventricular enlargement. Infants with galactokinase deficiency have significantly

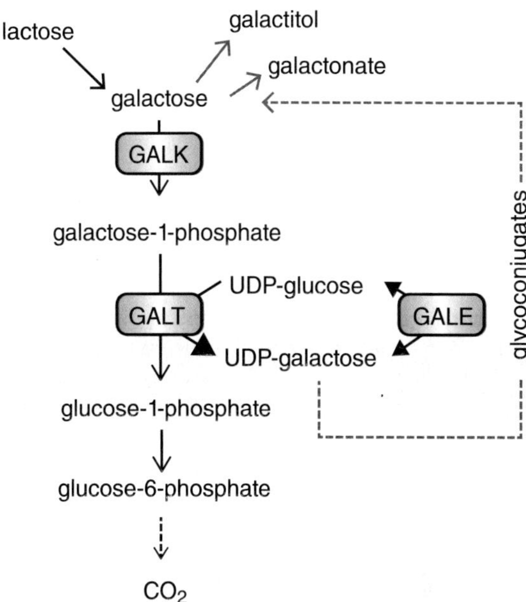

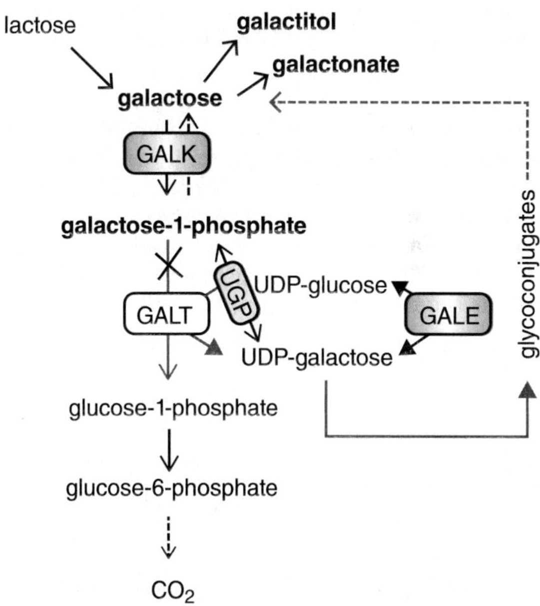

Fig. 75.4 Pathway for Galactose Metabolism and Galactose-1-Phosphate Uridylyltransferase (GALT) Deficiency–Associated Alteration. (A) The Leloir pathway is responsible for galactose metabolism. Dietary lactose is hydrolyzed in the intestinal tract, and subsequently the absorbed galactose is transported to the liver, where it is trapped as galactose-1-phosphate, the first step of the Leloir pathway. The enzyme that is deficient in classic galactosemia, GALT, subsequently converts the galactose-1-phosphate and urinie diphosphate (UDP)-glucose to UDP-galactose and glucose-1-phosphate, which may subsequently be converted to glucose-6-phosphate and enter the glycolytic pathway or be hydrolyzed for efflux out of the liver. The last enzyme in the Leloir pathway, uridine diphosphate galactose-4-epimerase (GALE) is very important in allowing UDP-galactose to be transformed into UDP-glucose and to maintain the steady-state UDP-galactose/UDP-glucose ratio in different cells, thus playing an important role in homeostasis of glycoconjugate formation. (B) Galactose metabolism in GALT deficiency. The absence of GALT enzyme activity causes accumulation of galactose-1-phosphate, a biomarker for GALT deficiency. Galactose, galactitol, and galactonate levels are also elevated. Although not very active, the UDP-glucose pyrophosphorylase (UGP) enzyme can convert galactose-1-phosphate to UDP-galactose. *GALT,* Galactose-1-phosphate uridylyltransferase. (Reproduced with permission and with minor modifications from Demirbas et al. Hereditary galactosemia. *Metabolism.* 2018;83:188–196.)

fewer clinical signs of disease; only cataracts, typically not present in the newborn, become apparent later in infancy, and these infants have fewer neurodevelopmental disabilities.[19]

The severity of symptoms is related to whether the enzyme deficiency is generalized in erythrocytes and all other tissues or only in erythrocytes. Infants with variant galactosemia may tolerate the typical milk diet of early infancy but often develop elevated galactose and galactitol levels when more solid foods are introduced.

Diagnosis

The metabolic pathway of galactose and defects associated with GALT deficiency are described in Fig. 75.2. Galactosemia is diagnosed in routine NBS, either with a low GALT level or elevated galactose levels in blood or increased reducing substances such as galactose and galactitol in urine. The urinary tests can be false positive and need further confirmation. NBS is typically performed by measuring GALT activity in erythrocytes or galactose levels (if greater than 14.5 mg/dL [0.8 mmol/L]) in whole blood. Elevated galactose levels are suggestive, but the infant has to have adequate enteral intake of lactose-containing feeds (human milk or standard infant formula). Abnormal tests should trigger removal of lactose-containing fluid or feeds until further genetic testing confirms the diagnosis.

Prenatal diagnosis during pregnancy can be performed with the GALT assay in fibroblasts from amniotic fluid or with a chorionic villus biopsy (CVB), or a mutation analysis of DNA extracted from a CVB, if the genotype of the parent or the affected infant is known.

Treatment

The immediate intervention is to immediately remove lactose-containing feedings (human milk or standard formula) and to replace these with a soy-based formula; these changes need to be made even before confirmatory testing is complete. Other therapies should be provided as clinically indicated, such as phototherapy, antibiotics, or intravenous fluids. Symptoms may resolve quickly after appropriate dietary interventions are provided. Early diagnosis usually reduces the mortality of galactosemia, but it may not alter the long-term neurodevelopmental outcome.

Phenylketonuria

Introduction

Phenylketonuria (PKU) is a rare AR disorder of phenylalanine (Phe) metabolism caused by mutations in the gene encoding phenylalanine hydroxylase (*PAH*). The condition is associated with Phe accumulation in the brain and other organs (Fig. 75.5). More than 950 *PAH* variants are known to be associated with PKU.[20]

Hyperphenylalaninemia can also occur due to defects in the regeneration or biosynthesis of the PAH cofactor tetrahydrobiopterin (BH4).[20] If untreated or undiagnosed, the neurotoxic effects of excess phenylalanine can lead to impaired postnatal cognitive development. Both types of hyperphenylalaninemia (PAH and BH4 deficient) are thought to be heterogeneous disorders that vary from severe (for example, classic PKU) to mild, benign, and transient forms. Enzyme deficiency yields a spectrum of disorders such as mild hyperphenylalaninemia, mild phenylketonuria, and classic phenylketonuria.[21,22]

The prevalence of PKU varies worldwide. In Europe, the mean prevalence is approximately 1 per 10,000 newborns, with a higher rate in some countries such as Ireland and Turkey and a very low rate in Finland.

Clinical Features

NBS has permitted early identification of infants with PKU, and very few are now seen with clinical signs and symptoms. The classic signs were microcephaly, hypotonia, motor deficits, eczematous rash, autism, seizures, and developmental problems.

Many infants with milder symptoms may present in later infancy with seizures, tremors, stunted growth, hyperactivity, eczema, or a musty odor of their breath, skin, or urine. If undiagnosed at birth and if treatment is not started quickly, the disorder can cause irreversible brain damage and intellectual disabilities.

Diagnosis

In the 1960s, Guthrie developed a simple test to detect hyperphenylalaninemia in large populations. Prenatal genetic testing is available in families known to have carriers of the disease. A

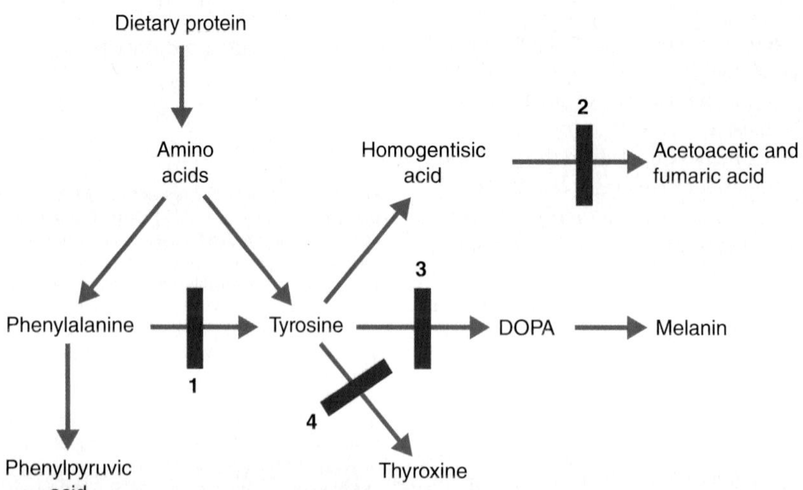

Fig. 75.5 Inborn Errors of Metabolism in the Phenylalanine/Tyrosine Pathway. (1) Phenylketonuria. Lack of phenylalanine hydroxylase blocks conversion of phenylalanine to tyrosine; phenylalanine and phenylpyruvic acid appear in the urine. (2) Alkaptonuria. Lack of homogentisic acid oxidase causes accumulation of homogentisic acid. (3) Albinism. Lack of the enzyme tyrosinase prevents conversion of tyrosine via dihydroxyphenylalanine (DOPA) to melanin. (4) Familial hypothyroidism. Deficiency of any one of several enzymes impairs iodination of tyrosine in the formation of thyroid hormone. (Reproduced with permission and minor modifications from Morley. Disorders of metabolism and homeostasis. *Underwood's Pathology*, 6, 95–114.)

symptomatic infant with a positive NBS result should be referred to a specialized metabolic center to ensure the best outcome of PKU. Tandem mass spectrometry can be useful in analysis of amino acid profiles of blood samples taken beyond 24 hours after birth. Infants with blood Phe concentrations >600 μmol/L should be treated. No immediate treatment is recommended if untreated blood Phe levels are <360 μmol/L.[23] PKU is an AR condition with more than 400 gene variants that are known to be pathogenic. Most patients are heterozygous carriers. Genetic testing is not mandatory for diagnosis, but it may help catalog the likely severity of disease because there is a good correlation between the genotype and clinical phenotypes.[24]

Treatment

Immediate initiation of treatment is essential to prevent neurologic damage, preferably before the age of 10 days. The cornerstone of PKU treatment is a low Phe diet in combination with Phe-free L-amino acid supplements for life. Some PKU centers use casein glycomacropeptide or large neutral amino acids as alternative dietary supplements. Certain patients are responsive to and are treated with BH4 acting as a pharmaceutical chaperone (prescribed as sapropterin dihydrochloride). Possible future treatments include enzyme substitution and gene therapy. Patients with an untreated Phe concentration of 360 to 600 μmol/L should be treated and followed up.[24]

Maple Syrup Urine Disease

Introduction

Maple syrup urine disease (MSUD) is an AR inherited disorder caused by deficiency of the branched-chain alpha-keto acid dehydrogenase (BCKD) complex (Fig. 75.6). Deficient BCKD complex activity can cause accumulation of the branched-chain amino acids (BCAAs; leucine, valine, and isoleucine). The incidence of MSUD is approximately 1 per 185,000 births worldwide, ranging between 1 per 26,000 and 1 per 1,000,000 live births.[25]

There are five phenotypes of MSUD, with different clinical presentations. Four are caused by mutations in BCKD: a classic variant with three milder variants, an intermediate, an intermittent, and a thiamine-responsive subset. A fifth phenotype is caused by dihydrolipoyl dehydrogenase (E3)-deficiency.[26]

Clinical Features

The clinical presentation depends on the severity of the underlying disorder and metabolic decompensation, ranging from intermittent symptoms of various degrees, such as hypotonia and failure to thrive, to acute life-threatening encephalopathy.

The classic MSUD is the most severe phenotype and accounts for nearly 75% of all cases. These patients have less than 3% of the normal BCKD complex activity. Neonates with classic MSUD are born asymptomatic but typically present within the first few weeks of life. The most common clinical features are feeding intolerance, a maple syrup urine odor, seizures, coma, and death. Patients with the variant phenotypes have higher residual enzyme activity and may have normal leucine levels during anabolic states. Under severe catabolic stress, these patients can experience severe metabolic decompensations with increased leucine concentrations.

Diagnosis

Metabolic pathways for BCAAs are described in Fig. 75.4. MSUD is included in many NBS programs, which may enable detection before the onset of severe symptoms. The tandem mass-spectrometry can detect BCAAs and alloisoleucine in dried blood spots. Before the widespread availability of screening, many infants were diagnosed based on the clinical manifestation and the characteristic maple syrup odor of the urine.

The diagnosis of MSUD can occur with mutations in the following genes:

1. Type 1A mutations occur in the branched-chain α-keto acid dehydrogenase, E1α subunit (*BCKDHA*).
2. Type 1B mutations occur in the branched-chain α-keto acid dehydrogenase, E1β subunit (*BCKDHB*).
3. Type II mutations affect the E2 subunit (*DBT*).
4. Type III mutations occur in the E3 subunit (*DLD*).[26]

Prenatal diagnosis during pregnancy can be performed in fibroblasts from amniotic fluid or a CVB or by a mutation analysis of DNA extracted from a CVB if the pathogenic variants of the parent or the affected infant are known.

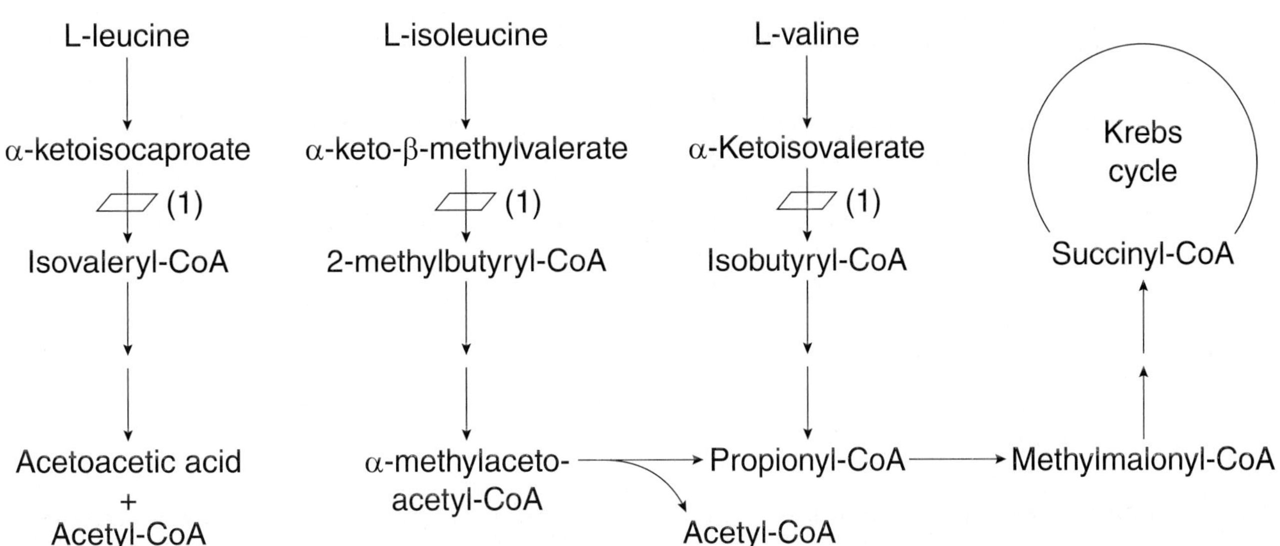

Fig. 75.6 Abbreviated Pathway for the Metabolism of the Branched-Chain Amino Acids. The known enzyme defect affecting the amino acid metabolism is (1) branched-chain ketoacid dehydrogenase, causing maple syrup urine disease. *CoA*, Coenzyme A. (Reproduced with permission and minor modifications from Sanchez-Russo and Wilcox. Amino acid metabolism. *Emery and Rimoin's Principles and Practice of Medical Genetics and Genomics: Metabolic Disorders*, 3, 49–104.)

Treatment

MSUD can cause severe neurologic deterioration unless an early diagnosis is made and immediate treatment initiated by dietary restriction of BCAAs. The treatment for MSUD includes low-protein diet supplementation with BCAA-free formula, symptomatic treatment during metabolic crises, and frequent clinical and biochemical monitoring. Acute metabolic decompensation is corrected by treating the precipitating stress while delivering sufficient calories, insulin, free amino acids, isoleucine, and valine to achieve sustained net protein synthesis in tissues.[25]

Some centers use hemodialysis/hemofiltration to remove BCAAs from the extracellular compartment. Brain edema is a common complication of metabolic encephalopathy and requires careful intensive care management. Transplantation of allogeneic liver tissue can allow unrestricted diets and protect the patient from metabolic crises, but it does not reverse preexisting psychomotor disability or mental illness.

Medium-chain Acyl-CoA Dehydrogenase Deficiency

Introduction

Medium-chain acyl-CoA dehydrogenase (MCAD) deficiency is an AR defect of fatty acid β-oxidation disorders. MCAD is caused by mutations in the acyl-CoA dehydrogenase medium-chain gene (*ACADM*).[27] The prevalence of MCAD varies by ethnicity, ranging from 1 per 5000 to 1 per 20,000 live births. The carrier frequency in some countries may be high as 1 in 70.[12]

The MCAD enzyme converts medium-chain fatty acyl-CoA into short-chain fatty acyl-CoA and acetyl CoA to generate energy via ketones during times of fasting (Fig. 75.7). During these periods of fasting, gluconeogenesis is used via MCAD to maintain blood glucose levels via the production of ketone bodies as acetyl-CoA accumulates.[28]

Clinical Features

The wide availability of newborn screens has reduced the acute crises from MCAD deficiency. Breastfeeding infants are at particularly high risk in the first 72 hours, depending on maternal breast milk supply. If supply is low, then neonates may experience prolonged periods of fasting, resulting in an early presentation of metabolic crisis. Presenting symptoms can include altered mental status, lethargy, seizures, emesis, and even death in about 20% of patients with an initial crisis.[29] On physical exam, hepatomegaly may be noted. The disorder is seen in neonates, although the presentation can be delayed to childhood or later depending on the exact mutations.[30]

Diagnosis

MCAD is included in many NBS programs, which may enable early detection prior to the onset of severe symptoms. A positive NBS screening with elevated acylcarnitines may help early identification. The diagnosis can then be confirmed by urine organic acid analysis, plasma acylcarnitine profiling, and testing for mutations in the *ACADM* gene.[30] Prenatal diagnosis is feasible.

Treatment

Early diagnosis and treatment can avoid possible death or disability. Management is by reducing times of fasting and ensuring nutrition intake to meet metabolic demands; infants have lower tolerance for fasting, and it decreases even further during critical illness. These

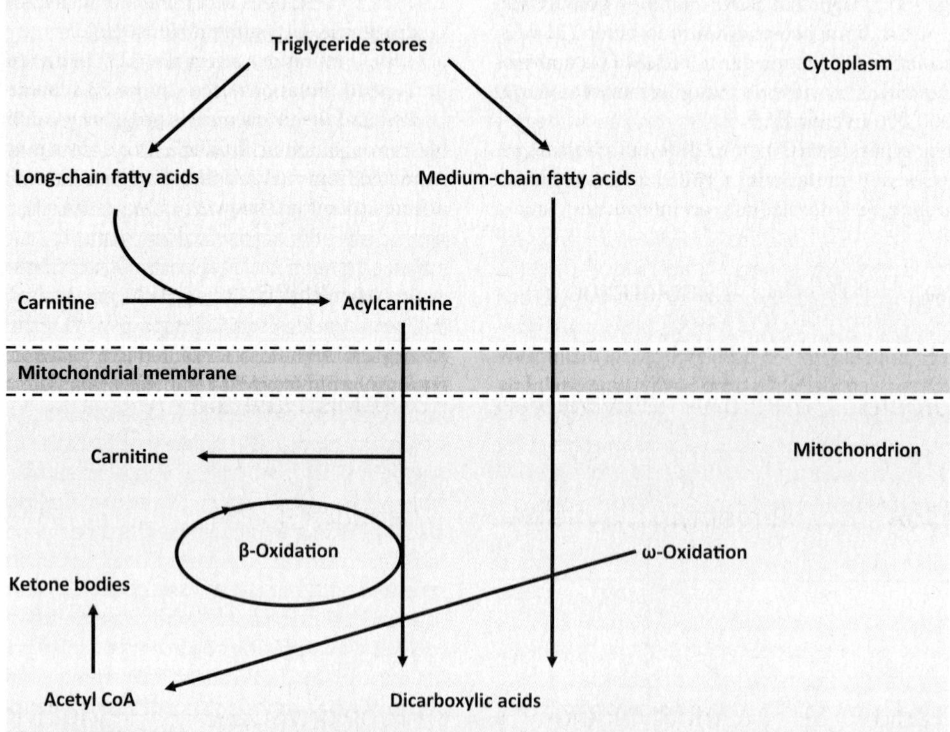

Fig. 75.7 Fatty Acid Oxidation. Triglycerides are mainly composed of long-chain fatty acids, which require transfer across the mitochondrial membrane as an acylcarnitine. Medium-chain fatty acids can cross the mitochondrial membrane directly. Within the mitochondrion, fatty acids then undergo β-oxidation, in which the fatty acid molecule is sequentially shortened by two carbon units, releasing acetyl-coenzyme A (CoA). Certain enzymes involved in β-oxidation, including medium-chain acyl-CoA dehydrogenase, are chain-length specific. Deficiency of this enzyme prevents the normal catabolism of both long- and medium-chain fatty acids and results in an increase in medium-chain acylcarnitines in blood, increased ω-oxidation to form dicarboxylic acids, and a reduction in ketone-body production. (Reproduced with permission and minor modifications from Jameson and Walter. Medium-chain acyl-CoA dehydrogenase deficiency—A review. *Paediatrics and Child Health*. 2011;21:90–93.)

infants can be treated with a high-carbohydrate and low-fat diet, avoiding medium-chain triglycerides. Patients with carnitine transport deficiency may benefit from carnitine supplementation to enhance fatty acid beta-oxidation.

Citrullinemia

Introduction

Citrullinemia is an AR disorder of the urea cycle caused by mutations in the argininosuccinate synthetase (*ASS1*) and *SLC25A13* genes. The lack of this enzyme results in hyperammonemia; affected infants show increased serum ammonia (1000–3000 μmol/L, compared with normal values <100 μmol/L).[31]

There are two forms of citrullinemia:

1. Type 1, "classic/neonatal" citrullinemia, presents within the first few days of life. Affected infants appear normal at birth but become symptomatic as blood ammonia levels rise. Type 1 affects approximately 1 per 17,000 to 55,000 infants worldwide and is associated with mutations in *ASS1*.
2. Type 2 citrullinemia, also known as "citrin deficiency," is caused by mutations in *SLC25A13*. This defect can present with classic hyperammonemia in the newborn, cholestasis, and fatty liver. Many infants present with insidious neurologic findings, hyperammonemia, hypercitrullinemia, and hyperlipidemia. The condition also has an adult-onset form.

Clinical Features

Newborns typically appear healthy for the first 24 hours of life. Tachypnea and respiratory alkalosis are early findings, but if untreated, these infants develop worsening lethargy, seizures, coma, hepatomegaly with increased transaminases, and eventually death. MRI can show extensive changes (Fig. 75.8). There is also a late-onset form that presents in later infancy with episodic hyperammonemia and cognitive impairment.

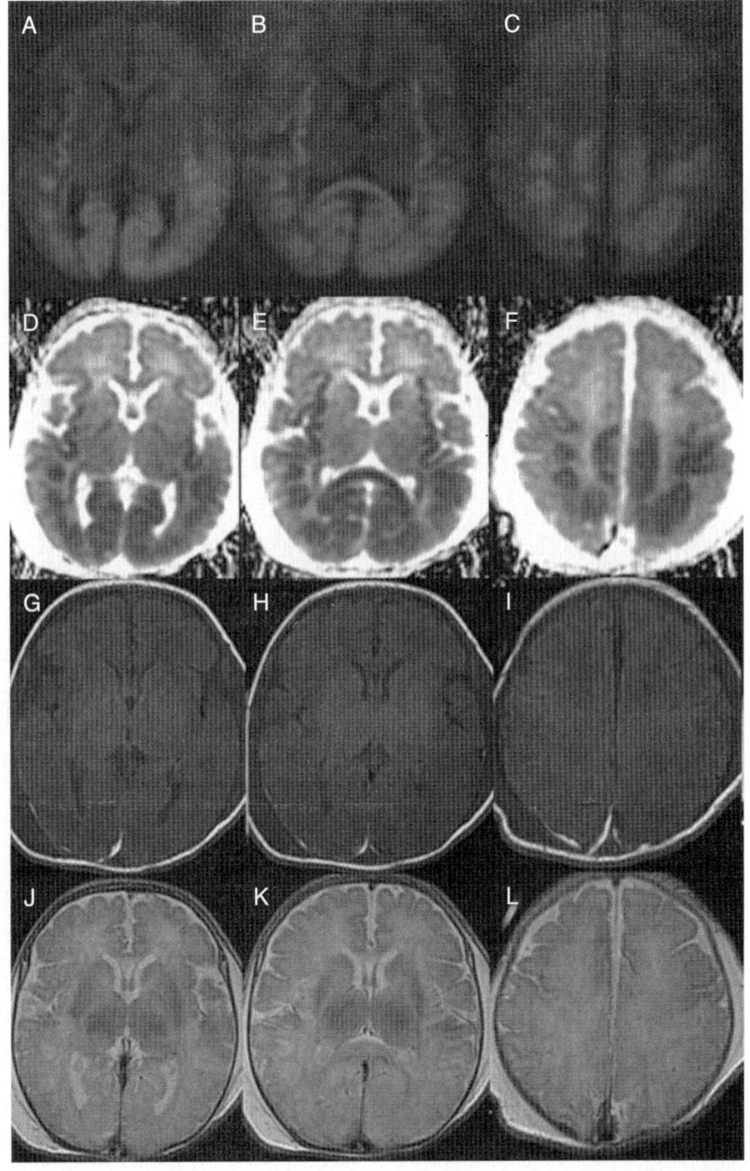

Fig. 75.8 Classic Citrullinemia Type I. (A–C) Diffusion-weighted magnetic resonance imaging (DWI). (D–F) apparent diffusion coefficient (ADC) maps. (G–I) T1. (J–L) T2. In a 7-day-old female with seizures and citrullinemia, reduced diffusivity is seen predominantly in the cortex, in both cerebral hemispheres, and in the splenium of the corpus callosum, with T1 and T2 prolongation in these same areas. Small bilateral parieto-occipital acute subdural hematomas and subgaleal hematomas with caput succedaneum are also observed. (Reproduced with permission and minor modifications from Rodrigues and Grant. Diffusion-weighted imaging in neonates. *Neuroimaging Clin N Am*. 2011;21(1):127–151.)

Diagnosis

The diagnosis is confirmed by measuring amino-acid levels in blood and urine. Blood gas analysis can be used to analyze pH, CO_2, the anion gap, and blood lactate. Plasma acyl carnitine, plasma and urine, amino acids, and determination of orotic acid can be useful. Elevated plasma ammonia levels of 150 μmol/L or higher in neonates, associated with a normal anion gap and a normal blood glucose level, should lead to specific testing for a urea-cycle defect. Orotic acid levels will be elevated in the urine. Citrulline levels will be elevated in the blood, whereas arginine levels will be low. DNA molecular testing of the *ASS* gene and enzymatic studies may also be helpful in confirming the diagnosis.

Genetic testing is now widely available. The findings of hyperammonemia and elevated citrulline in the newborn dried blood screening can suggest one of two metabolic defects: the deficiency of argininosuccinic acid synthetase (citrullinemia) or argininosuccinate lyase (associated with argininosuccinic aciduria). The diagnosis can be confirmed by directed assays in cultured fibroblasts or by genetic testing. Prenatal diagnosis is possible by assay of enzyme activity in amniotic fluid or by mutation analysis of cultured chorionic villus cells.

Treatment

In most cases, treatment needs to be instituted empirically before a specific diagnosis is confirmed. The metabolic screen helps to broadly categorize the patient's IEM, on the basis of which empirical treatment can be instituted. A timely diagnosis and initiation of therapy to lower ammonia levels are vital for prognosis.

Treatment includes immediate, specific management. Emergency management includes the administration of dextrose/electrolyte fluids to mitigate catabolism and dehydration, establishment of central venous access, and provision of other physiologic support. Specific medications for hyperammonemia include sodium benzoate and phenylacetate. Sodium benzoate combines with glycine to make hippuric acid and sodium phenylacetate combines with glutamine to make phenylacetylglutamine, which are excreted in the urine. Arginine must also be administered because it replenishes circulating amino acid levels. A higher dose is required in the management of citrullinemia. Fluid and electrolytes should be optimized to maintain normal intracranial pressure. Dialysis if medical management fails is very effective for the removal of ammonia. Exchange transfusion is not usually recommended because it removes ammonia only from the intravascular compartment.

After stabilization, nutritional management takes precedence. A low-protein diet and special medical formulae are often recommended, with emphasis on other nonprotein caloric sources. These infants need to be closely monitored. A biochemical genetics specialist and a metabolic genetics dietitian should coordinate the treatment.

CHAPTER 76

Screening Programs for Early Detection of Inborn Errors of Metabolism in Neonates

Amarilis Sanchez-Valle

KEY POINTS

1. Should protein in the diet be limited while waiting for results? No. It is not recommended to change the diet to a specialized diet without confirmation of results. However, if the baby is critically ill, it may be recommended to stop feeds due to instability. It is not recommended to stop all protein for more than 24 to 48 hours in patients with inborn errors of metabolism, due to the risk of catabolism. It is imperative to work fast to confirm the newborn screen results and be able to appropriately manage the baby.
2. Is carnitine added to total parenteral nutrition (TPN) adequate as a supplement? The amount added to TPN is below the recommended dosage for carnitine uptake deficiency. It may be sufficient to affect newborn screen results. Therefore it is sometimes recommended to stop TPN for hours before sending testing.
3. How long to hold TPN prior to blood or urine collection? There is no evidence-based literature on the perfect timing. Many state labs will recommend waiting for 48 hours after TPN has been discontinued. However, many labs will recommend to provide Intravenous Fluids (IVF) without amino acids for 3 to 4 hours prior to drawing confirmatory testing.
4. Can the baby be discharged before the results come back? It depends on the disorder for which the baby is being evaluated. It is best to communicate with the referral center prior to discharging baby.

Introduction

In this chapter, we are going to discuss the origins of the newborn screening program in the United States. We are going to learn about the process of selection of disorders to the newborn screen program. The chapter will describe the process of evaluating a baby with an abnormal newborn screen and the next steps to take. The purpose of the chapter is to familiarize the neonatologist with the newborn screening program and disorders. The chapter includes special considerations that can affect the newborn screening results, specifically in the neonatal intensive care unit (NICU).

Background

In the United States, a program was established in the 1960s to screen all neonates for the detection of classic phenylketonuria (PKU).[1] To this day, newborn screening is considered one of the most successful public health programs due to its ability to screen large populations, identify babies at risk of fatal illnesses, and prevent their death or severe comorbidities. It was developed by Dr. Robert Guthrie with the purpose of identifying babies who had PKU to prevent intellectual disability by starting a special diet at birth. The newborn screen started with a simple method of adding a few drops of blood to a filter card and testing it with a bacterial inhibition assay to determine the amount of phenylalanine in a baby's blood. The filter card used was known as the PKU card, and when babies had abnormalities, it was called having an abnormal PKU test. Even though we have been screening for many more disorders since the 1990s, the name of the PKU test remains, creating confusion for parents. The author of this chapter feels strongly that healthcare providers should use the terminology "newborn screen test results" when discussing findings with parents or other healthcare providers.

Although technology changed in 1990 with the addition of tandem mass spectroscopy, we continue to use a filter card for blood collection. Nowadays, we also use gene sequencing as part of the newborn screening. The goals of the newborn screen are to prevent or minimize significant morbidity and mortality associated with various disorders.[2]

Selection of Disorders

In 1968, Wilson and Jungner wrote a report to the World Health Organization proposing screening criteria (Box 76.1).[3] In 2006 the Maternal and Child Health Bureau commissioned the American College of Medical Genetics (ACMG) to develop a uniform screening panel and system.[4] Their selection criteria stated that a condition should meet the following minimal criteria: it can be identified at a time (24–48 hours after birth) at which it would not ordinarily be detected clinically; a test with appropriate sensitivity and specificity is available for it; and there are demonstrated benefits of early detection, timely intervention, and efficacious treatment of the condition.

The Advisory Committee on Heritable Disorders in Newborns and Children has the purpose of evaluating disorders and making recommendations to the U.S. Department of Health and Human Services. The Recommended Uniform Screening Panel (RUSP) is the final list recommended by the U.S. Department of Health and Human Services. After a new disorder is proposed to the committee, the selection to add it to the RUSP is based on evidence-based literature. The recommendations are independent of financial support, and each state has the autonomy to decide which disorders it will screen for and how to support its program. Initially in 2006, the RUSP included 29 conditions that were mandated and an additional 25 conditions that were part of the differential diagnosis of a core panel of conditions, were clinically significant, and were revealed with the screening

■ Box 76.1 Wilson and Jungner Classic Screening Criteria[1]

1. The condition sought should be an important health problem.
2. There should be an accepted treatment for patients with recognized disease.
3. Facilities for diagnosis and treatment should be available.
4. There should be a recognizable latent or early symptomatic stage.
5. There should be a suitable test or examination.
6. The test should be acceptable to the population.
7. The natural history of the condition, including development from latent to declared disease, should be adequately understood.
8. There should be an agreed policy on whom to treat as patients.
9. The cost of case-finding (including diagnosis and treatment of patients diagnosed) should be economically balanced in relation to possible expenditure on medical care as a whole.
10. Case-finding should be a continuing process and not a "once and for all" project.

technology but lacked efficacious treatment or were incidental findings with potential clinical significance. Currently, the RUSP includes 37 core conditions and 26 secondary conditions (as of February 2023).[5] The core and secondary conditions can be classified as organic acidemias, fatty acid oxidation disorders (FAOD), amino acid disorders, endocrine disorders, hemoglobinopathies, and other genetic disorders (Fig. 76.1).

It is important to understand that although the United States are somewhat uniform in following the RUSP, they are not completely uniform, and some states take longer to implement new disorders into their programs. The RUSP list can be found at this website: https://www.hrsa.gov/advisory-committees/heritable-disorders/rusp/index.html.

Description of the Process

A filter card is collected at the birth place. The nurse or midwife has to perform a heelstick and fill five full circles with blood. The sample is then sent to the state lab. Every state has a different system; however, most states have carriers to pick up the filter cards daily and send them to their state lab.[6] There are a few states that do not have a state lab and have to send their filter cards to an adjacent state's lab. The speed of processing is of utmost importance because there are certain disorders that will present in the first few days of life. Every state must develop their reference ranges, and these are calibrated for newborns. There is no consent needed to obtain a filter card. Parents can refuse to have a filter card done. The recommendation is to obtain the filter card after 24 hours of life. There are states that recommend having a second newborn screen in the 2-week-old checkup.[7] NICUs have other recommendations due to the fragility of the population in those units. The recommendations for NICUs are to obtain the first newborn screen at birth in case there is an unexpected death. However, the screen must be repeated when the newborn is at least 48 to 72 hours of age. Another specimen is collected at 28 days of life and/or prior to discharge.

There are specific situations to be aware of in the NICU because some babies receive blood transfusions. Once a baby has had a red blood cell transfusion, certain disorders are not identified due to red blood cell enzymes, such as galactosemia and hemoglobinopathies. For these conditions, it is recommended to wait at least 120 days for enzyme testing. However, the physician can proceed with gene testing rather than waiting.

Another concerning reality is that there are extremely premature infants who spend more than 3 months in the NICU and have multiple newborn screens repeated. The reference ranges are meant for full-term newborns, which would result in abnormal newborn screens that are false-positive screens. Some researchers have published about the importance of using age-appropriate reference values when working with a prematurely born population.[8]

There are two disorders that are part of the RUSP that do not require blood collection: congenital hearing loss and critical congenital heart disease.

Congenital hearing loss screening has to include a one- or two-step validated protocol.[9] The most common protocol used is a two-step screening process that starts with otoacoustic emissions, followed by an auditory brainstem response if the first step is failed. Every baby should be screened for congenital hearing loss in the first month of life. If a baby is born at home or a birthing center, there should be a process established to refer the baby for screening in the first month of life.

Regarding critical congenital heart disease, the recommendations are to screen with pulse oximetry in a preductal and postductal position (right hand and a foot) after 24 hours of age. The baby should be off oxygen to perform the screening test. If the baby is unable to be weaned off oxygen for the test, an echocardiogram is recommended. If the screening test is positive (the baby has failed the screen), further tests are recommended. Fig. 76.2 shows the proposed algorithm (https://www.cdc.gov/ncbddd/heartdefects/hcp.html).[10]

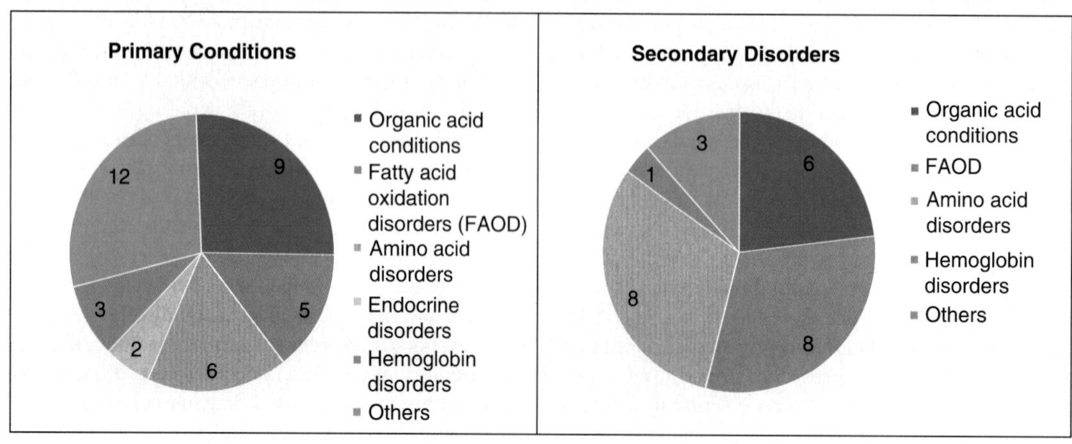

Fig. 76.1 Recommended Uniform Screening Panel.

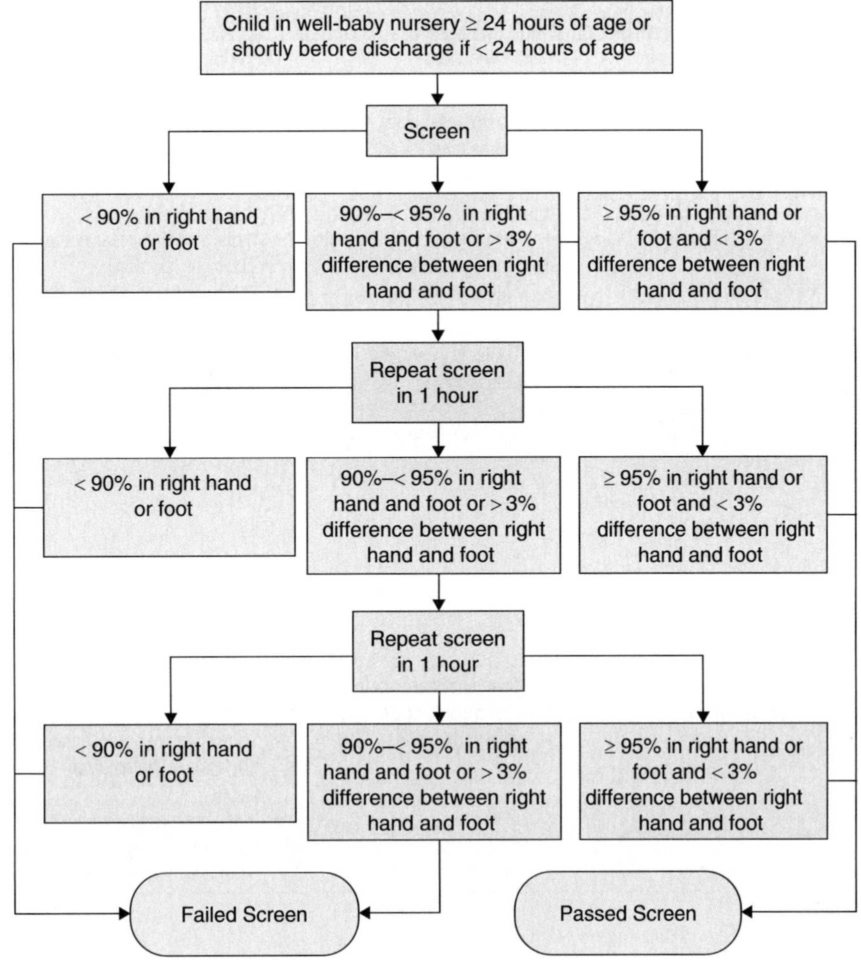

Fig. 76.2 Critical Congenital Heart Defect Newborn Screen Algorithm.

Abnormal Newborn Screen Results

For blood-tested disorders, once the filter card reaches the lab, it will be processed for the respective disorders included in that state's labs. There are certain conditions that require second-tier testing, and the results of those take longer, such as X-linked Adrenoleukodystrophy (XALD) and Mucopolysaccharidosis Type I (MPSI). Typically, the newborn screen results are available in the first 5 to 7 days of life. Every state has a process in place to manage abnormal newborn screen results. Neonatologists will encounter many abnormal newborn screens. The tables below summarize the first steps to take when encountering an abnormal newborn screen for one of the core disorders.

The ACMG prepared ACTion Sheets that provide information to the healthcare provider to give to families as well as algorithms to follow.[11] Tables 76.1 to 76.8 presented in this chapter are a summary of the ACT sheets posted at https://www.acmg.net/ACMG/Medical-Genetics-Practice-Resources/ACT_Sheets_and_Algorithms.aspx.

False-Positive/False-Negative Results

Total parenteral nutrition (TPN) can affect the concentrations of amino acids, commonly tyrosine or leucine. Carnitine can also be added to the TPN, which can affect newborn screen results for fatty acid oxidation disorders.[12] Medium-chain triglyceride oil is added to TPN or to milk as a caloric supplement, and it can affect the acylcarnitine species that are used for fatty acid oxidation screening (Table 76.9). Also, there are certain antibiotics (pivalic acid) that can affect the newborn screen results.[13,14] It is recommended in the premature or critically ill newborn to send the initial newborn screen prior to starting any treatment, which would typically be prior to 24 hours of life. It is important to keep in mind that when sending the sample prior to 24 hours of life, there is a higher risk for false-positive results for congenital hypothyroidism, congenital adrenal hyperplasia, and cystic fibrosis (CF) (screened by immunoreactive trypsinogen). There is also risk for false-negative results when sending an early sample. The conditions associated with false negatives are aminoacidopathies, organic acidemias, and congenital hypothyroidism (screened by thyroid stimulating hormone [TSH]). Prematurity is another factor for false positives due to factors such as liver immaturity, low birth weight with lack of normative reference ranges, fragility, and a low number of white blood cells (WBC).[12,15] Methionine, tyrosine, and branched-chain amino acid elevations can be seen in prematurity and liver disease.[16] Another situation seen in premature babies is multiple maternal antenatal courses of steroids (i.e., dexamethasone) for fetal lung maturation, which can result in false-negative results for congenital adrenal hyperplasia due to fetal adrenal suppression.

It is important to recognize that fatty acid oxidation disorders may present with abnormal biochemical findings during episodes of stress such as birth and the typical weight loss that happens after birth. Because NICU babies are typically treated quickly with TPN and adequate caloric supplementation, these disorders may be

Table 76.1 Organic Acidemias in the RUSP Core Disorders

Metabolite/Condition	Signs and Symptoms	First-Line Labs	Consider	Contact
C3 ↑ Propionic acidemia (PA)[a] Methylmalonic acidemia (MMA)[a] Cobalamin disorders[a]	• Poor feeding or vomiting • Lethargy • Tachypnea	• Plasma acylcarnitine profile • Urine organic acids • Plasma homocysteine	• If baby is ill: glucose, electrolytes, blood gas, ammonia, CBC and urine for ketones	Metabolic geneticist
C5 ↑[a] Isovaleric acidemia (IVA)[a] 2-Methylbutyrylglycinuria	• Poor feeding or vomiting • Lethargy • Tachypnea • Odor of sweaty feet[a]	• Plasma acylcarnitine profile • Urine organic acids • Urine acylglycines	• If baby is ill: glucose, electrolytes, blood gas, ammonia • False positive: antibiotic related (pivalic acid)	Metabolic geneticist
C5OH ↑[a] 3-Methylcrotonyl CoA carboxylase deficiency (3MCC)[a] 3-Hydroxy-3-methyglutaric aciduria (HMG CoA lyase deficiency)[a] Holocarboxylase synthase deficiency[a] β-Ketothiolase deficiency[a] 3-Methylglutaconic aciduria 2-Methyl-3-hydroxybutyric aciduria	• Poor feeding or vomiting • Lethargy • Hypoglycemia, ketonuria, metabolic acidosis	• Plasma acylcarnitine profile • Urine organic acids	• If baby is ill: glucose, electrolytes, blood gas, ammonia	Metabolic geneticist
C5DC ↑[a] Glutaric aciduria Type I (GAI)[a]	• Macrocephaly • Muscle hypotonia	• Plasma acylcarnitine profile • Urine organic acids • Urine acylcarnitine C5DC	• If baby is ill: glucose, electrolytes, blood gas • Baby at risk of neurodegenerative crisis with an intercurrent infectious illness • With appropriate treatment, 60%–70% of patients will not suffer neurodegenerative disease	Metabolic geneticist

[a]Core disorder.

C5DC, Glutarylcarnitine; *CBC,* cell blood count; *CoA,* coenzyme A; *RUSP,* recommended Uniform Screening Panel.

Table 76.2 Organic Acidemias and Fatty Acid Oxidation Disorders That Are in the RUSP as Secondary Conditions

Metabolite/Condition	Signs and Symptoms	First-Line Labs	Consider	Contact
C3DC ↑ Malonic acidemia	• Marked lethargy • Vomiting • Hypotonia • Hypoglycemia, lactic acidosis, and metabolic acidosis	• Plasma acylcarnitine profile • Plasma methylmalonic acid • Urine organic acids	• If baby is ill: glucose, electrolytes, blood gas • Other symptoms include seizures and cardiomyopathy	Metabolic geneticist
C4 ↑ Short-chain acyl-CoA dehydrogenase deficiency (SCAD) Isobutyrylglycinuria	• Poor feeding or vomiting • Lethargy • Hypoketotic hypoglycemia, metabolic acidosis	• Plasma acylcarnitine profile • Urine organic acids • Urine acylglycines • Urine acylcarnitine C4	• If baby is ill: glucose, electrolytes, blood gas, ammonia • Most neonates are asymptomatic • A neonate can be extremely ill with vomiting, lethargy, and seizures	Metabolic geneticist
C4-OH ↑ Medium/short-chain L-3-hydroxyacyl-CoA dehydrogenase deficiency (SCHAD)	• Poor feeding or vomiting • Lethargy • Hypoglycemia, metabolic acidosis	• Plasma acylcarnitine profile • Urine organic acids • Plasma insulin	• If baby is ill: glucose, electrolytes, blood gas, ammonia • Most neonates are asymptomatic • Severe hypoglycemia and severe hyperinsulinism may appear later • Sudden death in infancy has been reported	Metabolic geneticist

Table 76.2 Organic Acidemias and Fatty Acid Oxidation Disorders That Are in the RUSP as Secondary Conditions—cont'd

Metabolite/Condition	Signs and Symptoms	First-Line Labs	Consider	Contact
C4 ↑, C5 ↑ Glutaric acidemia type II (GAII)	• Poor feeding or vomiting • Lethargy • Odor of sweaty feet • Facial dysmorphism • Hypoketotic hypoglycemia, metabolic acidosis, hyperammonemia	• Plasma acylcarnitine profile • Urine organic acids • Urine acylglycines	• If baby is ill: glucose, electrolytes, blood gas, ammonia • Can have renal anomalies	Metabolic geneticist
C0/C16+C18 ↑ Carnitine palmitoyl transferase 1 deficiency (CPT1)	• Lethargy • Hepatomegaly • Seizures • Hypoketotic hypoglycemia	• Plasma free and total carnitine • Plasma acylcarnitine profile	• If baby is ill: glucose, electrolytes, blood gas, ammonia, LFTs	Metabolic geneticist
C16 ↑ **and/or C18:1 ↑** Carnitine palmitoyltransferase (CPT2) deficiency Carnitine acylcarnitine translocase (CACT) deficiency	• Poor feeding or vomiting • Lethargy • Dysmorphic facies • Hepatomegaly • Cardiac insufficiency • History of sudden unexpected death in a sibling	• Plasma acylcarnitine profile	• If baby is ill: glucose, electrolytes, blood gas, ammonia, LFTs, CPK • Neonatal form is associated with multiple congenital anomalies, profound illness with marked hypoglycemia, metabolic acidosis, cardiac arrhythmias, and facial dysmorphism	Metabolic geneticist

CPK, Creatine phosphokinase; *LFT,* liver function tests; *RUSP,* recommended Uniform Screening Panel.

Table 76.3 Fatty Acid Oxidation Disorders in the RUSP Core Disorders

Metabolite/Condition	Signs and Symptoms	First-Line Labs	Consider	Contact
C0 ↑ Carnitine uptake deficiency (CUD)	• Poor feeding • Lethargy • Tachypnea, tachycardia • Hepatomegaly • Hypotonia • Hypoglycemia	• Plasma free and total carnitine • Urine free and total carnitine	• If baby is ill: glucose, electrolytes, blood gas, ammonia, LFTs, CPK • Maternal carnitine deficiency (could be due to CUD or GA1) • Prematurity	Metabolic geneticist
C8 ↑ **C6 and C10 ↑** Medium-chain acyl-CoA dehydrogenase (MCAD) deficiency	• Poor feeding or vomiting • Lethargy • Hepatomegaly • Hypoglycemia, metabolic acidosis, hyperammonemia	• Plasma acylcarnitine profile • Urine organic acids • Urine acylglycines	• If baby is ill: glucose, electrolytes, blood gas, ammonia, LFTs • Avoid fasting • Hallmark features: vomiting, lethargy and hypoketotic hypoglycemia • Untreated MCAD deficiency is a significant cause of sudden death	Metabolic geneticist
C14:1 ↑ Very long–chain acyl-CoA dehydrogenase (VLCAD) deficiency	• Poor feeding or vomiting • Lethargy • Hypotonia • Hepatomegaly • Arrhythmia, evidence of cardiac decompensation • Hypoketotic hypoglycemia	• Plasma acylcarnitine profile	• If baby is ill: glucose, electrolytes, blood gas, ammonia, LFTs, CPK • Avoid fasting • Associated with high mortality unless treated promptly	Metabolic geneticist
C16-OH ↑ ± C18 ↑ Long-chain 3-hydroxyacyl-CoA dehydrogenase (LCHAD) deficiency Trifunctional protein (TFP) deficiency	• Poor feeding or vomiting • Lethargy • Hypoketotic hypoglycemia • Hepatomegaly • Cardiac insufficiency • History of sudden unexpected death in a sibling • Maternal liver disease during pregnancy	• Plasma acylcarnitine profile • Urine organic acids	• If baby is ill: glucose, electrolytes, blood gas, ammonia, LFTs, CPK, lactic acid • Avoid fasting • Associated with high mortality unless treated promptly • Hallmark features include hepatomegaly, cardiomyopathy, lethargy, hypoketotic hypoglycemia, elevated LFTs, and elevated CPK • Consider that cefotaxime treatment in the baby or mother may alter lab results	Metabolic geneticist

CPK, Creatine phosphokinase; *LFT,* liver function tests; *RUSP,* recommended Uniform Screening Panel.

Table 76.4 Amino Acid Disorders in the RUSP

Metabolite/Condition	Signs and Symptoms	First-Line Labs	Consider	Contact
Citrulline ↑[a] Argininosuccinic aciduria[a] Citrullinemia I[a] Citrullinemia II	• Poor feeding or vomiting • Lethargy, coma • Tachypnea • Hypotonia • Seizures • Signs of liver disease	• Ammonia (STAT on ice) • Plasma amino acids • Urine amino acids	• Differential diagnosis: citrulline: citrullinemia II (citrin deficiency), consider obtaining lactate for pyruvate carboxylase deficiency	Metabolic geneticist
Leucine ↑[a] Maple syrup urine disease[a]	• Poor feeding or vomiting • Lethargy • Tachypnea • Alternating hypertonia/hypotonia • Seizures	• Urine ketones • Plasma amino acids • Urine organic acids	• Differential diagnosis: hydroxyprolinemia (probably benign) • Maple syrup odor to urine and cerumen • Untreated, it will progress to irreversible intellectual disability, failure to thrive, seizures, coma, cerebral edema, and possibly death	Metabolic geneticist
Methionine ↑[a] Homocystinuria (CBS deficiency)[a] Hypermethioninemia	• Liver disease • Asymptomatic in the neonate	• Plasma amino acids • Plasma homocysteine • Plasma methylmalonic acid	• Differential diagnosis: hyperalimentation, liver disease • If untreated, may develop intellectual disability, ectopia lentis, a marfanoid appearance, osteoporosis, and thromboembolism	Metabolic geneticist
Phenylalanine ↑[a] Classic phenylketonuria[a] Hyperphenylalaninemia Biopterin defects	• Asymptomatic in the neonate	• Plasma amino acids	• Differential diagnosis: mild hyperphenylalaninemia; pterin defects; transient hyperphenylalaninemia • If untreated, PKU will cause irreversible intellectual disability and seizures	Metabolic geneticist
Tyrosine ↑[a] **Succinylacetone ↑**[a] Tyrosinemia type I[a] Tyrosinemia type II and III	• Asymptomatic in the neonate	• Plasma amino acids • Plasma AFP • Urine organic acids	• If baby is ill: glucose, electrolytes, LFTs • If untreated, it will cause liver disease and cirrhosis early in infancy	Metabolic geneticist
Arginine ↑ Argininemia	• Poor feeding or vomiting • Lethargy • Tachypnea • Usually, neonates are asymptomatic	• Ammonia (STAT on ice) • Plasma amino acids	• If untreated, can lead to intellectual disability, seizures, and spastic diplegia	Metabolic geneticist

[a]Core disorder.

AFP, Alpha fetoprotein; *CBS,* cystathionine beta-synthase; *LFT,* liver function tests; *PC,* pyruvate carboxylase; *PKU,* phyenyletonuria; *RUSP,* recommended Uniform Screening Panel.

Table 76.5 Endocrine Disorders and Galactosemia Disorders in the RUSP

Metabolite/Condition	Signs and Symptoms	First-Line Labs	Consider	Contact
TSH ↑[a] Primary congenital hypothyroidism[a]	• Most neonates are asymptomatic • May have prolonged jaundice, puffy facies, large fontanels, macroglossia, and umbilical hernia	• TSH • Free T4 • Repeat dried blood spot	• Transient congenital hypothyroidism • High-risk group: weight <1500 gm; NICU admission; same-sex twin; transfusion; congenital heart defect; other severe congenital anomaly; on dopamine, steroids, or iodine	Pediatric endocrinologist
17-Hydroxyprogesterone (17-OHP) ↑[a] Congenital adrenal hyperplasia (CAH)[a]	• Ambiguous genitalia or nonpalpable testes • Poor feeding • Vomiting	• If mild elevation and low suspicion: repeat newborn screen • If moderate/severe elevation and low suspicion: electrolytes, glucose, 17-OHP • If moderate/severe elevation and high suspicion: 21-OHD, ACTH stim, steroid profile, genotyping	• Stress, prematurity • At risk for life-threatening adrenal crises, shock, and death in males and females	Pediatric endocrinologist

Table 76.5 Endocrine Disorders and Galactosemia Disorders in the RUSP—cont'd

Metabolite/Condition	Signs and Symptoms	First-Line Labs	Consider	Contact
GALT ↓[a] Classic galactosemia[a] Galactoepimerase Galactokinase	• Jaundice • Poor feeding or vomiting • Lethargy • Bulging fontanel • Bleeding	• Quantitative RBC GALT assay • Please note that transfusions can invalidate results of RBC enzyme assays	• Stop breast or cow's milk and initiate nonlactose feeding • If baby is ill: check LFTs, quant RBC Gal-1-P, urine-reducing substance assay • False positive due to enzyme inactivation by high temperature and/or humidity • Presents in the first few days of life and may be fatal without treatment • Neonatal *Escherichia coli* sepsis can occur and is often fatal	Metabolic geneticist

[a]Primary disorder in the RUSP.

17-OHP, 17-Hydroxyprogesterone; *21-OHD,* 21-hydroxylase deficiency; *ACTH stim,* adrenocorticotropic hormone stimulation test; *GALT,* galactose-1-phosphate uridyl transferase; *LFT,* liver function test; *NICU,* neonatal intensive care unit; *RBC,* red blood cell; *RUSP,* Recommended Uniform Screening Panel; *steroid profile,* complete adrenal cortical hormone profile, e.g., by tandem mass spectrometry; *TSH,* thyroid stimulating hormone.

Table 76.6 Hemoglobinopathies and Immunodeficiency Disorders in the RUSP

Metabolite/Condition	Signs and Symptoms	First-Line Labs	Consider	Contact
Sickle cell anemia[a] Hemoglobin S/beta plus thalassemia (HbSβ+ disease)[a] Hemoglobin SC[a]	• Most neonates are asymptomatic • Splenomegaly	• CBC, retic count • Hb-hemoglobin profile analysis • Confirm by IEF, HPLC, electrophoresis, or DNA	• Initiate daily penicillin VK (125 mg po bid)[16a] prophylaxis and other treatment as recommended by the consultant	Pediatric hematologist
Severe combined immuno-deficiencies[a] T-cell related lymphocyte deficiencies	• Infections commonly occur starting by 2–4 months of life • Oral thrush may be seen	• CBC with differential and lymphocyte subset enumeration • Coordinate further testing, antibody levels, lymphocyte proliferation to mitogens, and molecular genetic testing as deemed appropriate	• Untreated patients develop life-threatening, infections due to bacteria, viruses, and fungi • If the infant requires transfusion of any blood product, be sure that only leukoreduced, irradiated products that are negative for cytomegaolovirus (CMV) are used • DO NOT give live attenuated rotavirus vaccine • Outcomes are best if this is performed within the first 3 months of life or before infections occur	Pediatric allergist/ immunologist and/or infectious disease specialist

[a]Primary disorder in the RUSP.

A, C, F, S, and *V,* Hemoglobins seen in neonatal screening; *CBC,* cell blood count; *HPLC,* high performance liquid chromatography; *IEF,* isoelectric focusing; *RUSP,* Recommended Uniform Screening Panel.

Table 76.7 Genetic Disorders in the RUSP

Metabolite/Condition	Signs and Symptoms	First-Line Labs	Consider	Contact
Biotinidase ↓ Biotinidase deficiency	• Poor feeding • Lethargy • Hypotonia • Neonates are usually asymptomatic	• If baby is ill: check glucose, electrolytes, blood gas, lactate, and ammonia • Serum biotinidase	• Processing/shipping can cause false positives • Episodic hypoglycemia, lethargy, hypotonia, and mild developmental delay can occur at any time from the neonatal period through childhood	Metabolic geneticist
Low oxygen Critical congenital heart disease (CCHD)	• Visible cyanosis, tachypnea • Murmur • Difficulty feeding	• Echocardiogram	• If untreated, CCHD may lead to significant morbidity or mortality	Pediatric cardiologist
Immunoreactive trypsinogen IRT ↑ ± DNA Cystic fibrosis (CF)	• Meconium ileus • Recurrent cough, wheezing	• Sweat chloride test • If only moderately elevated IRT, may repeat IRT	• Gastrointestinal abnormalities may cause elevation of IRT	Pediatric pulmonologist

Continued

Table 76.7 Genetic Disorders in the RUSP—cont'd

Metabolite/Condition	Signs and Symptoms	First-Line Labs	Consider	Contact
Hearing loss (>30 db)	• Neonates are usually asymptomatic	• Confirm by audiology evaluation • CMV testing	• If a baby does not pass a hearing screening, it is very important to get a full hearing test as soon as possible, but no later than 3 months of age	Geneticist Audiologist Otologist Early hearing detection and intervention (EHDI) program

CMV, Cytomegalovirus; *IRT,* immunoreactive trypsinogen; *RUSP,* Recommended Uniform Screening Panel.

Table 76.8 Most Recently Added Genetic Disorders in the RUSP

Condition	Signs and Symptoms	First-Line Labs	Consider	Contact
Pompe (glycogen storage disease type III)	• Muscle weakness or hypotonia • Feeding difficulties • Clinical evidence of heart disease	• Routine labs: CPK, LDH, AST, ALT • GAA enzyme activity • Urine hexose tetrasaccharide (Hex4)	• Uniformly fatal if untreated (infantile form)	Metabolic geneticist
Mucopolysaccharidosis type I (Hurler syndrome)	• Neonates are asymptomatic • Nonspecific findings include umbilical or inguinal hernia	• IDUA enzyme	• Mild dysostosis can be detected on radiographs at birth in severe disease	Metabolic geneticist
X-linked adrenoleukodystrophy	• Neonates are asymptomatic	• VLFCA	• Hemolysis or ketogenic diet can cause elevated VLCFA • Mustard seed oil can cause false-negative results	Metabolic geneticist Pediatric endocrinologist
Spinal muscular atrophy due to homozygous deletion of exon 7 in SMN1	• Hypotonia • Respiratory failure • Facial diplegia • Mild joint contractures • Poor suck reflex and swallow difficulties	• SMN1 gene testing	• May see tongue fasciculations	Metabolic geneticist Neuromuscular specialist
Mucopolysaccharidosis type II (Hunter syndrome)	• Neonates are asymptomatic; nonspecific findings include umbilical or inguinal hernia	• I2S enzyme	• Obtaining urine GAG which would reveal elevated dermatan and heparan sulfate	Metabolic geneticist

ALT, Alanine transaminase; *AST,* aspartate transaminase; *CPK,* creatine phosphokinase; *GAA,* acid alpha-glucosidase; *GAG,* glycosaminoglycans; *Hex4,* hexose tetrasaccharide, also called glucose tetrasaccharide; *I2S,* iduronate 2-sulfatase; *IDUA,* alpha-L-iduronidase; *LDH,* lactate dehydrogenase; *RUSP,* Recommended Uniform Screening Panel; *VLCFA,* very long chain fatty acids.

Table 76.9 Treatment and Screening Recommendations

Treatment	Best Time for Screening
RBC transfusion (includes in utero) Extracorporeal membrane oxygenation (ECMO)	120 days after RBC transfusion for hemoglobinopathies or GALT. May send DNA testing.
After total parenteral nutrition (TPN)	Most centers recommend to repeat newborn screen after 48 hours of stopping TPN. Some centers recommend interrupting TPN for 3 hours. No evidence-based medicine has been published.
Carnitine supplementation	After 4 days of discontinuation.
Medium-chain triglyceride supplementation	After 1 day of discontinuation.
Medications/antibiotics	After three half-lives of medication.

GALT, Galactose-1-phosphate uridyl transferase; *RBC,* red blood cell; *TPN,* total parenteral nutrition.

masked. It is important to proceed with confirmatory testing when there is an abnormal newborn screen and the baby has been referred for a suspected fatty acid oxidation disorder. If instead of sending confirmatory testing, a newborn screen is repeated, the baby may not show any biochemical abnormalities at the time, and the newborn screen will be a false negative.

The first-tier test for CF is immunoreactive trypsinogen (IRT), which can be affected by pancreatic damage such as hypoxic organ damage, resulting in a false-positive result for CF. However, a more serious consideration would be to have false-negative results due to not using age-adjusted cutoffs. All newborns with meconium ileus should be tested for CF, and they may not have elevated IRT, which would be a false-negative newborn screen.[17] Thus, they should have DNA testing and sweat chloride testing.

False-positive results are seen in biotinidase due to sample processing and due to the enzyme being thermolabile. Although the biotinidase enzyme is in the serum and should not be affected by a red blood cell transfusion, if the baby is on extracorporeal membrane oxygenation, the enzyme can be affected due to the large blood volume that is required. For galactosemia, a red blood cell transfusion would invalidate the newborn screen result.

Regarding endocrinopathies, we must consider that when using thyroxine (T4) as the screening tool for congenital hypothyroidism (CH), premature babies may have a false-negative result. Also, dopamine and steroids interrupt TSH release and may cause a false-negative result.[18] Many preterm babies will have a false-positive result for congenital adrenal hyperplasia (CAH).[19,20]

Thymectomy can result in secondary T-cell lymphopenia, which would result in a false-positive result for severe combined immunodeficiency (SCID).[21] Low numbers of white blood cells seen in preterm and low birth weight babies can cause low T cell receptor excision circles (TREC) concentrations and increase the likelihood of a false-positive result for SCID.

There are maternal factors that can also affect the newborn screen. If a mother is undergoing treatment for hyperthyroidism, the initial newborn screen can show transient hypothyroidism followed by a period of hyperthyroidism. On the other hand, if a mother has untreated hypothyroidism, the initial newborn screen will show elevated TSH and transient congenital hypothyroidism.[21]

It is important to obtain confirmatory testing after an abnormal newborn screen prior to changing diet or management, because the screen could be reflecting a maternal disorder. If a mother is affected by an inborn error of metabolism, the newborn screen of the baby may be a false positive for that particular disorder. One of the most common inborn errors of metabolism is PKU. If a mother has untreated PKU, the fetus is at risk for having maternal PKU syndrome, which presents with microcephaly, intrauterine growth restriction, and possible congenital heart defect.[22] Another common finding is an abnormal newborn screen that is concerning for PKU but that is actually a reflection of the mother's elevated phenylalanine level. Another common maternal finding that affects newborn screens is maternal vitamin B_{12} deficiency due to diet choices. The newborn screen for the baby typically will be flagged for elevated C3, which is due to a suspected methylmalonic acidemia or cobalamin disorder. However, it is only reflecting maternal B_{12} deficiency.

Mothers of babies with a fatty acid oxidation disorder have an increased chance of developing HELLP syndrome, specifically the long-chain disorders such as LCHAD deficiency.[23]

Common questions to the newborn screen program when managing an abnormal newborn screen result.

1. Should the protein in diet be limited while waiting for results? No. It is not recommended to change the diet to a specialized diet without confirmation of results. However, if baby is critically ill, it may be recommended to stop feeds due to instability. It is not recommended to stop all protein for more than 24-48 hours in patients with inborn errors of metabolism due to the risk of catabolism. It is imperative to work fast to confirm the newborn screen results and be able to appropriately manage the baby.
2. Is the Carnitine added to TPN adequate as a supplement? The amount added to TPN is below the recommended dosage for carnitine uptake deficiency. It may be sufficient to affect newborn screen results. Therefore, it is sometimes recommended to stop TPN for hours before sending testing.
3. How long to hold TPN prior to blood or urine collection? There is not evidence-based literature on the perfect timing. Many state labs will recommend waiting for 48 hours after TPN has been discontinued. However, many labs will recommend to provide IVFs without amino acids for 3-4 hours prior to drawing confirmatory testing.[24]
4. Can the baby be discharged before the results come back? It depends on the disorder that the baby is being evaluated for. It is best to communicate with the referral center prior to discharging baby.

SECTION 16

Genetic Conditions (Including Microarrays, Exome Sequencing)

OUTLINE

CHAPTER 77

An Overview of Genetic Testing

Wendy K. Chung, John P. Schacht, Haluk Kavus

KEY POINTS

1. Genomic medicine has emerged as a new discipline to analyze the human genome and genetic information as a part of clinical care.
2. There are various types of molecular techniques to detect various genetic variations. Each method has unique strengths and limitations, from conventional karyotyping to genome sequencing.
3. Clinicians needs to understand the limitations of the methods used in genetic testing to know what test to order and how to interpret a nondiagnostic test result.
4. Genomic testing ideally should be performed rapidly to have the greatest impact on neonatal management.

Diagnostic Techniques in Clinical Genetics

There are many methods used in clinical genetic testing, each of which has strengths and limitations.[1] These methods are applied to particular clinical-use cases such as newborn screening, carrier testing, noninvasive prenatal screening, presymptomatic testing, diagnostic testing, and pharmacogenomics.[2] Each method is optimized to address a specific type of genetic variation, and the methods are somewhat overlapping and largely complementary. Tandem mass spectrometry (MS) has a significant role in expansion of newborn screening. A karyotype is used to detect aneuploidies, large deletions or duplications, and chromosomal rearrangements. Fluorescence in situ hybridization (FISH) detects microdeletions and microduplications (although with less fidelity) but requires a correct hypothesis about which probe to use to detect the cytogenetic anomaly. By contrast, a chromosomal microarray (CMA) is hypothesis free and provides high resolution to detect small copy-number variants throughout the genome in a single test. Sanger sequencing was the traditional method to sequence and identify single-nucleotide variations and insertions/deletions of a few bases. With the development of next-generation sequencing (NGS) and massive parallel sequencing, the cost/base of sequencing decreased and throughput increased dramatically, making feasible the sequencing of panels of genes to diagnose genetically heterogeneous diseases for conditions such as cardiomyopathies and hereditary cancer.[3] Exome sequencing (ES) assesses only coding regions of most genes in the genome whereas genome sequencing (GS) assesses both coding and noncoding regions. ES and GS offer versatility and can be used to assess sequence-level variants and, with appropriate analysis copy number, variants and structural variants in the case of GS.

A summary comparing the different clinical genetic testing methods is provided in Table 77.1.

Chromosomal Disorders and Karyotyping

Chromosome disorders are an important category of genetic disease, occurring in approximately 1 of every 150 live births.[4] They are a common cause of intellectual disability and pregnancy loss. Chromosomal disorders can be divided into two groups: numerical and structural abnormalities. Numerical abnormalities result from the gain or loss of one or more chromosomes, referred to as an aneuploidy (e.g., trisomy, monosomy, or tetrasomy), or the addition of one or more complete haploid genomes, referred to as polyploidy (e.g., triploidy, tetraploidy).

Structural chromosome abnormalities can be unbalanced (the rearrangement causes a gain or loss of chromosomal material) or balanced (the rearrangement does not produce a loss or gain of chromosome material). Unbalanced abnormalities of chromosomes cause congenital anomalies and neurodevelopmental disorders more commonly than do balanced rearrangements. Structural alterations can be caused by translocations (reciprocal or Robertsonian translocations), ring chromosomes, insertions, deletions, or complex rearrangements.

Mosaicism

Mosaicism is the presence of at least two cell populations derived from the same zygote. Mitotic nondisjunction, trisomy rescue, or occurrence of a somatic new mutation can lead to the development of genetically different cell lines within the body. Mosaicism is possible for any type of genetic change, from a chromosome to a single nucleotide. Mosaicism can affect any cells or tissue within a developing embryo at any point after conception through adulthood. In gonadal mosaicism, the mosaic cells are restricted to the gonads and do not have a clinically observable phenotype but can be passed on to multiple progeny in the next generation. If the mosaic cells are found only in the placenta and absent in the embryo, this is known as confined placental mosaicism,[5] which may be detectable on a chorionic villus sample and may be associated with intrauterine growth restriction but not with congenital anomalies, neurodevelopmental disorders, or any other phenotype if the genetic anomaly is not present in the fetus.

Aneuploidy

Aneuploidy refers to missing or additional chromosomes that do not represent a multiple of 23 chromosomes. Trisomies of chromosomes 13, 18, and 21 are among the most clinically important chromosome

Table 77.1 Comparison of Clinical Genetic Testing Methods

	Karyotype	Chromosome SNP Microarray	FISH	Sanger Sequencing	Sequencing Panel	ES	GS
Single-nucleotide variations (SNVs)				X	X	X	X
Copy number variations (CNVs)		X	X			±	X
Balanced chromosomal rearrangement	X		X				±
Identification of new disease genes						X	X
Incidental findings						X	X
Cost	Low	Low	Low	Low	Low	High	High

ES, Exome sequencing; *FISH*, fluorescence in situ hybridization; *GS*, genome sequencing; *SNP*, single nucleotide polymorphism.

aneuploidies present in live-born infants. Monosomy (only one copy of a chromosome in an otherwise diploid cell) is much less common and more severe than trisomy (three copies of a chromosome) and is rarely viable. Nondisjunction causes errors in chromosome segregation and is the cause of aneuploidies. Multiple congenital anomalies, growth restriction, and intellectual disability are the most common phenotypes associated with trisomies.

Each of the common trisomies has a distinct neonatal phenotype that is recognizable by an experienced clinician. Trisomy 13 and 18 are both less common than trisomy 21, and survival beyond the first year is rare for trisomy 13 and 18. In contrast, individuals with Down syndrome usually have a life expectancy greater than 50 years. Most other autosomal trisomies result in early pregnancy loss, with trisomy 16 being a particularly common finding in first-trimester spontaneous miscarriages.

Trisomy 21, or Down syndrome, is the most common autosomal aneuploidy seen among live births. Approximately 95% of Down syndrome cases are caused by nondisjunction, and Robertsonian translocations cause most of the remainder. Mosaicism is seen in 2% to 4% of Down syndrome cases and is often associated with a milder phenotype. The most frequent cause of mosaicism in trisomies is a trisomic conception followed by loss of the extra chromosome during mitosis in some embryonic cells (trisomic rescue).

Trisomy 13 and 18 are sometimes compatible with survival to term, although 95% or more of affected fetuses are spontaneously aborted. These trisomies produce more severe disease than trisomy 21, with 90% to 95% mortality during the first year of life.

Turner syndrome is a sex chromosome aneuploidy and is most commonly associated with 45,X. Although this disorder is common at conception, it is relatively rare among live births, reflecting a high frequency of spontaneous abortion. Mosaicism increases the probability of survival to term. Klinefelter syndrome (47, XXY) is the most common disorder of sex chromosomes, with a prevalence of 1 in 500 in males. It is associated with mild phenotypic characteristics and infertility.[6] The most common features are summarized in Table 77.2.

Karyotype is a method of visualizing the chromosomes (Fig. 77.1A). There are many staining techniques, but Giemsa staining (G-banding) is the most common. The conventional metaphase karyotype has a resolution of 400 to 550 bands; however, a high-resolution prometaphase karyotype can resolve up to 860 bands. Imbalances greater than 5 to 10 Mb are generally visible on a karyotype. Chromosome structures such as supernumerary (marker) chromosomes (derivative chromosomes such as ring or isochromosomes) are most easily identified with karyotyping.

Fluorescence In Situ Hybridization

FISH is a technique to target specific chromosomal regions and visualize them in situ (Fig. 77.1B). Specific DNA probes are used for the hybridization to the targeted locus. Fluorophores allow visualization of the hybridized DNA to visualize subtle chromosome structural anomalies and detect targeted small deletions/duplications or count the total number of a specific chromosome. FISH can be performed rapidly and inexpensively (and therefore is often used prenatally) but requires an astute clinician to order the correct FISH test. CMA can simultaneously assess for copy number variations (CNVs) at thousands of loci and has become the most widely used test to detect genomic imbalances. However, CMA cannot detect balanced rearrangements such as inversions and translocations.

Table 77.2 Common Chromosomal Syndromes and Clinical Features

Syndrome	Karyotype	Main Clinical Features
Down	Trisomy 21	Single palmar crease, hypotonia, intellectual disability, open mouth with large tongue, upslanting palpebral fissures, epicanthal folds, depressed nasal bridge, short neck, congenital heart disease (atrioventricular canal defects)
Edwards	Trisomy 18	Clenched hands with overlapping fingers, prominent heels, prominent occiput, low-set malformed ears, micrognathia, small eyes, mouth, and nose, severe intellectual disability, congenital heart disease, horseshoe kidney
Patau	Trisomy 13	Cleft lip and/or palate, clenched hands, intellectual disability, polydactyly, congenital heart disease, midline brain anomalies, genitourinary abnormalities
Turner	45,X	Short stature, webbed neck, congenital heart disease (coarctation), widely spaced nipples, low hairline, premature ovarian failure
Klinefelter	47,XXY	Tall stature, small testes, azoospermia/infertility, gynecomastia
Triple X	47,XXX	Female with normal genitalia and fertility, at risk for educational and behavioral problems, early menopause

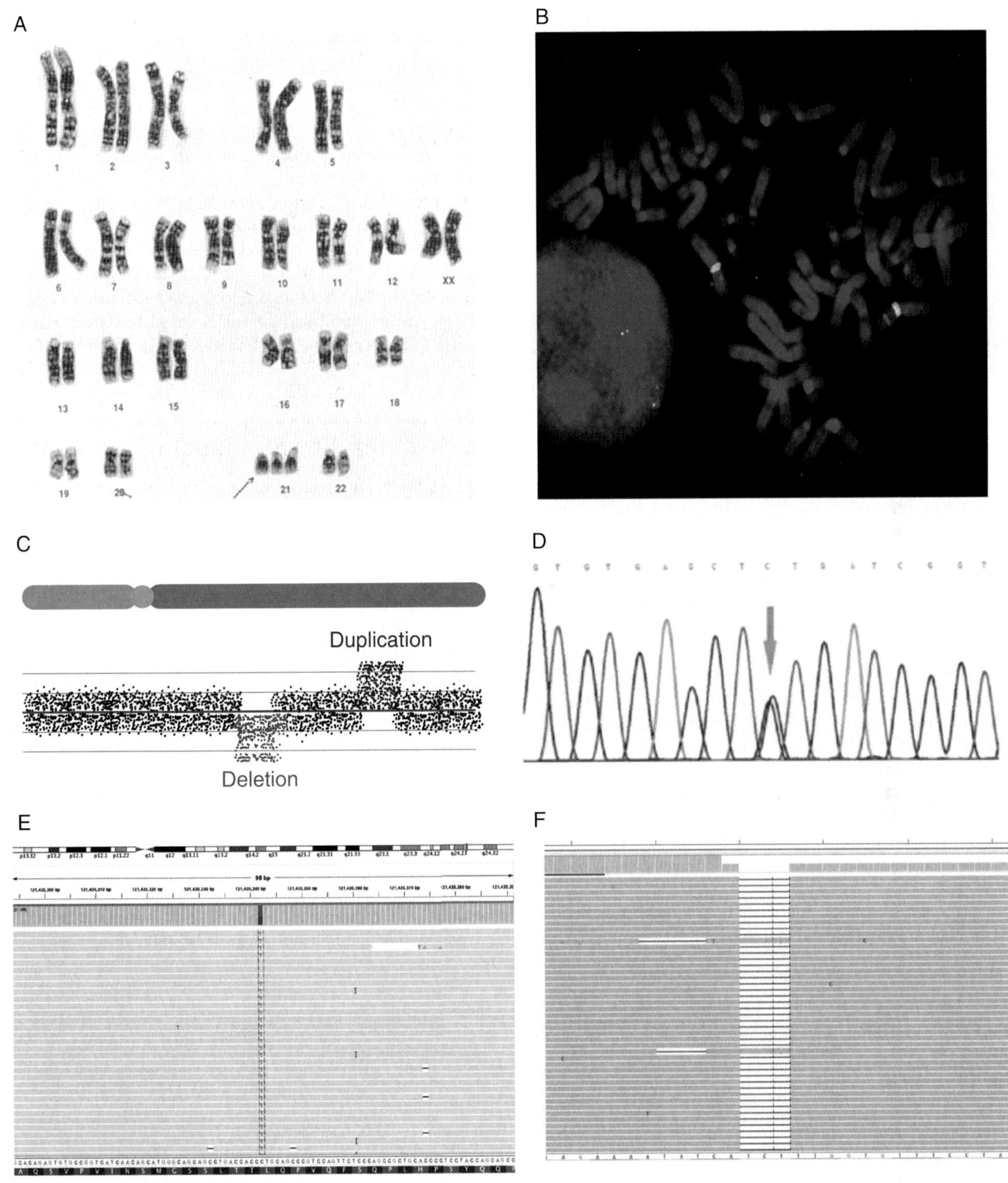

Fig. 77.1 Diagnostic Methods in Clinical Genetics. (A) Karyotyping image shows trisomy 21. (B) FISH image shows two red signals for the DMD gene and two green signals for the centromere of the X chromosome. (C) Chromosomal microarray illustration shows deletion (*red*) and duplication (*blue*) regions. (D) The Sanger sequencing illustration shows heterozygous single-nucleotide change. (E) Exome sequencing shows heterozygous single-nucleotide change. (F) The genome-sequencing illustration shows a deletion region of a chromosome. *FISH*, Fluorescence in situ hybridization. ([A] Image credit, Wessex Reg. Genetics Center, https://wellcomecollection.org; [B] image credit, Wessex Reg. Genetics Center, https://wellcomecollection.org.)

Chromosomal Microarray

Molecular methods including CMAs are often helpful to sensitively detect gains and losses that may be missed by standard karyotype alone (Fig. 77.1C). CMA has become a first-tier molecular cytogenetic diagnostic test for patients with unexplained developmental delay/ intellectual disability, autism spectrum disorders, or multiple congenital anomalies.[7] CMA is now routinely performed as oligoarrays with single-nucleotide polymorphism probes to provide high resolution for copy number variants and identify uniparental disomy and long stretches of homozygosity in families with consanguinity.[8]

There are regions of the genome with parent-of-origin effects as a result of genomic imprinting. Genomic imprinting is an epigenetic term describing monoallelic gene expression according to the parental origin. This epigenetic "mark" or imprint affects the chromatin structures and silences expression of the gene or genes that are imprinted. The imprint is maintained throughout the life of the organism, in virtually all tissues; however, germ cells erase and then reset imprints for transmission to the next generation. Imprinting disorders can be caused by:

1. sequence mutation in the relevant gene (*UBE3A* for Angelman syndrome);
2. deletion or duplication of imprinted genes;
3. uniparental disomy; or
4. epigenetic errors in imprinting centers, causing faulty imprinting.

Prader-Willi syndrome, Angelman syndrome, and Beckwith-Wiedemann syndrome are the well-studied examples of the role of genomic imprinting in human disease.

Uniparental disomy (UPD) refers to the presence of a disomic cell line containing two chromosomes that are inherited from only one parent rather than one chromosome being inherited from the mother and the other from the father. If the disomic chromosomes are received from identical sister chromatids, it is called isodisomy (the same copy of two chromosomes); if both homologs come from one parent, the situation is heterodisomy. Trisomy rescue is the mechanism of loss of a chromosome that restores a disomic state and escape from trisomy. If it happens, the resulting cell might show UPD.

If UPD occurs and includes a chromosome with an imprinted region such as chromosome 15, this may cause disease. For example, Angelman syndrome is due to mutations/deletions in the maternally expressed gene *UBE3A* or paternal UPD 15 such that there is no functional UBE3A allele because the maternal allele is missing. Angelman syndrome can also be due to epigenetic modifications of the imprinting center on chromosome 15q11, which results in loss of expression of *UBE3A*. These types of mechanisms explain most imprinting disorders reported to date.

Some of the most common microdeletion syndromes detectable by FISH or CMA are summarized in Table 77.3.

Sanger Sequencing

Sanger sequencing was once the primary method of sequencing (Fig. 77.1D); however, the decreased cost and increased throughput of massive parallel NGS has significantly increased the number of genes that can simultaneously be tested, up to an entire genome. Variants identified with NGS studies are routinely confirmed with Sanger sequencing. One large group of disorders called trinucleotide repeat expansion disorders includes Huntington disease, myotonic dystrophy, fragile X, and spinocerebellar ataxias. In this group, we need to find the exact number of the repeat count. Polymerase chain reaction–based methods can be used to detect the repeat number. Another technique called multiplex ligation-dependent probe amplification can be used to detect methylation status of the promoters, which is specifically important for fragile X syndrome.

Next-Generation Sequencing Technology

Genomic medicine is using advanced technologies to analyze individuals' genomic information and implement that information in clinical care.[9,10]

There are three main foci of sequencing for diagnostic purposes:

- Gene panels
- Exome sequencing
- Genome sequencing

Most sequencing methods are based on short-read technology and assess only 150 base-pair fragments (Fig. 77.2). This limits the types of mutations that can be detected and generally precludes the detection of triplet repeats and complex or large insertions/deletions in exome sequencing. Although sequence data generation is now relatively straightforward, interpretation of the variants is still complex. There are 30,000 to 50,000 variants in an exome and more than 1 million variants in a genome. There are different ways to filter variants based on allele frequency of the population, inheritance pattern, known mutations, predicted functional consequence of the variants, disease associations with the gene, and other, more advanced gene characteristics. Because our knowledge of variant

Table 77.3 Examples of Microdeletion Syndromes Detectable by FISH

Syndrome	Chromosomal Locus	Major Clinical Features
Deletion 1p36 syndrome	1p36	Intellectual disability, seizures, hearing loss, congenital heart disease, short stature, behavioral challenges
Wolf-Hirschhorn syndrome	4p16.3	Pre- and postnatal growth deficiency, iris coloboma, seizure, microcephaly
Cri-du-chat syndrome	5p	High-pitched cat-like cry, microcephaly, hypotonia, intellectual disability, low-set ears
Williams-Beuren syndrome	7q11.23	Supravalvular aortic stenosis, hypercalcemia, periorbital fullness, thick lips, friendly personality
WAGR syndrome	11p13	Wilms tumor, aniridia, genitourinary abnormalities, intellectual disability, obesity
Prader-Willi syndrome	15q11-q13 (imprinted region same as Angelman)	Intellectual disability, short stature, obesity, hypotonia, characteristic facies, small feet
Angelman syndrome	15q11-q13 (imprinted region same as Prader-Willi)	Intellectual disability, ataxia, behavioral abnormalities, seizures, hypotonia, wide-based gait
DiGeorge/VCF syndrome	22q11.2	Characteristic facies, cleft palate, heart defects, hypocalcemia, thymic hypoplasia

FISH, Fluorescence in situ hybridization; *VCF*, velocardiofacial.

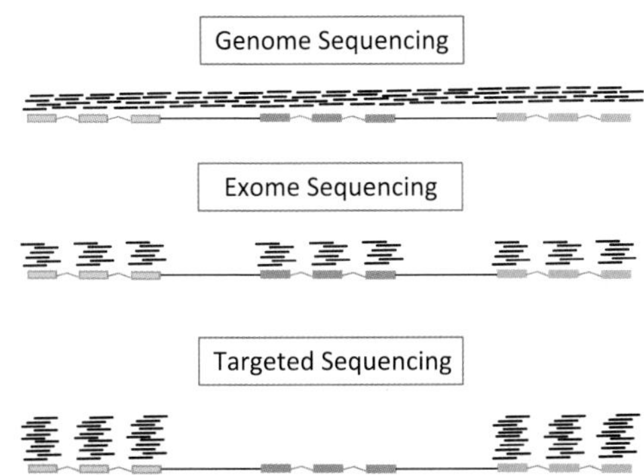

Fig. 77.2 Comparison of Genome Sequencing, Exome Sequencing, and Targeted Gene Panel Sequencing. Each gene is a different color, and each gene is made up of exons. Genome sequencing analyzes the entire genome, including genes and intergenic regions with the lowest read depth. Exome sequencing analyzes the exons of almost all genes. Targeted gene panel sequencing analyzes the exons of selected genes associated with the clinical indication and has the highest read depth when using short-read sequencing.

and gene functions is incomplete, the clinical sensitivity of trio-based exome/genome sequencing is only 40% to 60%,[1,11] and a normal test result reduces but does not eliminate the possibility that there is a genetic basis for the infant's disease.

In order to create a consensus and terminology between laboratories, the American College of Medical Genetics and Genomics (ACMG), the Association for Molecular Pathology (AMP), and the College of American Pathologists published a standards and guidelines for the interpretation of sequence variants report.[12] The ACMG and AMP recommend the use of specific standard terminology—"pathogenic," "likely pathogenic," "variant of uncertain significance," "likely benign," and "benign"—to describe variants identified in genes that cause Mendelian disorders. They also describe a process for classifying variants into these five categories based on criteria using types of evidence (e.g., population data, computational data, functional data, and segregation data).

As the amount of genetic data generated increases with genetic testing such as exome and genome sequencing, there is a chance of identifying genetic variants of clinical relevance that are not related to the primary indication for testing (incidental findings such as mutations for hereditary cancer or hereditary causes of sudden cardiac death). When the laboratory systematically and intentionally looks for variants in a prespecified set of genes unrelated to the primary indication, these are termed secondary findings. The consent process is important to determine which findings the patient would like to receive. Thus the generally accepted approach for incidental findings is to examine the exome/genome data for pathogenic/likely pathogenic variants in 59 medically actionable genes.[13]

The main uses of NGS methods related to human health are:

1. Diagnosis of single-gene diseases (Mendelian diseases);
2. Detection of the causative variant in patients with genetically heterogeneous conditions and incompletely genetically understood conditions such as congenital anomalies, intellectual disability, and autism spectrum disorder;
3. Simultaneous analysis of all disease-causing genes using panels for genetically heterogeneous diseases that are relatively well understood genetically (such as epilepsy, RASopathies, and maturity-onset diabetes of youth);
4. Detection of aneuploidy using cell-free fetal DNA in maternal blood;
5. Identification of new causal genes in Mendelian diseases; and
6. Testing of the mitochondrial genome for suspected mitochondrial diseases.

Gene Panel Testing

For conditions that are genetically heterogeneous, rather than selecting a single gene to test, it is now routine to test for a panel of genes causing the same phenotype/disease. The test is relatively fast (3–4 weeks) and cost effective to analyze all the known genes associated with the phenotype. Gene panels are available for sudden death, epilepsy, RASopathies (Noonan syndrome, cardiofaciocutaneous syndrome), congenital myopathy, and other clinically recognizable genetic disorders. It is even possible to combine all of the approximately 4800 disease-associated genes in one platform, called clinical Mendeliome.[14] However, as the number of genes in a panel increases, the number of variants of uncertain significance increases as well.

Gene panels are designed to provide complete coverage, with high sensitivity for the relevant regions of the targeted genes (Fig. 77.2). Gene panel coverage is close to 100% for relevant regions of selected genes, and any gaps in coverage with NGS are filled with Sanger sequencing. Another important advantage of gene panels is that read depth of the targeted regions is extremely high (1000 ×) and can be used to identify intragenic deletions/duplications. ES has lower average coverage of 80 ×, and GS has 30 × average.[15] The diagnostic rate of gene panels varies with phenotype. For narrow phenotypes such as retinal disease or monogenic diabetes, diagnostic rates are higher than for nonspecific phenotypes such as epilepsy or intellectual disability.[16,17] A subset of genes can be carved out from an exome analysis to create a virtual panel[18,19] and is used primarily for diseases for which new genes are routinely still being identified. Another heterogeneous group in which gene panel testing can be used is mitochondrial disorders. The mitochondrial DNA molecule is 16 kb in length and encodes 37 genes, all of which are fundamental for normal mitochondrial function and are also required for the function of ribosomal and transfer RNA molecules in the mitochondria. Mitochondrial encoded genes are solely inherited from the mother. It is possible to test mitochondrial disorders encoded by both nuclear and mitochondrial genes.

Exome Sequencing

ES (protein coding segments of almost all genes) is feasible and can be performed within 1 to 2 weeks (Fig. 77.1E). ES can be done only for the proband/affected individual or most effectively as a trio (parents and proband). Trio ES allows the lab to rapidly and sensitively detect de novo variants, significantly increasing the diagnostic yield. ES is a powerful diagnostic method for patients who have unexplained clinical findings. ES enables identification of new disease genes. The cost of ES is higher than that of gene panels but four to five times lower than that of GS. We do not yet have enough knowledge about most of the noncoding regions sequenced by GS to make GS worth the extra cost.

It is possible to detect dual diagnoses (two or more unrelated diagnoses) with ES, and the combination of two conditions often makes it clinically difficult to diagnose either one individually because the clinical characteristics may not be what are routinely

Table 77.4 Comparison of DNA Sequencing Methods

	Sequencing Panel	ES	GS
Variants detected	SNVs, deletion, duplications,	SNVs	SNVs, CNVs, noncoding variants
Variants per person	Depends on the panel size	30,000–50,000	>3 million
Read depth (average)	1000 ×	100 ×	30 ×
Coverage	≈100%	>92%	≈100%
Clinical sensitivity	Low-high Dependent on clinical condition assessed	High	High
Advantages	High coverage, good for some indications, least expensive	Cost-effective, allows for reanalysis as new genes are identified	Allows for reanalysis as new genes are identified; single test to capture whole genome for sequence variants, copy number variants, and structural variants

ES, Exome sequencing; *GS*, genome sequencing; *CNV*, copy number variation; *SNV*, single nucleotide variation.

observed for either individual diagnosis. Somatic mutations can be particularly difficult to detect by ES or GS and are more likely to be detected by panel gene tests based on differences in read depth.

A significant challenge associated with the clinical implementation of NGS for large panels and exomes/genome is the large number of variants identified. Distinguishing which of these variants is pathogenic is difficult because many of the variants identified are rare or novel and little is known about them. In addition, because not all genes for human diseases have yet been identified, variants that appear deleterious (de novo truncating variants) but are present in genes not currently associated with known diseases are termed genes of unknown significance. Furthermore, diagnoses may be missed despite comprehensive ES/GS because not all associations have been made between genes and diseases. Reevaluation of sequence data over time may yield additional diagnoses as scientific understanding of genetic variants and additional genetic conditions evolves. Thus reanalyzing and reinterpreting clinical sequence data can be valuable if the diagnosis was not made during the initial review. The ordering healthcare provider, clinical geneticist, clinical laboratory, and patient/family each may have a role in requesting reinterpretation or reanalysis of genetic results.[20,21] These expectations should be clearly outlined as part of the informed consent process.

Genome Sequencing

GS is the most comprehensive method to detect all types of genomic variations in the genome, including noncoding regions (Fig. 77.1F). It can detect copy number variations and structural variants. It is not routinely used in clinical diagnostics because the price is significantly higher than that of ES and the yield is not much higher. It can be useful for research purposes to define noncoding regions that are relevant to disease (Fig. 77.2). If GS prices come down with time, it may replace ES for diagnostic purposes (Table 77.4).

Making a genetic diagnosis earlier in life has a greater impact on medical care and may afford more effective treatment opportunities and minimize harm by decreasing the number of unnecessary diagnostic procedures or ineffective treatments. Pilot studies have been published to see how effective the newborn genomic sequencing is, both for well and ill newborns.[22] Rapid diagnosis in the neonatal or even prenatal period allows providers and parents to make better-informed decisions about care, get more accurate prognostic information, and draw upon experience with the genetic condition. Rapid genome sequencing of acutely ill patients in neonatal intensive care units is increasingly common and decreases costs and length of stay.[23]

CHAPTER 78

Genetics of Common Birth Defects in Newborns

Shannon N. Nees, Eric Jelin, Wendy K. Chung

KEY POINTS

1. Birth defects are among the leading causes of morbidity and mortality in children and are present in 3% to 6% of births.
2. The most common birth defects, which account for nearly half of the birth defects in the United States, are congenital heart disease, neural tube defects, oral facial clefts, and hypospadias.
3. Causes of birth defects include genetic causes such as chromosome disorders, copy number variants, monogenic disorders, epigenetics, and common variants, in addition to environmental contributions.
4. For each type of birth defect, there is a long list of possible genetic causes.
5. Many genetic variants can cause different birth defects or other associated medical or neurodevelopmental issues in different patients.
6. For syndromic birth defects, genetic testing should include chromosome microarray with reflex testing to exome sequencing.
7. For isolated birth defects in newborns, all the features may not yet be recognized. Chromosome microarray is routine, and exome sequencing is increasingly used as the cost of clinical sequencing decreases and as clinical utility is demonstrated.

Summary

Birth defects are among the leading causes of morbidity and mortality in children and are present in 3% to 6% of births. The majority of birth defects are thought to be isolated and nonsyndromic at birth; however, as the child grows and develops, many are appreciated to be associated with other medical problems, difficulty with growth, and/or neurodevelopmental and behavioral issues. The etiologies for most birth defects are unknown and are likely multifactorial. However, as genomic technologies have matured and been used to interrogate large cohorts of individuals with birth defects, a range of genetic causes have been identified, including chromosome disorders, copy number variants (CNVs), monogenic disorders, epigenetics, and common variants. In some cases, there may be contributions from both the maternal and fetal genomes because the mother's genotype influences the metabolism of cofactors such as folate that may be critical to certain birth defects including neural tube defects. A limitation to the systematic analysis of the etiology of birth defects has been the limited availability of unbiased prospective data from mothers during pregnancy along with birth and long-term outcomes paired with comprehensive genomic data to assess the contribution of genes and environment and their interactions. Advances in genomic tools have now made it possible to genomically assess fetuses and newborns with birth defects to diagnose the 20% to 30% of cases with identifiable genetic etiologies and provide more accurate prognostic information and tailored surveillance as well as intervention to those infants likely to have associated medical and neurodevelopmental issues. In addition to supporting the care of the infant, this genetic information can provide important information to parents to accurately estimate the risk of recurrence and provide families with informed reproductive strategies for future pregnancies.

Introduction

Nearly 8 million children are born each year with a serious birth defect worldwide.[1] The incidence of structural birth defects ranges from approximately 3% to 6% of all live births. Birth defects are a leading cause of infant mortality.[2] The most common birth defects, which account for nearly half of the birth defects in the United States, are congenital heart disease (CHD), neural tube defects, oral facial clefts, and hypospadias.[3] Most structural birth defects develop during the first trimester, and the majority of these defects are isolated and affect only one organ system. When birth defects are not isolated they are often referred to as syndromic, and in some but not all such cases, genetic etiologies can be identified. When birth defects are isolated, they are often termed nonsyndromic, and the etiology is more complex and thought to include an interaction between maternal and fetal genes and environment, including folic acid levels, maternal smoking, alcohol, obesity, diabetes, and teratogenic exposures.[4]

CHD is the most common type of birth defect and is present in approximately 1% of all live births.[5,6] CHD often requires at least one if not multiple surgeries. Neural tube defects result from incomplete closure of the vertebrae or skull, leading to exposed portions of the brain or spinal cord. The incidence of neural tube defects varies widely around the world, and the incidence has been decreased by folic acid supplementation. Oral facial clefts are a result of disturbed facial development, are present in approximately 2 in 1000 births, and are associated with problems feeding, speaking, and hearing. Hypospadias is present in approximately 3 in 1000 births and is often repaired by a simple surgical procedure.

Human development requires coordination of cell migration, proliferation, and cell death that ultimately determines embryonic form and function. The complexity of these developmental processes requires coordinated interaction of multiple genes in biologic pathways that can be disturbed by germline mutations, somatic mutations, epigenetics, stochastic events, and environmental agents. There are challenges to studying each of these mechanisms given that access to the appropriate cells or tissues at the appropriate time in development is often not possible in humans. Nonetheless, we have been able to advance our understanding of constitutional genomic causes of birth defects with advances in sequencing technology and capacity and the ability to readily identify de novo genetic events on a genome-wide basis.

In the following sections we will review the most common birth defect, CHD, as a representative birth defect. Other birth defects are similar in the types of genetic contributions, although the relative frequency of different classes of genetic variants and specific environmental exposures differ by birth defect.

Congenital Heart Disease

Evidence for the Genetic Basis of Congenital Heart Disease

The etiology of CHD is multifactorial. A genetic or environmental cause can be identified in about 20% to 30% of all cases, and that number is changing as new methods of testing become available.[7–10]

The overall incidence of CHD is similar between males and females; however, there are differences by type of CHD, with males having a slightly higher incidence of more severe lesions.[11,12] There are also differences in incidence of specific lesions based on race and ethnicity. Patent ductus arteriosus (PDA) and ventricular septal defects (VSDs) are more common in Europeans whereas atrial septal defects (ASDs) are more common in Hispanics.[13,14] The differences observed based on gender and ethnicity suggest that genetics play an important role in the development of specific types of CHD, with certain populations having increased genetic susceptibility.

The risk of CHD recurrence in the offspring of an affected parent is between 3% and 20%, depending on the lesion. Recurrence risk in the offspring of women with CHD is about twice as high as the recurrence in offspring of men with CHD.[15] Lesions with the highest recurrence risk are heterotaxy (HTX), right ventricular outflow tract obstruction, and left ventricular outflow tract obstruction.[16] Approximately half of siblings with recurrent CHD have a different lesion, supporting the theory that the etiology of CHD is multifactorial.[17]

Overall, twins have an increased risk of CHD compared with singleton pregnancies, which is thought to be due to vascular changes related to a shared placenta for monochorionic twins.[18–20] A population-based Taiwanese study calculated the adjusted risk ratio for CHD with an affected relative and found that it was 12.03 for a twin, 4.91 for a first-degree relative, and 1.21 for a second-degree relative.[21]

Genetic Testing in Congenital Heart Disease

Genetic testing for a fetus with CHD can start in the prenatal period with either chorionic villus sampling at 10 to 11 weeks' gestation or amniocentesis after 15 to 16 weeks' gestation to obtain placental/fetal DNA. More recently, noninvasive prenatal testing has been used to obtain fetal cell-free DNA from maternal blood to screen for aneuploidies and common deletions or duplications, most notably 22q11.2 deletion syndrome.[22–25] Noninvasive prenatal testing is a screening test, and abnormal findings require confirmatory testing using chorionic villi, amniocytes, or postnatal testing.

Clinical genetic testing in infants with CHD using karyotyping, fluorescence in situ hybridization (FISH), and chromosome microarray analysis (CMA) has an overall clinical yield of 15% to 25%, with a higher likelihood of finding a genetic diagnosis in patients with dysmorphic facial features and extracardiac anomalies.[26–31] Karyotyping allows for the identification of aneuploidies and large chromosomal rearrangements. CMA is used to detect CNVs across the genome and can reliably detect deletions or duplications as small as approximately 100,000 nucleotides. If a specific deletion or duplication syndrome is suspected, FISH can be used and allows for rapid turnaround and focused testing. It is most commonly used to test for 22q11.2 deletion.

Recent decreases in sequencing cost allow for more comprehensive assessment of the genome and have powered gene panel testing, exome sequencing (ES), and whole genome sequencing (WGS) in CHD. For each of these tests, significant bioinformatics analysis is required after sequencing to determine the significance of the variant in each individual patient, often using data from family members to assess for the inheritance status and segregation with CHD in the family. ES targets the protein-coding regions, which compose about 1.5% of the genome, and it has been particularly useful in assessing patients with CHD and extracardiac features.[32–36] ES is used increasingly in clinical practice because CHD is so genetically heterogeneous and because our knowledge of CHD genetics is incomplete.[37] The yield of ES for CHD in the clinical setting of a single large genetic reference laboratory was 28%.[38] WGS sequences the entire genome, including noncoding regions, but studies have not yet demonstrated the additional clinical utility of WGS in patients with CHD. WGS in CHD, however, remains an area of active investigation.

Chromosomal Aneuploidies

Aneuploidy is an abnormal number of chromosomes such as a trisomy. The risk of most aneuploidies increases with increasing maternal age. In the Baltimore–Washington Infant Study, chromosomal abnormalities were identified more than 100 times more frequently in patients with CHD compared with normal controls, with a total of 12.9% of CHD cases having chromosomal abnormalities.[39] The following sections review some of the most common aneuploidy syndromes associated with CHD. Table 78.1 contains further details on some of these syndromes.

Down Syndrome

Down syndrome is the most common chromosomal abnormality found in patients with CHD and is usually caused by complete trisomy 21.[40–42] CHD is found in 40% to 50% of patients with Down syndrome, most commonly atrioventricular septal defect (AVSD) in approximately 40% followed by VSD, ASD, PDA, and tetralogy of Fallot (TOF).[43,44] Down syndrome is also associated with a variety of other dysmorphic features and birth defects.

Trisomy 18 and 13

Many fetuses with trisomy 18 or 13 have multiple birth defects and do not survive to birth; however, among those who do, CHD is common. Ninety-five percent of patients with trisomy 18 have CHD, with PDA and VSD being the most common diagnoses. The majority of trisomy 13 patients have cardiac defects, with PDA, ASD, and VSD being the most common lesions.[45,46] Life expectancy is limited in both trisomy 18 and 13, and individuals generally die within the first year of life.

Turner Syndrome

Turner syndrome is a sex chromosome disorder that results from a complete or partial loss of an X chromosome, resulting in the 45, X karyotype. Those with mosaicism or structural abnormalities of the X chromosome tend to have less severe phenotypes compared with those with complete loss.[47,48] The most common cardiac lesions

Table 78.1 Common Aneuploidies and Copy Number Variants Associated With Syndromic Congenital Heart Disease[164]

Syndrome	Genetic Change	Prevalence in Live Births	Common Clinical Features	Associated Congenital Heart Disease	Patients With the Condition Who Have CHD, %	References
ANEUPLOIDIES						
Down syndrome	Trisomy 21	1 in 800	Hypotonia, flat facies, epicanthal folds, upslanting palpebral fissures, single palmar transverse crease, small ears, skeletal anomalies, intellectual disability	AVSD, VSD, ASD, PDA (less commonly TOF, D-TGA)	40–50	de Graaf et al.,[41,42] Allen et al.,[43] Bull et al.[165]
Patau syndrome	Trisomy 18	1 in 8000	Clenched hands, short sternum, limb anomalies, rocker-bottom feet, micrognathia, esophageal atresia, severe intellectual disability	PDA, ASD, VSD, AVSD, polyvalvular dysplasia, TOF, DORV	80–95	Musewe et al.,[45] Embleton et al.,[166,] Van Praagh et al.,[167] Springett et al.[168]
Edward syndrome	Trisomy 13	1 in 20,000	Midline facial defects, scalp defects, forebrain defects, polydactyly, hypotelorism, microcephaly, deafness, skin and nail defects, severe intellectual disability	PDA, ASD, VSD, HLHS, laterality defects	57–80	Musewe et al.,[45] Lin et al.,[46] Springett et al., [168] Wyllie et al.,[169] Goldstein et al.[170]
Turner syndrome	45, X	1 in 2500	Short stature, broad chest with wide-spaced nipples, webbed neck, congenital lymphedema, normal intelligence or mild learning disability	BAV, CoA, PAPVR, HLHS	35	Sybert et al.,[50] Gravholt et al.[171]
MICRODELETIONS/DUPLICATIONS						
Deletion 1p36 syndrome	1p36 deletion	1 in 5000	Growth deficiency, microcephaly, deep-set eyes, low-set ears, hearing loss, hypotonia, seizures, genital anomalies, intellectual disability	ASD, VSD, PDA, BAV, PS, MR, TOF, CoA, cardiomyopathy	70	Battaglia et al.[172]
1q21.1 deletion	1q21.1 deletion	Unknown (rare)	Short stature, cataracts, mood disorders, autism spectrum disorder, hypotonia	PDA, VSD, ASD, TOF, TA	33	Bernier et al.[173]
1q21.1 duplication	1q21.1 duplication	Unknown (rare)	Autism spectrum disorder, attention deficit hyperactivity disorder, intellectual disability, scoliosis, short stature, gastric ulcers	TOF, D-TGA,PS	27	Bernier et al.[173]
1q41q42 microdeletion	1q41q42 microdeletion	Unknown (rare)	Developmental delay, frontal bossing, deep-set eyes, broad nasal tip, cleft palate, clubfeet, seizure, short stature, congenital diaphragmatic hernia	BAV, ASD, VSD, TGA	40–50	Rosenfeld et al.[174]
2q31.1 microdeletion	2q31.1 microdeletion	Unknown (rare)	Growth retardation, microcephaly, craniosynostosis, cleft lip/palate, limb anomalies, genital anomalies	VSD, ASD, PDA, PS	38	Dimitrov et al.,[175] Mitter et al.[176]
2q37 microdeletion	2q37 microdeletion	Unknown (rare)	Short stature, obesity, intellectual disability, sparse hair, arched eyebrows, epicanthal folds, thin upper lip, small hands and feet, clinodactyly, central nervous system anomalies, ocular anomalies, gastrointestinal anomalies, renal anomalies, genitourinary anomalies	CoA, ASD, VSD	14–20	Casas et al.,[177] Falk et al.[178]
3p25 deletion	3p25 deletion	Unknown (rare)	Growth deficiency, microcephaly, hypotonia, polydactyly, renal anomalies, intellectual disability	AVSD, VSD	33	Shuib et al.[179]
Wolf-Hirschhorn syndrome	4p16.3 deletion	1 in 20,000 to 1 in 50,000	Feeding difficulty, seizures/epilepsy, microcephaly, wide spaced eyes, broad nasal bridge, intellectual disability	ASD, PS, VSD, PDA	50–65	Battaglia et al.[180]

Continued

Table 78.1 Common Aneuploidies and Copy Number Variants Associated With Syndromic Congenital Heart Disease—cont'd

Syndrome	Genetic Change	Prevalence in Live Births	Common Clinical Features	Associated Congenital Heart Disease	Patients With the Condition Who Have CHD, %	References
Deletion 4q	4q deletion	1 in 100,000	Growth deficiency, craniofacial anomalies, cleft palate, genitourinary defects, digital anomalies, intellectual disability	VSD, PDA, peripheral pulmonic stenosis, AS, ASD, TOF, CoA, tricuspid atresia	50	Xu et al.[181]
Cri-du-chat	5p deletion	1 in 15,000 to 1 in 50,000	Catlike cry, growth retardation, hypotonia, dysmorphic features, intellectual disability	PDA, VSD, ASD	15–20	Nguyen et al.,[182] Hills et al.[183]
Williams-Beuren syndrome	7q11,23 deletion (*ELN* gene)	1 in 20,000	Dysmorphic facial features, connective tissue abnormalities, skeletal and renal anomalies, cognitive defects, mild intellectual disability, growth and endocrine abnormalities including hypercalcemia in infancy	Supravalvar AS, supravalvar PS, branch pulmonary artery stenosis	50–80	Morris et al.,[66] Kececioglu et al.,[68] Morris[184]
8p23.1 deletion	8p23.1 deletion (including *GATA4*)	Unknown (rare)	Microcephaly, growth retardation, congenital diaphragmatic hernia, developmental delay, neuropsychiatric problems	AVSD, ASD, VSD, PS, TOF	50–75	Wat et al.[185]
Deletion 9p syndrome	9p deletion	Unknown (rare)	Trigonocephaly, midface hypoplasia, long philtrum, hypertelorism, up-slanting palpebral fissures, abnormal ears, abnormal external genitals, hypotonia, seizures, intellectual disability	PDA, VSD, ASD, CoA	45–50	Huret et al.,[186] Swinkels et al.[187]
Kleefstra syndrome	9q34.3 subtelomeric deletion (including *EHMT1*)	Unknown (rare)	Intellectual disability, delayed speech hypotonia, microcephaly, brachycephaly, hypertelorism, synophrys, midface hypoplasia, anteverted nares, prognathism, everted lips, macroglossia, behavioral problems, obesity	ASD, VSD, TOF, pulmonary arterial stenosis	30–47	Kleefstra et al.,[188] Kleefstra et al.[189]
Deletion 10p	10p deletion	Unknown (rare)	Hypoparathyroidism, immune deficiency, deafness, renal anomalies, intellectual disability	PS, BAV, ASD, VSD	42	Lindstrand et al.[190]
Duplication 10q24-qter	10q duplication	Unknown (rare)	Growth retardation, hypotonia, microcephaly, dysmorphic facies, kidney anomalies, limb anomalies, intellectual disability	TOF, AVSD, VSD	20–50	Aglan et al.,[191] Carter et al.[192]
Jacobsen syndrome	11q deletion	1 in 100,000	Growth retardation, developmental delay, thrombocytopenia, platelet dysfunction, wide-spaced eyes, strabismus, broad nasal bridge, thin upper lip, prominent forehead, intellectual disability, autism, immunodeficiency	VSD, HLHS, AS, CoA, Shone's complex	56	Grossfeld et al.[193]
15q24 microdeletion	15q24 microdeletion	Unknown (rare)	Growth retardation, intellectual disability, abnormal corpus callosum, microcephaly, abnormal ears, hearing loss, genital anomalies, digital anomalies	PDA, pulmonary arterial stenosis, PS	20–40	Mefford et al.[194]
Koolen-de Vries syndrome	17q21 microdeletion	1 in 16,000	Hypotonia, developmental delay, seizures, facial dysmorphisms, friendly behavior	ASD, VSD	27	Koolen et al.[195]
22q11.2 deletion syndrome (DiGeorge, velocardiofacial syndrome)	22q11.2 deletion	1 in 6000	Hypertelorism, broad nasal root, long and narrow face, long, slender fingers, hypocalcemia, immunodeficiency, behavioral problems, autism spectrum disorder, learning disability, psychiatric problems	IAA type B, TA, TOF, right aortic arch	75–80	Botto et al.,[196] Digilio et al.,[197] Peyvandi et al.[198]

Table 78.1 Common Aneuploidies and Copy Number Variants Associated With Syndromic Congenital Heart Disease—cont'd

Syndrome	Genetic Change	Prevalence in Live Births	Common Clinical Features	Associated Congenital Heart Disease	Patients With the Condition Who Have CHD, %	References
22q11.2 duplication	22q11.2 duplication	Unknown	Velopharyngeal insufficiency, cleft palate, hearing loss, facial anomalies, urogenital abnormalities, mild learning disability, hypotonia, scoliosis, frequent infections	VSD, aortic regurgitation, MVP, CoA, TOF, HLHS, IAA, TA, D-TGA	15	Portnoï[199]
Phelan-McDermid syndrome	22q13 microdeletion	Unknown (rare)	Developmental delay, intellectual disability, hypotonia, absent/delayed speech, autism spectrum disorder, long, narrow head, prominent ears, pointed chin, droopy eyebrows, deep-set eyes	TR, ASD, PDA, TAPVR	25	Phelan et al.[200]

[a]Jones KM, Jones MC, Del Campo M. P. Smith's recognizable patterns of human malformation. In: *Smith's Recognizable Patterns of Human Malformation.* 7th ed. Elsevier Inc; 2013:7–83.

AS, Aortic stenosis; *ASD,* atrial septal defect; *AVSD,* atrioventricular septal defect; *BAV,* bicuspid aortic valve; *CoA,* coarctation of the aorta; *DORV,* double outlet right ventricle; *D-TGA,* d-loop transposition of the great arteries; *HLHS,* hypoplastic left heart syndrome; *IAA,* interrupted aortic arch; *MR,* Mitral regurgitation; *MVP,* mitral valve prolapse; *PAPVR,* partial anomalous pulmonary venous return; *PDA,* patent ductus arteriosus; *PS,* pulmonary stenosis; *TA,* truncus arteriosus; *TAPVR,* total anomalous pulmonary venous return; *TOF,* tetralogy of Fallot; *TR,* tricuspid regurgitation, *VSD,* ventricular septal defect.

Adapted from Pierpont et al., 2018.

associated with Turner syndrome are left-sided lesions, including bicuspid aortic valve in 30% of patients and coarctation of the aorta in 10% of patients. More serious lesions such as partial anomalous pulmonary venous return and hypoplastic left heart syndrome are less common.[49,50]

Copy Number Variations

CNVs consist of deletions or duplications of contiguous regions of DNA that affect approximately 12% of the genome and can impact either a single gene or multiple contiguous genes.[51] Pathogenic CNVs tend to be *de novo* and large and to disrupt coding portions of genes that are dosage sensitive. These are found more frequently in patients with CHD compared with controls. CNVs are observed more frequently in patients with CHD and extracardiac features compared with those with isolated CHD.[52–55] In 2007, Thienpont et al. used array-comparative genomic hybridization in patients with CHD and associated extracardiac anomalies and identified likely pathogenic CNVs in 17% of patients.[56] In 2014, Glessner et al. performed whole exome sequencing (WES) in 538 patients with CHD and found that 9.8% of patients without a previous genetic diagnosis had a rare *de novo* CNV.[33] Table 78.1 lists several of the CNVs associated with CHD.

Recent data have demonstrated that CNVs are not only causative of CHD, but they also impact clinical outcomes. In 2013, Carey et al. compared neurocognitive and growth outcomes in patients with single-ventricle physiology and found that patients with pathogenic CNVs had decreased linear growth, and those with CNVs associated with known genomic disorders had the poorest neurocognitive and growth outcomes.[57] Kim et al. examined CNVs in 422 cases of nonsyndromic CHD and found that the presence of a likely pathogenic CNV was associated with significantly lower transplant-free survival after surgery.[58] The increased risk of morbidity in patients with large CNVs may be due to additional genes that are impacted or due to pleiotropic effects of single genes within the region. Some of the most common syndromes caused by CNVs and associated with CHD are described below.

22q11.2 Deletion Syndrome

22q11.2 deletion syndrome is the most common microdeletion syndrome associated with CHD. The majority of patients clinically diagnosed with DiGeorge or velocardiofacial syndrome have a microdeletion of 22q11.2. Of patients with 22q11.2 deletion, 75% to 80% have CHD, with conotruncal defects being the most common lesions.[59] The prevalence of 22q11.2 deletion in patients with CHD is highest in patients with type B interrupted aortic arch, truncus arteriosus, TOF, and isolated aortic arch anomalies.[60–64] Among patients with conotruncal lesions, up to 50% have a 22q11.2 deletion.[65]

Williams-Beuren Syndrome

Williams-Beuren syndrome, or Williams syndrome, is caused by a contiguous gene deletion at 7q11.23 that encompasses the elastin gene *ELN*.[66,67] Similar to 22q11.2 deletion syndrome, deletions are often sporadic but can be inherited. Between 50% and 80% of patients with Williams syndrome have CHD, most commonly supravalvar aortic stenosis, supravalvar pulmonic stenosis, and branch pulmonary artery stenosis.[68]

Mutations in *ELN*, a critical component of vascular tissue, are observed in patients with autosomal-dominant isolated supravalvar aortic stenosis, leading to the conclusion that haploinsufficiency of this gene is the etiology of CHD in patients with Williams syndrome.[67,69,70]

Single-Gene Defects

In addition to CNVs, *de novo* sequence variants in single genes have been identified using ES in patients with CHD, both in syndromic and nonsyndromic cases. Patients with CHD have an excess burden of *de novo* protein-altering variants in genes that are expressed during cardiac development.[71] A European study using ES in 1891 patients found that in patients with nonisolated CHD, there were an increased number of *de novo* protein-truncating variants and deleterious missense variants in known autosomal-dominant CHD-associated genes and in non-CHD genes associated with developmental delay. In patients with isolated CHD, there was a much lower frequency of *de novo* deleterious variants, but there was an increase in rare, inherited protein-truncating variants in CHD-associated genes, likely representing mutations that are incompletely penetrant.[32]

Monogenic Conditions Causing Syndromic CHD

As sequencing techniques have improved, the genetic causes of several well-characterized clinical syndromes have been discovered. The following section describes examples of the most common monogenic syndromes associated with CHD. These syndromes are inherited in an autosomal-dominant manner. Some are caused by variants in one gene and others are genetically heterogeneous. Table 78.2 contains additional details for selected syndromes.

Alagille Syndrome

Alagille syndrome is a condition consisting of CHD, hepatic complications including bile duct paucity and cholestasis, and skeletal and ophthalmologic anomalies. There is significant variability in its expression even within the same family, with some individuals displaying very mild features and others with severe CHD or liver disease leading to transplant or death.[72–75] More than 90% of patients with Alagille syndrome have cardiovascular involvement. The most common lesion is branch pulmonary artery stenosis.

Table 78.2 Common Monogenic Conditions Associated With Syndromic Congenital Heart Disease

Syndrome	Gene(s)	Loci	Live Birth Prevalence	Common Clinical Features	Associated Congenital Heart Disease	Patients With the Genetic Condition Who Have CHD, %	References
Adams-Oliver	*DLL4* *DOCK6* *EOGT* *NOTCH1*	15q15.1 19p13.2 3p14.1 9q34.3	Unknown (rare)	Aplasia cutis congenital, transverse terminal limb defects	BAV, PDA, PS, VSD, ASD, TOF	20	Hassed et al.[201]
Alagille	*JAG1* *NOTCH2*	20p12.2 1p12-p11	1 in 100,000	Bile duct paucity, cholestasis, posterior embryotoxin, butterfly vertebrae, renal defects	Branch pulmonary artery stenosis, TOF, PA	90–95	McElhinney et al.,[76] Emerick et al.,[77] McDaniell et al.,[78] Turnpenny et al.[202]
Axenfeld-Rieger	*FOXC1*	6p25.3	1 in 200,000	Ocular anomalies including glaucoma, dental anomalies, redundant periumbilical skin	ASD, AS, PS, TOF, BAV, TA	Unknown	Gripp et al.[203]
Baller-Gerold and Rothmund-Thomson	*RECQL4*	8q24.3	Unknown (rare)	Radial hypoplasia, craniosynostosis, poikiloderma, growth deficiency, malignancy	VSD, TOF, subaortic stenosis	25	Van Maldergem et al.,[204] Fradin et al.[205]
Bardet-Biedl	*BBS2* *BBS6*	16q13 20p12.2	1 in 100,000 to 1 in 160,000	Retinal dystrophy, polydactyly, obesity, genital anomalies, renal dysfunction, learning difficulties	AS, PS, PDA, cardiomyopathies	7–50	Forsythe et al.,[206] Suspitsin et al.[207]
Cantu	*ABCC9*	12p12.1	Unknown (rare)	Congenital hypertrichosis, osteochondroplasia, macrocephaly, coarse facial features	Cardiomegaly, ventricular hypertrophy, PDA, BAV	60–75	Grange et al.,[208] Scurr et al.[209]
Carpenter	*RAB23*	6p11.2	Unknown (rare)	Craniosynostosis, polysyndactyly, obesity	ASD, VSD, TOF, PDA, PS	18–50	Kadakia et al.,[210] Jenkins et al.[211]
Cardiofaciocutaneous	*BRAF* *KRAS* *MAP2K1* *MAP2K2*	7q34 12p12.1 15q22.31 19p13.3	1 in 810,000	Curly hair, sparse eyebrows, feeding difficulty, developmental delay	PS, ASD, VSD, HCM	75	Jhang et al.,[98] Pierpont et al.[107]
Congenital heart defects, dysmorphic facial features, and intellectual developmental disorder	*CDK13*	7p14.1	Unknown (rare)	Intellectual disability, hypertelorism, upslanted palpebral fissures, wide nasal bridge and narrow mouth, seizures	ASD, VSD, PS	56	Sifrim et al.,[32] Hamilton et al.,[212] Bostwick et al.[213]
Char	*TFAP2B*	6p12.3	Unknown (rare)	Dysmorphic facies, abnormal fifth digit, strabismus, hearing anomalies	PDA, VSD	26–75	Satoda et al.,[214] Satoda et al.[215]

Table 78.2 Common Monogenic Conditions Associated With Syndromic Congenital Heart Disease—cont'd

Syndrome	Gene(s)	Loci	Live Birth Prevalence	Common Clinical Features	Associated Congenital Heart Disease	Patients With the Genetic Condition Who Have CHD, %	References
CHARGE	*CHD7*	8q12	1 in 10,000 to 1 in 15,000	Coloboma, choanal atresia, growth retardation, genital hypoplasia, ear anomalies, intellectual disability	TOF, PDA, DORV, AVSD, VSD	75–85	Trider et al.,[216] Corsten-Janssen et al.[217]
Coffin-Siris	*ARID1B* *SMARCA4*	6q25 22q11	Unknown (rare)	Intellectual disability, feeding difficulty, coarse facies, hypoplastic distal phalanges, hypertrichosis	ASD, VSD, PS, AS, dextrocardia, CoA, PDA, TOF	44	Kosho et al.,[218] Nemani et al.[219]
Cornelia de Lange	*NIPBL*	5p13	1 in 10,000 to 1 in 30,000	Growth retardation, dysmorphic facies, hirsutism, limb deficiency	VSD, ASD, PS, PDA	13–70	Selicorni et al.[220]
Costello	*HRAS*	11p15.5	1 in 300,000 to 1 in 1,250,000	Short stature, feeding difficulties, coarse facial features, skin abnormalities, intellectual disability	PS, ASD, VSD, HCM, arrhythmias	50–60	Abe et al.,[106] Lin et al.[221]
Ellis–van Creveld	*EVC* *EVC2*	4p16.2 4p16.2	1 in 60,000 to 1 in 200,000	Short limbs, short ribs, postaxial polydactyly, dysplastic nails and teeth	Common atrium	60–75	O'Connor et al.,[222] Ruiz-Perez et al.,[223,224]
Fragile X	*FMR1*	Xq27.3	1 in 4000 males, 1 in 8000 females	Intellectual disability, autism spectrum disorder, macrocephaly, macroorchidism, seizures, prominent forehead, large ears, hyperflexibility	MVP, aortic dilation	10–20	Kidd et al.[225]
Genitopatellar or Ohdo/SBBYS	*KAT6B*	10q22.2	Unknown (rare)	Intellectual disability, genital and patellar anomalies	ASD, VSD, PFO	50	Campeau et al.[226]
Heterotaxy	*GDF1* *NODAL* *ZIC3*	19p13.11 10q22.1 Xq26.3	1 in 10,000	Biliary atresia, abdominal situs abnormality, spleen abnormality, isomerism of lungs and bronchi, systemic venous anomalies	Pulmonary venous anomalies, atrial anomalies, AVSD, PS, AS, conotruncal anomalies	>90	Belmont et al.,[110] Jin et al.,[120] Lin et al.[227]
Holt-Oram	*TBX5*	12q24.1	1 in 100,000	Upper limb anomalies	ASD, VSD, AVSD, conduction defects	75	McDermott et al.,[86] Basson et al.[90]
Johanson-Blizzard	*UBR1*	15q15.2	Unknown (rare)	Pancreatic insufficiency, hypoplastic/aplastic nasal alae, cutis aplasia, developmental delay, intellectual disability	Dysplastic mitral valve, PDA, VSD, ASD, dextrocardia	10	Alpay et al.,[228] Almashraki et al.[229]
Kabuki	*KDM6A* *KMT2D*	Xp11.3 12q13	1 in 32,000	Growth deficiency, wide palpebral fissures, arched eyebrows, protruding ears, clinodactyly, intellectual disability	CoA, BAV, VSD	30–50	Hannibal et al.,[230] Wessels et al.[231]

Continued

Table 78.2 Common Monogenic Conditions Associated With Syndromic Congenital Heart Disease—cont'd

Syndrome	Gene(s)	Loci	Live Birth Prevalence	Common Clinical Features	Associated Congenital Heart Disease	Patients With the Genetic Condition Who Have CHD, %	References
Kleefstra	*EHMT1*	9q34.3	Unknown (rare)	Microcephaly, hypotonia, neuropsychiatric anomalies, broad forehead, synophrys, midface hypoplasia, depressed nasal bridge, short nose, ear anomalies, intellectual disability	ASD, VSD, TOF, PDA, CoA, BAV	40–45	Kleefstra et al.,[189] Ciaccio et al.[232]
Koolen–De Vries	*KANSL1*	17q21.31	1 in 16,000	Hypotonia, friendly behavior, long face, upslanting palpebral fissures, narrow/short palpebral fissures, ptosis, epicanthal folds, bulbous nasal tip (88%), everted lower lip, large prominent ears, intellectual disability, epilepsy, kidney anomalies	ASD, VSD, PDA, BAV, PS	39	Koolen et al.[195,233]
Loeys-Dietz	*TGFBR1* *TGFBR2* *SMAD3*	9q22.33 3p24.1 15q22.33	Unknown (rare)	Aortic and peripheral arterial aneurysms, pectus excavatum, scoliosis, talipes equinovarus, hypertelorism, cleft palata/bifid uvula	BAV, PDA, ASD, MVP	30–50	MacCarrick et al.,[234] Loughborough et al.[235]
Mandibulofacial dysostosis, Guion-Almeida type	*EFTUD2*	17q21.31	Unknown (rare)	Microcephaly, midface hypoplasia, micrognathia, choanal atresia, hearing loss, cleft palateintellectual disability	ASD, VSD, PDA	30–60	Lines et al.,[236] Lehalle et al.[237]
Marfan	*FBN1*	15q21.1	1 in 5000	Ocular anomalies (ectopia lentis), skeletal anomalies (arachnodactyly, loose joints), vascular anomalies	AR, MVP	80	Thacoor [238]
Mental retardation, autosomal dominant	*KAT6A*	8p11.21	Unknown (rare)	Microcephaly, global developmental delay, craniofacial dysmorphism, hypotonia, feeding difficulty, ocular anomalies	PDA, ASD, VSD	Unknown	Tham et al.,[239] Arboleda et al.[240]
Mowat-Wilson	*ZEB2*	2q22.3	Unknown (rare)	Short stature, microcephaly, hypertelorism, pointed chin, Hirschsprung disease, intellectual disability, seizures	VSD, CoA, ASD, PDA, PS	50	Garavelli et al.,[241] Zweier et al.[242]
Myhre	*SMAD4*	18q21.2	Unknown (rare)	Short stature, dysmorphic facies, hearing loss, laryngeal anomalies, arthropathy, intellectual disability	ASD, VSD, PDA, PS, AS, CoA	60	Lin et al.[243]

Table 78.2 Common Monogenic Conditions Associated With Syndromic Congenital Heart Disease—cont'd

Syndrome	Gene(s)	Loci	Live Birth Prevalence	Common Clinical Features	Associated Congenital Heart Disease	Patients With the Genetic Condition Who Have CHD, %	References
Nephronophthisis and Meckel-Gruber–like syndrome	*NPHP3*	3q22.1	Unknown (rare)	Nephronoophthisis, CNS malformations, cystic kidneys, polydactyly, situs inversus	AS, ASD, PDA	20	Bergmann et al.,[244] Salonen et al.,[245] Tory et al.[246]
Neurofibromatosis	*NF1*	17q11.2	1 in 3000 to 1 in 4000	Changes in skin pigmentation, tumor growth, macrocephaly, scoliosis, hypertension	PS, CoA, MR, PDA, VSD, AS, AR, ASD	2–15	Incecik et al.,[247] Lin et al.,[248] Leppävirta et al.[249]
Noonan	*PTPN11* *SOS1* *RAF1* *KRAS* *NRAS* *RIT1* *SHOC2* *SOS2* *BRAF* *LZTR1*	12q24.13 2p22.1 3p25.2 12p12.1 1p13.2 1q22 10q25.2 14q21.3 7q34 22q11.21	1 in 1000 to 1 in 2500	Dysmorphic facies, short stature, chest deformities, lymphatic anomalies, skeletal anomalies, hematologic defects	PS, HCM, ASD, TOF, AVSD, VSD, PDA	75–90	Romano et al.,[95,] Marino et al.,[96] Jhang et al.[98]
Noonan syndrome with multiple lentigines	*PTPN11*	12q24.13	Unknown (rare)	Multiple lentigines, hearing loss, mild learning issues	HCM, conduction abnormalities	80	Aoki et al.,[105] Limongelli et al.,[250] Sarkozy et al.[251]
Oculofaciocardiodental (OFCD)	*BCOR*	Xp11.4	Unknown (rare)	Congenital cataracts, microphthalmia, dysmorphic features, dental anomalies, syndactyly, flexion deformities, intellectual disability	ASD, VSD, PS, AS, PDA, dextrocardia, DORV	66–74	Hilton et al.,[252] Horn et al.[253]
Orofaciodigital	*OFD1*	Xp22.2	Unknown (rare)	Ciliary defects, facial anomalies, abnormal digits, brain and kidney anomalies	ASD, AVSD, HLHS	33–100	Bouman et al.[254]
Peter's plus	*B3GLCT/ B3GALTL*	13q12.3	Unknown (rare)	Anterior eye anomalies, developmental delay, cleft lip and palate, short statues, broad hands and feet	ASD, VSD, PS, subvalvar AS	25–30	Lesnik et al.,[255] Maillette de Buy Wenniger-Prick [256]
Polycystic kidney disease, autosomal dominant	*PKD1*	16p13.3	1 in 1000	Polycystic kidneys, hypertension, extrarenal cysts	MVP, ASD, PDA	10–20	Dell,[257] Ivy et al.[258]
Renal-hepatic-pancreatic dysplasia/ nephronopthisis	*NEK8*	17q11.2	Unknown (rare)	Ciliary dysfunction, renal, hepatic and pancreatic anomalies	Cardiomegaly, HCM, septal defects, PDA	Unknown	Grampa et al.,[259] Rajagopalan et al.[260]
Roberts	*ESCO2*	8p21.1	Unknown (rare)	Growth retardation, cleft lip/palate, hypertelorism, sparse hair, symmetric limb reduction, cryptorchidism, intellectual disability	ASD, AS	20–50	Van Den Berg et al.,[261] Goh et al.[262]

Continued

Table 78.2 Common Monogenic Conditions Associated With Syndromic Congenital Heart Disease—cont'd

Syndrome	Gene(s)	Loci	Live Birth Prevalence	Common Clinical Features	Associated Congenital Heart Disease	Patients With the Genetic Condition Who Have CHD, %	References
Robinow	*ROR2*	9q22.31	Unknown (rare)	Mesomelic limb shortening, hypertelorism, nasal anomalies, midface hypoplasia, brachydactyly, clinodactyly, micropenis, short stature, scoliosis	PS, VSD, ASD, DORV, TOF, CoA, TA	15–30	Al-Ata et al.,[263] Mazzeu et al.[264]
Rubinstein-Taybi	*CBP* *EP300*	16p13.3 22q13.2	1 in 100,000 to 1 in 125,000	Growth retardation, microcephaly, highly arched eyebrows, long eyelashes, down-slanting palpebral fissures, broad nasal bridge, beaked nose, highly arched palate, broad thumbs, large toes, intellectual disability	PDA, VSD, ASD	30	Stevens et al.,[265] Hennekam[266]
Sifrim-Hitz-Weiss	*CHD4*	12p13.31	Unknown (rare)	Developmental delay, hearing loss, macrocephaly, palate abnormalities, ventriculomegaly, hypogonadism, intellectual disability	PDA, ASD, VSD, BAV, TOF, CoA	Unknown	Sifrim et al.,[32] Weiss et al.[267]
Smith-Lemli-Opitz	*DHCR7*	11q12–13	1 in 15,000 to 1 in 60,000	Growth retardation, dysmorphic facial features, genital anomalies, limb anomalies, intellectual disability	AVSD, ASD, VSD	50	Lin et al.,[268] Digilio et al.,[269] Waterham et al.[270]
Sotos	*NSD1*	5p35.3	1 in 10,000 to 1 in 50,000	Tall stature, macrocephaly, high anterior hairline, frontal bossing, thin face, downslanting palpebral fissures, advanced bone age, developmental delay	ASD, PDA, VSD	8–50	Leventopoulos et al.[271]
Syndromic microphthalmia/ pulmonary hypoplasia-diaphragmatic hernia-anophthalmia-cardiac defect (PDAC)	*STRA6*	15q24.1	Unknown (rare)	Pulmonary hypoplasia, diaphragmatic defects, bilateral anopthalmia, contractures, camptodactyly	ASD, VSD, PS, PDA, PA, TOF, CoA, TA	50	Marcadier et al.[272]
Townes-Brocks	*SALL1*	16p12.1	1 in 250,000	Imperforate anus, dysplastic ears, thumb malformations, renal agenesis, multicystic kidneys, microphthalmia	VSD, ASD, PA, TA	20–30	Liberalesso et al.,[273] Miller et al.[274]
Weill-Marchesani	*ADAMTS10*	19p13.2	Unknown (rare)	Short stature, brachydactyly, joint stiffness, microspherophakia, ectopia lentis	MVP, AS, PS	50	Dagoneau et al.,[275] Kojuri et al.[276]

AR, Aortic regurgitation; *AS*, aortic stenosis; *ASD*, atrial septal defect; *AVSD*, atrioventricular septal defect; *BAV*, bicuspid aortic valve; *CoA*, coarctation of the aorta; *DORV*, double outlet right ventricle; *HCM*, hypertrophic cardiomyopathy; *HLHS*, hypoplastic left heart syndrome; *MR*, mitral regurgitation; *MVP*, mitral valve prolapse; *PA*, pulmonary atresia; *PDA*, patent ductus arteriosus; *PFO*, patent foramen ovale; *PS*, pulmonary stenosis; *SBBYS*, Say-Barber-Biesecker-Young-Simpson syndrome; *TA*, truncus arteriosus; *TOF*, tetralogy of Fallot; *TR*, tricuspid regurgitation; *VSD*, ventricular septal defect.

More complex lesions include TOF with or without pulmonary atresia.[76,77]

Alagille syndrome is genetically heterogeneous; the two most commonly associated genes are *JAG1*, which encodes a ligand in the Notch signaling pathway, and *NOTCH2*, a Notch receptor.[78–81] The Notch signaling pathway is important for controlling cell fate during development, and mutations in this pathway are also associated with other cardiac diseases.[82] *JAG1* mutations are found in approximately 90% of individuals with clinical Alagille syndrome.[83] In addition, 3% to 7% of patients have deletions of chromosome 20p12, which contains *JAG1*. *NOTCH2* mutations are found in 1% to 2% of individuals with Alagille syndrome.[78,84]

Holt-Oram Syndrome

The two most common features of Holt-Oram syndrome are CHD and upper-extremity malformations.[85] All patients with Holt-Oram syndrome have some upper-limb anomaly, ranging from mild abnormalities of the carpal bone to complete phocomelia.[86] Among patients with Holt-Oram syndrome, 75% have CHD, and the most common types are ASDs and VSDs. More complex forms of CHD occur in approximately 15% to 25% of patients.[87–89] Patients are also at risk for cardiac conduction disease, which can be progressive and lead to complete heart block.[86,90]

Approximately 75% of cases of Holt-Oram syndrome are caused by mutations in *TBX5*, a member of the T-box family of transcription factors that plays a role in regulation of gene expression during embryogenesis.[91–93] In the remaining 25% of cases of Holt-Oram syndrome, no genetic etiology has been identified, although it is hypothesized that these patients may have mutations in regulatory domains of *TBX5* not included in routine sequencing.

Noonan Syndrome and RASopathies

Noonan syndrome and the RASopathies are a group of disorders with overlapping phenotypes including CHD, short stature, dysmorphic facial features, and abnormal neurodevelopment. These disorders are caused by mutations in genes that encode proteins involved in the RAS/MAPK pathway, a signal-transduction pathway important for cell growth, differentiation, senescence, and death.[94] Other than Noonan syndrome, disorders include cardiofaciocutaneous syndrome (CFC), Costello syndrome (CS), and Noonan syndrome with multiple lentigines.

Noonan syndrome is a disorder with both clinical and genetic heterogeneity consisting of characteristic facial features, short stature, CHD, cardiomyopathy, and chest deformities.[94,95] Eighty to ninety percent of individuals have cardiac involvement. The most common cardiovascular findings are pulmonic stenosis in 50% to 60% and hypertrophic cardiomyopathy (HCM) in 20%.[96–98] The presence of HCM contributes to significant mortality and tends to have earlier onset and be more rapidly progressive than other types of pediatric HCM.[99,100]

About half of the patients with Noonan syndrome have missense variants in *PTPN11*, which lead to activation of SHP2 and increased RAS/MAPK signaling.[101,102] Among those without *PTPN11* variants, 20% have variants in *SOS1*.[103] The cardiovascular manifestations of Noonan syndrome vary depending on the mutation. Mutations in *PTPN11* are more commonly associated with pulmonary stenosis (PS), whereas mutations in *RAF1* or *RIT1* are associated with high risk of HCM.[98,101,104,105]

The other RASopathies share some common features including developmental delays, short stature, ptosis, hypertelorism, and macrocephaly. Individuals with CFC and CS tend to have more severe cognitive impairment compared with individuals with Noonan syndrome.[106] Cardiac defects are found in approximately 75% of individuals with CFC, and similar to Noonan syndrome, the most common findings are pulmonary stenosis and HCM.[98,107]

Heterotaxy and Ciliopathies

The heart is an asymmetric organ, and left-right patterning is critical for normal cardiac development. Disorders of left-right patterning include HTX syndrome, in which there is abnormal sidedness of multiple organs and situs inversus totalis, in which the organs are in a mirror-image pattern. Data from the National Birth Defects Prevention Study demonstrated that among patients with laterality defects, 68% had complex CHD and another 9% has simple CHD. The association between CHD and laterality defects suggests a common developmental mechanism, perhaps due to defects in cilia as the primary cause of these abnormalities.

Cilia are organelles that have a crucial role in cellular signaling during development, particularly in the proper formation of the left-right axis in the developing embryo.[108] Abnormal ciliary structure or function is associated with syndromic ciliopathies, which include primary ciliary dyskinesia (PCD) and HTX, both of which are associated with CHD.[109]

HTX has a high risk of familial recurrence.[17] All types of inheritance, including X-linked, autosomal dominant, and autosomal recessive, have been described with multiple implicated genes including *LEFTYA*, *CRYPTIC*, and *ACVR2B*.[110] Pathogenic variants in *ZIC3*, a zinc-finger transcription factor involved in heart looping, are thought to contribute to approximately 5% of HTX cases in males.[111,112]

PCD is a disorder characterized by abnormal ciliary motility in the airway tract, which leads to frequent respiratory infections and complications.[113,114] HTX and associated CHDs are found in approximately 6% of patients with PCD, demonstrating the overlapping phenotypes and genetic etiologies of these conditions.[115]

There is evidence that mutations in cilia genes are also involved in isolated CHD, especially AVSDs and d-loop transposition of the great arteries.[116] In patients with CHD but no HTX, there is a high incidence of ciliary motion defects, up to 51% in one study.[117]

GDF1 and Founder Ashkenazi Mutation

Given the heterogeneity of CHD, there are likely to be genes involved in the pathogenesis of CHD in specific populations. One such gene is *GDF1*, which is associated with CHD in the Ashkenazi Jewish population. A study screening 375 unrelated patients with various forms of CHD identified loss-of-function mutations in *GDF1* among cases with various types of CHD, including conotruncal defects and atrioventricular canal defects. These were heterozygous mutations, and the researchers hypothesized that *GDF1* represented a susceptibility gene.[118] Linkage analysis in a family with right atrial isomerism led to the identification of compound heterozygous recessively inherited truncating mutations in *GDF1*.[119] A large study using ES data for 2871 CHD cases demonstrated an increase in homozygous mutations in *GDF1* among Ashkenazi Jewish cases. One specific mutation, c.1091T>C, accounted for approximately 5% of severe CHD cases among those with Ashkenazi descent.[120]

Monogenic Causes of Isolated CHD

In addition to the syndromes described above, variants in an increasing number of genes have been identified in individuals with isolated

CHD, initially through studies of familial CHD and later through the use of next-generation sequencing. Among the genes that have been identified, most fall into one of the following functional categories and play an important role in normal cardiac development: transcription factors, signaling molecules, and structural proteins.[121] Select examples in each of these functional categories are described below. Table 78.3 contains additional genes associated with isolated CHD. The list of genes associated with isolated CHD is rapidly expanding.

Transcription Factors

There is a set of highly conserved transcription factors that are critical for cardiac development.[122,123] In 1998, mutations in the homeobox transcription factor *NKX2-5* were reported in both familial and sporadic cases of CHD associated with conduction defects.[124] The most common phenotype in individuals with *NKX2-5* mutations is ASD with conduction delay.[125,126] Identification of *NKX2-5* mutations in individuals with these cardiac findings is clinically relevant because they are at increased risk of progressive conduction disease and sudden cardiac death, and the genetic information is considered in decision-making regarding pacemakers and implantable cardiac defibrillators.[127,128]

Other transcription factors that have been associated with structural heart disease in both human and mouse models include members of the GATA family[129–133] and members of the Tbox family, which have been implicated in both syndromic and isolated forms of CHD.[134–137] Recent work has identified *SOX17* as a contributor to CHD associated with pulmonary hypertension and isolated and familial pulmonary hypertension.[138] *SOX17* is a transcriptional target of GATA4, and it inhibits signaling in the Wnt/β-catenin pathway involved in cardiac development.[139,140]

Cell Signaling and Adhesion Models

Many signaling pathways are involved in cardiac development, and genes involved in these pathways are frequently disrupted in patients with CHD. Notch signaling is important for cellular differentiation and is involved in the pathogenesis of both isolated and syndromic CHD.[78,79,81,141,142] Mutations in *NOTCH1* have been identified in autosomal-dominantly inherited CHD consisting primarily of a bicuspid aortic valve and are associated with abnormalities of the outflow tracts and semilunar valves.[143–145] Mutations in *NOTCH1* in patients with isolated TOF were noted to be the most frequent site of genetic variants, accounting for 4.5% of patients.[146]

Another cell-signaling family that is crucial for cardiac development is the TGF-β cytokine superfamily. Several genes in this family are implicated in heart development, including *BMP-2*, *BMP-4*, *TGF-β 2*, and *TGF-β 3*.[147,148] The TGF-β superfamily also includes Nodal, a secreted signaling ligand that has been implicated in laterality

Table 78.3 Selected Monogenic Causes of Isolated Congenital Heart Disease

Gene	Loci	Mode of Inheritance	Cardiac Disease	References
ACTC1	15q14	AD	ASD, HCM, DCM, LVNC	Matsson et al.[155]
CITED2	6q24.1	AD	ASD, VSD	Sperling et al.[277]
CRELD1	3p25.3	AD	ASD, AVSD	Guo et al.[278]
GATA4	8p23.1	AD	ASD, VSD, AVSD, PS, TOF	Zhang et al.[279]
GATA5	20q13.33	AD/AR	ASD, BAV, TOF, VSD, DORV	Shan et al.,[280] Jiang et al.[281]
GATA6	18q11.2	AD	TA, TOF	Kodo et al.,[130] Xu et al.,[282] Zhang et al.[283]
HAND1	5q33.2	AD	SV, VSD	Reamon-Buettner et al.,[284,285]
HAND2	4q34.1	AD	PS, TOF, VSD	Sun et al.,[286] Shen et al.,[287] Töpf et al.[288]
MEIS2	15q14	AD	ASD, VSD, CoA	Verheije et al.[289]
MYBPC3	11p11.2	AD	ASD, PDA, VSD, MR	Wessels et al.,[290] Wells et al.[291]
MYH6	14q11.2	AD, AR	ASD, HCM, DCM, HLHS	Jin et al.,[120] Theis et al.[153]
MYH7	14q11.2	AD for CM	EA, LVNC, HCM, DCM	Hanchard et al.,[292] Postma et al.[154]
NODAL	10q22.1	AD	D-TGA, DORV, TOF, VSD	Mohapatra et al.,[149] Roessler et al.[150]
NOTCH1	9q34.3	AD	ASD, VSD, CoA, HLHS, DORV	Garg et al.,[145] Kerstjens-Frederikse et al.[143]
NKX2-5	5q35.1	AD	ASD, TOF, HLHS	Schott et al.,[124] Stallmeyer et al.,[125] Benson et al.[126]
NR2F2	15q26.2	AD	AVSD, AS, CoA, VSD, HLHS, TOF, DORV	Al Turki et al.,[28] Qiao et al.,[293] Bashamboo et al.[294]
SMAD2	18q21.1	AD	HTX, DORV, ASD, VSD, PDA	Zaidi et al.,[71] Granadillo et al.[295]
SMAD6	15q22.31	AD	BAV, CoA, AS	Grillis et al.[296]
TAB2	6q25.1	AD	BAV, AS, TOF	Thienpont et al.[297]
TBX1	22q11.2	AD	Conotruncal defects, VSD, IAA, ASD	Yagi et al.[298]
TBX5	12q24.1	AD	VSD, ASD, AVSD, conduction defects	Basson et al.[299]
TBX20	7p14.2	Unknown	ASD, VSD, MS, DCM	Kirk et al.[136]

Genes in this table are associated with congenital heart disease based on criteria established by Clinical Genome Resource.[178]

AS, Aortic stenosis; *ASD*, atrial septal defect; *AVSD*, atrioventricular septal defect; *BAV*, bicuspid aortic valve; *CoA*, coarctation of the aorta; *DCM*, dilated cardiomyopathy; *DORV*, double outlet right ventricle; *D-TGA*, d-loop transposition of the great arteries; *EA*, Ebstein's anomaly of the tricuspid valve; *HCM*, hypertrophic cardiomyopathy; *HLHS*, hypoplastic left heart syndrome; *HTX*, heterotaxy syndrome; *IAA*, interrupted aortic arch; *LVNC*, left ventricular noncompaction; *MR*, mitral regurgitation; *MS*, mitral stenosis; *PDA*, patent ductus arteriosus; *PS*, pulmonary stenosis; *SV*, single ventricle; *TA*, truncus arteriosus; *TOF*, tetralogy of Fallot; *VSD*, ventricular septal defect.

defects including HTX and isolated CHD.[149,150] Isolated CHD lesions associated with *NODAL* mutations include d-loop transposition of the great arteries, double outlet right ventricle, TOF, and isolated VSDs.

Structural Proteins

Mutations in structural cardiac proteins also contribute to CHD in some patients. Mutations in cardiac sarcomere proteins are associated with cardiomyopathies and recently have been reported in some types of CHD. *MYH6* encodes myosin heavy chain 6, and dominant mutations have been associated with ASDs in addition to dilated cardiomyopathy.[151,152] Recently, recessive *MYH6* missense mutations were identified in two patients with hypoplastic left heart syndrome and decreased ventricular function, suggesting a role in the development of the normal ventricular myocardium.[153] Mutations in *MYH7*, another sarcomeric protein, have been associated with Ebstein's anomaly of the tricuspid valve and left ventricular noncompaction.[154] *ACTC1* encodes a cardiac actin, and mutations have been identified in familial cases of ASDs without cardiac dysfunction.[155]

Histone Modifiers

ES has identified several monogenic causes of isolated and nonisolated CHD. Zaidi et al. used ES in 362 severe cases of CHD and demonstrated an excess of likely damaging *de novo* variants in genes expressed during cardiac development. This study demonstrated significant enrichment of genes involved in the modification of histone 3 lysine 4 (H34K).[71] Methylated H34K is an important regulator of developmental genes. Other genes in this pathway, including *MLL2, KDM6A,* and *CHD7,* have been previously associated with CHD.[156,157] Histone modifications are important regulators of gene expression. These data suggest that the H34K pathway is important for appropriate gene regulation during cardiac development and that other epigenetic mechanisms may play a role in the pathogenesis of CHD.

Common Variants and CHD

Given that the majority of CHD cases do not yet have a known genetic cause, several authors have hypothesized that common variants may play a role in the risk of CHD. Genome-wide association studies have been used to identify common variants associated with specific types of CHD. A large study of patients with CHD found a region on chromosome 4p16 that was associated with risk of ASD, and the genotype at this locus accounted for approximately 9% of the population-attributable risk.[158] A genome-wide association study in the Han Chinese population identified two loci, 1p12 and 4q13.1, associated with CHD. Another study in the Han Chinese using a compound heterozygous model identified four additional loci that explained 7.8% of the CHD variance in the population, suggesting that multiple modes of inheritance are contributing.[159] Several studies have examined specific groups of CHD, including left-sided lesions and TOF, and have identified susceptibility loci that account for a small proportion of the genetic variation in each case.[159] Although common variants likely have a role in CHD susceptibility, these account for only a small proportion of the genetic risk, and large studies of individuals with similar CHD lesions are needed to identify additional susceptibility loci.

Recommendations for Clinical Genetic Testing

Recommendations for clinical genetic testing for patients with birth defects are evolving. Any individual with features suggestive of a recognizable chromosomal condition should undergo focused testing. Because many syndromic forms of birth defects have variable presentations, patients with multiple birth defects and/or additional findings including dysmorphic features, growth deficiency, or developmental delay should be offered genetic testing. If there is a family history of congenital anomalies or multiple miscarriages, genetic testing should also be offered. In neonates and young infants, it can be difficult to appreciate dysmorphic features, cognitive delays, and extracardiac anomalies. For fetuses diagnosed with birth defects, there is a much higher chance of identifying genetic abnormalities, possibly due to high rates of intrauterine demise with certain conditions. For this reason, genetic testing and counseling should be offered in all cases of prenatally diagnosed birth defects, because a positive test may help identify additional anomalies and affect pregnancy management.[61,160,161]

CMA is the appropriate first-line test for most individuals and has been shown to be cost-effective.[162,163] In cases where rapid results will have a clinical benefit, FISH can be considered. The limitation of CMA is that balanced chromosomal rearrangements cannot be detected, and if this is suspected, a karyotype is needed. If CMA is negative and a genetic cause is strongly suspected, ES can be considered.

Conclusion

A given syndrome or genetic variant can cause different birth defects and types of CHD in different patients due to genetic modifiers. In addition, for each type of birth defect, there is a long list of possible genetic causes. As sequencing becomes more cost-effective, additional causes will certainly be identified, and we are just beginning to understand how genetics impact outcomes among patients with birth defects. For syndromic birth defects, CMA with reflex testing to ES is frequently performed. For isolated birth defects, CMA is often performed, and in newborns for whom all the features may not yet be recognized, ES may also become standard as the cost of clinical sequencing decreases and as clinical utility is demonstrated.

CHAPTER 79 Common Monogenetic Conditions in Newborns

Christine H. Umandap, Elaine M. Pereira

KEY POINTS

1. Considering and making a genetic diagnosis early can help direct evaluation and management in the newborn, leading to better patient care.
2. Significant renal disease and subsequent pulmonary disease are common in autosomal recessive kidney disease, requiring supportive care.
3. Newborns with achondroplasia should have specific imaging and studies to decrease the risk of neurocervical junction compromise.
4. RASopathies should be considered in newborns with cardiac abnormalities (pulmonary valve stenosis, hypertrophic cardiomyopathy) and certain facial characteristics; gene panel testing is recommended given the phenotypic overlap of many of the conditions.
5. Tuberous sclerosis complex can be diagnosed prenatally and in the newborn, requiring monitoring and management of seizures to decrease morbidity and mortality.
6. Spinal muscular atrophy is now on newborn screening panels in many states and has approved medications and gene therapy that will change the natural history of this condition.
7. Many newborns with congenital myotonic dystrophy type 1 require respiratory and nutritional support in the first year of life.

Genetic conditions involving aneuploidy (trisomy 21, trisomy 18, trisomy 13) are commonly considered in an infant with multiple congenital anomalies or dysmorphic features. Genetic syndromes caused by pathogenic changes in a specific gene or set of genes may have more subtle findings in the newborn period and could be overlooked. Although the conditions are easier to recognize as the patient gets older, considering them in the differential diagnosis during the neonatal period is essential to directing appropriate management. Establishing a genetic diagnosis can lead to more efficient use of resources and proper care for the neonate.

Autosomal Recessive Polycystic Kidney Disease

Autosomal recessive polycystic kidney disease (ARPKD) is one of the most common causes of neonatal cystic kidneys, with an incidence of 1 in 20,000 live births.[1] There is wide variability in disease severity in the newborn period.

Pathophysiology

The *PKHD1* gene encodes the protein fibrocystin, which is localized to the bile ducts, kidney, and pancreas. Fibrocystin is thought to play a role in primary cilia, which are important in kidney tubule and biliary cell function,[2] and disease is due to loss of fibrocystin function.

Clinical Features

In ARPKD, ultrasounds can identify increased echogenicity and renal size. Prenatal ultrasounds can also detect oligohydramnios, which leads to pulmonary hypoplasia. The oligohydramnios can lead to abnormal facial features, which include low-set ears; flattened facial features, especially the nose; epicanthal folds; and micrognathia. Given the renal and pulmonary abnormalities, systemic hypertension and chronic lung disease are common. ARPKD is characterized by congenital hepatic fibrosis, but its clinical manifestations, including hepatosplenomegaly and portal hypertension, take time to develop. These manifestations sometimes develop as early as infancy but are more commonly seen in childhood.[3]

Evaluation

To establish the ARPKD diagnosis, pathogenic mutations in both copies of the *PKHD1* or *DXIPIL* gene should be present, with renal cystic enlargement and congenital hepatic fibrosis. Although liver biopsies can diagnose ARPKD, noninvasive imaging is preferred. There are numerous mutations in the *PKHD1* gene, and to date there is no genotype-phenotype correlation that can help prognosticate the severity of the condition. Mutations in *DZIPIL*, which encodes a protein involved in ciliogenesis, can be considered if molecular testing for *PKHD1* is normal.

Given the risk of pulmonary hypoplasia, monitoring the neonate's respiratory status is critical. Regular lab work to access renal function and to ensure there are no serious electrolyte abnormalities is also important. Calcium, magnesium, sodium, chloride, potassium, liver function tests (albumin, prothrombin time [PT], and partial thromboplastin time [PTT]), vitamin E, 35-OH vitamin D, and fat-soluble vitamins need to be monitored to evaluate renal and hepatic function.[1]

Management

Treatment is based on clinical presentation. Given the extent of renal and hepatobiliary disease, nephrotoxic agents like aminoglycosides and nonsteroidal antiinflammatory drugs should be avoided. Respiratory distress from pulmonary hypoplasia may require mechanical ventilation. If the neonate has anuria or oliguria, dialysis is likely necessary. Fluid balance is important because dehydration is common. Angiotensin II receptor inhibitors and/or angiotensin-converting enzyme inhibitors are usually first-line treatments for hypertension, and alpha- and beta-adrenoreceptor agonists should be avoided. If the renal disease is severe, erythropoietin-stimulating agents or iron supplements may be needed for anemia. Since the liver can be affected, it is important to monitor the neonate's nutrition. Bile acid supplementation may be required if biliary dysfunction is significant with low serum levels of fat-soluble vitamins or if magnetic resonance cholangiopancreatography shows significant intrahepatic ductal dilation. Recurrent bacteremia can be a sign of bacterial cholangitis and should be treated aggressively with antibiotics. If portal hypertension is present, sclerotherapy can be used for esophageal varices. If the infant has feeding difficulties, feeding tubes or gastrostomy should be considered. Poor growth can result from chronic kidney disease, and growth hormone may be helpful, but this has not been rigorously demonstrated.[4] Ursodeoxycholic acid can be used to decrease gallstone formation. If the portal hypertension is severe, it is important to immunize against meningococcus, *Haemophilus influenzae* type B, strep pneumococcus, and other encapsulated bacteria. For chronic lung disease, palivizumab can be beneficial.

A phase 1 clinical trail was completed to assess the effect of the multikinase inhibitor tesevatinib on the progression of renal and hepatobiliary disease in ARPKD. Although the trial is for children 5 to 12 years old, the data may help with the care of neonates in the future. More recently, phase 3 trails are recruiting neonates and children with ARPKD to look at the safety of the vasopressin V2 receptors competitive antagonist Tolvaptan and possible delays in dialysis.

Long-Term Outcomes

Advancements in neonatal resuscitation and management have led to improved survival for neonates with ARPKD. However, mortality is still high, with approximately 30% of individuals dying in the first year from pulmonary complications. If the infant survives the first year, 10-year survival is approximately 82%. However, there is significant morbidity from progressive renal failure and hepatic fibrosis.[5] If the disease is extensive, a renal or renal-hepatic transplantation can be performed.[6]

Achondroplasia

Achondroplasia is the most common skeletal dysplasia, with an incidence of 1 in 25,000 to 30,000 live births.[7] This autosomal-dominant disorder has 100% penetrance.

Pathophysiology

The fibroblast growth factor receptor type 3 (*FGFR3*) gene produces a protein abundant in chondrocytes, the precursors of cartilaginous bone.[7] FGFR3 is a cell-surface receptor that plays a role in cell proliferation. Achondroplasia is caused by a single mutation (glycine to arginine at amino acid 380) in the *FGFR3* gene, which results in the continuous activation of the mitogen-activated protein kinase (MAPK)-extracellular signal-regulated kinase pathway in chondrocytes, which in turn inhibits endochondral ossification.[8]

Clinical Manifestations

Although achondroplasia can be suspected prenatally when shortened long bones are noted on third-trimester ultrasounds, many babies are not diagnosed until after birth. Skeletal findings include rhizomelic (proximal limb) shortening accompanied by redundant skin folds of the extremities and brachydactyly (shortened fingers) that may have a bifurcating appearance of the third and fourth fingers, giving a trident sign. Macrocephaly with frontal bossing and midface hypoplasia are common. A small and abnormally shaped foramen magnum is a notable finding in infants. As part of the skeletal dysplasia, the positioning and length of the Eustachian tube is altered, leading to an increased risk of otitis media. Because of the small chest size, some infants can develop restrictive pulmonary complications. Both central and obstructive sleep apnea can be seen in infants. Thoracolumbar kyphosis is seen in up to 95% of infants with achondroplasia.[7] Lower-extremity bowing secondary to knee instability, internal tibial torsion, and lateral bowing is seen in some individuals.[9] The proportionately large head size leads to delays in gross motor milestones.[10]

Table 79.1 Features of Achondroplasia and Hypochondroplasia

Features of Achondroplasia and Hypochondroplasia	Achondroplasia	Hypochondroplasia
CLINICAL FEATURES		
Macrocephaly	Present in both but generally more severe in achondroplasia	
Midfacial hypoplasia		
Rhizomelic limb shortening		
Redundant skin folds in the arms and legs		
Short chest		
Craniocervical junction problems	More common	Less common
Intelligence	Normal intellect	Some have cognitive problems
Seizures	Less common	More common p.Asn540Lys > p.Lys650Asn
RADIOLOGIC FEATURES		
Temporal lobe dysgenesis	Less common	More common p.Asn540Lys > p.Lys650Asn
GENETIC DIAGNOSIS		
FGFR3 mutation in chromosome 4p16.3	Substitution of glycine to arginine (p.Gly380Arg) > 80% of cases are *de novo* mutations	Substitution of asparagine to lysine (p.Asn540Lys)—most common Substitution of lysine to asparagine (p.Lys650Asn)—less common

Evaluation

Concerns for achondroplasia are normally raised after a thorough infant physical exam or from prenatal ultrasounds. *FGFR3* gene mutation testing should be performed to confirm the diagnosis. Normally, a skeletal survey is done to identify characteristic findings such as disproportionate shortening of the long bones, squaring off of the iliac bones, a round-shaped pelvis, flattening of the acetabulum and vertebrae, and sacrosciatic notch narrowing.[7,11,12] It is important to note that if *FGFR3* mutation testing for achondroplasia is negative, sequencing the gene may be warranted to rule out milder forms of *FGFR3*-related skeletal dysplasia such as hypochondroplasia (Table 79.1).

Management

Once the diagnosis has been established, neuroimaging should be performed as early as possible to assess the craniocervical junction. Narrowing of this area causes increased mortality in infancy[13] because vertebral arterial and spinal cord compression at the level of the foramen magnum can cause central sleep apnea, high cervical myelopathy, and even sudden death. Although brain computed

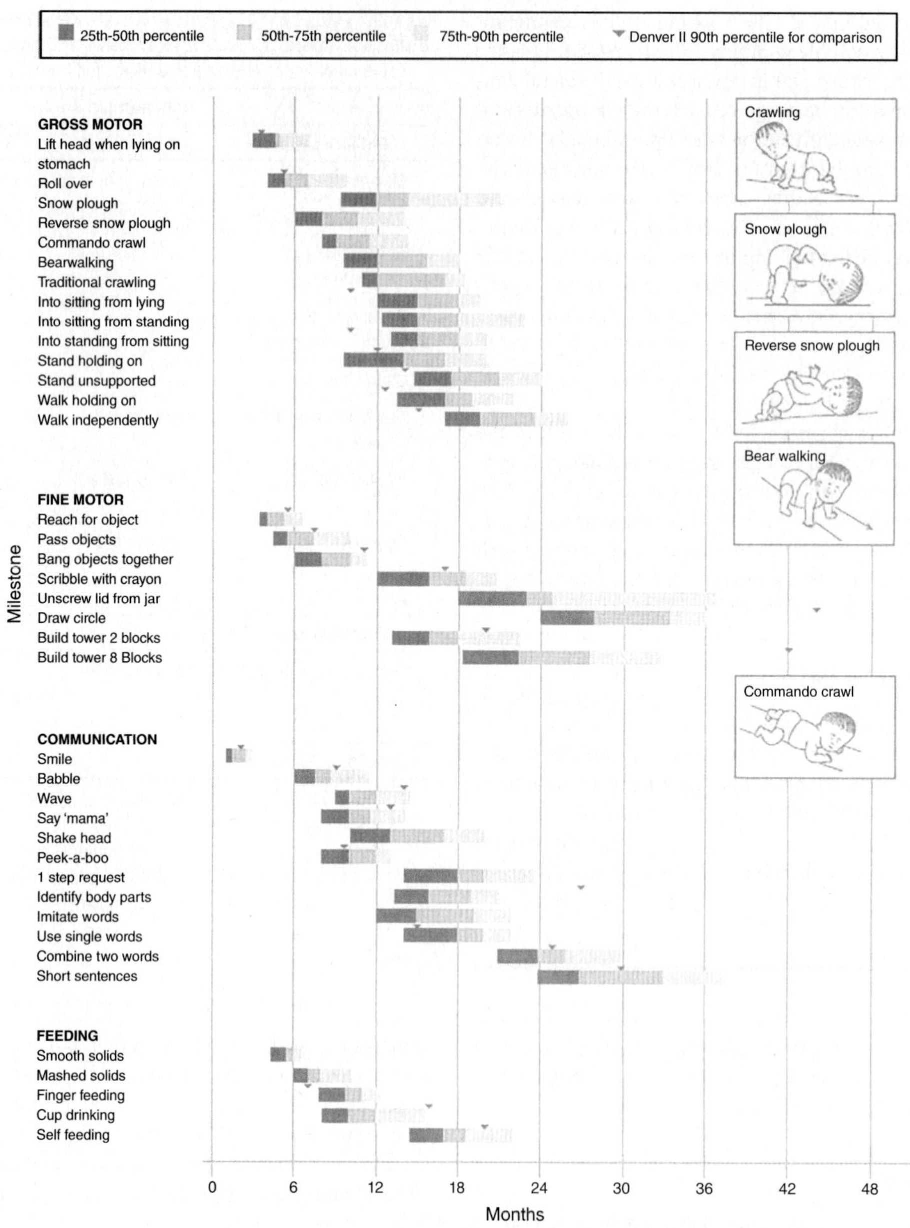

Fig. 79.1 Developmental Norms for Achondroplasia. (Created by Ireland et al. in 2011, this chart compares the Denver II Scale with what is normally seen in infants with achondroplasia.)

tomography has standard measurements for the foramen magnum in infants with achondroplasia, brain magnetic resonance imaging (MRI) will give better images of the cervical spinal cord and brainstem. A polysomnography is also recommended to assess for central sleep apnea and hypopnea. Because infants with achondroplasia have small chests and the ribs can have a paradoxical movement with inspiration, the infant can appear to have retractions and respiratory distress during normal respiration. Extraaxial fluid and ventriculomegaly are common in children with achondroplasia. It is also more common for these infants to sweat more that the general population. Therefore these findings alone should not prompt further evaluation. However, rapid increase in head circumference, hyperreflexia, reflex asymmetry, clonus, severe hypotonia, and desaturations to <85% should raise suspicions for increased intracranial pressure or craniocervical compression and should prompt immediate consultation with a pediatric neurosurgeon.[7]

For ongoing management, age- and sex-specific achondroplasia growth charts ensure the infant is growing at the appropriate velocity and not gaining excessive weight, which would exacerbate neurologic and orthopedic complications.[14,15] Additionally, infants can demonstrate unusual movements called preorthograde movements, which may raise concern in parents but are actually normal in achondroplasia. Given the common thoracolumbar kyphosis, activities that aggravate this, such as unsupported sitting or strollers with poor back support, should be avoided. Infants should be positioned prone during part of the waking day to increase muscle tone. If kyphosis worsens or does not spontaneously resolve when the child starts to walk, referral to a pediatric orthopedic surgeon is warranted to prevent neurologic complications. Because developmental delay is common, specific achondroplasia developmental norms were developed (Fig. 79.1).[10] Given that children with achondroplasia have expressive language delay, treatment of recurrent otitis media is recommended to reduce the possibility of conductive hearing loss.[7] For this reason, audiology exams should be repeated at 1 year old and if any concerns are raised about the child's hearing.

Because of the short stature, adaptive measures and occupational therapy are encouraged. Limb-lengthening is a surgical procedure to increase height in patients with achondroplasia but is controversial given the burden and complications. Growth hormone has been approved for achondrophasia. It results in increased growth velocity during the first 2 years of treatment, with an additional 3.5 cm in final height in males and 2.8 cm in final height in females, based on a long-term follow-up study.[16]

In 2021, the FDA approved vosoritide, a C-type natriuretic peptide (CNP) analog. Normally CNP inhibits the MAPK signaling pathway, which in turn leads to endochondrial ossification and bone growth promotion. This medication can given as a daily injection in children at least 5 years old until the growth plates close. Studies showed an increased height of 1.57 cm a year.[16a]

Long-Term Outcomes

With the management described above, early mortality in infants with achondroplasia has decreased. If there are no neurologic complications, intelligence is normal.[7,17] Those with achondroplasia have near normal to normal life expectancy. Without intervention, the average height is approximately 131 cm in males and 124 cm in females.

RASopathies

RASopathies describe a group of genetic conditions that affect the RAS/MAPK pathway. Combined, the RASopathies affect 1 in 1000 individuals.

Pathophysiology

The RAS/MAPK pathway is a signal transduction pathway. Mutations in genes in the RAS/MAPK pathway directly or indirectly lead to genetic disorders that are grouped as RASopathies (Fig. 79.2). A particular RASopathy can be caused by mutations in one of several genes. Similarly, different mutations in a single gene can lead to different RASopathies (Table 79.2).

The *PTPN11* gene produces a protein tyrosine phosphatase known as SHP2. Mutations in specific domains of the protein can cause SHP2 to constitutively activate signaling of the RAS/MAPK pathway. The *SOS1* gene helps keep RAS inactive. Mutations in the *SOS1* gene disrupt this inhibition, which in turn increases active RAS. The *RAF1* gene encodes the protein CRAF, which has a binding, phosphorylation, and kinase domain; a mutation affecting the kinase domain increases RAS signaling. Mutations in the *PTPN11* and *SOS1* genes account for the majority of Noonan syndrome cases. Mutations in the *PTPN11* and *RAF1* genes account for most cases of Noonan syndrome with multiple lentigines. Specific mutations in the *HRAS* gene in exon 2 cause the protein GTPase HRAS to remain active and increase RAS/MAPK signaling, causing Costello syndrome. The *BRAF*, *MAP2K1*, and *MAP2K2* genes make up proteins involved in the MAPK signaling pathway, and most mutations in these genes cause cardio-facio-cutaneous (CFC) syndrome by increasing kinase activity, which leads to increased MAPK pathway activation.[18]

Clinical Features

Because the RASopathies affect the same pathway, these genetic conditions have overlapping dysmorphic features and clinical manifestations (Table 79.3). Prenatally, cystic hygroma or increased nuchal translucency is commonly seen. Polyhydramnios is another

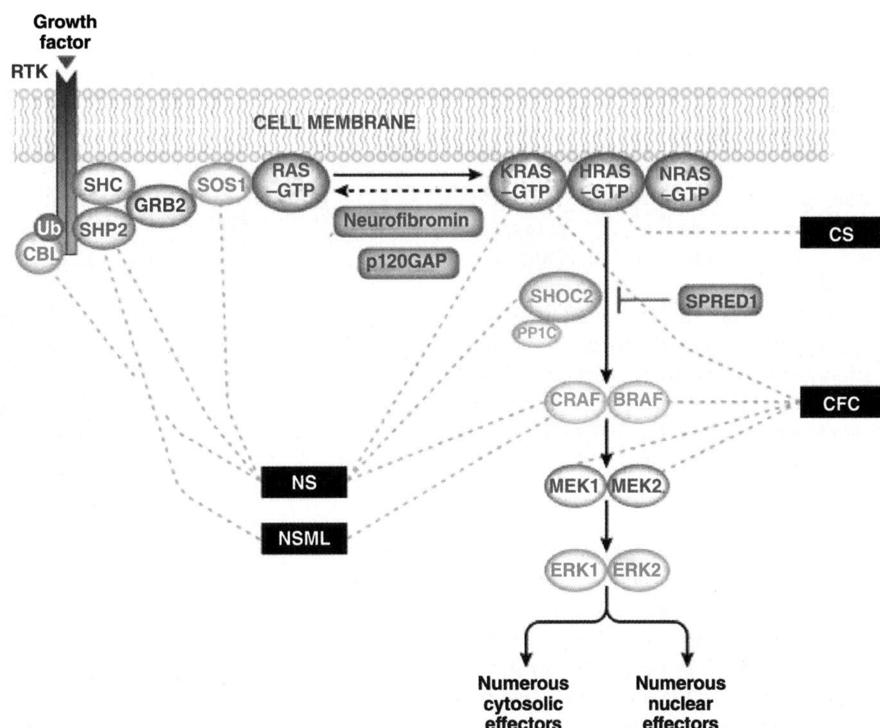

Fig. 79.2 The RAS/MAPK Signal Transduction Pathway Involves Many Proteins Which, if Mutated, Can Lead to RASopathies. *Dashed lines* represent the proteins that could be affected by the particular RASopathy. *CFC*, Cardio-facio-cutaneous syndrome; *CS*, Costello syndrome; *NS*, Noonan syndrome; *NSML*, Noonan syndrome with multiple lentigines. (Modified from Rauen KA. The RASopathies. *Annu Rev Genomics Hum Genet*. 2013;14:355–369.)

Table 79.2 RASopathy Syndromes and More Common Gene Associations

	RASopathy Syndromes			
	Noonan	NSML	Costello	CFC
Gene				
PTPN11	50%	90%		
SOS1	10%–13%			
KRAS	<5%			<2%
HRAS			100%	
RIT1	5%			
CRAF	5%	<5%		
BRAF	<2%			75%
MEK1	<2%			25%
MEK2				

CFC, Cardio-facio-cutaneous syndrome; *NSML*, Noonan syndrome with multiple lentigines.

Table 79.3 Common Features in RASopathy Syndromes

Features	Noonan	NSML	Costello	CFC
Prenatal	Cystic hygroma; nuchal translucency; polyhydramnios			
			Wrist ulnar deviation	
Craniofacial	Hypertelorism, downward slanting palpebral fissures, ptosis Low-set, posteriorly rotated ears			
		Milder		Coarser
Cardiac	Pulmonary valve stenosis; hypertrophic cardiomyopathy; arrythmia			
Chest	Widely spaced nipples; pectus abnormality			
GI	Feeding issues (resolve with time)		Feeding issues	
Renal	Mild structural change			
Urogenital	Cryptorchidism			
Heme	Coagulopathy			
Neurologic	Hypotonia			
	Developmental delay Learning issues	Mild intellectual disability	Developmental delay Intellectual disability	Seizures
ENT/ audiology	SNHL			Recurrent otitis media
Orthopedics	Short stature		Fingers: ulnar deviation	
Dermatologic	Follicular keratosis	Lentigines Café au lait	Papillomas Deep crease on palms and soles Loose skin	Sparse hair Keratosis pilaris Dystrophic nails

CFC, Cardio-facio-cutaneous syndrome; *GI*, gastrointestinal; *NSML*, Noonan syndrome with multiple lentigines; *SNHL*, sensorineural hearing loss.

Roberts AE, Allanson JE, Tartaglia M, Gelb BD. Noonan syndrome. *Lancet.* 2013;381(9863):333–342; van Trier DC, van der Burgt I, Draaijer RW, Cruysberg JRM, Noordam C, Draaisma JM. Ocular findings in Noonan syndrome: a retrospective cohort study of 105 patients. *Eur J Pediatr.* 2018;177(8):1293–1298; Bessis D, Morice-Picard F, Bourrat E, et al. Dermatological manifestations in cardiofaciocutaneous syndrome: a prospective multicentric study of 45 mutation-positive patients. *Br J Dermatol.* 2019;180(1):172–180; Pierpont ME, Magoulas PL, Adi S, et al. Cardio-facio-cutaneous syndrome: clinical features, diagnosis, and management guidelines. *Pediatrics.* 2014;134(4):e1149–1162; Romano AA, Allanson JE, Dahlgren J, et al. Noonan syndrome: clinical features, diagnosis, and management guidelines. *Pediatrics.* 2010;126(4):746–759.

typical prenatal ultrasound finding. Postnatally, individuals with RASopathies have unifying craniofacial characteristics. Eyes can be hyperteloric (widely spaced) with downward slanting palpebral fissures, epicanthal folds, and ptosis. Ears can be low set and posteriorly rotated, whereas the neck is often short with redundant skin and a lower posterior hairline. Facial features can be milder or coarser, depending on the specific RASopathy. Congenital heart conditions, specifically pulmonary valve stenosis, hypertrophic cardiomyopathy, and ventricular septal defects, are common.[19] Pectus abnormalities, wide-spaced nipples, cryptorchidism, hypotonia, and feeding difficulties can be observed. There is a spectrum of developmental delay, learning disabilities, and intellectual disability in these conditions. Approximately 50% of patients with CFC develop seizures, often starting in infancy. Although most cases develop after infancy, dermatologic manifestations can help distinguish between the various RASopathies. An exception is seen in Costello syndrome, with deep palmar creases and ulnar deviation of the fingers notable at birth.[20]

Evaluation

A multigene panel analyzing genes associated with the RAS/MAPK pathway is the preferred method for diagnosing a RASopathy. Once a specific diagnosis is made, an echocardiogram and renal ultrasound should be performed to evaluate for structural abnormalities. Abnormalities in the neurologic exam may warrant a brain MRI to rule out structural abnormalities. If hypotonia leads to feeding difficulties, an endocrinology evaluation should be initiated to assess for growth hormone deficiency as an etiology for failure to thrive. Individuals with Noonan syndrome need to be screened for coagulopathy with a CBC, PT, and PTT.

Management

Management guidelines have been established for many of the RASopathies.[21–23] There are specific growth charts for Noonan syndrome and Noonan syndrome with multiple lentigines. Decreased growth velocity warrants an endocrinology evaluation for growth hormone deficiency. A feeding evaluation is advised if there is poor weight gain in the first 2 years. Most infants with Costello syndrome have severe feeding issues that require a nasogastric tube or a gastrostomy tube. If hypotonia is present, evaluations for developmental services are important. Developmental services are especially important with Costello syndrome because developmental delay and intellectual disability are nearly always present.[24] Given that 50% of CFC individuals develop seizures, an electroencephalogram would be performed to assess for seizures.

Long-Term Outcomes

With Noonan syndrome, if untreated, final height will be less than the third percentile.[25] With growth hormone, final height is increased.[26] Individuals with Costello syndrome have an increased risk of tumors (15%) including rhabdomyosarcoma and neuroblastoma. Although transitional cell bladder carcinoma is normally seen in adults, it can be seen in preteens and adolescents.[27]

Tuberous Sclerosis Complex

Tuberous sclerosis complex (TSC) is an autosomal dominant neurocutaneous disorder with variable expressivity that affects multiple organ systems. The incidence is 1 in 6000 live births.

Pathophysiology

The *TSC1* and *TSC2* genes produce the proteins hamartin and tuberin, respectively, which form a heterodimer. This heterodimer complex inhibits the mTOR pathway, which is known to regulate cell growth, proliferation, metabolism, survival, aging, memory, and immunity. Therefore pathogenic mutations in either the *TSC1* or *TSC2* gene disrupt the heterodimer and lead to increased mTOR pathway activity, which then causes abnormal cell proliferation and overgrowth.[28]

Clinical Features

Many features of TSC can be seen prenatally or within the neonatal period. Cardiac rhabdomyomas are the common initial manifestation[29] and can be detected prenatally as early as 20 weeks' gestational age. These rhabdomyomas can grow throughout gestation and typically regress after birth.[30] Hypomelanotic macules, also known as "ash leaf spots," are another common finding in infants. The combination of cardiac rhabdomyomas and hypomelanotic macules are observed in 85% of infants with TSC. Cortical dysplasias (tubers and white-matter abnormalities in the brain) and subependymal nodules (benign tumors that arise from the ependymal cells lining the lateral and third ventricles) are reported in 94% and 90% of TSC1 and TCS2, respectively.[31] Given the structural brain abnormalities, seizures are commonly seen in TSC, including infantile seizures and focal epilepsy.[29] Renal cysts and angiomyolipomas are benign but can increase in number and size over the individual's life span and can lead to increased morbidity and mortality (see long-term outcomes). Retinal hamartomas (plaque-like lesions) are normally asymptomatic.

Over time, more skin findings develop (Table 79.4) in almost every patient with TSC. Small 1- to 3-mm hypopigmented macules called "confetti" lesions are common on the extremities. Facial angiofibromas are usually symmetric over the face, appearing before 5 years old. Shagreen patches are raised yellow-brown hamartomas normally found on the torso, commonly in the lumbosacral area, and develop during the childhood or preteenage years. Periungual and subungual fibromas develop in the preteenage years along the proximal nail folds and can often disrupt nail growth.[32]

Evaluation

A definite diagnosis of TSC is confirmed with a pathogenic mutation in the *TSC1* or *TSC2* gene when there are two major clinical features or when there is one major clinical feature plus at least two minor features (see Table 79.4). Diagnosis during infancy can be difficult because some of the findings do not develop until later in life (Fig. 79.3)[29]; molecular testing is important to confirm the diagnosis in this age group.

Once a diagnosis of TSC is confirmed, it is important to evaluate for the various manifestations of TSC. Evaluation should include an echocardiogram to evaluate cardiac rhabdomyomas in children under 3 years, an electrocardiogram to assess for arrhythmias that could

Table 79.4 2012 Updated Diagnostic Criteria for Tuberous Sclerosis Complex

Genetic diagnostic criteria

- Identification of a pathogenic mutation in *TSC1* or *TSC2* is sufficient to make a diagnosis of TS

Clinical diagnostic criteria

Definitive diagnosis
1. ≥2 Major features
2. ≥1 Major feature and ≥2 minor features
Possible diagnosis
1. ≥1 Major feature
2. ≥2 Minor features

Diagnostic Criteria	Age of Onset	Diagnostic Modalities
Cortical dysplasias	Appear prenatally or at birth	*Standard:* Brain MRI with and without gadolinium
Subependymal nodules		
Subependymal giant cell astrocytoma	Appear prenatally or at birth Also commonly seen during childhood or adolescent period	*Alternatives:* Head CT or head US (suboptimal results compared with MRI)
Cardiac rhabdomyoma • Well-circumscribed tumors, usually found in the ventricles of the heart	Appear prenatally or at birth	Echocardiogram (Echo)
≥3 Hypomelanotic macules at least 5 mm in diameter	At birth or during infancy	Physical exam
≥3 Angiofibromas or fibrous cephalic plaque	Appear starting 2–5 years old; increase in size and number during adolescence	
Multiple retinal hamartomas	May appear in young children	Ophthalmologic evaluation
Shagreen patch	Appear in the first decade of life	Physical exam
≥2 Ungual fibromas	Usually appear during adolescence/adulthood	
Lymphangioleiomyomatosis	Usually found in adults	Baseline pulmonary function test, 6-minute walk test, high-resolution CT scan, serum vascular endothelial growth factor type D (VEGF-D) level for patients ≥18 years of age
≥2 Angiomyolipomas		*Standard:* Abdomen MRI
		Alternatives: Abdomen CT or abdomen US (suboptimal results compared with MRI)

Continued

Table 79.4 2012 Updated Diagnostic Criteria for Tuberous Sclerosis Complex—cont'd

Diagnostic Criteria	Age of Onset	Diagnostic Modalities
"Confetti" skin lesions	Usually found in adults	Physical exam
>3 Dental enamel pits	Usually found in adults	
≥2 Intraoral fibromas	Fibromas in the gingiva, oral mucosa, and tongue Usually found in adults	
Retinal achromic patch	Rare, with incidence of 1/20,000 of the general population	Ophthalmologic evaluation
Multiple renal cysts	May be seen in patients with *TSC1* or *TSC2* mutations, or in patients with contiguous deletion of the *TSC2* and *PKD1* genes	*Standard:* Abdomen MRI *Alternatives:* Abdomen CT or abdomen US (suboptimal results compared with MRI)
Nonrenal hamartomas	Rare	

CT, Computed tomography; *MRI,* magnetic resonance imaging; *TS,* tuberous sclerosis; *US,* ultrasound.

Northrup and Krueger. Tuberous sclerosis complex diagnostic criteria update: Recommendations of the 2012 International Tuberous Sclerosis Complex Consensus Conference. *Pediatr Neurol.* 2013;49(4):243–254; Krueger and Northrup. Tuberous sclerosis complex surveillance and management: recommendations of the 2012 International Tuberous Sclerosis Complex Consensus Conference. *Pediatr Neurol.* 2013;49(4):255–265.)

arise from areas where a rhabdomyoma has regressed, and a brain MRI to assess for structural abnormalities or migrational defects. Given the increased incidence of seizures, an electroencephalogram should be done. Although an abdominal ultrasound can evaluate for renal cysts, an abdominal MRI can also detect angiomyolipomas that are fat-poor and can be missed on an ultrasound; if possible, the brain and abdominal MRI should be done simultaneously to minimize the contrast load and decrease the number of anesthetics. Blood pressure and renal function should be regularly assessed. A full ophthalmologic exam should be performed to evaluate for retinal abnormalities.[33]

Management

Recommendations for asymptomatic individuals are outlined below, with more frequent evaluations warranted if the patient becomes symptomatic.[33] Infants with cardiac rhabdomyomas should be followed by a pediatric cardiologist with an echocardiogram every 1 to 3 years until the lesions regress; more frequent follow-up is required if the infant is symptomatic. Electrocardiograms should be done at least every 3 to 5 years.[30,33] Brain MRIs are recommended every 1 to 3 years until the age of 25 years to monitor for subependymal giant cell astrocytoma growth. Routine electroencephalograms should be done if seizures are suspected. Blood pressure and renal function assessing glomerular filtration rate should be checked annually. An abdominal MRI is recommended every 1 to 3 years to assess for kidney abnormalities; contrast use is dependent on kidney function. Because repeated use of gadolinium-based contrast agents may cause organ deposits, the brain and abdominal MRI can be done simultaneously to limit contrast use. Skin evaluations should be done annually for lesions that are symptomatic, causing pain, bleeding, or disfiguring; in these cases treatment options in the form of surgical excision, laser therapy, or topical mTORC1 inhibitors may be pursued. If eye findings were noted on the initial evaluation, annual evaluations are recommended.

Medical management in TSC is often focused on epilepsy. Vigabatrin, a gamma-aminobutyric acid aminotransferase inhibitor, has been useful in controlling and preventing infantile spasms among infants with TSC and is therefore the first-line treatment. The exact mechanism of action in infantile spasms has not been fully elucidated but is thought to be inhibition of the mTOR pathway. Adrenocorticotropin hormone is the second-line treatment in patients who respond poorly to vigabatrin.[29,33] If seizures are too difficult to manage with medications, surgery is considered, ranging from excision of identified epileptic foci to wider resections.

Multiple clinical trials using mTOR inhibitors are ongoing to identify alternative medications for TSC. Rapamycin is currently

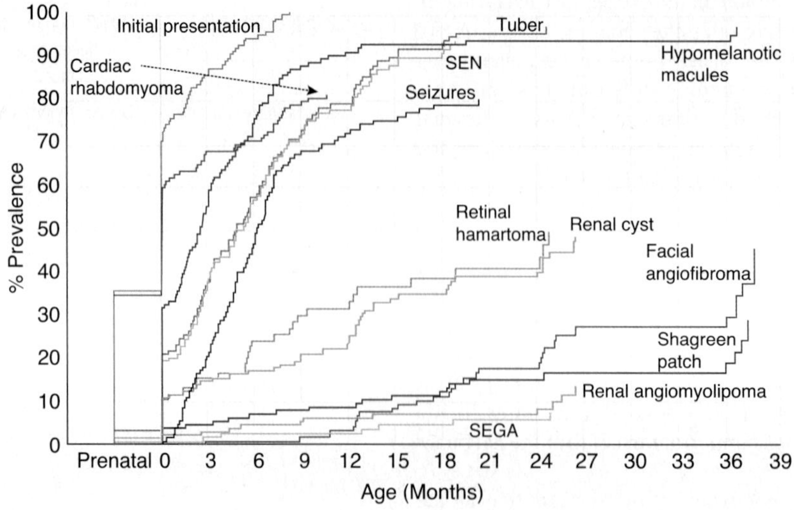

Fig. 79.3 Age of Symptom Presentation in Tuberous Sclerosis Complex. Cardiac rhabdomyomas, hypomelanotic macules, subependymal nodules, tubers, renal cysts, and retinal hamartomas can be seen during the neonatal period. *SEGA,* Subependymal giant cell astrocytomas; *SEN,* subependymal nodules. (Modified from Davis PE, Filip-Dhima R, Sideridis G, et al. Presentation and diagnosis of tuberous sclerosis complex in infants. *Pediatrics.* 2017;140(6).)

being studied in the treatment of angiomyolipomas and for angiofibromas. Everolimus has been shown to improve treatment-resistant seizures and angiolipomas.[34–36] Use of these medications in children less than 2 years old has been promising.[37] The FDA approved Epidiolex (cannabidiol) oral solution for treatment of tuberous sclerosis complex associated seizures in patients one year of age and older in 2020 38, and Hyftor (sirolimus topical gel) 0.2% with facial angiofibromas in patients 6 years of age and older in 2022.[37a,37b]

Long-Term Outcomes

Ninety percent of individuals with TSC have a TSC-associated neuropsychiatric disorder during their lifetime, including intellectual disabilities, behavioral problems, psychiatric problems, psychosocial difficulties, neuropsychological disorders, and academic problems.

There is significant morbidity associated with TSC. Complications from seizures including status epilepticus can decrease life expectancy. Angiomyolipomas can become malignant, and renal cell carcinoma is more common in patients with TSC than in the general population.

Spinal Muscular Atrophy

Spinal muscular atrophy (SMA) is a progressive neuromuscular disease with an incidence of 1 in 10,000 live births.

Pathophysiology

The *SMN1* gene produces survival motor neuron (SMN) protein, which is required for motor neuron function. The SMN protein helps regulate small nuclear ribonuclear proteins by assembling specific proteins on target RNAs. The SMN protein inhibits cell apoptosis.[38] If both copies of the *SMN1* gene have a pathogenic variant, the snRNP complexes are not assembled or moved properly, which in turn leads to splicing changes in the cell and inhibited cellular growth. The *SMN2* gene is similar to the *SMN1* gene except for a few nucleotides; a specific C-to-T nucleotide change creates an exon splicing suppressor that excludes exon 7, making a smaller, less stable SMN protein. The *SMN2* gene can create approximately 10% of full-length SMN protein. Although normally each individual has two copies of a gene, individuals can have zero to eight copies of the *SMN2* gene. Therefore in an individual with SMA, there may be some full-length SMN protein made from SMN2, which is correlated with *SMN2* copy number and a milder phenotype.[39]

Clinical Features

SMA should be suspected if there is symmetric weakness affecting proximal muscles more than distal muscles. With time, symptoms progress as brainstem nuclei and lower motor neurons from the spinal cord anterior horn cells degenerate, leading to muscle atrophy. SMA type 0 has a prenatal phenotype with limited fetal movement. These neonates have multiple contractures, poor respiratory effort, and extreme weakness. SMA type I presents before 6 months of age. Although the infant with SMA type I can have some contractures (especially in the knee), the main morbidity involves feeding and respiration. Without support, infants often fail to thrive and have respiratory insufficiency and recurrent infections that are often fatal. Although infants with SMA type I will not sit, those with SMA type II can sit independently but lose this ability later. If neonates live into childhood, scoliosis is frequent. Individuals with SMA type III develop variable symptoms later in childhood, whereas those with SMA type IV develop symptoms in adulthood (Table 79.5).

Table 79.5 Spinal Muscular Atrophy Subtypes

SMA Subtype	# SMN2 Copies Normally Seen	Age of Symptom Onset	Characteristics/Life Span Without Intervention
0	1	Prenatal	Severe hypotonia, facial diplegia, early respiratory failure, life span <6 months
I	2	<6 months	Mild joint contracture, suck and swallow deficits, sit with support, life span often <2 y
II	3	6–18 months	Sit independently, 70% live into mid-20s
III	3	>18 months	Independent ambulation, life span normal
IV	4	Adulthood	Muscle weakness in 20s to 30s, independent ambulation, life span normal

SMA, Spinal muscular atrophy.

Evaluation

SMA can be diagnosed with molecular testing. Ninety-six percent of individuals with SMA have exon 7 deletions from both copies of the *SMN1* gene, usually inherited from carrier parents.[40] Once a diagnosis of SMA is confirmed, it is important to evaluate the infant's respiratory status. Given bulbar dysfunction, it is important to check the infant's nutritional status. If there are contractures, physical therapy and orthopedic evaluation are warranted.

Management

Prior to 2017, mainstay treatment for SMA was based on symptoms. Infants with SMA I and SMA II have gastric dysmotility and gastroesophageal reflux. As a result, gastrostomy tubes were almost always needed in infants with SMA. Respiratory support for hypoventilation can range from using bilevel positive airway pressure (BiPAP) to mechanical ventilation. Because there is a poor gag reflex, suctioning and chest physiotherapy are important as well. The SMA Care group has diagnosis and management guidelines detailing pulmonary and acute care management.[41] If severe scoliosis occurs, surgical repair using a vertical expandable prosthetic titanium rib can be considered.[42] Although this procedure shows better forced vital capacity during pulmonary function studies, the predicted forced vital capacity decreases over time.[43]

The landscape of SMA management, particularly in SMA type I, changed dramatically in 2017 when the FDA approved nusinersen for clinical use. Nusinersen is an RNA antisense nucleotide that alters the *SMN2* transcript so exon 7 is included. This increases the amount of SMN protein.[44,45] The major limitation is that it can only be administered intrathecally and must be given in repeated regular intervals. Effective presymptomatic treatment options led to the addition of SMA to the Recommended Uniform Screening Panel for newborn screening in the USA.[46] Gene addition with adeno-associated virus-9 vectors containing the *SMN1* gene are given in a one-time intravenous infusion. Preliminary findings from treatment studies have been promising.[47] In June 2019, gene therapy (onasemnogene abeparvovec-xiol) was approved in the USA for treatment of children less than 2 years old with SMA who have two *SMN1* mutations and two or three copies of *SMN2*. Risdiplam, approved in August 2020, is similar to Nusinersen since it uses mRNA splicing. However, this medication is available orally and can be taken in any affected patient over 2 months of age.[47a]

Long-Term Outcomes

With SMA type I, survival was 8 months with death typically before 2 years of age.[48] As shown in Table 79.5, life expectancy increases with the number of *SMN2* copies. However, with nusinersen and gene replacement therapy, this landscape will change because life expectancy for SMA type I is likely to dramatically increase.

Congenital Myotonic Dystrophy Type 1

Myotonic dystrophy type 1 (MD1) has a wide spectrum of clinical findings depending on the exact mutation and repeat size. The most severe form, congenital MD1, has an incidence between 1 in 3500 and 1 in 16,000 live births, depending on the studied population.[49–51]

Pathophysiology

The *DMPK* gene encodes the myotonic dystrophy protein kinase (DMPK). Abnormal RNA transcript processing can lead to expansion of a C-T-G repeat in the 3′ untranslated region of the *DMPK* gene. Having more than 50 C-T-G repeats disrupts the normal function of the musclebind-like protein (MBNL) and CUG binding protein (CUGBP). Normally MBNL and CUGBP process RNA by mediating alternative splicing, including developmental regulation. When the *DMPK* gene with the expanded repeat is transcribed into mRNA, the MBNL protein binds to this CUG-rich region and is sequestered. This change in proteins available for alternative splicing leads to disruptions in many proteins including TNNT2, which affects the heart and skeletal muscle, and the insulin receptor. This causes inappropriate protein translation and causes many of the clinical features seen in the MD1.[52]

An interesting characteristic of the *DMPK* mutation is anticipation. When there are more than 34 C-T-G repeats, the gene becomes unstable and the repeats can expand in size during meiosis in the mother, leading to more C-T-G repeats in the offspring. The greater the number of repeats, the earlier the onset of clinical features. In congenital MD1, for which there are normally more than 1000 C-T-G repeats, most cases are due to anticipation from the maternally inherited *DMPK* gene.

Clinical Features

Prenatally there is concern for congenital MD1 with decreased fetal movement and polyhydramnios.[53] At birth, generalized hypotonia and weakness are prominent. There can be striking facial diplegia, which leads to a characteristic upper lip that resembles an inverted V or tenting. There can be significant feeding and swallowing difficulties. Weakness of the diaphragm and aspiration lead to respiratory distress in up to 25% to 50% of infants.[51] Tight heel cords and talipes equinovarus are also common.

Evaluation

To establish a diagnosis of congenital MD1, targeted testing is performed to assess the number of C-T-G repeats in the *DMPK* gene. Pulmonary function tests are important to assess respiratory capacity.

Management

Management is targeted to symptom severity.[54] Respiratory support may require mechanical ventilation. With hyptonia and weakened facial muscles, feeding is difficult and often requires feeding access. With feeding therapies and time, this can improve. To avoid contractures, occupational and physical therapy are beneficial. For the talipes equinovarus, serial casting or even surgery may be warranted. If the individual requires surgery, precautions should be taken due to increased complications with anesthesia.

Currently there is a clinical trial assessing the efficacy and safety of tideglusib, an inhibitor of glycogen synthase kinase 3, in MD1.

Long-Term Outcomes

Within the first month there is 20% mortality, mostly due to respiratory compromise. Requiring ventilatory support for more than 30 days is usually a poor prognosticator. For those who survive past infancy, myotonia will develop in time and is universal by 10 years of age. Facial weakness makes speech delay and subsequent dysarthria common. Vision can be compromised with hyperopia or astigmatism. Intellectual disabilities are commonly seen with congenital MD1, although the exact mechanism is unclear. Those with congenital MD1 can live into their mid-30s.[51]

CHAPTER 80

Common Chromosomal Conditions in Newborns

Marisa Gilstrop Thompson, Eric Jelin, Angie Jelin

KEY POINTS

1. Chromosomal abnormalities can be numerical abnormalities (aneuploidy), structural anomalies such as copy number variants (microdeletions or duplications), inversions, translocations, and the formation of isochromosomes or ring chromosomes.
2. Sex chromosome abnormalities such as Turner syndrome, triple X syndrome, and Klinefelter syndrome have been studied.
3. The most common prenatally diagnosed aneuploidies include trisomy 13, trisomy 18, and trisomy 21. Trisomy 13 and 18 can be diagnosed on prenatal ultrasound by multiple anomalies. Trisomy 21 is frequently seen and is characterized by a widely variable phenotype with intellectual disability and an average life span of 6 decades.
4. Microdeletion and microduplication syndromes include a host of phenotypes that typically involve some level of intellectual disability and characteristic physical features. DiGeorge syndrome has been studied extensively in view of its association with congenital cardiac defects. Other notable microdeletion/microduplication disorders include deletion 1p36, Wolf-Hirschhorn, cri-du-chat, Williams-Beuren, and WAGR (Wilms tumor–aniridia–genitourinary anomalies–retarded development) syndromes. All aneuploidies, microdeletions, and microduplications require testing through a chromosomal microarray.

Introduction

Chromosomal conditions affect 1 in 150 live births[1] and include numerical abnormalities (aneuploidy) and smaller chromosomal structural abnormalities such as copy number variants (CNVs) (microdeletions or duplications), inversions, translocations, and the formation of isochromosomes or ring chromosomes (Fig. 80.1).[2] In this chapter, we focus on some of the more frequently seen aneuploidies that affect the newborn and are often compatible with survival, such as Turner syndrome, triple X syndrome, Klinefelter syndrome, and trisomies of chromosomes 13, 18, and 21. The prognosis for aneuploidies varies widely and includes patients with trisomy 21 living into their 60s; patients with trisomy 13 or 18, rarely living beyond their first year; and most other autosomal trisomies resulting in early pregnancy losses. Unless there is mosaicism, trisomies such as those of chromosome 16, frequently result in first-trimester spontaneous miscarriages.

Most cases of aneuploidy are identified prenatally through screening with cell-free DNA and/or sonographic findings. Confirmatory diagnostic testing is performed prenatally via chorionic villus sampling or amniocentesis.[3] Postnatally, the diagnosis may be suspected based on an abnormal physical exam or laboratory test findings, and confirmatory testing is typically performed on blood. Standard karyotype techniques detect additional or absent chromosome material including chromosomal duplications and deletions greater than 5 to 10 Mb in size.[2] The karyotype can also be used to evaluate the chromosome configuration and identify translocated chromosomal material and ring chromosomes.

CNVs entail a large group of structural alterations within a chromosome resulting in extra or missing copies of specific regions of DNA and are typically detected via chromosomal microarray. They are classified as pathologic, benign, or of uncertain significance, and some CNVs have variable expressivity. The most common clinical feature of a CNV is intellectual disability.[4] The most well-known and well-described microdeletion syndrome is DiGeorge syndrome, a microdeletion in 22q11.2.[5] Family members affected with a pathogenic 22q11.2 deletion exhibit variable clinical severity; some require medical treatment and frequent hospitalization whereas others require no clinical interventions.

The pathogenicity of a CNV is dependent on whether it is a duplication or deletion, its size/length, whether it is of parental origin (such as in Prader-Willi syndrome [PWS] and Angelman syndrome), and the function of the genes involved within that segment. These details are best clarified by chromosomal microarray.[2] Possible results when testing for a CNV include "benign," with no disease-related changes seen in that patient's copy number compared with the general population; a "pathologic" result that indicates a change in the copy number compared with the general population and that is believed to contribute to a disease or disability; or a "variant of uncertain significance" result that indicates a change has been found compared with the general population, but with an uncertain relationship of this change to disease.[6] Patients who are interested in undergoing testing for CNVs should be counseled regarding their personal beliefs and attitudes about the potential outcome of having a child with disabilities. Furthermore, counseling should include the idea that identification of a variant may be associated with a variable phenotype and may be carried be one of the parents.[7]

Turner Syndrome (Monosomy X) and Triple X Syndrome (Trisomy X)

Turner syndrome is a sex-chromosome disorder resulting in a female phenotype with only one effective X chromosome. The hallmarks of this clinical syndrome include short stature, neck webbing, widely spaced nipples, cardiovascular disease, and ovarian failure (Fig. 80.2).[8] Prenatally, ultrasound findings may include increased nuchal translucency, cystic hygroma, cardiac anomalies including aortic coarctation, or fetal hydrops[9]; more than 95% of fetuses with

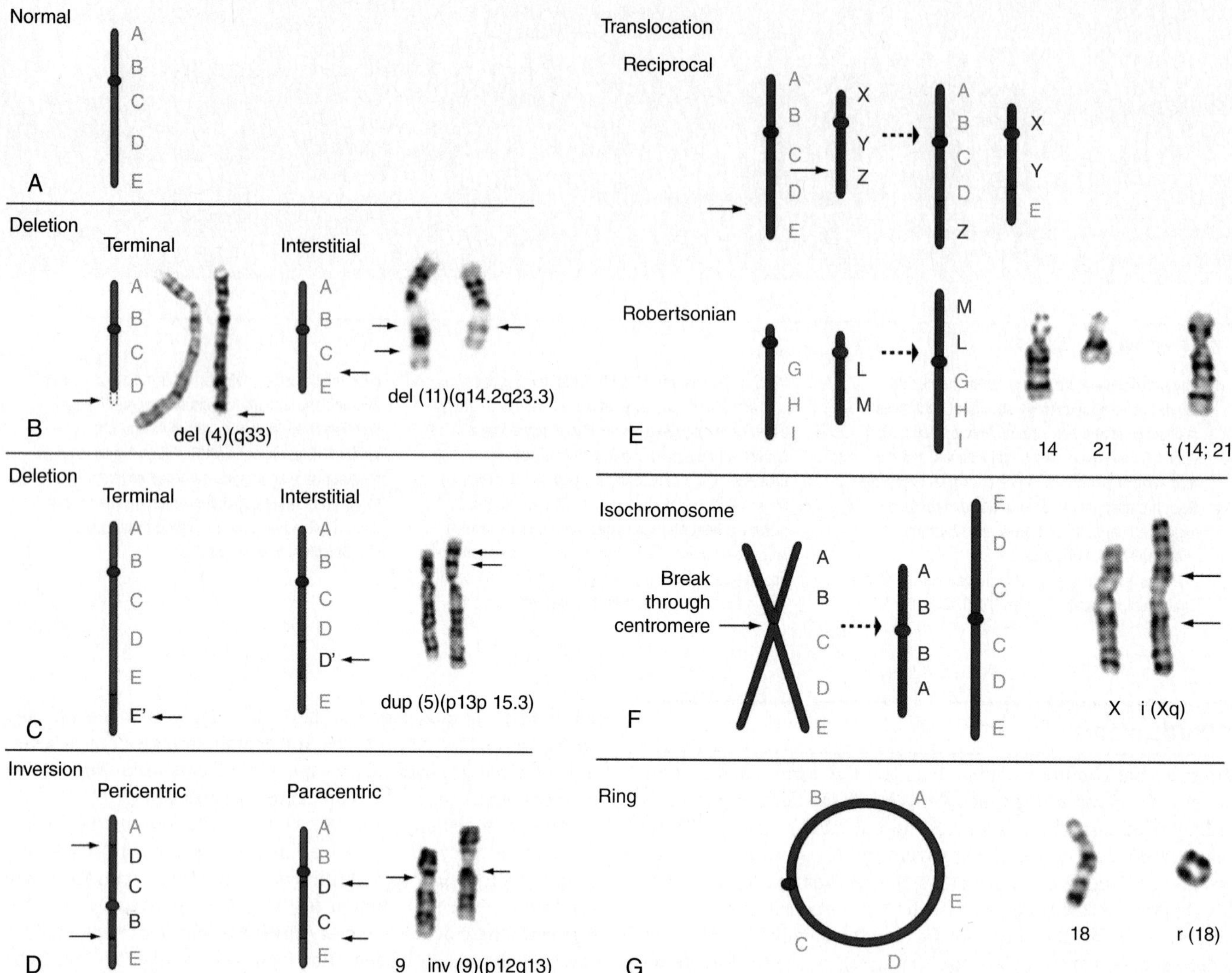

Fig. 80.1 Schematic Representation of the Most Frequent of the Structural Chromosome Anomalies. (A) The normal configuration of a generalized chromosome, where A to E represent different gene loci and the centromere is represented by a *dot* located between the B and C loci. (B) Deletion: Chromosome deletion showing terminal (loss of E locus) and interstitial (loss of D locus) configurations. Examples: Terminal deletion of the long arm of chromosome 4 and an interstitial deletion of the long arm of chromosome 11. (C) Duplication: Chromosome duplication showing terminal (gain of E′) and interstitial (gain of D′) configurations. Example: Terminal duplication of the short arm of chromosome 5 (*double arrows* indicate the duplicated band). (D) Inversion: Chromosome inversion showing pericentric and paracentric forms. Example: Pericentric inversion of chromosome 9 (*arrows* indicate centromeres). (E) Translocation: Reciprocal translocation, where the E and Z loci exchange places. The figure shows a Robertsonian translocation as the fusion of two acrocentric chromosomes at the centromere. Example: Chromosomes 14 and 21 followed by the 14;21 Robertsonian translocation. (F) Isochromosome: Results from a misdivision of the centromere, generating inverted duplications of the long and short arms of the original chromosome. Example: Isochromosome of the long arm of the X chromosome. (G) Ring chromosome. Example: Chromosome 18 and ring 18. (Reproduced with permission and minor modifications from Perle and Stein. Applications of cytogenetics in modern pathology. In: *Henry's Clinical Diagnosis and Management by Laboratory Methods*, 71, 1411–1433.e2.)

Turner syndrome end in a miscarriage.[10] If not identified prenatally, the diagnosis is most commonly suspected at birth due to lymphedema of the hands or feet, neck webbing, or nail dysplasia. Although Turner syndrome is thought to be the most common sex-chromosome abnormality in females, the true prevalence is difficult to determine due to those with a milder phenotype remaining undiagnosed.[11]

The majority of patients diagnosed with Turner syndrome are subsequently found to have monosomy X on testing. A subset of patients are found to have a mosaic complement,[12] with the remaining patients exhibiting a structural rearrangement that renders one X chromosome abnormal. Examples of these structural rearrangements include isochromosomes, ring chromosomes, or chromosomal deletions.[13]

The diagnosis of Turner syndrome is confirmed with karyotype. Both aneuploidy and structural rearrangements are readily identified by this method. After a confirmed diagnosis, patients need to be evaluated and monitored for associated anomalies including but not limited to cardiac disease, hearing and eye abnormalities, and learning disabilities.[11] As the patient ages, counseling should be performed regarding the differences in fertility compared with the general population. Overall mortality rates are increased approximately threefold for patients with Turner syndrome compared with the general population. This has been found at all ages and for many major causes of death.[14]

Triple X syndrome, defined as a female with a 47,XXX genotype, presents with a widely variable phenotype. Clinical features include taller height compared with their cohorts, some cognitive disability, psychological disorders, and/or a delay in motor milestones.[15]

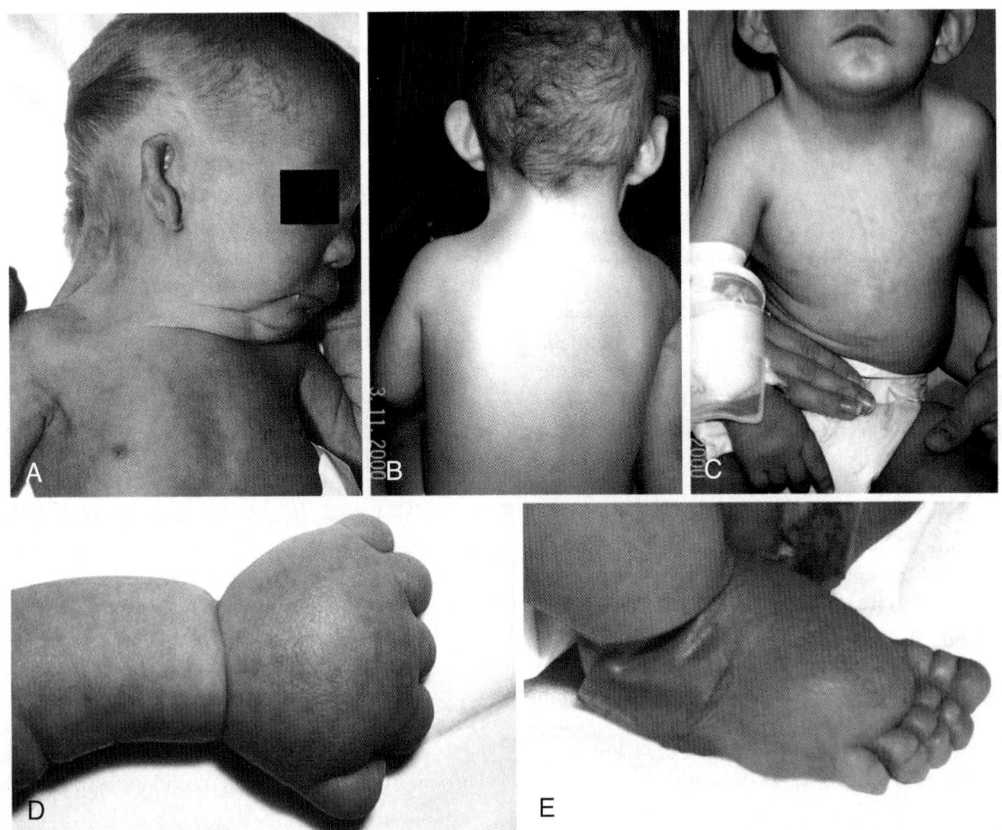

Fig. 80.2 Physical Manifestations Associated With Turner Syndrome. (A) Webbed neck with low hairline, shield chest with widely spaced nipples, abnormal ears, and micrognathia. (B) Low-set posterior hairline seen in an older child who also has protruding ears. (C) Mild webbing of the neck; prominent, low-set, forward-protruding ears; small, widely spaced nipples. The midline scar is from a prior cardiac surgery. (D, E) Prominent lymphedema of the hands and feet. (From Ferri. Turner syndrome. In: *Ferri's Clinical Advisor*, 2022:1532.e2–1532.e3.)

Puberty and fertility are generally unaffected, but some women are at risk for early menopause. This syndrome does not have any specific fetal markers notable on ultrasound and is rarely diagnosed prenatally. Many individuals are asymptomatic throughout their lives and remain undiagnosed.[16] The diagnosis of triple X syndrome is made via standard karyotype, in which the number of X chromosomes can be readily counted.

Turner syndrome and triple X syndrome are not typically inherited. The etiology of these syndromes, as with most aneuploidies, is due to nondisjunction of either the egg or sperm cells during meiosis. If nondisjunction occurs after conception, the patient may present with a mosaic version of these syndromes.[2]

Klinefelter Syndrome

Klinefelter syndrome is another sex-chromosome abnormality of a phenotypic male with an extra X chromosome. The most common clinical features include tall stature, small testes, and infertility. Although overall intelligence is typically within the normal range, learning difficulties may be present.[17] Many boys with Klinefelter syndrome do not show any obvious signs of the syndrome in infancy or childhood, and there are no specific sonographic findings noted prenatally. Some children may exhibit hypotonia and delayed motor milestones, with the average age of walking without therapeutic intervention documented at 18 months.[18]

There are some males with more than two X chromosomes. The greater the number of X chromosomes, the more severe the phenotype is.[19] Patients with greater numbers of X chromosomes may have lower IQs and more pronounced physical features or may exhibit congenital cardiac disease.

Similar to Turner and triple X syndrome, Klinefelter syndrome is diagnosed via standard karyotype. This provides the ability to determine the specific number of X chromosomes and subsequently to provide appropriate counseling for the patient. In general, patients with Klinefelter syndrome live a full life span compared with the general population. Counseling should include information that the incidence of breast cancer can be approximately 57 times higher in patients with Klinefelter compared with the general population.[20]

Jacobs Syndrome

Jacobs syndrome, also known as 47,XYY syndrome, is characterized by an extra copy of the Y chromosome in each of a male's cells. It is believed to occur in approximately 1 out of every 1000 boys.[21] On physical examination, males may be taller than their cohorts and have macrocephaly, clinodactyly, and hypertelorism.[22] There have been no associated findings of infertility or abnormal sexual development, but clinically, patients with Jacobs syndrome have been noted to have an increased risk of learning disabilities, language delays, motor delays, and behavioral disorders.[23] There are no specific prenatal findings for this disorder, and most prenatal diagnoses are made incidentally.

As with other sex-chromosome aneuploidies, Jacobs syndrome is best identified through standard karyotype to identify the number of Y chromosomes present. Nondisjunction during meiosis is the most common etiology for this karyotype, with postzygotic nondisjunction during mitosis being the cause of mosaic 46XY/47XYY patients.[24] Most patients with 47,XYY have a delayed diagnosis, with a median age of 17.1 years at diagnosis.[25] Counseling should include information regarding a decreased life expectancy, with cancer, pulmonary, and trauma etiologies being the main source of increased mortality rates for these patients.[21]

Trisomy 13 and Trisomy 18

Trisomy 13, also known as Patau syndrome, is a chromosomal condition defined by a karyotype with an additional copy (or portion) of chromosome 13. Clinical features of Patau syndrome include but are not limited to congenital heart anomalies, cleft lip/palate, hypotonia, and brain abnormalities (Fig. 80.3). All surviving individuals have severe intellectual disability. Trisomy 13 occurs in about 1 in 12,000 to 20,000 newborns, with an increased incidence in offspring of older women.[2] Trisomy 18, also known as Edwards syndrome, is a chromosomal condition defined by an additional copy (or portion) of chromosome 18. Similar to trisomy 13, patients with trisomy 18 may also have congenital heart and brain anomalies, with the distinction of overlapping/clenched fingers and growth restriction (Table 80.1; Fig. 80.4). Trisomy 18 occurs in approximately 1 in 6000 to 8000 newborns.[2] For both trisomies, less than 10% of patients survive beyond the first year of life due to the severe range of medical conditions associated with these disorders.

Trisomy 13 and trisomy 18 are often suspected in pregnancies based on results of abnormal first- or second-trimester screening tests or abnormal ultrasound findings. Diagnostic testing sent for karyotype on a chorionic villus sample or amniotic fluid is recommended.[26] Although cell-free fetal DNA is a highly sensitive screening test, it should not be used for diagnostic purposes.

Management of trisomy 13 and trisomy 18 largely depends on the individual patient's symptoms and severity of the condition. Common symptoms include apnea, feeding difficulties with or without cleft lip/palate, seizures, and heart anomalies. Because both trisomies 13 and 18 have low survival rates, in most centers management is largely centered on supportive care, and surgical interventions are generally withheld.[27,28] Multidisciplinary teams that include the newborn's parents have been found to be most beneficial in creating a treatment plan that balances each intervention with the limited potential of long-term survival.

In the majority of cases of trisomy 13 or 18, the causative event occurs during meiosis.[2] This event is usually an error in nondisjunction. This error has been found to occur more frequently in women's eggs as they age, creating an increased incidence of these conditions in offspring of older women.

Trisomy 21

Trisomy 21, also known as Down syndrome, is the most common chromosomal condition diagnosed in the United States, occurring in

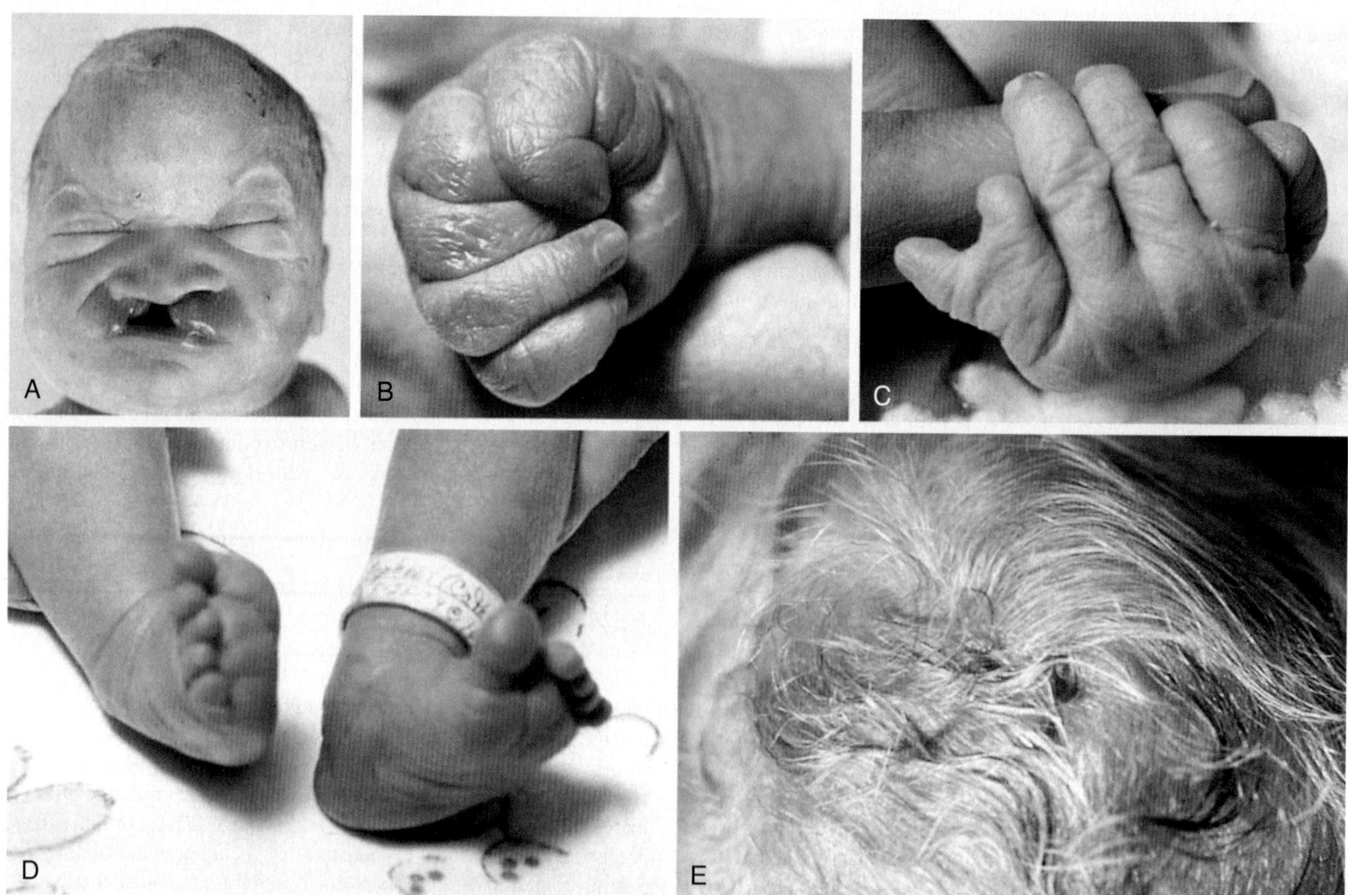

Fig. 80.3 Physical Manifestations Associated With Trisomy 13. (A) Facies showing midline defect. (B) Clenched hand with overlapping fingers. (C) Postaxial polydactyly. (D) Equinovarus deformity. (E) Typical punched-out scalp lesions of *aplasia cutis congenita*. (From Madan-Khetarpal et al. Genetic disorders and dysmorphic conditions. In: *Zitelli and Davis' Atlas of Pediatric Physical Diagnosis*, 2018.)

Table 80.1 Physical Abnormalities and the Frequency of Occurrence in Trisomy 13 and Trisomy 18 Syndromes[a]

Abnormality	Trisomy 13	Trisomy 18
Severe developmental retardation	++++	++++
Approximately 90% die within first year	++++	++++
Cryptorchidism in males	++++	++++
Low-set, malformed ears	++++	++++
Multiple major congenital anomalies	++++	++++
Prominent occiput	+	++++
Cleft lip and/or palate	+++	+
Micrognathia	++	+++
Microphthalmos	+++	++
Coloboma of iris	+++	+
Short sternum	+	+++
Rocker-bottom feet	++	+++
Congenital heart disease	++	++++
Scalp defects	+++	+
Flexion deformities of fingers	++	++++
Polydactyly	+++	+
Hypoplasia of nails	++	+++
Hypertonia in infancy	+	+++
Apneic spells in infancy	+++	+
Midline brain defects	+++	+
Horseshoe kidneys	+	+++

[a]The number of plus signs (+) indicates the relative frequency of each abnormality.

1 of 850 live births.[2] This syndrome is caused by extra material from chromosome 21 and results in a wide range of phenotypes. All patients with Down syndrome will have some form of intellectual disability but may also have heart anomalies, feeding difficulties, and a group of physical features that include a flattened face, almond-shaped eyes, and a single palmar crease (Fig. 80.5). The average life span for an individual with Down syndrome is 60 years.[29,30]

The cytogenetic arrangement by which the patient has extra material from chromosome 21 may be used to divide Down syndrome into "types." The *classic type* involves three separate copies of chromosome 21 in each cell instead of the typical two copies. This accounts for 95% of individuals diagnosed with Down syndrome. Approximately 3% of patients have an extra part of or a whole chromosome 21 attached to another chromosome, also known as a Robertsonian *translocation.* The remaining 2% of patients have *mosaic* Down syndrome, in which some cells have three copies of chromosome 21 and other cells have the typical two copies of chromosome 21.[31] These three types will all appear the same on non-invasive prenatal screening (NIPS) during pregnancy but can be differentiated through diagnostic testing via a karyotype obtained through chorionic villus sampling or an amniocentesis. Postnatally, a karyotype should be performed on peripheral blood, with specific tissue sampling if there is a negative blood test and a concern for mosaic Down syndrome.[32]

Similar to trisomy 13 or 18, management of trisomy 21 is largely dependent on the individual patient's symptoms and the severity of their condition. Unlike trisomies 13 and 18, patients with trisomy 21 are almost always offered life-saving or life-prolonging surgeries and interventions, because this condition is not associated with a high mortality rate. With Down syndrome being a very well-known condition, there are many services and groups available to help diagnosed children with management of their intellectual and

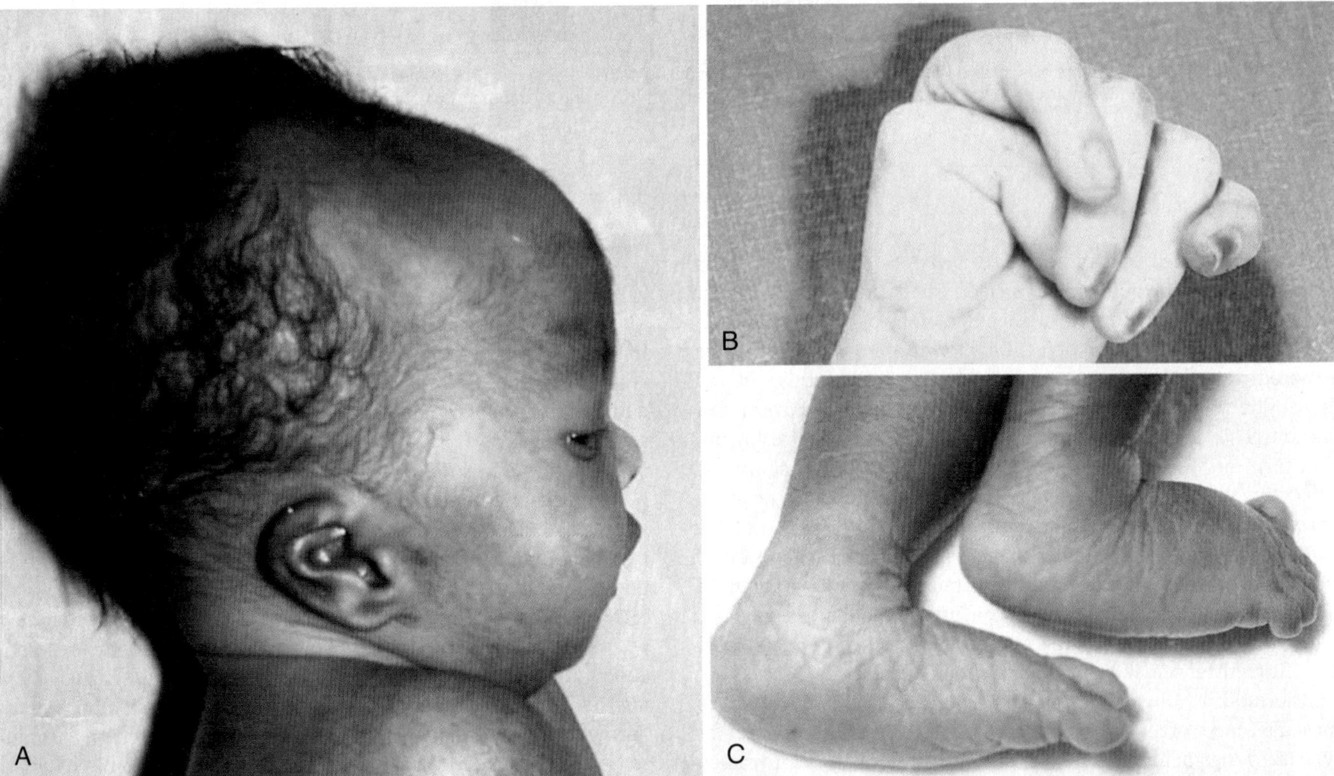

Fig. 80.4 Physical Manifestations Associated With Trisomy 18. (A) Prominent occiput and low-set, posteriorly rotated malformed auricles. (B) Clenched hand showing the typical pattern of overlapping fingers. (C) Rocker-bottom feet. (From: Madan-Khetarpal et al. Genetic disorders and dysmorphic conditions. In: *Zitelli and Davis' Atlas of Pediatric Physical Diagnosis*, 2018.)

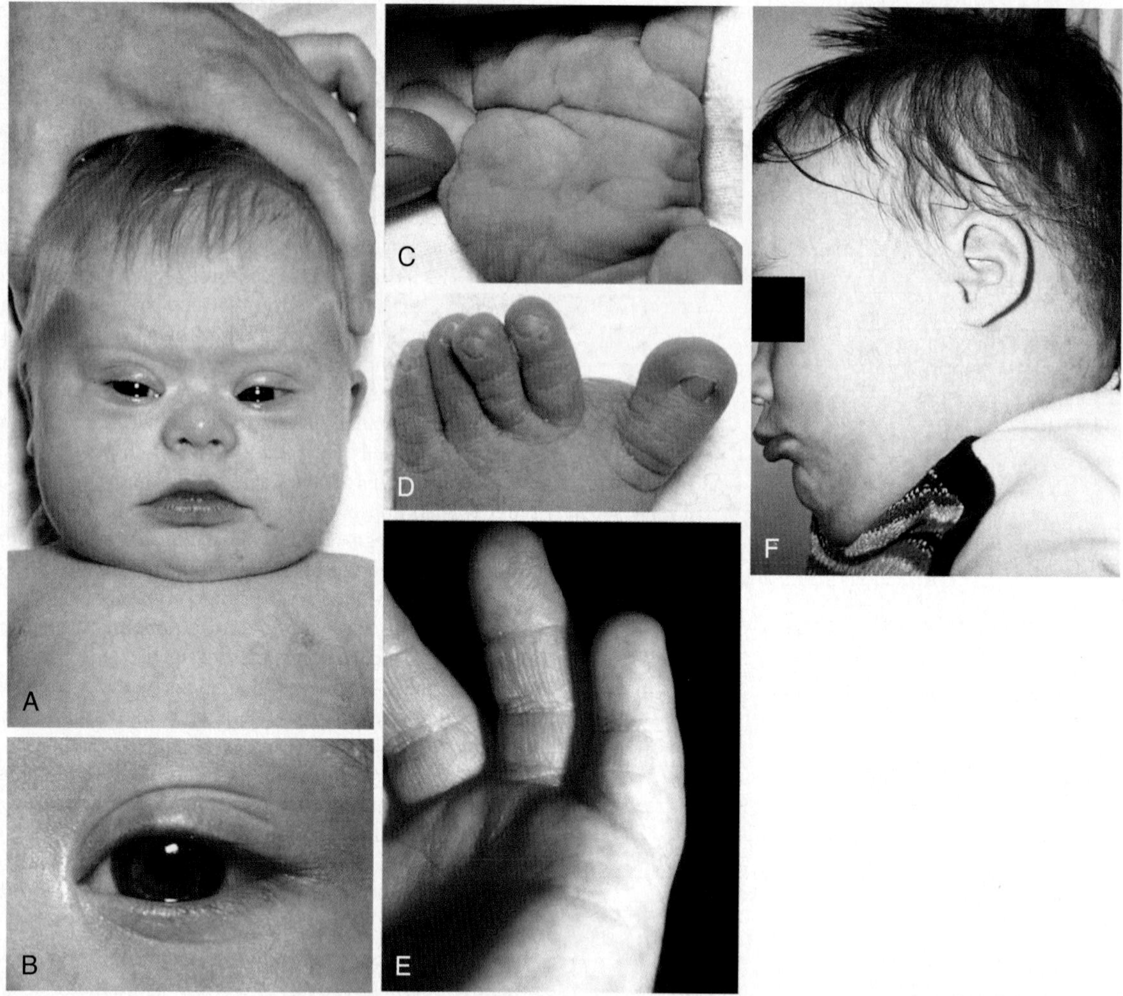

Fig. 80.5 Physical Manifestations Associated With Down Syndrome. (A) Upslanting palpebral fissures. (B) Brushfield spots. (C) Single palmar crease. (D) Sandal gap deformity. (E) Clinodactyly. (F) Brachycephaly. (From Madan-Khetarpal et al. Genetic disorders and dysmorphic conditions. In: *Zitelli and Davis' Atlas of Pediatric Physical Diagnosis*, 2018.)

physical disabilities. The American Academy of Pediatrics also offers a health supervision guideline to assist the pediatrician in caring for a child with Down syndrome at each age group.[33]

Similar to other aneuploidies, Down syndrome is thought to be a sporadic event during conception and is typically not considered to be inherited. Occasionally, unaffected parents may have a balanced translocation of chromosome 13, 18, or 21 which may result in a form of "inherited" trisomy 13, trisomy 18, or trisomy 21, respectively. A parent with a balanced translocation has an overall normal number of genes, collectively, but the configuration of the chromosomes results in a higher chance of passing on the rearranged "abnormal" chromosome to offspring. Parents with a known balanced translocation are at a higher risk of having subsequent pregnancies affected by a trisomy regardless of their age at conception, with the specific recurrence risk being dependent on which chromosomes are translocated. In Down syndrome, the translocation between chromosome 21 and other acrocentric chromosomes results in a particular type of arrangement called a Robertsonian translocation.[2] For women with a previous pregnancy affected by trisomy 21 who do not have a translocation, the recurrence risk is approximately 1% higher than their baseline age-associated risk.[31]

Microdeletion/Microduplication Syndromes

The phrase "microdeletion syndrome" is used to describe disorders in which one or more small segments of a chromosome are deleted, resulting in specific related clinical syndromes (Table 80.2).[34] The deletions are smaller than 5 million base pairs (5 Mb) and may span several genes that are too small to be detected by conventional cytogenetic methods or high-resolution karyotyping. One of the most recognized microdeletion disorders is DiGeorge syndrome, also known as 22q11.2 deletion syndrome. DiGeorge provides a classic representation of microdeletion syndromes in that it affects multiple body systems with high variability in expressivity. Also similar to many microdeletion syndromes, 22q11.2 syndrome can manifest with psychiatric symptoms or learning/developmental delays.[35] Other recognized examples of disorders commonly caused by a microdeletion are PWS and Angelman syndrome. Both of these syndromes are due to the loss of functioning genes located on chromosome 15 (15q11-q13). If the gene function is lost from the paternal copy of chromosome 15, it results in PWS, whereas if the gene loss comes from the maternal copy of chromosome 15, it results in Angelman syndrome.[36] Although there are different etiologies for the loss

Table 80.2 Syndromes Associated With Chromosomal Microdeletions

Syndrome	Major Findings	Comments
Cri-du-chat (deletion 5p15.2)	Microcephaly, round face, down-slanting palpebral fissures, epicanthal folds, hypertelorism, catlike cry in infancy	
Isolated lissencephaly	Lissencephaly (incomplete development of brain with smooth surface)	Approximately 30% have deletion 17p13.3
Miller-Dieker phenotype with lissencephaly	Microcephaly, lissencephaly, variable high forehead, vertical furrowing of central forehead, low-set ears, small nose with anteverted nostrils, congenital heart disease, poor feeding	Deletion 17p13.3 in vast majority

of these genes (including uniparental disomy), 70% of cases are due to a microdeletion.[37] Both disorders result in some form of intellectual disability. Patients with PWS are known for their overeating and short stature, and Angelman patients are known for their uncoordinated jerking movements and happy disposition. In the newborn period, patients with PWS typically present with poor feeding because of weak suck and low muscle tone, whereas patients with Angelman syndrome may not present until later in life with delayed milestones or seizures.

Additional well-described microdeletion syndromes to note include cri-du-chat, deletion 1p36, Wolf-Hirschhorn, Williams-Beuren, and Wilms tumor–aniridia–genitourinary anomalies–retarded development (WAGR) syndromes. Phenotypes for these syndromes range from the expected learning/intellectual disability found in almost all microdeletion syndromes to an increase in tumor susceptibility. Phenotypes are found to have highly variable expressivity. Cri-du-chat syndrome is known for the pathognomonic high-pitched cry, whereas Wolf-Hirchhorn patients have iris colobomas. Management of these syndromes involves individualized subspecialty care determined by the patient's symptoms.[38–40]

Microduplication syndromes involve disorders in which small chromosomal segments, typically one to three megabases (Mb) long, are duplicated.[41] These duplicated segments involve contiguous genes. As with microdeletion syndromes, these genetic changes are too small to be detected by conventional cytogenetic methods or high-resolution karyotyping and are diagnosed through microarray. The phenotype of microduplication syndromes are not as well-characterized as microdeletion syndromes but typically involve psychiatric manifestations or learning/developmental delays in addition to a specific constellation of physical exam findings.[42]

As with all chromosomal disorders, there is no treatment for microdeletion or microduplication syndromes. Management is focused on multidisciplinary teams that can concentrate on the individual symptoms the patient may have. Early interventions such as occupational and physical therapies are also recommended to assist in long-term planning of the child's needs.

SECTION

17 Neonatal Surgical Conditions

OUTLINE

CHAPTER 81

Necrotizing Enterocolitis

Jennine Weller, Maame E. S. Sampah, Andres J. Gonzalez Salazar, David J. Hackam

KEY POINTS

1. Necrotizing enterocolitis (NEC) is a disease of premature infants that results in life-threatening intestinal ischemia and necrosis.
2. Suspect NEC presents in a stable, formula-fed premature neonate who suddenly develops feeding intolerance and abdominal distention. Infants with suspected disease have abdominal distention, bilious emesis, and bloody stools but no specific radiographic features of NEC. Some of these infants may have temperature instability, apnea, bradycardia, or lethargy.
3. In infants with definite NEC, bowel ischemia becomes detectable on abdominal radiography with the presence of pneumatosis. Many have abdominal tenderness, cellulitis, metabolic acidosis, and thrombocytopenia.
4. Advanced NEC progresses to frank bowel wall necrosis causing intestinal perforation and pneumoperitoneum, peritonitis, septic shock, disseminated intravascular coagulation, and ultimately circulatory collapse.
5. Advances in circulating biomarkers and imaging may help in earlier diagnosis of NEC.
6. Medical management of NEC comprises bowel rest with gastrointestinal decompression, parenteral nutrition, careful administration of fluids, and broad-spectrum antibiotics.
7. Surgery is indicated in infants with pneumoperitoneum and/or portal venous gas. Infants with rapidly increasing clinical instability with extensive intestinal disease, severe thrombocytopenia, anemia, or metabolic acidosis may also benefit from surgical exploration.

Introduction

Necrotizing enterocolitis (NEC) is a disease of premature infants that results in life-threatening intestinal ischemia and necrosis. Approximately 1 to 3 per 1000 infants born in the United States will develop NEC,[1,2] and NEC is the leading cause of death due to gastrointestinal pathology in premature infants.[3] The incidence of NEC is inversely proportional to gestational age, making the disease relatively rare in full-term infants and more common in premature infants.[3] The incidence is as high as 13% in infants born at or before 33 weeks' gestation or weighing less than 2500 g.[3,4] Black and Hispanic infants also have higher incidence of and mortality from NEC, demonstrating that racial disparities exist for NEC care.[5–8]

The average mortality risk for NEC is 20% to 30%[9] but can approach 50% in patients with significant bowel injury.[10] Infants who survive NEC are also at risk for serious long-term morbidity. Damage to the brain and bowel from NEC causes lasting neurocognitive injury in 30% to 50% of survivors.[3,11] Intestinal strictures from ischemic injury occur in 12% to 35% of infants.[3,12] Complications also arise from the surgical management of NEC, with significant bowel resections resulting in short bowel syndrome (SBS) (20%–35%)[13] and growth delay (10%).[3,14]

Risk Factors

The etiology of NEC remains an active area of investigation. However, clinical and experimental data implicate immature immune signaling and abnormal microbial colonization of the intestinal mucosa. These factors contribute to the characteristic intestinal necrosis and inflammation associated with NEC.[3,15]

Clinically, the most significant risk factor for NEC is prematurity.[16,17] Formula feeding,[18] blood transfusions,[19] prolonged empiric antibiotics,[20] and use of antacids[21] are also known risk factors. From observational studies, maternal risk factors for NEC also exist and include prolonged rupture of membranes, maternal infection, Black race, preeclampsia, placental abruption, and intrauterine growth restriction.[17]

No single genetic determinant has been implicated in NEC pathogenesis, however results of twin studies suggest a familial predisposition.[18] As will be described in more detail below, NEC develops in response to the activation of the innate immune receptor, toll-like receptor 4 (TLR4), on the surface of the intestinal epithelium, which is expressed at high levels in premature compared with full-term infants.[22–24]

TLR4 activation in the intestinal epithelium leads to enterocyte death by apoptosis and necroptosis[25–28] and impaired healing via reduced proliferation and migration of enterocytes in the intestinal epithelium.[27,29,30] The reason that TLR4 is expressed at high levels in the intestinal epithelium of premature infants is found in the nonimmune role that TLR4 plays in the regulation of normal intestinal development through its activation of Wnt and Notch.[31] Thus in the presence of prematurity, when the intestinal lumen becomes colonized with microbes that express the TLR4 ligand lipopolysaccharide, TLR4 signaling switches from a developmental to an inflammatory role, and NEC develops. This "cross switching" hypothesis of NEC is fundamental to our understanding of disease pathogenesis and of our search for novel therapies.

In support of the clinical relevance of TLR4 signaling in the pathogenesis of NEC, mutations of the single immunoglobulin and toll-interleukin 1 receptor (SIGIRR) gene, an inhibitor of TLR4 activation, for instance, have been associated with NEC development.[32–35] Other gene polymorphisms under study for their association with NEC are proinflammatory cytokines such as tumor necrosis factor α,[36] interleukin (IL)–4 receptor α-chain,[37] IL-6,[38] IL-23 receptor and IL-17,[39] and vascular endothelial growth factor.[40]

The Five Clinical Presentations of NEC in Infants

NEC typically presents in a stable, formula-fed premature neonate who suddenly develops feeding intolerance and abdominal distention. NEC onset is dependent on an infant's gestational age at birth. Extremely premature infants (born at ≤27 weeks' gestation)

Table 81.1 Clinical Presentation of NEC

NEC Scenarios	Presentation	Labs and Imaging	Management	Operative Considerations
Textbook NEC	Premature infant starts formula and develops sudden abdominal distention, emesis, bloody stools *Textbook NEC* follows the classic progression through Bell's stages	• Normal leukocyte count • Mild bandemia • Stable hemoglobin • Thrombocytopenia • Pneumatosis, often in the right lower quadrant	• NPO • Medical therapy for NEC • Follow serial abdominal radiographs every 6–8 hours • Operate for progression to pneumoperitoneum	• Bowel has patchy ischemia with discrete necrotic foci • Resect all necrosed segments and evaluate for perforation • Perform a second-look procedure for all questionably viable bowel segments within 12–18 hours
NEC with refractory, nonprogressive pneumatosis	A variant of *textbook NEC* where the disease progression halts at Bell's stage II	• Persistent pneumatosis on abdominal radiograph despite maximum medical therapy • Slowly down-trending platelets and hemoglobin requiring intermittent transfusions	• Watch for alternative signs of bowel necrosis: worsening abdominal distention, ongoing transfusion requirements suggesting coagulative bowel necrosis, or increasing ventilatory/vasopressor support • Clearly communicate planned thresholds for surgery on a case-by-case basis	• The operative window is often missed, leading to extensive bowel necrosis, septic shock, coagulopathy, and circulatory collapse • Infants often benefit from reduction in intraabdominal pressure achieved with laparotomy
NEC with portal venous gas	A variant of *textbook NEC* that develops both pneumatosis and portal venous gas on abdominal radiograph	• Transient portal venous gas on an abdominal radiograph • Follow-up films often show "resolution" of portal venous gas but persistent pneumatosis	• Operate for all portal venous gas because it indicates advanced bowel necrosis	• Extent of bowel necrosis is variable • Portal venous gas does not indicate "resolved" intestinal injury; waiting to operate only worsens the extent of intestinal necrosis
Staccato NEC	An accelerated presentation compared with *textbook NEC* *Staccato NEC* presents within hours with a tense abdomen from severe ascites and rapid hemodynamic instability	• Severe thrombocytopenia, anemia, and metabolic acidosis • Extensive pneumatosis on abdominal radiographs	• Operate early on all infants with *staccato NEC*	• Expect severe ascites, extensive intestinal necrosis, and intraoperative hemodynamic instability • Waiting to operate for medical optimization only worsens the extent of intestinal necrosis • High morbidity and mortality
NEC totalis	An intraoperative finding of near-complete intestinal necrosis Can occur with any other NEC subtypes	• Severe thrombocytopenia, anemia, and metabolic acidosis • Radiographic findings are poorly sensitive for *NEC totalis*	• Continue with bowel resection unless there are major morbidities, brain injury, irreversible renal injury, fatal genetic anomaly, or informed parental choice	• *NEC totalis* alone is not a contraindication to definitive care; postoperative multidisciplinary intestinal management programs now facilitate enteral autonomy and good quality of life after extensive bowel resections

NEC, Necrotizing enterocolitis; *NPO*, nil per os (nothing by mouth).

typically develop NEC at 4 to 5 weeks of age, whereas NEC occurs within 2 weeks of age in full-term infants.[41] The inverse relationship between gestational age and NEC onset is potentially explained by the increased expression of TLR4 in the premature intestine, the delayed microbial colonization and altered T-cell–mediated adaptive immune response of the premature gut, and the frequent use of broad-spectrum antibiotics in neonatal intensive care.[3,42–44]

The presentation and progression of NEC is classically described by Bell's staging criteria, which categorize disease severity into suspected NEC (stage I), moderate NEC (stage II), and advanced NEC (stage III)[3,45] (Table 81.1). Infants with Bell's stage I disease have abdominal distention, bilious emesis, and bloody stools but no specific radiographic features of NEC.[3] Historically, high gastric residuals were also considered suspicious for NEC; however, this practice has fallen out of favor due to a lack of standardized protocols and frequent measurement error.[46] Neonates with suspected NEC may also have systemic inflammatory signs such as temperature instability, apnea, bradycardia, or lethargy.[47] When bowel ischemia from NEC becomes detectable on abdominal radiography with the presence of pneumatosis, infants are classified with Bell's stage II disease. They may also have abdominal tenderness, cellulitis, metabolic acidosis, and thrombocytopenia.[47] Finally, infants with Bell's stage III disease have progressed to frank bowel wall necrosis causing intestinal perforation and pneumoperitoneum, peritonitis, septic shock, disseminated intravascular coagulation, and ultimately circulatory collapse.[3,47]

Decades of clinical experience and a deeper understanding of the pathogenesis of NEC has taught us that NEC is not a homogeneous disease with a uniform clinical pattern but rather has several presentations that must be considered in order to appreciate a more complete understanding of how to successfully diagnose and treat this condition. We have recognized five presentations of NEC that include classic "textbook NEC," NEC that fails to improve after medical management, NEC with portal venous air, NEC *totalis*, and "staccato NEC."

Classic Textbook NEC

The classic "*textbook NEC*" presentation describes infants whose disease progression follows the classic Bell's staging descriptions, developing intestinal inflammation, ischemia, and ultimately necrosis with free air, as manifest by the presence of pneumoperitoneum on x-ray, during a 24- to 48-hour window.[48] Medical management can halt this progression in approximately 50% of infants, whereas the other half develop Bell's stage III with intestinal perforation that mandates surgical intervention.[49] However, many infants do not present with this classic "*textbook*" progression (see Table 81.1). The diagnosis of intestinal perforation is typically straightforward to establish, and surgical intervention is indicated after a period of resuscitation. We do not advocate delaying surgery while waiting for normalization of all lab values. It may be impossible to normalize the infant's physiology without resection of the diseased intestine, resulting in delayed surgery, more extensive disease, and worse outcome.

NEC That Fails to Improve After a Period of Medical Therapy

One of the most challenging diagnostic instances that occur in patients with NEC involves the child with medical disease (typically but not always with persistent pneumatosis) who fails to respond to medical therapy. These infants will typically start with *textbook NEC* that progresses to *pneumatosis* on abdominal radiograph. However, unlike *textbook NEC*, the disease will neither progress to intestinal perforation nor improve with maximal medical management. Radiographs may show persistent *pneumatosis*, persistent ileus, ascites, or some combination of these signs in the absence of free air.

Clinically, the child will display persistent abdominal fullness, with slowly down-trending platelets and hemoglobin, requiring intermittent transfusions. Platelet consumption is an important sign of coagulative necrosis of the small bowel and can be missed in the setting of transfusions that artificially stabilize thrombocytopenia.[50,51] Other concerning signs of bowel necrosis in these patients include increasing abdominal distention and increasing ventilatory or vasopressor support. In these patients, it is important to "set a line in the sand" in collaboration with the neonatology team. If the child fails to improve within 48 hours or if the child shows greater needs for ventilatory or inotropic support, for example, then surgical exploration of the abdomen is indicated.

NEC in the Presence of Portal Venous Gas

Portal venous gas is an important sign of severe NEC. In the patient who has abdominal distention and tenderness, the presence of *portal venous gas* generally indicates the presence of significant intestinal necrosis and mandates early exploration.[52] It is sufficient for the portal venous gas to be present on only a single film, because this finding may be fleeting despite the presence of extensive, irreversible intestinal damage,[52–55] and therefore its absence on later plain films does not imply resolution of bowel injury from NEC. Infants with a single radiograph showing *portal venous gas* should be treated as equivalent to those with *pneumoperitoneum* in the setting of appropriate clinical findings.

Staccato NEC

This presentation is known to all clinicians who care for infants with NEC, and it describes the child who has an extremely rapid course of deterioration. In "*staccato NEC*," patients manifest early deterioration as a reflection of progressive bowel necrosis. Within a few hours of presentation, infants with *staccato NEC* will have a tense abdomen from severe ascites, and abdominal radiographs will show some degree of *pneumatosis* with or without *portal venous gas. Staccato NEC* is associated with high mortality and is manifest by early hemodynamic instability, profound thrombocytopenia, and worsening respiratory distress due to progressive abdominal distention.[56]

NEC Totalis

NEC totalis refers to the most severe form of NEC, in which there is near-complete intestinal necrosis. Historically, *NEC totalis* was an indication for palliative care, with both surgeons and neonatologists adopting a fatalistic approach. However, with the dramatic improvements in management of patients with SBS and the dramatic success in achieving enteral autonomy as well as improvements in intestinal transplantation, the presence of *NEC totalis* need not be an immediate death sentence for a patient. Rather, in the appropriate setting, including the absence of major comorbitidies and a family that can partner and is willing to provide ongoing complex medical care, patients with *NEC totalis* can be offered intestinal resection and be considered salvageable.[57–59]

Differential Diagnoses

The initial presentation of NEC overlaps with other neonatal pathology, making early diagnosis a challenge. Signs of ileus and feeding intolerance seen at NEC onset are also present with anatomic intestinal obstructions (e.g., malrotation, intestinal atresia) or functional obstruction (e.g., Hirschsprung disease).[60] Septic ileus can mimic the hemodynamic instability and abdominal distention seen in later stages of NEC. Other causes of intestinal ischemia occur with volvulus or cardiac and hematologic disorders.[3,60] A milk protein allergy can also mimic the signs and symptoms of NEC, including radiographic features of *pneumatosis*, although this is a diagnosis of exclusion.[61]

NEC Versus Spontaneous Intestinal Perforation

It is especially important to distinguish NEC from spontaneous intestinal perforation (SIP), another disease of very low birth weight infants. SIP and NEC are different entities, although they overlap in presentation, and management strategies and prognoses markedly differ. SIP typically presents with sudden-onset pneumoperitoneum and peritonitis in the absence of bowel wall necrosis in a premature infant, usually within the first week of life.

SIP can be challenging to distinguish from NEC prior to laparotomy.[62] However, there are distinct differences in the risk factors, physical exam findings, and timing of disease onset that help distinguish between SIP and NEC. Unlike NEC, SIP is not associated with feeding onset and instead has distinct risk factors of indomethacin and postnatal steroid exposure.[63] Infants with SIP occasionally have a characteristic blue abdominal discoloration, whereas those with NEC classically have abdominal erythema and cellulitis.[62] In comparison with NEC, SIP occurs earlier: between days 7 and 10 of life in extremely low birth weight infants.[64] Patients with SIP do not display *pneumatosis intestinalis.*

Overall, distinguishing between NEC and SIP is imperative because patients with SIP can benefit from peritoneal drainage (PD) procedures whereas the ischemic bowel seen in NEC warrants

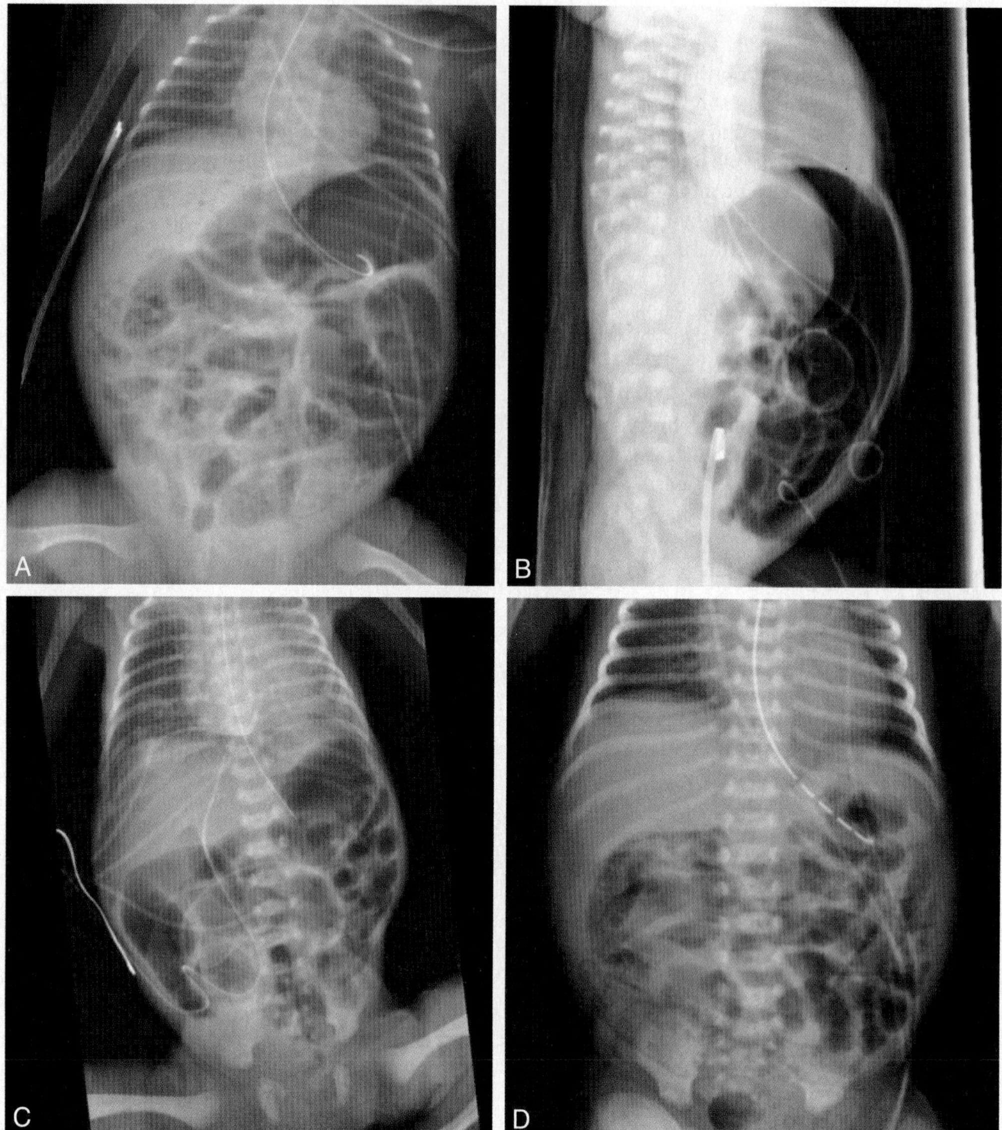

Fig. 81.1 (A) Portal venous air and pneumatosis intestinalis in necrotizing enterocolitis (NEC). (B) Pneumoperitoneum in a patient with severe NEC. (C) Intestinal ileus and pneumoperitoneum in NEC. (D) Significant pneumatosis intestinalis in necrotizing enterocolitis.

surgical exploration and bowel resection.[65] Outcomes of SIP are also better than those of NEC, and SIP does not result in long-term neurologic deficits.[66,67]

Diagnosis

Imaging

Upon clinical suspicion for NEC, serial anteroposterior and lateral abdominal radiographs every 6 to 8 hours are helpful to assess for disease progression.[68] Radiographs of early, suspected NEC frequently show nonspecific bowel distention.[47,69] As intestinal inflammation and ischemia develop, radiographs reveal focal distention of the bowel that progresses to bowel wall thickening and fixed intestinal loops.[69] A paucity of abdominal gas is also concerning for NEC.[47,70]

The hallmark diagnosis of NEC is radiographic evidence of *pneumatosis intestinalis* or portal venous gas (Fig. 81.1A, B). This extraluminal gas is a result of intestinal bacterial fermentation producing hydrogen gas, which then dissects the bowel wall and enters the portal venous system.[71,72] *Pneumatosis* and portal venous gas are highly specific (92%–100%) but poorly sensitive (34%–44%) for bowel injury that is due to NEC.[70]

As mentioned above, pneumoperitoneum is another diagnostic feature of radiographic NEC that requires prompt surgical intervention[72] (see Fig. 81.1C). Secondary to bowel perforation from intestinal necrosis, pneumoperitoneum may present with a large radiolucency over the abdomen, called the "football sign," or may be seen as air under the diaphragm. Although it has been reported that only approximately half of patients with perforated bowel from NEC have detectable pneumoperitoneum on imaging,[70] this figure is probably an overstatement. The message, though, is that the absence of pneumoperitoneum does not exclude the presence of intestinal perforation.

During the past decade, abdominal ultrasound has gained popularity as an alternative imaging modality for NEC.[68] Ultrasound enables visualization of early signs of NEC including decreased bowel peristalsis, intestinal wall thickening, and decreased bowel wall perfusion.[47] A recent meta-analysis showed that similar to abdominal radiographs, bowel ultrasound for NEC has low sensitivity but high specificity and is a reasonable adjunct for an NEC diagnosis.[73]

Biomarkers and Laboratory Parameters for the Diagnosis of NEC

There has been significant interest in identifying serum, fecal, and urine biomarkers that detect the intestinal inflammation and bowel wall injury seen in NEC.[74] Increases in acute-phase reactants such as C-reactive protein, serum amyloid A, chemokines, cytokines, and interleukins are nonspecific findings seen with NEC, yet they have been correlated with NEC severity and with need for surgery.[75,76] Markers for intestinal injury, such as intestinal fatty acid-binding protein (I-FABP),[77,78] fecal calprotectin,[79] and claudin-3,[80] can also assist the evaluation of patients with NEC. Trends in these markers may be more useful than any individual marker in isolation.

I-FABP is an enterocyte intracellular protein that is released with mucosal injury, and elevated levels in the urine and plasma are specific (91%) but not sensitive (64%) for diagnosing NEC.[77,81] Infants with elevated I-FABP at birth and during their first feeding are also more likely develop NEC.[82] Fecal calprotectin has high sensitivity (76%–100%) for bowel perforation and may have a role in differentiating Bell's stage IIB from stage III.[79,83,72] Urine claudin-3 is another potential biomarker for early detection of surgical NEC.[80]

Despite these findings, systematic reviews consistently report limited evidence for the utility of biomarkers for screening and diagnosis of NEC.[84–86] Therefore the current recommendation for NEC screening and management involves the evaluation of routine laboratory parameters in conjunction with imaging studies. Routine laboratory parameters assess disease severity and guide balanced fluid resuscitation in neonatal critical care.[87] Leukocytosis or leukopenia, thrombocytopenia, metabolic acidosis, glucose instability, and elevated C-reactive protein are frequently observed in infants with NEC.[50,86,88–90] Neutropenia, thrombocytopenia, and metabolic acidosis are associated with a poor prognosis and need for surgery, whereas a resolution of thrombocytopenia can indicate clinical improvement.[50,89,91] Therefore trending complete blood counts (CBC), serum chemistries, lactate, and blood gases are useful adjuncts to detect bowel ischemia, metabolic acidosis, and electrolyte derangements in the setting of diagnosed or suspected NEC.

Management

There are two fundamental pillars of NEC management:

1. Minimize NEC progression with medical management to prevent the development of intestinal necrosis.
2. Quickly identify and resect intestinal necrosis to obtain source control and limit the systemic inflammatory response.

Surgical exploration for pneumoperitoneum remains an absolute operative indication for infants with NEC.[92–94] However, infants with other presentations of NEC frequently require surgery (Table 81.2). As mentioned previously, *portal venous gas* in the presence of the appropriate clinical findings should be treated as equivalent to *pneumoperitoneum* and be a clear operative indication. Infants with rapidly progressive *staccato NEC* require early surgery for management of progressive clinical instability and extensive intestinal disease, even in the absence of other surgical indications. In the setting of severe thrombocytopenia, anemia, or metabolic acidosis, waiting to medically optimize these infants for surgery only results in worsening intestinal necrosis.[50,51,94]

Table 81.2 Operative Recommendations for NEC

- Infants with *textbook NEC* should undergo surgery for *pneumoperitoneum* on abdominal radiograph.
- Infants with *portal venous gas* or *staccato NEC* should receive early operations.
- Decisions to operate on NEC with *refractory, nonprogressive pneumatosis* are made case-by-case based on worsening clinical status.
- Infants with *NEC totalis* should receive definitive bowel resections and referral to multidisciplinary intestinal management programs.
- Peritoneal drainage is only indicated as a temporizing procedure in critically ill infants.

NEC, Necrotizing enterocolitis.

Infants who fail to respond to medical therapy can be a challenge to manage. These patients, who may have persistent *pneumatosis* or may have evidence of an ileus or ascites, require an individualized approach. Unfortunately, there are currently no accurate biomarkers or predictive scores that adequately identify bowel necrosis in these infants.[95] Therefore neonatology and pediatric surgical teams need to collaboratively establish clear thresholds for operative intervention. As mentioned above, one strategy is to draw a clinical "line in the sand," which when "crossed" will trigger surgery. Evidence that the clinical line has been crossed may include a significant increase in ventilatory support, persistent or ongoing transfusions, or escalation of inotropic support. Overall, we recommend a low threshold for operative intervention in infants with refractory, nonprogressive *pneumatosis* or other evidence of failure to improve with medical treatment.

When making the decision to operate, it is important to counsel families on short- and long-term outcomes including the risk of mortality and implications for long-term quality of life. Patients at higher risk for poor surgical outcomes include those with existing comorbidities such as congenital heart disease and those who have progressed to the point of multisystem organ failure, significant coagulopathy, intraventricular bleeds, or irreversible renal failure. The exclusion criteria in patients with an otherwise operative indication for NEC include major comorbidity that would not be expected to improve with resection of necrotic bowel.

Medical Management

Medical management of NEC should be instituted in all patients once NEC is diagnosed. This management consists of bowel rest with gastrointestinal decompression, parenteral nutrition, careful administration of fluids, and broad-spectrum antibiotics. Because infants with NEC often have hemodynamic instability and apnea, intensive monitoring is important to guide inotropic use, transfusion therapy, and the need for mechanical ventilation.[87] Medical management alone successfully treats NEC in approximately half of patients, recognizing that a significant number of patients who are treated with NEC may have Bell 1 NEC, and thus, potentially another, alternate diagnosis may be responsible for the patient's symptoms.[92,93]

Feeding and Parenteral Nutrition

Upon diagnosis of NEC, the infant is placed on bowel rest and gastric decompression is initiated via a nasogastric or orogastric tube. This approach provides management of ileus and minimizes bowel distention, which can worsen bowel ischemia. Parenteral nutrition is recommended to provide adequate protein for weight gain and facilitate tissue repair. However, supplemental parenteral nutrition at NEC onset is not associated with decreased rates of surgical intervention or mortality.[96,97]

Feeding should be reinstated as soon as possible based on clinical improvement and lack of *pneumatosis* and portal venous gas.[97] The best timing for reinitiating enteral feeds remains unclear. Retrospective studies suggest it is safe to restart enteral feeding within the first week after diagnosis,[98,99] and delaying feeding increases the risk of central line–associated bloodstream infections.[100] However, a meta-analysis comparing early versus late reinitiation of feeding showed no differences in NEC recurrence, catheter-related sepsis, or post-NEC strictures.[101,102]

Antibiotic Therapy

Broad-spectrum antibiotics are recommended to all patients with suspected and established NEC[103] because 20% to 30% will have bacteremia.[104,105] Current antibiotic regimens include coverage for gram-positive and gram-negative bacteria, whereas anaerobic coverage is included in the setting of advancing disease.[103,106]

Overall, antibiotic regimens should be decided based on susceptibility patterns of the neonatal intensive care unit (NICU) and the clinical status of the infant. Changes in antibiotics, the addition of antifungals or anaerobic coverage, and the duration of treatment should be adjusted based on an infant's clinical progression and culture results.[87]

Operative Management

Exploratory Laparotomy

Operating on an infant with NEC requires a clear set of goals (resection of necrotic bowel where possible, abdominal decompression with silo placement, etc), an experienced team, excellent communication between all members, appropriate anesthesia coverage, available blood products, warming devices, and a gentle and efficient operative touch. The choice of location (in the NICU versus in the operating room) can be varied based on the prevailing practices of the individual institution, but in general terms, if an infant is on a jet ventilator or oscillator, then surgery in the NICU will be required, whereas in most other cases, surgery in the operating room is preferable. There is not a clear "lower weight" limit for surgery for NEC, because operations can be performed safely and efficiently in even the smallest of infants.

Surgery for NEC begins with an exploratory laparotomy performed through a transverse abdominal incision at approximately the level of the umbilicus, oriented to either the right or the left based on the location of the tenderness or the findings of pneumatosis on the abdominal films (Fig. 81.1D). When in doubt, orient the incision to the right, because the terminal ileum is the most common site of disease.

During initial entry into the peritoneal cavity, the surgeon takes care to avoid the low-lying liver in a premature infant's abdomen. All segments of bowel are then carefully exteriorized and assessed for inflammation and necrosis. It is essential that the bowel and mesentery be handled with extreme care, because even minimal tugging can cause retroperitoneal bleeding. If necrotic bowel is identified, a bowel resection is performed. The mesentery can be divided using cautery alone, although the use of ties may be more hemostatic in the child with significant coagulopathy. If there is a question of bowel viability, the bowel segment may be left in situ and a silo placed to allow for reassessment of bowel viability within 24 to 48 hours.[107]

Our general approach is to perform a resection with creation of an ostomy and mucus fistula. In some cases, especially if short segments are involved, some surgeons advocate for primary anastomosis, although this significantly increases the risk of postoperative morbidity from anastomotic leak. Whereas a primary anastomosis could avoid risks of fluid and electrolyte derangments that may be associated with a very proximal stoma, such risks are minimized with a practice of early closure and/or distal refeeding of collected stoma effluent from the proximal bowel.[108,109]

If the infant is hemodynamically unstable, the surgeon may resect bowel segments with definite necrosis and place a silo to allow for resuscitation followed by a second look; in these cases, abdominal decompression may be sufficient to allow for physiologic recovery. A proximal enterostomy may be performed when a phlegmonous mass is identified, in order to avoid complications associated with dissection in an inflamed field.

An enterostomy should be reversed after at least 6 weeks have passed from the initial surgery and the infant is clinically stable. We recommend a contrast study to evaluate for intestinal stricture prior to an ostomy-reversal procedure.[110,111]

Peritoneal Drainage

Current thinking indicates that exploratory laparotomy for NEC allows for resection of necrotic bowel and abdominal decompression and improves both short- and long-term outcomes. There have been studies of PD for NEC that showed equivalence to operative surgery.[112,113] Such studies were contaminated by a significant number of patients who were nonrandomized to either group and on closer analysis mainly fell into the operative group, suggesting that the individual surgeons knew what was indicated. Moreover, these trials were also complicated by the presence of patients who never were fed or who did not have pneumotisis, suggesting that they had SIP and not NEC.

Because of the high risk of bias in these studies and the poor effectiveness of PD for treatment of NEC, we recommend that all patients with surgical disease undergo an exploratory laparotomy with bowel resection. Although PD may serve as a temporizing measure in an unstable patient, it is unlikely to provide definitive treatment for a patient with NEC. By contrast, drain placement is often sufficient for a patient with SIP, although the child needs to be monitored very closely for signs of improvement versus deterioration.

When indicated, placement of a PD can be performed at bedside with appropriate intravenous sedation and local anesthesia. To place a PD, the surgeon makes a small transverse incision in the right lower quadrant and bluntly dissects through the abdominal wall to access the peritoneal cavity. A rush of air with efflux of meconium may be noted, but often not. A hemostat or tonsil clamp is then passed transabdominally while hugging the anterior abdominal wall, taking care not to damage the bladder, and a Penrose drain or vessel loop is withdrawn back and secured.

Complications From NEC

Postoperative Complications

Infants with NEC who require surgery have mortality rates up to 50%,[10] and those who survive face a 70% risk of postoperative complications.[114,115] These complications include intraoperative hepatic parenchymal bleeding, recurrent NEC, postoperative intestinal strictures, wound or enterostomy complications, SBS, and neurodevelopmental impairment.

Liver Bleeding

Liver bleeding can be fatal and occurs due to direct liver injury during abdominal entry or dissection of the hepatic flexure of the colon. It can also occur from shear force trauma with liver retraction. The treatment is surgical control of bleeding.[116,117]

Recurrent NEC

The incidence of recurrent NEC is 5% to 10%.[87,118] It typically occurs approximately 30 days after onset of the first NEC episode, regardless of that episode's severity or management. Mortality and management of recurrent NEC is the same as for the first incidence of NEC.[119,120]

Intestinal Strictures

Intestinal strictures are a common complication after NEC, occurring in 12% to 35% of infants.[3,12] Strictures occur at sites of pathologic bowel inflammation or intestinal anastomoses after bowel resection.[121] Strictures result in bowel obstruction, presenting as abdominal distention and multiple dilated intestinal loops on abdominal radiograph. An upper and lower gastrointestinal study with contrast can aid diagnosis, and surgical resection or stricturoplasty is warranted.

Wound Complications

Wound complications are common in preterm infants and include surgical site infections, superficial separation of the skin, and fascial dehiscence.[114,115,118,122] Wounds should be carefully examined for evidence of skin breakdown, erythema, or purulent and ascitic discharge. Treatment involves antibiotics, wound care, and occasionally surgical management. Careful closure of the skin, particularly around a stoma, can help minimize these wound complications.

Enterostomy Complications

Enterostomies in neonates are prone to prolapse, stenosis, and side-fistulas. They can also cause electrolyte imbalances, malnutrition, dehydration, failure to thrive, and neurodevelopmental impairment.[123] Enterostomy complications have a combined incidence of 6% to 42% in infants.[115,118] Prevention of these complications starts in the operating room with selection of healthy-appearing bowel that should be brought up to the abdominal wall with minimal tension. Prolapse and skin irritation may require local wound management, and stenosis or spontaneous closure of a stoma may require surgical revision. Metabolic and fluid-balance complications are initially treated with supportive care, but early restoration of continuity is the definitive management.

Short Bowel Syndrome

NEC is the most common cause of SBS in children, accounting for more than 35% of all SBS cases.[124] Childhood SBS is accompanied by significant morbidity due to intestinal failure–associated liver disease, small bowel bacterial overgrowth, nephrocalcinosis, cholelithiasis, and metabolic bone disease.[125] The severity of malabsorption seen in SBS depends on the extent of intestinal injury caused by NEC and the length and location of bowel resected. Poor intestinal absorptive capacity is seen with resection of the majority of the small bowel, resection of the ileocecal valve, and poor intestinal motility.[126]

Although children with SBS historically have had high mortality due to intestinal failure–associated liver disease and nutritional-line infections, current multidisciplinary intestinal rehabilitation programs have greatly improved survival and quality of life for children with SBS. These programs use hepatoprotective total parenteral nutrition strategies and protocols to prevent central line–associated bloodstream infections.[127] Today, overall survival to adolescence in children with SBS from NEC is more than 90%, and 50% to 70% of children achieve enteral autonomy.[126]

Intestinal transplantation has also improved quality of life for children with SBS. Historically, intestinal transplantation had poor outcomes, but there have been recent improvements in 1-year survival rates, which are now up to 80%.[128] Intestinal transplant recipients achieve enteral autonomy in 95% of cases[128]; however, ongoing concerns include the risk for chronic rejection, sepsis, chronic renal disease, and posttransplant lymphoproliferative disorder. Currently, the indications for intestinal transplant in the setting of SBS from NEC remain under review.[129]

Based on the current success in management of patients with SBS and the positive outcomes after tranplantion of the intestine, surgery should be offered to patients with *NEC totalis*, provided that parental wishes are respected and that an informed decision can be made. It is particularly important that the care team is aware of the excellent outcomes that can be achieved in patients with SBS in reaching enteral autonomy either through medical management or through the receipt of an intestinal transplant.

Neurodevelopmental Complications of NEC

Poor neurodevelopmental outcomes are a significant and frequent long-term complication of NEC and occur in 30% to 50% of NEC survivors.[3,11] Our group has shown that inflammation from the intestine can have a direct effect on the brain, through activation of microglia and recruitment of proinflammatory lymphocytes.[130,131] There is a direct association between the severity of NEC and the risk of future neurodevelopmental delay. Infants with significant disease, defined as those who require surgical resection, have a twofold increased risk of neurodevelopmental impairment compared with those treated medically.[123,132] Our improved understanding of the mechanisms of NEC-associated brain injury have led us to adopt a strategy of performing early resection of diseased bowel to limit the severity and duration of the systemic inflammatory response seen in NEC.

Outcomes and Prevention in Patients Undergoing Surgery for NEC

The overall mortality from NEC has improved over time and is currently estimated between 20% and 30%,[49,93] compared with approximately 50% in the 1970s.[133] This improvement is primarily attributed to the successful reduction of NEC incidence through unit education and standardized protocols.[134] The most significant measure for NEC prevention is the administration of human breast milk.[135–137] Others include implementing strict feeding protocols,[138] limiting exposure to antacids or antibiotics, and use of specific probiotics.[139,140]

Despite these efforts, infants with advanced surgical disease and those born extremely prematurely, with congenital heart defects, or with chromosomal abnormalities still face an increased risk of mortality from NEC.[141] Currently, compared with medically managed NEC, advanced disease that requires surgery has increased mortality (35% versus 21%),[49] longer hospital lengths of stay,[142] worse short-term growth delay (61% versus 56%),[142] and worse long-term neurodevelopmental impairment and severe disability.[14,142] There is still a great need for interventions that halt the progression of NEC and minimize the need for surgical intervention.

Summary

NEC is a major disease that affects premature infants and requires a collaborative approach between the NICU team, the family, and the pediatric surgeons. It is important to recognize the five presentations of NEC (*textbook NEC*, failure to medically improve, portal venous gas, *staccato NEC*, and *NEC totalis*) in order to gauge the appropriate intervention. Exploratory laparotomy is performed to remove necrotic bowel, decompress the abdomen, and prevent long-term neurologic sequelae and is thus superior to the placement of a small drain, which accomplishes none of these goals. Patients with NEC must be distinguished from those with SIP, which does respond to drainage alone and which has an overall improved prognosis. A greater understanding of the pathogenesis of this disease will lead to earlier diagnosis, specific therapies, and improved outcomes.

CHAPTER 82

Extracorporeal Membrane Oxygenation in Neonates

Eric W. Etchill, Alejandro V. Garcia

KEY POINTS

1. Extracorporeal membrane oxygenation (ECMO) is a potentially life-saving technology for newborns with refractory cardiopulmonary failure of reversible etiology.
2. ECMO involves draining deoxygenated venous blood, extracorporeal oxygenation and removal of carbon dioxide from the blood, and returning the blood via an infusion cannula either into a vein or artery.
3. Cannulation can either be peripheral, via the neck or femoral vessels, or centrally, via the right atrium and ascending aorta.
4. The most frequent respiratory indications for ECMO include congenital diaphragmatic hernias and meconium aspiration syndrome. It has also been long used for neonates with congenital diaphragmatic hernia refractory to maximal conventional therapy. In severe cases of persistent pulmonary hypertension of the newborn (up to 40%) that fail to respond to medical therapy including the use of vasodilatory agents, ECMO may be used to provide adequate gas exchange.
5. ECMO is frequently needed in neonates with congenital cardiac defects such as hypoplastic left heart syndrome, cyanotic defects with decreased or shunted pulmonary flow, left or right ventricular outflow tract obstruction, and septal defects with refractory cardiac arrest. ECMO support prior to definitive repair can improve survival.
6. Extracorporeal cardiopulmonary resuscitation is rapid deployment of venoarterial ECMO to provide circulatory support in patients in whom conventional cardiopulmonary resuscitation for 20 consecutive minutes is unsuccessful in achieving sustained return of spontaneous circulation. This can improve outcomes.

Introduction

Extracorporeal membrane oxygenation (ECMO) is a potentially life-saving technology for newborns with refractory cardiopulmonary failure of reversible etiology. ECMO involves draining deoxygenated venous blood, extracorporeal gas exchange thereby oxygenating and removing carbon dioxide from the blood, and returning the blood via an infusion cannula either into a vein (venovenous ECMO) or artery (venoarterial ECMO; Fig. 82.1). Cannulation can be either peripheral, most commonly via the neck or femoral vessels, or central, usually via the right atrium and ascending aorta (Fig. 82.2). In neonates, peripheral cannulation usually occurs via the internal jugular vein and carotid artery, because the femoral vessels are diminutive, technically challenging, and associated with greater complications. Dual lumen single-stage cannulas also exist, which have two separate lumens for infusion and drainage and are usually placed in the neck under fluoroscopic or echocardiographic guidance.

The use of ECMO in the neonatal population has expanded significantly since its inception in the early 1970s, due to a combination of improved technology, the expanding role of ECMO, and its encouraging outcomes. Indications for ECMO in the neonate can be broadly grouped into those that are intended to manage primary respiratory failure or cardiac failure or those following refractory cardiac arrest (extracorporeal cardiopulmonary resuscitation [ECPR]). This chapter uses the most recent literature to review current indications, applications, complications, and outcomes for ECMO in the neonate and discusses current controversies with respect to patient selection and ECMO management in this critically ill population.

Epidemiology

The use of ECMO has increased substantially in children and neonates during the past 3 decades, with roughly 3000 children placed on ECMO in 2019 according to the Extracorporeal Life Support Organization (ELSO) database.[1] Among all children, roughly 800 neonates were cannulated onto ECMO for respiratory disease in 2019, an overall decrease from 1300 to 1500 neonates cannulated onto ECMO for respiratory disease annually from 1990 to 1994. Survival of neonates placed on ECMO for respiratory disease has decreased from roughly 80% in 1990 to 60%-65% in 2020, thought to be largely a result of expanding indications and placing sicker children on ECMO as technology continues to improve and ECMO management continues to evolve. From 2014 through 2020, the overall survival to discharge for neonates on ECMO for pulmonary indications was approximately 68%. Similarly, the use of ECMO has increased overall in neonates with cardiac disease, from less than 100 patients in the early 1990s to approximately 450 patients annually from 2015 to 2020. Survival in this population has ranged from 32% to 50% annually, with an overall similar survival-to-discharge rate of 50%, similar to the 1990s survival rate. As with neonates with respiratory disease, this relatively stagnant survival among patients with cardiac disease cannulated onto ECMO was thought to be due to increasing medical complexity of the underlying cardiac disease and associated comorbidities. For neonates cannulated onto ECMO for cardiopulmonary resuscitation (CPR), overall survival to discharge is roughly 40% to 45%.[1]

ECMO—Respiratory

Cannulation for respiratory failure composes approximately 20% to 30% of all neonatal ECMO cannulations and usually occurs in the setting of pulmonary hypertension or persistent fetal circulation. ECMO for respiratory support of the neonate is associated with the highest survival percentage among all neonatal and pediatric ECMO support, with 65% to 70% survival to hospital discharge. In terms of specific disease processes, roughly one-third of all neonatal ECMO cannulations for respiratory failure are due to congenital

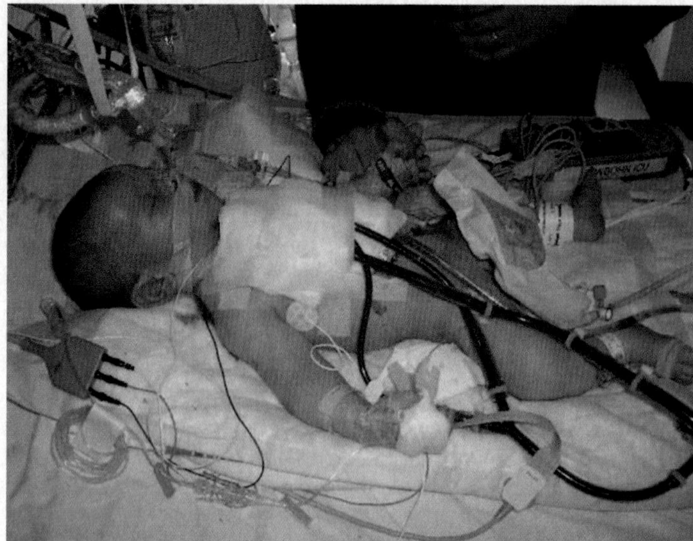

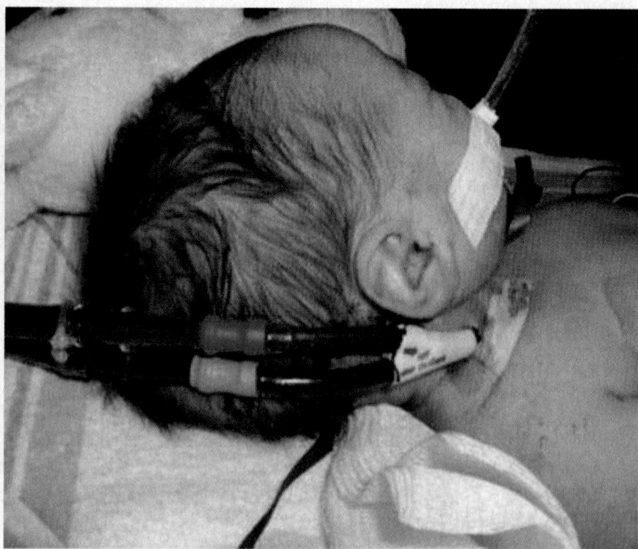

Fig. 82.1 A Patient With a Life-Threatening Congenital Cardiac Anomaly Being Treated With Veno-Arterial Extracorporeal Membrane Oxygenation.

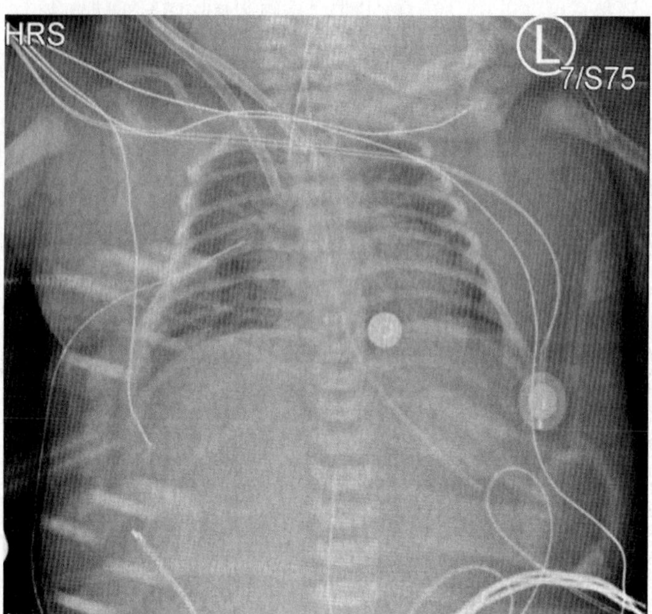

Fig. 82.2 Chest X-Ray of a Neonate Being Treated With Extracorporeal Membrane Oxygenation. Cannulas are seen in the right atrium and in the ascending aorta.

diaphragmatic hernias, which have an average ECMO duration of 12 days and a 50% rate of survival to hospital discharge. Meconium aspiration syndrome represents the second-highest proportion (roughly 25%) of indications for neonatal ECMO, has an average ECMO run of 6 days, and is associated with greater than 90% survival to hospital discharge. Primary pulmonary hypertension represents roughly 20% of all neonatal ECMO cannulations for respiratory failure, has a 7-day average run duration, and is associated with roughly 75% survival to hospital discharge.[2]

Physiologic indications for ECMO cannulation in neonatal respiratory failure include an oxygen index (defined as [mean airway pressure × fraction of inspired oxygen (FiO_2)]/[postductal partial pressure of arterial blood oxygen (PaO_2)] × 100) greater than 40 for more than 4 hours, failure to wean from 100% oxygen despite prolonged (greater than 48 hours) maximal medical therapy for persistent episodes of decompensation, severe refractory hypoxic respiratory failure with acute decompensation (PaO_2 less than 40), severe pulmonary hypertension with evidence of right ventricular and/or left ventricular dysfunction, and hypotension resistant to vasopressors or inotropic medications. Absolute contraindications include lethal chromosomal disorders or other lethal anomalies, irreversible brain damage, uncontrolled bleeding, and grade 3 or greater intraventricular hemorrhage. Relative contraindications include a gestational age of less than 34 weeks, birth weight loss of 2 kg, and mechanical ventilation for more than 10 to 14 days.

Complications suffered during ECMO are associated with greater mortality and can roughly be broken down into biomechanical, hemorrhagic, neurologic, cardiovascular, pulmonary, limb, and infectious complications. Among infants undergoing ECMO for respiratory support, 17% experience clots in the oxygenator and an additional 30% experience clots elsewhere in the circuit, 14% have separate cannulation site or surgical site bleeding, nearly 11% undergo significant hemolysis, disseminated intravascular coagulation occurs in 3%, and 1.7% of infants experience gastrointestinal hemorrhage. Fifteen percent of infants experience a neurologic injury, with 7% experiencing infarct and 7.5% experiencing hemorrhage. An additional 7% suffer cardiac tamponade, 4.5% suffer a pulmonary hemorrhage, and less than 1% suffer limb ischemia.

Congenital Diaphragmatic Hernia

ECMO has long been used for neonates with congenital diaphragmatic hernias (CDHs) refractory to maximal conventional therapy. Although criteria for patient selection can be institution-specific, in general, ECMO is used for patients with CDHs who otherwise would not survive due to severe pulmonary hypertension. Criteria that ECMO centers may use to decide whether an infant with a CDH is a candidate for ECMO include an inability to maintain preductal oxygen saturations above 80%, refractory hypotension, persistent metabolic acidosis or lactatemia, peak inspiratory pressures greater than 28 to 30 cm H_2O, or mean airway pressures greater than 15 cm H_2O.

As with other indications for ECMO due to respiratory failure, relative exclusions may include patients with a gestational age less than 34 weeks or weight less than 2 kg, and absolute exclusions may include patients with legal chromosomal abnormalities and those with irreversible multiorgan failure and severe intracranial hemorrhage. Because improvements in pulmonary hypertension and CDH can take several weeks and may be independent of surgical repair, patients may have prolonged, complicated courses of ECMO and are at increased risk of complications as the duration of the ECMO run increases. Routine neurologic monitoring is indicated, and discussions regarding the futility of care and potential withdrawal of support are indicated in the setting of significant intracranial hemorrhage, worsening clinical status, multiorgan failure, or failure of clinical improvement despite adequate surgical repair and otherwise optimal medical therapy.

Persistent Pulmonary Hypertension of the Newborn

Persistent pulmonary hypertension of the newborn (PPHN) is a disease process characterized by abnormally increased pulmonary vascular resistance soon after birth, with subsequent right-to-left shunting of blood through the fetal circulatory system resulting in severe hypoxemia that is commonly refractory to conventional respiratory support. In severe cases of PPHN (up to 40%) that fail to respond to medical therapy including the use of vasodilatory agents, ECMO may be used to provide adequate gas exchange and prevent or mitigate irreversible lung injury until pulmonary vascular resistance decreases and pulmonary hypertension resolves. Criteria for ECMO in this setting generally consist of an oxygenation index greater than or equal to 40. Patients who are cannulated on ECMO for PPHN have an excellent prognosis, with survival rates exceeding 80%. Shorter duration of ECMO support is associated with improved survival. Prematurity, pre-ECMO pH less than 7.2, pre-ECMO arterial blood oxygen saturation (Sao_2) less than 65%, and ECMO duration greater than or equal to 7 days were independently associated with mortality in this patient population.[3]

Meconium Aspiration Syndrome

For patients with meconium aspiration syndrome refractory to conventional medical therapy, ECMO may be an otherwise lifesaving therapy because it provides cardiopulmonary support while the underlying pulmonary disease process resolves.[4,5] ECMO is indicated in approximately 1.5% of all patients who are admitted to the neonatal intensive care unit with meconium aspiration syndrome. The use of ECMO in this setting is associated with a favorable prognosis (greater than 90% survival to discharge), because patients tend to do well once the reversible sequela of the aspiration syndrome resolve, the lungs improve, and the child is able to successfully wean from the ECMO circuit and survive to discharge.

ECMO—Cardiac

Congenital heart disease is the most common reason neonates are cannulated on ECMO for cardiac failure. Hypoplastic left heart syndrome, cyanotic defects with decreased or shunted pulmonary flow, left or right ventricular outflow tract obstruction, and septal defects can all result in refractory cardiac arrest in which ECMO support prior to definitive repair is associated with increased survival. The average ECMO run duration for congenital heart disease is 6 days, and 40% to 50% of all patients supported on ECMO in the setting of congenital heart disease survive to hospital discharge. Additional indications for cardiac ECMO include myocarditis, cardiomyopathy, cardiogenic shock, and cardiac arrest, which together compose less than 10% of all neonatal cardiac ECMO runs and are associated with a 40% to 50% rate of survival to hospital discharge.[2]

As with ECMO in the setting of respiratory failure, physiologic indications exist for cardiac ECMO and include refractory cardiogenic shock (generally seen in the setting of cardiomyopathy, acute myocarditis, or cardiac dysfunction and severe sepsis), postoperative refractory cardiac failure (such as postcardiotomy shock when neonates fail to wean from cardiopulmonary bypass, postoperative low cardiac output syndrome, refractory cardiac arrhythmias, and pulmonary retention), cardiac arrest refractory to conventional CPR (ECPR; see next section), procedural support (during heart or lung transplantation), or as a bridge to heart or lung transplantation or durable mechanical circulatory support such as a ventricular assist device. No absolute contraindications exist specific to cardiac ECMO, but relative contraindications, which significantly overlap with those for ECMO and respiratory failure, include end-stage primary disease or incurable malignancy with poor prognosis, multiorgan failure, severe neurologic injury or intracranial hemorrhage, uncontrolled visceral bleeding, prematurity (less than 34 weeks' gestational age), small size (less than 2 kg), chromosomal abnormalities, and patient care directives specifying against or limiting ECMO use. ECMO is also generally not recommended in this population if the neonate has or will have significant residual lesions after cardiac surgery or is unlikely to be a transplant candidate.

In addition to characteristics that are relative contraindications to cannulation, several patient- and disease-specific characteristics are associated with mortality in neonatal patients supported by ECMO for cardiac failure. Prior to cannulation, patients with single-ventricle physiology, myocarditis, or cardiomyopathy, patients requiring high levels of inotropes or with profound acidosis (pH less than 7.2) or high lactate, patients requiring CPR, and neonates with evidence of renal failure or fluid overload are likely to suffer higher mortality once cannulated onto ECMO. Once on ECMO, patients who fail to clear lactate within 24 hours, remain fluid overloaded, experience bleeding complications, suffer extracardiac complications including stroke, intracranial hemorrhage, or renal failure, or remain on ECMO for more than 7 days, experience significantly high mortality.[6]

Conversely, several characteristics prior to ECMO cannulation exist that are associated with lower mortality. Neonates with larger body weights (greater than 3.3 kg), without chromosomal abnormalities, with two-ventricle physiology, with low inotropic requirements, with a duration of ventilation less than 14 days prior to ECMO, and without significant acidosis or elevated lactates as well as who do not require CPR and do not have renal failure or extracardiac involvement prior to ECMO experience lower mortality. Similarly, neonates who clear lactate within 24 hours of being cannulated onto ECMO, those who do not suffer the above-mentioned bleeding or extracardiac systemic complications, and those who have a duration of ECMO support less than 5 days are more likely to survive until hospital discharge.[6]

Among all neonates supported by ECMO for cardiac failure, approximately 1% experience oxygenator clots, with an additional 25% to 30% experiencing clots elsewhere in the ECMO circuit. Compared with patients supported for respiratory failure, a much higher proportion experience surgical site bleeding (30% versus 6%) and cannulation site bleeding (11% versus 8%), 11% experience significant hemolysis, and 4% suffer disseminated intravascular coagulation; gastrointestinal hemorrhage occurs in 1%. Additionally, infants supported on ECMO for cardiac failure experience high rates of intracranial hemorrhage (11% versus 7.5%) and lower rates of intracranial infarction (3% versus 7%) compared with neonates supported for respiratory failure; 6% experience additional cardiac complications, 5% experience pulmonary hemorrhage, and 0.2% develop limb ischemia.

ECMO—ECPR

Extracorporeal cardiopulmonary resuscitation, or ECPR, is defined as the rapid deployment of venoarterial ECMO to provide circulatory support in patients in whom conventional CPR is unsuccessful in achieving sustained return of spontaneous circulation, which is deemed to have occurred when chest compressions are not required for 20 consecutive minutes and signs of circulation persist.[6a] ECPR is different than venoarterial ECMO in that with ECPR, ECMO is in the setting of conventional CPR, whereas venoarterial ECMO is initiated for low cardiac output either without cardiac arrest or following sustained return of spontaneous circulation. Neonatal ECPR is associated with a 35% to 45% rate of survival to hospital discharge.

Survival among neonates who suffer out-of-hospital cardiac arrest is more favorable compared with those who suffer in-hospital cardiac arrest. According to American Heart Association guidelines, there currently is insufficient evidence for or against the use of ECPR for infants with noncardiac diagnoses who suffer in-hospital cardiac arrest.[7,8] However, ECPR may be considered for infants with cardiac diagnoses who have in-hospital cardiac arrest and for institutions in settings with existing ECMO protocols, expertise, and equipment (class IIb).[9,10] In a study looking at outcomes of 593 cases of pediatric ECPR in the setting of in-hospital cardiac arrest at 32 hospitals between 2010 and 2014, mortality remained relatively constant, with overall mortality of 59% (60% survival to ECMO decannulation and 41% survival to hospital discharge).[11] Neonates composed more than one-third of the study population.[11]

Those who survive are more likely to have a primary medical or surgical etiology of cardiac arrest and have a shorter duration of arrest (42 minutes for survivors of hospital discharge versus 51 minutes for nonsurvivors). Additionally, odds of death increase with the presence of renal insufficiency and any adverse events or complications during ECMO and with an increasing number of adverse events during ECMO. Neurologic injury is the complication most associated with mortality; patients who suffer neurologic complications have nearly three times the odds of death compared with those who do not. The time of day (weekday versus weekend) of the arrest, the location of in-hospital arrest, whether the arrest was witnessed or not, and the first documented rhythm are not associated with survival.[11] Among those who survive, the average duration is 4 days, and more than 80% of patients experience an adverse event (compared with 90% of nonsurvivors). These complications include cardiovascular (56%), hemorrhagic (33%), metabolic (26%), and renal (25%) complications, seizures (10%), intracranial hemorrhage (8%), cerebral infarction (3%), infections (6%), and pulmonary complications (4%). However, among those who do survive, 93% have a favorable neurologic outcome at hospital discharge.[11,12] In a study looking at up to 1-year survival and neurobehavioral outcomes among infants and children who were supported with ECPR after undergoing in-hospital cardiac arrest, 85% had a preexisting cardiac condition, 51% had postcardiac surgery, 57% were less than 1 year of age, 78% had a CPR duration greater than 30 minutes, more than 40% survived to 12 months after hospital discharge, and 30% survived to 12 months with a favorable neuropsychological outcome.[13]

Neurologic Outcomes

As previously mentioned, neurologic complications among neonates supported by ECMO are common and associated with worse prognoses. Acute neurologic injury, which includes hypoxic-ischemic injury, intracranial hemorrhage, ischemic stroke, and clinical or electroencephalographic evidence of seizures, occurs in 10% to 35% of infants and increases mortality by roughly 100%.[12,14,15] Furthermore, infant and child ECMO survivors suffer lasting neurologic outcomes. A systematic review of neurologic outcomes after ECMO in children ages 0 to 18 years looked at studies consisting of patients with CDHs, cardiac disease, cardiac arrest, and next populations and found that 10% to 50% of children's performed more than two standard deviations below the mean on cognitive testing.[12] The brain is particularly susceptible to injury during ECMO due to the pre-ECMO hypoxic-ischemic injury suffered during cardiopulmonary failure cardiac arrest, combined with the inflammatory state of the ECMO circuit and the need for systemic anticoagulation. As such, accurate and timely neuromonitoring is particularly important. Neuromonitoring can be done via a variety of modalities, including cross-sectional imaging, Doppler ultrasound, electroencephalography, cerebral oximetry, and awake neuromonitoring, which is more common in neonates than in children or adults.[16]

Controversies and Ethical Considerations

As previously discussed, gestational age <34 weeks and weight <2 kg have historically been contraindications to ECMO cannulation, due in part to technical challenges as well as to overall poor prognoses including increased risk of intraventricular hemorrhage and death. However, recent studies have challenged these criteria. A study by Church et al. looking at outcomes of patients with a gestational age of 34 weeks or less cannulated onto ECMO found no difference in intracranial hemorrhage between patients with a gestational age of 29 to 33 weeks compared with 34 weeks (21% versus 17%). However, there was a statistically significant higher incidence of cerebral infarct (22% versus 16%; $P = .03$) and overall lower survival among patients of 29 to 33 weeks' gestational age compared with 34 weeks (48% versus 58%; $P = .05$). Intracranial hemorrhage and survival were not associated with gestational age during logistic regression analysis. The authors concluded that the modestly worse differences seen in the cohort of lower gestational age may be clinically acceptable, arguing against using a gestational age of <34 weeks as an absolute contraindication to ECMO.[17]

In a retrospective study of the ELSO database looking at infants weighing less than or greater than 2 kg at the time of ECMO cannulation, Rozmiarek et al. found that although overall survival was lower in patients weighing less than 2 kg (53% versus 77%; $P < .001$), a survival rate of 40% or greater could be achieved in infants who weighed as little as 1.6 kg. Judicious use of anticoagulation in this population could also improve survival, because bleeding was associated with a significantly lower survival rate.[18] In a separate study looking at extremely low birth weight infants with congenital diaphragmatic hernias supported with ECMO, Delaplain et al. found increased mortality among infants who weighed less than 2 kg but not among those less than 34 weeks' gestational age.[19]

There is no shortage of ethical considerations related to the deployment and use of ECMO, particularly in infants. Because ECMO is a highly resource-intensive therapy, deliberate and thoughtful consideration should be made for each potential infant that could potentially benefit from ECMO. We recommend a multidisciplinary group of clinicians and stakeholders for consideration and routine reviewing of ECMO candidates and institutional criteria for cannulation, with liberal use of ethics committees when deemed appropriate.[20]

Once infants are cannulated onto ECMO, decisions related to withdrawal of support can be particularly challenging. Early and frequent discussions of the family's specific goals and frequent evaluation and reevaluation of the abilities of ECMO to meet those goals throughout the patient's ECMO course are particularly important. Additional ethical considerations include expanding ECMO to broader indications and expanded patient populations despite a lack of clear evidence regarding prognosis and outcomes; the role of ECMO in brain-dead potential organ donors; the role of regional ECMO centers; and decisions surrounding futility or continuation of ongoing care and/or ECMO support.[20,21]

CHAPTER 83 Intestinal Surgery in the Newborn—Atresias, Volvulus, and Everything Else

Ross M. Beckman, Daniel S. Rhee

KEY POINTS

1. The processes leading to duodenal atresia and distal atresia are unknown but reflect a general defect in intestinal development. In the past, duodenal atresia was thought to result from failure of recanalization of the duodenal lumen, but there is little basis to support this theory. In animals, vascular occlusion causes intestinal changes that look similar to intestinal atresia, but there is little evidence to indicate that intestinal atresia in humans follows vascular accidents. For reasons that are unknown, duodenal atresia has a high association with other congenital anomalies.
2. A "double bubble" sign seen on x-ray (which reflects air within the stomach and duodenum) or on prenatal ultrasound (which reflects accumulated fluid within these two compartments) can be diagnostic for duodenal atresia. Presence of distal air can distinguish complete versus partial obstruction.
3. Bilious emesis in the newborn should raise immediate suspicion for malrotation and requires prompt evaluation and intervention.
4. The upper gastrointestinal series is the accepted standard for diagnosis of malrotation; however, if midgut volvulus is suspected, emergent surgery without imaging is warranted.
5. Abdominal wall defects can be diagnosed prenatally and should be referred to tertiary care centers where immediate access to pediatric surgical consultation is available.
6. Omphaloceles are highly associated with congenital anomalies, particularly cardiac and chromosomal, whereas gastroschisis is not.

Introduction

Disorders of the intestine that require surgery in the newborn may evolve from an array of congenital or functional disorders. These often present as complete or partial obstructions, which may result from intrinsic and extrinsic pathology. Findings such as bilious emesis, abdominal distention, or failure to pass meconium are signs of obstruction, and learning to quickly identify the location and underlying nature of these disorders is essential, because conditions such as volvulus may require emergent surgery. In addition, disorders of the abdominal wall present unique challenges in surgical and medical management. This chapter focuses on the more common indications for intestinal surgery in the newborn, specifically intestinal atresia, malrotation, meconium ileus, and duplication cysts as well as abdominal wall defects, gastroschisis, and omphalocele.

Intestinal Atresia

Pathophysiology

Intestinal atresia is the most common cause of obstruction in the neonate, affecting approximately 1.6 per 10,000 newborns, with duodenal atresia making up approximately 60%.[1] Although all forms of intestinal atresia result from some anomaly in normal embryonic development, the clinical implications vary based on their anatomic locations.

Duodenal atresia occurs most commonly as an error in early embryonic development. In the past, it was thought that duodenal development required a series of complex proliferation followed by recanalization steps and that failure to recanalize in the proximal gut results in the obstruction or stenosis.[2] However, there is little evidence to support this notion, and it is more likely that duodenal atresia reflects an error in the complex steps that underlie normal intestinal development. For reasons that are not well understood, there is a high association with cardiac and urogenital anomalies, VACTERL (vertebral defects, anal atresia, cardiac defects, tracheo-esophageal fistula, renal anomalies, and limb abnormalities), and other GI anomalies such as malrotation, annular pancreas, esophageal atresia, and imperforate anus. Approximately 30% of cases are associated with trisomy 21, and 3% to 8% of trisomy 21 patients are born with atresia.[2,3] Duodenal atresia is classified into three main categories, shown in Table 83.1.

Jejunoileal atresia may occur anywhere in the remainder of the small bowel. In elegant experiments on dogs, vascular occlusion resulted in the development of intestinal changes that mimic atresia, although there is little evidence that ischemic insult acquired in utero during fetal development occurs in patients with atresia. Although some researchers have hypothesized that the affected bowel becomes necrotic and subsequently involutes and resorbs, leaving blind proximal and distal ends with a widely varied extent of involved or absent bowel, there is no evidence for necrosis or involution in patients with atresia. In-utero volvulus, internal hernia, and even in-utero intussusception may occur, leading to broad disruption of the gastrointestinal (GI) tract, but these are distinct entities from the commonly seen instances of intestinal atresia. In select cases, arterial vasoconstriction or thrombosis precipitated by maternal smoking, drug use, medications, or inherited thrombophilias have been thought to play a role, although the vast majority of cases of intestinal atresia lack any identifiable risk factor for thromboembolic disease.[2] Similar to duodenal atresia, patterns of jejunoileal atresia have been classified into four main groups (see Table 83.1).

Table 83.1 Classification Systems for Duodenal and Jejunoileal Atresia

	Duodenal Atresia	Jejunoileal Atresia
Type 1	A mucosal membrane occludes the duodenal lumen, usually at or near the level of the ampulla of Vater. It can be completely occlusive (1A); fenestrated, allowing passage of air and contrast distal to the second "bubble" (1B); or a variant in which the membrane is elongated with the apex located distal to its origin, known as a "windsock anomaly" (1C).	A mucosal web forms within the bowel, causing luminal obstruction. No resulting loss of intestinal length.
Type 2	Proximal and distal duodenal segments end blindly with an intervening fibrous cord connecting them.	There is a gap in luminal continuity with a connecting cord-like scar or band connecting the proximal and distal bowel. The mesentery remains intact between the discontinuous bowel.
Type 3	Type 3 is the rarest subtype, often associated with annular pancreas; the atretic proximal and distal ends end blindly with absence of intervening mesentery.[4]	In type 3, a gap exists between the proximal and distal small intestine and there is a mesenteric defect.
Type 3b		In type 3b, a large section of bowel supplied by the distal superior mesenteric artery is absent and the distal section of ileum is shortened and coiled in a spiral around a vascular stalk from the ileocolic artery—so-called apple peel atresia. It usually results from a midgut volvulus in the setting of intestinal malrotation[5]
Type 4		Multiple gaps in intestinal continuity exist, often a combination of type 2 and type 3 defects. This can result in a very short length of functional small bowel.

Colonic atresia is the least common location, and its etiology is unknown. It may be seen in conjunction with small-intestinal atresia and can be associated with Hirschsprung disease and gastroschisis.

Clinical Features

Prenatal diagnosis of intestinal atresia is increasingly common with improvements in sensitivity of ultrasound; however, fewer than half of patients are diagnosed before birth. Sonographic signs include polyhydramnios and dilatation of the proximal small bowel with distal decompression. Sensitivity increases with more proximal lesions, because the bowel becomes more distended with swallowed amniotic fluid that the short proximal segment is unable to fully absorb. Duodenal atresia classically exhibits a "double bubble" sign with distention of the stomach and first portion of the duodenum and is the most commonly discovered prenatally, whereas colonic atresia is infrequently prenatally diagnosed unless more proximal involvement is also present.[6,7]

Postnatally, infants will present with signs of intestinal obstruction including persistent or forceful emesis and abdominal distention; however, this varies by location and extent of involved bowel. Duodenal atresia will result in gastric distention and early emesis that may be bilious depending on the location of the atresia in relation to the ampulla of Vater. Passage of meconium is common in these infants. Neonates with jejunoileal atresia will typically have increased abdominal distention and bilious emesis within the first 2 days of life and usually will not pass meconium. Colonic atresia exhibits the most distended abdomen because the entire bowel may fill with air and enteric contents, and it tends to present the latest.

Evaluation

Prenatal suspicion (polyhydramnios, sonographic double bubble) or postnatal signs of obstruction (persistent emesis, abdominal distention) should trigger further evaluation for intestinal atresia including history, physical exam, and family history of associated congenital anomalies. The timing and onset of distention and emesis, presence or absence of bilious emesis, and passage of meconium should be noted and the abdomen assessed for tenderness and distention. Peritonitis may suggest the presence of intestinal perforation or compromised bowel. Inspection for associated congenital anomalies should be performed. Basic chemistry labs may reveal associated metabolic derangements secondary to persistent emesis.

Abdominal x-ray is generally the first imaging study to further assess the extent and pattern of intestinal dilatation and presence of free air or pneumatosis, which would prompt urgent operative exploration. The "double bubble" sign on plain film with gasless distal bowel is again seen in duodenal obstruction due to air-filled gastric and duodenal dilatation; however, this may not be seen in very proximal atresia. Findings of distal gas with a "double bubble" sign are more consistent with a partial duodenal obstruction or more rarely can be seen with anomalous bile duct anatomy. More distal obstruction will again exhibit a dilated proximal bowel with air fluid levels and decompressed gasless distal bowel. Colonic atresia will show dilated colonic loops, often with a ground-glass or soap-bubble appearance on plain radiograph. Preoperative screening echocardiography and head and abdominal ultrasound are performed to assess for associated anomalies that may affect timing of any planned intervention. Malrotation with or without midgut volvulus can mimic atresia, and an upper GI water-soluble contrast study should be performed emergently if the diagnosis is in doubt. This test may also demonstrate the location of atresia for preoperative planning. Contrast enema may also be performed to elucidate the extent and location of distal atresia and will often demonstrate a microcolon due to lack of use, as well as inability to advance contrast into the dilated proximal loops.

Management

Antenatal suspicion for intestinal atresia warrants transfer of care to a center with availability of pediatric surgical consultation. Initial postnatal management includes withholding of feeds and prompt placement of a decompressive nasogastric tube to prevent aspiration. Infants with significant emesis or enteric tube output are susceptible to dehydration and electrolyte abnormalities and should receive intravenous resuscitation and electrolyte replacement. Broad-spectrum intravenous antibiotics are started for sepsis prophylaxis against GI bacterial translocation and for perioperative prophylaxis.

Definitive management is surgical in all types of intestinal atresia, with the principles being relief of obstruction and restoration of continuity while preserving functional bowel and minimizing long-term complications. The operative approach differs by anatomic location and subtype, however. Multiple techniques have been described to repair duodenal atresia since its initial report by Ladd in 1931,[8] including duodenojejunostomy, side-to-side duodenoduodenostomy, and partial web excision; however, the current standard described by Kimura is the diamond-shaped duodenoduodenostomy. The dilated duodenum is mobilized, and a handsewn anastomosis is performed between a transverse incision in the dilated proximal duodenum and a longitudinal incision in the distal duodenum. This technique was found to have earlier anastomotic function and lower long-term stricture rates.[9] Certain cases of type 1 duodenal atresia may be amenable to simple excision of the duodenal web through an anterior duodenotomy; however, great care must be taken to identify and preserve the ampulla of Vater, as it is generally located at the same level as the web. Gentle compression of the gallbladder may aid in identification of the ampulla by visualization of bilious output in the duodenum.[10] Some infants—typically those with extremely low birth weight—may benefit from a duodenojejunostomy due to its relative technical ease,[10] and this is our strong preference. Laparoscopic repair of duodenal atresia is increasingly being used, and in experienced hands, long-term outcomes compared with open have been similar and with shorter hospital stays and time to advancement to full feeds.[11]

Atresia of the jejunum is less amenable to laparoscopic repair due to obscuring distention of multiple loops of small bowel and is generally treated with an open approach. The atretic area or areas are identified and resected with primary end-to-end or end-to-side anastomosis. In very small or unstable infants with distal small bowel atresia, an end ileostomy or jejunostomy with mucous fistula may be performed with subsequent delayed bowel anastomosis at 2 to 4 months of age. Primary web excision through an enterotomy for type 1 lesions are seldom performed given the risk for recurrence and stricture.[3]

Colonic atresia may develop into a closed loop obstruction if an intact ileocecal valve is present, and emergent surgical consultation is necessary. Colonic atresia is mostly treated with resection of atretic bowel and either primary anastomosis or staged anastomosis depending on the overall stability of the patient.[3]

Due to the increased risk of multiple sites of atresia, saline or air should be injected intraoperatively into the distal bowel to detect additional sites of obstruction. Size mismatch of proximal and distal segments is an expected occurrence that may complicate primary anastomosis and lead to dysmotility. It is important to resect the proximal bowel for some distance to optimize motility and function. Tapering enteroplasty may be used in cases in which the intestine is very dilated, and it involves a longitudinal resection of the antimesenteric portion of the proximal dilated bowel to equilibrate the two sides of the anastomosis. We perform the tapering enteroplasty over a large red rubber catheter and use stapling devices to remove the antimesenteric dilated bowel. Concomitant anomalies requiring additional procedures at the time of the initial operation are also common. Those infants with intestinal malrotation should undergo a Ladd's procedure with appendectomy at initial presentation, and those with imperforate anus should undergo initial temporary colostomy.

Long-Term Outcomes

Although postoperative complications are common after correction of intestinal atresia, overall long-term outcomes are quite good if treated promptly and appropriately. Postoperative adhesive bowel obstructions and anastomotic strictures can occur and may warrant reoperation. Other common perioperative complications include prolonged ileus, anastomotic leak, wound infection, late adhesive bowel obstruction, and colostomy prolapse and retraction. Duodenal atresia has 0% to 4% operative mortality and up to 10% overall mortality, mostly attributable to comorbid congenital anomalies including complex cardiac anomalies.[3,12] Jejunoileal atresia has a low association with complex cardiac malformations and therefore has low early mortality (<1%); however, it has greater overall major morbidity and mortality (16% overall in-hospital mortality) related to an increased extent of resection and complications of intestinal failure and sepsis.[3,12] Colonic atresia, if diagnosed early, has excellent prognosis with survival to discharge approaching 100%[3]; however, outcomes become significantly worse with delayed diagnosis and progression to gangrene and perforation. In long-term follow-up, patients with intestinal atresia grow up to have quality of life similar to that of healthy controls, with major differences attributed largely to associated conditions such as trisomy 21 and not to decreased GI quality of life.[13]

Malrotation and Volvulus

Pathophysiology

Intestinal malrotation results from an arrest in the normal rotation of the gut during embryonic development. The GI tract undergoes rapid growth and expands outside of the coelom into the yolk stalk during weeks 4 to 8. It begins its normal rotation with a 90-degree counterclockwise turn about the axis of the superior mesenteric artery and then returns to the abdominal cavity in the 8th to 10th week of gestation to continue a further 180-degree rotation before its fixation to the posterior abdomen. The end result of this 270-degree turn is the cecum fixed in the right lower abdomen and the duodenum fixed in the left upper abdomen with a broad base of mesentery separating the two fixation points.

Various errors in normal rotation may occur, from complete nonrotation to reverse rotation of part or all of the embryonic gut. Complete nonrotation leaves the small intestine on the right side of the abdomen and the colon on the left, leaving a wide mesenteric base, and therefore there is low risk of volvulus. Malrotation, however, results in a nonrotated duodenojejunal limb with partial rotation of the cecum located in the upper mid-abdomen with a narrow mesenteric base that is susceptible to midgut volvulus and strangulation, its most feared complication. The cecum also has peritoneal attachments, called Ladd's bands, to the right lateral abdominal wall that overlie and compress the duodenum, causing duodenal obstruction.

Clinical Features

Intestinal malrotation is thought to occur in 1 in 500 live births based on autopsy studies; however, only 1 in 6000 lead to clinical presentation. The true incidence is unknown because many remain asymptomatic. Those that do present with symptoms may do so at any time from infancy to adulthood; however, approximately 30% to 50% occur within the first month of life and 70% within the first year of life.[14–16] Intestinal volvulus is the most feared complication and can result in life-threatening intestinal ischemia and necrosis; however, more benign presentation with duodenal obstruction due to compression from overlying Ladd's bands may occur. Bilious emesis is typically the first sign in infants[14] and should trigger immediate suspicion for malrotation, but nonbilious emesis may also occur, especially with proximal duodenal obstruction. Abdominal distention and tenderness may be present with midgut volvulus and may progress to hemodynamic instability, peritonitis, and hematochezia in cases of threatened or necrotic bowel. Patients with malrotation may have associated congenital anomalies, most commonly diaphragmatic hernia, complex cardiac anomalies, and abdominal wall disorders. Heterotaxia disorders have associated malrotation in 40% to 90% of cases.[16,17] Older children may present with acute volvulus as well but often have a more insidious onset of chronic abdominal pain, intermittent bilious or nonbilious emesis, failure to thrive, malabsorption, motility disorders, or chylous ascites.[14]

Evaluation

Due to the potential for life-threatening intestinal volvulus, clinicians must have a high level of suspicion for any of the signs of malrotation mentioned above. Any infant with bilious emesis, duodenal obstruction, or abdominal tenderness with hemodynamic changes or with nonbilious emesis in the setting of a known associated congenital anomaly should be treated as having intestinal volvulus until proven otherwise and undergo emergent evaluation and/or intervention. Hemodynamic instability with peritonitis requires no further workup and should undergo emergent surgical exploration to address potential threatened or necrotic bowel. In the absence of such hard signs, workup should begin with a plain abdominal film, which is nonspecific for malrotation, but it will show the bowel gas pattern and evaluate for free intraperitoneal air. Additionally, plain film may show a nasoenteric tube placed in a malpositioned duodenum or a double bubble sign indicating duodenal obstruction. In the hemodynamically stable infant, a fluoroscopic upper GI series with small bowel follow-through remains the imaging gold standard for diagnosis of malrotation. A misplaced duodenum with the ligament of Treitz to the right of midline and a corkscrew appearance of the proximal bowel is suggestive of malrotation; however, any abnormal placement of the duodenojejunal junction can be suspicious for malrotation. Duodenal obstruction seen on upper GI may mimic duodenal atresia; however, a tapering bird's beak at the point of obstruction is suggestive of volvulus. In centers with experienced radiologists, upper GI studies have sensitivity up to 96% for detecting malrotation[18]; however, results may be subtle or inconclusive, with a false-positive rate up to 15%.[19] Useful radiologic studies to assist in diagnosis include ultrasound to assess the location of the duodenum in relation to the mesenteric vessels and "swirling" of the vessels in cases of volvulus. The location of the cecum may not correlate with disorders of rotation, although in the past, barium enema was used to assess the location of the cecum. Diagnostic laparoscopy or laparotomy may be required to make a definitive diagnosis in the absence of definitive radiologic studies if clinical suspicion is high enough.

Management

The definitive treatment for intestinal malrotation and associated intestinal volvulus and duodenal obstruction is the Ladd's procedure. Its goal is not to restore normal intestinal anatomy but rather to reduce the risk of obstruction, volvulus, and devastating intestinal necrosis. Preoperatively, the patient is resuscitated, a decompressive nasogastric tube is placed, and broad-spectrum perioperative antibiotics are administered. Symptomatic patients should be taken emergently to the operating room due to the risk of volvulus and its potentially devastating sequelae.

Ladd's procedure involves exploration of the abdominal cavity to confirm the abnormal anatomy, reduction of any volvulus if present, division of the Ladd's bands that tether the cecum to the right lateral abdominal wall and duodenum if present, widening the base of the mesentery by incising the peritoneum to gain length between the arcades of the superior mesenteric artery, and prophylactic appendectomy due to the abnormal position of the appendix and the risk for subsequent atypical presentation of appendicitis.[20] The bowel must be fully examined for areas of injury or necrosis, with resection and possible ostomy versus primary anastomosis if nonviable bowel is found. Temporary closure may be employed with subsequent return for a second look if areas of questionable viability are present. Complete nonrotation of the intestine carries a low risk of volvulus because the mesenteric base is typically wide; however, distinguishing nonrotation from malrotation is difficult without direct visualization, so exploration and appendectomy are indicated in most cases.

Historically, the open laparotomy with the Ladd's procedure was felt necessary for formation of adhesions to secure the bowel in a position of nonrotation to prevent recurrent volvulus. Newer evidence has since emerged supporting the role of laparoscopic Ladd's procedure in the treatment of malrotation.[20,21] Operative times and rates of recurrent volvulus appear to be equivalent between open and laparoscopic approaches, and laparoscopy is associated with lower rates of postoperative bowel obstruction and overall complication rates as well as a shorter hospital stay. The laparoscopic approach to Ladd's procedure is a safe and effective option in experienced hands.

The approach to the asymptomatic child with radiographic signs of intestinal malrotation remains controversial, especially when discovered outside the neonatal period. Elective exploration is generally indicated in cases of incidentally diagnosed malrotation in a neonate due to the high morbidity associated with potential volvulus. Most cases of volvulus occur in infancy and the risk is thought to decrease with age, but the true natural history of the disease is not well known because many patients remain asymptomatic for life.[14] In the presence of a documented malrotation, diagnostic laparoscopy with Ladd's procedure is a safe and effective option.

Long-Term Outcomes

Outcomes after Ladd's procedure for malrotation are largely dependent on the presence of volvulus and necrotic bowel. Those without necrotic bowel have an excellent prognosis with survival approaching 100%, and most deaths are associated with congenital cardiac disease. Of the 40% of neonates who present with midgut volvulus requiring intestinal resection, long-term outcomes are based on the extent of resection and remaining bowel function. Those requiring >75% resection of small bowel are at high risk of subsequent intestinal failure and mortality.[22] Additional morbidity after Ladd's procedure include postoperative ileus, adhesive small bowel obstruction, and anastomotic leak and stricture. Rates of recurrent volvulus are low (approximately 0%–5%) and do not appear to be different in a laparoscopic versus open approach.[19,21]

Meconium Ileus

Meconium ileus (MI) is a cause of neonatal bowel obstruction primarily seen in patients with cystic fibrosis (CF). It is the earliest manifestation of CF and results from luminal obstruction by inspissated meconium that adheres to the wall of the bowel, typically in the distal ileum, although the entire intestinal tract may be involved. Mutations in the CF transmembrane conductance regulator gene (*CFTR*) result in desiccation and thickening of intraluminal mucus due to errors in electrolyte transport across the mucous membrane. The majority of cases of MI are CF related; however, some isolated series report rates as high as 46% without positive CF testing, signifying additional contributors that may also influence this disease process.[23,24]

Clinical presentation typically includes abdominal distention, feeding intolerance, emesis, and failure to pass meconium within 24 to 48 hours. MI is classified as complex if there are associated GI complications including bowel necrosis, intestinal perforation, meconium peritonitis, atresia, or volvulus. Up to 40% of patients with CF present with complex disease, whereas it is exceedingly rare in non-CF patients.[24]

As CF carrier testing becomes more common and fetal ultrasound improves, prenatal diagnosis of MI has become more common. Ultrasound findings include dilated small bowel, hyperechoic intraluminal meconium masses, or peritoneal calcifications in the case of perforation and meconium peritonitis. Suspicious ultrasound findings should prompt parental CF screening, and those with confirmation of CF or continued abnormal ultrasound findings should be referred to a tertiary pediatric care center with pediatric surgical expertise. Postnatally, abdominal x-ray will also reveal dilated intestinal loops, possible signs of perforation such as free air, or peritoneal calcifications. Contrast enema is the next step in evaluation for patients without signs of perforation and may show diminutive colon and meconium pellets in the distal ileum. Infants with suspected MI should undergo definitive testing for CF.[25]

As in any case of neonatal bowel obstruction, initial management includes fluid and electrolyte resuscitation, nasogastric decompression, and prophylactic broad-spectrum antibiotics. Preservation of intestinal function and nutritional support is of critical importance for CF patients, and a conservative first-line approach in management in MI is recommended. Infants with simple MI confirmed on diagnostic enema should undergo therapeutic enema using hyperosmotic contrast under fluoroscopic guidance, which may be performed serially, drawing fluid into the lumen to soften and break up inspissated meconium. Addition of N-acetylcysteine may increase efficacy. Operative intervention is indicated for infants with complex MI or those who fail nonoperative management, with goals of disimpaction of inspissated meconium, restoration of luminal continuity, and conservation of functional bowel length. Several approaches have been employed to allow for continued postoperative irrigation, including tube enterostomy, proximal or distal chimney enterostomy, and Mikulicz double-barreled enterostomy, with resection of any necrotic or nonfunctional bowel if necessary. Resection with intraoperative meconium evacuation and primary anastomosis is also an option; it immediately restores full bowel continuity but does not allow further local irrigation and may have higher leak rates.[25] Postoperatively, enteral feeds should be advanced as soon as tolerated, with pancreatic enzyme replacement therapy in patients with pancreatic dysfunction. Ostomy reversal is generally performed by 6 weeks to 2 months from the time of surgery but is dependent on the patient's clinical status.[25]

With improvements in neonatal intensive care, nutritional support, infection prevention, and nonoperative and operative interventions, prognosis has become quite good for patients with MI, with survival approaching 100%. Long-term pulmonary outcomes and overall survival are equivalent between patients with CF and without MI and between those treated for complex versus simple disease.[25]

Meconium plug syndrome is a disease process that also presents in the neonatal period with obstruction due to inspissated thickened meconium; however, it is considered to be a separate entity from MI. Meconium plugs generally occur in the colon rather than the ileum, and approximately 30% resolve without any intervention whereas nearly all (97%) resolve with hyperosmotic contrast enema. It is associated with Hirschsprung disease in up to 38% of cases, and although there does appear to be an association with CF, it is highly variable in the literature (0%–43%) with possible confusion in discriminating plug from ileus in older data.[26,27]

Duplication Cysts

Duplication cysts are cystic or tubular structures composed of intestinal remnants that share a muscular layer and mesenteric blood supply with the adjacent bowel but have separate mucosal layers. These contain epithelium of the associated bowel, or ectopic (gastric) or respiratory epithelium. Duplication cysts are uncommon, reported in 1 in 4500 by autopsy reports.[28] The exact etiology is unknown, but one prominent theory is the split notochord theory. During the third week of gestation, the notochord appears and grows cephalad with the endoderm. As the notochord separates from the endoderm, a band between them causes a traction diverticulum, which develops into the duplication cyst.[29] These can occur anywhere along the alimentary tract from the mouth to the anus but most commonly occur in the small intestine.[30]

Clinical presentation is widely variable based on size, location, and presence of gastric mucosa. These can cause obstructive symptoms through external compression or as lead points for intussusception or a segmental volvulus. Gastric duplications may present with vomiting or poor feeding. Duodenal duplications may cause jaundice or pancreatitis. Ectopic gastric mucosa can secrete acid, causing ulceration of adjacent bowel and leading to GI bleeding or perforation. Children with duplication cysts have a higher incidence of associated anomalies including spinal malformations, intestinal atresias, malrotation, or urinary tract anomalies in midgut and hindgut duplication cysts. This incidence is higher for those with multiple duplications.[30,31]

Duplication cysts can often be detected with pre- or postnatal ultrasound; however, determining the origin is not always possible. Computed tomography or magnetic resonance imaging are not generally indicated but are useful to further characterize duodenal duplications. If intestinal bleeding is present, a Meckel scan may be useful to identify ectopic gastric mucosa.

Surgical excision of duplication cysts is recommended to prevent complications of obstruction, bleeding, or infection. Complete resection is the goal; however, the size and location may prohibit complete resection without significant morbidity such as esophageal, gastric, duodenal, or long-segment intestinal lesions. Partial resection with stripping of the mucosa may be necessary in these cases. Duodenal lesions present a unique challenge because most are located on the medial side of the second portion of the duodenum, and intraoperative cholangiography with internal drainage may be indicated to avoid injury to the biliary system.[32] Cystic duplication cysts on the small intestine are located on the mesenteric border and require a segmental bowel resection with primary anastomosis. Examination for additional synchronous cysts should be performed, because synchronous duplication cysts can be seen in 20% of cases.[32] Tubular cysts on the small intestine can involve long segments, and complete resection would lead to short-gut syndrome. Partial resection of the seromuscular wall with stripping of the mucosa along the length of the duplication, or creating openings between the duplication cyst and adjacent bowel, are preferable alternatives to complete resection. Outcomes from duplication cyst resections are generally excellent but depend largely on the location and extent of the resection required. Recurrences can occur if the cysts were incompletely excised.

Abdominal Wall Defects

Pathophysiology

Omphalocele and gastroschisis are clinically distinct abdominal wall defects. Omphalocele results from an error in embryonic development leading to failure of the cephalic, caudal, and/or lateral folds to close the abdominal wall defect, typically by the 10th week of gestation.[33,34] Loops of intestine, stomach, and liver may herniate through the defect, but these are contained within a membranous sac (Fig. 83.1). There is a high association with other anomalies, particularly cardiac and chromosomal disorders. Failure of the cephalic fold is associated with pentalogy of Cantrell (cleft sternum, diaphragmatic defects, pericardial defects, cardiac anomalies, and omphalocele),[35] whereas failure of the caudal fold is associated with lower abdominal defects (bladder exstrophy, cloacal exstrophy, and imperforate anus).

The etiology of gastroschisis is not exactly clear but appears to result from dissociation of the right umbilical vein and subsequent weakness and rupture of the abdominal wall (Fig. 83.2).[33] The vast majority of all gastroschisis occurs to the right of the umbilicus. Gastroschisis is typically not associated with other developmental anomalies; however, intestinal atresia can be seen in up to 15% of cases, and there is a high association with intrauterine growth restriction.[36]

Clinical Features

Omphalocele

Omphalocele has a prevalence of 2.1 in 10,000 births and is associated with older mothers (>40 years) and maternal obesity.[36] Associated anomalies occur in up to 80% of patients, with the most common being cardiac defects (ventricular septal defect is most common) and chromosomal anomalies, the majority being trisomy 18, 13, and 21. Beckwith-Wiedemann syndrome is associated with fetal and early childhood overgrowth (macroglossia, hypoglycemia, and visceromegaly), with half of patients having an omphalocele.[37] At delivery, a central defect of the abdominal wall is easily seen with herniation of abdominal contents that are covered with a membranous sac. The umbilical cord inserts into the sac, and the herniated contents can contain intestine, stomach, or liver. Although rare, sac rupture can occur in utero. Pulmonary hypoplasia is also common.

Gastroschisis

The incidence of gastroschisis is increasing worldwide, from 2.3 cases per 10,000 live births in 1995 to 4.3 per 10,000 in 2016.[36] Young maternal age is a risk factor. After delivery, an abdominal wall defect with herniated exposed intestine is seen lateral to the umbilicus. Persistent exposure to amniotic fluid results in an intestinal peel, and the bowel may be thick and matted. Intestinal atresia may be seen, although this is not always apparent on initial exam. Prenatal volvulus or closing/vanishing gastroschisis are rare but can lead to severe intestinal loss.[38]

Evaluation

Prenatal ultrasound can readily detect and distinguish between omphalocele and gastroschisis. Prenatal findings for omphalocele will show a membrane covering the herniated contents with an umbilical cord inserting directly into the sac, whereas in gastroschisis, the umbilical cord insertion site is normal, and free-floating loops of intestine are seen herniating through a paramedian defect.[39] Elevated AFP is seen in both disorders; however, this is more common in gastroschisis.

Management

Antenatal detection of either omphalocele or gastroschisis warrants planned delivery at a pediatric tertiary center with immediate availability of neonatologists and pediatric surgical consultation. The need for cesarean section should be based on obstetric indications

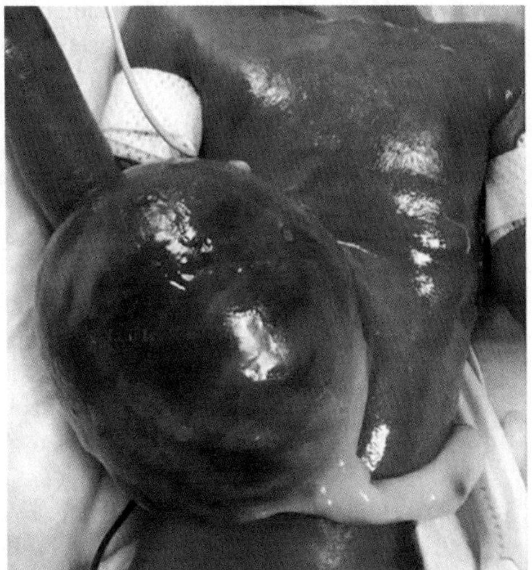

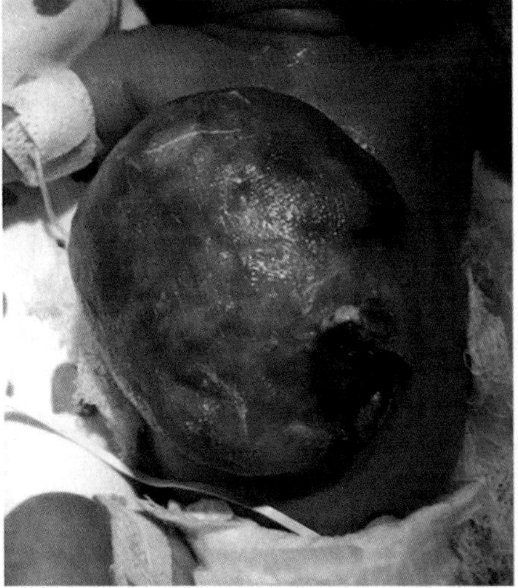

Fig. 83.1 Giant Omphalocele in a Newborn. (A) Giant omphalocele with an intact sac with a large portion of liver and intestine within the sac. Note that the umbilical cord inserts into the sac directly. (B) The same omphalocele at 3 weeks of life after painting of the sac with silvadene and betadine.

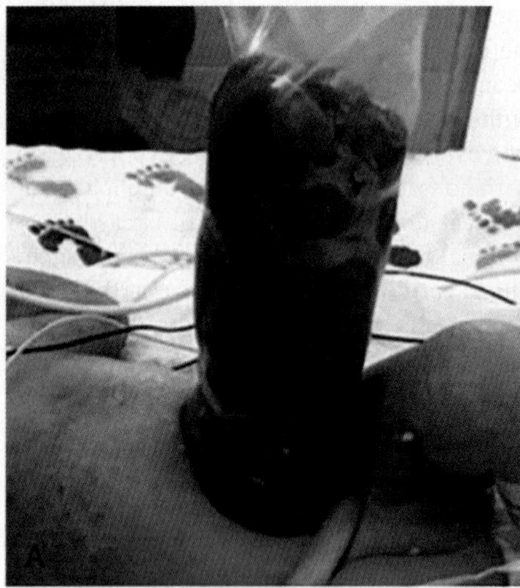

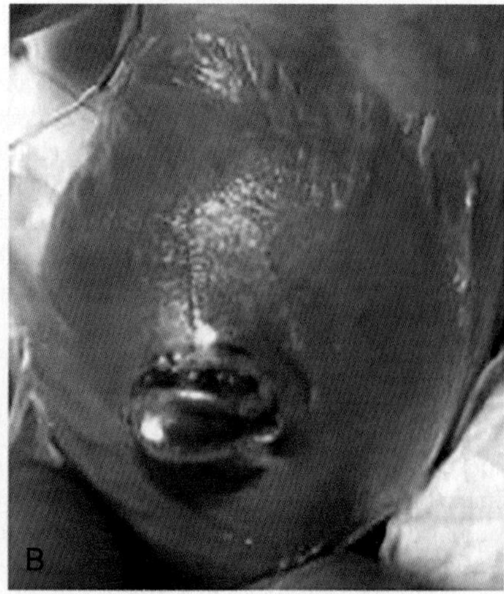

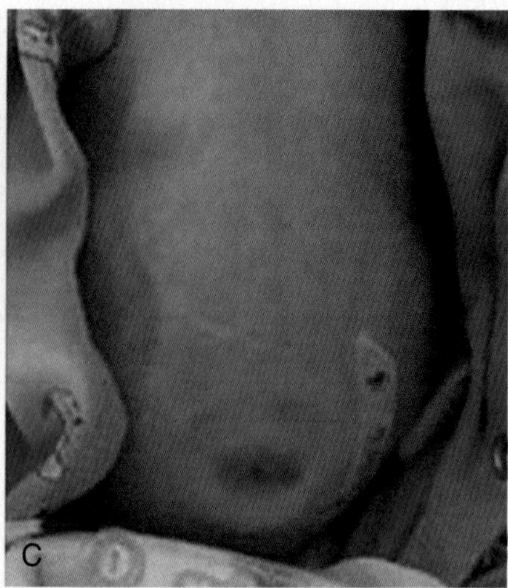

Fig. 83.2 Staged Sutureless Repair of Gastroschisis. (A) Placement of silo with intestine suspended above the patient. (B) After adequate reduction of bowel, the umbilical cord was placed over the defect and a clear plastic dressing was applied over the whole abdomen. (C) Final result with normal-appearing umbilicus.

because vaginal delivery has not been shown to adversely affect outcomes for gastroschisis or omphalocele.[36,40] However, some advocate for cesarian sections for giant omphaloceles due to risk of rupturing the sac during vaginal delivery.[41]

After delivery, the initial management of both defects is similar. The herniated abdominal contents are covered to minimize heat and fluid loss, typically using a bowel bag, but clear plastic wrap or warm saline-soaked gauze can be used for omphaloceles. The child may need positioning on the right side to avoid stretching or twisting of the mesenteric vessels. A nasogastric tube is placed and intravenous fluids are initiated. Broad-spectrum antibiotics are given. For omphaloceles, a thorough evaluation for associated anomalies should be carried out and include echocardiogram, plain chest, pelvis, and spine radiographs, renal ultrasound, and chromosomal analysis.

Omphalocele

Determining the optimal management of the omphalocele depends on the patient's gestational age and weight, the size of the omphalocele, liver involvement, and cardiac or other associated anomalies. Small- or medium-sized omphaloceles with adequate abdominal domain should be closed primarily if associated comorbidities allow. This involves excision of the sac, reduction of herniated contents, and closure of the fascia with or without a synthetic patch. For larger omphaloceles, returning the contents into the abdominal cavity may cause respiratory failure, especially with pulmonary hypoplasia, or abdominal compartment syndrome (ACS).[42] Use of a silo allows a staged repair and closure, typically over the course of 7 to 10 days. Patients with giant omphaloceles or with significant comorbidities can be managed initially with a "paint and wait" strategy, where the omphalocele sac is treated with silver sulfadiazine, diluted betadine, or other irritant that will cause eschar formation around the sac and eventual epithelialization. These patients can then undergo elective repair later in infancy or childhood.[41,43]

Gastroschisis

Closure of the gastroschisis is performed primarily or in a staged approach. Primary repair is preferred if it can be performed safely without resulting in high intraabdominal pressures and ACS. ACS may not be apparent until several hours and warrants close attention after the repair. For a staged approach, a spring-loaded Silastic silo device is placed at the bedside, and the bowel can be suspended in a column above the patient.[41,44,45] Sequential reductions of the bowel within the silo are performed over the course of the next several days until the bowel is reduced to the level of the fascia and subsequent repair can be successfully performed. Repair can be performed operatively by creating skin flaps and closing the abdominal wall fascia, or alternatively, by sutureless repair using the umbilical stalk as a cap over the defect. This latter technique can sometimes be performed without general anesthesia.[46]

Prolonged ileus is expected due to intestinal dysmotility, and parenteral nutrition is initiated early until full enteral feeds are achieved. Full tolerance of enteral feeds may take weeks to months. An associated intestinal atresia may not be diagnosed for weeks after abdominal wall closure and will require operative exploration, typically weeks after initial closure. In addition, necrotizing enterocolitis is seen in up to 15% of patients with gastroschisis.[47]

Long-Term Outcomes

For patients with omphalocele, the major sources of mortality are from the associated anomalies, particularly cardiac defects. Long-term survival has increased association with feeding difficulties, gastroesophageal reflux disease, pulmonary insufficiency, neurodevelopmental deficiencies, and concerns of cosmetic appearance.[48–50] Overall outcomes for children with gastroschisis have improved significantly, with survival rates exceeding 90%.[41] Gastroesophageal reflux disease is common, seen in 90% of patients, and cryptorchidism is seen in 38.7%. Ventral hernias are seen in 10% to 15%.

CHAPTER 84

Pulmonary Surgery in the Newborn

Andres J. Gonzalez Salazar, Carley Blevins, Eric Jelin

KEY POINTS

1. Neonatal respiratory disease that requires surgery can have devastating consequences. Care for patients with these conditions involves a multidisciplinary team including neonatologists, pediatric surgeons, nurses, and respiratory therapists.
2. These surgical respiratory defects include upper airway stenosis, laryngomalacia and tracheomalacia, congenital lung lesions, and the congenital defects of the diaphragm.
3. Stridor is the most characteristic finding of upper respiratory obstructions. Acute obstruction may be asymptomatic or present with stridor, tachypnea, fatigue, nasal flaring, cyanosis, drooling, and use of accessory muscles. Chronic obstruction may present as failure to thrive and poor weight gain due to poor coordination between swallowing and breathing.
4. Laryngomalacia is the most frequently seen congenital laryngeal anomaly and typically presents with stridor. It is characterized by an inward collapse of the supraglottic airway with inspiration. Laryngeal stenosis can occur in the supraglottic or the subglottic regions.
5. Tracheomalacia is characterized by an increased collapsibility of the trachea. This is caused by structural anomalies of the tracheal cartilage or posterior membrane or by external vascular compression. In congenital tracheal stenosis the trachea is narrow due to complete, abnormal cartilaginous rings that result in stenotic segments.
6. Abnormalities of the aortic arch and pulmonary vasculature can compress the airway and cause respiratory compromise. Patients present with noisy breathing, barking cough, recurrent respiratory tract infections, and dysphagia and may have episodes of apnea.
7. Congenital lung lesions are a spectrum of developmental anomalies such as congenital pulmonary airway malformations, bronchopulmonary sequestrations, and congenital lobar emphysema. Other malformations include bronchogenic cysts, lymphangiomas, and pleuropulmonary blastomas.
8. Congenital diaphragmatic hernia is a defect of the diaphragm through which any intraabdominal organ can protrude into the chest. It is intrinsically associated with lung hypoplasia and pulmonary hypertension beyond simple physical compression.
9. Diaphragmatic eventrations are marked by an abnormal elevation of the hemidiaphragm. These can be congenital or acquired. Congenital diaphragmatic eventrations result from incomplete development of the central tendon or the muscular portion of the diaphragm.

Upper Respiratory Airway Disease

Diseases of the upper respiratory airway in infants can be classified according to their etiology as congenital or acquired. Acquired disease is more common and primarily associated with prolonged intubation, whereas congenital disease is associated with a developmental defect during gestation.[1–3] In the neonate, this distinction may be hard to make because an acquired injury is commonly superimposed on a congenital abnormality.[1,4]

Anatomically, the pediatric upper airway is similar to an inverted cone, with the trachea fitting into the cricoid above it, the cricoid into the thyroid cartilage, and the thyroid cartilage into the hyoid space (Fig. 84.1).[4,5] The larynx of a term infant measures approximately 4.5 mm in the coronal plane and 7 mm in the sagittal plane. It allows for respiration and protection of the respiratory tract but also serves the secondary function of phonation through the use of the vocal cords. The narrowest point of the larynx is the subglottic space, measuring 4 mm across.[1]

Clinical Characteristics

The presentation of upper airway disease is highly variable. Patients may be asymptomatic or present with stridor, tachypnea, fatigue, nasal flaring, cyanosis, drooling, and use of accessory muscles. Chronic obstruction may present as failure to thrive and poor weight gain due to poor coordination between swallowing and breathing.[2]

Stridor is the most characteristic finding of upper respiratory obstructions. The types of stridor are based on the affected portion of the respiratory tree. Stridor during inspiration is characteristic of obstructions in the supraglottic region, whereas stridor during expiration is caused by lesions in the intrathoracic trachea or bronchi. Obstruction of the glottis or subglottis causes a biphasic stridor, heard during both inspiration and expiration. Emergent medical attention is warranted, because this form of stridor can quickly precede respiratory collapse.

Examination of a neonate in respiratory distress should begin with an evaluation for upper airway disease. The initial step is to access the acuity of respiratory compromise. If the airway is unstable, emergency airway access through endotracheal intubation or a surgical airway procedure (tracheostomy) is performed. If the child is stable, patient data can be gathered including history of prematurity, endotracheal intubation, or associated syndromes. Due to the location of the airway and gastrointestinal tract in relation to one another, difficulty swallowing or eating may be indicative of mediastinal masses, vascular rings, or other lesions such as a foreign body in the esophagus. Information concerning episodes of choking, coughing, or cyanotic spells during feeds also constitutes an important finding.[1,2]

Diagnosis

Endoscopy

Evaluation of the upper airway is done through direct visualization or with endoscopic equipment. It may be performed on an awake child, which allows for functional and dynamic assessment of the larynx and vocal cords, or it can be done under sedation or general

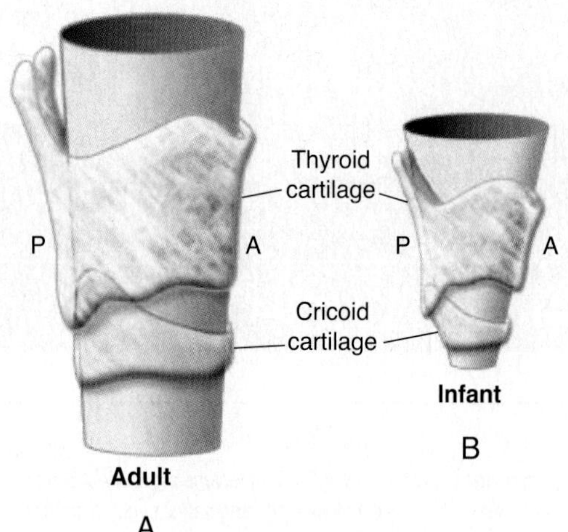

Fig. 84.1 Anatomic Differences Between the Adult (A) and Infant (B) Larynx. The infant larynx is an inverted cone with a larger difference between the top and the bottom radius. The subglottis is the narrowest point of the larynx. *A*, Anterior; *P*, posterior. (Obtained with permission from Fiadjoe JE, Litman RS, Serber JF, Stricker PA, Coté CJ. The pediatric airway. In: Coté CJ, Lerman J, Anderson BJ, eds. *A Practice of Anesthesia for Infants and Children*. Elsevier; 2019:297–339.e21. doi:10.1016/B978-0-323-42974-0.00014-8.)

anesthesia, which is better suited for obstructive lesions and those further down the respiratory tract.

Endoscopic airway evaluation is ideally done in a setting with ample cooperation between the anesthesiologist, a nurse or surgical assistant, a pulmonologist, and the surgeon (ear, nose and throat [ENT] and/or pediatric surgeon). Assessment in the setting of respiratory compromise should be done efficiently and carefully. Any forceful contact with the upper airway mucosa may easily worsen the respiratory status. Instruments for urgent airway access should be easily available.

The visualization of the larynx, or laryngoscopy, is categorized according to whether the provider is directly viewing the larynx (direct laryngoscopy) or is viewing the larynx through a mirror or camera (indirect laryngoscopy). Awake, flexible fiberoptic laryngoscopy allows for assessment of dynamic airway collapse and vocal cord mobility. It may help evaluate the sinonasal cavity (nasolacrimal duct cysts and polyps, nasoseptal deviation), nasopharynx (choanal atresia, nasopharyngeal stenosis, adenoid hypertrophy), oropharynx (tonsil hypertrophy, pharyngomalacia), and larynx (laryngomalacia, vocal cord immobility).[6]

Evaluation of the trachea and bronchi is performed with a bronchoscope. Flexible bronchoscopy allows for assessment of the distal airway. The standard pediatric flexible bronchoscope is 3.5 to 3.7 mm in diameter and can be used in patients who weigh as little as 700 g.[2] Some of them can pass through tracheostomy tubes or endotracheal tubes and still allow for ventilation. Flexible bronchoscopy can be performed through the mouth or nare. This provides the advantage of evaluating patients with anatomic anomalies or maxillofacial trauma.

Rigid bronchoscopy permits detailed examination of the trachea and proximal bronchi and allows for the use of instruments through its larger ports. However, it can only be performed through the mouth and thus requires neck hyperextension. Children with physical conditions that cause decreased width of the mouth opening or decreased neck mobility are at higher risk of complications.[7]

Endoscopic techniques are versatile procedures that not only allow for diagnosis through visual assessment, ultrasound evaluation, and biologic sampling but may also be therapeutic in certain situations. Laser fulguration with CO_2, respiratory secretion clearance, and stent deployment are some therapeutic techniques. Additionally, when patient have worsening respiratory status, endoscopy can provide assistance for quick intubation or safe surgical airway access.

Imaging

Radiographic imaging can be performed depending on symptoms and may aid in the differential diagnosis. The soft tissue of the neck and chest is viewed in lateral and anteroposterior radiographs during both inspiration and expiration. Computed tomography (CT) scans and magnetic resonance imaging (MRI) can be used to delineate the anatomy and with contrast enhancement can help evaluate vascular structures or masses that may be compressing the airway.

Laryngomalacia

Laryngomalacia is the most common congenital laryngeal anomaly and the most common cause of stridor in infants. It is characterized by an inward collapse of the supraglottic airway with inspiration.[8,9] Symptoms may start shortly after birth with an average age of presentation of 2 weeks.[10] Mild disease presents only as stridor, whereas moderate disease will also be accompanied by difficulty feeding. Ten percent of patients develop severe airway compromise, which requires surgical intervention.[9]

Laryngomalacia is associated with several neonatal conditions. Gastroesophageal reflux is the most frequently associated comorbidity, with reported rates of up to 66%.[11] Treatment for gastroesophageal reflux is therefore often required. Neurologic disease is also seen in 8% to 45% of children requiring operative management.[12]

Awake flexible fiberoptic laryngoscopy is the standard for diagnosis because it allows for direct and dynamic visualization of the supraglottic airway. Radiographic techniques have little use but may rule out other pulmonary conditions.

The majority of patients with laryngomalacia have resolution of their symptoms with conservative management (speech therapy, acid suppression, and food thickening), with reports showing 80% to 90% resolution of symptoms within 4 to 42 months.[13,14] As the child grows, the airway enlarges and symptoms decrease. For patient with severe symptoms, surgical management is required. Supraglottoplasty is the surgical procedure of choice. It involves removing prolapsing supraglottic tissue with surgical instruments or endoscopically with CO_2 laser.[15,16]

Laryngeal Stenosis

Stenosis of the larynx can be divided according to the area of involvement. It can occur in the supraglottis or the subglottis. The subglottis, the portion of the airway with the smallest diameter, is the most commonly involved. A lumen diameter less than 4 mm in full-term infants and less than 3 mm in preterm infants is considered stenotic.[1]

Subglottic stenosis is the third most common congenital laryngeal anomaly in the newborn, after laryngomalacia and vocal fold paralysis, and is the most common acquired laryngeal anomaly.[17,18] It is caused by failure of recanalization of the airway by the 10th week of gestation or by iatrogenic injury due to placement of a large endotracheal tube. It is associated with trisomy 21, CHARGE syndrome, and 22q11 deletion syndrome.[3,6]

As prolonged endotracheal intubation became more common for preterm infants, the incidence of subglottic stenosis increased.

Reports from the 1960s saw rates ranging from 12% to 20% among patient with prolonged periods of intubation.[19] Advances in intubation techniques and improved endotracheal tube care have decreased the incidence to 0.9% to 8.3%.[20–23]

Mild cases can be managed conservatively, with the majority of patients outgrowing the condition.[24] Severe cases require surgical intervention, usually by tracheostomy. Other management options include endoscopic balloon dilation and laryngotracheal reconstruction with cartilage graft.[25,26]

Laryngeal Webs and Laryngeal Atresia

Laryngeal or glottic webs may be congenital or acquired. Congenital webs are associated with deletions of chromosome 22q11.2, and acquired lesions are caused by injury to the larynx. Given syndromic associations, patients should undergo evaluation for other anomalies.[3]

Laryngeal webs are classified according to the degree of obstruction, with the most severe being total laryngeal atresia.[19] Hoarseness is the most common symptoms seen in webs, whereas aphonia and rapid asphyxia are seen with atresia. Diagnosis is initially clinical and confirmed with endoscopic techniques.

Management goals are to address the obstruction and preserve phonation. If severe airway obstruction is present, tracheostomy is mandated and definitive management delayed. For mild laryngeal webs, endoscopic lysis with topical mitomycin is sufficient,[27] but for more severe webs, laryngotracheal reconstruction may be required.[28] Total atresia of the larynx causes congenital high airway obstruction syndrome in utero. This syndrome is generally lethal, but some reports of survival with fetal intervention have been reported.[19,29]

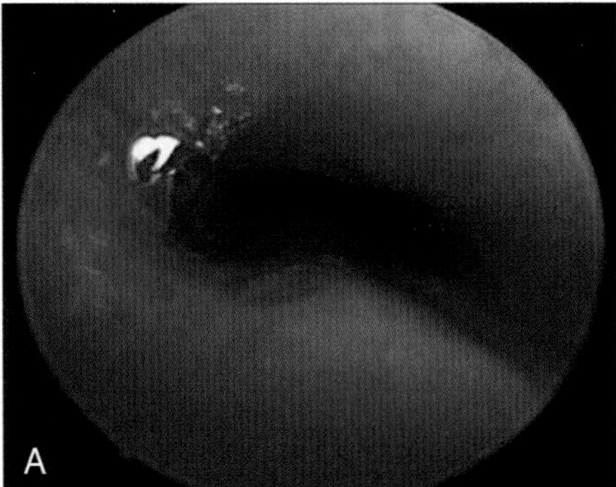

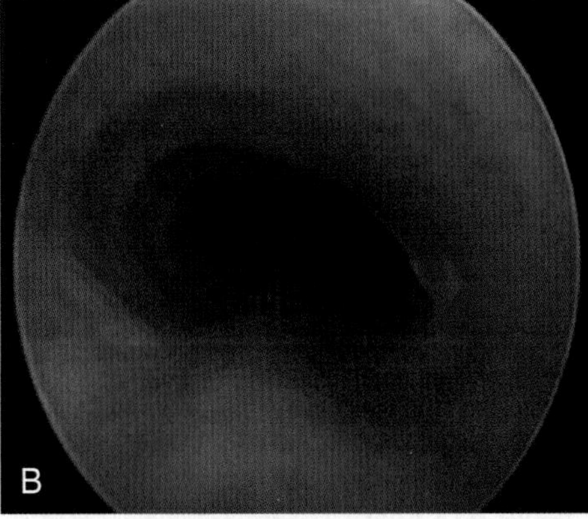

Fig. 84.2 Secondary Tracheomalacia Caused by Innominate Artery Compression. (A) Before aortopexy. (B) After aortopexy. (Obtained with permission from Thompson DM, Cotton RT. Lesions of the larynx, trachea, and upper airway. In: Grosfeld JL, O'Neill JA, Coran AG, Fonkalsrud EW, Caldamone AA, eds. *Pediatric Surgery*. Elsevier/Saunders; 2006: 1–2, 983–1000. doi:10.1016/B978-0-323-42974-0.00014-8.)

Tracheomalacia

Tracheomalacia is a condition characterized by an increased collapsibility of the trachea. This is caused by structural anomalies of the tracheal cartilage or posterior membrane or external vascular compression (Fig. 84.2). Patients with a history of tracheoesophageal fistula or those who undergo prolonged intubation have increased risk of developing this disease.[30,31]

Symptoms generally only occur during periods of high respiratory demand. These symptoms consist of a brassy cough, expiratory stridor, and "dying spells" that happen during or immediately after feeding. Direct visualization via endoscopy is the gold standard for diagnosis, but CT and MRI are used as complementary studies to assess for external compression.

Symptoms of mild cases of tracheomalacia improve and resolve over the first year of life. Medical treatment with hypertonic nebulizers, inhaled steroids, and bronchodilators help manage symptoms.[32] Continuous positive airway pressure is effective for moderate disease, and surgical interventions are reserved for patients with "dying spells," recurrent infection, or difficulty extubating.[30,33]

Historically, tracheostomy and mechanical ventilation were the mainstay treatment for patients with severe tracheomalacia. This approach has fallen out of favor due to the risks associated with long-term tracheostomy tube placement. Current management is individualized and depends on associated conditions (vascular compression, mediastinal masses, and presence of tracheoesophageal fistula). Surgical options include open or thoracoscopic aortopexy, tracheal resection with end-to-end anastomosis, slide tracheoplasty, and tracheopexy (Fig. 84.3).[30,34]

Intraluminal airway stenting has been used to decrease the effects of tracheal narrowing. Newer stents can be deployed into the airway endoscopically and require bronchoscopy and fluoroscopy to ensure the stent is appropriately placed to support the lumen best.[35] Although stents to treat tracheomalacia seem promising, potential complications such as stent migration causing erosion or obstruction may be significant.[35]

Tracheal Stenosis

The normal trachea has horseshoe-shaped cartilaginous rings and a posterior wall composed of connective tissue and the trachealis muscle. This morphology gives the trachea enough compliance to provide adequate ventilation. In congenital tracheal stenosis (CTS) the trachea is narrow due to complete, abnormal cartilaginous rings, which result in stenotic segments.[2,4,36] CTS is associated with congenital vascular and cardiac malformations in 25% to 70% of cases and with lung hypoplasia and total lung agenesis.[36]

Presentation of CTS is variable and depends on the degree of stenosis. It can present in the early neonatal period with stridor, cyanotic spells, and coarse cough or may develop later in childhood, associated with exercise-related respiratory difficulties.[37] The stenotic segment does not necessarily produce immediate respiratory distress, but in the setting of mucosal edema, it may lead to acute airway obstruction and require surgical intervention.[4]

Acquired tracheal stenosis is most frequently caused by an iatrogenic event that leads to inflammation, ulceration, and scarring.[4] This is common in patients with underlying CTS, where an

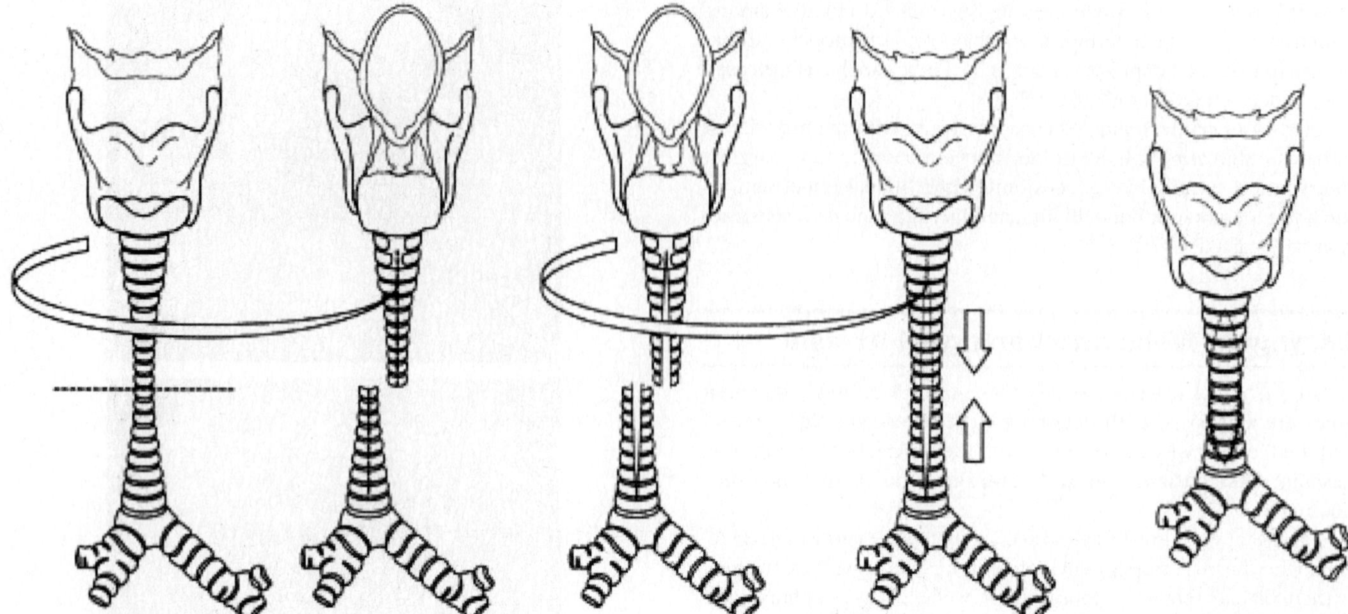

Fig. 84.3 Slide Tracheoplasty Technique. Transverse section of the trachea. The proximal segment is slid posteriorly and the distal segment anteriorly through the midline. The portions are slid together, doubling the circumference. (Obtained with permission from Thompson DM, Cotton RT. Lesions of the larynx, trachea, and upper airway. In: Grosfeld JL, O'Neill JA, Coran AG, Fonkalsrud EW, Caldamone AA, eds. *Pediatric Surgery*. Elsevier/Saunders; 2006: 1–2, 983–1000. doi:10.1016/B978-0-323-42974-0.00014-8.)

endotracheal tube of what would normally be an appropriate size for the age causes injury in a small airway.

Bronchoscopy yields a definitive diagnosis by confirming the presence of complete tracheal rings, whereas imaging techniques such as CT or MRI may provide information about the relationship of the mediastinal structures and the airway and can help rule out other diagnoses.[38]

Patients with minimal symptoms can be managed expectantly, and serial examinations are done to assess tracheal growth. For patients with persistent symptoms, operative management is indicated. Intervention includes tracheal resection with end-to-end anastomosis, patch tracheoplasty, and slide tracheoplasty.[39]

Vascular Compression of the Airway

Abnormalities of the aortic arch and pulmonary vasculature can cause compression of the airway and lead to respiratory compromise. Patients present with noisy breathing, barking cough, recurrent respiratory tract infections, and dysphagia and may have episodes of apnea. Diagnostic workup includes chest radiograph, CT scan with contrast enhancement, bronchoscopy, and echocardiogram. The most common causes of vascular airway compression are innominate artery compression syndrome and vascular rings.[40]

Innominate artery compression syndrome occurs when there is anterior compression of the trachea by the innominate artery as it crosses from left to right prior to originating from the aorta.[40] Surgical therapy for severe disease involves suspending the innominate artery anteriorly by suturing it against the posterior sternum. Improved diagnostic techniques have facilitated better patient selection and an overall decrease in the number of procedures performed, along with improved outcomes.[40]

The most common vascular rings are the double aortic arch, the right aortic arch, and the pulmonary artery sling. In a double aortic arch, the aorta divides into two branches, one anterior and one posterior to the esophagus and trachea, and these join posteriorly to form the descending aorta.[41] Patients with a right aortic arch have an aortic arch that courses to the right of the trachea and esophagus. The left subclavian artery arises posterior to the esophagus and a persistent ligamentum arteriosum connects to the descending aorta, coursing anterior to the trachea and forming a ring.[40] A pulmonary artery sling is formed by an anomalous course of the left pulmonary artery in which the artery arises from the right pulmonary artery and courses posterior to the right mainstem bronchus and trachea before reaching the left pulmonary hilum.[42] Treatment of vascular rings is surgical and commonly requires clamping, division, and reimplantation of these vessels by a pediatric cardiothoracic surgeon.[40]

Congenital Lung Lesions

Congenital lung lesions are a spectra of developmental anomalies of the bronchopulmonary unit.[43] Multiple variations exist including congenital pulmonary airway malformation (CPAM), bronchopulmonary sequestration (BPS), and congenital lobar emphysema (CLE). Other malformations include bronchogenic cysts, lymphangiomas, and pleuropulmonary blastomas.[43,44]

Clinical Characteristics

The majority of these lesions cause no impact on fetal development, they are diagnosed incidentally during routine prenatal evaluation and remain stable or regress.[45,46] Lesions that progressively enlarge may be associated with lung hypoplasia and mediastinal shift, which can lead to cardiac failure and subsequently to hydrops fetalis. Hydrops fetalis is the most important predictor of poor perinatal outcome in these patients.[47–49]

Delivery is usually uncomplicated, and more than 70% of neonates are asymptomatic.[50] Those few with symptoms may require ventilatory support. Although infrequent, symptoms beyond the neonatal period are related to recurrent respiratory tract infections, chronic cough, and wheezing. More severe variants may present as pneumothorax, hemothorax, air embolism, or high-output cardiac failure due to shunting via collaterals.[51]

Diagnosis

Prenatal

Serial fetal ultrasounds are done to assess the size, location, and progression of the lesion. These lesions are cystic or solid lesions and can be divided morphologically into two categories: (1) macrocystic lesions (with at least one cyst greater than 5 mm) and (2) microcystic lesions (seen as a solid mass) (Fig. 84.4).[47]

Additionally, ultrasound permits characterization of the lesion and fetus to predict prognosis. Prognostic ultrasound markers include mediastinal shift, diaphragmatic eversion, polyhydramnios, ascites, pleural effusion, and, importantly, lesion size.[52]

The size of the lesion is best understood in relationship to the size of the rest of the fetus. This is performed by comparing the volume of the lesion to the head circumference of the fetus, which is called the cyst volume-to-head circumference ratio (CVR). A CVR greater than 1.6 before 24 weeks of gestation has been associated with an 80% risk of developing hydrops fetalis. Prenatal characteristics of high risk include a CVR greater than 1.6, placentomegaly, abnormal fetal echocardiography, diaphragm eversion, or severe mediastinal shift.[52,53] Fetal MRI is currently used in some centers to describe the lesions and may also help characterize other associated findings such as pulmonary hypoplasia.[54]

Postnatal

Once the infant is born, a thorough physical exam is performed. Chest radiograph has a low sensitivity but may show a mediastinal or lung field mass.[46] CT scan and MRI with contrast enhancement may aid in identifying the anatomy and vasculature. Pathologic analysis after resection provides definitive diagnosis.

Management

Prenatal

Prenatal management of all congenital lung lesions follows the same algorithm. Management considers the viability of the fetus, gestational age, CVR, and risk of developing hydrops fetalis. For patients with a low risk of developing hydrops fetalis (CVR $\leq$ 1.6), serial ultrasound monitoring and elective resection after term delivery are indicated.

High-risk patients (CVR $>$ 1.6, placentomegaly, severe mediastinal shift, diaphragm eversion, or lung hypoplasia) are managed differently depending on the morphologic characteristics. If microcystic, administration of maternal betamethasone has shown to increase survival, reverse hydrops, and decrease fetal surgical interventions.[55,56] In contrast, macrocystic lesions have not been shown to benefit from maternal steroids treatment.[52]

Fetuses who despite conservative or medical management continue to have worsening CVR or hydrops fetalis progression may benefit from fetal interventions. These include prenatal cyst decompression or open fetal surgery. When patients have high postnatal survival probability or are born at more than 32 weeks of gestation, ex-utero intrapartum treatment (EXIT) procedure and resection after induced preterm delivery may be done.[43,52]

Prenatal cyst decompression is achieved by transamniotic needle decompression or thoracoamniotic shunt, with evidence suggesting improved survival.[57] Fetal lobectomy is a last-resort option for refractory lesions, with a few case series reporting resolution of hydrops and return of the mediastinum to midline after the procedure.[48] Survival in these series is a maximum of 50% but comes at the cost of significant maternal morbidity and prematurity.[55]

Postnatal

Postnatal management is determined based on time of diagnosis and symptom presentation. Initial management relies on ventilatory support for symptomatic patients and chest tube placement for pleural complications. Vasopressor support and/or extracorporeal membrane

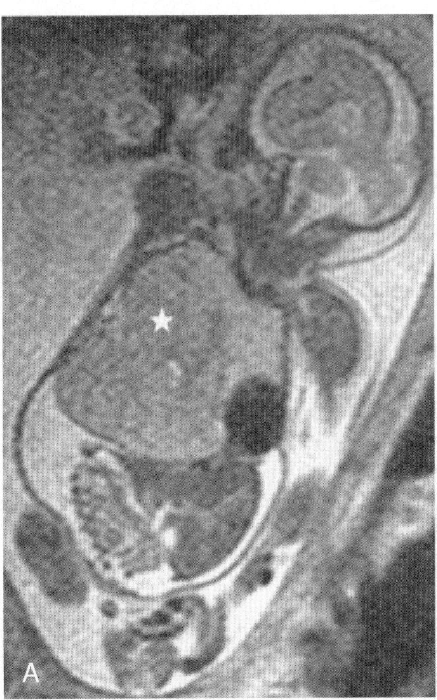

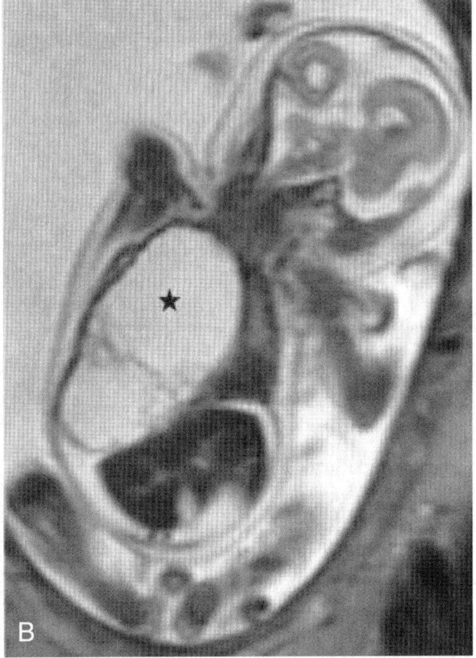

Fig. 84.4 Fetal Magnetic Resonance Imaging Showing a Microcystic Congenital Lung Lesion. Seen as a solid mass (A) and a macrocystic lesion (B) containing a large cyst *(marked by stars)*. (Obtained with permission from Pablo L, Flake AW. Congenital bronchopulmonary malformations. In: Holcomb GW III, Murphy JP, St. Peter SD, eds. *Ashcraft's Pediatric Surgery*. Elsevier; 2020:348–360. doi:10.1016/B978-1-4160-6127-4.00022-7.)

oxygenation (ECMO) are rarely required. When pulmonary hypoplasia is present, surgical intervention can be delayed until the patient is stable.

With a few exceptions, complete resection is the goal, and this can be accomplished via thoracotomy or video-assisted thoracoscopic surgery.[58] In a meta-analysis comparing thoracoscopic versus open resection, there were no significant differences in complication rates. Length of stay and chest tube duration were longer in the thoracotomy group.[59]

Lobectomy has been the standard technique for resection of congenital lung lesions. Lung-sparing resection techniques have been studied as a feasible and safe approach, but current evidence provides no information about benefits for long-term pulmonary function and superiority to standard lobectomy.[52,60–63] Wedge resection is considered in cases of bilateral or multiple lobe involvement.

Congenital Pulmonary Airway Malformation

CPAM is a developmental anomaly of the lower respiratory tract that has an unspecified origin and is relatively uncommon. Given advances in prenatal diagnosis, early and accurate identification is becoming more common, and some authors posit that the incidence will continue to rise.[64] Current studies show incidences between 1 in 7000 and 1 in 35,000.[58,64]

CPAMs are characterized by proliferation of immature bronchiolar structures localized to an area of the lung.[65] They have a small communication path with the tracheobronchial tree and receive and drain blood through the pulmonary circulation in most cases. Some may have an additional arterial supply from systemic branches, the most common being from the abdominal aorta. Lesions with combined pulmonary and systemic vasculature are called hybrid lesions.[58]

Lesions can affect any part of the lung and are found in the left and right sides equally. Unilobar cases account for 80% to 95% of presentations, with the remaining few being bilateral (2%) and even fewer involving more than one lobe of one or both lungs.[43]

Treatment of asymptomatic CPAM is controversial. Arguments in favor of early surgical treatment are higher rates of infection in patients with CPAM and an association with lung malignancies such as bronchoalveolar carcinoma and pleuropulmonary blastoma.[66–68] Conservative management relies on CT scans for monitoring increasing radiation exposure. A 2016 meta-analysis of retrospective studies comparing conservative management and surgical resection for asymptomatic CPAM concluded that resection was safe and prevented the risk of symptom development, albeit with increased morbidity compared with nonsurgically managed patients.[69] The treatment of choice for symptomatic CPAM is a lobectomy of the involved lobe.[70]

Bronchopulmonary Sequestration

Bronchopulmonary sequestrations represent 10% of diagnosed congenital lung lesions.[71] They are characterized by a lower respiratory tract mass that has no communication with the tracheobronchial tree and receives systemic arterial supply but may have systemic and/or pulmonary venous return.[43]

The two main forms of BPS are intralobar sequestration (iBPS) and extralobar sequestration (eBPS). iBPS (75% of cases) has venous return to the pulmonary veins and shares the same visceral pleura as its adjacent normal lung lobe, whereas eBPS (25% of cases) may have systemic or pulmonary venous return and has its own distinct pleura.[71] The etiology of eBPS differs from iBPS by arising from an abnormal budding in the early foregut development.

In a 2019 case series of 208 patients with BPS, eBPS was most frequently located in the paraspinal region and more commonly in the left lower thorax, although a few cases were located in the right side and middle or upper thorax, diaphragm, abdomen, and neck. iBPS was uniformly found in lower lobes.[72] This is consistent with previous literature.[73]

eBPS is managed differently than CPAM. Studies suggest that serially followed eBPS lesions decrease over time. They also have less reported infection incidence and malignancy risk; therefore it is safer to follow lesions without surgical intervention.[74,75] Surgical management of eBPS consists of ligation of the feeding vessel and removal of tissue via thoracoscopy.

Given that iBPS is more involved with the lung parenchyma, has high output physiology, and has a higher risk of infection, postnatal lobectomy is generally recommended.[43]

Congenital Lobar Emphysema

CLE is a rare (1 in 20,000 to 1 in 30,000 live births) anomalous lung development disease that results in hyperinflation of one or more lobes of the lung. It is more common in males than females in a ratio of 3:1.[58]

Although the developmental mechanism has not been completely defined, it seems that CLE arises from localized malformations that result in overinflation of the lung segment. Inappropriate bronchial valvular mechanisms (one-way valves), obstructive processes, or a polyalveolar lobe are possible explanatory causes.[43,58]

Obstruction of the airway during development is seen in 25% of cases. The obstruction results in air trapping and histologic changes of the alveolar distension without structural anomaly. CLE with a polyalveolar lobe occurs in up to one-third of cases and is characterized by a three- to five-fold increase in the number of alveoli without changes in the bronchial branches. Studies suggest that a polyalveolar lobe may be a normal reaction of the parenchyma distal to a complete bronchial obstruction during gestation.[76]

Upper lobe involvement occurs on the left in 40% to 50% of patients and on the right in 20%. The right middle lobe is involved in 25% to 30% of patients, and lower lobe involvement is extremely rare (2%–5%).[77,78]

Clinical Presentation

Many patients with CLE present with respiratory distress, although a significant number can also be asymptomatic or display evidence of mild tachypnea. Subtle signs of increased work of breathing can include feeding difficulties and poor weight gain. In patients who develop respiratory distress, symptoms occur immediately after birth or up to 4 months of age. Rapidly progressing respiratory failure is expected in symptomatic neonates and warrants emergency thoracotomy in 10% to 15% of cases.[58] Neonates can have a shift in apical cardiac impulse to the contralateral side, decreased breath sounds in the affected hemothorax, and hyperresonance to percussion.

Diagnosis

CLE is not associated with significant prenatal findings. Ultrasound may show retained fluid, which develops into trapped air postnatally. This can cause mediastinal shift.

Chest radiograph can show an opaque mass if there is an obstructive etiology, but it can also show an air-trapping pattern. Mediastinal and tracheal shift, compression and collapse of ipsilateral unaffected lobe(s), and flattening or inversion of the ipsilateral diaphragm may also be present.

Management

In asymptomatic patients, no resection is required and patients may be safely followed leading to spontaneous regression.[79–81] Surgical treatment is not warranted in cases where CLE is caused by cartilaginous weakness of lobar bronchus, cases of mucous plugs, or cases of viral bronchiolitis, because they can resolve spontaneously over time. When CLE is caused by a bronchogenic cyst, the cyst may be excised while retaining the affected lobe.[43]

Neonates with severe symptoms require immediate surgical intervention, while a delayed approach can be offered in those infants with milder manifestations. Surgery should be performed as soon as possible to avoid increased risk of infection or respiratory distress and to allow for maximum compensatory lung growth. The gold standard of surgical therapy is a formal lobectomy.[43]

Bronchogenic Cysts

Bronchogenic cysts originate from an abnormal budding of the fetal tracheal diverticulum or the primitive foregut. They may communicate with the tracheobronchial tree and may be located anywhere along the respiratory apparatus. They do not have bronchial vascular development. Histologically they have cartilage, smooth muscle, and epithelial glandular tissue. Enlargement of these cysts can cause bronchial obstruction and dilate the lung distally.[43]

Diagnosis

Prenatal diagnosis is infrequent but can potentially be seen as a unilocular fluid-filled cyst in the middle posterior portions of the mediastinum with distal lung dilation. Postnatal chest radiograph may show a mediastinal or lung mass. This can be followed up by a bronchoscopy and CT scan for further evaluation. Echocardiography should also be performed to eliminate other diagnoses including pericardial cyst.

Management

The goal of treatment is to decrease the risk of infection, airway compromise, and impingement on the trachea, bronchus, heart, or esophagus or if the etiology of the mass is unknown.

Surgical resection is performed based on the location of the cyst and adjacent structures. Cross-field ventilation or cardiopulmonary bypass is reserved in the case of cystic involvement with the trachea or mainstem bronchi, which is extremely rare. Thoracotomy or thoracoscopic excision of the cyst are the procedure of choice.[43]

Congenital Diaphragmatic Hernia

A congenital diaphragmatic hernia (CDH) is a defect of the diaphragm through which any intraabdominal organ can protrude into the chest. CDH is thought to be a systemic disease that involves a field defect of the diaphragm and/or lungs. It is intrinsically associated with lung hypoplasia and pulmonary hypertension (PHTN) beyond simple physical compression.[82] Furthermore, CDH is often part of a syndrome that involves multiple anomalies in other systems. Treatment is therefore complex and usually requires a multidisciplinary team to care for its components.

CDH occurs between 2.3 and 2.4 per 10,000 live births,[83,84] and despite advances during the past two decades, it continues to have mortality of 20% to 30%.[85–87] Nevertheless, recent data obtained from centers with focused CDH care report survival rates as high as 90% in severe cases, which emphasize the importance of standardizing care to achieve similar results in all centers.[88]

Anatomy and Embryology

The earliest evidence of a diaphragm precursor is seen during the fourth week of gestation. The diaphragm is thought to develop from the interaction of several embryonic components. The septum transversum is located ventrally; it is the precursor of the central tendon. Dorsolaterally are the pleuroperitoneal folds and dorsally, the crura of the esophageal mesentery. These form the crural and dorsal structures.[89,90]

These structures interact, surround the developing foregut, and start separating the pleuropericardial and peritoneal cavities to form the primitive diaphragm. At week 6, the communications between the pleural and peritoneal cavities begin to close as the pleuroperitoneal membranes develop. By week 8, the pleural and peritoneal cavities are separated. Muscularization then occurs, with migration of phrenic nerve axons and myoblasts from cervical segments to form the mature diaphragm.[91]

Current theories explaining the pathogenesis include failure of muscularization of the diaphragm prior to closure of the pleuroperitoneal canals; this causes a weakness in the diaphragm, protrusion of intraabdominal organs, and mechanical compression of the developing lung, leading to lung hypoplasia. Other authors have postulated that the abnormal lung development is part of an overall field defect and is not dependent on a mechanical effect of the bowel; this may lead to a weakened posthepatic mesenchymal plate and impaired diaphragm fusion. More recently, the role of the muscle connective tissue fibroblasts derived from the pleuroperitoneal folds has been associated with the morphogenesis of the diaphragm; mutations in these cells might contribute to abnormal diaphragmatic development.[82,91–93]

CDH affects the left side in 80% to 85% of cases and the right side in 10% to 15% of cases, with the remaining few cases being bilateral. Approximately 90% are posterolateral, passing through a defect caused by failure of fusion of the pleuroperitoneal folds and the transverse septum with the intercostal muscles, known as Bochdalek hernias. Ten percent are anterior and are caused by failure of fusion of the transverse septum and the lateral body wall; these are Morgagni hernias.[84,94,95]

Pathophysiology

The main pathophysiologic components of CDH are pulmonary hypoplasia and PHTN. Pulmonary hypoplasia is characterized by a uniform loss of pulmonary mass, bronchial branching, decreased alveolar to arteriolar ratios, abnormally thick-walled arterioles, and decreased vasoreactivity.[96] This is caused by arrest of alveolar development at the midcanalicular stage of lung embryogenesis and is directly related to mortality, long-term morbidity, and limited quality of outcome from CDH.[96]

The pulmonary vasculature during the last weeks of gestation is a high-resistance, low-flow system. As the child is born, it transitions into a low-resistance, high-flow system in the first months of life. In patients with CDH there is evidence of increased arteriolar muscularization and decreased pulmonary artery density, which causes persistence of the high pulmonary vascular resistance.[96] Severity of

CDH-associated PHTN tracks with overall morbidity and mortality. Some studies show that persistent suprasystemic pulmonary artery pressures after 3 weeks of life had a mortality rate of 100%.[97]

Diagnosis

Prenatal Diagnosis

Prenatal evaluation provides an important aspect of the care of patients with CDH. It estimates prognosis and is an adjunct to prenatal counseling, triage, and future management. Similar to other congenital diseases, a high index of suspicion for other anomalies should be considered and worked up.

Up to 40% of CDH cases have at least one additional congenital anomaly, and 30% have a causative genetic variation.[98,99] Thirty percent will present with cardiovascular anomalies, the most common being left ventricular hypoplasia, followed by atrial septal defect.[100] Eighteen percent will be urogenital, 15% musculoskeletal, and 10% neurological.[101] CDH is also associated with other gastrointestinal complications such as malrotation and accessory spleen.[101]

Although rare, hydrops can also develop from herniation of intraabdominal organs into the thorax by causing mediastinal shift and cardiac failure. Prognosis is poor for these patients.[102]

Fetal Ultrasound

Ultrasound is the standard modality for diagnosis of CDH. It can assess lung size, liver position, stomach position, and associated congenital anomalies. Recent data estimate that it has a prenatal detection rate of greater than 60%, with more severe forms having detection rates of up to 75% in high-volume centers.[103,104]

With current fetal ultrasound techniques, diaphragmatic hernias can be identified as early as 14 to 15 weeks of gestation.[94] Herniated bowel appears as heterogenous echoes in the thoracic cavity, and by week 18 it is possible to see an incomplete diaphragm. The presence of gastric bubbles above the diaphragm and a small abdominal circumference can also be detected.

Herniation of the stomach may lead to kinking and obstruction of the upper gastrointestinal tract, which can be seen as polyhydramnios. Mediastinal shift can also be present, and although it is not specific for CDH, it may help differentiate between left- and right-sided hernias.

Ultrasound plays an important role in risk stratification. The most common predictors of postnatal survival are liver herniation into the thorax and the fetal lung volume, which is assessed by measurement of the observed to expected lung-to-head circumference ratio (O/E LHR).[94,105]

The LHR is the ratio between the lung area and the head circumference. On ultrasound the lung area is measured in the hemithorax contralateral to the hernia at the level of a four-chamber view of the fetal heart in cross-section images. An O/E LHR less than 25% has a historically predicted survival rate from 12.5% to 30%, whereas an O/E LHR greater than 35% historically predicts a survival rate of 65% to 88%.[105–107]

Disadvantages of fetal ultrasound include its user dependence. Efforts are currently being made to standardize prenatal ultrasound assessment of the fetus.[108]

Fetal Magnetic Resonance Imaging

MRI has been shown to enhance prenatal evaluation. It is less user dependent and is less affected by maternal body habitus and fetal movements. It provides specific anatomic detail of the diaphragm defect, hernia location, hernia contents, and surrounding structures.[109,110]

Ultrafast fetal MRI has also proven useful in predicting outcomes for some patients with CDH. It provides accurate measurement of the liver-to-diaphragm ratio and may also assist in the quantification of pulmonary hypoplasia by measurement of the observed to expected total fetal lung volume.

The liver-to-diaphragm ratio is a surrogate for severity of herniation, and a high ratio is associated with worse outcomes.[111] Likewise, a 2017 meta-analysis showed statistical differences between the mean MRI-calculated total fetal lung volume for survivors with CDH versus those who did not survive.[105]

Postnatal Diagnosis

Respiratory distress is the most common symptom after birth, although some patients may be asymptomatic. The hypoxia does not progress over time but instead appears suddenly and rapidly after a period of good ventilation and oxygenation. As the neonate takes a breath, distension of the stomach and intestine occurs, causing compression of the thoracic cavity and mediastinum.

On physical exam, patients will have absent or decreased breath sounds on the ipsilateral side. Severe herniation of the abdominal viscera presents as a barrel chest with a scaphoid abdomen. The point of maximal cardiac impulse may be displaced if there is mediastinal shift.

Postnatal diagnostic confirmation is achieved by chest radiography to visualize the intrathoracic intestinal loops, nasogastric tube curled up in the chest, absence of a diaphragmatic shadow on the herniated side, mediastinal and cardiac shift toward the contralateral side, and possibly intrathoracic herniation of the left lobe of the liver.

Management

Prenatal Care

Patients with CDH should be managed by obstetricians in a tertiary perinatal center in consultation with both pediatric surgeons and neonatologists. Other specialists to include in the consultation process are geneticists, financial counselors, and social workers.

Once the diagnosis is made with a screening prenatal ultrasound, an advanced fetal ultrasound is carried out with assessment of morphologic parameters, associated anomalies, anatomic characteristics of the diaphragmatic hernia, and risk stratification.

Patients with isolated CDH have considerably higher survival rates than patients with associated anomalies.[88,112] Given the high association with chromosomal abnormalities, genetic consultation with karyotype analysis should be considered. Identification of a genetic component may provide important information regarding prognosis and future management. Chromosomal anomalies, lethal syndromes, and other negative predictors are to be identified and shared to allow parents to make an informed decision about their pregnancy.

Prenatal therapy with medications has been pursued with the hope of minimizing the development of lung hypoplpasia and pulmonary hypertension. Although there is evidence for the use of prenatal steroids for lung maturity and development in prematurity, this effect was not seen in CDH.[86,113] Sildenafil is a drug commonly used for the treatment of PHTN postnatally. It is currently in consideration for clinical trials in prenatal CDH.[114] Current studies are also targeting vitamin A, glucagon-like peptide-1 agonists, and tyrosine kinase inhibitors as potential therapeutic options.[115–118]

Prenatal Interventions

Current fetal interventions mainly target improving lung hypoplasia and PHTN and not in utero repair of the diaphragm. In the 1980s, open fetal diaphragmatic repair was performed with the hypothesis that fetal reduction and closure of the hernia before week 24 of gestation would improve lung development. Subsequent prospective studies showed that fetuses undergoing fetal repair had higher complication rates without improvements in survival compared with the standard postnatal care. These interventions are therefore currently not performed.[119,120]

Although open fetal surgery provided no benefits, minimally invasive procedures are currently being studied as possible options. Fetoscopic tracheal occlusion (FETO) was first conceptualized in the 1970s as a method of improving lung hypoplasia.[121] It is a technique that has evolved and currently involves use of single-port fetoscopy to deploy a detachable balloon endotracheally between weeks 27 and 32 of gestation. The LHR is monitored to assess for lung hypoplasia improvement, and the balloon is removed 5 to 7 weeks after placement. FETO increases tracheobronchial pressure, leading to increased lung-branching morphogenesis and inducing lung hyperplasia.[122]

The first experiences of outcomes for FETO show promising results. In patients with severe CDH with an expected survival of 0% to 24%, there were observed survival rates after intervention of 35% to 49% (LHR < 1.0).[123] Other studies showed survival rates of 73%, although expectant management achieved a survival rate of 77% (LHR < 1.4).[107] Refinements in patient selection and inclusion criteria may provide additional information about which patients can benefit from this procedure. The Tracheal Occlusion to Accelerate Lung Growth (TOTAL) trial, which started in 2011 and is still ongoing, aims to address these questions.

Postnatal Care

Immediate cardiopulmonary resuscitation is the initial postnatal goal. Priorities are maintaining adequate oxygenation and perfusion, minimizing acidosis, managing PHTN, and supporting cardiac output. Once the patient is stable, operative repair of the diaphragmatic hernia is performed.

Cardiopulmonary Resuscitation

Respiratory support is provided immediately with endotracheal intubation, mechanical ventilation, and placement of a nasogastric tube for foregut decompression. Preductal and postductal oxygenation monitoring allows for assessment of systemic and cerebral perfusion in the setting of persistent fetal circulation, and acid-base balance measurement assists in titration of mechanical ventilation.

The goal for mechanical ventilation is to maintain oxygenation while limiting the risks of ventilator-induced lung injury and alveolar instability. Fractional inspired oxygen is titrated to an oxygen saturation goal of above 80% and respiratory rates of 40 to 60 breaths per minute to target a partial pressure of CO_2 of less than 70 mm Hg and a pH above 7.2.[124] Low inspiratory peak airway pressures of less than 25 cm H_2O minimize volutrauma and barotrauma.[86,124]

High-frequency oscillatory ventilator (HFOV) strategies are employed when conventional ventilation does not reverse hypercapnia and hypoxemia. Nevertheless, a randomized controlled trial done in 2016 comparing HFOV and conventional mechanical ventilation showed no clear superiority between strategies, with small advantages toward conventional mechanical ventilation.[125]

Management of Pulmonary Hypertension

Gentle ventilatory parameters will help minimize hypoxia and acidosis, which are paramount for treating PHTN. Several studies outline the importance of prompt management of PHTN. Patients who developed normal pulmonary artery pressures of less than 50% systemic pressure by the first 3 weeks of life were found to have a 100% survival rate.[126] In the same vein, patients with PHTN at 4 weeks of age had a high risk of death.[97]

Assessment of PHTN and cardiac function is best done through the use of echocardiography. It is used to identify the presence of any cardiac anomalies and measure right and left ventricular function, pulmonary artery flow, and level of right-to-left shunt through a patent ductus arteriosus and patent foramen ovale. This provides information about the severity of PHTN and left ventricular function.

Strategies to improve PHTN include targeted vasodilation of the pulmonary vasculature and minimizing the pressure overload on the right ventricle.

Options that target pulmonary vasculature include inhaled nitric oxide (iNO) and sildenafil. A recent review for iNO showed no decreased mortality or need for ECMO in patients with CDH-associated PHTN, and therefore the study group recommended its use only in infants with hypoxic respiratory failure from etiologies other than CDH.[127] Sildenafil has shown evidence of improving oxygenation and avoiding ECMO in the setting of PHTN that is refractory to iNO therapy.[128] Bosentan, an endothelin-1 receptor antagonist, has been used for treatment of PHTN, but there is limited evidence of its efficacy in CDH.[129–131]

Closure of the ductus arteriosus in the setting of PHTN may cause an acute decrease in systemic perfusion of previously stable patients. The closure prevents offload of the right ventricle, leading to progressive right heart dysfunction. To decrease the right ventricle overload, prostaglandin E1 analogs may be used to reopen the ductus arteriosus and improve right ventricle pressures.[86]

In patients with left ventricular dysfunction, inotropic agents such as dopamine, dobutamine, epinephrine, and milrinone may increase left ventricular output and increase systemic pressure, minimizing right-to-left ductal shunting.

In patients with continued respiratory failure despite medical management, ECMO is a viable option. It is indicated for patients with continued respiratory failure, for prevention of ventilator-induced barotrauma, and for unstable patients with adequate lung parenchyma and potentially reversible PHTN. Venovenous or venoarterial ECMO are both equal options. Patients with CDH who undergo ECMO have survival rates of 30% to 50%.[132,133]

Surgical Management

There are several options for operative repair of CDH. It can be open or minimally invasive. A subcostal approach is the most common open repair, whereas a thoracoscopy is the most common minimally invasive approach (Fig. 84.5).[134] Comparing benefits of minimally invasive with open procedures proves difficult, because minimally invasive techniques are reserved for patients within a lower risk category, whereas open procedures are reserved for higher risk patients.[135] The approach mostly depends on center experience and careful patient selection.

Advantages of minimally invasive surgery (MIS) repair after risk stratification with multivariable regression analysis demonstrated a decrease in incidence of bowel obstruction and decreased length of stay but showed increased recurrence.[134]

Several studies reviewing early (less than 12 hours) versus later repair (after 24–96 hours) have noted no differences in survival.[136,137] More recently, and adjusting for severity of disease, no differences were seen in mortality among patients undergoing surgery between

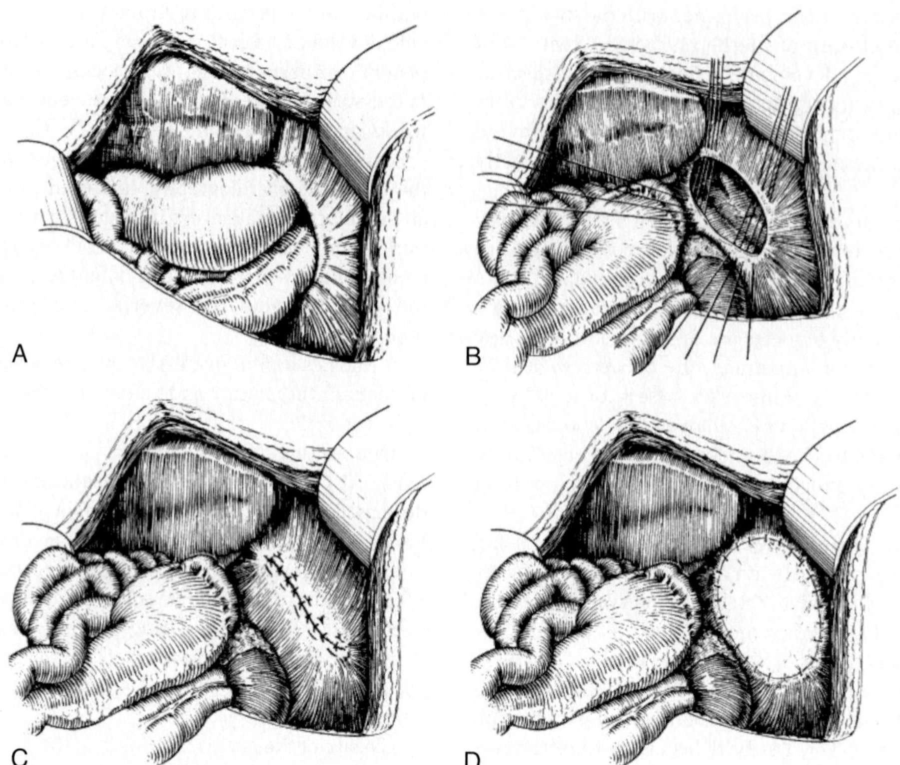

Fig. 84.5 Illustrated Representation of a Left Congenital Diaphragmatic Hernia Repair Via Left Open Subcostal Approach. (A) Unreduced left congenital diaphragmatic hernia. (B) Reduction of diaphragmatic hernia into the abdominal cavity. Sutures have been placed for primary repair. (C) Completed primary repair of left congenital diaphragmatic hernia. (D) Patch repair of left congenital diaphragmatic hernia. (Obtained with permission from Stolar CJH, Dillon PW. Congenital diaphragmatic hernia and eventration. In: Coran AG, ed. *Pediatric Surgery*. Elsevier; 2012:809–824. doi:10.1016/B978-0-323-07255-7.00063-5.)

0 and 3, 4 and 7, and more than 8 days of life.[137] To further complicate this quandary, patients on ECMO seem to have improved survival rates when repair is done within 3 days,[138,139] suggesting potential benefit of early repair in patients who will undergo ECMO or to allow for early decannulation once ECMO is instated.[140]

Given these findings, repair is recommended once the patient is stabilized from a cardiopulmonary perspective, and an earlier approach might prove beneficial for patients on ECMO.[86] Individualized care and risk stratification are key for the operative timing decision.

During surgery, patients undergo careful monitoring of blood pressure and pre- and postductal blood gases, a central line for central venous pressure, and intraabdominal pressure measurement via foley or nasogastric tube.

The goal of surgical repair is to achieve complete reduction of the intraabdominal viscera from the thorax and to provide a tension-free closure of the diaphragmatic hernia. Careful attention is paid to decreased respiratory compliance once abdominal closure is performed. Temporary abdominal wall closure (silo, vacuum-assisted closure, or skin-only closure) may be considered in cases with high intraabdominal peak inspiratory pressures.

A chest tube may or may not be placed to manage pneumothorax or pleural effusion. It is kept in a water seal to avoid lung injury and removed promptly to avoid infectious complications.[83,141]

Prosthetic replacement of the diaphragm is warranted in the case of large defects or agenesis. Prosthetic patches are anchored on the diaphragmatic border or on the anterior and posterior ribs. Patches used for closure can be synthetic (polytetrafluoroethylene [Gore-Tex] or composite polypropylene [Marlex]) or biosynthetic (bioengineered porcine intestinal submucosal matrix [Surgisis] or acellular porcine dermal collagen patch [Permacol]).

Diaphragmatic Eventration

A diaphragmatic eventration is a disease in which there is an abnormal elevation of the hemidiaphragm. It can be congenital or acquired. Congenital diaphragmatic eventrations results from incomplete development of the central tendon or the muscular portion of the diaphragm. Acquired eventrations are caused by injury to the phrenic nerve due to trauma during birth, cervical or thoracic procedures, tumor invasion, or infection resulting in paralysis of the diaphragm.[83]

Clinical Presentation

Diaphragmatic eventrations may be asymptomatic or cause acute respiratory distress. The underdeveloped or paralyzed diaphragm loses the inspiratory caudal movement necessary for complete ventilation and can interfere with the respiratory function.[142,143] Mediastinal shift is possible, resulting in tracheal shift and stridor. Associated gastrointestinal symptoms include dysphagia and reflux symptoms due to left-side eventration causing displacement of the stomach and esophagus.

Diagnosis

Eventrations can be identified using chest radiograph and further studied with ultrasound or fluoroscopy to note abnormal diaphragmatic movement. A CT scan or operative visualization is necessary to distinguish between extensive eventration and CDH.[143]

Management

Eventration can require mechanical ventilation. This is a clear indication for operative intervention. In most patients, however, the presentation is subtler and the decision to operate is made after all medical therapies exhausted. The goal of the surgical repair is to eliminate the paradoxical diaphragmatic movement and mediastinal shift by plicating the paralyzed or atrophic diaphragm in the low thoracic position. Sutures are placed to imbricate the diaphragm and prevent abnormal movement. Surgery may be done open, laparoscopically, or thoracoscopically.[144,145]

CHAPTER 85 Congenital Anorectal Malformations and Hirschsprung Disease in the Neonate

Isam W. Nasr, Eric W. Etchill

KEY POINTS

1. Congenital anorectal malformations and Hirschsprung disease present in neonates with symptoms of distal intestinal obstruction and distal gastrointestinal tract dysmotility.
2. Anorectal malformations are a congenital group of disorders that occur when the hindgut fails to develop in the appropriate anatomic position and with appropriate caliber. These malformations are associated with problems of fecal incontinence.
3. Hirschsprung disease is a congenital disorder of the enteric nervous system characterized by the absence of ganglion nerve cells, resulting in the inability of stool to pass through the colon and rectum.
4. Patients with anorectal malformations and Hirschsprung disease benefit from early diagnosis and generally require surgical intervention.
5. Long-term outcomes and quality of life are optimized through adequate follow-up, dietary adjustments, and an effective bowel management program.

Introduction

Congenital anorectal malformations (ARMs) and Hirschsprung disease (HSCR) are disorders that present in neonates with symptoms of intestinal obstruction and distal gastrointestinal tract dysmotility. ARMs compose a spectrum of congenital malformations that result in mechanical bowel obstruction, whereas HSCR is a disorder of the enteric nervous system that results in varying degrees of functional obstruction. Both ARMs and HSCR disorders are frequently associated with a variety of other disorders and syndromes.[1] Patients with either an ARM or HSCR benefit from early diagnosis and require surgical intervention, which generally provides improvement in bowel function and quality of life.

Anorectal Malformations

Pathophysiology of Anorectal Malformations

ARMs are a congenital group of disorders that occur when the hindgut fails to develop in the appropriate anatomic position and with appropriate caliber.[1] One out of every 4000 to 5000 newborns is born with a congenital ARM.[2] The incidence is slightly higher in males. Prenatal diagnosis is generally uncommon. A minority of cases present after the neonatal age, with the majority of patients developing symptoms in the first weeks of life.[3] Prompt, early diagnosis allows for appropriate counseling, operative planning, and overall management in the neonatal period. The goal of surgery is to restore normal anatomy and in so doing allow for normal function and motility with minimal long-term morbidity.

Normal Continence

The three primary components that maintain bowel continence are voluntary muscle constriction, anal canal sensation, and bowel motility.[4] Voluntary muscle structures include the levator muscles, the striated muscle complex, and the external sphincter. Neonates with ARMs will have varying degrees of hypodevelopment of these voluntary muscles. For these voluntary muscles to contract appropriately, sensation of the anal canal must be intact. In general, patients with ARMs are born without an anal canal or with a malformed anal canal, thus severely impairing sensation and inhibiting voluntary muscle contracture. Lastly, peristaltic contraction of the distal large bowel, the rectosigmoid, is usually felt prior to defecation. This leads to relaxation of the voluntary rectal muscles, which allows the contents within the rectum to be interrogated by the sensate anal canal. These voluntary muscles can either then push the rectal contents back into the sigmoid until the appropriate time for evacuation or, together with a Valsalva maneuver, evacuate the contents. Rectosigmoid motility is disrupted in ARMs, contributing to an inability to achieve appropriate continence.[5]

Clinical Features of Anorectal Malformations

As mentioned, ARMs compose a spectrum of disorders. Some disorders such as rectoperineal fistulas occur in both males and females, whereas other disorders are unique to each sex. Risk factors for the development of congenital ARMs include prematurity, being small for gestational age, and possibly maternal obesity and smoking.[6]

In general, ARMs can be classified according to whether the fistula or hindgut opening is "high" or "low."[1] Patients with "low" fistulas have anterior fistulas that open onto the perineal surface and are best treated with early surgical corrections. Repairs of low fistulas usually do not require diversion and can be repaired in a single-stage procedure.

In some patients, the fistula cannot be clearly visualized and the anatomy is not clearly delineated. This is because the fistula location is "high," occurring at the bladder or urethra (rectobladder neck or rectourethral) in males or at the posterior fourchette or within the introitus (rectovestibular fistula) in females. The most severe form, seen in females, is a cloaca in which the neonate has a single perineal orifice, with the rectum and genitourinary tract sharing a common channel. In other cases still, there may be normally developed anus and sphincter muscles without a fistula, yet the rectum is strictured or atretic.[7] In general, high fistulas are repaired in multiple stages

Table 85.1 Types of Anorectal Malformations According to Sex

Males	Females
Rectoperineal fistula	Rectoperineal fistula
Imperforate anus without fistula	Imperforate anus without fistula
Rectal atresia/rectal stenosis	Rectal atresia/rectal stenosis
Rectourethral bulbar fistula	Rectovestibular fistula
Rectourethral prostatic fistula	Rectovaginal fistula
Rectobladder neck fistula	Cloaca

to minimize risk of injury to neighboring structures and to allow for the delineation of the variant anatomy prior to definitive repair.[8]

Types of Anorectal Malformations

There are several types of ARMs, as described in Table 85.1. A rectoperineal fistula is an ARM that can occur in both males and females. In this defect the rectum is located close to the sphincter mechanism.[9] With rectoperineal fistulas, only the most distal aspect of the rectum is positioned anteriorly. Otherwise, most of the rectum appropriately lies within the muscle complex. These defects tend to have appropriate muscle quality and sacral development. Imperforate anus without fistula occurs when the anal opening is either absent or located in the wrong position.[10] There is an increased incidence of this malformation with Down syndrome.[11] Rectal stenosis or atresia is where the caliber of the rectum is too narrow to allow stool to pass.[12]

Although several ARMs are shared by both males and females, such as rectoperineal fistulas, each sex has specific defects unique to it. Male neonates can be born with rectourethral fistulas, where the rectum connects directly to the urethra, causing the two structures to share a common wall.[13] Rectourethral bulbar fistulas are the most common ARMs in males. With this defect, the rectum abnormally communicates with the lowest portion of the posterior urethra. In rectourethral prostatic fistulas, the fistula occurs at the more proximal prostatic urethra. In general, lower fistulas are associated with better sphincter muscle quality, a more fully developed sacrum, and a prominent midline groove. Classically, neonates with these defects will pass meconium through the urethra. Another defect seen exclusively in males is the rectobladder neck fistula. In this malformation, the rectum directly opens into the neck of the bladder. In general, these fistulas confer a poor prognosis for bowel control because they are associated with poorly developed levator muscles, a striated muscle complex, and an external sphincter. Further, neonates with this fistula tend to have poorly developed sacrums and flat perineums, further prohibiting adequate bowel continence.

Rectovestibular fistulas are the most common defects in females and occur when the rectum is displaced anteriorly, leading to a fistula between the rectum and the vulva vestibule. This causes an ectopic anus to open into the labia minora. These fistulas are associated with an overall excellent functional prognosis. A rectovaginal fistula occurs when the rectovestibular fistula occurs within the hymen and is a much rarer congenital defect.[14] A persistent cloaca, in which the distal vagina, rectum, and urinary tract all combine to form a single perineal channel, is another defect exclusive to females.[15] The length of this common channel is variable, ranging from 1 to 7 cm. Shorter channels, usually less than 3 cm, can be repaired with posterior sagittal anorectoplasty (PSARP) and confer a better prognosis than do longer channel defects. This is due to the difficulty in mobilizing the vagina with longer defects, which may ultimately lead to the need for vaginal replacement or a transabdominal approach due to the location of the rectal opening high in the vagina.

Fecal Control

As previously discussed, normal fecal continence relies on appropriate voluntary muscle constriction, anal canal sensation, and bowel motility. Factors are impacted by a multitude of issues including the type of ARM, type of operation, operative complications, quality of perineal muscles, sacral deformities, and spinal abnormalities. Rectal atresia or stenosis, a short cloaca less than 3 cm, and imperforate anus without fistula are defects that are associated with a good prognosis. Additional favorable prognostic factors include a normal sacrum, no presacral masses, a good buttock crease, and a good anal dimple. Long cloacal channels greater than 3 cm, higher fistulas such as rectoprostatic and rectobladder neck fistulas, the presence of myelomeningoceles, and sacral or spinal abnormalities are associated with poorer outcomes.

Evaluation of Anorectal Malformations

ARMs may be suspected prenatally if the presence of sacral, renal, or genitourinary anomalies is identified. However, the majority of ARMs are first detected on the initial neonatal examination. If meconium is present, it should be thoroughly cleaned away to enable complete examination of the perineum. Delayed diagnosis of ARMs, which occurs in up to 50% of cases, is associated with significant morbidity and mortality.[16] Of note, patients with rectal stenosis may have an unremarkable physical exam. If stenosis is suspected, a rectal catheter can be passed to evaluate luminal patency, and anal calibration with dilators can be useful in excluding stenosis. The presence of meconium in urine after 24 to 48 hours of life is indicative of a fistula with the urinary tract.[1] Clinical exam is generally sufficient for discriminating between low and high fistulas. To further delineate the anatomy, contrasted prone images can be taken after 24 hours of life once gas has had time to reach the distal bowel.[2]

Defects Associated With Anorectal Malformations

ARMs are frequently associated with VACTERL (vertebral, anorectal, cardiac, tracheoesophageal, renal, and limb) defects. In general, the higher the defect, the more likely that an associated VACTERL defect is present.[17,18] All patients with a confirmed or suspected ARM should undergo an investigation for VACTERL abnormalities.

Vertebral defects include sacral hypoplasia and a tethered cord. Sacral deformities are the most common defects associated with ARMs and are directly associated with the ability to achieve continence with either medical or surgical repair. For all patients with an ARM, plain radiographs should be obtained in the neonatal period. Having more than two absent sacral vertebrae is a poor prognostic sign for bowel continence. The sacral ratio, which is the ratio of the distance between the tip of the coccyx to the inferior point of the sacroiliac joint divided by the distance between the iliac crest to the inferior point of the sacroiliac joint, has been shown to be correlated with bowel function and fecal continence in patients with ARMs[19] (Fig. 85.1). A sacral ratio less than 0.7 is associated with poor bowel function, whereas a ratio less than 0.3 is associated with no chance for bowel control. A ratio greater than 0.7 is associated with good bowel control.

An association exists between rectal stenosis, sacral abnormalities, and presacral masses. Thus magnetic resonance imaging for presacral masses in patients with rectal stenosis should be considered.[12,20,21]

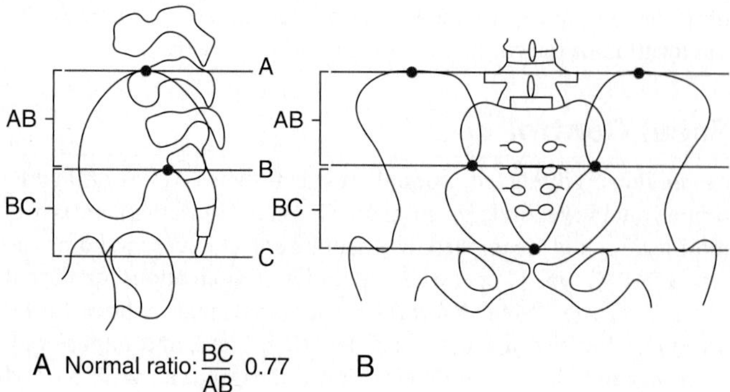

Fig. 85.1 Sacral Ratio. A sacral ratio of less than 0.3 portends poor ability for bowel control whereas a ratio greater than 0.7 suggests good bowel control.

A tethered cord is associated with higher defects that generally have a poorer prognosis. All patients with an ARM should have a spinal cord ultrasound within the first month of life, because it becomes difficult to visualize the spinal cord thereafter.[1,18] Releasing the tethered cord may improve urinary function, although there is no clear evidence that it improves bowel function.

A cardiac echocardiogram is recommended to evaluate structural cardiac anomalies, and any cardiac anomaly identified other than a patent ductus arteriosus or patent foramen ovale should be referred to a pediatric cardiac surgeon.[22,23] There is no association between cardiac defects and the ARM subtype.[24]

Patients with an ARM are also at increased risk of esophageal atresia or tracheoesophageal fistulas. If a nasogastric tube can be passed into the stomach and the neonate is feeding normally, esophageal atresia can be excluded and the chances of a tracheoesophageal fistula are minimal. If an H-type tracheoesophageal fistula (4%–5% of all tracheoesophageal fistulas) is suspected, an appropriate esophagogram and surgical referral should ensue.[24,25]

Renal and genitourinary defects are associated with the presence of ARMs, and anomalies of the upper urinary tract system are the most common defects present with VACTERL syndromes (>90%).[18,22] Vesicoureteral reflux is common, and there is evidence that prophylactic antibiotics should be administered until a urologic assessment including a renal ultrasound and a voiding cystourethrography is complete.[22] Generally, higher malformations have more frequent urologic abnormalities. Patients with low defects have a 10% chance of a genitourinary defect, whereas lower defects such as cloaca and rectobladder neck defects have a 90% chance of a genitourinary defect.[18,22] Early identification is essential for optimal treatment and long-term management.

Limb defects including polydactyly, syndactyly, hypoplastic thumbs, and radial aplasia are also more common in patients with ARMs, although these are less common than in HSCR.[18] If such defects are identified, referral should be made to a pediatric plastic or orthopedic surgeon. Additionally, nonfistula types of ARMs are strongly associated with Down syndrome.[26]

Management of Anorectal Malformations

Once the infant's ARM anatomy has been identified and the infant has been resuscitated and evaluated for associated anomalies, surgical planning should commence as appropriate. As mentioned, patients with low fistulas may be candidates for single-stage repair, whereas those with high fistulas are usually first managed with a diverting colostomy. For those with high fistulas who undergo a two-stage repair, contrast should be injected into the mucous fistula to appropriately distend the rectum, delineating the anatomy prior to definitive surgery. This assists with surgical planning by allowing for an understanding of the fistula position in relation to the urethra and the sacrum.

Generally, midline approaches to repairing high ARMs reduce the chance of injury to surrounding nerves or muscle. PSARP is the standard of care for high fistulas, including rectourethral fistulas and rectoprostatic fistulas.[27] The goal of repairing the ARM with this approach is to carefully dissect the fistula from the urethra and place it within the sphincter while minimizing damage to the surrounding structures and muscles. Because the fistula is often fused or intimately related to the rectum, often there is no clear surgical plane. This underscores the necessity of meticulous surgical dissection required for this crucial step. Laparoscopy may be useful for the dissection, particularly for higher defects. Once dissection is complete, the hindgut must be carefully and accurately placed within the sphincter mechanism. This can be aided by the use of a muscle stimulator.

The goal of PSARP when repairing cloacae, in which the rectum, vagina, and/or urinary tract fuse to form a common channel, is to safely separate the urogenital structures from the gastrointestinal tract. This may be best achieved through a multidisciplinary approach consisting of pediatric surgery, urology, and gynecology. Postoperative care after PSARP entails daily dilatations after 3 to 4 weeks to prevent stricturing and stenosis.

Long-Term Outcomes of Anorectal Malformations

A mechanism for long-term follow-up of patients undergoing surgical repair for ARMs is essential. Acquiring a good functional outcome is paramount, and this consists of allowing the child to begin school and live a normal social life with minimal difficulty. Problems with incontinence or constipation are relatively common and can be a source of major distress for the patients and their families; however, the majority of these symptoms can be controlled with adequate follow-up, dietary adjustments, and a good bowel management program. These patients typically follow up routinely with a surgeon to tailor the bowel regimen according to the needs of the individual patient. Daily enemas are often part of the regimen in patients who are unable to achieve continence and therefore rely on mechanical evacuation of stool on a daily basis. Osmotic laxatives such as polyglycol have been shown to exacerbate fecal incontinence in these patients, whereas stimulant laxatives in combination with a high-fiber diet are more efficacious.[9] Patients who are dependent on daily enemas may benefit from an antegrade enema procedure such as the antegrade continence enema. In an institutional study examining intermediate and long-term outcomes of a bowel management program for children with severe constipation of incontinence, more than one-third of postoperative patients had antegrade continence enema management, which was associated with successful treatment of their symptoms.[28] Additionally, evidence suggests that the outcomes among patients with nonfistula types of ARMs are similar to those of patients with fistula types of ARMs.[26]

Hirschprung Disease

Pathophysiology of Hirschsprung Disease

Hirschsprung disease (also known as HSCR, congenital megacolon, or colonic aganglionosis) is a congenital disorder of the enteric nervous system characterized by failed neural crest migration and subsequent absence of myenteric and submucosal ganglion nerve cells (Auerbach and Meissner plexuses) in a segment of distal bowel. This failed migration occurs during weeks 4 through 12 of gestation and results in spastic, uncoordinated muscle movement, preventing the ability of stool to pass through the colon and rectum.[29] This ineffective peristalsis leads to constipation and functional obstruction, putting the patient at risk for bowel perforation, enterocolitis, and serious bacterial infections, among other complications. Distally, the aganglionic bowel segment usually starts at the anus and extends most commonly to the rectosigmoid; however, long-segment disease has been reported, extending throughout the colon and sometimes into the small bowel.[30,31] Other variants include ultrashort disease and the controversial skipped-lesion pathology.[30,32,33]

HSCR is multifactorial and can be either familial or spontaneous.[29] Roughly 20% of all patients with HSCR have other neurologic, cardiovascular, urologic, or gastrointestinal abnormalities.[34] It is believed that isolated HSCR occurs due to mutations in two major groups of genes, the *RET* and *EDNRB* genes. Short-segment HSCR is associated with a *RET* proto-oncogene abnormality located on chromosome 10q11.2.[35] HSCR can also occur in the setting of chromosomal abnormalities or genetic syndromes. Down syndrome is the most common chromosomal abnormality associated with HSCR, present in roughly 10% of all patients.[36] Additional disorders associated with HSCR that are potentially linked to failed neural crest migration include congenital deafness, hydrocephalus, bladder diverticulum, Meckel diverticulum, imperforate anus, ventricular septal defects, renal agenesis, cryptorchidism, Waardenburg syndrome, Mowat-Wilson syndrome, Fryns syndrome, neonatal central hypoventilation syndrome, neuroblastoma, pheochromocytoma, multiple endocrine neoplasia type 2a, and familial medullary thyroid carcinoma.[29,34,37–39] Retrospective and prospective genetic analyses have demonstrated a potential benefit to systematic *RET* mutation screening in HSCR patients to identify preclinical medullary thyroid carcinoma.[40] Furthermore, in patients with multiple endocrine neoplasia type 2a who exhibit gastrointestinal symptoms, the threshold for investigation for HSCR should be very low.[41]

Clinical Features of Hirschsprung Disease

HSCR occurs in approximately 1 in 5000 infants and is three to four times more common in males than females. It is less common in premature infants compared with term infants.[42] It most commonly presents shortly after birth in the neonatal period, although it may present in older childhood or even in adulthood. In the majority (80%) of patients with HSCR, the colon or rectum is affected. Infants with an absence of ganglion cells in the rectum and sigmoid colon are said to have short-segment disease. Roughly 12% of infants have ganglion cells missing from the majority of the large intestine and have what is referred to as long-segment disease. Approximately 6% to 8% of infants will have ganglion cells missing throughout the entire colon and possibly part of the small intestine, referred to as total colonic HSCR. If there is an absence of ganglion cells throughout the entire small bowel and large bowel, this is referred to as total intestinal aganglionosis.

Enterocolitis and colonic perforation are the most serious complications associated with HSCR and the most common causes of HSCR-related mortality. Enterocolitis is the result of functional intestinal obstruction due to the absence of ganglion cells in the distal bowel. Early symptoms of enterocolitis include abdominal distention, foul-smelling watery diarrhea, poor feeding, and lethargy. Late symptoms include emesis, hematochezia, shock, and multiorgan failure.

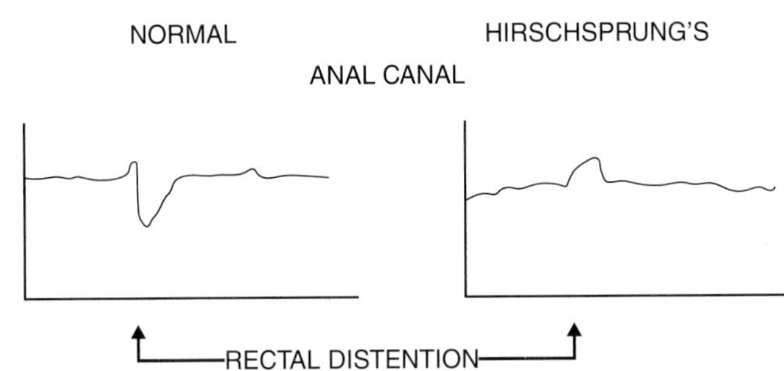

Fig. 85.2 Anal Manometry. Absence of relaxation reflex in response to dilatation may be diagnostic.

Once enterocolitis is suspected, prompt treatment should begin, which entails thorough rectal irrigation several times a day along with antibiotics. Oral Flagyl may be adequate for mild disease, whereas intravenous broad-spectrum antibiotics should be used for more severe disease. Rectal irrigation consists of repeatedly irrigating with 10 to 15 cc/kg warm normal saline through a large-caliber catheter as it is advanced proximally.

Evaluation of Hirschsprung Disease

The majority of patients with HSCR are diagnosed in infancy. Prompt diagnosis is essential to avoid potentially devastating complications including toxic megacolon and enterocolitis.[43] Integral to an accurate diagnosis is a complete patient and family history, a thorough physical examination, appropriate imaging, and a sufficient biopsy. HSCR should be suspected in any infant who fails to pass meconium within the first 24 to 48 hours of life, a finding present in 90% of all patients with HSCR. Associated additional signs and symptoms in the neonate include abdominal distention and pain, bilious emesis, jaundice, difficulty stooling, poor feeding, and a tight anal sphincter with an empty rectum or explosive diarrhea upon digital interrogation.[29] The differential diagnosis for HSCR should include ileal atresia, colonic atresia, malrotation with volvulus, meconium plug syndrome, meconium ileus, necrotizing enterocolitis, toxic megacolon, and sepsis.[1]

The initial recommended workup should include an abdominal x-ray, which may reveal a nonspecific bowel gas pattern or dilated proximal loops of bowel suggestive of obstruction. Anorectal manometry, which is used to test the rectoanal inhibitory reflex, has a negative predictive value up to 100% and may be employed as a screening test to reduce the number of negative biopsies[44,45] (Fig. 85.2). In patients with suspected HSCR, a Gastrografin contrast enema is recommended, with images taken immediately after contrast instillation and then 24 hours after the enema.[46] A pathognomonic finding on contrast enema for HSCR is the presence of a transition zone, where a marked change in caliber occurs with a dilated normal colon above and a narrowed aganglionic colon below. Additional features include a delay in contrast evacuation after 24 hours, a rectosigmoid index (the maximum width of the rectum divided by the maximum width of the sigmoid) less than 1, and irregularity or jejunization of the mucosa.[46–48] The 24-hour delayed film after the contrast enema has a high negative predictive value (>85%) and can be useful in ruling out disease if there is an absence of contrast in the colon.[47] The level of radiologic transition zone on the enema can also be useful for assessing the extent of disease involvement and can assist with operative planning.[47,49] A contrast enema should not be performed in patients with suspected enterocolitis due to the risk of perforation.

Although radiographic and manometric studies are useful in identifying patients either likely or not likely to have HSCR, a rectal biopsy with careful evaluation of the specimen by an experienced pathologist remains the gold standard and is generally recommended for disease confirmation in neonates suspected of having the disease.[43] These patients should be referred to pediatric surgeons for biopsy. The biopsy sample should be at least 1.5 cm above the dentate line, because the rectum distal to the dentate line does not contain ganglion cells.[43] A simple suction biopsy using one of several techniques in which two to three specimens are obtained to reduce the risk of a false-negative biopsy should be used. Suction biopsies are associated with a low risk of perforation and bleeding and are usually able to be performed at the bedside. An absence of ganglion cells in the colonic submucosa and the presence of hypertrophic nerve trunks are pathognomonic for HSCR.[29,43] If the biopsy demonstrated an absence of ganglion cells but no hypertrophic nerve trunks, a full-thickness biopsy or punch biopsy may be warranted.[43] These techniques require general anesthesia and are associated with increased rates of perforation, bleeding, and scarring.[43] Endoscopic biopsies using jumbo biopsy forceps have been performed with reported diagnostic accuracy matching or exceeding suction rectal biopsies.[50] However, endoscopic biopsies require procedural sedation, and it is unclear whether smaller endoscopic specimens are of adequate quality to reliably and consistently diagnose HSCR.[43]

Rectal biopsies are not recommended in premature infants due to both the difficulty in recognizing ganglion cells in premature children and the increased associated risks of biopsy-associated complications. Furthermore, because HSCR occurs much less frequently in premature infants compared with term infants, rectal suction biopsies should be used selectively, and alternative diagnoses should be explored when delayed stooling patterns are encountered.[42] If HSCR is suspected, the distal rectum should be decompressed using stimulation or irrigations until the infant is closer to term and a definitive biopsy can safely proceed.[43]

Management of Hirschsprung Disease

If not immediately diagnosed or treated, the affected infant's symptoms may progress to constipation, poor weight gain, delayed growth, enterocolitis, and death. Hirschsprung-associated enterocolitis is the most frequent complication of HSCR, occurring in 30% to 40% of individuals. It is associated with significant mortality and presents with fever, explosive diarrhea, abdominal distention, lethargy, and vomiting. Left untreated, it may progress to toxic megacolon, sepsis, and death. Any suspicion of Hirschsprung-associated enterocolitis warrants emergent evaluation and potential treatment as described.

Once a diagnosis of HSCR is confirmed, treatment nearly always requires surgery to resect the aganglionic portion of colon or rectum and to connect the healthy, normally innervated bowel to the anus. Prior to surgery, the neonate should be adequately and aggressively resuscitated. The infant should receive broad-spectrum antibiotics, have a nasogastric tube placed for proximal decompression, and undergo serial rectal irrigations to decompress the distal bowel and to reduce the risk of developing enterocolitis.

The standard surgical approach for short-segment HSCR in an otherwise healthy neonate with a nondistended colon is the ileoanal pull-through. Several variants of the pull-through procedure exist. Currently, most pull-through procedures are completed in a single stage, and sequential colonic biopsies are performed until healthy bowel with ganglion cells is identified. However, if a child has a severely low birth weight (less than 2 kg), Hirschsprung-associated enterocolitis, or a significantly dilated colon or is otherwise critically ill, the pull-through may be completed in multiple stages in an attempt to mitigate further morbidity. The multistaged approach includes creating a temporary diverting colostomy followed by a return to the operating room for a formal anastomosis several months later, once the child has grown or has been medically optimized. This approach was also commonly employed historically, given high rates of anastomotic leaks and strictures.

As mentioned, several one-stage pull-through techniques exist. All are generally considered to be highly successful with a low rate of complications. The single-stage Swenson operation is the original pull-through procedure and involves complete resection of the aganglionic colon, deep pelvic dissection, and creating an end-to-end anastomosis of the normal colon to the distal rectum (Fig. 85.3).[51] The patient is placed supine, and the affected colon and rectum are dissected down to the level of the internal sphincters. A perineal approach is used to create the coloanal anastomosis.

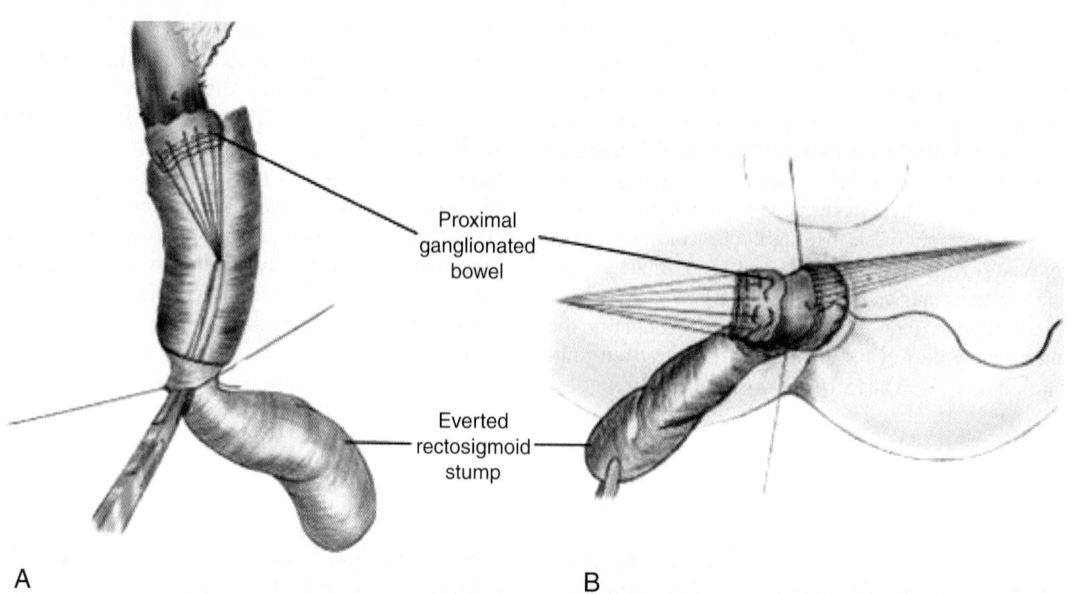

Fig. 85.3 Principles of the Swenson Pull-Through Procedure. (A) The proximal ganglionated bowel is grasped through an incision in the prolapsed rectosigmoid stump. (B) The ganglionated bowel is then sewn to the anus. (From Holcomb GW, Patrick Murphy J, Ostlie DJ. *Ashcraft's Pediatric Surgery E-Book.* Elsevier Health Sciences; 2014.)

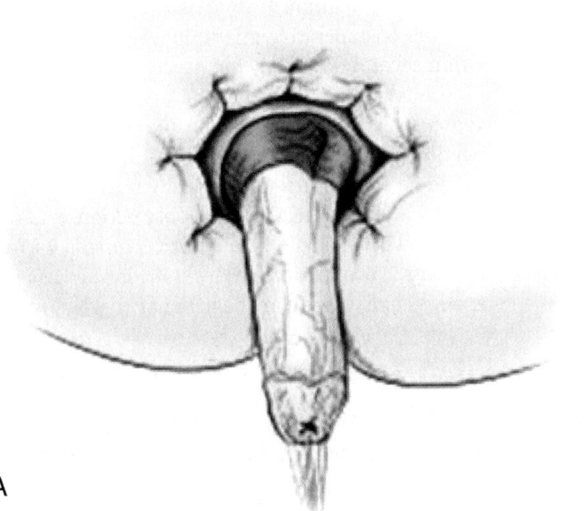

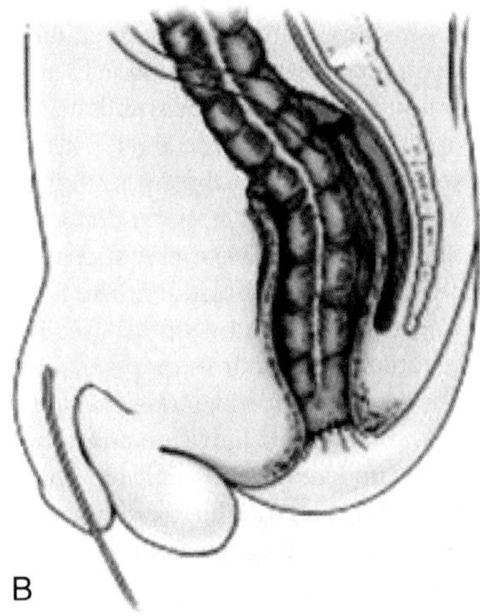

Fig. 85.4 (A) For the Soave operation, there is extramucosal dissection of the rectum after circumferential incision of the rectal mucosa. (B) The ganglionated colon is pulled through the aganglionic rectal cuff, and a coloanal anastomosis is performed. (From Holcomb GW, Patrick Murphy J, Ostlie DJ. *Ashcraft's Pediatric Surgery E-Book.* Elsevier Health Sciences; 2014.)

The Soave procedure attempts to mitigate injury to pelvic structures and consists of removing the rectal mucosa and submucosa, then anastomosing the pull-through portion of bowel within a cuff of aganglionic rectum (Fig. 85.4). The original procedure was performed in two stages, with the first being a pull-through extending out through the anus and the second for creating the anastomosis several weeks later. This procedure is now commonly employed as a one-stage approach.[52] Through a perineal approach, the submucosa is dissected endorectally starting 0.5 to 1 cm above the dentate line and extending to normal colon. The normal colon is then pulled through for the coloanal anastomosis, leaving a cuff of aganglionic muscle.

Another approach is the Duhamel procedure, which consists of resecting the aganglionic colon to the rectum and bringing normal proximal colon behind the rectum and anterior to the sacrum in an avascular space (Fig. 85.5). An end-to-side anastomosis with the posterior rectal wall is then performed using an endorectal stapler. This procedure leaves the rectum intact and is advantageous for infants with long-segment HSCR, requires less pelvic dissection, and reduces the risk of stricture because of the large anastomosis.[53,54] The Duhamel procedure has been adapted to a laparoscopic approach, and a meta-analysis of retrospective data suggests that it is superior to the open approach in terms of hospital stay, time to oral feeds, incontinence, and further intervention with no difference in constipation or enterocolitis.[53–55]

Like the Duhamel procedure, both the Swenson and Soave procedures have adapted to new technology and can both be completed via a transanal approach with or without laparoscopic assistance. These approaches have been shown to decrease length of stay and reduce complications compared with a laparotomy.[56] The laparoscopic-assisted approach consists of a laparoscopic mobilization of the rectum below the peritoneal reflection, combined with endoscopic dissection of the colon and rectum. The rectum is then prolapsed through the anus and the anastomosis is performed transanally. The transanal approach without laparoscopic assistance, known as the transanal endorectal pull through (TERPT), is performed entirely transanally without laparoscopic or open dissection. A submucosal dissection is performed proximal to the dentate line, and the rectal muscle is incised circumferentially. The entire rectum and distal sigmoid colon are delivered through the anus, allowing for the diseased bowel to be resected and the healthy bowel to be anastomosed. This approach is ideal for patients with more distal transition zones. Compared with the transanal Soave procedure, the transanal Swenson procedure may result in less blood loss, a shorter operation time, and fewer complications.[56]

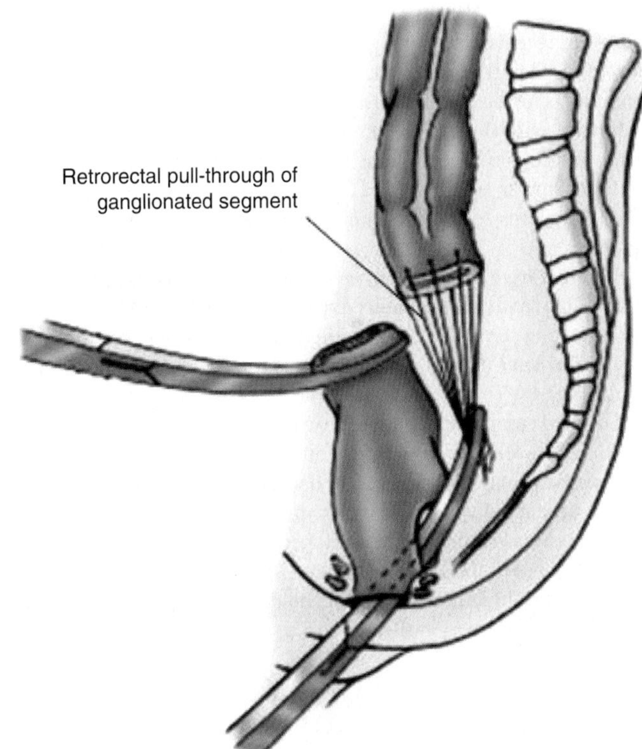

Fig. 85.5 With the Duhamel technique, the ganglionated bowel is delivered through an incision in the posterior aspect of the native aganglionic rectum and sewn to the anus. The septum between the ganglionated pull-through colon and the aganglionic native rectum is then divided using a stapler. (From Holcomb GW, Patrick Murphy J, Ostlie DJ. *Ashcraft's Pediatric Surgery E-Book.* Elsevier Health Sciences; 2014.)

Several recent studies have further compared the TERPT and transabdominal approaches. Two recent meta-analyses determined that a TERPT is associated with a shorter hospital length of stay, a shorter operative time, reduced postoperative incontinence, and less constipation compared with the transabdominal approach.[57,58] However, more robust controlled prospective trials are indicated, and it is generally recommended that the surgeon should perform the approach with which he or she is most familiar and comfortable.

Both the Duhamel and the Soave operations help preserve the nerve supply to the rectum and bladder. The Soave procedure is prone to stricture formation and generally requires anastomotic dilations for several months after the surgery. A more recent iteration of the Soave procedure is a one-stage transanal approach that eliminates the need for an abdominal incision and colostomy.

Most patients who undergo laparoscopic or TERPT procedures can be fed immediately after the procedure and discharged home within several days, once it is clear that the child is stooling regularly and that there is no skin breakdown. Failure to pass stool within 2 days from surgery is a cause for concern and should raise suspicion for anastomotic problems including stricture, leakage, or twist during the pull-through, as described below. One to two weeks after the operation, the anastomosis should be calibrated with a dilator. Historically, parents would then dilate the anastomosis daily to weekly for 1 to 2 months in the hopes of reducing the rate of anastomotic strictures. However, recent data suggest performing routine anal dilatations does not reduce the risk of developing anastomotic strictures or enterocolitis and may be associated with the development of late-onset strictures compared with those children with short-segment disease who did not undergo routine dilations or who underwent weekly calibration.[59,60] Barrier cream should be prescribed for the perineum and buttock regions to prevent skin breakdown secondary to frequent stooling.

Perioperative mortality rates for any of the surgical procedures is very low, and most patients experience significant improvement without long-term sequelae. Patients with long-segment HSCR or those who have HSCR in addition to other syndromes tend to do worse.

Surgical complications include wound infection, intraabdominal bleeding, bowel perforation, fecal incontinence, anastomotic dehiscence, strictures, rectal stenosis, or damage to surrounding structures including seminal vesicles, the urethra, or the vagina. When stenosis is present, this can usually be managed with serial dilation over the course of several weeks.[61] There can also be residual aganglionosis, which places the infant at risk for the development of enterocolitis and requires a redo pull-through procedure. Other long-term complications include persistent obstruction, incontinence, and chronic constipation.

If the postoperative infant does not have normal bowel function within several days after the procedure, a workup for surgical complications should commence. Plain x-rays can be helpful in assessing stool burden, and a contrast enema can evaluate the size, quality, and function of the remaining colon. The distal bowel and the anastomosis should be evaluated endoscopically under anesthesia to evaluate for stricture, dehiscence, twisting, obstruction, and overall appearance. A rectal biopsy should be obtained to assess for residual aganglionic segments. Constipation and fecal incontinence can be managed with laxatives and a bowel management program, respectively.

Long-Term Outcomes in Hirschprung Disease

With appropriate early diagnosis and treatment, most children (90%) with HSCR will go on to live normal, healthy lives. Children with long-segment disease, Down syndrome, and other major comorbidities tend to do worse. Up to 10% of patients may develop constipation with obstructive symptoms, and 1% may develop incontinence. Both constipation and incontinence can be managed with chronic bowel management and usually improve within the first 5 years of life. Enterocolitis can occur several years after surgery, usually due to residual aganglionic bowel. Most cases of postoperative enterocolitis occur within the first 2 years after surgery. Thus infants should be closely monitored for evidence of enterocolitis after surgery. In general, patients should generally be on a high-fiber diet after surgery to minimize bowel stasis and reduce the risk of enterocolitis.

Conclusions

ARMs and Hirschprung disease are congenital anorectal disorders best treated with surgical management. The defects range from minor and readily treatable to complex and associated with a poor prognosis. Timely recognition, diagnosis, and treatment remain the mainstays for optimum long-term outcomes. As diagnostic modalities and surgical interventions continue to evolve, physicians must continue to seek ways to improve functional outcomes and patients' quality of life. In patients who continue to suffer from sequelae of these diseases, most commonly due to fecal incontinence or constipation, the pediatric surgeon plays a pivotal role in the management of the patient through bowel management programs aimed at optimizing quality of life.

CHAPTER 86

Esophageal Surgery in Neonates: Esophageal Atresia, Gastroesophageal Reflux, and Other Congenital Anomalies

Mark L. Kovler, Shaun M. Kunisaki

KEY POINTS

1. Esophageal surgery in neonates includes the treatment of esophageal atresia, gastroesophageal reflux, congenital esophageal stenosis, esophageal duplication, and vascular rings.
2. Esophageal atresia, with or without tracheoesophageal atresia, is the most common congenital anomaly of the esophagus, occurring in 1 in 3500 live births.
3. The surgical treatment of esophageal atresia has undergone several advances including the introduction of thoracoscopic repair.
4. Management of long-gap esophageal atresia remains challenging even at high-volume centers.
5. Results from recent large, multicenter registries brought into question some aspects of traditional surgical management of esophageal atresia and are moving management toward an evidenced-based approach.

Introduction

Esophageal pathology in the newborn period represents a broad range of disorders that affect feeding, swallowing, and airway protection. These conditions require the multidisciplinary care of neonatologists, pediatric surgeons, aerodigestive specialists, and many others and are just a part of the complex care delivered to infants in modern neonatal intensive care units. A detailed understanding of the surgical considerations of infants with congenital and acquired esophageal pathologies is advantageous to those who are focused on these most fragile patients, because the respiratory and developmental morbidities associated with esophageal pathology can be significant. Herein, we review the principles of surgical management of esophageal pathology in the newborn, including esophageal atresia (EA) and tracheoesophageal fistula (TEF), gastroesophageal reflux disease, and other congenital anomalies, with a focus on the evidence-based clinical approaches and evaluation of outcomes.

EA and TEF

Pathophysiology

Embryology

EA occurs in approximately 1 in 3500 live births and is a congenital anomaly that develops in utero.[1] During normal development, the respiratory and digestive tracts separate into the anterior trachea and the posterior esophagus, a process that commences with the outgrowth of the trachea from the ventral foregut by the fourth week of gestation.[2,3] The precise mechanism by which EA/TEF occurs during organogenesis is incompletely understood, but several risk factors have been discovered that increase the odds of EA/TEF. EA occurs more commonly in twins, with a relative risk of EA in twins compared with singleton pregnancies of 2.56 (95% CI, 2.01–3.25).[2] EA is also seen in a number of other congenital associations and genetic syndromes. Up to one in four infants born with EA will have an associated nonrandom anomaly as part of the VACTERL association—a spectrum that includes vertebral, anorectal, cardiac, tracheal, esophageal, renal, and limb anomalies.[4,5] Additionally, genetic syndromes occur in 10% of infants with EA and include trisomy (chromosomes 13, 18, or 21) and single-gene disorders (CHARGE syndrome [coloboma, heart defects, atresia of the choanae, retardation of growth and mental development, genital underdevelopment, esophageal atresia], DiGeorge syndrome, Feingold syndrome, Opitz syndrome, and Fanconi anemia).[2]

Anatomy and Classification

A familiarity with the anatomic variations of EA/TEF is critical for the systematic assessment of an infant suspected of having the anomaly, an understanding of the physiologic consequences of uncorrected EA/TEF, and the formulation of a surgical strategy for correction. The most commonly used classification is that described by Gross,[6] but a simple description of the anatomy of each arrangement can be equally helpful in understanding the presenting features and pathophysiology associated with each (Fig. 86.1). Five common anatomic variants are described, in order of most to least frequent: (1) EA with distal TEF—Gross type C, (2) isolated EA with no fistula—Gross type A, (3) TEF with no EA—commonly referred to as "H" type fistula, (4) EA with a proximal TEF—Gross type B, and (5) EA with both proximal and distal TEFs—Gross type D.

The most common conformation, EA with distal TEF, occurs in 86% of cases.[7] In this arrangement, frequently referred to by its Gross classification "type C," the proximal esophagus ends in a blind pouch in the superior mediastinum, typically at the level of the third to fourth thoracic vertebra.[6,7] The fistula occurs between the distal esophagus and the posterior wall of the trachea, usually within centimeters of the carina. This anatomy allows for the passage of air from the trachea into the low-resistance distal esophagus and intraabdominal intestinal tract, and thus intraluminal abdominal gas will be appreciated on plain radiograph. Additionally, because a TEF does exist, there is risk for gastric contamination of the respiratory tract with subsequent pneumonitis.

The next most common configuration occurs far less frequently, in 8% of cases, and involves an isolated EA with no fistula (type A).[8]

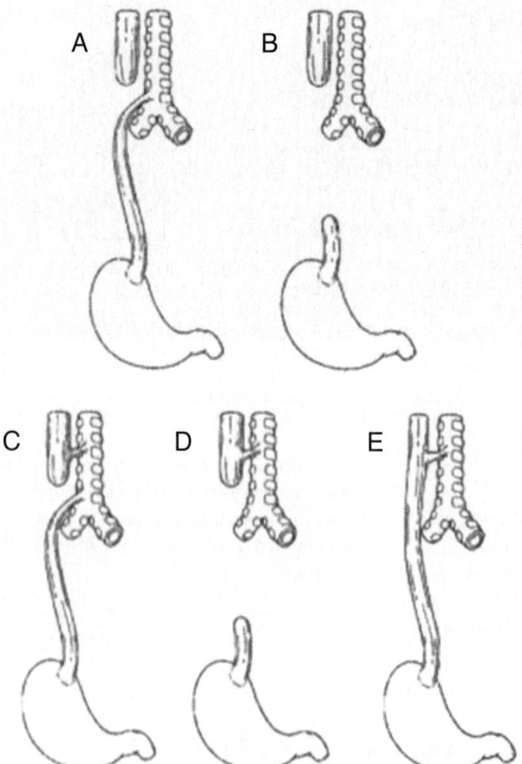

Fig. 86.1 The Five Described Anatomic Configurations of Esophageal Atresia and Tracheoesophageal Fistula. (A) Esophageal atresia with distal tracheoesophageal fistula. (B) Esophageal atresia without tracheoesophageal fistula. (C) Esophageal atresia with both proximal and distal tracheoesophageal fistula. (D) Esophageal atresia with proximal tracheoesophageal fistula. (E) Isolated tracheoesophageal fistula. (From Bruch SW, Coran AG. Congenital malformations of the esophagus. In: *Pediatric Gastrointestinal and Liver Disease* 4th ed. Philadelphia: Elsevier; 2011:222–231.)

The absence of a distal fistula will result in a gasless abdomen, which can be seen on radiograph. In contrast to the gap distance in the typical type C defect, the distance between the blind upper and lower ends of the esophagus in type A is relatively far in isolated EA, thereby often precluding the possibility for a primary anastomosis shortly after birth.[9]

The third most common type, TEF with no EA, occurs in only 4% of cases but presents some unique diagnostic challenges.[7,10] Although this is frequently referred to as an "H" type fistula, it has also been more accurately described as an "N" type due to the fistula running from the proximal orifice in the trachea to a distal orifice in the esophagus. Although there is no EA, most of these children can eat orally. The clinical presentation of this type is often more subtle and can involve difficulty feeding or, occasionally, excessive flatulence due to the increased passage of gas into the gastrointestinal tract. This condition can go undetected in the newborn period.[11]

Natural History

The abnormal anatomic arrangements that result from EA/TEF produce predictable physiologic patterns that are important to recognize and aid in operative planning. Without surgical repair or a temporizing operation, there is no spontaneous resolution of the pathophysiologic consequences of the enteral system discontinuity and/or fistulous connection between the aerodigestive tracts. Therefore, before surgical correction became a feasible operation, the condition was uniformly fatal.[12] In the modern era, up-front surgical correction is successful in most cases, and when not possible (due to comorbidities, extreme low birth weight, or long-gap atresia), temporizing strategies to manage the fistula and to provide enteric feeding access can be implemented.

Without continuity of the digestive tract, neonates with EA are unable to feed orally and thus will develop oral aversion. Although enteral access can be attained surgically, neonates with uncorrected EA are also unable to handle oral secretions, which increases the risk of recurrent oropharyngeal aspiration. Additionally, abnormal development of the trachea and aspiration of gastric contents through a fistulous tract leads to pneumonitis and respiratory compromise.

Clinical Features

Prenatal Diagnosis

Less than 20% of EA/TEF cases are detected prenatally.[13] The characteristic findings on prenatal ultrasound suggestive of EA/TEF are polyhydramnios, an absent or small stomach bubble, and a "pouch sign" in which a fluid-filled, blind-ending esophagus is seen during fetal swallowing.[13] However, these findings are usually not seen at the 20-week anatomic survey, are nonspecific, and can often be misleading, because there are several other and more common causes of polyhydramnios, and stomach size can vary even in cases of EA due to gastric secretion production. A recent meta-analysis of contemporary prenatal ultrasound estimated the sensitivity of detecting EA/TEF to be only 31.7%.[13] The addition of fetal magnetic resonance imaging (MRI) has somewhat improved the ability to diagnose EA/TEF prenatally. When performed for cases of suspected EA/TEF, fetal MRI has a sensitivity of 94.7% and a specificity of 89.3%.[13]

Clinical Presentation

The clinical presentation of a newborn with EA/TEF is well known to the experienced neonatologist and pediatric surgeon. EA with TEF typically presents just after birth with excessive drooling and the inability to tolerate feeding. It is not uncommon for the first attempt at feeding to result in coughing, choking, or cyanosis. All infants with these signs should be evaluated for EA with an attempt at careful placement of an esophageal feeding tube, which will meet resistance at the level of the atresia—most commonly approximately 10 cm from the lips. A plain chest radiograph will confirm the atresia when the tube is seen to be coiled in the upper esophageal pouch. In the extremely premature neonate, the only other esophageal disorder that should be considered in the differential diagnosis is an iatrogenic upper esophageal tear caused during orogastric tube placement. In these situations, an esophagram using a small volume of radiopaque contrast may be helpful to clarify the diagnosis.

If an abdominal radiograph demonstrates gas in the abdomen, in the presence of EA, it can be assumed that a distal TEF is also present (Fig. 86.2). A concomitant duodenal atresia is present in 2% to 5% of patients, in which abdominal radiograph will show a "double bubble" sign.[14] In contrast, if the abdomen is completely gasless, no such distal fistula is suspected. On physical examination, a scaphoid abdomen raises the suspicion for pure EA with no fistula, whereas a distended abdomen indicates the presence of a distal TEF.

The presentation of TEF without EA (H-type TEF) is not as obvious because the esophagus remains in continuity, which allows for clearance of saliva, the passage of an esophageal tube, and oral feeding. Furthermore, the presence of associated anomalies is less frequent, so suspicion for TEF may be underappreciated.[10] TEF without EA should be considered in infants with coughing and choking during feeding, which occurs due to aspiration through the fistula. Nevertheless, these symptoms are associated with a broad differential, and

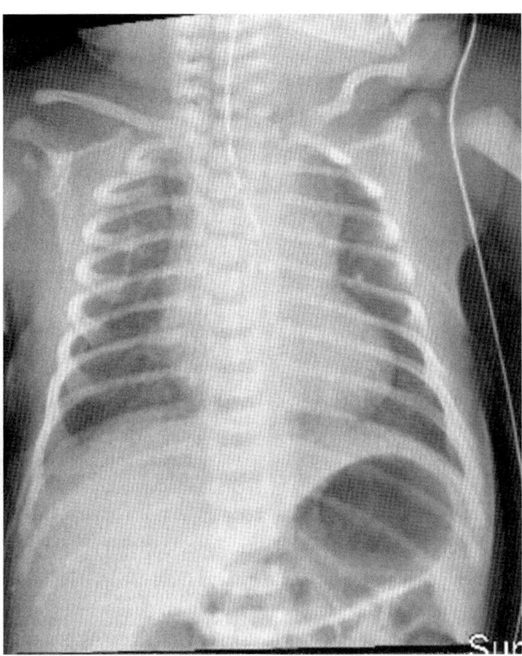

Fig. 86.2 Plain Radiograph Demonstrating an Enteric Tube Terminating in the Upper Mediastinum Indicating Esophageal Atresia, With Abdominal Gas Pattern Consistent With a Distal Tracheoesophageal Fistula.

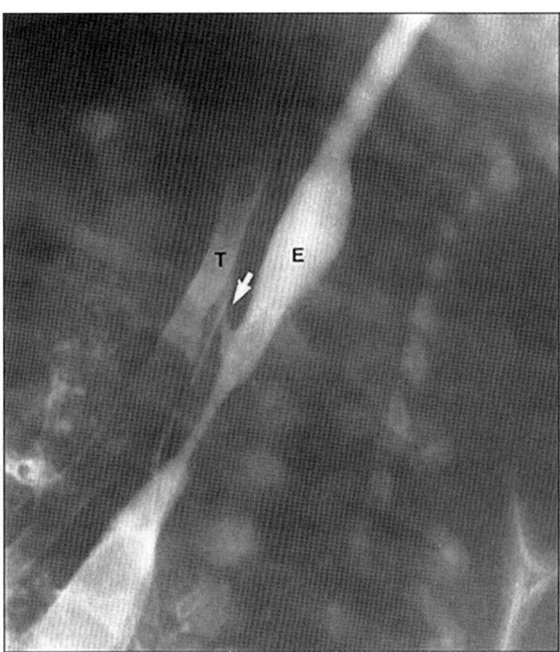

Fig. 86.3 Prone-Pullback Esophagram Showing the Esophagus (*E*) in Continuity, the Fistula (*arrow*), and the Trachea (*T*) in the "H-type" Tracheoesophageal Fistula. (From Gore RM, Levine MS. Esophageal atresia. *High-Yield Imaging: Gastrointestinal*. Philadelphia: Elsevier; 2010:816–818.)

the diagnosis of TEF without EA is elusive and can be missed in the neonatal period in up to one-third of cases.[10,11] If TEF without EA is suspected, it is best diagnosed with a prone pull-back esophagram and/or rigid bronchoscopy[10,15] (Fig. 86.3).

Evaluation

Evaluation of Associated Anomalies

Once EA/TEF is diagnosed, a comprehensive evaluation of the associated anatomic and chromosomal anomalies ensues to determine treatment priorities. The most common accompanying anomalies are part of the VACTERL (vertebral, anorectal, cardiac, tracheal, esophageal, renal, limb/laryngeal) association. Therefore a complete physical exam is performed with a special focus on the cardiac (30%–60%), anorectal (7%–12%), and limb (6%–10%) exams.[16–19]

The most urgent adjunct study is echocardiography to assess for congenital cardiac disease, which is a major driver of mortality.[1,16,17] The most common cardiac anomalies associated with EA/TEF are atrial septal defect, ventricular septal defect, and tetralogy of Fallot.[16,17] In addition to identification of cardiac anomalies that might require urgent treatment, echocardiography can identify anomalies of the upper mediastinal vessels that are important to operative planning. These occur in up to 18% of patients and include a right-sided aortic arch (2%–6%) and an aberrant right-sided subclavian artery (12%).[20] When a vascular anomaly is detected, cross-sectional imaging should be considered to optimize the operative approach.

Additional adjunct studies should be performed in all EA/TEF patients to rule out renal, limb, vertebral, and chromosomal abnormalities. Renal ultrasound will characterize the presence of the kidneys and any irregularities in renal development. Suspected radial limb anomalies on physical exam should be confirmed by plain radiography. Spinal radiography and ultrasound are used to look for vertebral anomalies and a tethered spinal cord, respectively. Any stigmata of chromosomal abnormalities should prompt a genetics consult.

Management

Preoperative Management

The goal of preoperative management of EA/TEF is to maintain cardiorespiratory stability and to provide hydration and nutrition until surgical repair is accomplished. To decrease oropharyngeal aspiration and respiratory tract contamination with gastroesophageal contents, newborns are made NPO (nil per os), and a large-bore oral esophageal sump drainage tube should be placed into the blind-ending esophageal pouch and put to continuous suction. A double lumen Replogle-type tube is best for drainage, and simple feeding catheters should be avoided. The head of the bed is elevated to 45 degrees and acid suppressive therapy is begun. Intravenous hydration is provided, and typically, a central venous catheter is placed for administration of parenteral nutrition because in most cases, it is anticipated that enteral feeding will not begin until 5 to 7 days after surgical repair.

The approach to respiratory management in neonates with a type C EA/TEF is based on avoidance of air flow preferentially through the fistula into the gastrointestinal tract. Excessive air entry into the stomach can cause gastric distension leading to further respiratory failure, an increase in reflux and aspiration through the fistula, and even gastric perforation. Spontaneous respiration is preferred and can be accomplished in most infants, especially those born at term. When mechanical ventilation is necessary, it should be undertaken judiciously and by a team experienced in the advanced respiratory support of neonates with EA/TEF. Also, a pediatric surgical team should be available should any emergent operative intervention be required.

During endotracheal intubation, care must be taken to avoid intubation of the fistula, which can lead to rapid decompensation.

Patients with EA/TEF are at an increased risk for laryngeal anomalies, which can result in a challenging airway.[21] The ideal positioning of the endotracheal tube when a TEF is present is to place the tip of the tube just below the level of the fistula,[22] and flexible bronchoscopy can be a valuable tool to confirm the position of the endotracheal tube in relation to the fistula. Once the airway is secured, lower ventilator pressures should be used, and high-frequency oscillator ventilation has been described as an approach to minimize gastric distension.[23]

In routine cases in otherwise healthy newborns, operative repair of a type C EA/TEF can take place within the first 24 to 48 hours of life to minimize aspiration and pulmonary soiling. Perioperative antibiotics are given to cover skin and upper gastrointestinal flora. Finally, EA/TEF repair is a major surgery, and preoperative optimization includes correction of any coagulopathy of the newborn, which is usually through vitamin K administration.

Operative Repair of EA/TEF

The goals of operative repair of any type C EA/TEF are twofold—division of the fistula and establishment of esophageal continuity. Once the airway is secured, rigid bronchoscopy is routinely performed to locate the TEF and to assess for the rare possibility of an additional proximal fistula. The operation is most commonly performed through a right thoracotomy incision. During dissection anterior to the proximal esophagus, care must be taken to avoid a posterior tracheal injury. Once sufficient esophageal length is attained, the two ends are sutured together by a single-layer end-to-end anastomosis. A chest tube is left in the extrapleural space adjacent to the anastomosis to control any potential anastomotic leak.

Traditionally, most surgeons have left a transanastomotic nasogastric feeding tube across the esophageal connection. Transanastomotic tubes have been reported to be used in almost three-fourths of cases in large academic medical centers.[24] The transanastomotic tube has been placed both for early feeding access while the anastomosis is healing and because some have thought the tube improves healing through stenting of the esophagus. However, these theoretical advantages have not been supported by recent studies, and the tube may induce a foreign-body reaction that might have negative implications. Strikingly, in recent studies, transanastomotic tubes were associated with an increased risk of stricture formation.[25,26] Therefore the routine use of transanastomotic feeding tubes after TEF repair for EA with distal TEF is no longer recommended. The association between transanastomotic tubes and stricture has been explained through animal models demonstrating an increased rate of stricture with mechanical shearing by a foreign body and increased exposure to gastric acid reflux, which can occur when a tube is placed across the gastroesophageal junction.[27]

Thoracotomy in infancy, even with a muscle-sparing approach, is associated with reported long-term morbidities including muscle weakness, winged scapula, and scoliosis.[28,29] Therefore a minimally invasive approach to repair using thoracoscopic surgery has been developed as an alternative to traditional thoracotomy. Additional potential benefits of thoracoscopy for EA/TEF repair include improved visualization of the posterior mediastinum and improved cosmesis.[30] However, thoracoscopic EA/TEF repair is technically challenging, and only between 10% and 20% of EA/TEF repairs in the United States are performed thoracoscopically.[31] When thoracoscopy is the selected approach, outcomes appear to be equivalent to open repair, with no differences in anastomotic leak or stricture rate.[30,32] However, there may be significant selection bias when comparing thoracoscopic with open EA/TEF repair.

Management of Long-Gap EA

Long-gap atresia is often defined when the distance between esophageal ends measures at least three vertebral bodies based on preoperative imaging studies.[33] Although the surgical management of most type C EA/TEF neonates is relatively straightforward, management of long-gap EA, usually type A EA, remains a significant challenge. These patients are best managed at a center of excellence with a multidisciplinary care team devoted to the care of these complex patients.

The initial management of long-gap EA consists of (1) feeding gastrostomy placement to allow for enteral feeds, (2) continuous suctioning of the upper esophageal pouch, and (3) serial imaging with contrast to determine gap distance. A baby with pure EA in the absence of a fistula is not at imminent risk of aspiration and pulmonary soiling. Therefore definitive repair can be delayed for 1 to 3 months to allow the gap the opportunity to spontaneously narrow over time. Cervical esophagostomy is strongly discouraged because it will make subsequent attempts at a delayed primary repair more difficult.

Gastrostomy placement in infants with pure EA can be challenging because the stomach is relatively small from disuse, and placement should be strategic to allow for use of the stomach as an esophageal replacement conduit in the future if needed. After a gastrostomy tube is placed, the infant is allowed to feed enterally and grow in the neonatal intensive care unit, with continued suction drainage of the proximal pouch. With bolus gastrostomy feeds, the distal esophageal pouch may grow and lengthen. The proximal pouch may also lengthen over time due to the swallowing reflex with sham feeds. In most cases, the gap will shorten by approximately two vertebral bodies, enabling a delayed primary anastomosis.[34–36]

Gap distance is assessed with serial gap studies, also referred to as "gapograms" (Fig. 86.4). The initial study is typically obtained once the gastrostomy site heals and is repeated at monthly intervals for up to 3 months.[34] It is most accurate to measure the gap length in terms of vertebral bodies rather than centimeters to account for

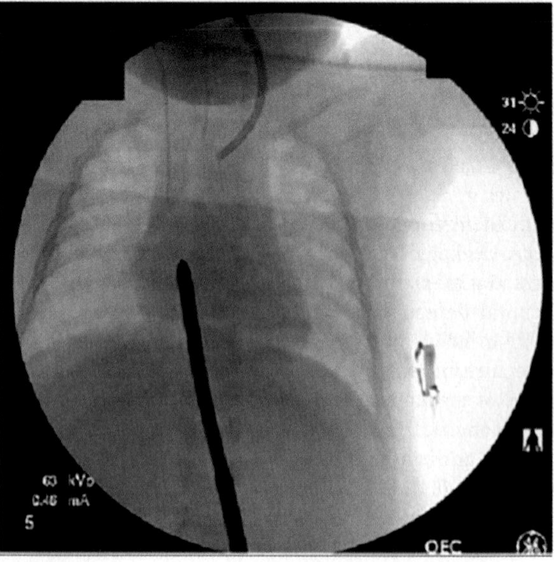

Fig. 86.4 Gap Study to Assess Length Between Ends of a Long-Gap Esophageal Atresia. Here the proximal pouch is demarcated with a small esophageal bougie passed through the mouth, and the extent of the distal pouch is seen by passage of an endoscope through the gastrostomy. (From Afridi FG, Shorter N, Vaughan R, Neptune S, Singh S. Primary repair of long gap esophageal atresia in a neonate employing circular myotomy on upper pouch and a novel hemicircular myotomy on the distal pouch. *J Pediatr Surg Case Reports.* 2019;44:101188.)

infant growth and variation in size over time.[8] Primary repair is usually attainable when the gap distance is less than two vertebral bodies.

For those patients who fail to gain adequate length for primary anastomosis, the options include growth induction under tension (Foker process) or esophageal replacement with an autologous conduit. The Foker process involves surgically applied tension on both ends of the esophagus through suture placement by either thoracotomy[37] or thoracoscopy.[38] Pledgeted horizontal mattress sutures are placed through the esophageal wall adjacent to the blind-ending pouches, and the sutures are then externalized through the posterior chest in a crossed fashion. Interval increases in the tension applied to the sutures externally can lead to growth during a period of several weeks, and this can be visualized on radiograph if the ends tied to the atretic esophagus are tagged with a radiopaque clip. Success rates at achieving primary esophagoesophagostomy with the Foker technique have been reported as high as 80%, but the procedure has not been widely embraced by the pediatric surgical community because it has been difficult to reproduce in low-volume centers and can lead to substantial complications, including lethal mediastinal sepsis if the sutures pull out inadvertently.[39] When the gap remains too long for primary connection, esophageal replacement with stomach, colon, or small intestine is the only reliable option for surgical reconstruction. Although not without some controversy, the gastric transposition procedure is the most straightforward and reproducible esophageal replacement procedure and is associated with acceptable outcomes.[40]

Postoperative Care

After operative repair of EA/TEF is completed, most infants return to the neonatal intensive care unit and remain intubated. To allow for the anastomosis to heal, central venous access is maintained for parenteral nutrition. The most critical component of immediate postoperative care in neonates after EA/TEF repair is airway control. Although most healthy infants can be extubated within 48 hours after the operation, early extubation should be undertaken judiciously to avoid the potential morbidity of reintubation. The operative dissection that occurs posterior to the trachea results in airway edema, and the delicately sutured tracheal repair is at risk for dehiscence should reintubation be required. Furthermore, the use of noninvasive positive pressure ventilation modes such as CPAP should be avoided after esophageal repair because of their tendency to put increased tension on the new anastomosis.

Gastroesophageal reflux should be prevented because it can theoretically increase anastomotic strictures. Infants with EA/TEF have poor esophageal motility, an incompetent gastroesophageal junction, and a relatively small stomach, all increasing the risk of esophageal reflux of gastric contents onto the fresh anastomosis. Elevating the head of the bed to 30 to 45 degrees and acid blockade with either proton pump inhibitors or H_2 blockers are the standard of care.[31] However, despite its nearly ubiquitous use, the benefit of acid blockade in the immediate postoperative period for preventing anastomotic stricture has not been clearly supported by the literature.[41] In contrast, acid blockade carries its own risks in the neonatal period, including increased rates of necrotizing enterocolitis, sepsis, and respiratory infections.[42,43] Therefore the utility of prophylactic acid suppression after EA/TEF repair remains in question, and further studies are needed.

A postoperative esophagram should be performed to assess for subclinical anastomotic leakage prior to initiation of oral feeds and removal of the chest tube. Conventionally, esophagrams are obtained around postoperative day 7; however, an early-esophagram approach on postoperative day 5 has been trialed and resulted in no adverse outcomes or missed leaks.[25]

Complications

Although morbidity is common, perioperative mortality is rare after surgery for EA/TEF and typically results in the setting of complex congenital heart disease.[31] However, complications after surgery for EA/TEF are actually the rule rather than the exception, with the majority of infants experiencing a manageable complication. Bleeding and surgical-site infections are rarely encountered and can be avoided with meticulous surgical technique, perioperative antibiotics, and the precautions previously discussed. More common complications specific to EA/TEF repair are anastomotic leak and stricture.

Anastomotic leaks occur in approximately 15% to 20% of cases.[31,44,45] Leaks occur due to technical errors in creation of the anastomosis, an excessive degree of tension across the connection, or ischemia after extensive mobilization, especially of the distal esophagus. The most significant independent risk factors for anastomotic leaks are long-gap atresia and the use of a prosthetic material interposition between the esophagus and tracheal suture lines, which is no longer recommended.[25,31] A leak is suspected by frothy salivary secretions from the chest tube or an unexpected pneumothorax, or it is seen on esophagram (Fig. 86.5). Most leaks are small and will close spontaneously with time if managed with antibiotics and chest tube drainage. An esophagram to confirm closure of the leak should be performed 1 week after prior imaging or when frothy secretions from the chest tube decrease significantly. Major leaks are rare but can lead to uncontrolled sepsis due to overwhelming mediastinitis. When a severe disruption causes sepsis and clinical instability, diversion with cervical esophagostomy may be required.

An additional complication that occurs with frustrating frequency is anastomotic stricture. A stricture requiring intervention occurs in approximately 40% of cases, and as discussed, the major modifiable risk factor for stricture formation is the use of a transanastomotic feeding tube.[25,31,46] Initial treatment of an anastomotic stricture is endoscopic dilation, which can be performed safely as early as 2 to 3 weeks after the initial operation when the stricture is identified. Most surgeons perform endoscopic dilation using a balloon dilating catheter placed and inflated under fluoroscopic guidance.[24] Although strictures are common, they are manageable with repeat dilations, and resolution occurs in up to 90% of cases.[47] Patients with recalcitrant strictures should be evaluated and treated for any ongoing gastroesophageal reflux. If symptoms persist, there may be a need for other treatment options, including intralesional steroid injection, topical mitomycin C, stricturoplasty, and stricture resection,[48] before resorting to esophageal replacement. Although self-expandable intraluminal stents are an attractive option due to their success in the management of benign strictures in adults, recent experience has shown these devices to be associated with high complication rates and near universal stricture recurrence after stent removal in children.[49]

Special Situations in the NICU

Emergency Management of Respiratory Failure in the TEF Neonate

Infants who suffer significant respiratory failure in the setting of a distal TEF pose a unique physiologic challenge. Typically, these patients are premature neonates who may require endotracheal intubation with significant positive-pressure ventilatory support. Because lung compliance is often poor in these patients, the

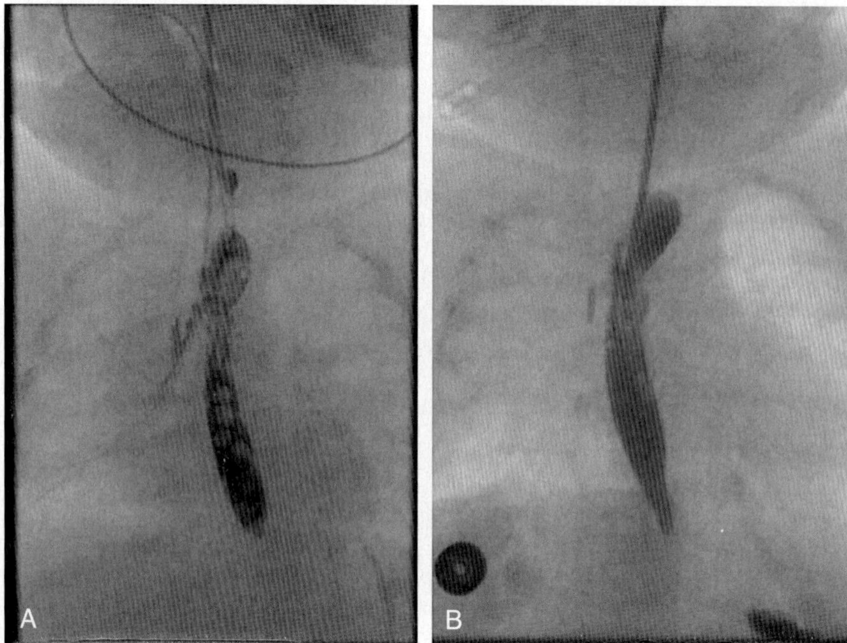

Fig. 86.5 (A) Esophagram demonstrating a leak after esophageal atresia/tracheoesophageal fistula repair. The leak is controlled by an adjacent chest tube left in place postoperatively. (B) Seven days later, esophagram showing resolution of the leak.

gastrointestinal tract provides a lower-pressure system during ventilation, and thus a significant portion of each breath passes through the distal TEF rather than into the lungs. This can lead to significant gastric and abdominal distension, which further compromises ventilation through high abdominal pressures on the diaphragm, and gastric perforation has also been described.[50] The physiologic insult caused by gastric distension further exacerbates the problem, and the cycle continues unless the physiology is disrupted.

The first and least-invasive maneuver to disrupt this cycle is a change to a high-frequency jet ventilator, which can decrease airway pressures and shunting across the fistula.[23,51] If a significant portion of each tidal volume continues to pass across the fistula, the endotracheal tube can be advanced in an attempt to bypass the fistula, usually into the right or left mainstem bronchus.[23] Placement of a cuffed endotracheal tube can also assist in blocking the fistula.[23] Another approach to occlusion of the fistula is to use bronchoscopy to place a small Fogarty catheter through the fistula with inflation of the balloon tip for occlusion.[52]

From the abdomen, bedside gastric decompression with a percutaneously placed gastrostomy tube placed to water seal allows for egress of air from the stomach and also increases the resistance of the gastrointestinal tract to further insufflation.[53] It is critical that the gastrostomy be placed to a chest tube canister with underwater seal settings. Otherwise, the resistance across the gastrointestinal tract will actually drop, leading to increased shunting of air across the fistula and severe rapid respiratory compromise.[54]

In patients who fail conservative measures, emergent operative therapy is indicated. In those too unstable for thoracotomy, laparotomy with temporary exclusion of the gastrointestinal tract from the esophagus at the gastroesophageal junction can be performed.[55] In those stable for transfer to the operating room, emergent thoracotomy with immediate control of the fistula is effective (Fig. 86.6). If fistula control results in respiratory and hemodynamic stability at that point in the operation, the surgeon can proceed with formal esophageal repair. However, if the infant continues to be unstable, the distal esophagus should be sutured to the prevertebral fascia in preparation for a staged esophageal repair. The chest is then closed, and a gastrostomy tube is placed through an abdominal incision. Delayed repair of the esophagus with reasonable outcomes has been reported once infants are stabilized and weigh more than 1.5 kg.[56]

Management of H-Type TEF

As discussed, the diagnosis of "H-type" TEF is challenging due to esophageal continuity. Additionally, the surgical approach to these fistulas differs from the more common conformations because the fistula is usually located in the cervical region and the repair does not require an esophageal anastomosis. Most H-type TEFs can be repaired through the right neck as opposed to the right chest.[11] Preoperative localization of the fistula is essential. One common localization technique is to pass a guidewire or catheter across the fistula by rigid bronchoscopy. A right-neck exploration is then performed through an incision just above the clavicle. Outcomes from H-type TEF are better than from other types because esophageal motility is relatively normal and there is no circumferential anastomosis, decreasing the risk of leak and stricture.[10] However, more than 20% of cases result in recurrent laryngeal nerve injury, owing to the location of the nerve in close proximity to the fistula.[10]

Long-Term Outcomes

Survival for neonates born with EA/TEF depends on their degree of prematurity, associated congenital cardiac anomalies, and chromosomal abnormalities. The first survival risk stratification was done by Waterston in the 1960s and updated by Spitz in 1994.[57] The Spitz classification remains broadly used, although birth weight has become a less significant risk factor during the past 2 decades due to improvements in neonatal care for very low birth weight infants.[7,57,58] In the Spitz classification, the infants with the highest survival (97%) are those with no cardiac anomaly and birth weight greater than 1500 g. Infants without a cardiac anomaly but birth weight less than 1500 g have a 59% survival rate, and infants

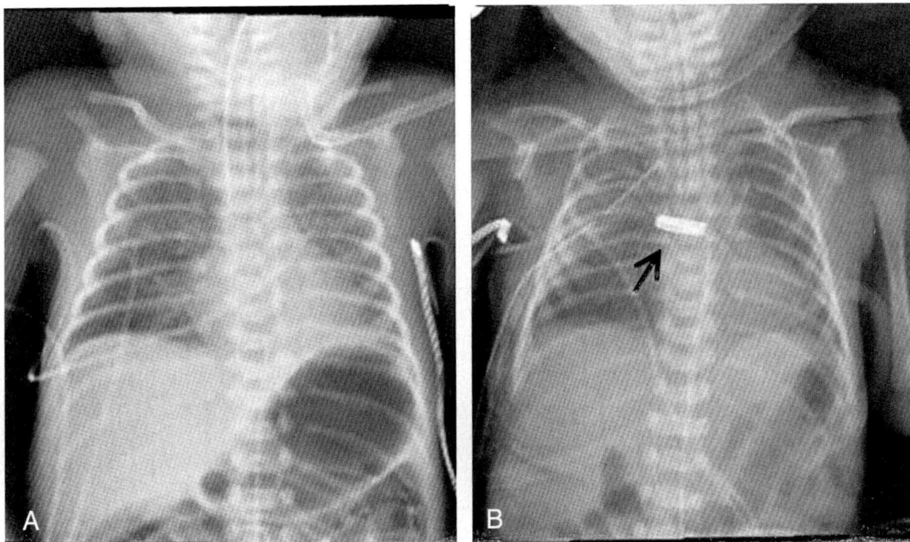

Fig. 86.6 (A) A premature infant with esophageal atresia and distal tracheoesophageal fistula who developed gastric distension and respiratory compromise. (B) Resolution of gastric distension after emergent fistula control with surgical clips (*arrow*) and gastrostomy placement.

with both birth weight less than 1500 g and a cardiac anomaly have the worst prognosis with survival of 22%.[57]

Despite low mortality, the long-term morbidity associated with EA/TEF is significant. Children and adults who were born with EA/TEF are more likely to suffer from reactive airway disease, bronchitis, recurrent pneumonias, and upper gastrointestinal complaints, particularly dysphagia and reflux.[59,60] Dysphagia and reflux have been reported in more than half of patients who are over 10 years of age with a history of EA/TEF, and they seem to persist into adulthood.[61,62] Upper gastrointestinal complaints in these patients could be secondary to a congenital abnormality in the innervation of the native esophagus or due to extensive surgical mobilization that disrupts neural networks.[63] Late-onset esophageal complications include an increased risk of Barrett's esophagus, and eight cases of cancer at the esophageal anastomosis have been reported.[64] It is unclear how frequently patients with a history of EA/TEF should undergo endoscopic surveillance for these complications, and large-scale studies are needed. Long-term respiratory symptoms after EA/TEF occur in three categories: obstructive defects, airway hyperresponsiveness, and restrictive defects.[65] Wheezing is the most common complaint and is seen in 35% of patients at least 10 years out from EA/TEF repair, and recurrent respiratory tract infections and diagnosed asthma occur in nearly one-fourth of patients.[61] Although respiratory symptoms also persist into adulthood,[66] they are more mild, and most can be managed without medications.[65,67]

Surgery for Other Esophageal Pathology in Neonates

Surgery for Gastroesophageal Reflux Disease

GERD is common in neonates because of an immature lower esophageal sphincter, and many congenital anomalies such as EA and congenital diaphragmatic hernia predispose to reflux.[41,68] The presentation of GERD in infants is well known to the neonatologist and pediatrician and includes frequent emesis, poor weight gain, and food intolerance. Pulmonary symptoms such as wheezing, choking, and apneic events are also seen, especially in neonates. The diagnosis of GERD can be made based on clinical symptoms and a variety of tests demonstrating pathologic reflux. Esophageal pH monitoring is the gold standard for diagnosis[69] but is limited by the need to withhold acid suppressive therapy in order to obtain an accurate reading. Furthermore, the applicability of pH monitoring in preterm infants is variable because of their high baseline gastric pH.[70] Therefore the addition of impedance monitoring is frequently used to aid in the diagnosis of pathologic GERD in neonates.

Surgery for gastroesophageal reflux in infants is reserved for patients who fail medical management or those who have life-threatening complications of reflux.[71] These patients typically fall into one of the three categories: patients with frequent regurgitation and oral intolerance who fail to gain weight due to gastrointestinal symptoms, patients with significant pulmonary comorbidity for whom soiling of the respiratory tract with regurgitated gastric contents is particularly detrimental, and those with neurologic disorders who require enteral access and are unlikely to feed by the oral enteral route. Patients with an apparent life-threatening event attributed to reflux may also proceed to surgery without documentation of GERD.[68] Because the literature regarding the role of surgery for reflux is limited, there is no broad consensus on the precise indications for surgery. Thus the decision to proceed to surgery is based on local practice patterns and multidisciplinary discussion, with wide practice variation nationally.[71] As a general rule, infants less than 6 months of age have a high likelihood of reflux symptoms resolving spontaneously by 12 to 18 months of age; therefore surgery for reflux in the neonatal population should be reserved for those with serious complications, as described.[72]

The most widely performed operation for reflux in infants is Nissen fundoplication with gastrostomy tube placement. A Nissen fundoplication is a 360-degree posterior wrap of the fundus around the esophagus. The operation can be performed using either an open or laparoscopic approach. Usually, a gastrostomy tube is placed for feeding access. Three randomized controlled trials have compared laparoscopic and open Nissen fundoplication, none demonstrating a clear advantage of one over the other.[73–75]

After Nissen fundoplication, the infant is returned to the neonatal intensive care unit and can be extubated as soon as the respiratory status allows. Initially, the gastrostomy tube is left to straight drainage to avoid gastric distension in the immediate postoperative period. Within 24 hours, enteral feeds can often be started through the gastrostomy and advanced as tolerated. Complications after Nissen fundoplication are uncommon but may include intraoperative technical problems (e.g., bleeding, vagus nerve injury, pneumothorax), postoperative complications (dysphagia and bloating), and failure of the fundoplication with recurrence of reflux. Recurrence of reflux is uncommon, but patients who undergo the operation at a younger age and those with neurologic impairment are at increased risk.[76]

An alternative option for larger infants with GERD refractory to medical management who also have oropharyngeal dysphagia is surgical placement of a gastrostomy tube with later exchange for a transpyloric gastrojejunostomy tube for feeding access. Although perceived to be less invasive than Nissen fundoplication because it preserves native anatomy, gastrojejunostomy tube placement does not allow for bolus feeds and has a high rate of dislodgement requiring procedural replacement.[77] Direct comparison between this approach and Nissen fundoplication has not been studied adequately to determine the optimal surgical treatment of GERD in neonates.[78]

Congenital Esophageal Stenosis, Duplication Cysts, and Vascular Rings

Several additional congenital anomalies of the esophagus can present in the neonatal population but are more often seen in older infants. Congenital esophageal stenosis can present similarly to EA, with vomiting and dysphagia with the introduction of feeds. However, there is rarely a complete obstruction, so an esophageal tube will pass and the anomaly may not have clinical symptoms present until the introduction of solid foods later in infancy.[79] Most lesions can be treated with a trial of esophageal dilation, with operative repair reserved for persistent stenosis. Surgery may involve myotomy or segmental resection of the stenosis with anastomosis.[80]

Congenital esophageal duplication occurs from vacuolization of the esophagus during the first trimester of gestation and can present with respiratory symptoms, vomiting, regurgitation, and occasionally a palpable neck mass.[79] Although sometimes detected in the neonatal period, esophageal duplication cysts are frequently identified for the first time in childhood and adulthood.[81] Operative resection is the treatment for congenital esophageal duplication to prevent growth and subsequent compression of surrounding structures.

Finally, several vascular anomalies of the mediastinum can cause esophageal rings with compression and upper gastrointestinal symptoms. These include anomalies of the aortic arch with aberrant subclavian arteries and pulmonary arterial slings.[82] In addition to dysphagia, they may present with respiratory symptoms including wheezing, stridor, and cyanosis with feeding. Surgical repair can range from ligation of aberrant vessels to extensive vascular reconstruction. Cross-sectional imaging and consultation with a pediatric cardiac surgeon are recommended.

Summary

Congenital esophageal anomalies represent an important and complex set of disorders affecting newborns managed in neonatal intensive care units worldwide. Although great strides have been made in survival of patients with these disorders, significant morbidity continues to occur beyond the neonatal period. An increased understanding of the developmental events that result in esophageal anomalies and large prospective studies on their management are needed to continue to improve the health of these most fragile patients.

SECTION 18

Current State of Neonatal Palliative Care

OUTLINE

CHAPTER 87 Caring for Families Who Have Previously Endured Multiple Perinatal Losses

Kathryn Grauerholz, Michaelene Fredenburg, Shandeigh N. Berry, DiAnn Ecret

KEY POINTS

1. Parents with a history of multiple previous fetal/neonatal losses may find it difficult to care for a critically ill newborn infant. The fear of losing yet another child can be heartrending and traumatic.
2. An individual's fundamental beliefs about themselves and their future children are not only disrupted by a pregnancy loss or undesirable perinatal diagnosis, but are often accompanied by psychological sequelae.
3. Cultural silence and the disenfranchised nature of the repeated losses of children contribute to prolonged, amplified, and sometimes, delayed grief reactions.
4. Neonatologists and other healthcare providers often feel ill-equipped to address the emotional and grief aspects of reproductive loss.
5. A well-informed team of clinical care providers with basic knowledge about the unique aspects of perinatal loss coupled with an understanding of the grieving process and beneficial communication modalities can lay the foundation for a healthy grieving trajectory for families enduring a reproductive loss.

Reproductive Story

Reproductive psychologists Jaffe and Diamond[1] observed that individuals envision their future family with an array of hopes and dreams long before conception, and the trauma occurs when those expectations fail to come to fruition. They found that individuals' fundamental beliefs about themselves and their offspring is disrupted by the experience of perinatal morbidity or mortality, which can be devastating. Although the grief trajectory is highly individual, Jaffe and Diamond found the following themes to be consistent among those grieving a reproductive loss: not only has the child died, but a part of them has died as well; there is a loss of hopes and dreams for themselves and the child; and there are feelings of failure at the most basic level. The extent of loss can be multilayered. Neonatologists and all care providers in neonatal intensive care units (NICUs) live this story repeatedly with the families they care for. For parents who have had a history of multiple fetal/neonatal losses, caring for a critically ill newborn infant can abrade and reopen all the wounds that had seemingly healed over time. The fear of losing yet another child can be heartrending and traumatic; it can reaggravate all the previous trauma and nightmares that they believed had subsided.

Ontological Death

In an ontological death, that which "dies" is not a physical entity but rather the *meaning* in one's life. This type of death accompanies great personal loss and often results in a loss of identity, because the roles and practices in which self-identity were constructed have been damaged. Perinatal loss results in an ontological death through the collapse of previously understood or taken-for-granted meanings of what it is to be pregnant. Viewing the loss of a young infant to a life-limiting diagnosis, severe disability, or extended stay in the neonatal unit through the lens of an ontological death provides insight into how parents might reconstruct meaning and identity from this experience.

When considering the complex issues surrounding the loss of a newborn infant soon after birth, the model of an ontological death may guide healthcare professionals in adopting a holistic approach that cares for the social, psychological, emotional, and spiritual needs of parents in addition to the immediate physical needs. This model also illustrates the importance of providing ongoing follow-up care as parents reconstruct their understanding of how the world works, who they are in this world, and how to continue living in their new reality. This is also where an individual begins to rewrite their reproductive story. Put another way, based on their new lived experiences and reconstructed identity, the reproductive story evolves.

Complexity of the Loss of Young Infants

As previously stated, the experience of having lost a young infant is typically not limited to perinatal death or the fear for the future of a fragile infant. Families confronted with a life-limiting fetal diagnosis, fragile infancy, or reproductive loss often present a complex response that may encompass a variety of emotions such as fear, shock, anger, anxiety, sadness, guilt, even jealousy of other parents with healthy babies.[2–4] For parents with a very low birth weight infant in comparison to parents with babies of normal birth weight, studies indicated a five times higher risk for severe psychological distress manifested as depression, anxiety, and obsessive-compulsive behaviors.[5,6] Additionally, factors that can overwhelm the parent's ability to cope include financial strain, travel expenses, long commutes, and time away from other family members.[6] Without the assistance of multidisciplinary planning and support, reproductive bereavement can be replete with isolation, secrecy, ambivalence, and shame.

Reproductive and early infant loss in its various forms is prevalent, impacting tens of millions of couples worldwide each year, yet the reaction and trajectory for these couples is highly individualized. The researchers who developed and conducted a body of research using the Perinatal Grief Scale classified reactions to perinatal loss in three progressive subscales: active grief, difficulty coping, and despair (Fig. 87.1).[6a,7] They found a wide range of emotions and no clearly delineated time frame or pattern. Perinatal grief was found to linger for long periods of time. It was truly difficult. Similar immediate or delayed grief reactions were seen in the partners of those who had physically lost the infant. At 24 months the partners were actually scoring higher in the subset of "despair," with more intense feelings of worthlessness and hopelessness than the mother herself.

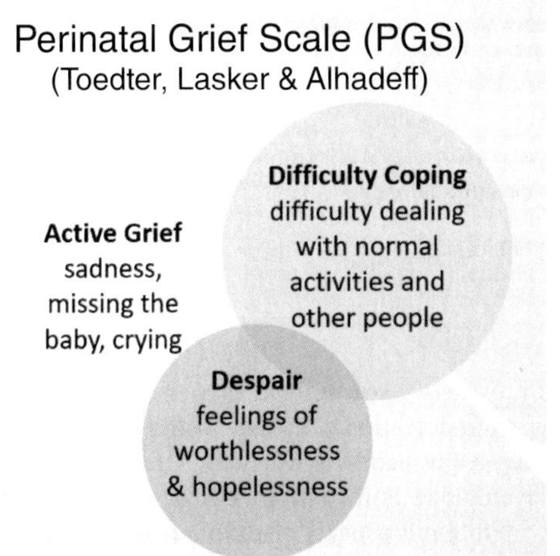

Fig. 87.1 Subcategories of Perinatal Grief Identified in Studies Utilizing the Perinatal Grief Scale.

Disenfranchised Grief

Studies have found that perinatal death and illness are as emotionally painful as the loss of an older child or adult family member and are associated with a grief trajectory that is culturally disenfranchised.[8] In our experience, the loss of a newborn or a young infant can be even more traumatic. The grief trajectory may be prolonged and complicated due to lack of support, disenfranchisement, and the ambiguous nature of the loss.[8–10,10a] Doka (2002), introduced the concept of disenfranchised grief, which he described as an experience that "is not openly acknowledged, socially validated, or publicly observed (p. 5)." Secrecy and/or shame contribute to disenfranchised grief, and individuals do not feel entitled to grieve. Parents enduring a perinatal loss or that of a young infant can find themselves traversing a grieving trajectory that has not been sufficiently established by society and can be likened to an unworn path of bereavement.

Disenfranchised grief may also impact one's mental health. It would be erroneous to assume everyone has a difficult or negative reaction to their loss. Sometimes a loss can have an impact on mental and physical health. Sometimes not. However, that does not mean it is a "nonevent." Everyone is impacted differently, and one's reaction can change or intensify over time. Trauma is associated with long-term biopsychosocial consequences that impact the capacity to learn, cope, and adapt, which can lead to chronic maladaptive dysregulation of sympathetic nervous system activation.[11]

The natural responses associated with the protection and survival of children are likely to trigger maladaptive stress response states associated with trauma, which can ultimately result in numerous long-term physical and psychological harms. If someone is hurting and not being allowed to express that grief or pain, it can impact mental health and potentially contribute to anxiety, depression, substance misuse, eating disorder, or complicated grief.[12–14] If the behavior is constant or long term, it can have a severe impact. Your interaction and attention to the grief can potentially mitigate these detrimental repercussions.

Impact of Previous Losses During Pregnancy or Early Infancy

The loss of a fetus or young infant is distinctly different from experiences surrounding the loss of a parent, spouse, friend, or even an older child. Because perinatal loss cannot be compared with other socially experienced losses, it is easy to misunderstand the meaning or fear of such a loss. Parents' experiences do not always align with societal expectations.

Prenatal attachment does not dissolve immediately when a fetal/newborn loss occurs. Although society expects parents to quickly move on, parents may continue to grieve deeply for long periods of time.[12,15] The paradox of such a loss contributes to disenfranchised grief, especially if the meaning of the loss is not understood or acknowledged.[16] Interacting with and treating parents according to a socially accepted expectation of the perinatal loss experience contrasts with parents' needs. Recognizing our own assumptions of what parents need or how we think they should respond is equally important. The acknowledgment and attention to the holistic emotional, spiritual, and behavioral needs that a person requires to affirm intrinsic meaning and purpose must be integrated into the plan of care. Healing-centered engagement seeks to affirm and "authentically" dignify human experiences of loss rather than to oversimplify them as a problem to be solved biologically.[17] This helps us as healthcare professionals to mitigate the risk of further disenfranchising parents' grief.

Grief

Attention to parental grief has been shown to be highly beneficial to parent–provider/staff interactions in the NICU (91% of study respondents), second only to frequent family meetings (94% of study respondents).[18] Kübler-Ross[19] pioneered grief therapy in the 1980s and authored her observations of five stages of grief. These stages have been recognized by several theorists, but the basic RABDA paradigm (*r*eject, *a*nger, *b*argaining, *d*epression, and *a*cceptance) is shared. Their purpose was intended to describe the journey of individuals coping with a terminal diagnosis and was not necessarily meant to be generalized for all loss experiences. Although the stages of grief helped to understand the nature of grief, they did not offer practical applications for professionals to provide grief assistance.

Worden[20] noted that stages of grief may not always follow a linear pattern to a point of resolution. He introduced a series of tasks that need to be worked on throughout the grieving process (Fig. 87.2). The tasks are not meant to be presented in a particular order, and the bereaved often move in and out of the different tasks as they grieve. Working through the tasks of grief is an onward journey of self-discovery or rediscovery. There may be triggers of painful

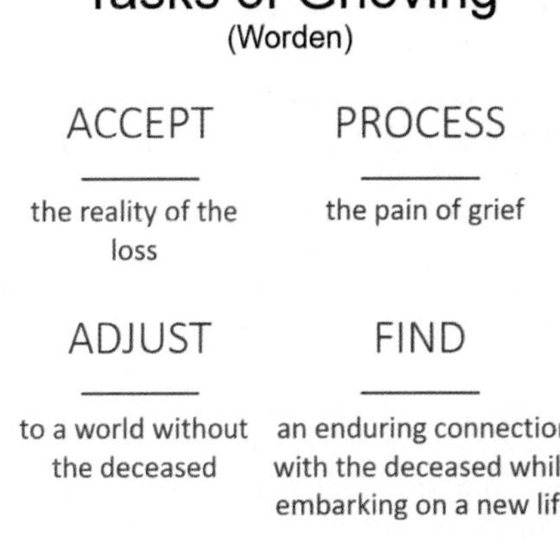

Fig. 87.2 Tasks Identified to Facilitate Normal Grieving.

Principles of Care	
1. Validate the loss and legitimize grief	6. Be open and listen with intent
2. Encourage patients to share their feelings	7. Be empathetic
3. Acknowledge patients' feelings	8. Be honest and realistic
4. Assess level of patients' knowledge	9. Provide reassurance where appropriate
5. Provide additional information	10. Maintain confidentiality

Fig. 87.3 Principles of impactful grief care. (Provincial Council for Maternal Child Health. *Early Pregnancy Loss in the Emergency Department: Recommendations for the Provision of Compassionate Care*. Toronto, Ontario, Canada: Provincial Council for Maternal Child Health; 2017.)

recollection, such as previously shared places, holidays, or anniversaries. The loss is not forgotten, but rather incorporated into the individual's conceptualization of their new self.

One of the tasks of grieving is accepting the reality of the loss. Grief is often multifaceted, impacting many aspects of life, and the bereaved will need to come to terms with the full impact of loss. It is a process that may include a change in relationships (spouse, parents, God), lifestyle, role, or dreams. This task is difficult to work through if the loss is unacknowledged or disenfranchised.

A task that is often worked on in tandem with accepting the reality of the loss is processing the pain of grief. Each loss experience will mean working through a range of different emotions: sadness, fear, despair, guilt, shame, relief, and many others. The emotions need to be acknowledged and discussed to begin to understand and work through them. Avoidance and denial of the emotional experience can lead to unhealthy behaviors. Providing the opportunity to express a variety of emotions—some of which may seem contradictory (i.e., feeling both relieved and sad)—is of great value to families enduring reproductive loss.

Another task is adjusting to the world without the deceased, which can be understood within the ontological death concept. A grieving individual will have to adjust and recreate their self-concept answering the question, "What does my world look like without that person or that child?" Despite the tendency to return to what was familiar, the individual cannot go back to the same way it was before.

The individual grappling with the loss will need to find an enduring connection to the person who has died. Allowing for thoughts and memories and engaging in memorialization is an important aspect of healing. The ambiguous nature of reproductive loss makes this task particularly challenging. Frequently the only reported connection to a pregnancy loss is pain or guilt. Often people will cling to the guilt or pain because they fear their child will be forgotten. Memorializing the loss is helpful and crucial to assisting those grappling with reproductive loss. Healthcare professionals are able to assist with memorialization by providing photos and tokens (the infant's cap, hospital band, and identification card) and facilitating the disposition of the fetal or infant remains.

Role of the Healthcare Professional

Research indicates that inadequate bereavement support in neonatal settings has been attributed to a lack of education and training.[2,21–24] Farren and her colleagues[25] extrapolated on the reasons for dismissal of the presence of parental grief: "Exposure to [pregnancy loss] on a daily basis may lead clinicians to normalize the experience and overlook the possible profound psychological sequelae" (p. 8). In one study, perinatal palliative and end-of-life training was perceived to be of benefit by most (91.8%) of the neonatologists.[22] In other studies, providing professionals with bereavement and end-of-life training not only resulted in improved patient and family outcomes, but care providers also exhibited better emotional coping.[23,26,27,27a] Effective communication provided to those encountering a severe or life-threatening neonatal illness or reproductive loss have been shown to enhance both patient efficacy and professional confidence.[18,28,29] Integral aspects of refining communication related to care delivery include improving eye contact and body language, increasing self-awareness, using reflective listening, and practicing specific responses via role-play activities.

The role of the care provider is critical, and limited time is a frequently cited barrier to the provision of healthcare. Intentionally engaging simple communicative modalities, applying practical applications, engaging interdisciplinary assistance, and providing resources are some simple actions that can be done that do not require extra time but can have a positive impact (Fig. 87.3)[30]. Acknowledging the loss is paramount for normalizing grief reactions and initiating a healthy grief trajectory (Fig. 87.4). An intentional effort to be present and actively listen even when time is limited enfranchises the emotional reaction to the loss.

The NURSE mnemonic can be a helpful strategy for conveying empathy for those enduring a reproductive loss: (N)ame or state the emotion, (U)nderstand their reaction, (R)espect or praise their strengths given the situation, (S)upport is conveyed, and (E)xplore or ask patient to elaborate on the emotions shared.[31]

It is important to recognize that everyone grieves differently even within the same family. Some may find it challenging not to judge, criticize, or wonder about another's grief or lack of grief. It is imperative to understand that there is not a clear directive on how to grieve or how long to grieve. Grief is better described as a process or a journey. Reactions can intensify or evolve over time with no point of resolution. Gently educating parents about the uniqueness of grief reactions will assist them in their grieving journey both individually and as a family.

Responses provided for other types of losses are also appropriate for reproductive loss. Reactions may include saying, "I am sorry. You're not alone. How are you doing?" Receptivity of emotions and

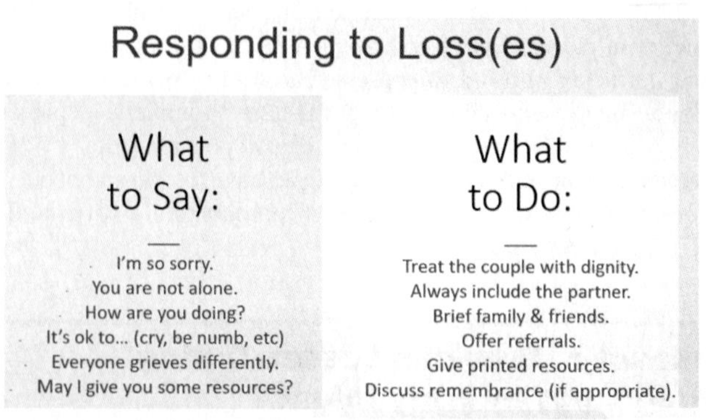

Responding to Loss(es)
What to Say:
I'm so sorry.
You are not alone.
How are you doing?
It's ok to... (cry, be numb, etc)
Everyone grieves differently.
May I give you some resources?
What to Do:
Treat the couple with dignity.
Always include the partner.
Brief family & friends.
Offer referrals.
Give printed resources.
Discuss remembrance (if appropriate).

Fig. 87.4 Practical Examples of Supportive Responses to a Reproductive Loss.

mixed reactions with statements such as "It's okay to {cry, be angry, feel numb}" can help normalize a person's response to the loss. The bereaved person or partner should be treated with dignity regardless of the current situation with their infant or the manner in which the loss took place. The care provider can offer resources including patient information sheets and memorializing options. By empathetically engaging with those grieving a reproductive loss and providing an individualized framework for grief, the provider essentially gives those impacted permission to grieve.

Other family members and friends can also be directed as to how they can support the couple when confidentiality regulations permit. The provider can let supportive person(s) know that it is important to acknowledge the loss and for them to tell the bereaved that they are sorry for the loss. Suggesting expressions of support such as providing meals or giving the couple memorial items such as sympathy cards, candles, or pieces of jewelry can also be appropriate. If the family embraces certain rituals or spiritual practices, family members or friends can be encouraged to assist with planning and preparation.

Finally, an interdisciplinary team approach that includes a social worker and chaplain allows for holistic care that takes into consideration the family's social, psychological, emotional, and spiritual needs. This team approach also helps to overcome time constraints and provides emotional support for healthcare providers within the unit. Furthermore, opportunities to debrief and a culture that encourages self-care is paramount in the high-intensity atmosphere of the neonatal unit—especially as the team authentically attends to the needs of grieving parents and their families.

CHAPTER 88 Current State of Perinatal Palliative Care: Clinical Practice, Training, and Research

Renee Boss, Sara Munoz-Blanco, Steven Leuthner

KEY POINTS

1. Perinatal palliative care (PPC) programs are increasing across the U.S. These services exist in a wide variety of settings from health care institutions to community- or faith-based organizations, have varying levels of ability and comfort in providing PPC for different clinical scenarios and levels of diagnostic certainty, and varying access to multi-disciplinary specialists and variable missions and visions of the program.
2. PPC is evolving beyond providing supportive end of life care only, and can provide an extra layer of support to infants, families and clinicians while medical treatments are attempted for serious diagnoses that may not necessarily pose a high risk of death.
3. In comparison to the evidence for palliative care for older children and adults, there remain basic and unanswered questions related to palliative care for infants.
4. A growing body of research is dedicated to symptom control for the actively dying infant, ranging from optimal medication titration to the ethical complexity of double effect where medications for symptom management could shorten life.
5. A challenging limitation of PPC research is the difficulty in accurately and adequately defining the outcomes that matter to infants, families, staff, and health systems.

Introduction

Palliative care is specialized medical care targeting quality of life for patients with serious illness and their families. The practice grew out of the hospice movement and became a board-certified medical subspecialty in 2006.[1] Although hospice focuses on end-of-life care, palliative care can begin at the time of a serious diagnosis. In 2000 the American Academy of Pediatrics recommended "clinical policies and minimum standards that promote the welfare of infants and children living with life-threatening or terminal conditions, with the goal of providing equitable and effective support for curative, life-prolonging and palliative care."[2]

Palliative care for neonates may be termed *perinatal palliative care* (PPC), encompassing prenatal/ postnatal care by inpatient and outpatient palliative care providers; *perinatal hospice*, referring to prenatal/postnatal care from hospice providers; or *neonatal palliative care*, or simply pediatric palliative care. Here we use the phrases "perinatal palliative care" and "perinatal hospice" to include prenatal and postnatal services.

Primary palliative care can be delivered by any interdisciplinary provider as a matter of the routine management of seriously ill patients, as when obstetric social workers provide grief counseling, when neonatologists manage infant pain, or when nurses promote nonnutritive breastfeeding for maternal-infant bonding (Fig. 88.1). Subspecialty palliative care is provided by interdisciplinary clinicians with additional training and certification in pain and symptom management, holistic family supports, and communication. Importantly, these services can span the inpatient/outpatient settings and often include extended bereavement support. Access to subspecialty PPC is growing across the United States.[3]

Perinatal hospice may include a physical inpatient setting for infants receiving complex medications or technologies or who are actively dying. Perinatal hospice is also delivered at home. After a prenatal diagnosis of a serious fetal condition, perinatal hospice nurses, social workers, chaplains, child life specialists, or others can visit the family home to assist with birth plans, counseling, sibling supports, and preparation for end-of-life care. After birth, if infants are able to be discharged home, home hospice provides continuity of these services via intermittent home visits and 24/7 phone support. For families comfortable with death at home, hospice providers can provide comfort interventions for the infant, be present for the death, and initiate postmortem activities including death certificates and funeral details. Perinatal hospice providers also provide longitudinal bereavement support, sometimes with enhanced support during common trigger experiences such as additional pregnancies.

The core of all PPC and hospice is an interdisciplinary team that draws on the unique expertise of individual providers and prioritizes coordination and continuity to support families (Fig. 88.2). Although referrals for perinatal hospice are based on expectations for death in infancy (e.g., within 6 months of hospice enrollment), there is greater variability in PPC referrals. Some centers use "trigger diagnoses," for example, all infants born at <24 weeks' gestation. Local palliative care resources must be adequate to support this approach. In centers without triggers, palliative care referral may be limited to patients with clearly life-threatening conditions or may include patients with complex chronic conditions that are debilitating yet not immediately life threatening, for example, infants with severe bronchopulmonary dysplasia and tracheostomy/ventilator dependence.

In this chapter we will review the existing evidence to support PPC clinical practices, education, and research.

The Clinical Practice of Perinatal Palliative Care

Availability of Perinatal Palliative Care Across the United States

Although pregnancy and childbirth have always included high mortality, the first publications regarding the concept of PPC programs were from Whitfield and Mangurten.[4,5] Whitfield et al. described

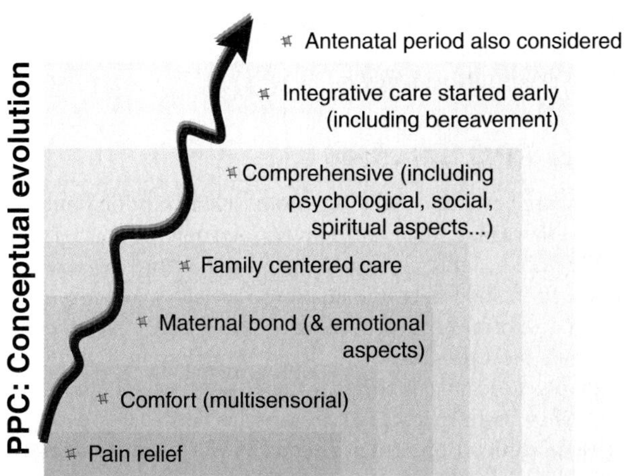

Fig. 88.1 Conceptual Evolution of Perinatal Palliative Care. (Reproduced with permission from Jackson and Vasudevan. *Paediatrics and Child Health*, 2020;4:124–128.)

the application of hospice concepts to neonatal care, including the family room or essentially the physical environment, the involvement of family in the decision-making process, and the hospice training of neonatal intensive care (NICU) nurses. Mangurten described a series of six infants and their process for medical care and death at home. The term *perinatal hospice* was first used in the obstetric literature, essentially describing it as an alternative to termination of pregnancy.[6] That same decade, publications emerged describing the development and outcomes of neonatal and perinatal palliative services and end-of-life care.[7–13] The provision of perinatal bereavement practices in birth centers and NICUs has subsequently become more standard, and continuing education in this specialty is available. For example, Resolve Through Sharing (resolvethroughsharing.org) offers three training programs that include palliative care: perinatal bereavement (PPC), neonatal and pediatric bereavement, and adult bereavement (adult palliative care).

A recent survey of PPC programs reported there are perinatal services in at least 30 states, with 70% of them being less than 10 years old.[3,14] These services exist in a wide variety of settings, from healthcare institutions to community- or faith-based organizations. It makes sense that programs may have varying levels of ability and comfort in providing PPC for different clinical scenarios and levels of diagnostic certainty, with varying access to multidisciplinary specialists and variable missions and visions of the program. The growth of PPC programs is exemplified by the ever-increasing number of professional publications.[3,10,14]

Triggers to Identify Eligible Patients

Identification of which infants and families might benefit from PPC often involves specific fetal/neonatal diagnoses (Table 88.1). Catlin and Carter first described clinical situations in which one should consider neonatal palliative care, coming up with three generalizable categories: (1) newborns at the limits of viability, (2) newborns with congenital anomalies considered incompatible with prolonged life, and (3) newborns with overwhelming illness.[9] The question then became whether these categories could be reasonably predicted prenatally when the disease or condition was diagnosed in utero.[11] Choices about whether to incorporate PPC before birth relies on the degree of diagnostic and prognostic certainty and the meaning of the prognosis to the prospective parents. "Meaning" reflects the

Table 88.1 Categories of Neonates Eligible for Perinatal Palliative Care

Category 1	**Life-threatening conditions for which curative treatment may be feasible but can fail** Involving palliative care services may be necessary when treatment fails or is expected to fail. After successful curative treatment or clinical stability, there may no longer be a need for palliative care services. *Examples of conditions: extreme prematurity, congenital heart disease, severe PPHN*
Category 2	**Conditions in which premature death is inevitable** Long periods of intense treatment or intensive care provision may be delivered with the aim of prolonging life and allowing some participation in normal activity. *Examples of conditions: chromosomal abnormalities, bilateral renal agenesis*
Category 3	**Progressive conditions without curative treatment options** Treatment is exclusively palliative and may commonly extend over many months or years. *Examples of conditions: spinal muscular atrophy, mitochondrial disorders*
Category 4	**Irreversible but nonprogressive conditions causing severe disability, leading to susceptibility to health complications and likelihood of premature death** *Examples of conditions: severe hypoxic ischemic encephalopathy*

Reproduced with permission and minor modifications from Jackson and Vasudevan. Palliative care in the neonatal intensive care unit. *Paediatrics and Child Health*, 2020; 30:124–128.

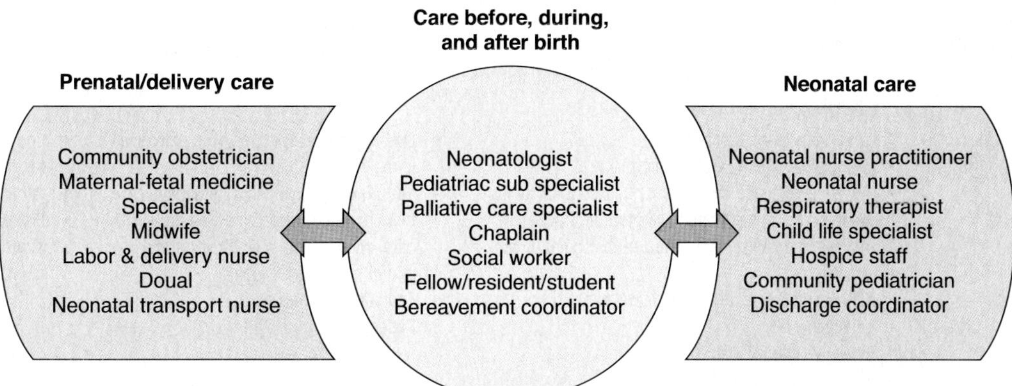

Fig. 88.2 Potential Interdisciplinary Team Members. There is a constant need for clear communication and consensual decision-making when caring for infants at high-risk of mortality. (From Boss et al. Prenatal and neonatal palliative care. *Textbook of Interdisciplinary Pediatric Palliative Care*, 37, 387–401.)

ethical principle of family values about what they believe is in the infant's best interest.[11,12]

Historically, PPC was most commonly applied in cases in which the fetus was deemed to have a lethal condition. Other "trigger criteria" for PPC involvement have included diagnoses such as anencephaly, skeletal dysplasia, renal agenesis, and certain chromosomal defects.[9,11,12] Over time, however, PPC has evolved and the lists of relevant diagnoses are changing. Some of this evolution has come from changing values, whereas others are from advances in medical technology. For example, trisomy 18 had been considered a lethal condition; however, some advocates have demanded more aggressive care, making it difficult to declare a case definitively lethal, although these children still have a life-limiting disorder.[15–17] Fetal interventions are also changing "lethal" diagnoses, as with amnioinfusion for fetal renal agenesis, which may be able to preserve fetal lung development to permit live birth and eventual dialysis and renal transplant.[18]

PPC is evolving beyond providing supportive end-of-life care only and can provide an extra layer of support to infants, families, and clinicians while medical treatments are attempted for serious diagnoses that may not necessarily pose a high risk of death.

Timing of PPC Integration

The concept of palliative care for patients of any age has advanced from being a hospice model of care to an integrated model of support from the time of diagnosis.[19] The concept of introducing palliative care at the time of diagnosis and providing integrated palliative and curative treatments has been described in the oncology literature.[2,20] This model of concurrent care is evolving in the perinatal world as well and needs further study.[10]

Typical PPC Services

Primary care providers including obstetricians, certified nurse midwives, pediatricians, labor and delivery, and newborn nursery nurses should be able to offer essential, core-component PPC services for families, to include decision support, pain and symptom management, and referral to local resources (Table 88.2). As reported by Wool et al., most programs offer some form of a care coordinator to provide psychosocial support, spiritual resources, and bereavement care.[14] When more specialized services are needed, for example, in the case of difficult-to-treat symptoms or diagnostic ambiguity, an interdisciplinary PPC team consultation is warranted. The type of PPC services a palliative care team can provide are dependent on the program location and resources. PPC providers can get to know parents so as to better assist them with goals of care and decision-making. This might include decisions about termination, fetal therapy, comfort care after birth, or planning for nonescalation if an infant does poorly after initial resuscitation. PPC teams may also offer longitudinal psychosocial, spiritual, and bereavement supports for families that may begin prenatally and last as long as years after birth. PPC teams can also assist with end-of-life care including memory making, legacy planning, hospice transition, and symptom management.

Table 88.2 Scope of Perinatal Palliative Care Services

Perinatal Palliative Care Services Level	Services and Skills	Providers	Education
Primary—offered within any community Cases require certainty of lethality (e.g., anencephaly)	Basic skills: • Recognize the need for PPC • Access fetal/infant/family needs • Psychosocial support • Spiritual support • Bereavement support • Recognize need for referral	• Primary obstetrician, certified nurse midwife, pediatrician and/or family practice provider • Labor and delivery nursing staff and/or care coordinator • Hospital chaplain and social work services • Access to bereavement care in community	• Key staff member training in perinatal bereavement with continuing education
Secondary—needed in cases of more diagnostic ambiguity and prognostic uncertainty and for rare disorders the community is uncomfortable with (e.g., HLHS or trisomy 18 with plans for PPC)	Additional midlevel skills and competencies: • Interdisciplinary team care coordination • Disease-specific management, including pain and symptom management • Documentation of advance care planning/ directives • Basic hospice and home health regulation and practice • Psychological and spiritual support of parent and siblings	• Primary subspecialists (e.g., maternal fetal medicine, neonatologist, other pediatric subspecialists) • Care coordinator • Access to social and spiritual care providers with pediatric experience • Access to a consultant in palliative care	• Majority of staff having some training in perinatal bereavement through continuing education • Key staff with advanced training and certification to coordinate care
Tertiary—more complex situation including trial of therapies and fetal interventions	Advanced skills and competencies: • Complex advance care planning • Advanced disease-specific management, including trials, limits, and pain and symptom management • Advanced hospice and home health regulation and practice • Ethics and law related to perinatal care and death and dying • Palliative care research • Palliative care education • Palliative care advocacy	• On-site specialist in pediatric palliative care • Complex interdisciplinary palliative care team (e.g., social services, spiritual care, child life for siblings, maternal and/or child psychology) • Education support staff • Research support staff	• Continuous education in the field • Participation in research • Provision of education, modeling, training of others

HLDS, Hypoplastic left heart syndrome; *PPC*, perinatal palliative care.

Location of Care/Systems Issues for PPC

The location of care for these patients will be dictated by where the family lives, the clinical situation, and the decision a family makes. Cases deemed to be lethal, by disease diagnosis and/or parental decision on level of care, could be managed at a community hospital if there are perinatal and pediatric providers who feel comfortable serving as a resource, if the hospital has supportive resources (e.g., chaplaincy), and if there is a hospice or palliative care team in the area that can provide perinatal services. There can, unfortunately, be discomfort among either providers or organizations and thus there are limitations to these resources in many communities.[21] To overcome this issue, systemic changes through education and training are required; resources are provided below.

When the comfort level or resources are limited or when the case is more clinically complex in care and decision-making, an interdisciplinary team in a tertiary care institution is required. In these instances, there may still be a variety of locations where PPC and hospice may occur. These areas include maternal fetal medicine clinics, fetal centers, labor and delivery (including possibly cesarean section rooms), the newborn nursery, and the NICU. A health system sensitive to PPC should have resources to support families and staff in all these areas.

Primary and Subspecialty Perinatal Palliative Care Training

The Interdisciplinary Team

The interdisciplinary team is the foundation of good PPC. Primary palliative care is delivered in the course of the usual care delivered by physicians, nurses, therapists, and social workers who come from obstetrics/maternal-fetal medicine or the NICU, pediatric subspecialists (cardiology, surgery, etc.), and general pediatrics. In addition, the subspecialty PPC team may comprise physicians, nurse practitioners, nurses, social workers, chaplains, child life specialists, and pharmacists, each with unique expertise and perspectives in the care of patients with serious illness and their families. With so many interdisciplinary clinicians involved in care for a patient, there is the potential for poorly coordinated care; it is clear that poor interactions with families can have long-term adverse consequences for their mental health and bereavement.[22] Intentional interdisciplinary team collaboration strives for consistent care and requires clinicians to be trained to provide it.

The Institute of Medicine's 2014 report delineated three major barriers to palliative care implementation: educational silos, lack of training in communication skills, and a dearth of palliative care curricula in medical and nursing education.[23] Although any infant with a potential life-limiting condition should receive PPC, limited and/or variable education makes this impossible.[13]

Palliative Care Training

Subspecialty palliative care is a relatively young field, recognized by the American Board of Medicine in 2006.[1] Pediatric palliative care is an even younger field, with fewer than 20 training programs across the United States at the time of this writing. Currently, Accreditation Council for Graduate Medical Education requirements for palliative care subspecialty training do not include experience in PPC. Developing and including this PPC content in palliative care subspecialty training should be a priority. Physicians dually trained in neonatology and palliative care are ideal candidates to provide PPC; however, such dually trained clinicians are scarce.

Table 88.3 Training for Perinatal Palliative Care and Hospice
Resolve Through Sharing Bereavement Services
Pregnancy Loss and Infant Death Alliance (PLIDA)
Center for Advancement of Palliative Care (CAPC) modules
End-of-Life Nursing Education Consortium (ELNEC)
Perinatal and Neonatal Palliative Care module
Hospice and Palliative Nurses Association (HPNA)
Certification for Perinatal Loss Care
When Hello Means Goodbye: An Exploration into Perinatal Palliative Care
National Hospice and Palliative Care Organization (NHPCO)
Evidence-Based Neonatal and Perinatal Palliative Care With Brian Carter, MD
Education in Palliative and End-of-Life Care (EPEC)–Pediatrics
International Children's Palliative Care Network e-learning course
Royal College of Midwives (UK)
Perinatal Palliative Care: The midwives' role

Data from perinatalhospice.org.

Expanding access to PPC for families across the United States clearly relies on routine training in primary palliative care practices for any clinician involved in perinatal care. Primary PPC training should include pain and symptom management, communication skills, interprofessional collaboration, successful identification of family values and goals of care, end-of-life care, and bereavement.[24] Educational needs may vary by specialty and provider role. For example, in addition to communication difficulties, trainees in neonatal medicine specifically experience challenges around prognostic uncertainty, ethical complexity, and limited exposure to pediatric/neonatal palliative care teams.[25] Furthermore, in a study of NICU clinicians in Taiwan, doctors desired more communication training, whereas nurses wanted more training about symptom management.[26] Thus, it is imperative to consider both key topics and audience.

Few evidence-based models of primary PPC education for non-palliative care subspecialists have been described (Table 88.3). Several authors have compared different education techniques, such as simulation versus lectures, for general palliative care principles. Some studies target pediatric content, but only a few are specific to PPC. Two studies are worth mentioning. O'Shea et al. found that nursing students' knowledge of perinatal and pediatric palliative care increased by integrating the evidence-based End-of-Life Nursing Education Consortium (ELNEC) curriculum modules into nursing education.[27] Sessions were led by faculty trained in ELNEC Core Curriculum for Pediatric and Perinatal Palliative and End-of-Life Care. The course included lectures, case studies, and simulations. LoGiudice and O'Shea explored integration of PPC into midwifery education, including topics such as rights of the dying neonate, birth plans, cultural and religious considerations of perinatal death, death in the NICU, and perinatal bereavement, all of which meet midwifery competencies and maternal health needs.[28] The authors suggest that sustainability of such a model requires access to educators who can provide content in a variety of settings (i.e., lectures and simulation) and partnering with institutional palliative care resources.

Data regarding the impact of such primary palliative care training on clinical practice and outcomes is also sparse. Common forms of pediatric palliative care education evaluation include pre– and post–self-assessment surveys, feedback from external reviewers during simulation training, and use of surveys and scales such as the End-of-Life Professional Caregiver Survey and the Self-efficacy for Inter-Professional Experience Learning Scale.[29–31] Simulation-based training can increase palliative care consult rates. Brock et al. demonstrated a 64% increase in consults 6 months after pediatric cardiology, hematology/oncology, intensive care, and neonatology fellows participated in simulation-based training.[30] In addition, a train-the-trainer approach using the Education in Palliative and End-of-Life Care for Pediatrics curriculum led to quality-improvement interventions at most participating sites, including increasing the number of days from both palliative care referral to death and from documentation of advance care planning to death.[32] Other clinical outcome measures to show the impact of primary palliative care training are lacking, however. Future quality-improvement and research efforts should focus on this area (i.e., patient/family feedback, standardization of care delivery measures, hospitalization rates, enrollment on hospice, etc.).[33]

Progress in Perinatal Palliative Care Research

Research relevant to PPC from the past 2 decades mirrors other advances in fetal and neonatal basic and clinical research but also integrates empirical work in social sciences, psychology, and bioethics. The evidence base for pain and symptom management, for example, draws on a foundation of animal and fetal research regarding the pathophysiology of pain and discomfort, along with studies regarding NICU clinicians' ability to detect, treat, and monitor symptoms and studies of the impact that infant suffering has on medical decision-making and parent coping. A growing body of research is dedicated to symptom control for the actively dying infant, ranging from optimal medication titration to the ethical complexity of a double effect where medications for symptom management could shorten life. Much research relevant to PPC has explored counseling and decision-making for periviable infants, infants with "lethal" conditions, and infants with very poor neurologic prognosis. Again, this work has evolved as basic science and clinical research have expanded gestational viability, improved outcomes from bronchopulmonary dysplasia, and reduced brain injury via therapeutic hypothermia. Palliative care research also tracks parent and extended-family experiences of serious neonatal illness, NICU admission, and bereavement. Finally, as palliative care services become more available in the perinatal period, research is growing about palliative care provision by NICU clinicians, use of subspecialty palliative care consultations, and the impact of these services on patients, families, clinicians, and health systems.

Coming chapters address these content areas in depth and catalog existing studies. The number of studies, especially those with robust statistical power and representative populations, is relatively small compared with some other areas of neonatal research. It is important to recognize the unique challenges relevant to building a robust body of research regarding PPC. First, palliative care as a medical specialty is just over 10 years old, and the physician fellowship does not include a research requirement; this means that there are still few clinician-researchers trained in this area. Some conclusions about PPC outcomes must therefore be derived from studies with related research questions or study samples (e.g., older children or adults). This limitation will improve over time as more palliative care researchers are trained.

Defining Outcomes

A more challenging limitation of PPC research is the difficulty in accurately and adequately defining the outcomes that matter to infants, families, staff, and health systems. Palliative care outcomes that are essential for older patients, for example, are poorly defined for infants: anxiety, nausea, cold, pruritus, suffering, and dignity. For studies of parents, researchers must adapt methods from social science and psychology to define outcomes of interest such as trust, values,

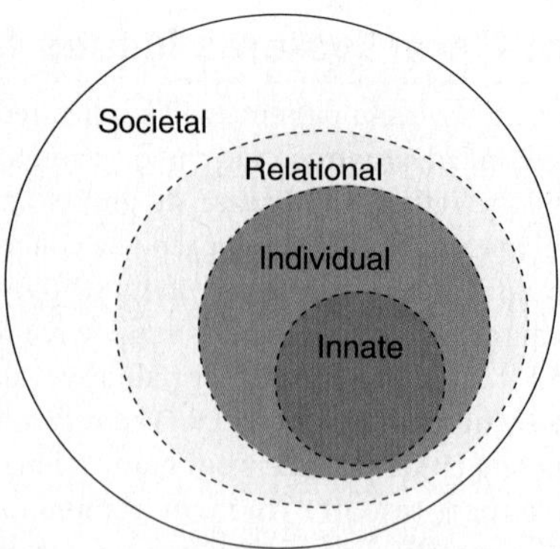

Fig. 88.3 Krishna's Ring Theory of Personhood (RToP). Evidenced in Palliative Medicine, the RToP suggests that caring for critically ill patients has diverse effects on doctors' and nurses' values, beliefs, ideals, motivations, actions, relationships, and on how they perceive their roles and responsibilities within society. The impact on healthcare professionals can be better understood in terms of four dynamically interlinked domains. Depicted as four concentric rings, these four key aspects of personhood are composed of the innate, individual, relational and societal domains.

emotions, and spirituality. And while NICU staff outcomes are uncommonly targeted in neonatology research, staff distress, burnout, skills in communication and human interactions, and values are often relevant to the care received by seriously ill infants and their families (Fig. 88.3). System-level outcomes of palliative care practices are also challenging; because palliative interventions often decrease ICU days and surgical interventions, this may reduce hospital revenue. Finally, perinatal/neonatal researchers face challenges in defining what overall "good" outcomes are for palliative care, especially when infant outcomes, family outcomes, and system outcomes may conflict, as when prolonging an infant's ICU dependence for weeks to months given the parents' goal of time with their child. All of these research outcomes are important to the care of infants with serious and life-threatening conditions; defining them requires ongoing academic rigor.

Methodological Challenges

Methodological complexities also pervade PPC studies that attempt to measure the above outcomes. The number of infants receiving palliative care is much smaller than the adult population, undermining statistical power. Another obvious challenge is recruiting and obtaining informed consent from parents who are emotionally overwhelmed and whose time with their infant may be limited.[34] Such challenges mean that many studies about end-of-life care use retrospective chart review, which inherently distorts the variables that can be tracked.[7,8,35] And while communication and decision-making are key aspects of palliative care, the methodologies to meaningfully study conversations and human interactions remain modest. Published studies of decisions about resuscitation of periviable infants, for instance, often rely on parents' or clinicians' recollections of a prior conversation and rarely account for longitudinal discussions with shifting members of a large, interdisciplinary NICU team. Even when conversations can be recorded for research, analytic methodologies are incomplete. Quantitative analytic software simply counts instances of particular phrases or behaviors (e.g., assessing parent understanding), which is just a portion of what we need to know about what makes conversations successful.[36] Qualitative analysis of conversations is more nuanced but typically involves small samples and parents who are naturally inclined to reflect on and share their narratives; data from parents without advanced degrees, fathers, and nonwhite families are underrepresented in qualitative work. Table 88.4 characterizes existing data about collaborative decision-making between parents and clinicians

Table 88.4 Summary of Studies of Periviable Counseling Practices: Methodology and Primary Outcomes

Authors, Year	Methodology	Primary Outcome(s) Relevant to Periviable Counseling	Study Population, No.
CLINICIAN SURVEY OR INTERVIEW			
Survey Done in United States			
Bastek et al., 2005,[38] Peerzada et al., 2004[39]	Survey of neonatologists across 6 US states	Attitudes and practices	149
Doron et al., 1998[40]	Survey of US neonatologists on day of delivery and infant chart review	Impact of parent versus physician preferences on neonatal resuscitation	42 charts, 6 neonatologists
Singh et al., 2007[41]	Survey of US neonatologists	Resuscitation preferences at 22–26 weeks and delivery room prognostic abilities	666
International Survey			
De Leeuw et al., 2000[42]	Survey of neonatal physicians and nurses from 11 countries	Hypothetical treatment approach	1401 MDs, 3425 nurses
Martinez et al., 2005[43]	Survey of neonatologists across 6 Pacific Rim countries	Impact of parent beliefs, physician opinions, and local resources on decisions	318
Interviews/Focus Groups			
Geurtzen et al., 2018[44]	Focus groups with Dutch perinatal professionals	Preferences for content, organization, and decision-making during counseling	35 obstetricians and neonatologists
Haward et al., 2017[45]	Interviews with "expert" neonatologists	Perspectives on counseling and decision-making	22
PARENT SURVEY OR INTERVIEW			
Survey/Interview in United States			
Boss et al., 2008[46]	Qualitative interviews, median 3 years after infant death	Parent understanding of resuscitation options and desired role in decisions	26 mothers
Kaempf et al., 2009[47]	Retrospective chart review and maternal interview immediately and again 6–18 months after counseling	Experience with consensus staff guidelines for periviable management	260 charts, 50 mothers
Tucker Edmonds et al., 2019[48]	Qualitative interviews immediately after counseling	Parent desired role in decisions; values used to make decisions	54 parents
International Survey/Interview			
Geurtzen et al., 2018[49]	Retrospective survey of Dutch parents of ELBW infants	Experience of counseling	61
Partridge et al., 2005[50]	Retrospective survey of parents of ELBW infants; interviews with subset of parents from across 6 Pacific Rim countries and California	Variability in parent recall of counseling	327
MATCHED CLINICIAN/PARENT DATA			
Grobman et al., 2010[51]	Qualitative interviews, before and after delivery	Preferred approaches to counseling	54 parents, 52 clinicians
Payot et al., 2007[52]	Qualitative survey of parents and neonatologists immediately after prenatal consult at 23–25 weeks	Process of sharing decisions	12 parents, 12 neonatologists
Streiner et al., 2001[53]	Retrospective survey during longitudinal study of ELBW outcomes	Attitudes about viability and treatment decisions	169 parents, 98 neonatologists, 99 nurses
Studer et al., 2016[54]	Audiotaped prenatal consultation followed by parent and neonatologist survey	Content of counseling and satisfaction	17 conversations
Zupancic et al., 2002[55]	Questionnaire within 24 hours of counseling at 22–30 weeks	Parent desire for participation in decisions and understanding of management plan	49 mothers, number of clinicians not stated
OTHER			
Boss et al., 2012[56]	Simulation	Analysis of counseling of simulated parents of ELBW patients	10 neonatologists
Moro et al., 2011[57]	Case study	Description of parent decision-making about life support for ELBW patients from prenatal to end-of-life	5 cases
Tucker Edmonds et al., 2014[58]	Simulation	Impact of maternal race and insurer on periviable shared decisions	16 obstetricians, 15 neonatologists

for periviable infants, highlighting the near total lack of empirical evidence about these conversations in the form of audiorecordings. The shortcomings of these evolving methodologies, combined with a research focus on parent-driven outcomes, can undermine competing for research dollars from typical funders of perinatal and neonatal research. Together, these challenges further reduce study scope and slow the progress of academic work in PPC.

Future Research

In comparison with the evidence for palliative care for older children and adults, there remain basic and unanswered questions related to palliative care for infants. As palliative care services expand their availability beyond end-of-life care, for instance, it is unclear which infants and families benefit most from this expansion—infants who are chronically critically ill, those who will have home medical technology, or those who have severe neurologic injury?[37] Neonatal advance directives are also poorly studied, as are family preferences regarding organ donation. It is unclear how many parents prefer for their infants to die at home versus in the hospital; this is typically desired for older pediatric and adult patients, but bringing an infant home to die who has not previously lived in the family home raises unique logistical and family issues. These basic questions require robust inquiry.

CHAPTER 89

Serious Communication in the Neonatal Intensive Care Unit: Evidence for Strategies and Training

Stephanie K. Kukora, Naomi T. Laventhal

KEY POINTS

1. With a high incidence of morbidity and mortality, the care of critically ill newborns brings unique complexities in communication between the care providers and families.
2. Because newborns cannot make their wishes known, surrogates, generally parents, collaborate with physicians to determine appropriate goals of care. These decisions entail discussions of sophisticated information about the disease process, available therapies, known risks and outcomes, and personal values. The discussions are frequently complicated by strong parental emotions, stemming from altered expectations for their child's future and the fear of loss.
3. The stressful, emotionally charged nature of decision-making can sometimes lead to conflict and mistrust between families and providers and to disagreements about the best course of action.
4. Sharing bad news is stressful for both the clinicians and the families and can hinder important goals-of-care discussions or even lead to avoidance of these conversations.
5. A number of guidelines and recommendations exist to assist neonatologists and other care providers in the care of these patients. The importance of shared decision-making in this setting cannot be emphasized enough.

Communication in the Neonatal Intensive Care Unit

Although challenges in communication exist in all areas of medicine, the anticipation and care of critically ill newborns imparts unique communication complexities. More than 20,000 infants die in the newborn period annually in the United States, with the highest rates of mortality arising from complications of prematurity, congenital anomalies, and genetic disorders.[1] Technological advancements in newborn critical care have improved survival of infants with these conditions during the past several decades, but prognostication regarding which of these infants will not survive and which survivors will have life-long developmental impairment remains imperfect. In these situations of expected poor prognosis and marked uncertainty, high-stakes decisions regarding which interventions to provide must be made. Because newborns cannot make their wishes known, surrogates, generally parents, collaborate with physicians to determine appropriate goals of care. These decisions entail discussions of sophisticated information about pathophysiology, medical technology and therapies, statistical risks and outcomes, and personal values. They are also often complicated by strong emotions on the part of parents, stemming from altered expectations for their child's future and the experience of loss that has become increasingly uncommon in our society and is rarely discussed.[2]

Because of the stressful and emotionally charged nature of decision-making in this context, conflict within and between families and providers is not uncommon in the neonatal intensive care unit (NICU).[3–6] Disagreements about which course of action best promotes the best interests of the infant are escalated by poor communication in these highly sensitive situations.[6] Sharing bad news is stressful for clinicians and may lead to avoidance of these conversations. Likewise, failure to listen and engage in discussion around disparate perspectives and values in goals-of-care discussions not only can lead to mistrust of the care team by parents but also can preference misdiagnosis and a treatment or outcome that does not align with parents' wishes.[7] These communication problems negatively impact parents' NICU experience and perhaps their only memories of their child alive and have serious long-term implications for parents, including grief, decisional conflict, and regret.[8,9] Additionally, difficulties with communication, particularly about goals of care, and values differences can contribute to moral distress and burnout among caregivers.[10–13]

Although the communication challenges arising in the neonatal intensive care setting can seem overwhelming, empiric evidence exists for identifying where and how communication problems arise and strategies to mitigate them. This chapter will explore serious communication in the NICU, including advantages and disadvantages of current physician approaches to challenging conversations, how these differ from what parents desire for these conversations, and how to advance practices to improve communication. Two specific examples of challenging, serious communication situations—antenatal consultation for life-threatening diagnoses and goals of care in critical illness and end-of-life decision-making—will be explored, as will teaching these communication skills to clinicians and trainees.

What Clinicians Should Do

Guidelines

A number of guidelines and recommendations exist to assist neonatologists and other care providers in the sensitive discussions that arise in antenatal consultation and end-of-life care.[14–25] In these situations, neonatal healthcare professionals have the complicated task of determining whether the medical situation warrants shared decision-making or whether the prognosis is so good that resuscitative care is obligated or is so poor that comfort care is the only medically appropriate choice.[26] Prediction of a high likelihood of intact survival necessitates provision of intensive care in the best interests of the infant; likewise, a certain prognosis of nonsurvivability necessitates comfort care (Fig. 89.1).[27] In these situations, parents should be involved in close, sensitive communication about what to expect but should not be presented with options that are ethically impermissible.

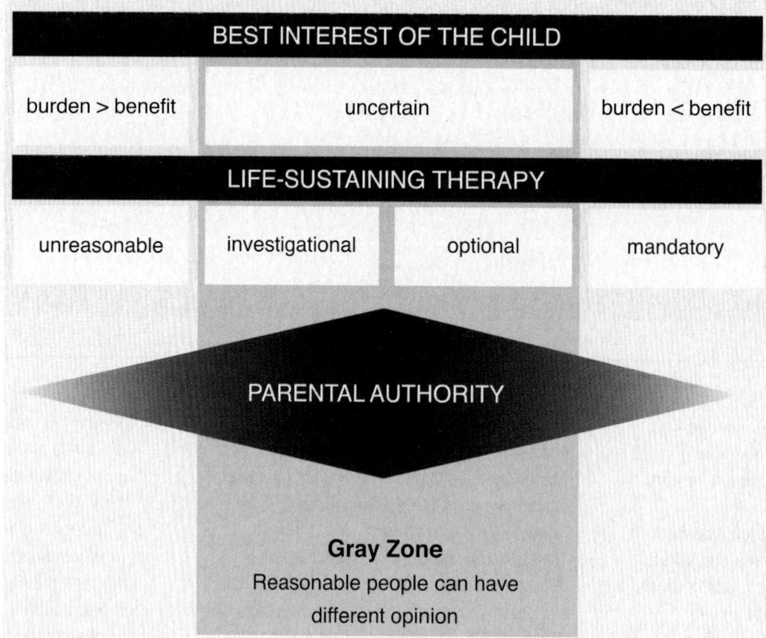

Fig. 89.1 In the Gray Zone of Neonatal Ethical Decision-Making, Parental Authority Drives Decisions Because the Best Interest of the Infant May Be Unclear and Proposed Treatments Can Be Classified as Investigational or Optional. Outside the borders of the gray zone, parental authority is limited, and treatments are considered unreasonable when burden clearly outweighs benefit or mandatory when benefit clearly outweighs burden. (Adapted from Berger TM. Decisions in the gray zone: evidence-based or culture-based? *J Pediatr.* 2010;156:7–9, Fig. 1, p. 8.)

When prognosis is uncertain, however, and death or disability is likely, medical facts alone cannot inform which option is in the clear best interest of the infant. In these cases, multiple different goals of care might be appropriate, and decisions should be based on the parents' values that frame their perceptions of the possible outcomes.[28]

In situations of anticipated extreme prematurity, the delineations of when intensive therapy is obligated, recommended, optional, or inappropriate are seemingly clearer than for antenatal decisions for fetal anomalies and genetic conditions. Epidemiologic outcome data exist for infants born at these gestational ages, and professional society guidelines have recommended gestational age thresholds bounding parental authority based on these statistics.[15,18,19] Debate exists, however, about whether simplistic rules are appropriate for determining ethically permissible care options.[29] Although this gestational age approach facilitates standardization in counseling, gestational dating is imprecise, and other factors impact morbidity and mortality, including sex, fetal weight, plurality, administration of antenatal steroids, and reason for delivery.[30] Individual characteristics of the infant, mother, and medical provider may be difficult to quantify but nevertheless cannot be ignored in considering therapeutic options.

For antenatal consultation for a serious fetal anomaly or genetic condition, neonatal providers must also determine where the ethical boundaries of resuscitation options fall, although epidemiologic data are usually unavailable.[17,31,32] Variability in the types, combinations, and degree of severity of anomalies, particularly if complicated by growth restriction or the heightened risk of premature delivery, make prognostication difficult.[33–37] Additionally, existing survival data for many of these conditions are potentially biased by the "self-fulfilling prophecy," in which life-saving interventions are categorically withheld, reinforcing the perception that the condition is uniformly lethal.[38] Clinicians often must rely on available information from obstetric imaging and experiential knowledge of outcomes for this population, an approach that is inherently imperfect.[39] Although some condition-specific recommendations for antenatal counseling exist,[40–43] contemporary care practices have shifted during the past 15 years toward deferring to parents' values to guide resuscitation decisions for infants with uncertain prognoses or who have conditions with a high risk of morbidity and mortality, such as trisomy 13 and trisomy 18.[44–46]

Professional society statements for management of end-of-life care provide guidance for clinicians on withdrawing or forgoing therapies such as artificial nutrition or other supportive interventions when these treatments are felt to be nonbeneficial or will not achieve a desirable outcome in terms of length or quality of life.[20,20,25,47] These guidelines do not prescribe clear thresholds of when life-prolonging care may be appropriately withheld or withdrawn but rather encourage shared decision-making between parents and healthcare professionals in these situations. Clear communication, particularly about code status and expectations for ongoing interventions, is strongly endorsed, although specific guidance on how to engage in these conversations is not explicitly provided.

Shared Decision-Making

Although the shared decision-making approach is ubiquitously championed for communication about resuscitation and end-of-life care for all patients, what shared decision-making entails and how to best employ it in practice remains elusive for critically ill newborns. In an American College of Critical Care Medicine and American Thoracic Society policy statement, Kon and coauthors[48] define shared decision-making as "a collaborative process that allows patients, or surrogates, and clinicians to make healthcare decisions together, taking into account the best scientific evidence available, as well as the patient's values, goals, and preferences." In the NICU, these decisions are typically shared between clinicians and parents/families because these patients cannot make their wishes known. Three

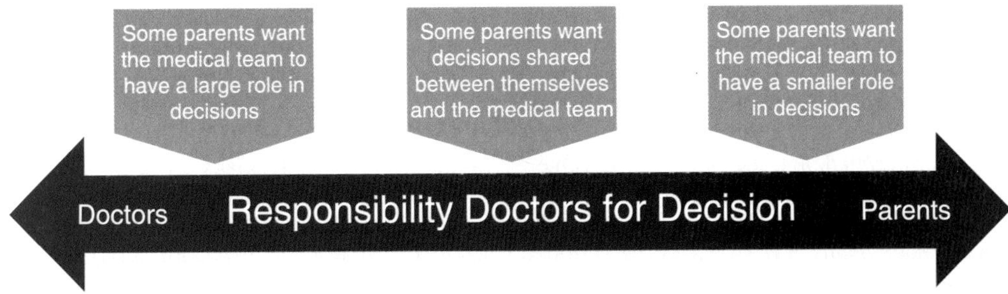

Fig. 89.2 The Spectrum of Decisional Authority. Parent preferences for the degree of responsibility for decisions varies between specific decisions and decision-makers. Decisional responsibility can be equally shared between clinicians and patients/families, or more or less control may be ceded to the medical team based on the patient's or family's preferences.

key procedural stages are recommended. The first is information exchange, in which clinicians share medical information and parents share their values, goals, and preferences. This is followed by a period of deliberation, in which opinions are shared, questions are asked, and misconceptions are corrected by both parties in determining the most appropriate treatment option for the patient. Finally, the care team and parents agree on a treatment decision based on the most preferable option.[48]

Tailoring the process to specific needs of the decision-makers is emphasized in this statement, because families' desire for decisional authority is variable between families and in different decision contexts. Although most prefer that decisional responsibility be shared equally or nearly equally with clinicians, a nontrivial minority wish to have significantly more or less control in the decision-making process.[49] It is therefore appropriate that when a family clearly understands their values and is comfortable assuming greater independence, allowing them to choose from among the medically acceptable options may be appropriate. Conversely, if the patient or parent/surrogate has been emotionally or psychologically averse to assuming a strong role in decision-making, a higher degree of clinician involvement in the decision may be warranted (Fig. 89.2).[48] Parents' preferences for decisional authority may also change over time, based on changes in the patient's clinical status, familiarity with medical information and decisions made, and trust in the care team.[48]

The *Shared Decision-Making in ICUs Policy Statement* also notes the importance of communication, both for explaining medical facts and for eliciting families' values.[48] Providers are encouraged to explain medical options in understandable terms and ask for families to explain back their understanding. Likewise, facilitating dialogue in which families consider and share their values is an essential skill for healthcare professionals, because these values may conflict, be difficult to articulate, and change over time.[28] The recommendations also highlight providing emotional support to families by acknowledging strong emotions and expressing empathy, although specific behaviors to employ these skills in practice are not described. Although basic components of good communication, such as ensuring adequate seating for all participants, moving the discussion away from the bedside when surrogate families are making decisions for incapacitated patients, using the patient's name, and minimizing distractions can be modified, none of these strategies teach a clinician to authentically feel empathy. Although continued research in this area has the potential to support practice, role-modeling, and education, no single approach can account for fundamental variation among providers, and the expectation of a single standardized method for conducting these conversations is not realistic.

What Clinicians Do

Numerous studies of neonatal providers have identified opportunities to improve communication and shared decision-making in practice. Surveys of neonatal clinicians and patients, as well as recording and videotaping of real and simulated encounters, have shed light on suboptimal communication practices and have laid a foundation for ongoing efforts to enhance this aspect of neonatal intensive care.

Practice Variation

Clinicians self-report wide practice variations in their approach to resuscitating critically ill infants,[50–55] which may be attributable to variations in regional or national guidelines[56] and cultures between institutions and sites of training.[57] This nonuniformity may bias clinical decision-making by way of shaping which treatment options are offered to parents,[58,59] and it likely impacts the ultimate survival of these infants.[60] Standardization of guidelines within and across institutions has been proposed as a way of ensuring a just approach to counseling[61]; however, debate remains regarding what level of standardization would be optimal[62] or whether standardization would even be appropriate.[29,63,64]

Engaging Parents

Neonatologists also report divergent attitudes about whether to involve parents in decision-making and to what degree.[51–53,65–67] Likewise, in practice, they struggle to identify parents' desired degree of decisional authority and to appropriately engage parents at this level.[68,69] In one survey, the majority of neonatologists identified providing information to expectant parents in antenatal consultation to be central to their role, but far fewer felt weighing the risks and benefits of the treatment options with parents was.[65] Engaging in personal discussions about perceptions of death and quality of life or religious/spiritual views with parents is uncomfortable for clinicians in antenatal consultations and NICU settings and may be avoided in these contexts.[65,70] This may be related to insufficient attention to teaching these aspects of communication in subspecialty training.[70,71]

Provision of Information

When providing parents with information, neonatal providers frequently discuss potential morbidity and mortality outcomes to guide decision-making.[65,72] Several studies have shown, however, that the information they provide is often inaccurate and more pessimistic than is warranted by the epidemiologic data.[73–76] To combat the misinformation, the National Institute of Child Health and Human Development (NICHD) developed an online calculator in 2008,[77] and the vast majority of neonatologists report reliance on this or similar tools for counseling.[78] The accuracy of the outcome probabilities predicted by these tools is limited by both the data itself, which may reflect a prior epoch of therapeutic interventions, and the precision with which characteristics such as gestational age and fetal weight can be measured. Although parents desire individualized outcome information, clinicians often quote the statistical outcome data,[78,79] which may be difficult for parents with poor health literacy and numeracy to understand.[80] Additionally, how clinicians present this information, including message framing or default options, may influence parents' decisions.[81,82] Decision aids have been proposed as a strategy to impart outcome information to parents in a way that is clear and comprehensible.[83–85] Although these strategies have demonstrated utility in increasing parental knowledge, it remains unclear whether this is helpful to parents' decision-making.[83] The outcomes clinicians report to parents are generally derived from research studies evaluating treatments and may not be meaningful to parents making these decisions.[86] Instead, parents may consider statistical information to frame their expectations rather than to guide decisions.[87] Additionally, when neonatal healthcare professionals discuss possible outcomes, they tend to focus on the medical outcome of the infant rather than the broader implications of the potential outcomes in relation to the family.[88,89]

Values

Several studies have also suggested that clinicians' approaches to shared decision-making may be influenced by their personal values. Neonatologists' attitudes about death have been found to correlate with how they approach end-of-life decisions for their patients,[90] and a study of pediatric ICU providers identified that their personal values impacted life-supportive treatment options that they offer and recommend to families.[91] This is particularly concerning because providers' views differ from those of parents. Neonatologists are more likely than parents to rate states of disability as worse than death[92] and are less likely to save infants at all costs.[92,93] In the prenatal period, clinicians encourage pregnancy termination in situations of an anticipated nonsurvivable prognosis rather than approaching the decision neutrally,[94] and many would choose termination themselves if facing a serious diagnosis.[95] Clinicians are particularly pessimistic toward premature infants, choosing to forgo resuscitation of these patients more frequently than in older patients with similar prognoses.[96,97] This pessimism toward infants with poor prognoses likely begins in training. Although nearly all pediatrics residents in one survey felt it was a social responsibility to care for severely disabled children, more than two-thirds felt frustrated about providing care to infants with no hope of cure or independent functioning and questioned the care in these cases.[98] Pediatrics residents, like attending physicians, overestimate disability and death in very premature infants,[57,99] are reluctant to initiate resuscitation for depressed premature infants,[57] and express attitudes that the gestational age thresholds for resuscitation are too low.[100] Although it is not realistic for clinicians to clear their minds of personal values and beliefs, recognition of the impact of values and differences in values on communication is paramount; clinicians should be mindful of their own visceral and emotional responses to charged clinical scenarios and cultivate a thoughtful and proactive approach to mitigating potential bias and imposition of values.

What Parents Want

In this section, the available evidence that informs communication in two commonly encountered, difficult clinical scenarios will be reviewed: antenatal counseling and end-of-life conversations. For each, dominant themes and goals are presented, with review of the evidence that supports their importance and of evidence-based approaches for the clinician.

Antenatal Counseling

To address some of the many pitfalls of counseling for infants with extreme prematurity, genetic conditions, or major anomalies, a number of studies have investigated parents' attitudes toward antenatal consultation and needs for decision-making in this context. Kharrat et al. reported in a systematic review of parents' communication needs in counseling for prematurity that parents report clear preferences for when and where they wish for consultation to occur, what information they want presented and in what manner, and how they wish to be involved in the decision-making.[72] Although there are differences in the nature of consultation for prematurity compared with other conditions, many of the overarching themes identified are consistent with studies of parents who have undergone antenatal consultation for anomalies and genetic disorders.

Empathetic Communication

Receiving a diagnosis of a congenital anomaly,[101,102] genetic disorder,[103] or threatened extreme premature delivery[104,105] is a stressful and traumatic event. Parents anticipating an uneventful pregnancy and healthy child are suddenly faced with a myriad of difficult decisions such as whether to continue or terminate the pregnancy, what (if any) fetal monitoring is appropriate, when to deliver the infant and by what route, and which resuscitative interventions to provide at delivery. Parents have made clear that although expectations for their child are changed by the diagnosis, their child's personhood has not. Using the infant's name in discussions, as well as focusing on their infant as a baby and not a diagnosis, is valuable to parents in this context.[106] Likewise, listening, asking about the infant and family, answering parents' questions, and acknowledging their emotions can help reduce parental anxiety and establish trust.[107,108] Specific behaviors including making visual contact, using gentle touch, and pacing the conversation to parents' needs can also facilitate parent participation in these conversations.[107]

Consultation Setting

Another aspect of empathetic communication is choosing the appropriate setting for the antenatal consultation. Although truly emergent deliveries impede counselors' ability to control the timing and environment of the consultation, a quiet, private setting with adequate seating and space is preferable for these conversations.[109] The timing of the conversation is also important to parents. For parents threatened with extreme prematurity, admission to the hospital may occur at any time of day or night, and maternal labor or medications may be distracting or interfere with cognition and comprehension. Finding a time when the mother is alert and attentive, the consultation not rushed, and there is time for parents to process information before delivery is challenging but appreciated by parents.[72,107] Delaying the consultation to allow support people to be present is also important to parents.[110] These considerations must be balanced against the risk of imminent delivery—in some cases the window of opportunity to meet with the expectant parents before delivery is quite narrow.

For consultations for anomalies and genetic disorders, often in the outpatient setting, the timing is typically less urgent but still a significant consideration. Repeat visits for additional imaging and meetings with subspecialty consultants are often required. Meeting with subspecialists as a group in consultation so that all care-team members can participate in the same conversation reduces conflicting information and parents' anxiety levels.[111] Parents facing any of these diagnoses report benefit from multiple, repeated consultations, because this allows time for processing information and reflection on values.[72,110,112,113]

Engaging Expectant Parents in Decision-Making

In consultations in which the anticipated prognosis of the infant is poor, parents typically wish to be involved in decisions regarding which therapies to provide at the time of delivery.[69,72,107,114,115] What level of decisional authority individual parents desire and how much they wish to cede to clinicians in resuscitation decisions vary between parents.[69,72] Some parents feel that it is their parental responsibility to make the final decision independently, and others would prefer that the providers carry the burden of this difficult choice. Most parents, however, prefer a shared decision-making approach, with the clinicians providing relevant medical information that is pertinent to decision-making and with some degree of recommendation from the healthcare professional based on the medical information of the case and the values they have shared. Tailoring the antenatal consultation to meet parents' needs is clearly desirable, but this requires the counselor to have the time to sit and identify what the parents need *and* to be knowledgeable and flexible enough to change the approach to the encounter on the spot. Haward et al. described a practice they dub "controlled improvisation" to support appropriately individualized consultation.[108]

Providing Information

To participate meaningfully in consultation and decision-making, parents report that medical information provided by the medical team is essential. For diverse diagnoses warranting antenatal goals of care decision-making, parents desire information about the prognosis, specifically in regard to likelihood of survival and risks of long-term developmental impairment.[72,105,113,116,117] This information should be presented clearly, in terms that are understandable to parents. Caution should be used in quoting numerical statistical information from large epidemiologic studies to parents, because they are not only difficult for parents to comprehend[80] but also may not accurately reflect the prognosis of the particular infants' situation.[89] Consultation based on a monologue-style listing of potential poor outcomes with numeric estimates of their frequency (e.g., "your baby has a 72% chance of moderate or severe impairment consisting of cognitive motor scores 1 or 2 standard deviations below the mean, respectively, measured at 2 years of age") may have the allure of seeming impartial and comprehensive but might not be helpful to expectant parents anticipating the birth of *their* baby, and it conflates population estimates with an individual's chance of a particular outcome. Instead, presenting individualized information based on the unique characteristics of the infant and specific circumstances of the pregnancy and delivery is more helpful to parents.[107,113,116,117] For example, "in large groups of babies like Sophie, many surviving infants go on to have significant long-term problems with brain development. We can talk more about what that might mean for Sophie and your family if that would be helpful to you" broadly addresses the limitations of population-based outcome data for individual prognostication and invites parents to help the counselor understand their own values and/or to request more granular information if they feel it will be helpful to them. Although clinicians may perceive that prognostic predictions without exact numerical probabilities are less scientific and sophisticated, parents are less inclined to make decisions based on survival estimates than their own values.[86]

In situations of poor prognosis, parents wish to be informed of the risks of morbidity and mortality, even when this information is emotionally distressing[72,113]; however, parents find this information more helpful in preparing to participate in their infant's care than in making decisions to provide or withhold supportive therapies.[72,109] Excessively pessimistic framings of survival and impairment information, even when prognosis is poor, dashes parents' hope and is unhelpful both in parents' coping and in fostering trust and rapport in the care team.[86,118] When prognosis is uncertain, parents wish for this to be honestly discussed. Both over- and understatement of certainty can have serious consequences. Having an infant survive after being told excessively negative prognostic information was reported by parents as irrevocably damaging to their trust in their care team.[118] However, using the guise of uncertainty to avoid sharing bad news leaves parents without adequate information for decision-making.

In addition to prognosis, parents want information during antenatal consultation that focuses on the anticipated medical course, potential treatments and interventions, and how they can take an active role in their infant's care after delivery.[107,115,117,119] Many parents are unfamiliar with the NICU environment; helping them form expectations of what their child's life will be like and what technology they are anticipated to need are helpful in mitigating anxiety.[120] Tours of the NICU and delivery area are also often helpful to parents,[121] and resource/veteran parents offering peer-to-peer support may also be valuable.[122,123]

Values

Parents' values are critically important in how they consider major decisions about their infants, perhaps more so than prediction of survival.[86] Unlike the quantitative way clinicians historically have approached these decisions, parents approach these situations based on emotions rather than rationality.[67,124] Hope and spirituality were overarching themes in multiple studies of parents facing extreme prematurity,[72,86,113,118] and considerations around religion and faith influence parents' decision-making.[86,125] Even when the chance of survival is slim, giving their child a "fighting chance" and not squandering an opportunity for survival is important to many parents.[86,118,125] Parents also tend to view neurodevelopmental impairment differently than clinicians do; in a large, longitudinal study, parents of surviving extremely premature infants rated their quality of life better than their physicians did.[126–128]

Parents facing diagnoses of genetic disorders and severe congenital anomalies report similar values in their decision-making. Parents of surviving children with trisomy 13 and 18 perceive that their children are happy and enrich their families.[129] These parents do consider issues of suffering and quality of life in making decisions about interventions to provide at delivery. Their expectations are not unrealistically focused on intact survival but rather on achievable goals such as having the ability to meet their child, bring their child home, and give their child a happy life.[130] Even when medical providers predict a lethal diagnosis, some parents choose to continue the pregnancy and do so based on their beliefs, values, and experiences.[116,131] Parents have described wanting their child to be treated as a person and discussed by name, and they express hopes like wanting to meet their child alive.[106,116]

End-of-Life Conversations

After a critically ill infant is delivered and is in the NICU, parents and clinicians may again be faced with decision-making around goals of care. These decisions, like resuscitation decisions in the antenatal period, are emotionally challenging. There are many opportunities for improvement in communication between healthcare professionals and parents in this context, and a number of studies of parents have revealed how clinicians can better support decision-making.[8,70,88,115,118,132–160]

As is the case for antenatal consultations, conversations to discuss redirection of care goals for critically ill infants are quite sensitive. An empathetic approach is essential to supporting parents, including thoughtful consideration of the language, information, timing, and environment of the communication. Parents have detailed recollection of how bad news was delivered even years later, and their perceptions of the situation affect their long-term well-being.[152,160,161]

A private, quiet setting is helpful in conversations around end-of-life decisions for infants, ideally away from the infant's bedside, allowing parents to listen without distractions.[138,141] Likewise, the number of people present should be carefully considered. Although it may be advantageous for parents to be able to speak with different subspecialists involved in the infant's care simultaneously, these conversations can be overwhelmed with excessive medical staff and trainees.[162] Obtaining pertinent information and recommendations from care-team members who are not essential to the meeting can be done by the primary team in anticipation of these discussions. Parents clearly value a nursing presence in these meetings, especially nurses with preexisting relationships with the family.[115,118,139,150,163] Timing of decision-making conversations for dying infants is also important, because time pressure has the potential to impact the decisions that are made. Parents who are rushed with urgent decisions often opt for prolonging life.[147] Importantly, time to process and come to terms with the situation at each stage impacts parents' coping.[148]

Empathetic Language and Trust

Empathetic language and behaviors by medical team members are important to parents in conversations about and provision of end-of-life care. Numerous studies of parents with infants in a NICU have found that there are opportunities to improve communication, regardless of the infant's diagnosis and prognosis. When an infant is critically ill or dying, however, communication challenges are particularly problematic. Parents of dying infants report that avoidance or abandonment by staff,[143,155,156] along with perceived stalling and avoidance of giving bad news that ultimately delay disclosure, are upsetting.[152] Likewise, behaviors like speaking abruptly, seeming cold and insensitive to the family's situation, and laughing or joking outside the dying child's room are detrimental to parental coping.[136] When care providers dismiss parents' observations and concerns, parents question the honesty of the providers.[157] Mistrust in clinicians leads parents to doubt the truthfulness of medical information provided, including the prognosis,[157,159] which creates conflict in decision-making.[4,5] Distrust in the medical facts can in turn lead to distrust in the care team's recommendation for redirection of care and may contribute to decision regret, even when parents to accede to recommendations to withhold or withdraw life-prolonging interventions.

Clinician behaviors that parents report foster trust in the medical team include discussing information in an unrushed, compassionate, and sensitive manner.[160] Clinicians should be thoughtful not only of specific language used in discussions but also of tone of voice and body language.[159] Acknowledging the difficulty of the situation[156] and addressing parents with humility and understanding also facilitates communication.[8,135,156,159] Sensitivity to the power differential between clinicians and patients as well as racial, language, and cultural barriers is also paramount.[141,144,151,164]

Decisional Authority

Parents of critically ill infants in the NICU wish to be involved in decisions about their child's care, particularly for decisions that are high-stakes and values-based.[165] Numerous studies of parents have shown that parents desire some degree of participation in decisions about end-of-life care, but preferences range from receiving information and having little to no decisional responsibility to complete control.[67,86,115,136,137,140,148,150,153,157,166] Most parents in NICU studies endorse a shared approach to these decisions, which is consistent with evidence from parents facing similar decisions in the pediatric ICU[49,167,168] and pediatric oncology.[169,170] Engaging parents in end-of-life decisions for their infant in a way that aligns with their desired level of decisional authority is important to their long-term well-being, because their perception of their role in the decision impacts grief and coping.[137,156,160] Parents, much more so than clinicians, have to live with the emotional consequences of these decisions.[140] When parents of infants who die in the NICU feel that physicians made the decision to discontinue supportive therapies alone, they experience more grief than those who felt the decision was shared; those who believe they have borne the burden of the decision alone experience the most grief.[137] Parents who are given information without recommendation or guidance by their care team also experience more feelings of anxiety and abandonment on later reflection.[8]

Information

For parents to be involved in goals-of-care decisions, particularly about the end of life, medical information regarding the condition, prognosis, and possible treatments for their infant is necessary[154]; however, this information alone is not sufficient to support their needs.[109] Clinicians need to also discuss the broader implications of these decisions and what this could mean for the child and the family in the short- and long-term. Parents vary in the quantity of information they desire in these conversations[154] but benefit most when they perceive it is personalized and complete but not excessive.[146,159,160] Parents appreciate clarity in communication of factual medical information, including avoidance of jargon or overly technical terms and avoidance of ambiguity.[157,159,160] Divergent opinions from different members of the care team should be limited, because this can be confusing and distressing to parents.[150,159,160,171,172] In discussions of prognosis specifically, parents report wanting to hear clear, objective evidence when the anticipated outcome is poor with certainty.[148] When prognosis is uncertain, however, honest, factual discussion of the medical information and disclosure of the uncertainty is valued.[136,148,154,157,159,160] Withholding information, as well as presenting unfounded, overly optimistic or pessimistic survival predictions, has the potential to undermine trust in the clinician if parents feel they are being manipulated.[136,157,160]

Values

As in antenatal resuscitation decisions, parents may have values in making decisions about end-of-life care for their child that differ from those held by their providers. These values appear to be ethnoculturally derived and based on personal philosophic principles more than past experiences.[144,151] For parents, concerns about suffering and quality of life[140,145,147,167] are tempered against hope[150,158,160] and the desire for more time with their child.[134,140,147,164] Many parents choose to pursue all therapies that preserve an

Prenatal Consultation Checklist __/__/__ Mother's name: ______ ID: ______

Reason for consultation: ______ OB name: ______
☐ Communication with OB team: ______ Joint consultation with OB: ☐ yes ☐ no
Parent told about consultation: ☐ yes ☐ no Significant person present: ______

Allow enough time / Limit interruptions (phone/pager) / Ensure privacy (# people) / Sit down

Establish trust with parents
☐ Neonatologist introduction / role
☐ NICU team introduction
☐ Ask about the baby
"Do you have a name?" ______
"Tell me about your baby" ______
"Does he/she have siblings?" ______
☐ Ask and Listen to parents' main concerns
- "What is your greatest fear?"
- "What is most important to you as a family?"
- "Is anything worrying you at home or work?"
- "What do you expect from this consultation?"
- "What can I do for you?"

Address personalized parental concerns & questions
☐ Ask parents if they prefer statistical data, general terms, or both
☐ Discuss potential complications of prematurity relevant to them
☐ Explain their role as parents of a premature baby
- Parental roles: touching, talking, family attachment
- Baby appearance and behavior
- Parent as caregiver: feeding/breastfeeding, clothing
- Parental involvement in future decisions
☐ Explain how the NICU works
- NICU visit offered ☐yes ☐no date: __/__/__
- Allied HCP visit offered ☐yes ☐no

Comments: ______

NICU team members (Name, role): ______

Follow-up
☐ NICU visit done (Date: __/__/__)
☐ Allied HCPs consulted (Role & date): ______

☐ Follow-up visit (ideally) by same neonatologist
- Date: __/__/__, GA: ______
☐ Written documents given
Further comments: ______

Fig. 89.3 Suggested Template for Parent-Centered Antenatal Consultation Form, Part 1. (Adapted from Haward MF, Gaucher N, Payot A, Robson K, Janvier, A. Personalized decision making: practical recommendations for antenatal counseling for fragile neonates. *Clin Perinatol.* 2017;44:429–445, Fig. 1, p. 435.)

opportunity for survival, because they perceive that giving up a chance at life would be unacceptable[135,155]; parents have expressed that the knowledge that "everything" was tried was comforting to them in their bereavement.[136] Memory-making[133,141,145,156,173] and cultural/religious practices are important to parents when death is inevitable,[141,151,164] and it is likely that NICU parents, like parents of older children in the ICU, consider "being a good parent" as influential in their decision-making.[174] Physical proximity to the dying child has been noted in ICU studies of older children to be important as well.[164,175]

Despite this emphasis on eliciting, understanding, and taking into account parents' values in end-of-life decision-making, doing so is challenging. Parents may struggle to identify, understand, and articulate their own values.[142] Even if they find their values unclear, parents rarely regret the decisions made when they feel they were adequately involved in the decision process,[132–134,142,158] although some report regrets about how their time was spent while their child was living.[133] In some studies, however, a proportion of parents felt that their expectations were not met or their wishes were not respected.[141,150]

Recommendations for Practice

Parents have repeatedly indicated that communication with the medical team colors their perceptions of this extraordinarily difficult situation. Although neonatal healthcare providers who occupy this professional space may hone their communication skills and become adept at supporting parents in high-stakes decisions before and after birth of the infant, the detachment necessary to engage in these encounters routinely has the potential to widen the divide between clinicians and parents, who are the least oriented to the process but the most affected by it.

1. Individualize information to meet parents' needs: Possession of all the relevant facts is an essential component of informed consent and supports parental authority in these decisions. Facts that are not understood are unhelpful to meaningful informed consent. The clinician should anticipate being in possession of wider and deeper knowledge that will necessarily be shared; the quality of communication need not be measured by the volume of information transferred from the clinician to the parent. Neonatal healthcare professionals should use available tools to elicit informational needs and share information in a contextually appropriate way (Figs. 89.3 and 89.4).
2. Involve and empower families: As the natural surrogate decision-makers for children, who inherently exist in their family's shared culture and values, parents have a fundamental authority to act in their children's well-being and should be engaged in decision-making in the role of *parents* (rather than *ad hoc* medical providers); life-and-death decisions parents make before and after birth are *parenting* decisions. Parents should be encouraged to ask questions about their child's condition, medical support needs, and how they can be involved in daily care. For parents who may be overwhelmed and unsure what questions to ask, clinicians may suggest example questions that parents commonly want to know[176] (Table 89.1).
3. Base decisions on parents' values: Elicitation of parental values is the lynchpin of shared decision-making for infants. Parents' values are not uniform but often diverge from medical providers,

Date: __/__/__ OB Name:____________________ Reason for consultation: Prematurity Other __________		Mother's Name: __________ DOB: __/__/__ Room nr.:__________ Hosp. ID:__________

BABY GA:________ (U/S ________ LMP________) Singleton Twin ______ EFW:__________ (__/__/__) Gender:________ β-methasone __/__/__ __/__/__ __/__/__	**MOTHER** Age:______ G ___ P___ A___ Blood Gr:___ Serol.:__________ Habits: __________ Medications: __________ PMH: __________ OBST, H:__________

CURRENT PREGNANCY

T1 ______________________________

T1 U/S(__/__/__/)______________________

T2 ______________________________

T2 U/S(__/__/__/)______________________

T3 ______________________________

T3 U/S(__/__/__/)______________________

DISCUSSION Mother Father Other significant: __________

OB present: __________ NICU Team: __________

Baby's name:__________ __________

Parents' main concerns: ______________________________

Family situation: ______________________________

Information discussed relative to parents' needs: Complications of prematurity Parental roles

How NICU works

☐ NICU visit offered Written documentation provided: ☐ yes ☐ no

Follow-up ☐ NICU visit done (Date: __/__/____/) ☐ Allied HCPs consulted (Role & date): __________ ☐ Follow-up visit by neonatologist: __________ Date: __/__/__ , GA:______	Neonatologist Name: __________ Signature:__________ Date: __/__/____

Fig. 89.4 Suggested Template for Parent-Centered Antenatal Consultation Form, Part 2. (Adapted from Haward MF, Gaucher N, Payot A, Robson K, Janvier A. Personalized decision making: practical recommendations for antenatal counseling for fragile neonates. *Clin Perinatol.* 2017;44:429–445, Fig. 2, p. 440.)

whose experience of critical neonatal illness differs greatly from their own. Parents' values are not inherently illogical, and parents who base decisions on values rarely regret their choices (Fig. 89.5).

4. Foster trust through empathy: Although step-by-step instructions for good communication are limited in their ability to foster authentic empathy, neonatologists who have experienced the NICU from a parent's perspective recommend strategies for supporting parents in these situations[177] (Table 89.2).
5. Balance developing the ownership and individual skill needed to support parents through high-stakes decision-making with the need to provide families with what they need in the moment: Consider consultation with perinatal hospice/pediatric palliative care if the parents' needs exceed the team's abilities to provide

Table 89.1 Types and Examples of Common Parent Questions

Types of Questions Parents May Have	Examples of Parent Questions
Communication with medical care team	Should I join daily rounds? Can I join virtually or by phone? How can I be involved in the care plan decisions?
Getting updates about their child's condition	What are the roles of clinicians on my care team? How do I reach them to get information about my baby when I cannot attend rounds?
Use of a pulse oximeter and other bedside monitoring devices	Can someone teach me about what this device is measuring? What level on the monitor means my baby has a safe level of oxygen?
Changes in clinical condition	How will I know if my baby is getting sicker? What are signs that I should be worried?
Feeding devices such as a nasogastric tube	How long will my baby be expected to need this device? Can someone start teaching me about how I can work on feeding skills with my baby?
Decision-making in "gray" areas	How will I know when there is a decision to be made and what the treatment options are? Can someone help me understand the risks and benefits of each option?
Long-term outcomes	What types of outcomes are possible for a child with medical conditions like mine has? What outcomes are most likely?
Preparing for life after discharge	Can someone start teaching me about anticipated after-discharge needs? Can I get information about things I can do to promote my baby's development?
Tracheostomy or other long-term supportive technology	How long is my child expected to have this type of support? What will life be like at home with this these care needs? How have other families adjusted to the changes of having a child receiving this kind of support? Can someone start teaching me how to care for my child with these devices?

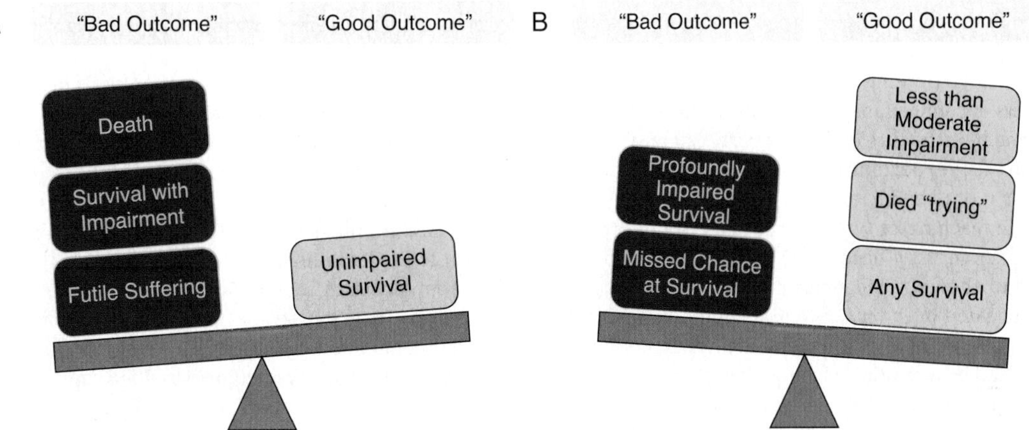

Fig. 89.5 (A) Clinicians may perceive a high likelihood of nonsurvival paired with a high chance of moderate to severe impairment among survivors as dismal, with only a very low chance of the "desired" outcome of intact survival. Given the statistical probabilities, the burdens of infant suffering and societal cost may appear to outweigh the benefit of therapy, and comfort care is logically recommended. (B) Parents may view these outcomes differently. If any survival, even with impairment, is seen as a desirable outcome, the probability of a "good" outcome increases. If having a surviving very impaired child is considered the most undesirable outcome, the risk of this is low, because many of the sickest infants die. Finally, if dying after intensive care is perceived as favorable compared with possibly missing an opportunity to have an intact survivor, the risk of the unfavorable outcome falls to zero if an attempt at resuscitation is made. (Adapted from Kukora SK, Boss RD. Values-based shared decision-making in the antenatal period. *Semin Fetal Neonatal Med.* 2017. doi:10.1016/j.siny.2017.09.003. Fig. 4, p. 22.)

coordinated and comprehensive end-of-life care or complex decision-making.

Communication Education

Although the literature suggests approaches to engaging parents in serious communication in antenatal counseling and neonatal end-of-life care, written recommendations are difficult to translate into clinical practice. Only a few of the suggested interventions are specific and modifiable. Some require additional mindfulness on the part of the clinician, such as choosing an appropriate environment for the communication; others require attention to changes to behaviors that may not be conscious or natural, such as body language and eye contact. Much of the guidance for these conversations, however, is vague. Instructing clinicians to be sensitive and empathetic or to elicit parents' values and desired level of decisional authority is unhelpful without telling them how to do so. Although some of the approaches recommend specific language or phrasing to initiate shared decision making[176] or tools to support and facilitate communication,[84,108] the skills to partake in these discussions effectively cannot be learned from reading alone.

Approaches to teaching clinician trainees how to deliver serious, life-altering news have been well studied, but there is no consensus on the most effective way to impart these skills. Clinicians in a variety of specialties find these emotional conversations stressful and feel that they have been inadequately trained to engage in them.[178–181] Anxiety about their patients' and their own emotional reactions may lead providers toward emotional avoidance rather than empathy and engagement.[180] Unfortunately, time in practice and experience with bad-news conversations does not improve distress in these clinical contexts.[180]

Table 89.2 Recommendations to Clinicians

- NICU care providers need to be cognizant of parents' emotional needs, which can have both negative and positive impacts after discharge. Such experiences can manifest with sleep disorders, dysfunction at work, periodic anxiety, and even reactive depression.
- Neonatal care is not an exact science. Care providers must remain humble. Avoid framing parents' decisions and actions negatively, such as: "Parents don't understand" or "If I were in their situation, I would not..." Too often, it is providers, not parents, who do not have a panoramic view.
- Update parents on all possible risks, but also give a positive outlook by recalling success stories.
- Remind parents that the infant's illness was not caused by something that they did. Recall that clinicians rarely know the etiopathogenesis of most neonatal disorders.
- Remind parents that the child is so fortunate in having parents who care. Help them to prioritize their energy and well-being, get enough rest and sleep, continue to attend to their other children, and recognize what they can and cannot control. Encourage them to let go where they can.
- Remind parents that life will change after the infant recovers from the current clinical instability, and once she/he is discharged from the NICU, they will be able to hold her/him with all the parental affection and care. It will get better.

NICU, Neonatal intensive care unit.
Summarized from Janvier et al., 177.

To address this need, educators have developed a number of in-person communication trainings focused on task-specific practices to address bad-news encounters, particularly for medical trainees.[178] The specific content and structure of these educational interventions are variable, but the experiential nature of active learning approaches appear more beneficial in imparting these skills compared with didactic teaching or written materials alone. For these programs to be effective, they necessitate that sessions be at least several hours long to allow sufficient participation opportunity, and they are ideally repeated over time.[182] While approaches featuring intensive communication practice and simulated patient scenarios reinforce this essential experiential learning, they are often resource intensive and their effects are difficult to evaluate.[178]

Fellows graduating from neonatal-perinatal training programs report that although they have received extensive education on medical management of critically ill neonates, they do not feel adequately trained to engage in complex communication with parents.[71] Conversations about end-of-life care and values such as religion and spirituality were among the most uncomfortable for fellows, and the majority perceive that they prioritize communication education in these situations over their supervising faculty.[71] Likewise, communication training in antenatal counseling is not universal in fellowship training programs, with the majority of programs lacking formalized curricula.[183] Although program directors acknowledge the importance of perinatal decision-making in clinical practice, many report their graduating fellows are not adequately trained or only somewhat competent in this domain.[183] When fellows are evaluated for antenatal counseling proficiency, neonatology training programs often focus on the information delivery as the goal, rather than the experience of parents.[184] Perceptions of fellows' performance by the actor parents in simulations do not align with assessments of faculty, because they report feeling overwhelmed and bullied with the excessive information.[184]

Despite the need for training programs focusing on the specific communication challenges of neonatal care provision, very few have been reported in the literature. The Neonatal Critical Care Communication (NC3) training reported by Boss et al.[185] is a 3-day intensive communication skills module for fellows and nurse practitioners. In this session, participants were given didactic overviews of evidence-based frameworks for complex conversations in the NICU, then engaged in small-group role-playing sessions with actors playing family members. The cases used for role-playing focused on common NICU situations that fostered participants' interaction longitudinally in three stages of conversation: disclosing bad news, negotiating care goals, and end-of-life discussion. The fellows and practitioners were given feedback during these interactions and were subsequently encouraged to informally practice additional challenging scenarios they had encountered. The training was rated favorably by participants on surveys following the program, and all reported increased confidence in their skills.

The Relational Learning approach described by Meyer et al.[186] involved more diverse interprofessional providers participating in 6-hour workshops. The workshops began with collaborative exercises, an educational film, and a brief didactic presentation highlighting the challenges of communication in the NICU context. Participants then engaged in role-playing cases with professional actors portraying family members, with subsequent reflection and feedback. The session concluded with group discussion, sharing the practical applications learned in the role plays and the potential application to practice. This training was also rated highly by participants on a posttraining and follow-up survey, with the majority reporting improvement in at least one category on self-appraisal.

Virtual standardized patient training has also been proposed as a method for teaching communication skills in antenatal counseling. Motz et al.[187] demonstrated utility and feasibility in using a simulator programmed to display emotions through facial expressions and body language to assess participants' skills in identifying emotions and selecting empathetic responses. Whether these virtual simulator-based trainings translate to improvements in clinical behaviors is yet to be determined.

Approaches to communication education using techniques from improvisational theater, or "medical improv," have also been piloted in the neonatal setting. Improv exercises from improvisational theater are being increasingly integrated to build communication in a variety of professional education settings, including medical training.[188] These exercises emphasize skills that are foundational to serious conversations, including listening, adaptability, fluidity of thought, cooperation, empathy, and spontaneity. Stokes et al.[184] noted that neonatology fellows and attending physicians participating in a 3-hour workshop targeting skills necessary in antenatal counseling identified thoughtful insights about their behaviors in these conversations that could be applied to clinical practice. Likewise, Sawyer et al.[189] reported results from a 90-minute workshop for neonatologists and fellows focusing on verbal and non-verbal behaviors affecting interpersonal communication. The authors compare the prevailing educational model for antenatal counseling to emerging models, including medical improvisation, noting that newer approaches may better teach learners to express empathy in challenging conversations. Participants in a postworkshop questionnaire and follow-up survey indicated on self-reflection measures that the workshop had improved the quality of their antenatal counseling, ability to connect emotionally with parents, listening and observation skills, flexibility, bedside manner, and empathy.[189]

While these experiential, neonatology-specific communication trainings are promising, they have been piloted on small sample sizes and have relied largely on self-reported subjective measures of performance. Participants in these interventions were usually self-selected, creating considerable potential for bias because clinicians desiring to enhance these communication skills may be more willing to attend, participate meaningfully, and evaluate these programs highly. Further research exploring these training methodologies with diverse interprofessional neonatology providers and measuring the impact on behaviors in practice and families' experiences is warranted.

Conclusion

How best to engage in clear, effective, and compassionate serious conversation in NICU settings is informed by an abundance of empirical work, both specific to the NICU context and more broadly. The importance of research on what healthcare professionals do, what parents experience and want, and how best to develop and teach communication skills cannot be overstated. Although ethical paradigms can *and have* shifted, requiring adjustment in individual providers' attitudes and approaches over years of practice, these shifts are in large part attributable to rigorous empirical study. Some aspects of good communication, such as adequate time, space, and infrastructural resources, must be provided by institutions, and clinicians should work within their organization to foster a culture of expectation and insistence on these resources. Other aspects such as empathy, kindness, and interpersonal skill must be cultivated over a lifetime, beginning much earlier than medical/professional school or postgraduate training, but all neonatal providers have an obligation to be mindful of these essential aspects of care.

CHAPTER

90 Pain and Symptom Management in Newborns Receiving Palliative and End-of-Life Care

Kelstan Ellis, Brian S. Carter

KEY POINTS

1. Perinatal palliative care is specialized medical care for fetuses/infants with life-threatening or terminal conditions, with the goal of providing equitable and effective support for curative, life-prolonging, and palliative care for patients and their families.
2. Perinatal hospice may include care of infants diagnosed with a serious medical condition in a physical inpatient setting or at home.
3. Perinatal palliative care is a difficult situation for both families and care providers and needs inputs from multiple disciplines such as perinatal hospice nurses, social workers, chaplains, child life specialists, or others who can assist with birth plans, counseling, sibling support, and preparation for end-of-life care.
4. The scope of perinatal palliative care services may include (1) primary care offered within any community, for lethal conditions such as anencephaly; (2) secondary care, for conditions with diagnostic ambiguity or prognostic uncertainty and rare disorders with which medical services and the community are uncomfortable (examples may include trisomy 18 and complex congenital cardiac defects), and (3) tertiary care, which includes more complex situations that may require fetal interventions and trials of therapies.

Introduction

The provision of end-of-life (EOL) palliative care to critically ill fetuses or newborn infants is difficult for both the families and the care providers. In many infants, the need for EOL care may arise suddenly, following a catastrophic change in condition or following a complication. In extremely premature infants with a difficult clinical course, the transition to palliative care may be gradual as more organ-specific complications are recognized. In these two groups, bereavement is a distinct phase. The situation may be more complex in a third group, who may have short phases of curing and healing that bring joy, such as infants with difficult-to-treat genetic conditions, but these phases may be mixed with periods when the baseline diagnosis again becomes prominent and brings resignation (Fig. 90.1). In other lines of thinking, the temporal course has been considered to be primary variable (Fig. 90.2). There has also been some recognition of the epochs of EOL care (Fig. 90.3).

One of the primary goals of EOL care is controlling distressing symptoms. Both clinician and parental perception of adequate control of symptoms including pain, agitation, and air hunger is a central component of the EOL experience. However, the newborn patient population poses unique challenges to symptom palliation, because infants are nonverbal and symptoms may present differently than in older patients (Fig. 90.4). There is limited research in the assessment of many symptoms, such as delirium and air hunger, whereas other symptoms, such as pain, have a multitude of measures. Numerous pain scales exist, and most use both a physiologic and a behavioral assessment that might be characterized as subjective.[1] For other symptoms, the lack of widely accepted and validated assessment measures may cause clinicians to be less confident or aggressive in their management of symptoms such as agitation, delirium, or air hunger. However, professionals in the healing arts have an ethical and moral responsibility to alleviate suffering. Hence, despite these challenges, it remains the responsibility of the treatment team to minimize, and to alleviate as much as possible, neonatal patient suffering. This chapter will present interventions, both pharmacologic and nonpharmacologic, that can optimize comfort during the EOL period.

Although many of these therapies have overlapping indications for curative interventions, the focus of this chapter will be to outline management of the symptoms frequently experienced by infants in the EOL period. As with most comfort-focused care plans, all interventions should be considered in the context of the family's goals and wishes for the child.

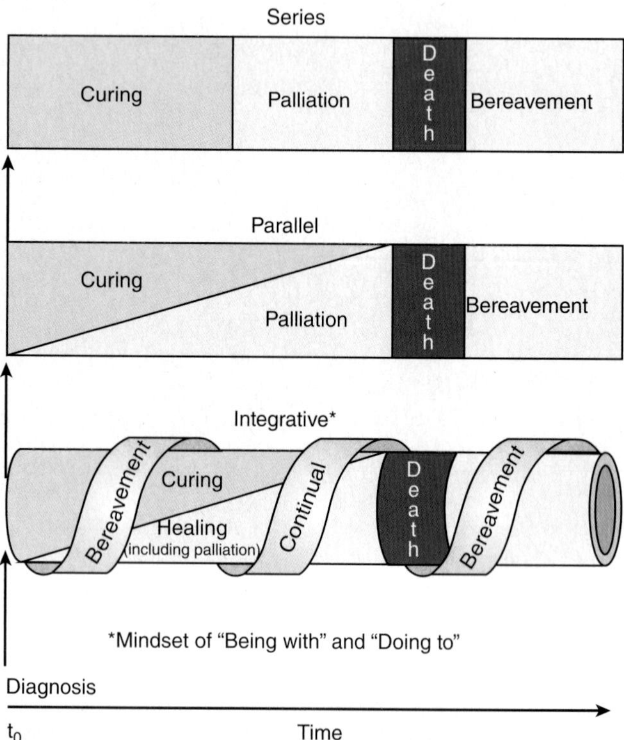

Fig. 90.1 Various Models for Providing Palliative Care. (Reproduced after modifications from Cortezzo and Carter. Palliative care. *Avery's Diseases of the Newborn*, 35, 446–452.e2.)

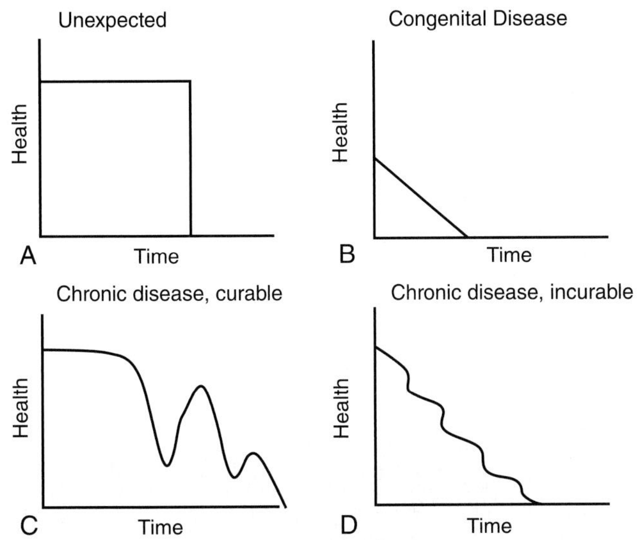

Fig. 90.2 Death Trajectories in Neonatal Intensive Care Units. Although losing a baby is always a tragedy, death can follow several different trajectories: (A) sudden, unexpected death, (B) death from a lethal congenital anomaly, (C) death from a potentially curable disease, and (D) death from chronic, terminal disease. (Reproduced after modifications from Basu RK. End-of-life care in pediatrics. *Pediatr Clin N Am.* 2013;60:725–739.)

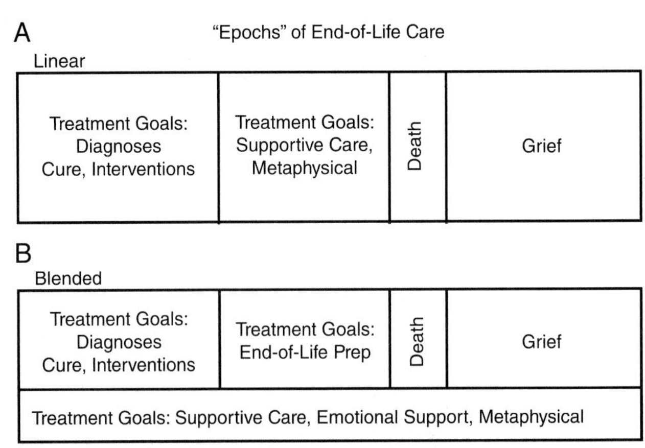

Fig. 90.3 Epochs of End-of-Life Care Can Change Care Delivery. In the intensive care unit, treatment goals do not easily fit a linear construct (A) where treatment goals fit into distinct "epochs." A more realistic and appropriate care construct is blended (B), where treatment directed at cure and supportive care are intertwined throughout the entire period of a child's dying process. (Reproduced after modifications from Basu RK. End-of-life care in pediatrics. *Pediatr Clin N Am.* 2013;60:725–739.)

Palliative Care Time Line
Care directed at underlying illness and physical, emotional, social, and spiritual needs of the child and family
End-of-life care
Grief Care
Enhancing quality of life and death
Finding comfort, meaning, and support

Fig. 90.4 Palliative Care Encompasses the Entire Duration of the Dying Process. Palliative care should start early if needed. If disease progresses and the focus of medical treatment needs to shift, the goals of palliative care should be directed toward comforting the infants and family. The care needs to continue after death. (Reproduced after modifications from Basu RK. End-of-life care in pediatrics. *Pediatr Clin N Am.* 2013; 60:725–739.)

Pain

Aggressive treatment of pain in the dying neonate may make some caregivers uncomfortable. Given the multitude of modalities to address pain, leaving it untreated is ethically indefensible, especially in the EOL setting. Historically, there were incorrect or incomplete understandings of how newborns experienced of pain.[2] It was not until the 1980s that the medical field had a major paradigm shift to acknowledge and subsequently treat neonatal pain. Despite the now well-accepted understanding of neonatal pain, there remain concerns that pain is still inconsistently treated, including in the EOL period.[3] Contributing to this inconsistent treatment or undertreatment of pain at the EOL may be a concern that achieving adequate pain control may hasten death. However, evidence demonstrates that infants with adequate pain control live longer than do those with uncontrolled pain and agitation.[4] Additionally, there is evidence that exposure to analgesic and anxiolytic medications in infants who die in intensive care units has increased significantly during the past 15 years.[5] Treatment of pain is a vital component of a palliative care plan.

The first step in achieving adequate pain control is determining how to assess pain. Recent studies evaluating pain scales in the neonatal palliative care population found that there is not sufficient evidence to conclude that one scale is superior to others.[1,6] The importance of using the same scale consistently, with frequent assessment and documentation, has been well described. Tables 90.1 and 90.2

Table 90.1 Common Pain Assessment Tools Used in Neonates

Assessment Tool	Indicators	Gestational Age (wk)
Neonatal Facial Coding System (NFCS)	Brow lowering Eye squeeze Nasolabial furrowing Lip opening Vertical mouth stretch Horizontal mouth stretch Taut tongue Chin quiver Lip pursing	24–32
Premature Infant Pain Profile (PIPP)	Gestational age Behavioral state Maximum heart rate Percentage decrease in O_2 saturation Brow bulge Eye squeeze Nasolabial furrowing	28–40
Neonatal Pain Agitation and Sedation Scale (NPASS)	Crying Behavioral state Facial expressions Extremities/ton Vital signs	23–40
Behavioral Indicators of Infant Pain (BIIP)	Behavioral state Facial expressions Hand movements	24–32
Douleur Aiguë du Nouveau-né (DAN)	Facial movements Limb movements Vocal expressions	24–41
Premature Infant Pain Profile-Revised (PIPP-R)	Maximum heart rate Percentage decrease in O_2 sat Brow bulge Eye squeeze Nasolabial furrowing Gestational age and behavioral state	25–40
Faceless Acute Neonatal Pain Scale (FANS)	Change in heart rate Bradycardia, desaturation (acute discomfort) Limb movements Vocal expressions	30–35
Neonatal Infant Pain Scale (NIPS)	Facial expressions Crying Breathing patterns Arm movements Leg movements State of arousal	26–47
Crying Requires Increased Oxygen Administration, Increased Vital Signs, Expression, Sleeplessness (CRIES)	Crying Fio_2 requirement Increased blood pressure and heart rate Facial expressions Sleep state	32–60
COMFORTneo	Alertness Calmness/agitation Respiratory response (ventilated patients) Crying (spontaneously breathing patients) Body movement Facial tension Body muscle tone	24.6–42.6
COVERS Neonatal Pain Scale	Crying Fio_2 requirement Vital signs Facial expressions Resting state Body movement	27–40
Pain Assessment in Neonates (PAIN)	Crying Breathing patterns Extremity movement State of arousal Fio_2 requirement Increase in heart rate	26–47
Pain Assessment Tool (PAT)	Posture/tone Crying Sleep pattern Facial expressions Heart rate O_2 saturation Blood pressure Nurse perception	27–40
Scale for Use in Newborns (SUN)	CNS state Breathing patterns Movement Tone Facial expressions Heart rate Blood pressure	24–40
Echelle Douleur Inconfort Nouveau-né (EDIN)	Facial activity Body movement Quality of sleep Quality of contact with nurses Consolability	25–36
Bernese Pain Scale for Neonates (BPSN)	Alertness Duration of crying Time to calm Skin color Eyebrow bulge with eye squeeze Posture/tone Breathing patterns	27–41

CNS, Central nervous system.

Table 90.2 Comparison of Indicated Use for Neonatal Pain Assessments

Scale	Acute Pain	Prolonged Pain	Postoperative Pain	Level of Sedation
NFCS	X	X	X	
PIPP	X			
PIPP-R	X			
NPASS	X	X		X
BIIP	X			
DAN	X*			
FANS	X			
NIPS	X		X	
CRIES		X	X	
COMFORTNeo		X		X
COVERS	X			
PAIN	X			
PAT		X		
SUN	X			
EDIN		X		
BPSN	X			

BIIP, Behavioral Indicators of Infant Pain; *BPSN*, Bernese Pain Scale for Neonates; *COVERS*, COVERS Neonatal Pain Scale; *CRIES*, Crying Requires Increased Oxygen Administration, Increased Vital Signs, Expression, Sleeplessness; *DAN*, Douleur Aiguë de Nouveau-né; *EDIN*, Echelle Douleur Inconfort Nouveau-né; *FANS*, Faceless Acute Neonatal Pain Scale; *NFCS*, Neonatal Facial Coding System; *NIPS*, Neonatal Infant Pain Scale; *NPASS*, Neonatal Pain Agitation and Sedation Scale; *PAIN*, Pain Assessment in Neonates; *PAT*, Pain Assessment Tool; *PIPP*, Premature Infant Pain Profile; *PIPP-R*, Premature Infant Pain Profile-Revised; *SUN*, Scale for Use in Newborns.

are compiled from numerous published references that outline pain assessment tools for neonates.[1]

Opioids

The opioid class of medications has been used worldwide for the treatment of pain. These medications bind to opioid receptors (mu, kappa, delta, and sigma) in the central nervous system and can act in a variety of ways including as agonists, antagonists, mixed agonist-antagonists, or partial agonists.

Clinicians in the neonatal intensive care unit (NICU) and other EOL settings are likely familiar with the administration of opioids to achieve pain control in the newborn patient—most notably morphine and fentanyl. In addition to the choice of specific medication, the dose, route of administration, and attention to potential adverse effects require attention. In EOL circumstances, traditional and convenient intravenous routes of administration such as central lines or peripheral intravenous lines (IVs) may have been removed to allow for a more natural death. The benefit and need for pain control may merit discussion of maintaining IV access. However, there are alternative dosing routes, including oral/buccal, enteral, and intranasal, that may allow for continued pain control without the need for an IV.

Fentanyl is roughly 100 times more potent than morphine, with a shorter onset of action and shorter half-life. Fentanyl is only available in IV and intranasal routes. Although evidence is limited, intranasal fentanyl appears to be effective and safe in achieving pain control in the newborn.[7] There is a known risk of chest wall rigidity with fentanyl, occurring in $<10\%$ of patients and seen with large bolus doses that are rapidly administered.[8] Additionally, increased frequency of apneas may occur with a bolus compared with continuous dosing of fentanyl.[9]

Morphine is widely used in palliative care across all patient populations and remains an excellent choice in the EOL setting because it is widely available, economically favorable, and can be administered enterally or parenterally. Continuous morphine infusion may increase the risk of a patient developing hyperalgesia, myoclonic movements, or pruritus, which can increase distress in the EOL period.[10] If hyperalgesia is suspected or there is continued or increased pain despite escalating doses of morphine, opioid rotation should be considered in addition to concomitant treatment with clonidine.[11] Hydromorphone may be an acceptable and available alternative.

Respiratory depression is a potential adverse effect of all opioid medications, but evidence indicates that this occurs less frequently with morphine than fentanyl. Multiple studies have shown that morphine administration is not likely to hasten patient death.[12,13] Additionally, opioids have a known potential to increase sedation, which may be desirable in the EOL setting. Literature suggests that morphine remains an excellent choice for pain control in the neonatal patient population because it may alleviate additional symptoms such as dyspnea.

Clear communication regarding the potential for respiratory depression and sedation should be maintained between the medical team (physicians, nurses, trainees, etc.) and the family when prescribing opioids. This may be most likely with an escalation of opioid dosing, the use of two opioids at the same time, or the concomitant use of other adjunctive medications such as benzodiazepines or barbiturates in managing pain, anxiety, or seizures, because these all can result in respiratory depression. The ethical principle of double effect is often applicable here, where the intention to treat pain may have foreseeable but undesirable effects.[14] This doctrine allows for aggressive management of symptoms even to the point of sedation, respiratory depression, or death, with the understanding that these "side effects" are not the intention. If traditionally accepted treatment methods are not adequately relieving the symptoms, higher doses and/or addition of secondary agents should be considered. The goal of escalating medications in such scenarios must be to minimize unrelenting suffering rather than to hasten death. Some practitioners remain uncomfortable with this, even in the EOL setting. Regardless, it remains important to families for their child to not experience pain during the dying process. Therefore, if the goal is to minimize suffering in the dying patient, subsequent, unintended respiratory depression is ethically permissible.

Additional Medications for Pain Control

Benzodiazepines can be used in conjunction with opioids to improve pain control. Midazolam and lorazepam are frequently used in this newborn population, particularly in the EOL setting. In addition to pain control, these medications can reduce agitation and anxiety, although validated means of measuring these symptoms are not readily available for the neonatal population. It is noteworthy that a relatively high number of neonates (up to 10%) receiving benzodiazepines might experience myoclonic jerking.[15] This may be related to neurologic immaturity or ischemic injury. Benzodiazepines should not be used as a single agent for pain control but are a good adjunct to opioid medications. Additionally, they can be administered in a variety of routes, making them desirable in the EOL setting. Intranasal midazolam can also be used to aid in seizure control, which may be a concern in some patients.

Barbiturates can also be beneficial for the treatment of anxiety and agitation. Although these drugs (pentobarbital or phenobarbital) are good sedatives, they are not analgesics. Their role in neonatal EOL care will be discussed later in this chapter.

Dexmedetomidine and propofol have become widely accepted in postoperative and sedation protocols and may be helpful agents in the EOL setting, particularly if opioid-associated respiratory depression is a concern. Dexmedetomidine requires intravenous access and has a relatively short half-life (2 hours). Clonidine, like dexmedetomidine, is an alpha-2 agonist. It has been used to aid in weaning patients off pain and sedation medications.[16] Its use in pediatric EOL care is not yet well described in the literature. Propofol can be administered intranasally or intravenously. In limited studies there has been notable variability in response to bolus dosing.[17] Unfortunately, no studies to date have been performed regarding the use of dexmedetomidine or propofol in the EOL setting, so no specific recommendations can be made at this time.

When considering pain management, the source and the type of pain should be considered. Specifically, neuropathic pain requires medications that work through a different mechanism than the antinociception opioid medications already discussed. One of the most commonly used medications in this arena is gabapentin, a gamma-aminobutyric acid analog thought to inhibit pain via voltage-dependent calcium ion channels in the central nervous system. Gabapentin has been demonstrated to reduce opioid and sedative medication use.[18] This medication can be particularly useful in infants with neuro-irritability, chronic pain, and suspected viscera-hyperalgesia. Additionally, a recent study has demonstrated the effectiveness of gabapentin as an adjunct to morphine, yielding improved pain control compared with the use of morphine alone in pediatric patients.[19] Gabapentin has a relatively low side-effect profile, and dosing can be escalated quickly. There is potential for withdrawal, although this has not been well studied in the newborn population.

Acetaminophen may be used orally or rectally for mild-to-moderate pain or as an antipyretic in the EOL period. There is evidence that IV paracetamol (the prodrug of acetaminophen) is an effective opioid adjunct in the postoperative management of neonatal pain.[20] Data on use of nonsteroidal antiinflammatory drugs (e.g., ibuprofen, naproxen) at the EOL in the newborn population remain lacking.

Ketamine has garnered attention in recent years. It has multiple desirable properties including anxiolysis, analgesia, and amnesia. To date, it has not been routinely used or well studied in the EOL setting in neonates. Typically, it is administered via IV, although there is emerging evidence of its efficacy when administered intranasally.[21,22]

There are a multitude of nonpharmacologic interventions that can and should be used to minimize pain in the EOL period. These will be discussed in a later section of this chapter, because in addition to treating pain, the majority of these are used to mitigate generalized suffering.

Nonpain Symptoms

Anxiety and Agitation

A great deal of anxiety and agitation in the EOL context can be mitigated by achieving adequate pain control and minimizing noxious or invasive interventions. These symptoms can be related to pain but have also been recognized as individual symptoms meriting additional interventions beyond pain control. As seen in the pain scales discussed above, many symptoms include agitation as a component. For intubated patients, security of the airway, suctioning of secretions, and appropriate depth of the endotracheal tube are all fundamental assessments that merit attention and correction before using medication. Similarly, environmental stimuli should be reduced. In the NICU this often includes a reduction in laboratory testing (heel pricks, phlebotomy, or arterial sticks), imaging studies, and exposure to bright light and noise. As discussed in the previous section on pain, benzodiazepines are the most commonly used medications in this context. This class of drugs reduces anxiety and effects muscle relaxation through the central nervous system, thereby reducing agitation, and in reducing these phenomena, these drugs reduce the augmentation or potentiation of pain. However, nonpharmacologic measures should also be employed (see the subsequent section).

Additionally, barbiturates have been used historically in the NICU to treat agitation and seizures. Phenobarbital has not been studied in the EOL context and may be less desirable for acute symptom management due to its long half-life, making dose adjustment difficult. Pentobarbital can be given orally or intravenously; it demonstrates more profound effects than phenobarbital and is shorter acting. Pentobarbital administration may cause some practitioners unease due to its historical use in euthanasia protocols. Clear and consistent communication about pentobarbital's indication for use, as well as frequent monitoring, should be used, and there should be a shared understanding and agreement for its rationale by caregivers and families. Lastly, barbiturates have been demonstrated to be effective as a sole agent for sedation in some patients in whom tolerance to opioids and benzodiazepines has developed after long-term use.[23,24]

Delirium

Delirium is becoming an increasingly recognized symptom of patients in the NICU. The Cornell Assessment of Pediatric Delirium can be used in the neonatal population and is tied to developmental "anchor points" that can be used in infants.[25] Harris et al. described the overlap between delirium, pain, and other potential contributing and compounding factors in their European Society of Paediatric and Neonatal Intensive Care (ESPNIC) position statement in 2016.[26] The most common signs of pain in infants include tachycardia, tachypnea, vigorous body movements, increased muscle tension, and inconsolable crying. Other patients may show agitation, inconsolability, and altered sleep-wake cycle. Delirium is associated most frequently with lethargy and altered consciousness. Drug withdrawal may manifest with tremors, fever, sweating, and in some infants, persistent vomiting and/or diarrhea.

Although literature evidence specific to the neonatal population is scant, assessment tools and treatments used for infants in the pediatric or pediatric cardiac ICU may be helpful, and delirium should be considered and consultation with pediatric psychiatry sought. This may be especially true when an older infant in the NICU (e.g., 2 months of age or older) who has been on assisted ventilation for a lengthy time or has been a surgical patient is demonstrating symptoms despite the use of opioids and benzodiazepines.[27–29] The use of dexmedetomidine in infants requiring cardiac surgery does not minimize delirium in that population.[30] Although not well described in randomized controlled trials or comparative effectiveness studies in the neonatology literature, there is some evidence indicating effective treatment of neonatal delirium with haloperidol or atypical antipsychotic drugs such as risperidone or quetiapine.[27,29–31] In addition to neuroleptic initiation, attempts to improve delirium typically include weaning from continuous infusions of benzodiazepines and opioids and transitioning to lower doses of sedation and analgesic agents in bolus dosing.

Dyspnea

"Air hunger" is a common symptom of concern in EOL across the age spectrum. NICU patients at risk of dyspnea include those who are ventilator dependent. Although a curative plan of care is in place, the mainstay of treatment for dyspnea is to provide additional respiratory support while balancing the risks of oxygen exposure. The patient most likely to need medical dyspnea symptom management is the actively dying neonate, especially one who has been managed on positive pressure or has had an fraction of inspired oxygen (FiO_2) of >0.40 for a lengthy period. The approach to treatment in the newborn population is similar to that for older patients. Opioid medications remain the mainstay of treatment for dyspnea in the dying newborn. In addition to the opioid medications already discussed here, intranasal fentanyl offers quick onset and does not require IV access. Sublingual morphine can also be used for dyspnea, but there are some concerns for adequate absorption, and the time to absorption can be greater than 2 hours. Prompt relief of air hunger is desirable and should be pursued. Like most facets of symptom management at the end of a newborn's life, additional research would be beneficial.

Sialorrhea

Secretions can be problematic and cause a "death rattle" that is distressing to families and loved ones of a dying neonate. Deep suctioning can be traumatic to patients, but alleviation of some secretions through clinician or parental oral and pharyngeal suctioning is acceptable. In older pediatric patients, atropine drops administered sublingually have been shown to effectively decrease secretions,[32] and transdermal scopolamine is frequently used in the adult hospice population.[33] However, neither of these has been studied in the newborn population, and therefore they have not been accepted into common practice.

Myoclonus

Myoclonic jerking may occur in the neonate as a result of hypoxic ischemic brain damage or an immature central nervous system or as a side effect from another medication that is being used in the treatment of agitation or pain—frequently opioids, most classically morphine. Myoclonus can be a distressing symptom, particularly to family members of infants at the EOL. Management should be focused on reversing the underlying cause if possible, i.e., stopping medications that may contribute to myoclonic jerking. If the jerking is not determined to be the side effect of a medication, discussion with the family and reassurance may be helpful. Avoid using neuromuscular blocking agents simply to mask myoclonus, because this only introduces additional concerns, including a need for complete ventilator support (and again, this may make some clinicians uneasy because this class of agents has been used in euthanasia).

Seizures

If a patient is known to have an underlying seizure disorder, any established anticonvulsant medications should be continued. Hypoxia at the EOL may result in seizures, and maintaining a route to easily administer additional anticonvulsant medications may be desirable. Although any uncontrolled symptom can be difficult to witness in a dying child, seizures are particularly distressing for families. This is likely due to the physical manifestations of convulsing as visible evidence of suffering. As previously mentioned, some benzodiazepines including lorazepam and midazolam are frequently used as pain adjuncts and anxiolytics at the EOL. These conceivably may also aid in seizure control, because both have been used for refractory seizures in the critically ill neonate. Midazolam has also been studied in the palliative care setting.[34]

Nonpharmacologic Interventions

Although medical management is extremely valuable in the relief of symptoms, nonpharmacologic interventions for pain and anxiolysis are effective and convenient and may be considered primary interventions from which to start. They are safe and often allow for less "technical" interventions—allowing family caregivers to contribute to the care and management of their loved one at the EOL. Interventions that have been studied and shown to reduce pain in neonates in the ICU include facilitated tuck/swaddling, skin to skin (also called kangaroo care), holding, sucrose administration, massage, breastfeeding, and nonnutritive sucking.[35,36] A recent study demonstrated decreased pain scores in infants exposed to the diffused odor of their mother's breast milk.[37] The majority of these interventions have been studied in procedural pain, and extensive literature in the palliative care context does not exist. However, because of the high potential for benefit with minimal to no risk, it may be reasonable to recommend any or all of these to aid in comfort at a neonate's EOL. Studies have demonstrated that parents recognize the environment as an important component of the EOL experience, both positive and negative.[38] Having family rooms, spaces for parents to sleep, etc. were shown to be positive associations. Bright lights, noise, and technology were suggested to be negative associations. Parents of a dying infant should be allowed and encouraged to hold their child, skin to skin or swaddled as desired, and incorporate comforting touch, soothing sounds, and suckling. Notably, parents also express that the location of death was not as important as the people who were present for the death of their child.

Symptom Management in the Actively Dying Neonate

The circumstances surrounding the actively dying infant require special consideration. There should be efforts made, ideally prior to the final days or hours of a child's life, to determine the family's goals, hopes, and wishes for the dying process. Helping families achieve these goals may require a skilled interdisciplinary team. Healthcare professionals who work in the NICU typically have experience and some training in EOL management. However, when there are symptoms that are difficult to control, when there is distress among the medical team and/or family, or when additional support is needed, subspecialty consultation can be beneficial. For example, if medications that are considered the standard of care for management of newborn distress are insufficient for pain/symptom control and additional agents are being considered, pain management or palliative care teams may be helpful. Some families may desire religious rituals to be performed, photographs taken, and many other important experiences. Medical management and adequate symptom control play an important role in creating a peaceful environment for the EOL.

To help facilitate the appropriate environment for the dying process, unnecessary procedures and interventions such as lab draws and monitoring of vital signs should be reduced. These can cause additional patient pain, exacerbate symptoms, and contribute to caregiver distress (both parents and staff). Additional considerations should include the location of death (in the NICU or a rooming-in room, on a hospital ward, in a palliative care suite, or at home), understanding that there may be specific circumstances, logistics, or safety concerns that affect each of these choices. It is typically very comforting for both the baby and family to allow patient holding, but this too may require special or unique considerations to respect safety and minimize any associated decompensation during the process.

As the EOL approaches, it is the responsibility of the healthcare team to provide continual assessment and management of the patient's and family's needs. Informed clinicians should strive for open communication and can both lead and partner with parents in advocating for adequate symptom management. Additionally, these clinicians can provide anticipatory guidance about the dying process, including decreasing tone, perfusion, and temperature; changes in color; waning responsiveness; and changes in the respiratory pattern. The progression to death may also be impacted by the need to withdraw life-supporting medical technology. Clinicians should be prepared to counsel families on how each step of procedures and removal of medical equipment and devices will impact the patient and any expected changes that may be observed.

Conclusion

The death of a neonate is always a tragedy. Similarly distressing are uncontrolled symptoms, particularly in this exceptionally vulnerable population. It is the goal of the medical team, including NICU staff and subspecialty teams, to provide care to these patients even through their deaths by minimizing suffering and maximizing comfort. This chapter has laid out a variety of pharmacologic and nonpharmacologic interventions that should be considered and used in the NICU when a patient is receiving palliative care and particularly in the period surrounding the EOL.

CHAPTER 91

Palliative Care Family Support in Neonatology

Erin R. Currie, Hema Navaneethan, Meaghann S. Weaver

KEY POINTS

1. Neonatal intensive care unit (NICU) admission rates have increased over time, with a consequent increase in the number of extremely premature and critically ill infants who are at risk of chronic illness and mortality.
2. The death of an infant is one of the most devastating and difficult experiences in life. Parents of seriously ill infants bear many roles such as caregiver, advocate, and decision-maker while maintaining hope and managing uncertainty related to their infant's prognosis.
3. Palliative care requires interdisciplinary specialty groups who seek to work with seriously ill infants and their families to provide comprehensive treatment of suffering.
4. Families' spiritual needs to be considered. End-of-life care is extremely important to bereaved NICU parents as they cling to the limited memories of their deceased infant.
5. Family bereavement supports may include individual/family counseling, spiritual support, efforts to encourage verbal and/or nonverbal expression in parent groups, family camps, longitudinal staff remembrances, and follow-up meetings.

In this chapter we will describe the evidence for palliative care family support beginning in the prenatal period and extending to acute and chronic neonatal intensive care unit (NICU) care and finally to bereavement. Neonatal providers have the unique opportunity to improve family-centered care for patients and families experiencing serious illness in the NICU and to make a long-term impact on NICU families' lives (Fig. 91.1). For infants who do not survive, neonatal providers may improve the care leading up to death and affect parent grief experiences by facilitating an interdisciplinary palliative approach and supporting families to create meaningful and positive memories despite the limitations of an intensive care unit (ICU) environment. However, there are challenges to implementing this palliative approach and providing care that is concordant with family wishes (Fig. 91.2). Perinatal palliative care (PPC) as an additional layer of family support is often delayed until death is imminent, preventing families from experiencing the full range of this layer of support. Beginning with a fetal diagnosis, families require intensive support given the extremely difficult decisions they must make in the event of a life-limiting or life-threatening diagnosis. During a NICU hospitalization, the infant's state of clinical uncertainty and unknown survival makes decision-making very difficult for families, and they require intensive support to balance their new identity as a "NICU parent" with life and other demands outside of the hospital. Medical advancements have decreased the number of perinatal and infant deaths over time; however, there are now more infants surviving with chronic critical illness, and families continue to require support as their goals of care shift.

Prenatal Phase

Clinical Case Report

Cynthia is a 26-year-old woman from Mississippi who is pregnant with her third child. Cynthia and the child's father are no longer together; the father of the baby is involved but lives in another city 45 minutes away. Cynthia currently lives in a small town and travels nearly 2 hours to the nearest tertiary care hospital for the majority of her medical care.

Cynthia arrives at her 20-week ultrasound appointment. During the ultrasound, Cynthia can tell something is wrong. Her worries are confirmed when she and her mother are unexpectedly asked to meet with a maternal-fetal medicine specialist after the ultrasound. Cynthia is heartbroken as she learns her baby, a boy, has multiple congenital malformations. Although the maternal-fetal medicine specialist states that additional testing is needed, she explains to Cynthia that she will likely have difficult decisions to make soon. The specialist predicts the fetus may survive until delivery, but it is unclear how long he may survive after birth. If he

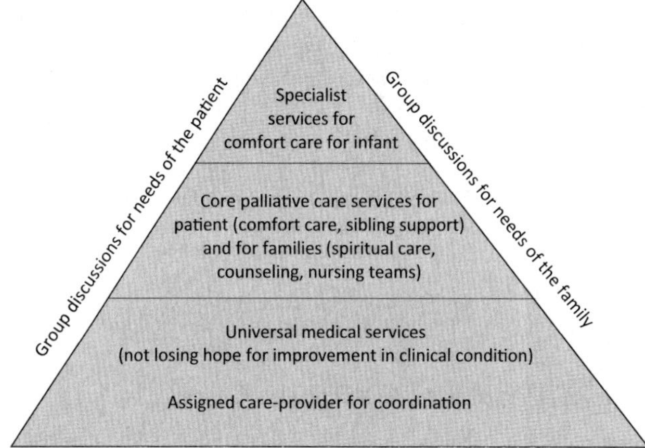

Fig. 91.1 Care of Critically Ill Infants and Their Families. Support for patients and families should be integrated with ongoing medical care.

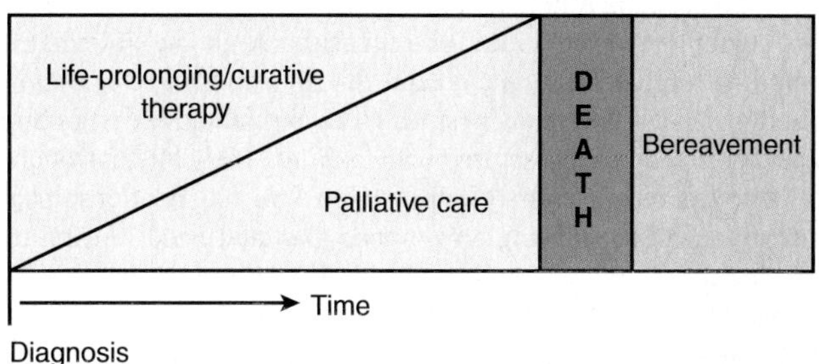

Fig. 91.2 Current Accepted Model for Care of Infants at Serious Risk of Mortality. (Reproduced with permission and modifications from Natbony. Palliative care. In: *Harriet Lane Handbook*, ch. 23, 566–573.e1.)

survives, the specialist worries he will never breathe on his own and will have severe delays in development. The specialist shares with Cynthia that there are multiple care pathways to consider at this time, but given the severity of the anomalies, she encourages Cynthia to think about termination of the pregnancy.

Cynthia is overcome with sadness and grief. Cynthia has a strong faith tradition and fears judgment for even considering termination of the pregnancy. She is torn because she also worries her child will not have the quality of life she would want for him. Cynthia is left feeling completely overwhelmed and is unsure how to proceed.

Epidemiology of Perinatal Death and Parent Outcomes

With advancements in perinatal medicine, perinatal mortality has steadily declined during the past several decades, although it has begun to plateau in more recent years.[1,2] In 2016, the perinatal mortality rate in the United States was 6.0 deaths per 1000 live births.[2] Although there have been overall declines in perinatal mortality rates, a large disparity remains in outcomes related to race and geography. The mortality rate of infants born to non-Hispanic Black women is more than twice that of non-Hispanic White women, and the southern states of Mississippi and Alabama have consistently had worse outcomes than the rest of the country.[2]

It is important to recognize that perinatal loss is a traumatic event with long-lasting parental effects. Gold et al.[3] found that after a perinatal loss, bereaved mothers had four times higher odds of depressive symptoms and seven times higher odds of posttraumatic stress disorder symptoms. Although no differences in symptom levels were noted among races, disparities in treatment were noted. African American mothers who screened positive for posttraumatic stress disorder or depression were much less likely to receive treatment.[3] Perinatal loss also affects the marital dyad. Couples who had stillbirths were at higher risk of dissolution of their relationship in the decade following the death compared with those who did not have a fetal loss.[3]

In 2017, congenital malformations were the most common cause of infant mortality in the United States.[4] Many advancements in perinatal medicine have led to earlier and more accurate fetal diagnoses. Although these early forms of screening can provide families and clinicians with beneficial information regarding the health of the mother and fetus, parents are often not prepared for a potentially life-threatening or life-limiting diagnosis for their child.[6]

Role of Perinatal Palliative Care

Parents who have received news of a life-limiting or life-threatening fetal diagnosis describe "grieving multiple losses," including the loss of their healthy baby, the loss of a normal pregnancy, and the loss of future parenting.[7] After the diagnosis of a life-limiting or life-threatening fetal diagnosis, the American College of Obstetricians and Gynecologists committee on ethics and the American Academy of Pediatrics committee on bioethics recommend that the "full range of options, including fetal intervention, postnatal therapy, palliative care or pregnancy termination" be discussed with families.[8] Early PPC, introduced at the time of diagnosis, may help develop a trusting relationship and can guide decision-making and support parental needs during this complex time. PPC brings the interdisciplinary approach into the prenatal period and the immediate postnatal period (see Fig. 91.1). An interdisciplinary approach is vital to palliative care principles and should be integrated throughout the care of the patient and family.[5,6] For example, social workers often work with the PPC team to identify financial or counseling resources, child life specialists can assist with preparing siblings for the birth and possibly death of a newborn, and lactation specialists may assist the mothers with either weaning off of breast milk or donating their breast milk.

Spiritual and Cultural Considerations

A family's spiritual needs and wishes should be considered at all points in care. Parents may struggle with existential questions after the diagnosis of a life-limiting condition. In a study evaluating values applied to parental decision-making in delivery room resuscitations, family decision-making was largely steered by religion, spirituality, and hope as opposed to the medical information presented.[7] Wishes for spiritual or cultural rituals should be coordinated whenever possible. The care team should be aware of any culture-specific customs or practices and honor them whenever able.[7,8]

Communication

After news of a life-limiting or life-threatening diagnosis, parents are often forced to make difficult and often time-sensitive decisions regarding multiple aspects of care for their child. Communication and information delivery during this prenatal time is crucial. In a study of 19 families given the prenatal diagnosis of trisomy 18, the majority of parents felt they were not appropriately informed about the potential diagnosis during the screening process and believed ultrasound findings were poorly communicated.[9] From the same study, empathic communication was found to be essential in parents' overall satisfaction with care.[9] It is important to recognize that a family's communication needs may vary. Whereas some families may choose to seek out additional information regarding the diagnosis, others may avoid it as a method of coping.[10] Dialogue with parents about their preferred communication styles and approach to receiving information is important in making sure parental needs are being met.

Prenatal consultation with neonatologists provides parents with the opportunity to discuss care and talk through decisions specific to their child and family. Miquel-Verges et al. conducted interviews with 22 women after a diagnosis of congenital anomalies and discovered parents valued five major themes in prenatal consultation.[11] Parents valued the opportunity to feel prepared, have a knowledgeable physician, have a caring physician, have the opportunity to allow hope, and spend time with the physician. Parents also felt touring the NICU beforehand equipped them with additional knowledge and helped them feel more prepared for a transition to NICU care.[12]

Prenatal Decisions: Termination, Imaging, Monitoring

After a discussion of possible options, some parents face the difficult decision of continuation or termination of the pregnancy. In a study by Breeze et al., the median time for parents to decide on termination or continuation of pregnancy was 1.5 days (range, 0–8 days), illustrating the urgent nature in which this decision must sometimes be made.[12] Parents' decision to continue or terminate a pregnancy may be multifactorial. In a study by Guon et al. of 332 parents who chose continuation of pregnancy in the setting of a trisomy 13 or trisomy 18 diagnosis, themes of moral beliefs and child-centered reasons such as love for their child, the value of their child, and uncertain outcomes affected their decision to continue the pregnancy.[13] Families who choose continuation of pregnancy often hear messaging to terminate the pregnancy or face feeling unsupported by their medical team.[14]

Ongoing maternal and fetal care, including potential interventions and monitoring, should be discussed and individualized to facilitate plans matching parental goals.[15] Offering families routine fetal surveillance may provide reassurance and add a sense of normalcy to the pregnancy.[15] Routine surveillance and standardized testing such as ultrasounds can also promote memory-making and bonding. In a qualitative study, seven parents were interviewed who received life-threatening fetal diagnoses, and all parents expressed their desire to hear the fetal heartbeat and see ultrasound images as a chance to "get to know their baby."[16]

Delivery Decisions: Location, Mode, and Infant Care

Parental preferences surrounding intrapartum care should be discussed in conjunction with the obstetrician and neonatologist or pediatrician (see Fig. 91.2). Parents who reported struggling for control over prenatal and delivery options were reported to have lower levels of satisfaction with care.[9] The location of delivery is one component that should be reviewed. Based on parental goals, some families may choose to deliver within their community to be closer to home and familiar supports. Some families may plan for delivery in a larger, tertiary care center with additional access to neonatology and potential life-sustaining measures.[9] The mode of delivery is another key component to be evaluated. Although vaginal delivery has been previously considered the recommended mode of delivery in the setting of a lethal diagnosis, a cesarean section may be considered in some situations. Women may request a cesarean section with the goal of delivering a live infant.[14,15] Parents were noted to be dissatisfied with care in situations where physicians declined to perform a cesarean section when requested at the time of delivery.[9]

Reviewing steps of resuscitation with the family and determining how these potential actions and interventions fit with their goals should be completed prenatally whenever possible. For families planning on a focus on comfort after delivery, it is important to discuss anticipated symptom management needs.[8,15] Plans for memory-making activities such as photographs, hand and foot prints, and molds may also be coordinated prior to delivery when possible. Communication of intrapartum plans should be shared with all members of the care team who may participate in the delivery and provide ongoing care to ensure parental wishes are met.[15]

Ongoing Decisions: The Unexpected and the Uncertain

Recognizing the limitations of prognostication that remain despite technological advancements, preparing families for unexpected outcomes is an important step (Table 91.1). Introducing families to potential decisional points they may face in the future allows parents the opportunity to consider these complex choices in a more controlled setting. This may include reviewing potential ongoing interventions or familial wishes for discharge with hospice support if feasible.[18,19] Diagnosis of a life-limiting or life-threatening prenatal diagnosis forces parents to make complex and often unexpected choices regarding the care of their child. Palliative care provides longitudinal and interdisciplinary support to families and individualized guidance centered on goals of care throughout the decision-making process.[9,11,15,18,19]

Table 91.1 Prenatal Diagnoses in Which Palliative Care Should Be Considered

1. Genetic abnormalities
   a. Trisomy 13, 15, or 18
   b. Triploidy
   c. Thanatophoric dwarfism or lethal forms of osteogenesis imperfecta
   d. Some inborn errors of metabolism
2. Renal abnormalities
   a. Potter's syndrome/renal agenesis with severe lung hypoplasia
   b. Some cases of polycystic kidney disease or renal failure requiring dialysis
3. Central nervous system abnormalities
   a. Anencephaly/acrania
   b. Holoprosencephaly
   c. Some complex or severe cases of meningomyelocele or large encephalocele
   d. Hydranencephaly
   e. Congenital severe hydrocephalus with absent/minimal brain growth
   f. Neurodegenerative diseases requiring ventilation
4. Heart defects
   a. Acardia
   b. Inoperable cardiac anomalies
   c. Hypoplastic left heart syndrome
   d. Ectopia cordis
5. Structural anomalies
   a. Some cases of giant omphalocele
   b. Severe congenital diaphragmatic hernia with lung hypoplasia
   c. Inoperable conjoined twins

From Catlin A, Carter B. Creation of a neonatal end-of-life palliative care protocol. *J Perinatol.* 2002;22(3):184.

Acute Neonatal Intensive Care Phase

Continuation of Clinical Case Report

Cynthia decides to maintain her pregnancy and delivers her baby boy, named Jacob, at 28 weeks' gestation. Upon birth, Jacob's multiple congenital anomalies are confirmed, and he is intubated, stabilized, and transferred 2 hours away to the only specialized children's hospital in the state. During Jacob's first week of life, he is extubated and placed on nasal continuous positive airway pressure, and feedings are started via nasogastric tube. Cynthia is still recovering from childbirth and is relieved that Jacob is stable. However, she is struggling to care for herself, Jacob, and her other two children, who are temporarily staying with her mother 2 hours away. She is on the waiting list for a room at the Ronald McDonald house and is currently residing in the NICU at the bedside. The palliative care team is now involved and is starting to talk to her about her goals of care given Jacob's life-limiting prognosis and the likely need for chronic feeding and respiratory support. On day of life 8, Jacob develops a distended abdomen, and a necrotizing enterocolitis diagnosis is confirmed. His congenital anomalies are now complicated by surgical resection of the bowel and short-gut syndrome. Cynthia was just beginning to accept the reality of a complex, chronic illness and was hopeful to have time at home with Jacob and her family. Now, she is struggling to make decisions given the sudden change in Jacob's clinical course.

NICU Hospitalizations and Infant Death in the United States

NICU admission rates have steadily increased over time.[17] In 2012, there were 77.9 NICU admissions per 1000 live births and a substantial increase in admissions for infants born weighing at least 2500 g. Therefore more and more parents are experiencing the stress of a NICU hospitalization. In 2017 more than 22,000 infants died in the United States, with the majority of infant deaths occurring in an intensive care setting.[18] As with perinatal mortality, there are known racial disparities within infant mortality. Parents of non-Hispanic Black infants were twice as likely to suffer from infant mortality (11.4 per 1000 births) than were parents of non-Hispanic White infants (4.9 per 1000 births).[19] These significant disparities must be addressed in the provision of culturally appropriate palliative and end-of-life care for families in the NICU. Clearly, NICU parents are a growing group within NICU family-centered care who require intensive support throughout a NICU admission.

Parent Experiences and Needs in an Uncertain NICU Environment

NICU patients commonly oscillate between periods of stability and then intense periods of uncertain survival. During the ups and downs of NICU illness trajectories, parents of seriously ill infants bear many roles such as caregiver, advocate, and decision-maker, while maintaining hope and managing uncertainty related to their infant's prognosis.[20,21] Parents of infants in the NICU are heavily burdened psychologically, psychosocially, financially, spiritually, and physically because of the heavy demands associated with caring for a seriously ill infant and maintaining life outside of the NICU.[20] These demands place parents of infants in the NICU at a higher risk for and prevalence of anxiety, depression, stress, acute stress disorder, and posttraumatic stress disorder.[22] Therefore, it is critical to understand how neonatal healthcare providers may better support parents of seriously ill infants, and in particular, those infants and parents who receive end-of-life care.

Parent Support Needs

Parents of seriously ill NICU patients experience unique needs in order to develop their identity as a parent and meaningful memories as a family.[23] Because of the inherent uncertainty in NICU patient survival and discharge to a home setting, NICU providers should optimize the quality of time and provide opportunities for memory making regardless of prognosis. For infants who die in the NICU, these patients and families experience life together within the intensive or acute care setting.[18,24] This presents limitations for parents who wish to involve other children and extended family members in their infant's care, because there are often NICU policies preventing young children or numerous family members from visiting the NICU. Privacy is a priority for parents as they anticipate the death of their infant and wish to make the most of the limited time they have together.[25] If the NICU is an open unit with multiple bed spaces in one room, transferring the patient to a private room where the restrictions on visitors are not as rigid may be an appropriate alternative for inpatient end-of-life care.

Developing and maintaining the parent role in an unnatural setting such as the NICU requires careful consideration and communication from the neonatal medical team.[23] Providing "normal" parenting opportunities through end-of-life care, such as holding the infant and providing hands-on care,is extremely important to bereaved NICU parents as they cling to the limited memories of their infant after death.[20,23] Parents of seriously ill infants prefer communication from healthcare providers that is compassionate, sensitive, kind, sincere, nonjudgmental, and sympathetic to the stresses parents must manage while their infant is hospitalized in the ICU.[25–30] Parents of infants in the NICU also reported the need for healthcare providers to take care of parents during the NICU admission by giving "permission" to leave the bedside and engage in self-care without feeling like a bad parent.[20,28] Outside of the neonatal medical team, bereaved parents have reported friends, family, and religious or community groups as supportive.[20] However, other NICU parents are seen as especially supportive because of the ability to express empathy and seek support from those who "know their road."[20]

Cultural Differences in Parent End-of-Life Experiences

Because of the known racial disparities in perinatal and infant mortality,[4] it is critical to understand cultural preferences in the NICU. Brooten et al.[27] found racial differences in what parents did not find helpful from healthcare providers near their child's death. White and Hispanic parents reported insensitive and nonsupportive staff as the most unhelpful characteristics, whereas Black parents reported conflict between providers and parents as the least helpful.[27] Davies et al.[31] explored the palliative care experiences of Mexican and Chinese American parents and found less optimal patterns of communication, including no information or basic information regarding prognosis of the child's health status. This resulted in parent frustration, anger, and sadness.[31] If interpretation is required, the interpreter must be trained to provide accurate information to the families, even if it is "bad news." Providing honest, compassionate communication to families is essential to build trust between the medical team and the family. Lack of accurate interpretation could result in the perpetuation of cultural barriers and make the already tragic experience worse for these vulnerable parents.

Decision-Making: Central Role for Parents in the NICU

Decision-making is often shared between the parents and neonatal medical team. High-quality communication from the medical team is critical for parents to join in informed, goal-concordant decisions. Parents of infants hospitalized in a NICU preferred straightforward information that was presented in a positive way due to parental beliefs of medical miracles and the importance of maintaining hope in the decision-making process.[30,32] However, the fast-paced clinical changes and urgent nature of decisions make this a difficult process for clinicians and parents. Parents often receive updates and prognostic information in clinician-parent conferences. During these conferences, parents are presented with complex clinical information and sometimes uncertain prognoses.[33]

Conflicts Between the Healthcare Team and Parents

Parents often have different opinions and beliefs about survival of preterm infants than their neonatal providers do. Boulais et al.[34] conducted a study comparing concern for infant mortality among perinatal and neonatal physicians and parents of infants who were discharged alive from the NICU. Physicians believed that parental concern for mortality increased with decreased gestational age.[34] However, parents were just as worried for their infants no matter the gestational age of their infant. [34] Parental concern for mortality was, however, associated with infant length of stay and the documentation of at least one discussion regarding infant mortality with physicians.[34] It is clear that conversations with clinicians have an impact on family understanding; thus the first step to getting families and clinicians on the same page about mortality is to talk about it.

Determining prognostic information in the neonatal population is difficult for providers because they must forecast survival and quality of life without reliable data. However, neonatal providers are tasked with delivering prognostic information to families and predicting the infant's prognosis, short- and long-term outcomes, and quality-of-life issues.[35] Boss et al.[35] recorded and analyzed 16 parent-clinician conferences that discussed "difficult news" (e.g., severe intracranial hemorrhage, cardiopulmonary resuscitation decisions, or genetic diagnoses). Prognostic information was shared in most care conferences, and prognosis discussions were initiated by the provider. However, this prognostic information was delivered broadly rather than as detailed information related to the prognosis. Without detailed information, broad statements may be subject to different interpretations. Also, clinicians in this study explained that less than 25% of the cases discussed had a chance of surviving without serious complications; however, clinicians were twice as likely to be optimistic versus pessimistic when explaining the prognosis to parents. Parents and clinicians often walked away from these care conferences with different interpretations of the infant's prognosis and quality of life, with parents having more of an optimistic view of their infant's survival and quality of life.

Decision-Making at the End-of-Life

Parents describe an infant's death as the most devastating and difficult experience they have faced.[36] Parents may see their infant suffering from invasive procedures that are deemed futile and decide to limit medical treatment, withdraw life-sustaining technology (e.g., compassionate extubation), or use home hospice services. After infant death, parents must decide to see or hold their infant, donate organs, agree to an autopsy, and make funeral arrangements. These end-of-life decisions are particularly stressful, partly because they are often made in a NICU environment with unfamiliar people and noises, little privacy, and impending loss of their identity as a parent and the parent caretaking role.[25] Neonatologists may support parents by offering to discuss the autopsy and organ donation processes with them before a precipitous decision must be made.

Parents often struggle with the "what-ifs" after infant death. That is, parents may report feeling at peace with the death but continue to wonder what the outcome would have been if different interventions were attempted at different times.[20] Brooten et al.[37] explored parents' retrospective reflections on what they had wished was done or not done during their child's death in the NICU or pediatric intensive care unit. Mothers wished to have spent more time with the child, held the child more, and selected a different treatment course. Fathers wished to have spent more time with their child and monitored their child more closely.[37] These regrets emphasize the importance of providing high-quality, supportive communication surrounding decision-making, recognizing the importance of the parent role, and creating meaningful opportunities for parents to develop memories with their infant in the NICU. Neonatologists may also support parents by providing a post-death conference and discussing autopsy reports and the events leading up to their infant's death to clarify any questions and provide an element of clarity to the parents' grief process.[25,28,38,39]

Sources of Support for Parents During End-of-Life Decision Making

Use of a Question Prompt List to Empower Parents

The use of a question prompt list (QPL) in the processes of information gathering and informed decision-making is one strategy to engage parents in informed decision-making and provide goal-concordant care. A QPL is a suggested list of questions for the patient or caregiver that guides communication with the healthcare team. Lemmon et al.[40] developed a QPL for NICU families to use in preparation for clinician-parent care conferences. This QPL was developed using audio-recorded NICU care conferences with parents of infants treated for therapeutic hypothermia and was universally accepted by NICU clinicians and parents.[40] An example QPL item on being a NICU parent is the following: "What is the best way for me to participate when the team makes the plan for the day (rounds)?"[40] Parents who used a QPL found that it was useful and facilitated more prepared answers from their neonatology team.[41] Implementing decision-making supports such as a QPL may empower parents to ask questions that are most important to them during a time when they may be too overwhelmed to develop a list of questions on their own.

Perinatal Palliative Care as an Added Layer of Support in the NICU

Palliative care is an interdisciplinary specialty that aims to provide the best possible quality of life for seriously ill infants and their families and involves comprehensive treatment of suffering.[42] By definition, serious illness is "a health condition that carries a high risk of mortality and either negatively impacts a person's daily function or quality of life, or excessively strains their caregivers."[43] There are three general categories of patients who receive PPC in the NICU: (1) newborns born at the threshold of viability, (2) newborns or infants born with birth anomalies that may threaten vital functions, and (3) newborns or infants who are receiving intensive care but become burdened with interventions that no longer seem beneficial and are instead only prolonging the infant's dying or causing suffering.[44] For infants and their parents to receive the maximum benefit, PPC should be initiated at the time of diagnosis and provided concurrently with curative efforts.[42,45] Early integration of PPC is a great opportunity to build trust with the medical team, and PPC support may assist parents with eliciting goals of care and planning questions and discussions with the neonatal medical team during care conferences. Palliative providers specialize in eliciting care preferences by using excellent communication skills, supporting the decision-making process, managing distressing symptoms, helping to increase the continuity of care, providing family support, and enhancing quality of life in all realms of suffering including physical, spiritual, psychological, and psychosocial suffering.[46] PPC may facilitate the opportunities for parents to make memories with their infant by coordinating resources, eliciting parent preferences for care, aligning care with their preferences, and facilitating cultural rituals that are important to families.

However, PPC is commonly avoided in the NICU or integrated only near the end of life when death is imminent. One common explanation for the avoidance of PPC in the NICU is the misconception that palliative care means giving up on aggressive treatment and transitioning to exclusive end-of-life or comfort care.[20] However, bereaved parents have reported positive experiences with PPC teams before infant death in the NICU. For example, parents wished they had involved the PPC team earlier and more often because the palliative care team acted as a sounding board for their questions and concerns and orchestrated meaningful opportunities for them to create memories with their infant when survival was uncertain.[20] For NICU patients who did receive PPC, PPC teams were most often consulted for communication needs or aligning care with the goals of care and wishes of the family.[47] Neonatologists have reported the value of communication expertise that palliative care providers brought to their complex clinical cases.

Chronic Critical Illness Phase

Continuation of Clinical Case Report

Cynthia has returned to work part-time. She and Baby Jacob's siblings faithfully visit the NICU every weekend because of work schedules and financial hardships associated with the 2-hour commute to the hospital. Baby Jacob is recovering from acute necrotizing enterocolitis. His feeds are through a gastrostomy tube. Due to having undergone multiple bowel surgeries and a subsequent short gut, he receives calories through total parental nutrition in a central line despite multiple attempts to advance to full feeds. Cynthia expresses disappointment that he isn't able to "enjoy eating" or "receive comfort from either breastfeeding or even a bottle." He depends on a tracheostomy with a back-up ventilator rate for respiratory support. Due to the home health nursing shortage in his community, Baby Jacob remains in the hospital setting for his first 11 months of life. Cynthia is struggling with the reality that he may reach his first birthday never having been home. His siblings continue to ask, "When will Baby Jacob come home?"

Table 91.2 Neonatal/Pediatric Chronic Critical Illness (CCI)

Prolonged hospitalization	Hospitalization in an intensive care unit (ICU) for >28 days after term corrected age. In some hospitals, many such infants may be transferred to pediatric intensive care units (PICU) and if so, the hospitalization would be considered prolonged with PICU stays >14 consecutive days. CCI is defined as a history of prolonged ICU stay and/or 2 or more acute care or ICU admissions within 12 months.
Prolonged dependence on technology	Dependence on one or more support systems, including respiratory support with tracheostomy, mechanical ventilation, non-invasive positive-pressure ventilation, or continuous positive airway pressure; feeding assistance through a gastrostomy/jejunostomy; renal replacement therapy; or support for other vital organs.

Epidemiology and Definition of Chronic Critical Illness

Advances in medicine and development of biomedical technology have dramatically shifted the epidemiology of pediatric outcomes in the past 2 to 3 decades.[48] Life-prolonging interventions have resulted in the survival of infants with previously terminal medical conditions. Infants are now surviving with chronic critical illness, often through the support of multiple advanced medical technologies and extended hospitalizations to include intensive-care stays (Table 91.2).[51] Although less than 1% of the United States pediatric population consists of children with medical complexity, this population accounts for as much as one-third of total pediatric healthcare spending and almost half of pediatric hospital charges.[49,50]

Children with medical complexity are noted to be lifelong high users of healthcare, warranting service coordination among multiple subspecialists and interdisciplinary team members. In a recent study quantifying the time invested by multidisciplinary care team members to perform nonreimbursable care coordination activities for children with medical complexity, the median time spent in nonreimbursed care coordination was 2.3 hours (interquartile range, 0.8–6.8 hours) per child per month.[52] This translates into the need for case managers in NICU settings and the need to proactively help families with discharge planning and preparatory care coordination even in a busy NICU setting.

The location of care for children with complex, chronic medical conditions is often limited to inpatient hospital settings or skilled nursing facilities due to gaps in home service provisions. The longitudinal relationships and developmental stimulation deserved by children is often beyond that which is currently offered in biomedical-focused critical care settings.[53] Enabling factors and barriers to the empowerment of home as a feasible care location are listed in Table 91.3. The concept of home as a feasible, viable, and livable location requires "intentional care models."[54]

Lack of home-care nursing was recognized as the most frequent cause of discharge delay for technology-dependent children in hospital settings, "directly accounting for an average length of stay increase of 53.9 days (range: 4–204) and 35.7 days (3–63) for new and existing patients, respectively."[55] Respiratory technology, younger age of the child, and lack of insurance plan coverage are consistently cited as reasons for discharge delays.[55,56] NICU providers and interdisciplinary team members need to prepare families of children with chronic critical illness for potential loss of parental employment due to lack of access to home nursing and long-term hands-on medical needs for children.

Table 91.3 Facilitators and Barriers to Home as a Feasible Care Setting for Children With Chronic, Critical Illness

Facilitators	Barriers
Communication and coordination of healthcare teams across care settings	Gaps in pediatric home health nursing
Early and longitudinal family education and inclusion	Lack of coverage for home-based durable medical supplies and equipment for children
State-supported case management with tangible transition models	Inconsistent family support
Home-based interdisciplinary care services	Care model centralization to inpatient hospital services
Empowerment of general pediatric medical homes	Minimal reimbursement for home-based services

Table 91.4 Model of Exploring Medical Technology's Decisional Impact on Lived Experience

Medical Technology	Lived Experience Inquiries
Central line	1. Family access to a sterile environment for dressing changes 2. Impact on the bathing routine or water play 3. Risk of infection and change in urgency level with fevers when an outpatient
Gastrostomy tube	1. Cultural or familial interpretation of nutrition 2. Implications of the role of food for pleasure and social interaction versus for caloric intake
Tracheostomy with ventilator	1. Escalation of care may shift the child's ability to discharge to a home setting 2. Meaning of the expansion of medical technologies to sustain or maintain life

Early and longitudinal palliative care integration for babies with complex health needs is noted to be formative in decision-making and family support. For a baby such as Jacob, the palliative care team could help the NICU providers with decisional assessment for each escalation of care technology to include informational case management and translation of each decision into the family's "lived experience." Palliative care teams can help extend family-centered care to address sibling, paternal, and grandparent factors.[57,58] An example of a model for decisional impact of escalation of medical technologies is provided as Table 91.4.

Bereavement Phase

Continuation of Clinical Case Report

Baby Jacob is noted to have increased secretions and work of breathing. Cynthia is tearful at his bedside, recognizing Baby Jacob is less alert to her voice and touch. Despite maximal medical management, Baby Jacob continues to worsen, requires more hemodynamic and respiratory support, and is steadily less responsive to provider interventions and to maternal presence. He undergoes a code event. Cynthia, the baby's father, Steven, and Cynthia's mother meet with the palliative care team and decide to compassionately discontinue artificial technologies and allow natural death. Jacob is held by his mother, who is comforted by his grandmother's singing in his hospital room at the time of death. Baby Jacob has never been in his home nursery, so the family brings his nursery bedding to the intensive care unit and his home lamp to surround him with physical reminders of comfort. After Jacob's death, Cynthia struggles to make decisions about an autopsy and the disposition of Jacob's body. She is now planning Jacob's funeral with financial assistance from the hospital pastoral care department. Cynthia is struggling with talking to her surviving children about Jacob's death and adjusting to a new family routine without Jacob.

Bereaved Parent Health Epidemiology

Bereaved parents describe their child's death as a life-changing event.[36] The complex grief process bereaved parents endure places them at risk for poor health. Bereaved parents are at an increased risk for mortality,[59] psychiatric hospitalizations,[60] and morbidity including cancer[61,62] and type 2 diabetes[63] compared with parents who have not lost a child. Parents who lost their only child were at the highest risk for psychiatric hospitalizations.[62] Specifically, parents report frequent acute illness episodes and hospitalization in the first 13 months following an infant/child death in the NICU or pediatric intensive care unit.[64,65] It is critical to acknowledge the grief experiences of bereaved parents of NICU infants and develop effective support to facilitate healthy coping and grief outcomes in this population.

Parent Grief Experiences

Memories from the ICU remain with parents for years after their infants' death[66] and may affect their grief experiences.[67] Thus it is critical to facilitate families' preferences for the sometimes brief moments they have with their infants. Currie et al.[36] conducted a qualitative study exploring parent grief and coping experiences after infant death in the NICU. Parents reported changing levels of grief over time, with grief symptoms waxing and waning in the first year of life and eventually decreasing over time. However, the grief never completely dissipated; rather, the type of emotions and intensity of grief symptoms shifted. Personal growth was also reported and was manifested by new insights that brought positive meaning to their lives. Some parents suffered from spiritual or existential distress but also reported spiritual growth over time, becoming "closer to God."[36] These parents' coping styles also evolved over time. Some of the barriers parents reported to coping with grief were different coping styles between the mother and father, lack of accessible grief counseling, and hurtful communication from friends, family, and community members.[36] In contrast, helpful coping strategies were remembering their infant through traditions or physical keepsakes, developing a support network with other parents who could emphasize with their grief and experiences, spending time making sense of the loss through researching their infant's medical condition, and cognitive distraction by staying busy with new hobbies.[36]

Grief as a Shared Family Experience

Grief for families of children with serious illness begins at the moment of diagnosis (including fetal diagnosis), fluctuates with remissions and exacerbations of the illness, escalates at the time of death (although feelings of relief and guilt may interplay), and continues at varying levels for years afterward. Parental impact from infant death is notably prolonged and not easily measured by calendar chronology. Families never "get over" the death of their child and move on; instead, they learn to move through and with the experience as they integrate the memories of their child into a "new normal" of family life. The goal of the grief trajectory, if adequately supported, is to eventually enter into a season of posttraumatic growth. The loss of a child impacts not only parents but also siblings, grandparents, and the community at large.

Sibling bereavement needs to include clear communication in a developmentally relevant format.[68] Child life specialists may serve as resources to help families understand how and when children grieve, include siblings in remembering their sibling, and validate inclusion of siblings in the end-of-life and bereavement process.[69] Depending on their developmental stage, siblings may appreciate being offered memory-making ideas such as making artwork to remember their sibling, receiving footprints and handprints of their sibling, or putting special mementos in a memory box to honor their sibling's life.[70]

Grandparent bereavement is unique in that grandparents are often "double-grievers" in mourning the loss for their adult child and mourning the loss of their grandchild.[71] Grandparents have been termed "forgotten grievers" despite their "cumulative pain," because they are often positioned to care for their adult children's grief while also grieving their own loss.[72] The roles of grandparents in a family structure and even the amount of access a grandparent has been granted to medical information by their adult child impacts the grandparent experience.[73]

Historically, the NICU and palliative care literature focused on maternal grief in a way that has not fully acknowledged the paternal experience of neonatal life or loss.[74] Qualitative literature on the grief experience for fathers after the death of a child has highlighted themes of grief denial, lonely grief, bottled feelings, and an abrupt return to work or activity to distract and cope.[75] Grief patterns may not coincide in chronology, in intensity, or in expression.[76] How a dad experiences infant life and loss is highly related to how a dad defines his father role,[74,77] warranting interdisciplinary father-specific grief attentiveness rather than a "one size fits all" grief model for parents. Grief support is ideally individualized to parent identity and parents' perception of their role.

Family bereavement supports may include the following:

1. Individual or family counseling[78,79]
2. Moderated parent support group [80,81]
3. Bibliotherapy resources[82]
4. Chaplain/spiritual ministry[83]
5. Art therapy or legacy-intervention such as digital storytelling[74]
6. Family camps[84]
7. Child life inclusion or sibling legacy experiences[85,86]
8. Longitudinal staff remembrances in the form of cards or personalized contact[87]
9. Offering a follow-up meeting with the infant's medical team to discuss autopsy results and events leading up to infant death[88]

Staff Remembering

Whether in the form of attendance at a memorial service, a personalized sympathy card about their child, a remembrance card for their child, or a coordinated grief counseling phone call, bereaved families have described feeling supported by commemorative events and supportive gestures by staff.[89] Individual staff members may feel at a loss for what to say or how to say it to a bereaved family, warranting a team approach to coordinated bereavement.[90] Although the death of a child is always tragic, professional meaning can be derived from knowing the child's comfort and function were maximized throughout his or her lifetime because of palliative interventions; that the family's grief and distress were lessened; and that a peaceful death, if it occurs, was achieved. A family-centered palliative care approach supports families experiencing serious illness in the NICU and loss from the time of diagnosis through the time of discharge or bereavement.[91]

SECTION

19 Follow-Up

OUTLINE

CHAPTER 92

Early Diagnosis and Intervention in Neonatal Intensive Care Units

Naveen Jain

KEY POINTS

1. Most infants who develop neurodevelopmental disability (NDD) are normal on examination at birth.
2. Surveillance for NDD must start with neurologic examination in the neonatal intensive care unit and continue through childhood, because early diagnosis and intervention may be beneficial.
3. A tailored care plan should guide healthcare professionals and parents to best practices that support intact outcomes from birth to childhood.
4. Estimation of the risk of NDD is based on the severity of perinatal factors; promotion of early and guided parent participation; optimization of nutrition, such as with the use of mother's own milk (such interventions should be evaluated with anthropometric follow-up, with head growth interpreted in the context of weight and length centiles); infrastructure changes and training of staff, including physicians, nurses, and therapists (occupational, physical, and speech) to promote developmentally sensitive care; early screening for retinopathy of prematurity, hearing, hypothyroidism, and neurosonographical abnormalities; and standardization of a protocol-based discharge planning process.

Except for a small proportion of babies with genetic disorders, preterm babies (or other sick babies) are born "normal." Most neurodevelopmental disorders (NDDs) seem to be acquired due to severe medical morbidities that necessitate intensive care, an experience that, despite best efforts, is quite unlike the in-utero environment. Providing a child the opportunity to achieve full potential is the prime responsibility of perinatal healthcare professionals. Now that neonatal care has grown "beyond survival," the priorities have moved to the intactness and quality of survival (good neurodevelopment outcome).

Neonatal intensive care unit (NICU) graduates have high rates of NDDs, and many of these disorders (poor scholastic performance, behavioral issues, and adaptation to society) are more frequent than cerebral palsy, blindness, and deafness put together (disabilities that are measured in our current protocols). Efforts to improve the disruptive NICU environment with developmentally supportive care (DSC), combined with continued surveillance for NDDs through childhood, would be logical. Early detection of suboptimal neurodevelopmental performance deviating toward an NDD, and timely institution of DSC, will very likely improve outcomes.

The pursuit for a perfect diagnostic tool to predict NDDs in the early neonatal period may not be the best approach. The aim of early detection is to identify at-risk infants who may benefit from early intervention, to prevent rather than confirm the presence of NDDs. Early referral and scientifically appropriate therapies with good interprofessional coordination must be offered as a seamless care plan to parents before discharging the infants from the NICU.

The search for suboptimal behaviors starts at birth and continues even after discharge from the NICU; this is collectively called as "follow-up of NICU graduates."[1] The earlier an at-risk infant can be identified, the greater the likelihood of a good outcome without an NDD may be.[2] In the NICU, the care providers are constantly focused on preventing mortality in an infant being cared for with multiple life-support systems. The availability of well-organized, validated algorithms for management of respiratory supports, circulation, fluid and electrolytes, nutrition, jaundice, and infection control ensure minimum errors. Now, we need to develop similar, meticulously developed care bundles for early detection, referral, and intervention to optimize neurodevelopment. To optimize DSC practices and surveillance alongside medical care, we have developed a checklist model in our NICU that we call the "blue book," which begins on the first postnatal day and continues through discharge (Fig. 92.1). The "follow-up" after discharge into childhood will be discussed in the next chapter. In the following sections, we propose a simple process map, as a time-line checklist, that will help care-providers to incorporate neurodevelopment follow-up with medical care.

Days 1 to 3 of Life

Step 1: Assign Risk of NDD Based on Perinatal Factor Severity

The severity of a perinatal risk factor has a greater association with NDDs than its mere presence. The lowest gestations (<28 weeks), a need for extensive resuscitation (chest compression/medications), symptomatic hypoglycemia (seizures), prolonged ventilation, or abnormal neurosonogram (ventriculomegaly, periventricular leukomalacia [PVL] or grade 3 intraventricular hemorrhage [IVH]) were found to be independent risk factors in a study that included babies born at <34 weeks.[3] Babies with two or more of these risk factors were noted in 12% of the population and had higher risk of an NDD at 1 year of age (17% versus 4%) than did those with one or none of these factors. This intuitive model of risk assignment allows a large proportion of NICU babies to be sent back to a community pediatrician. The risk-stratification tool was evaluated in a small sample of 225 babies, and multiple perinatal factors were evaluated. The study also had limitations innate to retrospective studies and has not been evaluated for external validity. However, the simplicity of the model clearly supported by biologic plausibility allows constructing regionally adapted risk-stratification strategies. The potential risk factors for NDD are arranged in ascending order of severity across the rows. If any of the risk factors is assigned to the high-risk category (right column), the baby becomes a candidate for intense follow-up and early intervention.

Of course, all NICU babies are at risk of neurodevelopment deviation and should be offered DSC. However, it is particularly important to identify the babies at highest risk. This can help the medical teams and parents prepare and act timely. This reduces the bulk of the workload on the specialist follow-up service, allowing better resource use. An equally important benefit of stratification to a

Neurodevelopment Assessment & Development Supportive Care	
DAY 1	Parental counseling and Early Parent Participation Program (EPPP) Medical risk factors recorded in risk stratification chart Encourage mother for expressed breast milk
DAY 3-7	Screening for congenital hypothyroidism Occipitofrontal circumference(OFC) Medical risk factors recorded in risk stratification chart Early stimulation once hemodynamically stable Parents touch and talk to baby, get involved in care of baby Infant position Assessment tool
1-2 WEEK	Neurosonogram OFC Repeat Thyroid screening Multivitamin, human-milk fortifier (HMF) (or calcium phosphate) once on full feed Medical risk factors recorded in risk stratification chart Early stimulation once hemodynamically stable: kangaroo mother care (KMC), non-nutritive sucking (NNS) NNS may be started as soon as baby is on full feeds (use oral stimulation when oro-gastric feeds are given), put to breast after expressing milk. May try direct breastfeeding/and paladai feeding at 32-34 weeks Oromotor stimulation Early Intervention
2-3 WEEK	Retinopathy of prematurity (ROP) screening for those at risk of aggressive posterior-retinopathy of prematurity (AP-ROP) OFC Weight (should have regained birth weight) Oil massaging
1 MONTH	ROP screening-subsequent visits based on Ophthalmologist's opinion till 44 week Phosphorus/alkaline phosphatase/hemoglobin OFC Weight Serum ferritin, start iron supplement
6-8 WEEKS	Vaccination Neurobehavior OFC Weight Early stimulation

Fig. 92.1 Checklist for Neurodevelopmental Assessment and Focused Efforts to Support Development.

relatively lower risk group is reduced emotional drain and socioeconomic burden on the family. Babies previously considered as low risk may have pointers to NDDs that evolve during follow-up; they must be referred by the community (family) pediatrician to specialized follow-up services.

Table 92.1 may be adapted to suit the regional needs of the clinical service. Tertiary-care NICUs may use the model that follows.

Step 2: Early Parent Participation (Enriched Environment)

Parents must participate in the care of sick babies in the NICU from the start. The father must visit and touch the baby immediately after admission to the NICU, and the mother must participate as soon her health permits. They must have unlimited access to the baby. They must be empowered as partners in DSC through structured education and training.

Multiple studies have demonstrated the most obvious fact—that parents are critical to the healthy development of a baby, and from the start! (Fig. 92.2).[4] Strangely, the role of parents in many NICUs is still limited to seeing the baby during the visiting hours. Family-integrated care aims at minimizing parent-infant separation.[5] Better breast milk feeding rates, appropriate growth, and lower parent stress are consistently demonstrated in the family-integrated care (FIC) model of care; each of these have definite positive influences on neurodevelopment. In a large, multisite randomized controlled trial conducted in Australia, Canada, and New Zealand, parents participated at least 6 hours a day in care of stable (no or low respiratory support) babies born at less than 33 weeks.[6] A decrease in anxiety and depressive symptoms in

Table 92.1 Risk Stratification for NDD for NICU Infants

Factors	At-Risk Community Follow-Up	High-Risk Specialized Follow-Up
Gestation	>26 weeks	≤26 weeks
Birth weight	>1000 g	≤1000 g
Fetal growth	>10th centile	≤10th centile for gestation
Antenatal risk factors		Abruptio placenta Death of MC twin A/R EDF Severe eclampsia
Resuscitation at birth		Chest compression, medications Moderate/severe HIE
Perfusion		Shock requiring inotropes PDA requiring medical/surgical treatment
Respiratory care	Noninvasive ventilation Short-duration ventilation	>7 days of invasive ventilation Pneumothorax Inhaled nitric oxide Need for high-frequency ventilation
Infection		Chorio-amnionitis Culture-positive sepsis Meningitis
Bilirubin-induced neuronal damage		Exchange transfusion for severe hyperbilirubinemia
Neonatal encephalopathy		Encephalopathy (any cause) lasting >24 hours Seizures

A/R EDF, Absence/reversal of end-diastolic flow; *HIE*, hypoxic ischemic encephalopathy; *MC*, monochorionic twins; *NDD*, neurodevelopmental disability; *NICU*, neonatal intensive care unit; *PDA*, patent ductus arteriosus.

infants proved that the presence of parents mitigates the negative influences of pain associated with diagnostic and therapeutic procedures and stressful environments. Also, parents and families who were allowed FIC experienced less strain.

Parents are traditionally involved in care only after babies are medically stable, often a few days before discharge from the NICU. This obviously is too late! A recently published randomized controlled trial from India demonstrated that parent involvement very early (from day 1) is safe and beneficial.[7] Preterm babies (born between 28 and 33 weeks) had lesser events of physiologic instability (apnea, feed intolerance) if they were cared for by parents early. Breast milk feeding rates were also higher in the early parent participation group. In a similar study from Hong Kong, decreases in severe retinopathy of prematurity (ROP) rates were demonstrated.

COVID 19 significantly restricted the number of parents in NICUs and posed new challenges. There has been a temporary setback to FIC. Evidence supports breastfeeding and benefits of avoiding separation of the mother and baby, despite COVID.[8]

Step 3: Mother's Own Milk

Efforts to maximize feeding with mother's own milk should start with antenatal counseling.[9] Immediately after delivery, the mother is advised to express breast milk frequently, either manually or using a breast pump. Pain relief must be combined with minimizing emotional stress by honest updates on the baby's health and opportunities to touch the baby. Galactagogues may be required if mother's own milk is not available despite best efforts at the end of 1 to 2 weeks after the birth of the baby. Breast milk feeding is associated with better neurodevelopment.[10]

Days 3 to 7 of Life in the NICU

Step 4: Track Head Circumference

Head circumference measurement should be started at 2 to 3 days of life. A weekly plot of head circumference must continue until discharge from the NICU and at every visit thereafter until 2 years age. Look for slow head growth (risk of an NDD) or rapid head growth (points to hydrocephalus). Head circumference is best interpreted in relation to length and weight centiles. Serial measurements have greater prognostic value than does a single point measure.

Population studies from Canada have shown that poor head growth *between birth and discharge* from the NICU was associated with poor motor and cognitive outcomes in preterm babies (<29 weeks).[11] The outcomes were poorer in infants whose head growth *failed to catch up* after discharge from the NICU.

Head circumference at birth (reflection of fetal growth) was associated with poor development outcomes at 2 years among infants born at <34 weeks. In a study from France, infants who had a *catch down growth* from birth to discharge also had poor outcomes.[12] A synergistic negative effect was noted when both poor fetal growth and postnatal growth of the head were present.

There can be inherent errors in head measurement. Also, isolated slow growth of the head is not always predictive. Small head circumference was noted at 2 years of age in 12% of NICU survivors from a NICU in the United States,[13] but a small head was predictive of poor developmental outcomes only when associated with epilepsy.

Step 5: Compliance With Core Elements of Developmentally Supportive Care[14]

1. Engineering/infrastructure optimization to provide a DSC environment.
2. Staff awareness of DSC.
3. Attention to the position in which the baby is nursed, synchronizing care with optimal behavioral states, ensuring protected sleep, and minimizing negative sensations such as pain, noise, and excess light.
4. Parent education: Parents must be supported throughout the NICU stay by a structured transfer of knowledge and skills through printed leaflets, group teaching, and videos or online classes.
5. Various early intervention programs are practiced across NICUs. A recent systematic review found the Newborn Individualized Developmental Care and Assessment Program was proven to be beneficial.[15]

Step 6: Role of Neonatal Therapy in the NICU

Neonatal therapy is provided by occupational therapists, physical therapists, and speech therapists. Their role in the NICU includes positioning of babies, passive stretch, hand function, neck control, sensory integrations, oral stimulation, and much more; they also help families to cope better. The need for full-time services of each type of therapist has been defined by recent recommendations.[16]

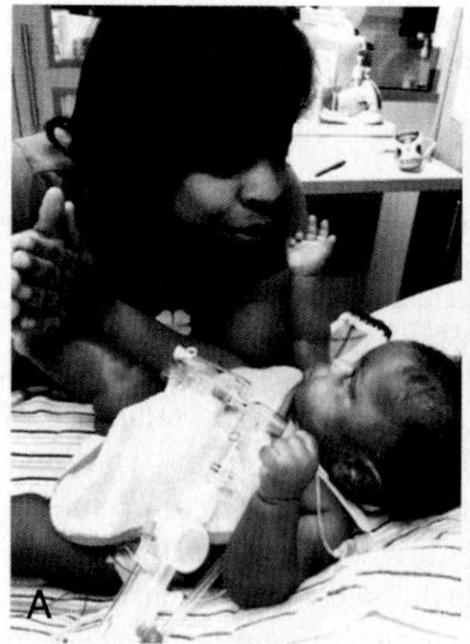

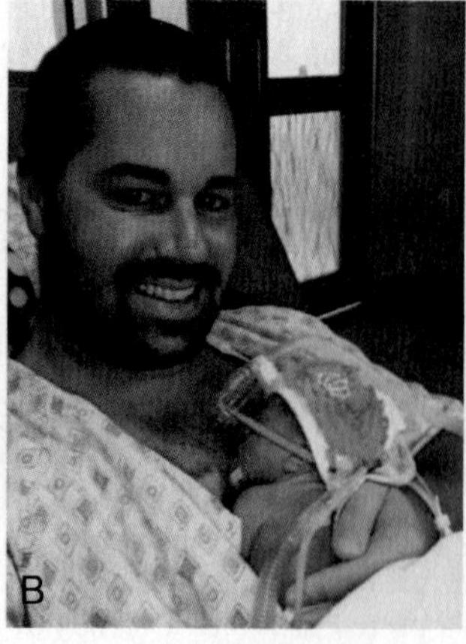

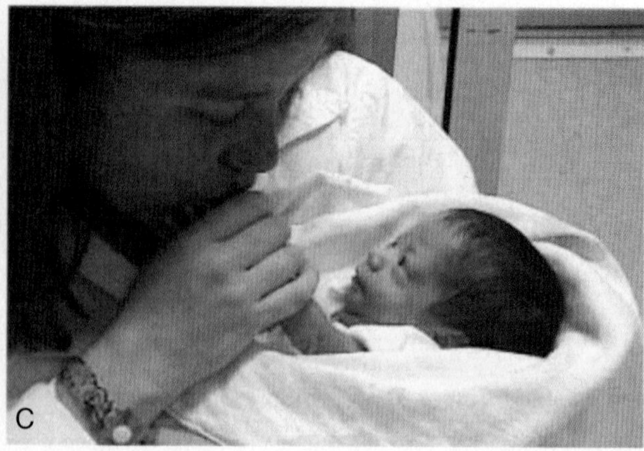

Fig. 92.2 Bonding Opportunities With Parents Are Important in Developmental Care. (A) Infant interacting with the mother. Mutual reciprocity is promoted during massage and social engagement opportunities. (B) Dad and daughter engaged in skin-to-skin care. (C) The infant's response to maternal affection is evident in the intent gaze. Parent-infant interaction can promote individualized developmental care for high-risk newborns in the neonatal intensive care unit. (A and B were reproduced with permission and minor modifications from Ricciardi and Blatz. Developmental care—understanding and applying the science. In: *Klaus and Fanaroff's Care of the High-Risk Neonate*, 8, 171–189.e7; C was reproduced with permission from Vandenberg KA. *Early Hum Dev.* 2007;83:433–442.)

Step 7: Screening

Screening for congenital hypothyroidism must be initiated at day 3 to 7 of life and then followed by a repeat test in preterm infants at 2 to 4 weeks and 6 to 8 weeks of life, nearing an estimated term age.[17]

Days 7 to 14

Neurosonograms: Most NICUs recommend at least 2 neurosonograms, the first at 7 to 14 days of life and the second at 36 to 40 weeks of life.

Third to Fourth Week

1. ROP screening must be initiated and continued as per protocol.
2. Repeat a thyroid function test.
3. Hearing screening must include automated brainstem evoked audiometry (screening by otoacoustic emissions (OAE) alone will miss sensorineural impairment).
4. A neurosonogram done at 36 to 40 weeks' postmenstrual age has higher predictive ability than an early scan.
5. Routine use of magnetic resonance imaging at estimated term age is not recommended.

Prior to Discharge From the NICU

Step 8: Neurologic Examination

Classify the baby's behavior as optimal or suboptimal after a neurologic examination.

Suboptimal behavior is associated with a higher risk of NDDs; these babies will benefit from closer follow-up and a more intense intervention program. The negative predictive value of neurologic examination is good; a normal report indicates that the baby is at a low risk of NDDs and can be followed up with a community facility. The positive predictive values are fortunately low, so most babies, despite suboptimal neurologic findings, will eventually be normal.

Neonates have well-organized brain structure and function from very early life.[18] As early as 23 weeks' gestation, preterm neonates have consistent responses to most stimuli, and neurologic examination uses these to classify babies' behavior as optimal or suboptimal.

The General Movement Assessment tool is a very reliable tool but requires training and experience to interpret, limiting its widespread use. The Hammersmith Neonatal Neurological Examination (HNNE) is easy to perform and requires no additional training. The shorter version of the HNNE takes less than 10 minutes to complete. The HNNE assesses orientation of the baby to vision and hearing; the ease with which one can arouse and console are a measure of higher functions. The baby's tone is assessed systematically as head and neck, trunk, upper limbs, and lower limbs. Spontaneous movements, reflexes, and abnormal signs are elicited. The HNNE has been found to have reasonable predictive ability, compared with magnetic resonance imaging, in predicting outcomes.[19] The HNNE has recently been evaluated for use earlier than term gestation (Fig. 92.3).[20] The HNNE performed early (HNNE PE) was used before discharge of the preterm baby from birth admission, at a median gestation of 36 weeks. The diagnostic accuracy was similar to that of an HNNE performed at estimated term age. Besides the greater benefit of early detection of neonates at higher risk, the neurologic examination was easier to perform on a baby still admitted to the hospital than on an outpatient basis.

The Premie-Neuro tool evaluated neurobehavior of preterm infants even earlier, at 30 weeks' postmenstrual age, and found it to predict reliably adverse neurobehavior at later ages.[21] Reliable evaluation of neurobehavior in preterm infants may be performed by the NICU Network Neurobehavioral Scale, Neurobehavioral Assessment of the Preterm Infant, and Assessment of Preterm Infants' Behavior.[22,23]

Step 9: Discharge Planning[24]

Discharge planning starts with admission; the medical care team must inform the family about a tentative date of discharge (this date may be revised as the health condition evolves). Family-centered care throughout the NICU stay facilitates a smooth transition to home. The discharge planning meeting must happen at least a few days prior to discharge, allowing sufficient time to the family.

Standardization reduces inadvertent misses. The cost of care and hospital stay are also reduced.

	Warning signs				Warning signs
POSTURE	arms & legs extended or very slightly flexed	legs slightly flexed For 25-27 weekers only	leg well-flexed but not adducted	leg well-flexed & adducted near abdomen	abnormal posture: a) opistotonus b) arm flexed, leg extended
ARM TRACTION	arms remain straight; no resistance	arms flex slightly or some resistance felt	arms flex well till shoulder lifts, then straighten	arms flex at approx 100° & mantained as shoulder lifts	flexion of arms <100°; mantained when body lifts up
LEG TRACTION	legs straight - no resistance	knees flex slightly or some resistance felt	knees flex well till bottom lifts up	knees flex and remain flexed when bottom up	knee flexion stays when back+bottom up
HEAD CONTROL (1)	no attempt to raise head	infant tries; effort better felt than seen	raised head but drops forward or back	raises head: remains vertical; it may wobble	
HEAD CONTROL (2)	no attempt to raise head	infant tries: effort better felt than seen For 25-29 weekers only	raises head but drops forward or back	raises head: remains vertical: it may wobble	head remains upright or neck extended; connot be passively flexed
HEAD LAG	head drops & stays back	tries to lift head but it drops back	able to lift head slightly	lifts head in line with body	head in front of line of body
VENTRAL SUSPENSION	back curved, head & limbs hang straight	back curved; head ↓, limbs slightly flexed	back slightly curved, limbs flexed	back straight, head in line with back, limbs flexed	back straight, head above line of body
SPONT. MOVEMENT (quality)	only stretches	stretches and rendom abrupt movements; some smooth movements	fluent movements but monotonous	fluent alternating movements of arms + legs; good variability	• cramped synchronised; • mouthing • jerky or other abnormal movement
TREMOR		no tremor or tremor only when crying	tremor only after Moro or occasionally when awake	frequent tremors when awake	continuous tremors
MORO RESPONSE	no response or opening of hands only	full abduction at shoulder and extension of the arms; no adduction	full abduction but only delayed or partial adduction	partial abduction at shoulder and extension of arms followed by smooth adduction	• no abduction or adduction • only forword extension of arms from the shoulders • marked adduction only
VISUAL ORIENTATION	does not follow/follows briefly to the side but loses stimuli B T	follows horizontally and vertically; no head turn B T	follows horizontally and vertically: turns head B T	follows in a circle B T	

ABNORMAL SIGNS	Facial Palsy	Abn Eye Movements	Sunset Sign	Fisted hand(s)	Clonus
	Y N	Y N	Y N	Y N	Y N

Fig. 92.3 Neurologic assessment of preterm infants at term corrected gestational age. (Reproduced with permission and after minor modifications from Romeo DM et al. Neurologic assessment tool for screening preterm infants at term age. *J Pediatr*. 2012 Dec 1;161(6):1166–1168.)

Components of Discharge Readiness (With Relevance to Neurodevelopment)

1. Knowledge of parents (and primary caregivers)—have they attended all the education sessions pertaining to developmental follow-up (ROP, hearing, and neurodevelopmental follow-up until 6 years of age)?
2. Skills of care—DSC, kangaroo mother care (KMC), and early stimulation.
3. Follow-up schedule—ensure coordination with subspecialists; caretakers must be informed about details of each visit, duration at the hospital, etc.
4. Community-connect—written and verbal transfer of the neurodevelopmental follow-up plan to a pediatric facility near the home or to the family doctor.
5. Individual medical care plan for neonates with special needs (such as oxygen, gastrostomy, or tracheostomy).
6. Assessment and documentation of parent coping (including mother's medical health, immunization of parents and family [cocoon vaccination], and mental health assessment).
7. Address cultural and religious needs (e.g., timing of circumcision, ceremonies with larger attendance, etc.) and identify socioeconomic vulnerability (single parent, lack of healthcare access near to home, poor internet access limiting tele-health, etc.).

Checklist—Predischarge (With Relevance to Neurodevelopment)

1. Parents have attended all education sessions
2. Weight tracking on growth chart
3. Head growth tracking on growth chart
4. Physical examination
5. Medication plan
6. ROP findings and next date
7. Hearing screen report and follow-up date
8. Neuroimaging reports and follow-up (if necessary)/other imaging (such as renal)
9. Neurologic examination
10. Specific mention of risks to neurodevelopment
11. Early intervention—examples: KMC, occupational therapy
12. Parental coping

Hand Over to Parents and Primary Care Physician

Introduce follow-up service locations and processes.

1. Detailed and organized discharge summary—diagnosis; therapies; pending reports; plan for care and follow-up; reports of ROP, hearing, and neurologic examinations; lab tests; neuroimaging; and special needs.
2. Verbal (telephonic) transfer of important details.

Step 10: Registration for Quality Assurance

The translation of best science to best practice requires a structured plan, a communication plan to the team, and a periodic audit of compliance and outcomes. Web-based models have been used to improve compliance with follow-up and early referral.[25] A printed, simple checklist (blue book) has been practiced in the author's unit for 20 years; this has been adapted across more than 250 NICUs in India. We register every high-risk pregnancy in a "blue book." The parents carry over the book to the NICU. The book has a day-wise checklist, mentioned through the chapter as must-do activities. The book stays with the family at discharge of the baby and is designed to incorporate all specialists' notes (ROP, hearing, imaging, therapists, development assessments) and medical care including immunization, thus achieving the desirable goal of integrating medical care with developmental care.

CHAPTER 93

Early Diagnosis and Intervention—On Neonatal Follow-Up

Naveen Jain

KEY POINTS

1. The care of a sick infant must continue into childhood, and families must be guided just as diligently after discharge as they were during intensive care.
2. A continuum of care after discharge, involving dedicated multidisciplinary teams, is important for early intervention and meticulous follow-up.
3. During developmental surveillance, uniform application of one well-validated tool is important for consistency in early intervention and/or referral. Several such test batteries are available, including the Bayley Scale of Infant Development, Hammersmith Neonatal Neurological Examination, Hammersmith Infant Neonatal Neurological Examination, Alberta Infant Motor Scale, and/or Milani-Comparetti Motor Development Screening Test, all of which show a fairly high degree of correlation. There is also a need for early evaluation of vision and of hearing and language.
4. Timely referral and interprofessional integration with occupational health, speech, and physical therapy are needed.
5. The availability of supportive services has been shown to be important not only for high-risk infants but also for the well-being of the parents and other family members.

Infants discharged from the neonatal intensive care unit (NICU) are at higher risk of medical and neurodevelopmental disorders and will benefit from well-defined clinical care protocols on "care after discharge." There are several important considerations: (1) there is a need for a process map to address the complex needs of the infants and families sent home from NICU; (2) parental dissatisfaction has been noted in both the developed and the developing parts of the world on access to guidance and care after discharge from a relatively structured NICU protocol life; and (3) most parents encountered delays in diagnosis, referral, and inappropriate communication of information. In this chapter, we seek to outline the core principles in designing a structured follow-up program for babies discharged from the NICU. Several indicators for the quality of care are available that can be used as a template to organize medical and developmental care of babies discharged from the NICU. There is a need for follow up-schedules and services tailored for individual infants based on their needs, and the systems also need to be adapted as per regional resources.

Ensuring Continuity and Compliance After Discharge From the NICU

Healthy child and adult outcomes must be planned from birth. The team coordinating developmental assessment and therapy must participate in care from day 1 of the baby's life in the NICU. This early relationship is beneficial to both the family and the development coordinators. The developmental services must be placed at par with lifesaving intensive care.

A development coordinator must be a part of NICU service rounds. The development services team gathers information on the education, occupation, and economic and emotional status of the caregivers and the medical team records the perinatal biologic risk factors, both in the same blue book. Through a modular "early parent participation program," parents are guided to the need and processes of developmental services. This includes introduction to the NICU and lactation support in the first week of the NICU stay; by the second week, when the baby is medically stable, the development coordinator introduces to the family the need for and protocols of retinopathy of prematurity (ROP), hearing, and neurosonogram screening. During the next sessions, the need for long-term follow-up including assessment of refraction, early language milestones, and early detection and mitigation of motor, cognitive, behavioral, and scholastic disabilities is shared. This ensures that the family is informed, before discharge from the NICU, about the need for and logistics of follow-up until school entry. The role and financial feasibility of development therapists into the NICU team from the start have been demonstrated in the Baby Bridge program in the United States.[1–6] Nurse-driven guided participation that included updates on the condition of the baby and education at periodic intervals in the NICU showed significant improvement in parent satisfaction, and perceived stress was less.[7] By using principles of quality improvement, there was a clear increase in compliance with follow-up and early referral, the most critical step in minimizing disability (loss of function and participation in activities of living) in children with early pointers to brain injury.[8]

Role of Developmental Follow-Up Services

Many allied health professionals (occupational therapists, speech therapists, and physical therapists) work together with the intensive care team to ensure intact neurodevelopment of the vulnerable infant.[9–11] In the NICU, there are several important considerations:

- Early intervention in the NICU—ensuring core principles of developmental supportive care with early participation of the parents;
- Education of parents on the need for screening and follow-up;
- Evaluation of neurobehavior of the baby in the NICU and recognition of suboptimal behaviors after discharge;
- Developmental surveillance and growth monitoring after discharge from the NICU;
- Early initiation of developmental therapy for motor, cognitive, and behavior disorders and speech delay;
- Coordination between specialists, therapists, and family physicians during postdischarge follow-up;
- Coordination of routine medical care and immunization;
- Establishment of links with community resources;
- Recognition and timely initiation of parental stress; and
- Recognition of financial and social issues.

Such a multidisciplinary follow-up team may include a developmental pediatrician, therapist, or nurse with at least 1 year of exposure in an NICU.

Developmental Surveillance—After Discharge From the NICU

1. Address medical concerns and *assess parents' coping as independent caregivers.* The first question asked is "How are you both? Mother (father) and baby?" Healthy parenting has a definite impact on infant behavior and future neurodevelopmental outcomes (Fig. 93.1).
2. Quickly review neurodevelopment in the NICU: the risk stratification chart; predischarge checklist; growth of head and weight; neuroimaging; screening reports for ROP, hearing, and thyroid levels; and neurobehavior and examination before discharge from the NICU.
3. Assess clues to suboptimal neurobehavior: choking during feeding (with loss of tone, going blue or pale, or violent coughing), very slow feeding (taking much longer than 20–30 minutes to finish a feed), clinical pointers (abnormal sucking in preterm infants[12]), excessive crying, and a poor sleep-wake rhythm.
4. Assess growth and nutrition: head growth (serial monitoring) and trajectory in relation to weight/length, weight gain (growth [weight] is an indirect measure of neurodevelopment and has associations with ROP), and specific nutrients (iron, iodine, and zinc have a possible influence on development).
5. Perform formal tests to assess neurobehavior of the NICU baby at term age for preterm babies and in the first weeks for a term-born baby: the best tool should be accurate in prediction of disability (need for intervention), should be easy to perform, and should be locally adapted (Fig. 93.2). Several test batteries are available; however, uniform application of one well-validated tool is highly important for consistency in early intervention and/or timely referral. These tests include the Bayley Scale of Infant Development (BSID), Hammersmith Neonatal Neurological Examination, Hammersmith Infant Neonatal Neurological Examination (HNNE), Alberta Infant Motor Scale, and/or Milani-Comparetti Motor Development Screening Test, all of which show a fairly high degree of correlation. There is also a need for early evaluation of vision and of hearing and language.

The Hammersmith Neonatal Neurological Examination can be performed with minimal training and requires only 10 to 15 minutes to complete. The General Movement Assessment is another well-known, accurate tool for the prediction of cerebral palsy (CP). The "nonintrusive" test can be performed without touching the infant (only a video needs to be shot, by even the parent at home); however, it does require some training and experience (several hundred babies) before a reliable report can be made. The NICU Network Neurobehavioral Scale, with 128 items, can provide an elaborate assessment of neurobehavior but requires training and time.

Beyond Early Infancy

The most accurate tools must be reserved for research purposes or for developing an individualized childcare plan. In busy office practice settings, most pediatricians may not be able to evaluate high-risk children for want of time and not having enough knowledge of formal development assessment tools; compliance was less than 50% in

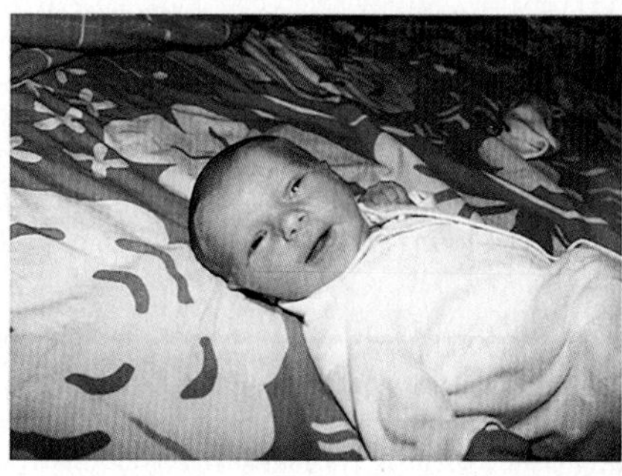
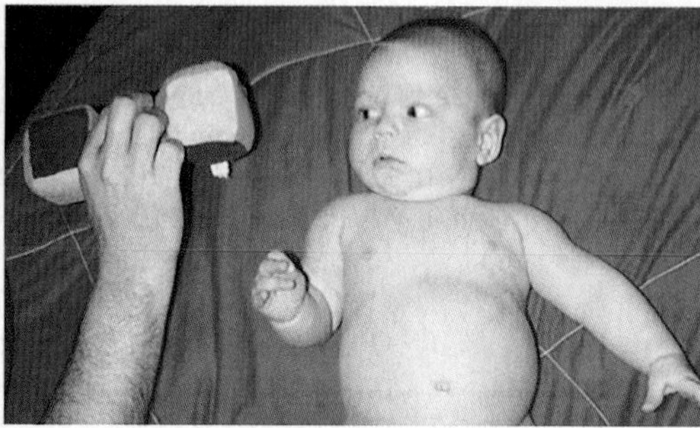

Fig. 93.1 (A) Early smiling. A 19-day-old infant smiles for her parents. (B) Localizing sound. A 3-month-old infant responds to interesting sounds by looking in the direction of the sound. (A, Reproduced with permission and minor modifications from Feldman and Chaves-Gnecco. Developmental/behavioral pediatrics. In: *Zitelli and Davis' Atlas of Pediatric Physical Diagnosis*, 3, 71–100. B, Reproduced with permission and minor modifications from Scalise-Smith and Umphred. *Umphred's Neurological Rehabilitation*, 2, 15–50.e6.)

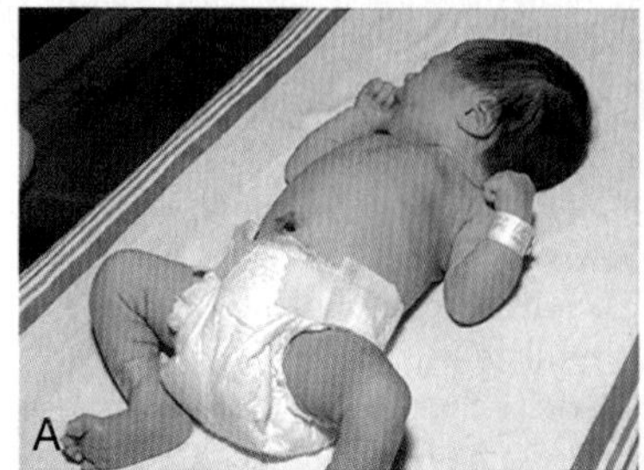

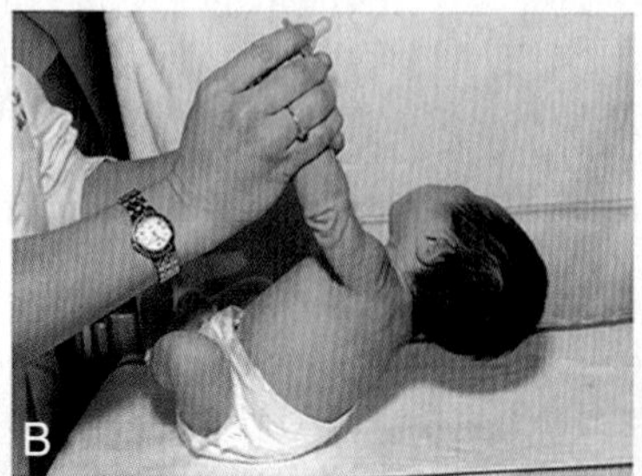

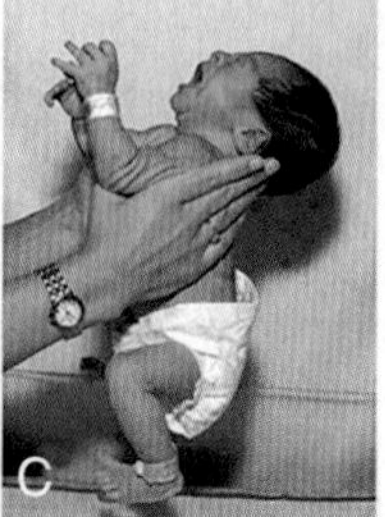

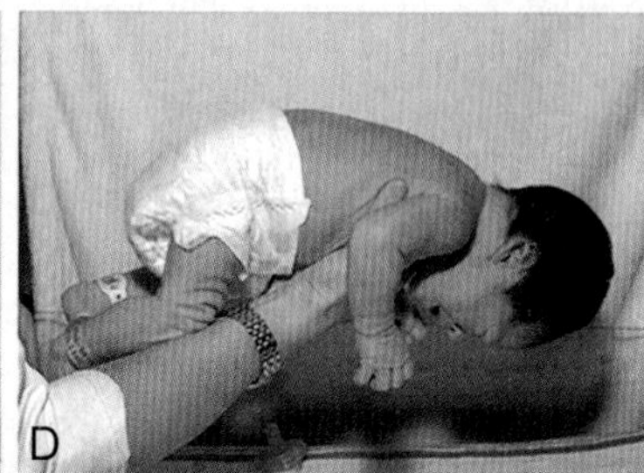

Fig. 93.2 Normal Tone in a Full-Term Neonate. (A) Flexed resting posture. (B) Traction response. (C) Vertical suspension. (D) Horizontal suspension. (Reproduced with permission and minor modification from Schor. Neurologic evaluation. In: *Nelson Textbook of Pediatrics*, ch. 608, 3053–3063.e1.)

high-risk children in a study from New Zealand.[13] The reasons cited by pediatricians include lack of time and clear protocols.

Neurologic examination using a standardized test battery is important for early diagnosis of CP. In Australia, studies showed that the BSID, HNNE, general movements assessment (GMA) Test of Infant Motor Performance scales, and imaging were all able to diagnose CP very early (before the age of 5 months) in infants discharged from the NICU.[14] Community-level screening must use tools that are easy to administer and can be completed in a short duration. Many tools have been evaluated for community screening in low- and middle-income countries.[15–24]

Vision

- Parents must be guided to ensure follow-up if the screening for ROP is not completed at the time of discharge from the NICU.
- Infants need timely referral if they show poor face regard, nystagmus at any age, or poor social smile by 2 months' corrected age. Those with squint (strabismus) persisting after the age of 4 months also need evaluation.
- Infants need screening for refractory errors (starting at 6–9 months of age and then annually until 6 years of age).
- Cortical visual dysfunction, such as with poor fixation, following, or in interaction with parents despite a "normal" eye report, needs evaluation.
- The role of an experienced optometrist who can prescribe spectacles or eye patches or provide other forms of intervention cannot be overemphasized.

Hearing and Language

- Infants discharged from the NICU are at a higher risk of sensorineural hearing impairment; they must be screened by brainstem evoked audiometry even if they have a normal otoacoustic emissions evaluation. Sequential evaluation with a brainstem evoked response evaluation may not be sufficient in infants who fail the otoacoustic emissions evaluation. Timely access to a hearing aid or cochlear implant may be very important for hearing and global development.
- Parents and pediatricians must be educated about early language milestones to detect any communication disorder.
- Speech/articulation disorders result from anatomic/coordination disorders of sound production; language disorders include problems arising from difficulty with hearing, comprehension at the cortical level, and expression.
- Clinicians should evaluate the environment (opportunities to speak) at home before looking for biologic causes of language delays.
- Importantly, language disorders can be a part of global developmental delay (cognitive disorder). A timely referral to a speech and language therapist is important.

Referral: Timely Specific Interventions and Interprofessional Integration

Developmental surveillance must be coupled with referral to scientifically proven therapies. Use of early intervention services is hugely dependent on the primary care physician's knowledge of scope and potential benefits, the access to resources, and interprofessional coordination.

Role of Pediatricians

Pediatricians have a very important, central role in the care of these at-risk infants. They are the guides on nutrition, monitoring for faltering growth, immunization, early detection of illnesses that can worsen developmental milestones, timely referral to specialists, and coordination of care for complex medical issues (Fig. 93.3).

Role of Developmental Specialists

Behavioral/developmental subspecialists are important for the evaluation of toddlers and children for behavioral disorders, autism spectrum disorders, and poor scholastic performance and for coordination of multidisciplinary care of children with established developmental disorders.

Role of Pediatric Neurologists

Neurologists recognize and treat developmental disorders. They have an important role in timely evaluation with neuroimaging, electroencephalography, or other specialized investigations including genetic testing. They also coordinate pharmacotherapy for seizures, hypertonia, hyperactivity, abnormal movements, and sleep disorders. Many infants with spasticity could benefit from novel therapeutic interventions such as the administration of botulinum toxin A or surgical dorsal rhizotomy, and they need evaluation and referral.

Role of Orthopedics

Orthopedicians play important roles in surveillance and management of gait disorders, hip abnormalities, and scoliosis, and they can help by timely application of appropriate orthoses and, if needed, surgical intervention (e.g., tenotomy for Achilles tendon contracture, hip surgery, or correction of scoliosis) and subsequent follow-up.

Neurosurgery

The importance of neurosurgical interventions such as selective dorsal rhizotomy for reduction of spasticity or shunt surgery for hydrocephalus (posthemorrhagic) is well known.

Role of Psychologists

Psychologists may be needed for the management of primary or secondary psychiatric manifestations in children with disability or for the support of parents.

Role of Therapists

1. **Occupational therapists** can help affected children to be able to participate in activities of daily living and play.[24] Pediatric occupational therapies have been shown to benefit children with disabilities[25–30] (Table 93.1).
2. **Speech therapists** can assist children who have swallowing dysfunction or language and speech disorders or those who need rehabilitation after the institution of a hearing aid or a cochlear implant.
3. **Physiotherapists** can institute and promote early intervention beginning in the NICU, with positioning and passive movements to prevent tone abnormalities. Physiotherapy is often the first referral for most children with motor disability.[28] Massage therapy can help in parent-infant bonding, and although unproven,

NEURODEVELOPMENTAL FOLLOW-UP

Age					
Date					
CDC grading					
AT angles					
DDST GM					
DDST FM					
DDST (L)					
DDST (PS)					
BSID					
Motor composite					
Lauguage composite					
Cognitive composite					
Functional assessment					
Vision					
Hearing					
Interpretation					
Development intervention					
Referral					
Feed back from specialist					

Fig. 93.3 Checklist for Neurodevelopmental Assessment and Focused Efforts to Support Development During Outpatient Follow-Up. *AT*, Amiel-Tison; *BSID*, Bayley Scale of Infant Development; *CDC*, Centers for Disease Control and follow-up; *DDST*, Denver Development Screening Test; *FM*, fine motor; *L*, language; *GM*, gross motor; *PS*, personal-social.

possibly with some improvement in posture and muscle tone in children with CP. The therapies can be offered as group therapy, individualized guided therapy, or home care based on the needs of the child.

Health Needs of Parents

Assessment of parental coping and timely referral is important. Parents of NICU graduates have higher stress and psychological manifestations, besides physical exhaustion. They cope with difficulties related to prolonged hospitalization of the child, fear of death or disability, financial aspects, and social conflicts. These challenges may manifest as anxiety and depression.

Audits and Process of Improvement

Research on the efficacy of coordinated follow-up and on predictors of intact outcomes versus disability can help children and also the medical care team. Children clearly benefit from being a part of systematic care; continuous feedback on outcomes of children at risk and those with disabilities allows improvement in science and the

Table 93.1 Occupational Therapies Associated With Improved Function in Children

Motor	Autism	Behavior	Feeding
Goal-directed training for children with CP: We decide on a specific set of goals for activities of daily life (wearing clothes, socks, buttoning)	Advanced behavior analysis (ABA), focusing on promoting healthy behavior	Positive Parenting Programs for children with behavior disorders to promote positive relationships and conduct	Standardized, protocol-driven introduction of oral feedings within 48 hours of reaching full orogastric feeds; shortens transition to total oral feeding
Home program for developmentally delayed infants: Careful monitoring of movement, activities, and functional tasks	Shared parent-medical attention to interactive tasks such as pointing to objects and coordinating looks at persons and objects	Token-economy contracts for appropriate behavior—token points are awarded for good behaviors; tokens could be exchanged for items/privileges	Sensorimotor-oral stimulation can improve oral feeding; such protocols may include stroking perioral and intraoral structures with a gloved finger for a specified time, pacifier sucking before feeding, stroking the cheeks, and providing cheek and chin/jaw support
Kinesio tape: This specialized elastic tape is made of latex-free cotton fibers; its elasticity is similar to that of muscle, skin, and fascia, and when properly applied, it does not restrict soft tissues but supports the weaker muscles in movements	Coaching parents of at-risk children to promote development, recognize their priorities, and create their own solutions; such coordination can promote developmentally appropriate function and behavior in these children	Cog-Fun program for attention-deficit and hyperactivity disorder (ADHD) may promote executive strategies through play	Flexed neck and reclined trunk positioning can minimize aspiration in at-risk children
In some infants, repeated administration of botulinum toxin-A/ occupational therapy (OT) can be superior to OT alone			Strategies such as using a squeezable bottle with a smooth flow or a rigid bottle with a crosscut-nipple can help feed infants with cleft palate
Bimanual occupational therapy focused on activities for both upper limbs			Parent education and feeding interventions
Counselor-assisted problem-solving (CAPS) for children with brain injury to improve executive function			
Cognitive orientation to occupational performance in children with developmental coordination disorders			
Constraint-induced movement therapy to promote the use of weak limb(s)			
Context-focused learning to help identify tasks of interest to the child and improve functional motor performance			

process of care delivery. The follow-up data can help develop information that serves as anticipatory guidance to parents. The research also allows scientific evaluation of intensive-care and follow-up therapies. Systematic follow-up research has modified many intensive-care practices such as the administration of caffeine for apnea; postnatal short-course, low-dose steroids for ventilator-dependent infants with chronic lung disease; indomethacin for patent ductus arteriosus; and use of therapeutic hypothermia. Also, many tools such as the "good enough draw-a-man test" have been questioned for validity, and conventional therapies such as harnesses for developmental dysplasia of the hip, routine physiotherapy, and neurodevelopmental therapy have not received sufficient support from evidence.

Prevention of disability at all levels must be a constant endeavor. If the neonate survives with a risk of disability, then early diagnosis and intervention must be initiated to modify the risk. In case the child has disabilities, the pediatrician, with the help of a team, must be as prepared as for the management of respiratory distress syndrome (RDS) shock, or neonatal jaundice. All members of the team should be able to guide the family through purposive and meaningful healthcare.

The template of the blue book, a checklist model on follow-up, and a comprehensive list of systematic reviews on infant and child development have been included in the revised edition of Illingworth's textbook[31] on development.

CHAPTER 94 Early Detection of Cerebral Palsy

Betsy E. Ostrander, Nathalie L. Maitre, Andrea F. Duncan

KEY POINTS

1. Cerebral Palsy (CP) originates from an injury or abnormality in the developing brain, resulting in abnormal muscle tone, and consequently, in altered movement, posture, and motor function.
2. Tools used to accurately detect CP in the first year of life include a combination of Prechtl General Movement Assessment (GMA), clinical history, standardized neurological exam, brain imaging, and an assessment of motor function.
3. The diagnosis of CP should be made as early as possible so that families may receive necessary support, infants may receive therapies specific to the diagnosis, and surveillance for co-morbidities can be intiated.
4. CP is often accompanied by other neurodevelopmental impairments, including orthopedic problems, epilepsy, and impaired cognition, perception, communication, and behavior.

Introduction

The inclusion of a chapter on early detection of Cerebral Palsy (CP) in a volume on evidence-based neonatology demonstrates a shift which started in the mid 2010's in the practice of neonatal follow-up. For several decades prior, neonatal intensive care units (NICUs) primarily leveraged follow-up programs to document the outcomes of their perinatal interventions.[1,2] At worst, NICU follow-up was seen as a necessary financial burden in order to have "long-term" outcomes for randomized controlled trials, with a single assessment visit at the age of 2 to administer Bayley Scale(s) of Infant and Toddler Development[3] assessment and a neurological exam.[4–9] At best, these programs functioned as strong reminders of the consequences of neonatal care and of neonatologists'[10,11] responsibilities that extended beyond saving patients' lives. The late Dr. Maureen Hack was the leader of a movement promoting standardized NICU follow-up at 2 years of age,[12–17] and influenced a generation of physicians to see detection of CP at this 2-year visit as an essential check-and-balance to the care provided in the NICU.[13] Most studies of outcomes after NICU care, whether clinical trials or not, started at the 2-year mark (18–22 or 22–26 months) and included some type of standardized neurological examination. Examiners, many of them without a strong neurological background, were tasked with attributing a diagnosis of CP based on algorithms for this exam.[6,9,10,18] Sometimes, infants with the worst types of neurological insults had already received a diagnosis by a neurologist. This was especially true if they had associated comorbidities such as seizures or coagulopathies. In this case, the follow-up physicians confirmed their colleagues' observations. Overall, the reported mean age at CP diagnosis in the 1990s ranged from 1 to 8 years, in the 2000's from 1 to 8 years and in the 2010's from 0 to 5 years.[19–21]

Studies of NICU graduates conducted in the 1990's and early 2000's showed a binary presence/absence of CP at 2 years after birth. Some studies measured the severity, and categorized the patients as having mild, moderate, or severe disability. More recently, the Gross Motor Function Classification System (GMFCS)[22] was adopted in many NICU follow-up studies to standardize and refine the description of CP[23,24] (Table 94.1). When reporting outcomes, children with a GMFCS level of 1 (i.e., those with the least gross motor impairment) were grouped with those without CP,[25,26] intimating that both populations had no impairment. This disregarded the very poor stability of the GMFCS at 2 years of age, especially when trying to predict outcomes into childhood or adulthood.[27] It also did not account for the numerous co-morbidities of CP that may impact children's ability to function far more than walking independently by the age of 2.[28,29] Most of all, it overlooked the well-documented concerns and frustrations of parents whose children had CP—whether with a GMFCS of 1 or 5—at waiting until the age of 2 to obtain a diagnosis.[28,30] Consequences of parental dissatisfaction range from mistrust of the healthcare system to depression and anxiety, with long-term adverse effects on their well-being and ability to advocate for the best care for their children.[28,31,32] Studies of parent perceptions surrounding the diagnosis clearly demonstrate their wishes to have an honest and direct conversation as early as possible. They accept the uncertainties inherent to such an early diagnosis and are also content with a classification of "high-risk for CP", but find delays in surveillance and counseling unacceptable.[31]

These concerns, as well as the initiatives of an international expert group, prompted a world summit in Vienna Austria, in July, 2014. The working group was composed of medical specialists in all disciplines broadly related to CP, including allied health professionals, researchers, community stakeholders, and parents. After a systematic review of the evidence, recommendations for early detection based on the Grading of Recommendations Assessment, Development and Evaluation (GRADE) system[33–37] were established and ultimately published in 2017.[30] Two types of patients were identified in whom CP could and should be detected before 2 years of age and preferably by 5 months. Those with *attributable risks* have known risk factors in the perinatal period that fit with the referral criteria for most NICU follow-up programs. They are preterm or have various types of pre- or postnatal insults, ranging from the macrostuctural (malformations, hemorrhage, ischemia, or thrombosis) to the microstructural (encephalopathy of prematurity, inflammation, infections). In these infants, a set of assessment tools can be used to make a diagnosis with predictive values for instruments ranging from 80%–98%.[38–46] Overall accuracy increases when several instruments

Table 94.1	Gross Motor Function Classification System (GMFCS)
Level I:	Walks without restrictions; limitations in more advanced gross motor skills
Level II:	Walks without assistive devices; limitations in walking outdoors in the community
Level III:	Walks with assistive mobility devices; limitations in walking outdoors and in the community
Level IV:	Self-mobility with limitations; children are transported or use power mobility outdoors and in the community
Level V:	Self-mobility is severely limited even with the use of assistive technology

Palisano R, Rosenbaum P, Walter S, Russell D, Wood E, Galuppi B. Development and reliability of a system to classify gross motor function in children with cerebral palsy. *Dev Med Child Neurol.* 1997;39(4): 214–223. doi:10.1111/j.1469-8749.1997.tb07414.x.

are used concurrently. For instance, increased predictive accuracy for CP at 3–4 months was obtained when absent fidgety movement patterns on the General Movements Assessment (GMA) were combined with term-equivalent age magnetic resonance imaging (MRI) results and Hammersmith Infant Neurological examination scores.[47] However, the authors of this report acknowledge that the precision obtained in prediction was balanced by the fact that the GMA and MRI readers were all expert level researchers in the field. The positive predictive value of assessments performed by trained researchers in high-risk population, in contrast to that of clinicians in an outpatient setting with a more diverse patient base remains an issue. In a study of two different countries' high-risk follow-up programs that included infants with congenital abnormalities or infections, the specificity of the GMA decreased to the mid-80s.[48] Regardless of the setting, the fact remains that a set of best-evidence guidelines, with GRADE recommendations for moderate-to-high quality exists to allow early detection and diagnosis of CP in high-risk infants.

More recently, as awareness of these guidelines has increased, a separate and confounding issue has occurred in neonatology. As advances in neonatal care, such as systematic use of antenatal steroids or of postnatal caffeine, have improved the developmental outcomes of preterm infants, the overall prevalence of severe forms of CP may be decreasing. Reports indicate that in some developed countries the overall incidence of CP may be decreasing, while severity remains constant.[49,50] However, reports in North America indicate that overall incidence may be increasing, as severity decreases.[51–53] Differences may be due to cohort characteristics or reporting and assessment methodologies. In either scenario, early detection may be more difficult than originally anticipated. The systematic application of guidelines for early detection of CP then becomes a necessary first step to best practice, and an essential next step is improvement of these guidelines in the face of a changing clinical picture for the next decade of NICU care.

The goal of this section is to help guide neurodevelopmental practitioners in their clinical practice by describing how the pathophysiological processes associated with development of CP can be identified in the perinatal period, what clinical features and assessments can support our best efforts at surveillance, which outcomes can help guide prognostic conversations with families, and why optimal management early on can lead to best outcomes for young patients in the future.

Pathophysiology

By definition, CP originates from an injury to or abnormality in the developing brain resulting in abnormal muscle tone which leads to impairment of motor function. To understand the pathophysiology of CP, it is helpful to understand the progression of fetal brain development which begins in the 3rd week of gestation. At 2 to 4 months, neuronal prolifieration occurs with rapid growth of subplate neurons which are the main neuronal components of the cerebral white matter. This is followed by neuronal migration from 3 to 5 months during which time there is also axonal and dendritic growth and synaptogenesis. Neuronal organization and myelination begin in the 3rd trimester and continues well after delivery, though the most rapid period of myelination occurs in the first 2 years of life. Injury to or maldevelopment of the developing brain causes specific brain injury patterns reflecting the disturbance of brain development during critical time windows. However, in many cases CP may not derive from a single cause but rather from a complex cascade of events.

Congentital Abnormalities

Congenital anomalies are found in 15%–19% of children with CP. Cerebral anomalies are the most common and may result from interruption of neuronal proliferation, migration, and differentiation during the first and second trimester.[54–56] Aberrancy of these developmental processes may lead to cortical malformations including polymicrogyria, lissencephaly, and pachygyria. Malformations of grey matter development accounts for approximately 10% of children with CP.[55] Other malformations such as hydranencephaly or schizencephaly may be secondary to infections during pregnancy or a vascular insult during periods of neuronal migration in the second trimester. Microcephaly and hydrocephalus are two of the most frequent cerebral anomalies in children with CP.[54] These may be secondary to abnormal brain development such as in Dandy Walker malformation or aqueductal stenosis, but may also be secondary to intrauterine insults such as a fetal intraventricular hemorrhage resulting in post-hemorrhagic hydrocephalus or intrauterine ischemic injury causing suboptimal brain growth. Congenital abnormalities of brain development are more common in term than preterm infants with CP (16% vs 2.5%) and more frequently associated with spastic quadriparesis or ataxic CP than hemiparetic or dystonic CP.[54,55] The prevalence of non-cerebral anomalies is also higher in children with CP than in the general population and include cardiac, musculoskeletal, and urinary abnormalities.[57]

Prematurity

Twenty-five thousand extremely-low-birth-weight (ELBW; birth weight less than 1000 grams) infants are born in the U.S. each year. Seventeen thousand are born at less than 28 weeks and considered extremely premature; these infants are at a higher risk of disability as the risk of CP is inversely correlated with birth weight and gestational age.[58] The prevalence of CP in children born extremely preterm is 5%–15%.[59–62] As survival in the very-low-birth-weight (VLBW; birth weight less than 1500 grams) population has improved in recent years, this has resulted in more children with long-term disabilities.[63] These include deficits in motor skills, cognition, language, behavior, and attention.[64,65] The pathogenesis of brain injury in this group is a combination of ischemia, hemorrhage, and inflammation damaging the cerebral cortex, white matter, thalamus, basal ganglia, and cerebellum. There are three main patterns of brain injury in preterm infants associated with long-term neuromotor impairments: periventricular leukomalacia (PVL), overall decrease in brain volume, and severe germinal matrix hemorrhage-intraventricular hemorrhage (GMH-IVH). Severe GMH-IVH is particularly likely to be associated with neuromotor impairments when accompanied by periventricular hemorrhagic infarction (PVHI).[5,66]

PVL is the most common injury of white matter in the premature infant. The pathogenesis of PVL is a combination of ischemia and inflammation during the period of rapid axonal and dendritic growth. Ischemia injures premyelinating oligodendrocytes resulting in hypomyelination and damages subplate neurons, likely via apoptosis.[67] The combination of ischemia and inflammation causes decrease in neuronal growth, axonal development and myelination, which can further lead to an overall decrease in volume of the thalamus, basal ganglia, cortex, corpus callosum, and cerebellum. There is both focal and diffuse necrosis which can be visualized macroscopically on head ultrasound as cystic PVL. The less obvious glial scarring only becomes evident after several weeks and requires MRI to visualize. Up to 50% of VLBW infants demonstrate findings of PVL on MRI but with advances in management of the critically-ill VLBW infant, the rates of cystic PVL have decreased to 4%, accounting for only a small percentage of overall infants with white matter injury.[61,68] Rates of CP in cystic PVL range from 52%–100% with the pattern of spastic diplegia being most common.[69–71]

GMH-IVH and periventricular hemorrhagic infarction (PVHI) cause injury via some of the same mechanisms resulting in PVL. The germinal matrix is the primary source of proliferation of oligodendrocyte progenitor cells. Hemorrhage in this area leads to the loss of myelin-producing cells, resulting in decreased myelination and lack of axonal development. There can be direct injury to GABAergic neurons (neurons that secrete gamma-amino butyric acid [GABA], the primary inhibitory neutrotransmitter in the brain), leading to decreased volume of the cerebral cortex and thalamus. These injuries may be exacerbated if post hemorrhagic hydrocephalus develops; this further impairs oligodendrocyte growth and myelination and results in axonal loss. The younger the infant, the greater the risk of severe hemorrhage.

Long-term motor deficits after PVHI correlate with topography of the parenchymal lesions with resultant spastic hemiparesis or asymmetrical spastic quadriparesis being most common. Laterality of PVHI also impacts outcomes, with 50%–67% of infants with unilateral PVHI developing CP, and up to 90% of infants with bilateral PVHI developing CP.[70,72–74]

Perinatal Stroke

Perinatal stroke is a group of cerebrovascular disorders which occur in the developing brain between 20 weeks of fetal life and 28 days postnatal life.[75] This is the highest risk period in childhood for arterial ischemic stroke and occurs in 1:4000 live births.[76] Perinatal stroke is the most common cause of hemiplegic cerebral palsy,[77] and 68% of children with perinatal stroke develop cerebral palsy.[78] The days before and after birth are a period of increased stroke risk for both mother and baby. This may be related to activation of coagulation in both mothers and newborns.[79] There are six subtypes of perinatal stroke, three of which are detected due to acute symptomatic presentation in the neonatal period, most often presenting as seizures. These include (a) neonatal arterial ischemic stroke (NAIS); (b) neonatal cerebral sinovenous thrombosis; and (c) neonatal hemorrhagic stroke. The other three subtypes of perinatal stroke are detected during evaluation of infant or child with hemiparetic CP or other neurological exam abnormalities and include (d) arterial presumed perinatal ischemic stroke; (e) periventricular venous infarction; and (f) presumed perinatal hemorrhagic stroke.

NAIS is the most common type of acute neonatal stroke. The majority involve the anterior circulation—specifically the middle cerebral artery (MCA) territory—and are more common on the left side.[80–82] Injury to the MCA territory can result in upper motor neuron injury in the cerebral cortex and descending corticospinal tracts at the levels of the posterior limb of the internal capsule and cerebral peduncle. These in addition to basal ganglia injury are associated with contralateral hemiparesis.[83–85]

A specific etiology is detected in less than 20% of cases of perinatal stroke.[81] Numerous risk factors have been identified, including placental disease,[86] fetal heart rate abnormalities, emergency caesarean section, need for resuscitation and 5-minute Apgar score less than 7.[82] Intrauterine growth restriction and small for gestational age are also associated with neonatal arterial ischemic stroke.[82,87] Though nulliparity, pre-eclampsia and gestational diabetes have been proposed to increase risk of perinatal stroke, these associations have been inconsistent across studies.

Infection

Both maternal and neonatal infections increase the risk of CP, though the mechanism is not well understood. Maternal chorioamnionitis has been documented in several studies to be associated with increased risk of CP in the child[88]; an increasing body of literature associates inflammatory markers with increased risk. In a large California population-based study, extra-uterine maternal infections also increased the risk of CP in the child.[88–90] This was true both for infections detected prenatally and perinatally.

Neonatal infection also increases the risk of CP, with higher infection rates noted in preterm children. In children born term, those with neonatal infection are more likely to have white matter injury (odds ratio [OR] 2.2) and develop spastic diplegia (OR 1.6) while children born pre-term were more likely to have white matter and cortical injury (OR 4.1) and develop spastic triplegia or quadriplegia (OR 2.4).[91]

Hypoxic-Ischemic Encephalopathy

Hypoxic-ischemic injury in the perinatal period accounts for up to 10% of cases of CP. Ischemia leads to neuronal necrosis and apoptosis as well as injury to oligodendrocytes and impaired cerebrovascular autoregulation.[68,92] The two predominant patterns of injury in neonatal hypoxic ischemic encephalopathy (HIE) are watershed injury (involving vascular boundary zone white matter and cortical grey matter) and deep grey matter nuclei which includes the basal ganglia and thalamus.[93,94] Injuries to the thalamus, basal ganglia, and posterior limb of the internal capsule are associated with worse developmental outcomes. Thirty-six percent to 44% of children with moderate to severe HIE were diagnosed with CP by 2 years of age,[95,96] with moderate to severe basal ganglia lesions the best predictor of CP.

Genetic Associations

The commonly held belief that CP does not run in families and is therefore not inherited has long been questioned because of the increased incidence of cerebral and non-cerebral congenital anomalies in children with CP. Controversy exists surrounding diagnosis of CP in infants with identified genetic anomalies, with some seeing these as distinct entities from CP. However, recent advances in identifying genetic disturbances in infants with CP supports instead that the presence of a genetic anomaly is the etiology of phenotypic presentation of the child, rather than an exclusionary criterion. The advent of DNA sequencing has allowed the identification of likely pathogenic variants. Mutations have been noted in KANK1, AP4M1,

AP4B1, APFS1, GAD1, ZC4H2, ADD3, and NKX2-1 genes.[97] Previously only 2% of CP cases were thought to be genetic. With the use of whole exome and whole genome sequencing, that has increased with up to 15% of cases suspected of having a genetic component.[97,98]

Postnatal Injury

While most cases of CP are caused by prenatal or perinatal events, postnatal injury does account for approximately 10%–20% of cases, particularly when these insults occur in infants or young children.[99] The most common causes of acquired injury include childhood stroke, trauma (including abusive head trauma or motor vehicle accidents), severe hypoxic events such as near-drowning, and infections (particularly meningitis) occurring in the first or second year of life.

Clinical Features and Evaluation of Cerebral Palsy

Early evaluation and recognition of the clinical features of CP are critical to early diagnosis and management. Cerebral palsy is a disorder defined by its phenotype, and clinical diagnosis requires a medical history, evaluation of neuroimaging, and use of standardized neurological and motor assessments.[30] Ruling out progressive disorders which may have treatable causes is also essential.

Altered movement and posture are key characteristics of CP, and it is classified principally by the motor abnormality found on neurological examination.[100] There are three types of motor abnormalities in CP: spasticity, dyskinesia, and ataxia. Though hypotonia is the predominant pattern of some children with motor impairments secondary to injury or abnormalities in the developing brain, there is not a consensus on whether hypotonic CP represents a distinct type of CP or represents a separate type of motor dysfunction. Dyskinetic CP is categorized into dystonic or choreoathetotic. The type is based upon the most prevalent motor feature.[101] Children may be classified as having 'mixed' CP if one motor disorder does not predominate. The spastic type of CP is most common. Spastic CP is categorized by topographical location as unilateral (hemiplegic) or bilateral. Bilateral CP includes diplegia—defined by the lower limbs being affected more than the upper limbs—and quadriplegia, which is defined by the trunk and all four limbs being affected (Novak 2017) though the involvement in the limbs may be asymmetrical. Dyskinetic and ataxic CP usually involve all four extremities. The extent of activity restriction is considered a part of the CP diagnosis, and children without activity restriction should not be considered to have CP.[101] The functional consequences of deficits should be considered and separately classified using validated scales such as the Gross Motor Function Classification System (GMFCS).[101] Children with quadriplegia are most likely to have a GMFCS of 2 or greater.[23]

During evaluation of CP, four components need specific evluation[101]: (a) the motor abnormality; (b) anatomical and neuroimaging findings; (c) functional impairments; and (d) information about the causation and timing. The description of the motor abnormality seen should include identification of abnormalities in tone, whether decreased or increased, in addition to any movement disorder(s) such as spasticity or dystonia. The anatomical distribution of motor deficits should be included, which might be unilateral or bilateral, and may show trunk, bulbar, and/or extremity involvement. There might be multiple neuroimaging findings such as intraventricular hemorrhage or white matter loss. Accompanying impairments may be age-dependent and can include seizures or vision impairment, in addition to other impairments known to be associated with CP.[102] The time frame during which the etiologic injury occurred should also be included if known.

Providers must recognize that the clinical characteristics of CP may change across childhood, and it may be difficult to characterize the type of CP during the first 1 year of life.[30] It is therefore appropriate to diagnose an infant with CP without attempting classification during infancy. An inability to provide certain classification, however; should not preclude an early diagnosis of CP.

Magnetic Resonance Imaging can aid classification. Neuroimaging abnormalities are seen in more than 80% of cases of CP. Most will show isolated white matter damage. Injury to the grey and white matter is most commonly associated with hemiplegic CP. Lesions that are pyramidal are more likely to be associated with hypertonia, spasticity, and brisk reflexes that may be diffuse. Extrapyramidal abnormalities are more often associated with dyskinesia and choreoathetosis.[103] In addition to motor abnormalities, PVL in particular has been associated with cognitive impairment and psychosocial deficits.[100] As slowly-progressive inborn errors of metabolism may mimic CP, metabolic investigations should be considered when diagnosing CP.[104,105] When documenting the CP diagnosis and classification, neuroimaging documentation as well as all metabolic investigations performed or in progress should be included.[101]

Clinicians should consider CP as not merely a motor syndrome, but a neurological impairment with numerous manifestations that may result from the primary disturbance that resulted in CP or from decreased perceptual experiences secondary to activity limitations.[106] CP is often accompanied by other neurodevelopmental impairments that can be debilitating, including secondary muscular problems such as hip displacement, seizures, and disorders of cognition, perception, communication, and behavior.[103] Seizures may be seen in up to 50% of children with hemiplegic CP. Autism screens show abnormalities in nearly 20% of preterm children with CP.[23,107,108] These patients must be evaluated for various comorbid conditions, and many of these issues seem to become more prominent at different ages. Hearing and vision should be assessed, if they have not already, when a diagnosis of CP is made. Epilepsy and cognitive impairment are more likely in children with quadriplegia.[107] Intellectual disabilities are seen more frequently in children who have CP and seizures.

Clinical findings associated with CP will differ based on gestational age at birth, age at assessment, the underlying disease process and the distribution of brain lesion(s)[107] (Figure 94.1). During the first 6 months after birth, CP may be difficult to distinguish from a global developmental delay. The first clinical signs of CP may be poor oromotor skills which may be noted even before a delay in developmental milestones is evident. The classic motor signs of CP recognized in older children and adults, such as spasticity, may not be present in young infants. Indeed, further myelination and basal ganglia maturation often must occur following the original injury in order for abnormal tone to develop. A child initially noted to have hyper- or hypotonicity on clinical examination in the first months of life may develop spasticity or dyskinesia over the first 2 years of life.[107] CP should therefore be considered in children with abnormal motor examinations that do not include spasticity or dyskinesia. During the first year after birth, maintenance of primitive reflexes beyond the accepted age of extinction should raise clinical concern for CP. Other clinical findings that should warrant early, standardized assessment for CP by experts include inability to sit independently by 9 months of age, hand function asymmetry or inability to bear weight in the heel and forefoot.

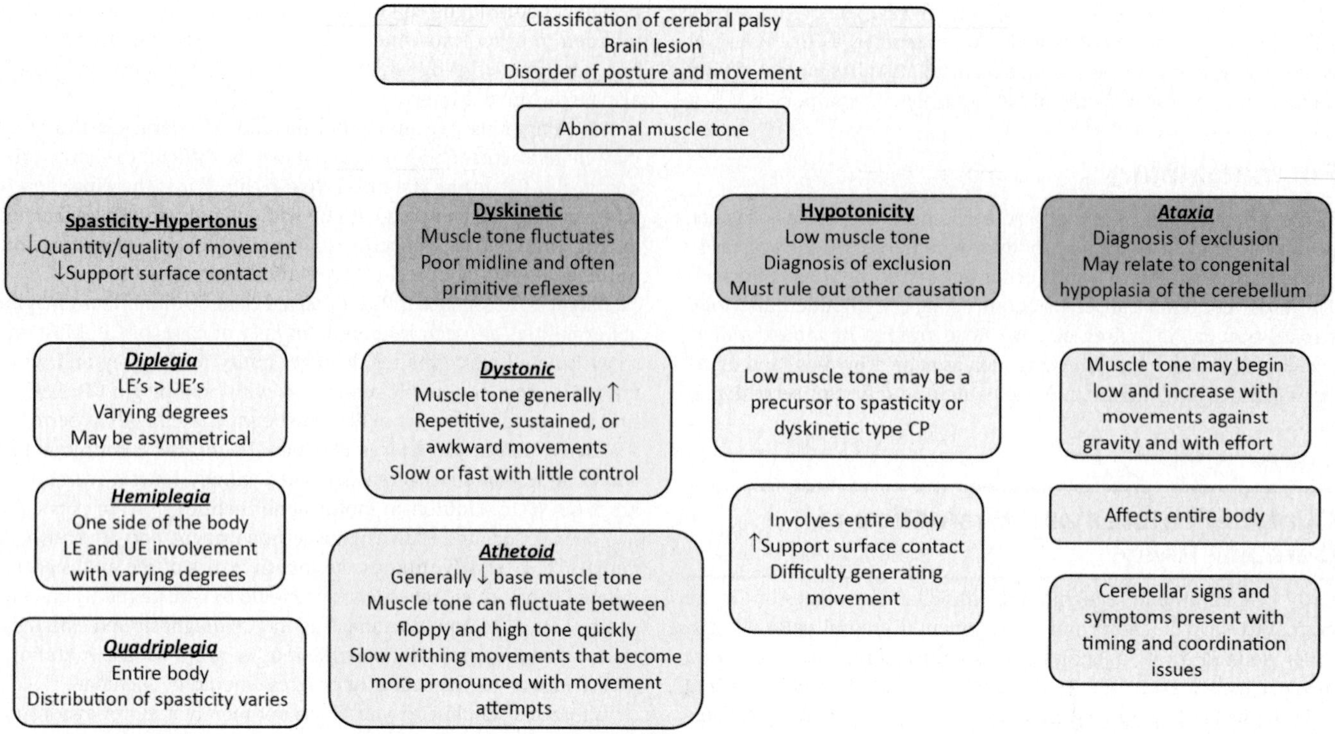

Classification of cerebral palsy
Brain lesion
Disorder of posture and movement

Abnormal muscle tone

Spasticity-Hypertonus
↓Quantity/quality of movement
↓Support surface contact

Diplegia
LE's > UE's
Varying degrees
May be asymmetrical

Hemiplegia
One side of the body
LE and UE involvement with varying degrees

Quadriplegia
Entire body
Distribution of spasticity varies

Dyskinetic
Muscle tone fluctuates
Poor midline and often primitive reflexes

Dystonic
Muscle tone generally ↑
Repetitive, sustained, or awkward movements
Slow or fast with little control

Athetoid
Generally ↓ base muscle tone
Muscle tone can fluctuate between floppy and high tone quickly
Slow writhing movements that become more pronounced with movement attempts

Hypotonicity
Low muscle tone
Diagnosis of exclusion
Must rule out other causation

Low muscle tone may be a precursor to spasticity or dyskinetic type CP

Involves entire body
↑Support surface contact
Difficulty generating movement

Ataxia
Diagnosis of exclusion
May relate to congenital hypoplasia of the cerebellum

Muscle tone may begin low and increase with movements against gravity and with effort

Affects entire body

Cerebellar signs and symptoms present with timing and coordination issues

Fig. 94.1 Classification of Cerebral Palsy. *CP*, Cerebral palsy; *LEs*, lower extremities; *UEs*, upper extremities. (Senesac and McAhren. Management of clinical problems of children with cerebral palsy. In: Umphred's Neurological Rehabilitation, 10, 246–284.e7.)

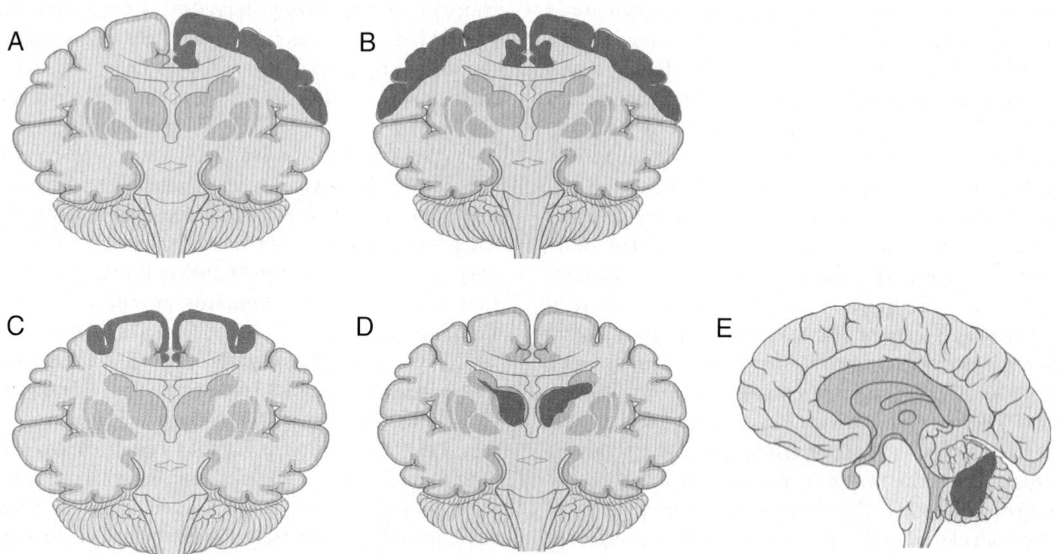

Fig. 94.2 Neurological Lesions Associated With Various Types of Cerebral Palsy (CP). Although there is some overlap in terminology used by various authors, CP can be classified according to distribution (regional versus global involvement, hemiplegic, diplegic, quadriplegic), physiologic type (spastic, dyskinetic/dystonic, dyskinetic/athetoid, ataxic), or by presumed neurological substrate (pyramidal, extrapyramidal). Above schematic figures show lesions (*grey*) associated with the broad categories of CP: (A) unilateral cortical lesions associated with hemiplegia; (B) bilateral lesions associated with quadriplegia; (C) bilateral, but relatively limited lesions in infants with spastic diplegia; (D) lesions in basal ganglia associated with athetoid and dystonic cerebral palsy; and (E) cerebellar lesions seen with infants with ataxia.

Guidelines for Diagnosis

In 2017, Novak et al.[30] published guidelines for early diagnosis of CP, including best evidence for assessments at various ages (Figure 94.2). According to the guidelines, the diagnosis of CP requires motor dysfunction (essential criterion) along with at least one of the following additional criteria: abnormal neuroimaging or clinical history indicating risk for CP. They noted that, in order to make a diagnosis prior to 6 months of corrected age, an experienced clinical team should utilize a combination of standardized tools with strong predictive validity in conjunction with clinical interpretation. Based on the best-available observational data (Figure 94.3), an algorithm for the early diagnosis of CP or

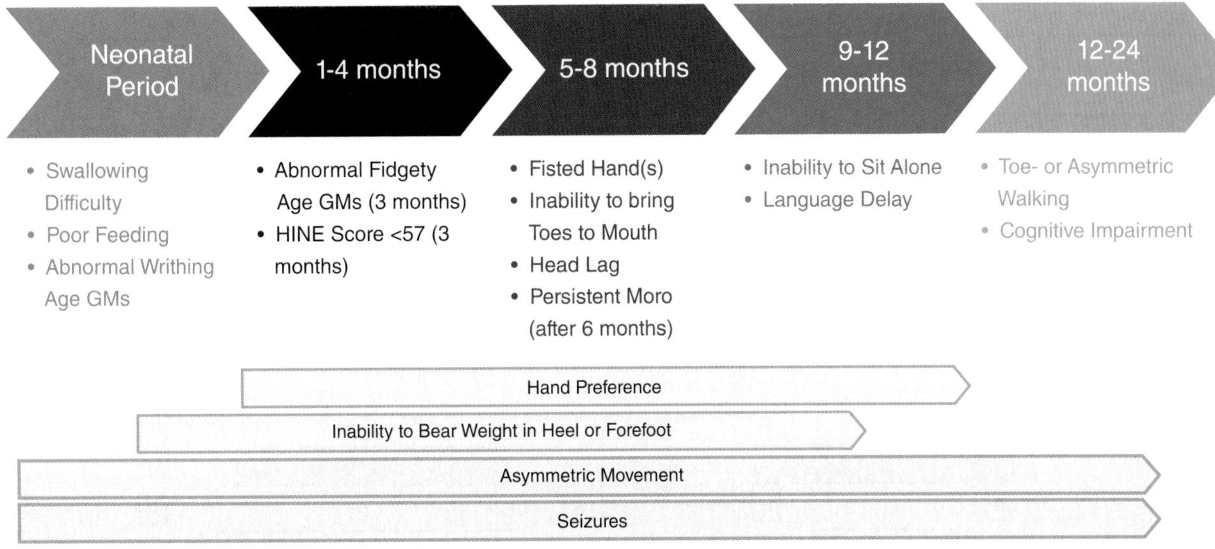

Fig. 94.3 Emergence of Clinical Signs Concerning for Cerebral Palsy.

high-risk of CP is being developed based on newborn-attributable risk categories around the corrected age less or more than 5 months (Figure 94.4). The authors of these guidelines recognized that all tools are not available to all practitioners, therefore, for each age, two pathways were provided—an ideal pathway based on the best evidence, and a 'next best' approach when the tools noted in the ideal pathway are not available. Importantly, when the diagnosis of CP is suspected but not certain, a designation of "high-risk of cerebral palsy" and referral for CP-specific therapies was recommended until the diagnosis is certain. The diagnosis should be made as early as possible, however, not only so that the infant may receive therapies specific to the diagnosis, but so that the parents may receive any supports necessary.

Infants with concern or newborn-attributable risk factors such as prematurity should be assessed for CP prior to 5 months' corrected age. The most accurate method for early detection of CP in children with newborn-detectable risks is a combination of the Prechtl Qualitative Assessment of General Movements (GMA; 98% sensitivity), MRI (86%–89% sensitivity), and clinical history. The GMA may be performed during the NICU stay at writhing age (term age to 2 months post-term) and again at fidgety age (6–9 weeks post-term age). If the GMA or MRI is not available, a standardized neurological assessment (the Hammersmith Infant Neurological Examination [HINE]), and a standardized motor assessment (the Test of Infant Motor Performance [TIMP]) are recommended. A score of < 57 on the HINE at 3 months' corrected age is 96% predictive of CP. Further, multiple GMAs or HINE scores combined with abnormal MRI examination are even more accurate than individual assessments.[30]

Following 5 months of age, different tools are used for early detection of CP. The most accurate method for detection of CP in infants older than 5 months' corrected age is a combination of the HINE, neuroimaging, a standardized motor assessment, and clinical history. As the majority of children with CP are born full-term and may not have a medical history indicating increased risk, it is critical that subspecialty as well as primary care providers recognize the early motor signs of CP. Once CP is identified, the motor severity can be established very well after the age of 2 years using the Gross Motor Function Classification System (GMFCS). Prior to that age, the GMFCS is less reliable.[109,110]

Long-Term Outcomes

Motor Outcomes

"Will my child walk?" is often one of the first questions parents ask after they find out their infant has a brain injury. When discussing prognosis for motor development during infancy, it is difficult to predict when or if children will develop functional ambulation. Prognosis for motor development depends on the type and severity of CP, intellectual ability, visual and sensory as well as social-emotional development. A large cohort of more than 50,000 individuals with CP in California demonstrated the wide range of severity: 6% of individuals with CP were unable to lift their head when lying in the prone position while 59% of individuals over 4 years old with CP walked without a supportive aid and 31% walked unaided for at least 20 feet with good balance.[111]

The subtypes of CP are also an important determinant of the motor outcome. Spastic quadriplegic, hypotonic, and ataxic subtypes are associated with non-independent ambulation whereas almost all children with hemiplegic CP achieve independent ambulation. Probability of independent walking was quite variable in spastic diplegic and dyskinetic CP.

It is only with time that a child's developmental trajectory comes into focus. On average, children reach about 90% of their motor function by 5 years old depending on their GMFCS level. The more severe the motor disability (GMFCS level IV and V), the younger the age at which the child will reach their motor potential.[27,101,106] Among children with CP who were not yet walking at 2 years of age, only 10% were able to walk independently by 6–7 years, and 17% were able to walk independently at a later age.[112] Factors associated with a good prognosis to achieve independent ambulation include ability to sit unsupported by 2 years of age. If a toddler can sit and pull to a stand by 2 years, they have a 76% chance of independent walking by 6 years.[112] Factors associated with a poor prognosis for achieving independent walking include inability to to sit or maintain head control by 2 years of age and persistence of primitive reflexes beyond 2 years.[112–114]

Early diagnosis of CP may allow for earlier focused interventions that may subsequently improve motor outcomes, and as new therapies emerge, patterns of motor development may change. Though

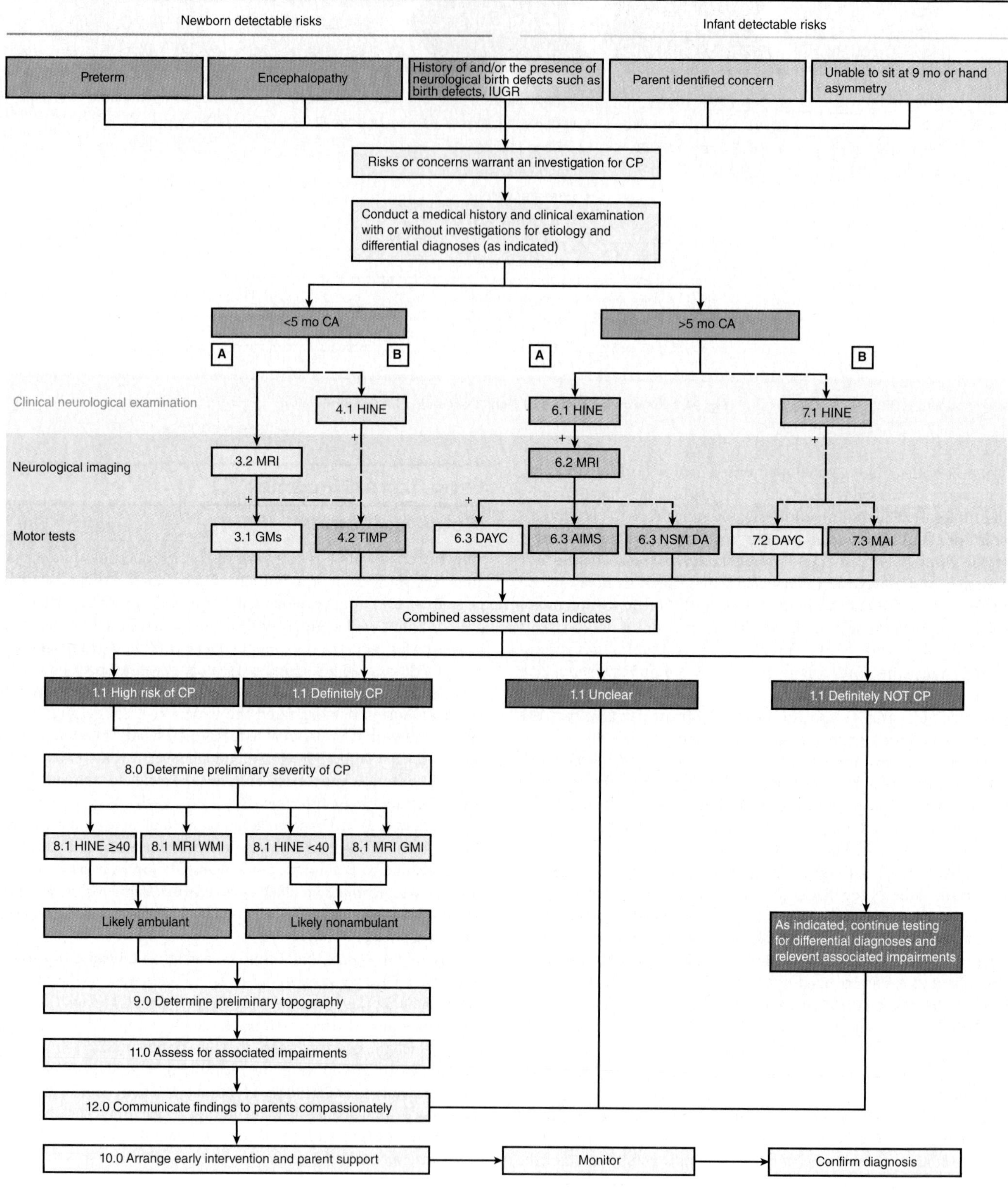
Algorithm for Early Diagnosis of Cerebral Palsy or High Risk of Cerebral Palsy
Newborn detectable risks
Infant detectable risks
Preterm
Encephalopathy
History of and/or the presence of neurological birth defects such as birth defects, IUGR
Parent identified concern
Unable to sit at 9 mo or hand asymmetry
Risks or concerns warrant an investigation for CP
Conduct a medical history and clinical examination with or without investigations for etiology and differential diagnoses (as indicated)
<5 mo CA
>5 mo CA
A
B
A
B
Clinical neurological examination
Neurological imaging
Motor tests
4.1 HINE
6.1 HINE
7.1 HINE
3.2 MRI
6.2 MRI
3.1 GMs
4.2 TIMP
6.3 DAYC
6.3 AIMS
6.3 NSM DA
7.2 DAYC
7.3 MAI
Combined assessment data indicates
1.1 High risk of CP
1.1 Definitely CP
1.1 Unclear
1.1 Definitely NOT CP
8.0 Determine preliminary severity of CP
8.1 HINE ≥40
8.1 MRI WMI
8.1 HINE <40
8.1 MRI GMI
Likely ambulant
Likely nonambulant
As indicated, continue testing for differential diagnoses and relevent associated impairments
9.0 Determine preliminary topography
11.0 Assess for associated impairments
12.0 Communicate findings to parents compassionately
10.0 Arrange early intervention and parent support
Monitor
Confirm diagnosis
A indicates the best available evidence pathway. B indicates the next best available evidence pathway when some tools for evaluation shown in pathway A are not available. AIMS, Alberta Infant Motor Scale; CA, corrected age; CP, cerebral palsy; DAYC, Developmental Assessment of Young Children; GMs, Prechtl Qualitative Assessment of General Movements; HINE, Hammersmith Infant Neurological Examination; IUGR, interuterine growth restriction; MAI, Motor Assessment of Infants; MRI, magnetic resonance imaging; NSMDA, Neuro Sensory Motor Development Assessment; TIMP, Test of Infant Motor Performance; WMI, white matter injury.

Fig. 94.4 Early Detection Pathway. (Reproduced from Novak et al. Early, accurate diagnosis and early intervention in cerebral palsy: advances in diagnosis and treatment. In: *JAMA Pediatr.* 2017;171:897–907.)

most children reach their motor potential by 5–7 years, continued efforts by parents, therapists, physicians, and educators should be made to promote independence and participation.

Nonmotor Outcomes

Increasing GMFCS level is also associated with an increased risk of comorbidities.[29] Children who are unable to ambulate (GMFCS Level IV or V) are more likely to have visual impairment, severe cognitive impairment, limited communication ability, and feeding difficulties. Pain and behavior are the exceptions to this general rule, with pain present at all levels of physical disability and behavioral deficits more common in children with milder physical disability.[28]

Survival

Mortality is highest in the first 5 years of life with severe intellectual disability, severe motor impairment, poor head control, and tube feeding the strongest predictors of early death.[111,115,116] The severity of overall disability is the most important predictor of long-term survival. Most children with mild CP (GMFCS levels I–II) survive into adulthood though life expectancy is generally lower for individuals with CP than the general population. From the Western Australian CP registry study, for those with mild disability who survived past 5 years, life expectancy was 62.5 years compared with 39.6 years for those with more severe disability. Respiratory illness—often aspiration pneumonia—was the most common cause of death.[116] With improvements in diagnosis and management, age and disability-specific mortality rates have declined in children with CP over the last 30 years.[111]

Prognosis

Predicting long-term outcomes for families whose children are at risk for CP is very challenging and can be stressful for families. Providers are often at a loss to answer specific questions parents have about the anticipated neurological function of their child in 5–10 years. Though 80% of children with CP have an abnormal MRI and the location and type of brain abnormality correlates generally with the subtype of CP, there are still significant limitations in the ability to predict outcomes for individual children. Other tools such as the Hammersmith Infant Neurological Examination can help predict asymmetrical CP with high predictive value. Despite this, it is important to provide parents with the range of outcomes and, when possible, the most likely outcome for their child. This will not only inform decision-making about care, but also encourage early identification of at-risk children and provision of targeted interventions when available.

Management

In neonatal follow-up clinics, the mainstay of management is prompt and accurate referral for evidence-based diagnostics and treatments. The strength and quality of evidence for assessments and interventions for infants at high-risk or with CP vary greatly between domains. Published systematic reviews of various topics can be found on most topics, and if not specific to infants with CP, they often target specific co-morbidities common to high-risk infants. In the absence of evidence, it is often inaccurate to extrapolate from interventions that have been successful in older children or adults, because infants seen neonatal follow-up are still in heightened phases of neuroplasticity.

Neuroplasticity, a term used to describe the ability of the developing brain to form new neural connections, pathways, and associations through neurotransmitter potentiation of more frequently generated action-potentials, is often touted as a mechanism to recover function in infants with brain insults. While animal research and limited human pediatric studies have demonstrated that effective compensatory or adaptive plasticity can occur, there are also an equal number reports of maladaptive neuroplasticity or of microstructural changes that do not reflect functional improvements. Plasticity is dependent not only on physiological conditions at the time of intervention, but also on genetically programmed windows of development and the molecular substrate at the time of insult. This is increasingly recognized as genetically-controlled or inherited. While the safety of interventions leveraging plasticity has been carefully studied for medical interventions such as adjuvants to hypothermia or emerging nanoparticle-antioxidant combinations, this has not been the case for developmental interventions. This is in contrast to an extensive body of literature on psychological and behavioral research that has demonstrated that potential for harm exists, regardless of delivery model or intent. The assumption for allied health interventions has mostly been that parent- or therapist-delivered strategies can only be beneficial, and at worst, ineffectual. However, extensive research in ophthalmological neuroscience has demonstrated that behavioral interventions delivered in very early time windows can actually result in permanent loss of visual function. Conversely, neuroplasticity in infants with amblyopia can result in compensatory decreased function in the less affected eye. Other examples of maladaptive plasticity resulting from early interventions exists in auditory and somatosensory systems, making the choice of intervention referral an important one in infants newly diagnosed with CP.

To assist neonatal follow-up practitioners in evaluation of assessment and intervention referrals, newer systematic reviews have adopted a GRADE system of recommendations to assess the quality of the evidence, values and preferences regarding a tool, balance of benefits versus disadvantages, amount of resource use, recommendation direction and overall strength of the recommendation. These elements can help providers establish guidelines for their setting and practice that can be tailored to their specific population. With regard to assessments in infants newly diagnosed with CP, neonatal follow-clinics have highly variable practices depending on whether they routinely follow all high-risk infants or only those in research studies, whether they focus on primary care or developmental trajectories, and whether they have access to multidisciplinary providers or primarily refer to other specialty settings. The age of the child at diagnosis and the potential comorbidities should guide assessment for referrals. In general, evaluation of systematic reviews and updates to these reviews are recommended to ensure continued improvement in clinical management of infants diagnosed early with CP.

Motor

For the past decades, NICU follow-up programs primarily diagnosed CP at or after the age of 2, with a justification that all patients received early intervention through state or federal programs regardless of diagnosis.[116a] While early intervention programs can result in short-term improvements and promote enriched environments, parent education, and awareness of longitudinal development under 3 years, most are not targeted to CP. This contrasts with autism, for which early intervention programs often require specially trained providers, utilize evidence-based approaches, and include strong parent education components.[117,118] However, recent research advances allow more targeted approaches to CP in the early years.

Systematic reviews of interventions to improve motor function in children with CP under two have allowed establishment of key principles for intervention design: motor strategies should start as early as possible, occur as frequently as possible when incorporated into daily routines, adapt to infant attention and endurance spans, be infant-initiated, and goal-directed.[30,39,119–121] New promising clinical trials of interventions for infants with CP are in progress or have concluded with exciting results.[122–126] For infants with CP and asymmetrical hand use starting as early as 6 months, combinations of bimanual and soft-constraint therapy can improve reach, fine motor skills, and even tactile function.[126] In those with the highest GMFCS levels, new trials have examined the effects of therapy dosing in improving the acquisition of gross motor skills.[119,127,128] Even head control may be improved, a critical function that differentiates GMFCS Levels IV and V levels, and allows the improvement of respiratory, language, and social-emotional skills, among others. New trials of parent-based upper extremity training, technology-assisted developmental milestone acquisition and goal-oriented, activity-based, environmental enrichment therapy are currently ongoing in infants with CP.[119]

Sensory

Sensory systems are the earliest to develop in fetal life and all infants at high-risk or with CP benefit from regular specialty examinations by audiologists[129,130] and ophthalmologists[131,132] in the first years. While these examinations have primarily been validated for clinical purposes such as hearing and vision evaluations, some, such as auditory or visual evoked potentials measured by electroencephalogram, allow a more in depth assessment of sensorineural function.[133–135] Most of these have high levels of internal and external validity and are not specific to CP. A battery of behavioral visual assessments was developed specifically for high-risk infants and allows more targeted evaluation of suspected low-vision impairments and tailoring of environmental supports. However, at this time the entire battery is not always included in routine ophthalmlogic exams throughout the world and may need to be specifically requested. Assessment of audiological function using behavioral tests can be challenging in young infants with CP, and evaluations of pathway integrity from the cochlea to the cortex may need to be performed under anesthesia to provide accurate results. For both vision[136–140] and hearing,[129,141–143] effective interventions ranging from surgery to augmentation can result in excellent outcomes preserving infants' ability to interact with their environment and family. Currently, a randomized clinical trial is studying the effect of a parent-supported intervention in improving vision in infants with CP who also suffer from cerebral visual impairment.[123] Less is known about somatosensory systems, but new interventions emphasizing increased and graduated exposures to tactile stimuli also show promise in improving neural responses.[126] Finally, while good assessments of multisensory reactivity in clinic or home environments can be performed by occupational therapists, the evidence for sensory integration therapies in infants is of very poor quality at this time and no recommendations with regards to safety or efficacy can be made.

Cognition

While the prevalence of cognitive and executive function impairments has been studied in older children with CP, little is known about the early years.[144] This is in great part due to the paucity of assessments that can accurately evaluate cognition in children with motor impairments. The cognitive domain of the Bayley Scales of Infant and Toddler Development[3] relies heavily on fine motor abilities and on postural control in sitting. While recommendations are made for adapting it to low vision and low hearing situations, little is known about standardization in cases of disordered or impaired movement. The Fourth edition of the Bayley[3] incorporates parent questionnaires and has adaptive administration components which may facilitate more accurate evaluation of cognition in NICU follow-up settings. Currently, the Mullen Scales of Early Learning[145] is the only test with some evidence of responsivity to intervention in infants with CP,[146] while the Mayes Motor-Free Compilation,[147] Fagan Test of Infant Intelligence,[148] and Bayley-III Low Motor/Vision[149,150] have some predictive and/or discriminative psychometric properties.[151] Evaluation of cognition and effectiveness of cognitive interventions in NICU follow-up is further complicated by numerous studies demonstrating that parental, genetic, socioeconomic factors explain upwards of 50% of variability in developmental outcomes of preterm infants. Until interventions are targeted specifically to CP, early intervention programs remain the mainstay of educating parents on development, responsivity, and enriched environments, although none of these have been shown to have effects lasting until school-age.

Sleep, Pain, Spasticity

Disorders of sleep are understudied in infants at high-risk or with CP under the age of 2, primarily due to the lack of easily-available measures in preverbal-populations.[152,153] Therefore, most studies have relied on parent-report behavioral questionnaires[154,155] such as the Brief Infant Sleep Questionnaire[156] or clinical sleep studies with or without electroencephalography.[157–159] Developmental progression of sleep from the preterm period onwards may influence frequently-measured outcomes such as cognition, language, motor, and behaviors/emotions. In NICU graduates, complicating pulmonary factors such as obstructive apnea or bronchopulmonary dysplasia may contribute to sleep disturbances related to other common conditions in infants with CP[160] such as seizures,[161] spasticity,[162] and pain.[163] There is some evidence to suggest that children with CP frequently experience behavioral sleep disturbances (17%–35% at preschool age)[154,155,164] and these are later associated with other neurodevelopmental problems such as cognitive impairments or tendencies to externalizing or internalizing behaviors.[154,165,166] Management of sleep problems specifically targeted to those with CP may therefore overlap with treatment of contributing co-morbidities. Evidence for sleep interventions in children with developmental disabilities suggests a role for parenting styles, emphasizing warmth, structure, and sleep hygiene (regularity of schedules, removal of televisions, or distractors in the sleep environment, and routines).[153,167–169] For children with CP, limited evidence suggests promotion of circadian cycle regularity through the use of environmental supports[168] and possibly, melatonin.[153]

Tone and movement disorders can significantly impact motor function, but also participation in family life and establishment of typical routines and sleep. Because of the lack of pain-report measures validated for children under 2, inferences about the links between spasticity and pain are derived from studies in older children.[170,171] Absence of typical pain manifestations in the early months after injury is a poor indicator of lack of pain, as studies comparing behavioral signs to brain-based measures have demonstrated.[172,173] In NICU follow-up settings, the safest practice may be to assume that if parents report perceiving pain in their infant with spasticity, the infant is experiencing pain. Management of spasticity can help relieve pain; positive parenting strategies, environmental adaptations, physical and occupational therapy practice can moderate spasticity and pain (Triple-P).[174,175] However, no studies have compared the effectiveness or safety of various anti-spasmodic agents in children under 2. Treatment is based on case reports, expert opinion or extrapolations from studies of older children.[121,162,176] In general, referral to physical medicine specialists or neurologists may be helpful if all non-medical interventions have proved ineffective. Interventions with the fewest safety concerns such as baclofen should be considered first, which may be followed by a benzodiazepine or carbidopa/levodopa, and only then most invasive and expensive ones such as botulinum toxin injections or surgery should be introduced.

Behavioral

Children with CP are at higher risk of having behavioral problems, including difficulties with peers, emotional problems, hyperactivity and problems with conduct.[23,30,101,155,177] Novak et al.[30] showed that 1 in 4 children with CP have behavioral abnormalities, a much-higher incidene of 1 in 10 in typically-developing children. Interventions targeting parenting, such as the multilevel Positive Parenting Program (Triple-P) intervention, have been demonstrated to be effective in improving behavior in children who are typically developing. A variant of Triple P, entitled Stepping Stones Triple P (SSTP),[174] has been designed for children with disabilities. The SSTP and Acceptance and Commitment Therapy are parent-targeted interventions that have been associated with decreased hyperactivity and improved child behavior in a randomized trial of children with CP at a mean age of 5 years.[178] Stepping Stones Triple P is largely group-based, and includes supporting parents to encourage desirable behavior in their child, teach their child new skills, and manage misbehavior in their children. Acceptance and Commitment Therapy involves two group sessions focused upon mindfulness, cognitive defusion, acceptance of emotions, identifying values, and making goals.[178] Though this trial was performed in children who were early school age, studies of behavioral interventions in younger children with CP are in progress.

Parents and Parenting

Parent well-being is beneficial to child development, and following the stress of the NICU, parents are at high risk for deficits in mental health. Coping with a diagnosis of CP is difficult, and the loss parents feel may contribute to elevated levels of parental stress.[30] Given this, close follow-up and family-centered surveillance and support are vital. It is critical that therapeutic support is provided at the time of diagnosis and beyond, given the importance of parental involvement in improving outcomes of children with CP.

Receiving the CP diagnosis as early as possible is a parent priority.[31] Most parents want to work collaboratively with the children's health-care providers in making treatment decisions and implementing a flexible, individualized plan of care.[52] The relational competencies parents identify as critical to having truly collaborative relationships with healthcare providers are caring (providing personalized care, being compassionate and respectful); open communication with parents; and interacting with children.[52] Communication of a CP diagnosis should occur over multiple, well-planned conversations. These conversations should be face-to-face, private, culturally sensitive, free of jargon, honest, and ideally should include both caregivers. The provider should outline the child and family's strengths and should be followed by provision of written communication and educational materials. The family should be invited to discuss their feelings and ask questions.[30]

The Triple P and SSTP parent interventions significantly improve parenting practices, parenting efficacy, parental adjustment, the coparental relationship, and satisfaction.[174,175] When combined with Acceptance and Commitment Therapy, a decrease in parental depression and anxiety have also been shown.[177]

Conclusion

Early identification of CP in NICU follow-up using best-practice guidelines derived from a systematic review of the evidence is now possible. Implementation of the early detection guidelines has started on a large scale clinically in the U.S. and North America. Efforts to accomplish this in Europe and Australia are forthcoming, as well as initiatives to translate these guidelines into practice in developing countries where NICU care and neonatal follow-up pose distinct challenges. The ultimate goal of early detection of CP is the design of effective interventions to change developmental trajectories when infants and families can benefit most from them, in order to maximize future participation in family and societal life, physical and mental health. Without early identification and vigilant, standardized surveillance, research in new treatments is almost impossible unless it occurs solely in research settings. Evidence-based clinical practice in NICU follow-up can ensure that all infants with CP benefit from this research, through broadly available and feasible initiatives in quality improvement, knowledge translation, and implementation science. Early detection and intervention for infants with CP is transforming neonatal follow-up from a clinical and ethical check-and-balance system for NICU care to an active and transformative care system for patients and their parents.

Section 19

CHAPTER

95 Use of Neuroimaging to Predict Adverse Developmental Outcomes in High-Risk Infants

Gayatri Athalye-Jape

KEY POINTS

1. Nearly half of all very low birth weight infants may have had brain injury due to hypoxia-ischemia, arterial ischemic stroke(s), inflammation, infection, and intraventricular hemorrhages (IVHs).
2. Neuroimaging is increasingly seen in a "biomarker-like role," where it can add to the information to develop and tailor the clinical developmental screening programs. Cranial ultrasound has been the modality of first choice to screen for brain injury because it enables the assessment of the temporal evolution of brain injury. Magnetic resonance imaging, with its noninvasive neuroimaging protocols, has defined the morphometric alterations in brain injury.
3. White matter injury (WMI) is the most common type of brain injury in preterm infants, seen with or without IVH. WMI can been seen in several neuropathological patterns, including cystic WMI with macroscopic focal necrosis evolving to cysts and noncystic WMI with multiple focal necrotic areas evolving to glial scars and diffuse astrogliosis without focal necrosis.
4. IVH is an important determinant of neurodevelopmental outcome. High-grade IVH that is seen in more than half of the ventricular volume or extending into the surrounding brain parenchyma is a reasonable predictor of neuromotor impairment including cerebral palsy.
5. Cerebellar hemorrhages are frequently seen in infants with IVH or periventricular hemorrhagic infarctions, and even isolated lesions have been associated with cognitive, learning, and behavioral deficits impacting quality of life and daily function.
6. Imaging abnormalities have been noted in severely ill neonates with multisystem organ failure, who are at risk of neurodevelopmental abnormalities. These infants may benefit from repeat imaging studies and early clinical intervention during follow-up.

Introduction

Advances in obstetric and neonatal care during the past 3 decades have significantly reduced mortality in very preterm (VP) infants.[1,2] However, up to 50% of the surviving very low birth weight infants (born with birth weights <1500 g) may have had brain injury, secondary to hypoxia-ischemia, arterial ischemic stroke(s), inflammation, infection, and intraventricular hemorrhages (IVHs) followed by posthemorrhagic ventricular dilatation (PHVD) and periventricular venous hemorrhagic infarction (PVHI).[3,11] Intracranial hemorrhage and white matter (WM) abnormalities are frequently seen in infants with earlier brain injury.[4–6] Such neurologic damage can cause life-long disabilities such as epilepsy, cerebral palsy (CP), motor dysfunction, neurosensory impairment, cognitive and language impairment, behavioral disorders such as attention deficit-hyperactivity disorder (ADHD), autism-spectrum disorders (ASDs), and even increased medium- and long-term mortality.[3,7–11]

Neuroimaging is increasingly seen in a "biomarker-like role," where it can add to the information to develop and tailor clinical developmental screening programs and improve our ability to define the exact type and extent of brain injury a neonate may have endured. In this context, the advances in precision medicine may be further helpful; applied machine learning and computational data analysis, neurocritical monitoring, neuroimaging, and the modern omics technologies may help in developing individualized programs.[12] This chapter is focused on current and ongoing advances in neuroimaging to expedite early diagnosis, measure structural brain damage, and track long-term neurodevelopmental outcomes. With continuing concerns about the short- and long-term impacts of radiation on the developing brain, it has been cranial ultrasound (cUS) and magnetic resonance imaging (MRI), not computed tomography, that have been used most frequently to image the neonatal brain. In the following sections, we first briefly introduce these two modalities; the remaining part of chapter is then organized based on the anatomic localization of the lesions.

Imaging of the Neonatal Central Nervous System

Cranial Ultrasound

cUS has been the modality of first choice to screen for brain injury in neonates since the 1970s because it enables temporal assessment of the evolution of brain injury and the overall growth and maturation of the central nervous system.[13,14] Advances in the resolution and

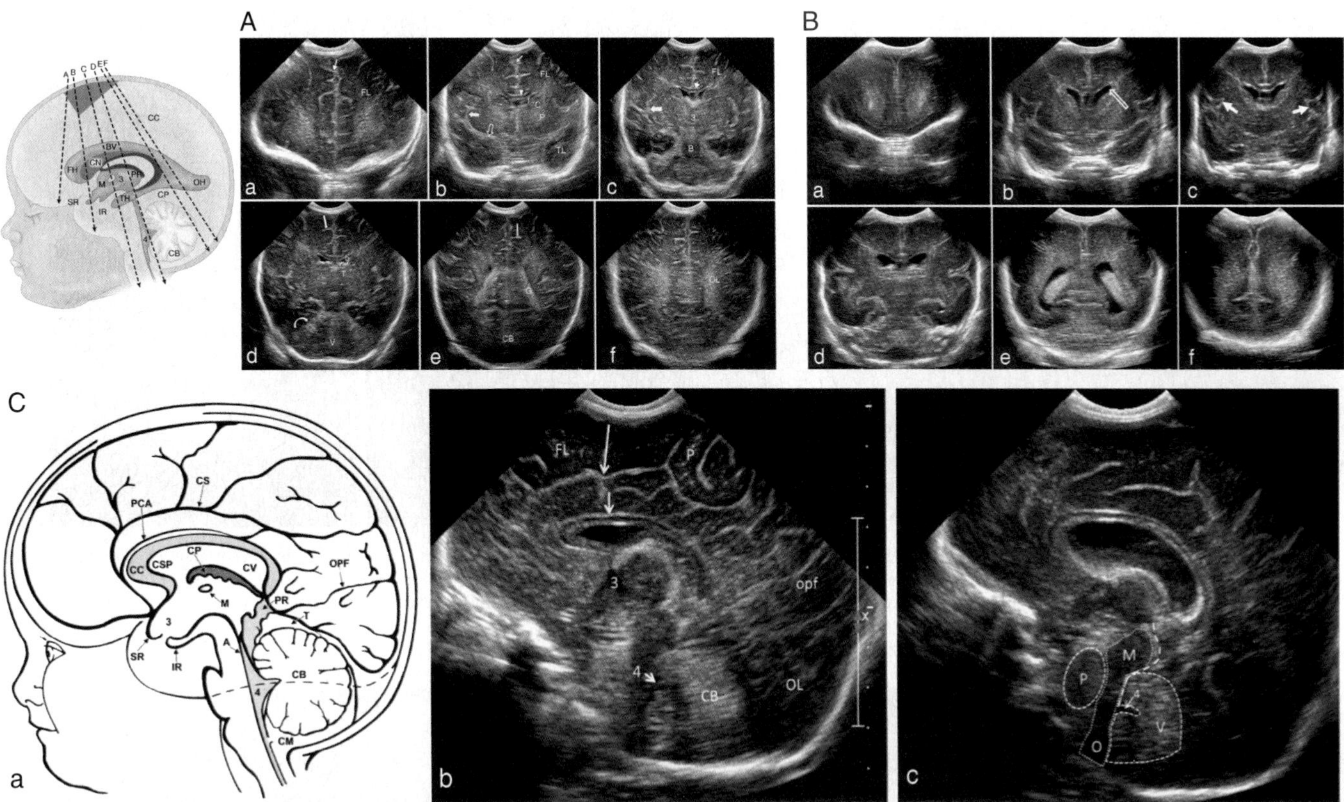

Fig. 95.1 Coronal Brain Ultrasound Planes Through Anterior Fontanelle in a Term (A) and a Preterm (B) Infant. (A) Parts a to f show the planes for imaging from front to back. *3*, Third ventricle; *4*, fourth ventricle; *BV*, body of lateral ventricle; *CB*, cerebellum; *CC*, cerebral cortex; *CN*, caudate nucleus; *CP*, choroid plexus; *FH*, frontal horn; *IR*, infundibular recess; *M*, massa intermedia; *OH*, occipital horn; *PR*, pineal recess; *SR*, supraoptic recess; *TH*, temporal horn. Images on the right show (a) *FL*, Frontal lobes; *small white arrow* in b, interhemispheric fissure. (b) *C*, Caudate nucleus; *f*, frontal horn of lateral ventricle (*thin arrow*); *P*, putamen; *TL*, temporal lobe; *arrowhead*, corpus callosum; *closed arrow*, sylvian fissure; *open arrow*, bifurcation of internal carotid artery. (c) *3*, Location of third ventricle; *B*, brainstem; *FL*, frontal lobe; *arrowhead*, corpus callosum. (d) *b*, Body of lateral ventricle; *c*, choroid plexus; *T*, thalamus; *V*, vermis of cerebellum; *curved arrow*, tentorium cerebelli; *straight arrow*, cingulate sulcus. (e) *CB*, Cerebellum; *G*, glomus of choroid plexus; *arrow*, cingulate sulcus. (f) *OL*, Occipital lobe. (B) In extremely premature infants, ventricles can be larger (*hollow arrow*). Sylvian fissures (*arrows*) may appear boxlike. (C) Normal midline sagittal anatomy. (a) Schematic drawing. *3*, Third ventricle; *4*, fourth ventricle; *A*, aqueduct; *CB*, cerebellum (vermis); *CC*, corpus callosum; *CM*, cisterna magna; *CP*, choroid plexus; *CS*, cingulate sulcus; *CSP*, cavum septi pellucidi; *CV*, cavum vergae; *IR*, infundibular recess; *M*, massa intermedia; *OPF*, occipitoparietal fissure; *PCA*, pericallosal artery; *PR*, pineal recess; *SR*, supraoptic recess; *T*, tentorium. (b) Normal midline sagittal ultrasound brain scan. *3*, Third ventricle; *4*, fourth ventricle; *CB*, cerebellar vermis; *FL*, frontal lobe; *OL*, occipital lobe; *opf*, occipitoparietal fissure; *P*, parietal lobe; *long arrow*, cingulate sulcus; *short arrow*, corpus callosum. (c) Sagittal midline sonogram. *4*, Fourth ventricle; *M*, midbrain; *O*, medulla oblongata; *P*, pons; *V*, cerebellar vermis; *dotted line*, aqueduct of Sylvius. (Reproduced after permission and minor modifications from Rumack and Auckland. *Diagnostic Ultrasound*, ch. 45, 1511–1572.)

image processing speed of cUS during the past decades have improved detection of WM abnormalities and have facilitated the diagnosis of cystic WM injury (WMI), the detection of cerebellar lesions and supratentorial WM cystic lesions,[13] and the evolution of germinal matrix hemorrhage-intraventicular hemorrhage (GMH-IVH).[15] Unfortunately, cUS cannot detect subtle lesions or diffuse gray matter (GM) and WMI. Fig. 95.1 shows the normal anatomy through coronal images from full-term (see Fig. 95.1A), premature (see Fig. 95.1A), and term sagittal views (see Fig. 95.1C). Fig. 95.2 shows the images through the occipital horn, and Fig. 95.3 shows the images seen through the mastoid fontanelle at the level of the fourth ventricle.

MRI

MRI, with its noninvasive neuroimaging protocols, has defined the morphometric alterations in brain injury. It has also helped identify predictors of neurodevelopmental outcome. Standard T1- and T2-weighted images are helpful in reviewing the anatomy of the developing brain. Common neurologic conditions such as hypoxic-ischemic brain injury, perinatal stroke, IVH-PVHI, central nervous system infections, and congenital cerebral malformations are easily detected on standard sequences. Advanced techniques such as brain morphometry, diffusion MRI, volumetric MRI, magnetic resonance spectroscopy (MRS), inversion recovery/fluid attenuated inversion recovery (FLAIR), and functional MRI at term-equivalent age (TEA) assist with prediction of developmental abnormalities.[16] Ultrafast/haste MRI sequences are useful for monitoring the progression of PHVD and to confirm shunt placement. Qualitative MRI helps with numerical measurements and enables construction of quantitative maps and complex brain images.[17] MRI outlines the appropriate burden of ventriculomegaly through a detailed presentation of the third and fourth ventricles, posterior fossa structures, and fourth ventricle outflow tract obstruction. Quantitative MRI supports volumetric assessments (myelinated and unmyelinated WM, cortical and deep GM, brainstem, cerebellum, and cerebrospinal fluid [CSF]) where volume is recorded in volumetric pixels or voxels. Higher ventricle volumes were associated with decreased cognitive performance in preterm children with IVH and other brain injury.[18,19] Bora et al.[20] reported that VP infants (born at 28–32 weeks) with ADHD had 4% less total cerebral volume and 36% more CSF than preterm comparators and 8% less total brain tissue and 144% more CSF volume compared with full-term children without attentional issues, even after adjusting for intracranial cavity volumes. Table 95.1

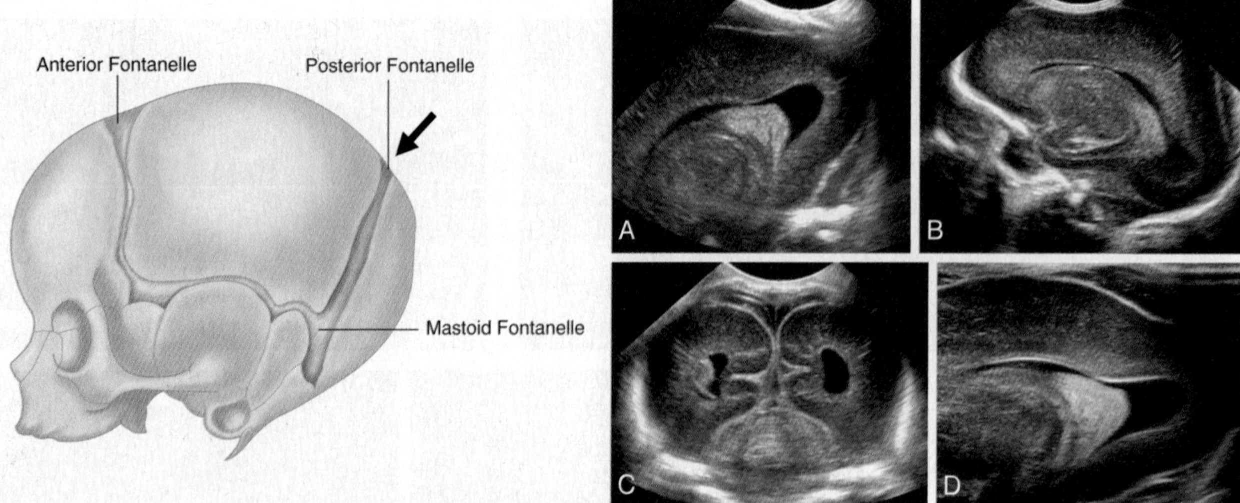

Fig. 95.2 Normal Brain Images of the Occipital Horn Obtained Through the Posterior Fontanelle (*Arrow*). (A) The sagittal occipital horn from the posterior fontanelle. (B) The same sagittal occipital horn from the anterior fontanelle. (C) Coronal occipital horns from the posterior fontanelle; an echogenic clot is visible in the right occipital horn. (D) The same occipital horn; the linear transducer shows increased resolution. (Reproduced after permission and minor modifications from Rumack and Auckland. *Diagnostic Ultrasound*, ch. 45, 1511–1572.)

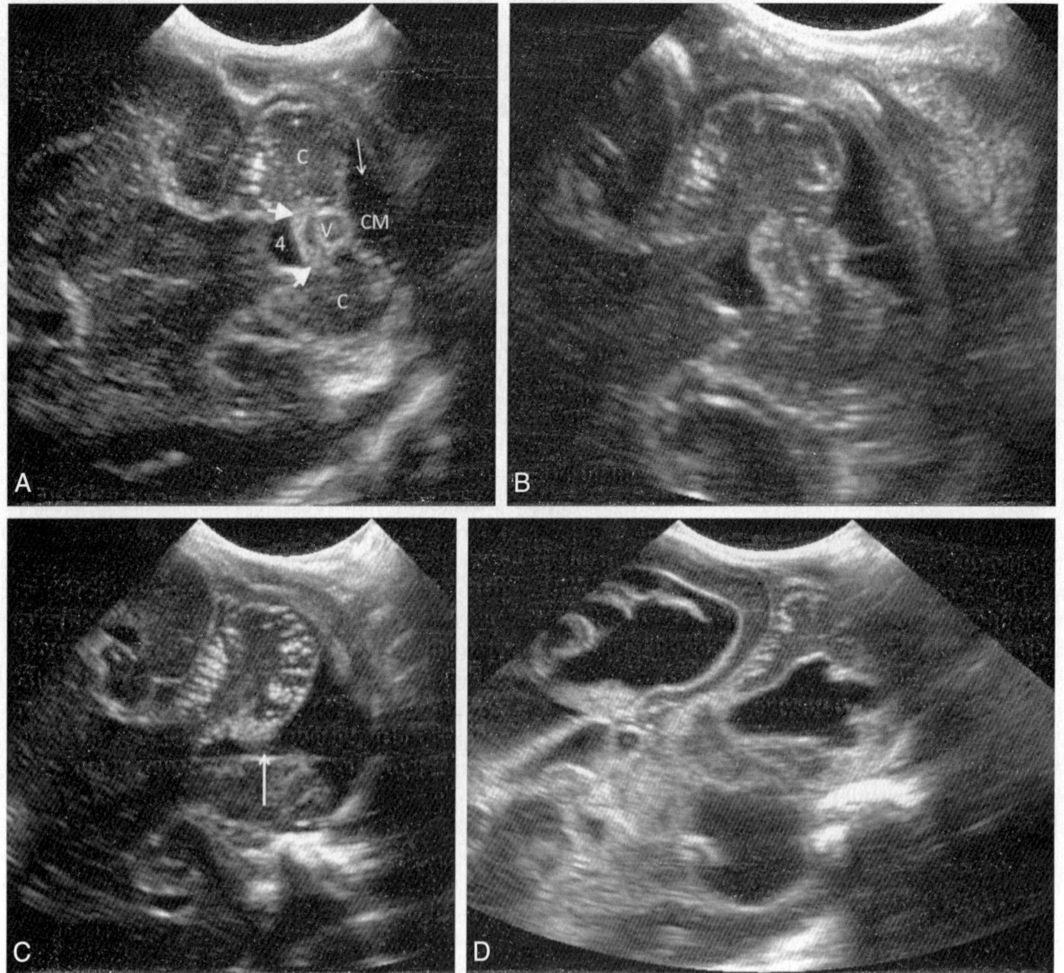

Fig. 95.3 Mastoid Fontanelle Images at the Fourth Ventricle Level in the Posterior Fossa. (A) Normal cerebellar hemispheres. Cisterna magna septa (*arrow*); choroid plexus in the roof of the fourth ventricle (*arrowheads*). (B) Normal axial cisterna magna. Note the radiating folia of the cerebellar hemispheres that contain relatively hypoechoic neural tissue and are surrounded by echogenic leptomeninges in the multiple cerebellar fissures. (C) Low posterior fossa view through the vallecula: deep groove between the cerebellar hemispheres which is occupied by the tonsil and inferior vermis (*arrow*). (D) Severe enlargement of the fourth ventricle in an infant with posthemorrhagic hydrocephalus. *4*, Fourth ventricle; *C*, cerebellar hemispheres; *CM*, cisterna magna; *V*, cerebellar vermis. (Reproduced after permission and minor modifications from Rumack and Auckland. *Diagnostic Ultrasound*, ch. 45, 1511–1572.)

Table 95.1 Variables Assessed by Clinical MRI at Term-Equivalent Age

Cerebral WM	Cysts ± signal abnormality, myelination of PLIC and corona radiata, size and morphology of corpus callosum (CC) and lateral ventricles, volume of periventricular WM
Cortical GM	Signal abnormality, cortical fold maturation, size of extracerebral space
Subcortical GM	Signal abnormality, symmetry and size of basal ganglia and thalamus
Cerebellum	Signal abnormality, symmetry, and size of hemispheres

GM, Gray matter; *MRI*, magnetic resonance imaging; *PLIC*, posterior limb of internal capsule; *WM*, white matter.

highlights the important variables assessed at TEA by MRI (adapted from Inder [2003], Woodward [2006], Nguyen [2009], Kidokoro [2013], and Walsh [2014]). Table 95.2 provides an overview of cUS and MRI as neuroimaging modalities (adapted from Sewell et al. [2018]).

Types of Brain Injury in the Neonatal Period

Preterm WMI

WMI is the most common type of brain injury in preterm infants and is seen with or without IVH (Fig. 95.4). Romero-Guzman et al. showed that the visible prevalence of preterm WMI (cystic and noncystic) was 14.7% on cUS and 32.8% on MRI. Prevalence increased with decreasing gestation: 39.6% in extremely preterm (EP) infants (<28 weeks), 27.4% in VP infants (<32 weeks), and 7.3% in infants <37 weeks. Known clinical risk factors were perinatal hypoxia, hypotension (ischemia), intrauterine infections, late onset bacteremia, and necrotizing enterocolitis.[21] The neuropathological patterns of WMI were cystic WMI with macroscopic focal necrosis evolving to cysts, noncystic WMI with multiple focal necrotic areas evolving to glial scars, and diffuse astrogliosis without focal necrosis.[22,23] Although classic cystic WMI is associated with spastic bilateral CP, diffuse cerebral WMI is associated with cognitive impairment or issues with behavior, attention, social interaction, hearing, and visual impairment.[24] The constellation of WMI and secondary trophic GM damage leads to altered cortical and thalamic development and is labeled *encephalopathy of prematurity*.[25] Reduced cerebral cortical and deep gray nuclei volumes, delayed cortical folding, and abnormal myelination are frequently reported at term-equivalent MRI (TE-MRI) in preterm infants with WMI.[26] Table 95.3 summarizes the common neuropathology patterns in preterm infants with brain injury. Impaired neurodevelopment at 2 years (cognitive delay in 23% and motor delay in 26%) may be seen in many preterm infants with normal cUS.[27]

Structural MRI is highly sensitive in detecting preterm WMI (Fig. 95.5). TE-MRI showing WMI was highly predictive of motor impairment and was inversely related to Bayley scores after controlling for confounders including gestation and sepsis.[28-30] WMI on

Table 95.2 Variables Assessed by Clinical MRI at Term-Equivalent Age

Modality	Anatomic Areas Visualized	Advantages	Disadvantages	Clinical Application	Recent Advances
CRANIAL ULTRASOUND (cUS)					
1. Anterior fontanelle views in coronal and sagittal sections	Ventricular systems, periventricular white matter, deep gray matter	• Cost-effective • Noninvasive • Portable • No need for sedation • Accurate diagnosis of IVH, cystic WM injury, ventriculomegaly, substantial arterial ischemic stroke, regional blood flow	• Interoperator variability • Variability between interpreters, for minor lesions • Less sensitive in detection of cystic WM injury, posterior fossa lesions, myelination, extraaxial lesions, cerebral ischemia, intraparenchymal hemorrhage, metabolic disturbances	• Well established, extensively used • Ideal for screening and serial imaging in unstable neonates	Improved resolution and image processing speed has improved detection of WM abnormalities associated with preterm brain injury
2. Posterior fossa views through mastoid and posterior fontanelles	Cerebellar hemispheres, cerebellar vermis, cisterna magna, fourth ventricle				
3. Color Doppler	Visualization of venous flow in transverse and sigmoid sinuses				
MAGNETIC RESONANCE IMAGING (MRI)					
1. Standard T1- and T2- weighted imaging for qualitative assessment of abnormal anatomy or myelination	• Ventricular systems, periventricular WM and deep GM • Cerebellar hemispheres, cerebellar vermis, cisterna magna, fourth ventricle and its plexus	• Better structural evaluation, particularly peripheral cerebral WM and GM, and posterior fossa	• Expensive • Needs technical and clinical expert interpretation • Availability • Need for specialized equipment • Nonportable so limited use in critically unwell neonates • Need for transport and sedation	• Can be used in high-risk neonates	Quantitative MRI techniques predict neurodevelopmental delay, language, executive function, behavioral issues
2. Advanced MRI techniques focused on quantitative analysis					

GM, Gray matter; *GMH*, germinal matrix hemorrhage; *IVH*, intraventricular hemorrhage; *WM*, white matter; *GM*, gray matter.

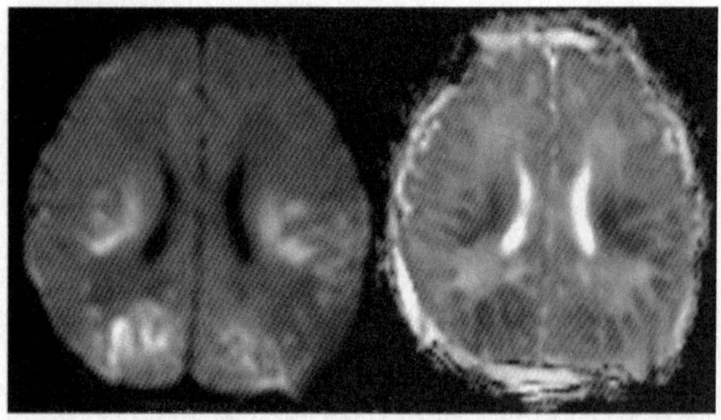

Fig. 95.4 Preterm Periventricular White Matter Leukomalacia/Injury (PVL). Diffusion-weighted imaging (*left*) and the apparent diffusion coefficient (*right*) show diffusion restriction within the periventricular white matter bilaterally. A similar injury pattern is also present in the bilateral posterior parietal subcortical white matter and cortical gray matter. Although white matter injury is more commonly visible in preterm infants, gray matter injury is also occasionally present. (Reproduced after permission and minor modifications from Miller et al. *Seminars in Pediatric Neurology*. 2020;33:100796.)

TE-MRI increased the risk of motor impairment (odds ratio [OR], 10) and cognitive impairment with intelligence quotient <70 at the age of 9 years (OR, 8.3); these persisted through school age.[4,31–33] Punctate WM lesions or diffuse excessive high signal intensity (DEHSI) were not predictive of significant cognitive or mental disability or CP in early childhood.[34,35] The value of MRI compared with cUS for prognostication of motor deficits is unclear; however, MRI may be superior to cUS for prediction of cognitive and behavioral issues.[36] Campbell et al. reported higher cognitive impairment (OR, 3.5; 95% CI, 1.7–7.4), CP (OR, 14.3; 95% CI, 6.5–31.5), and epilepsy (OR, 6.9; 95% CI, 2.9–16.8) in a cohort of 889 EP infants at 10 years whose cUS showed WMI without IVH. Similar associations were seen in WMI with IVH. Interestingly, the authors did not report adverse outcomes with isolated IVH.[37] Arulkumaran et al.[26] reported on TE-MRI findings in a cohort of 504 VP infants; 76% had acquired lesions, which included periventricular leukomalacia (PVL), hemorrhagic parenchymal infarction, GMH-IVH, punctate WM lesions, cerebellar hemorrhage (CBH), and subependymal cysts. All infants with PVL and 60% of those with hemorrhagic parenchymal infarction

Table 95.3 Neuroimaging Findings of Preterm Brain Injury and Clinical Outcomes

Neuroimaging Findings	Best Diagnostic Modality	Neuropathological Findings	Clinical Outcomes
Cystic WM abnormalities	cUS, MRI	Cystic PVL/cPVL (bilateral cysts) PVHI evolving to porencephalic cyst (usually unilateral)	Diplegic (RR, 5), hemiplegic (RR, 29), or quadriplegic (RR, 24) CP Location and size dependent (≥3 mm in parieto-occipital periventricular WM are highest risk) Hemiplegic CP with motor cortex involvement 10% with grade I PVL diagnosed with spastic diplegic CP by school age, ≈50% for those with cPVL Visual impairment with severe cPVL
Gray matter abnormalities	MRI	Neuronal loss and GM gliosis Subcortical GM and cerebellar involvement	Cognitive impairment, behavioral issues
Diffuse WM abnormalities	MRI	Diffuse cPVL (moderate-severe WM abnormality) Noncystic PVL (mild-moderate WM abnormality) Diffuse WM gliosis (normal-mild WM abnormality)	Cognitive impairment, behavioral issues Unclear
GMH-IVH Posthemorrhagic ventricular dilatation (PHVD)	cUS, MRI	Rupture of germinal matrix vessels	Location and severity dependent, grade III/PVHI associated with quadriplegic (RR, 5.1), diplegic (RR, 2.3), or hemiplegic (RR, 5.8) CP, cognitive and behavioral issues, and blindness Bilateral IVH with PHVD needing a shunt is associated with the highest rates of CP (80% prevalence) 50%–80% with PHVI are diagnosed with intellectual disability and behavioral issues at school age Bilateral PVHI: worst cognitive outcomes, grade III IVH and PVHI; need for education support in reading, mathematics, and writing
Punctate WM lesions	MRI	Ischemic lesion Hemorrhage/medullary venous congestion	Unclear, may have cognitive or behavioral issues
Diffuse excessive high signal intensity (DEHSI)	MRI	Unknown	No association between DEHSI and abnormal neurodevelopment
Encephalopathy of prematurity	MRI	PVL, neuronal/axonal loss	CP, autism, motor, cognitive, attention, behavioral, and social interaction issues
Ventriculomegaly: moderate (1–1.5 cm), severe (>1.5 cm)	cUS, MRI	Gliosis, demyelination, axonal degeneration	Quadriplegic (RR, 17), hemiplegic (RR, 17), or diplegic (RR, 5.7) CP Moderate-severe ventriculomegaly: 2- to 3-fold increase in cognitive delay and low IQ

CP, Cerebral palsy; *cPVL*, cystic periventricular leukomalacia; *cUS*, cranial ultrasound; *GM*, gray matter; *GMH*, germinal matrix hemorrhage; *IVH*, intraventricular hemorrhage; *MRI*, magnetic resonance imaging; *PVL*, periventricular leukomalacia; *PVHI*, periventricular hemorrhagic infarction; *RR*, risk ratio; *WM*, white matter.

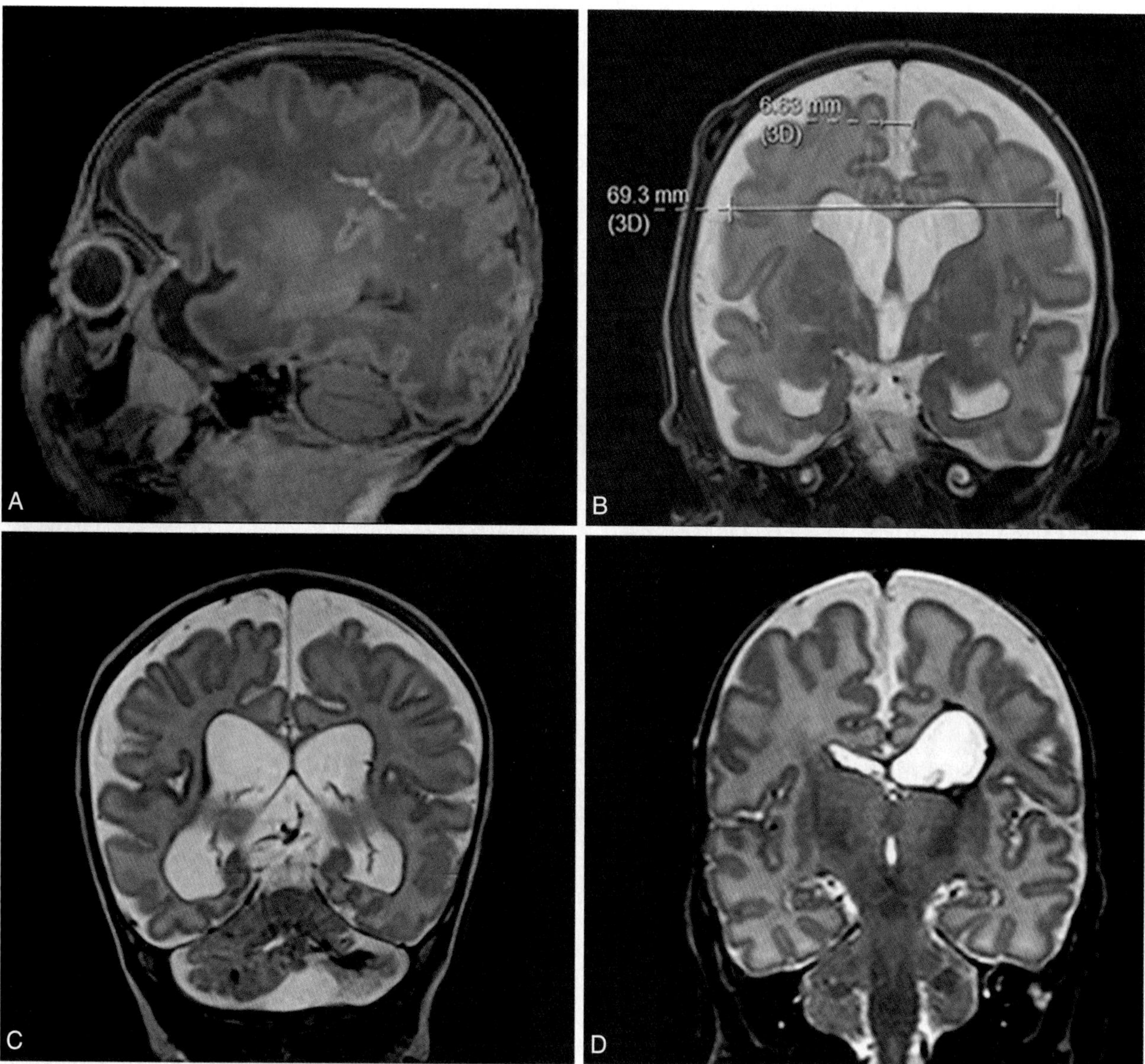

Fig. 95.5 Term-Equivalent Age Magnetic Resonance Imaging of the Preterm Infant. (A) Representative imaging of preterm infants with periventricular white matter lesions (PVWLs). (B) Metrics of biparietal width and interhemispheric diameter in a preterm infant with prominent extraaxial space and poor brain growth with diffuse loss of white matter volume and ex-vacuo ventricular dilatation. (C) Bilateral cerebellar hemorrhage. (D) Periventricular hemorrhagic infarction evolution with ex-vacuo ventricular dilatation and blood products lining the ventricle and interruption of the posterior limb of the internal capsule on the side of the injury. (Reproduced after permission and minor modifications from Inder et al. Neuroimaging of the preterm brain: review and recommendations. *J Pediatr*. 2021; in press.)

had abnormal motor outcomes. Routine 3T MRI at TEA demonstrated that an absence of focal lesions was 45% sensitive and 61% specific for normal neurodevelopment at 20 months and 17% sensitive and 94% specific for a normal motor outcome.[26] In their systematic review, Gotardo et al. concluded that children with any degree of IVH (relative risk [RR], 3.4; 95% CI, 1.6–7.22), cystic PVL (RR, 19.12; 95% CI, 4.57–79.9), and noncystic PVL (RR, 9.27; 95% CI, 5.93–14.5) were at increased risk of CP. Cystic PVL also increased risk of visual and hearing impairment.[38]

IVH and PHVD

IVH and PHVD (Figs. 95.6 and 95.7) are recognized, important determinants of neurodevelopmental outcome. High-grade IVH (grades 3 and 4), as per Papile grading, is a reasonable predictor of neuromotor impairment including CP.[38,39] Abnormal motor development at 2 years was reported with grade III (26%) and grade IV (53%) IVH.[40] A large grade III or IV IVH (PVHI) was associated with a four-fold increased risk of adverse outcomes (moderate to severe CP, cognitive delay, or severe visual or hearing impairment) compared with no IVH.[40] Recent studies have shown that the risk of adverse outcomes (neurosensory impairment, delayed development, CP, and deafness) was increased 1.5 times even with mild IVH.[38,40,41] In an Australian population-based cohort study focusing on 546 surviving EP infants, Hollebrandse et al. reported a trend for increased motor dysfunction with increasing severity of all grades of IVH, from 24% with no IVH to 92% with grade IV IVH. Children with grade I or II IVH were at higher risk of developing CP than were those without IVH (OR, 2.24; 95% CI, 1.21–4.16). Increased rates of impairment in intellectual ability and academic skills were observed with higher grades of IVH, but not for grades I and II. Low-grade IVH was associated with higher rates of CP in

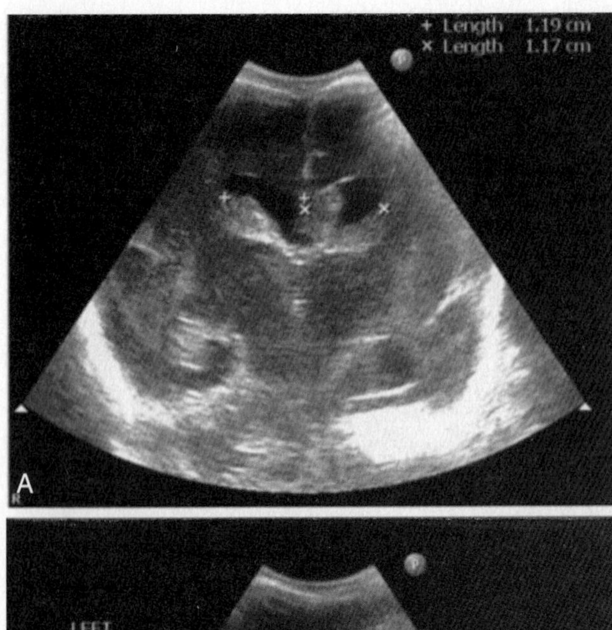

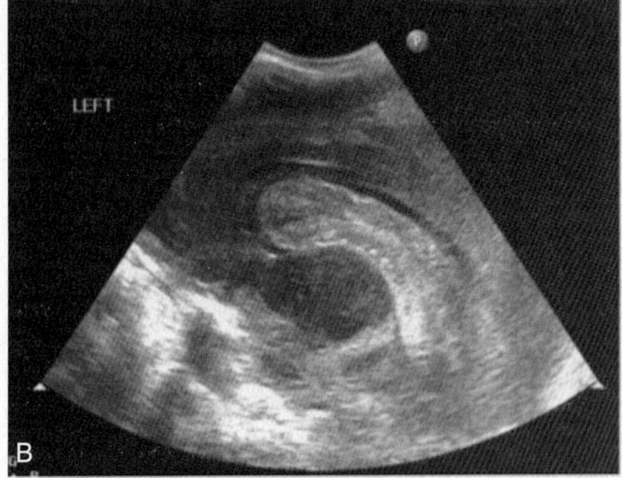

Fig. 95.6 Cranial Ultrasound Scans Show Intraventricular Hemorrhage. (A) Midcoronal view obtained on day 3, showing hemorrhage in both lateral ventricles. (B) Left parasagittal view, obtained on day 3, showing an extensive blood clot within the left lateral ventricle. (Reproduced after permission and minor modifications from Whitelaw A. In: *Neurology—Neonatology Questions and Controversies; Posthemorrhagic Hydrocephalus Management Strategies*, ch. 3, 47–62.)

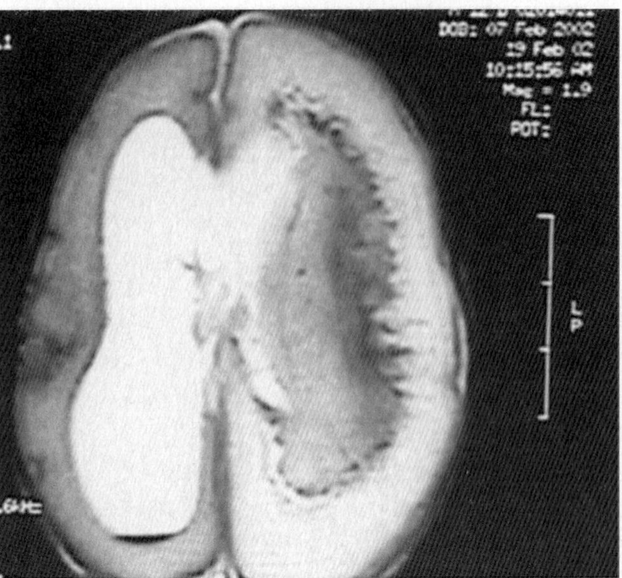

Fig. 95.7 T2-Weighted Magnetic Resonance Images of an Infant With Posthemorrhagic Ventricular Dilation. (A) The image shows extensive intraventricular debris, parenchymal injury and edema of the left ventricle, and gravitation of blood to the occipital pole of the right ventricle. (Reproduced after permission and minor modifications from Whitelaw A. In: *Neurology—Neonatology Questions and Controversies; Posthemorrhagic Hydrocephalus Management Strategies*, ch. 3, 47–62.)

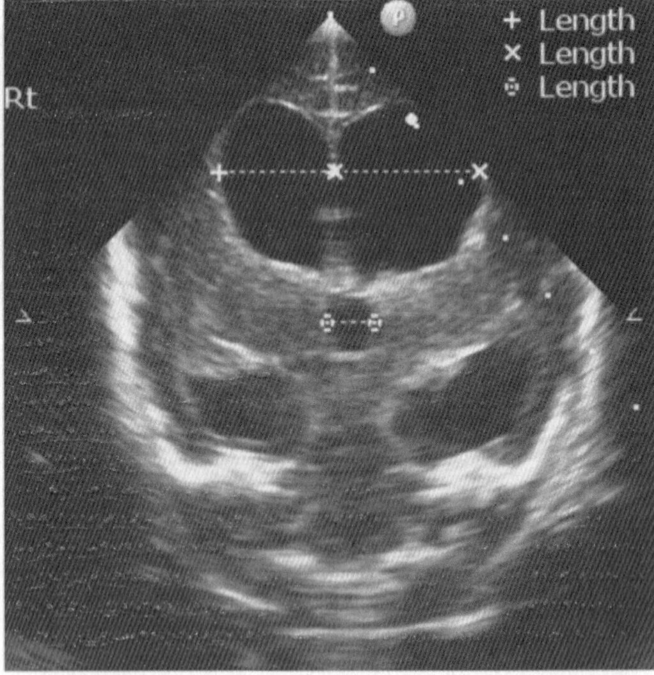

Fig. 95.8 Posthemorrhagic Ventricular Enlargement. Midcoronal view, obtained on day 18, showing enlargement of both lateral ventricles and the third ventricle. This infant had a bilateral intraventricular hemorrhage on postnatal day 3. (Reproduced after permission and minor modifications from Whitelaw A. In: *Neurology—Neonatology Questions and Controversies; Posthemorrhagic Hydrocephalus Management Strategies*, ch. 3, 47–62.)

school-aged children born EP but not with intellectual ability, executive function, academic skills, or overall motor function.[42]

For infants who develop PHVD (Fig. 95.8), the risk of delayed motor, visual, language, and problem-solving is higher.[43,44] PHVD impacts WM loss, and increased intracranial pressure compounds this effect. Ventriculomegaly is associated with gliosis, demyelination, and axonal degeneration. Periventricular WM damage reduces cortical volume further, which damages tracts responsible for memory, executive function, and language. The most anterior and posterior parts of the corpus callosum, which are actively involved in neuronal organization and premyelination, are damaged in PHVD. GM volume also reduces with IVH and PHVD. WMI is associated with a reduction in lentiform nuclear and thalamic volumes. PHVD impacts cerebellar volumes through diaschisis after parenchymal brain injury, free radical damage, or inflammatory response to blood products in the CSF.[45] Parenchymal injury may predict adverse neurodevelopmental outcomes (NDO) compared with ventricular size alone. The role of early compared with standard treatment of PHVD and its impact on cognitive outcomes is still being debated.[46–48]

MRI of preterm infants needing a shunt for PHVD show reduced total brain volumes and larger ventricular volumes. Risk of neurodevelopmental delay is higher with a lower baseline MRI score (lower total brain tissue, cerebrum, frontal lobes, basal ganglia, thalamus, and cerebellum and high ventricular volume).[49] Table 95.3

summarizes the neuroimaging findings of preterm brain injury and associated clinical outcomes.

Cerebellar Injury

The cerebellum is the "neuronal learning machine." CBHs are commonly seen with severe IVH/PVHI, although isolated ones have been reported to be associated with cognitive, learning, and behavioral deficits impacting quality of life and daily function.[45,50] In 67% of preterm infants with large CBHs compared with those with no CBHs (5%), abnormal neurodevelopment (increased tone and abnormal deep tendon reflexes, gait pattern, and ophthalmologic findings) at 2.5 years was reported.[50] Although posterior fossa views on cUS target infratentorial structures, MRI offers superior detection of cerebellar injury.[45,50] Tam et al. reported a five-fold increase in abnormal neurologic examination at 3 to 6 years of age in preterm infants with cerebellar lesions only detected on MRI.[45] Furthermore, impairment in cognition and learning and a short attention span that persist through school age have been reported.[33,49] Garfinkle et al. studied the association between CBH size and location on MRI and preschool-age neurodevelopment in 221 VP infants (median gestational age, 27.9 weeks). Thirty-six neonates had CBH: 14 (6%) with only punctate CBH and 22 (10%) with ≥1 larger CBH. CBH occurred most commonly in the inferior aspect of the posterior lobes. The CBH total volume was independently associated with motor scores at 4.5 years, whereas the CBH size was similarly associated with visuomotor integration and externalizing behavior but not cognition. Deeper extension of the CBH predicted adverse motor, visuomotor, and behavioral outcomes.[51]

Structural and functional cerebellar anomalies correlate with core autism behaviors. Hypoplasia of the posterior vermis was one of the first documented brain abnormalities in ASD, and decreased cerebellar cortical volume is seen in children with ASD. Cerebellar GM reductions (right crus I, left lobule VIII, and medial IX) may have functional impacts on specific cerebro-cerebellar circuits (e.g., reduced functional connectivity between right crus I and left-hemisphere language regions in language-impaired children with ASD). Both input and output pathways maybe disrupted due to structural differences in the cerebellar peduncles. Similar impairments have been reported with ADHD and learning difficulties.[52]

Hypoxic Ischemic Encephalopathy

Prior to the widespread adoption of therapeutic hypothermia for hypoxic ischemic encephalopathy (HIE), abnormalities on cUS were predictive of adverse outcomes in neonatal encephalopathy. Siegel et al. reported increased mortality in 50% of infants with periventricular echogenicity due to perinatal hypoxia-ischemia and residual neurologic deficits in 80% of survivors.[53] Babcock and Ball showed motor or developmental delay at 4 months in infants with HIE and cerebral atrophy or cystic encephalomalacia on cUS.[54] Abnormally low or high resistive indices on cUS Doppler were predictive of poor outcomes.[55] MRI is now the preferred neuroimaging of choice to define cerebral injury after HIE (Figs. 95.9–95.11). Both NICHD and clinical trials using therapeutic hypothermia showed that in cooled infants, the severity and pattern of brain injury on MRI are predictive of death or intellectual disability (IQ <70) at 18 to 24 months, and these persist through school age.[56,57] Advanced MRI

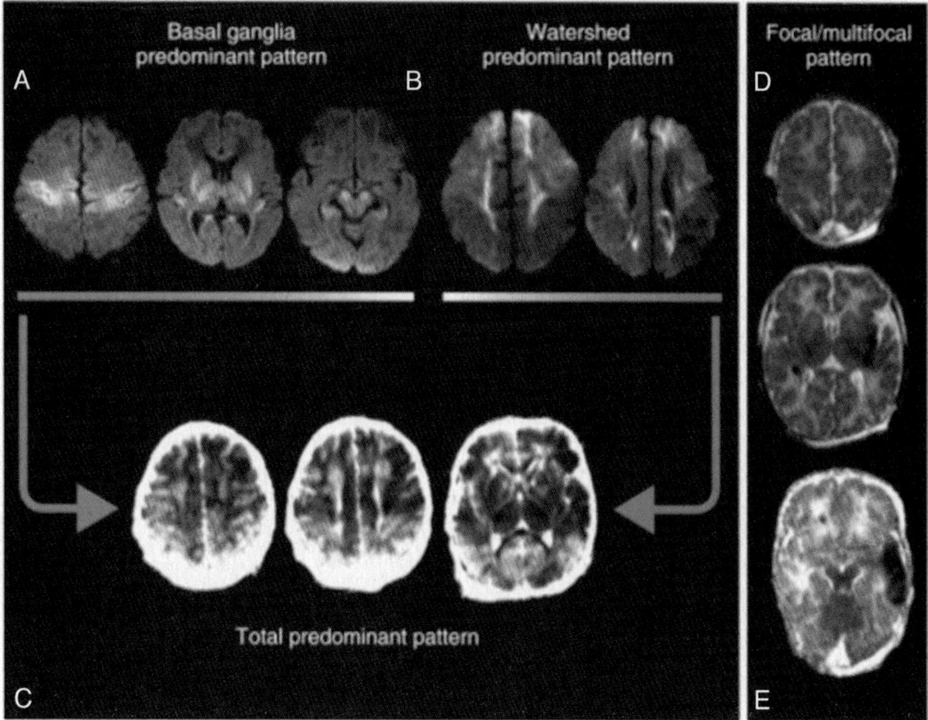

Fig. 95.9 Predominant Patterns of Brain Injury in Term Hypoxic-Ischemic Encephalopathy. (A) Basal-ganglia–predominant pattern of injury in a newborn with perinatal asphyxia imaged on the third day of life. Brain injury is demonstrated on diffusion-weighted imaging (DWI) as areas of restricted diffusion (hyperintense, bright areas) in the motor cortex around the central sulcus, thalami, basal ganglia, optic radiations, hippocampi, and midbrain. (B) Watershed-predominant pattern of injury in a newborn with perinatal asphyxia imaged on the third day of life. Cortical and subcortical brain injury is demonstrated on DWI in the watershed regions, affecting both the cortex and the white matter. Both the basal-nuclei–predominant and watershed-predominant patterns can lead to the total predominant pattern (C) if severe enough, as shown on these apparent diffusion coefficient (ADC) maps as areas of restricted diffusion (hypointense, dark areas). (D) Multifocal white-matter injury in the periventricular and subcortical white matter in a newborn, seen as areas of restricted diffusion identified by *arrows* (hypointense, dark areas) on the ADC maps. (E) Stroke: Focal infarct in the left middle cerebral artery territory in the same newborn with perinatal asphyxia, demonstrated on the ADC as an area of restricted diffusion marked by the *star* (hypointense, dark areas). (Reproduced after permission and minor modifications from Chau et al. Hypoxic-ischemic brain injury in the term newborn. In: *Swaiman's Pediatric Neurology*, 19, e331–e348.)

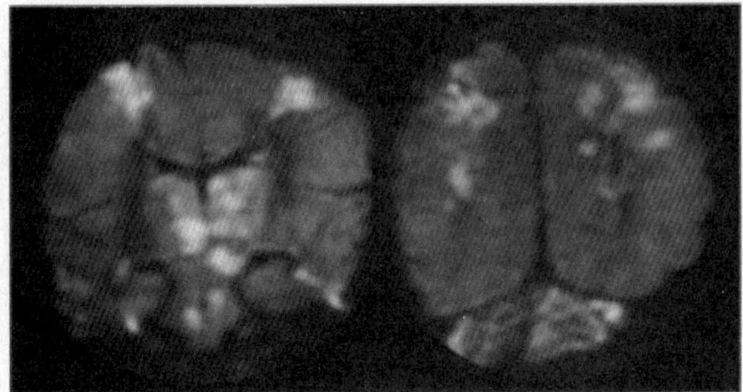

Fig. 95.10 Gray Matter Injury in a Term Infant. Extensive restricted diffusion on diffusion-weighted imaging in multiple gray matter containing regions of the brain including the "watershed" cortex, deep nuclear gray matter, brainstem, and cerebellum. (Reproduced after permission and minor modifications from Miller et al. *Seminars in Pediatric Neurology*. 2020;33:100796.)

techniques such as diffusion-weighted (DW) MRI add prognostic value to routine MRI. MR spectroscopy showing increased perfusion in the basal ganglia and thalamus may predict death or CP at 9 to 18 months of age.[58] MRS further highlights the role of lactate and N-acetyl aspartate to predict moderate to severe disability in infancy.[59]

Respiratory Failure Needing Extracorporeal Membrane Oxygenation

Rollins et al. reported that MRI identified significantly more abnormalities compared with routine cUS after neonatal extracorporeal membrane oxygenation (ECMO). However, neither MRI nor cUS findings were correlated with early neurodevelopmental outcome. Feeding ability at discharge was the overall best predictor of neurologic impairment in survivors. Fifty neonates had MRI (venoarterial, 37; venovenous, 13) after ECMO; 26 infants attended follow-up. cUS was abnormal in 24%, whereas MRI was abnormal in 62%. All infants

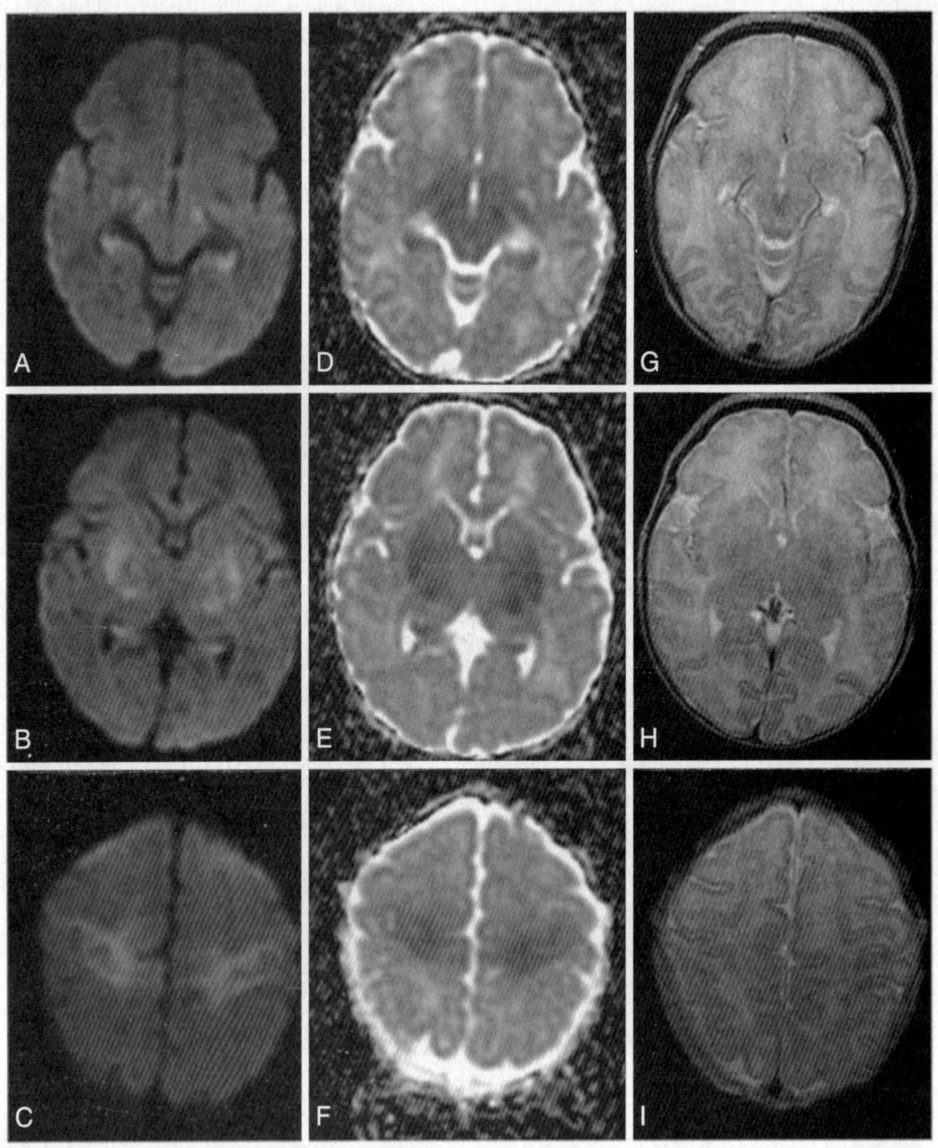

Fig. 95.11 Hypoxic-Ischemic Injury Central Pattern. (A–C) Echo planar imaging diffusion-weighted imaging (DWI); (D–F) apparent diffusion coefficient (ADC) maps; (G–I) T2-spin echo. A 3-day-old female term baby with a history of hypoxic-ischemic encephalopathy and neonatal seizures. DWI and ADC maps show reduced diffusion bilaterally in the putamina, ventral lateral thalami, hippocampi, corticospinal tracts, and perirolandic cortex. T2-weighted imaging (T2-WI) and T1-WI demonstrate abnormal signal in these same distributions. (Reproduced after permission and minor modifications from Rodrigues and Grant. Diffusion-weighted imaging in neonates. *Neuroimaging Clin N Am*. 2011;21:127–151.)

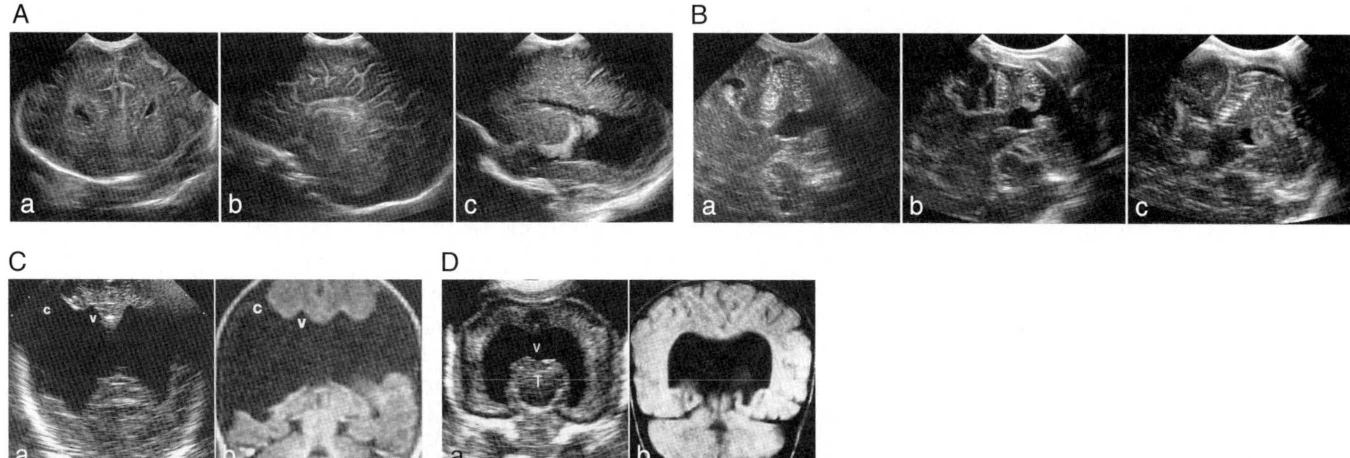

Fig. 95.12 Congenital Anomalies of the Central Nervous System. (A) Agenesis of the corpus callosum: (a) small frontal horns are widely separated; (b) sulci radiate in a sunburst pattern in parasagittal just off midline view; and (c) colpocephaly seen in parasagittal view of lateral ventricle. (B) Dandy-Walker complex compared with normal posterior fossa. (A) and (B) Axial posterior fossa sonograms in two infants with Dandy-Walker complex show a wide continuity between the fourth ventricle and the cisterna magna. (C) Normal axial sonogram of the fourth ventricle and slightly echogenic cerebellar vermis. (C) Open-lip schizencephaly. Coronal sonogram (a) and coronal MRI (b) show bilateral clefts. (D) Alobar holoprosencephaly. (a) Coronal sonogram shows single central ventricle (V) and fused thalami (T). No falx or interhemispheric fissure is present. (b) Coronal MRI. (A, Reproduced after permission and minor modifications from Rumack and Auckland. *Diagnostic Ultrasound*, ch. 45, 1511–1572; B, reproduced after permission and minor modifications from Rumack and Auckland. *Diagnostic Ultrasound*, ch. 45, 1511–1572; C, both figures reproduced after permission and minor modifications from Rumack and Auckland. *Diagnostic Ultrasound*, ch. 45, 1511–1572.)

with an abnormal cUS had an abnormal MRI, but an additional 50% of patients with a normal cUS had an abnormal MRI. Venoarterial ECMO was significantly associated with an abnormal MRI.[60]

Neonatal Arterial Ischemic Stroke

MRI is superior to cUS in diagnosing focal ischemic stroke. The left middle cerebral artery territory is commonly affected and is associated with motor asymmetry and contralateral hemiplegia. Visual deficits at school age, such as abnormal acuity, visual field deficits, and stereopsis, are not uncommon in middle cerebral artery strokes and seem to be associated with hemiplegia and more extensive lesions. The impact on cognitive outcomes in unclear. However, quantitative assessments, specifically volumetric delineation of stroke-related injury, may predict cognitive outcome. Furthermore, DW MRI to quantitatively assess corticospinal tracts may provide additional information on short-term motor outcomes, including mild motor disabilities.[61]

Congenital Heart Disease

Impaired neurodevelopmental outcomes including motor, cognitive, and sensory domains have been reported in survivors of critical congenital heart disease (CHD). These deficits may extend into adolescence and early adulthood. These are multifactorial in origin and include infant-specific risk factors, cardiac anatomy and physiology, and brain changes seen on MRI. Advances in imaging techniques have identified delayed brain development in the neonate with critical CHD and acquired brain injury. Some of these abnormalities can be detected preoperatively.[62]

Small for Gestational Age Due to Intrauterine Growth Restriction

Intrauterine growth restriction is associated with increased perinatal morbidity and mortality and adverse long-term neurodevelopmental sequelae. Twenty VP infants who were small for gestational age (SGA) were compared with age-matched infants who were appropriate for gestational age (AGA). Cerebral ventricular volumes were assessed using 3-dimensional ultrasound. The Prechtl General Movement Assessment was performed at 4 to 6 weeks after birth. The Test of Infant Motor Performance (TIMP) to measure functional motor behavior was performed at 4 to 6 and at 12 to 14 weeks' corrected age. The combined cerebral ventricular volumes between the two groups (SGA, 0.81 ± 0.42 cm^3 versus AGA, 0.72 ± 0.38 cm^3; $P = .4$) were comparable. TIMP assessment at 12 to 14 weeks' term-corrected age demonstrated significantly lower scores (worse performance) in SGA infants compared with the AGA cohort (regression coefficient, –7.74; 95% CI, –16.06 to 0.57; $P = .07$). A significant correlation between greater ventricular volume and lower TIMP scores in the cohorts was noted individually and also overall (SGA: r, –0.5; $P = .06$; AGA: r, –0.62; $P = .007$; overall, r, –0.53; $P = .001$).[63] Advanced MRI techniques in growth-restricted newborn lambs have shown macrostructural deficits in WM.[64] Batalle et al. demonstrated increased network infrastructure and raw efficiencies but reduced efficiency after normalization, demonstrating hyperconnected but suboptimally organized intrauterine growth restriction functional brain networks. They also reported a significant association between network features and neurobehavioral scores.[65]

Congenital Brain Anomalies

Many central nervous malformations can be recognized on imaging, such as agenesis of the corpus callosum (Fig. 95.12A), encephaloceles, Dandy-Walker malformation (see Fig. 95.12B), and severe malformations such as schizencephaly (see Fig. 95.12C) and holoprosencephaly (see Fig. 95.12D). Other malformations such as Walker-Warburg syndrome and severe lissencephaly can also be identified.[66]

Metabolic Disorders

Disorders with early presentation (usually in the first 48 hours after birth) include glycine encephalopathy (nonketotic hyperglycinemia), molybdenum cofactor deficiency, isolated sulfite oxidase deficiency, pyridoxine-dependent epilepsy, some mitochondrial disorders (pyruvate dehydrogenase deficiency), and some peroxisomal disorders

Table 95.4 Neurodevelopmental Correlates of Conventional MRI Volumetric Assessments

Neuroimaging Findings	Clinical Outcomes
Larger total brain tissue volumes	Higher cognitive and language scores
Higher WM volume	Improved motor outcome and processing speed
Volume reduction of the dorsolateral prefrontal cortex, sensorimotor, parietooccipital, and premotor cortices	Impaired working memory
Posterior cortical mantle thinning, decreased CC and white matter tract area, and greater posterior CSF percentages	Poorer visuospatial skills and nonverbal intelligence
Significantly reduced cortical and deep nuclear gray matter volumes[a]	Moderate to severe neurodevelopmental disability at 1 year
Higher cortical gray matter volumes[a]	Worse motor performance and cognition at 24 months, lower developmental quotients at age 3.5 years (Keunen 2016)
Lower cerebellar volumes	Poor executive function and motor skills Lower cognitive and language scores at 2 years
WM microstructure (cingulum, body, and splenium of the corpus callosum, middle cerebellar peduncle, left and right uncinate fasciculi, and right portion of the pathway between the premotor and primary motor cortices)	Improved expressive language and social-emotional scores

[a]Contradictory findings.

CC, Corpus callosum; *CF*, cerebrospinal fluid; *WM*, white matter.

Dorner 2019, Lean 2019, Young 2020, and Lee 2021.

(Zellweger syndrome, neonatal adrenoleukodystrophy). Clinical features and neuroimaging findings assist with targeted genetic and metabolic testing to determine the underlying diagnosis.[66]

Comparison of TE-cUS and TE-MRI for Predicting Neurodevelopmental Outcomes

Burkitt et al. investigated the accuracy of different grades of brain injuries on serial and TEA-cUS compared with TE-MRI in EP infants (<28 weeks) and determined the predictive value of imaging abnormalities on neurodevelopmental outcome at 1 and 3 years. Seventy-five infants were included in the study. Severe TEA-cUS injury had 100% positive predictive value (PPV) for predicting severe MRI injury compared with mild-to-moderate TEA-cUS injury or severe injury on the worst cUS scan. Absence of moderate to severe injury on TEA cUS or worst serial cUS was a good predictor of a normal MRI (negative predictive values [NPVs] >93%). Severe grade III injuries on TEA-cUS had high predictive values in predicting abnormal neurodevelopment at both 1 and 3 years of age (PPV, 100%). All grades of MRI and the worst serial cUS injuries poorly predicted abnormal neurodevelopment at 1 and 3 years. Absence of an injury either on a cUS or MRI did not predict a normal outcome. Multiple logistic regression did not show a significant correlation between imaging injury and neurodevelopmental outcomes.[67] Zhang et al.[68] assessed the accuracy of cUS grading to determine brain injury, investigated the relationship between serial cUS and neurodevelopment (mental development index and physical development index) in 129 EP infants. They reported mild CP (20.9%) and severe CP (5.8%–6.9%) in 86 survivors. TE-cUS and TE-MRI were 88% consistent with each other. Grade II and III IVH at the first cUS were associated with adverse mental (ORs, 3.2 and 3.78, respectively) and motor (ORs, 2.25 and 2.59, respectively) development. cUS classification demonstrated high sensitivity (79%–96%). Among all cUS classifications, the specificity of the first cUS was the lowest and that of TE-cUS was the highest (57% for the physical development index and 48% for the mental development index).The authors concluded that cUS classification had high sensitivity and high specificity for the prediction of CP, especially in TEA-cUS.

Advanced MRI Techniques

Advanced MRI techniques including resting-state, functional, and diffusion MRI have been increasingly used to demonstrate clinically relevant alterations in key WM tracts and the motor network in prematurely born infants and children. The importance of cerebral volumetric assessments is also being increasingly recognized (Table 95.4). Altered WM microstructural abnormalities in preterm infants have been shown to be associated with poor cognitive, language, social-emotional, and behavioral outcomes.[69,70] Janjic et al.[71] evaluated the ability of feed-forward neural networks (fNNs) to predict NDO of VP infants at 12 months using cerebral MR proton spectroscopy biomarkers (^{1}H-MRS) and diffusion tensor imaging (DTI) at TEA in their prospective study. TEA MRIs of 127 VP infants were included. The final data sets included 103 (for motor delay) and 115 (for cognitive delay) VP infants. Five metabolite ratios and two DTI characteristics in six different brain areas were evaluated. A feature selection algorithm was developed for receiving a subset of characteristics prevalent for the VP infants with a developmental delay. Finally, the predictors were constructed using multiple fNNs and four-fold cross-validation. They reported predicted cognitive delays of VP infants with 85.7% sensitivity, 100% specificity, 100% PPV, and 99.1% NPV using the constructed fNN predictors. They also reported 76.9% sensitivity, 98.9% specificity, a PPV of 90.9%, and an NPV of 96.7% for predicting motor outcomes. FNNs might be able to predict motor and cognitive development of VP infants at 12 months' corrected age by combining biomarkers of cerebral ^{1}H-MRS and DTI quantified at TEA.

Conclusions

Neurodevelopmental delay after brain injury in neonates contributes to significant morbidity and mortality in addition to an increased socioeconomic, psychological, and healthcare burden. Cranial ultrasound and MRI at term-equivalent age improve prediction of neurodevelopmental outcomes, most accurately for HIE, stroke, and white and gray matter injury.

CHAPTER 96

Neurodevelopmental Impairment in Specific Neonatal Disorders

Vinayak Mishra, Brian Sims, Margaret Kuper-Sassé, Akhil Maheshwari

KEY POINTS

1. Neonatal intensive care unit graduates are at risk of neurodevelopmental impairment (NDI).
2. NDI can occur in cognitive, motor, vision, hearing, or language domains and can seriously impair the child's social, academic, and behavioral functioning.
3. Periventricular white matter injury is the leading cause of long-term NDI, especially motor impairment in preterm infants.
4. Infants with hypoxic-ischemic encephalopathy, bronchopulmonary dysplasia, necrotizing enterocolitis, intraventricular hemorrhage, and sepsis are at high risk of NDI.

Introduction

Neurodevelopmental impairment (NDI) is an important long-term complication for neonatal intensive care unit (NICU) graduates.[1] Neonates admitted to the NICU are undergoing a critical period of neurologic development, and any insult to the brain could lead to detrimental neurodevelopmental outcomes. The improvement in high-risk neonates' survival rates due to neonatal care advancements has highlighted the importance of studying long-term neurologic prognosis. NDI can occur in cognitive, motor, vision, hearing, or language domains and can seriously impair the child's social, academic, and behavioral functioning.[2] To optimize outcomes, there should be a obligation to follow-up and ameliorate the neurodevelopmental outcomes of the NICU survivors.

This chapter discusses the epidemiology and pathophysiology of NDI in the context of five conditions frequently seen in the NICU. These are hypoxic-ischemic encephalopathy (HIE), bronchopulmonary dysplasia (BPD), necrotizing enterocolitis (NEC), intraventricular hemorrhage (IVH), and sepsis. This review includes evidence from our own quality-improvement studies and an extensive literature review of the PubMed, Embase, and Scopus databases. To avoid bias in identifying studies, keywords were short-listed *a priori* from anecdotal experience and PubMed's Medical Subject Heading thesaurus. In this review, considerable overlap is demonstrated in the neurodevelopmental manifestations and neurologic abnormalities among neonatal conditions, which indicates multifactorial pathogenesis of NDI.

Pathophysiology

The underlying mechanism of NDI in preterm NICU infants could be related to anatomic and physiologic vascular abnormalities associated with the relative immaturity of the brain (Fig. 96.1). Cerebral white matter is especially susceptible to prematurity-related vascular insults.[3] Periventricular white matter injury (PWMI) such as that seen in the lesions in Figs. 96.2 and 96.3 is a leading cause of long-term NDI.[3,4] These lesions frequently lead to motor impairment. PWMI is attributed to cerebral white matter blood flow interference because of the immature vasculature; ischemic white matter is vulnerable to free radical–mediated injury to the oligodendrocyte progenitors.[3] The severity of white matter abnormality in neonatal sepsis depends on the timing (postmenstrual age) of diagnosis, with more severe pathology in infants developing sepsis before 28 weeks.[5] Figs. 96.4 and 96.5 show the evolution of white matter lesions over longer periods of time.

Oligodendrocyte progenitors are particularly susceptible to ischemia and inflammation in the process of preterm encephalopathy.[6] The loss of lineage-specific progenitors and the consequent reduction in the number of mature oligodendrocytes can impair cerebral myelination. In animal models, cerebral hypoperfusion and hypoxia-ischemia have shown abnormalities in oligodendrocyte progenitor cells, periventricular white matter, and cortical gray matter.[7] Along similar lines, excessive glutamate release during neonatal stress in the NICU could lead to excitotoxic damage to the oligodendrocyte progenitors and cause PWMI. In addition, cerebral maturation is impeded in NEC, as evidenced by a lower rate of increase of the N-acetyl cysteine–choline ratio in affected infants than in unaffected controls.[8] Periventricular injuries could also be a consequence of moderate-severe IVH.

Intestinal inflammation could directly affect the severity of neuroinflammation (Fig. 96.6). Immunogenic systemic inflammatory reaction with an increase in cytokines such as tumor necrosis factor might contribute to the pathogenesis of PWMI.[9] Elevated plasma and cerebrospinal fluid interleukin-1 beta and tumor necrosis factor-alpha increase the risk for white matter injury in preterm neonates with early-onset sepsis.[9] Biouss et al. reported that neonatal mice with NEC had reduced cortical girth, abnormal cell apoptosis, a decreased population of mature neurons and oligodendrocytes, and defective development of neural progenitor cells.[10] Two other experimental models showed that animal neonates with NEC develop

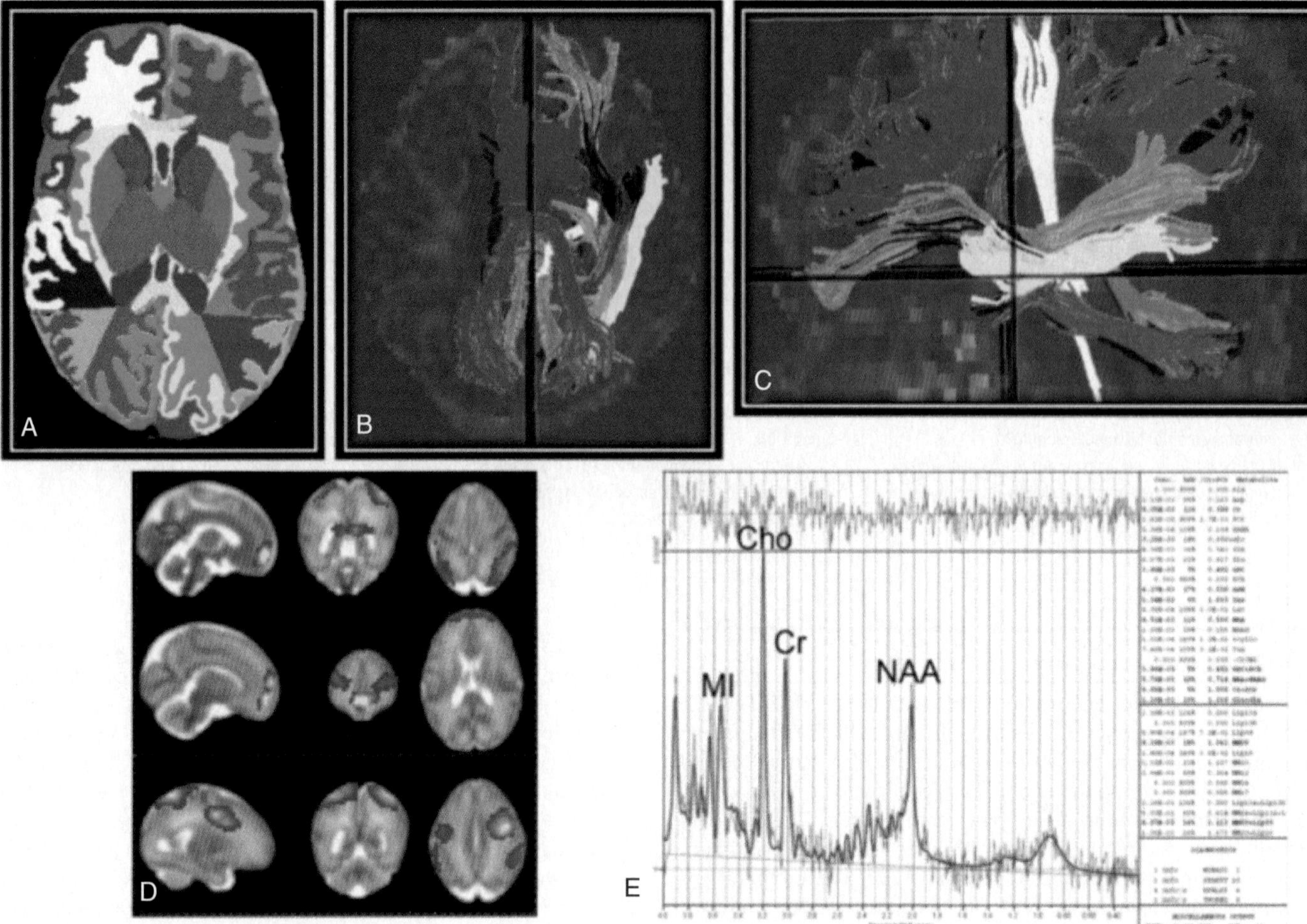

Fig. 96.1 (A) Brain-advanced magnetic resonance imaging (MRI) measurements including morphometry. (B and C) Diffusion tractography. (D) Functional connectivity MRI. (E) Magnetic resonance spectroscopy. Representative advanced MRI examples of an extremely low birth weight infant's brain at term-equivalent age display that was segmented into tissue classes, subcortical structures, and lobes (A); 10 white matter tracts, displayed in axial and sagittal orientations (B and C); panel D shows blood-oxygen level–dependent activations in the default mode (top panel), executive control (middle panel), and frontoparietal networks (bottom panel); and panel E is a processed proton magnetic resonance spectroscopy spectrum displaying the four main metabolites, including N-acetylaspartate (NAA), creatine (Cr), choline (Cho), and myo-inositol (MI). (With permission from Parikh NA. Advanced neuroimaging and its role in predicting neurodevelopmental outcomes in very preterm infants. *Semin Perinatol*. 2016;40(8):530-541; Reproduced with permission and minor modifications from Hintz and Parikh. The role of neonatal neuroimaging in predicting neurodevelopmental outcomes of preterm neonates. In: *Fanaroff and Martin's Neonatal-Perinatal Medicine*, 61, 1110–1122.)

neuroinflammation associated with altered hippocampal gene expression, abnormal myelination, and cognitive deficits due to activation of microglial cells.[11,12]

Furthermore, Niño et al.[12] explained that inflamed intestinal tissue in NEC releases toll-like receptor 4 activators such as lipopolysaccharides that propagate neuroinflammation and promote oxidative stress; this, as a result, leads to reduced myelination in the hippocampus, midbrain, and corpus callosum. Haynes et al.[13] hypothesized that free-radical oxidative and nitrative (due to nitric oxide) damage to oligodendrocyte progenitor cells contributes to PWMI. The studies described above indicate that early surgical removal of necrotic intestinal tissue in NEC could lower the severity of neuroinflammatory response in the brain, supporting a dose-related effect.

Other potential pathogenic mechanisms contribute to NDI development in NICU infants; poor nutrition and decreased growth associated with a prolonged stay in a NICU and exposure to surgery and anesthetics could contribute to abnormal neurologic development.[14–17] Ehrenkranz et al.[14] demonstrated that growth velocity during NICU admission was inversely associated with cerebral palsy (CP) and NDI incidence in extremely low birth weight (ELBW) infants. Besides, poor nutrition and inadequate caloric intake in preterm infants can lead to poor head growth, representing poor neurologic development.[15] It is important to note that antenatal steroids reduce the risk of NDI in extremely preterm infants partially by reducing the incidence of IVH and cystic periventricular leukomalacia.[18] A summary of the most frequently seen magnetic resonance imaging (MRI) prognostic biomarkers is shown in Tables 96.1 and 96.2.

Hypoxic-Ischemic Encephalopathy

Structural Abnormalities on Neuroimaging

MRI is better than cranial ultrasound at assessing cerebral parenchymal abnormalities. Cerebral MRI proves valuable in predicting neurodevelopmental outcomes (in motor, language, and cognition domains) in HIE infants; it had 95% sensitivity and 94% specificity in predicting neurodevelopment.[19] There are 6.23 times higher odds for NDI in the form of delayed development if MRI and magnetic resonance spectroscopy findings suggest HIE in the first week of life.[20] Cerebral MRI and magnetic resonance spectroscopy are validated biomarkers for predicting neurodevelopmental outcomes and evaluating the neurologic response to therapeutic hypothermia.[21]

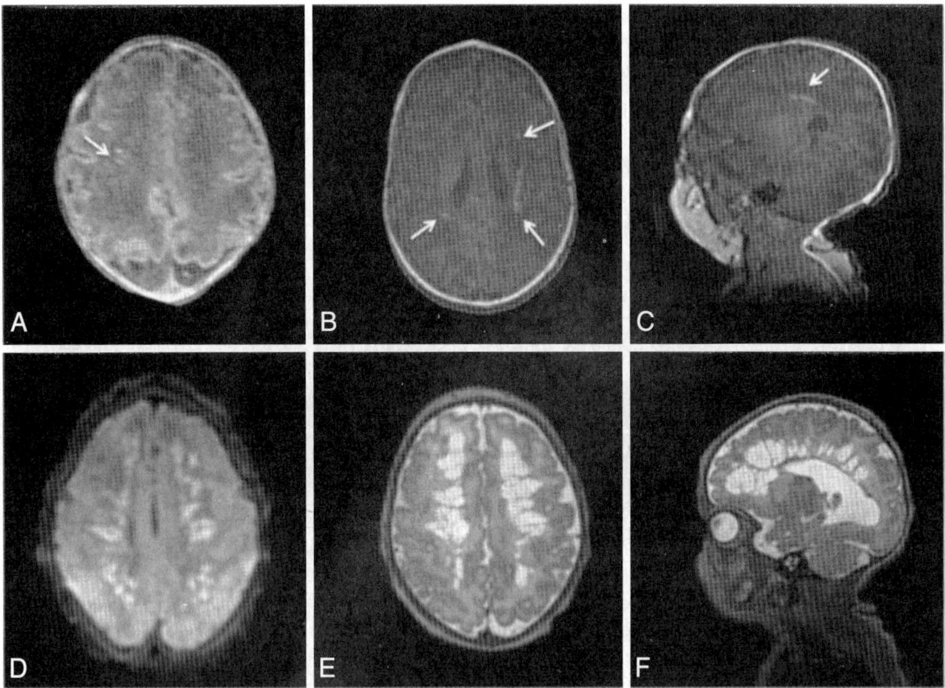

Fig. 96.2 White Matter Injury (WMI) of Prematurity. (A–C) Axial and sagittal T1-weighted magnetic resonance imaging (MRI) scans showing minimal WMI in the form of punctate lesions in a preterm infant of 29 weeks' gestation imaged at 38 weeks (A) and an infant with >20 punctate lesions clustered in the region of the upper corticospinal tracts on imaging obtained at 40 weeks (B and C). The infant in A had a normal outcome assessed at 4.5 years. The infant in B and C had the following Bayley Scales of Infant and Toddler Development, Third Edition (BSIC-III) scores at 18 months corrected age: motor, 96; cognitive, 103; and language, 101. (D–F) Evolving cystic WMI in a 34 weeks' gestation infant with perinatal hypoxic-ischemic encephalopathy secondary to placental abruption. (D) Axial diffusion-weighted imaging on day 5 after birth showing extensive diffusion restriction in the centrum semiovale. (E and F) Axial and sagittal T2-weighted magnetic resonance imaging obtained 3 weeks later showing interval evolution of extensive cystic WMI. The infant had spastic quadriplegia, cerebral visual impairment, cognitive delay, and language delay at 12 months' CA. (Reproduced with permission and after minor modifications from Gano et al. Cerebral palsy after very preterm birth—an imaging perspective. *Semin Fetal Neonatal Med*. 2020;25:101106.)

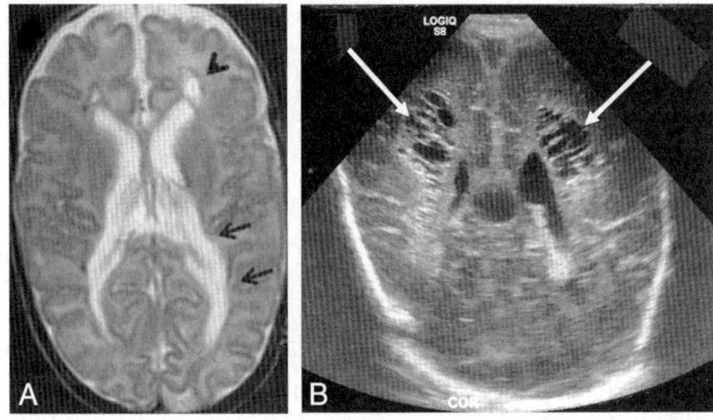

Fig. 96.3 Examples of Brain Injury in Premature Neonates. (A) Brain magnetic resonance imaging in a 2.5-month-old infant who was born at 30 weeks' gestational age. T2-weighted axial image demonstrates thinning of the periventricular white matter with regular outline of the lateral ventricles. (B) Cranial ultrasonographic scan obtained on day-of-life 15 demonstrating bilateral periventricular cystic changes in the white matter (*arrows*) after a preterm birth with histologic chorioamnionitis and funisitis and with an unremarkable early neonatal intensive care unit course. (A, Gunny et al. Paediatric neuroradiology. In: *Grainger & Allison's Diagnostic Radiology*, 76, 1984-2045; B, from Yap and Perlman. Mechanisms of brain injury in newborn infants associated with the fetal inflammatory response syndrome. *Semin Fetal Neonatal Med*. 2020;25:101110.)

Doppler ultrasound of the anterior or middle cerebral artery can be helpful; increased diastolic blood flow is correlated with NDI. Annink et al. studied 10-year-old children with HIE and showed mammillary bodies and hippocampi structural defects on MRI and diffusion tensor imaging (DTI) scans associated with memory problems and cognitive deficits.[22] An alteration or reversal of the white matter signal in the posterior limb of the internal capsule during the first week of life has a high sensitivity (92%) and a high positive predictive value (88%) for severe motor impairment at 2 years of age.[23] Besides, basal ganglia-thalamic lesions in HIE have an 89% predictive accuracy for severe motor impairment.[23] Other prominent injury sites are the cortical gray matter, brainstem, and cerebellar white matter, which are also associated with motor or cognitive NDI.[24] Diffusion-weighted imaging can detect basal ganglia–thalami lesions in the first week of life, and a low apparent diffusion coefficient and high lactate/N-acetyl aspartate ratio can prognosticate poor neurologic outcomes.[25,26]

Clinical Outcomes

HIE continues to be a major cause of NDI despite advancements in therapeutic hypothermia. HIE is one of the most common causes of CP; the other manifestations include epilepsy, global developmental delay, motor impairment, language delay, and cognitive impairment.[27,28] Neurologic prognosis depends on the severity of HIE; neonates with an initial cord blood pH <6.7 have a 90% risk for death or severe NDI at 18 months of age. In addition, Apgar scores of 0 to 3 at 5 minutes, a base deficit >20 mmol/L, decerebrate posture, lack of spontaneous activity, apnea, absence of oculocephalic reflexes, and refractory seizures increase the risk and severity of NDI. HIE is also associated with defects in visual function.[29]

The hypothermia protocol in HIE states that therapeutic hypothermia should be initiated in neonates who are born at >36 weeks' gestation and have evidence of HIE or moderate to severe encephalopathy. However, a systematic review by Conway et al. showed that 25% of infants with mild HIE had poor neurodevelopmental

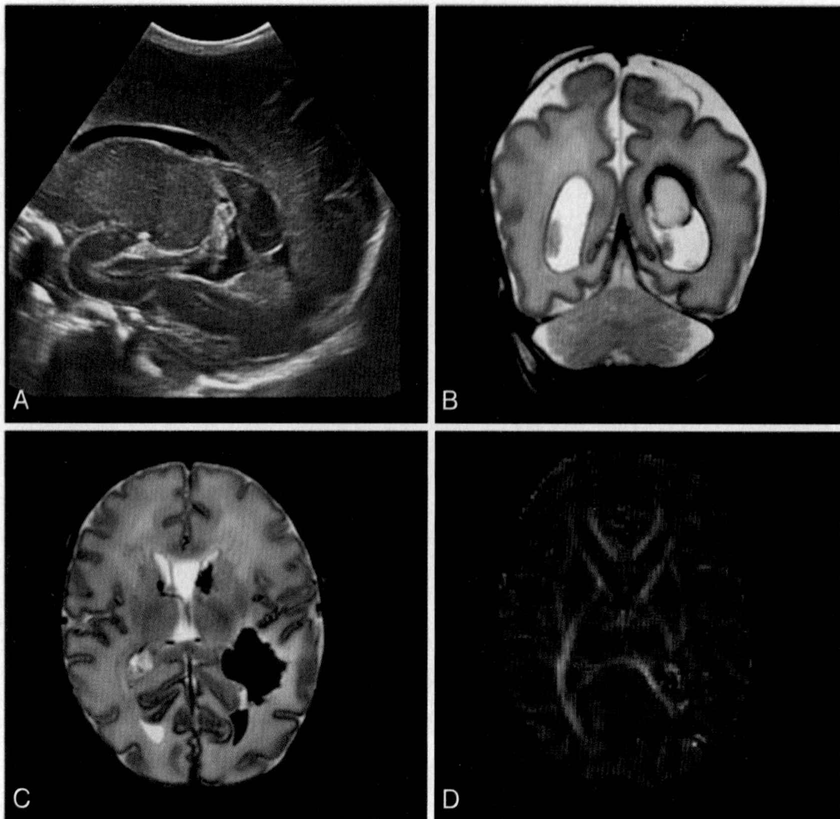

Fig. 96.4 Long-term Consequences of Moderate-Severe Intraventricular Hemorrhage (IVH). (A) Parasagittal cranial ultrasound scan on day 5 in a preterm infant of 26 weeks' gestation, showing a large IVH dilating the posterior part of the lateral ventricle. These abnormalities were confirmed on a coronal T2-weighted magnetic resonance imaging (MRI) sequence at 31 weeks' postmenstrual age. (B) The Bayley Scales of Infant and Toddler Development, Third Edition (BSIC-III) score at 24 months corrected age was borderline (87 for both composite cognitive and motor score). No neurosurgical intervention was required. (C) Axial T2-weighted MRI sequence in a preterm infant of 33 weeks' gestation showing a temporal periventricular hemorrhagic infarction (PVHI). (D) The direction encoded color map shows asymmetry of the optic radiation. The child attended mainstream school; at 5 years no cerebral palsy or visual field defect was detected, but the movement Assessment Battery for Children-II (ABC-II) score was in the 5th centile. (Reproduced with permission and after minor modifications from Gano et al. Cerebral palsy after very preterm birth—An imaging perspective. *Semin Fetal Neonatal Med*. 2020;25:101106.)

outcomes at 8 months or older.[30] Therapeutic hypothermia can decrease the incidence of CP and developmental delay.[27] Edmonds et al. [27a] showed that therapeutic hypothermia prevented NDI in 75.5% of neonates in their study sample; 12.1% of children developed minor neurologic signs and were at a higher risk for cognitive and behavioral defects.

Intraventricular Hemorrhage

Structural Abnormalities on Neuroimaging

Data on long-term neurologic and developmental follow-up of neonates with IVH are primarily based on cranial ultrasonography. However, cerebral MRI is more sensitive than ultrasound at identifying subtle parenchymal abnormalities associated with IVH—for instance, periventricular leukomalacia. IVH damages the germinal matrix and glial precursor cells and can thereby adversely affect cortical development. Vasileiadis et al. used three-dimensional volumetric imaging in preterm neonates to document a 16% reduction in cortical gray matter volume at near-term age.[31] Tract-based spatial statistics analysis of DTI results showed lower fractional anisotropy and higher radial and mean diffusivity of the corpus callosum, limbic pathway, and cerebellar white matter in neonates with IVH, which indicates white matter microstructural defects.[32] White matter microstructural defects can lead to NDI at 24 months of age.[32] Generally, ventriculomegaly present at term can heighten the risk of a poor neurodevelopmental outcome, because it is associated with periventricular parenchymal damage.

Clinical Outcomes

IVH is an independent risk factor for poor neurodevelopmental outcomes among high-risk NICU survivors.[33] Both low-grade (grade I-II) and severe IVH (grade III-IV) predispose to NDI.[33,34] Bolisetty et al., in their cohort study of 1472 preterm NICU survivors, showed that preterm infants with severe IVH had increased rates of CP (30%), developmental delay (17.5%), deafness (8.6%), and blindness (2.2%).[35] Preterm infants with low-grade IVH had higher rates of CP (10.4% vs. 6.5%), developmental delay (7.8% vs. 3.4%), and deafness (6.0% vs. 2.3%) than the group without IVH.[35]

ELBW infants with low-grade IVH had significantly higher rates of NDI (47% versus 28%), low Bayley Mental Development Index scores (<70) (45% versus 25%), and major neurologic defects (13% versus 5%) compared with infants with normal cranial ultrasound at 20 months' corrected age.[36] However, Payne et al. found that low-grade periventricular IVH in infants does not increase the risk of NDI significantly compared with infants without hemorrhage.[37] The laterality of severe IVH determines the extent of NDI in ELBW infants; infants with bilateral grade IV IVH had more severe NDI than those with unilateral grade IV IVH, whereas NDI associated with grades I-III IVH did not differ based on laterality.[38] The severity of NDI related to IVH does not depend on gender differences.[39]

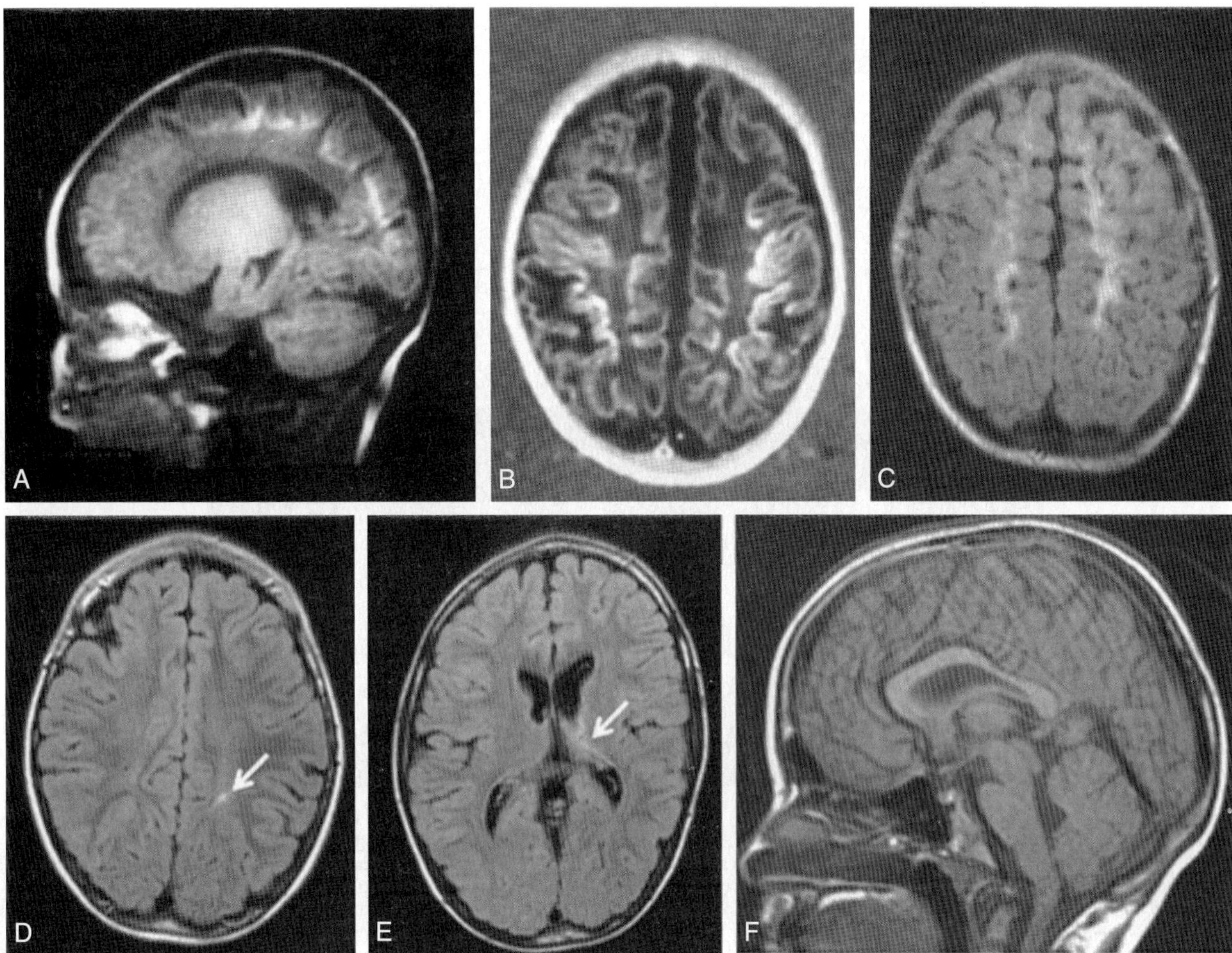

Fig. 96.5 Evolution of Neonatal Cerebral Injury Over a Decade. (A and B) Changes during the neonatal period. (A) Sagittal T1-weighted sequence showing extensive cortical highlighting. (B) Axial magnetic resonance imaging, inversion recovery sequence at the level of the centrum semiovale, showing extensive cortical highlighting and low signal intensity of the subcortical white matter. (C–F) Changes at 10 years of age. (C) fluid-attenuated inversion recovery (FLAIR) sequence of the same child at 10 years of age, showing high signal intensity changes, suggestive of gliosis with the same distribution; "watershed injury." (D) Axial FLAIR sequence at 10 years of age showing a single focal high-signal-intensity lesion; "mild WM lesion." (E) Axial FLAIR sequence at 10 years of age showing unilateral thalamic signal intensity changes; "basal ganglia/thalamus lesion." (F) Midsagittal T1-weighted sequence at 10 years of age, showing focal thinning of the corpus callosum; "WM lesion." (Reproduced with permission and minor modifications from van Kooij et al. Serial MRI and neurodevelopmental outcome in 9- to 10-year-old children with neonatal encephalopathy. *J Pediatr*. 2010;157:221–227.)

Bronchopulmonary Dysplasia

Structural Abnormalities on Neuroimaging

Cerebral MRI has provided a way to describe the anatomic abnormalities and predict neurodevelopmental outcomes in specific neonatal disorders. BPD is associated with defects in cortical maturation in preterm infants; it increases the risk for reduced cerebral surface and abnormal gyrification index on neuroimaging.[40] Neubauer et al. demonstrated that BPD is a significant predictor for abnormal cortical maturation and increases the probability of neurodevelopmental delay four-fold.[41] On DTI, the anisotropy score was lower, and the apparent diffusion coefficient was higher in the white matter of the internal capsule, corpus callosum, and cerebellum, suggesting abnormal white matter development.[42] The cerebral white matter volume in the corpus callosum, superior cerebellar peduncle, and corpus callosum were lower in BPD survivors than in infants without BPD.[43]

Clinical Outcomes

BPD is strongly linked with poor neurodevelopmental outcomes, especially in preterm children.[44] The incidence of CP is higher in neonatal BPD survivors than in gestational age–matched controls; the odds ratio for CP in BPD survivors was 1.66 (95% confidence interval, 1.01–2.74) in a retrospective study on preterm neonates by Hintz et al.[45] Natarajan et al. evaluated BPD survivors at 18 to 22 months' corrected age using the Bayley III assessment and concluded that cognitive impairment was more prevalent in those with BPD.[46] They also demonstrated that moderate to severe CP (Gross Motor Function Classification System level 2 or higher) (7.0% versus 2.1%), spastic diplegia (7.8% versus 4.1%), and quadriplegia (3.9% versus 0.9%) were more common in the BPD group than the non-BPD group.[46,47]

Majnemer et al. showed a 71% prevalence of neurodevelopmental defects, including microcephaly, gross and fine motor deficits, and behavioral difficulties, in the BPD group.[44,47a] Gross and fine motor deficits, blindness, deafness, language delay, and learning disabilities are more prevalent in BPD survivors than non-BPD children.[42,43] BPD children exhibited poorer speech and language outcomes at 8 years of age, with poorer articulation, intelligence quotient (IQ), and receptive language skills.[48] BPD survivors have lower full-scale IQ, performance IQ, verbal IQ, and reading and math grades than non-BPD students.[49,50] These findings highlight the importance of prevention and rehabilitation efforts for BPD survivors.

Neonates with BPD have recurrent episodes of hypoxia that can precipitate hypoxic brain injury. Increased severity of BPD, with a

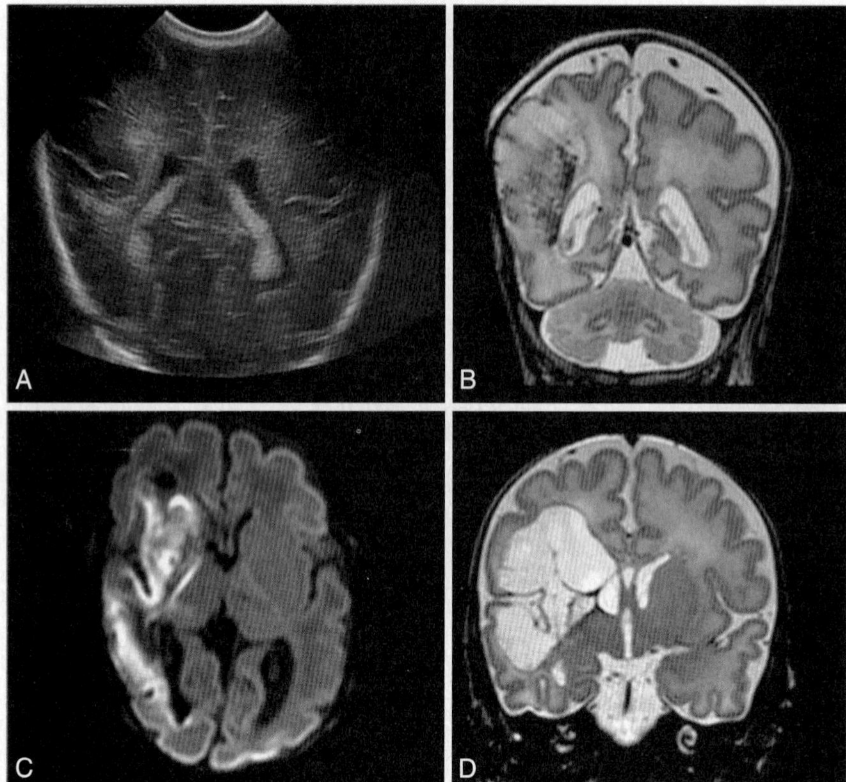

Fig. 96.6 Infants With Severe Systemic Illness Such as Necrotizing Enterocolitis (NEC) Can Develop Cerebral Changes. (A) Cranial ultrasound scan 2 days after surgery for NEC at 34 weeks' postmenstrual age in a preterm infant of 26 weeks' gestation, showing increased echogenicity in the white matter in the right hemisphere. (B) Coronal T2-weighted magnetic resonance imaging (MRI) performed a few days later shows a right-sided middle cerebral artery territory infarction, with partial loss of the cortical ribbon and areas of low signal intensity suggestive of hemorrhage, confirmed on a susceptibility weighted imaging (SWL). (C) Axial diffusion weighted image shows diffusion restriction with partial cortical sparing and involvement of the posterior limb of the internal capsule (PLIC). (D) Coronal T2-weighted MRI at term equivalent age showing extensive cystic evolution. The child developed unilateral hypsarrhythmia, and functional hemispherotomy was required to control the epilepsy. He had a hemiplegia (but was able to walk unaided at 30 months), hemianopia, and cognitive delay (cognitive composite score of 63 at 30 months' corrected age). (Reproduced with permission and after minor modifications from Gano et al. Cerebral palsy after very preterm birth—an imaging perspective. *Semin Fetal Neonatal Med*. 2020;25:101106.)

Table 96.1 Summary of Important Findings From Advanced Magnetic Resonance Imaging (MRI) Prognostic Biomarkers

Most common cerebral quantitative measurements	(1) Regional brain diameter or volume on structural MRI; (2) fractional anisotropy and/or mean diffusivity on dMRI; (3) brain metabolites, most commonly N-acetylaspartate (NAA)/choline ratio on MRS
Brain regions most predictive of neurodevelopmental impairment (identified in three or more studies)	Corpus callosum; centrum semiovale; sensorimotor cortex; subcortical gray matter; posterior limb of the internal capsule; cerebellum
Predicted outcomes examined	Cerebral palsy; minor motor abnormalities; permanent hearing loss; cognitive deficits; working memory; executive function; psychological/behavioral abnormalities

dMRI (N = 25); morphometric studies (N = 25); magnetic resonance spectroscopy (MRS) (N = 5).

Reproduced with permission and minor modification from Hintz and Parikh. The role of neonatal neuroimaging in predicting neurodevelopmental outcomes of preterm neonates. *Fanaroff and Martin's Neonatal-Perinatal Medicine*, 61, 1110–1122.

dMRI, diffusion Magnetic Resonance Imaging.

longer duration of hospitalization and home oxygen treatment, is associated with poorer neurodevelopmental outcomes.[51] One such report is summarized in Table 96.3. Short et al. found that children with more severe BPD had worse neurodevelopmental outcomes, with lower IQ, poorer Bayley mental and psychomotor development index scores, and less developed language abilities at 3 years.[52] The presence of pulmonary hypertension in BPD neonates aggravated NDI and growth parameters.[53]

Necrotizing Enterocolitis

Structural Abnormalities on Neuroimaging

Neuroimaging is helpful to establish a link between neurodevelopmental outcomes and cerebral injury patterns. A randomized controlled trial by Hintz et al. found the importance of near-term cranial ultrasound and MRI in prognosticating the neurodevelopmental outcomes in extremely preterm infants.[54] Woodward et al. also established the predictive value of term MRI in very preterm infants for NDI at 2 years of age.[55] Merhar et al. used MRI of the brain to demonstrate more severe brain injury in infants with surgical NEC than in those with medical NEC; brain injury was graded using a white matter injury scoring system, which was modified to include IVH and cerebellar hemorrhage.[56]

Various studies have used cranial ultrasound and MRI to evaluate and grade brain parenchymal abnormalities. An MRI brain scan can quantitatively assess the degree of brain maturation in preterm neonates.[57] Cranial ultrasound is more easily accessible and is used more than MRI in preterm infants.[58] Cranial ultrasound can accurately detect germinal layer hemorrhage, IVH, hemorrhagic parenchymal

Table 96.2 Clinical Outcomes in Major Illnesses Seen in Premature and Critically Ill Infants

Condition	Structural Abnormalities	Clinical Outcomes	References
Hypoxic-ischemic encephalopathy	• Cerebral edema • Intracranial calcification • Structural defects in cortical gray matter, basal ganglia, thalami, hippocampus, and mammillary bodies • White matter abnormalities	• Cerebral palsy • Epilepsy • Global developmental delay • Language delay • Cognitive impairment • Visual defects • Behavioral abnormalities • Learning disabilities • Memory and attention deficits	19–33
Intraventricular hemorrhage	• Subependymal hemorrhage • Intraparenchymal hemorrhage • Periventricular leukomalacia • Reduction in cortical gray matter volume • Ventriculomegaly	• Cerebral palsy • Developmental delay • Deafness • Visual defects • Cognitive impairment • Memory and attention deficits	34–47
Bronchopulmonary dysplasia	• Reduced cerebral surface • Abnormal cerebral gyrification • White matter abnormalities in the internal capsule, corpus callosum, superior cerebellar peduncle, and cerebellum	• Cerebral palsy • Cognitive impairment • Gross and fine motor deficits • Behavioral abnormalities • Language delay • Visual defects • Deafness • Learning disabilities	48–61
Necrotizing enterocolitis	• Intraventricular hemorrhage • Cerebellar hemorrhage • Hemorrhagic parenchymal infarction • Periventricular leukomalacia • Cortical gray matter abnormalities	• Cerebral palsy • Cognitive defects • Visual impairment • Deafness • Functional impairment • Memory and attention deficits • Language delay • Speech impairment	62–76
Neonatal sepsis	• Cerebral edema • Ventriculitis • Cerebritis • Brain abscess • Hydrocephalus • Cerebral infarction • Subdural empyema • Periventricular leukomalacia • Choroid plexus engorgement • Intraventricular debris accumulation	• Cerebral palsy • Neuropsychiatric conditions • Abnormal psychomotor development • Cognitive deficits • Language delays	77–85

infarction, and periventricular leukomalacia; however, its accuracy diminishes when identifying white matter injury patterns.[59] MRI is a better imaging modality than ultrasound to define the extent of cerebral and cerebellar white matter and gray matter abnormalities.[59,60] Neuroimaging needs to be further studied in the context of long-term neurodevelopmental follow-up of NEC survivors to advance its utility in predicting poor outcomes.

Clinical Outcomes

About 50% of NEC survivors have significant long-term morbidity, including gastrointestinal complications, growth impairment, and disrupted neurologic development.[61,62] NDI primarily occurs as CP, cognitive defects, visual impairment, and deafness.[63,64] NEC survivors are twice as likely to develop NDI than are infants without NEC, according to three systematic reviews.[63–65] According to a systematic review and meta-analysis by Matei et al., the overall NDI incidence in preterm infants with NEC is 40%, and the risk of NDI is significantly higher in NEC infants than in age-matched controls without NEC.[65] Pike et al. followed NEC survivors until 7 years and reported long-term functional impairment using the Health Utilities Index 3.[62]

NDI is a broad term that encompasses entities such as CP, blindness, deafness, and cognitive defects. CP is the most common NDI in preterm infants with NEC, with an incidence of approximately 17%.[65] In addition, blindness and deafness, both having an incidence of approximately 3%, were also more common in infants with NEC than in age-matched controls.[65] Preterm very low birth weight (VLBW) infants with NEC also have a higher probability of developing attention deficit hyperactivity disorder, especially parent-reported, during the early and middle childhood periods.[62,66,67] In a study of NEC infants by Stanford et al., 28% needed special education provision in school, and 21% required speech therapy.[68] In addition, NEC infants also have a higher likelihood of developing a poor cognitive index, language and speech impairment, behavioral disorders, memory and attention deficits, and overall poor educational results.[69–71] Table 96.4 shows the details of another such study that showed adverse neurodevelopmental outcomes in infants with surgical NEC.

Table 96.3 Bronchopulmonary Dysplasia (BPD) Increased the risk of Adverse Neurodevelopmental Outcome

	Severity Groups of BPD			
	Mild	Moderate	Severe	Non-BPD
Infants, No.	47	19	13	79
Normal cognitive development, No. (%)	32 (68.1)	7[a] (36.8)	4[a] (30.8)	66 (83.5)
Borderline cognitive development, No. (%)	8 (17.0)	**6[a] (31.6)**	**6[a] (46.2)**	7 (8.9)
Cognitive impairment, No. (%)	7 (15.0)	**6[a] (31.6)**	3 (23.1)	6 (7.6)
OR [95% CI]	**2.38[a] [1.0–5.6]**	**8.70[a] [2.9–26.3]**	**11.42[a] [3.1–42.7]**	
Corrected OR [95% CI]	1.85 [0.7–4.8]	**7.88[a] [2.4–26.4]**	**8.53[a] [1.9–37.7]**	
Normal motor development, No. (%)	36 (76.6)	13 (68.4)	**7[a] (53.8)**	65 (82.3)
MND, No. (%)	6 (12.8)	**5[a] (26.3)**	**5[a] (38.5)**	6 (7.6)
CP, No. (%)	5 (10.6)	1 (5.3)	1 (7.7)	7 (8.9)
OR [95% CI]	1.53 [0.6–3.7]	2.31 [0.7–7.2]	**5.83[a] [1.7–20.2]**	
Corrected OR [95% CI]	0.70 [0.2–2.5]	2.20 [0.5–9.7]	3.30 [0.5–20.9]	
Normal hearing, No. (%)	42 (89.4)	**14[a] (73.7)**	10 (76.9)	75 (94.9)
Hearing loss, No. (%)	5 (10.6)	**5[a] (26.3)**	3 (23.1)	4 (5.1)
Severe hearing loss, No. (%)	2 (4.3)	1 (5.3)	1 (7.7)	1 (1.3)
OR [95% CI]	2.74 [0.7–10.3]	**5.0[a] [1.7–20.2]**	**8.30[a] [1.8–39.2]**	
Corrected OR [95% CI]	2.16 [0.5–9.0]	4.05 [0.8–21.1]	5.08 [0.8–30.7]	
Normal sight, No. (%)	**18[a] (38.3)**	**8[a] (42.1)**	**2[a] (15.4)**	58 (73.4)
Refraction defects/strabismus, No. (%)	**17[a] (36.2)**	3 (15.8)	5 (38.5)	13 (16.5)
Blindness/residual vision, No. (%)	**12[a] (25.5)**	**8[a] (42.1)**	**6[a] (46.2)**	8 (10.1)
OR [95% CI]	**4.45[a] [2.1–9.6]**	**3.80[a] [1.3–10.7]**	**15.20[a] [3.1–74.3]**	
Corrected OR [95% CI]	2.51 [0.97–6.5]	1.83 [0.5–6.4]	**11.52[a] [1.2–109.7]**	
No disability, No. (%)	25 (53.2)	8 (42.1)	5 (38.5)	52 (65.8)
Mild disability, No. (%)	9 (19.1)	2 (10.5)	2 (15.4)	13 (16.5)
Moderate/severe disability, No. (%)	13 (27.7)	**9[a] (47.4)**	**5[a] (38.5)**	15 (19.0)
OR [95% CI]	1.70 [0.8–3.5]	2.65 [0.95–7.4]	3.08 [0.9–10.3]	
Corrected OR [95% CI]	0.71 [0.3–1.9]	1.30 [0.4–4.4]	2.88 [0.16–4.8]	

Psychological/behavioral abnormalitiesartate (NAA)/choline ratio on MR.

[a]Bronchopulmonary dysplasia (BPD) increased ls.

The authors reported mean values and odds ratio of the total DQ and Griffiths' Mental Developmental subscales for all study groups. Mean values were obtained not considering survived infants who unfortunately were not able to complete the assessment because of cerebral palsy, blindness, severe hearing loss, or other severe disabilities. Among excluded infants, 15 belonged to the control group, 13 to the mild, 9 to the moderate, and 5 to the severe group. Therefore DQ was evaluated in 64 infants without BPD and in 52 infants with BPD (34 mild, 10 moderate, and 8 severe).

Reproduced with permission and minor modifications from Callini et al. Neurodevelopmental outcomes in very preterm infants: the role of severity of bronchopulmonary dysplasia. *Early Hum Dev.* 2021;152:105275.

CP, Cerebral palsy; *MND*, motor neuron deficit; *NAA*, behavioral abnormalities N-acetyl aspartate; *OR*, odds ratio.

Neonatal Sepsis

Structural Abnormalities on Neuroimaging

Neurologic complications of neonatal sepsis include cerebral edema, ventriculitis, cerebritis, hydrocephalus, brain abscess, cerebral infarction, and subdural empyema.[72] White matter involvement, commonly in the form of periventricular leukomalacia, often occurs in sepsis due to a rise in proinflammatory cytokines. Neuroimaging in neonatal sepsis frequently displays choroid plexus engorgement, intraventricular debris accumulation, and contrast-enhancement of the ependyma.[73] Cranial ultrasound can identify cystic periventricular leukomalacia, hydrocephalus, and ventriculomegaly due to white matter loss in neonatal sepsis. MRI can delineate diffuse or subtle white matter loss using a three-dimensional volumetric technique. White matter abnormalities predispose to motor impairment and developmental delay, psychomotor abnormalities, and cognitive deficits. MRI can also recognize cerebellar involvement in neonatal sepsis, and it has been associated with abnormal motor, cognitive, and behavioral developmental parameters.[74]

Clinical Outcomes

Neonatal sepsis is a common cause of prolonged NICU admission and is especially prevalent in preterm VLBW neonates. A systematic review and meta-analysis of 15,331 VLBW infants showed that sepsis increases the risk for NDI (odds ratio, 2.09; 95% confidence interval, 1.65–2.65) and CP (odds ratio, 2.09; 95% confidence interval, 1.78–2.45).[75] A cohort study of VLBW infants in Cuba revealed that in infants with neonatal sepsis, the risk of NDI was heightened (47.1% versus 17.1%; odds ratio, 4.0; confidence interval, 1.1–14.3) compared with those without sepsis at 2 years.[76] There was no correlation with poor neurodevelopmental outcomes in case of suspected sepsis without microbiological evidence of infection.[77]

Table 96.4 Surgical Necrotizing Enterocolitis (NEC) With Late Bacteremia Increased the Risk of Each Adverse Neurodevelopmental Outcome[a]

Neurodevelopmental Correlate/Diagnosis	Surgical NEC and Late Bacteremia (n = 14)	Surgical NEC Only (n = 28)	Late Bacteremia Only (n = 245)	Neither (n = 809)
Quadriparetic CP	—	1.1 (0.2, 5.2)	1.4 (0.7, 2.7)	1.0
Diparetic CP	**8.4 (1.9, 39)**	1.3 (0.1, 11)	0.9 (0.4, 2.4)	1.0
GMFCS 2+	—	0.7 (0.1, 5.9)	1.5 (0.8, 2.9)	1.0
Bayley MDI < 70	2.7 (0.8, 8.9)	2.2 (0.9, 5.2)	**1.5 (1.05, 2.2)**	1.0
Bayley PDI < 70	2.1 (0.6, 7.1)	**2.7 (1.2, 6.4)**	1.3 (0.9, 1.9)	1.0
HC z score < −2	**9.3 (2.2, 40)**	1.4 (0.3, 5.9)	1.5 (0.9, 2.6)	1.0
HC z score ≥ −2, < −1	2.6 (0.5, 13)	1.9 (0.7, 5.4)	1.5 (0.98, 2.3)	1.0

[a]All models are adjusted for public insurance, maternal or fetal initiator for delivery, gestational age (23–24, 25–26, or 27 weeks), birth weight z score from thrombosis of the fetal stem vessels of the placenta and include a random effect cluster term for birth hospital. The table shows odds ratios and 95% confidence intervals from multivariable logistic regression models. Each outcome is a dichotomy. For quadriparesis and diparesis, the reference group is "no cerebral palsy." For head circumference *z* score < confidence intervals from multivariable logistic regression models t, 2021-01-01, Volume 152, Article 1

Reproduced with permission and minor modifications from Martin et al. Neurodevelopment of extremely preterm infants who had necrotizing enterocolitis with or without late bacteremia. *J Pediatr.* 2010;157:751.

CP, Cerebral palsy; *HC*, head circumference; *MDI*, mental developmental index; *PDI*, psychomotor developmental index.

Apart from motor abnormalities such as CP, neonatal sepsis also increases the risk for minor neurologic abnormalities associated with neuropsychiatric conditions.[78] It is also related to abnormal psychomotor development, cognitive deficits, and language delays. The degree of NDI is not affected by the bacterial pathogen, gram-positive or gram-negative; however, NDI is often more severe in nosocomial multidrug-resistant gram-negative and fungal infections.[79,80] The risk for NDI does not differ between early-onset sepsis and late-onset sepsis; however, the risk is increased if both are present together.[81]

Follow-Up of NICU Survivors

Much research is being conducted on understanding the pathogenesis and primary prevention of neonatal complications, including NDI. While these mechanisms are elucidated, the primary focus must be on close monitoring of NICU survivors, early detection of complications, and prompt interventions.[58] Ramel et al. concluded that the linear length of an infant determines the cognitive development parameters.[82] They also reported that in preterm infants, an increase in fat-free mass during hospitalization improved neurodevelopmental parameters at 12 months' corrected age.[83] Anthropometric measurements such as linear growth and head circumference correlate indirectly with brain growth and assess neurodevelopment in infants.[82] These measurements are easily obtainable, allow early identification of growth failure, and facilitate prompt intervention.

The Bayley Scales of Infant Development (BSID) is widely used to evaluate an infant's mental and psychomotor development and detect any degree of NDI. However, there have been reports that this standardized instrument has a few limitations.[58] Hack et al. assessed the BSID II Mental Development Index's validity and found that it poorly predicts cognitive function at school age.[84] Similarly, the Bayley Scales of Infant and Toddler Development (Bayley-III) failed to accurately estimate the developmental delay in 2-year-old toddlers.[85] BSID should be performed serially and supplemented with a detailed developmental assessment during the follow-up of preterm NICU survivors. Registration and monitoring of NDI in children with a history of an NICU stay should be made compulsory for NICU departments.

SECTION

20 Designing Clinical Trials in Neonatology

OUTLINE

CHAPTER 97

Quality Improvement in Neonatal Care

Colleen A. Hughes Driscoll

KEY POINTS

1. The quality of clinical care and improvement is typically measured in six areas: safety, effectiveness, patient-centeredness, timeliness, efficiency, and equality.
2. Healthcare administered during pregnancy, labor, and childbirth continues to show considerable center-to-center variability and needs careful study both for improving outcomes and also to reduce the possibility of harm.
3. The care of premature and critically ill infants in neonatal intensive care units involves high-risk skilled procedures that need careful analysis.
4. Quality improvement (QI) priorities need to be relevant to ill infants. The plan-do-study-act methodology is important to evaluate and refine treatment efforts.
5. The distinction between research and QI needs to be understood, with a clear distinction between activities that aim to improve the quality of care delivered to patients and those that may improve quality of care by contributing to generalizable knowledge.

General Considerations

Quality improvement (QI) has become a well-accepted science for improving healthcare quality across all settings.[1] The Institute of Medicine's six aims for a healthcare system have influenced QI efforts in the hospital environment, and neonatal intensive care units (NICUs) are poised to facilitate QI projects that promote safety, effectiveness, patient-centeredness, timeliness, efficiency, and equality.[2] Several aspects of newborn care combine to form ideal conditions for the application of continuous quality improvement (CQI):

- Healthcare administered during pregnancy, labor, and childbirth encompasses some of the most common processes of care delivery in the hospital setting.[3] The consistent need for maternal and newborn care during the perinatal period lends itself to the systematic testing of rapid cycle changes of CQI.
- Pregnancy and delivery involve the interaction between two distinct but dependent patients whose health and safety require unique consideration. Therefore, close collaboration and communication between maternal and neonatal providers is essential for care optimization.[4]
- NICUs are complex organizations with providers from various specialties. NICU care involves high-risk skilled procedures, specialized equipment, and relative uncertainty of patient clinical status in the immediate postpartum period. Patient safety can be adversely impacted in this type of environment if processes are not reliable.[1]
- Despite evidence to support best practices for pregnancy, labor, delivery, and neonatal care, notable variation in practice exists among hospitals.[5–8]
- Malpractice claims involving obstetric and pediatric care more commonly lead to higher awards than for other medical specialties.[9] Interventions that can improve healthcare delivery while reducing patient harm present an opportunity to reduce malpractice costs.

Methodology

The methods used to guide systematic rapid cycle changes in the NICU have a long history in industries outside of healthcare. Modern healthcare improvement draws on prior quality work developed in industries such as telecommunication, automotives, and manufacturing.[10] The commonly used plan-do-study-act (PDSA) cycle (Fig. 97.1), which has evolved during the course of the century, remains the cornerstone of QI methodology. Although there are several approaches and philosophies used in QI work in general, all of these techniques use the PDSA cycle at their core. The Associates in Process Improvement have adapted the PDSA cycle in their Model for Improvement approach, an approach championed by the Institute for Healthcare Improvement and adopted by many in healthcare QI work.[11]

In addition to having a working knowledge of PDSA cycles, the following factors should be considered in any QI project.[11]

Defining and Selecting the Problem to be Addressed

Having a clearly defined problem is an essential element of QI work. Defining the problem will allow project teams to describe shared missions and targets, focus ongoing work, and allow the team to determine whether the goals were met. One example of planning QI project(s) is shown in Fig. 97.2. There are many potential problems that a healthcare team may encounter every day during routine care delivery, and leaders must prioritize the problems to be addressed through QI work. The severity of the problem, the impact expected from a potential solution, and the anticipated effort to solve the problem should all be considered when prioritizing problems.

Establishing a Project Team

Project teams should be established early in the QI project and should minimally include, or be endorsed by, a leader who can ensure that changes are implemented. Given that NICU care is provided by a wide range of medical specialists and support staff, it is important to consider who is impacted by the problem and who would be impacted by the changes that may occur as a result of the QI work. The project team should include representation from the

A

Step	Description
PLAN	Determine root cause of problem and plan a change
DO	Carry out the change, preferably on a small scale
STUDY (CHECK)*	Study to see if the desired result was achieved, what went wrong, and what was learnerd
ACT	Adopt the change if the desired result was achieved and implement it on a large scale. If not, repeat the cycle using knowledge learned from the previous cycle

* The problem solving process usually begins at the STUDY step. This is where current performance is measured and compared with target performance. When the results indicate a gap that requires action, the Model for Improvement may be applied.

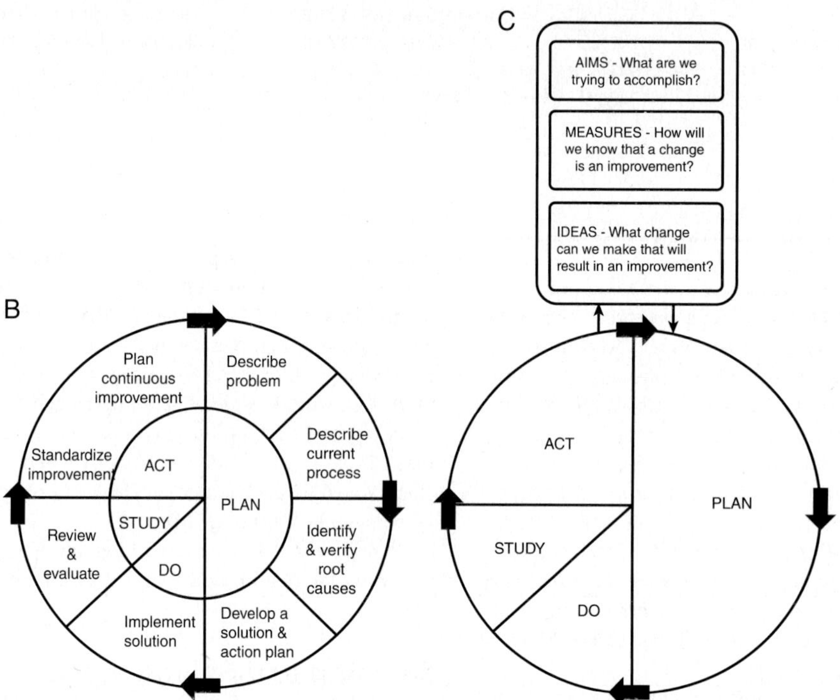

Fig. 97.1 The Plan-Do-Study-Act (PDSA) Cycle. (A) Overview of the steps of the PDSA cycle. (B) In the seven-step PDSA cycle, the "plan step" comprises 4 parts: (1) describe the problem, (2) describe the current process, (3) identify and verify root causes, and (4) develop a solution and action plan. In the "act step," the change is adopted and implemented on a large scale if the desired result was achieved. If not, the PDSA cycle is repeated using the newly acquired knowledge. The "act step" also includes plans for sustaining and monitoring the implemented change and planning new quality-improvement projects. (C) The Model for Improvement has an inquiry component composed of AIMS, MEASURES, and IDEAS and an activity component, which is the PDSA cycle. (Reproduced with permission from Eslamy et al. *Seminars in Ultrasound, CT, and MRI*. 2014;35:608–626.)

aforementioned groups. As the team examines the processes associated with the problem to be addressed, additional impacted groups may be identified and added to the project team. Project team members should have unique and well-defined responsibilities to prevent the team from becoming unnecessarily large or inefficient.

Establishing a Mission and Target

Developing a mission statement at the start of a QI project can be a way to disseminate the purpose of the QI work among front-line staff, who may not be part of the project team. Mission statements can be less specific than target statements, with the intention of uniting individuals around the project. An example might be "to reduce noise in the NICU for patients, families and staff." Targets are considerably more specific and should be constructed in a way that addresses the current and a desired state (Fig. 97.3). A timeline also needs to be defined. To continue the example, a workable target statement might be "to reduce the number of nonactionable patient alarms from 80 alarms per 12-hour shift to 70 alarms per 12-hours shift over the course of 4 weeks by modification of the programmed alarm limits." When developing targets, consideration should be given to how realistic it is to achieve the desired state, to alter the involved processes, and to achieve the goal desired state within the specified time frame.

Measures

To determine both the current state and changes to the current state, valid and consistent measurement is needed. Relying on measurements that are difficult to obtain can be prohibitive to a successful QI project. In the example of trying to reduce the number of nonactionable patient alarms, it would be virtually impossible to determine the frequency of alarms by direct, real-time observation. However, if one could easily query the patient monitors' alarm history on a

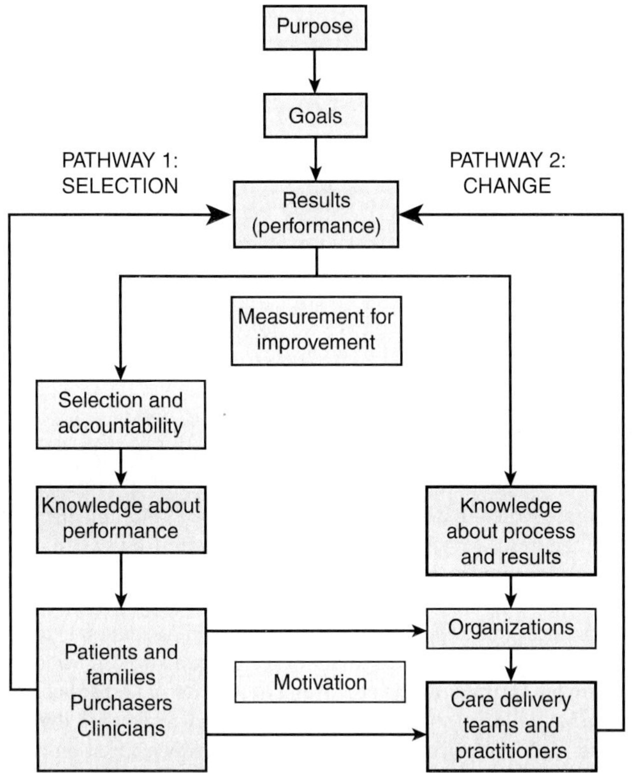

Fig. 97.2 Pathways to Quality Improvement. (Reproduced with permission from Profit et al. *Fanaroff and Martin's Neonatal-Perinatal Medicine*, 5, 67-101.)

daily basis and dissect the data into 12-hour shifts the project becomes more feasible. Additionally, it is important that project teams consider all potentially relevant measures including process measures, outcome measures, and balance measures from the start. Evaluating these measures in the context of time through the use of annotated run charts or statistical process control charts will help identify significant changes in relation to interventions.

Prioritizing Changes

Processes associated with healthcare delivery are frequently complex and should be clearly delineated before intervening. There are often a multitude of potential changes that can be made to a process, or its subprocesses, when evaluating for improvements. There may also be a need to stratify the needed changes to narrow disparities (Fig. 97.4). Team members may disagree on which changes will lead to the best outcome. Alternatively, team members may be overwhelmed by the magnitude of the process and have difficulty developing change ideas. When deliberating change ideas, consideration should be given to whether a reactive or fundamental change is needed, whether a change was tried and failed in the past, understanding the reason for prior failures, the time and effort required to implement the change, the potential for adversely impacting competing processes, the anticipated benefit gained from the change, and whether similar changes have been successful in similar environments.[12] Tools such as driver diagrams, Pareto charts, cause and effect diagrams, flow diagrams, impact effort matrices, and others can help teams develop and organize potential changes to a process.

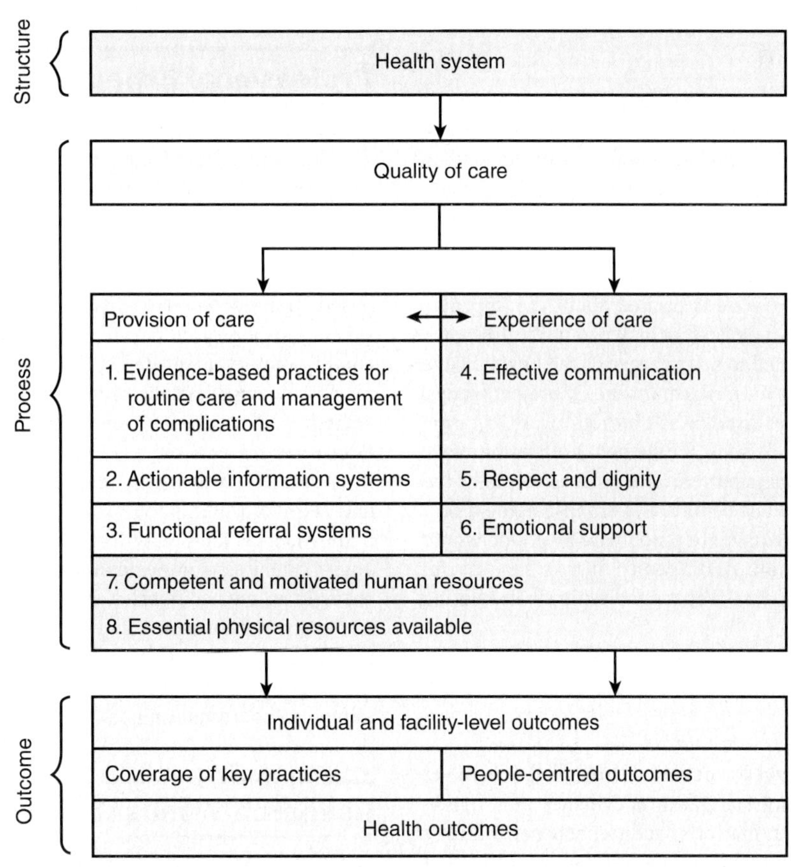

Fig. 97.3 World Health Organization Framework for the Quality of Maternal and Newborn Healthcare. (Reproduced with permission from Brizuela et al. *Lancet Global Health*. 2019;7:e624–e632.)

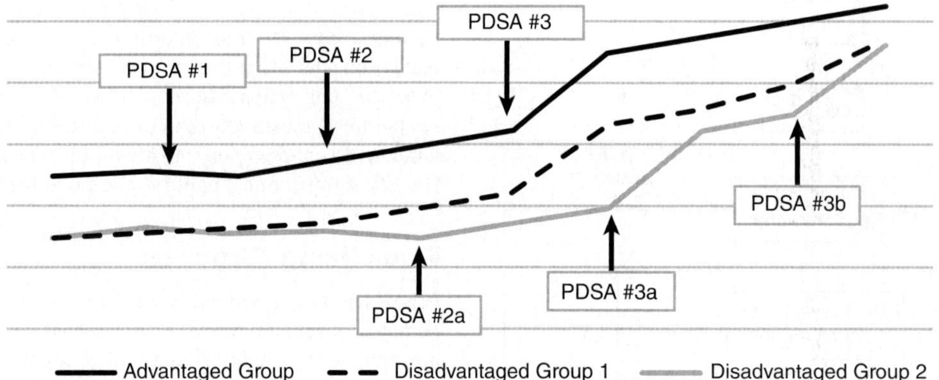

Fig. 97.4 Pathways to Quality Improvement. *PDSA*, Plan-do-study-act. (Reproduced with permission from Reichman et al. *Seminars in Fetal and Neonatal Medicine*. 2021;26:101–198.)

Communication

When changes are implemented in a clinical workflow, undoubtedly there will be a variety of responses from individual front-line staff. Although some individuals within an organization are likely to rapidly adopt new ideas into practice, others may hesitate or even resist change. Identifying early adopters of change can help project teams capitalize on their enthusiasm and promote full cultural adoption.[12] Effective and transparent communication of project goals, the rationale for change, and project outcomes can help staff members become more engaged in a QI project. Similarly, front-line staff should be provided with a clear mechanism to communicate any input to the project team, including concerns related to proposed changes.

Maintaining the Gain

When improvements occur after change implementations, focus should be placed on how to sustain that change within a process or system. For example, suppose the implementation of a morning team huddle with a physician, charge nurse, social worker, and case manager resulted in earlier NICU discharges. The discharges are now occurring 6.5 hours earlier on average, and the subsequent bed availability for new patients has resulted in significant financial gains for the hospital. Although everyone is excited about the improvements, the case manager finds it difficult to arrive to the huddle each day because her office is located in a far corner of the hospital. We might anticipate that as initial enthusiasm for the QI project wanes, the case manager may view the distance as a barrier to participation in the huddle and stop participating altogether. Rather than risk losing the case manager's participation, alternatives to make the huddle more sustainable would be beneficial. Perhaps having a conference call line for the case manager to participate by phone would support continued participation. Additionally, it may be a useful mechanism for other participants who find the physical meeting somewhat challenging.

Quality Networks

Whereas CQI projects should have an organized structure that involves not just leadership but front-line staff, there is evidence that organization through quality networks may offer additional benefits during CQI over projects done in isolation.[13,14] Networks may be formed at a national or regional level, may be voluntary or mandated, can have selected or open participation, or may be the result of a shared corporate structure among medical institutions.[15] Multiple networks have demonstrated significant improvements in neonatal outcomes across participating hospitals; however, the overall impact of network-based QI initiatives are mixed, and the sustainability of such outcomes is unclear.[4,15–17] Potential benefits of participation in quality networks include real-time guidance for hospitals whose leadership has limited QI training; the opportunity to learn from other hospitals' successes, failures, and challenges; allowing for structured data collection and analysis; and the opportunity to reduce variation within and between participating hospitals. Regardless of whether process or outcome measures improve as a result of participation in QI networks, the experience and knowledge gained from guided improvement methodology may be beneficial for individual hospitals.

Professional Expectations for QI

Governing bodies for both healthcare agencies and medical providers are increasingly requiring participation and experience in QI activities. Starting in 2010, the American Board of Pediatrics (ABP) incorporated a Performance In Practice component to its maintenance-of-certification program for diplomates.[18] This component requires diplomates to earn point values for either completing web-based QI activities, participating in an ongoing ABP-approved collaborative QI project, or publishing an article meeting Standards for Quality Improvement Reporting Excellence (SQUIRE) guidelines in a peer-reviewed journal within a 5-year cycle.[19] Training programs accredited through the Accreditation Council for Graduate Medical Education are now required to ensure trainees actively participate in patient-safety systems, receive formal patient-safety education, and receive training and experience in QI processes.[20] Accrediting bodies such as the Center for Medicare & Medicaid Services and the Joint Commission on Accreditation of Healthcare Organizations have strongly influenced hospital standards with respect to patient safety and quality improvement, with public transparency of outcomes further driving performance improvement.[21] Health departments at the state level also encourage quality and safety of NICUs by maintaining standards and supervising perinatal regionalization of care.[22]

Research Versus Quality Improvement

The distinction between activities that aim to improve the quality of care delivered to patients and those that may improve quality of care by contributing to generalizable knowledge can be unclear at times.[23] Understanding the ways in which QI and human subjects research differ is necessary to prevent potential patient harm. Human subjects research is a systematic investigation designed to develop or contribute to generalizable knowledge, and the research involves obtaining information about living individuals.[24] The overarching purpose of human subjects research in medicine is to improve health. QI efforts are also intended to improve health through systematic investigation; however, the investigation may or may not involve obtaining information from living individuals, and the results are not intended to be generalizable. There are many potential scenarios in which the lines between human subjects research and QI are blurred.

A very clear example of human subjects research would be a randomized controlled trial comparing two different surfactant products to determine which lowers lung compliance more rapidly in preterm infants. The study is designed to determine which drug is superior for a specific outcome and would provide information that could benefit a large number of physicians and preterm infants outside of the study. Because it is unknown whether one product has superior efficacy or one product imposes an increased risk of side effects, patients open themselves to potential inferior treatment by participation. As such, they deserve to have a clear understanding of the potential risks and benefits of participation. In this situation, an institutional review board (IRB) must ensure to the best of its ability that the potential knowledge gained by execution of the study warrants the risks to patients, that the patients are adequately informed of the risks and benefits, and that patients are able to maintain their autonomy.

Alternatively, there are many QI initiatives that clearly do not involve humans. For example, suppose a newborn, delivered by emergent cesarean section, was harmed when the newborn resuscitation team was not present at the time of birth and effective resuscitation was delayed. A root cause analysis revealed that the resuscitation team spent a considerable amount of time waiting for an elevator to bring them from the neonatal intensive care unit to the operative suite. These elevators were routinely used by the team because they were the closet elevators to the intensive care unit and operative suites. Unfortunately, they were one of the busiest sets of elevators and were slow to arrive when called. To allow for faster arrival of the resuscitation team to the operative suites, the resuscitation team was given an override key that would expedite the movement of the elevator car to the intensive care unit when the resuscitation team was needed in the operative suites. The project leadership tracked response times of the resuscitation team and the elevator movement before and after the change in practice. In this scenario, no living human data are being collected, and information gained during the investigation is not generalizable outside of this specific clinical workflow. Given that the presence of skilled newborn resuscitation providers at the time of an emergent delivery is overall beneficial to a depressed newborn, it is hard to imagine that this change in practice would lead to patient harm, and potential benefits are more obvious. In this situation, the change in workflow is intended to support the best-practice evidence. The intent of the project is to make the delivery of appropriate care more efficient—a clear example of quality improvement. The role for IRB oversight in such a situation is far less obvious.

There are times when systematic changes are made in a practice with a goal of improving the quality of care, yet risks to a patient may exist. Suppose a NICU would like to reduce the frequency of unplanned extubations among the patient population. Unplanned extubations are a known patient-safety issue that can result in increased morbidities in the NICU population.[25] The QI team makes several process interventions to standardize endotracheal tube care and then decides to analyze specific patient factors that may contribute to repeated unplanned extubations. Patient data, including outcome data and patient-specific clinical information, are being used to identify potential strategies for reducing repeated extubations. In this CQI project, patients may be at risk for breech of privacy. Additionally, might the interventions implemented to standardize care result in unintended negative consequences for a patient? Ideally, the interventions would have an evidence base or be part of an accepted standard of care. However, many times in neonatal care, the best practice is unknown. For improvement projects such as this, anticipating and tracking unintended consequences is important, and review by an IRB may be beneficial.

The absence of patient-specific data during an investigation is not by itself a qualifier for a project to be considered QI. Imagine that an investigator would like to assess for metabolites of environmental toxins in the urine of NICU patients. The investigator is concerned that commonly used NICU equipment and devices may expose infants to toxins. The urine samples would be collected from diapers that would otherwise be thrown away, and the samples would not contain any identifying information. There would be no interaction with the patient to obtain the sample. Although the intent is to improve the health of patients in the NICU, the investigator does not have the immediate ability to improve the outcome (reduce patient exposure to toxins), because there would not be an alternative set of equipment for use in the patient population. The information gained from this study is likely to contribute to general knowledge, because all patients in this population would have a risk of toxin exposure. Any potential benefits from this investigation would only benefit future patients, following the development of toxin-free equipment. Review by an IRB could help appropriately characterize this investigation and avoid its misclassification as QI.

Recurring examples throughout history have demonstrated that human subjects need protection from any risks incurred by study involvement. There is a wide range of potential risks to human subjects, ranging from severe (e.g., potential increased risk of death) to seemingly minor (e.g., reduced privacy). IRBs are necessary to provide independent oversight for human subjects research and to ensure that the research design has minimized risk and is likely to bring meaningful knowledge. However, IRB oversight is intended to protect research subjects, and there is not at this time any standardized mechanism available to protect patients who are the end-recipients of healthcare delivery QI efforts. Although IRBs can help investigators determine whether their work is or is not human subjects research, not all healthcare entities have ready access to an independent review, and an IRB review would not necessarily be an appropriate mechanism for QI oversight.[26] The obligation of healthcare agencies to provide safe, equitable, and effective care to their patients generally aligns with a patient's best interest; however, the method for achieving this care must also align. Unfortunately, considerable debate on how best to achieve this is ongoing.[23,26,27]

CHAPTER

98 Neonatal Randomized Controlled Trials

Gerri Baer, Norma Terrin, Donna Snyder, Jonathan M. Davis

KEY POINTS

1. Neonates and infants often are treated with medicines that have not been approved by regulatory authorities for use in this age group.
2. The inclusion of infants in drug development studies and clinical trials is limited by difficulties in enrollment, concerns for adverse effects due to developmental limitations, and the lack of universally accepted response variables in many conditions.
3. Neonatal randomized controlled trials (RCTs) are needed to evaluate the impact of interventions, from practice standards to devices to novel therapies or therapies that were developed for nonneonatal indications.
4. There is a need for RCTs not only to assess effectiveness and safety of neonatal therapies but also to focus on operational issues and outcomes for regulatory consideration.
5. Clinical investigations that evaluate interventions/procedures that present the prospect of direct benefit but carry a possibility of greater than minimal risk need review by institutional review boards. There is a need to ensure that the benefit-risk assessment is more favorable than that with alternative approaches.

Introduction

Neonates and infants often are treated with medicines that have not been approved by any regulatory authorities for use in this population.[1] High-risk neonates and children in general are seen as vulnerable, with their participation in drug development and clinical trials limited by numerous factors. Some of the reasons that so few products have been developed for neonates and children include gaps in understanding complex pathophysiology, a small market with many conditions involving rare diseases, challenges in the design and execution of clinical trials (including the need to wait for long periods of time to assess some clinical outcomes), and difficulties with the assessment of safety and efficacy. This has resulted in children being referred to as "therapeutic orphans."

This chapter will review fundamentals of the design and conduct of clinical trials in neonates and young infants. Although randomized controlled trials (RCTs) are considered the "gold standard," the use of alternative designs (e.g., cluster randomized trials) will also be discussed (Fig. 98.1). Ethical considerations, including issues related to informed consent, will be presented along with the need for engagement of parents and neonatal intensive care unit (NICU) staff in the trial design process.

Clinical Trial Designs

The likelihood that a clinical study will answer the research questions posed in a reliable manner, meaningful for decision makers and patients, while preventing important errors, can be dramatically improved through prospective attention to the design of all components of the study protocol, procedures and associated operational plans.[2]

—From the International Council for Harmonisation (ICH) E8(R1) Draft Guideline

Randomized, double-masked or blinded, placebo- or standard of care–controlled clinical trials have provided many of the key advances in neonatal therapeutics. Surfactant replacement for respiratory distress syndrome, caffeine for apnea of prematurity, therapeutic hypothermia for hypoxic-ischemic encephalopathy, and inhaled nitric oxide for persistent pulmonary hypertension of the newborn are among the most significant therapeutic successes in neonatology. Despite these successes, RCTs of preventive agents or therapies for conditions such as bronchopulmonary dysplasia and neonatal hypotension have not produced clear evidence of clinically meaningful benefit for any of the therapies studied.

RCTs remain an essential tool for assessing the effectiveness and safety of neonatal therapies, both novel therapies and those whose efficacy and/or safety may be unclear. It has been recognized that clinical trials may either fail to show an effect or fail to provide useful data due to problems with elements of design and implementation.[3] "Quality by design" is an approach that relies on sound prospective design and execution plans such as (1) focusing on protecting human subjects, (2) determining predefined objectives, (3) selecting appropriate study participants, (4) minimizing bias, (5) controlling confounding, (6) choosing measurable and well-defined study endpoints and methods of assessment, and (7) addressing operational and feasibility criteria.[2,4]

Human Subjects Protections and Neonatal Clinical Trials

The U.S. Department of Health and Human Services (HHS) and the Food and Drug Administration (FDA) require special protections for the inclusion of children in research. These protections are defined under HHS 21CFR§50, Subpart D, as the "Additional Safeguards for Children in Clinical Investigations" and under FDA 45CFR§46, Subpart D, as the "Additional Protections for Children Involved as Subjects in Research." The principles are the same, but the HHS and FDA Subpart D guidelines

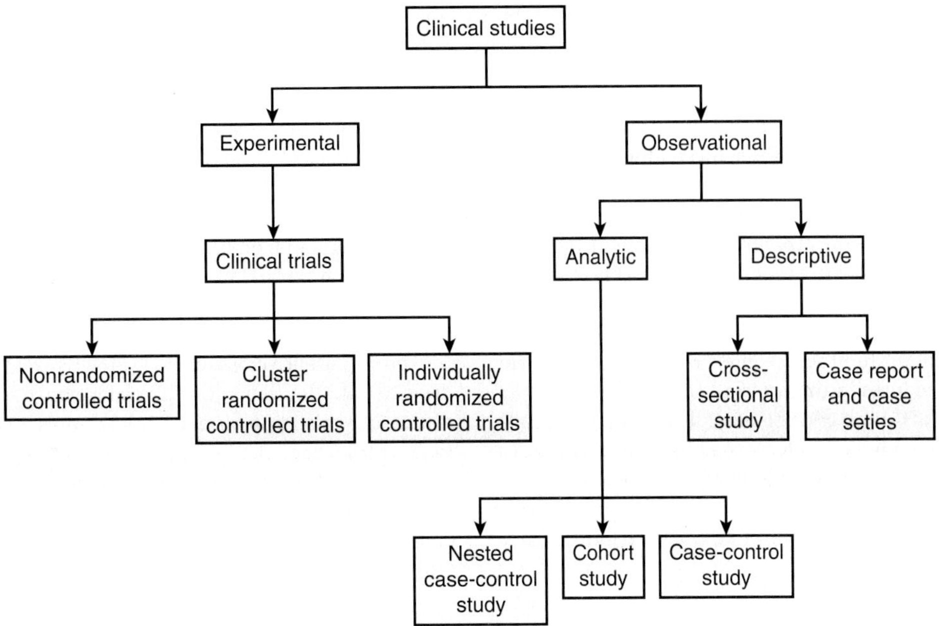

Fig. 98.1 Classification of Clinical Study Designs. (From Vetter T, Chou R. Clinical trial design methodology for outcome studies. *Practical Management of Pain.* 2014;80:1057-1065.e3.)

differ slightly in scope. The HHS regulation applies to "all research involving children as subjects, conducted or supported by HHS,"[5] whereas the FDA regulation applies only to studies of an FDA-regulated product.[6]

Under Subpart D, an institutional review board (IRB) can approve clinical investigations involving children that fall into the following categories:

1. not greater than minimal risk,
2. greater than minimal risk but presenting the prospect of direct benefit to individual subjects, or
3. greater than minimal risk and no prospect of direct benefit to individual subjects but likely to yield generalizable knowledge about the subjects' disorder or condition.

An IRB may determine that a study presents no more than minimal risk if all the interventions or procedures within the clinical investigation do not exceed minimal risk. Such studies may proceed with the permission of one parent or guardian. Minimal risk is difficult to define but is indexed to the risks for the population in their daily life, including routine examinations.[7] In the case of hospitalized neonates, a single blood draw (preferably with routine labs), bagged urine specimen, or a single chest radiograph may be considered minimal risk.

Interventions or procedures within a clinical investigation that convey greater than minimal risk but present the prospect of direct benefit (PDB) are reviewed by IRBs to ensure that the risk is justified by the anticipated benefit and that the benefit-risk assessment is at least as favorable to participants as would be available with alternative approaches. Permission of one parent or guardian must also be obtained for research approved under this category.[8] Protocols should clearly describe available alternatives to the investigational therapy and any adverse events and long-term consequences if known. A comprehensive understanding of therapeutic alternatives is critical to benefit-risk assessments for IRBs and regulators. An example of a study in this category may include evaluation of a novel therapy in a pediatric population for which the PDB to the child has been established and justifies the risk of exposure. Such an assessment should include whether there is adequate evidence to establish proof of concept to support a benefit and whether the proposed dose and duration of therapy are sufficient to offer a potential clinical benefit (Table 98.1).[9–11]

Table 98.1 Assessment of a Novel Therapy to Support a Prospect of Direct Benefit (PDB) and Minimize Potential Risks

Factors That May Support a Prospect of Benefit for a Novel Therapy	Tools to Support Benefit and Minimize Burdens/Risks
EVIDENCE TO SUPPORT PROOF OF CONCEPT	
Biological plausibility and scientific justification for the proposed mechanism of action and its expected effect in the condition of interest	Evaluate existing scientific rationale, summarize available experimental and observational data
Nonclinical evidence (*in-vitro* mechanistic studies, *in-vivo* studies in animal models)	*In vivo* data in animal models of disease can provide insight into the impact of the intervention on pathophysiology as well as dosing strategy
Clinical evidence in adults or older children with similar and/or relevant conditions	Efficacy responses may support benefit and data on adverse effects can provide important information to guide monitoring in a neonatal clinical trial
STRUCTURE OF THE STUDY INTERVENTION	
Dosing justification including evidence to support that the proposed doses are likely to have the intended treatment effect	• Modeling and simulation based on adult, pediatric, and/or nonclinical data can aid in dose selection based on predicted exposure-response relationship • Adaptive trial designs may allow for dose exploration and optimization within the context of a trial designed to offer PDB
Trial duration	• Consider treatment duration in the context of clinical practice • Measure intermediate/surrogate endpoints and clinically meaningful endpoints

Adapted from Bhatnagar M, Sheehan S, Sharma I, et al. Prospect of direct benefit in pediatric trials: practical challenges and potential solutions. *Pediatrics.* 2021;147(5):e2020049602.

Interventions or procedures in a clinical investigation that pose greater than minimal risk (referred to as a "minor increase over minimal risk") without a PDB for individual subjects but that is likely to yield important, generalizable knowledge about the participant's condition may be approvable if the minor increase is commensurate with expected medical experiences for the subject. Clinical investigations approved under this category require permission of both parents.

An example of a clinical investigation that might be allowed to proceed with a minor increase over minimal risk would be the evaluation of a single dose of an investigational product solely to collect pharmacokinetic data for which adequate safety data exist to characterize the risk as no more than a minor increase over minimal risk. For a clinical investigation to proceed under this category, all the interventions and procedures in the protocol (e.g., blood draws or any diagnostic testing) also need to be no more than a minor increase over minimal risk. This analysis is called a *component analysis of risk*, used to determine the overall acceptability of the clinical investigation including the risks and anticipated benefits of the interventions that are listed in the protocol (which must be analyzed individually as well as collectively).[12,13]

Selection of Study Population

For RCTs of interventions to *treat* a disease or condition, study participants should have the disease or condition with clear and reproducible diagnostic criteria. If the disease or condition is ill-defined either physiologically or clinically, enrolled patients may be a heterogeneous group. Identifying a potential treatment effect may be impossible in a study that enrolls patients with variable manifestations of a condition.

For RCTs of interventions to *prevent* a disease or condition, study participants must be at significant risk for developing that disease or condition. When the risk of a disease is low in a given population, participants could be enrolled in a study and exposed to an experimental intervention to prevent an infrequent outcome. In this scenario, understanding the safety of the study intervention is critical to any benefit-risk assessment. Strategies to identify a population at higher risk of the condition should reduce the proportion of enrolled neonates who would likely not have developed the condition. Enrichment strategies may include well-evaluated biomarkers and/or risk scores that are derived from clinical data.

Inclusion and exclusion criteria should be clearly defined and used to capture the population for whom the intervention is intended. Early-phase studies of a novel therapy in neonates may require study in a relatively homogeneous population to balance the unknown risks with the potential for individual benefit. Once more is known about the product's safety profile, later-phase RCTs may be able to enroll a more heterogeneous sample of patients that is similar to the intended use population.[2]

Therapeutic Intervention

Neonatal RCTs may evaluate the impact of interventions, from practice standards to devices to novel therapies or therapies that were developed for nonneonatal indications.[14] Subpart D guidelines, as discussed above, help guide the benefit-risk assessment for a trial protocol. An intervention that conveys more than a minor increase over minimal risk must provide a PDB to participants, with rare exceptions. In this category, clinical equipoise is assumed—the "honest, professional disagreement among expert clinicians about the preferred treatment"[15] and IRBs must determine whether the potential benefit justifies the risks.[8] PDB can be established based on information from the literature, animal models,[16] other nonclinical studies, and/or proof-of-concept studies in humans. Study protocols should include all available nonclinical and clinical evidence to support both PDB and safety to inform IRBs and regulatory bodies.

Nonclinical toxicology studies that support drug approval in adults or older children may not be sufficient to inform the safety of a treatment in the neonatal period. When a drug's impact on developing organ systems is unknown, juvenile animal studies can inform safety and/or dosing parameters.[17] Safety and tolerability information from healthy adult volunteer studies may also be needed to support neonatal studies if the drug has not been previously given to humans.[18]

The importance of establishing effective and safe dosing strategies prior to initiation of large RCTs cannot be overstated.[19] Thoroughly evaluating existing pharmacokinetic information and drug absorption, distribution, metabolism, and excretion data is critical to optimizing the dosing strategy and reducing the chance of trial failure due to suboptimal dosing.[20] Although dose selection is typically confirmed in phase 2 studies, later RCTs may incorporate more than one dosing regimen for confirmation.

Choice of Endpoint or Response Variable

The choice of a primary endpoint is fundamental to the quality of the study. The primary endpoint should be the variable capable of providing the most clinically meaningful and convincing evidence directly related to the primary objective of the trial.[21] The outcome that parents, neonatologists, and clinical staff most desire is a healthy child with optimal long-term cognitive, social, and physical abilities. Unfortunately, these efficacy objectives may be too distant to feasibly measure for most interventional trials, and there are numerous intervening factors between the NICU hospitalization and later childhood that may influence the effects of any neonatal intervention.

The prespecified primary endpoint should be well-defined in the protocol and its rationale explained. If there are several coequal primary outcomes, then the sample size calculation and analysis plan must account for multiplicity by controlling the type I error rate (the probability of rejecting at least one null hypothesis if the treatment has no benefit). If the sample size is not sufficient for testing more than one primary outcome, then the other measures of interest can be captured as secondary endpoints and may be supportive to the primary endpoint.

It is rare in neonates to be able to design a trial with a simple primary efficacy endpoint. In studies enrolling neonates of extremely low gestational age or other high-risk patients, death is a competing outcome that must be analyzed. The difference between two groups' proportions of a composite of "death before 36 weeks' postmenstrual age or morbidity" is a straightforward endpoint for powering an RCT, but results may be difficult to interpret if the two elements of the composite go in opposite directions. An alternative approach would be a composite that ranks the potential outcomes from best to worst (or worst to best), incorporating the input of family members as well as clinicians and researchers.[14] If the two elements were death and morbidity, then stakeholders would most likely rank death as the worst outcome, followed by surviving with morbidity, and finally surviving without morbidity (best). This approach can be extended to scenarios in which data collection is richer, such as when survival is captured as a time-to-event outcome and/or morbidity is measured longitudinally.[22]

Other composite endpoints, made up of multiple variables, have been used to assess a group of undesired outcomes, any one of which would constitute a negative result. Morbidity counts could provide an additional way to differentiate negative outcomes.[23] One caveat is that composites can be challenging to apply clinically, because a result for the composite does not imply a result for the individual elements. An alternative to composites is to collect and analyze mortality and morbidity as time-to-event outcomes. Then, hazard ratios and cumulative incidence functions *can* be estimated for the individual elements, accounting for the competing risk.[24] The illness-death model (also called the semicompeting risk model) is an extension of the competing risk model and may be used if a patient could die before or after developing the morbidity of interest.[24]

Biomarkers, or surrogate endpoints, can be useful in assessing pharmacodynamic effects in a proof-of-concept trial prior to designing a fully powered RCT to evaluate clinically meaningful endpoints. Biomarkers to help establish proof of concept could include imaging studies or laboratory tests. In rare cases in neonatology, a biomarker may be used as a primary efficacy endpoint. Continuous video electroencephalogram monitoring to evaluate reduction in seizure burden was accepted by a data-driven, expert consensus as a primary endpoint for neonatal seizure trials.[25] Additional biomarkers developed using clinical data and consensus processes will streamline clinical trials for other neonatal conditions.

Collection of Adverse Event Information

Adverse events (AEs) must be systematically collected in neonatal clinical trials in a similar fashion to other populations. AEs may be difficult to distinguish from typical neonatal complications and morbidities, especially in extremely preterm neonates and those with complicated disease processes. Nonetheless, RCTs provide an important opportunity to investigate differences in the frequency of AEs between active treatments or between treatment and placebo. Understanding background rates of morbidities can provide a critically important perspective when trial rates of specific neonatal morbidities are assessed.

Investigators and sponsors are responsible for collecting and reviewing serious AEs and keeping track of other sources of relevant data on the study intervention. RCT protocols must include a prospective plan for the monitoring and reporting of AEs. Regulatory authorities require timely reporting of serious and unexpected AEs for review.[26] An AE severity scale specific to neonatal clinical trials has been developed and is undergoing validation.[27] Consistent and standardized laboratory values have been established for trials for older children[28] and adults, but standardized neonatal laboratory values do not exist and are urgently needed.

Selection of the Control Group

The purpose of a control group is to allow the researcher to determine whether a difference in outcome between groups is caused by the intervention itself and not due to other factors (natural history, other treatments, comorbidities, etc.).[29] Randomized trials may be designed with a placebo control arm, a standard-of-care control arm without placebo, an active control arm, or a dose-response concurrent control arm.[2] In special cases such as rare and ultrarare diseases, external or historical (nonconcurrent) controls may be considered.

The advantages of placebo- or standard of care–controlled trials, when well blinded or masked, are well understood; with effective randomization, a difference in effect between the intervention arm and the control arm should be attributable to the intervention.[29] When a condition is usually treated with a standard therapy that is thought to be effective, and withholding that therapy would be considered unethical, an active control arm or an add-on design may be used if scientifically appropriate. In an add-on design, both arms receive the standard therapy with the investigational arm also receiving the treatment being evaluated.

Randomization

Randomization helps to ensure that the treatment and control arms are comparable, with similar background characteristics and prognostic factors (whether the factors are measured or not). Randomization also mitigates potential biases that may occur when assigning patients to the intervention group or the control group.[29] Biases may be either conscious or subconscious and may relate to a participant's prognosis or the investigator's assumptions about a participant or a treatment. When allocation is biased, the comparison between arms is easily invalidated. Theoretically, if the sample size is large enough, all variables will have the same distribution in each of the study arms. However, due to finite sample size, imbalance is common. Therefore investigators should stratify the randomization on key factors (to the extent possible—see below), check for imbalance between groups, and adjust the analyses for baseline variables that may be related to outcomes and are found to differ between groups (Table 98.2).

Most trials are randomized with a 1:1 ratio of patients to the intervention or control arms. This is generally the most efficient design, but there are sometimes reasons for using an alternative schema. For example, allocating more patients to the active intervention arm can improve power for detecting AEs, or it may be desirable to compare nonrandomized groups within an arm of an RCT, such as in a surgery arm that incorporates more than one surgical technique.

Block randomization is usually used instead of simple randomization to ensure approximately equal sample size across study arms. Stratification of the randomization on important prognostic factors ensures balance on those factors across study arms. The selection of factors to stratify on depends on the specific study design, outcomes,

Table 98.2 Examples of Randomization Strategies

Strategy	How It Works	Advantages	Limitations
1:1 randomization	Participants are randomized 1 to 1 to intervention or control	Efficiency and simplicity	Potential imbalance in important variables
2 (or more):1 randomization	Participants are randomized 2 (or more) to 1 to intervention or control	More participants receiving the intervention may improve detection of adverse events	Requires more complex statistical analysis
Block or stratified randomization	Participants are randomized with equal probability in small groups (e.g., 4, 6, 8); may be assigned by key prognostic variable	Helps achieve balance between arms on factors that may change during the course of enrollment (e.g., severity of illness)	Too many strata relative to sample size may not be balanced; requires adjustment for the stratification variable in the analysis
Cluster randomization	Randomization occurs at the level of the clinical setting (unit or practice) or cluster	Eliminates contamination; able to assess effectiveness in practice	Similarity of patients in a cluster or center to one another; may require complex balancing techniques

and sample size. Typical factors include sex and gestational age, and stratification by site can eliminate any influence of site effects on trial results. Any variable used for stratifying the randomization should be adjusted for in the analysis. If the number of strata is large relative to the sample size, stratification may not achieve balance on all factors. In that case, covariate adaptive randomization may be used instead of block randomization.

Two interventions can be tested in the same study using a 2 × 2 factorial design such as testing both a nutritional and a drug intervention for a specific condition. The trial would have four arms (nutrition and drug; nutrition and no drug; no nutrition and drug; no nutrition and no drug) and would be conducted similarly to a four-arm RCT. The effect of each intervention, the additive effect of the interventions, and the interaction of the interventions could be tested. This depends on the study objectives and hypotheses and assumes a sample size that accounts for multiple testing.

Cluster-randomized controlled trials (C-RCTs) are randomized at the level of the cluster or clinical setting. In the case of neonatal trials, the cluster likely represents the neonatal intensive care unit or nursery, depending on the intervention. A C-RCT design can eliminate contamination, which can occur when patients in the control group are inadvertently exposed to the intervention. Even when patients are randomized in an RCT to test efficacy, the trial may be followed by a separate trial to examine effectiveness. This process can assess whether the treatment that was tested in a highly controlled environment maintains its effectiveness under less stringent conditions, such as heterogeneous practice settings.[30] The cluster effect (that is, the tendency of patients in a cluster to be more similar to each other than to patients in other clusters) must be accounted for when determining sample size or analyzing a C-RCT. Achieving balance through allocation of clusters to study arms may require techniques that are more complex than block randomization or stratification, such as minimization or covariate constrained randomization.[31]

Adaptive Strategies

The term "adaptive design" can have numerous definitions. However, there are several common strategies that may be used to adjust a study protocol to incorporate information that was not available at the start of the trial.[32] Adaptive trial strategies should be anticipated prospectively and described clearly in the protocol. Potential advantages of adaptive designs include improved statistical efficiency (modification of sample size or group sequential design), improved understanding of drug effects (adaptive enrichment), ethical considerations (stopping rules), and/or acceptability to stakeholders due to added flexibility. Limitations of adaptive trial designs include the requirement for special analytical methods to avoid introducing bias or making erroneous conclusions, challenges in anticipating all potential outcomes, logistics of maintaining trial integrity, and difficulty with interpretability.[32]

Blinding or Masking of Assignment

Conscious or unconscious biases during the conduct and analysis of a clinical trial may be curbed by masking or blinding the participants' assigned treatment arms, although the possibility of bias is never eliminated entirely. In the case of neonatal RCTs, the investigators and clinical staff as well as family members should be blinded whenever possible.[33] If a treatment is unable to be adequately blinded or masked, elements of study conduct, including clinical care guidelines (e.g., threshold values for tapering or increasing treatment), ascertainment of endpoints, and reporting safety outcomes, must be clearly specified in the protocol.[2]

Informed Consent

Obtaining informed consent for participation in a research study is a legal, ethical, and regulatory requirement. Inherent in the consent process is the obligation to provide potential subjects or their proxies with adequate information regarding the study to ensure that their permission has been appropriately obtained. Inherent to informed consent in children are certain important concepts: (1) the parent(s)/guardian(s) must have the capacity to decide that their child can participate in a research study; (2) there should be full disclosure of all relevant information, especially the risks and benefits; (3) the study should be presented in the simplest way possible; (4) the decision to participate must be voluntary; and (5) informed consent should be a comprehensive communication process that is not limited to simply reviewing the informed consent form (ICF).[34] Informed consent is even more complicated and necessary in vulnerable populations such as critically ill neonates and children.[35]

Although a comprehensive consent process is important, previous studies have shown that researchers often fall short of developing appropriate ICFs.[36–38] For example, the length of the ICF has nearly tripled during the past 20 years (along with the complexity of study protocols), primarily due to institutional language relating to legal, ethical, insurance, and financial matters.[39] There is no evidence that these longer ICFs have led to a better understanding of study procedures, risks, or benefits or have improved the safety of research subjects.[40] ICF language continues to be problematic, especially in view of significant health literacy issues in the United States.[41] Finally, although diverse populations must be included in clinical trials, it may be impossible to translate the ICF into enough languages to meet the needs of a clinical trial.

The utility and potential advantage of a more concise and functional ICF was studied by Murray and colleagues in parents whose children had previously participated in or had been eligible to participate in a pediatric clinical trial.[42] The experimental ICF (with key information up front in a two-page summary and the rest of the required information in an appendix) was developed from a previous conventional ICF for a neonatal study. Either the more concise or the conventional ICF was randomly distributed to members of two parental advocacy groups, with 72% (59–82) responding. Significantly more parents in the more concise ICF group found the form "short and to the point" but thought it did not provide enough information. However, there was no evidence that understanding of key study components was impacted by how the information was presented.

The HHS recently revised the Common Rule, a set of federal regulations (Fed Reg) for ethical conduct of human-subjects research. One of the important changes is that similar to the Murray study, key information that is most relevant to a person's decision to participate is presented up front in the ICF in a concise and focused way.[43] This more concise ICF might also prompt enriched discussion between the investigator and participant, an approach that has been shown to increase research participants' understanding of study-related material.[37,44] It will be important to study parent or guardian comprehension using this new ICF in actual randomized controlled trials.

Other innovative approaches to improving informed consent have been developed. Rosenfeld and associates used visual aids in the consent process and found these had a strong influence on parental comprehension.[45] Multimedia patient educational interventions have also been found to be more effective when added to the traditional informed consent process.[46] Clinical investigators should continue to explore alternative methods of providing enhanced informed consent while maintaining equipoise regarding the range of outcomes that the intervention should be designed to achieve.

Recruitment and Retention of Trial Participants

Clinical trials are becoming increasingly complex, and there are multiple opportunities for failure throughout the lifecycle. Failure can arise from a variety of causes including (1) lack of efficacy, (2) issues related to safety, (3) inadequate funding, (4) inability to maintain strict manufacturing protocols, (5) regulatory issues, (6) a poorly trained workforce, (7) overly restrictive inclusion/exclusion criteria, and (8) problems with patient recruitment, enrollment, and retention.[47] In fact, most clinical trials fail due to the inability to recruit the projected number of subjects (based on sample size calculations) and are unable to enroll a diverse and representative population.

Adequate representation must be included in all National Institutes of Health (NIH)-supported research studies, because the effects of a drug may vary significantly in different gender, racial, and/or ethnic groups. Despite this, many pediatric clinical trials do not report the racial and ethnic composition of their study populations.[48] Nicholson and associates analyzed 165 clinical trials published between 2004 and 2014 and identified barriers to recruitment and retention of underrepresented populations, including language, trust/mistrust of the medical system, inclusion/exclusion criteria, socioeconomic status, and others.[49]

Strategies to improve recruitment include proactive or direct (face-to-face) communication, reactive or indirect (word of mouth, printed material, or broadcast media) communication, and/or multifaceted strategies such as compensation, flexibility, building rapport and trust, and employing an ethnically and culturally diverse research staff.[50] Building trust through community-based participatory research strategies is associated with higher enrollment of potential subjects.[49] There is also increasing use of social media to improve recruitment of eligible study participants. These approaches allow investigators to consider the voices of many key stakeholders such as patients, physicians, disease advocates, disease foundations, researchers, and medical centers, who may all have social media pages and accounts. Topolovec-Vranic and Natarajan reviewed 30 studies that described the use of various recruitment strategies and found in 12 studies that social media was the most effective recruitment approach, especially for hard-to-reach populations and observational studies.[51]

Once neonates are enrolled in a trial, it is essential to maintain the family's engagement in order to obtain complete and high-quality longitudinal data to support safety and/or efficacy of an intervention. Strategies that have been used to optimize retention efforts in longitudinal clinical trials include (1) incentives (financial), (2) a personal approach (birthday cards), (3) a dedicated phone line (providing cell phones), (4) project identity and logos, (5) participant convenience, and (6) repeated contact with participants.[52]

Long-Term Follow-Up in Neonatal RCTs

"Long-term" is an ill-defined term in neonatal and pediatric research. In neonatal RCTs, long-term is generally considered to be an evaluation at a minimum of 12 months' corrected gestational age (CGA). The National Institute of Child Health and Development's Neonatal Research Network has conducted multiple studies evaluating developmental milestones at 18 to 24 months' CGA using gold-standard examiners.[53] There are other research networks worldwide that evaluate long-term follow-up, particularly for extremely preterm neonates (<28 weeks' gestation at birth).

Long-term follow-up evaluations may be conducted to evaluate the safety of a study intervention or to evaluate its efficacy. When the primary objective of a trial is to study neuroprotection, neurodevelopmental evaluation at ≥2 years of age is likely to be the primary endpoint for the trial. The multicenter RCTs that established therapeutic hypothermia as the standard of care for moderate-severe neonatal hypoxic-ischemic encephalopathy measured their primary endpoints of death or moderate to severe disability at 18 to 22 months' CGA.[54,55]

In other cases, post-NICU discharge outcomes may be assessed to establish the durability of the effect or the impact of the therapy on outcomes that are clinically significant.[56,57] Trialists should seek to understand whether a therapy that improves physiologic parameters in the short-term has either a neutral, positive, or negative long-term impact on later clinical outcomes. However, in many neonatal trials, the primary endpoint will have been measured sooner than 18 to 22 months' CGA, with long-term evaluations primarily focused on a safety assessment of the therapeutic product or intervention.[58] Evaluations must be tailored to the study intervention and may include not only neurologic and developmental testing but social and behavioral testing and organ-specific evaluation.[59]

The Caffeine for Apnea of Prematurity (CAP) trial[60] was designed to evaluate a composite primary efficacy endpoint of death, cerebral palsy, cognitive delay, deafness, or blindness at 18 to 21 months' CGA.[61] Participants in the caffeine arm were less likely to experience the composite endpoint, chiefly driven by decreased rates of cerebral palsy and cognitive delay. The investigators continued long-term follow-up evaluations of the participants to ages 5 and 11. By age 5, the differences between caffeine and placebo arms had disappeared.[62] Academic and behavioral performance were again similar at age 11, but caffeine was associated with a lower rate of motor impairment.[63] These long-term follow-up studies provided support for the safety of this widely used therapy.

Stakeholder Engagement in Neonatal RCT Design

RCTs need to be designed with the rigor required to answer questions that are important to clinicians and families while remaining feasible and acceptable. For this to occur, the voices of parents, nursing and other clinical staff, and when possible, NICU graduates should be included in the design of neonatal trials. Families and patients have lived the short-term and long-term consequences of the neonatal conditions under evaluation.[64] Their experiences may be systematically gathered to help understand how parents would prefer to be approached for trial enrollment, what study procedures will be acceptable, and what endpoints are important to them.[65] Nurses, respiratory therapists, and social workers also provide unique perspectives about families in times of distress and uncertainty.

To develop the tools, standards, and approaches needed to accelerate drug development in neonates and children, the FDA and the Critical Path Institute, with support from the pharmaceutical industry, established the International Neonatal Consortium (INC) in 2015. This organization represents a unique public-private partnership that brings together global regulators (FDA, European meadicines agency [EMA], Health Canada, and pharmaceuticals and medical devices agency [PMDA]), neonatologists, nurses, pharmaceutical companies, funding organizations, and parent/patient advocacy groups to develop tools to address the unmet therapeutic needs of neonates.[66] The INC also established a clear path forward by focusing on parental input in the development of clinical trial protocols, developing master protocols and other tools to streamline clinical trials, and training investigators to conduct high-quality neonatal clinical trials. Operating in the precompetitive space, the INC addresses the need for measurement and assessment of clinical outcomes in neonates through teams that share data and expertise to advance regulatory science. Consortia such as INC have played a key role in addressing the shortfalls of neonatal drug development and clinical trials and have helped design a path forward.

Summary Conclusions

Planning and conducting neonatal RCTs is a complicated, expensive, and labor-intensive process, yet RCTs remain a critical tool for developing and evaluating effective and safe treatments for neonates. Understanding and using the framework of human subject protections and the components of "quality by design" in planning RCTs will help ensure that neonates are not subjected to undue risks without potential benefit. Neonates should only be enrolled in studies that are carefully designed with (1) a well-defined, at-risk population, (2) a clearly defined and clinically meaningful primary endpoint, (3) an evidence-based dosing strategy, (4) a feasible sample size, and (5) clear guidelines for AE collection and reporting. Input from families, nurses, physicians, and other clinical staff should be sought when developing research questions and protocol elements to ensure meaningfulness and feasibility.

Acknowledgment

The authors would like to acknowledge Susan McCune, MD, for her thorough, insightful review of this chapter.

CHAPTER 99

Designing Clinical Trials in Neonatology—International Trials

Marc Beltempo, Prakesh S. Shah

KEY POINTS

1. Assessing therapeutic safety and efficacy of a drug/device or technology requires carefully designed trials that are sufficiently powered to detect differences in outcomes.
2. International trials can help reduce the time required for the study and improve generalizability of the findings.
3. Variations in regulations for clinical trials between jurisdictions can significantly prolong the time required to conduct the trial.
4. Anticipating challenges by obtaining local expertise and buy-in from collaborators are keys to the success of international trials.

Introduction

In the past decades, the development and the study of drugs, technology, and interventions has moved from national and regionally centered activities to a global collaborative effort. This shift has occurred in all areas of medicine, including neonatology. Assessing therapeutic safety and efficacy of a drug/device or technology requires carefully designed trials that are sufficiently powered to detect differences in outcomes. This can be a particular challenge when studying interventions for a rare genetic disease, when the disease prevalence is relatively low (such as neonatal hypoxic ischemic encephalopathy), or when outcomes are rare. To complete a trial in a timely matter and recruit sufficient patients in a shorter time frame, multicenter, international trials have increased in the past 2 decades.[1]

Although international trials enhance external validity of the findings, there are several issues that need to be considered before embarking on such trials. These include variations in population demographics, racial and ethnic variation in propensity for complications, genetic differences between populations, and country-specific variations in health services organization.[2,3] Moreover, variations in care practice between countries can be a significant issue when it comes to evaluating therapeutic interventions, because differences in co-interventions could be extremely challenging.[4–6] The desire to enhance the generalizability of a trial's findings and the need for larger sample sizes recruited over short periods of time have led to an increase in international collaborations.[7] An international trial is a clinical trial that is conducted in two or more countries and uses a common study protocol. International trials can be completed faster and more efficiently than even a multicenter trial in a single country. International trials can also contribute to our knowledge base from a global health perspective when certain types of trials are conducted in countries that would not otherwise have access to a specific intervention or health program. Whether an international trial involves low- or high-income countries, it requires careful consideration and planning. This chapter focuses on specific opportunities and challenges that arise when conducting research in more than one country and how to address them (Fig. 99.1).

Building a Shared Vision of the Purpose of the Study

Careful planning of the trial is the most crucial initial step. Establishing a common understanding with potential collaborators about the health impacts of the disease and how the intervention can potentially improve a process or outcome or the health of participants is an essential first step to obtain buy-in to move forward. During the planning phase, careful attention must be paid to having clearly predefined study objectives that address a primary scientific question, the selection of appropriate subjects, the ability of the study design to appropriately address the research question, and having measurable and clinically important outcomes.

Once the need for a trial has been established, designing the trial is the next opportunity to have co-investigators actively contribute and continue to build engagement. This inherently leads to changes in the various design elements of the study, but this should be viewed as a unique opportunity to consolidate buy-in and participation of site investigators. Multicenter trial planning can be complex due to organizational differences between units. Mapping out how an intervention will be implemented in each unit is critical to troubleshoot and anticipate hurdles. International trials have added complexity due to between-country variations in roles of healthcare professionals, standards of care, cultural practices, and regulations that may impact the implementation of the protocol. Having local experts in trial design in each country can provide anticipatory guidance.

During the study design, the selection of participating sites will usually depend on disease prevalence at the institute, local expertise, availability of research infrastructure including administrative staff and clinical staff, a track record of implementing similar trials, and

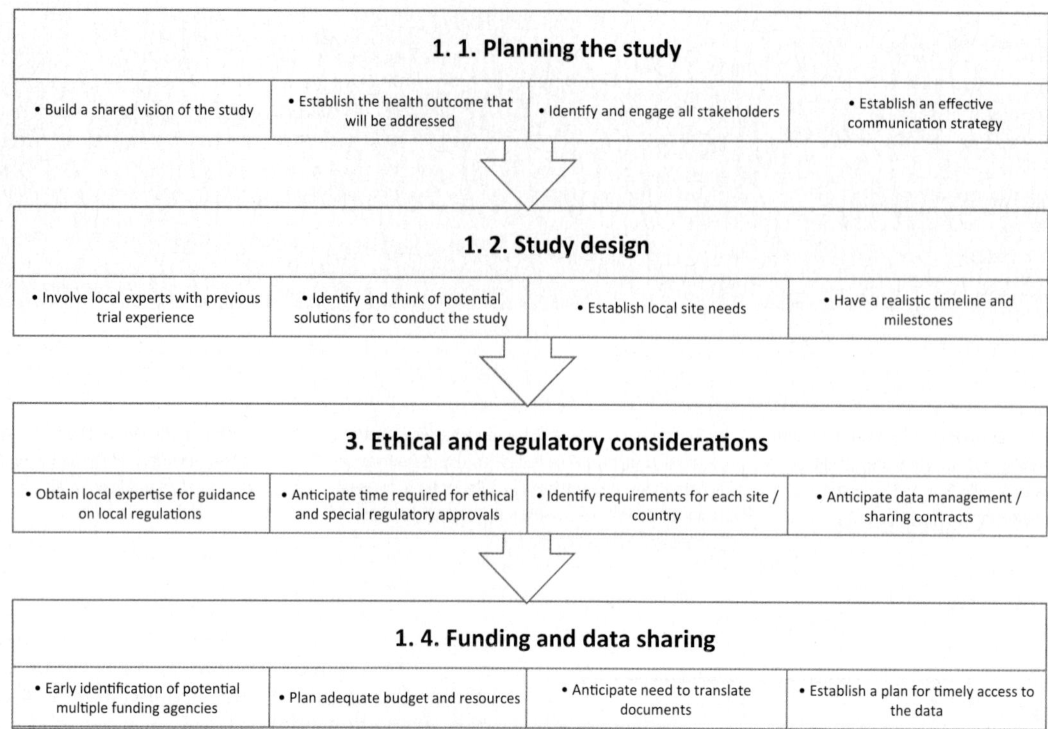

Fig. 99.1 Framework for the Design of International Clinical Trials in Neonatology.

the willingness of the center to participate. Practical aspects of such organization include a meeting of potential site investigators either face to face or via use of technologies (video/teleconferencing). During these meetings, the principal investigator(s) should explicitly list the time and resources required to participate to help potential sites assess their capacity to enroll.

How to Encourage Local Buy-in and Participation

Early involvement of all stakeholders in the study design and during each and every step of the preparation is the most important consideration. To achieve effective engagement, establishing effective communications is key. Successful communication strategies include regular tele/videoconferences, in-person meetings if possible, and regular electronic communications by e-mail or newsletters.[8,9] The essence of success will include incorporation of views from all stakeholders to the extent possible and feasible. Supporting and creating an environment for open dialogue will lead to development of a culture that values and encourages critical thinking about the quality of the trial. For the sites that are passive participants, actively seeking feedback would uncover some issues that would best be addressed in advance.

Regulatory and Ethical Considerations

It is relatively easy to conduct a single-center trial, from the perspectives of ethical and regulatory oversight. However, when a trial extends to either multiple centers within one jurisdiction or country or internationally within multiple jurisdictions and regulatory organizations, the complexity increases immensely. A majority of countries have their own agencies for oversight and regulations and guidelines for conducting clinical trials (e.g., the U.S. Food and Drug Administration, Health Canada, the European Medicines Agency, the UK Medicines and Healthcare Products Regulatory Agency, etc.). Regulations for the conduct of clinical trials refer to the rules and requirements for ethical and safe conduct of clinical trials.

To conduct clinical trials, investigators must obtain approval from an ethical board, also known as an institutional review board, research and ethics board, independent ethics committee, or ethical review board. Ethics boards are meant to apply ethical and regulatory frameworks that aim to minimize risks, have an optimal risk-benefit ratio, ensure informed consent is obtained, ensure that patients are recruited and compensated fairly, protect privacy, and ensure a methodologically rigorous approach.[10,11] Three basic ethical principles guide ethics boards: respect for participants, beneficence, and justice.[12] The ethics board is usually composed of a multidisciplinary panel of scientific peers, researchers, experts in bioethics and law, and representatives of the lay community. Typically, in the United States, a trial's coordinating center will obtain ethical board approval for the trial, and each participating center will need to obtain approval from their local ethical board before recruitment can start in their center. This process can vary based on the country.

Individual institutional ethics board review is based on the regulatory framework applied in the institution's jurisdiction. Some countries have attempted to harmonize these regulations to minimize variations. For example, in Europe, trials have to adhere to the European Union Clinical Trials Directive and European Union Good Clinical Practice Directive. However, interpretation and applications of these directives can vary.[13] Several different aspects of regulations need to be considered in international trials, such as the ethics board review process, regulations regarding the intervention, data sharing, data monitoring, contracts, and consent for participants.

Ethics Board Review Process

Despite similar frameworks and guiding ethical principles, each country, health region, and institution may have different ethics board requirements. This can mean having a single ethics board application for a single region or country or having to apply to the ethics board of each institution.[14] For example, a single ethics board review is required for nationwide clinical trials in the United Kingdom, France, and Australia, whereas individual institution review is required in countries such as Canada and the United States.

There are currently efforts to streamline the approach in the United States with the proposed revisions to the Common Rule, which is the regulation that guides federally supported human research in the United States.[15] Although the European Union Clinical Trials Regulation includes provisions for low-risk intervention trials and cluster randomized trials, the International Council for Harmonization of Good Clinical Practice guideline does not currently address these issues.[16,17] In Canada, attempts are underway to allow one ethics board to be the board of record; review from that ethics board will be acceptable to other ethics boards within the jurisdiction and would require only an administrative review. However, these are still local/regional initiatives, and national harmonization is lacking.

The variations in the ethics board review process can significantly affect the time required to obtain ethics board approval. For example, in a recent multicenter study in Canada involving 16 sites, the ethics board approval took a median time of 42 days (range, 4–443 days).[18] The investigators reported that the main issues raised by the ethics boards were different interpretations of privacy rules and language of the consent.

Sufficient time must be allocated for the ethics board applications, considering the process will vary based on institutions despite being in the same country and operating under the same regulations.[11] Variability in local requirements may include variations in assessment of the project itself, assessment of the level of risk of participation, privacy concerns, and the assessment of local resource availability to perform the research.[18,19] Strategies to mitigate delays include having collaborators with expertise in running clinical trials in each jurisdiction involved and consulting the ethics board at the time of trial design. It is often helpful to submit previous correspondence with the ethics board that has already granted approval along with a new ethics application for the same trial to another ethics board.

Regulations Affecting the Intervention Itself

Generally, an intervention being studied can be drug/device/technology. This may involve a new indication for an existing drug or a completely new molecule being tested. For a device or technology, it also could be a refined use for a different indication or a completely new technology. Based on the nature of the intervention being studied, regulations that apply will vary from one country to another.

When the intervention is a drug or device, a separate approval from each country's drug or medical device regulating agency is required, even for investigational purposes. Investigators must ensure that the drug/device can be studied in the participating country. The regulations regarding certain products vary between countries; an intervention that may be allowed to be tested in human studies in one country may not be permitted by another country at all. Clarification and proper documentation are necessary initial steps before embarking on a trial. Instances of inability to test specific modes of ventilation on new or existing ventilators have arisen when a specific ventilator was not approved or used in certain countries.

Data Sharing and Data Transfer Agreements

Once investigators have obtained ethics board approval from individual sites, the next step will be to finalize data sharing agreements between the data-receiving site and the data-transferring site. These agreements/contracts need to be signed between the coordinating site and each participating site. In a majority of cases, these contracts are initiated by the host site, which will receive the data. Legal support services are involved on either side, and they ensure that privacy, confidentiality, and security of data are taken care of by the receiving sites. Each jurisdiction may have different interpretations and concerns for privacy and confidentiality. For example, some institutions will not allow sharing of the exact date/time of birth of patients, whereas others will allow it with specific security measures. This step could be time consuming, laborious, and frustrating for clinical investigators who would like to initiate the trial and start recruitment. Personal experience indicates that at times, this step alone could take a few months if the study involves multiple centers. We recently spent 20 months to finalize a data-sharing agreement between Canada, Australia, and France for a retrospective study. For example, dealing with different health data protection regimes across European states could lead to challenges in accessing and sharing health data within Europe. It is hoped that implementation of the General Data Protection and Regulation framework will help with alignment of regulatory requirements.[20]

Investigators should preemptively think about primary and secondary use of data and the possibility that they may want access to data beyond the initial approval or contract period. It may be even more beneficial if the consent obtained from participants allows for secondary use of data if such approach is allowed by local ethics boards. The drafting of these agreements and what is included in consent is becoming increasingly more important because there is now a move toward public data sharing from studies/trials.[21] Many journals are now asking for data repository statements and data access arrangements. These issues should be carefully considered prior to initiation of international studies.

Data and Safety Monitoring Board

During the trial design, investigators need to determine whether the trial will require a data and safety monitoring board. A data and safety monitoring board is a group of independent individuals, external to the trial, who are experts in relevant areas. They review the accumulated data from the trial on a regular basis and advise the sponsor about the continued safety of trial participants, the continued validity of the trial, and the continued scientific merit of the trial. The need for a data and safety monitoring board for a trial will vary based on the type of intervention, size of the trial, potential risks for participants, and outcome measures. Several funding agencies such as the National Institutes of Health have developed guidelines on how to run data and safety monitoring boards (available at www.grants.nih.gov).[22,23]

In the context of an international trial with a data and safety monitoring board, it is important to make sure the data upload is done in a timely fashion. Strategies to improve timeliness include using a web-based system to allow to real-time data entry, monitoring of data quality, and continuous reporting and tracking of the study progress. Another consideration for a data and safety monitoring board in international studies is the potential need to translate data and safety monitoring board reports and communications with each ethics board.

Differences in Healthcare Systems and Insurance Structures

One increasingly recognized aspect of participation in trials is the insurance coverage of participants. Individual patient insurance coverage can affect their inclusion in a trial. Consequently, a country's healthcare insurance policy (universal vs. private) and the organization of its healthcare system (private vs. public hospitals) need to be considered prior to site enrollment.

Additionally, there are variations in insurance requirements and coverage for conducting research between countries. Clinical trials liability insurance that provides coverage for investigators in the event of harm caused to participants and subsequent compensation is often required. Increasingly, trials are asked to obtain insurance from private companies to ensure that if participants incur any unintended or previously unknown harm due to participation in trials, they are covered to receive appropriate medical care. A clinical trials liability insurance policy ensures that the investigators are adequately covered in case of harm incurred by patients. In general, clinical trials liability insurance is required for trials using medications/devices in humans and may be required for other clinical interventions. Additional loss or damage incurred by a drug/device developer may require a commercial general liability insurance policy.[24]

Financial Contracts

Participating sites are often compensated for patient enrollment, trial participation, and data collection. Typically, the coordinating center oversees the contracts with each participating site. This can be complex and time-consuming and can only be initiated after ethics approvals are obtained. Furthermore, contracts may need to be translated to another language. Investigators at the coordinating center should meet as early as possible with their grant and contracts office to review the contracting process and estimated timeline. Potential issues between countries include translation of contracts, currency, and indirect cost recovery.

Payment mechanisms can vary between trials. Compensation may be awarded per patient, as a lump-sum pay-for-participation for each site, or as compensation for each step, such as the research and ethics board (REB) application, study initiation, etc. Payment per patient enrolled tends to encourage sites to recruit more patients compared with a lump-sum site payment for participation. Payments per patient enrolled rewards sites that recruit more patients by creating a financial incentive to recruit. However, payments per patient enrolled can be more complex to negotiate with the contracts office and requires tracking of patient enrollment, tracking of data transfer, and constant communication between the coordinating site and each site investigator. Strategies to simplify the process include having the coordinating site prepare the invoice template for each local site at predefined times in the year (annually or biannually). Additional considerations need to be given on the mode of payments (wire transfer vs. check) and the currency used. Paper checks can be costly to send and may not even be accepted in different countries. Financial arrangement is an important step for the smooth conduct of a trial to ensure that sites are compensated adequately, to build site enthusiasm, and to keep the overall budget in control.

Informed Consent

Informed consent is an essential component of recognizing patient autonomy and respect for a person's right to make decisions about their participation in a clinical trial. Neonatal research is made complex because it requires proxy consent. Although requirements for consent can be cumbersome and create challenges when studies address interventions done emergently,[25] information required is generally similar between jurisdictions and relates to the information required for families to make properly informed decisions (level of risk, description of the intervention, and other therapeutic options). Some study designs, such as those assessing interventions in the delivery room, may require waived consent or deferred consent. Criteria for waived and deferred consent may vary according to the institution. Regardless of the method used to obtain consent, researchers should strive to be transparent with patients and families by providing information on the ongoing study and should return a summary of the results to the community and to individual participants.

Patient Reimbursement and Compensation

Variations exist between countries as to how patients/legal representatives can be reimbursed for their participation in clinical research. For example, some countries have regulations that prohibit incentives for parents/legal guardians in pediatrics trials whereas others allow it.[16,26] Additional considerations should be given when compensation is offered to families in vulnerable settings or in developing countries.[27] Investigators should be attentive to the sums of money and value of nonmonetary incentives used, which may seem coercive for patients living in a low-income setting.

Language and Translation of Documents

Although most investigators may speak a common language, some ethics boards and contracts offices may not accept documents such as the study protocol and contracts in English, depending on the country's official communication language. Time and funding must be allocated to translating these documents when required. Obtaining information on local ethics board communication language and requirements during the study design from local site investigators can help plan for these tasks. Additional considerations need to be given to translation of patient information pamphlets and patient consent forms, because these may introduce recruitment bias.[28] For example, although English may be an official language in a country, there may be cultural minorities that exclusively speak another language, which would exclude them from participating in the study and would lead to selection bias.[29] Anticipating the need to translate patient forms with site investigators during the design of the consent forms will reduce unnecessary delays at the time of ethics board approval.

Strategies to Navigate Regulatory Issues

The overall regulatory process needs to be overseen and followed by the coordinating center. Some departments or agencies may approve the substitution of another country's regulations governing protection of human subjects if they are at least equivalent to those of the other country. Several agencies already have arrangements to recognize their regulation process as comparable, such as the US Food and Drug Administration and Health Canada. Exemptions from such drug regulations typically involve research on clinical practice, educational practices, quality improvement trials, survey procedures, interviews, etc.[15] Mapping out the application process at the time of trial design is an essential part of reducing the time required for the application process.

Contract research organizations are companies that provide support to investigators and/or sponsors in the form of research services outsourced on a contract basis. They offer comprehensive services for all aspects of the study, including applying to ethics boards, obtaining contracts, patient recruitment, and data collection. They range from large, international, full-service organizations to

Table 99.1 Select List of Organizations and Websites Providing Guidelines for Clinical Trials[a]

Organization	Website
European Medicines Agency	https://www.ema.europa.eu/en
European Commission Pharmaceutical Unit	https://ec.europa.eu/health/human-use_en
Food and Drug Administration	https://www.fda.gov/home
Good Clinical Practice `Network	https://ichgcp.net
International Council for Harmonisation	https://www.ich.org
Legislation and guidance documents in the European Union governing medicinal products	https://ec.europa.eu/health/human-use/legal-framework_en
World Health Organization	https://www.who.int

[a]Placed in alphabetical order.

Table 99.2 Select List of Funding Agencies for International Trials[a]

Organization	Website
Bill and Melinda Gates Foundation	https://gcgh.grandchallenges.org
Canadian Institutes of Health Research	https://cihr-irsc.gc.ca
March of Dimes	http://www.marchofdimes.org
Medical Research Council	https://mrc.ukri.org
National Institutes of Health	https://www.nih.gov
National Institute for Health and Care Research (United Kingdom)	https://www.nihr.ac.uk
Patient-Centered Outcomes Research Institute	https://www.pcori.org
Thrasher Research Fund	https://www.thrasherresearch.org/
Wellcome	https://wellcome.ac.uk

[a]Placed in alphabetical order.

small, specialized groups. Local contract research organizations can facilitate navigating local regulations in a timely fashion but will add to the financial burden of the trial.

Guidelines for the Conduct of International Clinical Trials

There are three generic international guidelines for conducting clinical trials in human subjects.

1. The World Health Organization (WHO) guidelines for good clinical practice for trials on pharmaceutical products[30]
2. The International Ethical Guidelines for Biomedical Research Involving Human Subjects, by the Council for International Organizations of Medical Sciences[31]
3. The International Council for (formerly Conference on) Harmonization of Good Clinical Practice Guidelines[32]

The WHO guidelines concern all WHO member states but do not supersede local regulations. Each country may have adopted, modified, or developed their own specific guidelines. Consequently, during the trial design, it is relevant to identify which countries will participate and which guidelines will apply. As previously mentioned, even if a single guideline is followed within a country, interpretation may vary according to the institution. The Council of International Organizations of Medical Sciences is an international nongovernment organization with official relations with the WHO. Their guidelines focus on the ethical principles that guide medical research in low-resource countries and take into consideration the cultural and socioeconomic context and local laws. The International Council for Harmonization of Good Clinical Practice Guidelines is a joint collaborative with expertise from Europe, Japan, Canada, Australia, and the United States and partners from the pharmaceutical industry. Today, the International Council for Harmonization of Good Clinical Practice Guidelines has been implemented in most jurisdictions and is reasonably similar. The guidelines were originally intended for trials using pharmaceutical interventions but are now used beyond their original scope.

Each country has some specific regulations that may need to be addressed, but the main objective of the International Council for Harmonization of Good Clinical Practice Guidelines is to harmonize the application process and reduce delays. Table 99.1 provides a list of relevant websites for additional guidelines. A limitation of many of these guidelines is that they were not specifically developed for research in neonatology and may not include considerations for rare disease, deferred consent, or consent by a legal guardian.

Potential Sources of Funding

Funding of international trials can be a challenge. Each national agency has different regulations on what can be paid and who can be paid. The funding agency may have additional requirements prior to sending funds outside the country. For example, for studies led in the United States, all countries outside the United States that contain a participating site must be formally cleared though the US State Department before federal funds from the sponsor may be transferred for research activities. To reduce delays, a list of participating countries should be sent to the sponsor with the original protocol to allow for timely approval. Another funding strategy to obtain funding includes having investigators from each country apply to their national funding agencies. However, timing of funding applications and varying success rates can create a challenge to manage. Table 99.2 provides a nonexhaustive list of national and international funding agencies that support international research.

Conclusion

International trials have the potential to provide new scientific knowledge efficiently, and that knowledge can be generalizable to a wider population. International trials have the potential to address interventions for which the target population is small within a single country. However, an international trial requires consideration for variations in regulatory, ethical, and contractual obligations. These challenges can add to the time and costs required to run the trial. Early anticipation of these challenges with proper preparation, seeking adequate expertise, and securing sufficient funding can help reduce undesired delays and increase the probability of success.

SECTION

21 Healthcare Leadership

OUTLINE

CHAPTER 100

Organization of Neonatal Intensive Care

Prabhu S. Parimi, Guilherme M. Sant'Anna, Alvaro Dendi, Martin Antelo, Sundos Khuder, Jargalsaikhan Badarch, Mohammad M. Rahman, Ashok Kumar, Akhil Maheshwari

KEY POINTS

1. Neonatal intensive care units (NICUs) are organized for the clinical care of premature and critically ill newborn infants.
2. Healthcare centers require a well-considered structure to enable collaborative decision-making to provide family-centered, high-value care to the mother-infant dyad.
3. In most parts of the world, NICUs are designated per the infrastructural levels and the severity of illness of infants receiving care in the units.
4. With increasing information on the determinants of outcomes, specialized, disease-focused level IV NICUs are in development, such as small-baby units, neuroneonatal intensive care units (ICUs), congenital diaphragmatic ICUs, esophageal airway and trachea programs, and neonatal surgical units.
5. NICUs care for the most vulnerable patients receiving multisystem support, multiple medications, indwelling central catheters, parenteral nutrition, and various other clinical interventions. In this complex paradigm, a central philosophy of "zero harm" has been emphasized.
6. Care coordination and communication are key for a safe discharge process and optimal outcomes.

Neonatal Intensive Care Units

Neonatal intensive care units (NICUs) care for vulnerable patient populations, and there is a need to staff these in-patient hospital sections with an appropriate complement of medical, nursing, and support staff (healthcare professionals).[1] Medical and hospital leaders both need to work together to ensure efficient, seamless operations to provide the highest-value care to infants admitted to the NICUs and to their families. In most parts of the world, the NICUs are designated per the recommendations of the American Academy of Pediatrics in the United States and those of comparable national organizations, which closely resemble each other. This need to designate NICUs is indeed important, and these decisions have to be based on the complexity of medical conditions treated, the risk of mortality, and the average daily patient census in these units.

In the United States, there has been considerable discussion about the best strategies to improve neonatal care. The nurse-to-patient ratio, when analyzed in the context of illness acuity tools, is an important marker. There is also a need for continuous improvement in the utilization and education of the trainee workforce (physician residents, fellows, trainee nurses, and students in various auxiliary services). There are important recommendations from the Accreditation Council for Graduate Medical Education (https://www.acgme.org/) and comparable global organizations. These recommendations combine our current understanding of the impact of the skill sets of trainees and the staffing priorities in the newborn nurseries/NICUs. The goal of developing these collaborative healthcare teams is to provide safe, efficient, timely, and effective care based on current evidence. All these considerations require effective leadership, optimal communication, understanding of our goals, and coordinated care.

Leadership Structure

Healthcare centers require a well-considered structure to enable collaborative decision-making to provide family-centered, high-value care to the mother-infant dyad. This is a priority, and this change in focus contrasts with traditional leadership models that drew primarily on industrial structures that were recognized as financially efficient. It is now recognized that the medical director and the nurse manager need to work with all the other key leaders in the newborn nursery and the hospital to oversee policies and procedures and ensure constant availability of behavioral competencies, cognitive abilities, and technical skills in order to provide safe, effective, and evidence-based care. Obviously, they need to track clinical, quality, and revenue outcomes, but these goals need to be expanded. In this regard, the designation of NICUs by expert groups such as the American Academy of Pediatrics Committee on the Fetus and Newborn provides a framework with appropriate leadership structures to provide high-value patient care. Indeed, these designations are gradually being adopted worldwide.[2] For level I newborn nurseries, a designated pediatrician can serve as the medical director and collaborate with the nurse manager to provide care to healthy late preterm and term infants. This team can also treat a selected population of newborn infants with medical issues of relatively lower complexity seen in the first few days after delivery, such as establishing maternal feeding, preventing hypoglycemia, ensuring that infants with known high-risk factors do not have actual neonatal sepsis, observation of transient heart murmurs, and monitoring of physiologic hyperbilirubinemia. In this period, close medial-nursing teamwork will ensure appropriate transitional care, and if needed, a smooth transition to higher-intensity clinical management in level II–IV NICUs. All stakeholders will need to work together as a team to meet the needs of patients/families and also to ensure work-life balance for all care providers.

Table 100.1 Levels of Newborn Care

Level of Newborn Care	Scope
Level I	Care for healthy, full-term babies. The focus is to stabilize babies born at or near full term for discharge or ensure timely, safe transfer to facilities that provide advanced care.
Level II	Provide advanced newborn care to infants born at greater than 32 weeks' gestation or who are recovering from more serious conditions.
Level III	Provide subspecialty newborn care to infants born at less than 32 weeks' gestation and to those born with critical illness at all gestational ages. These facilities offer a full range of respiratory support and advanced imaging and can provide prompt and readily available access to a full range of pediatric medical subspecialties, pediatric surgeons, and pediatric anesthesiologists. There is a need to transfer infants with critical congenital heart defects or those who may need extracorporeal membrane oxygenation.
Level IV	Provide the highest-level, most acute care. These nurseries are located in hospitals that can provide surgical repair of complex congenital or acquired conditions and have a full range of pediatric medical and surgical subspecialties and pediatric anesthesiologists on site. Level IV neonatal intensive care units also facilitate transport and provide education outreach.

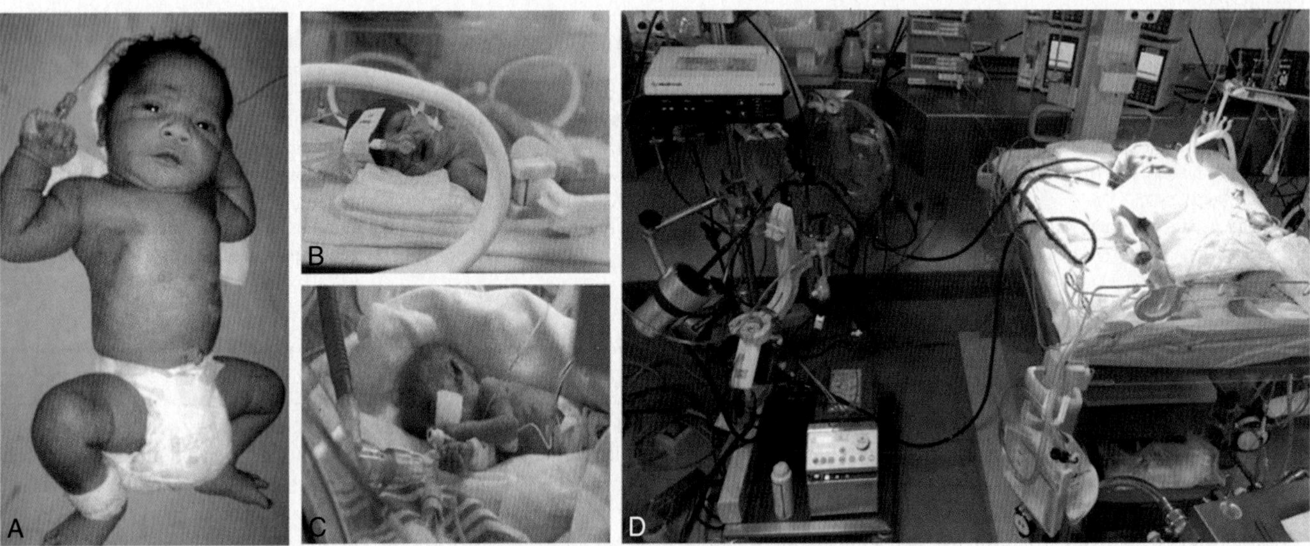

Fig. 100.1 (A) Term infant in a level I nursery (sick newborn care unit) in India recovering from transient tachypnea. (B) A 34 weeks' gestation premature infant with mild respiratory distress syndrome (RDS) receiving continuous positive airway pressure support in a level II neonatal intensive care unit (NICU) in Iraq. (C) A 27 weeks' gestation premature infant with moderately severe RDS on assisted ventilation in a level III NICU in the United States. (D) A term infant with a congenital cardiac defect being supported with extracorporeal membrane oxygenation in a level IV NICU in Uruguay.

Medical Staff

The composition of the care-provider workforce is usually based on the intensity- and complexity-based designation of the NICUs (Table 100.1, Fig. 100.1).[3]

Most level I nurseries are managed by pediatricians and experienced nurses. Other medical providers, such as pediatric and/or family practice nurse practitioners, physician assistants, and pediatric resident trainees may be involved. However, the numerical adequacy of care providers often varies between nurseries and may depend on the geographic location, the relative size of the medical center, the availability of resources, the number of births, and various other responsibilities entrusted to the providers. Ideally, a consistent, dedicated group of medical providers in the newborn nursery would facilitate seamless, high-value care, effective collaboration among staff, and overall satisfaction of mothers and families.[4] In many countries, these neonatal units have been provided the basic infrastructure to treat mild illnesses and avoid the need for long-distance transfers. One such example is the creation of sick newborn care units in India, which has helped lower the mortality rates in many parts of the country.

Level II nurseries have been successful in lowering infant mortality, but the levels of staffing remain variable. Studies show that the size of these nurseries is often dependent on operational revenues, requests by obstetricians, and the availability of experienced staff in the specific geographic location. Many level II NICUs are still managed by only a minimal number of neonatologist(s) available in the region, who work with advanced-practice providers (such as experienced midwives, advanced nurse practitioners, or physician assistants who have some experience in newborn care). The accreditation committees have emphasized that these level II nurseries need to have a skilled neonatal provider in house 24/7 to attend high-risk deliveries in a timely manner, and these recommendations have facilitated the development of an appropriate provider workforce. There is still a considerable shortage of adequately trained neonatal nurse practitioners across the world. Consequently, there is a desperate need for pediatricians with interest and expertise in neonatology (neonatal hospitalists) to maintain the workflow.

In level III and level IV NICUs, the staffing situation is slightly better. The medical provider workforce has evolved during the past 2 decades based on cohort-based care models and other specific areas of expertise. The medical provider groups in most level III and level IV

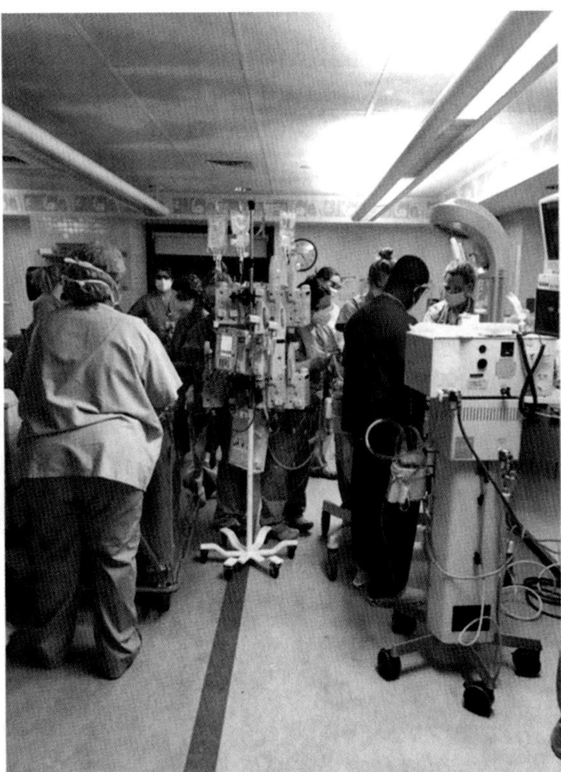

Fig. 100.2 Level IV Neonatal Intensive Care Units Coordinate Multispecialty Care of Critically Ill Infants. This photograph shows a team of multiple specialists resuscitating an infant with respiratory failure due to congenital diaphragmatic hernia.

NICUs are composed of neonatologists, neonatology fellows, pediatric residents, and advanced-practice providers (neonatal nurse practitioners and/or physician assistants). The staffing models in level III NICUs depend on whether there is a requirement for the neonatologists to be in house to render timely and in-person supervision of the trainee and/or auxiliary staff. The organizations make these operational decisions based on the need to hire neonatologists to provide in-house coverage and its financial implications. There is an ongoing debate on whether level III NICUs need 24/7 neonatologist coverage, because the impact on clinical outcomes remains unclear.

We do not anticipate major changes in the immediate future in the medical provider workforce in level III NICUs, but there is a possibility of a significant shift in care models in level IV NICUs. Children's hospitals, where most of the best-equipped level IV NICUs are located, are developing specialized, disease-focused units within the NICUs; these facilities include small-baby units, neuroneonatal intensive care units (ICUs), congenital diaphragmatic ICUs (Fig. 100.2), esophageal airway and trachea programs, and neonatal surgical units.[4,5] These specialized programs add to the complexities in the development of leadership, operations, medical provider staffing, and challenges in allocations of revenue and personnel. To find some solutions, many units are training the most-motivated personnel for collaborative functioning and leadership. There is a major need for committed medical providers, who can/will help plan and develop condition-specific clinical programs. These consolidated cohorts are already beginning to show improved expertise and clinical outcomes, timely referrals, allocation of resources, and the development of focused translational and clinical research. All these developments show exciting feed-forward loops with support from all constituents, be it physicians, hospitals, or the local administration. This may potentially bring a true change in the outlook for infants with problems that were hitherto considered to be lethal in most patients.

Nursing and Ancillary Staff

Due to their clinical complexity, patients in NICUs require highly trained, experienced nurses.[6] The role of experienced nurses extends beyond clinical care; these professionals are the ones who are in direct contact with the families for most the day and bring comfort and hope to the families with critically ill infants.

Currently there is no clear guidance regarding the most optimal nurse-to-infant ratios, which makes implementation in practice settings potentially difficult. These difficulties may contribute to suboptimal patient outcomes due to variations in nursing staffing patterns. The Institute of Medicine has called for reliable and valid measures to determine patient acuity (*Keeping Patients Safe*, 2003) and for using acuity measures and several other approaches to determine nursing staffing levels. In NICUs, the traditional considerations for determining the number of infants assigned to the nurse have been related to the patient (acuity score), nurse (assignments, qualifications, and nonnurse tasks), and various other characteristics of the facility. Similar to the considerations in the other parts of the hospital, the acuity of illness of a newborn infant has a significant bearing on the nurse-to-infant ratio. Infants in the highest acuity category have been treated with a 1:1 nurse-to-patient ratio, whereas the lower acuity levels have had each nurse caring for two to three infants. The allocation of an appropriate nurse-to-patient ratio depending on the acuity of patients is a reliable tool for determining the nursing workload. Specialized units within the NICU also requires highly skilled nurses to leverage their expertise in improving short- and long-term clinical outcomes.

There have been concerns about the addition of tasks other than those related to direct patient care to the workload of nurses. Neonatal patients, even when not apparently ill, have a high complexity in care because of the need to achieve feeding and other developmentally appropriate milestones within a critical temporal phase in the postnatal period. There is a need to recognize that a team-based approach is needed to leverage the skills of trained speech language pathologists, occupational therapists, physical therapists, and other ancillary staff members. There is a need to recognize the central role that nurses play in coordination of infant care.

Data, Quality, and Safety Staff

NICUs care for the most vulnerable patients receiving multisystem support, multiple medications, indwelling central catheters, parenteral nutrition, and various other clinical interventions. In this complex paradigm, a central philosophy of "zero harm" has been emphasized in various philosophy statements focused on quality-improvement (Fig. 100.3).[7] Studies have examined adverse outcomes such as medication errors, central line–associated bloodstream infections, surgical errors, unintended extubations, and the frequency of chronic lung disease (as an indirect measure of lung injury due to ventilatory support), and several approaches have also been examined to reduce the incidence of these events. Unfortunately, most NICUs all over the world have had to struggle with not having sufficient resources to examine these adverse outcomes in detail, develop protocols/guidelines to standardize care, and monitor safety data. To eliminate serious harm across individual hospitals and NICUs, several ICU conglomerations have defined high-reliability

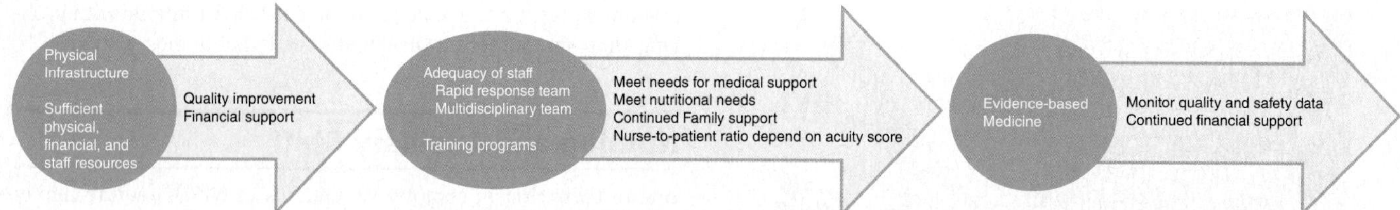

Fig. 100.3 Schematic Summarizing Aims for High-level Neonatal Intensive Care With *Zero Harm*.

principles and quality-improvement methods based on evidence-based care bundles. Many organizations are also trying to build infrastructure to collect and analyze data and to share and learn from other centers. The Neonatal Research Network in the United States (https://neonatal.rti.org/), the Institute of Health Policy, Management and Evaluation in Canada (https://ihpme.utoronto.ca/), and the more recent efforts to develop a Global Newborn Society network (https://www.globalnewbornsociety.org/resources) are some examples. The formation of NICU patient safety and quality committees, development of NICU-specific prospective databases, and training of medical, nursing, and advanced-practice providers are important investments toward providing high-value care.

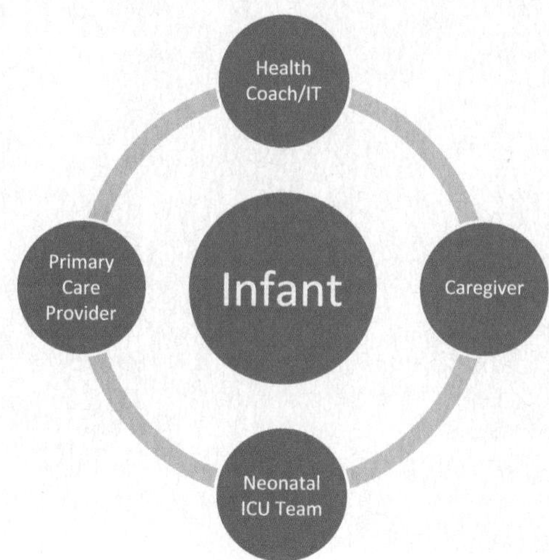

Fig. 100.4 Care Coordination and Communication Are Key for a Safe Discharge Process.

NICU Provider Workforce Shortages and Strategies

Concurrent implementation of strategies to improve patient care and the provider workforce can possibly improve outcomes by reducing the overall acuity of patient illness in NICUs, and this could also reduce the workload of NICU providers. Several patient-specific strategies have reduced the rates of NICU admissions and consequently have reduced the workload in these units. Some notable examples include the limitation of elective cesarean section deliveries to 39 weeks, standardized management of neonatal opioid withdrawal syndrome, and optimized duration of antibiotic therapy in infants suspected to have sepsis, which have reduced the length of hospital stay. Considering the significant shortages of auxiliary care providers such as nurse practitioners and physician assistants, hospitals and neonatal care programs have intensified efforts to identify and recruit these professionals, offset tuition costs, and offer other incentives to enable them to transition to these enhanced patient-care roles. Online educational programs have also enabled many nurses to continue with their primary jobs as a nurse while pursing these certifications without unduly impacting their financial position. In some programs, pediatricians with interest in newborn care can join neonatal programs and train to function as neonatal hospitalists. They can then work in NICUs under the supervision of the neonatologists.

Currently, the healthcare system has considerable unfilled needs in the neonatal provider workforce; every hospital offers comprehensive care to women, including obstetric and neonatal services, but the number of professionals to take care of infants is not sufficient. There are needs for establishing criteria for NICU admissions, adopting standardized care strategies for neonates, and recruiting and retaining auxiliary professionals. NICUs also need to commit time and resources to analyze data for patient safety and quality of care.

Transition to Home

In the United States, nearly 400,000 infants are admitted to NICUs every year. Apart from growing premature infants, patients with opioid withdrawal syndrome, gastrointestinal anomalies, hypoxemic ischemic encephalopathy, and critical congenital heart disease are at enhanced risk of rehospitalizations within 7 to 30 days. There is a need for a well-coordinated discharge process to optimize outcomes.[8] The discharge process can be smoothed if the primary caregivers can acquire appropriate skills and knowledge, emotional comfort, and confidence with the care of the infant. Many families may need training for the use of some medical equipment that they may need to use at home after hospital discharge.

Care coordination and communication are key for a safe discharge process and optimal outcomes (Fig. 100.4). Training such as in the *Health Coach Programs* in the NICU allows safe transition to home and seamless follow-up by the primary/subspecialist providers in the ambulatory setting.[8,9] The essential components of these programs focus on (1) teaching primary caregivers about care coordination to achieve independence; (2) standardizing the discharge process, including the use of handouts with specific instructions to respond appropriately to frequently seen problems (these materials can be tailored to the patient's specific condition); and (3) leveraging electronic communication with caregivers and primary care providers. The development of effective discharge processes can promote a safe, seamless transition in care; compliance with follow-up visits; fewer emergency room visits; and enhanced confidence and satisfaction in caregivers.

System Resources

The identification and recruitment of a health coach and a superuser to assist the NICU team to develop an electronic discharge checklist can facilitate an efficient and effective discharge process.[10] An experienced NICU nurse can assume this role to prepare families to gain competence and confidence to care for their infant. The health coach can enhance (1) sensitivity to the family's needs; (2) coaching of families to advocate for the needs of their infant and to participate in family-centered rounds; (3) accessibility to the NICU team; (4) communication to educate families about their infants' clinical condition; (5) development of individualized discharge plans; (6) development of appropriate, patient-specific educational materials; (7) assistance in scheduling educational classes (cardiopulmonary resuscitation), postdischarge appointments, and if needed, transportation; (8) coordination of postdischarge care; and (9) transmission of all the relevant information to the primary care provider.

NICU Team

The NICU clinical team must lead the effort in safe transition to care at home after discharge from the hospital. The discharge process should be conceptualized at the time of admission to the NICU, discussed during weekly multidisciplinary discharge huddles, and actively started 1 to 2 weeks prior to discharge. Collaborations with the health coach are important. The electronic health record designee should develop an electronic discharge checklist/template; focus on special needs such as apnea monitors, pulse oximeters, or gastrostomy tubes; participate in family education; provide any needed education materials to the primary care provider(s); and identify a NICU team member to serve as a liaison to assist the primary care provider after discharge.

Caregiver

At the time of discharge, the primary caregivers should receive easily understood information written at a fifth-grade level and should also be provided material important for the infant's special needs. The topics during the NICU stay cover clinical conditions specific to the baby, procedures, medications, and durable medical equipment. Recently, many institutions have begun incorporating simulations for patients being discharged home on CR monitors, gastrostomy tubes, and tracheostomy tubes with home ventilators. These novel strategies provide caregivers the necessary skillset, boost confidence to manage their infants at home, and prevent unindicated visits to the emergency room, thereby decreasing healthcare-associated costs. Shortly before transition to home, the primary caregivers need to receive educational materials on indications to seek medical help, medications and immunizations, feeding, managing breathing problems, support services, and contact numbers of the primary care provider and subspecialist office, as applicable.

Effective Communication

Strategies to develop effective communication with the primary care provider and the subspecialist are a vital component of the discharge process.[10,11] In this process, the discharge template/checklist and the electronic discharge summary are paramount. It is crucial to share the relevant clinical materials of each patient with the primary care provider. The NICU team members need to have at their disposal educational materials on anemia of prematurity, apnea of prematurity, bronchopulmonary dysplasia, gastroesophageal reflux, vision screening and retinopathy of prematurity, common discharge medications, feeding information, and other relevant information.[12] The American Academy of Pediatrics has recently proposed a "hybrid medical home model," whereby the high-risk NICU graduates are managed in the primary care provider's office with active assistance from the neonatologists and the subspecialists by adopting the process as described in this section.

There is a need for periodic electronic surveys to identify the needs of local primary care providers and for continuous improvement in patient care. Possible solutions for patient safety that consider both the transition to home and the continuum of care in the ambulatory setting should be identified. A well-orchestrated, systematic, and multidisciplinary approach that begins at the time of admission will facilitate a seamless and safe transition to home. The development of care-transitioning teams that include the hospital leadership, experts who manage and can analyze electronic health records, leaders from the NICU, case managers, social workers, and primary care providers in the region will promote safe transition of the patients from the hospital to their homes and provide value to all the involved stakeholders.

CHAPTER 101 Leadership and Organizational Culture in Healthcare

Prabhu S. Parimi, Jorge Fabres, Yahya Ethawi, Jubara Alallah, Michaelene Fredenburg, Rajesh Jain, Mohammad M. Rahman, Kei Lui, Arūnas Liubšys, Mimi L. Mynak, Barton Goldenberg, Giuseppe Buonocore, Akhil Maheshwari

KEY POINTS

1. All organizations, be it in healthcare or in any other sector(s) of society, strive for effective, potentially transformational leadership.
2. In any health-care system, infants receiving care in neonatal intensive care units are often the most vulnerable patients, with very high severity levels of illness.
3. The first step in analyzing the impact of leadership in any organization is to observe the interactions of the leaders and the workforce in that specific microenvironment.
4. The skill sets of a leader have a significant bearing on his/her ability to deliver safe, effective, integrated, and well-coordinated care.
5. We describe various leadership styles, which can be authoritative, transformational (collaborative), transactional, contingent, and participative. In our own review and discussions, we noted that a "SEAT" paradigm may be something to consider—there may be four main options available to a leader: to support, entrust, administer, and train.
6. We have also summarized workplace cultures, challenges, communication needs, and practice models for large organizations, including those focused on healthcare.

In any healthcare system, infants receiving care in neonatal intensive care units (NICUs) are often the most vulnerable patients, with very high severity levels of illness.[1] Consequently, the staff members working in these sections of hospitals work under high levels of stress.[2] To provide the best possible clinical care and to retain the most skilled professionals, there is a need for careful, continuous examination of not only the policies and procedures but also the work environment in these units.[3] The leadership and organizational culture are important determinants to ascertain that medical, nursing, and other professionals can work together to achieve these goals. Interestingly, the principles of leadership are similar across any sector, be it in healthcare or in industries with large-sized workforces.[4] In this chapter, we discuss the traits needed for effective leadership, the leadership styles seen in these high-risk operations, and the importance of maintaining an organizational culture that would be most conducive for retaining the best staff members and improving the quality of care. In addition to our own experience, we have drawn from an extensive literature search in the databases PubMed, Embase, and Scopus. To avoid bias in the identification of studies, keywords were short-listed *a priori* both from anecdotal experience and PubMed's Medical Subject Heading thesaurus.

Leadership

The first step in analyzing the impact of leadership on the work culture in any organization is to observe the interactions of both in that specific microenvironment. In healthcare, including in NICUs, these steps will enable the evaluation of patient safety and quality, staff well-being, and health outcomes. A leader, as defined by Peter Drucker, is "someone who has followers." Leadership may need larger goals; it may entail the virtue of navigating through turbulent times.[5] Interestingly, it may require a modified catechistic approach with prudence to see ahead, justice in dealing with others, fortitude with brave endurance, temperance to bring down the expectations for immediate gains, faith in the abilities of the team, humility, authenticity, maintaining the hope of eventual success, and charity to forgive errors when charting new territories.[6]

Warren Bennis defined leadership as a "function of knowing yourself, having a vision that is well articulated, building trust in colleagues, and taking effective action to realize your own leadership potential." A leader who demonstrates these abilities needs to take a preeminent role to shape the culture, defined as "the values, behaviors, goals, attitudes, practices and beliefs shared across an entire organization." At a panoramic level, the executive leadership with expertise and specialized training can promote the organizational culture by clearly defining and authentically living out the mission, vision, and values.[7] However, the microenvironment in the individual units may also affect the outcomes positively or negatively, be it on patient outcomes, perceptions of staff, or in their emotional well-being.

As in any specialized, critically important units in an organization, a NICU is a complex microenvironment that provides care for high-risk patients. The staff members interface with a host of specialists from various disciplines ranging from obstetrics, maternal-fetal medicine, pediatric subspecialists, members of palliative care teams, and others. Many other streams of staff members with different levels of experience, including nurses, pediatric resident trainees, nurse practitioners, physician-assistants, and neonatologists, are also involved. In this paradigm, the basic tenet of a physician leader with the overall responsibility in the unit is to involve/engage the team to render targeted, safe, effective, efficient, and timely care to optimize outcomes. The most important questions about the type of leadership and skill sets remain.

Leadership Types

Just as in any complex organizational microenvironment, the skill sets of a leader in a NICU have a significant bearing on his/her ability to deliver safe, effective, integrated, and well-coordinated care to the patients and their families. There are also new, evolving needs, and a leader today should be able to create a social culture of trust and consensus about the needs of tiny babies with involvement of other health systems and social media.

Physician leaders need different types of leadership styles depending on the context, and they need flexibility to adapt in a timely fashion. In the literature, six different leadership styles have been described. We have expanded on three styles that seemed most relevant to healthcare. The other three did not seem to be as pertinent/applicable in the NICU environment, so we mention those only briefly. As we developed this section, we reached out to leaders in various sectors of society; the needs to chart out the plans, inspire, evaluate, and intervene are similar.

Authoritative Leadership

Authoritative leadership involves the leader laying down expectations, clear guidelines, and defined outcomes. This model can be successful if the leader is a renowned, respected expert and facilitates efficiency in tasks that require quick turnarounds with few mistakes in implementation. However, it does not promote the growth of associates, and there may be less creativity and synergy. Leaders who base their leadership style solely on personal attributes such as appeal, intellect, and knowledge may lack empathy, emotional intelligence, and situational and social awareness (Great man theory).[8] In some situations, there may be higher dissatisfaction in the group and higher turnover rates of subordinates.

Transformational (Collaborative) Leadership

Transformational (collaborative) leadership is where a leader motivates team members through vision, shares control, serves as a change agent, exhibits concern and development of others, highly engages the team, delegates others to lead a process change, embraces resistance and proposes ways to deal with it, shows emotional intelligence, leads by example, and supports a nurturing and developing culture in the unit (Fig. 101.1).[9] Transformational leadership, particularly when it is character-based, may also include elements of both authentic leadership and servant leadership.[10] The behavior of authentic leaders is congruent with their beliefs—beliefs that prize high moral and ethical standards. Additionally, they are willing to let their colleagues view their flaws. Servant leadership encompasses authentic leadership with the added components of self-sacrifice and service to others. The concept of servant leadership was popularized by Robert Greenleaf in the 1970s. Since that time numerous books and articles have been written about the topic, and research has been conducted that has shown a positive correlation between servant leadership, employer satisfaction, and customer/patient loyalty.[10] A bedside nurse leading patient safety and quality initiatives, a neonatal nurse practitioner responsible for central line insertion and maintenance, a trainee developing clinical practice guidelines to reduce the variation in clinical practice, and a neonatologist leading the team are all examples of a transformational leader.

Transactional Leadership

Transactional leadership seeks to meet operational and financial targets and may leverage reward or punitive measures to achieve the desired goal. The resources for the reward may include verbal praise and recognition (intangible) and could include annual monetary incentives for meeting quality metrics. Negative feedback could include disciplinary actions that progressively increase with the frequency or implications of a specific act of commission/omission.[11] The role of transactional leadership in service improvement is limited.

Contingent Leadership

Contingent leadership varies depending on the context, needs, and attributes of the team members, which has been described as being based on the Trait Theory. Many experts have described this model as based on delegative "laissez-faire" interaction. Effective leaders take into consideration not only the situation but important qualities of each team member to make informed decisions regarding the role he/she needs to play.[12] They may delegate, support, coach, direct, or use other strategies based on the motivation and competency of the team member. It works well in a group that is limited in size and is composed of friendly experts who have worked together for some time. If it works, it can promote innovation and creativity. However, disagreements among senior experts may also cause loss of harmony and morale. This is a difficult model to use in the present day because workplaces are progressively becoming more complex, with increasing emphasis on financial and temporal efficiency.

Participative Leadership

Participative leadership is rooted in democratic models and can work well in a relatively small team of well-engaged, equally qualified experts who may have to deal with unexpected situations (situational

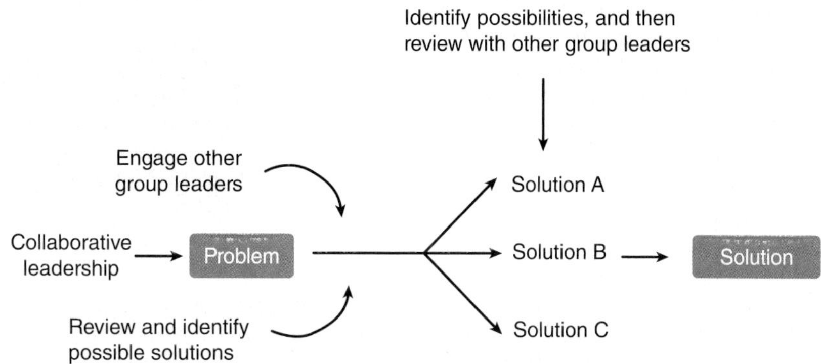

Fig. 101.1 Transformational (Collaborative) Approach to Problem Solving. A team of selected, most-experienced leaders identifies a few possible options for solutions and then picks one. This model is held in high regard and can be highly successful in established organizations with experienced leadership.

Support High Competency, Low Motivation	**Entrust** High Competency, High Motivation
Administer Low Competency, High Motivation	**Train** Low Competency, Low Motivation

Fig. 101.2 The SEAT Paradigm in Contingent Leadership. The leader has the options to *support*, when the workforce is competent but is not motivated; *entrust*, an easy option when a highly competent and motivated team is available; *administer*, when the team is motivated but does not have all the necessary expertise; or *train*, which is a slower option but may be the only possibility when the workforce is neither very competent nor very highly motivated.

theory).[13] It builds an engaging environment in the medium- and long-term, but the implementation of tasks can be time-consuming with the need for consensus development. This model may not work well with relatively less well-trained employees because there may be an appearance of a lack of consistency, and this may make it harder for them to project the most likely path that will be taken.

We have observed our own teams, and after extensive review and discussions, we found that we use an administrative strategy that could be named the "SEAT" paradigm, with four main options available to a leader: to support, entrust, administer, or train (Fig. 101.2). This strategy combines elements from different models because we have found qualified leaders in our team in some but not in all situations. In each of these possibilities, the leader is ultimately responsible for the outcome and needs to continuously observe the team for single-time-point events and for longitudinal patterns in performance.

Significance of Specific Leadership Styles

The impact of leadership style in healthcare has been studied most frequently in the United States and Canada and in the inpatient care setting. The three most common leadership styles described above (transformational, transactional, and contingent) are known to have improved the quality of care and reduced errors. The transformational style of leadership has had a very significant impact on patient safety and delivery of a high quality of care. Most of the data about the effect of the leadership style on organizational culture come from nursing literature. A transformational leader can improve organization, continuous learning, and effective communication, improve teamwork, and receive feedback as part of the development process. Studies have shown this style of leadership to reduce nursing turnover, improve staff satisfaction, and increase the retention of team members. This is particularly relevant to high-intensity settings such as the NICU. The shared leadership between the physician and nursing executives promotes a healthy work environment and high-value care to the critically ill infants and their families. However, these opinions are based on observation; there is a need to formally study these leadership styles and assess the impact on patient outcomes and the satisfaction levels among the patient-families and staff members.

Challenges

Most physician and nursing leaders have not received formal leadership training, and many of those who have been trained may not necessarily be able to translate the learning from didactic/simulated sessions into real-life scenarios. These leaders may benefit from self- or joint efforts at reflection through validated tools, which can promote insights into strengths and weaknesses in team management. Targeted and focused leadership development courses, such as in coaching, mentoring, and obtaining feedback from peers, subordinates, and superiors, may help. Development of standardized measurement tools could facilitate formal, more reliable identification of the most effective strategies. A more forward-looking approach would be to introduce leadership development focusing on handling change and conflict management education during medical school training, aiming to identify and prepare emerging physician leaders.

Organizational Culture

Organizational culture refers to values, behaviors, goals, attitudes, practices, and beliefs shared across an entire organization.[14] It is particularly relevant to the provider workforce and helps identify the work culture at the unit level. Understanding these variables can help identify hitherto unidentified determinants of health outcomes, morale, and well-being of staff members. Unlike many other sectors, such as industry, that function with large workforces, not many of these studies have been conducted in healthcare. The competing-values framework of organizational culture (Fig. 101.3) takes into consideration specific behaviors and practices. Understanding the prevailing culture at the unit level will allow critical assessment and appropriate adaptation with a goal to provide high-value care to the infants and their families and to care for unit team members. We have been evaluating and studying work cultures over time, and we classify various behavioral patterns in a four-group paradigm. To emphasize our belief in working together with mutual respect and recognition, we use the acronym *ROSE* to classify various possibilities.

As the name implies, the culture ROSE includes four approaches. **Reason** is focused on discussion, teamwork, and participation and aims to develop cohesiveness and team morale. The emphasis on **Order** (rank) creates a formal culture that focuses on an individual's relative position in an organization. These professional groups use

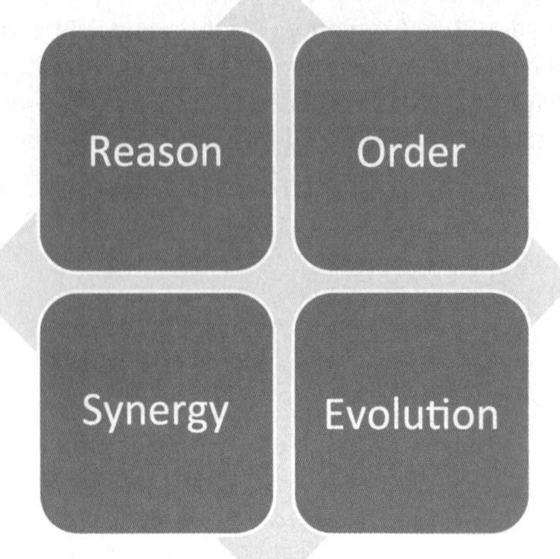

Fig. 101.3 "ROSE" Classification to Study Work Cultures in Various Organizations. The culture *Reason* focuses on discussion, *Order* on formal ranking, and *Synergy* on subgroups working together. *Evolution* takes a long-term view and rewards novelty and transformation. We chose this acronym to recognize the importance of softer aspects of human relationships such as care, compassion, and respect in the growth of organizations.

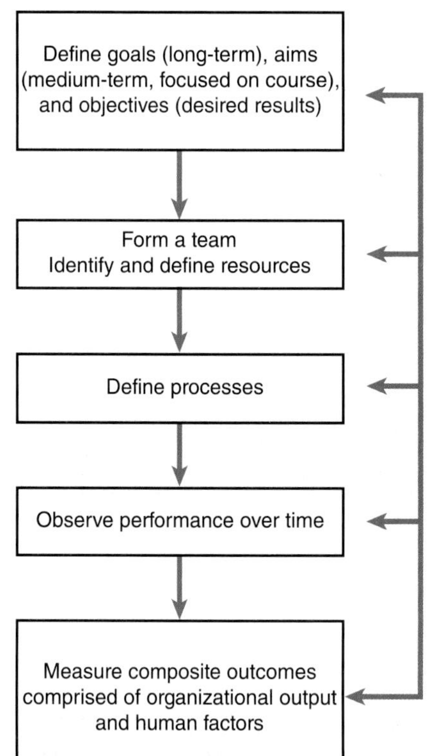

Team development must focus on:

- Avoidance of excessive workload situations by a carefully planned work-floor
- Careful consideration of the time-course needed to achieve the objectives
- Formation of a team that is adequate in skill-sets and availability of time
- Defining the tasks for the work-teams
- Eliminating distractions, and designating exact tasks to individuals
- Recognition of worker achievement, which could be on an everyday basis for dedication, periodically (monthly/quarterly) for objectives, and annually for achievement of aims.

A leader needs to find a balance:

- Balancing safety, a responsibility of the leader, and efficiency, a need for the organization
- Use of pre-decided policies and procedures to avoid undue production pressures
- Monitor that thoroughness is not being compromised to achieve efficiency
- Monitor for any signals indicating loss of safety
- Monitor for signals of production, to maintain efficiency.

Every newly-diagnosed difficulty needs careful evaluation. Important considerations are communication, situation awareness, decision-making, task-management, and teamwork.

Fig. 101.4 Balance Theory in Work Systems. We have used the "Balance Theory in Work Systems" to integrate knowledge about the impact of job/organizational design and goals, human factors, and job stress. There is increasing recognition of four important areas for improvement: (1) impact of the work system on worker performance, (2) multilevel analysis of the work system, (3) understanding the nonwork sphere, and (4) application to healthcare and patient safety, also known as the Systems Engineering Initiative for Patient Safety model of work system and patient safety.

written policies, procedures, rules, and regulations and emphasize stability and control. Such a culture is effective in the short term but may not always promote growth and innovation. Recognition of **Synergy** rewards teams working together to optimize results. It encourages efficiency and productivity to gain competitive advantage. Finally, the culture that stresses **Evolution** takes a longer-term view and encourages transformation, novelty, risk-taking, and flexibility with a goal toward growth.

Mahl and colleagues (Further Reading reference 8) examined the relationship between organizational culture, implementation of quality improvement (QI) efforts, and neonatal outcomes in 18 level III NICUs in Canada. They showed that the two most frequently seen cultures either emphasize teamwork or stress hierarchy. The NICU management team (physician and nursing leaders) rated QI implementation higher relative to nurses, nurse practitioners, and respiratory therapists. Hierarchical cultures and higher QI scores were associated with higher rates of survival without major morbidity. The favorable outcomes in these cultures can be promoted by developing optimal team function (Fig. 101.4) with standardization of practice. We believe that this work culture may be most effective in short-term observations. A combination of establishing clearly defined protocols, but at the same time, encouraging open discussions and recognizing thought leaders who can engage the teams may be the best strategy to improve outcomes. Continued training is also needed to maintain a highly skilled and motivated workforce.

Although the importance of workplace culture in QI and clinical outcomes is evident, there are concerns about professionalism in medical teams. There are implications in the provision of appropriate patient care, synergy and morale of team members, effectiveness of the unit/organization, and associated tangible and intangible costs. The idea of professionalism infers deep commitment to the profession, patients, and other healthcare providers, but inappropriate verbal or nonverbal communication may indicate low professional respect that results in an unpleasant work culture. Intensive care units have a stressful work environment, and there is a need to emphasize workplace civility. Both medical trainees (60%) and staff physicians (30%) report experiencing uncivil/unprofessional behavior in the workplace, a prevalence that is alarming and requires implementation of proactive strategies to promote a healthy work environment.

To develop proactive strategies, it is important to identify organizational factors that can help promote a pleasant work environment. Communication is a key element in developing a successful team (Fig. 101.5). Most NICUs are closed units with a neonatologist serving as the team leader. However, large multidisciplinary teams are always at risk of inadvertent creation of "silos" that may contribute to inappropriate interactions and subtle disrespectful behaviors. Many professionals work at more than one clinical site; this may result in their perceiving or being perceived as not working at a "home" site, which may put them at risk of being subject to disciplinary actions at lower thresholds. Finally, the leaders' reluctance/inability to recognize, acknowledge, and prevent or correct workplace disrespect or underrecognition can contribute to a "culture of silence" or even a hostile work environment that contributes to or exacerbates compassion fatigue.

Healthcare leaders must focus on developing a healthy workplace environment. There are several leadership practice models that can

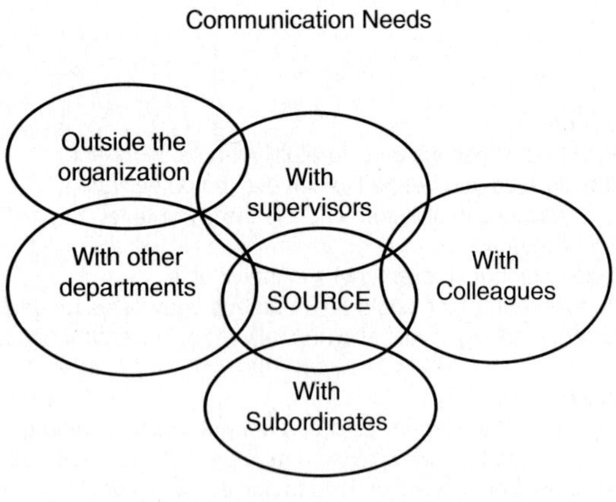

Fig. 101.5 Communication Needs. A central coordinator (source) should lead communication with various groups through multiple means, often with some redundancy, to ensure registration.

- Organizations need both top-down (for understanding of goals, aim, and objectives), and floor-up communication (for understanding of difficulties in access to technological, human, and organizational assets)
- Communication needs to be both (a) verbal, to ensure comprehension, because the written work can be easily misinterpreted; and (b) written, because the series of verbal expression, auditory registration, and comprehension, is not always guaranteed. Large organizations usually need multiple means of communication, sometimes with even some redundancy, to ensure registration.
- Safety attitudes may compete against economic thinking and thoroughness. The pressure for throughput, or the attempt to make up time by skipping essential procedures can erode safety and lead to a normalization of deviance.
- An incident reporting system is needed. Incoming reports should be deidentified, analyzed in a transparent fashion by a multi-professional team, and the recommendations should be communicated to the management of the organization.

Table 101.1 Practice Models

Practice Modes	Definition
Protocol-based	• Written definitions with interventions for procedures, targets, or timelines • Included in projected needs and expected outcomes; unique to each facility • Timeline can be expressed as outcomes, time, or both
Best practices	• Describes approaches proven effective in other organizations • Developed by experts in the field of work • Shared through databases and conferences
Consensus statement	• State-of-the-information statement form with implications for practice • Independent panels of experts resolves problems based on given intervention • Addresses organizational efficacy, risk, and projected needs
Outcomes management	• Multidisciplinary team critically reviews data and defines outcomes • Integrates services, care components, and providers with the goal of collaboration • Focused on defined needs; links care settings and timelines to outcomes
Evidence-based	• Framework to apply research in the setting • Study available data that has been evaluated for the specific application • Findings integrated with expectations and values

carry direct benefits with improved patient care and bring in subtle improvements by helping consolidate teams (Table 101.1).

They could help educate staff members, which can both improve skill sets and promote team development. In time, with increased confidence and harmony, the issues of uncivil behaviors can be handled more directly without disrupting the teams. Senior staff members can be trained to role-model professional behaviors and empowered to hold each other accountable. The medical and hospital leadership can be convinced to include citizenship as a key component in decisions to reward, promote, and recognize staff members. In this same scheme, many centers have very successfully incorporated 360-degree feedback from peers and anonymous feedback from trainees. Team development and synergy, including cultivation of self-care, are perhaps the most important determinants for improvement in patient outcomes, retention of experienced staff members, the development of a healthy work environment, and increased organizational effectiveness. Last but not least, the involvement of health systems and governments is mandatory to reach the goal to give to the newborn the best cure and care, wherever she/he may have been born.

FURTHER READING

Braithwaite J, Herkes J, Ludlow K, et al. Association between organizational and workplace cultures, and patient outcomes. Systematic review. *BMJ Open*. 2017;7:e017708.

Collins J. *Good to great and the social sector: A monograph to accompany good to great*. Boulder, CO: Collins; 2005.

Collins J. *Good to great: Why some companies make the leap…and others don't*. New York, NY: Harper Collins; 2001.

Fletcher K, Friedman A, Piedimonte G. Transformational and transactional leadership in health care seen through the lens of pediatrics. *J Pediatr*. 2019;204:7–9.

Hughes RL, Ginnett RC, Curphy GL. *Leadership: Enhancing the lessons of experience*. 8th ed. New York, NY: McGraw Hill Education; 2015.

Kumar R. Leadership in healthcare. *Anaesth Intensive Care Med*. 2013;14(1):39–41.

Mahl S, Lee SK, Baker R, et al. The association of organizational culture and quality improvement implementation with neonatal outcomes in the NICU. *J Pediatr Healthcare*. 2015;29(5):435–441.

Pattani R, Ginsburg S, Johnson AM, et al. Organizational factors contributing to incivility at an academic medical center and system-based solutions: A qualitative study. *Acad Med*. 2018;93(10):1569–1575.

Robbins B, Davidhizar R. Transformational leadership in healthcare today. *Health Care Manag*. 2020;39(3):117–121.

Sfantou DF, Laliotis A, Patelarou AE, et al. Importance of leadership style towards quality-of-care measure in healthcare settings: a systematic review. *HealthCare*. 2017;5(73):1–17.

Gabel S. Transformational leadership and healthcare. *Med Sci Educ*. 2013;23(1):55–60.

Xu JH. Leadership theory in clinical practice. *Chin Nurs Res*. 2017;4:155–157.

SECTION

22 Neonatal Dermatology

OUTLINE

CHAPTER 102 Skin Disorders in Newborn Infants

Shaifali Bhatia, Akhil Maheshwari

KEY POINTS

1. Neonatal skin matures with gestational age with increasing thickness, less permeability, and higher density of sweat and sebaceous glands. Keratinization begins at 24 weeks and matures near term.
2. Cold stress is an important risk to preterm infants. Lower skin thickness, less subcutaneous fat, and immaturity of the nervous system predisposes to heat loss.
3. Several minor congenital anomalies may predominantly involve the skin; these include dimpling, periauricular sinuses, pits, tags, cysts, supernumerary digits, supernumerary nipples, umbilical granulomas, and umbilical polyps.
4. Neonatal intensive care may leave skin lesions such as surgical scars, chemical and thermal burns, and scars from arterial catheters and repeated heal-sticks. Exposure to various infections and drugs may cause erythema multiforme, erythema nodosum, urticaria, and vasculitis.
5. Several congenital disorders of skin structure may be seen in newborn infants, such as epidermolysis bullosa, aplasia cutis congenita, mastocytosis, incontinentia pigmenti, nevi/birthmarks, and vascular anomalies.
6. Inflammatory disorders seen in the neonatal skin include diaper dermatitis, allergic contact dermatitis, seborrheic dermatitis, neonatal psoriasis, Langerhans cell histiocytosis, and benign cephalic histiocytosis.
7. Scaling abnormalities seen in the newborn skin include those seen in collodion babies and various forms of ichthyosis. Ichthyotic changes can also be seen as a part of many complex multisystem syndromes.
8. Transient cutaneous eruptions seen in neonates range from transient vascular phenomena, benign pustular dermatoses, erythema toxicum neonatorum, transient neonatal pustular melanosis, acropustulosis of infancy, eosinophilic pustular folliculitis, benign pustular dermatoses, sebaceous gland hyperplasia, miliaria, milia, infantile acne, subcutaneous fat necrosis, and neonatal lupus erythematosus to annular erythema of infancy.
9. Cutaneous infections in neonates include candidiasis, syphilis, herpes simplex, congenital and neonatal varicella, impetigo and staphylococcal scalded-skin syndrome, and scabies.
10. Several cutaneous neoplasms can be seen in neonates. These include infantile hemangiomas, hamartomatous nevi, epidermal nevi, sebaceous nevi, smooth muscle and pilar hamartomas, connective tissue nevi, congenital melanocytic nevi, giant congenital pigmented nevi, juvenile xanthogranulomas, dermoid cysts, recurrent infantile digital fibromas, congenital or infantile myofibromatosis, and in some cases, malignant tumors.

Newborn skin differs from that of adults in several ways. The following sections summarize developmental changes, transient cutaneous changes seen in neonates and young infants, congenital disorders of skin structure, inflammatory disorders, scaling abnormalities, skin infections, and cutaneous neoplasms. The information is summarized from our own clinical experience and from information mined from PubMed, Embase, and Scopus.

Immaturity of the Skin in Newborn Infants

Development

Neonatal skin matures with gestational age in terms of increasing thickness, reduced permeability, and the density of sweat and sebaceous glands.[1] At 30 weeks of gestational age, the skin thickness of about 27.4 μm is only half that of adults. There are fewer intercellular attachments, resulting in higher permeability and transepidermal water losses, and also a higher risk of blistering upon exposure to heat or chemical irritants. Percutaneous absorption of toxic substances is higher. Keratinization begins at 24 weeks and matures near term. An overview of the structure of the neonatal skin is shown in Fig. 102.1.

At birth, the skin is covered with *vernix caseosa*, a greasy white material of pH 6.7 to 7.4 containing lipids, protein, lanugo hair, shed skin cells, and water (Fig. 102.2A).[2] Beneath the vernix, the skin has a pH of 5.5 to 6.0. Overwashing, particularly with harsh soaps, may result in irritation and damage the normal barrier function. Some scaling may be normally seen on the trunk and on the hands and feet during the neonatal period (Fig. 102.2B).

Transient Cutaneous Changes Seen in Newborn Infants

Newborn infants frequently show many benign, transient skin findings that may be a source of parental anxiety. Early recognition is important to enable appropriate counseling to parents.

Unique physiologic changes such as the Harlequin change[3] are seen in approximately 10% of newborn infants between 2 to 5 days after birth. There is a benign, transient red color change lasting 30 seconds to 20 minutes in half of the body demarcated at the midline (Fig. 102.3).

Cold stress is an important risk to preterm infants. Thinner skin layers, less subcutaneous fat, and immaturity of the nervous system predispose to increased heat losses from evaporation, radiation, and conduction. When exposed to cold temperatures, some infants show acrocyanosis with bluish discoloration of hands and feet. There is no edema or other cutaneous changes. Careful examination can help differentiate it from central cyanosis seen on the lips, face, and/or trunk in pulmonary or cardiac disease.

Many infants show *cutis marmorata* after hypothermia; it is a diffuse, reticulated erythema with bluish-red marbling of the skin on the trunk and extremities (Fig. 102.4A). The changes of *cutis marmorata* may persist beyond the neonatal period in infants with trisomy 18 or 21, *Cornelia de Lange* syndrome, hypothyroidism, or

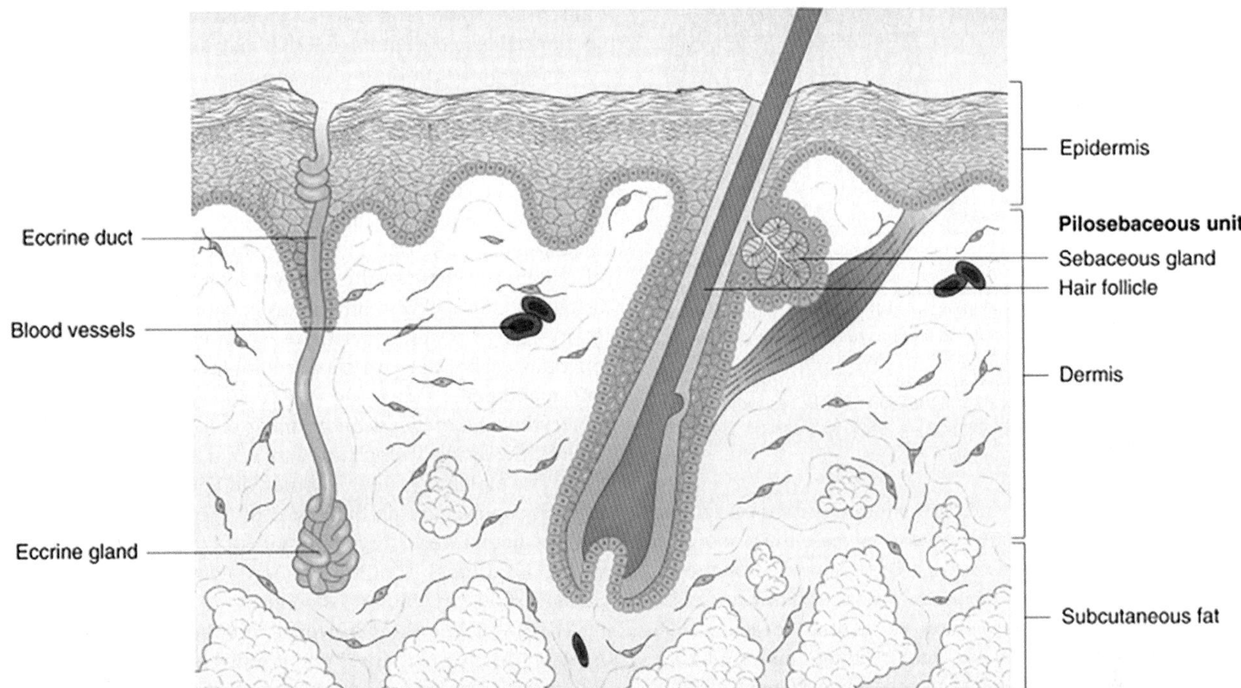

Fig. 102.1 Structure of Newborn Skin. The skin has three major divisions: epidermis, dermis, and subcutaneous fat. Adnexal structures include pilosebaceous units and eccrine ducts and glands (shown) and apocrine glands (not shown). (Reproduced with permission and minor modifications from Mancini AJ, Lawley LP. *Neonatal and Infant Dermatology*. 2015:14–23.e4.)

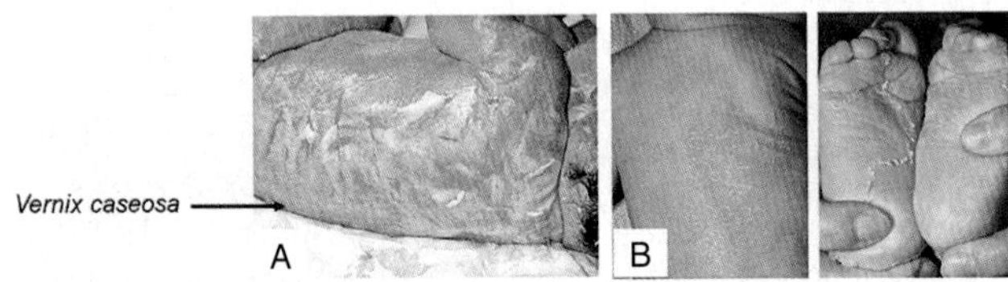

Fig. 102.2 Normal Postnatal Changes in Skin. (A) Vernix caseosa often covers the skin surface of healthy full-term newborn infants at delivery. (B) Minor scaling in a 1-week-old healthy infant on the back (*left*) and on the soles. (Reproduced with permission and minor modifications from Püttgen KB, Cohen BA. Neonatal dermatology. In: *Pediatric Dermatology*. 2:14–67.)

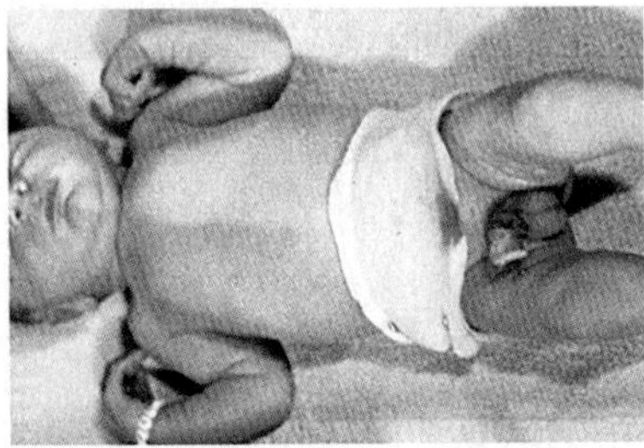

Fig. 102.3 Harlequin Color Change With the Dependent Side Transiently Acquiring a Bright Red Color. (Reproduced with permission and minor modifications from Püttgen KB, Cohen BA. Neonatal dermatology. In: *Pediatric Dermatology*. 2:14– 67.)

some central nervous system disorders. These changes need careful differentiation from *cutis marmorata telangiectatica congenita* or congenital phlebectasia (Fig. 102.4B).[4] These latter two conditions may be localized to patches on the trunk or extremities or extend in a Blaschkoid pattern (lines of Blaschko are pathways of epidermal cell migration and proliferation during the development of the fetus).[5]

Hyperthermia can also be a problem in growing infants with insulated clothing. Sweat glands may appear anatomically well-formed at 28 weeks' gestation, but the functional maturity is attained only beyond the first month after birth. Older phototherapy units increased the risk of hyperthermia, although this problem has been resolved with light-emitting diode lights.

Photosensitivity: Melanocytes begin synthesizing and transferring pigment to epidermal keratinocytes by 20 to 24 weeks' gestation, but the skin surface tends to be less pigmented during the first few postnatal months. Consequently, neonates and young infants have less natural protection from sunlight and are more likely to develop sunburn. Sun avoidance and protective clothing can be effective barriers to excessive sun exposure.[6]

Some disorders increase the risk of sunburns in infants. Hereditary porphyrias (Fig. 102.5A), xeroderma pigmentosum, Bloom syndrome,

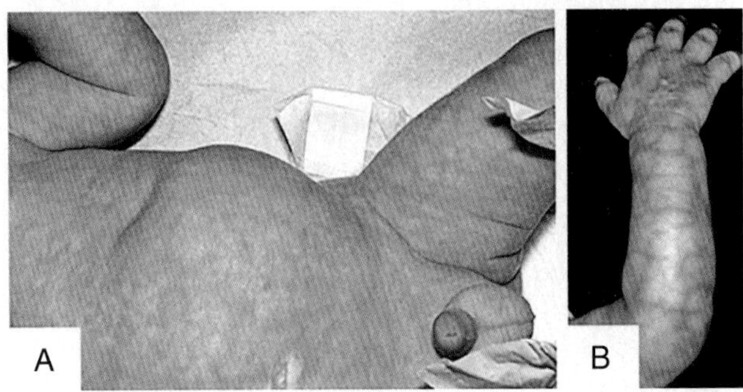

Fig. 102.4 (A) Cutis marmorata. The diffuse, reticulated erythema disappeared with warming of this newborn. (B) In differential diagnosis, *cutis marmorata telangiectatica congenita* should be considered. These are localized reticulated vascular malformations. (A, Reproduced with permission and minor modifications from Püttgen KB, Cohen BA. Neonatal dermatology. In: *Pediatric Dermatology*. 2:14–67; B, reproduced with permission and minor modifications from James et al. Dermal and subcutaneous tumors. In: *Andrews' Diseases of the Skin*, 28:587–635.e7.)

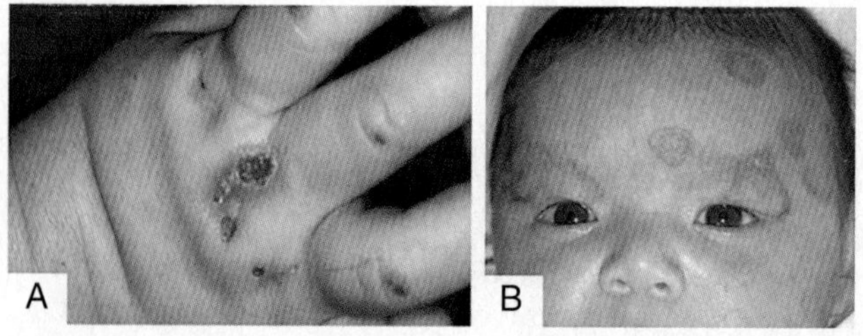

Fig. 102.5 Some Photosensitive Conditions. (A) Congenital erythropoietic porphyria. Crusted ulcerations, bullae, and erosions seen in areas exposed to ultraviolet or visible light. (B) Neonatal lupus erythematosus. Annular erythematous plaques on the forehead and scalp. The lesions resemble the annular form of subacute cutaneous lupus erythematosus. (A, Reproduced with permission and minor modifications from Bender NR and Chiu YE. Photosensitivity. In: *Nelson Textbook of Pediatrics*, ch. 675, 3496–3501.e1; B, reproduced with permission and minor modifications from Lee LA, Werth VP. Lupus erythematosus. *Dermatology*. 41:662–680.)

and Cockayne syndrome may increase photosensitivity. Neonatal lupus erythematosus (Fig. 102.5B) can also increase the risk of skin rashes after sun exposure.[6] Sunscreens are not approved by the US Food and Drug Administration for use in neonates, but if sun exposure cannot be strictly avoided, products with protective factors >30 can be protective for occasional use. Photoreactions may still occur with wavelengths of light that are not absorbed by currently available sunscreens. Some products that contain inert blocking agents such as zinc oxide and titanium dioxide may be helpful.

Benign pustular dermatoses include several innocent pustular eruptions that must be differentiated from infectious dermatoses. On biopsy, benign pustular dermatoses can be differentiated from herpes simplex lesions by the absence of multinucleated giant cells on Wright-stained smears of pustular contents. Negative Gram-stain and potassium hydroxide preparations can exclude bacterial and candidal infection. Viral and bacterial cultures may also help. Serologic studies for syphilis and scrapings for ectoparasites exclude syphilis and scabies in children with acropustulosis. Many benign pustular dermatoses can be confused with papulopustular rashes seen in sebaceous gland hyperplasia, miliaria, milia, and acne.

Erythema toxicum neonatorum is seen in up to 70% of full-term infants; the lesions, which are 2 to 3 mm in diameter, are erythematous and blotchy macules, papules, and pustules (Fig. 102.6A) that typically appear during the first 2 to 3 weeks after birth and then fade in about a week.[7] A Wright stain of the pustule contents reveals sheets of eosinophils and occasional neutrophils; 15% to 20% of patients show circulating eosinophilia.

Transient neonatal pustular melanosis is seen in <5% of African American infants. Lesions may be seen at birth as pustules 2 to 5 mm in diameter on a nonerythematous base (Fig. 102.6B)

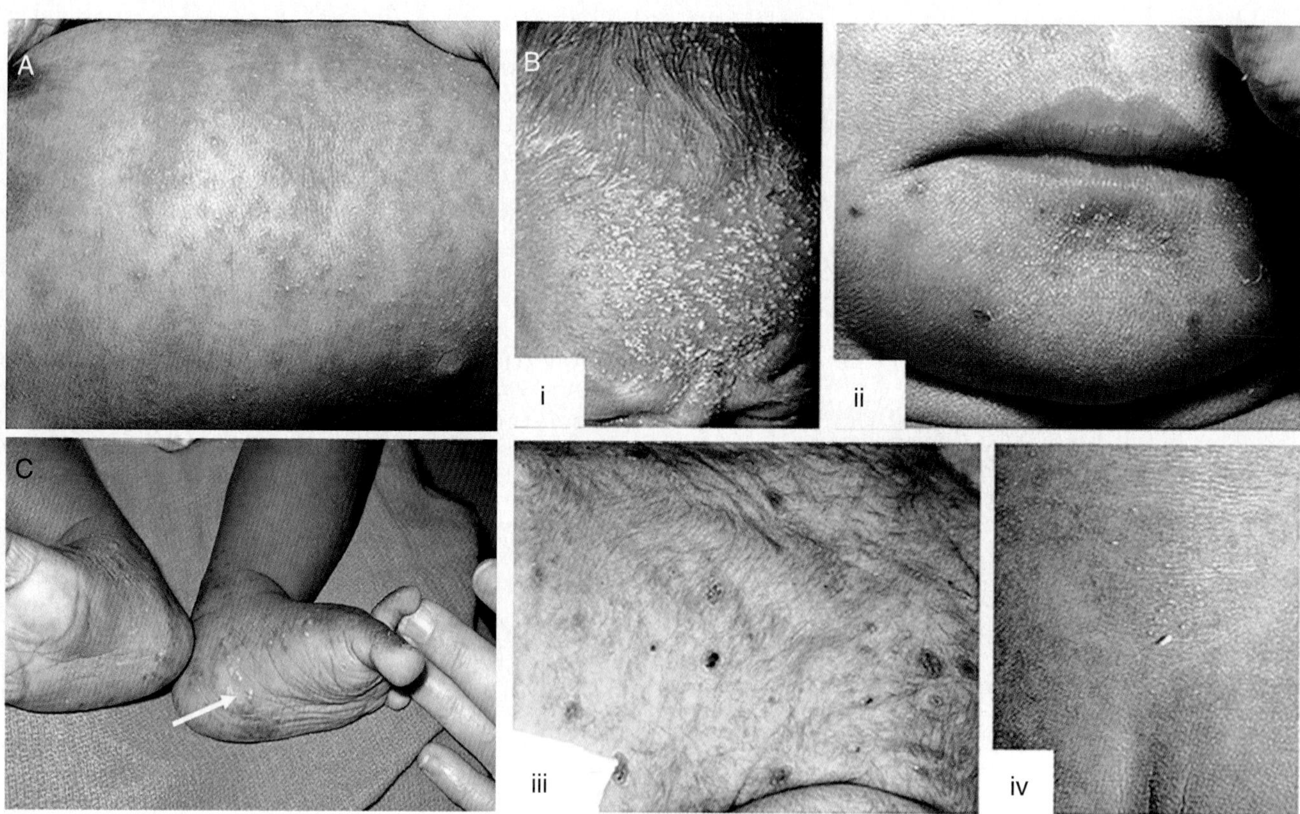

Fig. 102.6 (A) Erythema toxicum neonatorum. Numerous yellow papules and pustules are surrounded by large, intensely erythematous rings on the trunk of this infant. (B) Transient neonatal pustular melanosis. (i) Numerous tiny pustules dot the forehead and scalp of this light-pigmented neonate. (ii) Healing pustules leave marked hyperpigmentation and scales on the chin of this dark-pigmented baby. (iii) Dry, hyperpigmented crusts cover the back of this Asian newborn. (iv) Healing pustules and brown macules dot the lower back and sacrum of this child at birth. Note the Mongolian spot on his gluteal cleft. (C) Acropustulosis of infancy. Multiple 2- to 3-mm pustules covered the hands and feet of this otherwise healthy infant. Lesions recurred episodically until this child was 3 years old. (A, Reproduced with permission and minor modifications from Püttgen KB, Cohen BA. Neonatal dermatology. In: *Pediatric Dermatology*. 2:14-67; B, reproduced with permission and minor modifications from Püttgen KB, Cohen BA. Neonatal dermatology. In: *Pediatric Dermatology*. 2:14–67; C, reproduced with permission and minor modifications from Püttgen KB, Cohen BA. Neonatal dermatology. In: *Pediatric Dermatology*. 2:14–67.)

on the chin, neck, upper chest, sacrum, abdomen, and thighs. A central crust appears in a few days, which then desquamates to leave a hyperpigmented macule with a collarette of fine scale. Often, only brown macules with a rim of scale may be seen at birth. In lightly pigmented newborns, little or no hyperpigmentation remains. A Wright stain shows neutrophils and rare eosinophils.[8]

Acropustulosis of infancy is a chronic, recurrent, pustular, pruritic eruption that appears on the palms and soles (Fig. 102.6C) but may also involve the scalp, trunk, buttocks, and extremities. The lesions may first appear during the newborn period for 1 to 3 weeks, and episodes may recur until 2 to 3 years of age.[9] The cause is unknown; some infants have had scabies infestations prior to the onset of these lesions. Histopathology shows sterile, intraepidermal pustules with neutrophils and occasional eosinophils. Oral dapsone (2 mg/kg/day) can suppress symptoms in 24 to 48 hours. Topical application of high-potency corticosteroids on the palms and soles can also help.

Eosinophilic pustular folliculitis (Ofuji disease) is a rare, self-limiting vesiculopustular eruption on the scalp and forehead characterized by recurrent, follicular white vesicles and pustules 2 to 3 mm in diameter on an erythematous base. The disease typically affects young children but has also been noted in a few neonates. The lesions are marked by intense pruritus. The lesions contain large numbers of eosinophils, but no microorganisms have been seen. In some cases, eosinophilic pustular folliculitis may precede a fully evident hyperimmunoglobulin E syndrome. Topical corticosteroids, oral erythromycin, dapsone, colchicine, indomethacin, and cyclosporine may be helpful.[10]

Sebaceous gland hyperplasia is seen over the nose and cheeks of term infants. Lesions consist of multiple yellow papules 1 to 2 mm in diameter resulting from maternal or endogenous androgenic stimulation of sebaceous glands (Fig. 102.7). The eruption resolves within 4 to 6 months.[11]

Milia lesions are pearly, yellow papules 1 to 3 mm in diameter on the face, chin, and forehead of about half of all newborns (Fig. 102.8).[12] Similar lesions can occasionally be seen on the trunk and extremities. Most lesions resolve during the first month without treatment. Histology shows miniature epidermal inclusion cysts arising from the pilosebaceous appendages of vellus hair.

Miliaria results from obstruction and consequent rupture of eccrine sweat ducts. In term and preterm infants, miliaria occurs after the first week after birth in response to thermal stress. Lesions are seen in intertriginous areas and the scalp, face, and trunk.[13] In *miliaria crystallina*, superficial vesicles 1 to 2 mm in diameter appear on noninflamed skin due to blockage of ducts in the *stratum corneum* (Fig. 102.9A).[14] Small papules and pustules are typical of *miliaria rubra* (prickly heat), in which the obstruction occurs in the midepidermis (Fig. 102.9B). Deep-seated papulopustular lesions of *miliaria profunda* occur only rarely in infancy, when the duct ruptures at the dermal-epidermal junction. Cooling the skin and loosening clothing promotes resolution of the rash.

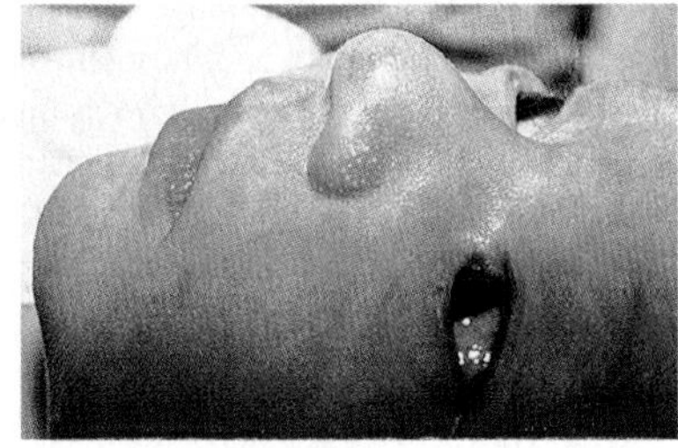

Fig. 102.7 Sebaceous Gland Hyperplasia. Note the yellow papules on the nose, forehead, and cheeks of this healthy newborn who also had a nodule that demonstrated the typical changes of Langerhans cell histiocytosis on histopathology. He had no evidence of systemic disease, and the nodule resolved without treatment over the first month of life. (Reproduced with permission and minor modifications from Püttgen KB, Cohen BA. Neonatal dermatology. In: *Pediatric Dermatology*. 2:14–67.)

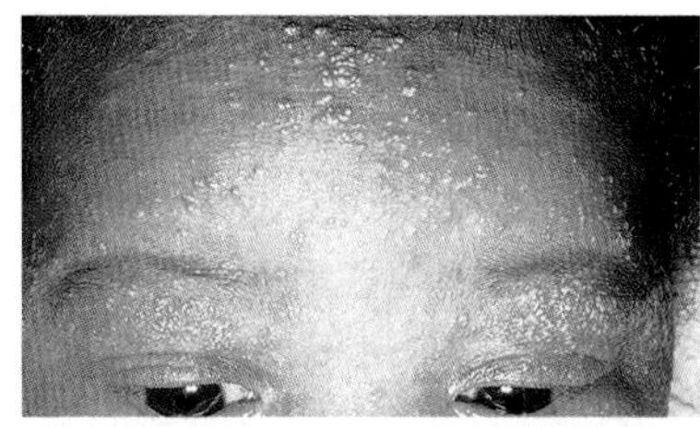

Fig. 102.8 Milia. Numerous pale small spherical lesion on the forehead and eyelids of a neonate. Cheek is another characteristic site. Reproduced with permission and minor modifications from Puttgen KB, et al. Neonatal dermatology. In: Pediatric Dermatology. Puttgen and Cohen, Eds. Published December 31, 2021. Pages 14-67.

Neonatal acne occurs in up to 20% of newborns; lesions may be present at birth, but the average onset is at 3 weeks. Inflammatory red papules and pustules predominate, and cysts may be seen. Unlike adolescent acne, no comedones are seen (Fig. 102.10).[15] The etiopathogenesis was believed to be related to stimulation of sebaceous glands by maternal androgens, but recent evidence suggests that these lesions may be an inflammatory reaction to colonizing *Malassezia* species.[16] Treatment is usually unnecessary because lesions involute spontaneously within 1 to 3 months. Ketoconazole cream may help in severe cases.

Subcutaneous fat necrosis is a rare, self-limited process that usually occurs in otherwise healthy full-term and postmature infants (Fig. 102.11). It has been reported to occur after total body cooling for treatment of hypoxic-ischemic encephalopathy. Discrete, tender, firm, red or hemorrhagic nodules and plaques up to 3 cm diameter appear on the cheeks, back, buttocks, arms, and thighs during the first few weeks of life.[8] The cause is unknown, but there may be a role of mechanical, cold, and hypoxic injury to fat. These nodules usually resolve without scarring in 1 to 2 months. Some lesions can get calcified. Many infants can develop nephrocalcinosis, poor weight gain, irritability, and seizures. Calcium should be monitored for the first 4 to 6 months after birth.[17] In some infants, thrombocytopenia, hyperlipidemia, and hyperglycemia may occur. Histopathology demonstrates fat necrosis with a foreign-body, giant-cell reaction. Remaining fat cells contain needle-shaped clefts, and calcium deposits are scattered throughout the subcutis.

Neonatal lupus erythematosus occurs with annular erythematous plaques 0.5 to 3 cm in diameter on the scalp, face, neck, upper trunk, and upper extremities (see Fig. 102.5B). A central scale, telangiectasias, atrophy, and pigmentary changes may be seen.[18] Some affected infants may show hepatosplenomegaly, anemia, leukopenia, thrombocytopenia, and lymphadenopathy. The disorder has been associated with transplacentally acquired anti-SS-A (Ro) and anti-SS-B (La) antibodies. Topical corticosteroids can expedite the resolution of inflammation in skin lesions, although atrophy, telangiectasias, and pigmentary changes may persist. The use of sunscreens and avoidance of direct sun exposure for a few months can help.

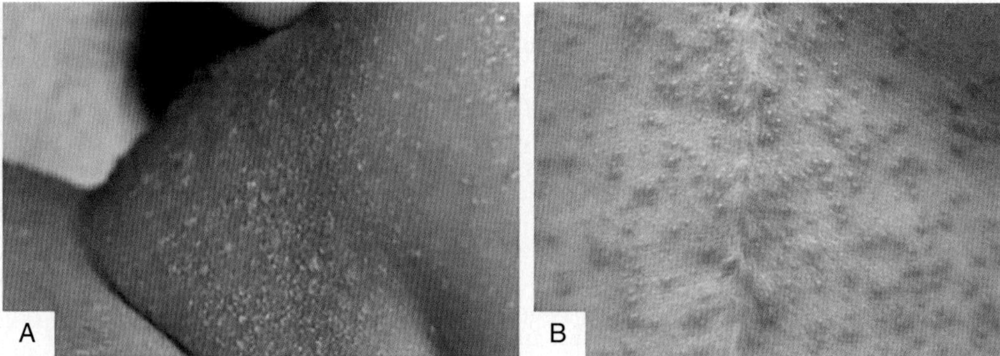

Fig. 102.9 Miliaria. (A) *Miliaria crystallina*. These tiny, thin-walled vesicles typically desquamate rapidly once the infant is moved to a cooler environment. (B) *Miliaria rubra*. Discrete, pruritic, erythematous papulovesicles. These lesions sometimes become confluent on an erythematous base. (A, Reproduced with permission and minor modifications from Miliaria crystallina. In: Fanaroff and Martin's Neonatal-Perinatal Medicine. Published December 31, 2019. Pages 1898-1932; B, reproduced with permission and minor modifications from James et al. Dermatoses Resulting From Physical Factors. In: *Andrews' Diseases of the Skin*, 3, 18–45.e3.)

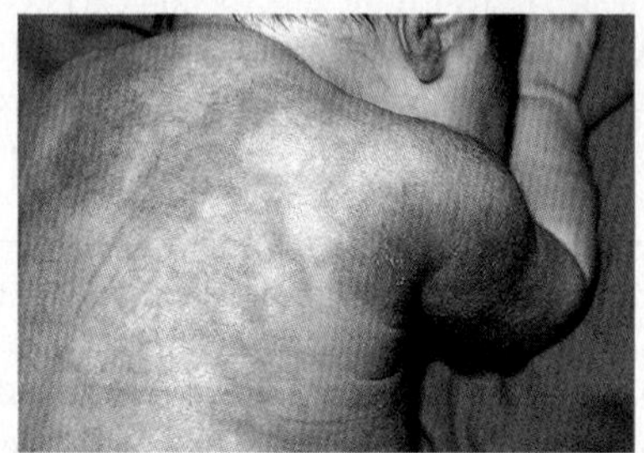

Fig. 102.10 Annular Erythema of Infancy. This eruption persisted for months on the trunk and extremities of an otherwise healthy infant. (Reproduced with permission and minor modifications from Püttgen KB, Cohen BA. Neonatal dermatology. In: *Pediatric Dermatology*. 2:14–67.)

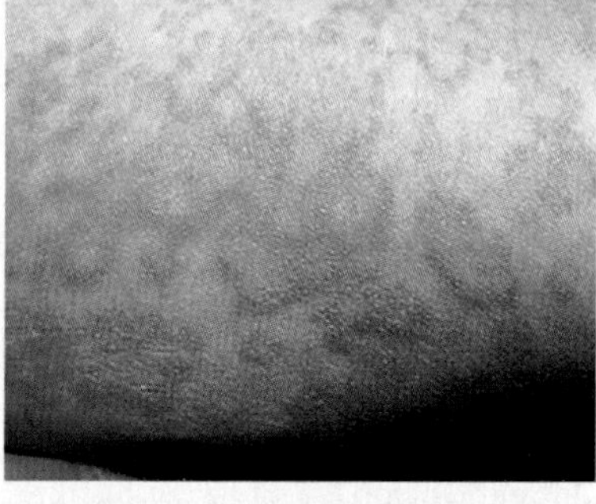

Fig. 102.12 Subcutaneous Fat Necrosis. Indurated, erythematous nodules and plaques on the shoulders and back. (Paller AS, Mancini AJ. Cutaneous disorders of the newborn. In: *Paller and Mancini—Hurwitz Clinical Pediatric Dermatology*. 2:11–41.e5.)

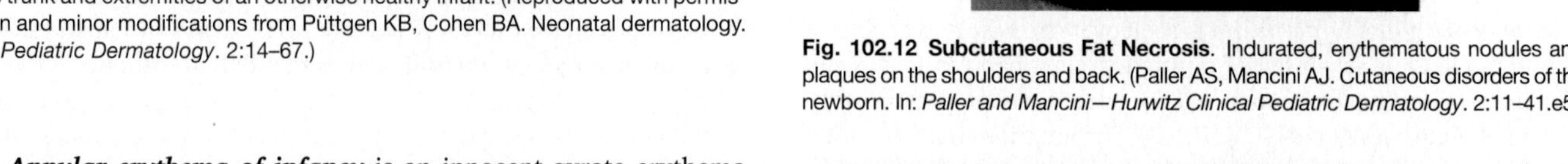

Annular erythema of infancy is an innocent gyrate erythema with red papules/plaques. Lesions may show a dusky center and may exceed 10 cm in diameter over 1 to 3 weeks (Fig. 102.12).[19] This reaction may be triggered by infections and drugs. Fortunately, these infants generally continue to thrive, and most lesions eventually resolve without treatment.

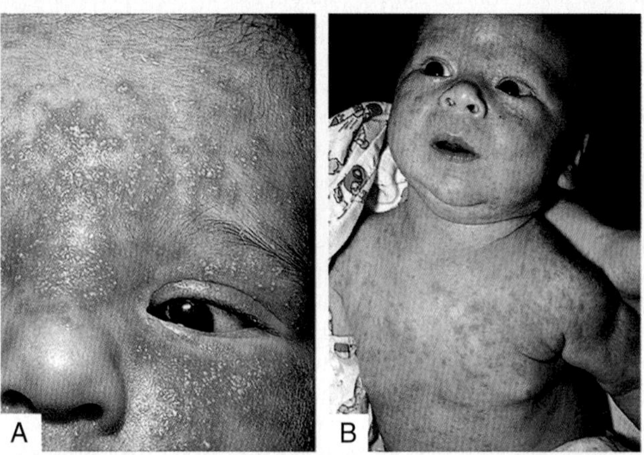

Fig. 102.11 Neonatal Acne. (A) Red papules and pustules covered the face of this 4-week-old boy. (B) Acne spread to the trunk of this healthy infant. In both children, the eruption resolved by 4 months of age. (Reproduced with permission and minor modifications from Püttgen KB, Cohen BA. Neonatal dermatology. In: *Pediatric Dermatology*. 2:14–67.)

Minor Congenital Anomalies That Predominantly Involve the Skin

Dimpling is frequently seen over bony prominences, particularly in the sacral area (Fig. 102.13A). Skin dimples may be the first sign of several dysmorphic syndromes, but most such lesions are usually of only cosmetic consequence. Spinal anomalies should be excluded when deep dimples, sinus tracts, or other cutaneous lesions such as lipomas, hemangiomas, nevi, and tufts of hair are seen over the lumbosacral spine. This area is readily visualized by ultrasound during the first 8 to 12 weeks after conception. Magnetic resonance imaging may provide more details.[20]

Periauricular sinuses, pits, tags/tragi, and cysts occur when brachial arches or clefts fail to fuse or close normally. These lesions develop between the preauricular area to the corner of the mouth (Fig. 102.13B).[21] Defects may be unilateral or bilateral and are occasionally associated with other facial or more complex malformation syndromes such as Goldenhar (oculoauriculovertebral) syndrome or branchio-oto-renal syndrome.[22,23] Most lesions are excised during childhood.[24]

Digital Abnormalities

Supernumerary digits are rudimentary structures at the base of the thumb or ulnar side of the fifth finger.[25] These are usually familial and asymptomatic. Histology shows nerve bundles and dermal connective tissue. A good cosmetic result is best achieved by local surgical excision. Syndactyly shows fused fingers. The fingers can be normal or anomalous; the number of affected fingers can differ (Fig. 102.13C).

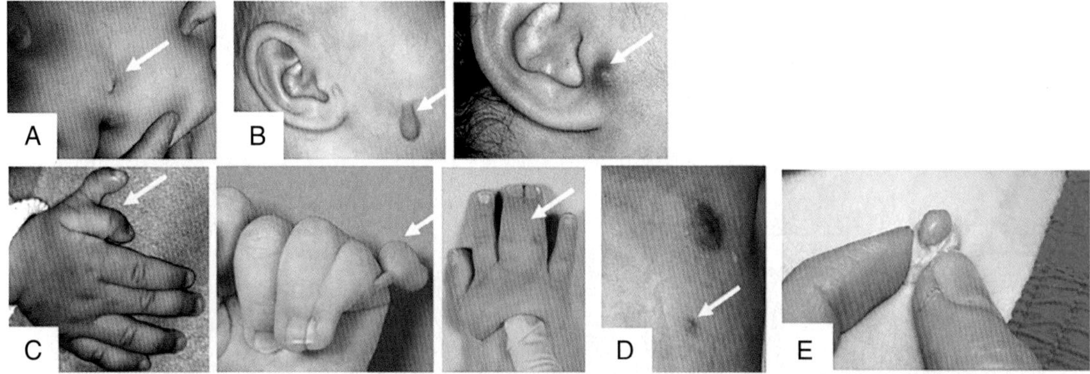

Fig. 102.13 Minor Congenital Anomalies. (A) Midline deep sacral dimple. The dimple was located above the gluteal cleft in association with a small tail. In contrast, a shallow dimple within the gluteal cleft is a common finding and not a sign of spinal dysraphism. (B) Accessory skin tag on cheek. Image on the right shows a congenital cyst in the preauricular area. (C) Supernumerary thumb, postaxial polydactyly, and syndactyly. (D) Supernumerary nipple with a surrounding areola. (E) An umbilical granuloma that responded to shave removal with light cautery. (A, Reproduced with permission and minor modifications from Abidi NY, Martin KL. Cutaneous defects. In: *Nelson Textbook of Pediatrics*, ch. 667, pp. 3456–3459 e1; B, reproduced with permission and minor modifications from Abidi NY, Martin KL. Cutaneous defects. In: *Nelson Textbook of Pediatrics*, ch. 667, pp. 3456–3459 e1, and image on the right reproduced with permission and minor modifications from Neonatal dermatology. In: Püttgen KB, Cohen, BA. *Pediatric Dermatology*. 2021: 14–67; C, the three images were reproduced with permission and minor modifications from Congenital hand IV: Syndactyly, synostosis, polydactyly, camptodactyly, and clinodactyly. In: Hovius SER, van Nieuwenhoven CA. *Plastic Surgery: Volume 6: Hand and Upper Extremity*. 2017:624–655.e4; D, panels G and H reproduced with permission and minor modifications from Developmental anomalies. In: Antaya RJ and Schaffer JV. *Dermatology*. 64:1057–1074; E, reproduced with permission and minor modifications from Püttgen KB, Cohen BA. Neonatal dermatology. In: *Pediatric Dermatology*. 2:14–67.)

Supernumerary nipples may be seen anywhere from the midaxilla to the inguinal area (Fig. 102.13D).[26] Some lesions lack areolae. Malignant degeneration is rare; excision is primarily for cosmetic purposes.

Umbilical granulomas and polyps are seen in infants in whom the cord separation gets delayed beyond the normal 7 to 14 days after birth (Fig. 102.13E).[24] Excessive moisture and low-grade infection may enhance the growth of granulation tissue. Cauterization with silver nitrate or desiccation with isopropyl alcohol promotes healing.

Umbilical polyps may result from persistence of the omphalomesenteric duct or urachus and may be seen as a red polyp with histopathological evidence of gastrointestinal or urinary mucosa. A mucoid discharge may occur at the tip. Surgical excision is necessary.[24]

Complications Associated With Neonatal Intensive Care

Reactive erythema with erythematous macules, plaques, and nodules can be triggered by various endogenous and environmental factors. In infants, erythema multiforme, erythema nodosum, urticaria, and vasculitis can occur after exposure to various infections and drugs. Management of affected infants involves identification and elimination of the offending agent.

Arterial catheters can cause local scarring (Fig. 102.14A) and distal ischemic damage. Umbilical arterial catheters can also cause vasospasm or thromboembolism, with resulting ischemia and necrosis of the genital and buttock skin (Fig. 102.14B). These ulcerations may take months to heal and require surgical repair. Radial artery catheters can also cause digital necrosis. In some infants, subtle findings such as discrepancies in hand size can become noticeable over time.

Vascular lines: Sites of insertion of subclavian and jugular venous lines can show small scars, but most fade away during infancy. There may be some dimpling at suture lines. Chest tube placement sites can show adhesions, scars, or injury to sensitive breast tissue. Most lesions fade away with time. Lateral placement beyond the breast tissue may reduce cosmetic damage.

Repeated heel-sticks for blood sampling can induce nodule formation (Fig. 102.14C), some of which can become calcified or turn into scars. Lesions are noticeable but usually not symptomatic.

Irritant, chemical, and thermal burns: Solutions containing topical iodophors (Fig. 102.14D) or irritant solvents can produce an erosive irritant dermatitis (Fig. 102.14E).[27] Repeated trauma from removal of monitor leads can cause skin atrophy at the sites where the electrodes were attached (Fig. 102.14F). Blocked intravascular catheters and soft-tissue infiltration by intravenous fluids can cause cutaneous inflammation. Hypertonic fluids can cause tissue damage.[28] Such lesions heal slowly and can even damage local tendons and joints.

Congenital Disorders of Skin Structure Seen in Newborn Infants

Epidermolysis bullosa (EB) dermatoses are blistering disorders marked by the development of skin lesions after trauma (Table 102.1, Fig. 102.15).[29] As described in this table, three types of EB can present in neonates.

The diagnosis of EB needs a detailed family history and a skin biopsy for immunofluorescent epitope mapping and/or electron microscopy. Prenatal diagnosis is possible using gene markers on amniocytes or electron microscopy on fetal skin biopsies. Infants with dystrophic EB may do well, whereas junctional disease may progressively worsen.

Treatment may need to be tailored according to the severity of disease.[30] In mild disease, trauma needs to be avoided to prevent the formation of bullae. Pain and progression of large blisters may be controlled by gently unroofing lesions or cutting a square skin window and covering with a topical antibiotic ointment and sterile gauze. Adhesives are applied from dressing to dressing and kept out of direct contact with the skin.

Severely afflicted infants need a multidisciplinary team for management, including a pediatrician, dermatologist, ophthalmologist, gastroenterologist, otolaryngologist, plastic surgeon, thoracic surgeon, and dentist, and a physical therapist may be needed. Preventive care includes avoidance of trauma to the skin and mucous membranes and early treatment of infection with topical and oral antibiotics. Iron may be required to replace chronic blood losses through the skin. Nonadhering dressings such as Vaseline gauze help retain moisture, reduce pain, and facilitate healing of erosions and ulcers.

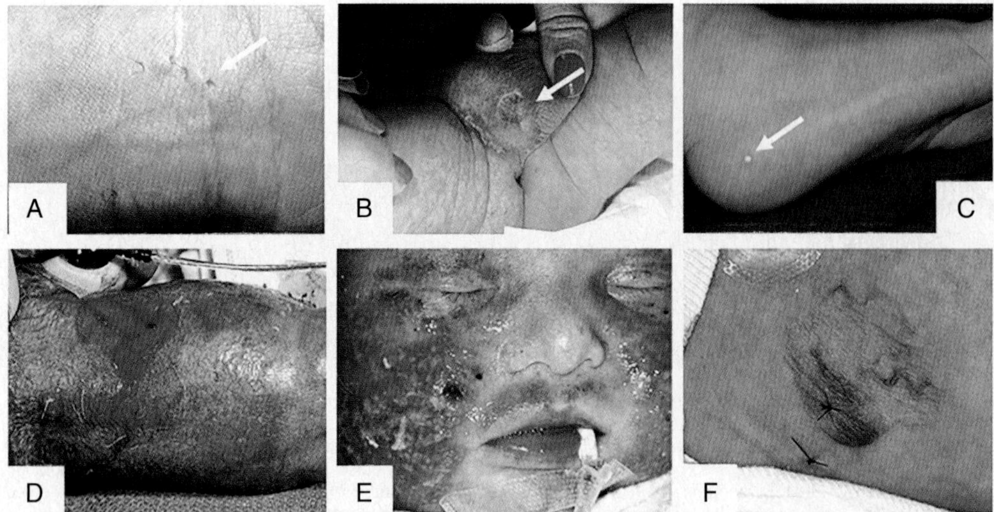

Fig. 102.14 Surgical Scars Due to Events During Intensive Care. (A) Scars at an arterial cut down site. (B) Umbilical artery catheter (UAC)-related injury. Several hours after a UAC was removed from this infant, a purple area developed unilaterally on the scrotum, perineum, and perirectal skin. After 1 day, the area became ulcerated. Note the formation of granulation tissue and early scarring 1 week later. (C) Heel-stick calcinosis. Firm, yellow-white papule on the lateral plantar heel of an infant who had multiple heel sticks as a newborn. (D) Application of a solution containing topical iodophor produced an erosive irritant dermatitis on the flank of a premature infant in the intensive care nursery. Fortunately, this area healed with only minimal scarring. (E) A chemical burn resulted from a solvent that was applied to this child's face to remove adhesive tape. Accidental thermal burns have been reported after exposure to heated water beds, radiant warmers, transcutaneous oxygen monitors, and heated, humidified air. Although cold stress must be minimized in the small premature infant, extensive burns that have cutaneous and airway involvement may be prevented by close monitoring of these devices. (F) Repeated trauma from removal of monitor leads produced a round, atrophic patch on the lower abdominal wall of this 29-week premature infant. Skin wrinkling, prominent vessels, and purpura are seen. (A, Reproduced with permission and minor modifications from Püttgen KB, Cohen BA. Neonatal dermatology. In: *Pediatric Dermatology*. 2:14–67; B, reproduced with permission and minor modifications from Püttgen KB, Cohen BA. Neonatal dermatology. In: *Pediatric Dermatology*. 2:14–67; C, reproduced with permission and minor modifications from Paller AS, Mancini AJ. Cutaneous disorders of the newborn. In: *Paller and Mancini—Hurwitz Clinical Pediatric Dermatology*. 2:11-41.e5; F, Panels d, e, and f were reproduced with permission and minor modifications from Püttgen KB, Cohen BA. Neonatal dermatology. In: *Pediatric Dermatology*. 2:14–67.)

Table 102.1 Epidermolysis Bullosa (EB) Variants That Can Present During the Neonatal Period

Type	Variant	Site of Blisters	Inheritance: Autosomal Dominant (AD) or Recessive (AR)	Molecular Defect	Clinical Features
Epidermolysis bullosa simplex (EBS)	EBS, Dowling–Meara	Basal layer for all EBS subtypes	AD	K5 (keratin 5), K14 (keratin 14)	Generalized blisters, grouped nail dystrophy, scarring; improve with age
	EBS, other generalized		AD	K5 (keratin 5), K14 (keratin 14)	Generalized blisters, nonscarring, worse on hands and feet
	EBS, muscular dystrophy		AR	PLEC1 (Plectin)	Generalized blisters; muscular dystrophy; granulation tissue in respiratory tract
	EBS, pyloric atresia		AR	*PLEC1 ITGA6, ITGB4* (α6β4-integrin)	Generalized blisters, aplasia cutis, pyloric atresia, deformities of pinnae and nasal alae, cryptorchidism
Junctional epidermolysis bullosa (JEB)	JEB–Herlitz	Lamina lucida for all JEB variants	AR	*LAMA3, LAMB3, LAMC2* (laminin-332)	Generalized blisters, nonscarring, nail dystrophy, oral-dental lesions; often lethal
	JEB–non-Herlitz			*LAMA3, LAMB3, LAMC2* (laminin-332)	Localized blistering of hands, feet; nail dystrophy; enamel dysplasia
	JEB–pyloric atresia			*ITGA6, ITGB4* (α6β4-integrin)	Generalized blisters, widespread aplasia cutis, genitourinary malformations, pyloric atresia
Dystrophic epidermolysis bullosa (DEB)	Generalized	Sublamina densa	AD	*COL7A1* (type VII collagen)	Albopapuloid skin lesions in some; mild esophageal and oral involvement
	Severe generalized			AR	Skin fragility; widespread blisters, scarring; nail dystrophy; risk of squamous cell carcinoma; severe oral, dental, esophageal, intestinal, and genitourinary involvement
	Generalized other			AR	Mild widespread lesions; mild oral involvement; normal life span

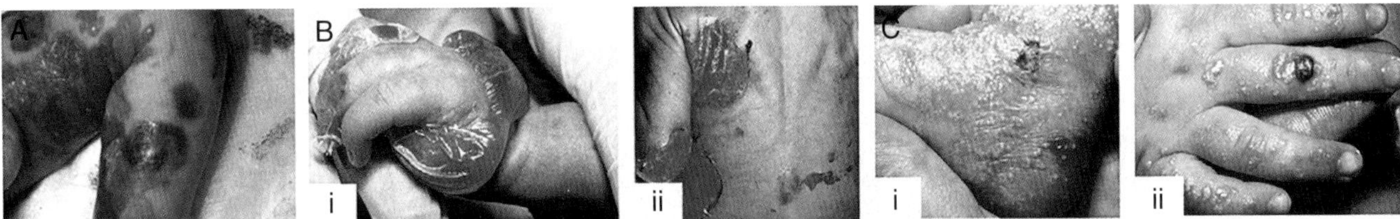

Fig. 102.15 Epidermolysis Bullosa. (A) *Epidermolysis bullosa simplex*. Numerous blisters form primarily in pressure areas on the hands and feet. (B) Junctional epidermolysis bullosa. Widespread involvement was seen in this infant at birth. (i) Note the erosions and the large, intact blister over the thumb and dorsum of the hand. (ii) Large, denuded areas occur over the back and buttocks. (C) Dystrophic epidermolysis bullosa. (i) Blisters, erosions, and hundreds of milia are seen on the foot and ankle and (ii) hand of this newborn. (A, Reproduced with permission and minor modifications from: Narendran V. The skin of the neonate. In: *Fanaroff and Martin's Neonatal-Perinatal Medicine*. 2019:1898–1932; B, reproduced with permission and minor modifications from: Püttgen KB, Cohen BA. Neonatal dermatology. In: *Pediatric Dermatology*, 2:14-67; C, reproduced with permission and minor modifications from: Püttgen KB, Cohen BA. Neonatal dermatology. In: *Pediatric Dermatology*, 2:14–67.)

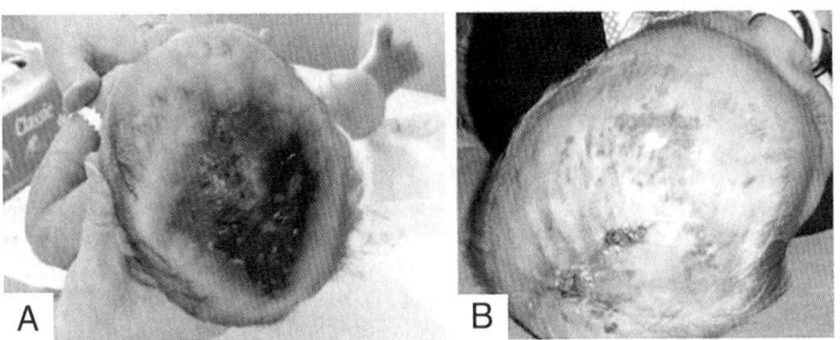

Fig. 102.16 Aplasia Cutis Congenita. Large, full-thickness scalp defects in neonates. (A) Scalp defect accompanied by a cranial bony defect. Conservative management without surgery led to complete bony recovery of the skull at 8 months of age. (B) Defect with residual scar alopecia and epithelialization of the skin defect with a hair collar. (Reproduced with permission and minor modifications from Narendran V. The skin of the neonate. In: *Fanaroff and Martin's Neonatal-Perinatal Medicine*. 2019;1898–1932.)

Aplasia cutis congenita is an idiopathic, heterogeneous group of disorders marked by congenital absence of the skin (Fig. 102.16).[31] The lesions appear as erosions or ulcerations covered with a crust or thin membrane, which heal with atrophic, hairless scars over the next few months, and involve the vertex of the scalp and sometimes the trunk and extremities.

Some congenital melanocytic nevi, nevoid malformations with hairless patches, perinatal trauma, scalp blood sampling, monitoring electrodes, and the application of forceps may also produce similar scalp ulcers. Magnetic resonance imaging (MRI) can help evaluate for connection to the underlying brain and bone. Uncomplicated lesions may be amenable to simple excisions or may need staged repair. Gentle normal saline compresses, topical antibiotics, and sterile dressings are adequate for most patients.

Mastocytosis can be seen at birth or in early infancy with one or more blistering cutaneous lesions or urticaria pigmentosa (cutaneous mastocytosis; Fig. 102.17).[32] The lesions show accumulated mast cells. Most cases are sporadic; some may have familial transmission.

Most lesions are seen on the trunk as macules, papules, and plaques, although other regions or organs such as the gastrointestinal tract, bone marrow, lungs, kidneys, and nervous system can be involved. Nonspecific physical stimuli can activate the mast cells and can trigger the appearance of urticarial lesions in the region. The Darier sign shows induction of hives upon stroking the affected skin.[33] The release of histamine and other vasoactive mediators from mast cells can trigger acute or chronic pruritus, diarrhea, gastric ulceration, bleeding, and hypotension.

Pruritus and systemic symptoms can usually be controlled with antihistamines and/or enteral cromolyn sodium 20 to 30 mg/kg/day divided in 4 doses. Severe cases can be treated with topical corticosteroids under occlusion, systemic corticosteroids, or photochemotherapy (psoralen-ultraviolet A light). The disease typically progresses for 1 to 2 years and then improves slowly.

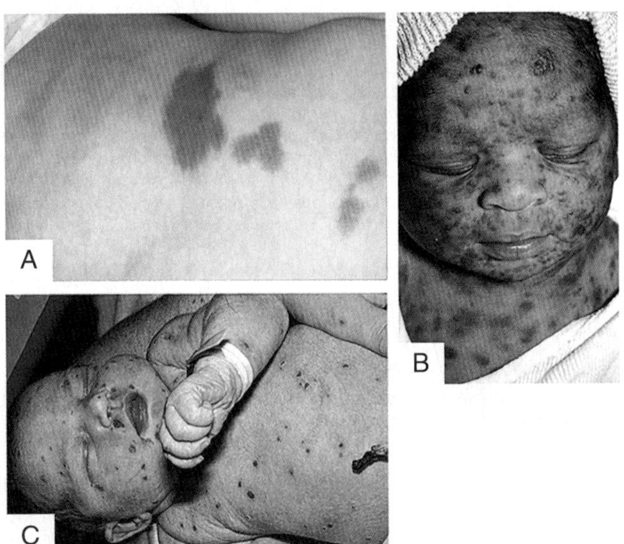

Fig. 102.17 Mastocytosis. (A) Urticaria pigmentosa. These solitary mastocytomas appear as red-brown plaques. (B) Hyperpigmentation is prominent in this healthy Black infant with urticaria pigmentosa. Note the blisters on her forehead. (C) Vesicles and crusted papules on a red urticarial base were present at birth in this asymptomatic newborn. After the crusts healed, no blisters recurred. (A, Reproduced with permission and minor modifications from Dinulos JGH. Urticaria, angioedema, and pruritus. In: *Habif's Clinical Dermatology*, ch. 6, 176–214.e1; B and C, reproduced with permission and minor modifications from Püttgen KB, Cohen BA. Neonatal dermatology. In: *Pediatric Dermatology*, 2:14–67.)

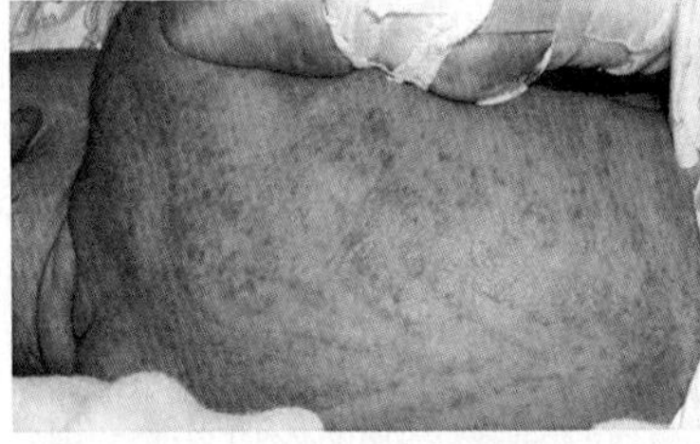

Fig. 102.18 Incontinentia Pigmenti. Erythematous vesicopapular lesions following the lines of Blaschko in a V-shaped configuration over the dorsal skin. Lesions typically evolve through verrucous, hyperpigmented stages to finally manifest hypopigmentation and dermal atrophy. (Reproduced with permission and minor modifications from Narendran V. The skin of the neonate. In: *Fanaroff and Martin's Neonatal-Perinatal Medicine*, 94:1898–1932.)

Incontinentia pigmenti is a neurocutaneous syndrome seen in neonates as patches of erythema and blisters on the trunk, scalp, and extremities, which are typically oriented in reticulated lines and swirls that follow the lines of Blaschko, special embryonic cleavage planes (Fig. 102.18). In later infancy, the lesions mature into hyperkeratotic, warty, marble-cake swirls and plaques.[34]

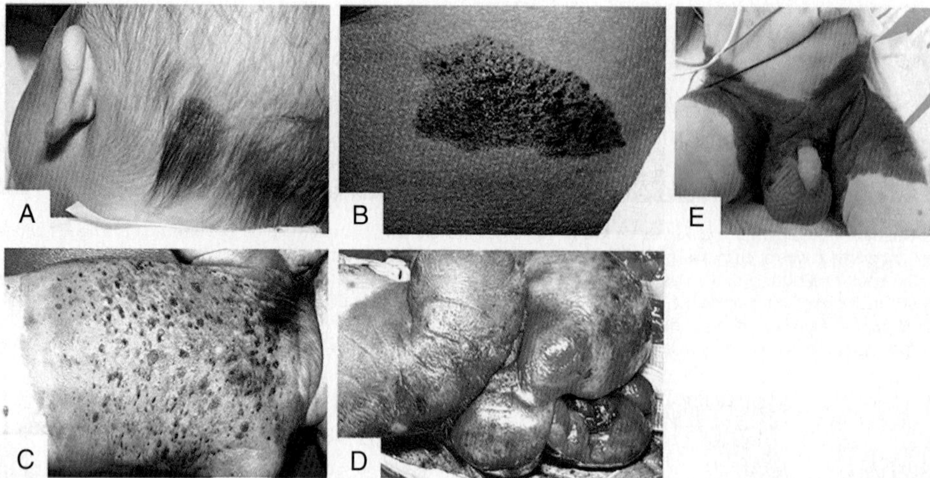

Fig. 102.19 **Congenital Pigmented Nevi**. (A) A small congenital pigmented nevus was associated with a tuft of dark hair on the scalp of an infant. (B) A medium-sized, 5-cm by 3-cm epidermal nevus uniformly studded with dark brown papules on the back. (C) A giant pigmented nevus contained numerous darkly pigmented nodules was associated with leptomeningeal involvement. (D) A large tumor developed within a giant pigmented nevus that involved the diaper area of this newborn. The tumor contained structures that arose from various neuroectodermal elements. The tumor was excised in several stages. (E) A relatively homogenous giant congenital melanocytic nevus involving the bathing trunk area with sparing of the genitalia. The skin was thickened with hypertrichosis. (D, Reproduced with permission and minor modifications from Püttgen KB, Cohen BA. Neonatal dermatology. In: *Pediatric Dermatology*, 2:14–67; E, reproduced with permission and minor modifications from Narendran V. The skin of the neonate. In: *Fanaroff and Martin's Neonatal-Perinatal Medicine*. 2019;1898–1932.)

Nevi/birthmarks: Nevi are hamartomatous skin lesions seen at birth or early infancy. These contain mature or nearly mature cutaneous epidermal or dermal elements (Fig. 102.19).[35]

Vascular anomalies: Infantile hemangiomas (IH) are vascular neoplasms seen in nearly 10% of all infants (Fig. 102.20). The details are included in the section focused on vascular malformations below. Many lesions regress during the second year (Fig. 102.21). The differential diagnosis includes the rare kaposiform hemangioendotheliomas and tufted angiomas, which may be associated with coagulopathy. Many of these rare hemangioma-like tumors have a bluish-purple appearance. These clinical features, temporal changes, and histopathological findings help differentiate these lesions.

IH need to be carefully differentiated from various vascular malformations (Table 102.2).[36] These vascular malformations are usually classified based on flow characteristics into slow-flow capillary, venous, and lymphatic malformations and fast-flow arterial or arteriovenous malformations.[37] Complex malformations may show characteristics of several different vascular structures.

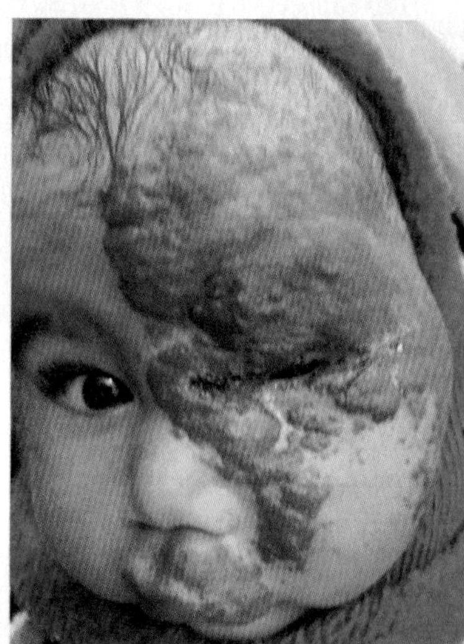

Fig. 102.20 Infantile Hemangioma Extending Into the Orbit. (Photograph provided by Dr. Devendra Panwar, Pediatric Surgeon, Jalandhar, India; Global Newborn Society.)

Vascular Malformations

Salmon patches (capillary ectasias, transient macular stains) are well-recognized capillary malformations that are typically seen on the nape of the neck ("stork bite"), glabella, forehead ("angel kiss"), upper eyelids, and sacrum (Fig. 102.22).[38] Some lesions fade during infancy or get camouflaged in normal pigmentation. Lesions on the neck and sacrum may be more persistent. The lesions may look more prominent during crying, breath holding, and physical exertion. These lesions do not usually require further evaluation.

Port-wine stains are capillary malformations that persist unchanged during childhood (Fig. 102.23).[39] These lesions are typically unilateral around the face, but other parts of the body can be involved. Such stains, particularly those that evolve into arteriovenous malformations, have been described in several genetic syndromes, so the patients need careful evaluation. Stains in the upper face may need evaluation for Sturge-Weber syndrome, which is associated with vascular malformations of the ipsilateral meninges, cerebral cortex, and eye. Superficial vascular lesions with limb or segmental trunk hypertrophy may be associated with Klippel–Trenaunay syndrome and may include capillary venous or capillary lymphatic venous malformations.

Venous malformations are slow-flow, dilated vascular channels in the deep dermis. The vessel walls are usually thin and fibrous. Superficial venous malformations may present as scattered or grouped blue or purple papules and nodules (Fig. 102.24), but deeper lesions may show a blue hue. Small localized lesions are often isolated. However, disseminated lesions may be associated with malformation syndromes such as blue rubber bleb nevus syndrome or Maffucci syndrome.

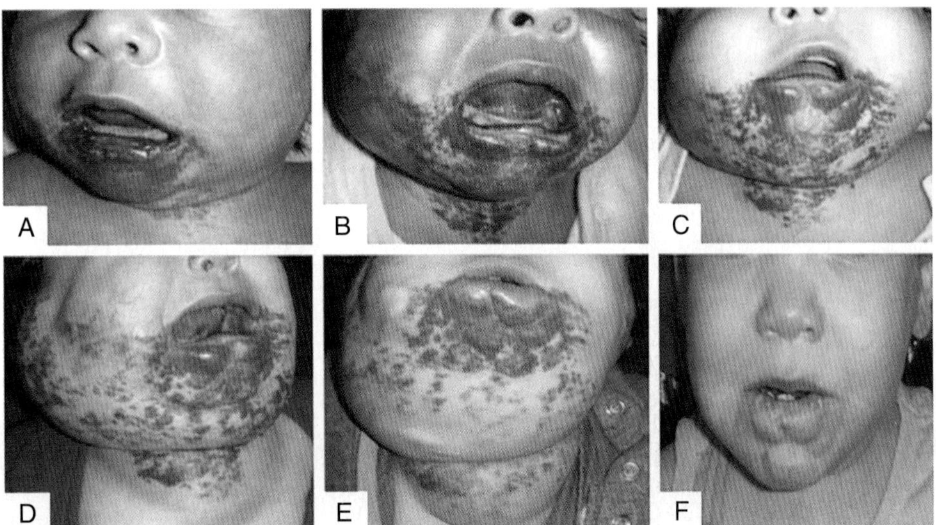

Fig. 102.21 Age-Related Regression in Infantile Hemangioma. (A) A lesion appeared on the lower face during the second postnatal week. Corticosteroid treatment was initiated. (B) An ulcerated area was noted on the lower lip at 4 weeks. (C) The ulcer began to heal at 2 months of age. (D) The hemangioma remained relatively stable for the next few months. Corticosteroid therapy was weaned, but the hemangioma began to grow again at age 11 months. (E) Propranolol therapy was initiated at 12 months. (F) Six months later, at 18 months of age, there was definite regression in the size of the hemangioma. (Reproduced with permission and minor modifications from Elsevier Point of Care, updated January 15, 2020.)

Table 102.2 Comparison of Hemangiomas and Vascular Malformations

	Hemangioma	Vascular Malformation
Clinical features	Subtle at birth; show rapid growth during infancy, and then regress spontaneously	Usually visible at birth; proportionate growth
Sex ratio	3:1 female predominance	1:1
Pathology	Proliferative neoplasm; hyperplastic endothelial cells	Flat endothelial cells form mature vascular structures; dysplastic vessels seen in proliferative, hyperplastic vascular tumors
Bone changes	Usually do not produce a mass effect	Variable distortion, thinning, invasion, rare destruction
Immunohistochemical markers	Markers of proliferative vascular tumors	No known markers
Coagulopathy	None; may be associated with vascular tumors such as tufted angiomas	Slow-flow venous, lymphatic, and combined lymphatic-venous malformations; may develop coagulopathy

Over time, venous malformations can induce distortions in underlying bones or joint damage with swelling, pain, and functional impairment.[40] Some lesions can be managed with conservative measures such as compression garments, but symptomatic lesions may need ablation with percutaneous sclerotherapy and/or surgical excision.

Lymphatic malformations are congenital malformations of the lymphatic system, many of which can be seen in newborn infants. Lesions are seen mostly on the head and neck. Histopathologically, there are large macrocystic lymphatic malformations containing lymph-filled spaces that show no connection with the rest of the lymphatic or venous system. Lesions with thrombosis or bleeding after trauma may show purple or black discoloration. Most lymphatic malformations involve skin and soft tissue; 10% involve viscera or bone.[41]

Lymphatic malformations may be seen in several syndromic conditions. In Proteus syndrome, dermal and subcutaneous lymphatic and venous malformations are associated with cutaneous port-wine stains, soft-tissue tumors, and epidermal nevi (Fig. 102.25).[42] Vascular malformations may extend into the mediastinum, peritoneum, retroperitoneal space, and viscera.

Surgical management of lymphatic malformations is difficult because they often extend around vital structures, and recurrence rates are high. Superficial lesions may be ablated with the carbon dioxide laser. Some of the deeper malformations may improve with sclerotherapy.

Arteriovenous malformations are fast-flow anomalies seen frequently on the head and neck (Fig. 102.26). Approximately half of the lesions are present at birth and appear similar to capillary or venous malformations; they may appear as tense vascular masses with a palpable thrill, bruit, and infiltration of the overlying skin.[37] Ultrasound and MRI studies can be useful in diagnosis.

Inflammatory Disorders of the Neonatal Skin

Acute inflammatory changes may include edema, erythema, and vesiculation; subacute/chronic changes may include scaling, lichenification, and altered pigmentation in the skin. Microscopically, the characteristics are epidermal thickening, leukocyte infiltration in the dermis, and scaling.

Diaper dermatitis is well recognized; red, scaly, and erosive lesions are seen in the perineum, lower abdomen, buttocks, and proximal thighs, but the intertriginous areas may be spared (Fig. 102.27A). The pathogenesis may involve contact dermatitis due to irritants.[43] The diaper area is at particular risk because of the

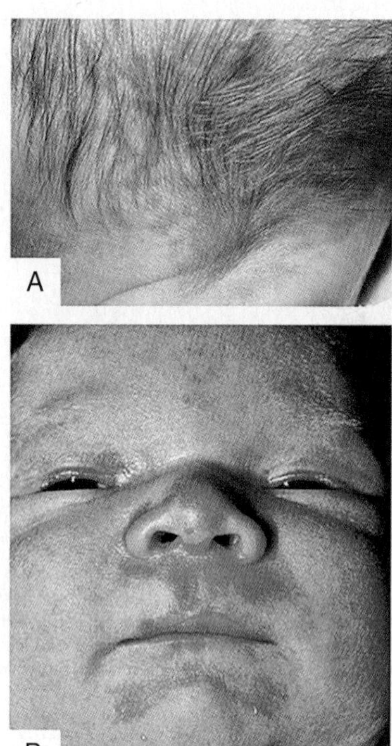

Fig. 102.22 Salmon Patches. (A) Typical, light-red, splotchy patch at the nape of the neck in a healthy newborn. (B) Similar patches were present on this child's eyelids, nose, upper lip, and chin. (Reproduced with permission and minor modifications from Püttgen KB, Cohen BA. Neonatal dermatology. In: *Pediatric Dermatology*, 2, 14-67.)

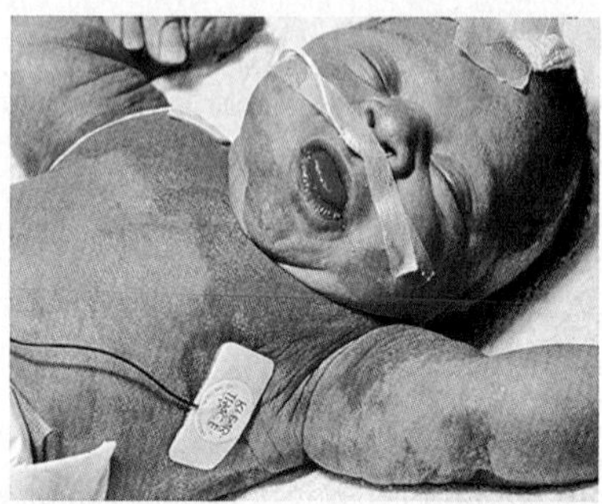

Fig. 102.23 Port-Wine Stains. This newborn had a port-wine stain involving his upper chest, neck, and portions of both arms that was associated with soft-tissue hypertrophy (Klippel-Trenaunay-Weber syndrome) and high-output cardiac failure. (Reproduced with permission and minor modifications from Püttgen KB, Cohen BA. Neonatal dermatology. In: *Pediatric Dermatology*, 2:14–67.)

continuous exposure to urine and feces. Irritants in powders and detergents and fecal bacteria may augment the inflammation.

Cleansing of the area, application of lubricants such as petrolatum, barrier pastes such as zinc oxide, and if possible, allowing the area to dry up using cloth diapers for a few days may be helpful. A few days of topical application of a low-potency topical corticosteroid such as hydrocortisone may expedite healing.

Allergic contact dermatitis may account for occasional diaper rashes (Fig. 102.27B).[44] Fragrances, preservatives, and emulsifiers in topical baby products and diapers may be associated with allergic reactions in the diaper area and on the face, trunk, and extremities. Cessation of the use of the offending agent, application of emollients, and treatment with a topical corticosteroid ointment such as hydrocortisone should solve the problem.

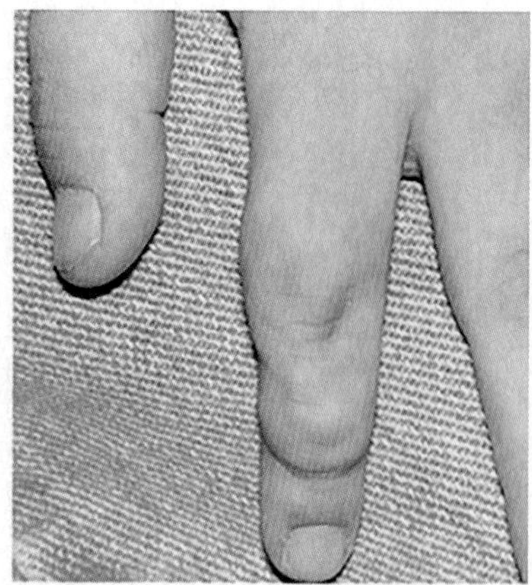

Fig. 102.24 Venous Malformation. A small subcutaneous congenital venous malformation on the right second finger was associated with aching pain, particularly after intense physical activity in this 6-year-old boy. (Reproduced with permission and minor modifications from Püttgen KB, Cohen BA. Neonatal dermatology. In: *Pediatric Dermatology*, 2:14–67.)

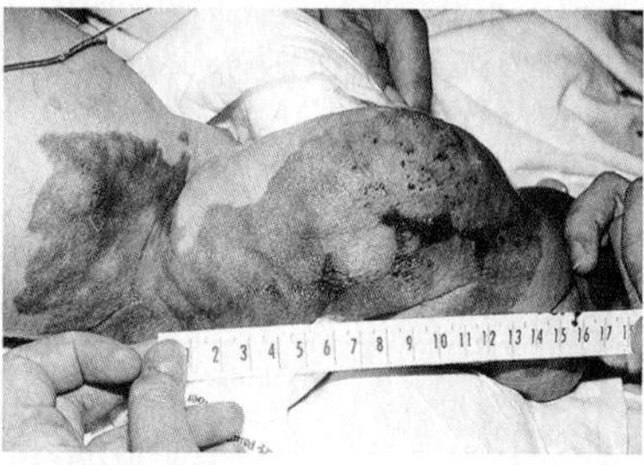

Fig. 102.25 Proteus Syndrome. Massive hypertrophy of the leg was associated with an extensive cutaneous port-wine stain, soft-tissue tumors, and a deep lymphangiohemangioma that involved the thigh, peritoneal cavity, and retroperitoneal space in this 1-month-old boy. These anomalies typically involve slow-flow vascular anomalies (capillary malformation, varicose veins, and macrocystic lymphatic malformations). (Reproduced with permission and minor modifications from Hook KP. Cutaneous vascular anomalies in the neonatal period. *Seminars in Perinatology*. 2013:37(1):40–48.)

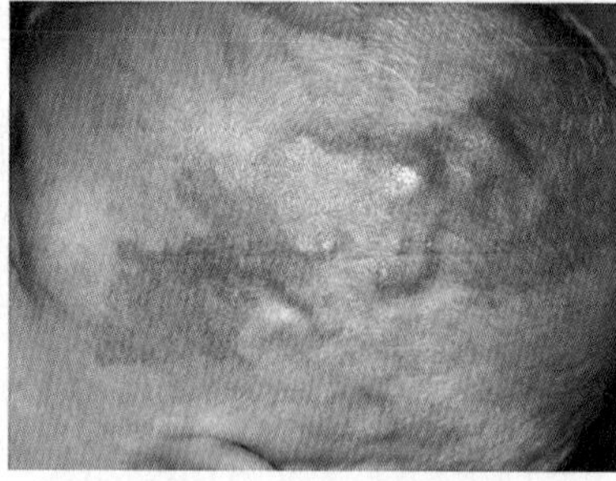

Fig. 102.26 Arteriovenous Malformation in Conjunction With a Port-Wine Stain of the Scalp of a Newborn. (Reproduced with permission and minor modifications from Martin KL. Vascular Disorders. In: *Nelson Textbook of Pediatrics*, ch. 669, 3461–3469.e1.)

Secondary infections in diaper rashes: In some cases, diaper dermatitis could become complicated by secondary staphylococcal infection, and pustules on an erythematous base may be seen (Fig. 102.27C).[44] Some ruptured lesions may show a collarette of scales around a red base. A Gram-stain/culture of pustule contents can confirm the diagnosis. In well-appearing full-term infants, topical antibiotics could be used, but in our experience, a few days of systemic antibiotics need strong consideration depending on the postnatal age. In other cases, candidal infections may occur (Fig. 102.27D).

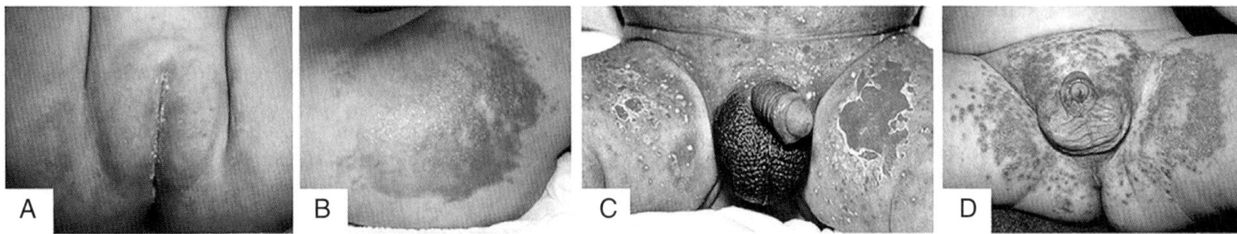

Fig. 102.27 Diaper Dermatitis. (A) Typically involves the convex surfaces and spares the creases in the diaper area. (B) Allergic contact diaper dermatitis due to disposable diaper components. Some infants develop secondary infections. (C) Staphylococcal diaper dermatitis. Numerous thin-walled pustules surrounded by red halos are seen, as well as multiple areas in which pustules have ruptured to leave a collarette of scaling around a denuded red base. (D) Diaper candidiasis. The eruption is bright red, with numerous pinpoint satellite papules and pustules. The urethra and intertriginous areas are prominently involved. (A, Reproduced with permission and minor modifications from *Diaper Dermatitis*. Elsevier Point of Care. Published May 23, 2016; updated January 20, 2021; B, Elsevier Point of Care, published May 23, 2016; from Krol AL et al. Diaper area eruptions. In: Eichenfield LF et al., eds. *Neonatal and Infant Dermatology*. 3rd ed. Philadelphia, PA: Elsevier; 2015:245–264.e2, Fig. 17.11; C and D, reproduced with permission and minor modifications from Püttgen KB, Cohen BA. Neonatal dermatology. In: *Pediatric Dermatology*, 2:14–67.)

Seborrheic dermatitis (Fig. 102.28) needs consideration as a diagnosis in infants with persistent diaper dermatitis. The diagnosis should be considered when the intertriginous areas are involved. Seborrheic dermatitis is marked by salmon-colored patches with greasy, yellow scale in the intertriginous areas, especially the diaper area, axillae, and scalp. Fissuring, maceration, and weeping may be seen.[45] The term "cradle cap" is used for thick, adherent scales around the occiput. Most patients with these lesions remain healthy. In many African American infants, transient postinflammatory hypopigmentation may be seen in the healing lesions. Some infants may also need careful evaluation for secondary candidiasis.

The cause of seborrheic dermatitis is unknown, although the yeast *Pityrosporum* has been suspected as a possible inducing agent.[46] Seborrheic dermatitis may clear spontaneously in a few weeks. Antiseborrheic shampoos containing mild keratolytics such as zinc pyrithione and salicylic acid, emollients, low-potency topical corticosteroids, or topical ketoconazole can help.

Neonatal psoriasis (Fig. 102.29) may occur in young infants, typically starting as a persistent diaper dermatitis. Some lesions may occur in the trunk and extremities. The lesions are typically bright red, scaly, and demarcated at the diaper line. Topical corticosteroids and/or calcineurin inhibitors approved for atopic dermatitis, pimecrolimus and tacrolimus, can help. Skin biopsy can help confirm the diagnosis. Treatment is guided by the severity of symptoms.[47]

Langerhans cell histiocytosis (LCH) may present with a severe seborrheic dermatitis-like eruption or as progressive diaper dermatitis (Fig. 102.30).[48] The lesions can appear hemorrhagic and erosive and then get scaly and crusted. Diagnostic skin biopsies demonstrate histiocytic infiltrates containing Langerhans cell (Birbeck) granules. Similar infiltrates may be seen in the bone marrow, liver, lungs, kidneys, and nervous system. Infants suspected of having LCH require a thorough work-up including full physical examination, skin biopsy, a laboratory work-up including complete blood count, a complete metabolic panel including liver function tests, serum osmolality, and urine osmolality, and initial imaging to include chest x-ray and skeletal survey. Early involvement of hematology/oncology and close follow-up are mandatory.

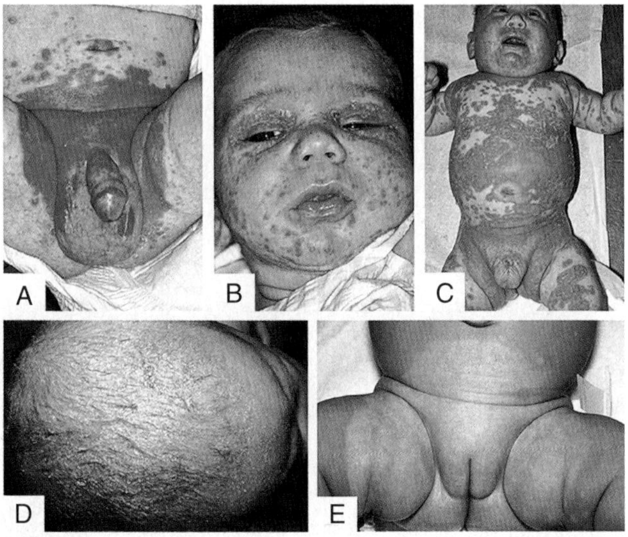

Fig. 102.28 Seborrheic Dermatitis. (A) Slightly greasy, red, scaling eruptions typically begin in the groin creases and spread throughout the diaper area. (B and C) In severely afflicted cases, the dermatitis may involve the trunk, face, and creases of the neck and extremities. (D) "Cradle cap" consists of thick, tenacious scaling of the scalp. (E) Postinflammatory hypopigmentation may be marked, particularly in darkly pigmented individuals. (Reproduced with permission and minor modifications from Püttgen KB, Cohen BA. Neonatal dermatology. In: *Pediatric Dermatology*, 2, 14-67.)

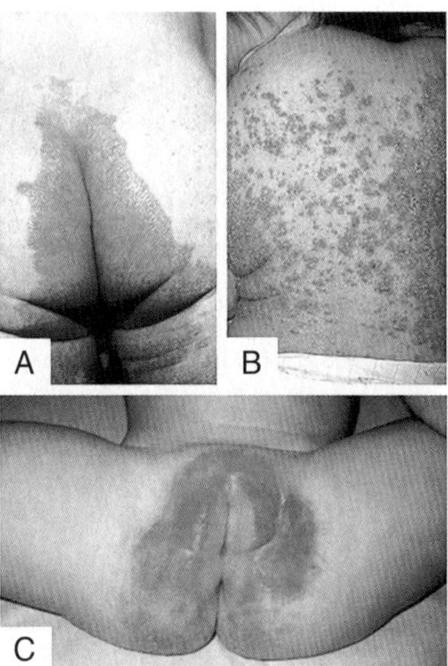

Fig. 102.29 Neonatal Psoriasis. This diaper dermatitis failed to respond to routine topical therapy. (A) A skin biopsy demonstrated histologic changes of psoriasis. (B) In some infants with psoriasis, thick, disseminated plaques appear. (C) Confluent, beefy red and pink plaques in the diaper area consistent with psoriasis; the eruption required short courses of mid- to high-potency topical steroids to control it. (Reproduced with permission and minor modifications from Püttgen KB, Cohen BA. Neonatal dermatology. In: *Pediatric Dermatology*, 2:14–67.)

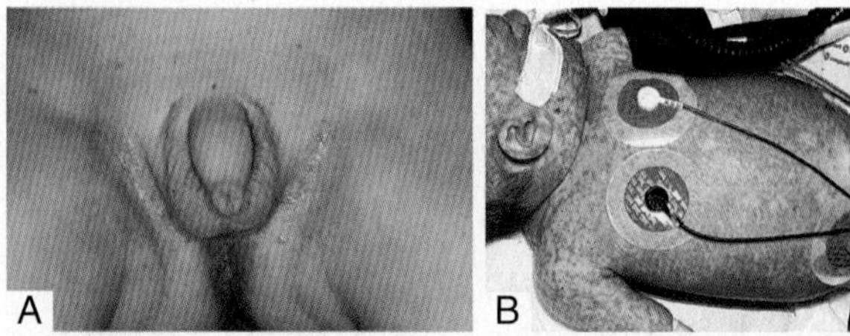

Fig. 102.30 Langerhans Cell Histiocytosis (LCH). (A) The lesions may first appear in the inguinal creases and then progress to multiorgan involvement. The skin lesions can be seen in the perineum and on the anterior scrotal surface. (B) In some infants, the diaper dermatitis can rapidly generalize to the entire skin surface. A photograph of a different 3-week-old infant shows a diffuse skin rash, which was associated with diarrhea, poor weight gain, lymphadenopathy, and hepatosplenomegaly. This child died of disseminated LCH at 6 weeks of age. (A, Reproduced with permission and minor modifications from Paller AS, Mancini AJ. Cutaneous disorders of the newborn. In: *Paller and Mancini—Hurwitz Clinical Pediatric Dermatology*, 2, 11–41.e5; B, reproduced with permission and minor modifications from Püttgen KB, Cohen BA. Neonatal dermatology. In: *Pediatric Dermatology*, 2, 14–67.)

Benign cephalic histiocytosis (BCH) is characterized by scattered yellow-brown papules and macules on the face, scalp, neck, and upper trunk in neonates and young infants (Fig. 102.31).[49] No systemic involvement occurs. It has been proposed that BCH may be an early-onset variant of juvenile xanthogranulomatosis. BCH lacks LCH markers such as S100 and Birbeck granules. No treatment is necessary because lesions regress over the first few years after birth.

Acrodermatitis enteropathica (AE) presents in neonates and young infants with an erosive diaper dermatitis, diarrhea, and hair loss. Weeping, crusted, erythematous patches also appear in a periorificial, acral, and intertriginous distribution (Fig. 102.32). Affected infants are irritable, grow poorly, and are prone to infection and septicemia.[50]

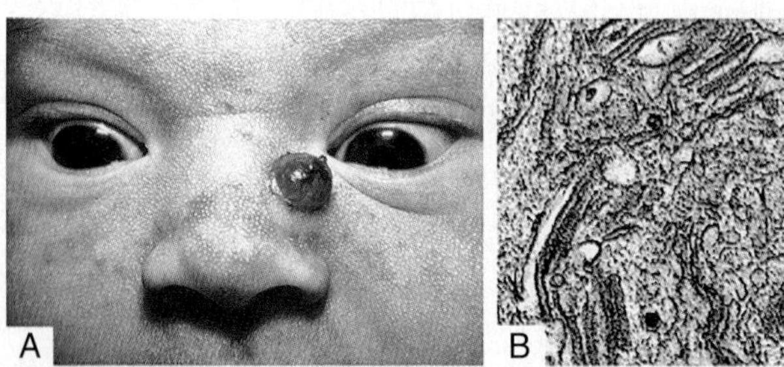

Fig. 102.31 Benign Cephalic Histiocytosis. (A) This healthy newborn with multiple congenital crusted papules was initially treated for herpes simplex infection. When the lesions did not respond to parenteral acyclovir, a skin biopsy that showed the typical changes of Langerhans cell histiocytosis (LCH) on routine pathology and (B) electron microscopy was performed. Note the tennis racket–shaped Birbeck granules diagnostic of LCH. The lesions resolved without treatment within 2 weeks. (Reproduced with permission and minor modifications from Püttgen KB, Cohen BA. Neonatal dermatology. In: *Pediatric Dermatology*, 2:14–67.)

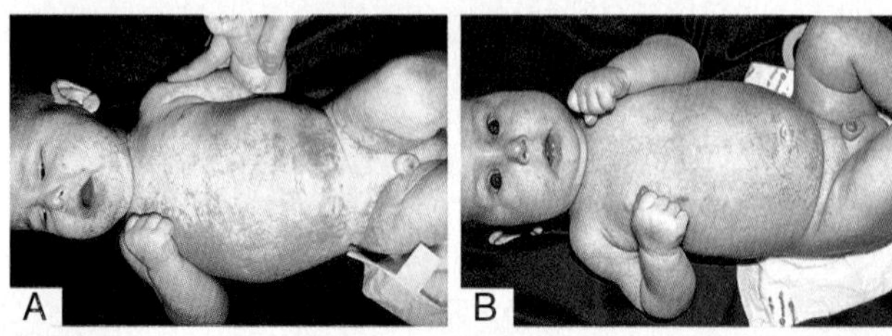

Fig. 102.32 Acrodermatitis Enteropathica. (A) A bright red, scaling dermatitis spread to the intertriginous areas, face, and extremities of this 4-week-old infant. (B) After 4 days of zinc supplementation, many lesions were healing with desquamation. (Reproduced with permission and minor modifications from Püttgen KB, Cohen BA. Neonatal dermatology. In: *Pediatric Dermatology*, 2:14–67.)

Some patients have branched-chain organic acid disorders, glutaric aciduria type I, or defects in the zinc-specific transporter gene *SLC39A4* that encodes an intestinal zinc transporter, Zip4. AE responds dramatically to high doses of oral or intravenous zinc. Some patients with genetic disorders require lifelong zinc supplements. AE-like rashes have also been noted in biotin deficiency, essential fatty acid deficiency, methylmalonic acidemia, propionic acidemia, type 1 glutaric aciduria, ornithine transcarbamylase deficiency, citrullinemia, maple syrup urine disease, and Hartnup disease. These conditions may need specific treatment.

Scaling Disorders

Collodion infants are born encased in a thick, tight, cellophane-like membrane (Fig. 102.33). The membrane may desquamate to leave normal skin in some, but more than two-thirds develop autosomal recessive congenital ichthyosis, which is most commonly lamellar ichthyosis.[51] In some infants, this membrane may indicate evaluation for conditions such as Netherton syndrome, Conradi–Hünermann syndrome, Sjögren–Larsson syndrome, or an ectodermal dysplasia.

The skin in collodion babies has impaired barrier function due to cracking and fissuring. They may have increased insensible water loss, heat loss, and risk of hypernatremic dehydration, cutaneous infection, and sepsis. Increased humidity (50%) and close thermal monitoring such as in an incubator may help. Topical applications should be restricted to bland emollients such as petrolatum. Desquamation is usually complete by 2 to 3 weeks of life. Cutaneous biopsies may be deferred until full desquamation.

Ichthyoses are a group of scaling disorders (Fig. 102.34). Table 102.3 summarizes the subtypes seen in neonates.[52] Table 102.4 lists syndromes with skin lesions resembling ichthyosis.

For treatment, mild scaling responds well to lubricants, urea-containing preparations, and α-hydroxy acids in emollients (lactic acid or glycolic acid). Topical retinoids such as adapalene, tretinoin, and tazarotene can be useful. Topical salicylic acid and urea preparations are not recommended for use in infants. Oral retinoids (isotretinoin, acitretin, and etretinate), calcipotriol, and N-acetylcysteine have shown promise in adults and need study. Clinical benefits must be weighed against the risk of systemic effects, particularly hepatic and skeletal toxicity.[53]

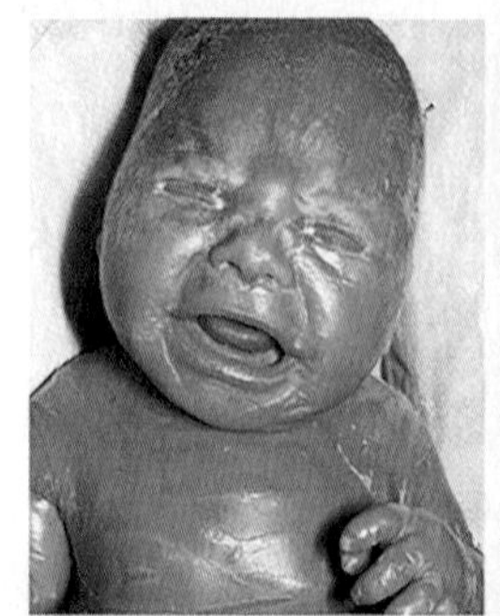

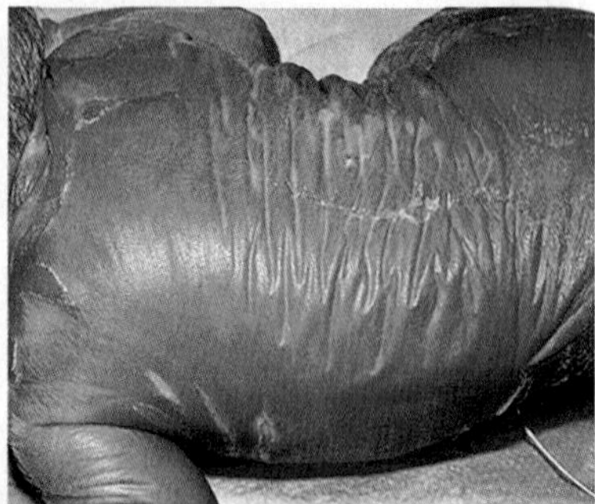

Fig. 102.33 Collodion Baby. A shiny, transparent membrane covered this baby at birth. She later developed lamellar ichthyosis. (Reproduced with permission and minor modifications from Püttgen KB, Cohen BA. Neonatal dermatology. In: *Pediatric Dermatology*, 2:14–67.)

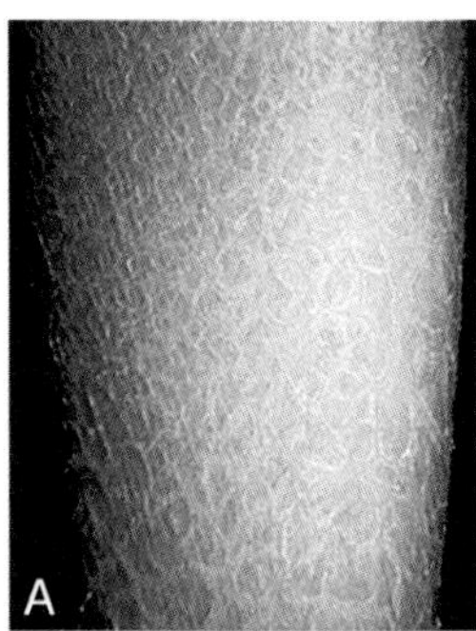

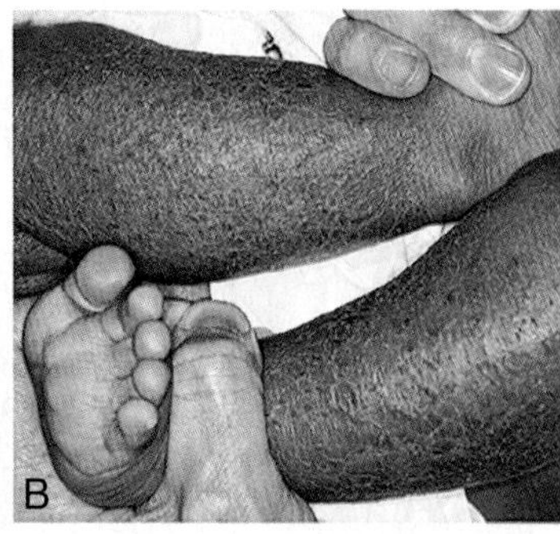

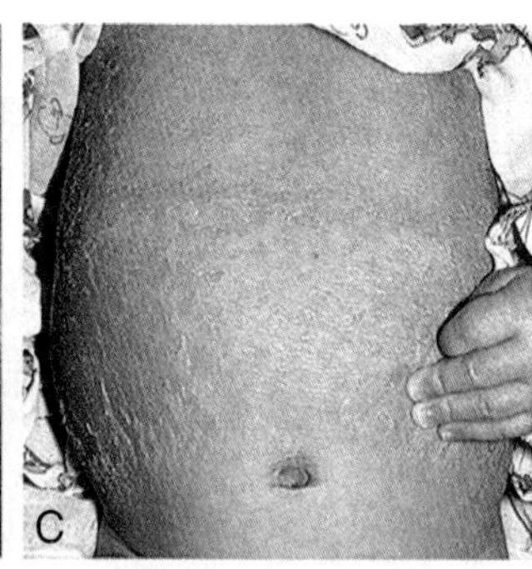

Fig. 102.34 Ichthyosis Vulgaris. (A) Typical fish-scale appearance on the lower extremities of a light-pigmented child. (B) The appearance on a dark-pigmented child. Both children had at least one parent with similar findings. (C) X-linked ichthyosis: "Dirty" tan scales on the trunk of this infant. (Reproduced with permission and minor modifications from Püttgen KB, Cohen BA. Neonatal dermatology. In: *Pediatric Dermatology*, 2:14–67.)

Table 102.3 Ichthyoses Seen During the Neonatal Period

Variant	Genetics	Incidence	Clinical Features
Congenital ichthyosiform erythroderma (MIM #242100; Fig. 102.35)	AR; associated genes: *TGM-1*, *ABCA12*, *NIPAL4* (ICHTHYIN), *ALOX12B*, *ALOXE3*	1/50 –1/100,000	Collodion baby; fine white scales on trunk, face, and scalp; large scales on legs; variable erythroderma
Lamellar ichthyosis (MIM #242300)	AR; associated genes: *TGM-1*, *ABCA12*, *NIPAL4* (ICHTHYIN), *CYP4F22*, *LIPN*	1/100,000	Collodion baby; generalized large, dark, plate-like scales; ectropion, eclabium; mild palmoplantar keratoderma
Epidermolytic hyperkeratosis (MIM #113800)	AD (most common); AR, sporadic; *KRT1*, *KRT10*	Rare	Widespread blisters at birth; increasing erythema, scales with age; marked scales in intertriginous areas, palms, soles; malodor from bacterial overgrowth
X-linked ichthyosis (MIM #308100)	X-linked recessive; steroid sulfatase gene	1/2000–1/6000 males	Large "dirty" scales on trunk and extremities, sparing flexures; variable in female carriers; corneal opacities in Descemet's membrane; cryptorchidism; placental sulfatase deficiency with prolonged maternal labor
Harlequin ichthyosis (MIM #242500; Fig. 102.36)	AR; abca12	Very rare	Thick plates of "armor"-like scales in neonates; survival about 50%; death can occur in first 3 months after birth

AD, Autosomal dominant; *AR*, autosomal recessive; *MIM*, Mendelian Inheritance in Man.

Table 102.4 Syndromes With Skin Lesions Resembling Ichthyosis

Syndrome/Disease	Genetics	Clinical Features
Netherton syndrome; MIM #256500	AR; *SPINK5*	Hair shaft anomaly (trichorrhexis invaginata most common), ichthyosis linearis circumflexa, atopic dermatitis, failure to thrive
Refsum disease, infantile (MIM #266510)	AR; associated genes: *PEX1*, *PXMP3*, *PEX26*	Retinitis pigmentosa, cerebellar ataxia, chronic polyneuritis with deafness, skin resembles ichthyosis vulgaris
Sjögren–Larsson syndrome (MIM #270200)	AR; *ALDH3A2* (fatty aldehyde dehydrogenase gene)	Spastic paralysis, mental retardation, seizures, glistening dots on retina, dental bone dysplasia, similar skin findings to congenital ichthyosiform erythroderma
Conradi–Hünermann syndrome (chondrodysplasia punctata type 2; MIM #302900)	X-linked dominant; EBP	Chondrodysplasia punctata, alopecia, skeletal anomalies, cataracts, dysmorphic facies, ichthyosiform erythroderma
KID (keratitis-ichthyosis-deafness) syndrome; MIM #148210	AD (sporadic); *GJB2* encoding connexin 26	Fixed keratotic plaques, keratoderma, atypical ichthyosis with prominent keratoses on extremities and head, neurosensory deafness, keratoconjunctivitis
CHILD syndrome; MIM #308050	X-linked recessive; *NSDHL*	Congenital hemidysplasia, unilateral ichthyosiform nevus (epidermal nevus), limb defects, cardiovascular and renal anomalies

AD, Autosomal dominant; *AR*, autosomal recessive; *CHILD*, congenital hemidysplasia with ichthyosiform erythroderma and limb defects; *EBP*, emopamil-binding protein (sterol isomerase; emopamil is a calcium channel blocker and a high-affinity ligand of human sterol isomerase); *MIM*, Mendelian Inheritance in Man.

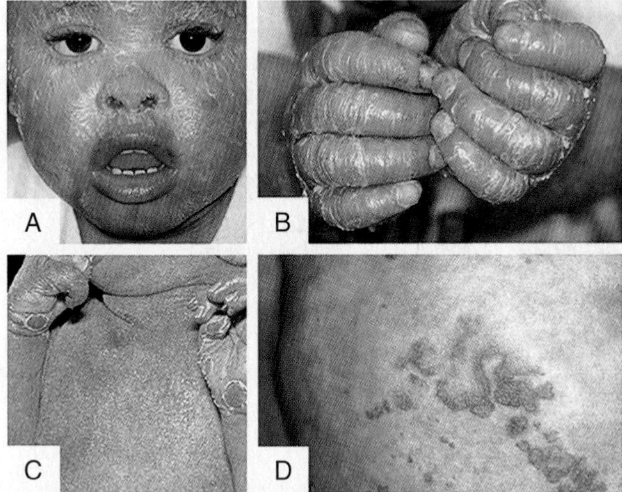

Fig. 102.35 Congenital Ichthyosiform Erythroderma. (A) Congenital erythroderma persisted in this child. (B) Note the marked scaling on her hands. (C) Generalized erythema with fine scaling was noted on the first day of life. (D) Shortly after his first birthday, this infant developed a new pattern of migrating, scaly, erythematous plaques typical of Netherton syndrome. Microscopic examination of his hair revealed trichorrhexis invaginata (bamboo hair). (Reproduced with permission and minor modifications from Püttgen KB, Cohen BA. Neonatal dermatology. In: *Pediatric Dermatology*, 2:14–67.)

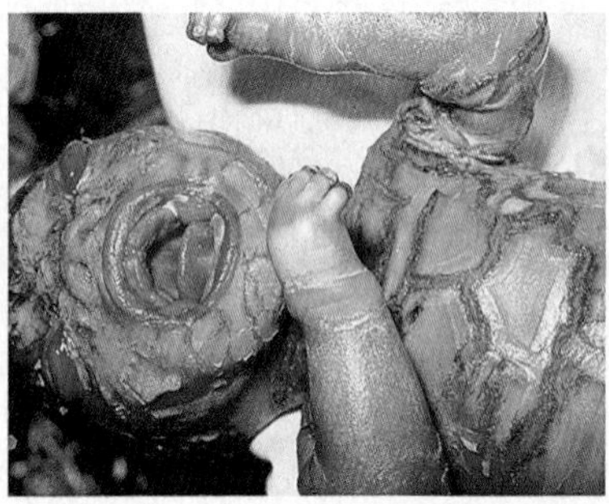

Fig. 102.36 Harlequin Ichthyosis. This baby developed thick, plate-like scales immediately after drying in the delivery room. Respiratory failure resulted in death during the first week. Note the ectropion and eclabium. (Reproduced with permission and minor modifications from Püttgen KB, Cohen BA. Neonatal dermatology. In: *Pediatric Dermatology*, 2:14–67.)

Cutaneous Infections

Please see specific chapters for candidiasis, congenital syphilis, and herpes simplex.

Congenital and neonatal varicella syndrome: Fetal infection during the first 20 weeks of gestation can present as neonatal varicella syndrome at birth with linear scars, limb anomalies, ocular defects, and central nervous system involvement (Fig. 102.37).[54]

Maternal infection during the first 3 weeks after delivery can cause neonatal varicella. Infection of the fetus/neonate in a 10-day period around delivery typically causes mild disease because of the presence of protective transplacental antibody. Infection acquired by the mother <5 days before delivery to 2 days after delivery, or lesions that develop in the newborn between days 5 and 10 of life, tend to have more severe infection and are at risk for dissemination with resulting pneumonitis, encephalitis, purpura fulminans, widespread bleeding, hypotension, and death.

Varicella-zoster immune globulin and parenteral acyclovir can improve outcomes if administered early in the course. Blister contents show multinucleated giant cells on Tzanck smears and can also be examined by culture, fluorescence studies, or polymerase chain reaction.

Impetigo and staphylococcal scalded-skin syndrome: Several common bacterial infections present with vesiculopustular eruptions in infancy. The rash tends to be localized in impetigo and generalized in staphylococcal scalded-skin syndrome (SSSS; Fig. 102.38).

In classic streptococcal impetigo, honey-colored crusts overlie infected insect bites, abrasions, and other skin rashes such as diaper dermatitis. Lesions may appear anywhere, although areas prone to trauma, such as the diaper area, circumcision wound, and umbilical stump, are frequent sites of primary infection.

Bullous impetigo shows slowly enlarging, blistering rings around central, umbilicated crusts.[55] These lesions are caused by epidermal toxin-producing types of *Staphylococci*, which produce exfoliative toxin A and exfoliative toxin B. In newborns and young infants, dissemination of the toxin may result in widespread erythema and blistering typical of SSSS. Gentle pressure on the skin causes the upper epidermis to slide off, leaving a denuded base (Nikolsky sign). In localized impetigo, bacteria are identified in Gram-stained material obtained directly from the rash. In SSSS, a primary cutaneous site of infection might not be identifiable, and noncutaneous sources

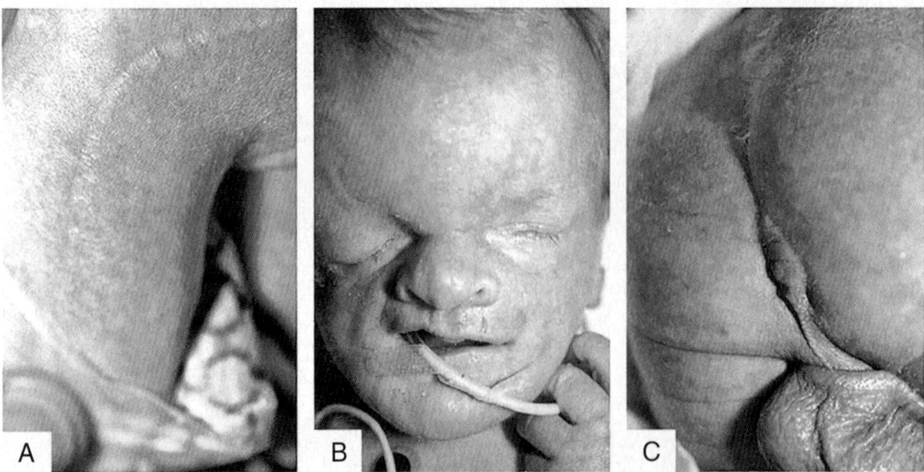

Fig. 102.37 Congenital Varicella. (A) A linear scar was evident on the arm of this newborn whose mother developed chickenpox during the first trimester. (B and C) This child also had multiple central nervous system, ocular, genitourinary, and gastrointestinal anomalies. Note the dysmorphic facies (B) and imperforate anus (C). (Reproduced with permission and minor modifications from Püttgen KB, Cohen BA. Neonatal dermatology. In: *Pediatric Dermatology*, 2:14–67.)

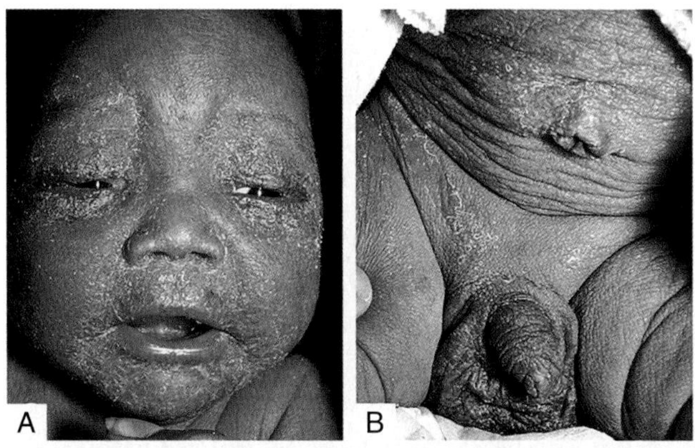

Fig. 102.38 Staphylococcal Scalded-Skin Syndrome in a Neonate Being Treated for Mastitis. Erosive patches were most marked on the (A) face and (B) diaper areas. (Reproduced with permission and minor modifications from Püttgen KB, Cohen BA. Neonatal dermatology. In: *Pediatric Dermatology*, 2:14–67.)

including lungs, bone, meninges, conjunctivae, and ears may need examination. Neonates usually need systemic antibiotics and need treatment per sepsis protocols.

Scabies is a well-characterized infection produced by the *Sarcoptes scabiei* mite. The impregnated female burrows through the outer epidermis and deposits her eggs. In infants, burrows are widespread with involvement of the trunk, scalp, and extremities, including the palms and soles. Infants may be otherwise healthy; chronic infestation may result in poor feeding, fussiness, and failure to thrive (Fig. 102.39).

The diagnosis should be considered for any infant with widespread dermatosis involving the palms and soles, particularly if other family members are involved. Permethrin 5% cream is first-line therapy for scabies.[56] Other agents are not recommended for young infants. The entire family should be treated. Lesions can reappear with reinfestation or inadequate therapy.

Cutaneous Neoplasms

IHs may be barely visible as telangiectasias or red macules in neonates but grow during infancy into bright red, partially compressible tumors (see Figs. 102.20 and 102.21). Many lesions may have a deep dermal or subcutaneous component. Histologically, rapidly growing lesions that appear early during infancy are highly cellular with small slit-like vascular lumina. As lesions mature, the vascular lumina become better defined, and the endothelial lining of vessels becomes flatter. Healing is mediated by apoptosis and decreasing cell proliferation. Regression is associated with fibrosis and replacement of the vascular tissue with fat.[36]

Prematurity is an important risk factor. There is a gender-based predilection, and IHs are three times more common in girls. IHs generally double in size in the first 2 months after birth and grow in an early proliferative phase in most lesions until 3 to 5 months of age; some lesions continue to grow at a slower rate until 12 months of age. Signs of early involution, such as graying of the surface and flattening of the deeper component, then appear. Regression occurs in approximately 25% by age 2 years, 40% to 50% by age 4 years, 60% to 75% by age 6 years, and 95% by adolescence. Some scarring, loose skin, or telangiectasias main remain visible.

A small group of congenital hemangiomas are fully formed at birth and are further classified into rapidly involuting congenital hemangiomas and noninvoluting congenital hemangiomas.[57] The majority of rapidly involuting congenital hemangiomas begin to regress shortly after birth, and many disappear in 12 to 18 months, whereas noninvoluting congenital hemangiomas persist indefinitely. Some authors suggest a third categorization of partially involuting congenital hemangiomas.

The treatment of IHs located near vital organs can be problematic.[58] Hemangiomas around the eye or extending into the orbit may cause obstruction amblyopia or damage the orbital contents. Multiple hemangiomas or single, large, rapidly growing lesions in young infants may be associated with high-output cardiac failure. Medical treatment is warranted and may involve propranolol, a nonselective beta blocker, as a first-line therapy; corticosteroids may be added. Hypoglycemia can be avoided by coinciding doses with feedings. Some small studies have evaluated atenolol, nadolol, or topical timolol. In lesions located near vital organs, intralesional steroids, early surgical excision, and/or pulsed-dye laser may need consideration.

Hamartomatous nevi include a number of birthmarks that contain various epidermal, dermal, and subcutaneous structures (see Fig. 102.19).[59]

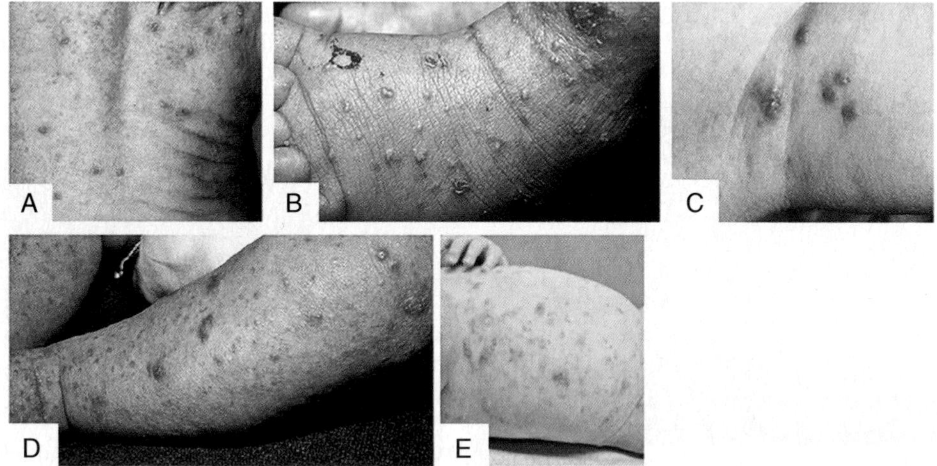

Fig. 102.39 Infants With Widespread Scabies. Burrows were present on (A) the trunk and (B) the feet. Nodules persisted on (C) the axillae and (D) the legs of these infants for 4 months. (E) This 10-week-old infant had been treated twice for scabies but continued to show evidence of burrows and papules until the entire family was treated. (Reproduced with permission and minor modifications from Püttgen KB, Cohen BA. Neonatal dermatology. In: *Pediatric Dermatology*, 2:14–67.)

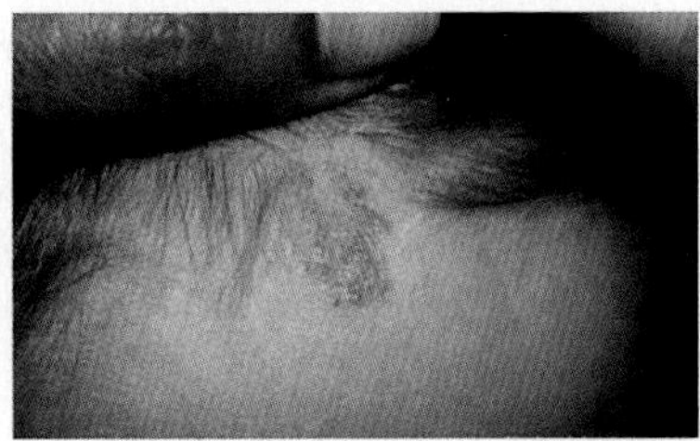

Fig. 102.40 Nevus Sebaceous. (Reproduced with permission and minor modifications from Prendiville JS. Lumps, bumps, and hamartomas. In: *Neonatal and Infant Dermatology*; 2015: 422–442.)

Epidermal nevi, typically seen in less than 1% of infants, are localized, linear, warty, hyperpigmented plaques of variable size (see Fig. 102.19).[59] The lesions can involve any cutaneous site or mucous membranes and consist of proliferating epidermal keratinocytes. Infants with large lesions need evaluation for seizures, developmental delay, and skeletal and ocular defects. Skin lesions may respond to topical retinoids or keratolytics such as lactic acid, salicylic acid, and urea. Small lesions can be excised or ablated by carbon dioxide laser.

Sebaceous nevi: Nevus sebaceous of Jadassohn is typically a linear, crescent-shaped, or round hairless, yellow, cobblestone-like plaque (Fig. 102.40).[60] Most lesions are seen on the head and neck but can occasionally appear on the trunk and extremities. Some lesions can show benign hypertrophy with warty nodules and plaques. Histology shows multiple sebaceous glands, ectopic apocrine glands, and primordial hair structures. Excision can be delayed until puberty.

Smooth muscle and pilar hamartomas contain smooth muscle bundles with prominent hair follicles. These nevi appear as minimally hyperpigmented, supple plaques 1 to 5 cm in diameter on the trunk (Fig. 102.41).[61] A pseudo-Darier sign or rippling of the skin occurs with rubbing.[62] These lesions do not pose a risk of malignancy.

Connective tissue nevi are hamartomas with increased dermal collagen and elastic tissue.[63] In neonates, plaques 1 to 10 cm in diameter with a *peau d'orange* texture may be seen on the trunk (Fig. 102.42). There may be radiographic densities in long bones. Some lesions may resemble shagreen patches of tuberous sclerosis, and there may be a need for investigation.

Congenital melanocytic nevi are pigmented macules/plaques, often with dense hair growth noted at birth or early infancy. The lesions may be lightly pigmented at birth and darken later.[35]

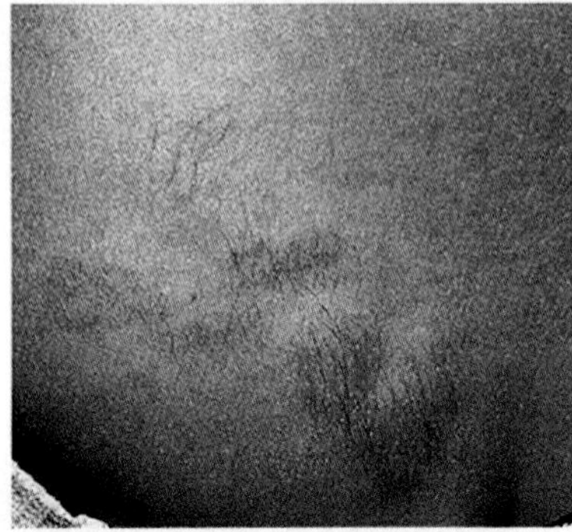

Fig. 102.41 Smooth Muscle and Pilar Hamartomas Contain Smooth Muscle Bundles With Prominent Hair Follicles. These nevi appear as minimally hyperpigmented. (Reproduced with permission and minor modifications from Neonatal dermatology. In: Püttgen and Cohen. *Pediatric Dermatology*, 2: 14–67.)

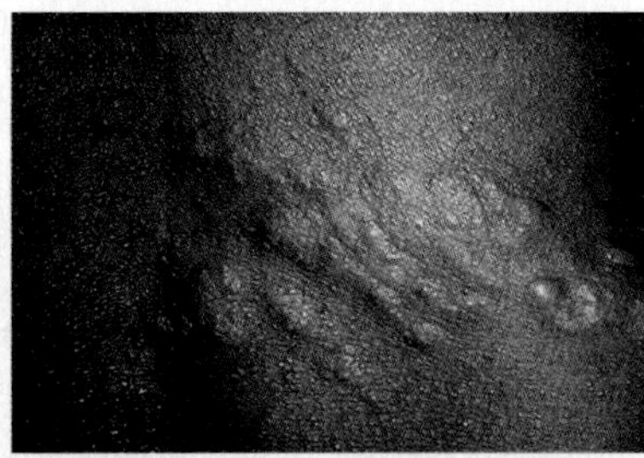

Fig. 102.42 Connective Tissue Nevi. Connective tissue nevi are uncommon lesions on the trunk that may present as isolated plaques, as multiple lesions (acquired or congenital), or as one finding in a more generalized disease. Biopsy findings include abnormal collagen bundles and altered amounts of elastin. (Reproduced with permission and minor modifications from James et al. Dermal and subcutaneous tumors. In: *Andrews' Diseases of the Skin*, 28:587–635.e7.)

Giant congenital pigmented nevi exceed 20 cm in diameter and are associated with a 2% to 6% lifetime risk of melanoma, which may occur prior to puberty. There is a need for monitoring with regular clinical evaluations and periodic MRI and/or radioimaging studies to examine the leptomeninges in the scalp, neck, and back. If there are possible malignant changes, surgical excision may need to be done in stages. Medium-sized (1.5–19.9 cm in diameter) and small (<1.5 cm in diameter) congenital pigmented nevi are also at risk of malignant changes, although these nevi can be removed during later childhood.[64]

Juvenile xanthogranulomas can be seen at birth or during early infancy as enlarging, pink to yellow papules, plaques, and nodules 0.5 to 4 cm in diameter, with overlying telangiectasias (Fig. 102.43). Most lesions are seen on the head, neck, and trunk and occasionally the extremities and are usually asymptomatic.[65] Biopsy shows characteristic lipid-laden histiocytes. Eye examinations may show spontaneous anterior chamber hemorrhage. Most infants do not need specific treatment, because the lesions typically regress during middle childhood.

Dermoid cysts (Fig. 102.44) are compressible or rubbery subcutaneous nodules 1 to 4 cm in diameter at the site of closure of embryonic clefts. Most lesions are seen on the forehead, periorbital area, midchest, sacrum, perineum, and scrotum during the neonatal period.[66] These cysts are lined by epidermis and contain mature adnexal structures, including sebaceous glands, eccrine glands, and apocrine glands. Dermoids that overlie the sacrum may be associated with occult defects of the vertebral column and spinal cord.[67] Midline lesions should be imaged; there is no risk of malignancy, but some lesions can erode the underlying bone and need excision.

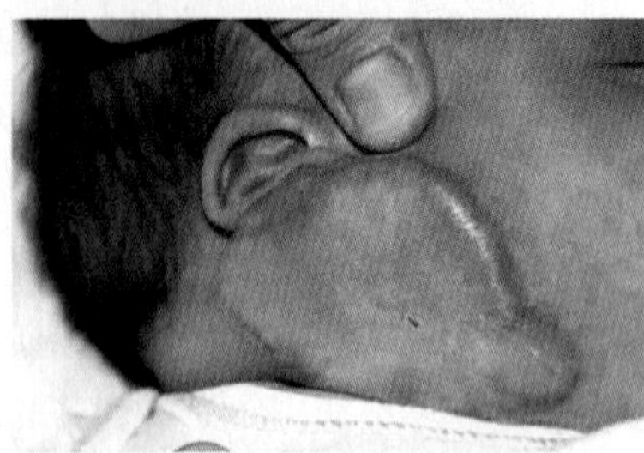

Fig. 102.43 Giant Congenital Juvenile Xanthogranuloma. Note the yellowish color of the plaque with an erythematous rim and peau d'orange surface. (Reproduced with permission and minor modifications from Narendran V. The skin of the neonate. In: *Fanaroff and Martin's Neonatal-Perinatal Medicine*. 2019;1898–1932.)

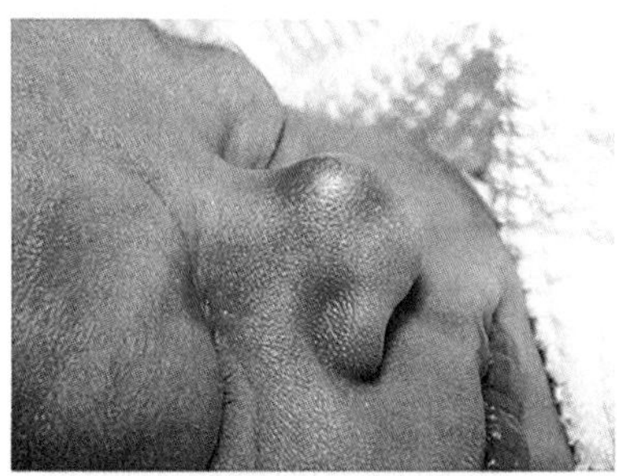

Fig. 102.44 Dermoid Cyst. This partially compressible mass was present on the nose at birth. A computed tomography scan of the head (to exclude a communication with the underlying central nervous system) was normal. (Reproduced with permission and minor modifications from Püttgen KB, Cohen BA. Neonatal dermatology. In: *Pediatric Dermatology*, 2:14–67.)

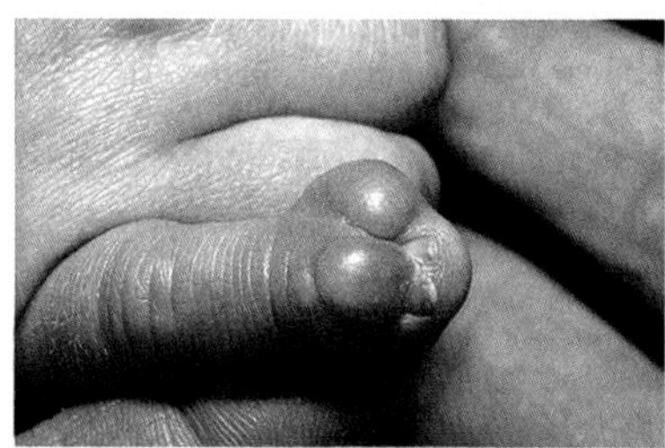

Fig. 102.45 Infantile Digital Fibroma. These tumors may only need close observation. After an initial growth phase, many can involute spontaneously. (Reproduced with permission and minor modifications from Püttgen KB, Cohen BA. Neonatal dermatology. In: *Pediatric Dermatology*, 2:14–67.)

Recurrent infantile digital fibromas are small (<2 cm) nodules on fingers and toes in infants (Fig. 102.45). Biopsy shows numerous fibroblasts and collagen bundles. Excision may be followed by recurrence, but most lesions finally involute spontaneously.[68]

Congenital or infantile myofibromatosis is characterized by subcutaneous, firm, red/blue nodules. Visceral lesions may be seen in the lungs.[69] Histologically, these tumors show fibroblasts and smooth muscle cells with no cytologic atypia. Most subcutaneous nodules involute spontaneously, and solitary lesions can be excised without recurrence.

Malignant tumors are uncommon in neonates. Cutaneous plaques and tumors may be seen in newborn infants with leukemia, rhabdomyosarcoma, lymphoma, and some carcinomas and sarcomas.[70–72] Most neuroblastomas are diagnosed later in infancy. Skin biopsy of rapidly growing or infiltrative lesions is required to confirm diagnosis and dictate therapy.

To conclude, the skin of a newborn infant differs from that of adults in many ways. This chapter has summarized various skin disorders seen in neonates, including congenital abnormalities, inflammatory conditions, infections, and neoplasms. As is evident in several sections, we still do not know the etiopathogenesis of many conditions. Further work is needed to improve our classifications for neonatal skin disorders, investigate the causes, standardize the treatment protocols, and understand the determinants of outcome.

Index

Note: Page number followed by *f*, *t* and *b* indicates figure, table and box respectively.